Prehospital EMERGENCY CARE

ninth edition

Joseph J. Mistovich, MEd, NREMT-P
Chairperson and Professor
Department of Health Professions
Youngstown State University
Youngstown, Ohio

Keith J. Karren, PhD, EMT-B
Professor
Department of Health Sciences
Brigham Young University
Provo, Utah

Medical Editor
Howard A. Werman, MD

Legacy Author
Brent Q. Hafen, PhD

Brady
is an imprint of

Pearson

Boston Columbus Indianapolis New York San Francisco Upper Saddle River
Amsterdam Cape Town Dubai London Madrid Milan Munich Paris Montreal Toronto
Delhi Mexico City Sao Paulo Sydney Hong Kong Seoul Singapore Taipei Tokyo

Library of Congress Cataloging-in-Publication Data
Mistovich, Joseph J.
Prehospital emergency care / Joseph J. Mistovich, Keith J. Karren ; medical editor, Howard A. Werman ; legacy author, Brent Q. Hafen. — 9th ed.
p. ; cm.
Includes bibliographical references and index.
ISBN-13: 978-0-13-502809-4
ISBN-10: 0-13-502809-4
1. Emergency medicine. 2. Emergency medical technicians. I. Karren, Keith J. II. Werman, Howard A. III. Hafen, Brent Q. IV. Title.
[DNLM: 1. Emergency Medical Services. 2. Emergencies. WX 215 M678p 2010]
RC86.7.H346 2010
616.02′5—dc22

2009015059

Publisher: Julie Levin Alexander
Publisher's Assistant: Regina Bruno
Editor-in-Chief: Marlene McHugh Pratt
Acquisitions Editor: Sladjana Repic
Senior Managing Editor for Development: Lois Berlowitz
Project Manager: Sandra Breuer
Editorial Assistant: Jonathan Cheung
Director of Marketing: Karen Allman
Executive Marketing Manager: Katrin Beacom
Marketing Specialist: Michael Sirinides
Marketing Assistant: Judy Noh
Managing Editor for Production: Patrick Walsh
Production Liaison: Faye Gemmellaro
Production Editor: Heather Willison, S4Carlisle Publishing Services
Manufacturing Manager: Ilene Sanford
Manufacturing Buyer: Pat Brown
Editorial Media Manager: Amy Peltier
Media Project Manager: Lorena Cerisano
Creative Director: John Christiana, Design Development Services
Interior and Cover Design: Kathy Mrozek, Design Development Services
Cover Image: Mark C. Ide
Managing Photography Editor: Michal Heron
Photographers: Michal Heron, Maria A.H. Lyle, Nathan Eldridge, Michael Gallitelli, Carl Leet, Ray Kemp/911 Imaging, and Kevin Link
Manager, Rights and Permissions: Zina Arabia
Manager, Visual Research: Beth Brenzel
Image Permission Coordinator: Vickie Menanteaux
Composition: S4Carlisle Publishing Services
Printer/Binder: Courier/Kendallville
Cover Printer: Lehigh-Phoenix Color/Hagerstown

Credits and acknowledgments borrowed from other sources and reproduced, with permission, in this textbook appear on the appropriate pages within the text.

Notice on Trademarks Many of the designations by manufacturers and sellers to distinguish their products are claimed as trademarks. Where those designations appear in this book, and the publisher was aware of a trademark claim, the designations have been printed in initial caps or all caps.

Notice on Care Procedures It is the intent of the authors and publisher that this textbook be used as part of a formal EMT education program taught by qualified instructors and supervised by a licensed physician. The procedures described in this textbook are based upon consultation with EMT and medical authorities. The authors and publisher have taken care to make certain that these procedures reflect currently accepted clinical practice; however, they cannot be considered absolute recommendations.

The material in this textbook contains the most current information available at the time of publication. However, federal, state, and local guidelines concerning clinical practices, including, without limitation, those governing infection control and universal precautions, change rapidly. The reader should note, therefore, that the new regulations may require changes in some procedures. It is the responsibility of the reader to become thoroughly familiar with the policies and procedures set by federal, state, and local agencies as well as the institution or agency where the reader is employed. The authors and the publisher of this textbook and the supplements written to accompany it disclaim any liability, loss, or risk resulting directly or indirectly from the suggested procedures and theory, from any undetected errors, or from the reader's misunderstanding of the text. It is the reader's responsibility to stay informed of any new changes or recommendations made by any federal, state, or local agency as well as by the reader's employing institution or agency.

Notice on Gender Usage The English language has historically given preference to the male gender. Among many words, the pronouns "he" and "his" are commonly used to describe both genders. Society evolves faster than language, and the male pronouns still predominate in our speech. The authors have made great effort to treat the two genders equally, recognizing that a significant percentage of EMTs are female. However, in some instances, male pronouns may be used to describe both males and females solely for the purpose of brevity. This is not intended to offend any readers of the female gender.

Notice on "Case Studies" The names used and situations depicted in the case studies throughout this text are fictitious.

Notice on Medications The authors and the publisher of this book have taken care to make certain that the equipment, doses of drugs, and schedules of treatment are correct and compatible with the standards generally accepted at the time of publication. Nevertheless, as new information becomes available, changes in treatment and in the use of equipment and drugs become necessary. The reader is advised to carefully consult the instruction and information material included in the page insert of each drug or therapeutic agent, piece of equipment, or device before administration. This advice is especially important when using new or infrequently used drugs. Prehospital care providers are warned that use of any drugs or techniques must be authorized by their medical director, in accord with local laws and regulations. The publisher disclaims any liability, loss, injury, or damage incurred as a consequence, directly or indirectly, of the use and application of any of the contents of this book.

Brady
is an imprint of

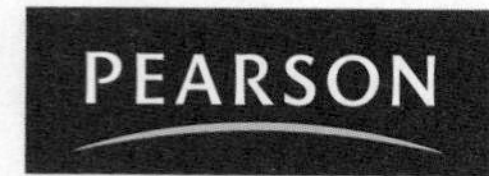

www.bradybooks.com

10 9 8 7
ISBN 13: 978-0-13-502809-4 (paper)
ISBN 10: 0-13-502809-4
ISBN 13: 978-0-13-502810-0 (case)
ISBN 10: 0-13-502810-8

Dedication

To my best friend and beautiful wife, Andrea, for her unconditional love and inspiration to pursue my dreams. To my daughters Katie, Kristyn, Chelsea, Morgan, and Kara, who are my never-ending sources of love, laughter, and adventure and remind me why life is so precious. I love you all! In memory of my father, Paul, who was a continuous source of encouragement and the epitome of perseverance. I have come to realize that he is my hero.

To Bill Brown, my EMS instructor, mentor, colleague, and most importantly my friend, an exemplary EMS educator, professional, and visionary, who instilled in me the meaning of commitment and a belief in excellence in emergency medical services.

JJM

To the new generation, who are just beginning their life experiences—specifically my grandchildren Joshua Keith, Kennedi, and Jackson David—and to all of the children whose educations will need excellent preparation.

KJK

Dr. Brent Hafen was a man of great conviction. He was dedicated to his church, his family, his values, his students, and to the field of EMS. Previous editions of this text and others coauthored by Dr. Hafen have had a tremendous influence on EMS training and education. He is deeply missed as a colleague and friend.

KJK and JJM

Brief Contents

PART 10

STANDARD Trauma 878

PART 11

STANDARD Special Patient Populations 1168

PART 12

STANDARD EMS Operations 1344

Detailed Contents

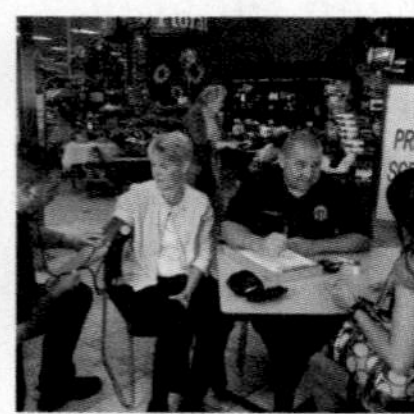

PART 1

CHAPTER 4 Documentation 68

CHAPTER 5 Communication 87

CHAPTER 6 Lifting and Moving Patients 110

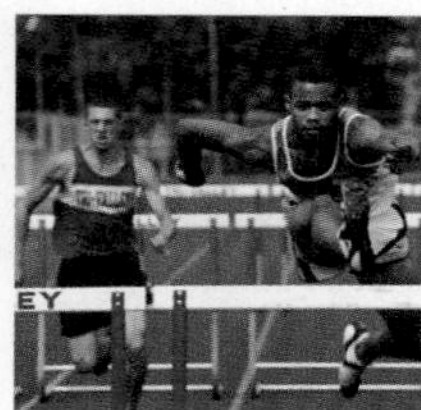

PART 2

STANDARD Anatomy and Physiology 142

STANDARD Medical Terminology 142

CHAPTER 7 Anatomy, Physiology, and Medical Terminology 144

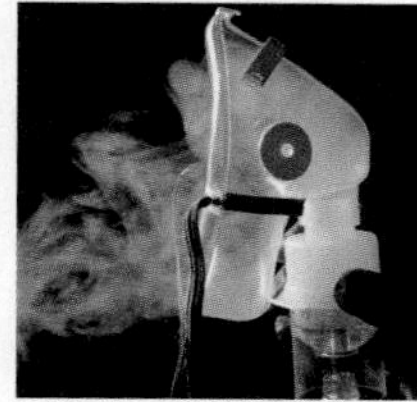

PART 3

STANDARD Pathophysiology 196

CHAPTER 8 Pathophysiology 198

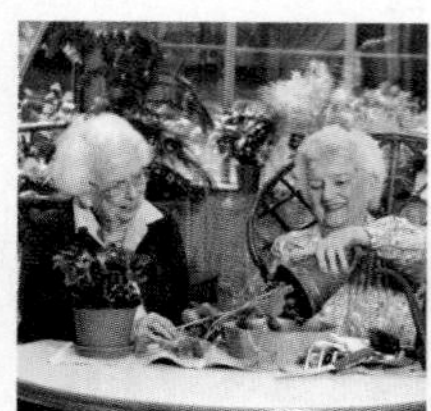

PART 4

STANDARD Life Span Development 228

CHAPTER 9 Life Span Development 230

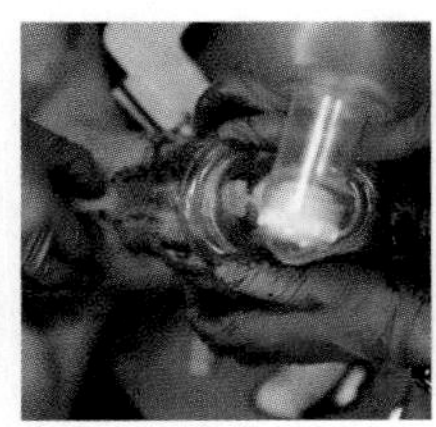

PART 5

STANDARD Airway Management, Respiration, and Artificial Ventilation 246

CHAPTER 10 Airway Management, Artificial Ventilation, and Oxygenation 248

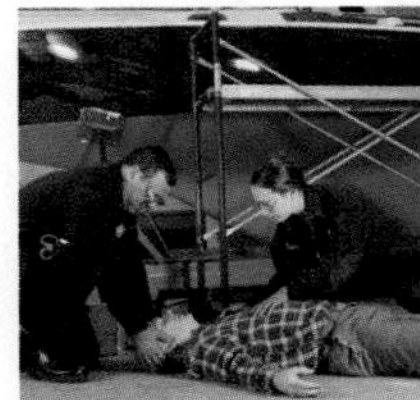

PART 6

STANDARD Assessment 314

CHAPTER 11 Baseline Vital Signs, Monitoring Devices, and History Taking 318

CHAPTER 12 Scene Size-Up 351

CHAPTER 13 Patient Assessment 373

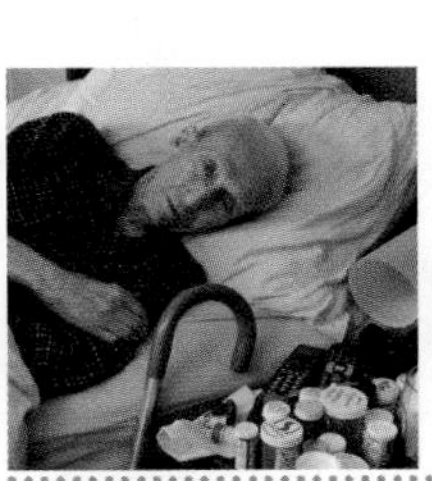

PART 7

STANDARD Pharmacology 470

CHAPTER 14 Pharmacology and Medication Administration 472

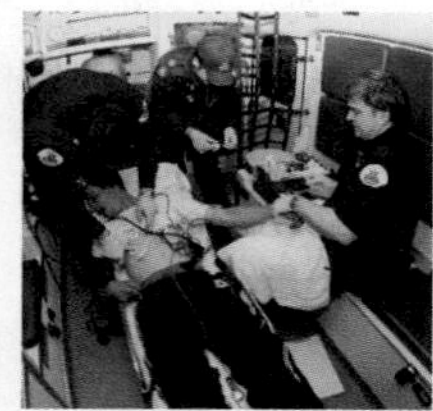

PART 8

STANDARD Shock and Resuscitation 488

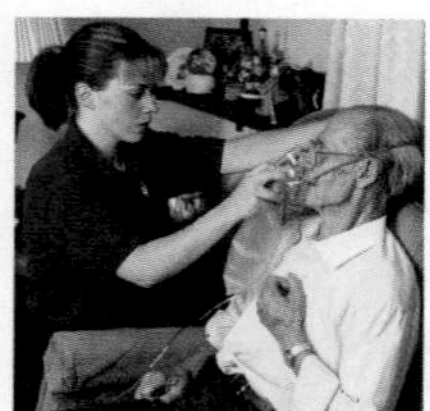

PART 9

STANDARD Medicine 532

CHAPTER 17 Cardiovascular Emergencies 582

CHAPTER 18 Altered Mental Status, Stroke, and Headache 620

CHAPTER 19 Seizures and Syncope 644

CHAPTER 20 Acute Diabetic Emergencies 662

CHAPTER 21 Anaphylactic Reactions 688

CHAPTER 22 Toxicologic Emergencies 711

CHAPTER 23 Abdominal, Gynecologic, Genitourinary, and Renal Emergencies 758

CHAPTER 24 Environmental Emergencies 793

CHAPTER 25 Submersion Incidents: Drowning and Diving Emergencies 836

CHAPTER 26 Behavioral Emergencies 857

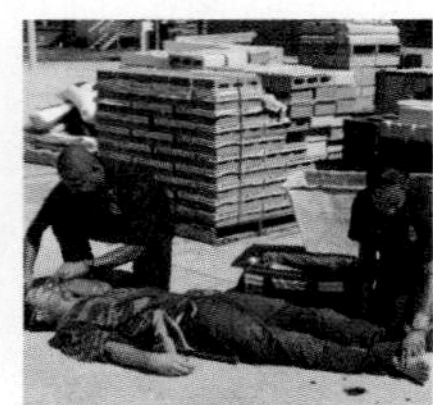

PART 10

STANDARD Trauma 878

CHAPTER 27 Trauma Overview: The Trauma Patient and the Trauma System 880

CHAPTER 28 Bleeding and Soft Tissue Trauma 906

CHAPTER 29 Burns 953

CHAPTER 30 Musculoskeletal Trauma 978

CHAPTER 31 Head Trauma 1013

CHAPTER 32 Spinal Column and Spinal Cord Trauma 1036

CHAPTER 33 Eye, Face, and Neck Trauma 1088

CHAPTER 34 Chest Trauma 1114

CHAPTER 35 Abdominal and Genitourinary Trauma 1138

CHAPTER 36 Multisystem Trauma and Trauma in Special Patient Populations 1152

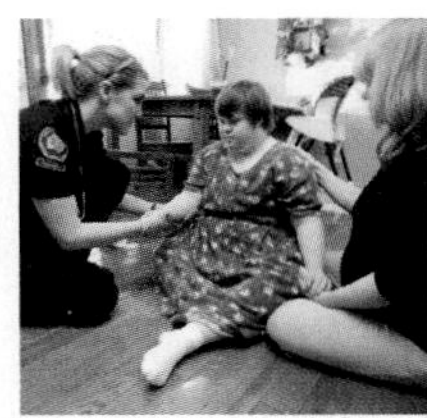

PART 11

STANDARD Special Patient Populations 1168

CHAPTER 37 Obstetrics and Care of the Newborn 1170

CHAPTER 38 Pediatrics 1212

CHAPTER 39 Geriatrics 1280

CHAPTER 40 Patients with Special Challenges 1309

CHAPTER 43 Hazardous Materials 1396

CHAPTER 44 Multiple-Casualty Incidents and Incident Management 1418

CHAPTER 45 EMS Response to Terrorism Involving Weapons of Mass Destruction 1440

Appendix 1 ALS-Assist Skills 1461

Appendix 2 Advanced Airway Management 1468

Key Features

Assessment Summaries

Emergency Care Protocols

Emergency Care Algorithms

EMT Skills

Preface

Prehospital Emergency Care, Ninth Edition, has been extensively revised to meet the National EMS Education Standards published by the National Highway Traffic Safety Administration in 2009 and to reflect the latest and best medical knowledge and practices in emergency medical services in the United States. Recognizing, as well, that equipment, standards, and practices vary from one state and local EMS service to another, the statement "follow local protocols" appears in numerous places throughout the text.

The content of *Prehospital Emergency Care,* Ninth Edition, is summarized here, with emphasis on "what's new" in this edition. One of the first things you will notice is that the text's table of contents has been newly organized to follow the National EMS Educational Standards, with segments designated as "Standards" replacing the "Modules" of prior editions.

STANDARD Preparatory

STANDARD Public Health

The chapters that fall under the first two standards, "Preparatory" and "Public Health," set the foundation for the chapters that follow with such basic topics as EMS systems; research; public health; workforce safety and wellness; medical, legal, and ethical issues; documentation; communication; and lifting and moving patients.

What's New in the "Preparatory" and "Public Health" Chapters?

- Chapter 1, "Emergency Medical Care Systems, Research, and Public Health," describes the **current levels of training**—Emergency Medical Responder (EMR), Emergency Medical Technician (EMT), Advanced Emergency Medical Technician (AEMT), and Paramedic. The new **NHSTA National EMS Education Standards** are noted, and the chapter includes new emphasis on research (in particular, **evidence-based medicine**) and the EMT's role in **public health**.
- Chapter 2, "Workforce Safety and Wellness of the EMT," includes a discussion of the recently approved federal requirements for **high-visibility apparel** to be worn by EMTs and other responders to roadway emergencies.
- Chapter 3, "Medical, Legal, and Ethical Issues," includes a new discussion of the concept of **involuntary consent** relative to mentally incompetent or incarcerated adults.
- Chapter 4, "Documentation," covers documentation of transfer of care and what can be done to provide the receiving facility with complete prehospital care and transfer of care reports **when there is no time to complete documentation before reporting back to service or no ability to print out a hard copy** at the receiving facility.
- Chapter 5, "Communication," includes updated information on **communications technology** and **cell phone communication,** communications involved in **transferring care** to another EMS provider, as well as **team communications** and **therapeutic communications**.
- Chapter 6, "Lifting and Moving Patients," offers a new list of **guidelines and indications for rapid extrication** and other urgent patient moves, new guidelines for **four-person and two-person stretcher carries** and for **carrying a supine patient on stairs**.

STANDARD Anatomy and Physiology

STANDARD Medical Terminology

These standards are covered in a single chapter, "Anatomy, Physiology, and Medical Terminology."

What's New in the Chapter on "Anatomy and Physiology" and "Medical Terminology"?

- Chapter 7, "Anatomy, Physiology, and Medical Terminology," along with expanded information on the mechanics and physiology of respiration, contains **more than 20 new anatomy and physiology illustrations**.

STANDARD Pathophysiology

This standard is covered in one chapter, "Pathophysiology."

What's New in the "Pathophysiology" Chapter?

- Chapter 8, "Pathophysiology," is **an entirely new chapter** in this edition, crafted to introduce the pathophysiological concepts included in the new NHTSA National EMS Education Standards—intended to provide EMTs with a more thorough conceptual knowledge of how the human body functions in the presence of illness and injury.

STANDARD Life Span Development

This standard is covered in one chapter, "Life Span Development."

What's New in the "Life Span Development" Chapter?

- Chapter 9, "Life Span Development," is basically unchanged from the prior edition, covering vital signs, physiological changes, and psychosocial changes that occur during the stages of life from birth through late adulthood.

STANDARD Airway Management, Respiration, and Artificial Ventilation

This standard is covered in one chapter, "Airway Management, Artificial Ventilation, and Oxygenation."

What's New in the "Airway/Respiration/Ventilation" Chapter?

- Chapter 10, "Airway Management, Artificial Ventilation, and Oxygenation," includes expanded information on the **components of respiration** (pulmonary ventilation, external and internal respiration, and cellular respiration and metabolism). There are enhanced discussions of **nervous control of respiration** and the **pathophysiology of disruptions to respiration and circulation** that can lead to cellular hypoxia. New sections discuss the differences in how the body responds to **positive pressure ventilation versus normal ventilation** and how and when to provide **positive pressure ventilation to a patient who is breathing spontaneously**.

STANDARD Assessment

The chapters that fall under the "Assessment" standard are those that detail baseline vital signs, monitoring devices, and history taking as well as scene size-up and the process of patient assessment.

What's New in the "Assessment" Chapters?

- Chapter 11, "Baseline Vital Signs, Monitoring Devices, and History Taking," provides increased emphasis on assessment of **adequate and inadequate breathing** and assessment of **pulses**. A new section on **noninvasive blood pressure monitors** has been added.
- Chapter 12, "Scene Size-Up," while still emphasizing the importance of analyzing the **mechanism of injury** in forming an index of suspicion for injury, now emphasizes **patient presentation** as being a more important indicator of patient condition and severity than mechanism of injury.
- Chapter 13, "Patient Assessment," now emphasizes basing oxygenation of a patient on the patient's presentation and SpO_2 (blood oxygen) levels rather than on predetermined formulas for oxygen concentration and flow—**a different approach to oxygenation** than in prior editions, based on the latest research. **Two approaches to the physical exam**—an **anatomical approach** and a **systems approach**—are introduced. In accordance with the NHTSA EMS Education Standards, the terms used for several of the steps of assessment are changed to **primary assessment, secondary assessment,** and **reassessment**.

STANDARD Pharmacology

This standard is covered in one chapter, "Pharmacology and Medication Administration."

What's New in the "Pharmacology" Chapter?

- Chapter 14, "Pharmacology and Medication Administration," now includes the **small-volume nebulizer** in addition to the metered-dose inhaler in the section on inhaled bronchodilators.

STANDARD Shock and Resuscitation

This standard is covered in one chapter, "Shock and Resuscitation."

What's New in the "Shock and Resuscitation" Chapter?

- Chapter 15, "Shock and Resuscitation," is **a new chapter** in this edition, to include the concepts of the most severe life threats, **shock** and **cardiac arrest**—their pathophysiology, assessment, and emergency medical treatment—in a single chapter.

STANDARD Medicine

The chapters within the "Medicine" standard are those on respiratory and cardiovascular emergencies; altered mental status, stroke, and headache; seizures and syncope; diabetic emergencies; anaphylactic reactions; toxicologic emergencies; abdominal, gynecologic, genitourinary, and renal emergencies; and environmental, drowning and diving, and behavioral emergencies.

What's New in the "Medicine" Chapters?

- Chapter 16, "Respiratory Emergencies," has expanded information on findings associated with respiratory distress. A new section on **small-volume nebulizers** has been included along with information on metered-dose inhalers as methods of administering bronchodilator medications.
- Chapter 17, "Cardiovascular Emergencies," has increased emphasis on the **pathophysiology** of conditions such as **angina pectoris, acute myocardial infarction, heart failure, and hypertensive emergencies**. Discussions of **special considerations in pediatric** and **geriatric** patients and the presentation of **acute coronary syndrome in females** have been expanded.
- Chapter 18, "Altered Mental Status, Stroke, and Headache," has expanded information on the **physiology and pathophysiology** of altered mental status including

discussion of the **reticular activating system**. There is special emphasis on the **pathophysiology, assessment, and emergency care for stroke**.

- Chapter 19, "Seizures and Syncope," has added information on the **pathophysiology** of seizures and syncope and a new section on **differentiating seizures from syncope**.
- Chapter 20, "Acute Diabetic Emergencies," includes expanded information on the pathophysiology of diabetes mellitus and additional information on the rationale and procedures for **testing blood glucose levels**.
- Chapter 21, "Anaphylactic Reactions," features a new emphasis on the **pathophysiology** of anaphylaxis and explanation of the **compensatory mechanisms that underlie specific signs and symptoms of anaphylactic reaction** as well as updated information on how to distinguish mild from severe allergic reactions.
- Chapter 22, "Toxicologic Emergencies," includes a new section on **amphetamines and methamphetamines** and, throughout the chapter, emphasizes basing oxygenation of a patient on the patient's presentation and SpO_2 (blood oxygen) levels rather than on predetermined formulas for oxygen concentration and flow.
- Chapter 23, "Abdominal, Gynecologic, Genitourinary, and Renal Emergencies," has included, for the first time, sections on **genitourinary and renal emergencies,** with detailed information on **kidney stones, kidney failure** and **dialysis, urinary tract infections,** and **urinary catheter management**.
- Chapter 24, "Environmental Emergencies," has expanded information on predisposing factors to generalized hypothermia and an extensive new section on various forms of **high altitude sickness**. This chapter was included in the "Medicine" standard due to the medical content.
- Chapter 25, "Submersion Incidents: Drowning and Diving Emergencies," includes new information on **conditions associated with drowning**, such as alcohol and drug use and trauma, **prognostic predictors** for outcomes from drowning, and the **pathophysiology** of drowning. This chapter was included in the "Medicine" standard due to the medical content.
- Chapter 26, "Behavioral Emergencies," includes new information on **medical causes of behavior changes** and additional **assessment guidelines**. There are new sections on **psychosis** and **agitated delirium** and expanded information on **techniques of dealing with behavioral emergency patients**.

STANDARD Trauma

The chapters within the "Trauma" standard include a trauma overview and chapters on bleeding and soft tissue trauma, burns, musculoskeletal trauma, trauma to the head, spinal column and spinal cord, eye, face, neck and chest, abdominal and genitourinary trauma, multisystem trauma, and trauma in special patient populations. Please note that chapters on "Environmental Emergencies" and "Submersion Incidents: Drowning and Diving Emergencies" were included in the "Medicine" standard due to the medical content.

What's New in the "Trauma" Chapters?

- Chapter 27, "Trauma Overview: The Trauma Patient and the Trauma System," includes new information on the **multisystem trauma patient** and a section on the **"golden period"** and why this concept has replaced the older "golden hour" concept. There are also new sections on **"Golden Principles** of Out-of-Hospital Trauma Care." and "**Special Considerations** in Trauma Care."
- Chapter 28, "Bleeding and Soft Tissue Trauma," provides new information on **classes of hemorrhage** and on the uses **tourniquets** and **hemostatic agents** in the control of bleeding. The section on **care for hypovolemic shock** has been extensively revised.
- Chapter 29, "Burns," includes expanded information regarding the **effects of burns on body systems** and a new list of **burn unit referral criteria** from the American College of Surgeons Committee on Trauma.
- Chapter 30, "Musculoskeletal Trauma," has added new information on **cartilage**, on the **functions of joints,** on **types of fractures, sprains, strains, and dislocations,** on **the six "Ps"** for assessment of possible fractures or dislocations, and on **formable splints**.
- Chapter 31, "Head Trauma," includes added information on **skull injuries, brain injuries,** and the **pathophysiology** of brain injury, and a new section on **brain herniation**.
- Chapter 32, "Spinal Column and Spinal Cord Trauma," has been extensively revised and includes new information on the **pain and light touch tracts** of the spinal cord and their relevance to assessment of spinal cord injury. New sections have been added or expanded on **complete cord injury, spinal shock,** and **incomplete cord injury,** including information on **central cord syndrome, anterior cord syndrome,** and **Brown-Séquard syndrome**.
- Chapter 33, "Eye, Face, and Neck Trauma," includes revised sections on **assessment** and a new section on care of an **avulsed tooth**.
- Chapter 34, "Chest Trauma," includes revised information on **open and closed chest injuries** and a new emphasis on keeping an **index of suspicion** for patients with **chest injuries that may not seem serious at first but then deteriorate rapidly** as well as for immediately life-threatening chest injuries.
- Chapter 35, "Abdominal and Genitourinary Trauma," has expanded information on **abdominal anatomy** and a new section on **reassessment of abdominal injuries** as well as revised information on **genitourinary trauma**.
- Chapter 36, "Multisystem Trauma and Trauma in Special Patient Populations," is **an entirely new chapter**. The opening section concerns the "golden principles" of **out-of-hospital multisystem trauma care**. The section on trauma in special patient populations discusses **trauma in pregnant patients, pediatric patients, geriatric patients,** and **cognitively impaired patients**.

STANDARD Special Patient Populations

The chapters that fall under the "Special Patient Populations" standard are chapters on obstetrics and newborn care, pediatrics, geriatrics, and patients with special challenges.

What's New in the "Special Patient Populations" Chapters?

- Chapter 37, "Obstetrics and Care of the Newborn," includes expanded information on the **anatomy and physiology of pregnancy**, new sections on the **menstrual cycle**, the **prenatal period**, and **physiological changes to various body systems in pregnancy**. There are also new sections on **post-term pregnancy** and **postpartum complications**, and the **American Heart Association algorithm on care of the newborn** is now included.
- Chapter 38, "Pediatrics," has been **entirely revised** to meet the new standards. Included are newly written sections on **developmental characteristics** of children; **assessment** of pediatric patients; **airway, respiratory,** and **cardiovascular conditions** in children; **other pediatric medical conditions; pediatric trauma;** and **child abuse and neglect**. Also included is a section on special considerations, including **Emergency Medical Services for Children (EMS-C), family-centered care**, and **EMT stress** associated with pediatric calls.
- Chapter 39, "Geriatrics," has expanded information on the geriatric **cardiovascular, respiratory, neurological, gastrointestinal, endocrine,** and **other body systems**. New sections have been added on **findings of trauma or shock** and **gastrointestinal bleeding**.
- Chapter 40, "Patients with Special Challenges," is **an entirely new chapter** that includes sections on **sensory impairments, cognitive and emotional impairments, paralysis, obesity, homelessness and poverty,** and **abuse**. There are also sections on technology dependence including **dependence on airway and respiratory devices, vascular access devices, dialysis, gastrointestinal and genitourinary devices,** and **intraventricular shunts**. A final section discusses dealing with **patients who are terminally ill**.

STANDARD EMS Operations

The chapters within the "EMS Operations" standard are chapters on ambulance and air medical operations, gaining access and patient extrication, hazardous materials, multiple-casualty incidents and incident management, and EMS response to terrorism and weapons of mass destruction.

What's New in the "EMS Operations" Chapters?

- Chapter 41, "Ambulance Operations and Air Medical Response," includes new sections under maintaining control of the ambulance on **driver distractions, driving alone, fatigue,** and **aggressive drivers**. Information on the recently approved federal requirements for **high-visibility apparel** has been added. There is an expanded discussion of **considerations for air medical transport**.
- Chapter 42, "Gaining Access and Patient Extrication," scene size-up information now includes performing a **360-degree assessment** and evaluating the **need for additional resources**. New sections discuss **alternative-fueled vehicles, undeployed air bags,** and **energy-absorbing bumpers**.
- Chapter 43, "Hazardous Materials," now introduces **the acronym *TRACEM*** (thermal, radiological, asphyxiation, chemical, etiological, and mechanical) for the types of damage that can be caused by hazardous materials.
- Chapter 44, "Multiple-Casualty Incidents and Incident Management," has included a feature on **planning** as part of the Incident Command System and expanded information on **staging and transport**.
- Chapter 45, "EMS Response to Terrorism Involving Weapons of Mass Destruction," has added a discussion of **applying the Incident Command System to a WMD situation** and a broader discussion of the **role of the EMT in a WMD incident**.

Appendices

The two appendices are Appendix 1, "ALS-Assist Skills," and Appendix 2, "Advanced Airway Management." The information in "ALS-Assist Skills" is basically unchanged from the prior edition. "Advanced Airway Management" was formerly a chapter, but because this topic is not included in the National EMS Education Standards for the EMT level, it is now included as an appendix. Information on "Basic Cardiac Life Support" and "Agricultural and Industrial Emergencies" can be found by accessing mybradykit for this title.

We Want to Hear from You

Many of the best ideas for improving our textbooks and training for future EMTs comes from the instructors and students who use our books and ancillary materials. If you have ideas to offer us or questions to ask, you can reach us at the addresses listed below.

Contact Joe Mistovich at:

jjmistovich@ysu.edu

Visit the Brady website at:

http://www.bradybooks.com

Acknowledgments

We wish to thank the following groups of people for their assistance in developing the Ninth Edition of *Prehospital Emergency Care.*

Medical Editor

Our special thanks to Howard A. Werman, MD, FACEP, Professor, Department of Emergency Medicine, and Medical Director, MedFlight, The Ohio State University College of Medicine and Public Health, Columbus, Ohio. Dr. Werman reviewed the entire manuscript to ensure that the highest degree of medical accuracy was attained. His insight and expertise were invaluable to the development of the text.

Contributing Writers

We would like to express special appreciation to the following specialists who contributed to chapter development in the Ninth Edition.

Randall W. Benner, MEd, MICP, NREMT-P
Director, Emergency Medical Technology
Instructor, Department of Health Professions
Youngstown State University
Youngstown, OH

Tom Brazelton, MD, MPH, FAAP
Associate Professor of Pediatrics
University of Wisconsin School of Medicine & Public Health
Medical Director, Pediatric Intensive Care Unit
American Family Children's Hospital
Madison, WI

Cornelia A. Bryan, BSAS, NREMT-P
Adjunct Faculty, Department of Health Professions
Youngstown State University
Youngstown, OH

William S. Krost, MBA, NREMTP
Director of Emergency Services & Health System Access
Blanchard Valley Health System Access
Findlay, OH

Glenn A. Miller, BSAS, NREMT-P
Emergency Preparedness Consultant
PMG Associates, LLC
Monroeville, PA

Reviewers

The following reviewers of Ninth Edition material provided invaluable feedback and suggestions:

Sandra (Sam) Bradley, EMT-P
Primary EMT Instructor/EMS Program Director
Los Medanos College
Pittsburg, CA

Greg Carlson, MS, BS, AAS, NREMT-P
EMS Teaching Specialist
Wisconsin Indianhead Technical College
New Richmond, WI

Christine Lee Clemens, EMT-P, BFA, MAED
EMS Program Coordinator
Edison State College
Ft. Myers, FL

Harvey Conner, AS, NREMT-P
Professor of EMS
Oklahoma City Community College
Oklahoma City, OK

Christopher Dunn, EMT-P
Lead Instructor
Northwest Community Hospital
Arlington Heights, IL

Phil Ester, BA, CCEMT-P, NREMT-P
EMS Instructor
High Plains Technology Center
Woodward, OK

Michael Fisher, BHS, NREMT-P
Professor, Director of Human Patient Simulation
STAT Center-Simulation Technologies and Training
Greenville Technical College
Greenville, SC

Greg Friese, MS, NREMT-P
President, Emergency Preparedness Systems LLC
Plover, WI

Holly Frost, MS, NREMT-P
Assistant Dean, EMS
Northern Virginia Community College
Springfield, VA

Dave Golding, EMT-P
Washington State Senior EMS Instructor
Aberdeen, WA

Jeff Harkcom, BS, EMT-P
EMT Program Coordinator/Adjunct Instructor
Indian River State College
Ft. Pierce, FL

Christopher E. Harris, MICT, I/C, BSHA
Captain
Sedgwick County EMS
Wichita, KS

James J. Hasson, BSAS, NREMT-P
Director
EMS Educational Institute
Sharon Regional Health System
Sharon, PA

Russell Hogue, EMT-P, EMT-I
Instructor
Yuba Community College
Marysville, CA

Scott C. Holliday, BS, EMT-P, CIC
Associate Director
St. John's University, Emergency Medical Service Institute
Meadows, NY

Sharon A. Ingram, NREMT-P
Training Officer
Stone Ambulance Service, Inc
Stuart, VA

Charlene Jansen, BS, EMT-P
EMS Programs Coordinator
St. Louis Community College
St. Louis, MO

Joe Kalilikani, Jr., EMT-B
Faculty
National Polytechnic College of Science
Los Angeles, CA

David Jay Kleiman, NREMT-P
Paramedic Instructor
North Metro Technical College
Acworth, GA

Sandra LeBlanc, BS, NREMT-P
Nunez Community College EMTP Coordinator
Chalmette, LA

Hal Lineback III, NREMT, PALS, ACLS Provider/ACLS Instr., AK EMT Instr. (Paramedic)
Adjunct Faculty
University of Alaska SE (Sitka)
Sitka, AK

Joseph McConomy Jr., MICP, EMT-B (I)
Senior EMT Instructor
Burlington County Emergency Services Training Center
Westampton, NJ

Nikhil Natarajan, BPS, NREMT-P, I/C
Adjunct Professor
SUNY Ulster
Stone Ridge, NY

Steve Nguyen, BS, NREMT-P
Tulsa Technology Center
Tulsa, OK

Donna Olafson
Director, EMT/MICT Program
Kansas City, Kansas Community College
Kansas City, KS

Gwendolyn (Gwen) M. Peel, NREMT-P, AAS
Emergency Services Management
DeKalb County Fire Rescue Academy
Tucker, GA

Warren J. Porter, MS, BA, LP, PNCCT
EMS Programs Manager
Garland Fire Department
Garland, TX

Bernard J. Schweter, PhD, MBA, EMSI, EMT-P
Clinical Preceptor/Instructor
Cuyahoga Community College
Cleveland, OH

Hezedean A. Smith, MA, BS, EMT-P
Professor of EMS, Valencia Community College
Lieutenant, Orlando Fire Department
Orlando, FL

David L. Sullivan, PhD, NREMT-P
Program Director
Saint Petersburg College
Pinellas Park, FL

Michael Thompson, EMT-B
EMS/Fire Instructor
CTEC at St. Cloud Technical College
St. Cloud, MN

Sedley A. Tomlinson, AAS, NREMT-B, I/C
Program Director
Air Evac Lifeteam
Little Rock, AR

Wayne D. Turner, EMT-P, EMSI
EMS Instructor
Cincinnati State EMS
Cincinnati, OH

Karyl White, MS, Paramedic/Instructor Coordinator
EMS Education Director
Barton County Community College
Great Bend, KS

We also wish to thank the EMS professionals in the following list who reviewed the eighth edition of *Prehospital Emergency Care*:

David K. Anderson, BS, EMT-P
Director of EMS Education
NW Regional Training Center
Vancouver, WA

Brenda M. Beasley, RN, BS, EMT-P
Department Chair Allied Health
Calhoun Community College
Wedowee, AL

John L. Beckman, AA
FF/EMT-P Instructor
Addison Fire Protection District
Fire Science Instructor
Technology Center of DuPage
Addison, IL

Richard J. Belle, BS, NREMT-P
Acadian Ambulance Service, Inc.
Lafayette, LA

Harvey Conner, AS, NREMT-P
Emergency Medical Sciences Program
Oklahoma City Community College
Oklahoma City, OK

Maylyn Geissler, NREMT-P
Louisiana EMS Quality Assurance
Education Coordinator
National EMS Academy
Slidell, LA

Barry Jensen, NREMT-P
Program Director
Center for Prehospital Care
UCLA School of Medicine
Los Angeles, CA

Greg Mullen, MS, NREMTP
National EMS Academy
Lafayette, LA

Michael Murrow
The George Washington University
Chesapeake Health & Safety
St. Mary's Advanced Life Support
Washington, DC

Douglas A. Paris, BS, NREMT-P
Department of Emergency Medical Technology
Greenville Technical College
Greenville, SC

Franco D. Piscitani, BSAS, NREMT-P
Affiliate Faculty
YSU Metro College
Youngstown, OH

Robert A. Schlussler, BE, NREMT-B
Paramedic Student
Seminole Community College
Sanford, FL

Brian J. Wilson, BA, NREMT-P
Division of Emergency Medical Services
Texas Tech School of Medicine
El Paso, TX

Jason P. Zielewicz, MS, NREMT-P
EMS Supervisor/Instructor
Office of EMS
The Pennsylvania State University
University Park, PA

Photo Acknowledgments

All photographs not credited adjacent to the photograph or in the photo credit section below were photographed on assignment for Brady/Pearson.

Photo Credits

Figures 15-20, 15-21, 22-08, 29-10, Scan 28-09A-G photographed for Pearson by Ray Kemp/911 Imaging

Photo Credits for Part Openers Part 02 © Michal Heron, Part 03 © Daniel Limmer, Part 04 © Michal Heron, Part 08 © Kevin Link, Part 11 © Kevin Link, Part 12 © Ray Kemp/911 Imaging

Photo Credits for Chapter Openers Chapter 07 © George Shelley/Masterfile, Chapter 09 © Royalty Free / Masterfile, Chapter 10 © Kevin Link, Chapter 14 © Daniel Limmer, Chapter 15 © Daniel Limmer, Chapters 27–36 © Mark C. Ide, Chapters 43–45 © Ed Kashi/Corbis

Organizations

We wish to thank the following organizations for their assistance in creating the photo program for this edition:

Columbus Division of Fire, Columbus, OH, Fire Chief Ned Pettus, Jr.

Delta Ambulance, Waterville, ME, Paul Thompson, EMT-P, Fleet Coordinator

Fairfield Fire Rescue, Fairfield, ME, Chief Duane Bickford

Falmouth Fire-EMS, Falmouth, ME, Asst. Chief Doug Patey, EMT-P, I/C

Kennebec Valley Emergency Medical Services Council, Winslow, ME, Rick Petrie, EMT-P

Kennebunk Fire and Rescue, Kennebunk, ME, Deputy Chief David Cluff

NorthStar Ambulance, Farmington, ME, Michael Senecal, EMT-P, Director

Norwich Township Fire Department, Hilliard, OH, Fire Chief David Long

Oakland Fire Rescue, Oakland, ME, Chief David Coughlin

Sanford Fire Department, Sanford, ME, Chief Raymond Parent, Regional Coordinator

Waterville Fire Department, Waterville, ME, Chief David Lafountain

Winslow Fire Department, Winslow, ME, Chief David Lafountain

Technical Advisors

Thanks to the following people for providing technical support during the photo shoots for this edition:

Technical Advisors in Ohio
Captain Shawn C. Koser, NREMT-P, CCEMT-P, AAS

Lisa K. Koser, MSN, RN, CEN, CCRN, EMT-P

Technical Advisors in Maine

Brian Chamberlin, EMT-P, KVEMSC/Augusta Rescue

Steven Diaz, MD, Maine General Medical Center & Maine EMS Medical Director

Carl French, CCEMTP/FF EMT-T, Sanford Fire Department, Sanford, ME

Judy French, EMT-I, Alfred Rescue, Alfred, ME

Lt. Paul Goldstein, FF/EMT

Mark King, EMT-P, KVEMSC/Winthrop Ambulance, Winthrop, ME

Marc Minkler, EMT-P, Portland Fire Department, Portland, ME

Asst. Chief Doug Patey, EMT-P, I/C, Falmouth Fire-EMS, Falmouth, ME

Rick Petrie, EMT-P, KVEMSC/United Ambulance, Winslow, ME

Carol Pillsbury, EMT-P, NorthStar Ambulance

Tiffany Stebbins, EMT-P, KVEMSC

Locations

Thanks to the following people and organizations who provided locations for our photographs:

Barry Acker, The Landing School, Arundel, ME

Colby College, Waterville, ME

David Cluff, Duffy's Tavern & Grill, Kennebunk, ME

Giant Eagle Corporation, Pittsburgh, PA

Giant Eagle Store, 6780 Hayden Run Rd., Hilliard, OH

Paul Goldstein, Falmouth, ME

David Groder, EMT-P, Oakland, ME

Jay Hallett, Handy Boat Yard, Falmouth, ME

Maineline Technology Group, Falmouth, ME

Allie Moore, EMT-B, Oakland, ME

OceanView at Falmouth, ME

Francis Pooler, Fairfield, ME

Sappi Fine Paper, Skowhegan, ME

Trinity Homes, 2700 E. Dublin Granville Rd., Columbus, OH

Erick and Kim Van Sickle, Leyland British Auto, Arundel, ME

Models

Thanks to the following people who portrayed patients and EMS providers in our photographs:

Models in Maine Richard Battle, Jessica Blomerth, Erica Bohlman, Jeremy R. Buzzell, Emily L. Carter, Brian Chamberlin, Eric Cheney, Vivian Chicoine, Amanda Chretien, Cody Chretien, Shanelle Coolidge, Stephanie Cordwell, Drew Corey, Gary H. Cushing, Jack Davis, Jonathan Denham, Diane Deyoe, Erin Deyoe, Shannon Deyoe, Steven Diaz, Thomas H. Doak, George Donovan, Paul J. Dubois, Casey Dugas, Chip Eames, Maurice Frappier, Jane Fenn, Regina M. Fife, Gary Foss, Robert G. Fox, Carl French, Judy French, Maurice Froppier, Sherry Given, Nancy Goldstein, Paul Goldstein, Jennifer L. Grey, Kristen Hagan, Ann E. Harrison-Billiat, Kevin L'Heureux, Helena Hollauer, Adolph Holmes, Alex Johnson, Mark King, Susan King, Rod Koehn, John Lacombe, Matthew Leach, Sarah Kaylee Leary, Travis Leary, Sarah K. Limmer, Kenneth Lovell, Kalem Malcolm, Allyson P. Moore, Gary Paradis, Thaddeus J. Pawlick, Jason C. Pfingst, Fran Pooler, Kathryn Pow, Nicole Prescott, Zachary Pushee, David Rackliffe, Gerald Roderick, Jim Scully, Stephen L. Smith, Kenneth Solorzano, McKenzie Stebbins, Andrew Stevenson, Edward Strapp, Todd Tracy, Eric Van Sickle, Kim Van Sickle, John G. Vatulas, Michelle Vrbanek, Llewellyn Wilson

Models in Ohio Ballard M. Armstrong, Norman Atwood, Thomas P. Bagley, Steven R. Basil, Joe Bauer, Rick Boerner, Douglas Brown, Marc P. Cain, Steven J. Chapman, Thad J. Cullison, Nicholas S. Daw, Herman Davis, Curt Dewey, Mark E. Dixon, Michael Donahoe, Patrick Dunbrack, Tim Durbin, Michael E. Ebets, Jeff Evans, Scott Ferguson, Donna Green, John Green, Brian W. Groff, Mark Howland, Michael Keller, Alex Koser, Jerrie Koser, John W. Koser, Ruth Koser, Shawn Koser, Stephen E. Koser, Rich Lawless, Tony Long, Craig McDonald, Angela Meeker, Robert Meeker, Ryan Moody, John Moore, Robert O'Neil, Matthew Parrish, Trina Patterson, Mike Powell, James R. Schiering III, Brenda Schultz, Arlene Sherer, Tasha Sherer, Buck Spangler, Jed Smith, Jeff Stanforth, Thomas Stermer, Lawrence Stevens, Leroy Stewart, Alex J. Sundberg, John Szymkowiak, Marsha Vayhinger, George Wallace, Chantal Weldon, Garrett Weldon, Donald Weldon, Kenneth Worley

Photo Coordinators

Thanks to the following for valuable assistance coordinating models, props, and locations for our photo shoots:

Judy French, EMT-I, Alfred Rescue

Kelly Roderick, KVEMSC

Brenda Schultz, Columbus Division of Fire

Photo Assistant and Digital Post-Production

Manjari Sharma

Authors' Letter to Students

Congratulations on your decision to undertake an EMT education program. The field of emergency medical services is extremely rewarding and will provide you with experiences you will find both challenging and gratifying.

Be Prepared

As an EMT student, you have a few pressing concerns. You want to be prepared:

- To pass your course exams
- To pass the credentialing exam that allows you to practice as an EMT
- To treat patients to the best of your ability
- To do well in all aspects of your job

As the authors, we want to assure you that *Prehospital Emergency Care,* Ninth Edition, is written to help you achieve those goals.

It All Makes Sense

The key to the above goals—passing your exams, providing excellent patient care, and doing well in your job—is understanding how everything fits together:

- A basic understanding of anatomy, physiology, and pathophysiology will allow you to better understand signs, symptoms, and emergency care.
- An anatomical and body systems approach to physical exam will link conditions to assessment findings.
- Knowledge of the presentations of common medical conditions and traumatic injuries encountered in the prehospital environment will enable you to perform efficient and accurate assessments.
- A diagnostic-based approach to patient assessment will allow you to form a differential field impression of the condition or injury.
- An assessment-based approach to patient assessment will allow you to identify and provide immediate emergency care for life-threatening conditions or injuries.
- You will learn how to provide the most efficient and effective emergency care.

The good news is that—although what you have to learn may seem daunting in the beginning—it all makes sense. In fact, that is the philosophy behind this textbook. Our purpose has been to show you at every step of your EMT education program how:

It all makes sense!

Features

All of the features in this textbook are designed to help you navigate through the anatomy, physiology, pathophysiology, assessment findings, medical conditions, traumatic injuries, and emergency care to best prepare you to provide excellent emergency medical services to the patient—beginning with the dispatch of the call, followed by assessment and management of the patient and delivery to the medical facility, through writing your prehospital care report. In addition to the 275 new photographs and 70 new illustrations, in the "clinical" chapters (on airway care, the medical chapters, and the trauma chapters) you will find:

- Assessment Tips
- Understanding Body Processes
- Drug Profiles
- Assessment Summaries
- Emergency Care Protocols
- Emergency Care Algorithms

And a special feature that appears throughout Chapter 13, "Patient Assessment":

- Critical Findings,

which explains, at every step of the assessment, critical conditions/signs/symptoms you may find . . . what might be causing them . . . and specifically what you should do when your assessment of the patient reveals one of these critical findings.

EMTs are often taught **WHAT** signs and symptoms they should expect to see in certain conditions and **WHAT** should be done; however, the **WHY** of assessment and emergency care is often not well addressed. Two of the features, "Understanding Body Processes" and "Assessment Tips"—in addition to expanded discussion within the chapters—provide you with a basic understanding so that you can better comprehend **WHY** you are seeing signs and symptoms and **WHY** you are providing specific emergency care.

The Assessment Summaries, Emergency Care Protocols, Emergency Care Algorithms, and Critical Findings features provide the most up-to-date strategies for providing competent care. These features and the entire text have been updated to conform to the latest American Heart Association guidelines.

In Your EMS Career

In your EMS career, you will respond to a variety of calls in uncontrolled environments requiring confidence, compassion, and a high degree of competence. As an EMT, you will be put to the test to think critically and respond instantaneously. The foundation for these skills will be provided in your education program; you will learn further and gain better clinical insight through patient contact, continuing education, and experience. Once you have read this textbook and complete your EMT program, you will have only begun your educational experience as an EMT. Every day you should strive to learn something new that may enhance your emergency patient care. Due to the dynamic nature of emergency medical services, you will become a lifelong learner.

Pathophysiology

As an EMT, you will be required to learn about many patient conditions and injuries that you will encounter in the prehospital environment. Identifying these conditions and injuries is most often based on the recognition of specific signs and symptoms and history findings. Not only is it difficult to memorize the myriad of signs and symptoms for each condition or injury, it is not desirable because not every patient presents with just one condition or injury or all of the same signs and symptoms. A good basic foundation of pathophysiology helps you to understand and explain the "why" behind the patient presentation. There is no need to memorize when you understand and can explain why each sign or symptom is occurring. Putting this together with a fundamental understanding of the pathophysiology of the conditions and a thorough approach to patient assessment will allow you to quickly recognize immediate life threats and provide excellent emergency care. Don't memorize, but understand. This is the foundation to making "it all make sense!"

The Importance of Patient Assessment

Patient assessment is one of the most important skills that an EMT performs, requiring good practical ability and also the capability to think critically. You must take each finding from the assessment, determine if an immediate lifesaving intervention is required, store the information learned in the back of your mind as you continue with the assessment, and finally put all the pieces of the assessment together to provide effective emergency medical care. The challenge is similar to putting a puzzle together. You start out with individual pieces of the puzzle that have to be connected together to form a meaningful picture. The pieces of the puzzle correlate to signs, symptoms, and other findings of the assessment. You must take the findings, consider them individually, and then put them together to form a whole picture of your patient. Specific findings are meaningless without fitting them into the entire picture.

Prehospital Emergency Care, Ninth Edition, provides a strong, comprehensive approach to patient assessment, which is reinforced at several points in the chapters—in the Case Study, chapter text, Assessment-Based Approach, Assessment Summaries, and Algorithms. This approach reinforces assessment information and also provides an alternative learning method. You will find the necessary clinical information integrated into the assessment approach for each section, unlike other sources that integrate the assessment information into the clinical information.

This textbook uses a two-tiered approach to teaching emergency medical care: assessment based and diagnostic based. An assessment-based approach to patient injuries and illnesses teaches you to identify life-threatening conditions and provide immediate interventions to reverse those problems. An assessment-based approach to acute patient care is followed no matter what level of care is provided. Once you have managed life-threatening conditions, you will then move to the next level of assessment, the diagnostic-based approach. The diagnostic-based approach entails putting the signs, symptoms, and other assessment findings together to come to a probability of what conditions the patient may be suffering from. Many EMS providers refer to this as their "differential field impression." *Prehospital Emergency Care,* Ninth Edition, presents the necessary information to move naturally, successfully, and effectively from the assessment-based approach to the diagnostic-based approach.

Using Medical Terminology

As you progress through your education program, you will learn a new system of communication that involves the use of appropriate medical terminology. It is important to establish a basic understanding of medical terminology so that you may communicate effectively, by both written and oral means, with other members of the medical team. *Prehospital Emergency Care,* Ninth Edition, addresses medical terminology within Chapter 7, "Anatomy, Physiology, and Medical Terminology," and has integrated a basic foundation of medical terminology into each chapter (see the terms in bold type and the glossary at the end of the book) that will help you to enhance your professional image and communication skills. You should expand your medical terminology base as you continue your education.

As You Begin Your EMS Career

We wish you the best of luck as you begin your career in emergency medical services. Our best piece of advice to you is to provide the best emergency care possible and always do what is right for the patient. This will allow you to contribute to the mission of emergency medical services.

Good luck and best wishes!

Joseph J. Mistovich
Keith J. Karren

About the Authors

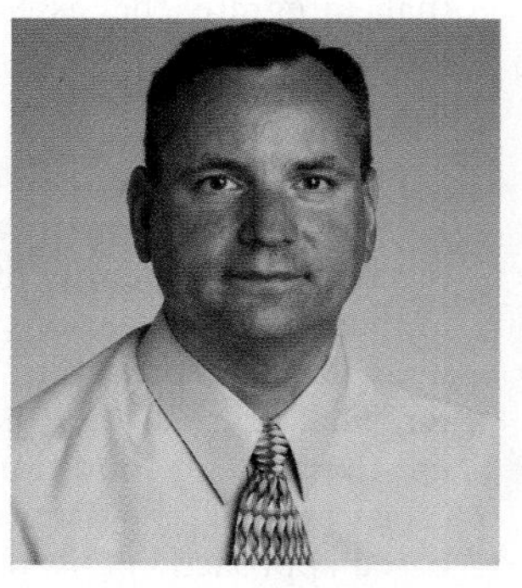

Joseph J. Mistovich, MEd, NREMT-P

Joseph Mistovich is Chairperson of the Department of Health Professions and a Professor at Youngstown State University in Youngstown, Ohio. He has more than 25 years of experience as an educator in emergency medical services.

Mr. Mistovich received his Master of Education degree in Community Health Education from Kent State University in 1988. He completed a Bachelor of Science in Applied Science degree with a major in Allied Health in 1985, and an Associate in Applied Science degree in Emergency Medical Technology in 1982 from Youngstown State University.

Mr. Mistovich is an author or coauthor of numerous EMS books and journal articles and is a frequent presenter at national and state EMS conferences.

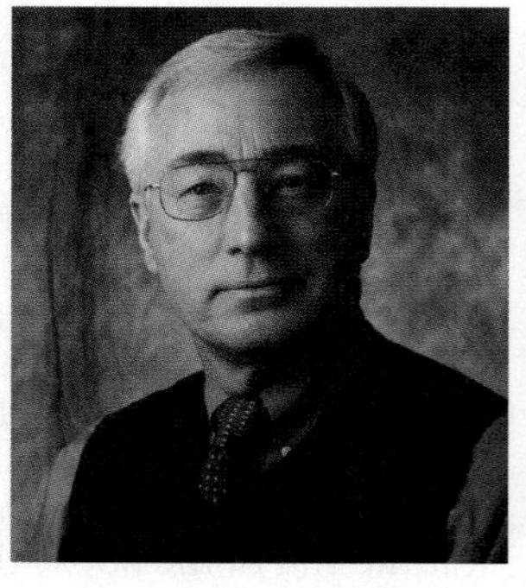

Keith J. Karren, PhD, EMT-B

Keith J. Karren is Professor and former Chairperson of the Department of Health Sciences at Brigham Young University in Provo, Utah. He has been a professional educator in health sciences and emergency medical services for more than 30 years. Dr. Karren received his Bachelor of Science and Master of Science degrees from Brigham Young University in 1969 and 1970, and his PhD in Health Science from Oregon State University in 1975. He graduated from one of the first EMT certification courses offered in Utah. Dr. Karren is the author or coauthor of numerous books on prehospital emergency care and health, including *First Aid for Colleges and Universities* and *First Responder: A Skills Approach.* He also directs the Prehospital Emergency Care and Crisis Intervention Conference, one of the premier EMS conferences in North America.

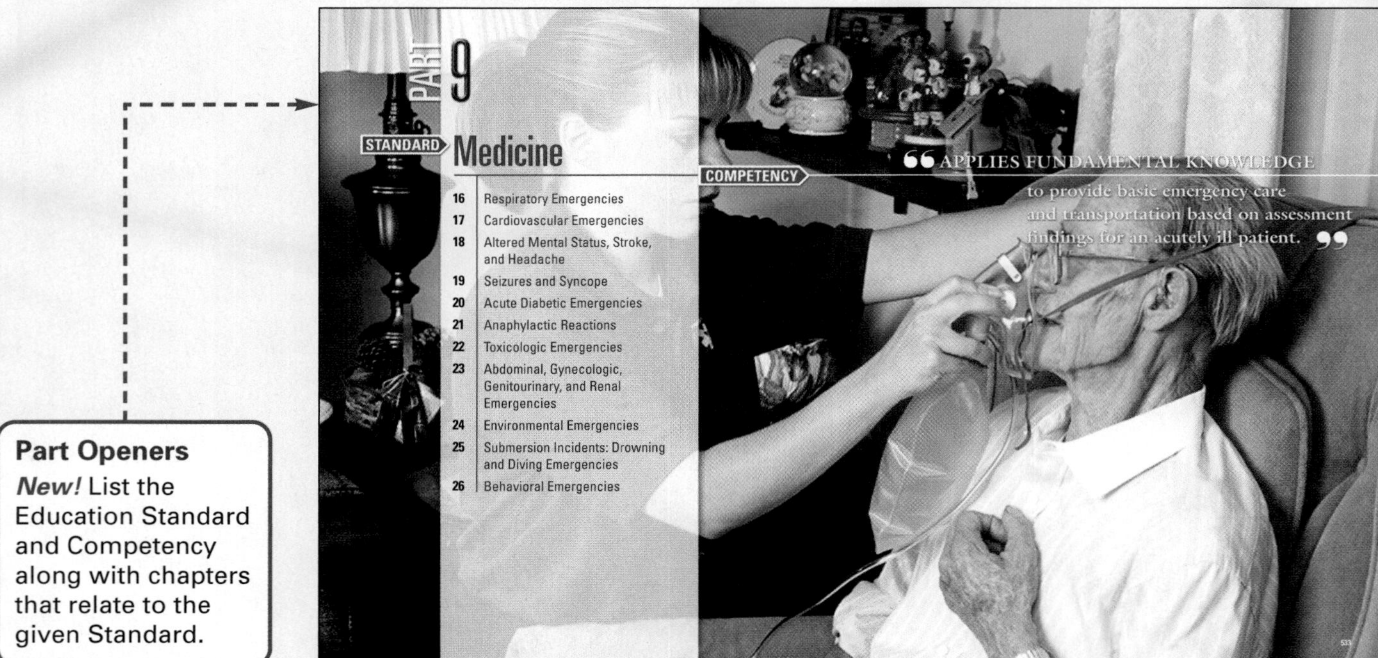

Part Openers
New! List the Education Standard and Competency along with chapters that relate to the given Standard.

Navigation Guide
New! This toolbox helps students navigate through the chapter materials. Placed at the beginning of each chapter, the Navigation Guide refers readers to the Education Standard, Competency, and Chapter Objectives, as well as to Key Terms, Media Resources, and the Chapter Case Study. These elements provide a foundation for learning chapter content.

Navigation Guide

The following items provide an overview to the purpose and content of this chapter. The Education Standard and Competency are from the new National EMS Education Standards.

STANDARD **Medicine** (Content Area: Respiratory)

COMPETENCY Applies fundamental knowledge to provide basic emergency care and transportation based on assessment findings for an acutely ill patient.

OBJECTIVES: After reading this chapter, you should be able to:

16-1. Define key terms introduced in this chapter.
16-2. Explain the importance of being able to quickly recognize and treat patients with respiratory emergencies.
16-3. Describe the structure and function of the respiratory system, including:
- **a.** Upper airway
- **b.** Lower airway
- **c.** Gas exchange
- **d.** Inspiratory and expiratory centers in the medulla and pons

16-4. Demonstrate the assessment of breath sounds.
16-5. Describe the characteristics of abnormal breath sounds, including:
- **a.** Wheezing
- **b.** Rhonchi
- **c.** Crackles (rales)

16-6. Explain the relationship between dyspnea and hypoxia.
16-7. Differentiate respiratory distress, respiratory failure, and respiratory arrest.
16-8. Describe the pathophysiology by which each of the following conditions leads to inadequate oxygenation:
- **a.** Obstructive pulmonary diseases: emphysema, chronic bronchitis, and asthma
- **b.** Pneumonia
- **c.** Pulmonary embolism
- **d.** Pulmonary edema
- **e.** Spontaneous pneumothorax
- **f.** Hyperventilation syndrome
- **g.** Epiglottitis
- **h.** Pertussis
- **i.** Cystic fibrosis
- **j.** Poisonous exposures
- **k.** Viral respiratory infections

16-9. As allowed by your scope of practice, demonstrate administering or assisting a patient with self-administration of bronchodilators by metered-dose inhaler and/or small-volume nebulizer.
16-10. Differentiate between short-acting beta$_2$ agonists appropriate for prehospital use and respiratory medications that are not intended for emergency use.
16-11. Describe special considerations in the assessment and management of pediatric and geriatric patients with respiratory emergencies, including:
- **a.** Differences in anatomy and physiology
- **b.** Causes of respiratory emergencies
- **c.** Differences in management

16-12. Employ an assessment-based approach in order to recognize indications for the following interventions in patients with respiratory complaints/emergencies:
- **a.** Establishing an airway
- **b.** Administration of oxygen
- **c.** Positive pressure ventilation
- **d.** Administration/assistance with self-administration of an inhaled beta$_2$ agonist
- **e.** Expedited transport
- **f.** ALS backup

16-13. Given a list of patient medications, recognize medications that are associated with respiratory disease.
16-14. Use reassessment to identify responses to treatment and changes in the conditions of patients presenting with respiratory complaints and emergencies.

Objectives
Objectives form the basis of each chapter and were developed around the Education Standards and Instructional Guidelines.

Key Terms

Page numbers identify where each key term first appears in the chapter.

Media Resources

Media exercises for weblinks, animations, and videos related to chapter content can be found under the mykit for this book at **www.bradybooks.com.**

Case Study and Follow-Up

Located at the end of the Chapter Navigation Guide, a Case Study draws students into the subject and creates a link between the text and real-life situations and experiences. The Case Study Follow-Up at the end of each chapter emphasizes key concepts learned and in-depth resolution.

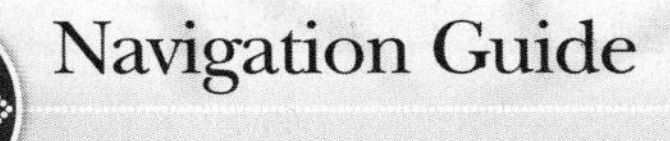

KEY TERMS: Page references indicate first major use in this chapter. For complete definitions, see the Glossary at the back of the book.

apnea p. 539
bronchoconstriction p. 539
bronchodilator p. 539
dyspnea p. 539
hypercarbia p. 540
hypoxemia p. 539
hypoxia p. 539
metered-dose inhaler (MDI) p. 554
pulsus paradoxus p. 568
respiratory arrest p. 540
respiratory distress p. 540
respiratory failure p. 540
small-volume nebulizer p. 555
spacer p. 555
tripod position p. 564

MEDIA RESOURCES: Please go to www.bradybooks.com to access mykit for this text. You will find quizzes, critical thinking scenarios, weblinks, animations, and videos related to this chapter—and much more. Look for online information on breath sounds and assessment tips. You will also find animations and video clips on asthma, tuberculosis, ARDS, and COPD.

CASE STUDY

The Dispatch

EMS Unit 106—respond to 1449 Porter Avenue, Apartment 322. You have a 31-year-old female patient complaining of respiratory distress. Time out is 1942 hours.

Upon Arrival

You and your partner arrive at the scene and are greeted at the curb by the husband of the patient. As you step out of the ambulance and begin to gather your equipment, you ask, "Did you place the call for EMS, sir?" He states very nervously, "Yes. It's my wife, Anna. She can't breathe. She really doesn't look good." As you and your partner begin walking toward the apartment complex, you ask, "What's your name?" His voice breaks as he tells you, "My name is John Sanders. We've only been married 2 months. Please—you've got to help my wife." You reply, "John, we'll take good care of your wife. But, you'll help us more if you can calm down."

As he leads you up narrow stairs to the third floor of the apartment complex, you scan the scene for safety hazards and note any obstacles that will make it difficult to extricate the patient from the building. Upon walking into the apartment, you note a young woman sitting upright on a kitchen chair, looking very scared, and leaning slightly forward with her arms locked in front of her to hold her up. Before you can even introduce yourself, she begins to speak one word at a time with a gasp for breath in between: "I—can't—breathe."

How Would You Proceed to Assess and Care for This Patient?

During this chapter you will learn about assessment and emergency care for a patient suffering from respiratory distress. Later, we will return to the case and apply the procedures learned.

Assessment Tips

Clinical insights that EMTs often learn over time. These enable the EMT to more accurately conduct an assessment and interpret the findings.

ASSESSMENT Tips

In any patient complaining of shortness of breath, assess for pain, redness, increased warmth, and swelling to the lower leg, especially at the calf. These are signs of a deep vein thrombosis (DVT), a blood clot in a vein of the lower leg that may have broken free, traveled to the lungs, and caused a pulmonary embolism. ■

Understanding Body Processes

This feature highlights the body processes that cause the conditions found by EMTs, creating the in-depth understanding that helps providers make the right decisions for patients.

Understanding BODY PROCESSES

The light-headedness, dizziness, or fainting experienced by the hyperventilating patient is caused by a drastic reduction of carbon dioxide (the rapid breathing blows off excessive amounts of carbon dioxide). This causes the cerebral arteries to constrict excessively, reducing blood flow to the brain tissue, causing the light-headedness, dizziness, and fainting. ■

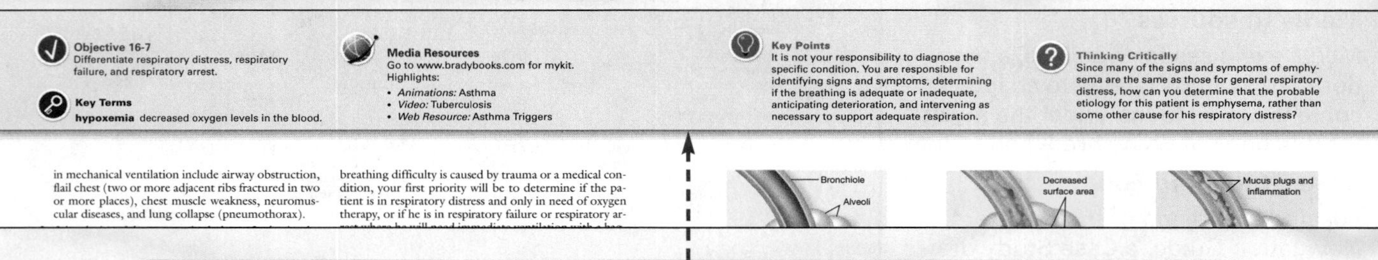

Navigation Bar
New! This feature runs across the top of many pages within the chapters. It reinforces and builds upon what is found in the Navigation Guide. It presents Objectives, Key Terms, Thinking Critically questions, and Key Points, and it highlights Media Resources for this book found through ***mybradykit.***

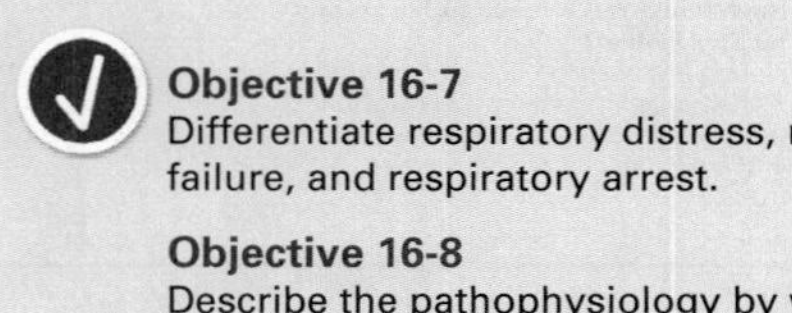

Objective 16-7
Differentiate respiratory distress, respiratory failure, and respiratory arrest.

Objective 16-8
Describe the pathophysiology by which various conditions lead to inadequate oxygenation.

Objectives
New! Objective references appear as close as possible to specific content being addressed.

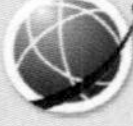

Media Resources
Go to www.bradybooks.com for mykit. Highlights:

- *Animation:* Asthma
- *Video:* Tuberculosis
- *Web Resource:* Asthma Triggers

Media Resources
New! Refers students to **www.bradybooks.com** to access a new resource—**mybradykit**—a one-stop shop for online chapter support materials. Includes specific references to animations, videos, weblinks, and much more.

Thinking Critically
Since many of the signs and symptoms of emphysema are the same as those for general respiratory distress, how can you determine that the probable etiology for this patient is emphysema, rather than some other cause for his respiratory distress?

Thinking Critically
New! Asks students to think critically and thoughtfully while applying their new knowledge.

Key Points
It is not your responsibility to diagnose the specific condition. You are responsible for identifying signs and symptoms, determining if the breathing is adequate or inadequate, anticipating deterioration, and intervening as necessary to support adequate respiration.

Key Points
New! These emphasize the text's core concepts.

Key Terms
hypoxemia decreased oxygen levels in the blood.

Key Terms
New! Boldfaced terms and their definitions are highlighted in the Navigation Bar.

Metered-Dose Inhaler (MDI) / Small-Volume Nebulizer (SVN)

Medication Name

Metered-dose inhalers contain medications with a variety of generic and trade names, including the following. (Note: Not all drugs that are packaged as an MDI are available for nebulization.)

Generic Name	Trade Name
Albuterol	Proventil®, Ventolin®
Metaproterenol	Metaprel®, Alupent®
Isoetharine	Bronkosol®
Bitolterol mesylate	Tornalate®
Salmeterol xinafoate	Serevent®
Ipratropium	Atrovent®
Levalbuterol	Xoponex
Pirbuterol	Maxair

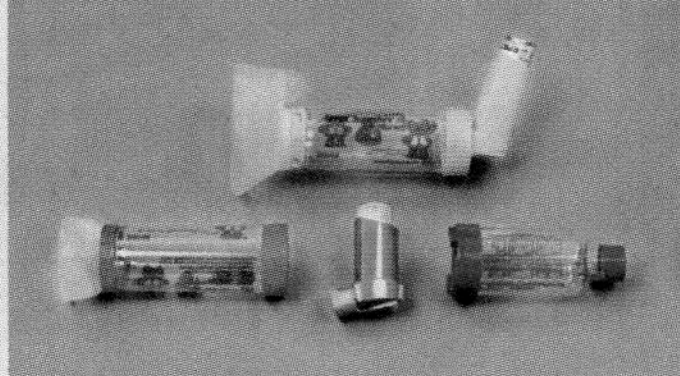
Meter-dosed inhaler.

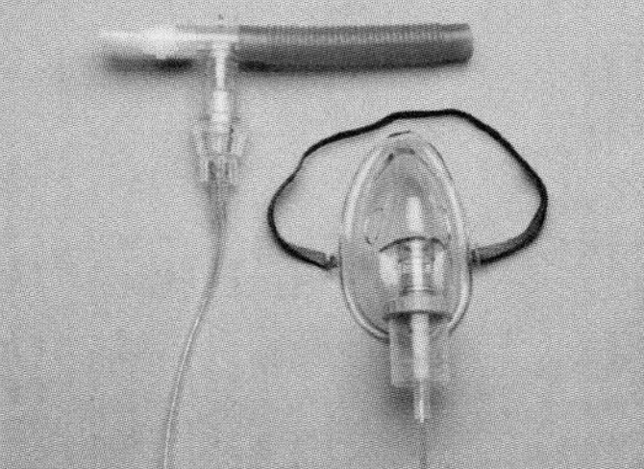
Small-volume nebulizer.
© Carl Leet, YSU

Indications

All of the following criteria must be met before an EMT administers a bronchodilator by metered-dose inhaler (MDI) or small-volume nebulizer (SVN) to a patient:

- The patient exhibits signs and symptoms of breathing difficulty (respiratory distress).
- The patient has a physician-prescribed metered-dose inhaler containing a medication specifically prepared to be delivered by nebulization.
- The EMT has received approval from medical direction, whether on-line or off-line, to administer the medication.

Contraindications

A bronchodilator by MDI or SVN should not be given if any of the following conditions exist:

- The patient is not responsive enough to use the MDI or SVN.
- The MDI or SVN is not prescribed for the patient.
- Medical direction has not granted permission.
- The patient has already taken the maximum allowed dose(s) prior to your arrival.

Medication Forms

Aerosolized medication in an MDI.

Liquid medication packaged to be poured directly into the nebulizer chamber of an SVN (see EMT Skills 16-4C).

Dosage

Each time an MDI is depressed, it delivers a precise dose of medication to the patient. The total number of times the medication can be administered is determined by medical direction. When using an SVN, it usually takes 5–10 minutes for the patient to inhale the medication, depending on the rate and depth of breathing. The medication should be inhaled until the SVN no longer produces a mist.

Administration

To administer a bronchodilator by MDI (EMT Skills 16-2):

1. Ensure right patient, right medication, right dose, right route, and right date. Determine if the patient is alert enough to use the inhaler and if any doses have already been administered prior to your arrival.
2. Obtain an order, either on-line or off-line, from medical direction to assist with the administration of the medication.
3. Ensure that the inhaler is at room temperature or warmer. Shake the canister vigorously for at least 30 seconds.

FIGURE 16-11 ✱ Metered-dose inhaler and small-volume nebulizer.

Drug Profiles

Provide medication name, indications, contraindications, medication form, dosage, administration, actions, side effects, and reassessment on medications commonly administered by EMTs.

Assessment Summary

RESPIRATORY DISTRESS

The following are findings that may be associated with breathing difficulty.

SCENE SIZE-UP

Is breathing difficulty due to a medical or a traumatic cause? Look for evidence of:

Mechanism of injury—collision, fall, guns, knives, bruising on chest
Home or portable oxygen tanks or concentrators indicating chronic respiratory problems
Alcohol or food that may indicate choking

Primary Assessment

General Impression

Position of patient:
Tripod
Lying flat

Circulation

Tachycardia (more typical in adult with hypoxia)
Bradycardia (more typical in infant or young child with hypoxia)
Cyanosis to mucous membranes, around nose and mouth, nail beds, chest, and neck

Status: Priority Patient

History and Secondary Assessment

History

Signs and symptoms:
Shortness of breath
Restlessness and anxiety
Difficulty in breathing while lying flat
Diaphoresis
Known allergies to medication or other substances
Medications for respiratory conditions
Home oxygen
Prescribed metered-dose inhaler (MDI)
Pre-existing respiratory or cardiac disease
Hospitalized for respiratory condition

Physical Exam

Head, neck, and face:
Cyanosis to face, neck, and mucous membranes
Jugular venous distention (may indicate heart failure or lung injury [tension pneumothorax])
Jugular vein engorgement on inhalation (Kussmaul sign)
Facial expression:
Agitated or confused
Speech:
Patient may gasp for breath between words.

Mental Status

Alert to unresponsive
Restlessness
Agitation
Disorientation

Airway

Inspect for incomplete or partial obstruction
Crowing and stridor (indicate partial obstruction)
Gurgling (indicates fluid in the airway; suction required)

Breathing

Signs of inadequate breathing, including poor chest rise and fall, poor volume heard and felt, diminished or absent breath sounds
Wheezing heard on auscultation
Nasal flaring
Pursed-lip breathing
Chest:
Retractions
Accessory muscle use
Wheezing
Productive cough
Barrel chest (indicates emphysema, a chronic respiratory condition)
Abdomen:
Use of abdominal muscles when breathing
Extremities:
Cyanosis to fingers and nail beds
Pale skin
Diaphoresis

Baseline Vital Signs

BP: normal
BP: sudden decrease in the systolic BP by 10 mmHg or greater with inhalation
HR: increased in adults; slow in infants and young children
Pulse: sudden decrease in the pulse amplitude with inhalation
RR: increased; may decrease with greater hypoxia
Skin: cyanosis, paleness, diaphoresis
Pupils: dilated; sluggish to respond to light
SpO_2: 95%

Assessment Summary

Assessment Summaries reinforce assessment steps and processes as well as key assessment findings for specific medical and trauma emergencies.

Emergency Care Algorithm
Emergency Care Algorithms are graphic pathways that visually summarize assessment and care steps for students.

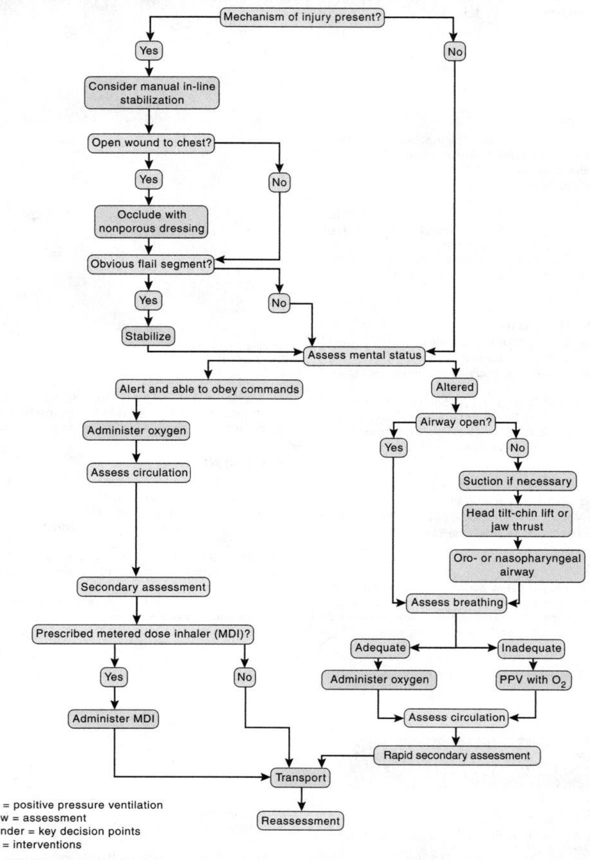

FIGURE 16-18 ✱ Emergency care algorithm: respiratory distress/failure/arrest.

Emergency Care Protocol
Emergency Care Protocols provide concise summaries of emergency care steps to be taken in medical and trauma emergencies.

Emergency Care Protocol

RESPIRATORY DISTRESS

1. Establish and maintain an open airway.
2. Suction secretions as necessary.
3. If breathing is inadequate, provide positive pressure ventilation with supplemental oxygen at a minimum rate of 10–12 ventilations/minute for an adult and 12–20 ventilations/minute for an infant or child.
4. If breathing is adequate, apply a nonrebreather mask at 15 lpm.
5. If the patient has signs and symptoms of breathing difficulty and has a prescribed metered-dose inhaler or a nebulization device, administer the beta 2-specific drug as appropriate according to medical direction:
   - Beta 2-specific drugs mimic the sympathetic nervous system and cause bronchodilation.
   - Dose is precisely delivered by the device.
   - Obtain an order from medical direction.
   - Ensure the "five rights" of medication administration.
   - Assemble the equipment (MDI or nebulizer) as discussed previously.
   - Place the device, and instruct the patient how to breathe.
   - Replace nonrebreather mask on patient.
   - Record time and reassess patient.
   - Beta 2 side effects:
     tachycardia
     tremors
     nervousness
     dry mouth
     nausea
6. Consider advanced life support if the condition does not improve.
7. Transport in a position of comfort.
8. Perform a reassessment of the patient's status every 5 minutes.
9. *Complete the secondary assessment.If your protocol allows, in cases of severe respiratory distress consider the use of continuous positive airway pressure (CPAP). Current studies show that patients in severe respiratory distress from a variety of conditions may benefit from CPAP. (See Chapter 10, "Airway Management, Artificial Ventilation, and Oxygenation."*

FIGURE 16-17b ✱ Emergency care protocol: respiratory distress.

EMT skills 16-2 Administering Medication by Metered-Dose Inhaler

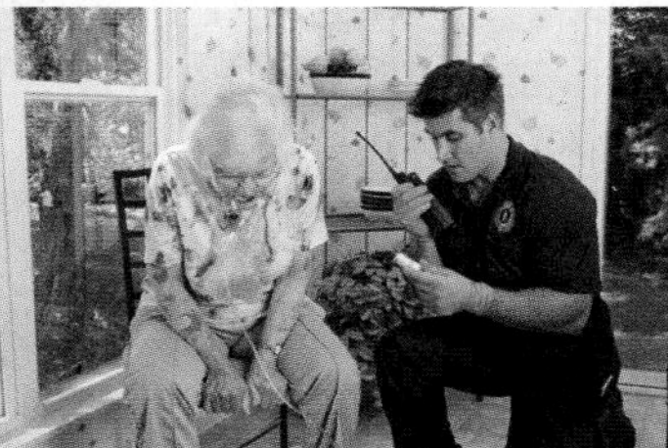
16-2A * Consult with medical direction for an order to administer the medication.

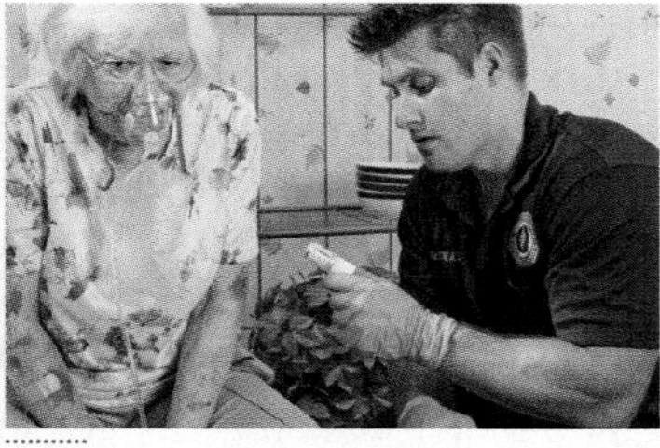
16-2B * Check to make sure the medication is for the patient, that it is the proper one to administer, and that it has not reached its expiration date.

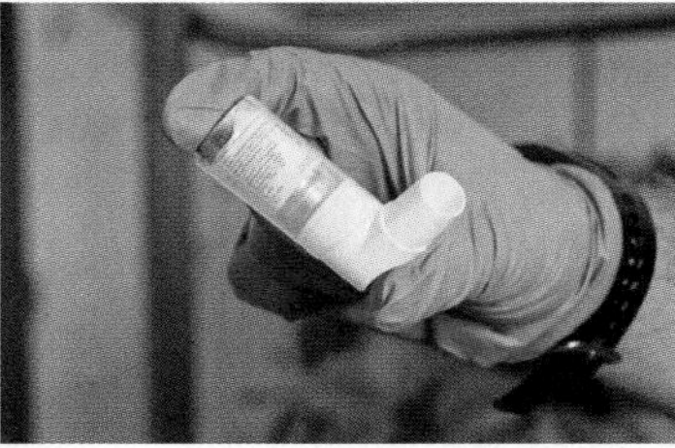
16-2C * Shake the inhaler vigorously for at least 30 seconds.

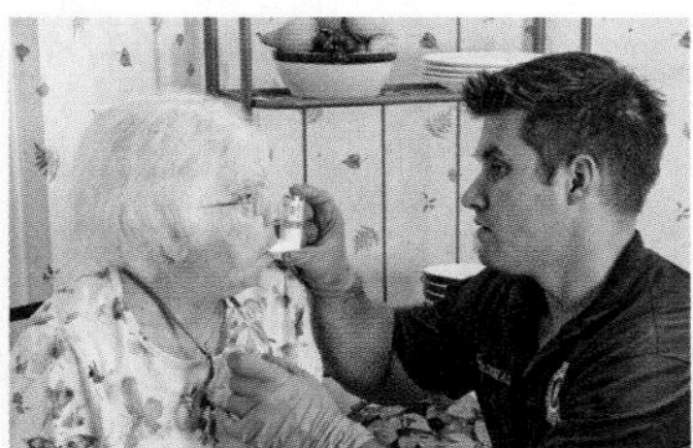
16-2D * Instruct the patient to inhale slowly and deeply for about 5 seconds. As the patient begins to inhale, depress the canister.

EMT Skills
Now all located at the end of each chapter before chapter review material, EMT Skills present key information and step-by-step procedures for easy reference.

CHAPTER REVIEW

SUMMARY

Respiratory emergencies can range from a patient experiencing respiratory distress to a patient who is in respiratory arrest. It is imperative to effectively assess the patient to determine if the condition is respiratory distress, respiratory failure, or respiratory arrest. The patient with breathing difficulty who is in respiratory distress is still able to compensate for the disturbance and needs supplemental oxygen to improve his oxygenation status. The patient in respiratory failure, as the name implies, has failed to continue to meet the metabolic demands of the body, and the respiratory rate or tidal volume is no longer adequate. This patient needs immediate ventilation with a bag-valve mask or other ventilation device and supplemental oxygen. A patient in respiratory arrest is no longer breathing and also needs immediate positive pressure ventilation.

A patient in respiratory distress who has a history of asthma, emphysema, or chronic bronchitis may have a metered-dose inhaler or home nebulizer unit that delivers a beta$_2$-specific drug. If so, you may assist the patient in using the device to relieve the bronchoconstriction that is impeding airflow into the alveoli.

Infants, children, and geriatric patients may present differently than adults when experiencing a respiratory emergency. Quick intervention is necessary since the most common cause of cardiac arrest in pediatric patients is from an airway or respiratory compromise, and geriatric patients may rapidly deteriorate because of poor compensatory mechanisms.

CASE STUDY FOLLOW-UP

SCENE SIZE-UP

You have been dispatched to a 31-year-old female patient complaining of difficulty in breathing. A man nervously greets you at the curb as you gather your equipment. He indicates that the patient is his wife, Anna Sanders, who is having an extremely hard time breathing. You are led up to the third floor of an apartment complex. You do not note any possible hazards, but are looking at how difficult the extrication might be. Upon walking into the apartment you note a young female patient sitting in a tripod position next to the kitchen table.

PRIMARY ASSESSMENT

As you start to introduce yourself, the patient begins to speak, gasping for her breath after each word. With great difficulty she states, "I—can't—breathe." Based on Mrs. Sanders's facial expression and posture, she appears to be in a great deal of distress. Her airway is open and her breathing is rapid and labored at a rate of 34 per minute. There are audible wheezes when she exhales. You immediately apply oxygen via a nonrebreather mask at 15 lpm. Her radial pulse is about 110 per minute. The skin is moist and slightly pale. You recognize the patient as a priority and signal your partner to get the stretcher while you continue with the secondary assessment.

SECONDARY ASSESSMENT

You begin to evaluate the difficulty in breathing using the OPQRST mnemonic. You ask Anna questions she can answer with a nod or a shake of her head to reduce her need to respond by speaking. Some questions you direct to her husband. You ascertain that the breathing difficulty began gradually about 2 hours ago and got progressively worse. She is unable to lie down because this causes her breathing to get much worse, although sitting up is not much better. She has had similar episodes in the past, but none seem to have been this severe. On a scale of 1 to 10, Mrs. Sanders indicates that her difficulty in breathing is about an 8 or 9.

You continue to obtain a history. The primary symptom is severe difficulty in breathing. Mrs. Sanders has an allergy to penicillin. When asked about medications that she takes, Mr. Sanders brings you a prescription of albuterol in a metered-dose inhaler. She is on no other medication. When asked if she has taken any of the albuterol, her husband says, "She took one puff about 15 minutes ago." She has a past medical history of asthma and suffers these attacks maybe once every 4 or 5 months. She has had nothing to eat for about 3 hours but drank a small glass of orange juice about an hour ago. She was cleaning the kitchen when the episode began.

You quickly perform a physical exam. You assess her neck for jugular vein distention. Inspection of her chest and abdomen reveals significant use of the abdominal muscles when exhaling. The breath sounds are diminished bilaterally and you hear wheezing even without using your stethoscope. Her fingertips are slightly cyanotic. You assess the baseline vital signs and find a blood pressure of 134/86; pulse of 118 per minute and regular; respirations at 32 per minute and labored with audible wheezing; the skin moist and slightly pale. Her SpO_2 reading is 88% prior to oxygen administration.

Chapter Review
The Chapter Summary, Case Study Follow-Up, In Review, and Critical Thinking questions comprise each chapter's review section, reinforcing the chapter's main points.

Mybradykit provides a one-stop shop for online chapter support materials and resources. You can prepare for class and exams with skills and objectives checklists, multiple-choice questions, case study activities, weblinks, animations, author podcasts, breath sounds, study aids, link to the Pearson eText, trauma gallery, chapter summaries in Spanish, and more! To access mybradykit, please visit **www.bradybooks.com**. A few key components are described here...

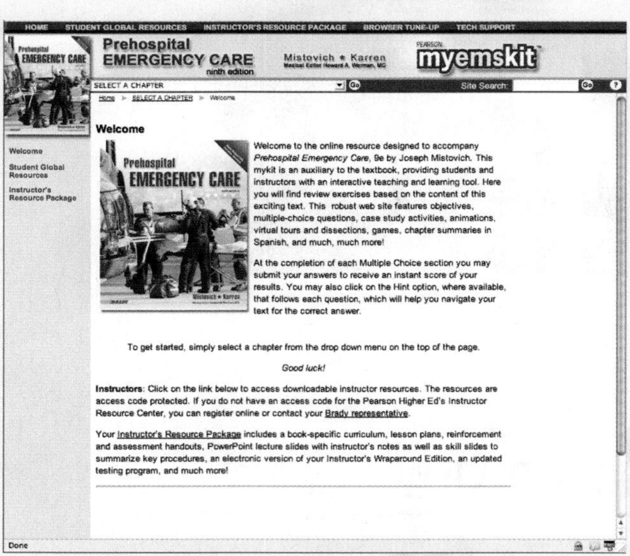

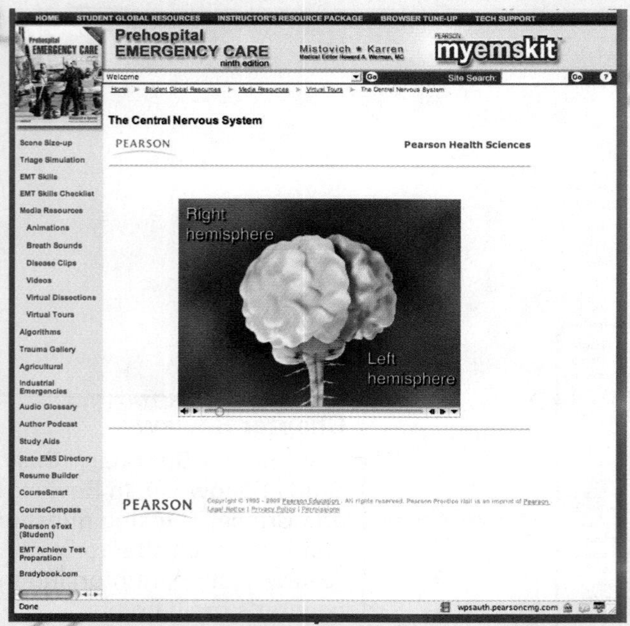

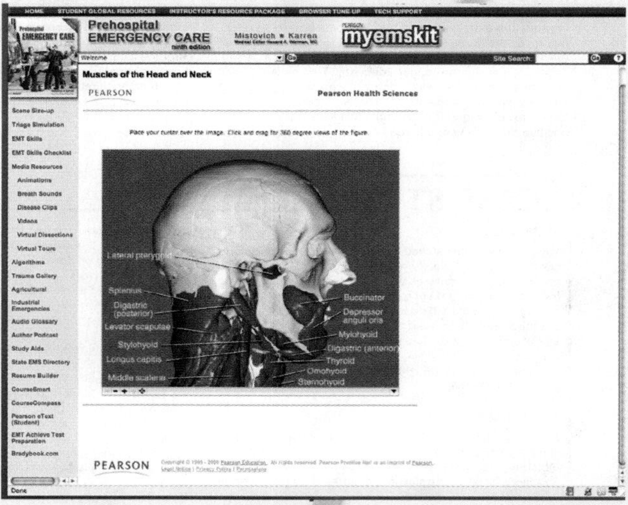

Virtual Tours

3D animations, including a Brain and Spinal Cord virtual tour, offer a deeper understanding and graphical view of difficult concepts.

Animations and Interactivities

Highly visual exercises enhance and reinforce anatomy, physiology, biology, and specific processes.

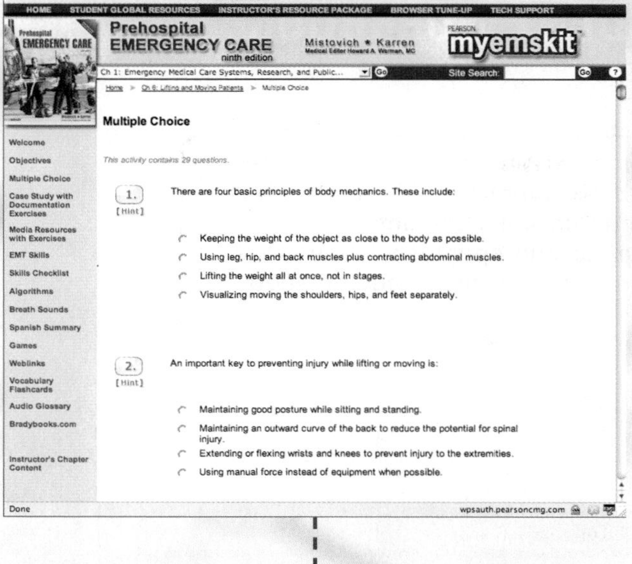

Chapter Quizzes
Chapter-specific multiple-choice quizzes reinforce and test knowledge.

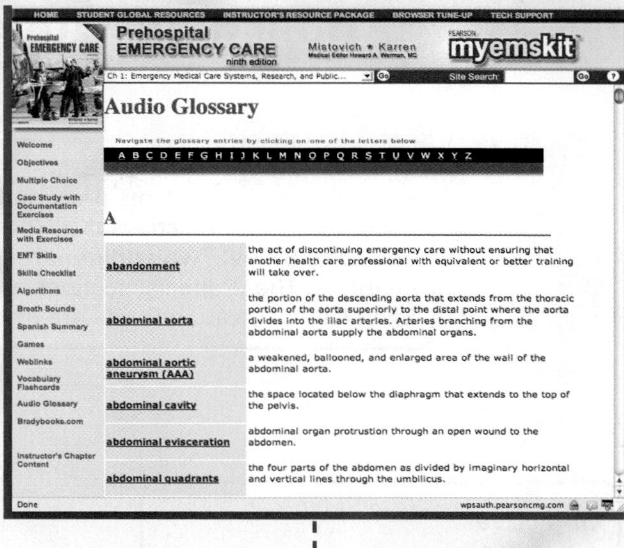

Glossary
This interactive glossary contains the definitions and audio pronunciations of key terms presented in the student text.

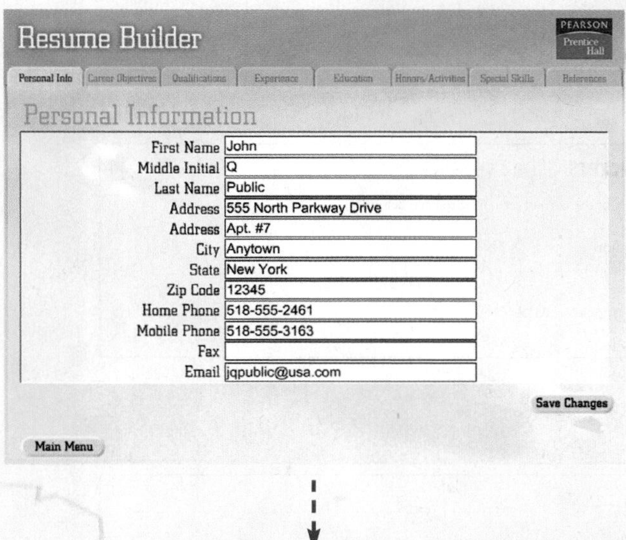

Resume Builder
This easy-to-use program helps create professional resumes and supporting documents. It includes four different resume styles, cover letters, reference lists, post-interview letters, and much more.

OTHER FEATURES

- **Anatomy Labeling Exercises**
  Drag-and-drop activities test knowledge of human anatomy.
- **Case Study with Documentation Exercise**
  Designed to develop critical thinking, each case study offers questions that help to hone the student's assessment skills.
- **Podcasts**
  Listen as Brady authors discuss key EMT topics.
- **Pearson eText**
  Get access to an electronic version of your textbook. This allows you to highlight and annotate key content.

The **Student Workbook** (ISBN 0-13-502809-4) is a self-instructional guide, written to reinforce key concepts presented in the textbook. Every chapter includes five basic sections: Objectives, Key Ideas, Terms and Concepts, Content Review, and Case Study. Two additional sections appear, as appropriate, in many of the chapters. These special sections are Medical Terminology and Documentation Exercise. Medication Cards are also provided.

Objectives
A list of objectives that form the basis of each chapter.

OBJECTIVES

After reading this chapter, you should be able to:

16-1. Define key terms introduced in this chapter.
16-2. Explain the importance of being able to quickly recognize and treat patients with respiratory emergencies.
16-3. Describe the structure and function of the respiratory system, including:
a. Upper airway
b. Lower airway
c. Gas exchange
d. Inspiratory and expiratory centers in the medulla and pons

Key Ideas
Summarize the chapter's key concepts.

KEY IDEAS

This chapter describes respiratory distress and respiratory failure. Emphasis is placed on ensuring an open airway and providing high-concentration oxygen or positive pressure ventilation, as needed, and not on trying to diagnose a specific underlying disease.

- There is a wide variety of signs and symptoms of respiratory distress. They may include any of these: shortness of breath; restlessness; increased pulse rate or breathing rate; decreased breathing rate; skin color changes; noisy breathing; inability to speak; retractions; shallow, slow, or irregular breathing; abdominal breathing; coughing; patient in a tripod position; unusual anatomy (barrel chest); altered mental status; nasal flaring; tracheal tugging or deviations; paradoxical motion; and/or pursed-lip breathing.

Terms and Concepts
Review major terms that are introduced in bold type in the textbook chapter and are listed and defined at the end of the book.

TERMS AND CONCEPTS

1. Write the number of the correct term next to each definition.
   1. Apnea
   2. Bronchodilator
   3. Bronchospasm
   4. Dyspnea
   5. Grunting
   6. Metered-dose inhaler (MDI)
   7. Respiratory arrest
   8. Respiratory failure

Content Review
Presents questions to review understanding of important information and concepts from the textbook chapter.

CONTENT REVIEW

1. Your patient is experiencing difficulty breathing but has adequate tidal volume and respiratory rate. This patient is said to be _____ and your treatment should include _____.
   a. in respiratory failure/ initiating immediate ventilation with BVM
   b. apneic/ beginning aggressive ventilation at once
   c. experiencing dyspnea/ administering oxygen at 6 liters per minute (lpm) via nasal cannula
   d. in respiratory distress/ administering oxygen via nonrebreather mask

CASE STUDY

It's 8:15 in the morning. You and your partner, Angie, have just received the report from the previous shift. With a cup of coffee in hand, you walk to the ambulance to inventory the supplies and equipment. The alerting system sounds: "Unit 105 respond to 155 Wick Avenue for an elderly patient complaining of difficulty breathing. Alert time 0816 hours." You and Angie get under way at once. En route, dispatch advises that they are on the phone with the son of the patient and that he is very apprehensive. You arrive at the scene and are met at the ambulance by the son. "Hurry! My mother is having trouble breathing." You quickly reassure him as he leads you to the patient. You find an elderly woman, Mrs. Frederick, sitting on the side of the bed, with slight use of accessory muscles. A quick survey of the house and room doesn't reveal indications of trauma. The patient's chest is rising and falling adequately. There is good air volume exchange. Auscultation of the lungs reveals breath sounds bilaterally with a slight wheezy sound. The respiratory rate is 20 per minute. The patient

Case Study
Presents one or more realistic scenarios and requires students to apply chapter information to solving patient management problems.

MEDICAL TERMINOLOGY

Term	Prefix	Word Root Combining Form	Suffix	Definition
apnea (AP-nee-ah)	a- (no, not, without, lack of)	pnea (to breathe or breathing)		Absence of breathing; respiratory arrest
bronchoconstriction (BRONG-koh-kun-STRIK-shun)		bronch/o (bronchi); constriction (narrowing an opening)		Constriction of the smooth muscles of the bronchi and bronchioles, causing a narrowing of the air passageways
bronchospasm (brong-koh-SPAZ-um)		bronch/o-(bronchi); spasm (constriction)		Spasm or constriction of the smooth muscles of the bronchi and bronchioles
dyspnea (DISP-nee-ah)	dys- (bad, difficult, painful)	pnea (to breathe or breathing)		Shortness of breath or perceived difficulty in breathing

Medical Terminology
Provides a chart of chapter-relevant medical terms that are frequently used in emergency care.

EMERGENCY TRIP SHEET

TRIP #
MEDIC #
BEGIN MILES
END MILES
CODE__/__ PAGE__/__
UNITS ON SCENE
NAME SEX M F DOB __/__/__
ADDRESS RACE
CITY STATE ZIP
PHONE ( ) - PCP DR.
RESPONDED FROM CITY
TAKEN FROM ZIP
DESTINATION REASON
SSN - - MEDICARE # MEDICAID #
INSURANCE CO INSURANCE # GROUP #
RESPONSIBLE PARTY ADDRESS
CITY STATE ZIP PHONE ( ) -
EMPLOYER

TIME	ON SCENE (1)	ON SCENE (2)	ON SCENE (3)	EN-ROUTE (1)	EN-ROUTE (2)	AT DESTINATION
BP						
PULSE						

BILLING USE ONLY
DAY
DATE
RECEIVED
DISPATCHED
EN-ROUTE
ON SCENE
TO HOSPITAL
AT HOSPITAL
IN-SERVICE

CREW	CERT	STATE #

IV THERAPY
SUCCESSFUL Y N # OF ATTEMPTS ____
ANGIO SIZE ____ ga.
SITE ____
TOTAL FLUID INFUSED ____ cc
BLOOD DRAW Y N INITIALS
INTUBATION INFORMATION

Documentation Exercise
Presents a real-life emergency-call scenario that is longer and more detailed than the Case Study scenarios, including detailed vital signs and other physical exam and patient history information that would be gathered on such a call.

ACTIVATED CHARCOAL

Medication Name: Activated charcoal, SuperChar, InstaChar, Actidose, LiquiChar.

Indications: Rarely used; may be ordered if it can be administered shortly after ingestion of opioids, anticholinergics, or medications with a sustained release.

Contraindications: (1) Altered mental status (not fully conscious). (2) Swallowed acids or alkalis. (3) Unable to swallow. (4) Cyanide overdose.

Medication Form: 12.5 grams premixed in water; powder form should be avoided.

Dosage: 1 gram of activated charcoal per kilogram of body weight; usual adult dose 25–50 grams, infants and children 12.5–25 grams.

(see over)

Medication Cards
Contains information about the medications that the EMT can administer or assist the patient in administering, with on-line or off-line approval from medical direction.

▶ EMT Achieve: Basic Test Preparation

(ISBN 0131136097)

This exciting program enables you to practice test-taking online. Tests contain questions across the major content found in national and state exams. All test questions have rationales and are reinforced with text, photo, illustrations, or video clips.

▶ Success! for the EMT, 2nd edition

(ISBN 0132253968)

This is the text to help you pass National Registry and other certification exams. All items are written and tested by educators and offer proven authoritative information. The text blends a comprehensive collection of practice exam questions with helpful test-taking tips and student hints. In-book CD-ROM contains practice tests.

▶ BLS Vital Signs (ISBN 0131748777)

Enables you to learn to take vital signs by practicing on a variety of patients in a variety of scenarios—mimicking what you'll see in the field. With two modes of use, practice and case studies, you can first practice the skills then apply them to simulated cases to test your understanding and enhance critical thinking skills.

▶ Active Learning Manual (ISBN 0131136291)

Is an accumulation of active learning exercises that extend beyond the classroom, encouraging students to develop a deeper understanding of both the knowledge and skills necessary to become an excellent EMT.

▶ Pocket Reference for BLS Providers

(ISBN 0131717309)

An essential resource, this handy pocket-sized field reference is written specifically for BLS providers. Skills checklist covers topics that include Airway Management and Breathing, Assessment, CPR, Shock Management, Immobilization, and Medical and Trauma Emergencies. Special skills pages are devoted to Pediatric Patients.

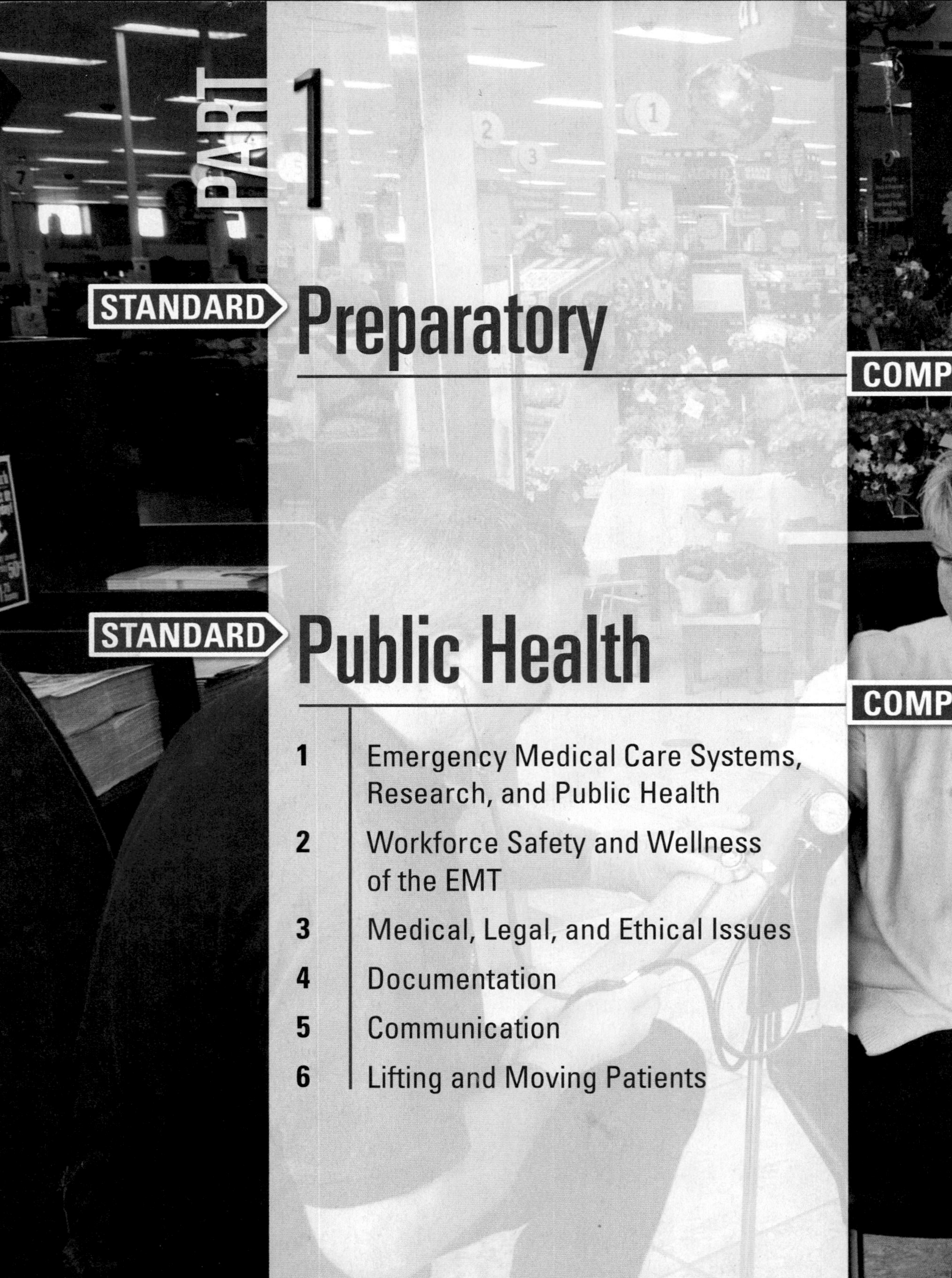

PART 1

STANDARD **Preparatory** COMPETENCY

STANDARD **Public Health** COMPETENCY

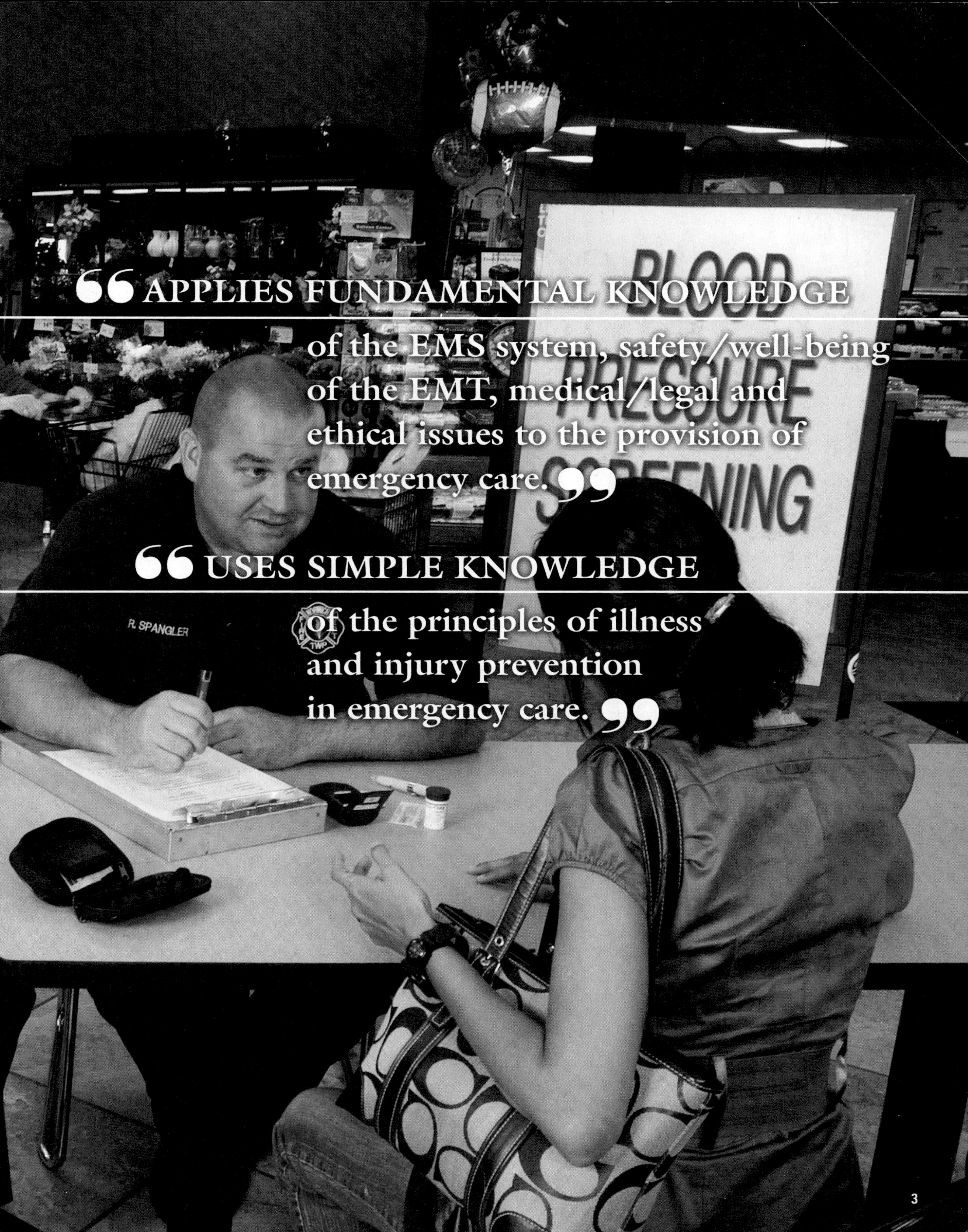

“APPLIES FUNDAMENTAL KNOWLEDGE of the EMS system, safety/well-being of the EMT, medical/legal and ethical issues to the provision of emergency care.”

“USES SIMPLE KNOWLEDGE of the principles of illness and injury prevention in emergency care.”

CHAPTER 1

Emergency Medical Care Systems, Research, and Public Health

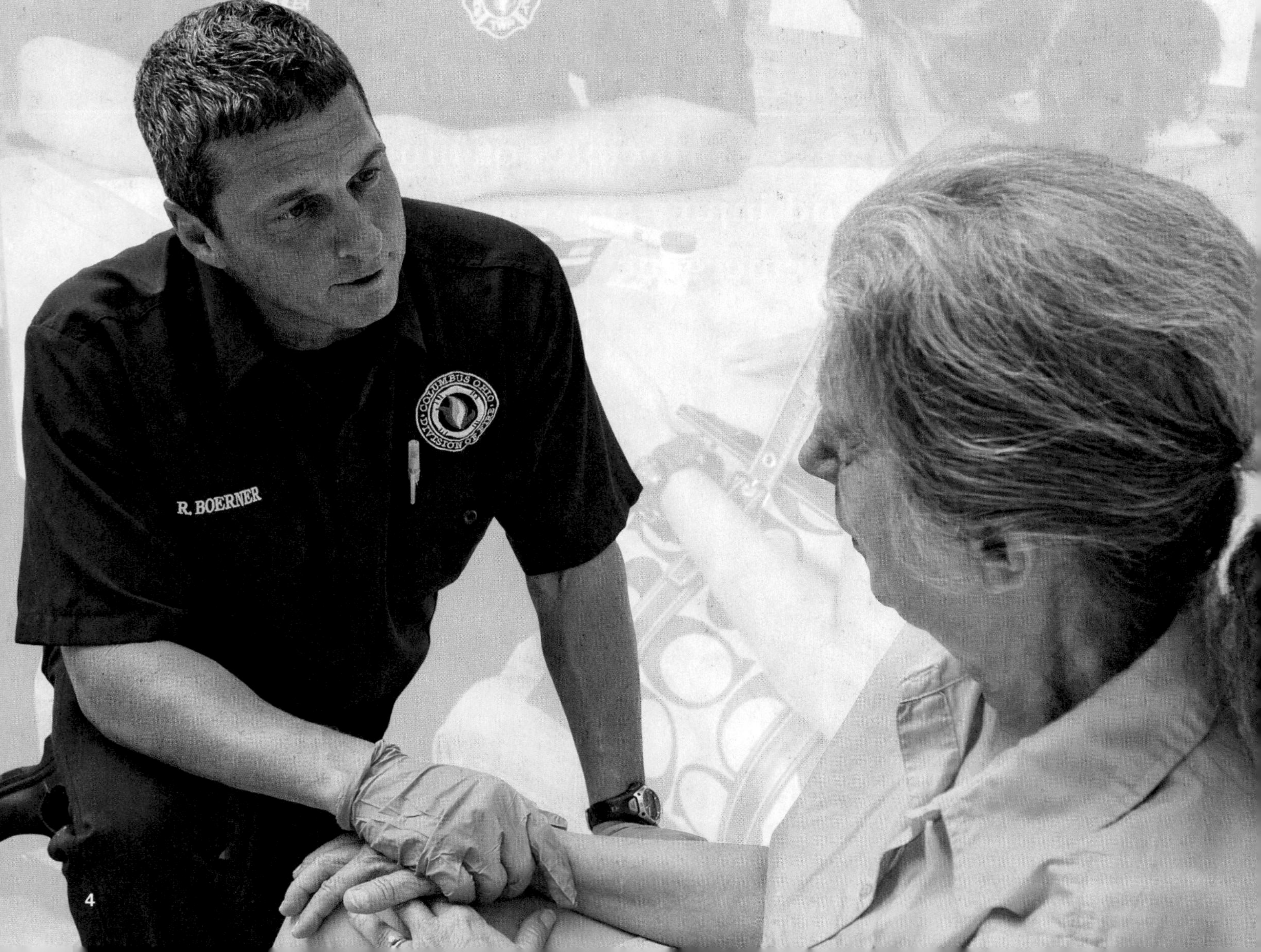

Navigation Guide

The following items provide an overview to the purpose and content of this chapter. The Education Standard and Competency are from the new National EMS Education Standards.

STANDARDS **Preparatory** (Content Areas: EMS Systems; Research); **Public Health**

COMPETENCIES Applies fundamental knowledge of the EMS system, safety/well-being of the EMT, medical/legal and ethical issues to the provision of emergency care.

Uses simple knowledge of the principles of illness and injury prevention to the provision of emergency care.

OBJECTIVES: After reading this chapter, you should be able to:

1-1. Define key terms introduced in this chapter.

1-2. Describe the key historical events that have shaped the development of the emergency medical services (EMS) system, including:
- **a.** Lessons learned in trauma care from experiences in the Korean and Vietnam conflicts
- **b.** Publication of *Accidental Death and Disability: The Neglected Disease of Modern Society*
- **c.** Highway Safety Act of 1966
- **d.** Emergency Medical Services System Act of 1973
- **e.** Public CPR courses
- **f.** Publication of the *National Emergency Medical Services Education and Practice Blueprint*
- **g.** Publication of *EMS Agenda for the Future* and *The EMS Education Agenda for the Future: A Systems Approach*
- **h.** Development of *National EMS Core Content*, *National EMS Scope of Practice Model*, and *National EMS Education Standards*
- **i.** The Institute of Medicine report *The Future of EMS Care: EMS at the Crossroads*

1-3. Briefly explain each of the components of the Technical Assistance Program Assessment Standards:
- **a.** Regulation and policy
- **b.** Resource management
- **c.** Human resources and training
- **d.** Transportation
- **e.** Facilities
- **f.** Communications
- **g.** Public information and education
- **h.** Medical direction
- **i.** Trauma systems
- **j.** Evaluation

1-4. Discuss the differences between 911 and non-911 EMS access systems, including the features and benefits of 911 systems.

1-5. Compare and contrast the scopes of practice of the following levels of EMS providers:
- **a.** Emergency Medical Responder (EMR)
- **b.** Emergency Medical Technician (EMT)
- **c.** Advanced Emergency Medical Technician (AEMT)
- **d.** Paramedic

1-6. Explain the importance of the EMT's understanding of the health care resources available in the community.

1-7. Give examples of how EMTs can carry out each of the following roles and responsibilities:
- **a.** Personal safety and the safety of others
- **b.** Patient assessment and emergency care
- **c.** Safe lifting and moving
- **d.** Transport and transfer of care
- **e.** Record keeping and data collection
- **f.** Patient advocacy

1-8. Describe the expectations of EMTs in terms of each of the following professional attributes:
- **a.** Appearance
- **b.** Knowledge and skills
- **c.** Physical demands
- **d.** Personal traits
- **e.** Maintaining certification and licensure

1-9. Discuss the purposes of medical direction/oversight in the EMS system.

1-10. Describe the purpose of quality improvement/continuous quality improvement programs in EMS.

1-11. Explain the EMT's roles and responsibilities in quality improvement.

1-12. Identify activities in EMS that pose a high risk of mistakes and injuries.

1-13. Discuss steps that you can take to minimize mistakes and injuries in EMS.

1-14. Discuss the steps of evidence-based decision making.

1-15. Explain the limitations of evidence-based decision making in EMS.

1-16. Describe the relationship between EMS and public health.

1-17. List the ten greatest public health achievements in the United States in the 20th century.

continued

Navigation Guide *continued*

KEY TERMS: Page references indicate first major use in this chapter. For complete definitions, see the Glossary at the back of the book.

Advanced Emergency Medical Technician (AEMT) p. 10
Americans with Disabilities Act (ADA) p. 12
Emergency Medical Responder (EMR) p. 9
Emergency Medical Technician (EMT) p. 9
EMS system p. 7
evidence-based medicine p. 18
medical direction p. 16
medical director p. 16
medical oversight p. 16
off-line medical direction p. 16
on-line medical direction p. 16
Paramedic p. 10
prehospital care p. 10
protocols p. 16
quality improvement (QI) p. 16
standing orders p. 16

MEDIA RESOURCES: Please go to www.bradybooks.com to access mykit for this text. You will find quizzes, critical thinking scenarios, weblinks, animations, and videos related to this chapter—and much more. Look for online information on the EMS Agenda for the Future. You will also find a video clip on EMS and the community.

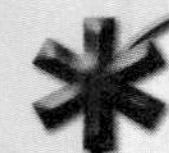

CASE STUDY

The Dispatch
EMS Unit 121—respond to 10915 Pine Lake Road in Perry Township—you have an elderly male at that location—victim of a fall—Perry Township Fire Department has been notified and is en route—time out 1032 hours.

En Route
While you confirm the address with dispatch, your partner pulls out the county map. "I know that location," he says. "Yes, here. We need to head north on Lincoln." You pull your unit out of the garage. Your partner operates the emergency lights and sirens. Within 8 minutes, you turn onto Pine Lake Road and spot a police car and a fire truck.

Upon Arrival
You position your ambulance in the driveway of the residence to afford an easy exit. As you leave the unit, the police officer—a First Responder who radioed for EMS help—tells you that a 65-year-old male fell about 30 feet down a very steep embankment behind his house. He's been at the bottom for about 30 minutes. The patient, Edgar Robinson, is conscious and is able to tell you that his right arm and leg are injured. The rescue squad from the fire department is preparing to rappel down the embankment to extricate the patient.

How Would You Proceed?
During this chapter, you will read about the roles and responsibilities of an EMT. Later, we will return to the case study and put in context some of the information you learned.

Introduction

One of the most critical health problems in the United States today is the sudden loss of life and disability caused by catastrophic accidents and illnesses. Every year thousands of people in this country die or suffer permanent harm because of the lack of adequate and available emergency medical services. As an Emergency Medical Technician (EMT), you can make a positive difference.

This course is designed to help you gain the knowledge, skills, and attitudes necessary to be a competent, productive, and valuable member of the Emergency Medical Services (EMS) team. As you begin, your instructor will provide the necessary paperwork, describe the expectations for the course and the job, inform you of required or available immunizations, and outline your state and local provisions for certification as an EMT.

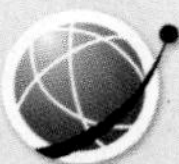

Media Resources
Go to www.bradybooks.com for mykit. Highlights:
- *Web Resource:* National Registry of EMTs
- *Web Resource:* EMS Agenda for the Future

Objective 1-2
Describe the key historical events that have shaped the development of the emergency medical services (EMS) system.

Key Terms
EMS system Emergency Medical Services system.

The Emergency Medical Services System

A Brief History

Emergency medical care has developed from the days when the local funeral home was the ambulance provider and patient care did not begin until arrival at the hospital. By contrast, the modern, sophisticated **EMS system** (Emergency Medical Services system) permits patient care to begin at the scene of the injury or illness, and EMS is part of a continuum of patient care that extends from the time of injury or illness until rehabilitation or discharge. Today, when a person becomes ill or suffers an injury, he has easy access to EMS by telephone, gets a prompt response, and can depend on getting high-quality prehospital emergency care from trained professionals.

What happens to an injured person before he reaches a hospital is of critical importance. Wars helped to teach us this lesson. During the Korean and Vietnam conflicts, for example, it became obvious that injured soldiers benefited from emergency care in the field prior to transport. This realization helped the civilian EMS system evolve from a mere provider of fast transport by poorly trained or untrained individuals who provided little or no care to a system where highly trained EMS personnel provide professional care at the scene and en route to the hospital. We continue to learn about trauma care from the wars in Iraq and Afghanistan and to implement changes in EMS practice based upon the outcomes of those patients.

The modern EMS system has evolved from its beginnings in the 1960s when the President's Committee for Traffic Safety identified a need to reduce the injuries and deaths related to highway crashes. In 1966, the National Academy of Sciences National Research Council published a report entitled *Accidental Death and Disability: The Neglected Disease of Modern Society.* This report became known as the "white paper," detailing the number of deaths and injuries related to traffic crashes in the United States. The "white paper" also identified severe deficiencies in the delivery of prehospital care in the United States and made recommendations intended to change ambulance systems, training requirements, and the provision of prehospital care. The following are some of the significant developments that have had a profound effect on emergency medical services:

- The Highway Safety Act of 1966 required each state to establish a highway safety program that met prescribed federal standards and included emergency services. The Department of Transportation, through its National Highway Traffic Safety Administration (NHTSA), took a leadership role in the development of emergency medical services. An early focus was improving the education of prehospital personnel. One initiative was the development of national standard curricula. The EMT programs of today have gradually evolved from this charge and continue to use a national standard curriculum.
- The Emergency Medical Services System Act of 1973 provided access to millions of dollars of funding geared to EMS system planning and implementation, personnel availability, and training.
- The American Heart Association began to teach cardiopulmonary resuscitation (CPR) and basic life support to the public. Completion of a CPR course is now a prerequisite to the EMT course.
- The National Registry of EMTs in 1993 released the *National Emergency Medical Services Education and Practice Blueprint,* which defined issues related to EMS training and education and was intended to guide the development of national training curricula.
- The National Highway Traffic Safety Administration in 1996 published the *EMS Agenda for the Future* document with the intent to make EMS a greater component in the health care system in the United States. In 2000, a follow-up document, *The EMS Education Agenda for the Future: A Systems Approach,* was released to address the issue of consistency in the education, training, and certification and licensure of entry-level EMS personnel nationally.
- The National Highway Traffic Safety Administration and Health Resources and Services Administration in 2005 published the *National EMS Core Content,* which defined the domain of knowledge found in the National EMS Scope of Practice Model. It promotes universal knowledge and skills for EMS personnel.
- The National Highway Traffic Safety Administration in 2006 published *The National EMS Scope of Practice Model,* which defines four levels of EMS licensure and the corresponding knowledge and skills necessary at each level. The Scope of Practice will be discussed later in the chapter.

Objective 1-3
Briefly explain each of the components of the Technical Assistance Program Assessment Standards.

Objective 1-4
Discuss the differences between 911 and non-911 EMS access systems, including the features and benefits of 911 systems.

- The Institute of Medicine report *The Future of EMS Care: EMS at the Crossroads* in 2006 recommended that all state governments adopt a common scope of practice that allows for reciprocity between states, national accreditation for all paramedic programs, and national certification as a prerequisite for state licensure and local credentialing.
- The National Highway Traffic Safety Administration's National EMS Education Standards outline the minimum terminal objectives for entry-level EMS personnel based on the National EMS Scope of Practice Model. The contents of this textbook are based on the National EMS Education Standards.

Advances continue to be made in emergency medical services design and response, equipment, research, and the education of EMTs. Many lives have been saved and unnecessary disabilities avoided because of these advances in emergency medical services.

Technical Assistance Program Assessment Standards

Each state has control of its own EMS system, independent of the federal government. However, the National Highway Traffic Safety Administration (NHTSA) provides a set of recommended standards called the "Technical Assistance Program Assessment Standards." A brief description of these standards follows. They will be discussed in much more detail throughout this text and in your EMT course.

- **Regulation and policy.** Each state must have laws, regulations, policies, and procedures that govern its EMS system. A state-level EMS agency is also required to provide leadership to local jurisdictions.
- **Resource management.** Each state must have central control of EMS resources so that each locality and all patients have equal access to acceptable emergency care.
- **Human resources and training.** All personnel who staff ambulances and transport patients must be trained to at least the EMT level.
- **Transportation.** Patients must be provided with safe, reliable transportation by ground or air ambulance.
- **Facilities.** Each seriously ill or injured patient must be delivered in a timely manner to an appropriate medical facility.
- **Communications.** A system of communications must be in place to provide public access to the system and communication among dispatcher, EMS personnel, and hospital.
- **Public information and education.** EMS personnel should participate in programs designed to educate the public in the prevention of injuries and how to properly and appropriately access the EMS system.
- **Medical direction.** Each EMS system must have a physician as a medical director to provide medical oversight that includes overseeing patient care and delegating appropriate medical practices to EMTs and other EMS personnel.
- **Trauma systems.** Each state must develop a system of specialized care for trauma patients, including one or more trauma centers and rehabilitation programs, plus systems for assigning and transporting patients to those facilities.
- **Evaluation.** Each state must have a quality improvement system for the continuing evaluation and upgrading of the system.

Access to the EMS System

There are two general systems by which the public can access emergency medical services: 911 and non-911.

Often referred to as the universal number, 911 is the phone number used nationwide to access emergency services, including police, fire, and EMS. The most common 911 system is enhanced. An enhanced 911 system, called E-911, provides automatic number identification (ANI) and automatic location identification (ALI), which indicate the exact address and phone number from which the call is being made. This information is automatically displayed on the computer screen of the call taker, even if the individual making the call hangs up. The main advantage of E-911 is that the address and phone number are automatically displayed, and an immediate response can be dispatched, even if the caller is unable to communicate effectively—for example, because of an injury or illness such as a stroke, or if he cannot recite his address in the confusion of the emergency, or if it is a child who cannot tell the call taker the address.

While exact procedures may vary, the basic process is the same. Calls are received by a public service answering point (PSAP) where a call taker collects, verifies, and records the information about the emergency, decides

Objective 1-5
Compare and contrast the scopes of practice of the four levels of EMS providers.

Key Terms
Emergency Medical Responder (EMR) EMS practitioner likely to be the first person on scene with emergency care training.

Key Terms
Emergency Medical Technician (EMT) EMS practitioner who provides basic emergency medical care.

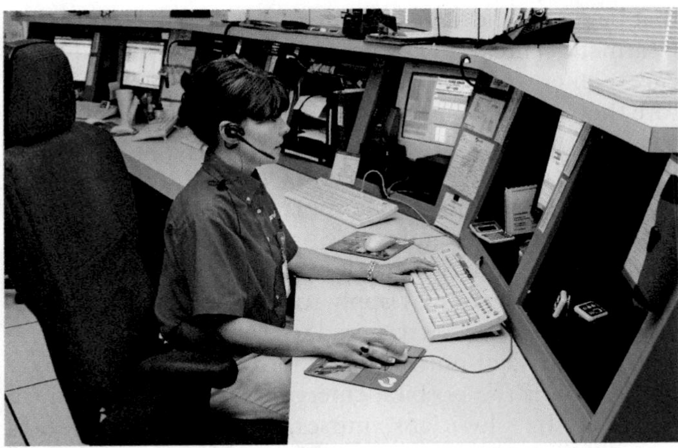

FIGURE 1-1 ✱ Communications play a vital role in the Emergency Medical Services (EMS) system.

which service must respond, and facilitates alerting the necessary service (Figure 1-1✱).

There are two main benefits to the 911 universal number:

- The public service answering point is generally staffed by trained communications personnel. Many are specially trained as Emergency Medical Dispatchers (EMDs), who not only take the call and facilitate the dispatch of emergency services but also provide instructions for lifesaving emergency care, such as bleeding control or CPR, that can be administered immediately by the caller or another person at the scene.
- The use of 911 reduces the time it takes the caller to access the emergency services system. The caller does not have to look up a ten-digit number to contact in the case of an emergency. The number is easy for young children to remember and dial. All three services—police, fire, and EMS—are accessible by dialing one number. Thus, all emergency resources can be dispatched simultaneously to a scene, for example, to a car crash that requires traffic control and investigation by the police, fire suppression and extrication by the fire service, and emergency medical care and transportation by EMS.

Cell phone technology when dialing 911 has made call delivery an issue in some areas. Traditionally, 911 systems were based on the geographic location of a phone number. That location is entered into a computer database that directs the call to the proper PSAP when 911 is dialed. Because cell phones use airwave transmission and are mobile, the phones are not able to be tracked in the same manner as the traditional phone line. When 911 is dialed on a cell phone, the call is often delivered to a central location or to the PSAP closest to the triggered call tower and is answered by a call taker who has nothing more than the caller's cell phone number. The call taker has no indication of the caller's location. The call taker must identify the location of the caller and get all of the necessary information. The call taker then must send the call to the appropriate PSAP. Thus, dialing 911 on a cell phone may lead to a delay in response. Some 911 systems have used cellular tower locations to route cell phone calls to the closest PSAP. This may not always get the caller to the needed emergency service. Technology to track the exact location of cell phone calls through global-positioning-satellite (GPS) has been developed and is now being used by many, but not yet all, EMS systems.

Levels of Training

The *National EMS Scope of Practice Model* released by the National Highway Traffic Safety Administration in 2005 was developed to bring a higher degree of consistency to EMS throughout the United States, improve patient care and safety, allow for easier reciprocity between states, and decrease public confusion by identifying specific national levels of EMS practitioners. The National Scope of Practice Model identifies the following four levels of EMS practitioners (Figure 1-2✱):

1. **Emergency Medical Responder (EMR),** which is similar to the First Responder level, provides immediate lifesaving care to patients who have accessed the EMS system and while awaiting response from a higher-level EMS practitioner. The EMR uses basic airway, ventilation, and oxygen therapy devices; takes patient vital signs; and provides stabilization of the spine and suspected extremity injuries, eye irrigation, bleeding control, emergency moves, CPR, automated external defibrillation, and emergency childbirth care.
2. **Emergency Medical Technician (EMT)** provides basic emergency medical care and transportation to patients who access the EMS system. The interventions provided by the EMT include those performed by the EMR but with basic equipment found on an ambulance. The EMT level is similar in scope to the EMT-Basic level with the addition of advanced oxygen

Key Terms

Advanced Emergency Medical Technician (AEMT) EMT with some additional qualifications for advanced care.

Paramedic EMS practitioner who provides the highest level of prehospital care.

Objective 1-6

Explain the importance of the EMT's understanding of the health care resources available in the community.

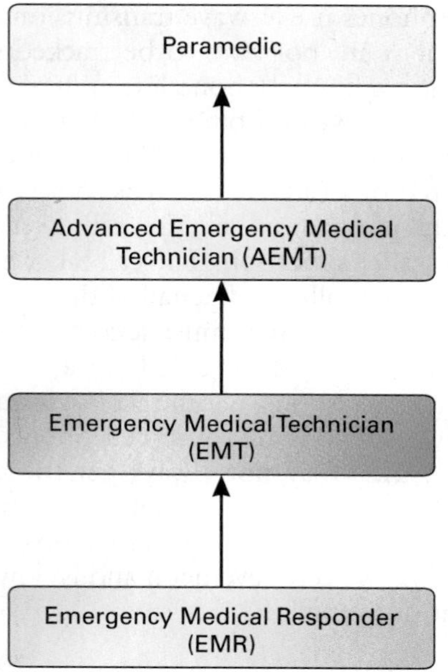

FIGURE 1-2 ✱ The four levels of EMS practitioners.

therapy and ventilation equipment, pulse oximetry, use of automatic blood pressure monitoring equipment, and limited medication administration.

3. **Advanced Emergency Medical Technician (AEMT)** provides both basic and limited advanced emergency medical care and transportation to patients in the prehospital environment. The AEMT provides all of the skills of the EMT with the addition of the use of advanced airway devices, monitoring of blood glucose levels, initiation of intravenous and intraosseous (in-the-bone) infusions, and administration of a select number of medications.
4. **Paramedic** scope of practice includes the skills performed by the EMT and AEMT with the addition of more advanced assessment and patient management skills and provision of the highest level of prehospital care. Paramedics perform advanced assessments, form a field impression, and provide invasive and drug interventions as well as transport. Their care is designed to reduce disability and death of patients who access the EMS system.

The Health Care System

First Responders and EMTs are an integral part of a community's health care system—a network of medical care that begins in the field and extends to hospitals and other treatment centers. In essence, EMTs provide **prehospital care**—emergency medical treatment given to patients before they are transported to a hospital or other facility. (In some areas the term *out-of-hospital care* is preferred, reflecting a trend toward providing care on the scene with or without subsequent transport to a hospital. Out-of-hospital care also includes care provided during interfacility transport. Your instructor can provide information on how or if this term may apply to your EMS system.)

The EMT may be required to decide on the facility to which the patient must be transported. The most familiar destination is the hospital emergency department, which is staffed by physicians, nurses, and others trained in emergency medical treatment. Here patients are stabilized and prepared for further care. Some patients may need to be transported to special facilities such as the following:

- ***Trauma center*** for rapid surgical intervention and specialized treatment of injuries that generally exceeds hospital emergency department capabilities (Figure 1-3✱)
- ***Burn center*** for specialized treatment of serious burns, often including long-term care and rehabilitation
- ***Obstetrical center*** for high-risk obstetric patients
- ***Pediatric center*** for specialized treatment of infants and children
- ***Poison center*** for specialized treatment of poisoning victims

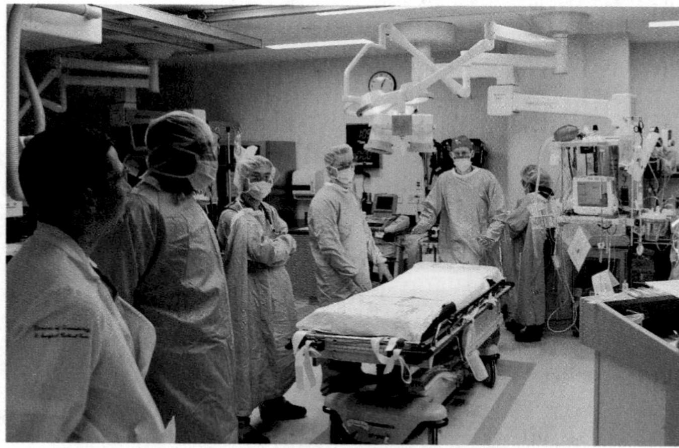

FIGURE 1-3 ✱ A trauma center can provide rapid surgical intervention and treatment of injuries that generally exceeds hospital emergency department capabilities. (© Edward T. Dickinson)

Key Terms
prehospital care emergency medical treatment given to patients before they are transported to a hospital or other facility.

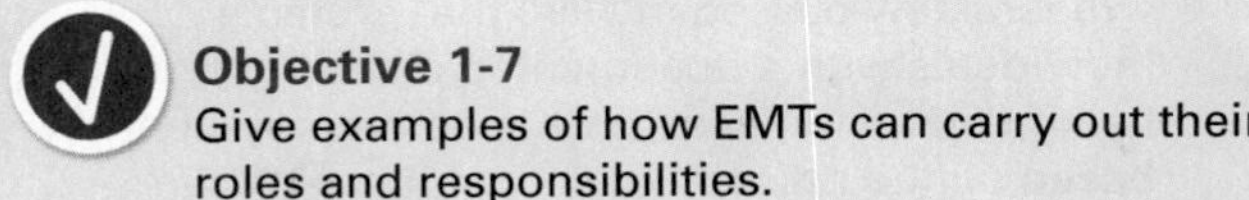

Objective 1-7
Give examples of how EMTs can carry out their roles and responsibilities.

- *Stroke center* to provide specialized care for specific acute stroke patients
- *Cardiac center* for the rapid and advanced management of patients suffering cardiac emergencies
- *Hyperbaric center* for the treatment of certain toxic exposures, diving emergencies, and other conditions
- *Spine injury center* for the management of patients with severe spine injuries
- *Psychiatric center* to care for patients with behavioral emergencies

You will often be called to emergencies where you and your partner are the only trained emergency personnel involved. At other times, two or more emergency services will be needed at the scene (Figure 1-4*). Specialized rescue teams and fire personnel, as well as law enforcement, all may be involved. As a member of the team that stabilizes and transports a patient (Figure 1-5*), you will be in a position to serve as the liaison between the community's medical services and those public safety workers.

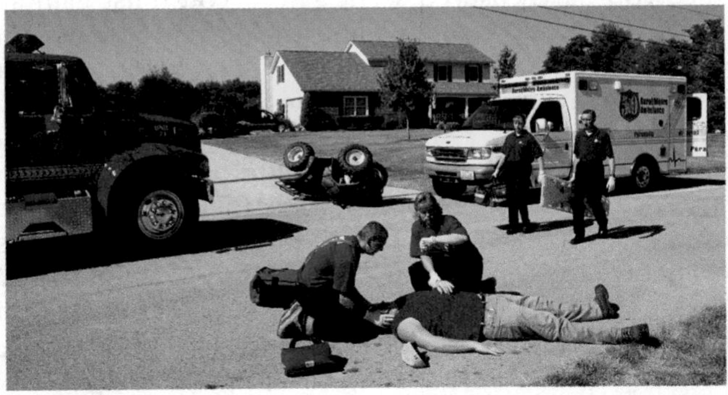

FIGURE 1-4 * The EMT works closely with other public safety personnel.

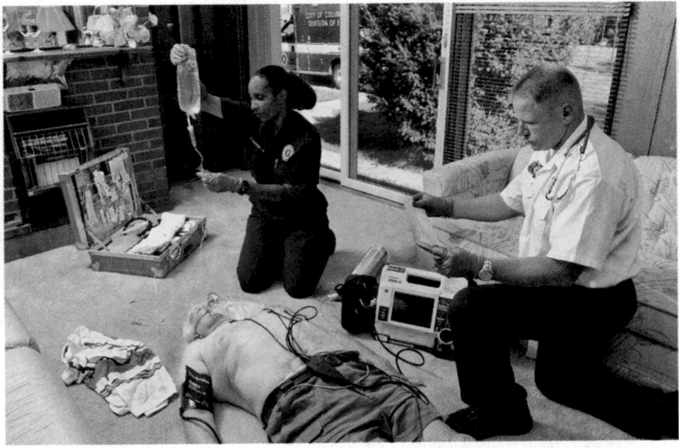

FIGURE 1-5 * You will often work as a team with paramedics and others.

The EMT

Roles and Responsibilities

While specific responsibilities may vary from one area to another, your general responsibilities as an EMT include personal safety and the safety of others, patient assessment and emergency medical care, safe lifting and moving, patient transport and transfer, record keeping and data collection, and patient advocacy. These and other responsibilities are found in Table 1-1. All of these will be covered in greater detail in later chapters.

TABLE 1-1 Roles and Responsibilities of the Emergency Medical Technician

- Maintain vehicle and equipment readiness.
- Ensure safety of the EMS crew, the patient, and bystanders at the scene.
- Operate the emergency vehicle.
- Assess the patient.
- Provide emergency care.
- Safely lift and move the patient.
- Prepare oral and written reports.
- Safely transport the patient.
- Transfer patient care.
- Perform record keeping and data collection.
- Serve as the patient's advocate.
- Provide emotional support to the patient, relatives, and others at the scene.
- Integrate the EMS service with other emergency and nonemergency services.
- Resolve the emergency incident.
- Maintain medical and legal standards.
- Provide administrative support.
- Enhance professional development.
- Develop and maintain community relations.

Key Terms

Americans with Disabilities Act (ADA) a federal law passed in 1990 that protects individuals with a documented disability from being denied initial or continued employment based on their disability.

Key Points

Your first and most important priority is to protect your own safety.

Thinking Critically

Why is your own safety your first and most important priority?

In light of these roles and responsibilities, the **Americans with Disabilities Act (ADA)** of 1990 protects individuals who have a documented disability from being denied initial or continued employment based on their disability. The employer must make necessary and reasonable adjustments so that individuals with disabilities are not precluded from employment. Check with your state EMS office and ADA representative to seek further information.

Personal Safety and the Safety of Others

Your first and most important priority is to protect your own safety (Figure 1-6*). Remember this rule: You cannot help the patient, other rescuers, or yourself if you are injured. You also do not want to endanger other rescuers by forcing them to rescue you—instead of the patient. Once scene safety is ensured, the patient's needs become your priority.

Drive safely at all times, using proper precautions to avoid traffic accidents. Use a seat belt whenever you drive or ride, unless you need to remove it to care for the patient. Remove yourself from potentially hazardous sites such as high-traffic areas, downed power lines, gasoline leaks, fires, chemical spills, radiation leaks, and so on. Never enter a volatile crowd situation, such as a riot, crime scene, or hostage situation, until it has been controlled by law enforcement. Take extra precautions when you suspect that a patient, relative, or bystander at the scene is under the influence of drugs or alcohol, has a behavioral disorder, or is emotionally charged, because these individuals have a tendency to suddenly change their behavior and may become a danger to you and your crew.

At the scene, follow directions from police, fire, utility, and other expert personnel. Create a safe area in which the patient can be treated (away from the threat of fire or explosion, for example). Redirect traffic for the safety of patients and bystanders.

Wear reflective emblems or clothing at night, and provide adequate lighting at an accident scene. Minimize personal injury from jagged metal or broken glass at an accident scene by wearing a helmet or hard hat, protective outerwear, eye protection, and leather gloves. In addition, wear protective gear, such as gloves, eye protection, mask, and gown, as necessary to avoid infectious diseases.

Patient Assessment and Emergency Care

Once you have ensured scene safety, you must gain access to patients, recognize and evaluate problems, and provide emergency care (Figure 1-7*)—often in situations that involve more than one patient. First, always perform a primary assessment to help you identify and care for immediately life-threatening problems, such as airway compromise, respiratory insufficiency, cardiac arrest, or severe bleeding. Then complete a secondary assessment, after which you can stabilize and treat other emergency injuries or conditions you discover or suspect. Work as quickly as possible while avoiding undue haste, carelessness, and mishandling of the patient. Always be aware of changing conditions and ensure that the scene remains safe.

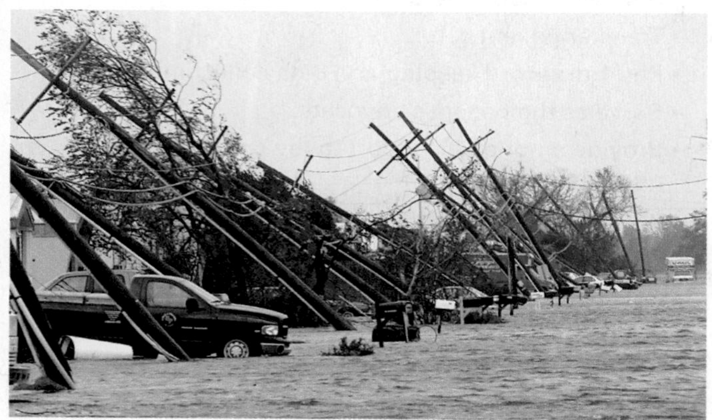

FIGURE 1-6 * The EMT must ensure personal safety at all times. (© Rick Wilking/Reuters/Corbis)

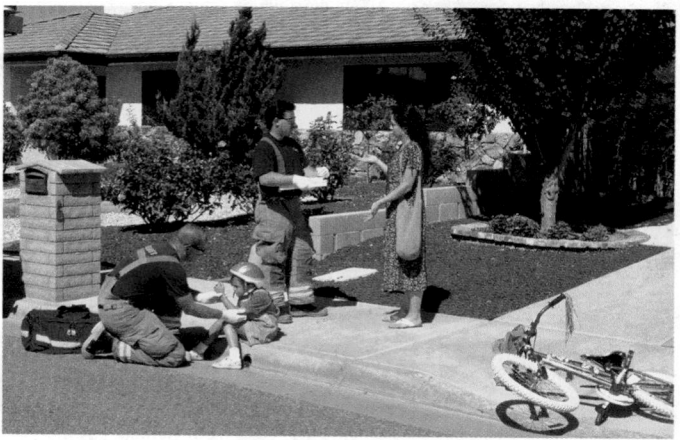

FIGURE 1-7 * The EMT is responsible for providing competent patient care.

Key Points
Always perform a primary assessment to identify and care for immediately life-threatening problems.

Thinking Critically
What are life-threatening problems you should treat immediately if found during your primary assessment of the patient ?

Key Points
Before leaving the hospital, or as soon as possible, complete the prehospital care report.

Safe Lifting and Moving

Prevent further injury of patients by always using the easiest and safest recommended emergency urgent or nonurgent moves and equipment. Prevent injuring yourself by always using proper body mechanics and by making sure you have sufficient help to lift and move patients and equipment.

Transport and Transfer of Care

Before leaving the scene, determine which facility (local emergency department, pediatric hospital, burn center, or other) will be most appropriate. Consider the patient's condition, the extent of injuries, prior health care contact, the relative locations, hospital staffing, and destination protocols when making transport decisions. Consult medical direction if necessary, and follow your local transport protocols.

Use the communications equipment available to you to notify the receiving facility of the number of patients, the destination(s), and the nature and extent of injuries. Alert the emergency department or receiving facility about high-priority patients and what will be needed immediately upon arrival, such as a trauma team or a stroke team. Report changes in the patient's condition, and consult medical direction during transport as appropriate and as required (Figures 1-8* and 1-9*).

Drive in a way that will minimize further injury and maximize patient comfort. Obey appropriate laws and regulations, and use lights and sirens properly. Realize that not all patients require the use of lights and sirens. Once you reach the destination, help remove the wheeled stretcher and maneuver it into the emergency department.

Report both verbally and in writing to the appropriate receiving facility personnel what injuries or conditions were identified, what care has been given to the patient, and the patient's response to treatment. Provide other assistance as needed and do not leave before the patient has been properly transferred to the care of the receiving facility personnel (Figure 1-10*).

Record Keeping and Data Collection

Throughout your shift, maintain an up-to-date log of calls, if required. Before leaving the hospital, or as soon as possible, complete the written or electronic prehospital care report (Figure 1-11*). A copy of this report will become part of the patient's medical record and part of your EMS system's permanent records.

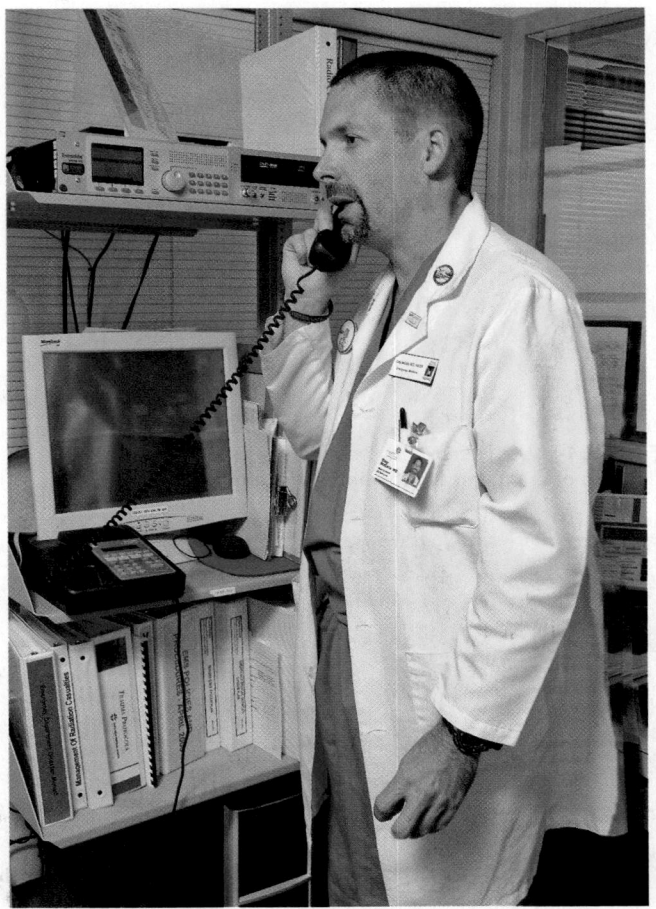

FIGURE 1-8 * The EMT can get on-line medical direction by telephone, cell phone, or radio.

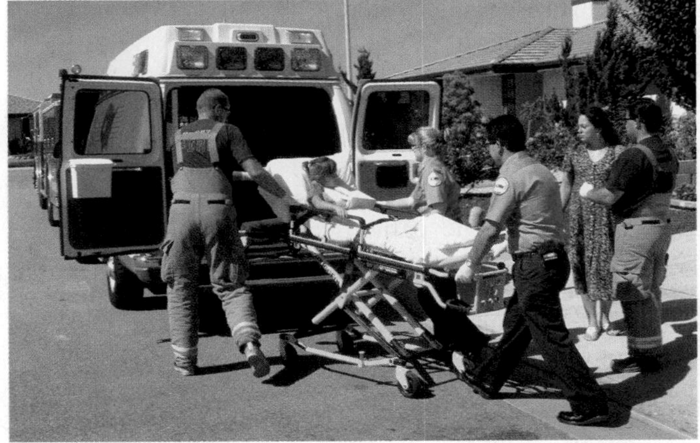

FIGURE 1-9 * Assessment and emergency care are continued en route to the medical facility.

Thinking Critically
What are some actions you might perform as the patient's advocate?

Objective 1-8
Describe the expectations of EMTs in terms of professional attributes.

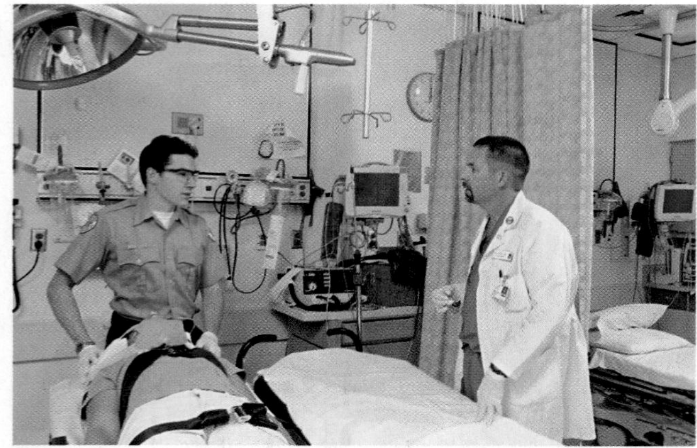

FIGURE 1-10 * The EMT is responsible for properly transferring the care of the patient to the appropriate medical personnel.

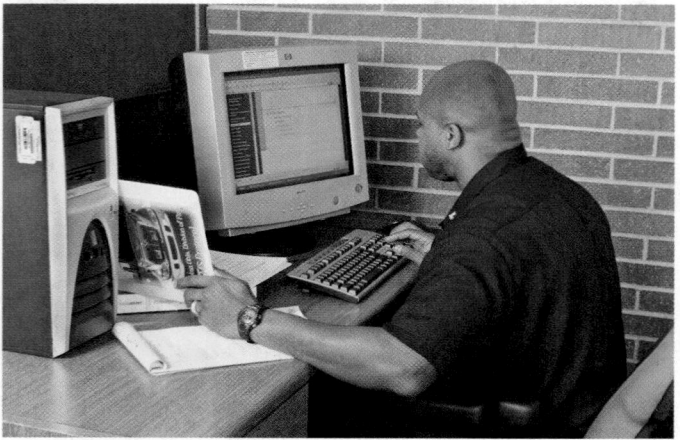

FIGURE 1-11 * As soon as possible, complete the written or electronic prehospital care report.

Patient Advocacy

As an emergency care provider, you are also responsible for protecting the patient's rights. At the scene, collect and safeguard a patient's valuables on his person, transport them with the patient, and document what was given to emergency department personnel. In the field, protect the patient's privacy, shield the patient as much as possible from curious bystanders, and answer questions truthfully. Conceal from curious onlookers the body of a patient who has died.

Make sure that the patient's friends or loved ones at the scene know how to get to the hospital or medical facility that you are transporting the patient to. In some systems a relative may be transported in the operator's section of the ambulance. At the receiving facility, act as the patient's advocate by making certain you have provided necessary information, especially about circumstances hospital personnel have not witnessed. Honor any patient requests that you reasonably can, such as notifying a relative or ensuring that the patient's home is secure. Be sure to adhere to all confidentiality rules when doing such activities.

Professional Attributes

A number of professional attributes are important to maximize your effectiveness as an EMT. They include appearance, knowledge, skills, the ability to meet physical demands, general interests and temperament, and maintenance of certification and licensure. See Table 1-2 for characteristics of professional behavior for EMTs.

Appearance

Excellent personal grooming and a neat, clean appearance help instill confidence in patients treated by EMTs—and help protect them from contamination that could be caused by dirty hands, dirty fingernails, or soiled clothing. Respond to the scene in complete uniform, or appropriate dress, to portray the positive image you want to communicate. Remember, you are on a medical team. Your appearance can send the message that you are competent and can be trusted to make the right decisions.

TABLE 1-2 Characteristics of Professional Behavior for EMTs

- Integrity
- Empathy
- Self-motivation
- Professional appearance and hygiene
- Self-confidence
- Effective time management
- Good verbal and written communication skills
- Teamwork and diplomacy
- Respect for patients, coworkers, and other health care professionals
- Patient advocate
- Careful delivery of service

Knowledge and Skills

To practice as an EMT, you need to successfully complete the basic training program for EMTs as outlined by the U.S. Department of Transportation. In addition to the required course work, you also need to know the following:

- ***Use and maintenance of common emergency equipment,*** such as suction machines, oxygen-delivery systems, airway adjuncts, automated external defibrillators, spinal immobilization equipment, splints, obstetrical kits, various types of patient-moving devices, and tools to gain access to the patient.
- ***Assistance with the administration of medications*** approved by medical direction.
- ***Cleaning, disinfection, and sterilization of nondisposable equipment.***
- ***Safety and security measures*** for yourself, your partner, and other rescuers, as well as for the patient and bystanders.
- ***Territory and terrain*** within the service area to allow expedient response to the scene and to the appropriate receiving facility.
- ***State and local traffic laws and ordinances*** concerning emergency transportation of the sick and injured. Ambulances are given certain privileges, but they are not immune from all traffic laws.

Use opportunities for continuing education to expand your knowledge and learn about advances in patient care, new equipment, or better ways of using existing equipment. Take refresher courses to renew your knowledge and skills. Finally, maintain up-to-date knowledge of local, state, and federal legislation, regulations, standards, guidelines, and issues that affect the emergency medical systems in your area.

Physical Demands

To be an EMT, you must be in good physical health. You must be able to lift and carry up to 125 pounds. Your eyesight must be good (correction by lenses is permitted), and you must have good color vision in order to properly assess a patient as well as for driving safely. Color vision is necessary to determine various changes in the color of the skin, nail beds, lips, and inside the mouth, which provide critical information about the severity and the possible condition the patient is experiencing. You must also be able to communicate effectively both orally and in writing. This will be necessary when communicating with patients, crew members, other emergency response personnel, and the medical staff. Your hearing must be good enough to accurately hear radio communications, patient and bystander responses, auscultated blood pressure, auscultated and other abnormal patient noises, communication from other crew members at the scene, and oral instructions.

Personal Traits

In times of crisis, patients will look toward someone to reestablish order in a suddenly chaotic world. Chances are that someone will be you. It can bring out the best in you as well as cause you a great deal of stress. To be effective as an EMT, you should have the following characteristics:

- **A calm and reassuring personality.** As an EMT you will often be required to perform skills and procedures while speaking in a reassuring and calming voice to a patient who may be agitated, in shock, or in a great deal of pain.
- **Leadership ability.** You must be able to assess a situation quickly, step forward to take control when appropriate, set action priorities, give clear and concise directions, be confident and persuasive enough to be obeyed, and carry through with what needs to be done.
- **Good judgment.** You must be able to make appropriate decisions quickly, often in unsafe or stressful situations involving human beings in crisis.
- **Good moral character.** While there are many legal constraints on the profession, you also have ethical obligations. You are in a position of public trust that can never be wholly defined by statute or case law alone.
- **Stability and adaptability.** Being an EMT can be quite stressful. Exhaustion, frustration, anger, and grief are part of the package. You must learn how to delay expressing your feelings until the emergency is over. Just as important, you must also understand that intense emotional reactions are normal and that seeking support from coworkers, counselors, friends, and family is an important aspect of keeping yourself mentally and physically fit.
- **Ability to listen.** You must be an effective listener when gathering information from patients and bystanders and when receiving orders from medical direction or others at the scene. You should exhibit empathy and compassion in your responses; however, you must always maintain a high degree of professionalism, confidence, and competence.
- **Resourcefulness and ability to improvise.** You will find yourself in some situations where a particular piece of equipment, tool, or technique doesn't quite work. You will need to be resourceful, quickly thinking and adapting to make things work for the best care for your patient. You will find yourself improvising to care for and move some patients. As an example, if a patient entrapped in an overturned vehicle needs immediate ventilation, you must determine the most effective method to gain entry to the vehicle, to provide ventilation with both you and the patient in an awkward and unusual position, and to continue to deliver ventilation while removing the patient from the wrecked vehicle. Each call, situation, and patient is different and requires quick

Objectives 1-9 and 1-10
Discuss medical direction/oversight and quality improvement in EMS.

Key Terms
medical director physician who is legally responsible for the **medical oversight** of an EMS system.

Key Terms
medical direction policies, procedures, and practices available either **off-line** (as **protocols** or **standing orders**) or **on-line** (by phone or radio).

thinking and resourcefulness to provide efficient and effective emergency care.

- **Cooperativeness.** Often your call may involve other emergency services, such as First Responders and the police. You must be able to act as a leader while fully cooperating with others at the scene to provide the best possible care to the patient.

Maintenance of Certification and Licensure

It is the personal responsibility of each EMT to maintain certification and licensure to practice. This involves meeting the necessary continuing education requirements, verifying skill competency, avoiding any criminal or unethical behavior, and submitting all fees necessary to maintain current certification and licensure.

Medical Direction/Medical Oversight

As an EMT, you are the designated agent of the physician medical director of your EMS system. The care you render to patients is considered an extension of the medical director's authority. (Learn your own state laws, statutes, and regulations in regard to medical direction.)

The **medical director** is a physician who is legally responsible for the clinical and patient care aspects of the EMS system. An EMS medical director is also involved in EMS education programs and refresher courses, overseeing and providing continuing education, and facilitating the quality improvement system. Every emergency medical service must have a medical director in order to provide any level of prehospital care.

The medical director is responsible for providing **medical direction.** A primary charge of medical direction is developing and establishing the guidelines under which the emergency medical service personnel function. These guidelines are referred to as **protocols.** Protocols comprise a full set of guidelines that define the entire scope of medical care (triage, treatment, transport, destination). Often referred to as orders, protocols may consist of both off-line and on-line medical direction.

Off-line medical direction is provided through a set of predetermined, written guidelines that allow EMTs to use their judgment to administer emergency medical care according to the written guidelines without having to contact a physician. **On-line medical direction** requires that the EMT acquire permission from a physician via cell phone, telephone, or radio communication prior to administering specific emergency care. As an example, the protocol for chest pain may read: (1) Administer oxygen via nonrebreather mask at 15 lpm; (2) place patient in position of comfort; (3) administer one patient-prescribed nitroglycerin tablet if systolic blood pressure is greater than 90 mmHg; (4) administer one 160–325 mg aspirin; (5) contact advanced life support; (6) if the patient does not experience relief of chest pain from one nitroglycerin tablet, contact medical direction to consider administering additional doses.

Items 1 through 5 are all off-line medical direction or standing orders. The EMT is expected to perform these treatments and activities for a patient having chest pain without having to contact the physician prior to treatment. However, in reference to item 6, if the patient is continuing to experience chest pain, the EMT must contact medical direction and receive permission to administer any additional doses of nitroglycerin. Because item 6 requires direct communication with the physician, it is considered on-line medical direction.

Standing orders are a subset of protocols that do not require real-time physician input. In some systems, the term is synonymous with off-line medical direction. In some systems, the term *standing orders* refers specifically to treatments that can be performed if communication cannot be established or is lost with medical direction.

Medical oversight is the emerging term that more comprehensively describes the EMS system medical director's responsibilities. These include all of the clinical and administrative functions and activities performed by the medical director as necessary to exercise ultimate responsibility for the emergency care provided by individual personnel and the entire EMS system.

Quality Improvement

Quality improvement (QI), also known as *continuous quality improvement (CQI),* is a system of internal and external reviews and audits of all aspects of an emergency medical system. To ensure that the public receives the highest quality of prehospital care, the goals of quality improvement are to identify those aspects of the system that can be improved and to implement plans and programs that will remedy any shortcomings. It is important to recognize that quality improvement is not designed to evaluate individual performance, but instead is intended to determine how effective the *system* is and to identify what improvements can be made to deliver a better service. Although quality improvement can identify an indi-

Key Terms

quality improvement (QI) a system of internal and external reviews and audits of an EMS system to ensure a high quality of care.

Objective 1-11

Explain the EMT's roles and responsibilities in quality improvement

Objective 1-12

Identify activities in EMS that pose a high risk of mistakes and injuries.

vidual with a poor performance that requires some type of corrective action or remedial work, as a general rule quality improvement should be used not as a penalty tool but as an evaluation system geared toward overall system improvement.

As an EMT, your role in quality improvement (Figure 1-12*) is to:

- **Document carefully.** Carefully and thoroughly document each call. Prehospital care reports that you prepare are studied by quality improvement committees to spot such things as excessive response times, which might be remedied by redeploying ambulances, or to identify seldom-used skills for refresher training.
- **Perform reviews and audits.** Become involved in the quality improvement process by volunteering for QI committee work or by critiquing the performance of other EMTs at the scene of a call.
- **Obtain feedback.** Gather feedback from patients, other EMS personnel, and hospital staff. This may be done formally through surveys distributed to patients and hospital staff members, or informally by seeking advice about your performance after a call from physicians, nurses, or other medical personnel.
- **Maintain equipment.** Conduct preventative maintenance on equipment and ensure it is in the proper working order.
- **Participate in continuing education.** Participate in refresher courses and continuing education to reinforce, update, and expand your knowledge and skills.
- **Maintain skills.** It is important to continuously practice your skills to a level of mastery.

Issues in Patient Safety

One of the most important issues that must be addressed when dealing with patients in the prehospital environment is safe delivery of care. There are some activities that are considered "high risk" and put the patient at greater risk for medical mistakes, injury, or exacerbating an existing injury. Some of these high-risk activities include:

- Transfer of care or "hand-off" at the scene between emergency responders or at the medical facility
- Poor communication that leads to misunderstanding and medical errors
- Carrying and moving patients in a manner that puts them at risk for being dropped

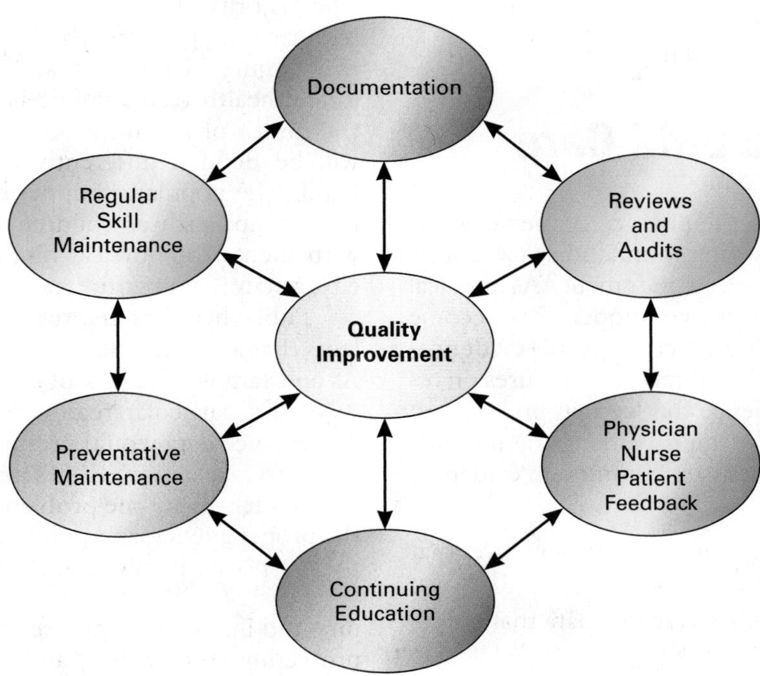

FIGURE 1-12 * The EMT takes an active role in quality improvement.

Objective 1-13
Discuss steps that you can take to minimize mistakes and injuries in EMS.

Key Terms

evidence-based medicine practice based on evidence that procedures, medications, and equipment improve patient outcome.

Objectives 1-14 and 1-15
Discuss the steps and the limitations of evidence-based decision making in EMS.

Objective 1-16
Describe the relationship between EMS and public health.

- Involvement in an ambulance crash while transporting the patient to a medical facility
- Lack of spinal immobilization or improper spinal immobilization procedures that increase the risk of converting a stable spinal column injury into an unstable spinal column injury, or improper immobilization that exacerbates the existing injury

Errors during patient care may also put the patient at risk. These errors usually result from failure of the EMT to properly perform a skill, failure of the rules the EMT must follow, or failure of the EMT to have obtained or retained the appropriate knowledge to perform patient care effectively.

You can take the following steps to prevent errors that may jeopardize the patient's safety:

- Develop clear protocols.
- Light the scene effectively.
- Try to minimize interruptions during assessment and emergency care.
- Clearly mark all drugs and packages so each is very distinct.
- Reflect on all actions.
- Question all assumptions.
- Use decision aids if necessary.
- Ask for assistance if you need it.

Research and EMS Care

The traditional approach to the practice of medicine involved a combination of a strong foundation of scientific knowledge, intuition, and good judgment. As medical practice has evolved, the science component has become more emphasized through the concept of **evidence-based medicine.** Evidence-based medicine focuses on research to provide clear evidence that certain procedures, medications, and equipment improve the patient's outcome. The following four steps are common in evidence-based decision making:

- Formulate a question about emergency care that needs to be answered.
- Search medical literature for research data that are related and applicable to the question.
- Appraise the evidence for validity and reliability.
- If the evidence supports a change in practice, change protocols and implement the change in prehospital emergency care.

Although an evidence-based approach appears to be extremely desirable in making decisions about prehospital patient management, very little research has so far been done regarding prehospital care. EMS has typically had to rely on research conducted for the hospital emergency department. Although hospital and prehospital emergency care are somewhat related, there are variables in the prehospital environment that are not encountered in the hospital setting; thus, it is often difficult to extrapolate and apply the results and conclusions of hospital emergency care research to prehospital practice.

Initiatives are under way to increase the amount of research conducted specifically to support or to change the delivery of prehospital emergency care. It is the responsibility of every EMT to participate in such research so that EMS can develop its own evidence-based practices to support and improve its profession.

Public Health

The majority of the EMT's responsibilities are concerned with treating patients who have a medical illness or traumatic injury. However, as an EMT you are also part of the public health team. Public health deals with protecting the health of an entire population. Specific populations will be defined differently depending on the issue at hand. The population under consideration may be a select group, such as children, elderly adults, individuals with mental or physical disabilities, a neighborhood, a city, a state, or an entire nation.

Public health is first responsible for identifying problems that affect the health of the population in question. As an example, the lack of the use of infant and child car seats in a particular region as identified through injury surveillance data would prompt the public health professional to take action. EMTs may be the frontline individuals in identifying the problem, reporting on the issue to the proper agency, and potentially providing education to those who are involved in the problem.

Public health attempts to reduce the incidence of injury and illness through preventative strategies geared at protecting, promoting, and improving the health of a population. This is typically achieved through research,

Thinking Critically
How would you describe the goals of public health? How can the EMT further those goals?

Objective 1-17
List the ten greatest public health achievements in the United States in the 20th century.

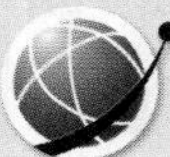

Media Resources
Go to www.bradybooks.com for mykit. Highlights:
- *Video:* EMS, the Community, and Children
- *Video:* Healthy People 2010

education, and health promotion. In published statements, the American Public Health Association has defined the vision of public health as "healthy people in healthy communities" and the mission of public health as "to promote physical and mental health and prevent disease, injury, and disability."

According to the Centers for Disease Control (CDC) *Morbidity and Mortality Weekly Report*, the ten greatest public health achievements in the United States in the 20th century were:

- ***Vaccinations*** to eliminate smallpox and polio, and to control measles, rubella, tetanus, diphtheria, *Haemophilus influenzae* type B, and other infectious diseases
- ***Motor-vehicle safety*** measures to reduce the number of motor-vehicle deaths
- ***Workplace safety*** measures to decrease the number of work-related deaths
- ***Control of infectious disease*** through clean water and sanitation and antimicrobial therapy
- ***Reduction in deaths from coronary heart disease and stroke*** related to the reduction in risk factors such as smoking and high blood pressure
- ***Safer and more healthful foods*** through controlling food contamination and ensuring the nutritional value of foods
- ***Decline in maternal and infant mortality*** through better hygiene, nutrition, antibiotics, access to health care, and technologic advances in maternal and infant care
- ***Use of barrier devices during sexual contacts*** to protect against pregnancy, HIV, and other sexually transmitted diseases
- ***Fluoridation of drinking water*** to prevent tooth decay and tooth loss
- ***Reduction in the use of tobacco products*** through promotion of cessation programs and reduction of second-hand smoke, resulting in improvement across a wide spectrum of health issues

Public health professionals may be involved in enforcing laws and regulations that protect the health and ensure the safety of the public. This may be achieved through legislation such as seat-belt and helmet laws.

EMS is part of the public health system and plays an integral role in carrying out its mission. Roles of EMS in public health include:

- Health prevention and promotion through primary prevention (vaccinations, education), secondary prevention of complications of disease, and health screening (Figures 1-13a and 1-13b*)
- Disease surveillance through identifying and reporting certain diseases or conditions that are identified as public health issues
- Injury prevention through education, promotion of the use of safety equipment (seat belt use, helmet use, falls prevention, fire prevention), and injury surveillance

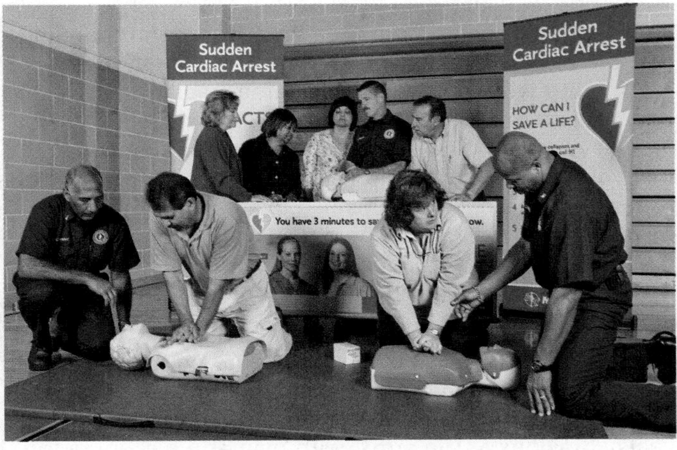

(a)

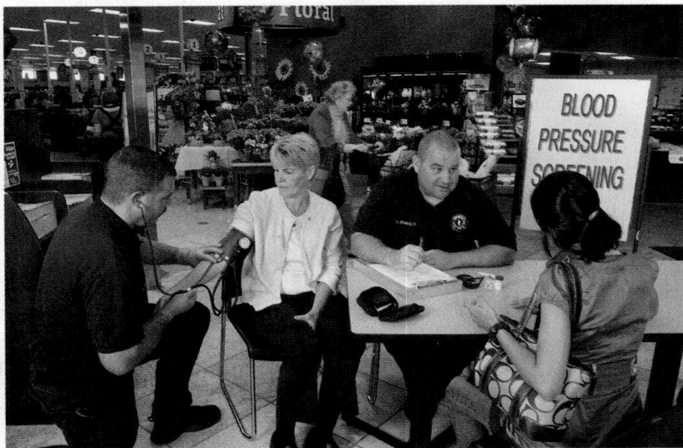

(b)

FIGURE 1-13 * The roles of the EMS in public health include participation in **(a)** public education programs and **(b)** health screenings.

CHAPTER REVIEW

SUMMARY

Emergency medical services systems have evolved dramatically from the days when the funeral home provided transportation of the sick and injured to the hospital as a courtesy. Many of the practices today have come from treating military casualties on the battlefield during various wars and conflicts. Because of the number of highway deaths associated with auto crashes, the Department of Transportation in the 1960s took a lead role in developing the education program for EMTs. Even though EMS systems are independent of federal government control, the National Highway Traffic Safety Administration (NHTSA) developed the Technical Assistance Program Assessment Standards as recommended guidelines for EMS systems.

Most EMS systems are accessed using the universal number 911. Quick access via this standardized number reduces response times. Enhanced 911 systems provide the name, geographic location, and phone number for the landline the call is being made from.

The levels of EMS training according to the National Scope of Practice Model are Emergency Medical Responder (EMR), Emergency Medical Technician (EMT), Advanced EMT (AEMT), and paramedic.

The EMT has many roles and responsibilities: safety, patient assessment and emergency care, transportation and transfer of care, patient advocacy, professional appearance, knowledge and skills, ability to handle physical demands, and positive personal traits. Many of these roles and responsibilities are essential to the function of the EMT.

Medical direction or medical oversight is a key component of any EMS system. An EMT is unable to function without medical direction. One responsibility of medical direction is to provide orders or protocols. Medical direction may be off-line, in the form of written patient care orders, or on-line, where you communicate directly with the physician or a designee for oral patient care orders.

To improve the EMS system, quality improvement (QI) must be performed to identify any weaknesses or inadequacies. QI is a continuous process that involves all aspects of the system, including the personnel who provide care.

Emergency care provided in the prehospital environment is continuously evolving based on current research. Treatments and techniques that were used in the past have been supported, changed, or eliminated based on evidence found in studies. New techniques and treatments are no longer implemented without adequate evidence to support their effectiveness. More research needs to be conducted that is specific to EMS.

Emergency medical services is part of the public health system, vision, and mission. EMS is on the frontline to reduce the incidence of injury and illness through preventative strategies that are geared toward protecting, promoting, and improving the health of a population. This is typically achieved through education, health and safety promotion, and research.

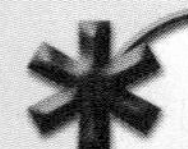

CASE STUDY FOLLOW-UP

SCENE SIZE-UP

You have been dispatched to a 65-year-old male, Edgar Robinson, who fell down a steep embankment behind his house. Although the rescue squad officer informs you that you will be in no personal danger, you and your partner are cautious as you carry your equipment closer to the embankment. As your partner takes the patient's wife, Mrs. Robinson, aside, the rescue squad officer tells you that his crew all have Emergency Medical Responder training and will immobilize Mr. Robinson on a backboard before bringing him up.

PRIMARY ASSESSMENT

One Emergency Medical Responder reports her observations of the patient to you as the others place the patient where you indicate. She tells you that the patient's chief complaint is of pain to his right wrist and right thigh and that the patient's airway is patent with respirations of 24 per minute with an adequate volume, radial pulse is 90 beats per minute and strong, and the skin is warm and dry.

As you begin your own primary assessment, you note that your general impression of Mr. Robinson is of an alert, robust older man. Mr. Robinson explains to you that while disposing of yard wastes, he got too close to the edge of the embankment and slipped.

SECONDARY ASSESSMENT

You perform a physical exam while your partner takes vital signs, which indicate no change from those reported by the Emergency Medical Responder. Your physical exam reveals abrasions to the arms, with pain and a slight deformity to the right wrist. There are also superficial abrasions to the right leg, with deformity, swelling, and pain to the right thigh. You discover that the patient cannot feel or move the toes of his right foot. However, pulses are present in the foot.

You initiate oxygen therapy via a nonrebreather mask.

The history you take, by asking questions of the patient, confirms sharp pain to the right wrist and thigh, which started immediately after he landed at the bottom of the embankment. Mr. Robinson also reports that he did not lose consciousness. He denies any other complaints but informs you that he is allergic to sulfa drugs and takes medication for high blood pressure.

After checking the immobilization of the patient, you enlist the Emergency Medical Responders to help you apply a traction splint to the right leg. Then you splint the injured wrist. During these procedures, you speak quietly and reassuringly to the patient.

REASSESSMENT

You move Mr. Robinson on the backboard to a wheeled stretcher, then transfer him to the ambulance. You notify the hospital that you are en route and give details of the patient's condition, then conduct a reassessment every 5 minutes to monitor his condition until you arrive at the hospital.

Upon arrival, you transfer care of the patient without incident to the emergency department staff and give your verbal report. You carefully complete your written prehospital care report and prepare the unit for the next call.

IN REVIEW

1. Describe the purpose of the modern EMS system.
2. Name two ways the public accesses the EMS system. Explain advantages or disadvantages of each.
3. List the four levels of prehospital emergency care training.
4. List six types of special facilities, other than a hospital emergency department, to which some patients may need to be transported.
5. List the general responsibilities of an EMT.
6. Describe at least five steps you can take to protect your own safety as an EMT.
7. Describe at least three ways you might act as the patient's advocate.
8. Describe the EMS physician medical director's primary responsibility.
9. List the goals of quality improvement.
10. Describe the EMT's role in quality improvement.
11. Describe evidence-based EMS care.
12. Explain the role of the EMT in public health.

CRITICAL THINKING

You are called to the residence of a 78-year-old male patient who appears to have suffered a stroke. The patient is unable to speak and appears agitated. The niece of the patient wants him transported to the small local hospital a few blocks from his house. A stroke center is approximately 20 minutes from your location.

1. What are your responsibilities while on this call?
2. How can you serve as the patient's advocate?
3. How can you use medical direction in this situation?

PEARSON

EXPLORE mybradykit™

Please go to **www.bradybooks.com** to access mykit for this text. You will find quizzes, critical thinking scenarios, weblinks, animations, and videos related to this chapter—and much more. Look for online information on the EMS Agenda for the Future. You will also find a video clip on EMS and the community.

Register your access code from the front of your book by going to **www.bradybooks.com** and selecting the mykit links.

Workforce Safety and Wellness of the EMT

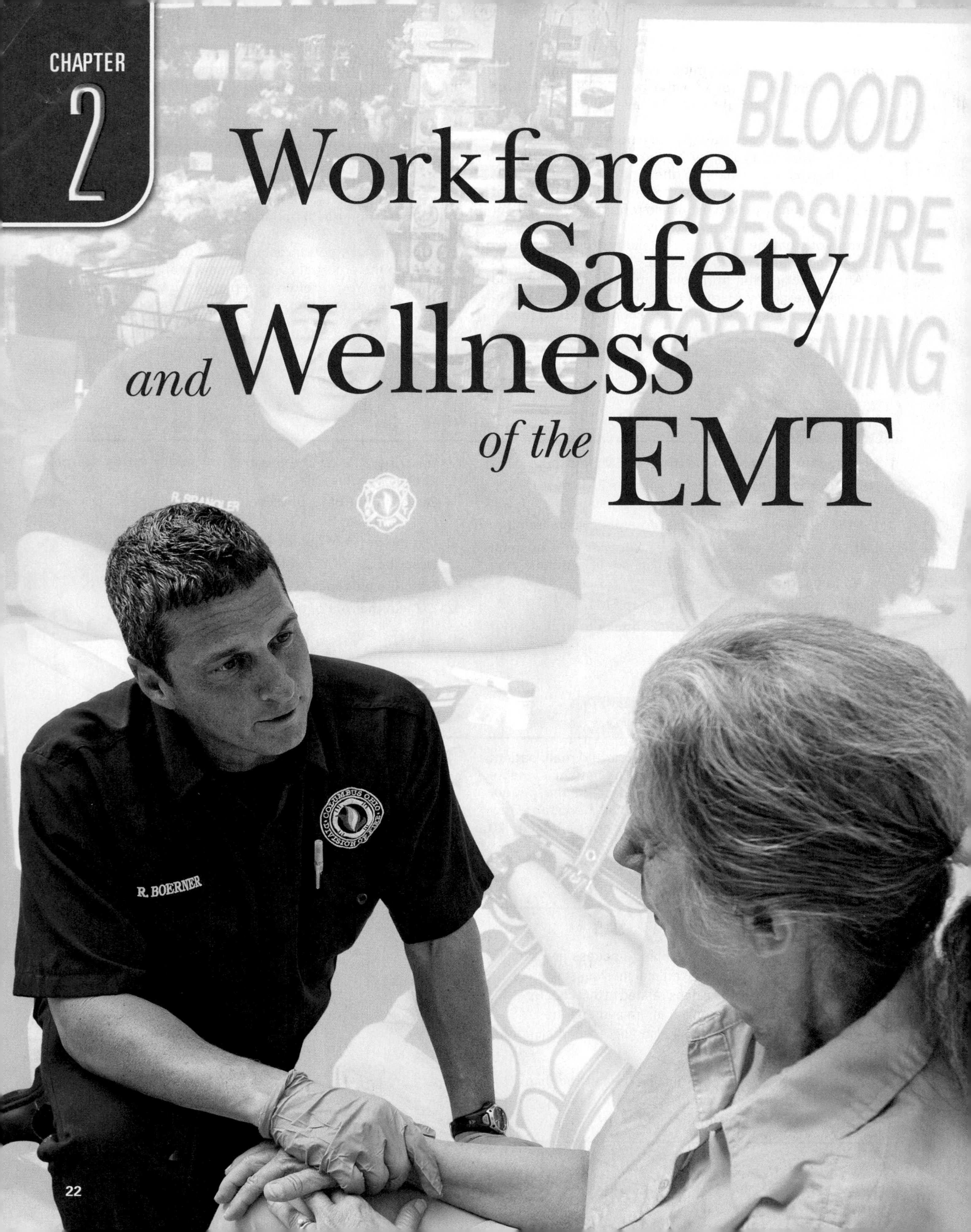

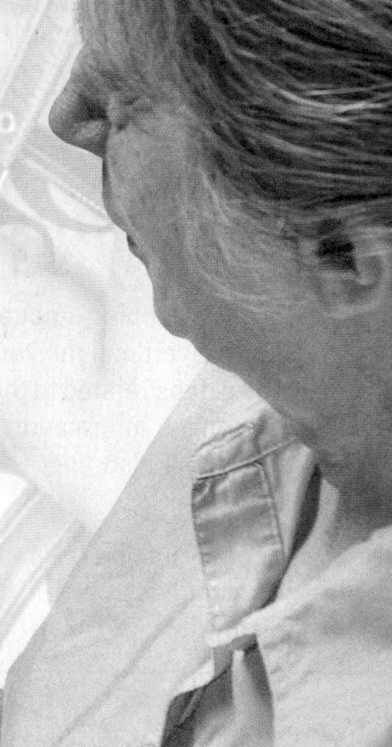

Navigation Guide

The following items provide an overview to the purpose and content of this chapter. The Education Standard and Competency are from the new National EMS Education Standards.

STANDARDS **Preparatory** (Content Areas: Workforce Safety and Wellness); **Medicine** (Infectious Diseases)

COMPETENCIES Applies fundamental knowledge of the EMS system, safety/well-being of the EMT, medical/legal and ethical issues to the provision of emergency care.

Applies fundamental knowledge to provide basic emergency care and transportation based on assessment findings for an acutely ill patient.

OBJECTIVES: After reading this chapter, you should be able to:

2-1. Define key terms introduced in this chapter.
2-2. Given a description of a patient or family member's behavior, identify the stage of grief it most likely represents.
2-3. Explain the principles for interacting with patients and family members in situations involving death and dying.
2-4. Give examples of situations that EMS providers may find stressful.
2-5. Compare and contrast the characteristics of acute, delayed, and cumulative stress reactions.
2-6. Recognize signs and symptoms of stress reactions.
2-7. Describe lifestyle changes you can make to help you deal with stress.
2-8. Describe responses your friends and family may have to your work in EMS.
2-9. Describe changes in the work environment that can help you manage job-related stress.
2-10. Discuss the components of a comprehensive system of critical incident stress management.
2-11. Describe measures you can take to protect yourself from exposure to diseases caused by pathogens and accidental and work-related injury.
2-12. Give examples of diseases caused by each of the different types of pathogens (bacteria, viruses, fungi, protozoa, and helminths).
2-13. Describe the Standard Precautions that must be taken to protect health care workers from exposure to infectious diseases.
2-14. Describe the personal protective equipment that may be used by EMS personnel.
2-15. Explain the role of immunizations and tuberculosis testing in maintaining good health.
2-16. Discuss the risks and preventive measures for specific infectious diseases of concern to EMTs, including:
  a. Hepatitis B
  b. Hepatitis C
  c. Tuberculosis
  d. Acquired immune deficiency syndrome
  e. Severe acute respiratory syndrome
  f. West Nile virus
  g. Infections due to multidrug-resistant organisms
2-17. Explain the risks and measures that can be taken to protect yourself against the following hazards:
  a. Hazardous materials
  b. Hazardous rescue situations
  c. Traffic-related injuries
  d. Violence and crime
2-18. Describe the components of physical and mental wellness.

KEY TERMS: Page references indicate first major use in this chapter. For complete definitions, see the Glossary at the back of the book.

burnout p. 27
cleaning p. 35
critical incident p. 29
critical incident stress debriefing (CISD) p. 29
defusing p. 30
disinfecting p. 35
pathogens p. 30
personal protective equipment (PPE) p. 32
purified protein derivative (PPD) tuberculin test p. 36
Standard Precautions p. 32
sterilization p. 35

MEDIA RESOURCES: Please go to www.bradybooks.com to access mykit for this text. You will find quizzes, critical thinking scenarios, weblinks, animations, and videos related to this chapter—and much more. Look for online information on stress management. You will also find a video clip on transmission and treatments for AIDS.

continued

CASE STUDY

The Dispatch

EMS Units 111 and 112—both units respond to 327 Manchester Avenue—possible domestic dispute with reported gunfire—called in by the police department—time out 1441 hours.

Upon Arrival

You immediately identify three city police cruisers outside the house. Patrol officers are kneeling behind their units with guns drawn and pointed at the house. One of the police officers is gesturing emphatically for you and your partner to keep back. Your partner stops the ambulance a good distance away. As you survey the scene with binoculars, you identify a downed police officer at the front door of the residence. He is not moving and seems to be bleeding profusely. You both hear gunfire.

How Would You Proceed?

During this chapter, you will learn about methods of safeguarding yourself from stress, body substances, and other hazards. Later, we will return to the case and apply the principles learned.

Introduction

As you proceed through your course and this text, you will study specific ways to safeguard your well-being—in the face of danger and under other high-stress circumstances. This chapter presents an overview. In it you will learn to recognize and deal with the stress that normally accompanies emergency work, to practice all appropriate Standard Precautions, to wear the appropriate personal protective equipment at the scene of accidents and illness, to recognize common infectious diseases, and to practice strategies to prevent work-related injuries.

Emotional Aspects of Emergency Care

In the course of providing emergency care, you will encounter family members, as well as patients, who are in distress—acute physical or mental suffering caused by pain, anxiety, strain, or sorrow. When such emotional pressures become too great for them to handle, emotional crisis occurs. The emergency care you provide can move those patients and family members toward re-establishing emotional equilibrium.

Death and Dying

Death and dying are inherent parts of emergency medical care. You must care for the dying patient's emotional needs, as well as his injuries or illnesses. If the patient has suffered a sudden death, you may also need to help the family or bystanders deal with the situation.

A study by Elizabeth Kübler-Ross on how people cope with death has identified five general stages that dying patients—and those close to them—will experience. However, each person is unique. Individuals will progress through the stages at their own rates and in their own ways. Although these stages usually apply to the dying patient, they also can apply to patients experiencing nonfatal emergencies. For example, a patient who loses both legs in an industrial accident will grieve the loss of the limbs.

Five Emotional Stages

Characteristically, you will not witness all five stages during emergency treatment. For example, the critically injured patient who is aware that death is imminent typically displays denial, bargaining, or depression. The terminally ill patient may be more prepared and display acceptance. The key for you is to accept all these emotions as real and necessary, and respond accordingly.

- **Denial ("Not me.").** At first, the patient may refuse to accept the possibility that death is near. This refusal, or denial, is a defense mechanism that creates a buffer between the shock of approaching death and the need to deal with the illness or injury.
- **Anger ("Why me?").** As the patient moves through denial, anger generally follows—and you may be the target. Do not become defensive. That kind of anger is an aspect of the grieving process both dying patients and their families go through. Be empathetic, and use your best listening and communication skills.

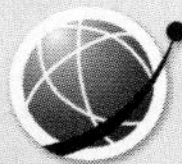

Media Resources

Go to www.bradybooks.com for mykit. Highlights:

- *Web Resource:* Hepatitis B and the Healthcare Worker
- *Web Resource:* Stress Management

Objective 2-2
Given a description of a patient or family behavior, identify their likely stage of grief.

Objective 2-3
Explain the principles for interacting with patients and family members in situations involving death and dying.

- **Bargaining ("Okay, but first let me . . .").** Following anger, the patient will likely try to "bargain," or make agreements that at least in the patient's mind will postpone death for a short time.
- **Depression ("Okay, but I haven't . . .").** As reality settles in, the patient may become silent, distant, sad, and despairing—usually about those he will leave behind and things left undone.
- **Acceptance ("Okay, I am not afraid.").** Finally, patients may appear to accept death, though not happy about it. At this stage, the family usually requires more support than the patient does.

Dealing with the Dying Patient, Family, and Bystanders

Although emergency care of the patient's illness or injury is your priority, you have an obligation to help patients and others through the grieving process. Keep in mind that patients, families, and bystanders may be progressing through the stages at different rates. Whatever stage they are in, their needs include dignity, respect, sharing, communication, privacy, and control. To help reduce their emotional burden:

- **Do everything possible to maintain the patient's dignity.** Avoid negative statements about the patient's condition. An unresponsive patient may hear what you say and feel the fear in your words. Even if the patient is unresponsive, talk to him as if he is fully alert and explain the care you are providing.
- **Show the greatest possible respect for the patient,** especially when death is imminent. Families will be extra sensitive to how the dying relative is treated. Even attitudes and unspoken messages are perceived. Allow family members to stay with the patient during resuscitation efforts, explain what you are doing, and assure them that you are making every possible effort to help the patient. It is important for the family to know with certainty that you never simply "gave up."
- **Communicate.** Help the patient become oriented to surroundings. Explain several times, if necessary, what has happened and where it has happened. Explain who you are and what you and others are planning to do. Assure the patient that you are doing everything possible and that you will see that the patient gets to a hospital as quickly as possible for further care. Without interrupting care for the patient, communicate the same message to the family. Explain any procedures you need to carry out. Give straightforward answers to questions. Report what you know to be true, but do not guess or make assumptions.
- **Allow family members to express themselves.** They should be able to scream, cry, or vent grief in a way that is not hazardous to you or others. This can help them progress through the stages of the grieving process. If they direct anger at you, remember not to take the attack personally. Be tolerant and avoid getting defensive.
- **Listen empathetically.** Many dying people want messages delivered to survivors. Take notes and assure the patient that you will do whatever you can to honor his requests. Then, follow through on your promise. If possible, you or a member of your team should stay with the family to listen to their concerns and answer their questions.
- **Do not give false assurances,** but let the patient know that everything that can be done to help will be done. Allow for some hope. Be honest but tactful. If the patient asks if he is dying, do not confirm it. Patients who do the most poorly are often the ones who feel hopeless. Instead, say something like "We are doing everything we can for you. We need you to help us by not giving up."
- **Use a gentle tone of voice with the patient and family.** Explain the scope of the injury or problem, the procedures you are doing, and related information as kindly as you can in terms the family can understand.
- **Take appropriate steps if the family wants to touch or hold the body after death.** If family members want to touch or hold the body after death (and if local protocol allows), arrange for it. Do what you can to improve the appearance of the body. Clean vomitus, blood, or secretions from the face and hands. Elevate the head for a few minutes to allow fluids to drain. If the body is mutilated, warn the family first, and explain that you have covered the badly injured parts. If a possible crime is involved, do not clean the patient or remove any blood. Do not allow the family to enter the crime scene or to touch the body until permission is granted by law enforcement, coroner, or medical examiner. It is vital that all crime scene evidence is preserved.

Key Points
You must care for not just the physical but also the emotional needs of the dying patient and his family.

Objective 2-4
Give examples of situations that EMS providers may find stressful.

Objective 2-5
Compare and contrast the characteristics of acute, delayed, and cumulative stress reactions.

- **Do what you can to comfort the family.** Offer help to family members who are at the scene. Even if death is imminent, arrange for them briefly to see and talk to the patient. This should not interrupt your emergency care or delay transport. Encourage the family to talk to an unresponsive patient. Explain that the patient may still hear and understand. If the patient is deceased and the family asks you to pray with them, do so if you feel comfortable about it. Stay with the family until the medical examiner or coroner arrives. Finally, if a family member asks to accompany the patient in the ambulance, make the arrangements if at all possible.

High-Stress Situations

Patients, families, and bystanders are not the only ones who experience extreme stress in an emergency situation. The EMT does too. Accepting and understanding that fact is the first step in learning how to handle it in healthy ways.

Stress is any change in the body's internal balance. It occurs when external demands become greater than personal resources. Top sources of stress for the EMT include long hours, boredom between calls, working too much and too hard, getting little recognition, having to respond instantly, making life-and-death decisions, fearing serious errors, dealing with dying people and grieving survivors, and being responsible for someone's life (Figure 2-1∗).

Many emergency calls may be considered "routine" with a minimal level of stress. However, the nature of some calls may produce extreme levels of stress. Some of these situations include:

- Multiple-casualty incidents (MCIs) involving multiple patients at a single scene
- Abuse and neglect of infants, children, adults, and the elderly
- Emergencies involving infants and children
- Injury or death of a coworker
- Responding and providing emergency care to a relative or bystander
- Severe traumatic injuries such as amputations

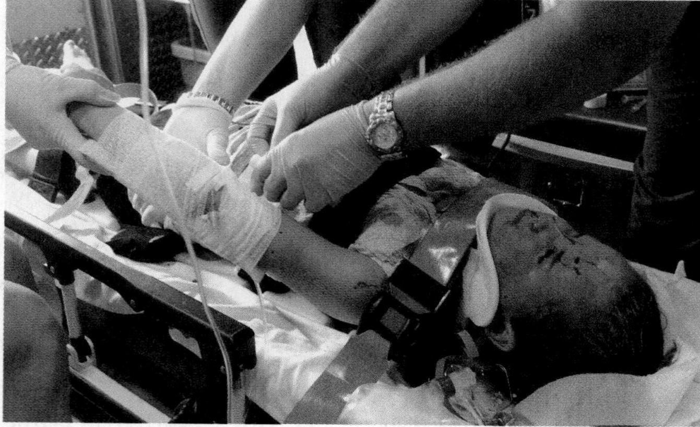

FIGURE 2-1 ∗ Responsibility for a life can be highly stressful. (© Mark C. Ide)

Stress Reactions

There are three basic types of stress reactions that the EMT may experience as a result of a high-stress incident or from constant exposure to stressful situations. The types of stress reactions are:

- **Acute stress reaction.** An acute stress reaction results from exposure to a high-stress situation. You may note the reaction not only in the patient or bystanders, but also in you, your partner, or other emergency service personnel at the scene of the high-stress incident. Signs and symptoms typically occur immediately or shortly after the incident and may involve cognitive, physical, behavioral, or psychological functions. If the patient is experiencing what appears to be a medical emergency, such as chest pain or shortness of breath, it may be necessary to provide emergency care and seek further medical treatment. If it is you, your partner, or another emergency worker with signs or symptoms of a possible medical emergency, seek immediate medical treatment.

  It is normal to experience some minor signs or symptoms associated with high-stress situations, such as nausea, elevated heart rate, sweating, tremors, loss of appetite or excessive eating, trouble concentrating, and inability to sleep. Some EMTs have none of these responses to the high-stress situation. This is also normal and is not an indication that they are stronger or better emergency care workers. It may be that they have different coping mechanisms to the stress situation.
- **Delayed stress reaction.** Posttraumatic stress disorder (PTSD) is a typical delayed stress reaction that occurs from exposure to a high-stress situation; however, the signs and symptoms are not evident imme-

Key Points
It is normal for EMTs to experience—or not to experience—signs or symptoms associated with high-stress situations. There is a wide range of normal coping mechanisms, and how you personally cope with stress has nothing to do with how good an EMT you are.

Key Terms
burnout a condition resulting from chronic job stress, characterized by a state of irritability and fatigue that can markedly decrease effectiveness.

Objective 2-6
Recognize signs and symptoms of stress reactions.

diately. It may be days, months, or even years before the patient begins to experience the signs and symptoms of stress. Since a period of time typically passes before the onset of signs and symptoms, it may be difficult to relate the stress reaction to the particular past incident that caused the condition, and the patient may not understand why he is experiencing it. PTSD typically produces nightmares, irritability, insomnia, inability to think clearly or concentrate, flashbacks, increased interpersonal conflicts, and a decreased ability to relate to others. People suffering from PTSD may seek relief through drug or alcohol use. A person experiencing PTSD needs to seek help from a mental health professional.

- **Cumulative stress reaction.** As the name implies, cumulative stress reaction is a result of constant exposure to stressful situations that build over time. This is a common cause of **burnout**—a state of exhaustion and irritability. Initially, the signs and symptoms are not well recognized and may include an increase in anxiety and irritability. As the stress progresses, a state of emotional exhaustion may be reached and the condition may progress to more severe physical ailments. It can markedly decrease an EMS provider's effectiveness in delivering emergency medical care. Some of the very best providers have had to leave the profession because of it. Many of the more severe signs and symptoms, listed next, are common in the cumulative stress reaction.

Common Signs and Symptoms of Stress Reactions

One of the best ways to prevent burnout is to recognize the warning signs of stress (Figure 2-2*). The earlier they are recognized, the easier they are to remedy. These warning signs include:

- Irritability with coworkers, family, and friends
- Inability to concentrate
- Difficulty sleeping and nightmares
- Anxiety
- Indecisiveness
- Guilt
- Loss of appetite

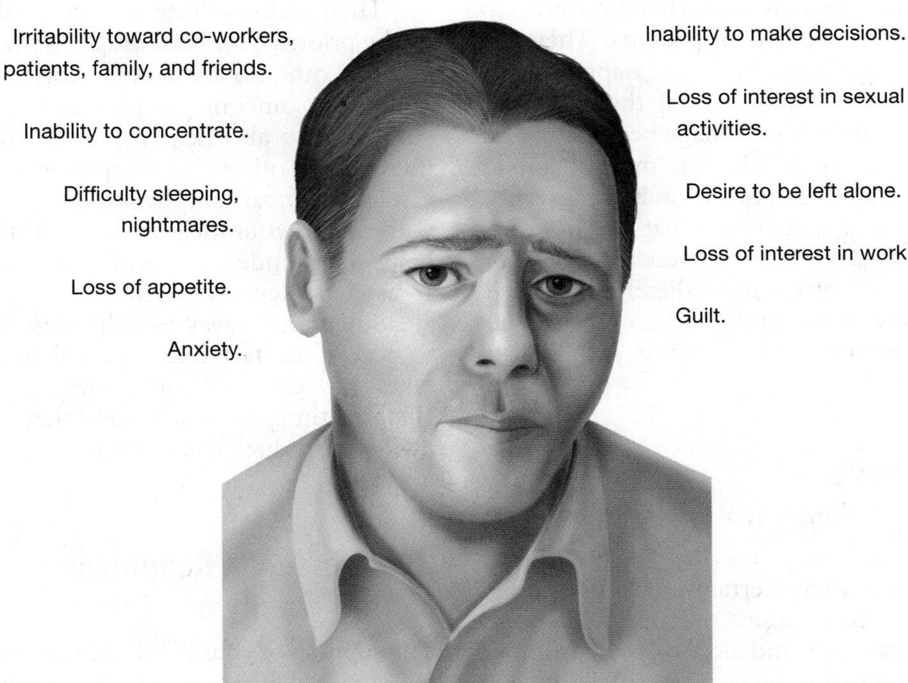
Irritability toward co-workers, patients, family, and friends.
Inability to concentrate.
Difficulty sleeping, nightmares.
Loss of appetite.
Anxiety.
Inability to make decisions.
Loss of interest in sexual activities.
Desire to be left alone.
Loss of interest in work.
Guilt.

FIGURE 2-2 * The warning signs of stress.

Thinking Critically
What is one step you could or would like to take that would improve the balance between work and other aspects of your life?

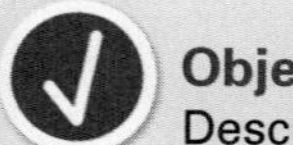

Objective 2-7
Describe lifestyle changes you can make to help you deal with stress.

Objective 2-8
Describe responses your friends and family may have to your work in EMS.

- Loss of sexual desire or interest
- Isolation
- Loss of interest in work

General categories of signs and symptoms also have been identified with stress. In addition to the warning signs just listed, these categories include:

- **Thinking.** Confusion, inability to make judgments or decisions, loss of motivation, chronic forgetfulness, loss of objectivity
- **Psychological.** Depression, excessive anger, negativism, hostility, defensiveness, mood swings, feelings of worthlessness
- **Physical.** Persistent exhaustion, headaches, gastrointestinal distress, dizziness, pounding heart
- **Behavioral.** Overeating, increased alcohol or drug use, grinding teeth, hyperactivity, lack of energy
- **Social.** Increased interpersonal conflicts, decreased ability to relate to patients as individuals

Stress Management

Many EMTs expose themselves to overwhelming stress in the desire to help meet the needs of patients. They feel completely responsible for everything that happens on a run, even things that are clearly out of their control. Some are so involved that their self-image becomes based on job performance. As an EMT, you must maintain good physical, emotional, social, behavioral, and psychological health. To this end, it is critical that you not only recognize the signs and symptoms of stress reactions but that you also manage the stress immediately—before it progresses and interferes with your ability to function effectively, in and out of the field. The next section lists ways to help you cope.

Make Lifestyle Changes

The following lifestyle changes can help you deal with stress:

- **Take a look at your diet.** Certain foods tend to increase the body's stress response. So cut down on the amount of sugar, caffeine, and alcohol you consume. Increase the amount of lean protein you eat, limit your carbohydrates, and decrease your saturated fat intake. While at work, eat frequently but in small amounts.
- **Exercise more often.** Exercise has all sorts of benefits. One of the greatest is that it provides a physical release for the pent-up emotions that accompany many crises. Another is that it helps to prevent injury.
- **Learn to relax.** Practice relaxation techniques, such as taking a deep breath, holding it, and blowing out forcefully. Meditation and visual imagery techniques are also helpful ways to relax. You may also wish to try temporary diversions, such as watching a funny movie, reading a good book, or going to a concert with a friend. Cut loose a little bit.
- **Avoid self-medication.** Reaching for a bottle—whether it is filled with alcohol or with pills—does not help you cope with stress. In fact, it will increase stress. Your problems are still there when you come out of the stupor, and they will probably be worse because you did not act on them immediately.

Keep Balance in Your Life

One way to keep a balance of work, recreation, family, health, and other interests is to assess your priorities. Take a few minutes to list all your activities on paper. Write "1" beside your first priority, "2" beside your second, and so on. Then address those activities—all of them—in order of the priority you have assigned them.

You can also share your worries with someone else. Talking to someone you trust and respect can help relieve stress. It can also help you to discover alternatives that might have otherwise escaped you. A good confidante can listen empathetically and ask questions that will help you explore your ideas honestly. Talking with loved ones helps them understand what you may be going through. It also lets them feel included.

Still another way to help keep balance in your life is to accept the fact that you will occasionally make mistakes. Honestly admit to yourself that no person is right all of the time, and understand that a mistake does not reduce your value. You do not have to be perfect to do a good job.

Recognize the Response of Your Family and Friends

The support of your family and friends is essential in helping you manage stress. However, you may find that they, too, suffer from a certain amount of stress as a result of your job. You may find:

Objective 2-9
Describe changes in the work environment that can help you manage job-related stress.

Key Terms
critical incident any situation that causes unusually strong emotions that interfere with the ability to function.

Key Terms
critical incident stress debriefing (CISD) a session where counselors help emergency personnel process emotions from a critical incident.

Objective 2-10
Discuss the components of a comprehensive system of critical incident stress management.

- **Lack of understanding.** Families typically have little if any knowledge about prehospital emergency care.
- **Fear of separation or of being ignored.** Long hours and demanding physical labor can take their toll and increase your family's distress over your absences. Typically you may hear: "Your job is more important to you than your family!"
- **Worry about on-call situations.** Stress at home may increase because your family may overemphasize or exaggerate the danger you face when you respond to emergency calls.
- **Inability to plan.** Family and friends may not understand why you cannot leave your call area or have to leave an event early. Typically you may hear: "You're not the only one on call. Let someone else go this time."
- **Frustrated desire to share.** You often find it too difficult to talk about what has happened during your shift. Your family and friends understand why, in a general way, but nevertheless feel frustrated in their desire to help and support you.

Help family and friends understand the nature of your work and what you do for patients. Talk to them. Describe how you feel about what you do. Answer their questions. Explaining the safety precautions you and coworkers take every day can ease their anxieties. Encouraging them to join you in staying fit (daily exercise and planning healthy meals, for example) also can help alleviate their concerns when you cannot be with them. Always include time with them on your list of priorities.

Make Changes in Your Work Environment

The following changes in your work environment can help you manage job-related stress:

- **Develop a "buddy" system with a coworker.** Keep an eye on each other, and suggest when relaxation or a diversion is advisable. Try a relaxation technique whenever you find your effectiveness diminishing.
- **Encourage and support your coworkers.** Make positive remarks, and resist the temptation to criticize or dwell on the negative.
- **Periodically take a break to get some exercise**—do some type of aerobic exercise, such as taking a brisk walk, riding an exercise bike, walking or running on a treadmill, using an elliptical machine, or a similar activity (Figure 2-3*).

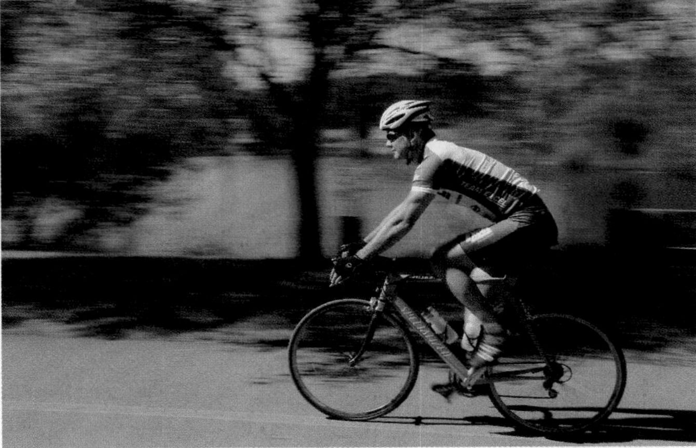

FIGURE 2-3 * Aerobic exercise is an effective way to relieve stress.

- **Request work shifts that allow you more time to relax** with your family and friends.
- **Request a rotation of duty assignment** to a less busy area or an area with a different type of call volume. As an example, move from a station that deals primarily with calls involving crime and violence, to a station that responds to more illnesses.

Seek Professional Help

You can also seek advice from mental health professionals, who can help you realize that your reactions are normal, mobilize your best coping strategies, and arm you with more effective ways to deal with stress in the future.

Critical Incident Stress Management

Emergency service personnel who suffer **critical incident** stress develop many of the signs and symptoms of burnout. They also may suffer from repeated mental images of the incident, fear of continuing in EMS work, and inability to function at the scene of subsequent emergencies. Critical incident stress management (CISM) is a process to deal with stress encountered by the EMT. It consists of two different approaches to stress management: critical incident stress debriefing and critical incident defusing.

A **critical incident stress debriefing (CISD)** is ideally held within 24 to 72 hours of a critical incident.

Key Terms
defusing an opportunity to vent emotions and get information before the CISD.

Key Terms
pathogens microorganisms such as bacteria and viruses that cause disease.

Objective 2-11
Describe measures you can take to protect yourself from exposure to diseases caused by pathogens and accidental and work-related injury.

During CISD, a team of peer counselors and mental health professionals help emergency service personnel work through seven phases. These phases are intended to allow the participants to review the facts of the event, share their feelings, identify signs and symptoms they are experiencing, sort through their feelings with the assistance of a mental health professional, receive suggestions for overcoming the stress, develop a plan of action for returning to the job, and be able to obtain follow-up assistance if lingering issues are present. CISD is not meant to assign blame. All information that is shared remains confidential.

CISD typically includes anyone involved in the incident—law enforcement personnel, firefighters, EMS personnel, communications personnel, and hospital emergency department personnel. In some cases, the debriefing may involve emergency service personnel family members, who are inevitably affected by the stress of the incident. In cases of multiple casualties, such as earthquakes, tornadoes, or severe hurricanes, a number of CISD meetings involving hundreds of people may need to be conducted.

Even if professional counselors are involved in sessions, CISD is not, in itself, professional counseling. Rather, it is a means to relieve stress.

Defusing is a version of CISD held within 1 to 4 hours following a critical incident. It is attended only by those most directly involved in the critical incident and lasts only 30 to 45 minutes. Less structured than a CISD meeting, defusing gives the smaller group of emergency service personnel an opportunity to vent their emotions and get information they may need before the larger group meets for CISD.

CISD has become controversial for many providers. The controversy stems from the need for scientific evidence that CISD truly assists emergency care personnel in resolving stress issues. It is important to keep current with the literature so that you may stay informed about the effectiveness of CISD. It is also important to recognize that a comprehensive critical stress management program involves more than CISD. Comprehensive critical incident stress management should include:

- Preincident stress education
- On-scene peer support
- One-on-one support
- Disaster support services
- Defusing
- CISD
- Follow-up services
- Spouse and family support
- Community outreach programs
- Other health and welfare programs

Scene Safety

Keeping yourself safe at the scene of an illness or injury involves taking appropriate measures to protect yourself from infectious disease, following proper rescue procedures, and knowing how to handle violence, especially at a crime scene. It is also important to be an advocate for these protective measures—to help keep fellow emergency service personnel, as well as yourself, safe and well.

Protecting Yourself from Disease

How Diseases Spread

Diseases are caused by **pathogens,** which are microorganisms that are typically visible only through a microscope and may be found in the environment around you and also residing on or within the patient you are assessing and treating. The most common pathogens you will encounter are bacteria, viruses, fungi, protozoa, and helminths.

- **Bacteria** are microscopic single-celled organisms that have the capability of reproducing on their own within a host (patient's body) that can provide a favorable environment and food supply. Common diseases produced by bacteria include sinus infection, ear infection, pneumonia (bacterial), strep throat, tuberculosis, and urinary tract infections. Bacterial infections typically respond to antibiotic treatment.
- **Viruses,** which are even smaller than bacteria, cannot grow on their own but require a host cell to reproduce. The virus invades a cell, reproduces, and then releases new virus particles that infect other cells. Those cells then produce more virus, spreading the infection throughout the body. Viruses are resistant to antibiotic treatment because they are located and unreachable within the host cell. Fortunately, most viruses are mild and self-limiting, such as the common cold or the flu. Conditions caused by viruses

Objective 2-12
Give examples of diseases caused by each of the different types of pathogens (bacteria, viruses, fungi, protozoa, and helminths).

Key Points
Pathogens can spread in a number of ways, including by way of blood and other body fluids or through the air.

include acquired immune deficiency syndrome (AIDS) from the human immunodeficiency virus (HIV), hepatitis (A, B, and C), pneumonia (viral), severe acute respiratory syndrome (SARS), chicken pox, and respiratory syncytial virus (RSV).

- **Fungi** are plantlike microorganisms that typically do not cause infection in a person with a normally functioning immune system. In a patient with a compromised immune system, fungi may cause diseases that would not be typically found, such as pneumonia in the HIV-infected person.
- **Protozoa** are single-celled organisms that are typically found in the soil and are able to move. Patients infected by protozoa often have a compromised immune system; however, some protozoa can cause infection in an uncompromised patient. The protozoa frequently enter the body through a fecal-oral route. Mosquitoes are carriers of protozoa that cause malaria. Some forms of gastroenteritis and vaginal infections are caused by protozoa in uncompromised immune systems.
- **Helminths** are parasitic worms, such as roundworms, flukes, and tapeworms, that cause infection. The helminth is typically introduced into the body by ingestion of worm eggs found in infected food or water or through the worm larvae invading through the skin. Hookworm, an example of a helminth infection, is a condition where the parasitic worm attaches to the patient's intestine, leading to blood loss and anemia.

Pathogens can spread in a number of ways, including by way of blood and other body fluids or through the air. An infectious disease is one that spreads from person to person (Table 2-1). It can spread directly through blood-to-blood contact, contact with open wounds and exposed tissue (Figure 2-4∗), and contact with the mucous membranes of the eyes and mouth. It can also spread indirectly by way of a contaminated object such as a needle. Airborne pathogens are spread by one person coughing, sneezing, or exhaling infected droplets that are then breathed into the respiratory tract of another person.

TABLE 2-1 Infectious Diseases, Transmission, and Personal Protective Measures

Disease	Transmission Mode	Incubation Period	Protective Measures
AIDS	Blood, semen, vaginal fluid, blood transfusion, needlestick, transplacental	Months	Gloves, eyewear, hand washing
Hepatitis B and C	Blood, semen, vaginal fluid, needlestick, transplacental, human bite, sexual contact (HBV)	Weeks or months	Gloves, eyewear, hand washing
Tuberculosis	Respiratory secretions, airborne or direct contact	2 to 6 weeks	Gloves, eyewear, HEPA or N-95 respirator, hand washing
Influenza	Airborne droplets, direct contact with body fluids	1 to 3 days	Gloves, surgical mask, hand washing
Chicken pox (varicella)	Airborne droplets, direct contact with open sores	11 to 21 days	Gloves, surgical mask, hand washing
Bacterial meningitis	Oral and nasal secretions	2 to 10 days	Gloves, surgical mask, hand washing
Pneumonia	Respiratory secretions and droplets	1 to 3 days	Gloves, surgical mask, hand washing
German measles (rubella)	Airborne droplets, transplacental	10 to 12 days	Gloves, surgical mask, hand washing
Whooping cough (pertussis)	Respiratory secretions, airborne droplets	6 to 20 days	Gloves, surgical mask, hand washing
Staphylococcal skin infection	Direct contact with infected lesion or contaminated object	1 to 3 days	Gloves, hand washing

Objectives 2-13 and 2-14
Describe Standard Precautions and personal protective equipment for EMS personnel.

Key Terms

Standard Precautions a method of preventing infection based on the concept that all blood and body fluids are infectious.

personal protective equipment (PPE) equipment worn to protect against injury and against spreading infectious disease.

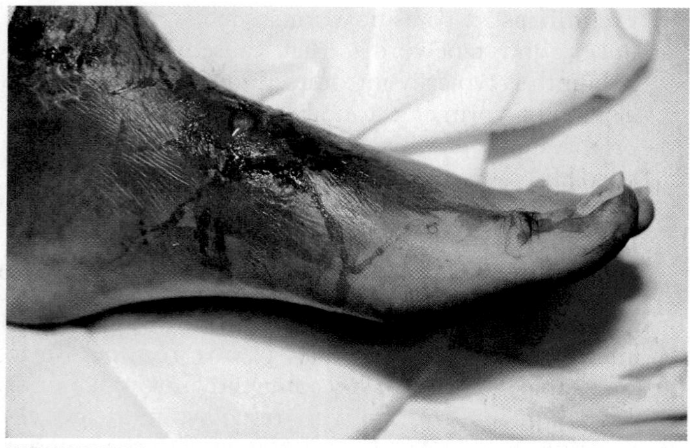

FIGURE 2-4 ∗ An open sore on the foot of an apparent drug user is an example of an open wound that has the potential to spread infection. (© Maria A. H. Lyle)

Standard Precautions

U.S. Department of Occupational Safety and Health Administration (OSHA) guidelines require emergency care personnel to take precautions against disease transmitted by blood and other potentially infectious substances or body fluids. Also, employers share the responsibility with the employee to ensure that the necessary equipment and procedures are in place to offer the necessary protection to emergency care personnel. Employers are responsible for developing a written exposure control plan and providing training, certain immunizations, and the proper equipment for protection against disease transmission. The employee must complete the training and follow the procedures outlined in the exposure control plan.

The employer is also responsible for developing and enforcing a written policy to be used in the case of an exposure of an employee to an infectious substance such as blood or other body fluids. Needlesticks or direct contact with potentially infectious body fluids must be properly documented. Some policies require baseline infection testing of the exposed worker immediately with subsequent testing at designated intervals. Federal legislation has been enacted to allow for notification of EMS personnel who have come in contact with a patient who is infected with a communicable disease such as HIV, hepatitis B virus (HBV), or tuberculosis bacterium (TB) (Figure 2-5∗).

Protecting yourself from disease transmission through exposure to blood and other body fluids was formerly referred to as body substance isolation (BSI); it is more recently called **Standard Precautions.** The equipment utilized for Standard Precautions is referred to as **personal protective equipment (PPE).** The following are guidelines for Standard Precautions.

Hand Washing *Hand washing is the single most important way you can prevent the spread of infection* (Figure 2-6∗). According to the U.S. Public Health Service, most contaminants can be removed from the skin with 10 to 15 seconds of vigorous lathering and scrubbing with plain soap. *Note: You should wash your hands even if you were wearing gloves.*

For maximum protection, begin by removing all jewelry from your hands and arms. Then proceed to vigorously lather and rub together all surfaces of your hands. Pay attention to creases, crevices, and the areas between your fingers. Use a brush to scrub under and around your fingernails. (It is recommended that you keep your nails short and unpolished.) If your hands are visibly soiled, spend more time washing them. Wash your wrists and forearms if they were exposed or possibly contaminated. Rinse thoroughly under a stream of running water. Dry well, using a disposable towel if you can.

If you do not have access to soap and running water in the field, you can temporarily use a foam or liquid washing agent that requires no water. Afterward, be sure to wash your hands again as soon as you can.

Personal Protective Equipment Always use PPE as a barrier against infection. It will help to prevent your skin and mucous membranes from coming in contact with a patient's blood and other body fluids. PPE includes eye protection, protective gloves, gowns, and masks (Figure 2-7∗).

- **Eye protection.** Use eye shields to protect against blood and other body fluids splashing into your eyes. Several types are available (Figure 2-8∗): clear plastic shields that cover the eyes or cover the whole face, protective eyewear (safety glasses) with side shields, and, if you wear prescription eyeglasses, there are removable side shields you can attach to your glasses. Form-fitting goggles also are available but are not required.
- **Protective gloves.** Wear high-quality vinyl, latex-free, or other synthetic gloves whenever you care for a patient. If a glove accidentally tears while in use, remove it as soon as you can do so safely. Then wash your hands and replace the glove with a new one. Never reuse gloves. Put on a new pair of gloves between contacts with different patients to avoid exposing one

INFECTIOUS DISEASE EXPOSURE PROCEDURE

Airborne Infection Such as TB (Tuberculosis)

1. You transport a patient who is infected with a life-threatening airborne disease, such as TB, but you are not aware that the patient is infected.
2. The medical facility diagnoses the disease in the patient you transported.
3. The medical facility must notify your designated officer within 48 hours.
4. Your designated officer notifies you that you have been exposed.
5. Your employer arranges for you to be evaluated and followed up by a doctor or other appropriate health care professional.

Bloodborne Infection Such as HIV (AIDS virus) or HBV (Hepatitis B virus)

1. You come into contact with blood or body fluids of a patient, and you wonder if that patient is infected with a life-threatening bloodborne disease such as HIV or HBV.
2. You seek immediate medical attention and document the incident for worker's compensation.
3. You ask your designated officer to determine if you have been exposed to an infectious disease.
4. Your designated officer (DO) must gather information and, if DO determines it is warranted, consult the medical facility to which the patient was transported.
5. The medical facility must gather information and report findings to your designated officer within 48 hours. Your DO notifies you of the findings. → (leads to: Your employer arranges for you to be evaluated and followed up by a doctor or other appropriate health care professional.)

FIGURE 2-5 ✱ Infectious disease exposure procedure.

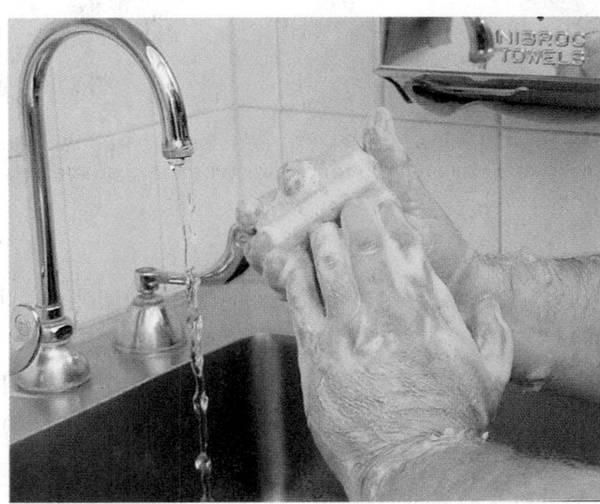

FIGURE 2-6 ✱ Thoroughly washing hands after patient contact is the first line of protection against infectious disease.

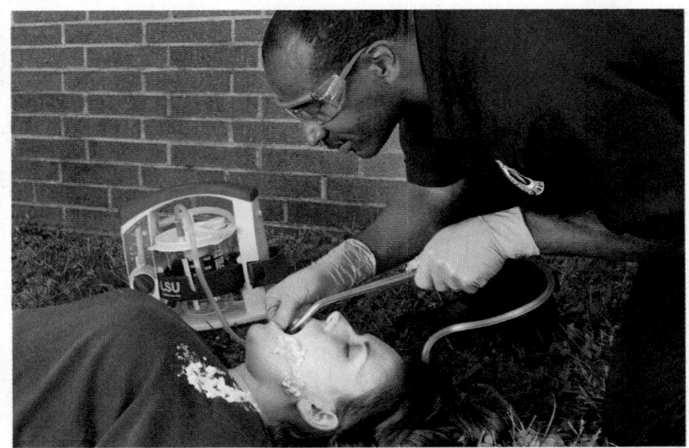

FIGURE 2-7 ✱ Wear a protective eyeshield and other personal protective equipment when suctioning a patient.

Thinking Critically
Have you ever neglected or rushed through any of the Standard Precautions that are intended to protect your health and that of your patients? What are some reasons why this might happen? What can you do make sure it doesn't?

Key Points
Whenever possible use—but never reuse—disposable equipment.

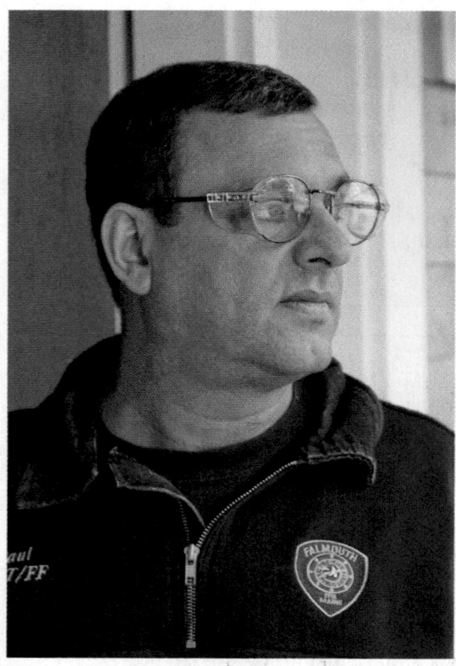

FIGURE 2-8 * Protective eyewear. Removable side shields are also available for prescription glasses.

patient to another's infection. Also, use a proper technique for removing contaminated gloves so that you do not accidentally expose yourself to any blood or other body fluids contained on the gloves' surface (EMT Skills 2-1). Upon glove removal, be sure to wash your hands thoroughly. In addition, wear a good pair of utility gloves when cleaning vehicles and equipment.

- **Gowns.** Wear a gown in any situation where there may be significant contact with blood or other body fluids, such as during childbirth or major trauma. If possible, use a disposable gown. If at all possible, also change your uniform after caring for a patient in a large-splash situation.
- **Masks.** Wear a disposable surgical-type face mask to prevent blood or other body fluids from being splashed into your nose or mouth. You may also put a surgical mask on the patient if an airborne disease is suspected (Figure 2-9*). If you are treating a patient suspected of having tuberculosis, you need additional protection. Wear a high-efficiency particulate air (HEPA) respirator or an N-95 respirator (Figure 2-10*).

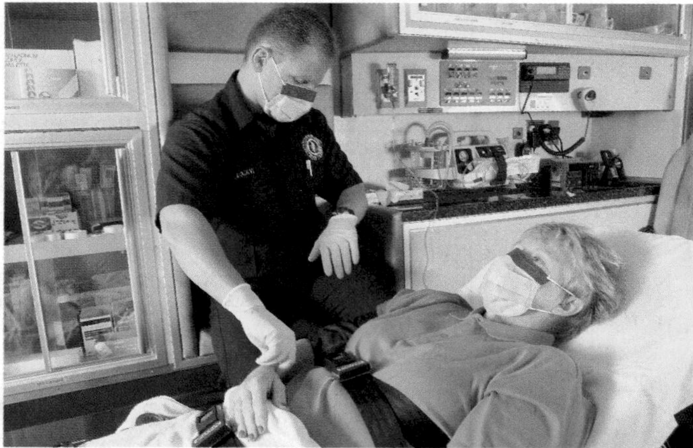

FIGURE 2-9 * Use surgical masks to protect against blood splatters or airborne disease.

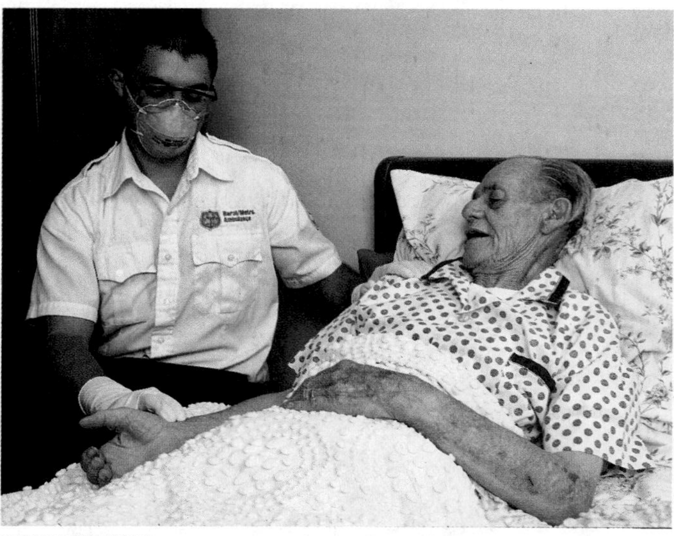

FIGURE 2-10 * Wear a special high-efficiency particulate air (HEPA) respirator or an N-95 respirator when you suspect tuberculosis.

Additional Guidelines The following guidelines should be observed as part of routine patient care:

- Whenever possible, use disposable equipment. Disinfect or sterilize nondisposable equipment according to local guidelines and protocols.
- Never reuse disposable equipment. Discard it after use with one patient. If you suspect that a patient may have an infectious disease, place used disposable

Key Terms

cleaning the process of washing a soiled object with soap and water.

Key Terms

disinfecting using a disinfectant such as alcohol or bleach to kill microorganisms.

sterilization subjecting an object to chemical or physical substances (typically, superheated steam in an autoclave) that kill all microorganisms.

equipment in a plastic bag clearly labeled as biohazardous or infectious waste. Then seal the bag. Equipment used with HIV, hepatitis B, or other infectious patients should be double-bagged.

- If your uniform gets soiled with body fluids, remove, bag, and label it. It should be washed in hot soapy water for at least 25 minutes. Take a hot shower yourself, and rinse thoroughly.
- After transferring care of a patient, gather all disposable equipment soiled by blood and other body fluids. Bag and seal it. Then label it as infectious waste (Figure 2-11*).
- Document in your logbook or on your flowsheet any contact with blood or other body fluids and any cleaning you have done as a result.
- Sponge, wipe, or wash noncritical items that do not ordinarily touch the patient or only touch intact skin (such as blood pressure cuffs). Rinse with clear water and allow to dry thoroughly.
- Patient care equipment that enters the body or that touches mucous membranes must be cleaned before each use with high-level disinfection or sterilization. Thoroughly clean to remove all blood, tissue, and other residue. Then follow local guidelines, local protocols, and manufacturer guidelines for disinfection or sterilization.
- Dispose of all needles or sharp instruments in a rigid, puncture-proof container ("sharps container") immediately after you use them. Do not recap needles (Figure 2-12*).
- Clean up blood and body fluids as soon as possible by routine cleaning with a hospital-grade disinfectant or a solution of household bleach and water.
- Walls, window coverings, and other nonhorizontal surfaces in the ambulance do not need routine cleaning, but should be cleaned if visibly soiled.
- Wash your hands thoroughly after cleaning the ambulance or disposing of equipment.

Cleaning, disinfecting, and sterilizing are all related terms. **Cleaning** is simply the process of washing a soiled object with soap and water. **Disinfecting** includes cleaning, but also involves using a hospital-grade disinfectant or germicide to kill many of the microorganisms that may be present on the surface of the object. **Sterilization** is the process by which an object is subject to a chemical or physical substance (such as superheated steam in an autoclave) that kills all microorganisms on the surface of an object. Generally, disinfection is used for items that will come in contact with the intact skin of a patient, such as backboards and splints. However, if the equipment will come in contact with mucous membranes or other open

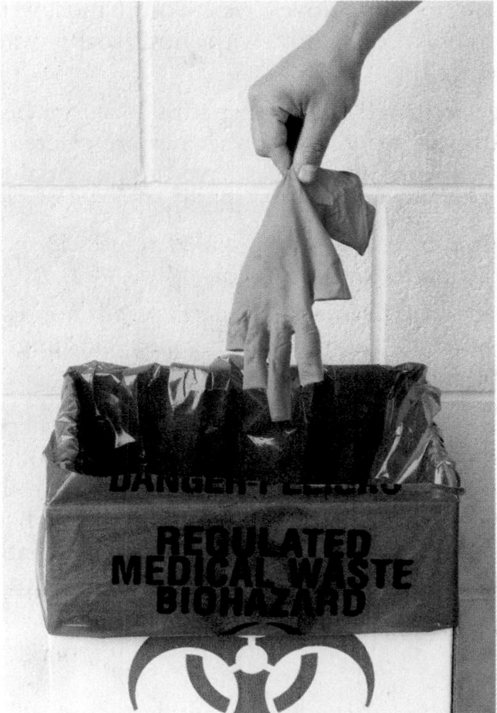

FIGURE 2-11 * Put items in a biohazard bag if infectious or contaminated with blood or other body fluids.

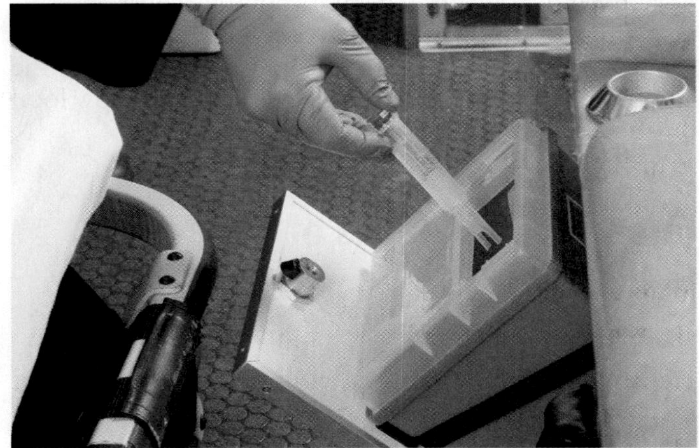

FIGURE 2-12 * Place all sharp instruments in a rigid, well-mounted, puncture-resistant container.

Key Terms

purified protein derivative (PPD) tuberculin test a test to determine the presence of a tuberculosis infection based on a person's positive reaction to tuberculin, a substance prepared from the tubercle bacillus.

Objective 2-15

Explain the role of immunizations and tuberculosis testing in maintaining good health.

or internal structures, it should be sterilized (laryngoscope blades, for example).

Immunizations Before you begin active duty, have a physician make sure you are adequately protected against common diseases. Have a **purified protein derivative (PPD) tuberculin test** to detect tuberculosis every year. This and the other immunizations listed here are recommended for active-duty EMTs:

- PPD tuberculin test (annually)
- Tetanus prophylaxis (every 10 years)
- Hepatitis B vaccine
- Influenza vaccine (annually)
- Polio immunization (if needed)
- Rubella (German measles) vaccine
- Measles vaccine (if needed)
- Mumps vaccine (if needed)
- Varicella vaccine (if needed)

Because some immunizations have been found to offer only partial protection, have your physician verify your immune status against rubella, measles, and mumps and obtain a hepatitis B titer. Although immunizations offer protection against many diseases, Standard Precautions must always be practiced, even by immunized EMTs.

Reporting Exposure State and local laws vary regarding the reporting of exposure to blood and other body fluids, especially if a patient is known to be HIV positive or have hepatitis B or is known to be in a high-risk category for infection. In general, promptly report any suspected exposure to your supervisor, including date and time of the exposure, type of body fluid involved, the amount of fluid, and details of the exposure. Follow local protocol and your service's exposure policies.

Infectious Diseases of Concern to the EMT

Hepatitis B

Hepatitis B is one of several viruses that directly affect the liver. A serious disease that can last for months, hepatitis B can be contracted through blood and body fluids. A major source of the virus is the chronic carrier, who usually has no signs or symptoms and is often unaware of being ill. These people can transmit the disease at any time.

The following are signs and symptoms of the hepatitis B virus:

- Fatigue
- Nausea and loss of appetite
- Abdominal pain
- Headache
- Fever
- Yellowish color of skin and whites of eyes (jaundice)
- Dark urine

Remember: Hepatitis B infection may not cause symptoms. You can be unaware of infection and still pass it on to others. Protective procedure recommendations include the following:

- Wear disposable protective gloves whenever you care for patients to prevent contact with blood and other body fluids. Make sure you have bandaged all cuts, lesions, scratches, hangnails, and any other open wound on your hands.
- After removing gloves, wash your hands, wrists, and forearms thoroughly with hot, soapy water and rinse well.
- Get vaccinated against hepatitis B before beginning EMS field work. These vaccines are offered by employers when employees have the potential to come in contact with blood and body fluids.
- Double-bag and seal all soiled refuse. Dispose of it according to local protocol.
- Clean and disinfect or sterilize all nondisposable equipment. Launder your soiled clothing in hot, soapy water and bleach.

If you suspect you have been exposed to hepatitis B, report the incident to your supervisor and follow your service's exposure policy. Care may include an injection of HBIG (hepatitis B immunoglobulin) immediately and again within a month if not previously vaccinated. You may also receive a vaccination, if you have not already had one.

Hepatitis C

Hepatitis C virus (HCV) infection has become the most common bloodborne infection in the United States.

Objective 2-16
Discuss the risks and preventive measures for specific infectious diseases of concern to EMTs.

Thinking Critically
Explain the best ways to prevent and/or respond to an exposure to hepatitis B, hepatitis C, tuberculosis, HIV/AIDS, SARS, West Nile virus, or multidrug-resistant organisms.

Fortunately, the risk of transmission through occupational exposure is relatively low since it requires introduction through the skin by needlestick. Transmission via the mucous membrane is rare. Testing of emergency personnel is recommended after exposure has occurred.

Approximately 80 percent of patients with HCV have no signs or symptoms. Those who are symptomatic typically present with the following:

- Jaundice (yellow color to skin and eyes)
- Fatigue
- Abdominal pain (may be located in right upper quadrant)
- Nausea
- Dark urine
- Loss of appetite

Unlike with hepatitis B, there is no vaccination to prevent hepatitis C infection. It is extremely important that you take Standard Precautions when dealing with exposure to body fluids, especially blood. Also be careful to avoid any sharps or needles with infected blood since this is the most significant route of HCV transmission for EMS personnel.

Tuberculosis

Tuberculosis almost vanished once, but it has made a dramatic comeback. In fact, researchers are worried because new drug-resistant strains are developing. The pathogen that causes tuberculosis is found in the lungs and other tissues of the infected patient. You can be infected by droplets from the cough of a patient and from the patient's infected sputum.

The main signs and symptoms of tuberculosis are as follows:

- Fever
- Cough (often coughing up blood)
- Night sweats
- Weight loss

OSHA has adopted protective procedure standards for rescuers. The standards include the use of special HEPA or N-95 respirators. Recommendations include the following:

- Wear disposable protective gloves to avoid contact with infected sputum or mucus.
- Wear a HEPA or N-95 (respirator) mask to avoid breathing infected droplets.
- Perform artificial ventilation with OSHA-approved equipment.
- After you remove your gloves, wash hands thoroughly with hot soapy water and rinse well.
- Disinfect all nondisposable equipment that was contaminated by the patient's body fluids with a hospital-grade disinfectant with a tuberculocidal agent. See that all linens and clothing are laundered in hot soapy water and bleach.

Acquired Immune Deficiency Syndrome (AIDS)

Fortunately, AIDS is not spread through casual contact. It cannot be transmitted by coughing, sneezing, sharing eating utensils, linens, skin contact, or such indirect exposures. It is more difficult to contract HIV (human immunodeficiency virus, the virus that causes AIDS) through occupational exposure than it is to contract the virus that causes hepatitis B. The identified modes of transmission include the following:

- Sexual contact involving the exchange of semen, blood, or through contact with vaginal or cervical secretions
- Infected needles
- Infected blood or blood products
- Mother–child transmission, which occurs when an infected mother passes the virus to her child, sometimes as early as the 12th week of gestation
- Contact with infected blood or secretions through mucous membranes or open skin

Simply stated, AIDS is a syndrome of medical problems caused by HIV, a virus that destroys the body's ability to fight infections. Many patients infected with HIV do not exhibit signs or symptoms and do not know they are infected. AIDS patients become infected with what are called opportunistic infections (infections that take advantage of the "opportunity" provided by the body's lack of ability to fight them). These infections are caused by viruses, bacteria, parasites, and fungi. They are serious illnesses that either do not occur or occur only in milder forms among people with healthy immune systems.

AIDS can involve many organs and systems of the body. This results in a countless array of signs and symptoms. The most common include the following:

- Persistent, low-grade fever
- Night sweats
- Swollen lymph glands
- Loss of appetite
- Nausea
- Persistent diarrhea
- Headache
- Sore throat
- Fatigue
- Weight loss
- Shortness of breath
- Mental status changes
- Muscle and joint aches
- Rash
- Various opportunistic infections

Remember—not everyone who is infected by HIV has yet developed, or even will develop, AIDS. However, people who carry HIV are still capable of spreading the infection to others, even if they have no signs or symptoms. Follow Standard Precautions at all times. They can significantly reduce your risk of becoming infected with HIV.

Severe Acute Respiratory Syndrome (SARS)

Severe acute respiratory syndrome (SARS) is a respiratory virus that was found in Asia in 2003. SARS cases have been identified worldwide, including in the United States and Canada. The virus is thought to be transmitted by close person-to-person contact by respiratory droplets produced by the infected person who coughs or sneezes. Close contact is generally defined as within 3 feet of the infected person. The respiratory droplets are then deposited on the mucous membranes of the mouth, nose, or eyes of the noninfected person. Also, the respiratory droplets may be deposited on an object that is touched by a noninfected person who then touches his eyes, inside his mouth, or his nose and subsequently becomes infected.

The following are signs and symptoms of SARS:

- A high fever of usually greater than 100°F (38°C)
- Headache and body ache
- General feeling of discomfort
- Respiratory symptoms
- Diarrhea
- Dry cough

Most patients with SARS will develop pneumonia. The patient may then present with more severe signs of respiratory distress.

The best protection for the EMT if SARS is suspected is to wear a surgical mask to avoid inhaling respiratory droplets, eye protection to avoid droplets entering the mucosa of the eyes, and gloves. Also place a surgical mask on the patient. When dealing with the patient or equipment used on the patient, do not touch your eyes, nose, or mouth with your gloved hands. Be sure to immediately remove the gloves after the patient exposure and wash your hands thoroughly. If you think you have been exposed, contact the person who manages infectious disease exposure at your EMS agency. Be alert for signs of fever and respiratory symptoms for 10 days after the exposure.

West Nile Virus

West Nile virus (WNV) is transmitted through the bite of an infected mosquito. Most mosquitoes are infected by feeding off an infected bird. Approximately 80 percent of the people infected with WNV will not show any signs or symptoms. However, some patients will present with severe to mild signs and symptoms. These include the following:

Severe Signs and Symptoms

- High fever
- Headache and stiff neck
- Confusion and disorientation to coma
- Seizures
- Muscle weakness
- Numbness
- Paralysis
- Vision loss

Mild Signs and Symptoms

- Fever
- Headache and body ache
- Nausea and vomiting
- Skin rash to chest, stomach, and back
- Soreness to neck from swollen lymph glands

The signs and symptoms of the severe cases may last for several weeks. Some of the signs and symptoms may be permanent. In mild cases, the signs and symptoms can last for only a few days to several weeks.

Standard Precautions will protect you from the virus. You are much more likely to contract the virus from a mosquito bite than through an occupational exposure from coming in contact with a patient who has the West Nile virus.

Multidrug-Resistant Organisms

Multidrug-resistant organisms are pathogens that have adapted to and developed the ability to resist standard antimicrobial drugs. As an EMT, you will likely come in

Objective 2-17
Explain the risks and measures that can be taken to protect yourself against various hazards.

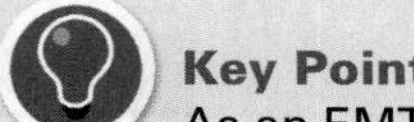

Key Points
As an EMT you must constantly be aware of the risk of potential injury associated with even the everyday aspects of the profession.

contact with these pathogens while transporting patients from hospitals, especially intensive care units and burn units, long-term care facilities, nursing homes, and other medical care facilities. They may also be found in patients who have chronic wounds or who frequently use health care facilities such as physicians' offices and hemodialysis centers. The most common types of pathogens are:

- Methicillin/oxacillin-resistant *Staphylococcus aureus* (MRSA)
- Vancomycin-resistant enterococci (VRE)
- Penicillin-resistant *Streptococcus pneumoniae* (PRSP)
- Drug-resistant *Streptococcus pneumoniae* (DRSP)

These organisms can produce many different types of infections that are resistant to standard antibiotic therapy. Patients may develop pneumonia, blood infections, ear infections, sinus infections, skin infections, and infections of the lining of the abdomen (peritonitis).

Transmission of the infection is usually through direct person-to-person contact. It is important that you follow the medical care facilities' instructions on personal protection when transporting these patients. At the minimum, follow your normal Standard Precautions and be sure to use good hand-washing procedures.

Protecting Yourself from Accidental and Work-Related Injury

As an EMT you must constantly be aware of the risk of potential injury associated with even the everyday aspects of the profession. Prevention of work-related injuries is addressed in many chapters throughout the book. Prevention strategies include the use of vehicle restraint systems, safe lifting and moving techniques, getting adequate sleep, physical fitness, proper nutrition, and practicing proper Standard Precautions against disease transmission.

You must also protect yourself during rescue operations involving hazardous materials, potentially life-threatening rescues, violence, and biological and chemical weapons of mass destruction. It is imperative that you not fall victim to the same hazards that affect your patients.

Hazardous Materials

Whenever you are called to a scene involving possible hazardous materials, use binoculars to try to identify the materials as hazardous before approaching. Look for signs or placards and compare them to those listed in the *Emergency Response Guidebook,* published by the U.S. Department of Transportation (Figures 2-13∗ and 2-14∗). A copy of the handbook should be in every emergency vehicle.

Rescuers trained in managing hazardous materials wear protective clothing at a hazardous materials emergency, including self-contained breathing apparatus and "hazmat" suits (Figures 2-15∗ and 2-16∗). Whenever possible, a specialized hazardous materials team should be called to control the scene before you enter. EMTs should provide emergency care only after the scene is safe, contamination is limited, and patient decontamination has been accomplished. See Chapter 43, "Hazardous Materials," for detailed discussion.

Rescue Situations

The following rescue situations involve potential threat to the life of both patients and emergency service personnel:

- Downed power lines or other potential for electrocution (Figure 2-17∗)
- Fire or threat of fire (including gasoline or chemical spills)
- Explosion or threat of explosion
- Hazardous materials
- Possible structural collapse
- Low oxygen levels in confined spaces
- Trenches that are not properly secured
- Biological, nuclear, and chemical weapons

Generally, you should call for assistance from specialized teams—from the power company or fire department, for example—before attempting rescue or patient treatment in a situation involving a life-threatening danger. If complex or extensive rescue is involved, also call for specialized rescue teams. Once a scene is controlled, follow local protocol in wearing the necessary personal protective equipment, such as turnout gear, puncture-proof gloves, helmet, and protective eyewear (Figure 2-18∗).

Plenty of rescues take place outdoors in the dark and in bad weather. If the rescue is being performed on a roadway, an essential for every rescuer is an ANSI/ISEA 107-2004 Class 2 or Class 3 approved high-visibility vest or 207-2006 public safety vest (PSV), as discussed in the next section. Depending on the situation, you might consider rubber or waterproof boots and slip-resistant

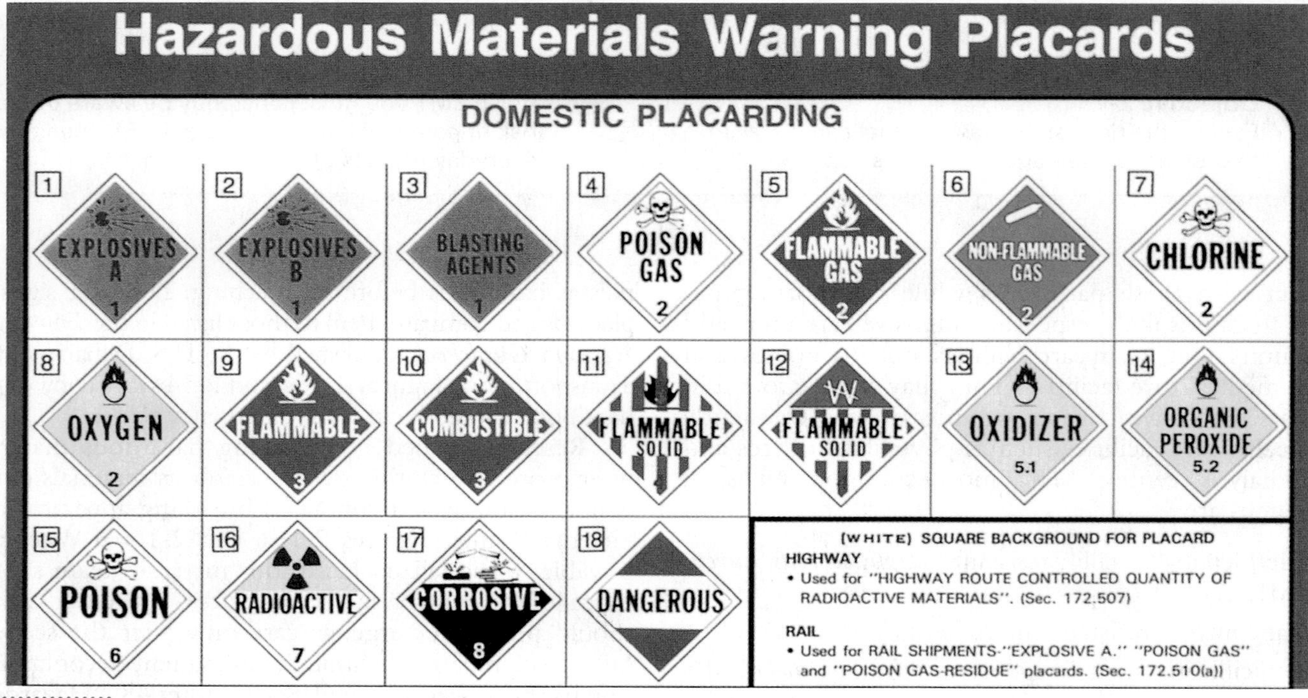

FIGURE 2-13 ✱ Examples of hazardous materials warning placards.

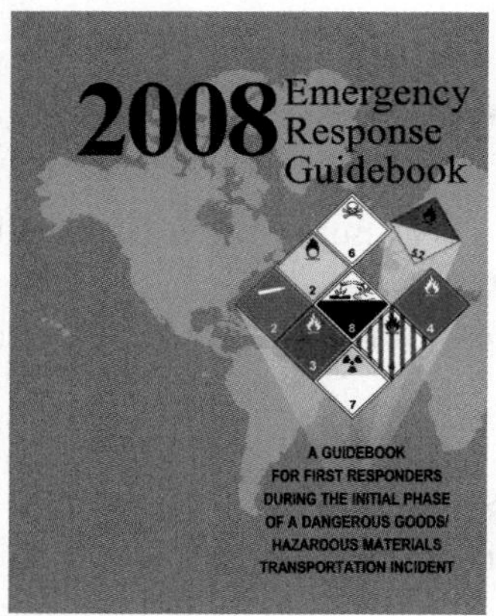

FIGURE 2-14 ✱ The *Emergency Response Guidebook* should be carried on all EMS vehicles.

waterproof gloves in wet weather. In cold weather, wear gloves, a warm hat, and long underwear, as well as several layers of clothing on your torso. In accidents involving grain, cement, or similar materials, wear a dust respirator. If there is any risk of falling debris, wear an impact-resistant protective helmet with reflective tape and a strap under the chin.

It is vital to your safety that you follow your system's protocols and policies on personal protection. A good rule is to be sure that you wear at least the protective equipment that others on the scene are required to wear. For example, if you are responding to a call at a factory and all the employees are required to wear a helmet while in the plant, the minimum protection you should wear is a helmet.

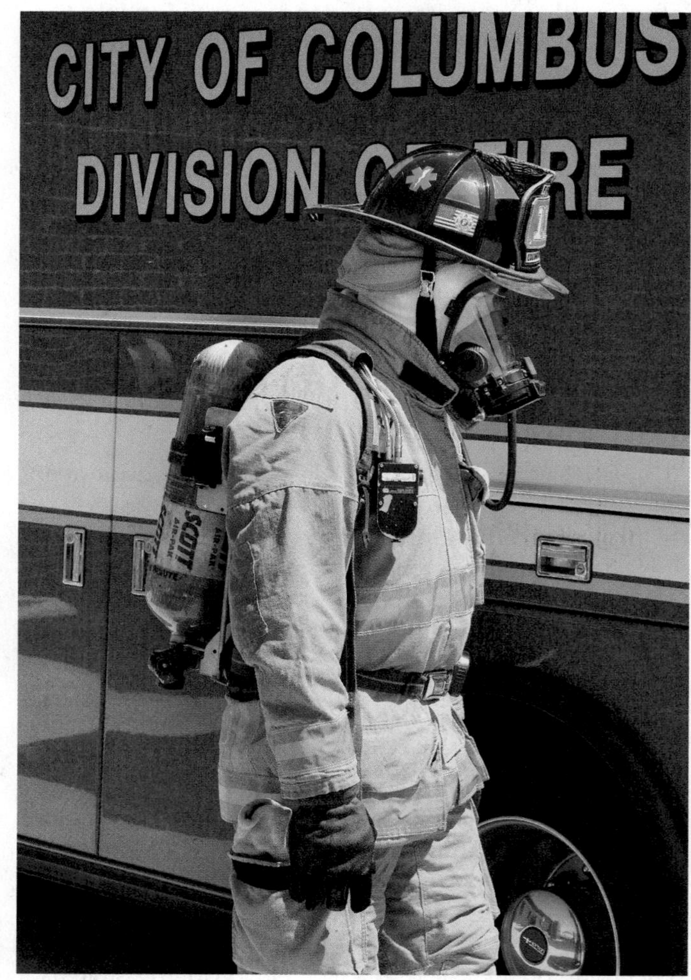

FIGURE 2-15 ✱ Self-contained breathing apparatus (SCBA).

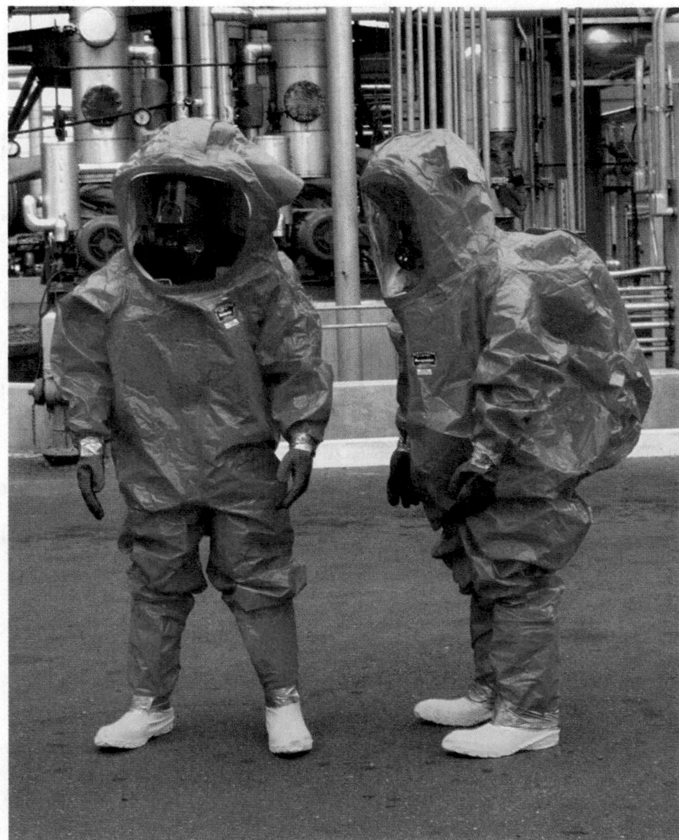

FIGURE 2-16 * Typical hazardous materials protective suits.

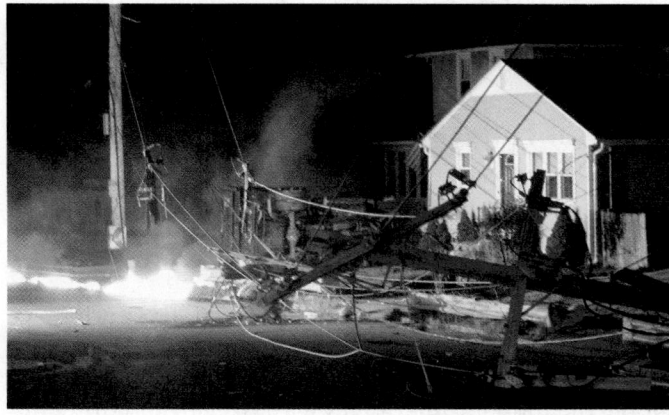

FIGURE 2-17 * Downed power lines pose a potential life threat for patients and rescuers. (© Mark C. Ide)

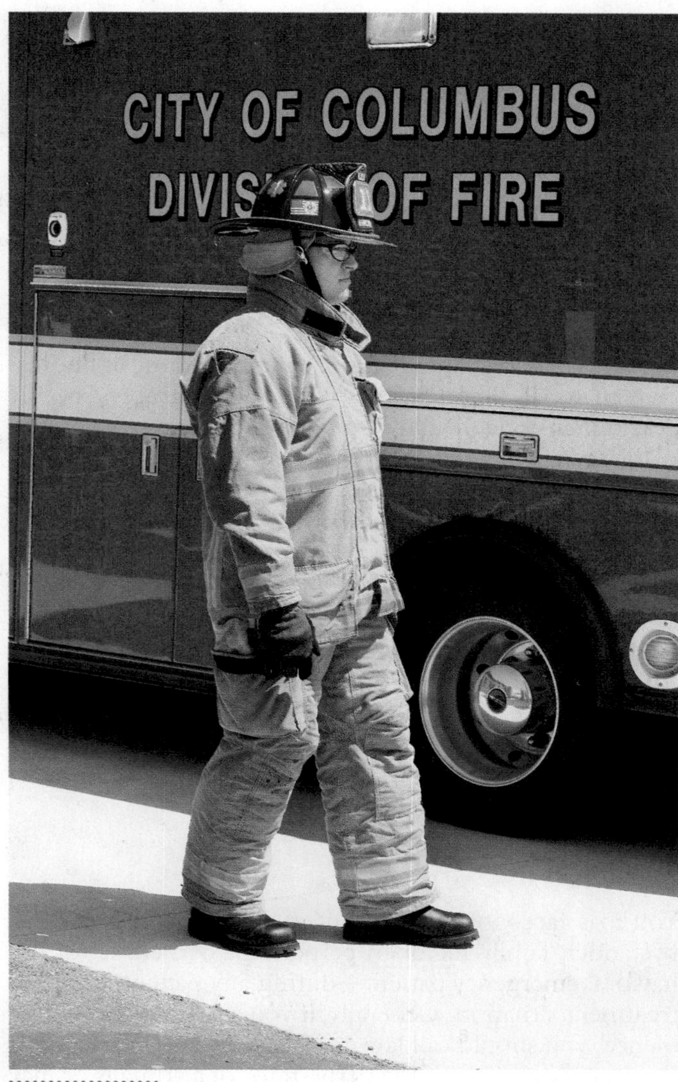

FIGURE 2-18 * Full protective gear, including eye protection, helmet, turnout gear, and gloves.

High-Visibility Vest A recently approved federal law requires all EMTs and other rescue personnel responding to accidents or other emergencies on or near a roadway to wear approved high-visibility apparel in an attempt to reduce the incidence of injury to emergency responders.

The American National Standards Institute (ANSI) and International Safety Equipment Association (ISEA) created the standard ANSI/ISEA 107-2004, American National Standard for High-Visibility Safety Apparel and Headwear. Three classes of garments were established:

Class 1—designed for workers in parking lots and other areas with traffic flow moving at less than 25 mph

Class 2—designed for personnel whose attention is diverted from traffic or where the traffic flow is moving at 25 mph or greater

Class 3—designed for personnel whose work greatly diverts their attention away from the roadway and where they are at serious risk from hazards created by moving vehicles

The ANSI/ISEA 207-2006 American National Standard for High-Visibility Public Safety Vests (PSV) was approved to increase the visibility of emergency personnel on the roadway and to reduce the incidence of roadway hazards. The newer standard made significant changes to

Key Points
Remaining well is essential in order for you to perform your responsibilities as an EMT to the best of your ability.

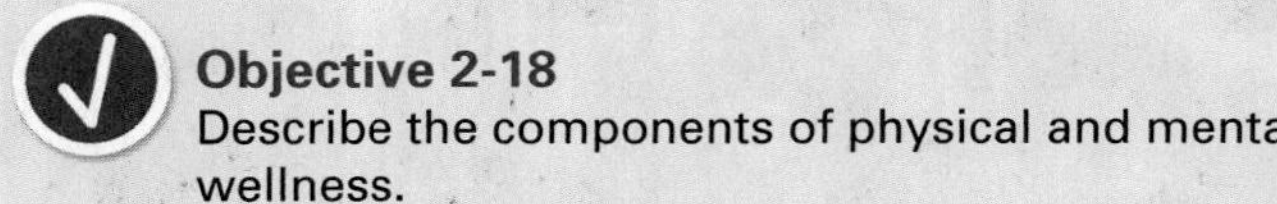

Objective 2-18
Describe the components of physical and mental wellness.

standard class garments to accommodate the public safety responder. The PSV has the same retro-reflective material as the Class 2 vest and nearly the same amount of fluorescent material. The PSV has breakaway features, specific vest dimensions to allow for fit over turnout gear, and color-specific markings to allow for differentiation between law enforcement, fire, and EMS personnel.

Currently, the Code of Federal Regulations requires all emergency personnel who are exposed to traffic within the right-of-way of a highway that receives federal funding to wear high-visibility safety apparel that meets the Class 2 or 3 standards of ANSI/ISEA 107-2004 or the Public Safety Vest standard ANSI/ISEA 207-2006. Additional information to protect emergency medical personnel while working on or near a roadway is found in Chapter 41, "Ambulance Operations and Air Medical Response."

Violence and Crime

You may face violence without warning—from a patient, bystander, family member, perpetrator of a crime, or behavioral emergency patient—during any patient rescue or treatment situation. Generally, if you suspect potential violence, you should call law enforcement before you enter the scene, especially if the perpetrator of a crime is or may still be present. Do not enter the scene to render patient care until it has been adequately controlled by law enforcement and until those with weapons (such as guns or knives) have been removed from the scene. Typical emergencies in which you should call law enforcement include domestic disputes, patients under the influence of drugs or alcohol who appear to be agitated or hostile, street or gang fights, bar fights, potential suicide, scenes with angry family members or angry bystanders, behavioral emergencies with hostile action or threats, and any type of crime scene.

Regardless of where you work, you may want to consider using body armor, sometimes called a "bullet-proof vest." Many metropolitan area EMS agencies issue body armor or provide some other means for personnel to be protected.

If you need to treat patients at a crime scene, take specific precautions to preserve the chain of evidence needed for investigation and prosecution. A general rule is to avoid disturbing the scene unless absolutely necessary for medical care. More specific details on crime scene behavior are listed in Chapter 3, "Medical, Legal, and Ethical Issues."

Wellness Principles

Remaining well is a fundamental aspect that allows you to perform your responsibilities as an EMT to the best of your ability. Wellness does not simply imply the lack of illness; it involves physical, intellectual, emotional, social, environmental, and spiritual dimensions. An imbalance in any of these dimensions could lead to a state of poor health. The following sections focus on the physical and mental components of wellness.

Physical Well-Being

Physical well-being focuses on the body and the ability to perform the physical demands of being an EMT. It includes physical fitness, adequate sleep, disease prevention, and injury prevention. Methods to reduce your incidence of acquiring an infectious disease and techniques to prevent injury from safety hazards have been discussed earlier in the chapter. Additional information regarding the prevention of injury associated with proper lifting and moving techniques will be discussed in Chapter 6, "Lifting and Moving Patients."

Physical Fitness

The core components to remaining physically fit and able to perform your job as an EMT are cardiovascular endurance, muscle strength, muscle endurance, muscle flexibility, and body composition.

Cardiovascular Endurance Cardiovascular endurance is gained through aerobic exercise that is geared toward improving the ability of the heart, lungs, and vessels to supply the muscles and organs with oxygen and other nutrients during prolonged periods of work. Walking, jogging, swimming, and using an elliptical or step machine can all help to strengthen the cardiovascular system. To obtain the benefits of cardiovascular exercise, it is necessary to reach and maintain your target heart rate for a period of time, often 30 to 40 minutes at least three days a week. Your target heart rate can be calculated by the following procedure:

1. Measure your resting heart rate.
2. Subtract your age from 220, which provides your estimated maximum heart rate.

Thinking Critically
Balanced nutrition and weight control are essential elements of physical fitness. What are some strategies you can use to maintain a reasonable diet while working as an EMT—a job that by its nature is seldom routine and often unpredictable?

Key Points
One of the keys to maintaining as near normal function as possible is getting an adequate amount of sleep.

3. Subtract your resting heart rate from your maximum heart rate, and then multiply that figure by 70% (0.70).
4. Add the final calculated number from step 3 to your resting heart rate.

The following is an example of calculating a target heart rate by this formula:

1. Resting heart rate is 62 beats per minute (bpm) for a 28-year-old.
2. Total estimated maximum heart rate is 192 bpm (220 – 28 = 192).
3. Total estimated maximum heart rate minus the resting heart rate is 130 bpm (192 − 62 = 130 bpm) multiplied by 70% = 91 bpm (130 × 0.70 = 91 bpm).
4. Target heart rate as calculated by adding the resting heart rate to the calculated figure in step 3 equals 153 bpm (91 + 62 = 153 bpm).

Muscle Strength Muscle strength is defined as the amount of force a muscle can produce through a single contraction. It is tested by the amount of weight that can be lifted. The primary way to build muscle strength is through weight lifting or other types of resistance exercises. Lifting heavy objects is a crucial and repetitive part of an EMT's job, including lifting patients and equipment.

Muscle Endurance Muscle endurance is defined as the ability of the muscle to function repeatedly without unwarranted fatigue. Improvement in muscle endurance is achieved by forcing the muscles to lift a greater weight than the muscle is used to. This, again, is achieved through weight training. Muscle endurance is necessary to be able to carry patients and equipment for long periods of time, such as from a bedroom to the ambulance.

Muscle Flexibility Muscle flexibility allows you to move your joints through the full range of motion. This is achieved primarily through stretching. Muscle flexibility is key to lifting and moving patients and equipment properly. Without adequate flexibility, you are prone to muscle and joint injury.

Body Composition Body composition is evaluated primarily by the ratio of body fat to total weight. A lower ratio of body fat is associated with a healthier individual. A higher ratio of body fat places the EMT at risk for chronic conditions such as heart disease, hypertension, and diabetes. Proper nutrition and exercise will help to reduce and/or maintain a proper ratio of body fat.

Adequate Sleep

EMS work is performed 24 hours a day, 7 days a week. When you work a shift that falls within a different span of the day than you are accustomed to being awake and alert, it interrupts your body's natural timing system, referred to as circadian rhythms. Interfering with your body's circadian rhythms makes you prone to difficulty with physical coordination, thought processes, and social functions.

One of the keys to maintaining as near normal function as possible is getting an adequate amount of sleep. Lack of sleep (sleep deprivation) puts you at risk for accidents and injury. It also puts your patients at risk of improper care resulting from your inability to function at the necessary mental and physical level. Individuals require a minimum of 8 to 10 hours of sleep each day. Studies have shown that a lack of regular sleep contributes to chronic diseases, such as heart disease, weight gain, and poor mental function. Methods to improve the quality and increase the number of hours of sleep include the following:

- Select an environment that mimics nighttime, such as one that is cool and dark.
- Select a regular time to sleep when a block of sleep can be achieved uninterrupted.
- Prepare yourself for sleep by not eating a heavy meal, drinking caffeine, nor exercising immediately before your sleep time.
- Reduce interruptions by turning off the phone ringer, shutting off pagers, turning cell phones to the silent mode, and posting a sign on your door indicating that you are sleeping.

Smoking Cessation

Smoking contributes dramatically to an unhealthy lifestyle. As an EMS professional, you are part of the public health system. One of your responsibilities is to promote a healthy lifestyle in the public to reduce the incidence of disease, illness, and injury. By smoking, you are violating this responsibility and increasing your own

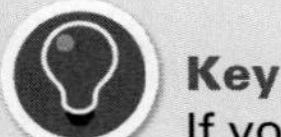

Key Points
If you or a fellow EMT is relying on drugs or alcohol, it is necessary to seek professional assistance.

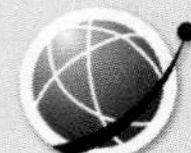

Media Resources
Go to www.bradybooks.com for mykit. Highlights:

- *Web Resource:* Hospice Foundation of America
- *Video:* Grief and a Child's Death

risk of cardiovascular and pulmonary disease, and cancer. There are a number of strategies available to quit smoking. By doing so, you will not only improve your public image but also greatly improve your health.

Alcohol- and Drug-Related Issues

Some EMS providers resort to the use of alcohol or drugs, prescription or illegal, in an attempt to reduce the mental and physical stress associated with the job. Overindulgence in alcohol to reduce or relieve stress is a practice that must be avoided. It has consequences for your health and mental function, and it does not get rid of the stress. Similarly, the use of medications or illegal drugs to cope with stress is a grave warning sign. If you or a fellow EMT is relying on drugs or alcohol, it is necessary to seek professional assistance. Many EMS agencies have employee assistance programs that are extremely beneficial in situations like these.

Mental Well-Being

Stress associated with EMS can easily affect your mental well-being. Over time, this can lead to the development of chronic physical illness as well as emotional issues. Individuals who are close to you and who are not involved in EMS may not understand the stresses of the job and what you are experiencing. This can contribute to difficulty in relationships and an imbalance in your personal life. It is important to talk to family members or those you are close to and explain how you are feeling. They may not completely understand; however, it is a step toward helping them understand. Exercise, relaxation, and engaging in something you enjoy, such as fishing or hiking, are great ways to reduce stress and improve your mental well-being.

If these methods are not enough to help you achieve a feeling of mental well-being, look into any employee assistance programs your agency may provide or seek out other sources of help, such as professional counseling.

Safe Glove Removal

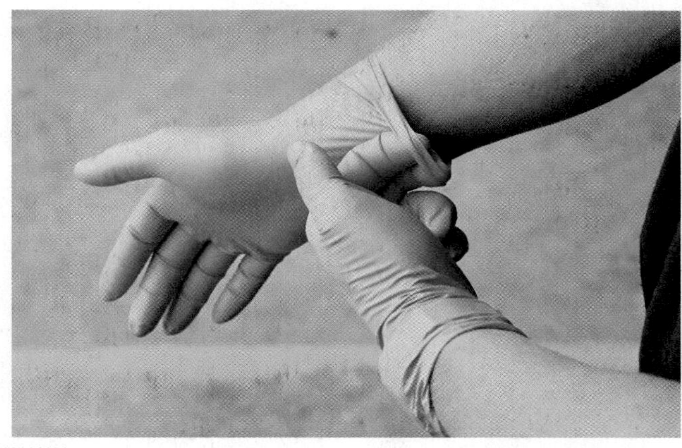

2-1A ✱ Follow a safe technique for removal of gloves. Use only contaminated glove surfaces to touch other contaminated glove surfaces, and use clean inside glove surfaces to touch other clean inside glove surfaces. Do not touch a contaminated surface with your bare hand or fingers.

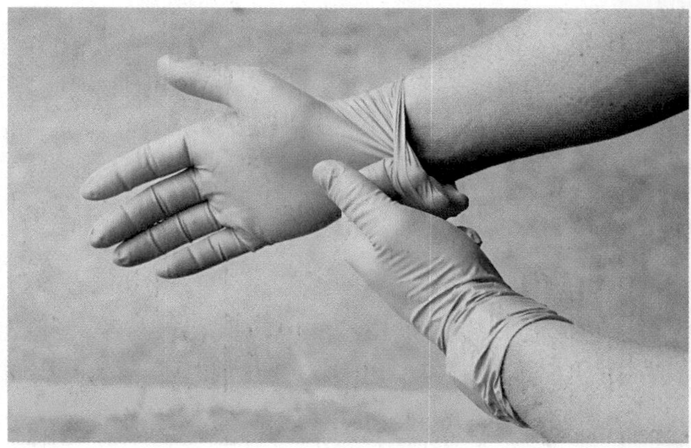

2-1B ✱ Use a gloved finger to pull a cuff out and down on the other glove. Do not touch the inside of the glove.

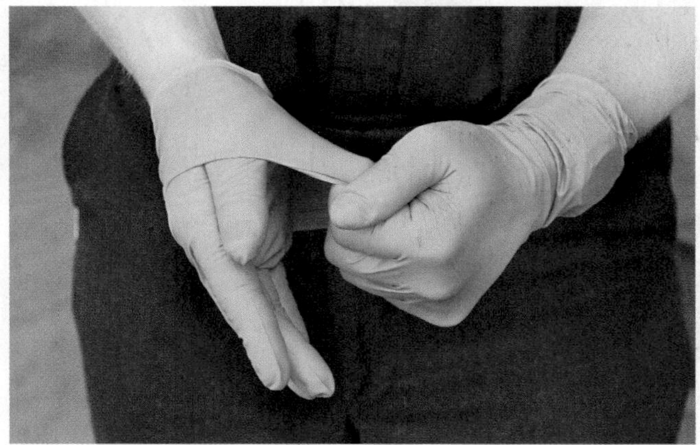

2-1C ✱ Without touching the inside of the glove, continue pulling it downward.

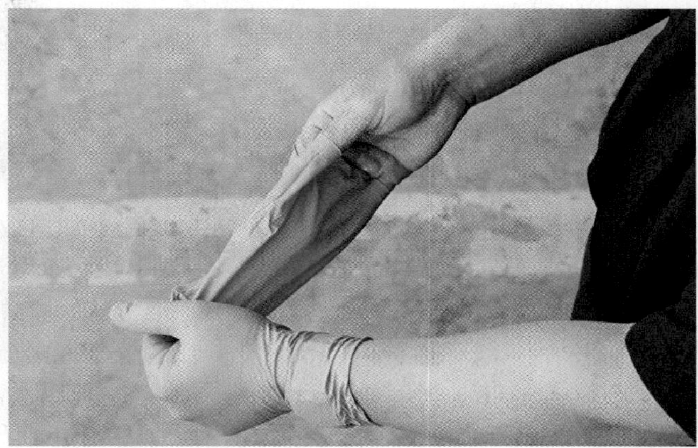

2-1D ✱ Pull until the glove is inside out and off all but the tips of the fingers and thumb.

continued

Safe Glove Removal *continued*

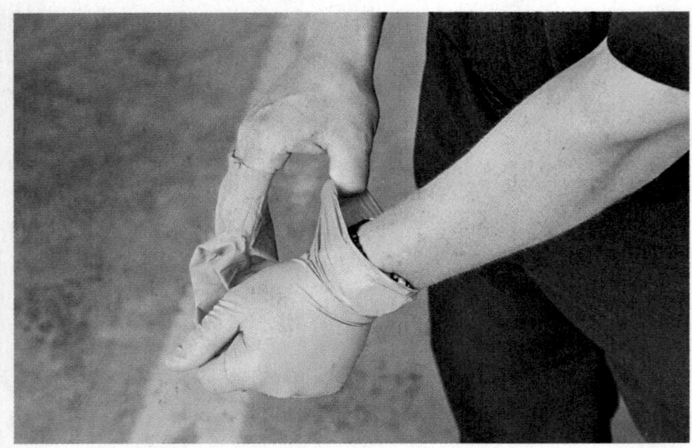

2-1E ✱ Hook the clean inside surface of the partially removed glove into the clean inside of the other glove.

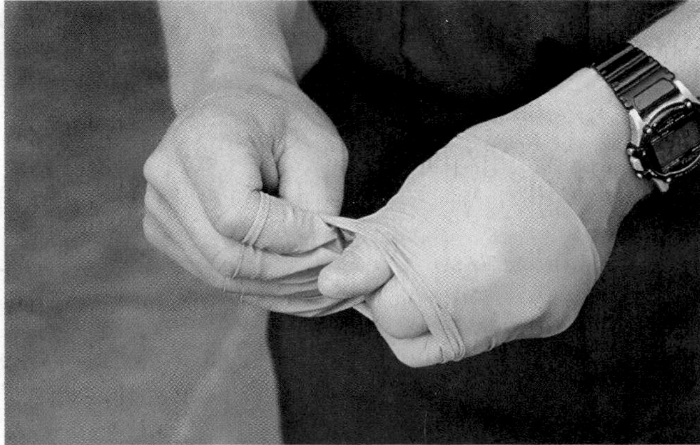

2-1F ✱ Use the clean inside surfaces of the partially removed glove to pinch and pull down on the other glove.

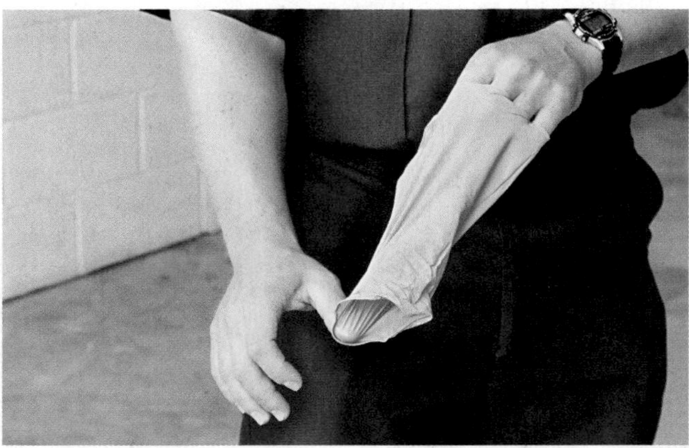

2-1G ✱ Finish pulling the second glove downward. Use the clean inside surfaces to finally pull off both gloves. Drop the contaminated gloves into a biohazard container.

CHAPTER REVIEW

SUMMARY

As an EMT, you will be faced with death and dying on a regular basis. It is likely that what you will experience in a short while most people will not experience in a lifetime. Some patients who are terminally ill will go through certain stages related to death and dying. Family members may go through the same stages but at different times. Be prepared to deal with these patients, their families, and their emotions.

Stress is inherent in emergency medical services and may have significant physical, emotional, psychological, and social impacts on your life. Be prepared to recognize the warning signs and symptoms of stress. Stress reactions may be acute, delayed, or cumulative. Once you have recognized stress, use effective methods to diminish or eliminate it.

One of the most important aspects of scene safety is protecting yourself against any hazards. This includes taking the necessary Standard Precautions against infectious disease. If responding to a scene that involves specialized rescue, such as for hazardous materials or swift water, do not attempt any type of rescue yourself unless you have received the necessary specialized training and have the proper equipment. Responding to scenes that involve violence and crime may present certain risks. Be sure to have the proper resources dispatched to secure the scene.

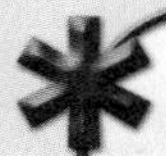

CASE STUDY FOLLOW-UP

SCENE SIZE-UP

You have been dispatched to the scene of a domestic dispute. You learn from the police that the husband is an unemployed alcoholic who is going through a "detox" program. He is holding his wife and two daughters hostage. An officer is already down, and a special tactics team is working to bring the situation under control.

Two hours later you are still not permitted to approach. The husband has released the two children and they are transported by another EMS unit. Suddenly there is a single gunshot. The husband appears at the front door, shooting randomly. The special tactics team returns fire. The man falls to the ground.

PATIENT ASSESSMENT

After the police secure the scene, you and your partner approach with Standard Precautions. Primary assessment shows that the downed police officer is dead, having received multiple gunshot wounds to the head and neck. The gunman is also dead, with multiple gunshot wounds to the head and chest. The wife inside the house is dead, shot once through the head. You and your partner return to the ambulance and notify dispatch that there will be no additional transports. The incident commander releases you and your partner from the scene.

CRITICAL INCIDENT FOLLOW-UP

During the drive back to the station, your partner is very quiet and tense. At the station, you try to get him to discuss the call. He responds angrily and tells you he is going to quit EMS. You both summon your supervisor, who recognizes the signs of acute stress reaction. The supervisor meets with the EMT and encourages him to contact the employee assistance program. He arranges to meet with a mental health professional to discuss the call. He returns to his next shift relaxed and confident that he can perform competently.

IN REVIEW

1. List the five stages through which a dying patient may pass.
2. Describe several things you can do—other than provide emergency medical care—to help dying patients.
3. List five of the signs and symptoms of chronic stress and burnout.
4. List four ways you can help deal with the stress in your life.
5. Identify some of the negative feelings families of EMTs may have in response to the job. Describe some of the ways you can help.
6. Describe the safety precautions an EMT can take to prevent the spread of infectious disease.
7. Discuss the responsibilities employers have, under OSHA guidelines, to protect emergency care personnel from transmission of infectious diseases.
8. Discuss the responsibilities emergency care employees have, under OSHA guidelines, for their own protection against transmission of infectious diseases.
9. List the personal protective equipment necessary for hazardous materials situations, rescue operations, and scenes of violence or crime.
10. List steps to prevent work-related injuries.
11. List common infectious diseases the EMT may encounter in the prehospital setting.
12. List strategies that contribute to physical and mental well-being.

CRITICAL THINKING

You are dispatched to the scene for a 3-year-old female child who was shot in the chest. As you arrive on the scene, you note blood covering the front porch and sidewalk.

1. What would you do to ensure scene safety?
2. What other resources should be requested?
3. Why is this a potential high-stress situation?
4. What can be done to reduce your stress associated with the call?

CHAPTER 3

Medical, Legal, and Ethical Issues

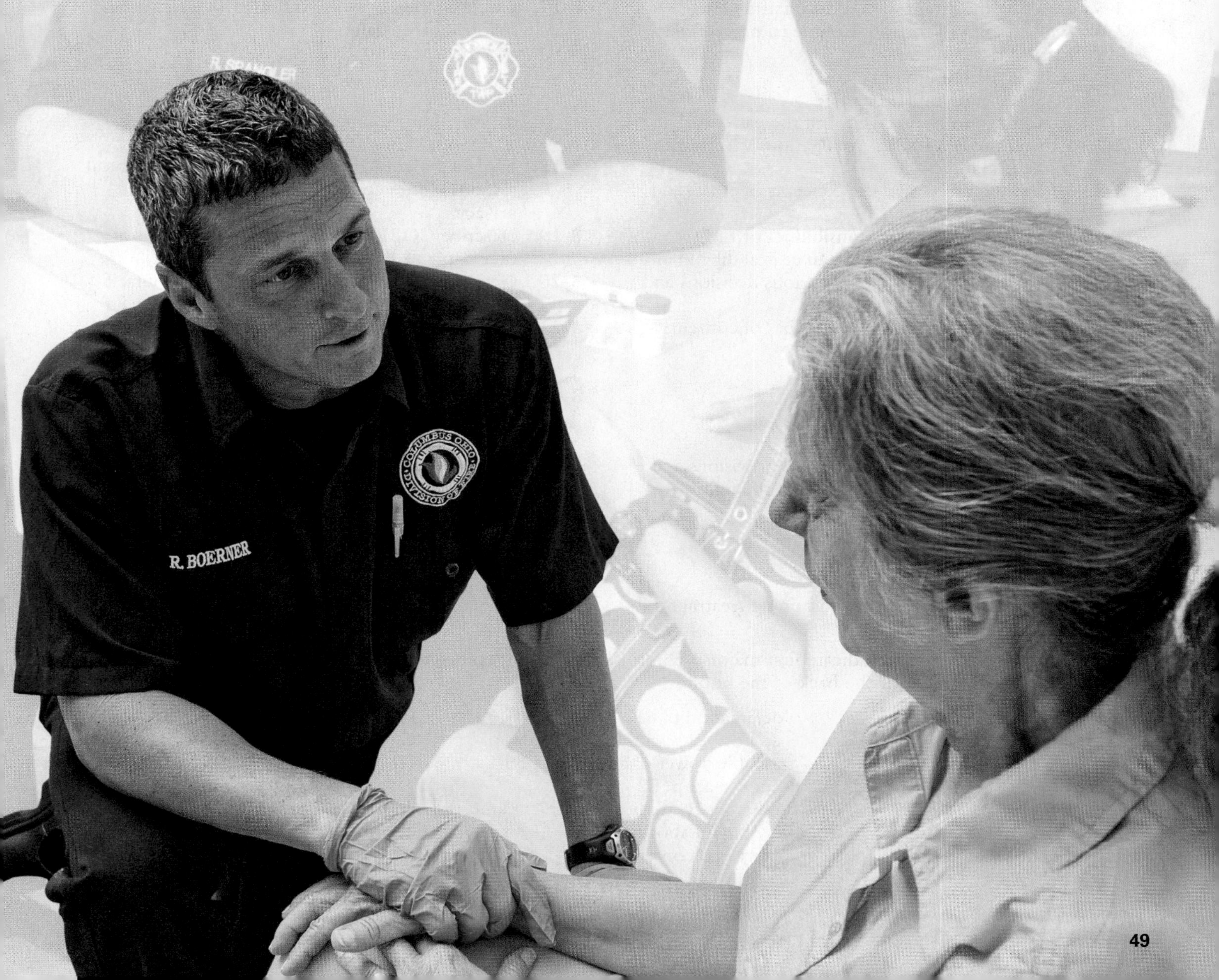

Navigation Guide

The following items provide an overview to the purpose and content of this chapter. The Education Standard and Competency are from the new National EMS Education Standards.

STANDARD **Preparatory** (Content Area: Medical/Legal and Ethical)

COMPETENCY Applies fundamental knowledge of the EMS system, safety/well-being of the EMT, medical/legal and ethical issues to the provision of emergency care.

OBJECTIVES: After reading this chapter, you should be able to:

3-1. Define key terms introduced in this chapter.

3-2. Differentiate between the concepts of *scope of practice* and *standard of care.*

3-3. Given a scenario, determine whether you would have a duty to act.

3-4. Explain your duties with respect to patients, your partner, yourself, and your equipment.

3-5. Describe the intent of Good Samaritan laws.

3-6. Explain each of the following legal protections for EMTs:
- **a.** Sovereign immunity
- **b.** Statutes of limitations
- **c.** Contributory negligence of the patient

3-7. Explain the EMT's legal obligations with respect to medical direction.

3-8. Differentiate between the concepts of ethics and morals.

3-9. Describe the ethical responsibilities of EMTs.

3-10. Given a scenario presenting an ethical dilemma, discuss the consequences of various decisions and actions.

3-11. Explain each of the following types of consent:
- **a.** Informed consent
- **b.** Expressed consent
- **c.** Implied consent
- **d.** Consent to treat minors
- **e.** Involuntary consent

3-12. Compare and contrast the typical provisions and prehospital applications of each of the following types of advance directives:
- **a.** Do not resuscitate order
- **b.** Living will
- **c.** Durable power of attorney
- **d.** Physican orders for life-sustaining treatment

3-13. Given a scenario in which a patient has an advance directive, determine the appropriate action to be taken.

3-14. Given a scenario in which a patient refuses care, discuss the actions you should take.

3-15. Differentiate between criminal and civil liability.

3-16. Explain the concept of negligence.

3-17. Give examples of ways you can avoid each of the following tort claims:
- **a.** Abandonment
- **b.** Assault
- **c.** Battery
- **d.** False imprisonment/kidnapping
- **e.** Defamation

3-18. Explain patients' rights and your legal and ethical responsibilities concerning confidentiality and privacy.

3-19. Describe COBRA and EMTALA provisions as they apply to EMS.

3-20. Give examples of ways you can protect yourself legally in transport and transfer situations.

3-21. Describe special considerations for patients who are potential organ donors.

3-22. Identify presumptive signs of death.

3-23. Identify situations in which law enforcement or the medical examiner's/coroner's office should be contacted.

3-24. Discuss special considerations in responding to potential crime scenes.

3-25. Describe situations in which the EMT may be mandated to make a report, such as suspected abuse, crimes, and infectious diseases.

KEY TERMS: Page references indicate first major use in this chapter. For complete definitions, see the Glossary at the back of the book.

abandonment p. 60
advance directive p. 55
assault p. 61
battery p. 61
consent p. 54
Consolidated Omnibus Budget Reconciliation Act (COBRA) p. 62
defamation p. 61
do not resuscitate (DNR) order p. 55
durable power of attorney p. 55
duty to act p. 52
Emergency Medical Treatment and Active Labor Act (EMTALA) p. 62
expressed consent p. 54
false imprisonment p. 61
Good Samaritan law p. 53
Health Insurance Portability and Accountability Act (HIPAA) p. 62
implied consent p. 54
informed consent p. 54
intentional tort p. 60

MEDIA RESOURCES: Please go to www.bradybooks.com to access mykit for this text. You will find quizzes, critical thinking scenarios, weblinks, animations, and videos related to this chapter—and much more. Look for online information on HIPAA and organ donation.

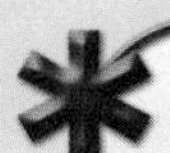

CASE STUDY

The Dispatch

EMS Unit 105—proceed to 733 East Third Street—you have an elderly male at that location with abdominal pain—time out 1430 hours.

Upon Arrival

An elderly woman, who tells you she is Mrs. Schuman, meets you and your partner on the front porch of the home. She is wearing only a nightgown, and the temperature is only 38°F. She says, "It's my husband. Something is wrong. I just can't handle him anymore."

You quickly usher Mrs. Schuman inside while you scan the scene for hazards. As soon as you enter you notice that the house is in shambles. The rooms are so cluttered that you and your partner can barely pass through. Mrs. Schuman leads you to the bedroom, where you find the patient lying on the bed. Mr. Schuman's eyes are open, and he's moaning softly. His bed sheets and undergarments are stained with dried urine. The odor is very strong, and the temperature inside the room is very cold.

How Would You Proceed with This Case?

During this chapter, you will learn about special legal and ethical considerations that have an impact on the medical care you administer to your patients. Later, we will return to the case and put in context some of the information you learned.

Introduction

Should you stop to treat an accident victim when you are off duty? May you treat a child when the parents are not present to give consent? Should you withhold cardiopulmonary resuscitation (CPR) if the patient's family asks you to? You will often need to act on medical, legal, and ethical issues such as these during your career as an EMT.

At times you may wonder if you can provide emergency care at all without being sued! You are unlikely to be sued successfully if you provide and carefully document care within your scope of practice and local protocols, with knowledge of such issues as patient consent and duty to act.

The Scope of Practice

Prehospital emergency care has changed significantly since its early days. One improvement has been in the quality of training that emergency medical personnel receive today. The public and the health care profession have come to expect a competent EMT who understands and accepts the legal and ethical responsibilities to the patient, to the medical director, and to the public.

Legal Duties

Typically, state laws identify the EMT's **scope of practice,** or the actions and care that EMTs are legally allowed to perform by the state in which they are providing emergency

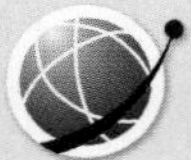

Media Resources
Go to www.bradybooks.com for mykit. Highlights:

- *Web Resource:* National EMS Education Standards
- *Web Resource:* EMT Code of Ethics

Key Terms
scope of practice the actions and care an EMT is legally allowed to perform.

Objective 3-2
Differentiate between the concepts of *scope of practice* and *standard of care.*

medical care. Scope of practice also identifies which activities would be deemed illegal if performed without licensure or certification and establishes boundaries among professionals. For example, providing oxygen under the appropriate circumstances is within the EMT's scope of practice. However, suturing a laceration is not and is therefore illegal—even if the EMT may actually know how to perform the skill.

Among the sources commonly used to define the EMT's scope of practice are the National Highway Traffic Safety Administration's *National EMS Scope of Practice Model* and the *National EMS Education Standards,* which reflect minimum training standards applied throughout the United States, as well as state laws, regulations, and policies. The scope of practice is not a practice guideline or protocol and does not define the standard of care. It is purely a definition of what actions can legally be performed by the EMT.

The **standard of care** would be defined as the care that is expected to be provided by an EMT with similar training when managing a patient in a similar situation. The concept of "the reasonable person standard" is applied. That is, what would a reasonably prudent EMT with similar training do in the same situation? Also, standard of care asks whether the EMT provided the care properly. Thus, standard of care deals with two principles: (1) Did the EMT provide the right assessment and emergency care for the patient? and (2) Did the EMT perform the assessment and emergency care properly?

The scope of practice asks: Was the EMT allowed by law to do what he did? Falling below the standard of care would constitute negligence. The following sources may be used to define the standard of care:

- Recognized and accepted EMT textbooks
- The care that would be expected by other EMTs in the community or region
- Local and state protocols
- National Highway Traffic Safety Administration's *National EMS Education Standards*
- The EMS system's operating policies and procedures

Duty to Act

The concept known as **duty to act** refers to your legal obligation to provide service, whether you think the patient needs an ambulance or not. Legally, while you are on duty you are obligated to care for a patient who requires and consents to it, rendering the necessary emergency care to the best of your ability and training. If you are off duty and not functioning in an EMS capacity, however, in most states you have no more legal obligation to act than any other citizen. While off duty in these states, you could legally do any of the following:

- Stop and help the accident victim at the scene.
- Pass the scene and call for help.
- Pass the scene and make no attempt to call for help.

Note, however, that some states *do* require EMTs to stop and render aid even when off duty.

Whether or not your state requires it, if you are off duty from your paid or volunteer service and publicly respond to a page for assistance at an emergency call, or if you come across a scene and decide to stop to provide emergency care, you will create a duty to act, even though you are off duty. The reason for this assumed duty to act is that others may not respond because they feel that your response has covered the call adequately and no other assistance is needed. If you begin emergency care and then decide to leave the scene, the patient could be placed in a situation that may be worse than if you had not responded at all. Once you do stop to help, thus creating the duty to act, you assume certain legal responsibilities. For example, once you have begun to provide care, you cannot leave until someone with the appropriate expertise—typically defined as one with an equal or higher level of training—takes over care. You are also legally responsible for any of the patient's personal property that you pick up.

One of the most important aspects of duty to your patient involves respecting the rights of the patient. It is your responsibility to serve as the patient's advocate and to protect and honor his rights. Part of that protection includes maintaining the privacy and confidentiality of the patient's medical status, history, and records. You are there to lessen the patient's suffering. You must also provide complete and competent care for your patient. This involves not only providing care for the physical injuries and illness, but also meeting the emotional needs of the patient. You must also do no further harm.

Your duty goes beyond accepting the responsibility to respond and provide emergency care to a patient. You also have a duty to self, a duty to your partner, and a duty to take responsibility for your equipment.

Objectives 3-3 and 3-4
Explain duty to act and your duties to patients, partner, self, and equipment.

Objectives 3-5 and 3-6
Explain Good Samaritan lawsand legal protections for EMTs.

Key Terms

standard of care care expected from any trained EMT under similar circumstances.

duty to act obligation to care for a patient.

Good Samaritan law provides liability immunity for emergency scene acts done in good faith.

Your duty to self requires that you obtain the necessary credentials to practice as an EMT, that you maintain your skills to a level of proficiency, that you maintain your mental health, and that you remain physically able to perform the duties of the job.

Your duty to your partner involves ensuring that he is physically and mentally fit to provide emergency medical care and other responsibilities of the job. If your partner reports for work under the influence of alcohol or drugs, you have a duty to report the situation to your supervisor. In the end, it protects you and protects the public.

Your duty regarding your equipment is vital. It is your legal responsibility as an EMT to ensure that all of your equipment is in proper working order. This is done at the beginning of each shift. If a piece of equipment malfunctions because of improper maintenance, or if you don't have a necessary piece of equipment to treat a patient, you are negligent in providing care to the patient.

Good Samaritan Laws

The first Good Samaritan law was enacted in 1959 in California specifically to protect from liability "persons licensed (such as a physician or surgeon) who in good faith render emergency care at the scene of the emergency . . . for civil damages as a result of any acts or omissions." Many states have immunity laws of their own, some of which specifically cover prehospital emergency care providers.

Generally, a **Good Samaritan law** protects a person who is not being paid for his services from liability for acts performed in good faith unless those acts constitute gross negligence. Therefore, the person suing must prove that the care provided was markedly below the standard of care and, in some cases, with willful or wanton intent to harm the patient.

Most states have specific laws authorizing EMTs to perform prehospital emergency medical procedures without a medical license. Most states also provide some form of immunity to nurses, physicians, supervisors, and other personnel who give directions to EMTs by cell phone, telephone, or radio. The laws governing private and public providers vary. Be sure to learn your local laws.

A Good Samaritan law does not prevent you from being sued, although it may provide you some protection against losing the lawsuit if you have performed according to the standard of care for an EMT. So while you are on duty or assisting off duty, your best defense to lawsuits is prevention. Always render care to the best of your ability, always work within your scope of practice and within the standard of care, always behave in a professional manner, and ensure that you are covered by adequate liability insurance. If you keep your patients' best interests in mind when rendering care, you will seldom, if ever, go wrong.

Other Legal Protections

Another type of immunity afforded to public or government emergency medical services is *sovereign immunity.* Sovereign immunity, also known as governmental immunity, prevents persons treated by governmentally operated EMS systems from suing the government for civil liability. Since private EMS companies are not government agencies, they are not protected under sovereign immunity.

Each state has determined an appropriate *statute of limitations* relative to negligence claims. This means that the patient has only a certain amount of time to file a negligence claim following either the event that caused the injury or illness or from the point of discovering that the problem existed. Statutes of limitations are typically measured in years.

If the patient contributed in any manner to his own injury or illness, and he chooses to file a negligence claim against an EMS provider, then the patient may be found guilty of *contributory negligence.* In other words, contributory negligence exists when there is a finding that the patient, through his own negligence, caused or contributed to the damage that was done to him.

Medical Direction

Your legal right to function as an EMT is contingent upon medical direction. When providing emergency care you should:

- Follow standing orders and protocols, as approved by medical direction.
- Establish cell phone, telephone, and radio communications with medical direction when appropriate.
- Communicate clearly and completely with medical direction, and follow orders medical direction gives in response.
- Any time there is a question about the scope or direction of care, consult medical direction.

Most areas also have protocols for cooperation between EMS personnel and other public safety services.

Objective 3-7
Explain the EMT's legal obligations with respect to medical direction.

Objectives 3-8 to 3-10
Differentiate ethics and morals and describe EMT ethical responsibilities and the consequences of ethical decisions.

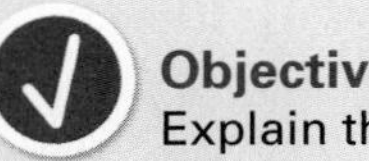

Objective 3-11
Explain the types of consent.

Key Terms
consent permission that must be obtained before care is rendered; types include **informed, expressed, implied, minor,** and **involuntary consent.**

Ethical Responsibilities

Ethics is a branch of philosophy specifically directed toward the study of morality, or morals. *Morals* are concepts of "right and wrong." A code of ethics is a list of rules of ideal conduct. A Code of Ethics for EMTs was issued by the National Association of Emergency Medical Technicians in 1978. Basically, if you place the welfare of the patient above all else when providing medical care, you will rarely commit an unethical act.

Your ethical responsibilities include these:

- Serve the needs of the patient with respect for human dignity, without regard to nationality, race, gender, creed, or status.
- Maintain skill mastery. Demonstrate respect for the competence of other medical professionals.
- Keep abreast of changes in EMS that affect patient care. Assume responsibility in defining and upholding professional standards.
- Critically review performances, seeking ways to improve response time, patient outcome, and communication. Assume responsibility for individual professional actions and judgment.
- Report with honesty. Hold in confidence all information obtained in the course of professional work unless required by law to divulge such information.
- Work harmoniously with other EMTs, nurses, physicians, and other members of the health care team.

Ethical and moral conflicts may sometimes arise during the performance of your duties. Such an ethical or moral issue may occur when, for example, you are responding to a terminally ill patient who is requesting that no treatment be rendered, and yet the do not resuscitate (DNR) orders presented to you have expired. Legally, you have an obligation to provide care, and yet you may feel an ethical obligation to honor the patient's wishes to receive no treatment, and a moral obligation to preserve life under any circumstances. In such a situation, obviously, legal and moral criteria would conflict with ethical criteria.

Other situations in which ethical and moral considerations may conflict include mass casualty events where medical care is being rationed as part of the triage process, and cardiac arrest in the wilderness where resources are limited and transportation time to definitive care is extended. The ethical and moral conflicts that arise as a result of situations like these can be very challenging. It is always best to remember that local protocols and applicable laws should be followed, and that medical direction can be contacted at any time to assist with decisions in these types of situations.

Issues of Patient Consent and Refusal

Types of Consent

Under the law, the conscious, competent, and rational patient has the right to accept or refuse emergency medical care. Therefore, it is necessary to obtain **consent**, or permission, before providing such care. Before emergency care is rendered, the patient must be informed of the care to be provided and the associated risks and consequences. Consent so obtained is termed **informed consent**.

After introducing yourself, you must indicate to the patient that you would like to perform an assessment to determine what his condition is, provide emergency care, and transport him to a medical facility. You must ask the patient if he understands and has any questions. Ask the patient for his explicit permission before proceeding, even if he was the one who placed the 911 call to EMS. This is particularly important if the assessment or treatment you are recommending is part of a research program in which the interventions in question have not yet been proven effective, which would complicate the process of ensuring that the patient is adequately informed.

Don't assume that the patient will always consent to all aspects of your assessment, care, and transport. Listen carefully to the patient's response so that you don't proceed without his consent. Even on the most routine of calls, if you were to touch a patient's body or clothing without first obtaining the proper consent, you could be charged with battery, or touching unlawfully. Battery applies to anyone who provides emergency care when the patient does not consent to the specific treatment. (Battery is discussed in more detail later in this chapter.)

In addition to informed consent, there are four other types of consent: **expressed consent**, **implied consent**, **minor consent**, and **involuntary consent**.

- ***Expressed consent*** must be obtained from every conscious, mentally competent adult before treatment is started. The patient must be of legal age, competent (meaning that the patient has the mental capacity to

Key Terms
advance directive instructions written in advance of care.

Objective 3-12
Compare types of advance directives.

Key Terms
do not resuscitate (DNR) order states which, if any, life-sustaining measures to take when vital functions cease.

living will delineates the signer's wishes about health care issues.

make a decision), able to make a rational decision, and informed of the assessment and procedures you will be performing and all related risks. Basically, the patient must receive—in terms the patient understands—all of the information that would affect a reasonable person's decision to accept or refuse treatment. Although a verbal confirmation of the patient's consent is preferable, nonverbal cues from the patient, such as nodding when asked if it is all right to perform an assessment, are acceptable as well. It is good practice to document the patient's approval.

- ***Implied consent***, also known as the *emergency doctrine*, occurs when you assume that a patient who is unresponsive or who is not competent or who is unable to make a rational decision (e.g., a patient who is disoriented because of a head injury) would consent to emergency care if he could. Implied consent also applies to the patient who initially refuses your care but then becomes unresponsive, incapacitated, or irrational because of illness or injury. In a true emergency where the patient is at significant risk of death, disability, or deterioration of condition, the law assumes that the unresponsive patient would give consent.
- ***Consent to treat a minor*** must be obtained from a parent, legal guardian, or other person who has been granted limited rights of decision making by the parent or guardian, such as a teacher, a stepparent, or another authorized caregiver. Depending on state law, a minor usually is any person under age 18 or 21. Minors are considered not legally competent to accept or refuse emergency care; however, if the parent or legal guardian is not present and cannot be reached to provide consent, the concept of implied consent, or the emergency doctrine, is used. It is assumed that the parent or legal guardian would consent to the care of the minor if they were present at the scene. It is imperative that you clearly document the circumstances in making the decision to render emergency care to the minor. You do not need consent of a parent or guardian to treat an emancipated minor—usually defined as a minor who is married, pregnant, a parent, a member of the armed forces, financially independent and living away from home, or one who has been declared emancipated by court decree.
- ***Involuntary consent*** can be applied when you are dealing with a mentally incompetent adult or with an individual who is in custody of law enforcement or is incarcerated. Gaining consent to assess and treat such individuals often involves a third party, such as a legal guardian, a law enforcement officer, or other officer of the court. If appropriately deemed to be incompetent or in legal custody, the patient does not have the legal right to determine his own care, which makes it necessary to gain consent from the appropriate individual with the legal authority to make decisions on that person's behalf.

Advance Directives

You may sometimes be called to treat terminally ill patients. In some cases, the patient may request—and a physician may order—that no resuscitation measures take place if the heart and lungs stop functioning. Legally, due in part to the federal Patient Self-Determination Act, the patient has a right to refuse resuscitative efforts. An **advance directive** (instructions written in advance) against resuscitation, signed by the patient, is a legally recognized document. This documents the wish of the chronically or terminally ill patient not to be resuscitated and legally allows the health care provider to withhold resuscitation.

Common types of advance directives are a do not resuscitate (DNR) order, a living will, a health care durable power of attorney, and physician orders for life-sustaining treatment (POLST). A **do not resuscitate (DNR) order** is a legal document or order that most often governs resuscitation issues only, whereas a **living will** is more often used to cover more general health care issues, including the use of long-term life support equipment such as ventilators and feeding tubes. A health care **durable power of attorney**, also known as a *health care proxy*, designates a person who is legally empowered to make health care decisions for the signer of the document if he is unable to do so for himself. Decisions by health care proxies usually pertain only to in-hospital or long-term care facility situations.

Physician orders for life-sustaining treatment (POLST) are used in patients with serious or terminal illness who are not expected to survive for longer than 1 year. Unlike a do not resuscitate order that is geared primarily to making a decision to resuscitate or not to resuscitate a patient, POLST is designed to allow the patient to choose and express the level of treatment he desires in the case of deterioration prior to the need for resuscitation. Thus, POLST implies the continuation of life-sustaining treatment with the potential for limitations.

Key Terms

durable power of attorney empowers someone to make health care decisions for the signer.

physician orders for life-sustaining treatment (POLST) identify desired level of life-sustaining treatment in patients with terminal or life-threatening illness.

Objectives 3-13 and 3-14

Given scenarios in which a patient has an advance directive or refuses care, determine the appropriate actions to be taken.

Key Points

If you place the welfare of the patient above all else, you will rarely commit an unethical act.

For example, the patient may choose the administration of medications but may refuse advanced airway procedures or defibrillation. The POLST is voluntary, not mandatory, for patients. You might find the POLST form in a health care facility, such as a nursing home or long-term care facility, or in a patient's home. One of the other types of advance directive may accompany the POLST form. The POLST form must be signed by a physician and include dates during which it is valid. The contact information for the physician must also be included. In some states, the POLST may be signed by a physician assistant (PA) or nurse practitioner (NP).

When you are presented with a DNR or POLST, you must determine to the best of your ability whether it is valid and interpret the manner in which the directive should be followed. Check to see that the physician's instructions are clear, concise, and unambiguous and typed or written in a clear hand on professional letterhead. Phrases like "no heroics" or "no extraordinary treatment" are not clear enough to meet legal requirements. In many jurisdictions and in some states, a standard legal form or varied legal forms are used for DNR orders (Figures 3-1∗ and 3-2∗). Be sure to learn the laws and protocols for the state you will function in, since they vary significantly. Some states require a written physician order; others have the patient wear a DNR bracelet. Most states require that the signed DNR or POLST order be present at the scene in order to withhold or limit treatment. Do not simply accept the word of the family. If the DNR or POLST order is not present, you are obligated to perform the resuscitation or needed treatment.

Some states have different degrees of DNR (different kinds of resuscitation treatments refused) and are based on various levels of chronic illness or terminal status. Some patients may request that only selected emergency care or comfort procedures be performed. Typically, oxygen administration is considered a standard comfort measure and should be provided for both the do-not-resuscitate and the modified-support patient. Be sure to learn your local protocol.

Advance directives may be filled with problems for prehospital providers. First, by its very nature, a living will is generally more useful in an institutional setting, such as a nursing home or hospital, where health care providers are aware of it and know the doctor who signed it. In addition, many advance directives require more than one physician to verify the patient's condition—a requirement that may be difficult to fulfill in the field, even if the advance directive is located. Finally, the time taken to scrutinize an advance directive can take precious moments away from providing resuscitative care.

Issues you may encounter at the scene regarding the DNR or POLST are questions about the validity of the document, interpretation of what care should or should not be provided, and a conflict between the DNR or POLST order and the wishes of a family member. To protect yourself, the best manner to proceed is to (1) consider initiating treatment immediately so that if the issue cannot be resolved you will not be held negligent for not providing care or delaying treatment, (2) contact medical direction for instructions on how to proceed, and (3) continue treatment until the problem has been resolved.

You will be in a much better position if you err by providing treatment rather than by withholding treatment when faced with questions about whether to provide care. In the absence of a valid DNR or POLST order and a physician's written instructions, you are obligated to begin full resuscitation or needed treatment immediately.

Refusing Treatment

Competency

The courts have ruled that a patient has the right to refuse care even if it results in the patient's death. In order for the patient to refuse care, it is vital that you first determine that the patient is competent. As noted earlier, a competent adult is one who is lucid and capable of making an informed decision. Typically, a patient is deemed to be lucid if he is able to accurately prove orientation to "person, place, and time." People who display an altered mental status or who are mentally ill or under the influence of drugs or alcohol may be considered not competent or incapacitated. Many states have laws that provide protection to members of EMS when implied consent to assess, treat, and transport an incapacitated patient. A competent adult has the right to refuse treatment—verbally, or by pulling away, shaking his head, gesturing you away, or pushing you away—or to withdraw from treatment after it has started.

Under the law, to refuse treatment or transport, a patient must be informed of and fully understand the treatment and all potential risks and consequences of refusal, up to and including the possibility of death if it is a potential risk. Have the patient explain to you what these potential consequences are if treatment is refused. If the patient does not understand the consequences, he would be deemed incompetent and treated under implied consent.

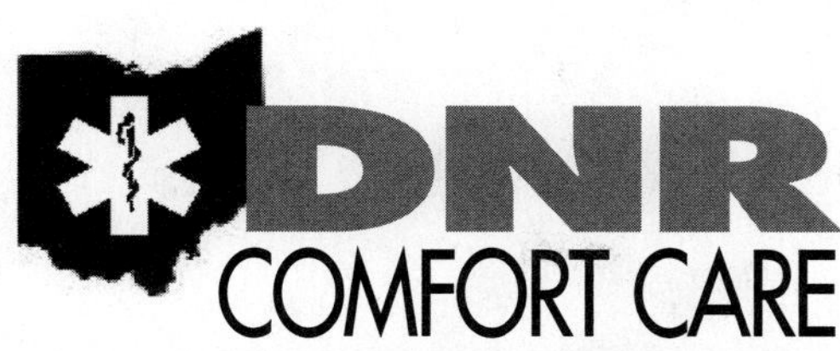

DNR IDENTIFICATION FORM

❑ **DNRCC**
(If this box is checked the DNR Comfort Care Protocol is activated immediately.)

❑ **DNRCC—Arrest**
(If this box is checked, the DNR Comfort Care Protocol is implemented in the event of a cardiac arrest or a respiratory arrest.)

Patient Name:____

Address:____

City________________________ State________ Zip________

Birthdate________________ Gender ❑ M ❑ F

Signature____________________________ (optional)

Certification of DNR Comfort Care Status (to be completed by the physician)*

(Check only one box)
❑ **Do-Not-Resuscitate Order**—My signature below constitutes and confirms a formal order to emergency medical services and other health care personnel that the person identified above is to be treated under the State of Ohio DNR Protocol. I affirm that this order is not contrary to reasonable medical standards or, to the best of my knowledge, contrary to the wishes of the person or of another person who is lawfully authorized to make informed medical decisions on the person's behalf. I also affirm that I have documented the grounds for this order in the person's medical record.

❑ **Living Will (Declaration) and Qualifying Condition**—The person identified above has a valid Ohio Living will (declaration) and has been certified by two physicians in accordance with Ohio law as being terminal or in a permanent unconscious state, or both.

Printed name of physician*:______________________________

Signature____________________ Date________________

Address:____________________ Phone________________

City/State____________________ Zip________________

* A DNR order may be issued by a certified nurse practitioner or clinical nurse specialist when authorized by section 2133.211 of the Ohio Revised Code.

See reverse side for DNR Protocol

Page 1 of 2

FIGURE 3-1 ✻ An Ohio EMS DNR identification form.

Once this has been accomplished, you must attempt to get the patient to sign an official "release from liability" form. The signed form—or a patient's witnessed refusal to sign the form—is only a part of the documentation of the case. You must document what you told the patient in regard to his condition and the potential consequences of refusing care as well as the patient's continued refusal. Basically, you must write down what you told the patient, and the patient's response. Be sure to get the patient and at least one witness, someone other than your partner, to sign the form.

When in doubt, always err in favor of providing care to the patient. If necessary, contact medical direction for advice.

Protecting Yourself in Refusal Situations

Complete and accurate documentation is a key factor in protecting yourself from liability for malpractice in the form of negligence or abandonment when a patient refuses treatment. Do the following before you leave the scene:

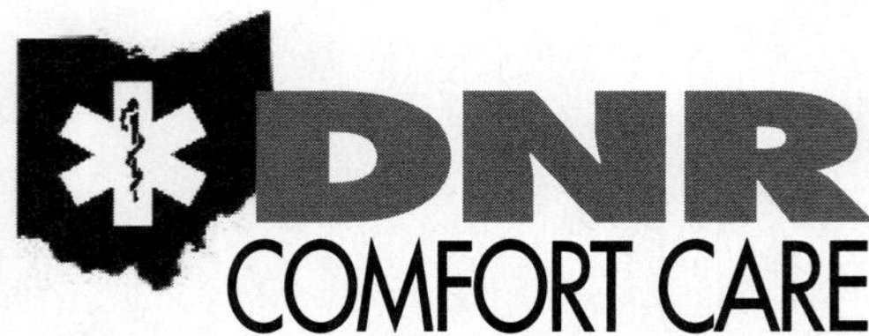

DO NOT RESUSCITATE COMFORT CARE PROTOCOL

After the State of Ohio DNR Protocol has been activated for a specific DNR Comfort Care patient, the Protocol specifies that emergency medical services and other health care workers are to do the following:

WILL:

- Suction the airway
- Administer oxygen
- Position for comfort
- Splint or immobilize
- Control bleeding
- Provide pain medication
- Provide emotional support
- Contact other appropriate health care providers such as hospice, home health, attending physician/CNS/CNP

WILL NOT:

- Administer chest compressions
- Insert artificial air way
- Administer resuscitative drugs
- Defibrillate or cardiovert
- Provide respiratory assistance (other than that listed above)
- Initiate resuscitative IV
- Initiate cardiac monitoring

If you have responded to an emergency situation by initiating any of the **WILL NOT** actions prior to confirming that the DNR Comfort Care Protocol should be activated, discontinue them when you activate the Protocol. You may continue respiratory assistance, IV medications, etc., that have been part of the patient's ongoing course of treatment for an underlying disease.

Page 2 of 2

FIGURE 3-1 ✻ An Ohio EMS DNR identification form. *continued*

- **Try again to persuade the patient to accept treatment or transport to a hospital.** Tell the patient why treatment or transport is essential. Be especially clear and diligent in explaining the possible consequences of refusal. Document your attempts to convince the patient as well as the consequences of refusal, and have the patient read aloud from the report to verify understanding.
- **Make sure the patient is competent and able to make a rational, informed decision.** A patient who is emotionally, intellectually, or physically impaired by illness or injury may not be capable of absorbing all the information you give. Make sure that the patient is not suicidal and not under the influence of drugs, alcohol, or other mind-altering substances.
- **Consult medical direction as needed, or as required by local protocol.**
- **If the patient still refuses, clearly document what was told to the patient, his response, and**

Thinking Critically

A family fight occurs over your terminally ill patient. His wife has a paper where the patient has scrawled "Don't revive me," his signature, and yesterday's date. His sister says "That's not legal. You have to keep him alive!" The patient goes into arrest. What should you do?

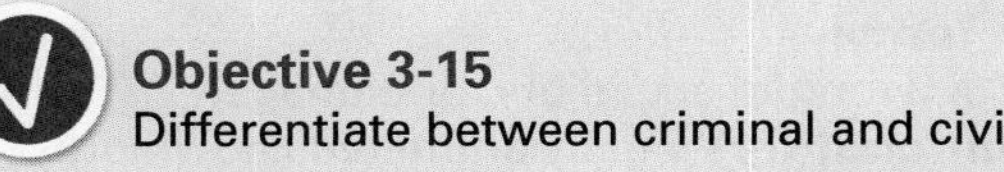

Objective 3-15

Differentiate between criminal and civil liability.

Objectives 3-16 and 3-17

Explain the concept of negligence and discuss ways to avoid various types of tort claims.

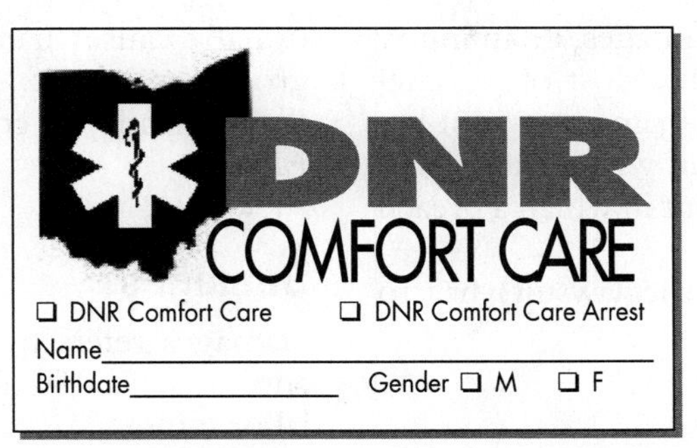

DNR
COMFORT CARE

☐ DNR Comfort Care ☐ DNR Comfort Care Arrest

Name____________________

Birthdate__________ Gender ☐ M ☐ F

Physician name____________________

Physician phone____________________

Other emergency phone____________________

The person named on the front of this card may revoke DNR Comfort Care status by destroying this card.

(a)

DNR COMFORT CARE

Name____________________ Gender__________

Physician's name____________________ Physician's Phone__________

☐ DNRCC ☐ DNRCC—ARREST

(b)

FIGURE 3-2 * DNR documents may also take alternative forms, as these examples from Ohio EMS show: **(a)** a DNR wallet card, and **(b)** a DNR hospital bracelet.

have him sign a refusal form. In some areas the form must be signed by witnesses (follow local protocol). If the patient refuses to sign the form, attempt to get signed statements of witnesses that the patient refused to sign. (How to document a patient refusal is discussed in greater detail in Chapter 4, "Documentation.")

- **Before you leave the scene, encourage the patient to seek help if certain symptoms develop.** If possible, be specific. Say things like "If you have a burning pain in your stomach" or "If you start seeing double." Avoid technical terms the patient might not understand. Document the fact that you encouraged the patient to seek help later.
- **If you are unsure whether the patient is able to make a rational decision, contact medical direction** for a consultation as to whether to treat and transport.

Other Legal Aspects of Emergency Care

Negligence

If you breach your legal duty, you create a liability. Two types of liability are criminal and civil. In a criminal liability case, the government, on behalf of the public, brings legal action against the EMT. This may result in a fine or even incarceration. In a civil action, an individual, known as the plaintiff, files a lawsuit against an individual EMT, the EMS agency or company, or others indirectly involved in the care of the patient, such as the supervisor or medical director. These latter individuals are known as the defendants. In a civil action, the defendant is accused of committing a **tort**, which is a wrongful act, injury, or damage. In civil or tort cases, the plaintiff usually seeks

Key Terms
tort a wrongful act, injury, or damage; **intentional tort** when committed knowingly.

negligence deviating from an accepted standard of care through carelessness, inattention, disregard, inadvertence, or oversight.

Key Terms
proximate cause when deviation from an accepted standard of care results in further injury to the patient.

abandonment discontinuing care without transferring care to a health care professional with equivalent or better training.

monetary compensation for an act, damages, or an injury that resulted from the EMT's actions. Most often, lawsuits against EMS involve negligence from a duty not being performed. **Negligence** is a tort in which there is no intent to do any harm to the patient but in which a breach in the duty to act occurred.

The plaintiff (person who files the lawsuit) has to prove the following four elements:

- The EMT had a duty to act.
- The EMT breached that duty to act.
- The patient suffered an injury or harm that is recognized by the law as a compensable injury.
- The injuries were the result of the breach of the duty (proximate cause).

If the plaintiff cannot prove all four of the elements, the suit will fail and no damages will be awarded.

Two common legal principles are often associated with negligence claims against EMS. The first is *res ipsa loquitur*, meaning "the thing speaks for itself." This concept is used in cases where a caregiver's inappropriate actions are obviously the cause of patient harm. The concept of *negligence per se* means that an act is considered to be negligent simply because it is in violation of a statute or regulation such as written EMS protocols or approved scope of practice.

Duty to Act

Duty to act, as described earlier in the chapter, is an obligation of the EMT to respond to the scene and to provide emergency care to the patient. Once a patient relationship has been established, which is simply done by the EMT making contact with the patient with the intent to provide emergency care, it cannot be terminated without the consent of the patient.

Breach of Duty to Act

A breach of the duty to act is when the EMT deviates from the standard of care. *Negligence* is a deviation from the standard of care. *Simple negligence* occurs when an EMT fails to perform care or when a mistake is made in the treatment. *Gross negligence* is willful, wanton, or extremely reckless patient care far beyond being negligent or careless. Gross negligence is care that is construed as being dangerous to the patient. An EMT who intentionally causes harm to a patient will be charged with gross negligence. Gross negligence may be so severe that it leads to criminal charges brought against the EMT.

Damages

Damages refers to injuries that are real, demonstrable, and recognizable by the law. The injuries cannot be trivial or minor.

Proximate Cause

It must be determined that the injuries suffered by the patient were the direct result of the EMT's negligence. This is referred to as **proximate cause** or causation. By contrast, the patient's injuries may be a result of the traumatic event or the underlying disease and not the negligence of the EMT.

Intentional Tort

An **intentional tort** is an action knowingly committed by an individual that is considered to be civilly wrong according to the law. Common intentional torts in EMS are abandonment, assault, battery, false imprisonment, and defamation. The primary difference between an intentional tort and negligence is that negligence is a failure to meet the standard of care that is typically permissible, whereas an intentional tort is knowingly committed.

Abandonment

If you stop treatment of the patient without transferring the care to another competent professional of an equal or higher level of training and certification or licensure, it would be considered **abandonment** (Figure 3-3*). Abandonment can occur in the emergency department if you do not officially transfer the care of the patient or if the transfer is to an inappropriate medical professional. For example, if you arrive at the emergency department, place the patient in an emergency department room, notify the ward clerk or secretary that the patient is there, and then leave the patient, you have just abandoned the patient. You must give an oral report to a physician, nurse, or other health care worker who is qualified to care for that patient and the injuries he has sustained or the

Key Terms

assault a threat to inflict harm on a person.

battery touching a person without his consent.

false imprisonment detention of a person without his consent or other legal authority.

Key Terms

defamation false communication that injures another person's reputation.

slander defaming through spoken statements with malicious intent or reckless disregard.

libel defaming through writing or mass media with malicious intent or reckless disregard.

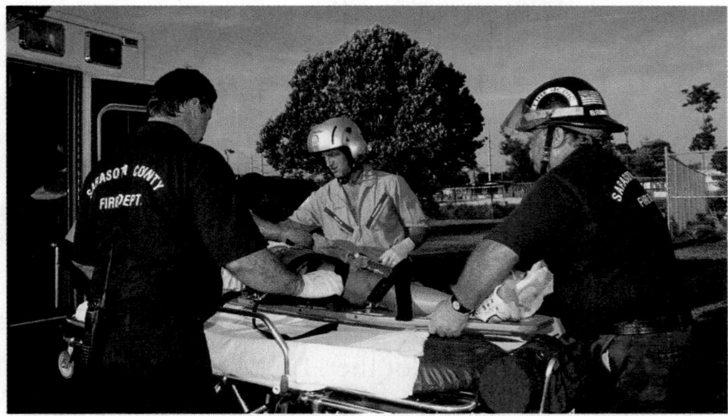

FIGURE 3-3 * EMTs transferring care to a flight crew for transport to a trauma center. You must always transfer care of the patient to a professional of equal or better training to avoid charges of abandonment. (© Maria A. H. Lyle)

condition he is suffering from. Simply moving the patient from your stretcher to the hospital bed does not constitute a patient transfer of care.

An EMT can fully assume the transfer of care of a patient at the scene from a paramedic or Advanced EMT only if the patient's condition or injuries can be managed by the EMT and no advanced life support skills are necessary. On the other hand, if the EMT transfers care of a multisystem trauma patient to a physician who is a dermatologist, the EMT has potentially abandoned the patient. Typically, a dermatologist is not qualified to manage a multisystem trauma patient.

Performing a thorough assessment and always providing care that is in the best interest of the patient will likely eliminate the risk of abandonment.

Assault

Assault is a willful threat to inflict harm on a patient. Assault can occur without actually touching the patient. If the patient has the apprehension of bodily harm and the EMT has the ability to do so, it would be considered assault. If the EMT threatens to stick the patient with an epinephrine auto-injector and holds it up in front of the patient, the EMT has potentially created a fear in the patient that the act will be committed.

Battery

Battery is the act of touching a patient unlawfully without his consent. If you don't seek and obtain consent, your emergency care might be construed as battery by the patient, even though your intention is good. Without consent, your touching of the patient is unlawful.

False Imprisonment or Kidnapping

If a patient is competent and refuses your assessment, treatment, and transport, you must obey his wishes. Taking the patient to the hospital or other medical care facility against his wishes may result in charges of **false imprisonment** or kidnapping. False imprisonment results from intentionally transporting a competent patient without his consent. It is not necessary that the patient is restrained, it is simply not allowing the competent patient to withdraw from treatment and transport when he desires to do so.

Defamation

If you release information to the public in either a written or spoken form that is construed to be damaging to that person's character, reputation, or standing within the community, you can be charged with **defamation**. The spoken form of defamation is **slander**. It is extremely important that you discuss patient, partner, and other emergency issues in a private setting and never in public. **Libel** is putting a false or damaging statement in written form or via mass media. Follow the correct policies and procedures for complaints against others so that you avoid any litigation involving defamation of character.

As an EMT, it is important to understand these components of a potential or real lawsuit. The best defense against such a suit is to provide emergency care to the best of your ability and to be sure that you understand clearly your scope of practice and the expected standard of care.

Confidentiality

While many jurisdictions do not have specific laws about confidentiality, laws do exist that prevent the invasion of a person's privacy. Some of them apply to cases involving emergency care, specifically to information obtained while getting a patient history, performing a physical assessment, and treating the patient. In many states, the deliberate invasion of a patient's privacy by an EMT may lead to loss of certification or licensure and other legal actions.

Do not speak to the press, your family, friends, or other members of the public about details of the emergency care

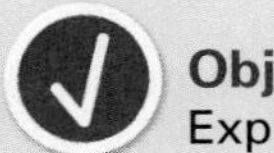

Objective 3-18
Explain patients' rights and your responsibilities re confidentiality and privacy.

Objective 3-19
Describe COBRA and EMTALA provisions as they apply to EMS.

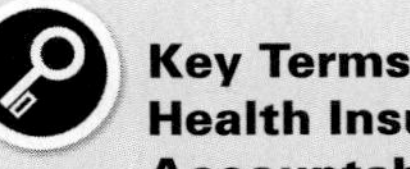

Key Terms
Health Insurance Portability and Accountability Act (HIPAA) protects the privacy of, and gives the patient control over, patient health care information.

you provided to a patient. If you speak about the emergency, you must not relate specifics about what a patient said, who the patient was with, and anything unusual about the patient's behavior or personal appearance. The same restrictions hold true of information you receive from another member of the EMS system. Confidentiality applies not only to cases of physical injury, but also to cases involving possible infectious diseases, illnesses, and emotional and psychological emergencies.

Releasing confidential information requires a written release form signed by the patient or a legal guardian. You should not release confidential written or spoken information about the patient to someone claiming to be a legal guardian until you have established legal guardianship. By law, you are allowed to release confidential patient information without a patient's or guardian's permission if:

- Another health care provider needs to know the information in order to continue medical care.
- An official public health or other governmental agency requires mandatory reporting of information related to your contact with the patient. State laws, for example, commonly require the reporting of incidents of rape, child abuse, elder abuse, neglect, domestic violence, certain communicable diseases, gunshots, stab wounds, animal bites, suspicious burns, and certain other crimes or conditions.
- You are requested by the police to provide the information as part of a potential criminal investigation.
- A third-party billing form requires the information.
- You are required by legal subpoena to provide the information in court.

Health Insurance Portability and Accountability Act (HIPAA)

The **Health Insurance Portability and Accountability Act (HIPAA)** of 1996 is a federal law that protects the privacy of patient health care information and gives the patient control over how the information is distributed and used. HIPAA requires strict adherence to policies and procedures regarding record keeping, storage, access, release, and discussion of patient medical records. EMS systems are required by federal law to have specific policies and procedures in place regarding confidentiality and privacy issues related to patient care records and information. Every person in the EMS system that comes into contact with patients or patient information must be aware of and understand these policies and procedures.

In regard to HIPAA and your practice as an EMT, you will find the following:

- You will be limited to discussing patient-specific information only with individuals with whom it is medically necessary to do so. You cannot go out into the ambulance bay area and begin to discuss your previous patient using specific patient information. There is no medical necessity in doing so and it can be construed as a violation of the HIPAA regulations.
- You will be trained on specific policies and procedures regarding privacy issues by your EMS agency.
- You and the patient will be provided with the patient privacy policies and procedures. It is your responsibility to obtain a signature from the patient acknowledging that he received the information. The form is often included with the insurance release form.
- Your EMS agency will have a designated Privacy Officer who will oversee HIPAA regulations. This is a good resource person to contact regarding issues related to patient-specific information.

If someone is requesting information from you, contact the person in your EMS system who is charged with the responsibility of managing and protecting confidential information. This is the most appropriate person to make the determination as to whether any information should be released and what information can be released and to whom without violating the privacy rights of the patient.

COBRA and EMTALA

The **Consolidated Omnibus Budget Reconciliation Act (COBRA)** and the **Emergency Medical Treatment and Active Labor Act (EMTALA)** are federal regulations that ensure the public's access to emergency health care regardless of ability to pay. They are intended to eliminate any discrimination in who is provided emergency medical care. The regulations prevent "patient dumping," in which a patient requiring medical care is turned away at the door or transferred to a public hospital because of inability to pay for the services. EMTALA is also known as the "anti-patient-dumping statute." EMTALA specifically deals with a patient seeking medical care for an emergency medical condition, whether it is due to an injury or an illness. Even though both regulations are primarily geared

Key Terms

Consolidated Omnibus Budget Reconciliation Act (COBRA) and **Emergency Medical Treatment and Active Labor Act (EMTALA)** regulations that ensure public access to emergency health care regardless of ability to pay.

Objective 3-20
Discuss how you can protect yourself legally in transport and transfer situations.

Objective 3-21
Describe special considerations for patients who are potential organ donors.

toward hospital treatment and transfer, EMS personnel are affected by certain aspects of the regulations, especially if the ambulance service is owned and operated by the hospital.

EMS becomes involved when patients are being transferred from a hospital to another medical facility. The key issue is the requirement of the transferring facility to ensure that the patient is stabilized to the best of the medical facility's ability prior to transfer. This does not mean that the patient cannot be a critical patient or would have no chance of deteriorating en route. However, the transferring facility must ensure that the ambulance crew performing the transfer is qualified and capable of managing the patient and his condition. For example, an EMT crew would not be able to perform a transfer of a patient requiring continuous electrocardiogram monitoring and intravenous infusion monitoring and drug therapy, because these skills are beyond an EMT's scope of practice. In this case, it would be the responsibility of the EMT to contact his supervisor or follow the EMS policies to notify the transferring facility that the EMT crew is not capable of doing the transfer. If the transfer is done, it could be an EMTALA violation. As an EMT, you have a responsibility to make sure that the patient is stable enough for transfer. If there is a question, it may be necessary for your EMS medical director to contact the transferring physician to discuss whether the EMS crew is capable of conducting the transfer. This must be done prior to loading the patient onto your cot and initiating the patient transfer.

If you are operating a hospital-based ambulance and make a decision to bypass your hospital, which is the closest appropriate medical facility, and take the patient to another medical facility because the patient does not have insurance nor the ability to pay for services, you can be charged with "patient dumping" under the EMTALA regulation.

Protecting Yourself in Transport and Transfer Situations

In an emergency transport to a medical facility, do not make a decision to transport to a specific medical facility based on the patient's ability to pay. Never report this information over the radio. Do not bypass a medical facility that is able to treat the patient, unless you are directed to do so by medical direction or the patient or predetermined protocol. Be sure to clearly document the reason for bypassing the medical facility.

If you are performing a transfer between hospitals or medical facilities:

- Get a full and clear report about the patient's condition.
- Ensure that you are able to provide the level of care necessary during the transport and it is within your scope of practice.
- Obtain the informed consent form signed by the patient or his legal guardian allowing for the transfer.
- Obtain the written certification of transfer that includes the transferring physician's name and address, facility receiving the patient, and the reason for the transfer.
- Know where you are going and take the quickest possible route.

Special Situations

Donors and Organ Harvesting

Organs can be donated only if there is a legal signed document giving permission to harvest the organs. A signed donor card is considered a legal document. A sticker affixed to the reverse side of a patient's driver's license, or an "organ donor" specification printed directly on the license, provides an intent to donate organs.

A potential organ donor should be treated no differently than any other patient requiring emergency care. The individual is a patient first, an organ donor last. In addition to providing appropriate care, you can assist the organ harvesting procedure as follows:

- Identify the patient as a potential donor based on the type of injuries or illness and treatment that was rendered. Patients who are about to die or who have died within hours are potential organ donors. In each case, however, hospital staff and the patient's family make the ultimate decision.
- Communicate with medical direction regarding the possibility of organ donation. You can initiate this process by alerting the receiving hospital's emergency department staff, who will in turn contact other necessary departments.
- Provide emergency care, such as CPR, that will help maintain vital organs in case harvesting is attempted. This is best accomplished by treating every patient equally well.

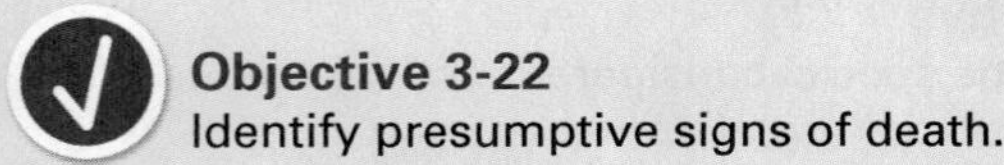

Objective 3-22
Identify presumptive signs of death.

Objective 3-23
Identify situations in which law enforcement or the medical examiner's/coroner's office should be contacted.

Medical Identification Insignia

A patient with a medical condition, such as an allergy, diabetes, or epilepsy, may be wearing or carrying a medical identification tag, such as a bracelet, necklace, or card (Figure 3-4*). Look for them during assessment. Note that medical identification insignia may also list a phone number you can call for specific treatment and medication requirements.

Recognizing Death in the Field

It is the ultimate responsibility of a physician to determine the cause of death. However, in some situations you may have to make a judgment as to whether to attempt resuscitation or not. As a general rule, if the patient is still warm and does not exhibit any obvious signs of death, begin resuscitation. An exception is hypothermia (low body temperature) where the patient's body is extremely cold and rigid. Hypothermic patients have survived long periods of cardiac arrest and cannot be considered dead until rewarmed.

When dealing with patients holding a DNR order or those with terminal illness, it is necessary to determine the presumptive signs of death. These include the following:

- Absence of a pulse, breathing, and breath sounds
- Complete unresponsiveness to any stimuli
- No eye movement or pupil response
- Absence of a blood pressure
- No reflexes

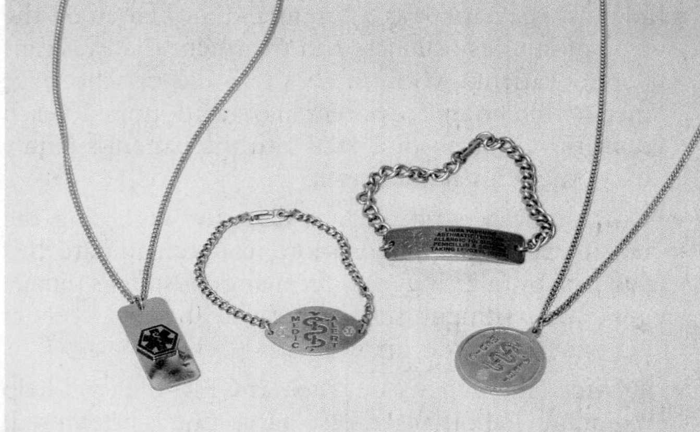

FIGURE 3-4 * Medical identification jewelry.

There are some situations in which signs of death are obvious and resuscitative efforts are not necessary. The obvious signs of death include:

- Decapitation
- Rigor mortis (body becomes stiff within 2–12 hours)
- Decomposition of the body
- Dependent lividity (discoloration of the skin from blood pooling that is effected by gravity) (Figure 3-5*)

Cases involving violent, unusual, or suspicious causes of death usually require investigation by the medical examiner or coroner. The medical examiner or coroner is usually called for:

- Homicides
- Suicides
- Violent deaths (including suspected child or elder abuse)
- Crash-related deaths (auto, motorcycle, all-terrain vehicle, snowmobile)
- Unusual scene characteristics (e.g., burns, electrocution)
- Sudden infant death syndrome (SIDS)
- Dead on arrival (depending on your local protocol)

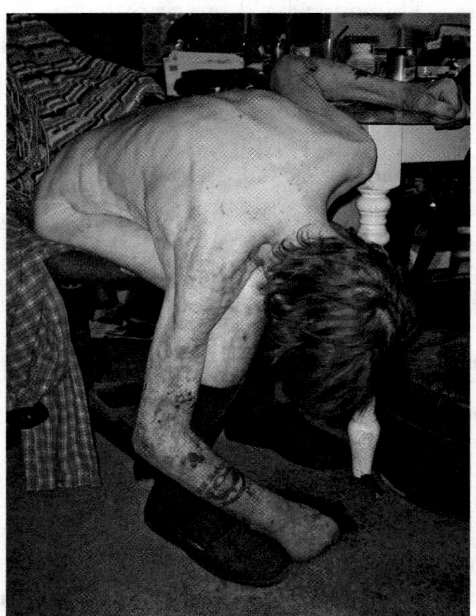

FIGURE 3-5 * Dependent lividity in a dead person. (© Skye Carpenter)

Objective 3-24
Discuss special considerations in responding to potential crime scenes.

Objective 3-25
Describe situations in which the EMT may be mandated to make a report, such as suspected abuse, crimes, and infectious diseases.

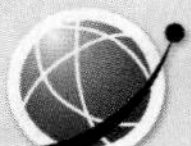

Media Resources
Go to www.bradybooks.com for mykit. Highlights:

- *Web Resource:* HIPAA Information
- *Web Resource:* Organ Donation

It is important to understand your local protocol related to death-in-the-field situations. It is better to err to benefit the patient and begin resuscitation if you have any doubt. Also, be sure you understand the situations in which the medical examiner or coroner must be called to investigate a field death.

Crime Scenes

Whenever an EMS is called to a potential crime scene, dispatch should also notify the police. Recognizing a possible crime scene requires a high index of suspicion. As a general guideline, a potential crime scene is any scene that may require police support, including a potential or actual suicide, homicide, drug overdose, domestic dispute, rape, abuse, hit-and-run accident, riot, robbery, gunfire, or potentially dangerous weapons.

Your first concern upon approaching a crime scene should be for your own safety. If you suspect that a crime is in progress or a criminal is still active at the scene, do not attempt to provide care to any patient. Wait until the police declare that the scene is safe. Keep in mind that even when the police declare the scene safe to enter, it can still be potentially dangerous.

Once the scene is secure, your priority is emergency care of the patient. However, also try to avoid disturbing anything that may be considered evidence:

- Take one way in and out.
- Touch only what you need to touch, and remember to tell a police officer if you move or touch anything.
- Move only what you need to move to protect the patient and to provide proper emergency care.
- Do not use a crime scene telephone unless the police give you permission to do so.
- In the absence of police permission, move the patient only if the patient is in danger or must be moved in order for you to provide care.
- Observe and document anything unusual.
- If possible, do not cut through holes in clothing possibly caused by bullets or stabbing.
- Do not cut through any knot in a rope or tie (a possible clue). Cut away from the knot. Do not cover the patient with a sheet.
- If the crime is rape, do not wash the patient or allow the patient to wash. Ask the patient not to change clothing, use the bathroom, or take anything by mouth, because doing so may destroy evidence. While you cannot force a person to avoid these activities, explain your reasons. Most will cooperate.

As an EMT, you may have a legal duty to report situations in which injury may have resulted from commission of a crime. Learn your local protocols.

Special Reporting Situations

You may be required to report certain conditions. Familiarize yourself with the requirements in your state. The following are commonly required reporting situations:

- **Abuse.** Many states require people to report suspected child abuse. Some states have very broad requirements, whereas others require reporting only from physicians. Such statutes frequently grant immunity from liability for libel, slander, or defamation of character as long as the report is made in good faith. In some states, laws also exist regarding the reporting of other kinds of abuse, such as abuse of the elderly and spousal abuse.
- **Crime.** Many states require EMTs to report an injury that may have resulted from a crime or to report injuries such as gunshot wounds, knife wounds, suspicious burns, and poisonings. Your state may also require you to report any injury that you suspect was caused by sexual assault.
- **Drug-related injuries.** Some states require you to report drug-related injuries. However, the U.S. Supreme Court has ruled that drug addiction—not drug possession—is an illness, not a crime.

Other situations you may be required to report include suspected infectious disease exposure, use of patient restraints to treat or transport patients against their will, cases in which a patient appears to be mentally incompetent or intoxicated, attempted suicides, and dog bites. Learn the laws in your state regarding situations you are required to report.

CHAPTER REVIEW

SUMMARY

Medical, legal, and ethical issues must always be considered when performing emergency care. EMTs must function within their scope of practice and to an acceptable standard of care. The scope of practice identifies what emergency care the EMT is legally able to perform, whereas the standard of care addresses whether the care was performed according to an accepted level of practice.

EMTs have a duty to act, that is, a legal obligation to respond and provide emergency care for the patient. However, your duty goes beyond providing emergency care. For example, you have a duty to remain up to date in all of your certifications and licensure, to check all equipment to ensure it is in working order, and to remain physically and emotionally fit to perform your job.

Medical direction provides the EMT with the legal right to function in the prehospital setting. Medical direction should be involved in providing medical oversight in all aspects of the emergency medical services system.

Before you assess the patient or provide emergency care, you must obtain consent from the patient. You must inform the patient of the assessment and emergency care to be provided and any consequences or risks associated with that care. Expressed consent involves the patient providing some type of acknowledgment or affirmation of the consent. Implied consent is used for patients who are unable to provide consent, such as a patient with an altered mental status but who, it is assumed, would provide consent if he were able to do so. Minor consent is a type of implied consent used when providing emergency care for minors whose parents or guardians are not present or able to give consent. Involuntary consent involves a third party and is used for those patients who are either mentally incapable or legally prevented from making their own health care decisions.

A competent patient has the right to refuse emergency care or to withdraw from emergency care or transport at any time. It is imperative that the patient is competent and able to make a rational decision before you accept his refusal. Clear and accurate documentation is the key to any patient refusal. Advance directives are predetermined orders that provide for refusal of care or resuscitation, commonly in terminally ill patients.

The most common type of lawsuit filed against an EMT is a tort. A tort is a civil action that often involves negligence. Four elements of negligence must be proven for the action to succeed: (1) that there was a duty to act, (2) that there was a breach in that duty, (3) that an injury occurred, and (4) that the injury resulted from the actions of the EMT. Other legal issues that the EMT must thoroughly understand are abandonment, battery, assault, false imprisonment, and defamation.

All information related to a patient on an EMS call must be held in the strictest confidence. Any information that could possibly identify the patient must not be released unless in certain legal and acceptable situations, such as to the medical staff to whom you are transferring care of the patient. The Health Insurance Portability and Accountability Act (HIPAA) has strict rules regarding the storage and release of patient information. You must clearly understand and abide by the policies of your EMS agency regarding patient information.

COBRA and EMTALA are federal regulations that have implications on the public's access to emergency health care. These regulations pertain primarily to medical facilities; however, EMS may be affected by these regulations when involved in transferring a patient to another medical facility.

Crime scenes warrant special attention by the EMT. The chain of evidence must not be disrupted and evidence must be preserved for law enforcement use. Disrupt a crime scene only if it is necessary to provide immediate emergency care to the patient. It is also important for you to be able to recognize patients who are obviously dead, whether as a result of crime or from natural causes.

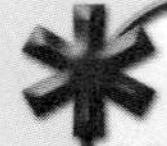

CASE STUDY FOLLOW-UP

SCENE SIZE-UP

You and your partner are dispatched to the scene of an elderly male complaining of abdominal pain. As you scan for hazards, you notice that there is clutter everywhere in the house and that the inside temperature is very cool. Although the patient's wife is alert, she seems confused. She changes the subject often and keeps asking your partner if she is her daughter Ellen.

PATIENT ASSESSMENT

Your general impression of Mr. Schuman is that he is conscious but disoriented and experiencing abdominal pain. His wife is unsure of his age, so you estimate that he is in his mid-80s. He responds to questions with unintelligible mumbled words. His airway is open; breathing and circulation appear normal. He does not appear to be in acute distress. Your partner applies an oxygen mask to provide

Mr. Schuman high-flow, high-concentration oxygen, which may help his mental condition as well as his apparent abdominal condition.

Trying to obtain a complete history is impossible, since the patient cannot respond coherently. Instead you perform a rapid assessment, a quick head-to-toe physical exam. Upon palpation of the abdomen, Mr. Schuman tries to force your hand away. If he were competent, you might take this gesture as a refusal of care. However, because of his disorientation, you continue providing care. You measure and record baseline vital signs—breathing rate; pulse; pupils; skin color, temperature, and condition; and blood pressure.

When you try to obtain a medical history from Mrs. Schuman, she does not understand. All she wants to do is show you her porcelain doll collection.

You prepare Mr. Schuman for transport and help his wife find a coat. During transport, you reassess the patient and find no change in his condition.

AN ETHICAL OBLIGATION

After transferring Mr. Schuman to hospital personnel, you contact the hospital's social service department, as you are required to do in case of elderly abuse or neglect. While you saw no signs of intentional abuse or neglect, you do believe that the Schumans are not capable of caring for themselves, and you are therefore ethically responsible to report the situation to ensure their safety after discharge.

Two weeks later you see the social worker who tells you that Mr. Schuman was diagnosed with a gastric ulcer and organic brain syndrome. Additionally, Mrs. Schuman has been diagnosed with Alzheimer disease. Both are now residents of a local extended-care nursing home, under 24-hour supervision. The social worker thanks you and your partner for bringing this case to his attention.

IN REVIEW

1. Define a "do not resuscitate (DNR)" order, and explain how an EMT should respond if presented with such an order.
2. Define three types of consent that must be obtained before emergency care is provided.
3. Explain how to handle a refusal of treatment.
4. Describe what must happen for the EMT to be liable for abandonment or negligence.
5. Describe what it means for an EMT to have a duty to act.
6. List the conditions under which an EMT may release confidential patient information.
7. List some ways in which an EMT can preserve evidence at a crime scene.
8. List situations that an EMT may be required to report.

CRITICAL THINKING

You are called to the scene for a 34-year-old female patient complaining of abdominal pain. Upon arrival, you find the patient lying in bed. She is alert and is holding her abdomen. She states that she is having bad "belly pain" that began about an hour prior to her calling 911. You perform an assessment, place the patient on oxygen, and prepare her for transport. The patient suddenly states, "I don't want to go to the hospital."

1. How would you initially gain consent in this patient?
2. How would you manage the patient's refusal to be transported?
3. What legal issues may you face if you continue with treatment and transport?

EXPLORE PEARSON **mybradykit**™

Please go to **www.bradybooks.com** to access mykit for this text. You will find quizzes, critical thinking scenarios, weblinks, animations, and videos related to this chapter—and much more. Look for online information on HIPAA and organ donation.

Register your access code from the front of your book by going to **www.bradybooks.com** and selecting the mykit links.

CHAPTER 4

Documentation

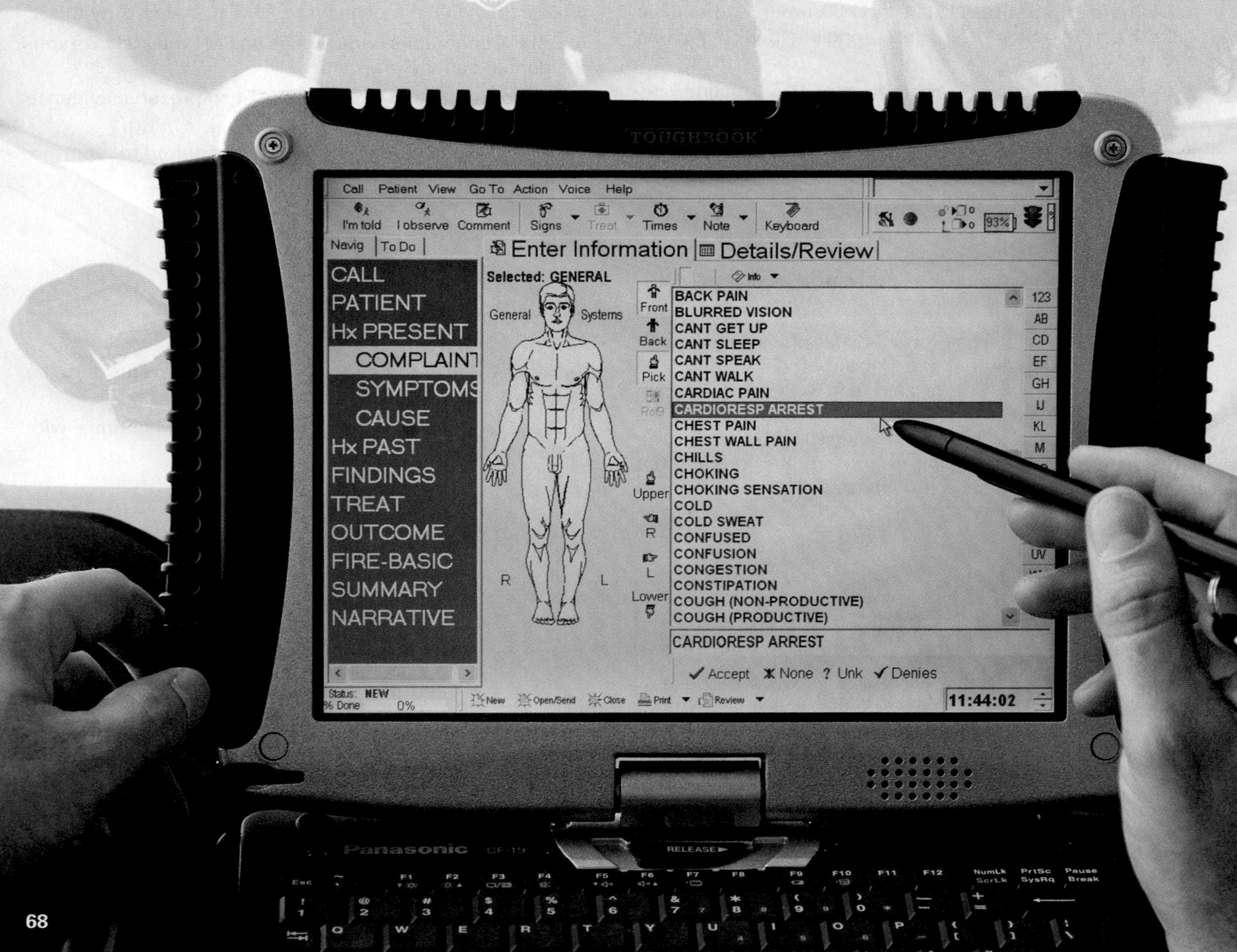

Navigation Guide

The following items provide an overview to the purpose and content of this chapter. The Education Standard and Competency are from the new National EMS Education Standards.

STANDARD **Preparatory** (Content Area: Documentation)

COMPETENCY Applies fundamental knowledge of the EMS system, safety/well-being of the EMT, medical/legal and ethical issues to the provision of emergency care.

OBJECTIVES: After reading this chapter, you should be able to:

4-1. Define key terms introduced in this chapter.
4-2. Describe each of the following purposes served by the prehospital care report (PCR):
  a. Continuity of patient care
  b. Administrative uses
  c. Legal document
  d. Education and research
  e. Evaluation and continuous quality improvement (CQI)
4-3. Describe characteristics, including advantages and disadvantages, of both paper and computer-based (electronic) PCR formats.
4-4. Explain the purposes of the U.S. Department of Transportation (DOT) minimum data set for PCRs.
4-5. List the elements of the DOT minimum data set for PCRs.
4-6. Describe the purpose and contents of each of the following sections of a PCR:
  a. Administrative data
  b. Patient demographics and other patient data
  c. Vital signs
  d. Narrative
  e. Treatment
4-7. Give examples of each of the following types of PCR narrative information:
  a. Chief complaint
  b. Pertinent history
  c. Subjective information
  d. Objective information
  e. Pertinent negatives
4-8. Use common abbreviations and medical terminology accurately in PCRs.
4-9. Explain each of the following legal concerns with respect to the PCR:
  a. Confidentiality
  b. Allowed distribution of the PCR or information included in it
  c. Documenting a patient's refusal of treatment
  d. Falsification of the PCR
  e. Correction of errors
4-10. Discuss how to handle each of the following situations with respect to the PCR:
  a. Transfer of patient care when returning to service prior to completing the PCR
  b. Multiple-casualty incidents (MCIs)
  c. Special reporting situations, such as infectious disease exposure and suspicion of abuse or neglect
4-11. Accurately and completely record pertinent patient and EMS call information using the SOAP, CHART, and CHEATED methods.

KEY TERMS: Page references indicate first major use in this chapter. For complete definitions, see the Glossary at the back of the book.

minimum data set p. 75
pertinent negatives p. 76
prehospital care report (PCR) p. 70
triage tag p. 83

MEDIA RESOURCES: Please go to www.bradybooks.com to access mykit for this text. You will find quizzes, critical thinking scenarios, weblinks, animations, and videos related to this chapter—and much more. Look for online information on the National EMS Information System and on the importance of good documentation.

continued

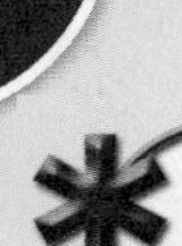

CASE STUDY

The Dispatch

EMS Unit 17—respond to 57 Vallejo Road. You have a man injured when his vehicle struck a parked car. Time out is 1321 hours.

Upon Arrival

You and your partner arrive at 1327 hours. As you drive up, you observe four people standing around two vehicles. As you get out of the ambulance, a woman walks over to you from the group. She says, "I called you. That's my van parked at the curb. I was in the house, heard a crash, looked out, and saw that that car had hit mine. The driver was slumped over the wheel, so I called 911 right away. When I came out of the house, though, he seemed to be all right. He's the one in the green shirt." She indicates a man who is pacing around inspecting the damage to the two vehicles.

You and your partner walk toward the man she points to, who appears to be in his mid-30s. He looks at you and says, "Great! As if I didn't have enough trouble today, I've got to deal with you guys! Go away. I don't need any help!"

How Would You Proceed to Assess, Care for, and Document This Patient Contact?

In this chapter, you will learn about the importance of documenting all your encounters with patients as well as the types of information that go into such documentation. Later, we will return to this case and apply what you have learned.

Introduction

Assessing a patient, treating him, and transporting him to a facility where he can receive necessary medical care are the most obvious parts of the EMT's job. But there is another function that you will have to perform as an EMT: documentation of data for each patient you come in contact with. That documentation, in the form of written or electronically generated records, will help ensure that the patient receives the best, most appropriate care at the facility to which he is transported. The most common type of record that is prepared and submitted is the **prehospital care report (PCR)**. The type of PCR varies widely among EMS systems and states; however, the information collected is basically the same. The documentation you generate and report via the PCR and other special reporting forms is important for other reasons as well, as you will learn in this chapter.

Functions of the Prehospital Care Report

The documentation you assemble and report via the prehospital care report serves a variety of functions. It can be helpful to the patient, to the medical personnel who treat him, to the organizations that have aided him, to scientists and researchers who may never come in actual contact with the patient, and also to you. These functions are discussed in the following paragraphs.

Continuity of Medical Care

The prime reason for high-quality documentation is, of course, high-quality patient care. Reporting the data you have obtained during your contact with a patient and recording, simply but completely, the emergency care rendered helps ensure continuity of care for the patient throughout his need for medical attention. Your documentation gives emergency department personnel the information they need to provide the most appropriate treatment in a timely manner.

When the emergency department staff study the description of a patient's mental status as well as the vital signs that you obtained and recorded during assessment and transport, they have a baseline against which that patient's improvement or deterioration can be measured. When they read your account of the patient's complaint and the signs and symptoms you have marked down, they have a clearer idea of what course they should follow in the treatment of that patient. When they note the interventions you have or have not performed, they know more clearly what measures to take and which would duplicate earlier efforts. In addition, your documentation will provide details from sources to which hospital personnel may have no access (e.g., bystanders, family, or awake patient).

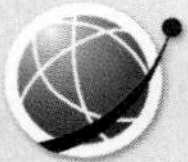

Media Resources
Go to www.bradybooks.com for mykit. Highlights:
- *Web Resource:* National EMS Information System

Key Terms
prehospital care report (PCR) documentation of an EMT's contact with a patient.

Objectives 4-2 and 4-3
Describe the purposes and formats of prehospital care reports (PCRs).

Administrative Uses

The documentation you provide typically becomes a part of the patient's permanent hospital record. It will be used in preparing bills and in submitting records to insurance companies. The information may also be used to contribute to statistics regarding the emergency medical service itself, such as the average response time, time on scene for critical trauma patients, or the number of cardiac arrest patients treated each year.

Legal Document

The medical documentation you prepare may also become a legal document. A run in which you were involved may have been the result of a crime. Or the incident may have led to a civil lawsuit. In either case, you may have to appear in court as a witness. Typically, the person who wrote the report will be the one called to testify in court. As such, you will refer to the documentation you generated for that run months or even years earlier. Legible, accurate, and complete documentation will be of major assistance in such cases. In addition, if you are the subject of a lawsuit, your documentation may be an essential element in your defense. Thus, it is important to clearly document objective and pertinent subjective findings, the status of the patient upon arrival on the scene, what emergency care was provided, when the emergency care was provided, and any changes in the patient's condition upon arrival at the medical facility.

Educational and Research Uses

Your documentation provides data for researchers studying a whole range of issues. Some researchers might be scientists looking to discover positive or negative effects of certain interventions at different stages of patient contact. Others might be experts in administration studying documentation in an effort to deliver services in a more timely or cost-effective manner. The PCR may be used to track or identify various patient presentations and conditions that may require additional education and training.

Evaluation and Continuous Quality Improvement

Reviews of documentation are an integral part of the quality improvement process. Remedial and continuing education courses for EMTs may be based on needs revealed by call documentation. PCRs are also used in medical oversight to determine if EMTs are adhering to protocols and the set standard of care for your area.

Collection of Data in Prehospital Care Reports

As you can see, the documentation you are responsible for (Figure 4-1*) has a variety of important uses. You should be as careful and thorough as possible when assembling it. The prehospital care report is a major piece of documentation you must provide for each patient encounter.

The PCR can have different names in different parts of the country, such as the run report or the trip sheet. The look of the PCR can also vary, depending on the format used for it and the information required on it.

PCR Formats

The most traditional format for the PCR is the written report. This format usually combines check boxes and write-on lines for vital signs and other information that can be entered briefly, along with areas for writing a fuller narrative account of the patient contact (Figure 4-2*).

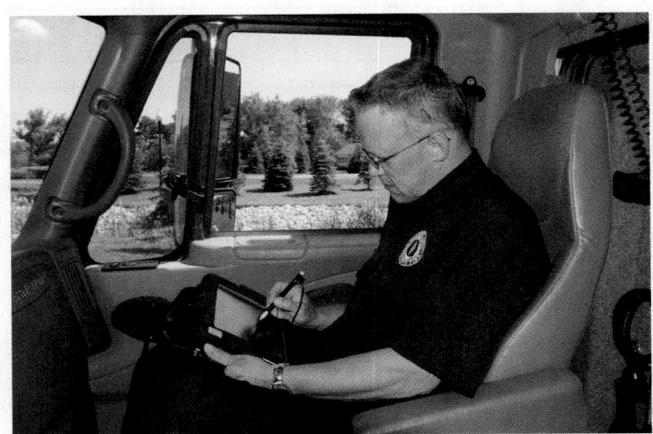

FIGURE 4-1 * Documentation has a variety of important uses.

TRIP#
MEDIC# LIC
BEGIN MILES
END MILES
CODE ___/___ PAGE ___/___
UNITS ON SCENE

Rural/Metro Ambulance
50 Years of Serving Others

PATIENT CARE REPORT

1-800-231-4872

❑ EMERGENCY DEPARTMENT
❑ INTER-FACILITY
❑ T-N-T REFUSAL/ STAND-BY

DAY
DATE
RECEIVED
DISPATCHED
EN-ROUTE
ON SCENE
PT. CONTACT
TO HOSPITAL
AT HOSPITAL
IN SERVICE

NAME (FIRST, MIDDLE, LAST) SEX M F DOB ___/___/___
ADDRESS WT. Kg RACE AGE
CITY STATE ZIP
PHONE ( ) PCP DR.
RESPONDED FROM CITY
ORIGIN CITY ZIP COUNTY
DESTINATION REASON
SSN MEDICARE# MEDICAID#
INSURANCE CO INSURANCE# GROUP#
RESPONSIBLE PARTY ADDRESS
CITY STATE ZIP PHONE ( )
RELATION TO PATIENT EMPLOYER

CREW	CERT	STATE#

CONDITION CODES EMD

TIME							
BP							
PULSE							
RESP							
GCS							
EKG							
PULSE OX	%	%	%	%	%	%	%
PAIN SCORE	/10	/10	/10	/10	/10	/10	/10

IV THERAPY – IV #1
SUCCESSFUL Y N # OF ATTEMPTS ___
ANGIO SIZE ___ ga.
SITE ___
TOTAL FLUID INFUSED ___ CC
BLOOD DRAW Y N INITIALS ___

IV THERAPY – IV #2
SUCCESSFUL Y N # OF ATTEMPTS ___
ANGIO SIZE ___ ga.
SITE ___
TOTAL FLUID INFUSED ___ CC
BLOOD DRAW Y N INITIALS ___

INTUBATION INFORMATION
SUCCESSFUL Y N # OF ATTEMPTS ___
TUBE SIZE ___ mm
TIME ___ INITIALS ___
END TITLE CO2 Y N EDD Y N
DEPT AT TEETH ___ cm

TIME	TREATMENT	DOSE	ROUTE	INIT

PAST MEDICAL HISTORY

MEDICATIONS

ALLERGIES

DISPATCHED FOR: C/C

HISTORY OF C/C

ASSESSMENT ALS ❑

TREATMENT

AUTHOR ❑ ALS ASSESSMENT PARTNER ❑ ALS ASSESSMENT ❑ OSHA

The Relizon Company CC756558-X (08/05) **ORIGINAL** AMB-001

FIGURE 4-2 ✱ Rural/Metro Ambulance Service, Youngstown, Ohio: prehospital care report.

An alternative format to the written report that is widely accepted and used is the computerized report (Figures 4-3a and 4-3b✱). The styles of computerized reports may vary. With some, the EMT fills in boxes on sheets of paper and the report is scanned by a computer. In others, data are entered directly into a laptop computer or a personal digital assistant (PDA) that is synchronized with a computer (Figures 4-4a and 4-4b✱).

A variation of the computerized report uses an electronic (computer) clipboard. In some "pen-based" computer systems, the computer clipboard has the capability of recognizing and interpreting the user's handwriting and converting the information he enters into an elec-

Medical Necessity may be satisfied if one or more of the following conditions are met:

	YES	NO
Did the patient require restraints?	❑	❑
Was the patient unconscious or in shock?	❑	❑
Did the patient require oxygen and could not self-administer?	❑	❑
Did the patient require any emergency treatment on the way to the destination? (Suctioning, Ventilation, etc.)	❑	❑
Did the patient need to remain immobile because of a fracture that had not been set or there was a possibility of a fracture?	❑	❑
Did the patient sustain an acute stroke or myocardial infarction?	❑	❑
Was the patient experiencing severe hemorrhaging?	❑	❑
Was the patient bed confined at the time of transport?	❑	❑
Was the patient only moveable by stretcher? (State reason(s) in narrative)	❑	❑

If this was an inter-facility transport, you must fully explain why the patient was transferred from one facility to another. All reasons MUST be fully documented on the PCR explaining why ambulance transport with EMS monitoring and care was required.

Why was patient at referring facility?

What's patient's medical condition requiring stretcher transportation?

How was the patient transferred to the stretcher?

❑ Stood with assistance & Pivoted ❑ Two person lift/carry ❑ Sheet transfer
❑ Other____

Upon patient contact, what treatment/services did the patient receive by EMS prior to departing referring facility?

❑ Suctioning ❑ Immobilization ❑ Sedation/Medication ❑ Restraints soft/chemical
❑ Other____

What medical interventions were required to complete the transport?

❑ Oxygen ❑ IV Therapy ❑ Restraints ❑ Cardiac Monitoring ❑ Airway Maintenance
❑ Medication Maintenance ❑ Other____

What treatment/services will patient receive at receiving facility?

How was the patient transferred from the stretcher?

❑ Stood with assistance & Pivoted ❑ Two person lift/carry ❑ Sheet transfer
❑ Other____

IV THERAPY
For Inter-facility Transports

ESTABLISHED BY FACILITY Y N
ANGIO SIZE____ga.
FLUID ADMINISTERING____
AMOUNT INFUSED
DURING TRANSPORT____CC

ALS+
MEDICATION (S) ORDER

____ml/hr.
Name Concentration Dose
____ml/hr.
Name Concentration Dose
____ml/hr.
Name Concentration Dose

❑ EKG ❑ Pulse OX
❑ O_2 ❑ Pump

I, the undersigned, hereby authorized all benefits to be made payable directly to Rural/Metro Ambulance. If I have Medicare, I permit a copy of this authorization to be used in place of the original, and I request that payment of authorized Medicare benefits be made on my behalf to Rural/Metro for any ambulance services provided to me by Rural/Metro Ambulance now or in the future. I hereby approve release of information including diagnosis, to Rural/Metro Ambulance, from any hospital, doctor, or other health care provider, for claims of insurance benefits. I authorize any holder of medical information or documentation about me to release it to the Medical Director of Rural/Metro Ambulance or their authorized agent for purposes of quality assurance or research. I understand I am financially responsible to Rural/Metro Ambulance for charges not covered by this authorization or denied by any insurance carrier and do hereby guarantee payment in full of this bill. I have been advised that this transport may be deemed not medically necessary and I accept responsibility for payment. I have been advised that I may be responsible for any unpaid portion of these charges not covered by Medicare, Medicaid, or other insurance. I further agree that if collection is made by suit or otherwise, I agree to pay all collection costs including reasonable attorney's fees.

I hereby acknowledge that I have been provided with a copy of Rural/Metro Corporation's Notice of Privacy Practices on this date.

Date____ Signature____

Notice of Privacy Practices delivered to patient ❑ Yes ❑ No ❑ Other____

If not delivered, state reason why.____

If signature was not obtained, state medical reason(s) ____

FIGURE 4-2 ✱ Rural/Metro Ambulance Service, Youngstown, Ohio: prehospital care report. *continued*

tronic format. Others offer selection items or lists that require little writing.

Computerized systems offer the promise of storing more information about a patient in a more legible format than written reports. They also allow greater efficiencies in storing, retrieving, and utilizing data the EMT collects. The EMT's computer can be linked to diagnostic and monitoring equipment; to electronic medical records; to computer-aided dispatch (CAD); and to computer systems handling fleet management, inventory control, e-mail, personnel, and payroll.

On a more basic level, a computerized system can check the EMT's spelling and use of abbreviations, ensuring a more accurate report. Such systems can also

Key Points
The information you enter in your PCR should provide a complete and accurate picture of your contact with the patient.

Thinking Critically
What is the meaning of the statement "If it wasn't written down, it wasn't done"?

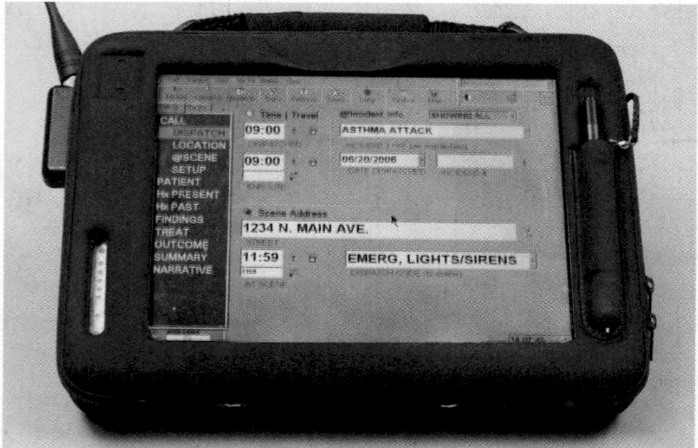

(a)

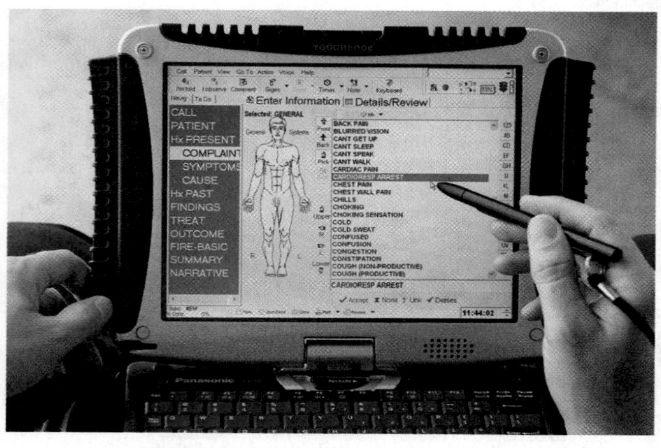

(b)

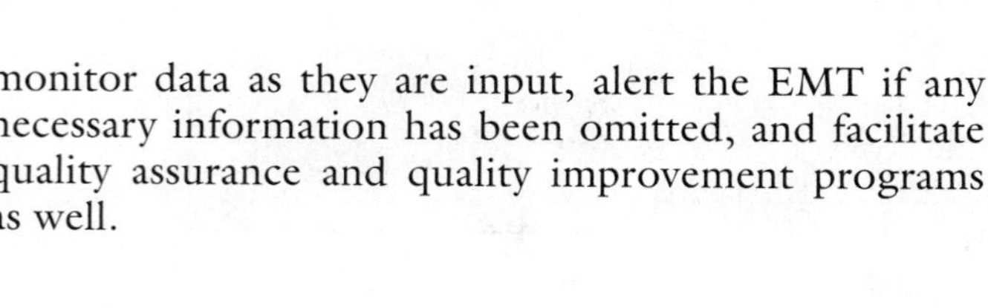

FIGURE 4-3 ✱ **(a)** A computerized PCR form. **(b)** A Toughbook computerized PCR form with patient figure on screen.

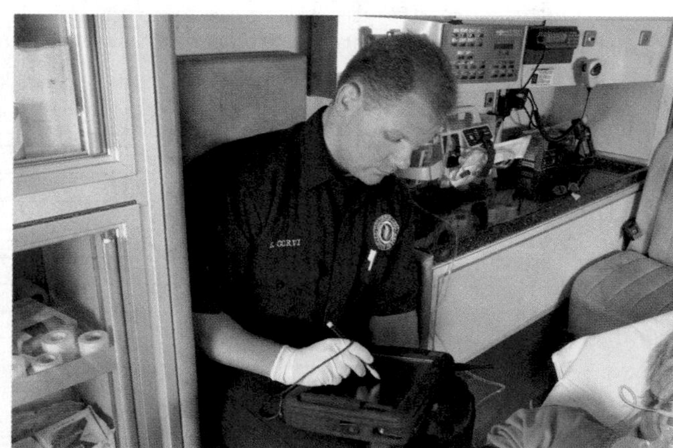

(a)

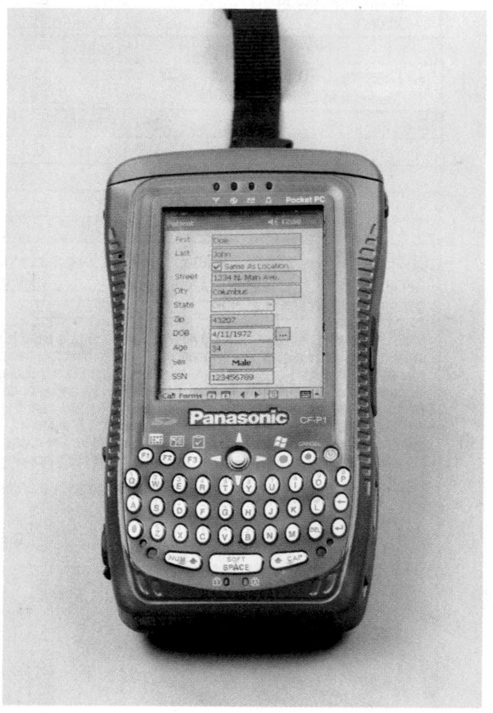

(b)

FIGURE 4-4 ✱ Information can be entered on a computerized form from **(a)** a laptop computer or, in some cases, from **(b)** an electronic personal data assistant (PDA).

monitor data as they are input, alert the EMT if any necessary information has been omitted, and facilitate quality assurance and quality improvement programs as well.

PCR Data

Of course, what makes the PCR useful is the information entered on it. That information should provide a complete and accurate picture of your contact with the patient. Remember these two basic rules when filling out any PCR: "If it wasn't written down, it wasn't done" (no one, including emergency department staff, will know it was done; and you won't be able to prove it was done, for example in a court of law) and "If it wasn't done, don't write it down" (which constitutes falsifying information).

Requirements for information on the PCR vary from system to system and state to state, but the types of information required and the sections of the PCR are generally quite similar.

Objectives 4-4 and 4-5
Explain the purposes and elements of the U.S. DOT minimum data set.

Objective 4-6
Describe the purpose and contents of each section of a PCR.

Key Terms
minimum data set the minimum information the U.S. Department of Transportation has determined should be included on all prehospital care reports.

The Minimum Data Set

The U.S. Department of Transportation (DOT) has made an effort to standardize the information collected on PCRs. Such standardization will, it is hoped, lead to a higher general level of patient care across the nation. It will also permit more meaningful comparison and analysis of data from various systems, which may speed the implementation of new and better methods of emergency care.

The DOT calls the information it wants on all PCRs the **minimum data set**. Following are the elements of information collected in the minimum data set:

Patient Information

- Chief complaint
- Level of responsiveness (AVPU)—mental status
- Blood pressure for patients greater than 3 years old
- Skin perfusion (capillary refill) for patients less than 6 years old
- Skin color, temperature, and condition
- Pulse rate
- Respiratory rate and effort
- Patient demographics (age, sex, race, weight)

Administrative Information

- Time the incident was reported
- Time the unit was notified
- Time of arrival at the patient
- Time the unit left the scene
- Time the unit arrived at its destination (hospital, etc.)
- Time of transfer of care

Another important element in establishing the minimum data set is the use of accurate and synchronous clocks. This means that all elements of an EMS system should use clocks or timekeeping devices that are accurately set and agree with each other. Dispatch's clock should not show one time, while the watches of the EMTs show another. Accurate timekeeping helps in the gathering of accurate medical information; for example, synchronous timekeeping by dispatch and the ambulance crew makes it easier to determine how long a patient has been in cardiac arrest before CPR or defibrillation was initiated. Accurate timekeeping can also be critical if administrative issues or legal questions over quality of care arise.

Many systems already require gathering the information included in the DOT's minimum data set. Such information is usually arranged in the following sections on the PCR.

Administrative Information

The administrative information section of the PCR is sometimes referred to as the run data. It usually includes the administrative information listed in the minimum data set. In addition, it may also include:

- The EMS unit number and the run or call number
- Names of crew members and their levels of certification
- The address to which the unit is dispatched

Patient Demographics and Other Patient Data

The next major section of the PCR contains primarily demographic patient information and other pertinent data about the patient. Most systems will require the following information:

- The patient's legal name, age, sex, race, birth date
- The patient's home address
- The insurance or billing information
- The location where the patient was found
- Any care given before the arrival of the EMTs

Vital Signs

A third major division of the PCR documents the patient's vital signs. On many forms, boxes are provided for checking off or writing in information. Computerized PCRs have drop-down menus that can be selected or data fields where the information can be entered. This section usually includes much of the patient information called for in the minimum data set. Various systems may also require additional data.

Ideally, at least two complete sets of vital signs should be taken and recorded. It is important to note the patient's position at the time the vital signs were taken (e.g., supine, standing, sitting). It is also critical to record the times at which the vital signs were obtained.

Patient Narrative

The next part of the PCR gives more detailed information about the patient and his problem than allowed for

Key Terms

pertinent negatives signs or symptoms that might be expected, based on the chief complaint, but are denied by the patient.

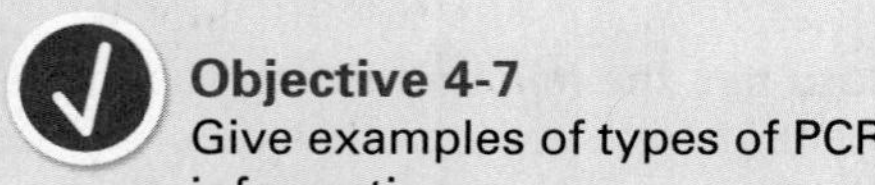

Objective 4-7
Give examples of types of PCR narrative information.

Objective 4-8
Use common abbreviations and medical terminology accurately in PCRs.

in check boxes or drop-down menus and limited data fields. This critical information sets the tone for the entire course of assessment, treatment, and documentation that will follow. This narrative section contains the following:

- The patient's chief complaint—This should be in the patient's own words or in the words of a bystander, if the patient is unresponsive. Put such statements in quotation marks ("My leg hurts") on the report.
- The patient's history or a description of the mechanism of injury—These data will include an account of when the chief complaint began and how it has progressed, along with other details of the patient history.

In this section of the PCR, you will create a brief but thorough picture of the patient and his problem. Remember that you are recording details for other medical personnel to use, not presenting your own conclusions about an incident. Careful observation of the patient and the scene as well as intelligent questioning of the patient and bystanders are essential. These methods will provide both *objective* and *pertinent subjective* information for the narrative section.

Objective information is measurable or verifiable in some way. It might be a reference to the patient's pulse rate or a statement that the patient has discoloration below both eyes. A sign is an objective observation.

Subjective information is based on an individual's perceptions or interpretations. Subjective information in the narrative section may come from either the patient or the EMT. For example, a patient might say, "I feel lightheaded." An EMT might observe, "The patient seems to be in pain." A symptom is a subjective finding.

Subjective information should be *pertinent;* that is, it should relate to the medical circumstances. It should not include attempts at diagnosis. Nor should it include irrelevant observations such as, "The patient's husband offered to transport the patient."

In questioning a patient, be alert to **pertinent negatives**. These are signs or symptoms that might be expected, based on the chief complaint, but that the patient denies having. A pertinent negative might be a patient's denial of pain after an automobile crash or a lack of difficulty in breathing in a case of chest pain. By noting the absence of pertinent signs and symptoms, you will provide the medical team that takes over care of the patient a fuller picture of his condition.

The narrative should briefly document the physical assessment in the order it was performed (i.e., head, neck, chest, and so on). Include pertinent information about the scene as well as about the patient. Note, for example, the presence of bottles of medication, a suicide note, or a collapsed ladder. If sensitive information is being reported, be sure to note the source of the information. As an example, if a wife states, "My husband is addicted to heroin," note the wife as the source of the highly sensitive but very important information.

Document the time and findings of each patient reassessment. This is especially important when attempting to identify trends in the patient's condition.

Write the narrative in a simple, direct style. Do not use radio codes or nonstandard abbreviations. Table 4-1 lists common standard abbreviations used by the EMT. A much more comprehensive list of abbreviations is found in Table 4-2.

TABLE 4-1 Commonly Accepted Abbreviations

a	before
c̄	with
NTG	nitroglycerin
O_2	oxygen
OB	obstetrics
P	after
PE	physical exam, pulmonary embolism
Po	orally, by mouth
Pt	patient
q	every
QID	four times a day
R/O	rule out
Rx	prescription
s̄	without
s/s	signs/symptoms
SIDS	sudden infant death syndrome
SL	sublingual
SOB	shortness of breath
stat	immediately
Sx	symptoms
TIA	transient ischemic attack
TID	three times a day
TKO	to keep open
Tx	treatment
X	times
y/o	years old
↑	increased
↓	decreased

TABLE 4-2 Standard Charting Abbreviations

Patient Information/Categories

African American	AA
Asian	A
Black	B
Chief complaint	CC
Complains of	c/o
Current health status	CHS
Date of birth	DOB
Differential diagnosis	DD or DDx
Estimated date of confinement	EDC
Family history	FH
Female	♀
Hispanic	H
History	Hx
History and physical	H&P
History of present illness	HPI or HOPI
Impression	IMP
Male	♂
Medications	Med
Newborn	NB
Past history	PH or PMH
Patient	Pt
Physical exam	PE
Private medical doctor	PMD
Signs and symptoms	S/S
Vital signs	VS
Weight	Wt
White	W
Year-old	y/o

Body Systems

Abdomen	Abd
Cardiovascular	CV
Central nervous system	CNS
Ear, nose, and throat	ENT
Gastrointestinal	GI
Genitourinary	GU
Gynecological	GYN
Head, eyes, ears, nose, and throat	HEENT
Musculoskeletal	M/S
Obstetrical	OB
Peripheral nervous system	PNS
Respiratory	Resp

Common Complaints

Abdominal pain	abd pn
Chest pain	CP
Dyspnea on exertion	DOE
Fever of unknown origin	FUO
Gunshot wound	GSW
Headache	H/A
Lower back pain	LBP
Nausea/vomiting	n/v
No apparent distress	NAD
Pain	pn
Shortness of breath	SOB
Substernal chest pain	sscp

Diagnoses

Abdominal aortic aneurysm	AAA
Abortion	Ab
Acute myocardial infarction	AMI
Adult respiratory distress syndrome	ARDS
Alcohol	ETOH
Atherosclerotic heart disease	ASHD
Chronic obstructive pulmonary disease	COPD
Chronic renal failure	CRF
Congestive heart failure	CHF
Coronary artery bypass graft	CABG
Coronary artery disease	CAD
Cystic fibrosis	CF
Dead on arrival	DOA
Delirium tremens	DTs
Deep vein thrombosis	DVT
Diabetes mellitus	DM
Dilation and curettage	D&C
Duodenal ulcer	DU
End-stage renal disease	ESRD
End-stage renal failure	ESRF
Epstein–Barr virus	EBV
Foreign body obstruction	FBO
Hepatitis B virus	HBV
Hiatal hernia	HH
Hypertension	HTN
Infectious disease	ID
Inferior wall myocardial infarction	IWMI
Insulin-dependent diabetes mellitus	IDDM
Intracranial pressure	ICP
Mass casualty incident	MCI
Mitral valve prolapse	MVP
Motor vehicle crash	MVC
Multiple sclerosis	MS
Non-insulin-dependent diabetes mellitus	NIDDM
Organic brain syndrome	OBS
Otitis media	OM
Overdose	OD
Paroxysmal nocturnal dyspnea	PND
Pelvic inflammatory disease	PID
Peptic ulcer disease	PUD
Pregnancies/births *(gravida/para)*	G/P
Pregnancy-induced hypertension	PIH
Pulmonary embolism	PE
Rheumatic heart disease	RHD
Sexually transmitted disease	STD
ST elevation myocardial infarction	STEMI
Transient ischemic attack	TIA
Tuberculosis	TB
Upper respiratory infection	URI
Urinary tract infection	UTI
Wolff–Parkinson–White syndrome (disease)	WPW

continued

TABLE 4-2 Standard Charting Abbreviations *continued*

Term	Abbreviation
Medications	
Angiotensin-converting enzyme	ACE
Aspirin	ASA
Bicarbonate	HCO_3^-
Birth control pills	BCP
Calcium	Ca^{++}
Calcium channel blocker	CCB
Calcium chloride	$CaCl_2$
Chloride	Cl^-
Digoxin	Dig
Dilantin (phenytoin sodium)	DPH
Diphenhydramine	DPHM
Diphtheria–Pertussis–Tetanus	DPT
Hydrochlorothiazide	HCTZ
Lactated Ringer's, Ringer's Lactate	LR, RL
Nitroglycerin	NTG
Nonsteroidal anti-inflammatory agent	NSAID
Normal saline	NS
Oral birth control pill	OBCP
Penicillin	PCN
Phenobarbital	PB
Potassium	K^+
Sodium bicarbonate	$NaHCO_3$
Sodium chloride	NaCl
Tylenol	APAP
Anatomy/Landmarks	
Abdomen	Abd
Antecubital	AC
Anterior axillary line	AAL
Anterior cruciate ligament	ACL
Anterior–posterior	A/P
Dorsalis pedis (pulse)	DP
Gallbladder	GB
Intercostal space	ICS
Lateral collateral ligament	LCL
Left lower lobe	LLL
Left lower quadrant	LLQ
Left upper lobe	LUL
Left upper quadrant	LUQ
Left ventricle	LV
Liver, spleen, and kidneys	LSK
Lymph node	LN
Midaxillary line	MAL
Posterior axillary line	PAL
Right lower lobe	RLL
Right lower quadrant	RLQ
Right middle lobe	RML
Right upper lobe	RUL
Right upper quadrant	RUQ
Temporomandibular joint	TMJ
Tympanic membrane	TM
Physical Exam/Findings	
Arterial blood gas	ABG
Bilateral breath sounds	BBS
Blood glucose level	BGL
Breath sounds	BS
Cerebrospinal fluid	CSF
Chest X-ray	CXR
Complete blood count	CBC
Computerized tomography	CT
Conscious, alert, and oriented	CAO
Costovertebral angle	CVA
Deep tendon reflexes	DTR
Dorsalis pedis (pulse)	DP
Electrocardiogram	EKG, ECG
Electroencephalogram	EEG
Expiratory	Exp
Extraocular movements (intact)	EOMI
Fetal heart tones	FHT
Full range of motion	FROM
Full-term normal delivery	FTND
Heart rate	HR
Heart sounds	HS
Hemoglobin	Hgb
Inspiratory	Insp
Jugular venous distention	JVD
Laceration	lac
Level of consciousness	LOC
Moves all extremities (well)	MAEW
Nontender	NT
Normal range of motion	NROM
Palpation	Palp
Passive range of motion	PROM
Point of maximal impulse	PMI
Posterior tibial (pulse)	PT
Pulse	P
Pupils equal and reactive to light	PEARL
Pupils equal, round, reactive to light and accommodation	PERRLA
Range of motion	ROM
Respirations	R
Temperature	T
Unconscious	unc
Urinary incontinence	UI
Miscellaneous Descriptors	
After (post-)	$\bar{p}$
After eating	pc
Alert and oriented	A/O
Anterior	ant.
Approximate	≈
As needed	prn
Before (ante-)	$\bar{a}$
Before eating (*ante cibum*, before meal)	a.c.
Body surface area (%)	BSA
Celsius	C°
Change	Δ
Decreased	↓
Equal	=
Fahrenheit	F°

TABLE 4-2 Standard Charting Abbreviations ***continued***

Term	Abbreviation
Immediately	stat
Increased	↑
Inferior	inf.
Left	Ⓛ
Less than	<
Moderate	mod.
More than	>
Negative	–
No, not, none	Ø
Not applicable	n/a
Number	No or #
Occasional	occ
Pack years	pk/yrs, p/y
Per	/
Positive	+
Posterior	post.
Postoperative	PO
Prior to arrival	PTA
Radiates to	→
Right	Ⓡ
Rule out	R/O
Secondary to	2°
Superior	sup.
Times (for 3 hours)	× (× 3h)
Unequal	≠
Warm and dry	W/D
While awake	WA
With (*cum*)	c̄
Within normal limits (*or* we never looked)	WNL
Without (*sine*)	s̄
Zero	0

Treatments/Dispositions

Term	Abbreviation
Advanced cardiac life support	ACLS
Advanced life support	ALS
Against medical advice	AMA
Automated external defibrillator	AED
Bag-valve mask	BVM
Basic life support	BLS
Cardiopulmonary resuscitation	CPR
Continuous positive airway pressure	CPAP
Do not resuscitate	DNR
Endotracheal tube	ETT
Estimated time of arrival	ETA
External cardiac pacing	ECP
Intermittent positive-pressure ventilation	IPPV
Long spine board	LSB
Nasal cannula	NC
Nasogastric	NG
Nasopharyngeal airway	NPA
No transport—refusal	NTR
Nonrebreather mask	NRM
Nothing by mouth	NPO
Oropharyngeal airway	OPA
Oxygen	O_2
Per square inch	psi
Physical therapy	PT
Positive end-expiratory pressure	PEEP
Short spine board	SSB
Therapy	Rx
Treatment	Tx
Turned over to	TOT
Verbal order	VO

Medication Administration/Metrics

Term	Abbreviation
Centimeter	cm
Cubic centimeter	cc
Deciliter	dL
Drop(s)	gtt(s)
Drops per minute	gtts/min
Every	q
Grain	gr
Gram	g, gm
Hour	h or hr
Hydrogen-ion concentration	pH
Intracardiac	IC
Intramuscular	IM
Intraosseous	IO
Intravenous	IV
Intravenous push	IVP
Joules	j
Keep vein open	KVO
Kilogram	kg
Liter	L
Liters per minute	LPM, L/min
Microgram	mcg
Milliequivalent	mEq
Milligram	mg
Milliliter	mL
Millimeter	mm
Millimeters of mercury	mmHg
Minute	min
Orally	po
Subcutaneous	SC, SQ
Sublingual	SL
To keep open	TKO

Cardiology

Term	Abbreviation
Atrial fibrillation	AF
Ventricular fibrillation	VF
Ventricular tachycardia	VT

Key Points

The narrative section of the PCR should create a brief but thorough picture of the patient and his problem for the purpose of helping other medical personnel understand the patient and his condition.

Thinking Critically

At home after your shift, your spouse says, "Hi honey. Anything interesting happen today?" What kind of information can you, or can't you, share without violating patient confidentiality or HIPAA?

Be especially careful in your use of medical terminology. Make sure you are using the proper term and that you are spelling it correctly. Look up spellings and definitions in a medical dictionary if you have any doubts. If you are still uneasy about the meaning of a term, or whether it applies to the situation you are describing, use everyday language instead. Mistakes in medical terminology can cause confusion and lead to delays or errors in treatment.

Treatment

The final information for entry on the PCR involves the treatment provided to the patient. This section should detail in chronological order all treatments you administer to a patient, what time they were administered, and indications of how the patient responded to that treatment. This information should be written in a clear narrative style, following the guidelines cited earlier in "Patient Narrative." An emergency physician, nurse, paramedic, or fellow EMT should, by reading your report, be able to learn what treatment was provided, the time it was provided, and whether the patient has improved or deteriorated since then.

It is important to include any other information that may be a local or state requirement. Specific data may be collected to enter into registries or other local or state databases for the purposes of research, education, or service performance.

▶ Legal Concerns

As noted earlier, the PCR is a legal document. Some legal issues involving documentation are discussed in the following sections.

Confidentiality

You must use care and discretion when handling any information about a patient. Remember that, as detailed in Chapter 3, "Medical, Legal, and Ethical Issues," confidentiality is the patient's legal right. The PCR and the information on it are considered confidential. Do not show the form or discuss the information on it with unauthorized individuals. Be familiar with the limitations of release of information mandated by the Health Insurance Portability and Accountability Act of 1996 (HIPAA).

Distribution

Follow state rules and local protocols in distributing the PCR and any additional information about a patient encounter. By law, you are generally permitted to provide confidential information about a patient to a health care provider who needs the information in order to continue care, to the police if they request information as part of a criminal investigation, to a third party if the information is required on a third-party billing form, or in court if required by a legal subpoena.

A copy of the PCR is generally left with the patient in the emergency department or receiving facility. The original is typically retained by the emergency medical services. A third copy may be forwarded to medical oversight or a quality improvement official. Electronic data may be transferred and distributed in a similar manner.

Refusal of Treatment

Chapter 3, "Medical, Legal, and Ethical Issues," discussed various issues that arise when a patient refuses treatment. As noted there, any competent adult has the right to refuse treatment. But legal questions often arise after the fact about whether the patient was truly competent. For this reason, you must make extra efforts with a patient who is refusing treatment to ensure that he fully understands what he is doing. You must also document your efforts completely.

1. When you encounter a patient who refuses treatment, try to perform as much of an assessment as possible. The extent of the examination will often depend on what the patient will allow you to do. Doing so may give you information to use in explaining what might happen if the patient continues to refuse treatment.
2. Before leaving the scene always try to make one more effort to persuade the patient to go to the hospital. Ensure that the patient can make a rational, informed decision and is not under the influence of alcohol or other mind-altering drugs, is not suffering from the effects of an illness or injury, and is not suicidal.
3. Inform the patient as clearly as possible why he should go to the hospital. Explain what may happen if he does not go. Discuss the possible consequences of delaying or refusing treatment. Confirm that the patient understands this information.

Objective 4-9
Explain the following legal concerns with respect to the PCR: confidentiality, allowed distribution of information, documenting refusal of treatment, falsification, and correction of errors.

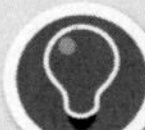

Key Points
Falsification of information on a PCR can compromise patient care and may lead to suspension, to revocation of certification or license, and potentially to criminal charges.

4. If the patient still refuses treatment, discuss the situation with medical direction as directed by local protocol. Such discussion can provide two major benefits. First, the patient may consider that the doctor's opinion carries more weight than the EMT's, so he may change his mind and accept treatment. Second, if the patient still refuses transport, the doctor can give the EMT direction in providing medical assistance at the scene.
5. If the patient still refuses to accept emergency care and/or transport, document in the PCR any assessment findings you have made, any emergency medical care you have given, and the explanation you gave the patient of the consequences of failing to accept care and/or transport (including potential death). Document if the patient refused to allow you to complete any or all of your assessment and if the patient refused any or all emergency care you intended to provide to him. You must document that the patient is alert and oriented to time, place, and person/self so there is no question that the patient understood the information and instructions you gave him. Then have the patient sign a refusal-of-care form (Figure 4-5∗). You should also have a family member, police officer, or bystander sign the form as a witness. If possible, obtain witnesses' addresses in case they must be contacted.
6. If the patient refuses to sign, have a family member, police officer, or bystander sign the form verifying that the patient refused. Each section of the refusal-of-care form must be completed.
7. Before leaving the scene, you should offer alternative methods of getting care (e.g., taking a taxi to a clinic or asking a friend or family member for help in seeing a doctor).
8. Finally, explain that you or another EMT crew will be happy to come back if the patient changes his mind and decides to accept treatment. It would be prudent to explain signs the patient may exhibit or symptoms he may complain of if the condition worsens.

Falsification

The PCR documents the nature and extent of emergency medical care an EMT provides. It is meant to be a thorough and accurate record. Any mistake in care must be highlighted on the PCR. In such a situation, the EMT might be tempted to falsify the PCR.

Such falsification of information on a PCR should never occur. When an error of omission or commission occurs, the EMT should not try to cover it up. Instead, the EMT should document exactly what did or did not happen and what steps were taken (if any) to correct the situation. False information may lead to suspension or revocation of EMT certification or license and, potentially, to criminal charges.

More importantly, falsification of patient data will compromise patient care. Other health care providers can

PATIENT REFUSAL

Patient ________ has been advised of the limitations of the prehospital evaluation and that the patient's illness or injury requires immediate medical evaluation and/or treatment.

Patient ________ has been advised in understandable terms that further harm could result without the proposed medical intervention and/or transportation to the hospital. The reasonable foreseeable risks are: ________. Transportation by means other than EMS providers could potentially place you or others at risk. At your request the EMS providers will return. EMS practitioners have spoken with Dr. ________ of ________ hospital to discuss pt. refusal of treatment and/or transportation to a hospital.

I, ________ (Print Name) have been advised by Rural/Metro Ambulance that my condition (or the condition of an individual that I am legally responsible for) is such that I (he or she) should be transported by ambulance to the nearest appropriate medical facility and be evaluated by a physician. Rural/Metro Ambulance has offered to provide such transportation. Notwithstanding Rural/Metro Ambulance's advice and offer to transport, I decline transport by Rural/Metro Ambulance.

I fully understand the nature of the proposed medical care and transportation and I fully comprehend the potential consequences of this refusal. I further attest that I am competent and authorized to make this refusal and I do forever release Rural/Metro Ambulance from any liability and give up any claim, demand or act on or against Rural/Metro Ambulance, its employees and any and all responding agencies. I understand that the patient is responsible for all charges incurred.

I understand that should my condition worsen in any way I should immediately seek medical attention at the nearest hospital emergency room or other Urgent Care facility. I understand that my refusal of transportation does not in any way affect my ability to call 911 or otherwise summon emergency help in order to obtain emergency medical services and transportation if my condition worsens.

I hereby acknowledge that I have been provided with a copy of Rural/Metro Corporation's Notice of Privacy Practices on this date.

TYPE OF REFUSAL (Patient Initial Below)
________ Refused All Care/Evaluation
________ Refused Transport

Signature ________
Date ________
Relationship to Patient (Responsible Party) ________
Signature (Witness) ________ Date ________

FIGURE 4-5 ∗ Rural/Metro Ambulance Service, Youngstown, Ohio: patient refusal form.

Thinking Critically
What's the harm in making up some earlier vital signs values that you forgot to measure or to enter on the PCR as long as the latest vitals you enter are correct?

Objective 4-10
Discuss how to handle these situations with respect to the PCR: transfer of patient care prior to completing the PCR; multiple-casualty incidents; and special reporting of infectious disease exposure and suspicion of abuse or neglect.

The ~~left~~ jm right pupil was fixed and dilated

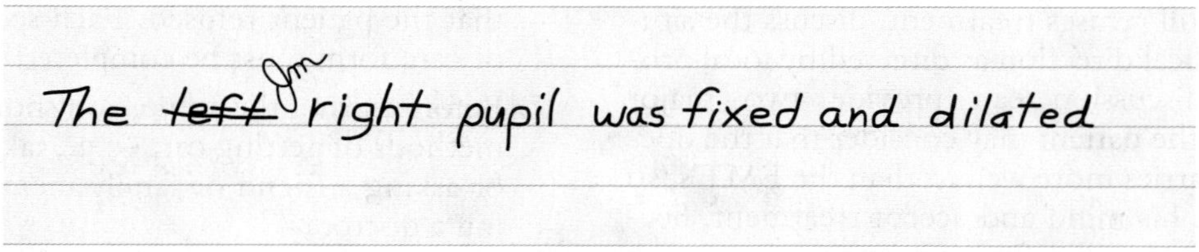

FIGURE 4-6 ✱ The proper way of correcting an error in a prehospital care report is to draw a single line through the error, initial it, and write the correct information beside it.

get an incorrect impression of the patient's condition from false assessment findings or a falsified report of treatment.

Certain areas of the PCR are more commonly falsified than others. One of those areas is vital signs. An EMT might, for some reason, neglect to take a set of vital signs and be tempted to make up numbers to cover the omission. Another area is treatment. An EMT might assist a patient in taking a medication without the approval of medical direction. Or he might have neglected to give oxygen to a patient complaining of chest pain. In the former case, the EMT might be tempted to leave out of the PCR the fact that he assisted in administration of medicine, while in the latter he might want to write in that oxygen was given. In none of these cases should the record be falsified. Although the changes might appear insignificant, they could have catastrophic results.

Correcting Errors

Even the most careful EMT will occasionally make errors in filling out the PCR. When such an error is discovered while a paper report is being written, draw a single horizontal line through the error, initial it, and write the correct information beside it (Figure 4-6✱). Do not try to erase or write over the error. Such actions could be interpreted as attempts to cover up a mistake or falsify the report.

When an error is discovered after the report form is submitted, draw a single horizontal line through the error, preferably using different-colored ink. Add a note with the correct information. Initial the entry and include the date and time of the correction. If information was omitted, the EMT should add a note with the correct information, the date, and the EMT's initials. Be sure to bring such changes to the attention of those to whom the incorrect report was submitted.

Most electronic PCR formats provide a method to amend the report if an error is discovered. If there is no way to electronically amend or submit an amended report, correct a printed copy using the traditional methods described for a paper report and resubmit the PCR as a corrected copy.

▶ Special Situations

There are certain circumstances in which the standard PCR will not be appropriate. Examples of such circumstances are discussed in the following sections.

Transfer-of-Care Report

Upon delivery of the patient in the medical facility, under ideal circumstances the EMT will complete a full PCR containing all of the patient data, obtain a transfer-of-care signature from the medical professional who is assuming patient care responsibility, and leave a copy of the full report with the facility. However, this ideal situation may not always exist. It may be necessary for your unit to return immediately to service to answer an additional call, precluding the EMT from submitting a full PCR until a later time.

Some computerized report formats do not provide the ability to print a hard-copy report to leave with the medical facility. Upon completion, the computerized report is downloaded into the EMS system's main computer and printed at a later time, then delivered or faxed to the medical facility.

In such cases, an abbreviated transfer-of-care form or "drop report" may be used to provide minimal patient data and collect a transfer-of-care signature. This abbreviated report can be used as a reference at a later time when completing the full PCR. A copy of the transfer report should be submitted with the full PCR.

Thinking Critically

If you don't have time to complete and submit your PCR form at the hospital before you are called to return to service, when and how should you complete a report? What interim reporting can you do before completing the full PCR?

Key Terms

triage tag information tag attached to a patient during a multiple-casualty incident.

Objective 4-11

Record call information using the SOAP, CHART, and CHEATED methods.

Multiple-Casualty Incidents

During multiple-casualty incidents (MCIs), such as plane crashes or multiple-vehicle collisions, rescuers are often overwhelmed with the number of patients requiring treatment. The needs of these patients can sometimes conflict with the need for complete documentation. In these cases, there may not be enough time to complete the standard PCR before turning to the next patient.

Each EMS system has its own MCI plan. Those plans should have some means of recording important medical information and keeping that information with the patient as he is moved for treatment. Often such basic information as chief complaint, vital signs, and treatment provided is recorded on a **triage tag** that is attached to the patient. Information from the tag can be used later to complete the PCR. In MCI situations, the PCRs will usually be less detailed than those of more typical, single-patient runs. Local plans should contain guidelines for what is expected in the PCRs in those situations. More information on MCI situations will be provided in Chapter 44, "Multiple-Casualty Incidents and Incident Management."

Special Reports

In some circumstances, EMTs must fill out special documentation other than the usual PCR. These cases require the notification of agencies and local authorities beyond the usual health care network. Such cases might include the following:

- Suspected abuse of a child or elderly person
- Possible exposure to an infectious disease (e.g., meningitis, hepatitis, TB, HIV)
- Injury to an EMS team member
- Other situations that the EMT feels might require special documentation or informing of another agency

State laws and local protocols usually outline the circumstances in which special reports are required and often provide a form for such reports. These special reports should be accurate, descriptive, and objective; should not lead to any conclusions; should contain the names of all individuals, services, and facilities involved; and should be submitted in a timely manner. Always keep a copy for your own agency's records. The procedure for distribution of such reports is also established by local protocol.

Alternative Documentation Methods

There are several alternative methods used to organize information on the prehospital care report. Three of these alternative methods are known by the mnemonics SOAP, CHART, and CHEATED—as described in the following sections.

SOAP

The mnemonic SOAP stands for subjective, objective, assessment, and plan. These components can be used to organize the information that needs to be documented on the prehospital care report.

S—subjective—refers to information that the patient must tell you. This is information or symptoms that you cannot see or feel during the physical exam. Symptoms are the patient's descriptions of how he is feeling. For example, the patient states, "I have terrible head pain." You have no physical evidence of the head pain, only the description provided by the patient.

O—objective—refers to information that you identify in the physical examination through inspection, palpation, and auscultation. Your sense of smell will also provide objective information. This kind of information is referred to as signs. For example, a large laceration is a sign of injury. Whether the patient complains of any pain or not, you are able to see the laceration and make an objective assumption that an injury has occurred.

A—assessment—refers to the field assessment, the general idea you form about the patient's condition on the basis of the information you have collected from the subjective and objective components, along with a scene assessment, the chief complaint, and any other information provided by bystanders or family. For example, you may surmise that a patient with a history of diabetes who is acting bizarrely, is not oriented, and has pale, cool, and clammy skin as well as tachycardia may be suffering from a low blood sugar level (hypoglycemia).

P—plan—refers to the plan of action and the emergency care provided to the patient. In the patient with diabetes, it may include the administration of oral glucose and oxygen and transportation to a medical facility.

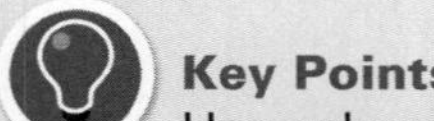

Key Points
Use only universally accepted medical abbreviations. Abbreviations that are made up or not universally understood can convey the wrong meaning or no meaning to other health care professionals who rely on your report as they care for the patient.

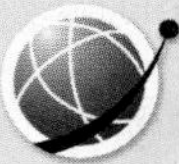

Media Resources
Go to www.bradybooks.com for mykit. Highlights:
- *Web Resource:* Documentation and the PCR

The SOAP method may be used by EMS systems as the basis for standard reporting practices. Some variations of the SOAP method exist and may be used to meet the specific needs of an EMS system. For example, the mnemonic SOAPIE may be used. The *I* refers to *intervention* and the *E* refers to *evaluation*. This would allow for a better account of the ongoing assessment that is conducted on the patient.

CHART

Another mnemonic used to organize documentation is CHART, which stands for the following:

C—chief complaint of the patient

H—history of the patient (including the SAMPLE history)

A—assessment findings gathered in the primary assessment, secondary assessment, detailed physical exam, and ongoing assessment

R—Rx for treatment that was provided to the patient

T—transport—any change in the patient's condition en route and the type of transport (e.g., emergency)

CHEATED

A more specific mnemonic used to organize documentation is CHEATED. This mnemonic organizes the documentation as follows:

C—chief complaint

H—history of the patient (including the SAMPLE history)

E—exam—information that was found in the physical examination of the patient

A—assessment—the field impression you derive by processing the history and physical exam findings and determining a condition the patient may be suffering from

T—treatment that was provided to the patient

E—evaluation—the information that is found during the ongoing assessment and any identified improvement or deterioration of the patient's condition

D—disposition—the transfer of patient care at the medical facility or to another health care provider

SOAP, CHART, and CHEATED represent different methods to organize the information expected to be documented on the prehospital care report. Whatever system is developed, it is important that it is used to ensure the most accurate documentation of the patient information.

Medical Abbreviations

Medical abbreviations can be used in your documentation on the prehospital care report. Abbreviations can save room and time when writing the PCR. However, it is extremely important that you use only universally accepted medical abbreviations and that you do not make up your own, because your made-up abbreviations might imply a different meaning or no meaning to other health care professionals who will read your report. Table 4-2 lists standard medical abbreviations.

CHAPTER REVIEW

SUMMARY

Documentation serves many functions in emergency medical services. It is used for the continuity of patient care, case reviews, a permanent record, legal purposes, and education and research. All documentation must be completely accurate and represent what truly occurred during the patient assessment and management. It must be legible and contain only acceptable objective and pertinent subjective information.

Documentation is also imperative in reporting refusal of care and transport. Your documentation may make the difference in proving that you fully informed the patient prior to his refusal. Because documentation is so vital to record keeping, and your PCR is a patient record, there is absolutely no tolerance for falsification of any information contained within the report. If an error is made, you must follow the recommended method for making corrections to the PCR.

CASE STUDY FOLLOW-UP

SCENE SIZE-UP

You have been dispatched to the scene of an automobile accident. As you pull up, you observe a group of people standing by two vehicles. You note that the left front end of one vehicle that is in the street, a midsize car, is dented in and the headlight is smashed. The right rear of the other, a minivan at the curb, is also dented and the light on that side is broken. A woman explains that the car struck her parked van while she was inside the house, and that she called 911. Your partner inspects the car for signs of damage and clues to mechanism of injury sustained during the collision. You note that the man who was driving the car is in his mid-30s and has a slight bruise on the left side of his forehead. Despite this evidence of trauma, he is on his feet. He angrily says he does not want your help.

PRIMARY ASSESSMENT

You remain calm and polite in spite of the driver's initial outburst. You and your partner introduce yourselves, and you say, "I understand that you've had some problems. We're certainly not here to give you any more trouble. We just want to make sure you're OK. Are you feeling all right? Do you have any pain, Mr . . .?"

"Makynen. Paul Makynen," he replies, appearing to grow calmer. "I'm sorry I flew off the handle, but it's been a bad day. I've been running late. I was on my way to see an important client when a dog ran out into the street. I braked and swerved. I missed it, but hit that van instead. I just bumped my forehead on the inside of the door frame. It's a little sore, I'm a little achy, but that's all. Look, I appreciate your coming out, but I'm OK, really. And I've got to get going."

You note from the patient's answer that he is alert, responsive, and having no difficulty in breathing. However, you recall that the woman who called 911 said that right after the collision Mr. Makynen was slumped over the wheel. You ask him if he thinks he lost consciousness, however briefly. He denies it and says, "Nah, I just put my head down on the wheel because I was disgusted." You see no signs of bleeding. His skin appears to be normal in color and dry. Mr. Makynen refuses your partner's attempt to provide manual stabilization of his head and neck but permits you to assess his radial pulse. You find that his pulse is slightly rapid but strong and regular and that his skin is warm to the touch.

SECONDARY ASSESSMENT

You explain to Mr. Makynen that you would like to do a physical exam to check for any signs of injury. He becomes angry again and says, "Come on. I'm okay. I don't need that." You ask if you can take his blood pressure and other vital signs, and he says, "No, no. Look, I really feel fine." He also refuses to answer any of the SAMPLE questions except to deny any pain or other symptoms. He rejects your suggestion that he be transported to the hospital.

You are not ready to give up yet. You tell Mr. Makynen that, because of the injury to the head, it would be best that he be checked by a doctor. You explain that head injuries often display no signs at first but can later develop into potentially life-threatening situations. He interrupts to say, "Fine, I'll take that chance, but I am leaving."

Your partner discreetly calls dispatch to say, "Patient is refusing emergency care and transport. We will inform you of our status shortly."

DOCUMENTATION

Meanwhile, recognizing that you are going to have no success in persuading Mr. Makynen to accept care, you explain to him that before he leaves he must sign a refusal-of-care form. You prepare the PCR and the refusal forms. On the PCR, you note the mechanism of injury, the bruise to the forehead, and your initial findings regarding his alert mental status, open airway, adequate breathing, absence of bleeding, pulse that is rapid but regular and strong, and skin color, temperature, and condition indicating adequate perfusion. You write that the patient denies pain and, although a witness reported that he was slumped over the wheel after the collision, the patient denies losing consciousness.

You document that, at this point, the patient refused further care. You also note your recommendation that the patient see a doctor and your explanation of the possible consequences. You add that the patient still refused further care.

You show the PCR to Mr. Makynen and allow him to read it and the refusal form. While he is doing so, your partner explains the situation to the owner of the van and another bystander and asks them to witness the refusal. They agree and, after Mr. Makynen signs the refusal form, they also sign where you indicate.

As Mr. Makynen gets into his car, you suggest again that he see his personal physician as soon as possible. You add that if he suddenly feels dizzy or in pain, he shouldn't hesitate to call 911 for assistance.

Your partner contacts dispatch and states that the patient has refused treatment and transport. Your unit is now clear and in service.

IN REVIEW

1. Explain the various uses of the documentation that the EMT generates after a patient contact.
2. Describe two common formats for the prehospital care report.
3. Explain the origin and purpose of the minimum data set.
4. Explain what the phrase "accurate and synchronous clocks" means and why they are important.
5. Define pertinent negatives.
6. List the steps you should take if a patient refuses treatment.
7. Explain the meaning and importance of the following two documentation rules: "If it wasn't written down, it wasn't done" and "If it wasn't done, don't write it down."
8. Describe how errors on PCRs should be corrected.
9. Explain how a multiple-casualty incident can affect EMT documentation.
10. Describe circumstances in which an EMT might be expected to file special reports with other agencies.

CRITICAL THINKING

You arrive on the scene and find a 36-year-old female patient who complains of severe abdominal pain. The patient is alert and oriented. Her vital signs are BP 88/64 mmHg; HR 128 bpm; R 24 and adequate chest rise; skin is pale, cool, and clammy; SpO_2 is 96% on room air. Her radial pulses are weak. She states the pain began suddenly about 4 hours ago and has progressively worsened. She was sitting on the couch watching television when it began. Nothing makes the pain better or worse. The pain is dull and aching, and it is intermittent. The pain does not radiate.

The patient rates the severity of her pain as 8 on a scale of 1 to 10. She states she feels light-headed and dizzy every time she stands up, and she also feels nauseated. She has no known allergies and takes over-the-counter Prilosec for heartburn. She has no pertinent medical history. She reports she had her tonsils removed when she was 10 years old. She has had nothing to eat or drink for about 7 hours. She states that she has "not felt real good" for a few days, and other than the time she has spent working at her desk at work, she has been at home on the couch. Her pupils are equal and sluggish to respond. She has no jugular venous distention (JVD). Her breath sounds are equal and clear bilaterally. Her abdomen is rigid and tender. There is no evidence of trauma to the abdomen. She has good motor and sensory function in all four extremities. Her peripheral pulses are very weak.

En route to the hospital, the patient begins to close her eyes. You must verbally instruct her to open her eyes. Her BP is 82/62 mmHg, HR 134 bpm, and R 26 with adequate chest rise. The pulse oximeter is providing an "error" reading. Her skin is more pale, cool, and clammy and her radial pulses are barely palpable.

When preparing to write the PCR, you note her name as Jennifer Sampson. She lives at 1321 Oakridge Drive in Smithville, Ohio.

1. What can this information be used for?
2. How will the medical personnel in the medical facility use the information?
3. What will your EMS use the information for?
4. What would you document in the patient information section of the minimum data set?
5. What would you document in the administrative section of the PCR?
6. What information would you write in the patient narrative section?
7. Should any of the information not be reported in the PCR?
8. If you were to make a mistake while writing the PCR, how would you correct it?
9. If the PCR contains a box for a third set of vital signs, what would you document in this patient?
10. How would you collect additional information needed for your PCR?

PEARSON
EXPLORE mybradykit™

Please go to **www.bradybooks.com** to access mykit for this text. You will find quizzes, critical thinking scenarios, weblinks, animations, and videos related to this chapter—and much more. Look for online information on the National EMS Information System and on the importance of good documentation.

Register your access code from the front of your book by going to **www.bradybooks.com** and selecting the mykit links.

CHAPTER

5

Communication

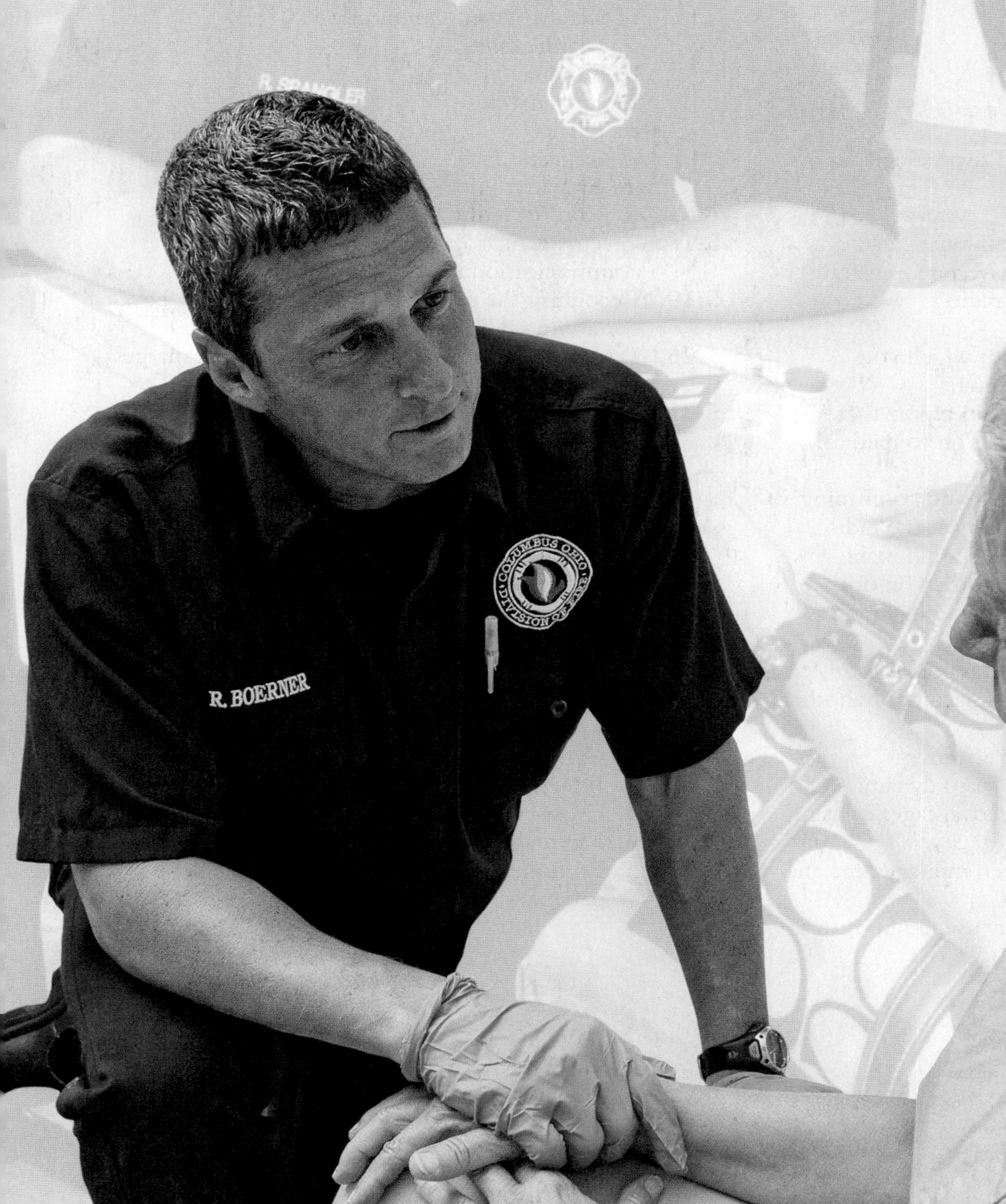

Navigation Guide

The following items provide an overview to the purpose and content of this chapter. The Education Standard and Competency are from the new National EMS Education Standards.

STANDARD **Preparatory** (Content Areas: EMS System Communication; Therapeutic Communication)

COMPETENCY Applies fundamental knowledge of the EMS system, safety/well-being of the EMT, medical/legal and ethical issues to the provision of emergency care.

OBJECTIVES: After reading this chapter, you should be able to:

5-1. Define key terms introduced in this chapter.

5-2. Discuss the purposes and characteristics of each of the following EMS system communication components:
- **a.** Base station
- **b.** Mobile radios
- **c.** Portable radios
- **d.** Digitalized radio equipment
- **e.** Mobile data terminals
- **f.** Cell phones

5-3. Describe the responsibilities of the Federal Communications Commission.

5-4. Explain the importance of EMS system communication equipment maintenance.

5-5. Given a radio transmitter/receiver, demonstrate the standard ground rules for radio communications.

5-6. List key points in an EMS call at which you should communicate with dispatch.

5-7. Deliver a concise, organized radio report that clearly conveys essential information to medical direction or the receiving facility.

5-8. Describe the process of receiving and confirming an order from medical direction over the radio.

5-9. Identify situations in which you should make additional contact with medical direction or the receiving facility after providing an initial radio report.

5-10. Given a scenario, deliver an oral report to transfer care of the patient to a receiving facility or another EMS provider.

5-11. Given a scenario, demonstrate effective communication that enhances team dynamics.

5-12. Discuss the advantages and disadvantages of using radio codes.

5-13. Convert back and forth between military time and standard clock times.

5-14. Communicate using commonly used radio terms.

5-15. Describe the components of the communication process.

5-16. Discuss factors that can enhance or interfere with effective communication.

5-17. Give examples of each of the following techniques of therapeutic communication:
- **a.** Clarification
- **b.** Summary
- **c.** Explanation
- **d.** Silence
- **e.** Reflection
- **f.** Empathy
- **g.** Confrontation

5-18. Given a scenario, engage in an effective communication process with a patient.

5-19. Recognize the potential messages that may be communicated via nonverbal behaviors.

5-20. Describe the uses, advantages, and disadvantages of open-ended and closed questions.

5-21. Analyze your communications with a patient in a scenario to recognize the following pitfalls in communication:
- **a.** Leading or biased questions
- **b.** Interrupting the patient
- **c.** Talking too much
- **d.** Providing false assurance
- **e.** Giving inappropriate advice
- **f.** Implying blame

5-22. Discuss considerations for each of the following situations:
- **a.** Communicating with a patient's family
- **b.** Getting a noncommunicative patient to talk
- **c.** Interviewing a hostile patient
- **d.** Cross-cultural communications
- **e.** Language barriers
- **f.** Communicating with children and elderly patients

Navigation Guide *continued*

KEY TERMS: Page references indicate first major use in this chapter. For complete definitions, see the Glossary at the back of the book.

base station p. 90
closed questions p. 104
communication p. 99
culture p. 105
decoder p. 91
decoding p. 99
defense mechanisms p. 101
encoder p. 91
encoding p. 99
ethnocentrism p. 106
feedback p. 99
gestures p. 103
haptics p. 103
intimate zone p. 103
leading questions p. 104
mobile data terminal p. 91
open-ended questions p. 104
repeaters p. 91
SBAR p. 96

MEDIA RESOURCES: Please go to www.bradybooks.com to access mykit for this text. You will find quizzes, critical thinking scenarios, weblinks, animations, and videos related to this chapter—and much more. Look for online information on effective communication. You will also find a video clip on nonverbal communication.

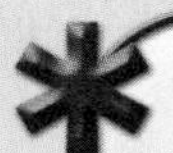

CASE STUDY

The Dispatch

EMS Unit 2—proceed to 101 Bate Road. You have a man bleeding heavily in the driveway there. Time out is 1128 hours.

"Dispatch, this is Unit 2," your partner radios back. We copy and are responding to 101 Bate Road. Our ETA is 10 minutes. Do you have any more information on the nature of the problem?"

Dispatch replies, "Unit 2, that is negative. The caller said he was bleeding and was in the driveway. That was all."

Upon Arrival

Bate Road is in a semirural area with houses widely spaced. Because the dispatch gave little information, you approach the scene with extreme caution, realizing that some act of violence may have led to the call. You park a short distance up the road from the house, which has an attached garage. There is one car in the driveway and only one person in sight, a man sitting on a bench next to the garage and clutching his hand. The scene appears secure, so you pull up and back into the driveway. Your partner radios, "Unit 2 to dispatch. We are on the scene at 101 Bate Road." Dispatch responds, "Unit 2 on the scene at 1137 hours."

Because the dispatch said there was bleeding at the scene, you and your partner put on gloves and protective eyewear. Your partner grabs the jump kit and you both step out. As you walk up the driveway, you scan the scene carefully, looking for any signs of possible danger. The garage door is open, and you can see a workbench at the back of it. No one else is in sight. Meanwhile, the man, who appears to be in his 40s, has gotten off the bench and is walking toward you. You note that his right hand is wrapped in a blood-soaked rag and that his shirt and pants are blood stained.

How Would You Proceed to Assess and Care for This Patient? How Would You Use Your Communications Skills and Equipment During Contact with the Patient?

During this chapter, you will learn about the elements of emergency prehospital care communications and communications systems. Later, we will return to the case and apply the procedures learned.

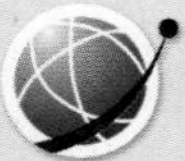

Media Resources

Go to www.bradybooks.com for mykit. Highlights:

- *Web Resource:* Effective Communication
- *Web Resource:* National Emergency Number Association

Key Terms

base station the central EMS dispatch and coordination area.

Objective 5-2

Discuss the purposes and characteristics of EMS system communication.

Introduction

Years ago, the job of ambulance crews was simply to transport patients to hospitals. The crews had no responsibility to provide emergency care to those patients. With such a limited role to perform, crews had no need for sophisticated communications systems.

Reliable communications systems are an essential part of EMS today. They permit EMTs to reach their patients more quickly and allow hospitals to prepare appropriately for the arrival of those patients. They allow EMTs to call for necessary resources and they also link EMTs in the field with doctors, enabling the EMTs to provide more lifesaving services than ever through contact with medical direction. For these reasons, understanding EMS communications skills and equipment is an essential part of the EMT's job.

In order to communicate effectively with a patient, it is important to understand the principles of therapeutic communication. EMTs should be able to communicate in a manner that establishes a positive relationship with their patients. EMTs must also be able to adjust the way they communicate with patients who have special needs.

EMS Communications System

Components of an Emergency Communications System

While emergency prehospital care communications systems vary considerably, many of them employ the components discussed in the next sections.

Base Station

The **base station** serves as a dispatch and coordination area and ideally is in contact with all other elements of the system (Figure 5-1*). The base should be located on a suitable terrain, preferably a hill, and be in proximity to the hospital that serves as a medical command center. Base stations generally use relatively high power output (80 to 150 watts) and should be equipped with a suitable antenna within a short distance. The antenna plays a critical part in transmission and reception efficiency.

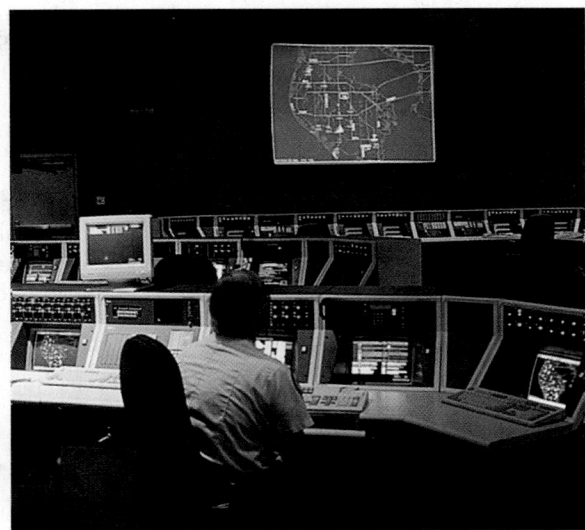

FIGURE 5-1 * EMS communications center.

Transmission power levels are limited by the Federal Communications Commission, and the minimum usable signal level for reception is limited by man-made noise. A good antenna system can compensate to some degree for these limitations.

Mobile Radios (Transmitter/Receivers)

Mobile radios (transmitter/receivers) are vehicle-mounted devices used to communicate within the EMS system. Mobile transmitters usually transmit effectively at lower power than base stations (typically 20 to 50 watts) (Figure 5-2*). Most mobile radios are able to transmit over a 10- to 15-mile range on average terrain. The transmission distance of a mobile radio is affected by the terrain and is reduced in mountainous areas or where there are many tall buildings. Mobile transmitters with higher outputs have proportionally greater transmission ranges than those with lower outputs.

Portable Radios (Transmitter/Receivers)

Portable, handheld transmitter/receivers are useful when you are out of your vehicle and must stay in communication with the base, with one another, and with medical direction (Figure 5-3*). Such portable units may also be used by medical direction when they are sta-

Key Terms

repeaters devices that receive transmissions from a low-powered source and rebroadcast them at another.

encoder device that breaks down sound waves into unique digital codes for radio transmission.

Key Terms

decoder device that recognizes and responds to certain codes imposed on radio broadcasts.

mobile data terminal device mounted in an ambulance cab that receives and displays information on a screen.

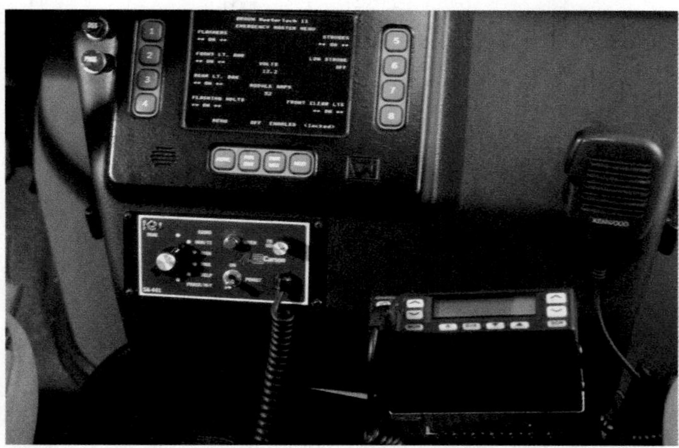

FIGURE 5-2 * A mobile two-way radio.

tioned at a hospital that has no radio. Portable units usually have power outputs ranging from 1 to 5 watts and thus have limited range, although the signal of a handheld transmitter may be boosted by retransmission through a repeater.

Repeaters

Repeaters are devices that receive transmissions from a relatively low-powered source such as a mobile or portable radio and rebroadcast them at another frequency and a higher power. Repeaters make communications possible in EMS systems that cover a wide area or where the terrain makes transmission and reception of signals difficult (Figure 5-4*). Repeaters can be located in emergency vehicles or at fixed sites throughout the area covered by the EMS system.

Digital Equipment

Digitalized radio equipment is common today. With such equipment, an **encoder** breaks down sound waves into unique digital codes, like those used in CD players, while a **decoder** recognizes and responds to only those codes. This equipment allows different mobile and base stations to operate on the same broadcast frequency, allowing more messages to be transmitted over those already crowded frequencies.

Included in digital communication is the use of a **mobile data terminal** that is mounted in the cab of the ambulance. Instead of a voice dispatch to a scene, the mobile data terminal receives a signal from the digital radio and displays the information on the terminal screen. Some equipment will also print the information on a hard copy. The EMT can reply to the dispatch by either hitting a designated button that indicates the unit is en route, or replying by voice communication. The data terminals are often installed to reduce the number of necessary radio transmissions. The EMT may also indicate that he is on the scene, en route to the hospital, at the hospital, and back in service by simply pushing a designated button. This is designed to facilitate communication and not replace voice communication.

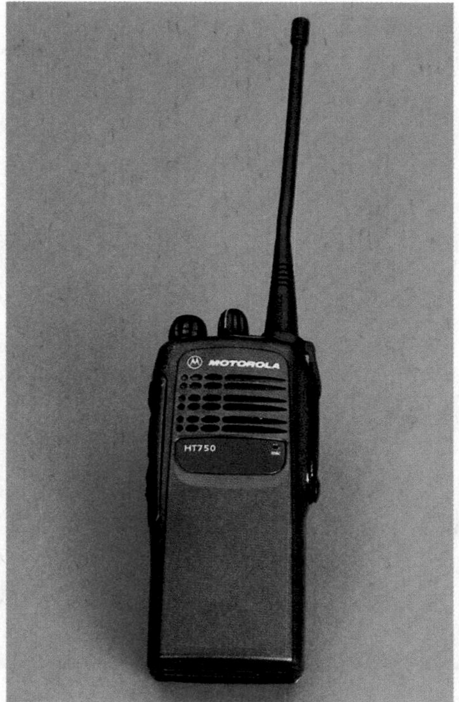

FIGURE 5-3 * A portable handheld radio.

Cell Phones

Some EMS communications systems use cell phones as a means of communication. Cell phones transmit and receive through the air rather than over wires (Figure 5-5*). They operate in the following manner: A particular geographical service area is divided into a network of slightly overlapping geographical cells that range from

Key Points
Cell phones have many advantages for EMS communications. Their chief disadvantage is that, as part of the public phone system, they can be overwhelmed during a disaster.

Objective 5-3
Describe the responsibilities of the Federal Communications Commission.

Objective 5-4
Explain the importance of EMS system communication equipment maintenance.

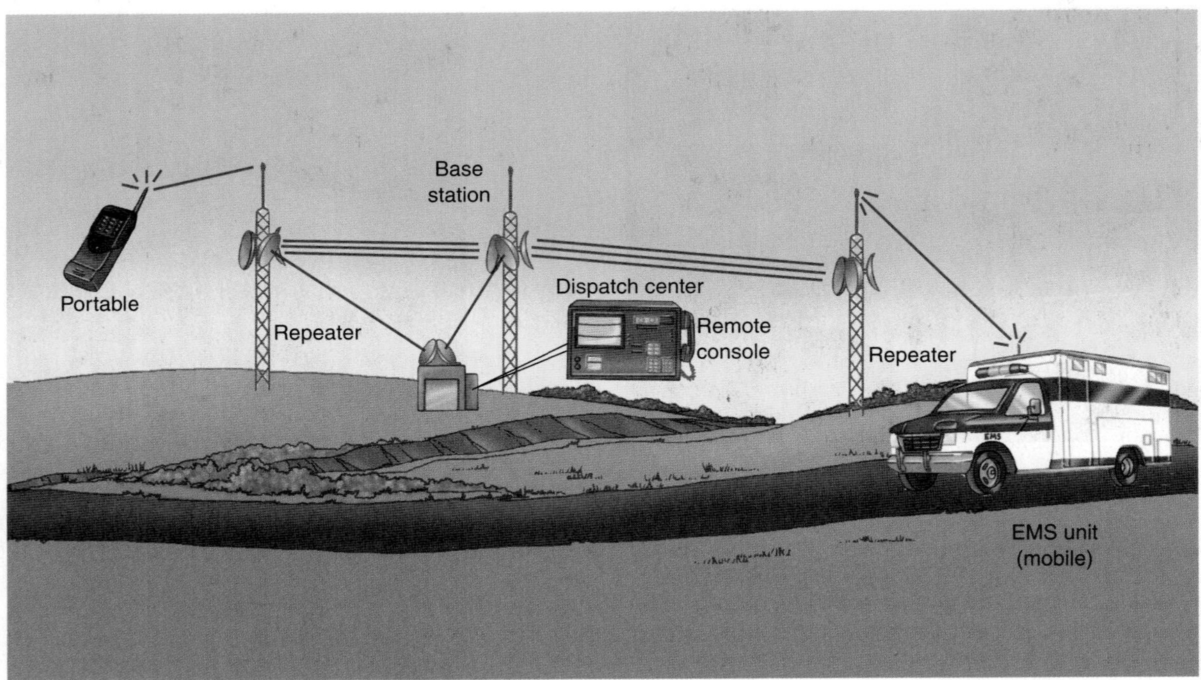

FIGURE 5-4 ✱ Example of an EMS communication system using repeaters.

2 to 40 square miles in size. The cells are the equivalent of radio base stations. When a telephone moves beyond one cell's range, service to it is automatically picked up by another cell.

Benefits of cell phones include excellent sound quality, availability of channels, easy maintenance, and, often, increased privacy of communications. They are often used as backups to an existing radio system or where the expense of establishing a radio system is too great. The major disadvantage of cellular phone systems for EMS use is that they are part of the public phone system and can easily be overwhelmed during multiple-casualty disasters.

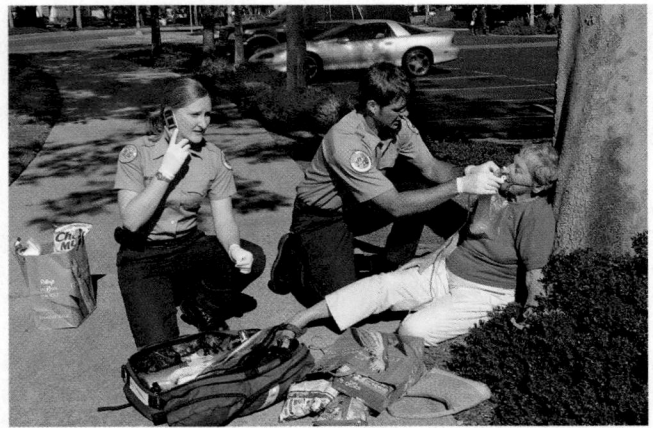

FIGURE 5-5 ✱ Cell phones are common in EMS communications.

Broadcast Regulations

The Federal Communications Commission (FCC) has jurisdiction over all radio operations in the United States, including those used by EMS systems. The FCC licenses individual base station operations, assigns radio call signs, approves equipment for use, establishes limitations for transmitter power output, assigns radio frequencies, and monitors field operations. The FCC has also set regulations to limit interference with emergency radio broadcasts and to bar the use of obscenity and profanity in broadcasts.

System Maintenance

Because a properly working communications system is at the heart of effective delivery of emergency medical services, regular maintenance of the system's equipment is a must. The equipment should not be mishandled or unnecessarily exposed to harsh environmental

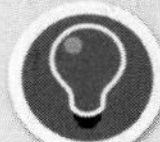

Key Points
Mobile and portable radios and telephones that operate on battery power should be checked every day and batteries replaced with freshly charged batteries.

Objective 5-5
Given a radio transmitter/receiver, demonstrate the standard ground rules for radio communications.

conditions. Regular cleaning with a damp cloth and a mild detergent should be part of the maintenance program. The communication equipment should also be checked to ensure that it is not drifting from its assigned frequency.

Mobile and portable radios and telephones that operate on battery power should be checked on a daily basis. Most equipment uses rechargeable batteries. Freshly charged batteries should be inserted every day, while the removed batteries are put in the recharger. In addition, a backup set of fully charged batteries should always be on hand.

EMTs need to be able to communicate with dispatch, contact one another, and consult medical direction. If the equipment is not functioning properly, these communications may be impaired and may cause significant problems within the system. Your service should have some provision for backing up its communications system. Such provisions might include the availability of emergency generators at the base and repeater stations in case of power failure or the supplying of cell phones to EMS units for use in cases of radio failure.

As technology changes, new equipment becomes available that may have a role within the EMS system. This new equipment may have benefits and features that currently do not exist in your present system and may eventually improve the quality of your EMS system's communication (Figure 5-6*).

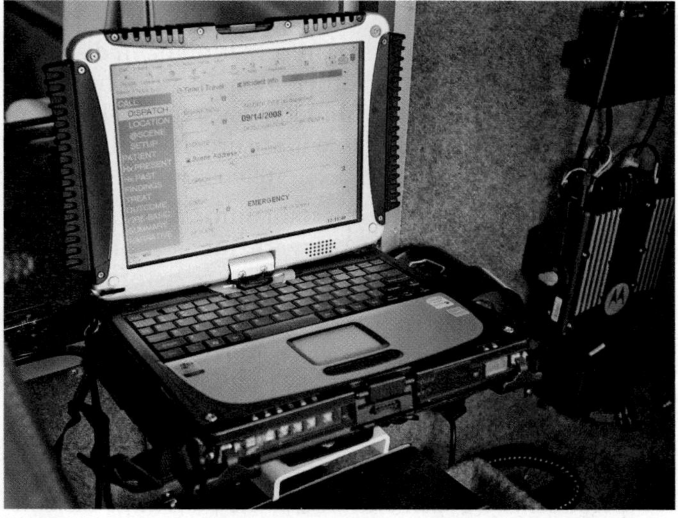

FIGURE 5-6 * Communication technologies continue to develop and change.

Communicating Within the System

As an EMT, you will be expected to communicate not just with your partners and patients but also with EMS dispatch, medical direction, and medical personnel at receiving facilities (Figure 5-7*). What follows are some guidelines for communication within the EMS system.

Ground Rules for Radio Communication

Whenever you are communicating via your radio to other members of the EMS system, there are some basic ground rules to keep in mind. These rules apply to your communications with any part of the EMS system and serve as a standard format for the transmission of information.

1. Turn on the radio and select the correct frequency. Use EMS frequencies only for EMS communication. Reduce background noise by closing your vehicle's windows.
2. Listen before transmitting. This ensures that the channel is clear of any other communications and avoids interruption of someone else's transmission. Adjust the radio to a proper volume.
3. Push the "press to talk" (PTT) button and wait 1 second before speaking. This will allow time for system repeaters to operate and will ensure that the initial part of your communication is not cut off.
4. Speak with your lips about 2 to 3 inches from the microphone. Speak clearly, calmly, and slowly in a monotone voice that can be completely understood (Figure 5-8*).
5. Address the unit being called by its name and number, and then identify your unit by name.
6. The unit being called will signal for you to begin transmission by saying "go ahead" or whatever is the standard in your system. If the unit being called responds with "stand by," that means wait to transmit until further notified.
7. Keep transmissions brief. If a transmission should take more than 30 seconds, pause for a few seconds to allow other units the chance to use the frequency for emergency transmissions.

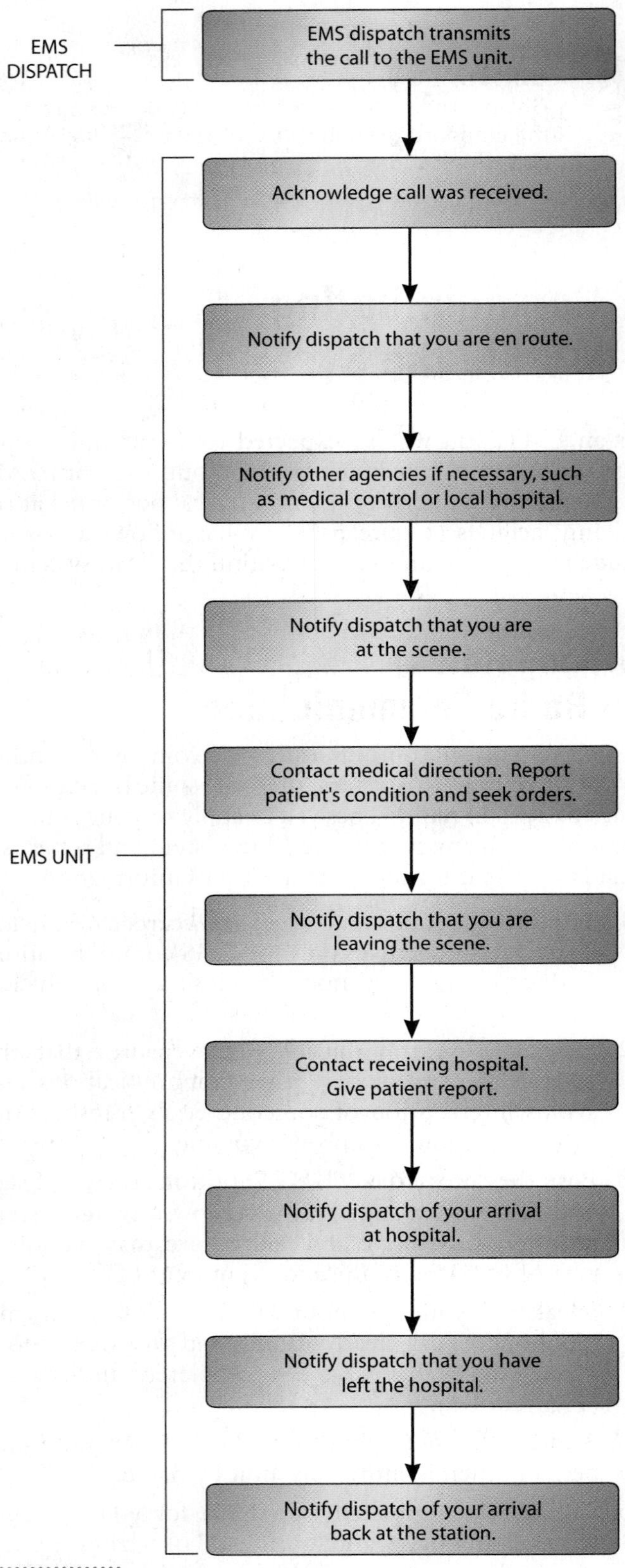
EMS
DISPATCH
EMS dispatch transmits the call to the EMS unit.
Acknowledge call was received.
Notify dispatch that you are en route.
Notify other agencies if necessary, such as medical control or local hospital.
Notify dispatch that you are at the scene.
Contact medical direction. Report patient's condition and seek orders.
EMS UNIT
Notify dispatch that you are leaving the scene.
Contact receiving hospital. Give patient report.
Notify dispatch of your arrival at hospital.
Notify dispatch that you have left the hospital.
Notify dispatch of your arrival back at the station.

FIGURE 5-7 ✱ Progression of radio transmissions.

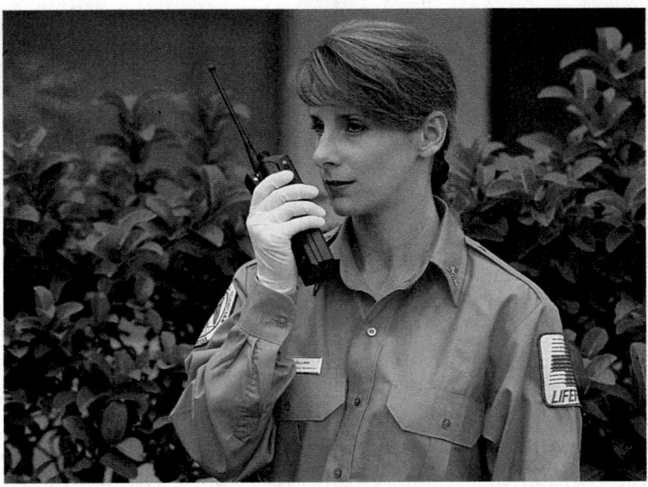

FIGURE 5-8 ✱ Hold the microphone about 2 inches from your lips as you speak into it.

8. Keep your transmission organized and to the point. Use plain English and clear text. Avoid slang and meaningless phrases such as "Be advised." Courtesy is assumed, so one should limit saying "Please," "Thank you," or "You're welcome." Also avoid codes or agency-specific terms unless their use is an accepted part of your system's communications.
9. When transmitting a number that might be confused with another (13 might be heard as 30), say the number ("thirteen"), then the individual digits that make it up ("one-three").
10. Avoid offering a diagnosis of the patient's problem. Instead, remain impartial and give only the objective information (observable, verifiable information such as vital signs, chief complaint, medications the patient has) and relevant subjective information (opinions or judgments such as, "The patient appears to be in extreme pain") that you have gathered during your patient assessment.
11. When receiving orders or information from dispatch, medical direction, or other medical personnel, use the "echo" method. Immediately repeat the order word for word. Doing so will ensure that you have received the information accurately and understand it.
12. Always write down important information, such as addresses, orders to assist with medication, and so forth that you receive from other parts of the EMS system.
13. The airwaves are public, and scanners, which are popular, can pick up radio and cell phone messages. Protect your patient's privacy by not using his name in your transmissions. Use objective, impartial language in describing the patient's condition. Do not make personalized comments about the patient or his condition; such statements could be grounds for a slander suit. Do not use profanity on the air.

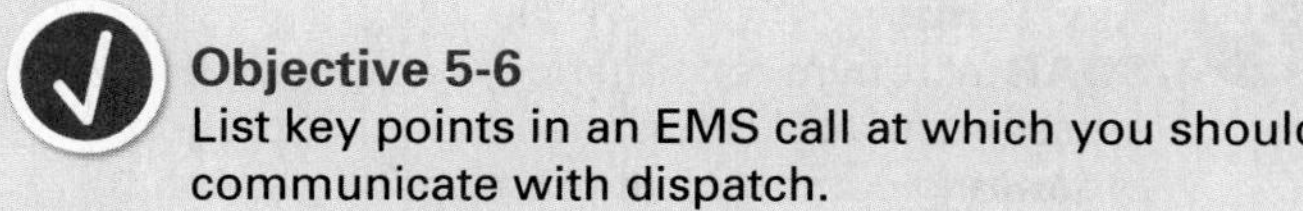

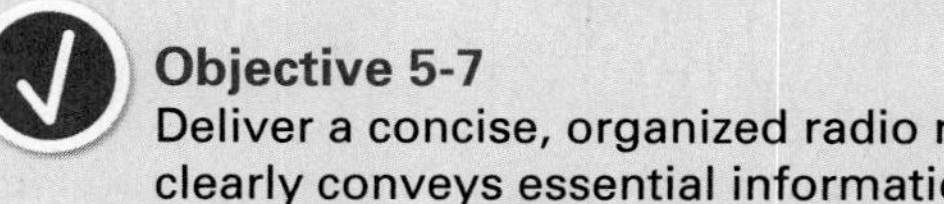

14. Use "we" rather than "I" in your transmissions; an EMT rarely acts alone.
15. Use "affirmative" and "negative" rather than "yes" and "no" in transmissions. The latter words can be difficult to hear.
16. When you are finished, say "Over." Wait for confirmation that the other unit has received your message and does not need to have anything repeated.

Phone/Cell Phone Communication

If your system utilizes phone or cell phone communications to deliver pertinent information, the content and format of the information should be treated similarly to that provided during radio communications. The EMT should be familiar with the cellular technology being used and should be aware of the cellular dead spots in the area. There should be another plan in place in case a cellular transmission fails while giving a report or communicating with another agency. The EMT should also be familiar with important and commonly utilized telephone numbers, such as those for medical direction, the local hospital emergency departments, and the dispatch centers.

Communicating with Dispatch

Your first contact on a run will probably be with your EMS system's dispatch—perhaps a certified Emergency Medical Dispatcher (EMD). Dispatch is the public's point of contact with the EMS system, usually through the phone system via the 911 universal emergency telephone number. It is the job of dispatch to obtain as much information as possible about an emergency, to direct the appropriate emergency service(s) to the scene, and to advise the caller on how to manage the situation until help arrives.

In many systems, dispatch records all conversations with initial callers, police, fire personnel, EMT units, and receiving facilities. These communications can all become part of the legal record if a call should eventually lead to a court case. This is another reason to be sure that your radio conversations are professional, concise, and accurate.

You will also note that dispatch gives the time after most communications with you. This will help you in providing times for your written report of a run. Accurate recording of time during a run can also be critical if the run should lead to a lawsuit.

The information that dispatch provides to you will assist you in doing your job. But remember that dispatch coordinates the different parts of the EMS system. Dispatch also needs information from you to ensure that all those parts work together efficiently. Communicate with dispatch at the following points:

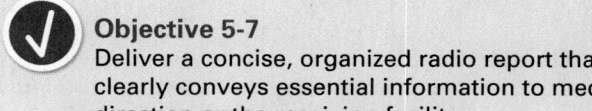

1. To acknowledge that the dispatched call information was received.
2. To advise dispatch when the unit is en route to the call.
3. To estimate your time of arrival at the scene while en route and to report any special road conditions, unusual delays, and so on.
4. To announce your unit's arrival on the scene, to request any needed additional resources, and to help coordinate the response. (In some systems, the unit must also report when they reach the patient after arriving on the scene.) Dispatch should be contacted if there is a prolonged on-scene time without communication.
5. To announce the unit's departure from the scene and to announce the destination hospital, number of patients transported (if more than one), and estimated time of arrival at the hospital.
6. To announce your arrival at the receiving hospital or other facility. If you were meeting at a rendezvous point, announce your arrival there.
7. To announce that you are "clear" and available for another assignment after the patient has been transferred.
8. To announce that you are leaving the hospital and are on your way back to the station.
9. To announce your arrival back at the station.

Communicating with Health Care Professionals

On a run, you may have to communicate with medical personnel at various times via your radio. The majority of these communications will be with your system's medical direction and with personnel at the facility to which you are transporting a patient. In some systems, you may need to communicate with other EMS providers to transfer care of the patient.

Communicating with Medical Direction

In some EMS systems, medical direction may be at your receiving facility. In others, it will be at a separate location.

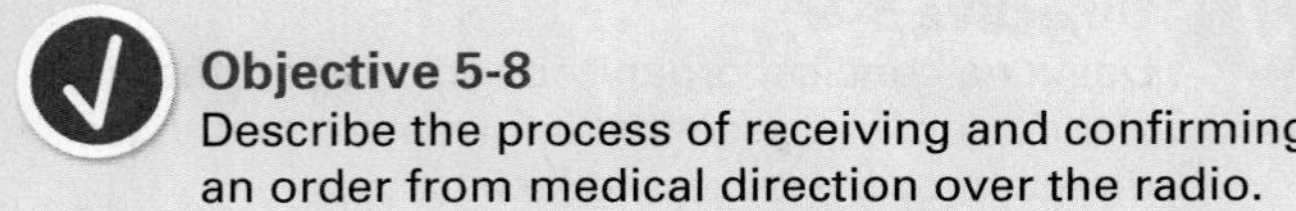

Objective 5-8
Describe the process of receiving and confirming an order from medical direction over the radio.

Key Terms
SBAR acronym for situation, background, assessment, and recommendation; a method of organizing communications about a patient.

You will often be expected to consult with medical direction on a run. There are cases in which medical direction may give you permission to assist in administering a patient's prescribed medication or may direct you to administer a medication from the ambulance's stock. Medical direction may also suggest procedures that you should follow with a patient or tell you not to perform other procedures.

Radio communications between EMTs in the field and their medical direction should be organized, concise, and pertinent. It is helpful to have an efficient and effective standard format for communicating patient information over the radio. This ensures that significant information is related in a consistent manner and that nothing is omitted. When communicating with medical direction, provide the following information:

1. Your unit's identification and its level of service: BLS (basic life support) or ALS (advanced life support). You may identify yourself as the provider giving the report.
2. The patient's age and sex.
3. The patient's chief complaint.
4. A brief, pertinent history of the present illness, including scene assessment and mechanism of injury.
5. Major past illnesses.
6. The patient's mental status.
7. The patient's baseline vital signs.
8. Pertinent findings of your physical examination of the patient.
9. Description of the emergency medical care you (and others) have given the patient.
10. The patient's response to the emergency medical care.
11. The patient's current condition.
12. Request for further actions/interventions at the receiving facility.
13. Estimated time of arrival.

To ensure that you have communicated accurately to medical direction and that you understand their directions completely, follow these additional guidelines:

- Be sure that the information you provide to medical direction is accurate and that you report it in a clear, understandable way. Remember that your patient's life may depend on the decisions that medical direction makes with that information.
- After receiving an order from medical direction to administer a medication or follow a procedure with a patient, repeat the order back word for word. This applies to things that medical direction tells you not to do as well.
- If you do not understand an order from medical direction, ask that it be repeated. Then repeat it back to medical direction word for word.
- If an order from medical direction appears to be inappropriate, question the order. Possibly medical direction misunderstood something in your description of the patient's condition or misspoke in prescribing a course of action. Asking questions may clarify the communication and may prevent the administration of a harmful medication or the application of an inappropriate procedure.

SBAR is method of organizing your communication into a standard format that would be particularly useful when communicating with medical direction, especially if you are seeking further orders. SBAR is an acronym for situation, background, assessment, and recommendation. *Situation* refers to the problem or reason why you are calling and the patient's chief complaint. *Background* is a concise description of the past medical history and the patient's response to treatment to that point. *Assessment* includes pertinent subjective and objective assessment findings such as mental status, vital signs, neurologic findings, blood glucose level, and Glasgow Coma Score. *Recommendation* is basically what you are requesting for the patient, such as an order to administer another nitroglycerin spray. The following is an example of the SBAR method of organizing communication:

Situation	Dr. White, this is EMT Stockdale. I have a 56-year-old male patient complaining of chest discomfort.
Background	He has a history of a previous MI and has a stent. His pain, which is typical of his previous MI, began 50 minutes ago. He experienced no relief of pain following administration of three nitroglycerin sprays or oxygen therapy. He was also given a 180 mg aspirin tablet.
Assessment	He is alert and his blood pressure is 168/98 mmHg. His heart rate is 108 bpm. He is very anxious.
Recommendation	I would like to administer another nitroglycerin spray.

Thinking Critically

Your elderly patient has suffered a fracture from a fall. You think you know why. In your radio report you say, "I think Grandpa was hitting the sauce today." Is it important to convey your suspicion that the patient is drunk? If so, how and when should you indicate this opinion?

Objective 5-9

Identify situations in which you should make additional contact with medical direction or the receiving facility after providing an initial radio report.

The primary advantage of using SBAR is that medical professionals involved in the communication have a certain expectation of what information will be given and how the information is to be communicated. This standard approach dramatically lessens the chance for miscommunication, lack of communication, or misunderstanding.

Communicating with the Receiving Facility

As an EMT, you will also be expected to communicate with medical personnel at the receiving facility to which you are transporting a patient. Staff at the facility need as much pertinent information about the incoming patient as possible to prepare for his arrival and to ensure continuity of care. Doctors and nurses may need to assign rooms and set aside equipment for your patient. They may need to request additional personnel to help with the patient upon your arrival. If, through your communication with the receiving facility, you provide an accurate picture of your patient's condition, the correct decisions about the assignment of resources can be made at the facility.

The information the EMT conveys to the receiving facility is quite similar to that given to medical direction. When you are about to leave the scene of a call and begin transport, contact the receiving facility with this information:

1. Your unit's identification and its level of service (BLS, ALS). You may identify yourself as the provider giving the report.
2. The patient's age and sex.
3. The patient's chief complaint.
4. A brief, pertinent history of the present illness, including scene assessment and mechanism of injury.
5. Major past illnesses.
6. The patient's mental status.
7. The patient's baseline vital signs.
8. Pertinent findings of your physical examination of the patient.
9. Description of the emergency medical care you (and Emergency Medical Responders) have given the patient.
10. The patient's response to the emergency medical care.
11. The patient's current condition.
12. Your estimated time of arrival at the facility.

As you transport the patient to the receiving facility, you will continue to reassess him and record your findings. Depending on your local protocol, you may be expected to communicate those findings, especially if the patient's condition is deteriorating, while you are en route. Make it a routine practice to report any deterioration or improvement to the receiving facility. In some systems, it may be necessary to notify the receiving hospital when you have arrived at their facility.

The Oral Report

Once you are at the facility and turning the patient over to staff there, you will deliver an oral report that takes into account your reassessment findings (Figure 5-9*). That oral report should summarize the information you already broadcast to the facility, along with updated information from your reassessment. Key items to include are the following:

- The patient's chief complaint
- The patient's vital signs taken en route
- Treatment given to the patient en route and his response to it
- Pertinent history not given in the earlier report to the facility

In addition to your oral reports to the receiving facility, both over the air and in person, you must also supply the facility with a copy of a written report. This document is known as the prehospital care report (PCR), as discussed in Chapter 4, "Documentation."

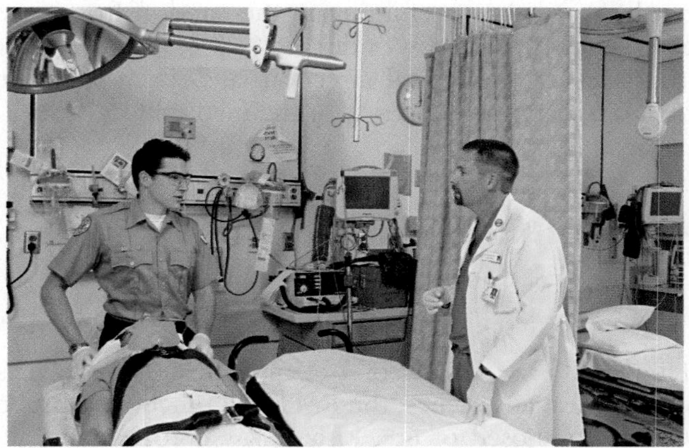

FIGURE 5-9 * You will deliver an oral report at the receiving facility.

Objective 5-10
Given a scenario, deliver an oral report to transfer care of the patient to a receiving facility or another EMS provider.

Key Points
As an EMT, you must be able to take charge confidently at the scene.

Objective 5-11
Given a scenario, demonstrate effective communication that enhances team dynamics.

Objective 5-12
Discuss the advantages and disadvantages of using radio codes.

Transferring Patient Care to Another EMS Provider

Sometimes it is necessary to transfer care of a patient from one EMT to another in the field. Make sure that you follow all your agency's policies and protocols when transferring patient care to another EMT or paramedic. When other EMS personnel arrive on the scene to take over patient care, it is important that you identify yourself and give them a verbal report. This report should include the following:

1. The patient's current condition
2. The patient's age and gender
3. The patient's chief complaint
4. A brief, pertinent history of what happened
5. A description of how you found the patient
6. Any major past illnesses
7. Vital signs you obtained from the patient
8. Pertinent findings of the physical exam
9. Any emergency medical care that was given
10. The patient's response to any emergency medical care that was provided

After giving your report, make sure you ask if they need any additional information before you leave the scene. Also, do not forget to obtain any information that you will need to complete your documentation of the call and transfer of care. Some agencies may request a copy of your documentation before you leave the scene so it can be included with their report to the facility.

The SBAR method of standardized communication can be particulary useful during the handoff from other emergency medical responders at the scene, when seeking orders from medical direction, and when providing the transfer report on arrival at the medical facility.

Team Communication and Dynamics

The EMT is a member of a team of health care professionals. At many scenes, the EMT will function as part of a team composed of fire, rescue, law enforcement, and other professionals. In these situations, the EMT is expected to communicate professionally with those working within the team as well as with others. Good team communication not only improves how the team accomplishes its goals, it also improves the quality of services provided to the patients and the community.

Taking Charge

It will be necessary for you as an EMT to take charge confidently at the scene to which you have been called. Your personal appearance and professional manner from the time of your arrival throughout your stay at the scene will help communicate to bystanders and family members, as well as to the patient, that you are in charge.

If you arrive on the scene and observe that the patient is alert and that no life-threatening conditions are present, it may be appropriate to be briefed—before you make direct contact with the patient—by the Emergency Medical Responder, whether that person is a police officer, a relative, or someone who has given first aid. This need not take more than a minute.

If the patient is unresponsive and life-threatening injuries are observed, go directly to the patient. Ask questions of the bystanders as you provide emergency care.

If a doctor is present or if fire-rescue personnel or police are also on the scene, an orderly transfer of authority must occur so that you are not simultaneously engaged in a dispute and attempting to care for the patient. Sometimes just asking a clear question like, "We're Emergency Medical Technicians. Is there anything we need to know before we provide emergency care?" will let rescue and police personnel brief you quickly and allow you to take over patient care. If a doctor is present, say, "We're certified EMTs, Doctor. How can we help?" In any situation, the EMT must be the advocate for good and proper patient care and not allow secondary issues to interfere with it.

Radio Codes

Some EMS systems use radio codes, either alone or in combination with messages in plain English. Radio codes can shorten radio air time and provide clear and concise information. They can also allow transmission of information in a format not understood by the patient, family members, or bystanders. There are, however, several disadvantages to the use of codes. First, the codes are useless unless everyone in the system understands them. Second, medical information is often too complex for

Objectives 5-13 and 5-14
Communicate using military time, standard clock times, and common radio terms.

Objectives 5-15 and 5-16
Describe the communication process and factors that can enhance or interfere with communication.

Key Terms

communication using verbal and nonverbal expressions as messages that are received and interpreted by others.

encoding process of converting information into a message.

codes. Third, some codes are infrequently used, so valuable time may be wasted looking up a code's meaning.

Some EMS services still use the Ten-Code system (for example, "10-4" meaning "received and understood"). Published by the Associated Public Safety Communications Officers (APCO), it is used primarily for dispatch and occasionally in EMS. Many EMS systems, however, have abandoned all codes in favor of standard English.

Times

U.S. Department of Transportation guidelines call for the use of accurate and synchronous clocks by EMTs. As an aid to ensuring such accuracy and synchronicity, most systems use military time rather than standard A.M. and P.M. designations in radio and written reports. Military time is a very simple system and correlates with standard time as follows:

1:00 A.M. to 12 Noon = 0100 to 1200 hours

1:00 P.M. to Midnight = 1300 to 2400 hours

Examples of the military time system include the following:

1427 hours is 2:27 P.M.

0030 hours is 30 minutes after midnight

Radio Terms

Radio conversations can be shortened by the use of one- or two-word phrases that are universally understood and employed. The following is a list of frequently used radio terms:

Break—afford a "pause" so that the hospital can respond or interrupt if necessary

Clear—end of transmission

Come in—requesting acknowledgment of transmission

Copy—message received and understood

ETA—estimated time of arrival

Go ahead—proceed with your message

Landline—refers to telephone communications

Over—end of message, awaiting reply

Repeat/say again—did not understand message

Spell out—asking sender to spell out phonetically words that are unclear

Stand by—please wait

10-4—acknowledging that message is received and understood

Therapeutic Communication

Principles of Patient Communication

Communication is an essential part of your job as an EMT. You must be able to communicate effectively with all those you come in contact with while you are on a call. Communication involves more than just what you say. Communication is a dynamic process that incorporates verbal and nonverbal expressions into meaningful messages that are received by others. These messages are composed of thoughts, ideas, information, and emotions that are sent by one person and interpreted by another. Many factors such as gender, culture, age, environment, and personal experience can influence how one sends and interprets these messages. As an EMT, you need to know how to communicate with patients in a manner that establishes a positive relationship. Once a positive relationship is formed, it becomes easier for you to get the information you need from the patient and to provide care.

The Communication Process

Communication begins when an individual, the *sender*, uses words and symbols to create a message. This process of converting information into a message is called **encoding.** The encoded message is sent to the *receiver*, the individual for whom the message is intended. To understand the message, the receiver must decode it. The process by which a message is translated and interpreted by the receiver is called **decoding.** Decoding is affected by the receiver's individual perceptions, values, and experiences. It is important that the intended meaning of the message be accurately decoded. The more closely the decoded message matches the intended meaning of the encoded message, the more effective the communication will be.

One way to ensure that the message is received as it was meant to be is through **feedback.** Feedback is any information that an individual receives about his behavior. It can be verbal or nonverbal, positive or negative. The receiver creates feedback to the message he received, then encodes that feedback to the original sender. The sender,

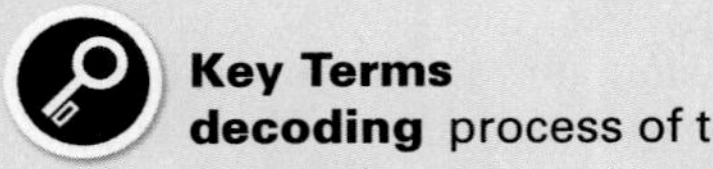

Key Terms

decoding process of translating and interpreting a message.

feedback any information that an individual receives about his behavior.

Objective 5-17
Give examples of clarification, summary, explanation, silence, reflection, empathy, and confrontation.

Objective 5-18
Given a scenario, engage in an effective communication process with a patient.

in turn, must decode the feedback in order to interpret it. Once again, decoding of the feedback message is affected by the decoder's personal perceptions, values, and experiences. This exchange of messages and feedback is repeated throughout the communication process.

Communication Responses

It is necessary to develop and establish a good rapport with your patients. Putting the patient and yourself at ease allows for better communication. If you treat your patients with respect, compassion, and empathy, your communication with them will be easier and more accurate.

As an EMT, you should understand that each patient will interpret your messages differently. You should also be aware that you need to interpret the patient's messages as closely as possible to the way he intends them. Actively listening to your patients will help you to accurately interpret what they mean to tell you and to understand what types of responses are most appropriate for each patient.

Some techniques that may facilitate communication with your patients are:

- **Clarification.** Sometimes it is necessary for the EMT to ask more questions in order to clarify the meaning of a message. Sometimes the patient may be so upset that he can't verbally express what he means to say. Let the patient know that you didn't understand what he meant, and ask him to say it again. If the message is not clear to you, communication will be impaired.
- **Summary.** It may be necessay for you to summarize your patient's messages in order to understand what he means. Rephrase what you have interpreted, and repeat it to the patient. You can ask if your summary is close to what he meant or felt. If your summary does not accurately represent the patient's feelings or ideas, ask for clarification.
- **Explanation.** As an EMT, you will have to explain many things in response to your patient's questions. You should present the information in way that he can understand it. Make sure you consider the patient's age and any language barriers when forming your response. You will also need to explain what he should expect to happen before it occurs. This will help establish trust and a good rapport between yourself and the patient. Watch for verbal and nonverbal clues that he does or does not understand your explanations.
- **Silence.** Sometimes what we don't say is more powerful than what we do say. Silence allows time to think and gain insight into what is occurring. It also allows time for patients who may be slow to answer because of language or other barriers to formulate an appropriate verbal response. Silence for an outgoing individual may be therapeutic, but for an individual coping with depression it may not be beneficial. As an EMT, you must consider your patient's needs when utilizing periods of silence.
- **Reflection.** This technique allows you to let the patient know that you understand what he said or feels. It redirects the patient's feelings and statements back to the patient in a way that promotes empathy, respect, and understanding.
- **Empathy.** Empathy is the ability to recognize and understand someone else's state of mind or feelings. It is the ability to put yourself in the patient's shoes. It is a characteristic that EMTs need to possess. Although you cannot actually experience what your patient has experienced, empathy enables you to understand how it has affected him.
- **Confrontation.** Sometimes it is necessary to confront a patient about discrepancies in his feelings, attitudes, beliefs, or behaviors. This is NOT to be accomplished through anger and aggression by the EMT. It may require an EMT to be more assertive than usual, but with the assertion comes a desire to help the patient overcome his crisis and understand his own feelings and behaviors. Even when you need to confront or challenge him, always respect the patient and act in the patient's best interest.
- **Facilitated communication.** Facilitated communication is done by supporting the patient's hand, wrist, arm, shoulder, or elbow so that he can select letters on a letterboard, electronic keyboard, or other communication device to communicate with you. People with certain developmental or sensory disabilities may require you to act as a facilitator. You must be careful not to influence what is being communicated by the patient to you.

Communicating with the Patient

When you arrive on a call, you may find the people at the scene injured, frightened, anxious, and possibly angry or in shock. These are all high-intensity emotions that can make getting information from and delivering information to

Thinking Critically
At a crash scene, everybody is hysterical including the trapped driver, his wife who managed to crawl out of the passenger side, and various bystanders. How would you go about establishing communication?

Key Terms
defense mechanisms psychological coping strategies individuals use to protect themselves from unwanted feelings or thoughts.

people difficult. To establish effective face-to-face communications with people in such circumstances, keep in mind the three Cs: competence, confidence, and compassion. If you convey these qualities in what you say and do, you will get better cooperation and have to deal with fewer hostile or irrational responses. As an EMT, it is important that you build a good rapport with your patient to promote trust. Patients expect that you will provide professional care and have a true concern for their needs.

Patient Contact

Developing rapport and communicating with your patient begins when you arrive on scene. It includes everything from how you present yourself physically to what you say and do from that first moment on. Follow these guidelines when communicating with the patient:

- First impressions are critical. Before you arrive on scene, make sure that your physical appearance positively reflects the health care professional you are. Just as your patient's appearance makes a first impression on you, your appearance makes an impression on your patient. Dress professionally and approach your patients with compassion and confidence.
- When you approach the patient, introduce yourself as you want to be called. Ask for the patient's name. Also ask what he wishes to be called. With older people, err on the side of formality—"Mrs. Lubeck" or "Mr. Perez"—since they may consider it disrespectful for a stranger to address them by their first name. Remember to continue to use the patient's name throughout your contact with him. This shows respect and conveys interest in the patient as an individual.
- Introduce the rest of your team to the patient. Although you may not be able to give the names of every responder on the call, make sure the patient knows which agencies and personnel are helping him. Your partner and anyone working closely with the patient should be identified by name.
- Be sure also to say, "I'm going to help you. Is that all right?" This will help in gaining consent for treatment as discussed in Chapter 3, "Medical, Legal, and Ethical Issues," and Chapter 4, "Documentation."
- Don't be surprised if a patient says, "No!" or "I'm okay!" when you ask about providing assistance. Usually the resistance will be a form of denial or another defense mechanism because he is simply frightened or confused. **Defense mechanisms** are psychological coping strategies the person may use to protect himself from unwanted feelings or thoughts. Although these defense mechanisms are used by patients to protect themselves, they can create barriers to communicating and interacting with them. Keep talking calmly and try to shift the patient's focus or use distraction by saying something like, "Looks like an accident happened here. I can see there's something wrong with your shoulder. Does it hurt?" or "Your husband called us because he's worried about you. Would it be all right if we talked about it for a minute or two?"
- Speak clearly, calmly, and slowly. People who are under stress or in medical shock process information more slowly. Speak distinctly and simply. Try to use language an average person will understand rather than medical terminology, codes, jargon, and abbreviations. Try to speak calmly and give orders quietly. Emotions can escalate quickly in tense situations.
- Use a professional tone of voice. Speak with concern and compassion. Modulate your voice if needed. Raise your voice only if the patient is hard of hearing. Avoid tones that might be perceived as flippant, sarcastic, angry, or otherwise unprofessional.
- Respect the patient's privacy. Try to limit the number of bystanders around the patient. Speak so the patient can hear you, but do not broadcast information to the rest of the crowd. Some patients may be reluctant to discuss their condition, even around friends or family, so try to interview the patient alone if possible.
- Limit interruptions when communicating with your patient. This will give you the chance to actively listen to your patient and help you communicate better with him. Allow interruptions only when absolutely necessary for the patient's care.
- Think about the position you assume in relation to the patient and be aware of your own body language. Be aware of the space between you and your patient.
- Try to control the physical environment. Make sure that the lighting is sufficient for you and the patient to see each other. Limit outside noise and interference so that you may actively listen to what your patient has to say. Turn off distracting equipment if it is not necessary for patient care. Ask for your patient's permission to turn off the television or other loud

Key Points
When you combine effective interviewing techniques with genuine compassion and concern, you will be able to gather the information you need to help your patients.

Objective 5-19
Recognize the potential messages that may be communicated via nonverbal behaviors.

devices if they interfere with your ability to hear and communicate.

- Be courteous. Patients and bystanders are often emotionally unstable. Explaining what you are doing, giving them choices when possible, being honest with them, and apologizing for necessary discomfort are ways of allowing them a sense of control in the situation.
- Actively listen to your patient. When a patient asks you questions, reply as fully as you can, explaining when you cannot answer a question. Also, give the patient ample time to answer a question before you ask another one.
- Be honest with the patient. If you are able to earn and maintain the patient's trust, it is often easier to provide the care that he needs. If that trust is lost, patient care may become more difficult to provide.

The Patient Interview

It is important to conduct an interview that will provide you with as much information as possible about your patient and the emergency. To do this, you need to know what types of questions to ask your patients and how to ask them. When you combine effective interviewing techniques with genuine compassion and concern, you will be able to gather the information you need to help your patients.

Nonverbal Communication

As stated earlier, your communication with the patient begins before you speak a word. Just as your physical appearance conveys professionalism, your nonverbal communication, or body language, conveys meaning too. Nonverbal communications such as those listed next speak just as strongly as, if not more strongly than, the words you say.

- **Posture.** The way you position yourself in relation to your patient will impact how you are perceived. Use your arms and body position effectively. Approach the patient with open arms, open hands, and relaxed shoulders. That will convey a message of concern, confidence, safety, and care. If you cross your arms, point your finger, clench your fists, or shake your head negatively, you signal that you are angry, hostile, disgusted, or uncomfortable around the patient (Figure 5-10a*). Such signals limit communication and often make the interviewing process uncomfortable and unproductive. Position yourself at the same level as your patient to indicate that you see the patient as your equal (Figure 5-10b*). If you stand over him, it suggests that you see yourself as an authority figure, which may be intimidating. An exception to

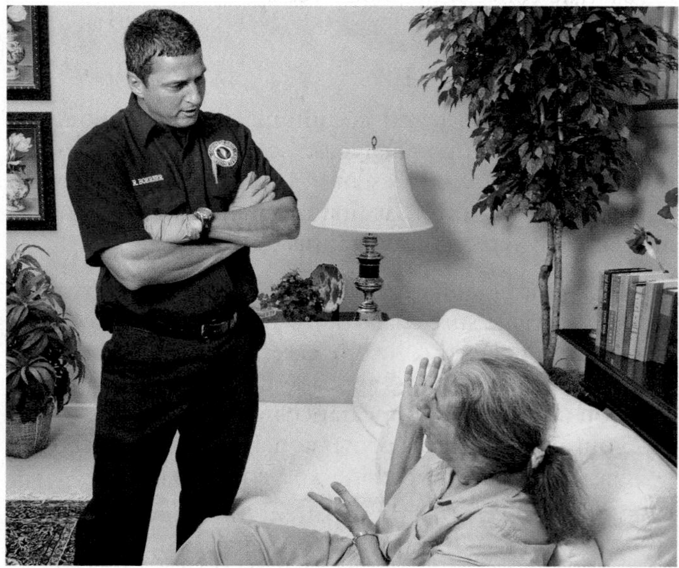

FIGURE 5-10a * Standing over a patient with crossed arms conveys an intimidating sense of yourself as an authority figure.

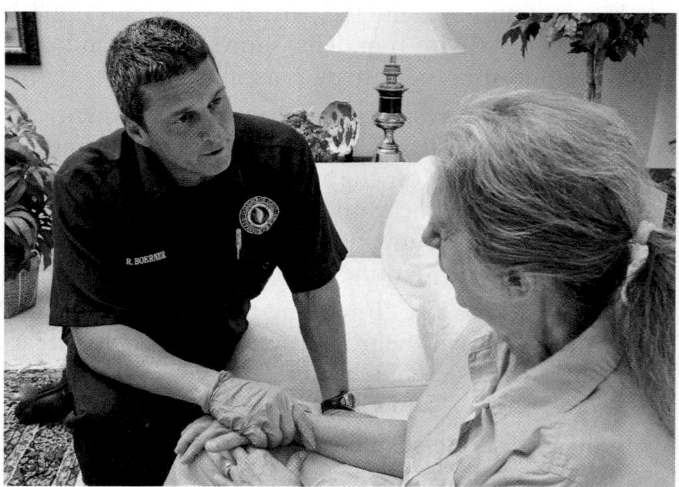

FIGURE 5-10b * Position yourself at the patient's eye level to indicate that you see the patient as your equal.

Key Terms

intimate zone in American culture, the space within less than 1½ feet of an individual.

gestures nonverbal body movements that convey meaning to others.

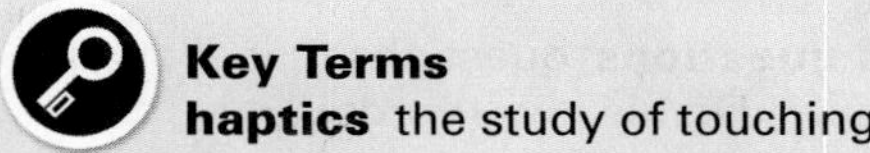

Key Terms

haptics the study of touching.

this is when a patient seems hostile or aggressive, in which case you may prefer to keep your eye level above his to assert your authority. When addressing children or the elderly, positioning yourself below their eye level may help them feel more comfortable and secure.

- **Distance.** Be aware of the distance between you and your patient. In American culture, the space within less than 1½ feet of an individual is called the **intimate zone.** Entering your patient's intimate zone may be seen as threatening, even though you have to be close in order to make a proper physical assessment. It is best to use a more personal distance of about 1 to 4 feet from your patient when you are communicating with him verbally. Ask and inform your patient about what you need to do before you enter his personal or intimate space. Most patients understand the need for you to enter this space. If you meet resistance, step back until you establish a better rapport and the patient trusts you to enter his space. An acceptable social distance to talk to another person without shouting would be about 4 to 12 feet. In public, most people will keep 12 feet or more between themselves and another person, but it sometimes cannot be done. Other cultures do not share the same spatial zones as Americans. Misunderstandings can occur when too much or too little space is used. Consider a patient's culture and nonverbal responses when invading his personal space. Observe your patient's eye contact and other reactions when you approach him. This may provide a guide as to how much distance to maintain between you.
- **Gestures. Gestures** are nonverbal body movements that convey meaning to others. They are composed of movements from any part of the body, including facial expressions. Facial expressions can include winking, smiling, rolling your eyes, pushing your eyebrows together, or any other expression that conveys an emotion. Your patient's facial expressions can indicate fear, anxiety, pain, sorrow, relief, or dismay. It is important that you watch and acknowledge your patient's expressions as indications of how he feels. A warm, kind smile indicates your concern and welcomes communication from your patient.
- **Eye contact.** Make and maintain eye contact when you are speaking with the patient. Doing so helps to communicate your interest and concern. However, you should be aware that some cultures (Asians, Native Americans, Indochinese, and Arabs, for example) consider direct eye contact impolite or aggressive; you may have to modify your behavior if you note that a patient is reluctant to make eye contact with you.
- **Haptics. Haptics** is the study of touching. Touch can be one of the most effective ways to help calm the patient and express your compassion and empathy. Holding a hand, patting a shoulder, giving a hug, or laying your hand on a forearm can be more powerful than words if done sincerely (Figure 5-11*). Most patients welcome a warm touch from the EMT who has come to help them. A patient's age, gender, culture, and experiences may influence how the touch is perceived. Maintaining eye contact can help you decide if the patient will allow you into his intimate space so that when you need to touch the person, that touch is not perceived as encroachment.

Both the EMT and the patient communicate verbally and nonverbally throughout the entire emergency call. Remember that nonverbal communication is individually interpreted by both of you and is exchanged just as verbal communication is. Culture, age, gender, and experience influence how nonverbal communication may be perceived. Sometimes, what is said verbally is contradicted by nonverbal expressions. When this contradiction occurs, the meaning of the message is primarily derived from what was expressed nonverbally.

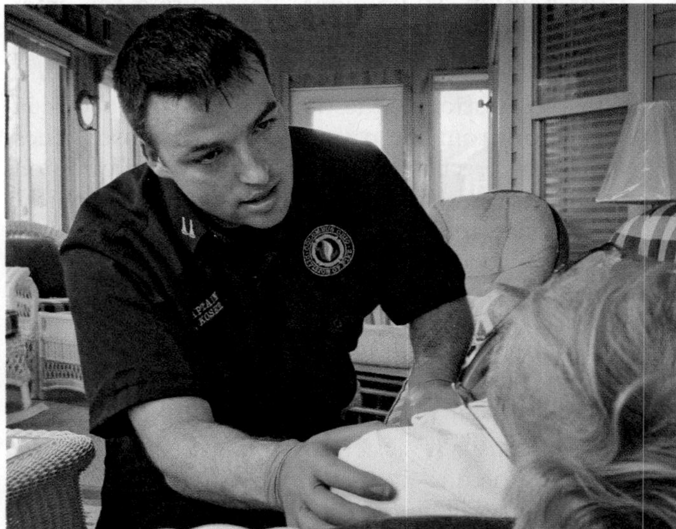

FIGURE 5-11 * Most patients welcome a warm, compassionate touch.

Objective 5-20
Describe the uses, advantages, and disadvantages of open-ended and closed questions.

Key Terms
open-ended questions questions that allow the patient to respond in his own words.

Key Terms
closed questions questions that call for specific information from the patient.

leading questions questions that suggest an answer.

Asking Questions

Most patients are more than willing to talk to you. Most will provide answers to the questions you ask without hesitation. Make sure that you ask one question at a time. Give the patient adequate time to respond to your question, and listen to his response before you ask another question. Choose language that the patient can understand. Avoid using professional jargon that your patient is not familiar with. Also, consider the patient's age and stage of development when asking a question. Adjust your communication strategies and techniques when interviewing children, elderly patients, patients with special needs, and patients from different cultures. Take notes, so that you can remember the information the patient provides to you. Different types of questions promote different responses from your patient.

- **Open-ended questions.** Questions that allow the patient to give a detailed response in his own words are called **open-ended questions.** This form of questioning will provide you with the most information. For example, when you arrive on scene you need to obtain the patient's chief complaint. If you ask "What seems to be the problem?" it allows the patient to state his chief complaint in his own way. "How are you feeling?" is another open-ended question that will provide significant information about your patient's condition. Keep in mind that some patients may not be able to provide a lot of detail because of their physical or emotional state during the emergency. If possible, however, ask open-ended questions throughout the patient interview.
- **Closed questions.** Questions that call for specific information from the patient are called **closed questions,** or direct questions. These types of questions are helpful when you need to get information quickly or to obtain additional information that may not have been provided from an open-ended response. They can be used to direct and control the flow of the interview. "What medications do you take?" and "When did the pain begin?" are examples of closed questions. The patient will normally respond with only the information you have asked for. These questions are usually easier for the patient to answer. Many of the questions that you ask during your history taking will be closed questions.

For more about questioning and history taking, see Chapter 13, "Patient Assessment."

Considerations in Interviewing

It is important to keep the patient interview moving in a therapeutic direction. Some considerations to keep in mind when you are interviewing the patient include the following:

- **Do not ask leading or biased questions. Leading questions** are questions that suggest an answer guided by the individual who is asking the question. An example of a leading question would be "So you're having chest pain. It really hurts badly doesn't it?" This type of question promotes answers that may not be accurate or beneficial to the patient interview and may lead the EMT to ask a series of questions that may not relate to the patient's actual complaint or symptoms.
- **Do not interrupt your patient when he is speaking.** You cannot listen or communicate effectively if you are not paying attention to what your patient is saying or doing. You may miss pertinent information that could affect your patient care if you do not allow the patient to finish his thoughts.
- **The patient or the EMT may talk too much.** When a patient is overly talkative, one way to help the interview progress is to ask more closed questions. This will help keep the answers shorter while still providing useful information. If you are overly talkative, you will not be able to actively listen to what your patient has to say.
- **Do not provide false assurance.** Never lie to your patient. Be honest but not heartless. Remember that most patients are overwhelmed by the emotions and situation they are enduring and look to you for safety, empathy, and assurance. If you genuinely address their concerns, they will typically feel more at ease.
- **Do not give inappropriate advice.** As a medical professional, you will be asked for advice by your patients. They want to have answers about their condition, but the best advice you can give them is to be evaluated by a physician at the hospital. You should not offer any form of diagnosis of your patient's condition, nor should you discourage your patient from receiving prompt medical treatment. Remember that you are an authority figure, and your opinion matters to your patients. Do not overstep or abuse the trust they have placed in you.
- **Do not ask "why" questions that imply blame.** Remain impartial and nonjudgmental at all times.

Thinking Critically

One lonely man is so glad to see you he talks your ear off. A woman at the next call won't look at you, mumbles replies, and volunteers nothing. How can you do the best possible interview with each of these difficult patients?

Objectives 5-21 and 5-22

Analyze your communications with patients with regard to questioning techniques, family issues, difficult patients, and culture or language issues.

Key Terms

culture the thoughts, communications, actions, and values of a racial, ethnic, religious, or social group.

Remember that your primary concern is for your patient. By asking questions like "Why did you do that?" you are creating an intimidating atmosphere that will impede both your communication and your patient care.

- **Family preference issues.** Although most family members are trying to help the patient, it is important to know your department's policies about interacting with family. Adults who are capable of providing their own informed consent are entitled to make their own decisions, regardless of their families' preferences. Explain the patient's rights to the family in an empathetic way. However, it is necessary to consider the families' preferences when treating and transporting children who require parental consent. Similarly, if the patient is mentally incompetent or is incapable of providing informed consent for any other reason, family preferences should be considered and honored if possible. (See Chapter 3, "Medical, Legal, and Ethical Issues," for a more detailed discussion of consent.) If, for whatever reason, the patient's situation dictates the use of a facility that is not preferred by the family or patient, explain kindly to the family why the facility you suggest is necessary. For example, if you have a major trauma patient but the family requests that you take the patient to a small local community emergency department, you can explain that the facility they want to go to may not have the staff or equipment to properly care for their loved one's injuries. Most patients and family members will be responsive to the change if you explain why it is in the patient's best interest.
- **Motivating the unmotivated patient to talk.** Start the interview in the normal way. Attempt to use open-ended questions to gain pertinent information. Make sure the patient understands the questions you are asking. Reassure him that you are there to help him. If your patient speaks a different language, you may choose to use a language line, which is an interpreter service provded by telephone. If the patient still has difficulty or refuses to answer your open-ended questions, ask closed questions instead. Provide positive feedback to any answers you receive and continue to build rapport. Continue to ask questions your patient can understand and continue to provide positive feedback to him. If your patient has any special needs, make sure you address them appropriately.
- **Interviewing a hostile patient.** Sometimes you must interview a patient who is hostile and does not want your help. Some patients may be under the influence of street drugs or alcohol while others may have psychological or other behavioral issues. Remember that if your safety is compromised, you must not approach the patient until the scene is safe. (See Chapter 12, "Scene Size-Up.") Request help from law enforcement if necessary. Some patients may require restraint. If they do, know your department's protocols and policies. It also may be necessary for you to have additional personnel available with you in case the patient becomes violent or makes false accusations. Once the scene is secured and safe, begin the interview as usual. To overcome some of the hostility, try to establish a good rapport with the patient. Make sure that you maintain a professional nonthreatening demeanor. Advise the patient that you are there to help him, and explain the benefits of having his cooperation. Inform your patient what conduct and behaviors are acceptable, and provide him with alternative ways to express himself. Then, conduct the interview in the same way that you would for any other unmotivated patient.

Special Circumstances

There are some categories of patients with whom you will have to make extra efforts to establish effective communications (Figure 5-12∗). You must adjust your communication strategies to meet the needs of your patients. Remember that, even when you are having problems communicating with someone, you should remain calm, confident, and caring. The following sections describe special communication circumstances that should be addressed by the EMT.

Transcultural Considerations

When providing care to a patient, the EMT should consider how the patient's culture will influence the dynamics of the call. **Culture** is composed of the thoughts, communications, actions, and values of a racial, ethnic, religious, or social group. It impacts how information is received, how illness is viewed, and what treatments are preferred by the individual patient. It is important to understand that both the EMT and the patient bring

Key Terms

ethnocentrism the view that one way of doing things is the right way and any other way is inferior.

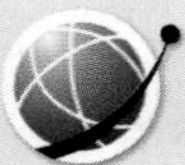

Media Resources

Go to www.bradybooks.com for mykit. Highlights:

- *Video:* Alternate Methods of Communication with Children
- *Video:* Nonverbal Communication

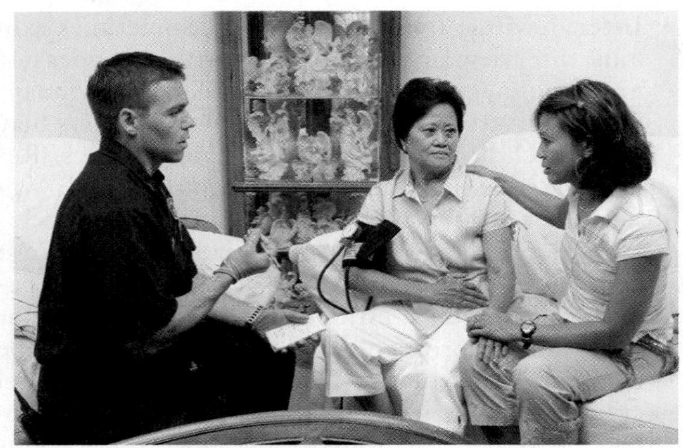

FIGURE 5-12 ✱ You may need to make a special effort to communicate with some patients, for example the elderly or those who don't speak English.

cultural stereotypes to a professional relationship. These stereotypes must be overcome to achieve a therapeutic relationship. **Ethnocentrism** is the view that one culture's way of doing things is the right way and any other way is inferior. EMTs should not view any culture as superior to another. It is important for the EMT to respect the patient's culture and avoid any cultural imposition. You should never impose your beliefs or values on your patients.

When addressing a patient from a different culture, you should begin by introducing yourself as you want to be called. Pay careful attention to the space between yourself and the patient. Remember that various cultures view space differently. Be sure to watch your patient for nonverbal signs that you are or are not maintaining an appropriate amount of space between you. In other cultures, many people accept the role of the sick person in different ways. Some of your patients may use established folk medicine practices before calling for your assistance.

Some patients may not speak English, and you may not speak their language, thus creating a language barrier between you and them. You can ask if relatives or bystanders can interpret for you. If no one at the scene can assist, check with dispatch or medical direction to see if they have anyone who can interpret for you over the radio. Toll-free interpreter lines are available. Remember to consider who has interpreted the information for you.

Considerations for Elderly Patients

Be prepared to take extra time in communicating with elderly people. Aging can bring with it potential problems with hearing and vision. Do not assume that all elderly patients have such problems, but if you detect signs of them, show understanding. Speak slowly, distinctly, and more loudly to such patients. Obtain their glasses or hearing aids for them. This will help in building a good rapport and communicating more effectively.

When dealing with a person who has a hearing problem, be sure your lips are visible as you speak. Make sure that you speak clearly, slowly, and distinctly. If a patient is deaf but indicates he can communicate through American Sign Language (ASL), check to see if relatives or bystanders can interpret for you. Also consider writing notes on a pad to communicate.

Never appear brusque or impatient, especially when helping an elderly patient. Always listen to the patient and allow ample time to answer your questions. Elderly patients may require extra assistance in collecting valuable information or their medications at the scene. Remember that these patients may easily become tired, and offer to help them get what you need for them. Many elderly patients resent being talked to as if they are children or mentally incapacitated. Make sure that you treat elderly patients, as you do for all patients, with respect and compassion and without condescension.

Considerations for Children

Working with children requires extra patience and effort. Having a child's parents present can aid in communicating with the child, but be sure the parents understand that they should remain calm and confident in front of the child. If they seem too frightened or disoriented by the situation, they will communicate those feelings to the child and complicate your ability to assist him.

Positioning yourself close to the patient's eye level is especially important with children. A uniformed figure towering overhead can be terribly upsetting to a child. Crouch down to the child's level or sit on the floor if the circumstances seem to suggest it. Maintain eye contact and speak calmly. Try to give clear explanations of what you are doing by using simple language and without talking down to the child. Always be honest with a child. If you lie to him, it will be extremely difficult to ever regain his trust. Communicating with the pediatric patient will be covered in detail in Chapter 38, "Pediatrics."

CHAPTER REVIEW

SUMMARY

Communication is one of the most fundamental functions performed in emergency medical services and is involved in all phases of a call. The call is initiated by communication between the patient, a relative, or a bystander, and the call taker. You are then notified by either verbal or digital communication to respond to the scene. At the scene and at the receiving facility, you will communicate with members of your team and with other health care professionals.

Communication during patient assessment and care is a primary means for gathering information from and about the patient and for providing appropriate emergency care to the patient. It should be performed in a manner that achieves a positive relationship with the patient and that will benefit the patient's outcome. You can adjust your communication strategies to develop a good rapport and facilitate communication with the broad variety of patients that you will encounter.

You will provide a verbal report to the receiving medical facility over the radio and finally in person. As communication systems continue to become more technologically sophisticated, you must refine your communication practices to meet the needs of the system.

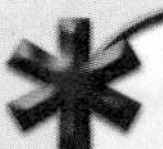

CASE STUDY FOLLOW-UP

SCENE SIZE-UP

You have been dispatched to 101 Bate Road with a report of a man bleeding. You approach the scene carefully, looking for any signs of danger. You see nothing that causes you concern, but you still exercise caution as you and your partner don gloves and protective eyewear and get out of the ambulance. As you do, a man who had been sitting next to the garage approaches you. He is holding a blood-soaked rag around his right hand. His shirt and pants are also blood stained. The man appears pale and seems to be sweating a little.

As you start toward him, the man says, "You guys got here fast. I'm glad to see you. I feel like an idiot having to call, but no one else was home and I felt a little dizzy seeing all the blood. The bleeding's almost stopped now, though. Oh, yeah. Hi. I'm Dave Behrens."

You introduce yourselves and lead Mr. Behrens to the ambulance where he can sit down. When he's seated, you ask, "How did you injure yourself, Mr. Behrens?" He replies, "I was cutting some molding with my saber saw at my workbench. That's in the garage. I think the cat must have gotten in and knocked over a bottle. Anyway, it startled me. I turned to look and ran my hand into the blade. Idiot."

PRIMARY ASSESSMENT

Your general impression of the patient is of a male in his mid-40s, injured, and alert. Because he responds fully to all questions, you see he has no breathing problems and his airway is patent. You assess his radial pulse on the uninjured side and find it to be slightly fast, but strong. The rag wrapped around the hand he says he injured is blood soaked, but no blood appears to be dripping from the wrapping now. Because the bleeding appears to be controlled and Mr. Behrens displays no signs or symptoms of shock, he is not considered a priority for rapid transport.

SECONDARY ASSESSMENT

Mr. Behrens has already given you the mechanism of injury, a cut from the blade of a saber saw. You now expose the injury, carefully removing the greasy rag in which he has wrapped the hand. The injury is an approximately 3-inch-long laceration across the base of the palm. The wound is now bleeding only minimally. You apply a sterile dressing to the wound and bandage it in place.

You assess distal perfusion by observing skin color, which appears normal, and by feeling the injured hand, which is warm and moist. You ask Mr. Behrens if he can gently wiggle the fingers of the injured hand and he does so. You then ask him to turn his head to one side and identify the fingers on the injured hand that you touch. He does so successfully.

You and your partner obtain a set of baseline vital signs. Mr. Behrens's blood pressure is 148/86 mmHg. His heart rate is 92 per minute. His respirations are 14 per minute, full and adequate. His skin is normal color, warm, and moist.

You take a history. It reveals the following: Mr. Behrens says the wound is causing slight pain; he has an allergy to penicillin; he is not currently taking any medications; he denies having any significant medical problems; he had a cup of coffee about 15 minutes before cutting himself; he denies that there were any strange or unusual problems prior to the accident.

You explain to Mr. Behrens that a doctor should look at and treat the cut and that you will transport him to the hospital. He refuses, however, to ride on the cot, saying, "It's bad enough that I had to call you for a dumb mistake. I'm not going to go in like something from *ER*." He agrees to ride on the jump seat and you secure him to it.

As you start off, you radio in a report: "Dispatch, this is Unit 2. We are en route to Columbia Memorial Hospital with a nonpriority patient." Dispatch replies, "Unit 2 en route to Columbia Memorial at 1143 hours."

REASSESSMENT

Your partner is riding in the back with Mr. Behrens. She performs the reassessment. She finds that Mr. Behrens remains completely alert and oriented. Blood has not soaked through the dressing, an indication that bleeding has been controlled. She takes another set of vital signs, then radios ahead to the hospital: "Columbia Memorial, this is Craryville BLS Unit 2 en route to you with an ETA of 10 minutes. We have a 46-year-old male with a 3-inch laceration of the right hand caused by a saber saw. The patient is alert and oriented. The patient says he is allergic to penicillin. His vital signs are blood pressure 146/84, radial pulse 80, respirations 14 and of good quality, skin normal, warm, and moist. We have dressed and bandaged the wound. Bleeding appears to have stopped and patient acknowledges only slight pain from the wound."

Your partner continues to monitor Mr. Behrens during transport, but notes no major changes in his condition other than that he now seems completely relaxed. As you pull up to the hospital, you radio this message: "Dispatch. This is Unit 2 arriving at Columbia Memorial." Dispatch acknowledges with "Unit 2 at Columbia Memorial at 1152 hours."

You and your partner assist Mr. Behrens from the ambulance and transfer him to the care of the hospital staff. Your partner says to the emergency department nurse, "This is Mr. David Behrens. He has a 3-inch laceration to the palm of his right hand from a saber saw. Mr. Behrens is allergic to penicillin. We applied a dressing and bandages to the wound and the bleeding appears to have stopped completely. His vitals are blood pressure 144/82 mmHg, pulse 80 bpm, respirations 14 per minute, skin color, temperature, and condition is normal."

The nurse takes charge of Mr. Behrens while your partner fills out the prehospital care report. You begin to straighten and clean the back of the ambulance. When your partner returns, you radio, "Dispatch, this is Unit 2. We are available for assignment." Dispatch replies, "Unit 2 available for assignment at 1207 hours." You then start back to base, remembering that you will radio dispatch upon your arrival there.

IN REVIEW

1. List the standard components of an EMS communications system.
2. Explain the function of a repeater.
3. Explain legal considerations that apply to EMS communications.
4. List the points at which EMTs on a run are expected to communicate with dispatch.
5. Explain the procedure that should be followed when medical direction orders an EMT to administer a medication or follow a designated procedure with a patient.
6. List the information that the EMT should provide to the receiving facility while en route with the patient.
7. List the information the EMT is expected to provide in the oral report when turning a patient over at a receiving facility.
8. Explain the importance of eye contact with a patient.
9. Explain the possible effects on communication with a patient of (a) the EMT's body position and (b) touch.
10. Explain what measures an EMT might take when trying to communicate with a patient who is deaf or hearing impaired.
11. Explain the process of communication.
12. Identify special interview situations that require communication adjustments.
13. Explain how culture can influence communication.
14. List hazards associated with interviewing patients.
15. Describe how to use questions to obtain specific information from a patient.
16. List possible types of responses that are common in communication.
17. Describe how to build a good rapport with a patient.

CRITICAL THINKING

You arrive on the scene and find a 36-year-old female patient who complains of severe abdominal pain. The patient is alert and oriented. Her vital signs are BP 88/64 mmHg; HR 128 bpm; R 24 and adequate chest rise; skin is pale, cool, and clammy; SpO_2 is 96% on room air. Her radial pulses are weak. She states the pain began suddenly about 4 hours ago and has progressively worsened. She was sitting on the couch watching television when it began. Nothing makes the pain better or worse. The pain is dull and aching, and it is intermittent. The pain does not radiate.

The patient rates the severity of her pain as 8 on a scale of 1 to 10. She states she feels light-headed and dizzy every time she stands up, and she also feels nauseated. She has no known allergies and takes over-the-counter Prilosec for heartburn. She has no pertinent medical history. She reports she had her tonsils removed when she was 10 years old. She has had nothing to eat or drink for about 7 hours. She states that she has "not felt real good" for a few days, and other than the time she has spent working at her desk at work, she has been at home on the couch. Her pupils are equal and sluggish to respond. She has no JVD. Her breath sounds are equal and clear bilaterally. Her abdomen is rigid and tender. There is no evidence of trauma to the abdomen. She has good motor and sensory function in all four extremities. Her peripheral pulses are very weak.

En route to the hospital, the patient begins to close her eyes. You must verbally instruct her to open her eyes. Her BP is 82/62 mmHg, HR 134 bpm, and R 26 with adequate chest rise. The pulse oximeter is providing an "error" reading. Her skin is more pale, cool, and clammy and her radial pulses are barely palpable. Your estimated time of arrival at the hospital is 7 minutes.

1. What techniques would you use to communicate with this patient?
2. Are there any special circumstances that you would consider when communicating with this patient?
3. Would you contact medical direction during your management of this patient?
4. What information is important to relay in the radio report to the receiving medical facility?
5. What information would you provide in your oral report to the medical personnel at the receiving medical facility during the transfer of care?
6. What information would you report regarding the change in the patient's condition?

EXPLORE PEARSON mybradykit™

Please go to **www.bradybooks.com** to access mykit for this text. You will find quizzes, critical thinking scenarios, weblinks, animations, and videos related to this chapter—and much more. Look for online information on effective communication. You will also find a video clip on nonverbal communication.

Register your access code from the front of your book by going to **www.bradybooks.com** and selecting the mykit links.

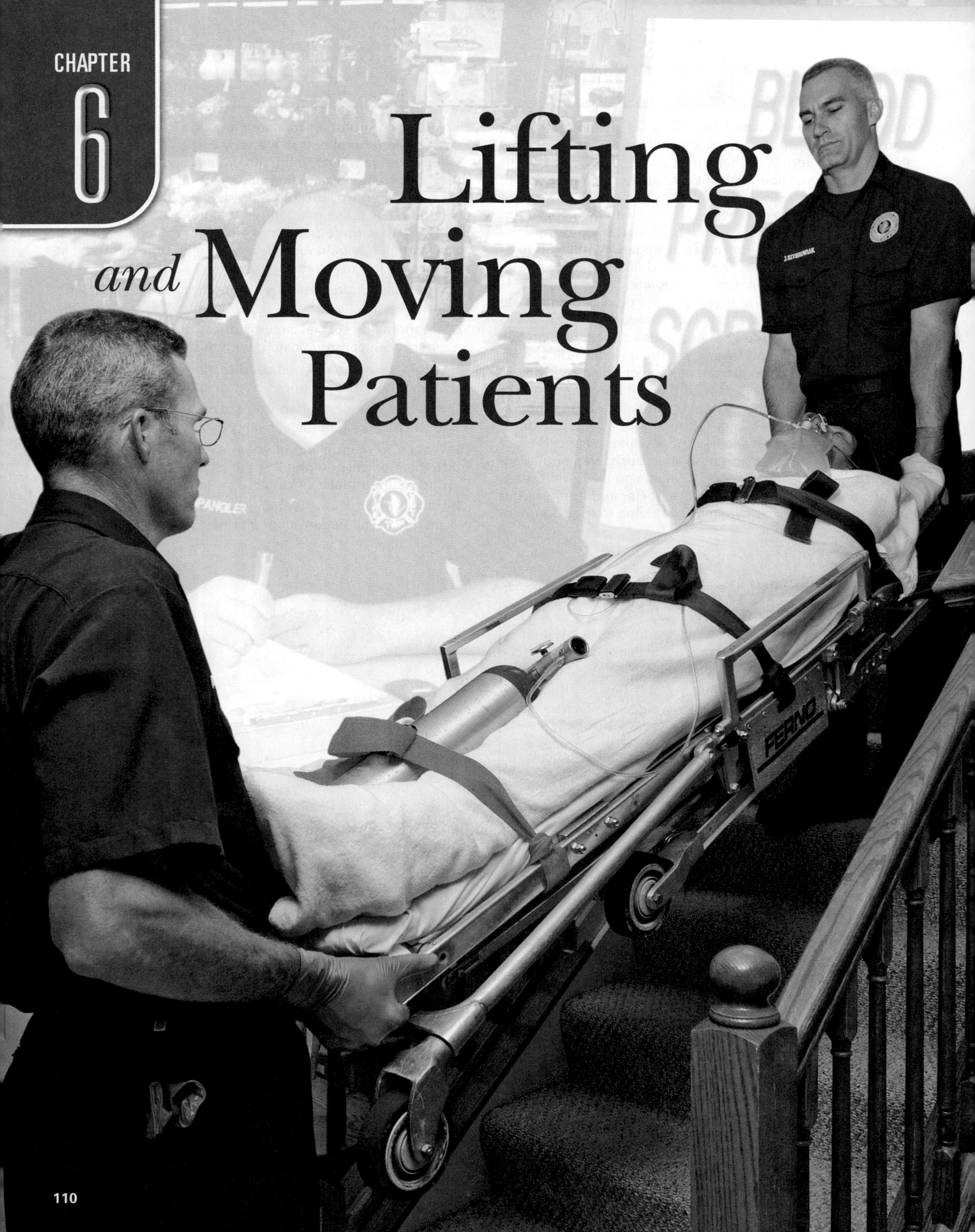

CHAPTER 6

Lifting and Moving Patients

Navigation Guide

The following items provide an overview to the purpose and content of this chapter. The Standard and Competency are from the new National EMS Education Standards.

STANDARD **Preparatory** (Content Areas: Workforce Safety and Wellness)

COMPETENCY Applies fundamental knowledge of the EMS system, safety/well-being of the EMT, medical/legal and ethical issues to the provision of emergency care.

OBJECTIVES: After reading this chapter, you should be able to:

6-1. Define key terms introduced in this chapter.
6-2. Explain the importance of always using proper techniques when lifting, carrying, and moving patients and equipment.
6-3. Define the term *body mechanics.*
6-4. Demonstrate each of the four principles of body mechanics listed in the text when lifting and moving patients and equipment.
6-5. Explain the roles of proper body posture and physical fitness in preventing injuries resulting from lifting and moving patients.
6-6. Describe considerations in teamwork and communication with partners and patients when lifting and moving patients.
6-7. Apply the general guidelines for lifting and moving patients that are described in the text.
6-8. Discuss the advantages, disadvantages, and steps of each of the following lifting and moving techniques and processes:
  a. Power lift
  b. Power grip
  c. Squat lift
  d. One-handed equipment carrying
  e. Reaching
  f. Log roll
  g. Pushing and pulling
6-9. Differentiate between scenarios in which emergency, urgent, and nonurgent moves are indicated.
6-10. Given a scenario, demonstrate an appropriate moving technique to be used, including:
  a. Armpit-forearm drag
  b. Shirt drag
  c. Blanket drag
  d. Rapid extrication
  e. Direct ground lift
  f. Extremity lift
  g. Direct carry
  h. Draw sheet method
6-11. Demonstrate the steps required to securely "package" a patient for transport.
6-12. Describe the proper use, advantages, disadvantages, and limitations of each of the following pieces of equipment used in lifting and moving patients:
  a. Wheeled stretcher
  b. Portable stretcher
  c. Stair chair
  d. Backboard
  e. Scoop stretcher
  f. Basket stretcher
  g. Flexible stretcher
  h. Devices for bariatric patients
6-13. Given a scenario involving any of the following types of patients, demonstrate proper positioning of the patient:
  a. Unresponsive patient
  b. Patient with chest pain or difficulty breathing
  c. Patient with known or suspected spinal injury
  d. Patient in shock
  e. Patient with nausea or vomiting
  f. Patient in third trimester of pregnancy
  g. Infant or toddler
  h. Elderly patient
  i. Patient with a physical disability
6-14. Discuss special considerations when preparing patients for air medical transport.
6-15. Discuss special considerations when using a neonatal isolette.

KEY TERMS: Page references indicate first major use in this chapter. For complete definitions, see the Glossary at the back of the book.

body mechanics p. 112
emergency move p. 117
kyphosis p. 113
lordosis p. 113
nonurgent move p. 117
power grip p. 115
power lift p. 115
urgent move p. 117

continued

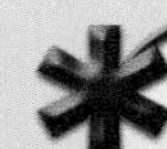

Navigation Guide *continued*

MEDIA RESOURCES: Please go to www.bradybooks.com to access mykit for this text. You will find quizzes, critical thinking scenarios, weblinks, animations, and videos related to this chapter—and much more. Look for online information on lifting bariatric patients.

CASE STUDY

The Dispatch

EMS Unit 101—proceed to 605 Lindsey Drive in Rockaway—a 72-year-old patient has a routine transfer to Dover General—time out is 0910 hours.

Upon Arrival

You are a probationary EMT accompanied by a training officer and an experienced EMT. Your training officer tells you that she knows the patient, Amanda Sanchez, and that this is one of three prescheduled visits Mrs. Sanchez takes to the hospital dialysis center every week. She tells you the patient cannot walk without assistance and will need help getting down one flight of stairs. As your partner parks the ambulance, he remarks that there is still snow and probably ice on the walk to the house.

How Would You Proceed to Package and Transport This Patient?

During this chapter, you will read about how to lift and move patients using good body mechanics and equipment designed to assist in patient movement. Later, we will return to the case study and apply the procedures learned.

▶ Introduction

A key skill that you will perform with almost every patient contact is the lifting and/or moving of a patient from where he is to your cot, then to the ambulance, and eventually to the hospital cot. Unfortunately, too many EMTs are injured every year because they attempt to lift patients or equipment improperly. The knowledge and use of proper body mechanics are a necessary foundation for your health, longevity, and effectiveness as an EMT.

The best way to move a patient in any circumstance is generally the easiest way that will not cause injury or pain to your patient or to yourself. Let your equipment do the work whenever possible. If you must lift, do it with a device designed for that purpose, if possible. As a rule, get as much help as you can to carry patients and equipment. Never risk falling or injuring yourself. And always follow the rules of body mechanics.

▶ Body Mechanics for Safe Lifting

As an EMT you are required to lift and carry patients and heavy equipment. If you perform these tasks improperly, bodily injury, strain, and lifelong pain can be the result. With conscious planning, good health, and skill, you can perform these tasks with minimum risk to yourself. Apply the principles and techniques of proper lifting and moving every day. Practice often enough for them to become automatic. Make them a habit that increases your safety and performance—even in the most stressful emergency situations.

Four Basic Principles

Body mechanics are defined as the safest and most efficient methods of using your body to gain a mechanical advantage. They are based on four simple principles:

- *Keep the weight of the object as close to the body as possible* (Figure 6-1∗). Back injury is much more likely to occur while reaching a great distance to lift a light object than while reaching a short distance to lift a heavy object.
- *To move a heavy object use the leg, hip, and gluteal (buttocks) muscles plus contracted abdominal muscles.* The use of these muscles will help you generate a huge amount of power safely. Always avoid using back muscles to move a heavy object.
- *"Stack."* Visualize the shoulders stacked on top of the hips, and the hips stacked on top of the feet (base).

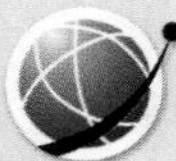

Media Resources

Go to www.bradybooks.com for mykit. Highlights:

- *Web Resource:* Lifting and Moving Patients
- *Web Resource:* Lifting Bariatric Patients

Key Terms

body mechanics applying safe methods of moving the body, correcting posture, and lifting.

Objectives 6-2 and 6-3

Explain the importance of proper lifting, carrying, and moving techniques, and define *body mechanics*.

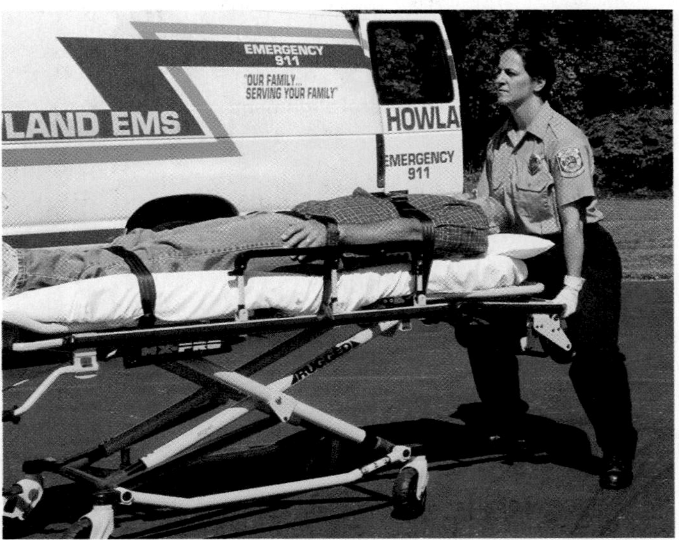

FIGURE 6-1 * Using proper body mechanics, the weight is kept close to the body as it is lifted.

Then move them as a unit. If any of the three are not aligned with the others, you can create twisting forces that are potentially harmful to the lower back.

- *Reduce the height or distance through which the object must be moved.* Get closer to the object or reposition it before lifting (Figure 6-2*). Lift in stages if necessary.

Lifting, carrying, moving, reaching, pushing, and pulling are all activities to which proper body mechanics should be applied. One important key to preventing injury is correct alignment of the spine. Maintaining a normal inward curve in the lower back significantly reduces the potential for spinal injury. Keeping wrists and knees in normal alignment can also help to prevent injury of the extremities. In addition, whenever possible, substitute equipment for manual force.

Posture and Fitness

One much-overlooked aspect of proper body mechanics is posture. Because you will spend a great deal of time sitting or standing, poor posture can easily fatigue back and abdominal muscles, thereby making you vulnerable to back injury.

One extreme of poor posture is the swayback, or excessive **lordosis**. In this posture the stomach is too anterior and the buttocks are too posterior, causing excessive stress on the lumbar region of the back. Another extreme is the slouch, or excessive **kyphosis**. In this posture the shoulders are rolled forward, which results in fatigue of the lower back and increases pressure on every region of the spine (Figure 6-3*).

Be aware of your posture. While standing, your ears, shoulders, and hips should be in vertical alignment, with knees slightly bent and pelvis slightly tucked forward (Figure 6-4*). In the proper sitting position, your weight should be evenly distributed on both ischia (lower portion of the pelvic bones), with your ears, shoulders, and hips in vertical alignment, and your feet should be flat on

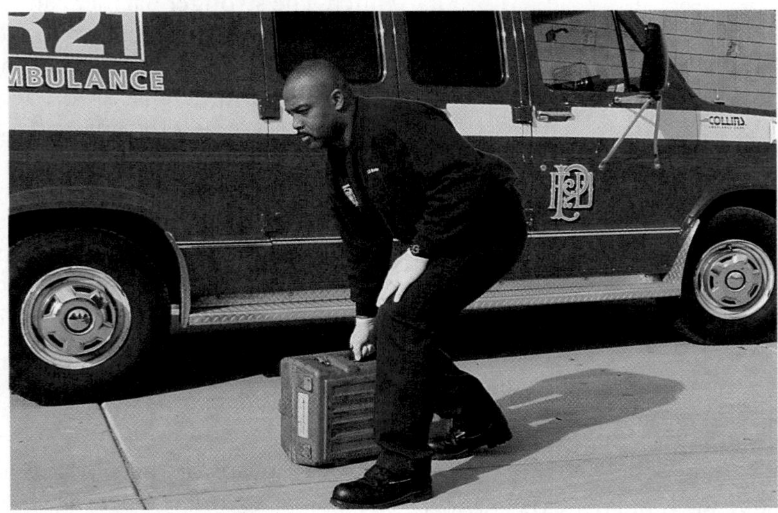

FIGURE 6-2 * Reduce the height or distance through which the object must be moved. Get closer, reposition it, or move it in stages.

Key Terms
lordosis abnormal anterior convexity of the spine. Also called *swayback.*

Objectives 6-4 and 6-5
Demonstrate the four principles of body mechanics and explain the roles of posture and fitness in preventing injuries resulting from lifting and moving.

Key Terms
kyphosis abnormal curvature of the spine with convexity backward. Also called *slouch.*

Objective 6-6
Describe considerations in teamwork and communication with partners and patients when lifting and moving patients.

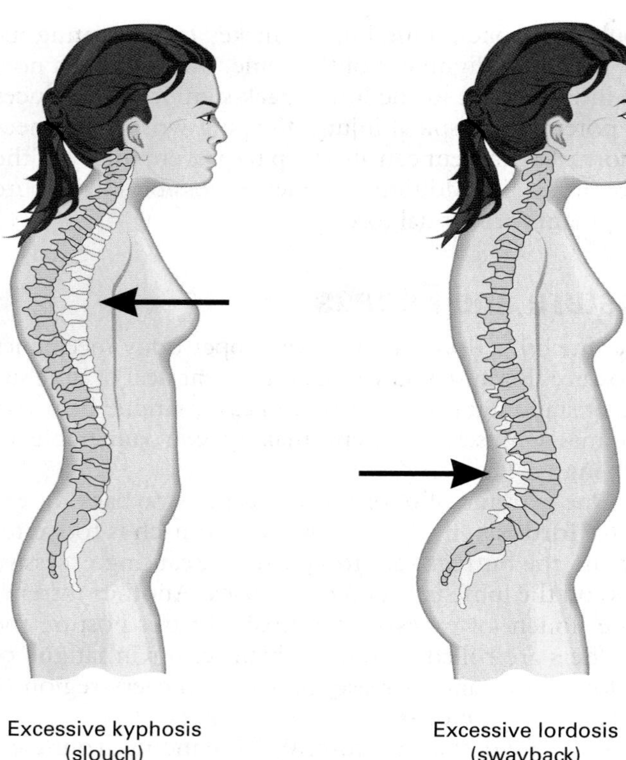

Excessive kyphosis (slouch)
Excessive lordosis (swayback)

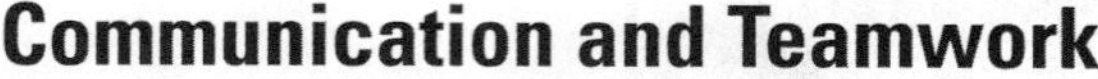

FIGURE 6-3 ✱ Extremes of poor posture are excessive lordosis (swayback) and excessive kyphosis (slouch).

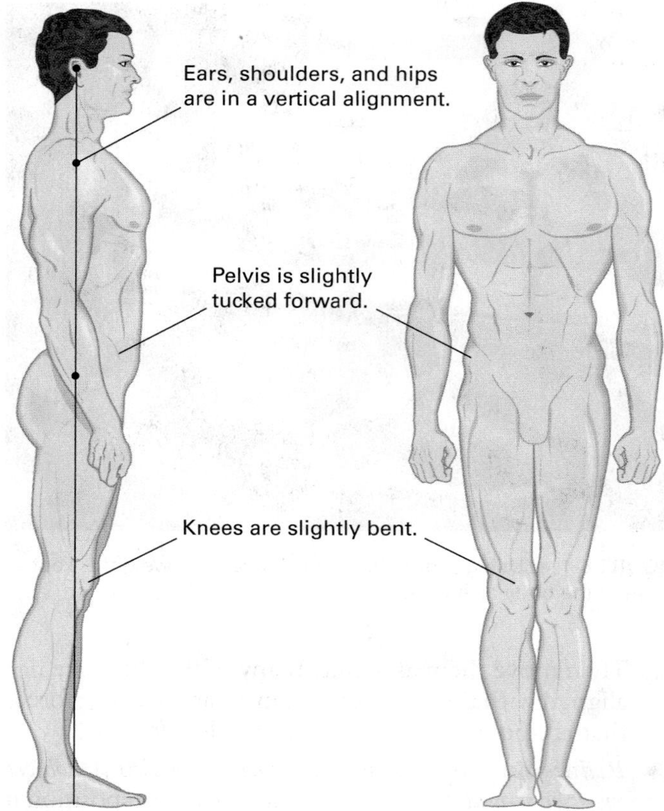

Ears, shoulders, and hips are in a vertical alignment.
Pelvis is slightly tucked forward.
Knees are slightly bent.

FIGURE 6-4 ✱ Proper standing posture.

the floor or crossed at your ankles. If possible, your lower back should be in contact with the support of the chair (Figure 6-5✱).

Proper body mechanics cannot sufficiently protect you if you are not physically fit. A proactive, well-balanced physical fitness program should include flexibility training, cardiovascular conditioning, strength training, and nutrition. Such a program can help you prevent injury, enhance performance, and manage stress.

Communication and Teamwork

In an emergency, teamwork and effective communication among team members are essential. Patients come in all sizes, shapes, and strengths. Just as a football coach positions players according to their abilities, rescuers should capitalize on their abilities to ensure the best outcome in an emergency.

All team members should be trained in the proper techniques. Problems can occur when partners are greatly mismatched, and not only to the overloaded weaker partner. The stronger partner can also be injured if the weaker one fails to lift. Ideally, partners in lifting and moving a patient or object should have adequate and equal strength and height. Two adequately strong but weaker rescuers are as efficient and safe as the pairing of two stronger rescuers.

In order for team members to work together effectively, they need to communicate throughout all lifting and moving tasks. Use commands that are easy for team members to understand. Verbally coordinate each lift from beginning to end. Good teamwork will also allow you to:

- Size up the scene immediately and accurately.
- Consider the weight of the patient and recognize the need for additional help.
- Be aware of the physical abilities and limitations of each team member.
- Select the most appropriate equipment for the job.

Objective 6-7
Apply the general guidelines for lifting and moving patients that are described in the text.

Objective 6-8
Discuss the advantages, disadvantages, and steps of the power lift, power grip, squat lift, one-handed carrying, reaching, log roll, pushing, and pulling.

Key Terms

power lift recommended technique for lifting. Feet are apart, knees bent, back and abdominal muscles tightened, back as straight as possible, lifting force driven through heels and arches, upper body rising before hips.

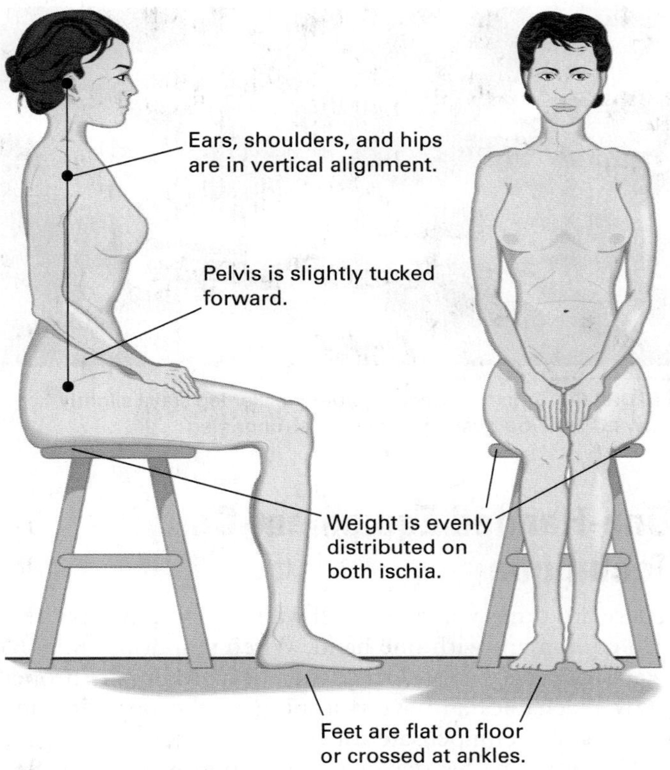
Ears, shoulders, and hips are in vertical alignment.
Pelvis is slightly tucked forward.
Weight is evenly distributed on both ischia.
Feet are flat on floor or crossed at ankles.

FIGURE 6-5 * Proper sitting posture.

Just as important as the communication between team members is the EMT's communication with the patient. If startled or frightened, the patient might shift body weight while you attempt the lift. Shifts in weight can cause disabling injury to rescuers as well as cause significant additional injury to the patient. Whenever a patient is able to understand, explain the plan before any action is taken. This will improve patient confidence and can engage the patient in assisting in his own rescue.

General Guidelines for Lifting and Moving

Know your own physical abilities and limitations. Do not overestimate yourself or other rescuers. Before lifting, know or find out the weight of the patient as well as the weight limitations of the equipment being used. Call for additional help whenever necessary. Even though your first impulse may be to jump in and help the patient, you must not proceed until you know you can do so safely.

Always try to use an even number of rescuers to maintain balance. Two-rescuer teams should carry heavy loads for 1 minute or less. More time can generate a high level of muscle fatigue, which can significantly increase the potential for injury. Whenever possible, transport patients and equipment on wheeled stretchers or other rolling devices.

When you must carry, keep the weight as close to your body as possible. Keep your back in a locked-in position. Do not hyperextend your back, or lean back from the waist. Refrain from twisting, and never lift and twist simultaneously. First lift, then turn as a unit.

The Power Lift

The **power lift** is the technique that offers you the best defense against injury and protects the patient with a safe and stable move. It also is a useful technique for rescuers with weak knees or thighs. In performing this technique, keep your back locked and avoid bending at the waist. Follow these steps (EMT Skills 6-1):

1. Place your feet a comfortable distance apart. For the average-sized person, this is usually about shoulder width. Taller rescuers might prefer a little wider stance since this brings them closer to the object to be lifted.
2. Turn your feet slightly outward. Most people find that this helps them feel more comfortable and more stable.
3. Bend your knees to bring your center of gravity closer to the object to be lifted. As you bend your knees, you should feel as though you are sitting down, not falling forward.
4. Tighten the muscles of your back and abdomen to splint the vulnerable lower back. The back should remain as straight as comfortable (there is normally a slight inward curve), with your head facing forward in a neutral position.
5. Straddle the object. Keep your feet flat with your weight evenly distributed and just forward of the heels.
6. Place your hands a comfortable distance from each other to provide balance to the object as it is lifted. This is usually at least 10 inches apart.
7. Always use a **power grip** to get maximum force from the hands (Figure 6-6*). That is, your palm and

Key Terms

power grip recommended gripping technique. The palm and fingers come in complete contact with the object and all fingers are bent at the same angle.

Key Points

Get as close as possible to the object you are going to lift. Do not reach or twist and lift at the same time.

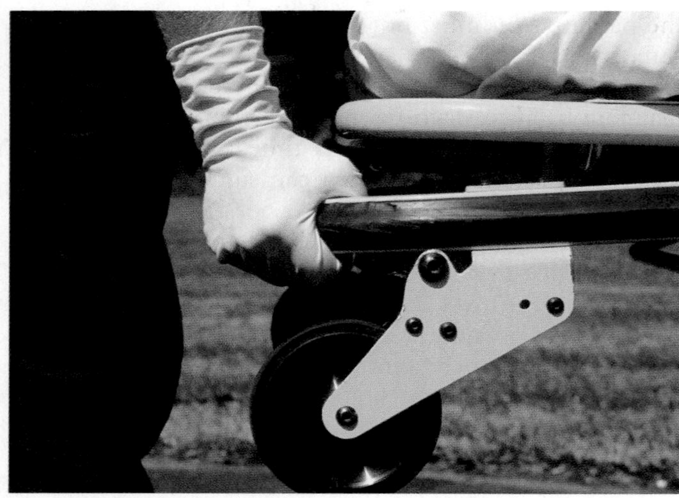

FIGURE 6-6 * In the power grip, palms and fingers should come in complete contact with the object and fingers should be bent at the same angle.

fingers should come in complete contact with the object and all fingers should be bent at the same angle.

8. As lifting begins, your back should remain locked in as the force is driven through the heels and arches of your feet. Your upper body should come up before the hips.
9. Reverse these steps to lower the wheeled stretcher or other object.

The Squat Lift

The squat lift is an alternative technique you can use if you have one weak leg, one weak ankle, or if both your knees and legs are strong and healthy (Figure 6-7*). In performing this technique, avoid bending at the waist.

1. Place your weaker leg slightly forward. This foot should stay flat on the ground throughout the lift.
2. Squat down until you can grasp the cot, stretcher, or other patient-moving device. Be sure to use the power grip.
3. Push yourself up with your stronger leg. Make sure your back is locked and your upper body goes up before your hips. Lead with your head.

While performing any lift, always remember to use your leg muscles—not your back—to lift, keep the weight as close to your body as possible, position yourself correctly, and communicate clearly and frequently with your partner.

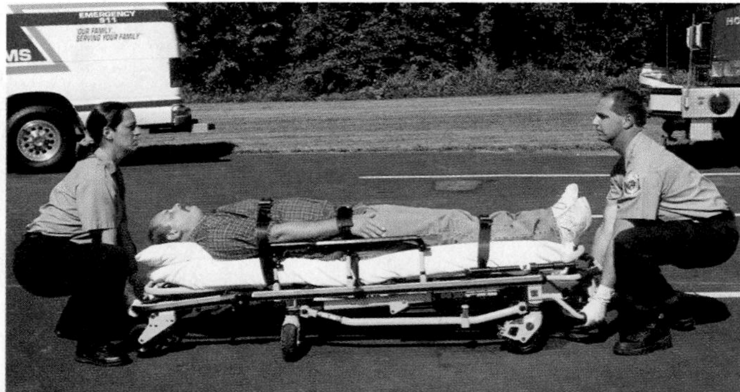

FIGURE 6-7 * In the squat lift, your weaker leg stays slightly forward and you push up with your stronger leg.

One-Handed Equipment-Carrying Technique

There are times when you will want to lift and carry certain equipment with one hand. When you do, be sure to keep your back in a locked position. Maintain proper body mechanics and avoid leaning to the opposite side too much to compensate for the imbalance.

To use a one-handed carrying technique (Figure 6-8*) to lift and move a patient-carrying device, first stagger your feet with one knee up and one knee pointing toward the ground. Bend at the hips, not the waist, and do not let your trunk go any farther forward than 45°. On command from the rescuer at the patient's head, simultaneously drive upward through the arch and heel of the front foot and the ball of the back foot.

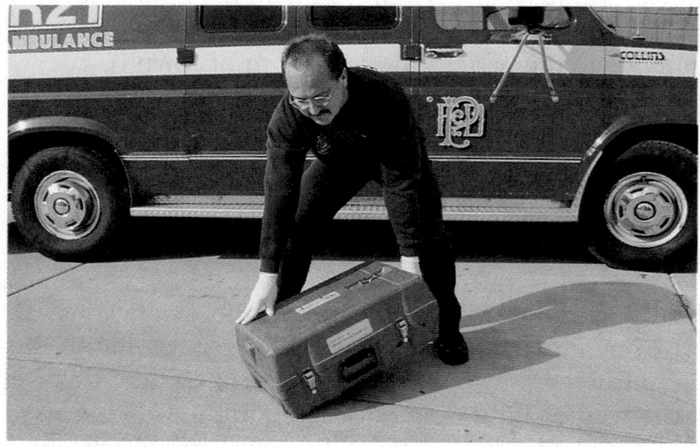

FIGURE 6-8 * One-handed carrying technique.

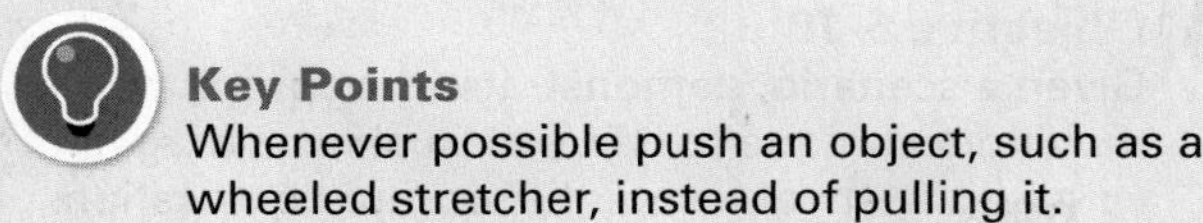

Key Points
Whenever possible push an object, such as a wheeled stretcher, instead of pulling it.

Key Points
The principles of proper body mechanics and lifting techniques must be applied to all situations in which the EMT has to lift patients or move equipment.

Reaching

Generally, a person can sustain a 100 percent effort for 6 seconds and a 50 percent effort for only 1 minute before becoming fatigued. After that minute, the potential for injury greatly increases. So, to minimize effort, whenever possible reposition the object or get closer to the object to avoid or reduce reaching and lifting. Especially avoid situations in which prolonged strenuous effort (more than 1 minute) is required.

Many times EMTs find it necessary to reach for equipment or for a patient (as in a log roll). When it is necessary, reach no more than 15–20 inches in front of the body. If an object is more than 20 inches away, move closer to it before attempting to reach and lift. When reaching, keep the back in a locked position. Do not twist. Use your free arm to support the weight of your upper body whenever possible. If you reach overhead, avoid hyperextending (that is, do not lean back from the waist).

When performing a log roll, lean from the hips, not the waist, and keep the back straight. Use the stronger shoulder muscles to assist whenever possible. (The log roll technique will be taught in Chapter 13, "Patient Assessment," and Chapter 32, "Spinal Column and Spinal Cord Trauma.")

Pushing and Pulling

Occasionally you will have to decide whether to push or pull an object. Whenever possible, push rather than pull (Figure 6-9*). If an object must be pulled, keep the load between your shoulders and hips and close to your body. Keep your back straight and slightly bend your knees. This will help to keep the line of pull through the center of your body.

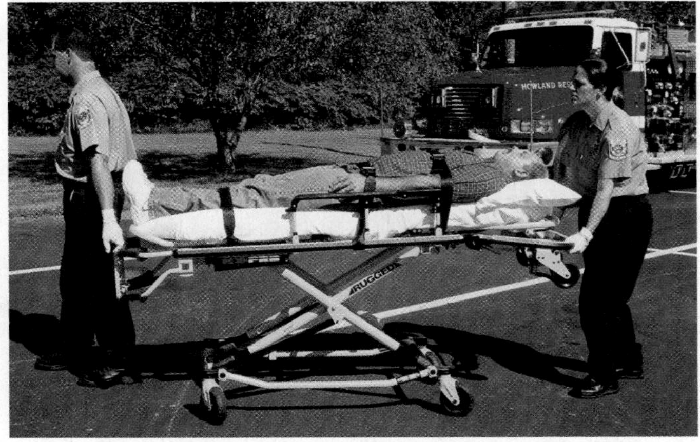

FIGURE 6-9 * Proper pulling and pushing.

When pushing, push from the areas between your waist and shoulders, if possible. If the weight is below waist level, use the kneeling position to avoid bending. Keep your elbows bent, with your arms close to the sides of your body. This will help to increase the force you can apply. Due to the inherent danger, even likelihood, of injury, avoid pushing or pulling an object that is overhead.

Lifting and Moving Patients

As mentioned at the beginning of the chapter, the principles of proper body mechanics and lifting techniques must be applied to all situations in which the EMT has to lift patients or move equipment. Although these principles are not expressly stated in the following discussions of specific lifting and moving techniques, it is expected that you, as an EMT, will always recall the principles of body mechanics to ensure your own safety and that of your partners and patients. Maintain a straight, rigid back by contracting the abdominal and gluteal muscles. Bend at the hips, not at the waist. Keep your head in a neutral position, not flexed forward or extended backward, and use your leg muscles, not your back, to lift, move, or drag the patient (Table 6-1).

There are three categories of patient moves: an emergency move, an urgent move, and a nonurgent move. In general, an **emergency move** should be performed when there is *immediate danger to the patient or to the rescuer.* An **urgent move** is performed when the patient is suffering an *immediate threat to life* and the patient must be moved quickly and transported for care. Finally, a **nonurgent move** is one in which *no immediate threat to life* exists and the patient can be moved in a normal manner when ready for transport.

Emergency Moves

The top priority in emergency care is to maintain the patient's airway, breathing, and circulation. The rule of thumb is to control any life-threatening problems and stabilize the patient before moving him. However, when the scene of an accident is unstable, or threatening to your life and the patient's, your priority changes. You must move the patient first. Make an emergency move only when no

Key Terms

emergency move made when there is immediate danger to the patient or to the rescuer.

Objective 6-9

Differentiate between scenarios in which emergency, urgent, and nonurgent moves are indicated.

Objective 6-10

Given a scenario, demonstrate an appropriate moving technique to be used, such as a drag, lift, carry, draw-sheet technique, or rapid extrication.

TABLE 6-1 Summary of Proper Body Mechanics

- Use teamwork, equipment, and imagination to make sure you are always in the position of using proper body mechanics.
- Use the power lift and power grip techniques as a best defense against injury.
- Reduce the height or distance through which an object must be moved. Lift in stages if necessary.
- Lift an object as close to your body as possible to avoid back injury.
- Avoid using back muscles to lift.
- Use legs, hips, and gluteal muscles plus abdominal muscles for safe, powerful lifts.
- While you are carrying an object, keep shoulders, hips, and feet in alignment.
- Use the proper posture—ears, shoulders, and hips in vertical alignment—when standing and sitting.
- Improve personal physical fitness to build strength and manage stress.

other options are available. Follow local protocol. Always take appropriate precautions to be sure you do not become an additional victim of the emergency.

In general, an emergency move should be performed when there is immediate danger to the patient or to the rescuer. Consider an emergency move under the following conditions:

- *Immediate environmental danger to the patient or rescuer,* such as:
  - *Fire or danger of fire.* Fire should always be considered a grave threat, not only to patients, but also to rescuers.
  - *Exposure to explosives or other hazardous materials.* When a patient is directly exposed to substances that can cause grave injury or death, move the patient immediately.
  - *Inability to protect the patient from other hazards at the scene.* Move the patient to safety when, for example, you haven't the resources to protect him from uncontrolled traffic, physically unstable surroundings, extreme weather conditions, or hostile crowds.
- *Inability to gain access to other patients who need lifesaving care.* In cases where more than one patient has been injured, you may need to move one in order to gain access to another. This may apply to moving a moderately injured person in order to gain access to one who has life-threatening injuries.
- *Inability to provide lifesaving care because of the patient's location or position.* There will be times when you need to change a patient's position, for instance to control hemorrhage, to defibrillate, or to perform CPR.

Remember: The greatest danger to the patient in any emergency move is the possibility of aggravating a spinal injury. Yet, it is impossible to move a patient quickly and still provide as much protection to the spine as would a spine board. In every such emergency, however, make every effort to provide as much protection to the spine as possible. And always make sure you pull the patient in the direction of the long axis of the body.

Three types of emergency moves are the armpit-forearm drag, the shirt drag, and the blanket drag.

The Armpit-Forearm Drag

In general, if the patient is on the floor or ground, you can move him by inserting your hands under the patient's armpits from the back. Grasp the patient's left forearm with your right hand, the right forearm with your left hand, and drag. Make sure you pull the patient in the direction of the long axis of the body (Figure 6-10*).

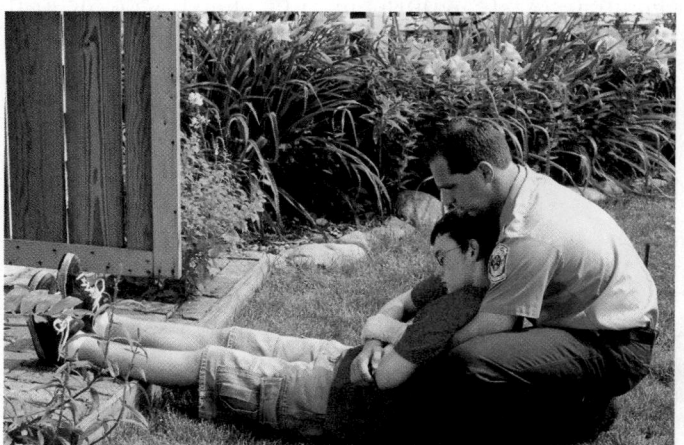

FIGURE 6-10 * The armpit-forearm drag. Slide your hands under the patient's armpits and grasp the forearms. Drag along the long axis of the patient's body.

Key Terms

urgent move made when there is an immediate threat to life because of the patient's condition and the patient must be moved quickly for transport.

nonurgent move made when no immediate threat to life exists.

Key Points

Rapid extrication should be used in patients with any abnormality of the airway, breathing, oxygenation, or circulation and for those with critical injuries or illnesses.

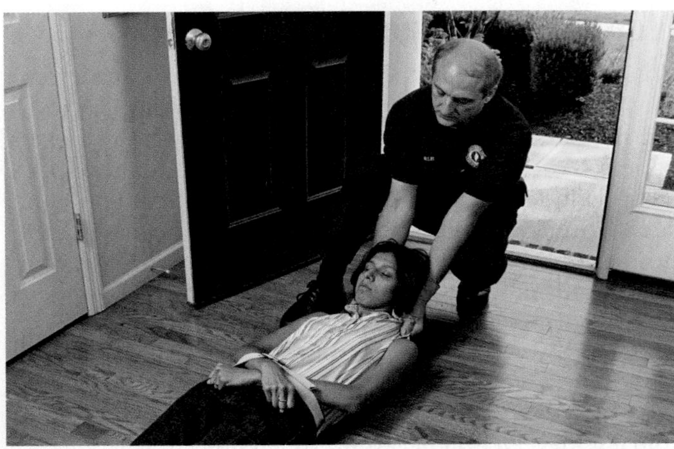

FIGURE 6-11 * The shirt drag.

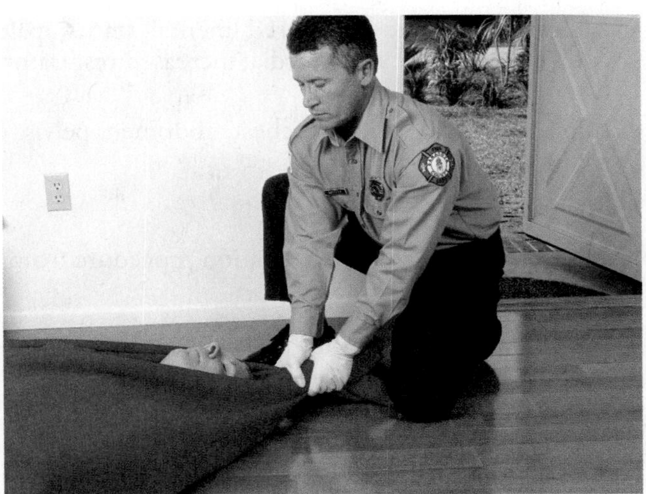

FIGURE 6-12 * The blanket drag.

The Shirt Drag

If the patient is wearing a shirt, you can use it to support the patient's head and pull (Figure 6-11*). Note that the shirt drag cannot be used if the patient is wearing only a T-shirt.

1. Fasten the patient's hands or wrists loosely together. If possible, link them to a belt or pants with a small Velcro strap or self-adherent bandage. This will serve to prevent the patient's arms from flopping or slipping out of the shirt.
2. Grasp the neck and shoulders of the shirt so that the patient's head rests on your fists.
3. Then using the shirt as a handle, pull the patient toward you. Be careful not to strangle the patient. The pulling power should engage the armpits, not the neck. Reposition your hands if you notice excessive pressure or strain from the shirt on the patient's neck.

The Blanket Drag

The blanket drag is an effective way for a single rescuer to move a patient to safety (Figure 6-12*). If you do not have a blanket, use a coat to drag the patient. Follow these steps:

1. Spread a blanket alongside the patient. Gather about half into lengthwise pleats.
2. Roll the patient away from you onto his side. Tuck the pleated part of the blanket as far beneath the patient as you can.
3. Roll the patient back onto the center of the blanket and onto his back.
4. Wrap the blanket securely around the patient.
5. Grab the part of the blanket that is beneath the patient's head, and drag the patient toward you.

Urgent Moves

Many times a patient in a motor vehicle collision must be quickly removed from the vehicle for emergency care and immediate transport, and the application of a short spine board or vest to immobilize the spine would take too much time. The rapid extrication move is designed for this situation. Medical patients may also require an urgent move. A patient in cardiac arrest who is found lying on the couch would need to immediately be placed on the floor or a hard surface to effectively carry out resuscitation.

Rapid Extrication

Rapid extrication should be used in patients with any abnormality of the airway, breathing, oxygenation, or circulation and for those with critical injuries and illnesses. See Chapter 32, "Spinal Column and Spinal Cord Trauma," for detailed discussion and illustrations of rapid extrication.

Indications for an urgent move using the rapid extrication technique include but are not limited to the following:

- Altered mental status
- Inadequate respiratory rate or tidal volume

Thinking Critically
During practice, a football player is tackled and can't get up. He's lying in the end zone about halfway between the uprights. Should you move him with a shoulder drag? A direct ground lift? Or a log roll onto a backboard? What precautions should you take?

- Indications of shock (altered mental status; pale, cool, clammy skin; tachycardia; increased respiratory rate)
- Injuries to the head, neck, chest, abdomen, pelvis
- Fracture of both femurs
- Major bleeding

A summary of the rapid extrication procedure from a motor vehicle follows:

1. One rescuer should bring the patient's head into a neutral in-line position and provide manual stabilization. This is best achieved from behind or to the side of the patient.
2. A second rescuer should apply a cervical-spine immobilization collar as a third places a long backboard near the door. The third rescuer should then move to the passenger seat.
3. The second rescuer should support the patient's thorax as the third frees the patient's legs from the pedals or from under the dashboard.
4. The second and the third rescuer rotate the patient in several short, coordinated moves until the patient's back is in the open doorway and his feet are on the seat.
5. Since the first rescuer can no longer support the patient's head, another rescuer should support the head until the first rescuer exits the vehicle and takes over supporting the head from the door opening.
6. The end of the long backboard is placed on the seat next to the patient's buttocks. Assistants support the other end of the board as the first and second rescuers lower the patient onto it, the first maintaining in-line stabilization of the head and neck.
7. The second and third rescuers should then slide the patient into the proper position on the board in short, coordinated moves as the first continues manual stabilization.

Several variations of this technique are possible. The most critical factor is that this procedure must be accomplished rapidly, but without any compromise to the patient's spine. In addition, operating inside a vehicle places the rescuer's lower back in a vulnerable position. Whenever possible, you should support your weight with a free arm or by resting your chest against the seat backs.

Nonurgent Moves

When there is no immediate threat to life, take the time to choose the best equipment and positioning for moving the patient safely. Generally, the best way to move a patient is the easiest way that will not cause injury or pain. That includes "walking" the patient, if he is able, while supporting him. Never walk a patient who becomes lightheaded or sweaty upon standing or who is having chest pain or respiratory problems, has an injured lower extremity, or has suspected spinal injury.

Whenever you move, lift, or carry a patient, remember to move him as a unit. Keep the patient's head and neck in a neutral position. If you suspect head, neck, or spinal injury, take all necessary spinal precautions. Be sure that all rescuers understand what is to be done before any move is attempted, and make one rescuer responsible for giving commands.

There are many ways to move patients. You are only limited by your imagination and the basic principles of body mechanics and patient safety and comfort. The direct ground lift, extremity lift, direct carry, and draw sheet methods are accepted nonurgent moves that provide the greatest safety to both you and the patient.

Direct Ground Lift

Note that the direct ground lift is not recommended for a heavier patient. When lifting a patient from the ground, it is usually safer and more mechanically efficient to use a long backboard. However, when this cannot be accomplished, follow these steps (EMT Skills 6-2):

1. Two or three rescuers should line up on the same side of the patient.
2. Each rescuer should kneel on one knee, preferably the same knee for all rescuers.
3. The second rescuer should place the patient's arms on the chest, if possible.
4. The first rescuer should then cradle the patient's head by placing one arm under the patient's neck and shoulder. Then he should place his other arm under the patient's lower back.
5. The second rescuer should place one arm under the patient's knees and one arm above the buttocks.
6. If a third rescuer is available, he should place both arms under the waist. The other two rescuers then

should slide their arms either up to the midback or down to the buttocks as appropriate.

7. On signal from the first rescuer, they should lift the patient to their knees and roll the patient in toward their chests.
8. On signal from the first rescuer, they should stand and move the patient to the stretcher or other patient-carrying device.
9. To lower the patient, the steps are reversed.

Remember that you should bend at the hips and not at the waist, your back should remain straight, and the lifting force should be generated from your legs and buttocks, not the back.

Extremity Lift

Use the extremity lift to move a patient from the ground to a patient-carrying device (EMT Skills 6-3). Note that this lift should not be used on a patient with suspected spinal or extremity injuries.

1. The first rescuer should kneel at the patient's head. A second rescuer should kneel at the patient's side by the knees.
2. The first rescuer should place one hand under each of the patient's shoulders, while the second rescuer grasps the patient's wrists.
3. The first rescuer should slip his hands under the patient's arms and grasp the patient's wrists.
4. The second rescuer can then slip his hands under the patient's knees.
5. Both rescuers should move up to a crouching position, keeping their backs straight and heads in neutral alignment.
6. On signal from the first rescuer, they should stand up simultaneously and move with the patient to a stretcher or other patient-carrying device.

While lifting the patient, each rescuer must maintain a straight back and contract the abdominal muscles. The rescuer's head must remain in line with the back. (If the head were to be extended backward, the rescuer would be forced to use the lower back muscles. Flexing the head forward would also put undue force on the lumbar disks.) When lifting the patient, the rescuer should drive upward with leg and gluteal muscles.

Direct Carry Method

The direct carry is one way of transferring a supine patient from a bed to a wheeled stretcher or from any patient-carrying device to another (EMT Skills 6-4):

1. Position the wheeled stretcher perpendicular to the bed, with the head of the device at the foot of the bed.
2. Prepare the wheeled stretcher by unbuckling straps and removing other items. Both rescuers should stand between the bed and stretcher, facing the patient.
3. The first rescuer then slides an arm under the patient's neck and cups the patient's shoulder.
4. After the second rescuer slides a hand under the patient's hip and lifts slightly, the first rescuer should slide an arm under the patient's back. The second rescuer then places his arms under the patient's hips and calves.
5. The rescuers slide the patient to the edge of the bed, lift and curl the patient to their chests, and then rotate and place the patient gently onto the wheeled stretcher.

Draw Sheet Method

Another way of transferring a supine patient from a bed to a wheeled stretcher or from any patient-carrying device to another is the draw sheet method (EMT Skills 6-5):

1. Loosen the bottom sheet of the bed.
2. Position the wheeled stretcher next to the bed. Prepare it by adjusting height, lowering rails, unbuckling straps, and so on.
3. Reach across the stretcher and grasp the sheet firmly at the patient's head, chest, hips, and knees. As you reach across the stretcher, use your hips to support yourself against the stretcher.
4. Slide the patient gently onto the wheeled stretcher. Be sure to contract your abdominal and gluteal muscles to splint the lower back.

Packaging for Transportation

Packaging simply means readying the patient for transport. That is, once the patient is stabilized and all interventions have been checked, you must select and prepare the appropriate carrying device, safely transfer and secure the patient to the carrying device, and finally move the patient and carrying device to the ambulance for loading and unloading.

Some general considerations: Make sure the carrying device is locked in the open position before positioning the patient. Use an appropriate lifting, moving, or carrying technique to place the patient on the carrying device. Generally, place a sheet or blanket on the carrying device and, when the patient is positioned, cover him as appropriate with sheets or blankets to maintain body temperature. Then secure him with straps. Make certain all straps and ties are tucked in or positioned so that they will not cause you to trip and fall. When the patient is placed in the ambulance, be sure both the patient and the carrying device are secured properly before the ambulance moves.

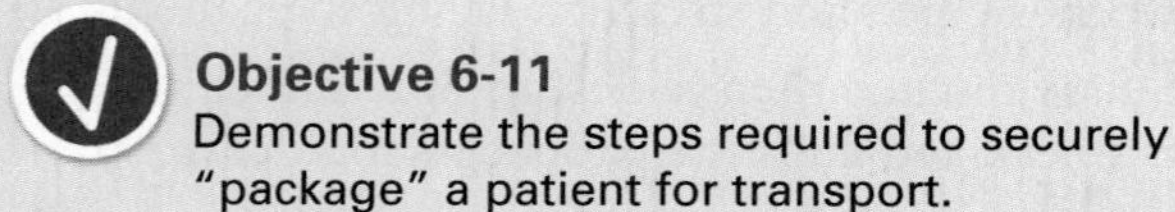

Objective 6-11
Demonstrate the steps required to securely "package" a patient for transport.

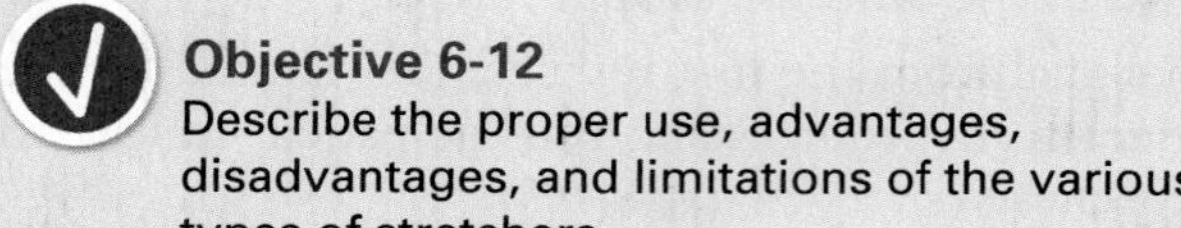

Objective 6-12
Describe the proper use, advantages, disadvantages, and limitations of the various types of stretchers.

Note: If you suspect head, neck, or spinal injury, take all necessary spinal precautions before, during, and after packaging.

Equipment

Both medical and trauma patients need to be moved, packaged, and transported in ways that will not make their conditions worse. To make the best choices of equipment for your patients, learn the advantages and disadvantages of each type (Table 6-2). Practice often, and follow manufacturer instructions for inspection, cleaning, repair, and upkeep.

Wheeled Stretcher

The wheeled stretcher (also called an ambulance gurney or cot) is the patient-carrying device most commonly used by rescue personnel (Figure 6-13*). It is also the safest and most comfortable means of transferring a patient. Most wheeled stretchers are designed to accommodate weights up to 400 pounds and can be adapted to almost any patient position. They also can serve as a means of securing and carrying equipment to the patient's location.

To roll a wheeled stretcher, the rescuer at the head pushes and the rescuer at the foot guides. One limitation of the device is that rolling is usually restricted to smooth

TABLE 6-2 Patient-Carrying Devices

Device	Advantages	Disadvantages
Wheeled stretcher	Enables movement without carrying Accommodates variety of positions, heights, and lengths Safe traversal of stairways and curbs Can be lifted or lowered from ends or sides Durable Mechanically simple Comfortable	X-ray opacity Difficult to maneuver over uneven ground Adds significant amount of weight when lifting is necessary
Portable stretcher	Lightweight Compact Excellent for use as auxiliary stretcher Can be used in spaces too confined or narrow for wheeled stretcher Some models have folding wheels and posts for easier movement Easily loaded and off-loaded Can be folded for storage	Must be carried Metal styles interfere with some X-rays
Stair chair	Good for use on stairways, narrow corridors and doorways, small elevators Some models can be converted into portable stretchers Newer models have tracks that eliminate carrying down steps	Must be carried (older models) Does not accommodate trauma patients Should not be used for patients with altered mental status or lower extremity injury Fairly complex Consumes considerable space

TABLE 6-2 Patient-Carrying Devices *continued*

Device	Advantages	Disadvantages
Backboard	Good spinal immobilizer Good lifting device Can float Lightweight Compact Can serve as CPR surface Mechanically simple X-ray translucency Can be carried and loaded from ends or sides Integrates well with various other equipment	Must be carried Usually must be left with patient Unstable for moves up or down inclines Uncomfortable
Scoop stretcher	Can be used in confined areas in which other stretchers will not fit Allows easy application of restraints Integrates well with various other equipment	Must be carried Requires padding of head and body prominences Metal scoop stretcher should be prewarmed if air temperature is cold Not recommended for patients with suspected spinal injury Consumes considerable space
Basket stretcher	Good for traversing rough terrain Can be fitted with flotation harness for water rescue Extremely durable Can be carried from sides or ends Integrates well with various other equipment	Must be carried Bulky High cost Usually must be left with patient Metal style interferes with some X-rays Needs special training for use in rope or ladder rescues
Flexible stretcher	Especially useful for narrow and restricted hallways Can be carried from sides or ends	Must be carried

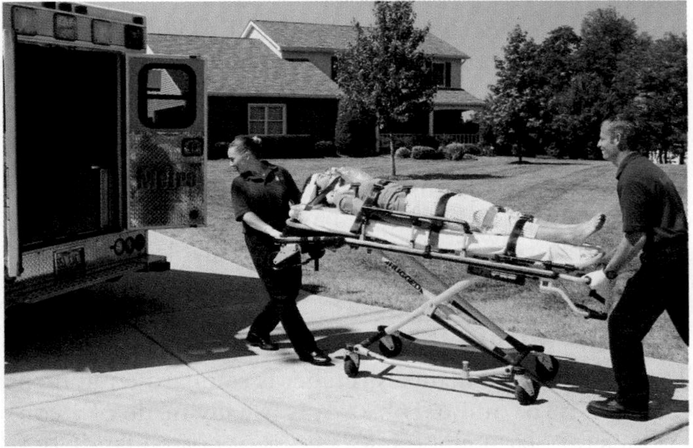

FIGURE 6-13 ✱ EMTs move a wheeled stretcher into position to load into the ambulance.

terrain. However, four rescuers—one at each corner—can keep it stable and move it over rough ground. Two rescuers can carry a wheeled stretcher in narrow spaces. However, they would need to face each other from opposite ends, the stretcher could be easily unbalanced, and the lift and carry would require considerable strength (Figures 6-14a and 6-14b✱).

There are two basic types of wheeled stretchers in the United States: the lift-in cot and the roll-in cot (Figures 6-15a and 6-15b✱). Each weighs about 70 pounds and is constructed of aluminum alloy. The lift-in cot requires two attendants, one on each side, when loading and unloading from the ambulance (EMT Skills 6-6). The roll-in cot uses special wheels at the head to simplify the loading and unloading procedure (EMT Skills 6-7). The roll-in type significantly reduces the amount of twisting and lifting that is required of rescuers. Some roll-in cots use pneumatic or electric devices to lift and lower the cot.

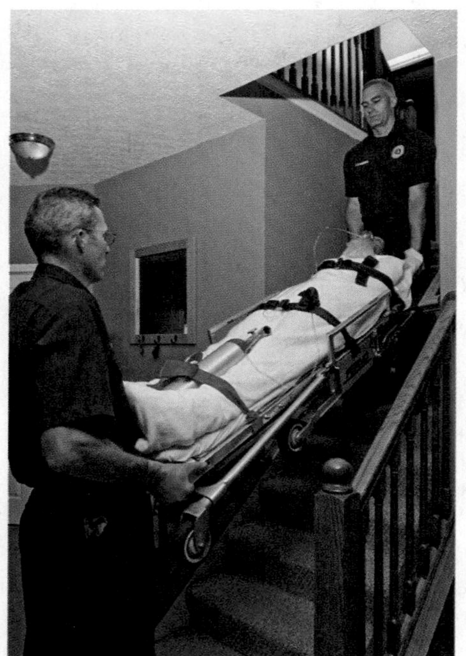

FIGURE 6-14a * Two-rescuer stretcher carry.

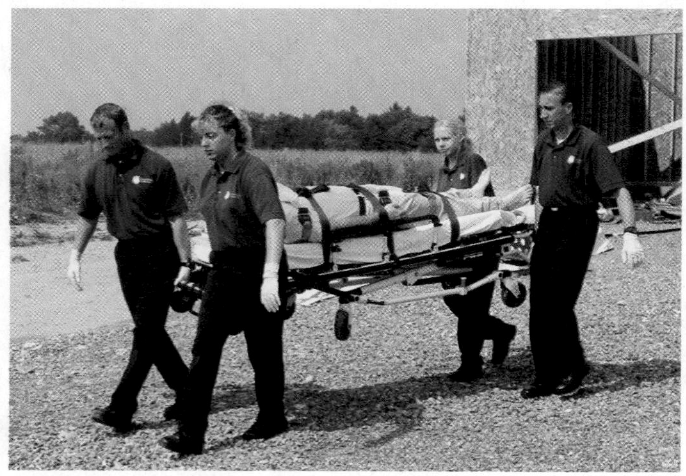

FIGURE 6-14b * Four-rescuer stretcher carry.

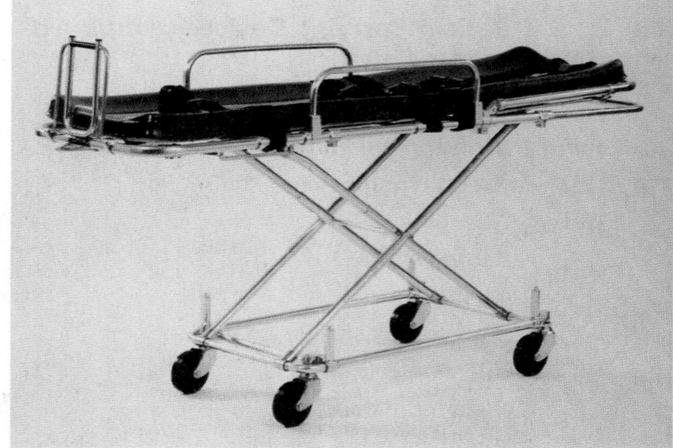

FIGURE 6-15a * Wheeled stretcher, lift-in type. (© Ferno Corporation)

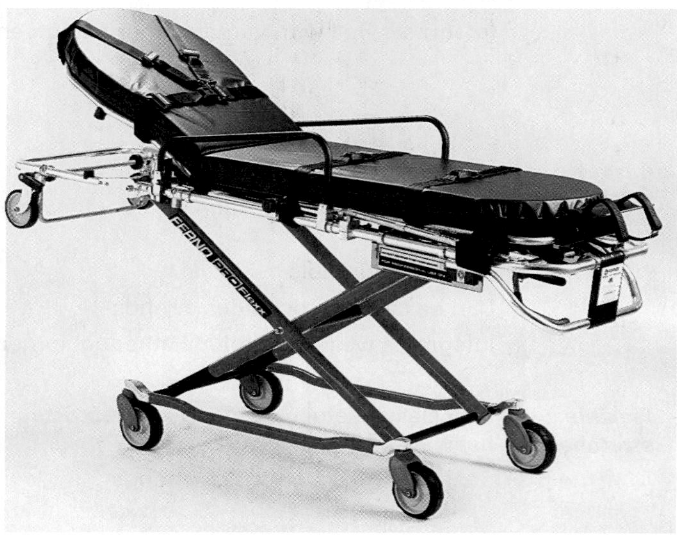

FIGURE 6-15b * Wheeled stretcher, roll-in type. (© Ferno Corporation)

Trained emergency personnel should stay with a patient on a wheeled stretcher at all times. The patient should never be left unattended, even when secured. Before loading a wheeled stretcher into the ambulance, be sure there is enough lifting power. Load hanging stretchers before wheeled stretchers. Once in the ambulance, be sure the stretchers and patients are secure before the ambulance moves.

Bariatric Stretchers and Devices

With an ever-growing overweight population, specialized stretchers and other devices have been designed to transport morbidly obese patients. These stretchers and devices are called *bariatric devices* (EMT Skills 6-8). Some bariatric stretchers are designed to hold patients up to 1,600 pounds in a wheels-down position. The stretchers have larger wheels for stability, wider cot dimensions, and more heavily constructed frames. Some stretchers are part of a bariatric transport system that includes an ambulance ramp and winch. There are even specialized bariatric transport ambulances now available.

Portable Stretcher

The portable ambulance stretcher is standard equipment (Figures 6-16a and 6-16b*). It is usually made of a continuous tubular metal frame, canvas or coated fabric bottom, and straps to secure the patient. It may also be referred to as a soft cot. It is a conventional carrying device that is particularly useful when the patient must be

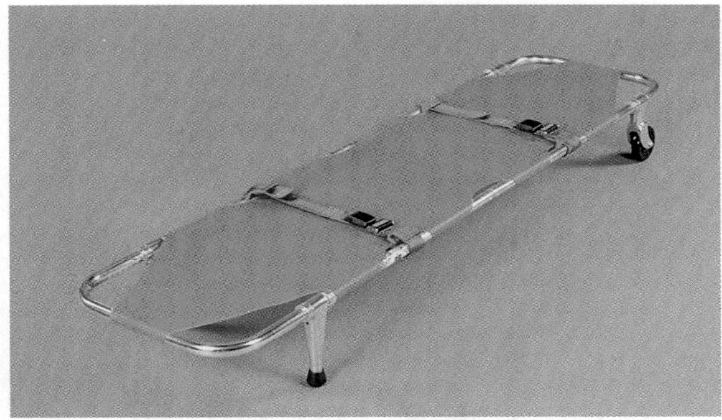

FIGURE 6-16a ✻ Portable ambulance stretcher with continuous tubular metal frame.

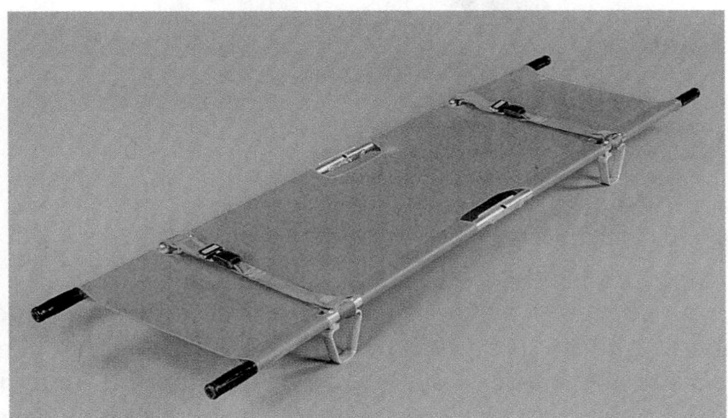

FIGURE 6-16b ✻ Pole stretcher, or canvas litter.

removed from a space too confined or narrow for a wheeled stretcher. It is often used as an auxiliary to the wheeled stretcher when there is more than one patient to transport. It can be loaded easily into an ambulance and off-loaded easily once in the ambulance.

The portable ambulance stretcher generally is available in three styles: the basic model, the basic with folding wheels and posts, and the breakaway. The basic model is used as an auxiliary stretcher, which can be placed on the squad bench or suspended from hanging hardware inside the ambulance. It is very light and, though it has a load capacity of up to 350 pounds, it is not recommended for that much weight. Most models can be folded in half for storage.

One type of portable stretcher is the pole stretcher or canvas litter (Figure 6-16b), which has been used worldwide for centuries. It is lightweight and folds compactly. The vinyl-coated model is easy to clean. It is comfortable for the patient, especially when the head is padded, though it should not be used when spinal immobilization is necessary unless it is used with a long backboard. One drawback is that care must be taken when placing the patient on rocky ground for any length of time. Soft tissue injury may result. When you are going to use the canvas pole stretcher to transport a patient, take care to see that the crosspieces are locked in place. When lifting a patient on a pole stretcher, it is preferable to have four or more rescuers.

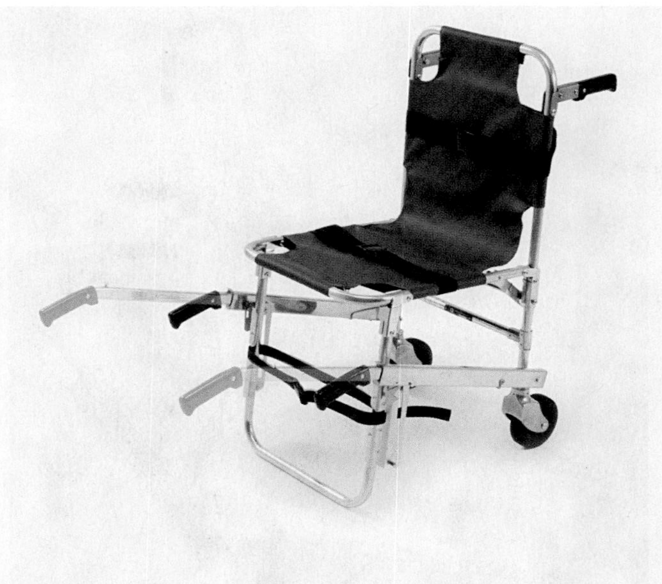

FIGURE 6-17 ✻ Stair chair. (© Ferno Corporation)

Stair Chair

A stair chair (Figure 6-17✻) is useful when a wheeled stretcher cannot traverse narrow corridors and doorways, small elevators, and stairways. Some models can be converted into portable stretchers. Do not use a stair chair when the patient has an altered mental status, suspected spinal injury, or injuries to the lower extremities.

To move a patient up or down stairs on a stair chair, explain to the patient everything you plan to do. Check to be sure all straps are secure. Then the rescuers should proceed with the following (EMT Skills 6-9):

1. One rescuer should stand behind the chair at the head, and another should stand at the foot facing the patient. A third rescuer, if available, should prepare to "spot" by standing behind the rescuer who will be moving backward (up or down the stairs). Instruct the patient not to reach out.
2. As the chair is tilted back by the rescuer at the head, the rescuer at the foot should grasp the chair by its legs.
3. Both rescuers should lift and begin to carry simultaneously. If the chair has wheels, they should not be allowed to touch the steps.
4. As the rescuers descend (or ascend) with the patient, the spotter should count out the steps and identify upcoming conditions.

Tracked Stair Chair A newer model stair chair is also available and is designed with a track that can be lowered behind where the patient is sitting (Figure 6-18✻). This track comes into contact with the steps as the patient is being moved down stairs, and allows the chair to glide down the steps with minimal effort exerted by the EMT. It still requires two rescuers, one at the head and one at the foot of the patient, for stabilization of the device.

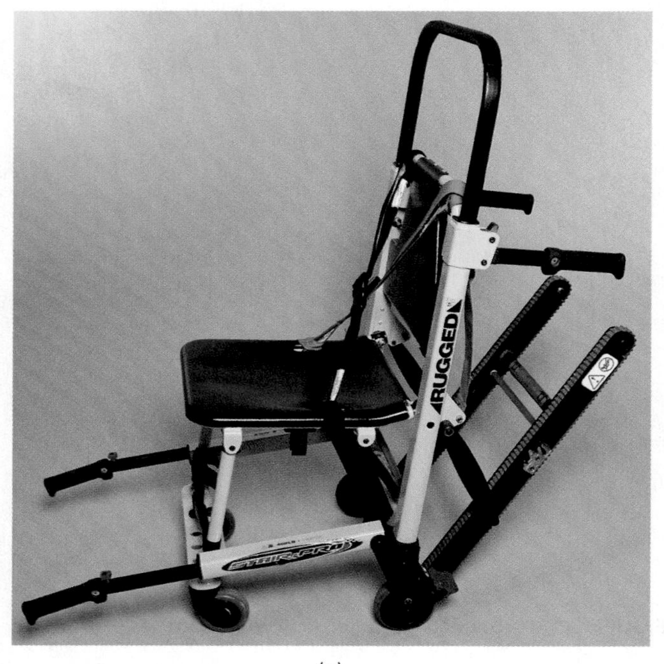

(a)

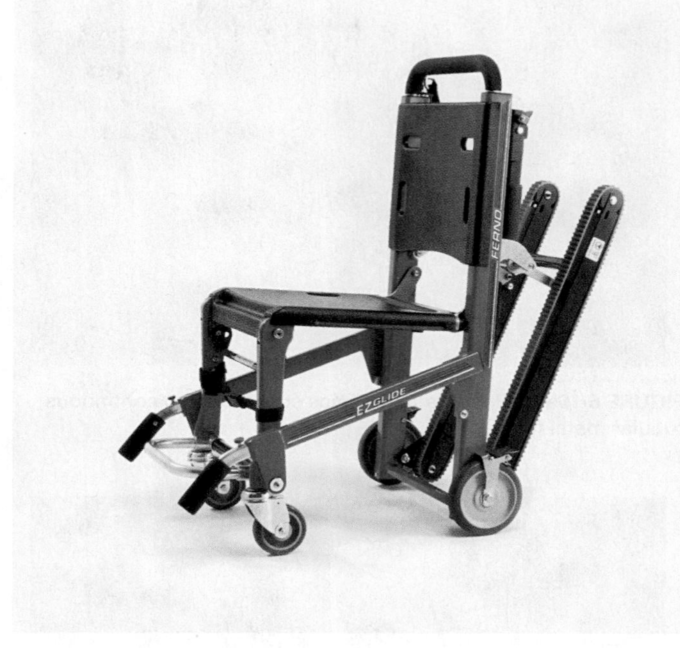

(b)

FIGURE 6-18 ✱ **(a)** and **(b)** A stair chair with a mechanical track allows easier patient movement over stairs. (© Ferno Corporation)

While this style chair still has all the same features as more common models, the new design eliminates the need to lift the chair while moving down the steps.

Backboards

Standard operating equipment in any emergency vehicle is the backboard (Figure 6-19a✱). It can protect the patient from rocky ground surfaces, and it acts as a spinal immobilizer. Straps and a head immobilizer device usually can be applied and secured without problems.

Long and short backboards are made of lightweight plastic or composite materials with molded handholds. Common styles are the Farrington (rectangular with round corners) and the Ohio (with mitered corners and tapering sides). The Ohio fits into most basket stretchers and can be more easily maneuvered in and out of cars. Long backboards may also be referred to as long spineboards.

Short backboards usually are used to immobilize noncritical sitting patients before moving them. One special type of short backboard is the vest-type or corset-type immobilizer such as the Ferno Kendrick Extrication Device (KED) (Figure 6-19b✱). Once a short backboard is applied, the patient should be placed on a long backboard. See Chapter 32, "Spinal Column and Spinal Cord Trauma."

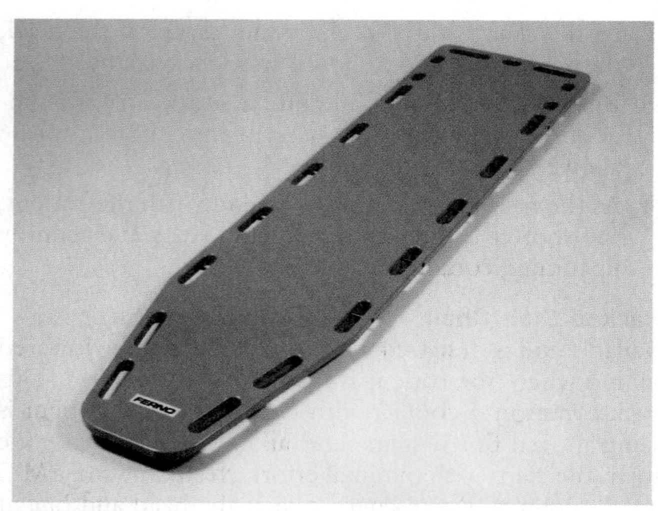

FIGURE 6-19a ✱ Long backboard.

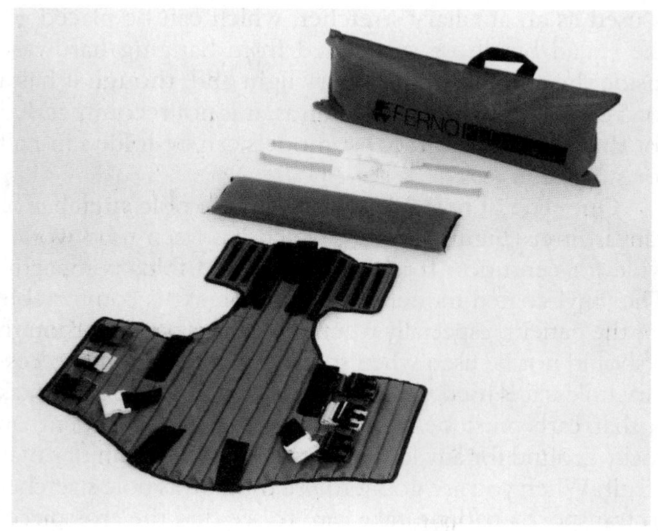

FIGURE 6-19b ✱ Kendrick Extrication Device (KED). (© Ferno Corporation)

Thinking Critically

A hiker who fell into a steep ravine has suffered a sprained ankle and can't climb out by himself. He is sitting up and alert and tells you he weighs about 275 pounds. He has no signs or symptoms of spinal injury. How would you move him to the ambulance?

Also available is a full body vacuum mattress that can be used as both a backboard and a moving device once the patient is placed on it (Figures 6-20a and 6-20b*). This design uses vacuum technology to conform the mattress into whatever shape is necessary given the patient. It eliminates the need to pad any extra voids between a traditional rigid backboard and the patient's body, and it becomes rigid enough after the vacuum has been applied to allow the two or more EMTs to lift and carry the patient. Several benefits of this equipment are that it is lightweight, it conforms to the patient's shape, it fits within a basket stretcher, and it is designed with several hand grips for the care providers to grasp when preparing to lift the patient.

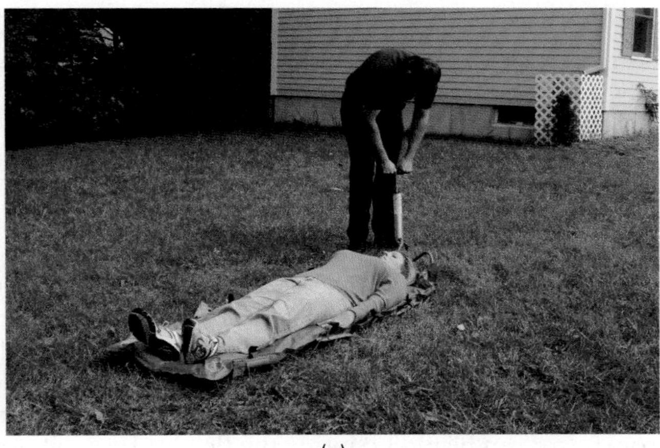

(a)

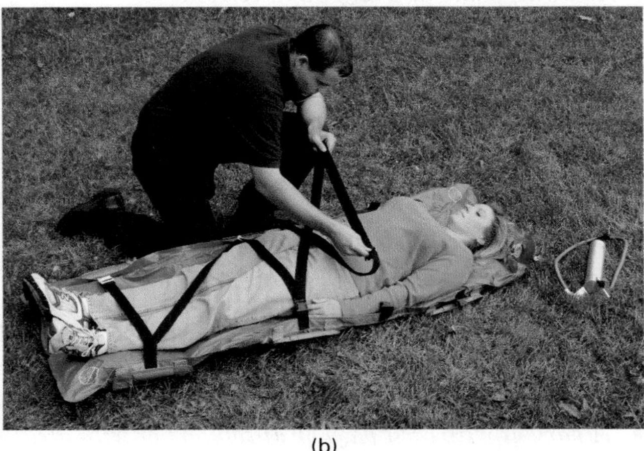

(b)

FIGURE 6-20 * Full body vacuum mattress can be used for immobilization or for moving the patient. **(a)** The device is shaped around the patient and air is withdrawn. **(b)** The patient is then secured to the rigid, conforming vacuum mattress.

Scoop Stretcher

Designed for patients weighing up to 300 pounds, the scoop or orthopedic stretcher is made to be assembled and disassembled around the patient (Figure 6-21*). An advantage is that it can be used in confined areas where other conventional stretchers will not fit. It can also be used for pelvic fractures or bilateral femur fractures to prevent further injury. A disadvantage is that some devices are constructed entirely of metal, which picks up the temperature of the environment. Note also that the scoop stretcher is not recommended for patients with suspected spinal injury.

To use a scoop stretcher properly, you must have access to the patient from all sides. At least two rescuers are required—one to prepare and position the stretcher and one to move the patient. Follow these steps (EMT Skills 6-10):

1. Adjust the stretcher to the length of the patient.
2. Separate the stretcher halves, and place one on each side of the patient. Keeping the patient's spine inline, gently roll the patient onto one side. Slide half of the stretcher under the patient.
3. If you have not been able to examine the patient's back before this time, do so now. Then return the patient to a supine position.
4. Assemble the head end of the scoop stretcher.
5. Roll the patient's body to the other side. Swing the remaining half of the stretcher into a closed (assembled) position. Latch the foot end of the stretcher.
6. Pad the patient's head and any bony prominence with a pillow or a folded sheet.
7. Secure the patient with at least three body straps.

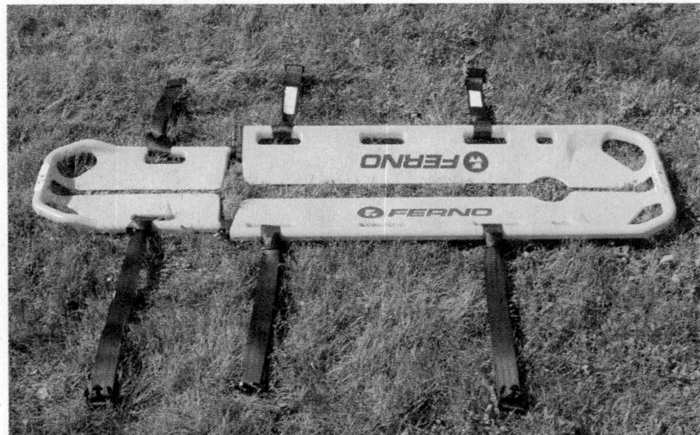

FIGURE 6-21 * Scoop stretcher.

Objective 6-13
Given a scenario involving a particular type of patient, demonstrate proper positioning of the patient.

Basket Stretcher

Most commonly called the Stokes basket, a basket stretcher is shaped like a long basket and comes in two basic styles (Figures 6-22a and 6-22b*). One style has a welded metal frame fitted with a contoured chicken-wire web. The other style has a tubular aluminum frame riveted to a molded polyethylene shell. Either will accommodate a scoop stretcher or Ohio-type backboard. Basket stretchers will fit onto wheeled stretchers which can be used to move the patient. Be sure to secure the basket to the wheeled stretcher prior to any movement.

A basket stretcher has the advantage of enabling you to completely immobilize a patient who is already on a backboard and to move him over any kind of terrain. The lightweight polyethylene style slides easily and smoothly over snow and rough terrain while protecting the patient from branches and twigs. Note: Do not move a patient in a basket stretcher by rope or ladder unless you have been specifically trained to do so.

Place the mattress from a wheeled stretcher into a basket stretcher to increase patient comfort and insulate him from the cold. If you choose not to use a mattress, be sure to pad the patient's head. If you anticipate especially rough transport, pad the edges of the patient's body with rolled blankets and strap him securely into place with nylon webbing.

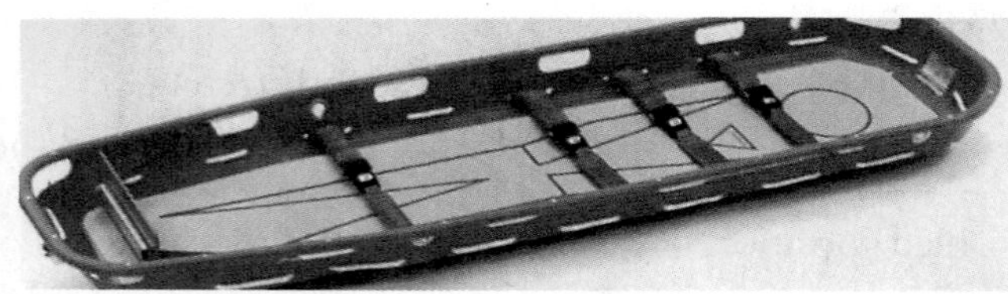

FIGURE 6-22a * Basket stretcher.

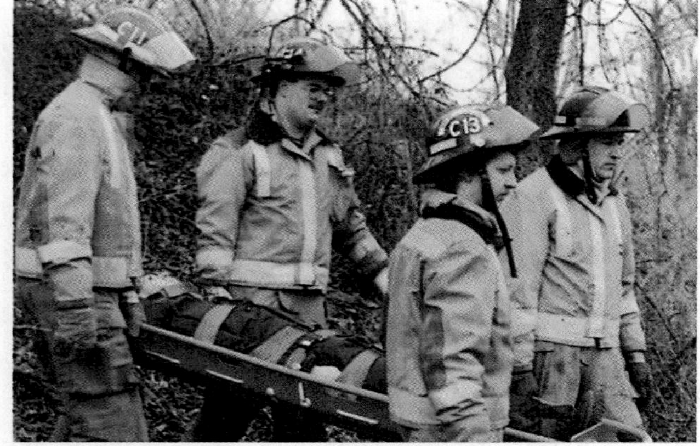

FIGURE 6-22b * Using a basket stretcher to move a patient over rough terrain.

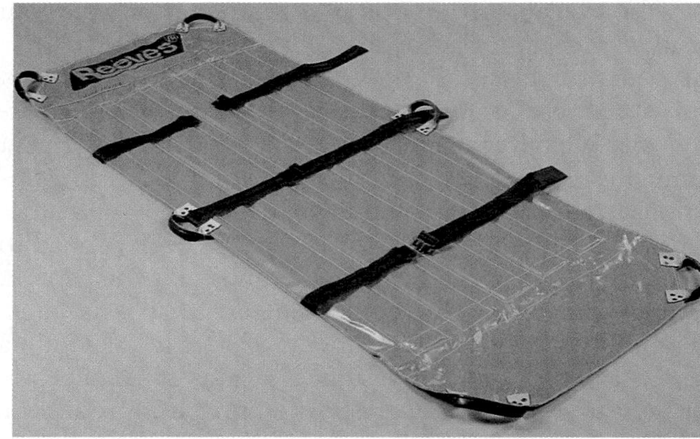

FIGURE 6-23 * Flexible stretcher.

Flexible Stretcher

A flexible (or Reeves) stretcher is a special transfer device made of canvas or synthetic materials (Figure 6-23*). It has six large lifting and carrying handles, three on each side. It is especially useful for narrow and restricted hallways such as those found in mobile homes. A patient on a backboard can be placed inside the flexible stretcher for moves down stairs or over rough terrain.

Patient Positioning

Generally, a patient is placed on a carrying device in a supine or sitting position, unless the patient's condition dictates otherwise.

- *An unresponsive patient with no suspected head, neck, or spinal injury* should be placed in a left lateral recumbent position (coma or recovery position) to face the rescuer once in the ambulance. This position aids in draining fluids or vomitus from the mouth and helps prevent aspiration into the lungs.
- *A patient with chest pain or discomfort or with breathing difficulties* should be placed in a position of comfort, usually sitting up, if hypotension is not present.
- *A patient with suspected spinal injury* should be immobilized on a long backboard. Once immobilized,

Key Points
A child's car seat should be used to transport the child only if it is not damaged.

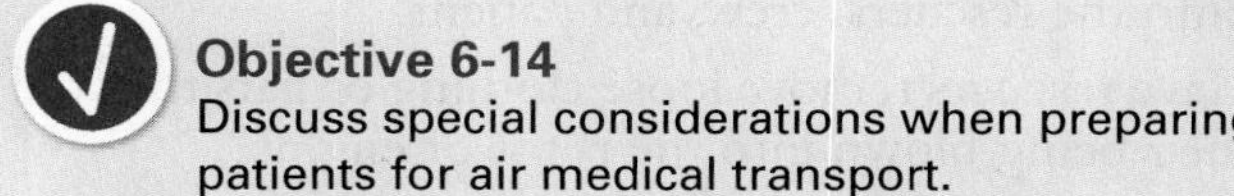

Objective 6-14
Discuss special considerations when preparing patients for air medical transport.

the patient and backboard can be tilted as a unit to place the patient on his left side for drainage from the mouth.

- *A patient in shock (hypoperfusion)* should be placed in a supine position unless your protocol indicates otherwise.
- *An alert patient who is nauseated or vomiting* should be transported in a sitting or a recovery position. That position should allow you to manage the patient's airway.
- *A pregnant patient in her third trimester* should be positioned on her left side.

Consider the following suggestions when moving and positioning patients with special needs:

- *Pregnant women.* A pregnant woman will probably feel more comfortable on her left side. That position takes the weight of the baby off the large blood vessels and nerves in the abdomen, preventing supine hypotensive syndrome (dizziness, drop in blood pressure, and decreased cardiac output). If there is excess vaginal bleeding, place the woman in a supine position. If you suspect a prolapsed umbilical cord, place the woman on her back and elevate her hips with a pillow. Follow local protocol. (See Chapter 37, "Obstetrics and Care of the Newborn," for details on these conditions.)
- *Infants and toddlers.* An infant or toddler who is not critically injured can usually be carried easily in an infant car seat. When possible, use the child's own car seat to reduce fear of being in an unfamiliar environment. You can also use the car seat as an immobilizer. Simply pack the space around the child with rolled towels or folded sheets taped as padding. Note that the car seat should be used only if it is not damaged. (See Chapter 38, "Pediatrics," for more information on immobilization of infants and toddlers.)
- *Elderly patients.* A possible limitation in an elderly patient is osteoporosis, a loss of mass that makes the bones extremely brittle and prone to fracture. In these cases, take extra care to avoid accidental injury. Make sure the patient understands what is happening and where you are taking her.
- *Patients with physical disabilities.* Use common sense in handling patients who have physical disabilities. The nature of the disability will let you know how to compensate. If, for example, the patient has fused joints or twisted limbs, position the patient to provide the greatest comfort. Take extra care in strapping. Whenever possible, use a rolled towel or other padding to support areas that might need it. Ask the patient to explain what positions are possible and comfortable for him.

Packaging Patients for Air Transport

When the distance to the appropriate hospital is great or the patient's condition is critical, the use of a helicopter or fixed-wing aircraft for patient transportation might be considered. (See Chapter 41, "Ambulance Operations and Air Medical Response," for more detail on helicopter transport.) In this situation, there are some special considerations in packaging the patient to ensure safety of the patient, rescuers, and helicopter crew. Follow local protocols for use of air ambulance service. Following are some basic guidelines for preparing a patient for air transport:

1. Be sure that a patient who has been contaminated by a hazardous material has been thoroughly decontaminated. Especially in the confined space of a helicopter, it is possible for the crew to be overcome by hazardous fumes and lose control of the craft.
2. If at all possible and appropriate, have the patient's airway managed with an endotracheal tube prior to the arrival of the aircraft.
3. Leave the chest accessible if the patient is intubated so the aircraft crew can assess the patient's breath sounds prior to transport.
4. If the patient is to be transported by helicopter and is immobilized on a backboard, be sure the board is one that can be accommodated in the model of helicopter that will respond.
5. Be sure the patient is well secured to the backboard so as not to be jostled while moving to the aircraft or in flight.
6. Secure all equipment, blankets, sheets, and so on with tape so they cannot blow off the patient and into the rotor or engine of the aircraft. Secure all loose equipment at the scene.
7. Communicate to the patient what you are doing and prepare him to expect the noise and rotor wash of an incoming helicopter.
8. Cover the patient's eyes, ears, and exposed wounds to protect them from the noise and rotor wash.

9. Consider having an engine company wet the landing zone to prevent dust and debris from being blown onto the rescuers, crew, and patient.
10. Have rescuers remove loose clothing or hats to avoid their being blown into the rotor or engine.
11. Do not approach the aircraft with the patient until instructed by the pilot or crew. Unless otherwise instructed, let the crew assist you in loading the aircraft. Stay well clear of the tail rotor, and observe all safety and danger placards. For everyone's safety, learn how to approach an aircraft BEFORE an emergency call.
12. When moving the patient to be loaded into a helicopter, lay an IV bag on the patient's chest instead of having it held up by a rescuer.
13. When loading a patient into a helicopter, minimize the number of people under the rotors at all times. Refer to local protocols and air transportation companies for further guidelines.

General Guidelines for Carrying a Patient Using a Backboard, Portable Stretcher, or Flexible Stretcher

As mentioned previously, a wheeled device should be your preference to move a patient whenever possible. However, there are many situations where the wheeled device is not feasible, such as moving a patient down or up steps, in a narrow hallway with angles, or over rough terrain. In those cases, you will use a backboard, portable stretcher, or flexible stretcher to move the patient either to the wheeled stretcher or directly to the back of the ambulance, depending on the situation. The method in which you position yourself to carry the patient is dependent on the number of EMTs or other emergency response personnel at the scene to assist with the lift and carry.

Some general guidelines for moving a patient on these devices are:

- Secure the patient to the device using a minimum of three straps.
- Secure the patient's hands in the device so they cannot reach out and grab you or your partner, a railing, or other objects that may throw you and your partner off balance.
- Always carry the device with the patient's feet first when going down steps or downhill.
- Always carry the device with the patient's head first when going up steps or uphill.
- Consider your and your partner's limitations as to weight and your ability to move the patient safely without further injury to the patient or yourselves.
- Know your limitations when considering moving patients from a unique situation such as a hillside, an unstable area, or a high angle, and seek assistance from properly trained rescuers.
- Constantly communicate with your partner or team to coordinate the move.
- Keep the patient's weight as close to your body as possible.

Two-Person Carry

If only you and your partner are available for a carry, one EMT is positioned at the head of the patient while the other is at the foot. The stronger person should be at the head since most of the weight is at that end. The EMT at the foot end faces the EMT at the head end. This requires the EMT at the foot end to walk backward.

Be extremely cautious when employing this type of carry. One problem is that the EMT at the foot end can lose his balance by tripping over an unseen object. If a third person is available, place him behind the person at the foot end to act as a spotter. This person will often grasp the belt of the EMT at the foot end to provide balance and stabilization to that EMT. He will also call out obstacles to the EMT at the foot end. Another problem in this situation is that there is no EMT or rescuer to provide stabilization at the sides of the patient, so the carrying device can easily become unbalanced from side to side. Additionally, because only two EMTs are carrying the entire weight of the patient, they can fatigue quickly, which places them and the patient at greater risk for injury.

Four-Person Carry

When four emergency personnel are available, a different carrying configuration is often used. One rescuer is placed at the patient's head. Another is placed at the foot end, facing forward with his hands behind his body to grasp the carrying device. The other two rescuers are placed at each side, facing forward and grasping the carrying device with the hand closest to the patient. This puts all rescuers facing forward, forming a diamond configuration.

An alternative rectangular configuration may be used when four rescuers are present. Two rescuers are placed on opposite sides of the carrying device on the head end and two rescuers on opposite sides at the foot end of the carrying device. All rescuers face forward and grasp the carrying device with the hand that is closest to the patient.

Carrying a Supine Patient on Stairs

A stair chair should be the device of choice to move a patient up or down stairs if the patient's mental status and

Thinking Critically
A woman has fallen down some steps and landed hard on the concrete cellar floor. The stairway is narrow and makes a right-angle turn at a small landing. What kind of carrying device would you use to remove her to the ambulance? What special precautions should you take?

Objective 6-15
Discuss special considerations when using a neonatal isolette.

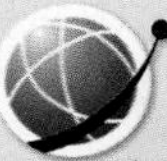

Media Resources
Go to www.bradybooks.com for mykit. Highlights:
- *Web Resource:* Lifting Information

condition allow it. If the patient must be placed in a supine position to be moved up or down stairs, be sure the patient is secured to the device so he cannot slide out from either the foot or head end of the device. Also, be sure to secure the patient's hands within the device so he cannot grab you, a railing, or any other object that could throw you off balance while carrying him.

When a supine patient is to be carried down stairs, typically one EMT is placed at the head end of the device facing the patient and the other is placed at the foot end of the device facing the patient with his back to the stairs. If possible, a spotter is placed behind the EMT at the foot end to provide guidance and stabilization and to count off the steps. The EMT at the foot end is first down the steps. This configuration is often used because of the limited width of a stairwell that doesn't allow EMTs to be on both sides of the patient.

When moving a patient up steps, the same EMT configuration is used. The patient is carried head first; therefore, the EMT at the head end moves backward up the steps. If available, the spotter will be ahead of and guiding the EMT at the head end.

Neonatal Isolette

You may be required to transport a neonate from one medical facility to another in a neonatal isolette. The isolette is designed to keep the neonate in a warm environment to prevent hypothermia. Isolettes are wheeled devices that engage the typical stretcher mounts in the ambulance. It is important to ensure that the isolette can be properly secured in the ambulance. The isolette is either lifted into the ambulance or rolled in up a ramp.

EMT skills 6-1 Power Lift

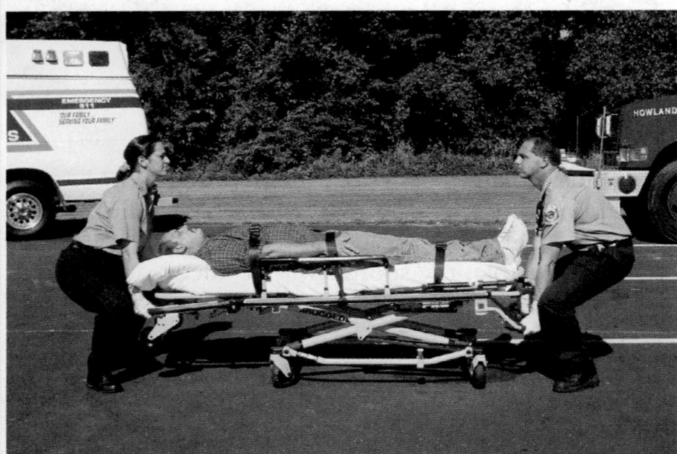

6-1A * Get in position. Your feet should be about shoulder width apart, turned slightly outward, and flat on the ground.

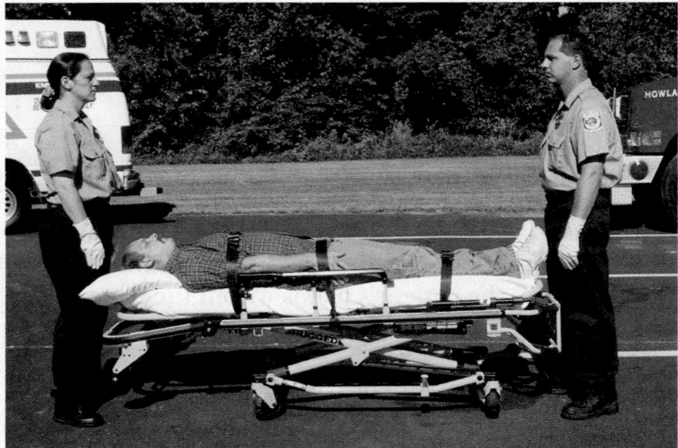

6-1B * As lifting begins, your back should remain locked and your feet should remain flat. Tighten the muscles of your back and abdomen to splint the lower back.

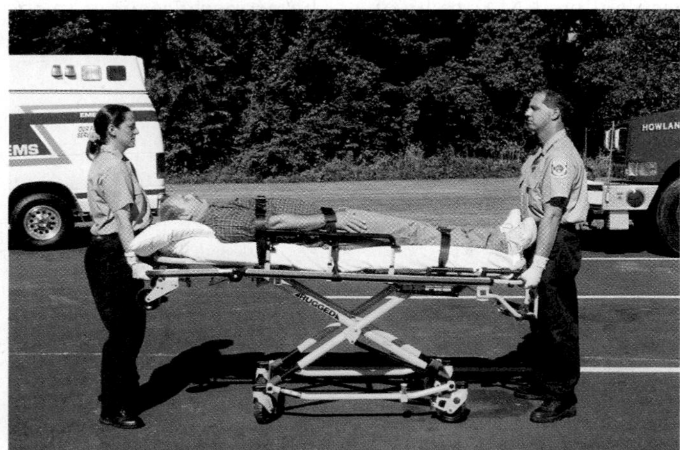

6-1C * As you return to a standing position, make sure your back is locked in and your upper body comes up before your hips.

EMT skills 6-2 Direct Ground Lift

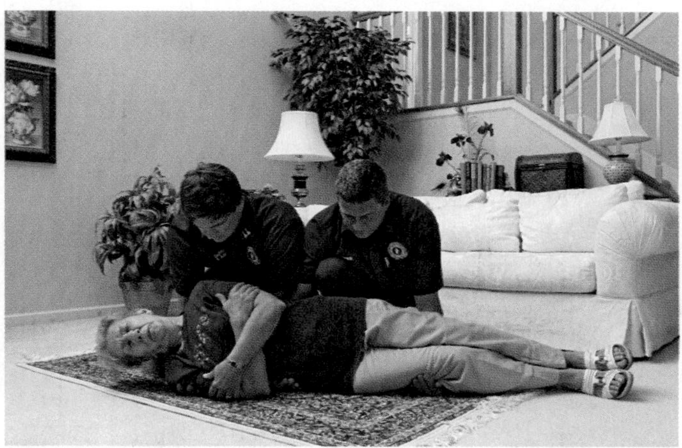

6-2A * Position your arms under the patient. Be sure to cradle the head. If a third rescuer is available, he should slide both arms under the waist while the first two rescuers move their arms up and down as appropriate.

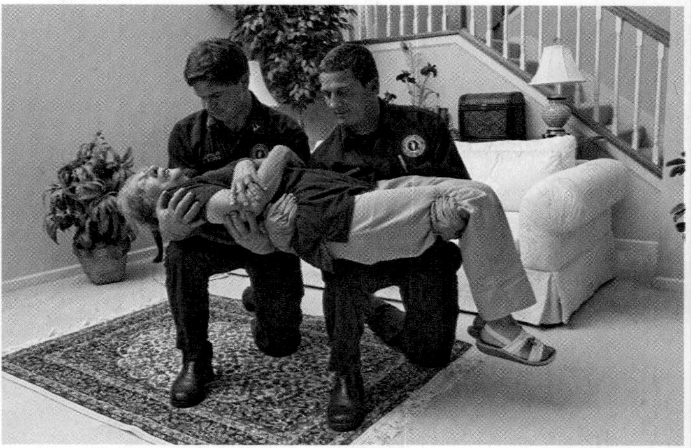

6-2B * Lift the patient to your knees and roll toward your chests.

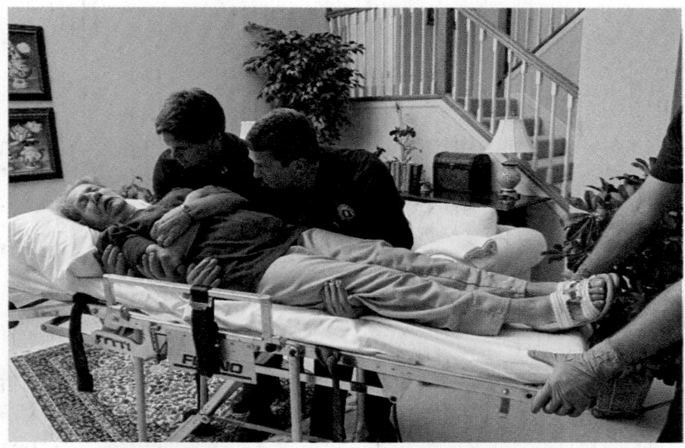

6-2C * On signal, move the patient to the carrying device.

EMT skills 6-3 Extremity Lift

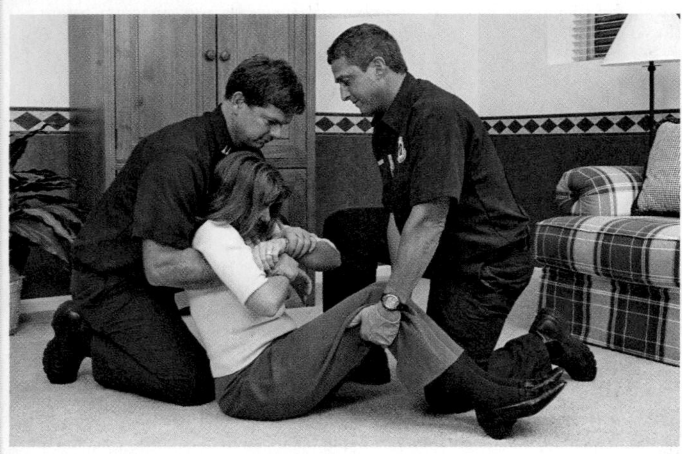

6-3A * One rescuer should put one hand under each arm and grasp the wrists. The other should slip hands under the knees.

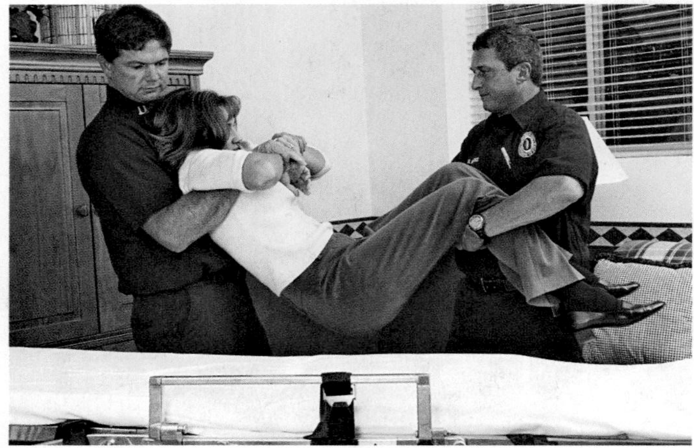

6-3B * Both rescuers should move up to a crouching and then standing position.

EMT skills 6-4 Direct Carry

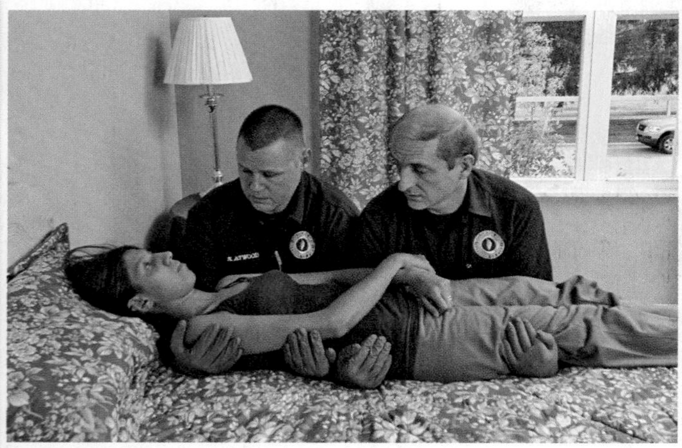

6-4A * Position your arms under the patient and slide the patient to the edge of the bed.

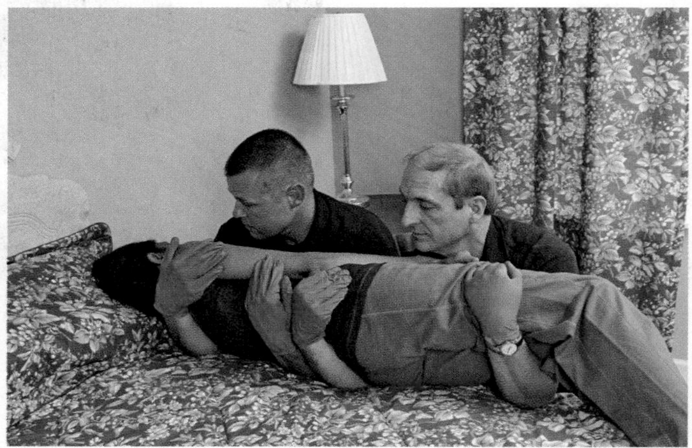

6-4B * Lift the patient and curl toward your chests.

EMT skills 6-4 Direct Carry *continued*

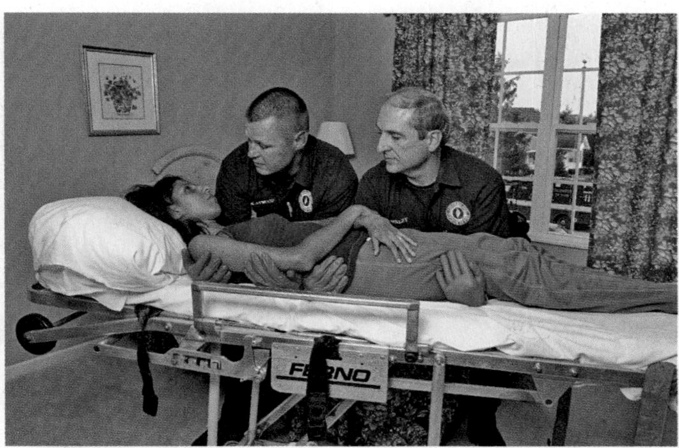

6-4C ✱ Rotate and place the patient gently on the carrying device.

EMT skills 6-5 Draw Sheet Method

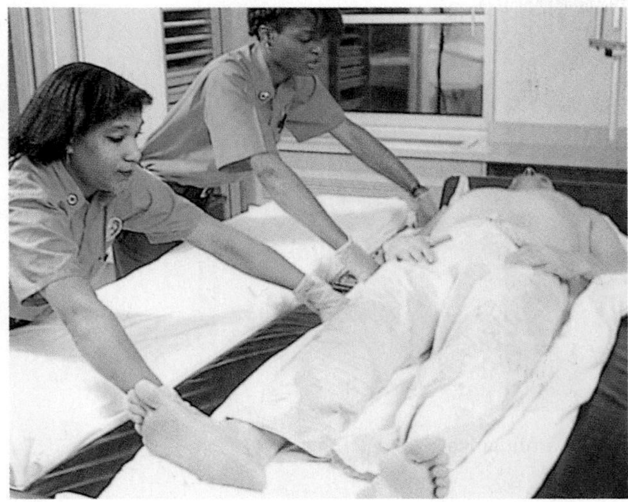

6-5A ✱ Reach across the stretcher and grasp the sheet firmly.

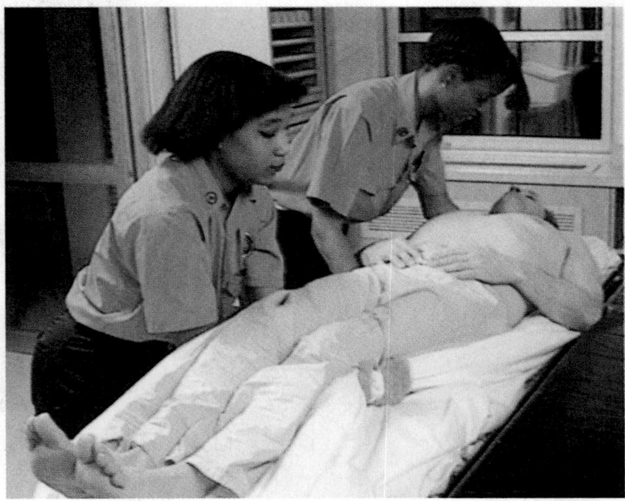

6-5B ✱ Slide the patient gently onto the carrying device.

EMT skills 6-6 Loading the Lift-In Wheeled Stretcher

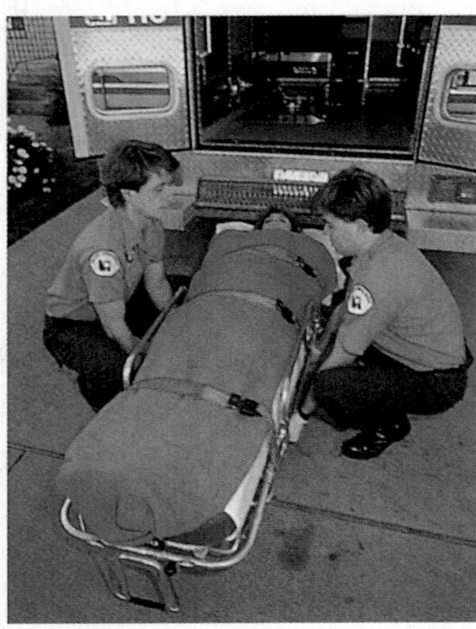

6-6A ✱ Using the principles of body mechanics, prepare to lift.

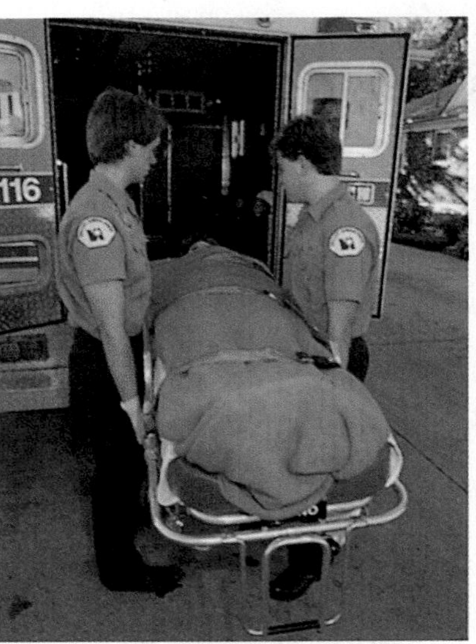

6-6B ✱ Lift the stretcher to standing position.

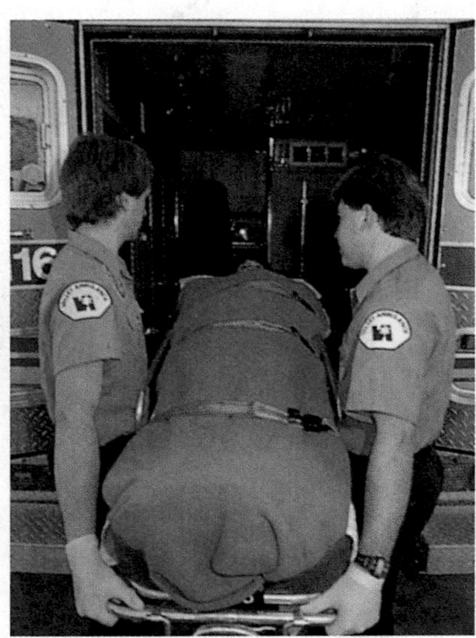

6-6C ✱ Move the patient and stretcher into the ambulance.

EMT skills 6-7 Loading the Roll-In Wheeled Stretcher

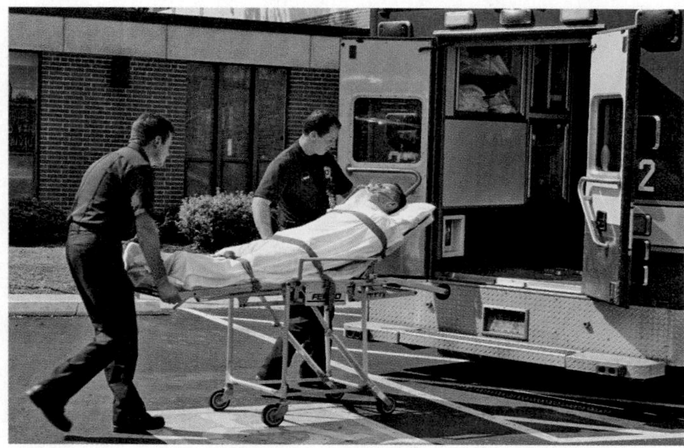

6-7A ✻ Roll the stretcher to the ambulance.

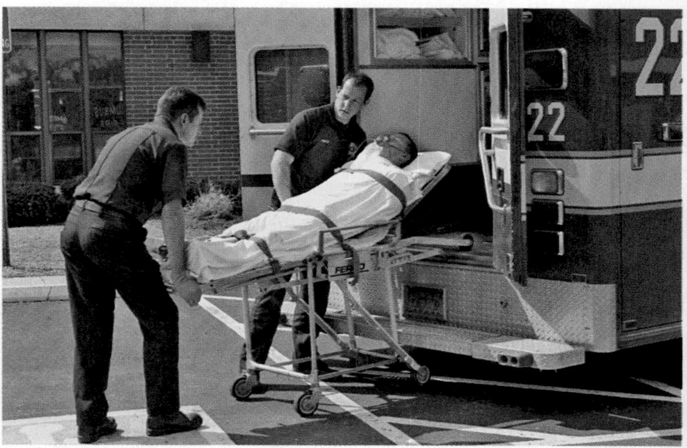

6-7B ✻ Roll the front of the stretcher into the ambulance until the safety mechanism engages.

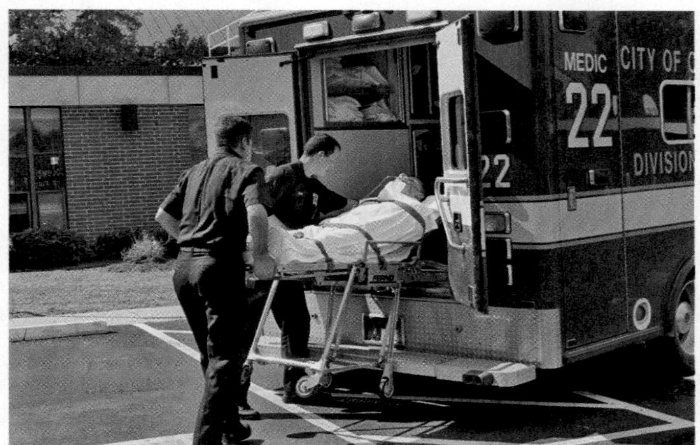

6-7C ✻ Disengage the carriage lock at the foot and roll the stretcher into the ambulance.

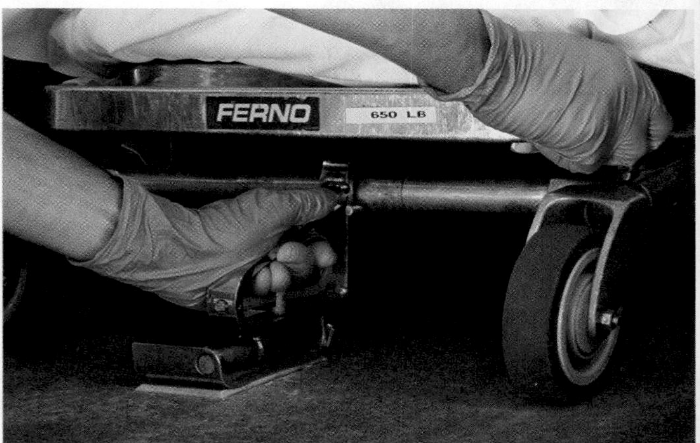

6-7D ✻ Lock the stretcher into position.

EMT skills 6-8 Bariatric Stretchers

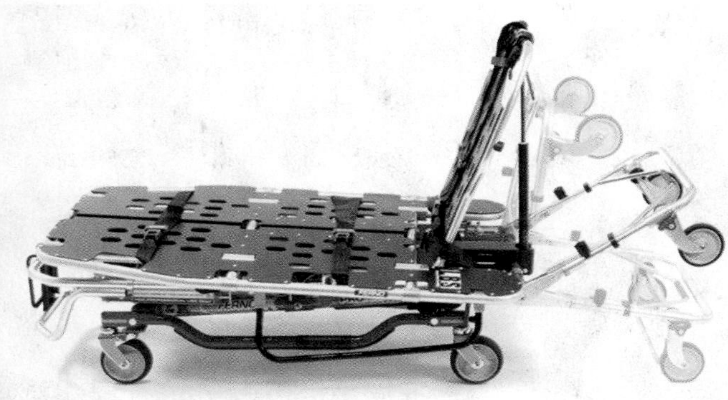

6-8A * The Ferno LBS (large body surface) board converts a Ferno cot into a bariatric cot handling up to 1,000 pounds. (© Ferno-Washington, Inc.)

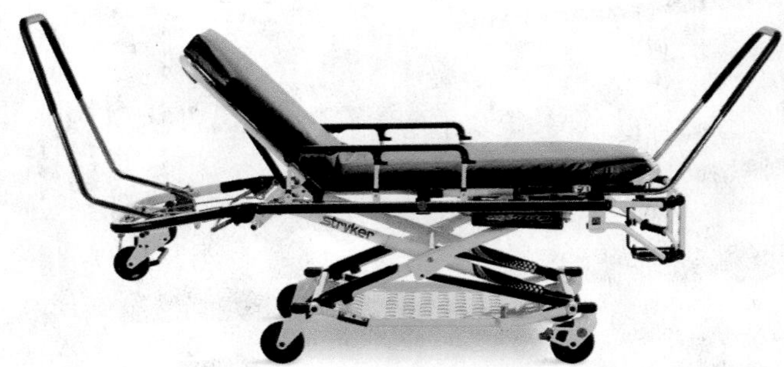

6-8B * The Stryker MX-PRO® Bariatric Transport cot will handle patients from 850 to 1,600 pounds and can be used with accessory winch and ramp loading devices. (© Stryker Corporation)

EMT skills 6-9 Moving a Patient on a Stair Chair

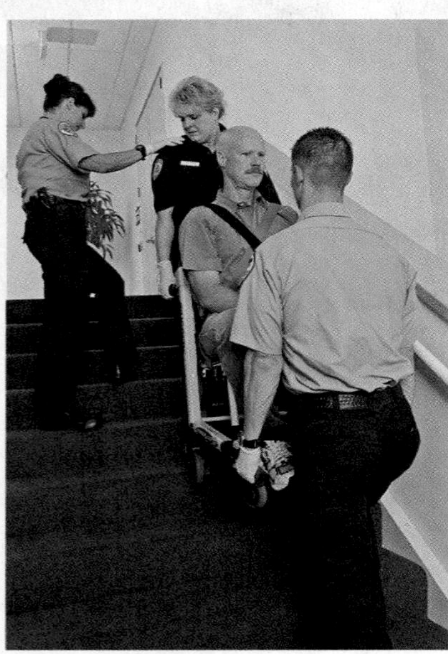

6-9A * Moving a patient up stairs in a stair chair—spotter above.

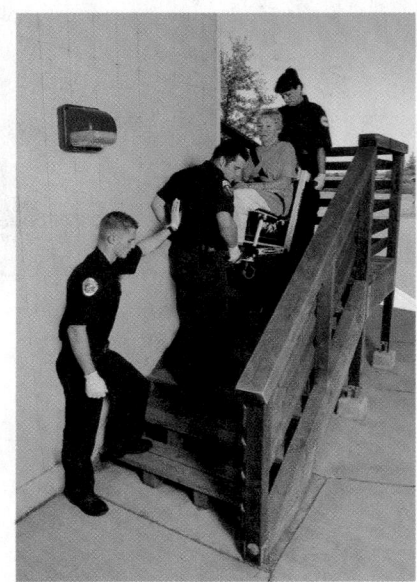

6-9B * Moving a patient down stairs in a stair chair—spotter below.

EMT skills 6-10 Applying the Scoop Stretcher

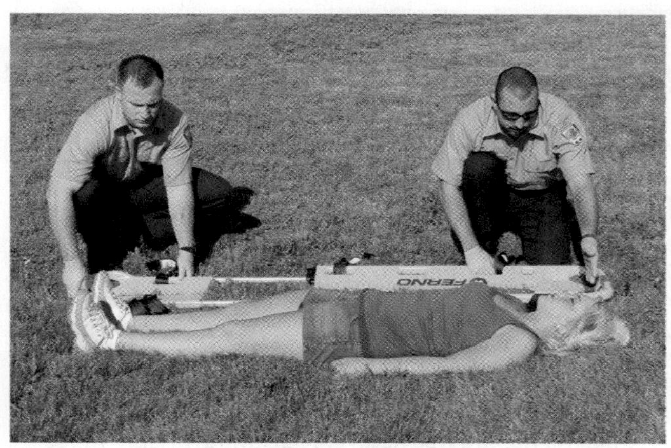

6-10A ✱ Adjust length of the scoop stretcher.

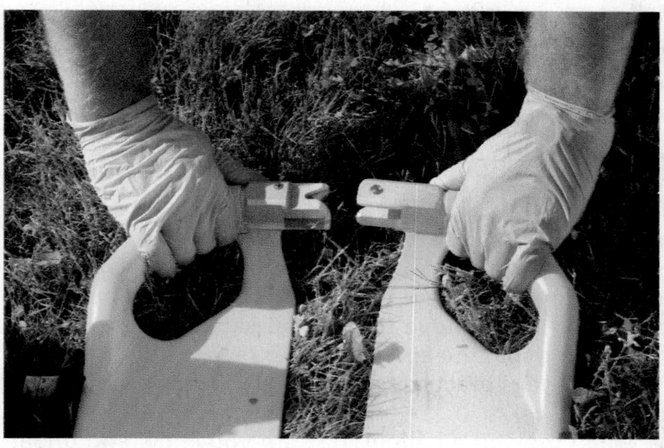

6-10B ✱ Separate the stretcher halves.

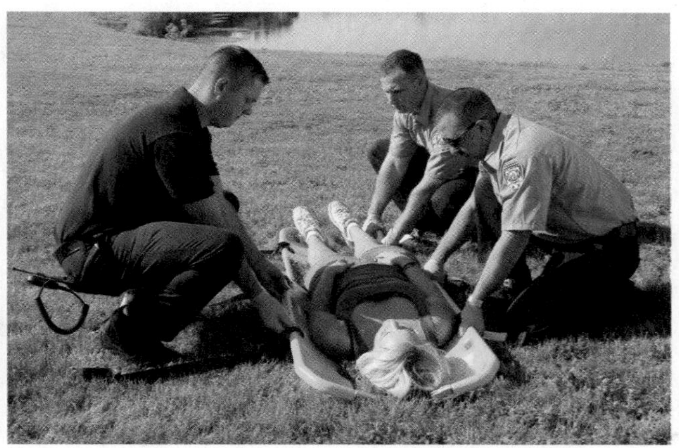

6-10C ✱ Gently slide half of the stretcher under the patient.

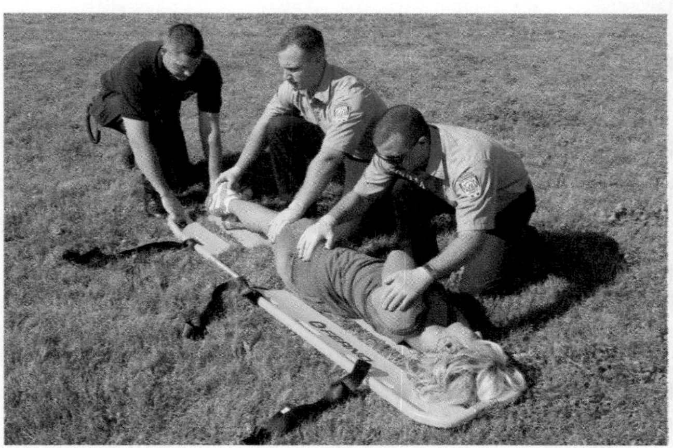

6-10D ✱ Swing the remaining half of the stretcher into a closed position.

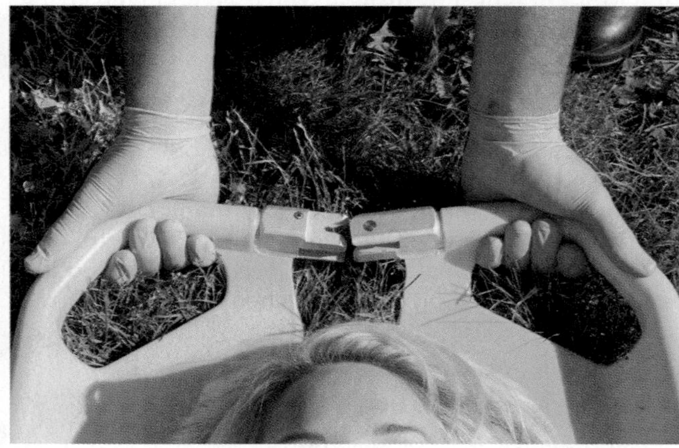

6-10E ✱ Close and lock the stretcher halves.

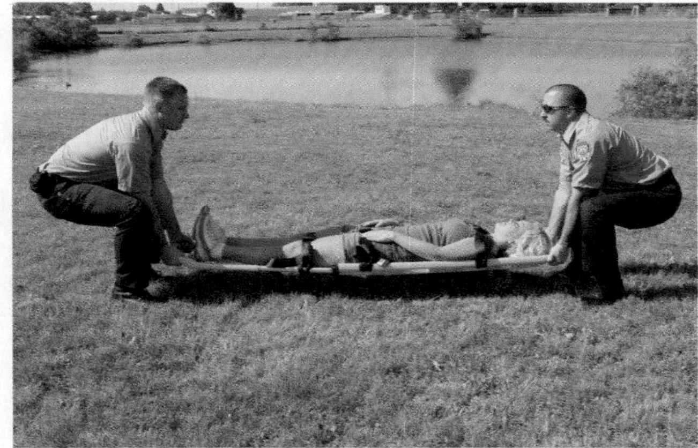

6-10F ✱ Lift the stretcher from its ends.

CHAPTER REVIEW

SUMMARY

Lifting and moving patients is a fundamental task performed by EMTs. Patients are often found on the second floor of a home, in a basement, around the corner in the bedroom, or down a narrow hallway—all of which require special techniques to move the patient safely to the wheeled stretcher and into the ambulance. To reduce your incidence of injury, always practice proper body mechanics and lifting techniques.

When moving a patient, be sure you know and understand how to perform the moves and what equipment is the safest for you and the patient. Always communicate with your team members and with the patient. Your priority is to avoid injury to you, your partner, other members of the emergency response team, and the patient. Select the best possible equipment to allow the patient to be moved in the safest manner, taking into consideration his condition. As an example, a patient with severe shortness of breath will not want to be moved lying supine. Thus, it may be necessary to use a stair chair to move him to the first floor.

Once the patient has been successfully moved, reassess the security of the straps and the device. Never leave the patient alone on the wheeled stretcher, especially if it is in a raised position.

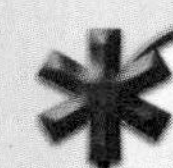

CASE STUDY FOLLOW-UP

SCENE SIZE-UP

You have been dispatched to a 72-year-old female patient, Amanda Sanchez, to take her on a routine transfer to the hospital dialysis center. As your partners unload the stair chair and blankets from the ambulance, you shovel the short walk to the front of the house and apply salt. While you are upstairs, the ice will have a chance to melt.

The patient's daughter opens the door and sends you up a flight of narrow stairs to the bedroom. Mrs. Sanchez greets you there, and you notice that she is using a walker. Your partners take in the stair chair and prepare it for the patient.

PATIENT ASSESSMENT

The training officer suggests that you practice taking a history and vital signs.

LIFTING AND MOVING THE PATIENT

After taking a history and vital signs, you listen as your training officer explains the procedure to the patient. She explains that you and your partner will place Mrs. Sanchez on the hospital blanket in the stair chair, tuck her in so she'll be warm, and secure her for a safe trip down the stairs.

Mrs. Sanchez asks if she will need her winter overcoat. Your partner explains that a warm hat and scarf would be okay, but the overcoat may be too bulky for the move. He promises her the blankets and the ambulance will keep her warm. He also says she can take the coat with her in case she needs it later. You and your partners then package the patient and move her to the stairwell.

At the top of the stairs, your training officer explains exactly what will be done next, while you and your partner quickly check the straps. When she's finished, the training officer says, "Mrs. Sanchez, remember? You may feel as if you're falling for a second. But you won't fall. We'll be holding you. Is it okay that we begin now?"

Mrs. Sanchez agrees, and you get behind the chair at the head. Your partner, who is taller than you, stands at the foot facing the patient. The training officer moves to the top of the steps to "spot." As you tilt the chair back, your partner grasps it by its legs. You then open the space between your feet, tighten your muscles to lock your back, make sure your hands and fingers are properly positioned, and bend from the hips to pick up the patient. You make sure you can keep the weight and arms as close to your body as possible. When you're both ready, you both say so.

Your training officer tells you how many steps there are ahead. Both of you start the descent. The trainer-spotter counts out the steps as you descend. You and the other carrier are keeping pace and checking in. The three of you sound like this:

One step. Okay. Okay.

Two step. Okay. Too fast, slow down.

Three step. Okay. Okay. (and so on)

You and your partner place the stair chair down at the bottom of the steps to rest for a minute. Mrs. Sanchez's daughter opens the front door, and the training officer checks to see that the walkway is clear of obstacles and ice. When you are all assured it is safe, you wheel the chair out to the ambulance and load the patient onto the ambulance cot.

REASSESSMENT

Inside the ambulance, you make certain the patient is comfortable, loosening her scarf and the blankets. You perform a reassessment en route and arrive at the hospital without any change in the patient's condition. You and your partners transfer Mrs. Sanchez to the hospital staff, complete the necessary paperwork, and then proceed to ready the ambulance for the next call.

IN REVIEW

1. List the four basic principles of body mechanics.
2. Explain how to perform the power grip, and when you should use it.
3. Explain how to perform the power lift, and when you should use it.
4. Name the three categories of patient moves, and explain when each should be used.
5. List some of the guidelines and safety precautions for carrying.
6. Explain, briefly, how to perform (a) a direct ground lift, (b) an extremity lift, (c) a direct carry, and (d) the draw sheet method.
7. Name the device that is recommended for carrying a patient up and down stairs, whenever possible, and explain the function of the spotter.
8. Name types of patient-carrying devices you would consider using if the spaces you need to traverse are too narrow or too confined for a wheeled stretcher.
9. Explain the proper body mechanics for reaching while doing a log roll.
10. Explain the safety guidelines for pushing and pulling.

CRITICAL THINKING

You are on the scene providing emergency care to a 76-year-old female patient who was found in bed on the second floor of her home. She is propped up in bed, using several pillows, and complains that she cannot breathe when lying flat. The bedroom is located down a narrow hallway.

1. What device should you use to move the patient to the ambulance?
2. What special circumstances should you consider when selecting the equipment?
3. How would you move the patient from the bed to the device being used to move her?
4. What body techniques will you use to prevent injury to yourself when performing the moves?

PEARSON

EXPLORE mybradykit™

Please go to **www.bradybooks.com** to access mykit for this text. You will find quizzes, critical thinking scenarios, weblinks, animations, and videos related to this chapter—and much more. Look for information on lifting bariatric patients.

Register your access code from the front of your book by going to **www.bradybooks.com** and selecting the mykit links.

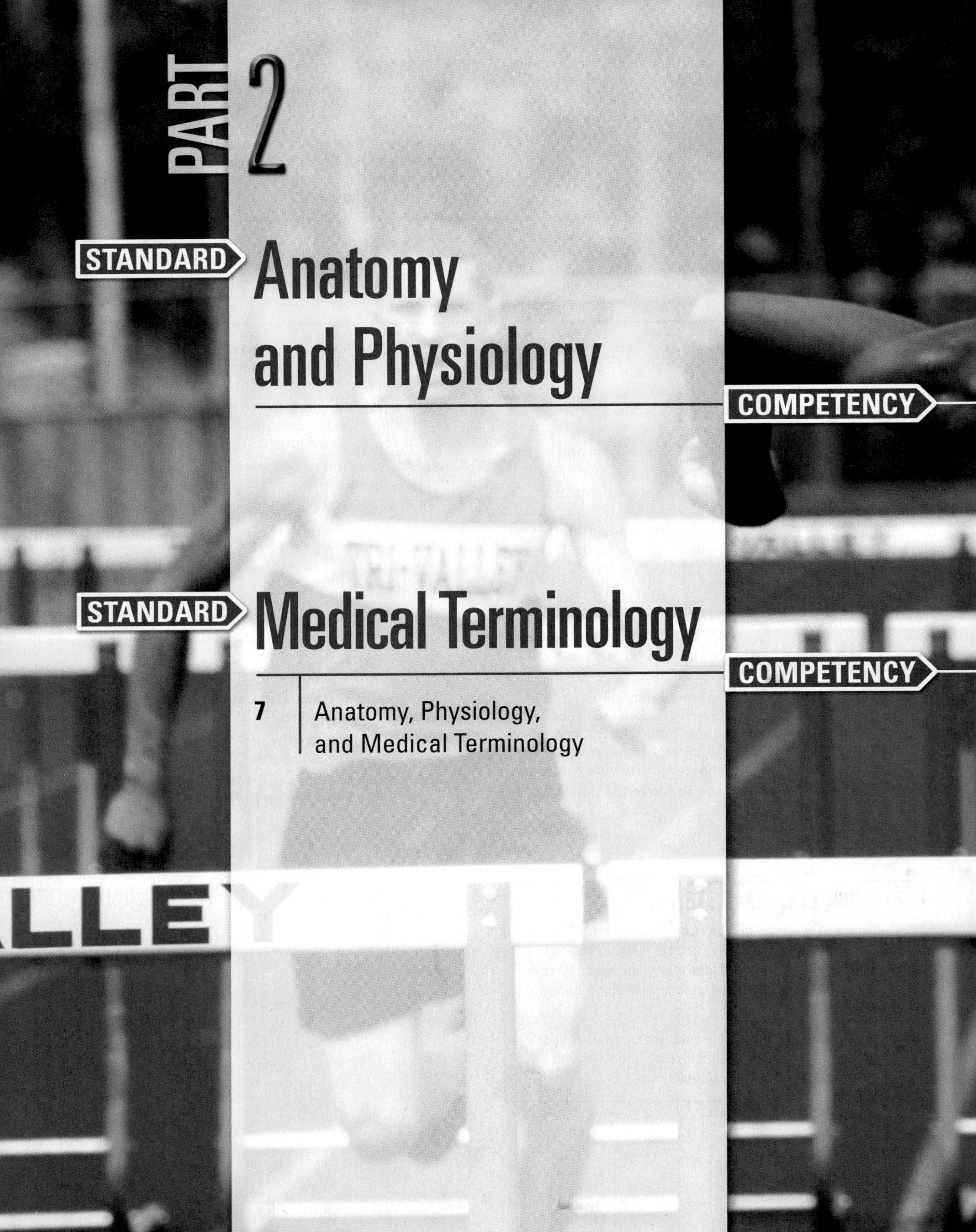

PART 2

STANDARD

Anatomy and Physiology

COMPETENCY

STANDARD

Medical Terminology

COMPETENCY

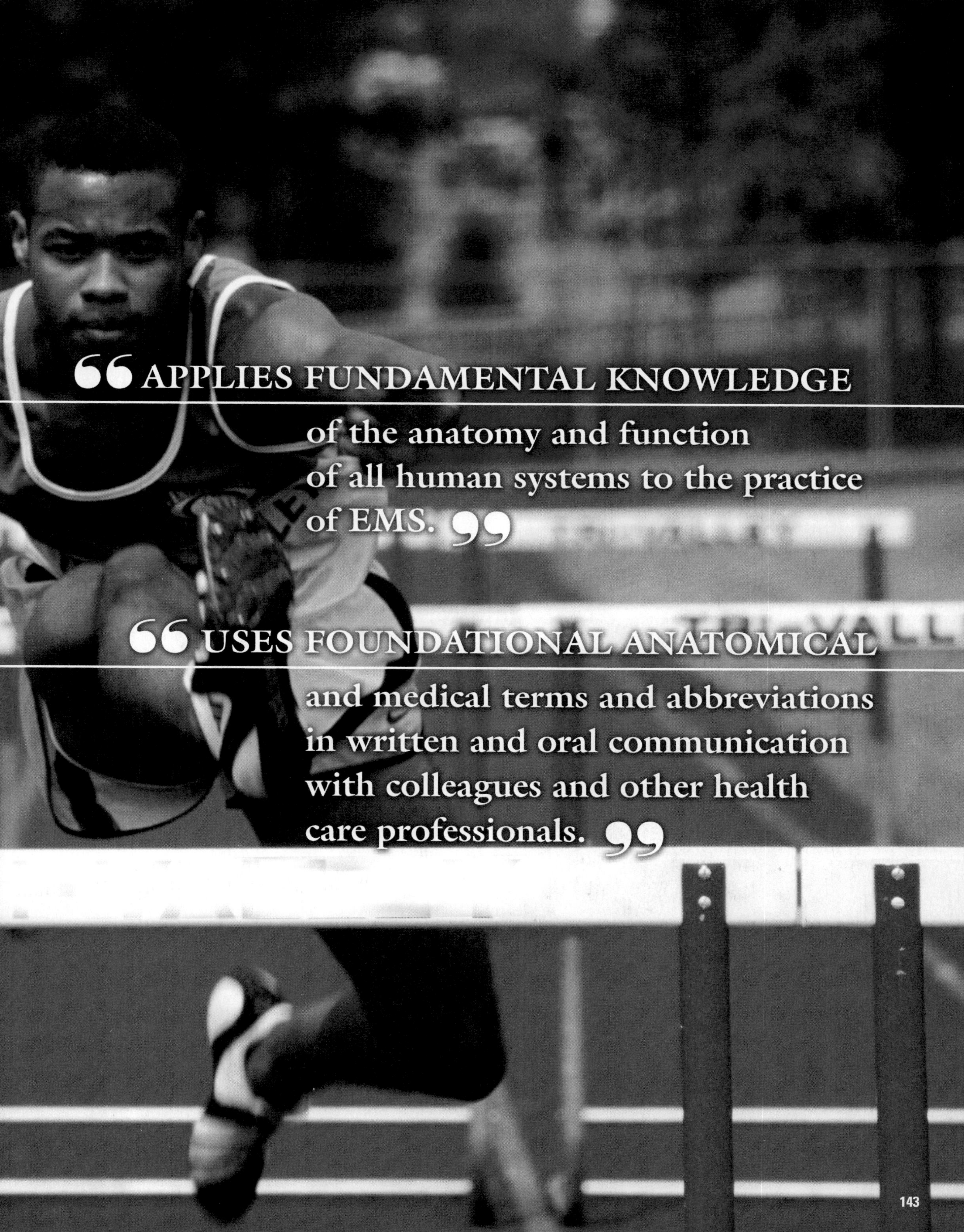
“APPLIES FUNDAMENTAL KNOWLEDGE
of the anatomy and function
of all human systems to the practice
of EMS.”
“USES FOUNDATIONAL ANATOMICAL
and medical terms and abbreviations
in written and oral communication
with colleagues and other health
care professionals.”

CHAPTER 7

Anatomy, Physiology, and Medical Terminology

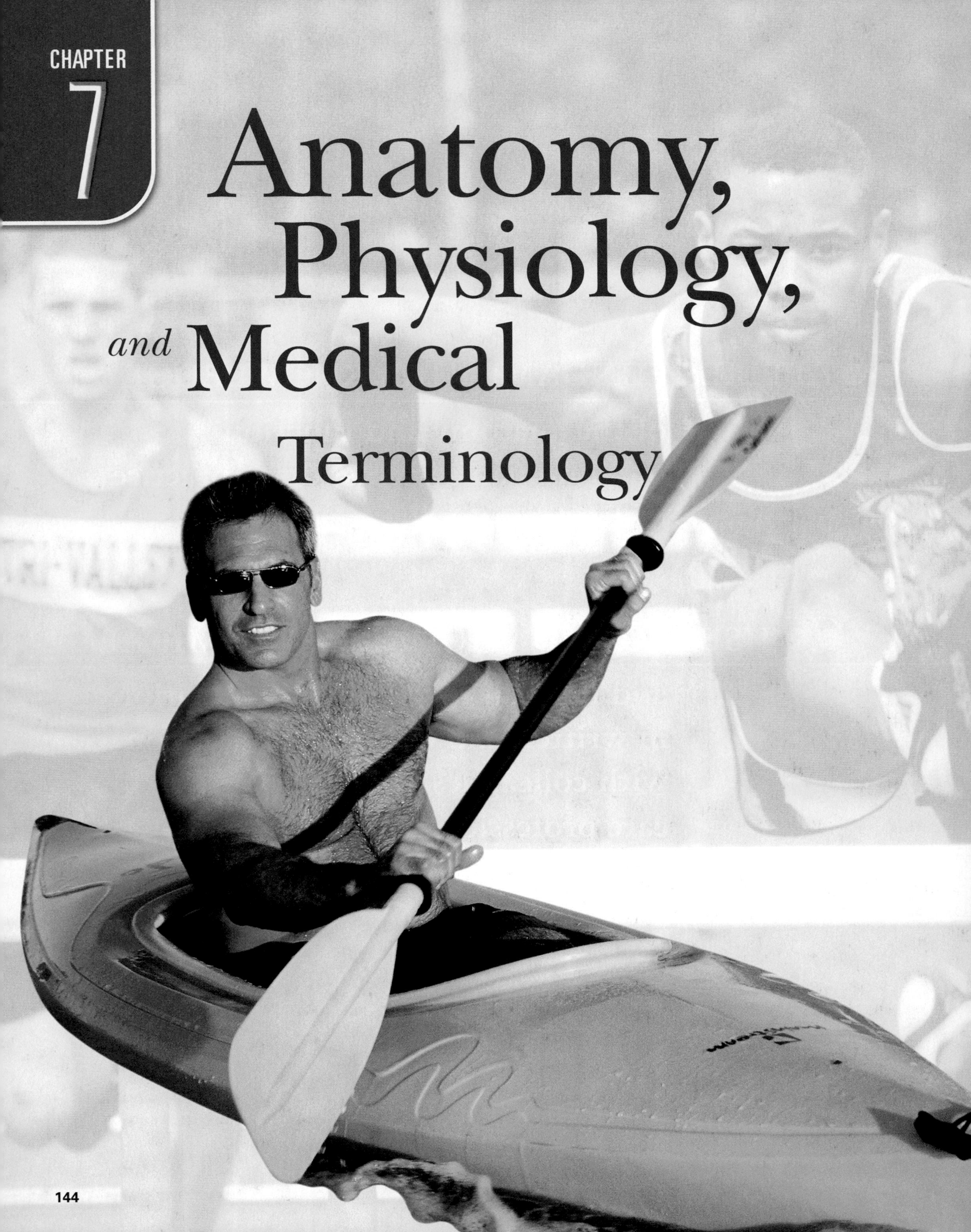

Navigation Guide

The following items provide an overview to the purpose and content of this chapter. The Standards and Competencies are from the new National EMS Education Standards.

STANDARDS **Anatomy and Physiology; Medical Terminology**

COMPETENCIES Applies fundamental knowledge of the anatomy and function of all human systems to the practice of EMS.

Uses foundational anatomical and medical terms and abbreviations in written and oral communication with colleagues and other health professionals.

OBJECTIVES: After reading this chapter, you should be able to:

7-1. Define key terms introduced in this chapter.
7-2. Explain the importance of knowledge of anatomy and physiology to patient assessment and care.
7-3. Define the terms *anatomy* and *physiology.*
7-4. Describe each of the following terms of position:
- **a.** Anatomical position
- **b.** Supine
- **c.** Prone
- **d.** Lateral recumbent
- **e.** Fowler position
- **f.** Semi-Fowler position
- **g.** Trendelenburg position
- **h.** Shock position

7-5. Identify each of the following anatomical terms:
- **a.** Midline
- **b.** Sagittal plane
- **c.** Frontal plane
- **d.** Transverse plane
- **e.** Midaxillary line
- **f.** Midclavicular line
- **g.** Anterior and posterior
- **h.** Dorsal and ventral
- **i.** Right and left
- **j.** Superior and inferior
- **k.** Medial and lateral
- **l.** Proximal and distal
- **m.** Plantar
- **n.** Palmar
- **o.** Abdominal quadrants: right upper quadrant, left upper quadrant, left lower quadrant, right lower quadrant

7-6. State the function of each of the following musculoskeletal system structures:
- **a.** Skeletal muscle
- **b.** Tendons
- **c.** Ligaments
- **d.** Bone

7-7. Describe each of the following components of the skeleton, including its location, the bones that make it up, and its function:
- **a.** Skull
  - **i.** Cranium
  - **ii.** Face
- **b.** Spinal column
  - **i.** Cervical spine
  - **ii.** Thoracic spine
  - **iii.** Lumbar spine
  - **iv.** Sacral spine
  - **v.** Coccyx
- **c.** Thorax
  - **i.** Sternum (including manubrium, body, and xiphoid process)
  - **ii.** Ribs
- **d.** Pelvis
  - **i.** Ilium and iliac crest
  - **ii.** Ischium
  - **iii.** Pubis
  - **iv.** Acetabulum
- **e.** Upper extremities
  - **i.** Clavicle
  - **ii.** Scapula, including acromion process
  - **iii.** Humerus
  - **iv.** Radius
  - **v.** Ulna, including olecranon process
  - **vi.** Carpals
  - **vii.** Metacarpals
  - **viii.** Phalanges
- **f.** Lower extremities
  - **i.** Femur
  - **ii.** Patella
  - **iii.** Tibia, including medial malleolus
  - **iv.** Fibula, including lateral malleolus
  - **v.** Tarsals, including the calcaneus
  - **vi.** Metatarsals
  - **vii.** Phalanges

7-8. Demonstrate each of the following joint movements:
- **a.** Flexion and extension
- **b.** Adduction and abduction
- **c.** Circumduction
- **d.** Pronation and supination

7-9. Describe each of the following types of joints:
- **a.** Ball-and-socket
- **b.** Hinge
- **c.** Pivot
- **d.** Gliding

continued

Navigation Guide *continued*

e. Saddle
f. Condyloid

7-10. Differentiate between skeletal (voluntary), smooth (involuntary), and cardiac muscle.

7-11. Identify the basic functions of the respiratory system:

7-12. Identify the following structures of the respiratory system:
a. Upper airway: nose, mouth, pharynx, nasopharynx, larynx
b. Lower airway: trachea, bronchi, bronchioles, alveoli
c. Epiglottis
d. Lungs
e. Pleura
f. Diaphragm

7-13. Identify important differences in respiratory system anatomy in children.

7-14. Describe the basic mechanics and physiology of normal ventilation, respiration, and oxygenation, including:
a. Inhalation and exhalation
b. Use of intercostal muscles and diaphragm
c. Negative and positive pressure
d. Nervous system control of respiration
e. Alveolar/capillary exchange of oxygen and carbon dioxide
f. Capillary/cell exchange of oxygen and carbon dioxide

7-15. Identify characteristics of both adequate and inadequate breathing.

7-16. List the functions of the circulatory (cardiovascular) system.

7-17. Describe the anatomy and physiology of the heart to include:
a. Location and size
b. Tissue layers
c. Chambers
d. Valves
e. Blood supply
f. Blood flow through the heart
g. Conduction system

7-18. Discuss the anatomy and physiology of the blood, circulation, perfusion, and metabolism to convey basic comprehension of:
a. Arteries and arterioles
b. Capillaries
c. Veins and venules
d. Blood composition
e. Perfusion and capillary exchange
f. Cell metabolism

7-19. Describe the basic functions of the nervous system.

7-20. Differentiate between the structural components and basic functions of the central nervous system and peripheral nervous system.

7-21. Differentiate between the functional divisions of the peripheral nervous system:
a. Voluntary (somatic) nervous system
b. Involuntary (autonomic) nervous system
  i. Sympathetic division
  ii. Parasympathetic division

7-22. Describe the basic role of the reticular activating system (RAS) and cerebral hemispheres in consciousness and unconsciousness.

7-23. Explain the overall function of the endocrine system.

7-24. Discuss the location and general function of each of the following components of the endocrine system:
a. Thyroid gland
b. Parathyroid glands
c. Adrenal glands
d. Gonads
e. Islets of Langerhans of the pancreas, insulin, and glucagon
f. Pituitary gland

7-25. Describe the general actions of epinephrine and norepinephrine on $beta_1$, $beta_2$, $alpha_1$, and $alpha_2$ receptors of the sympathetic nervous system.

7-26. List the general functions of the integumentary system.

7-27. Identify the structures of the integumentary system, including the epidermis, dermis, and subcutaneous layer.

7-28. Describe the basic anatomy and physiology of each of the following structures of the digestive system:
a. Stomach
b. Pancreas
c. Liver
d. Gallbladder
e. Small intestine (duodenum, jejunum, ileum)
f. Colon

7-29. List the basic structure and function of the organs of the urinary or renal system to include:
a. Kidneys
b. Ureters
c. Urinary bladder
d. Urethra

7-30. State the basic structure and function of the organs of the male and female reproductive systems:
a. Male
  i. Testes
  ii. Accessory glands
  iii. Penis

Navigation Guide *continued*

b. Female
  i. Ovaries
  ii. Fallopian tubes
  iii. Uterus
  iv. Vagina
  v. External genitalia

7-31. Explain the importance of knowledge of medical terminology in communication among health care team members.

7-32. Apply knowledge of common prefixes, suffixes, and roots to interpret medical terms.

KEY TERMS: Page references indicate first major use in this chapter. For complete definitions, see the Glossary at the back of the book.

anatomy p. 147
circulatory system p. 168
digestive system p. 182
endocrine system p. 178
integumentary system p. 181
musculoskeletal system p. 153
nervous system p. 175
physiology p. 147
reproductive system p. 184
respiratory system p. 162
urinary/renal system p. 184

MEDIA RESOURCES: Please go to www.bradybooks.com to access mykit for this text. You will find quizzes, critical thinking scenarios, weblinks, animations, and videos related to this chapter—and much more. Look for online information on identifying body systems. You will also find animations on the heart, endocrine system, and skeletal system.

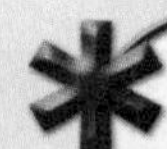

CASE STUDY

The Dispatch

EMS Unit 108—respond to Centennial Park on Highland Avenue—you have a female patient at that location who suffered a burn—time out 1306 hours.

Upon Arrival

After positioning the ambulance out of the flow of traffic, you scan the scene for hazards and exit. A woman runs up to you and says, "A woman over here was trying to refuel her son's model airplane when the gas tank blew up or something." You approach the patient and find that she is sitting on a patch of grass about 15 feet away from a smoldering model plane.

How Would You Proceed to Assess and Care for This Patient?

During this chapter, you will read a brief overview of the human body. Later, we will return to the case study and put in context some of the information you learned.

▶ Introduction

Knowledge of the human body and its systems is essential to high-quality patient assessment and emergency care. That understanding will help you recognize when the body is working as it should and when there are life-threatening deviations to normal function. Your ability to use proper terminology to describe the human body will also allow you to communicate patient information to other health care professionals concisely and accurately.

▶ Anatomical Terms

Basic knowledge of the human body includes the study of anatomy and physiology. The word **anatomy** refers to the structure of the body and the relationship of its parts to each other (how the body is made). The word **physiology** refers to the function of the living body and its parts (how the body works).

As you proceed through your course, you will encounter descriptive terms you may not have heard or used

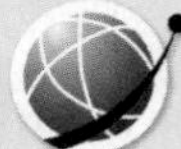

Media Resources

Go to www.bradybooks.com for mykit. Highlights:

- *Web Resource:* Online Human Anatomy
- *Web Resource:* Online Medical Dictionary

Objectives 7-2 to 7-5

Explain the importance of knowledge of anatomy and physiology.

before. Study and learn them. It is essential that you use them correctly to describe position, direction, and location of a patient and his illness or injury. Using correct terms minimizes confusion and helps to communicate the exact extent of a patient's problem based on a careful physical assessment.

One term that is essential for you to understand and use is the **anatomical position**. Unless otherwise indicated, all references to the human body assume the anatomical position: The patient is standing erect, facing forward, with arms down at the sides and palms forward. This basic position is used as the point of reference whenever terms of direction and location are used. Other terms of position include (Figures 7-1a to 7-1f✻):

- **Supine**. The patient is lying face up on his back.
- **Prone**. The patient is lying face down on his stomach.
- **Lateral recumbent (recovery) position**. The patient is lying on his left or right side. Be sure to place the patient on the side so that you can easily monitor the airway. Also, be careful not to allow excessive pressure on the chest that might impair the breathing

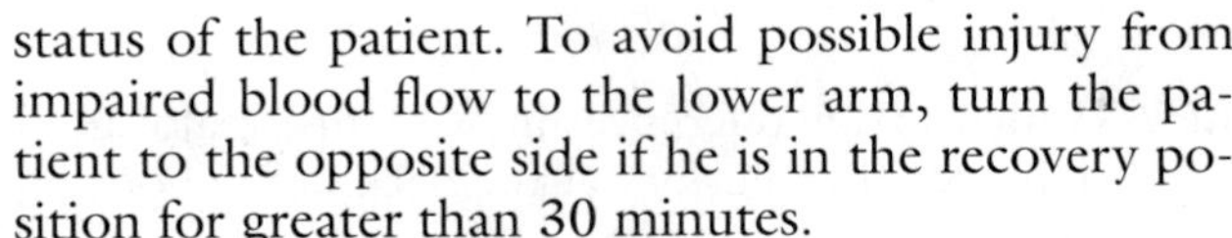

status of the patient. To avoid possible injury from impaired blood flow to the lower arm, turn the patient to the opposite side if he is in the recovery position for greater than 30 minutes.
- **Fowler position**. The patient is lying on his back with his upper body elevated at a 45° to 60° angle.
- **Semi-Fowler position**. The patient is lying on his back with the upper body elevated at an angle less than 45°.
- **Trendelenburg position**. The patient is lying on his back with the legs elevated higher than the head and body on an inclined plane (head down, legs up). *This position, which was once used in the management of shock, is no longer recommended.* With the patient in the Trendelenburg position, the abdominal organs may be pushed up against the diaphragm, from gravity, and make breathing more difficult for the patient. It may also increase the pressure inside the skull in patients with a head injury. *It is definitely contraindicated in a patient with a suspected spine injury.*

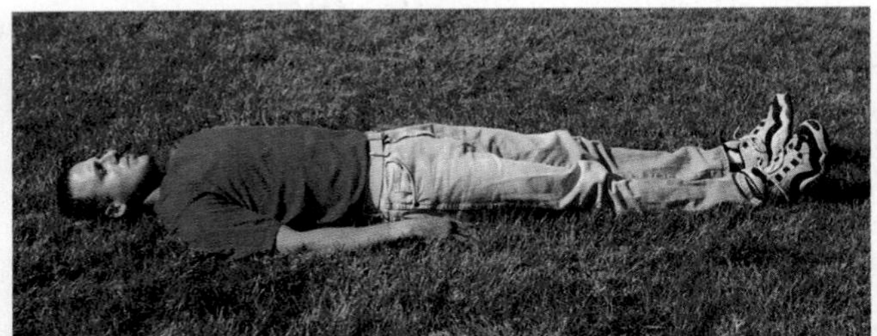

FIGURE 7-1a ✻ Supine position.

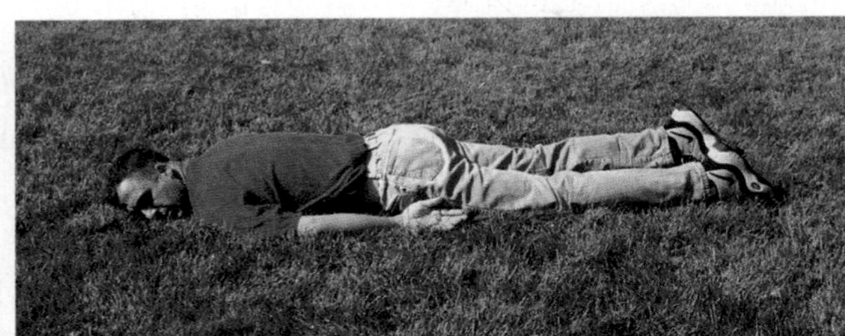

FIGURE 7-1b ✻ Prone position.

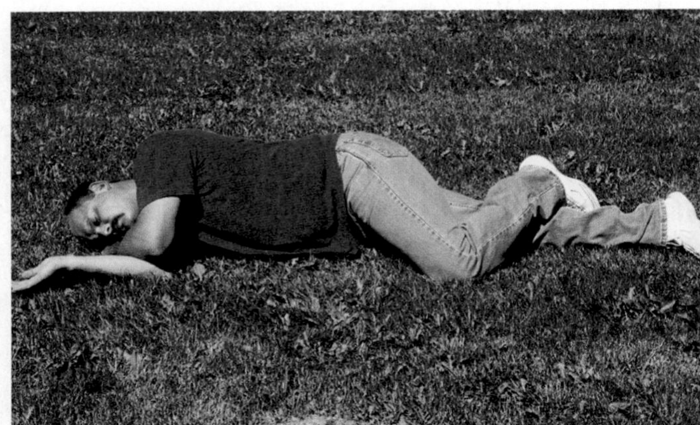

FIGURE 7-1c ✻ Right lateral recumbent position.

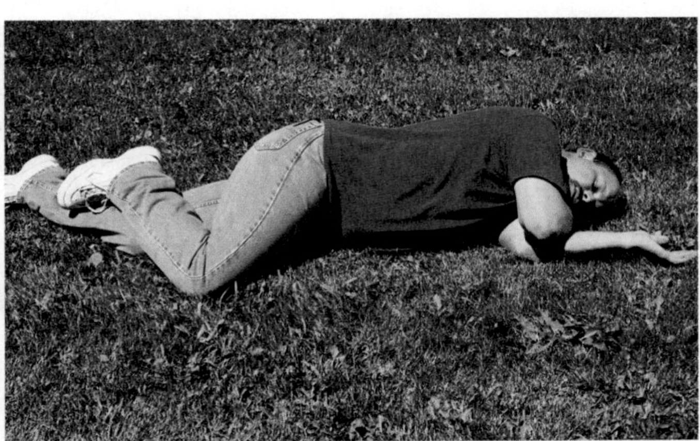

FIGURE 7-1d ✻ Left lateral recumbent position.

Key Terms

anatomy the study of the structure of the body and the relationship of its parts to each other.

physiology the study of the function of the living body and its parts.

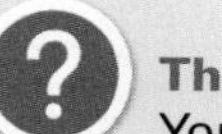

Thinking Critically

Your patient is bleeding profusely and, you figure, is going into shock. As a result, vital body system functions will be impaired and you must intervene to support them. Mentally, you say "thanks" for all those hours you spent studying anatomy and physiology. Why?

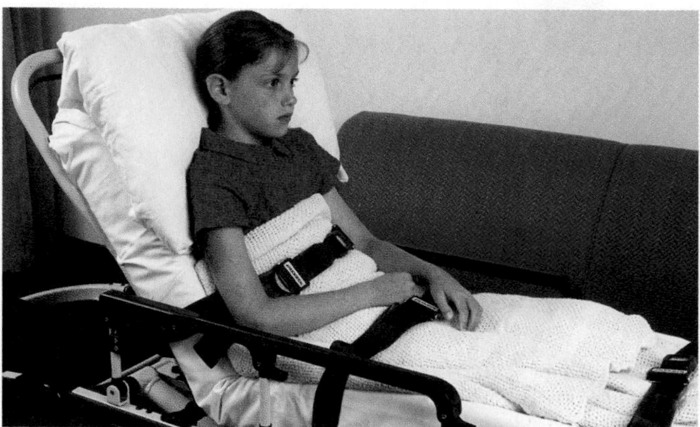

FIGURE 7-1e * Fowler position.

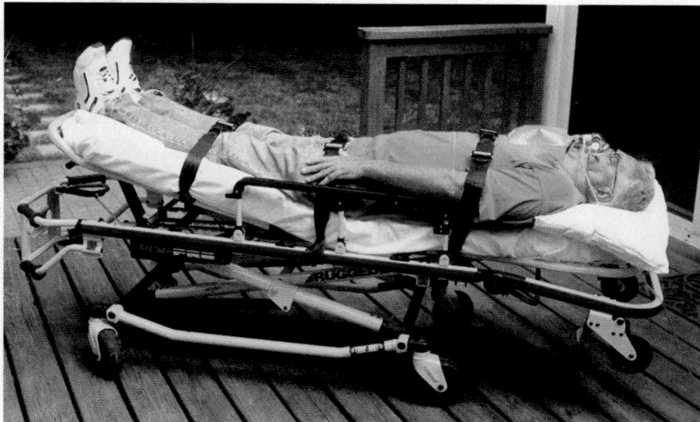

FIGURE 7-1f * Trendelenburg position.

- **Shock position**. This is an alternative to the Trendelenburg position, where only the feet and legs are elevated approximately 12 inches. *Like the Trendelenburg position, the shock position is no longer recommended in the treatment of shock. This position is also contraindicated in a patient with a suspected spine injury.* You may find this position still used for the patient who has suffered a simple faint.

In assessing a patient's condition, it is important to know certain external and internal landmarks, or the anatomical regions of the body and related parts (Figures 7-2* through 7-9*). Referring to these landmarks makes your description of the patient's condition more understandable, especially when you are seeking on-line medical direction.

Imaginary divisions of the body are called **anatomical planes**. There are also anatomical lines used to reference points on the body. These planes and lines indicate the internal body structure and the relationship of different groups of organs to others. Anatomical planes and lines are delineated by the following (Figures 7-2* and 7-3*):

- **Sagittal plane**. The sagittal plane, or median plane, is a vertical plane that runs lengthwise and divides the body into right and left segments. The segments do not have to be equal. If the plane divides the body into two equal halves it would be referred to as the **midsagittal plane**.
- **Frontal or coronal plane**. The frontal or coronal plane divides the body into front and back halves.
- **Transverse or horizontal plane**. The transverse or horizontal plane is parallel with the ground and divides

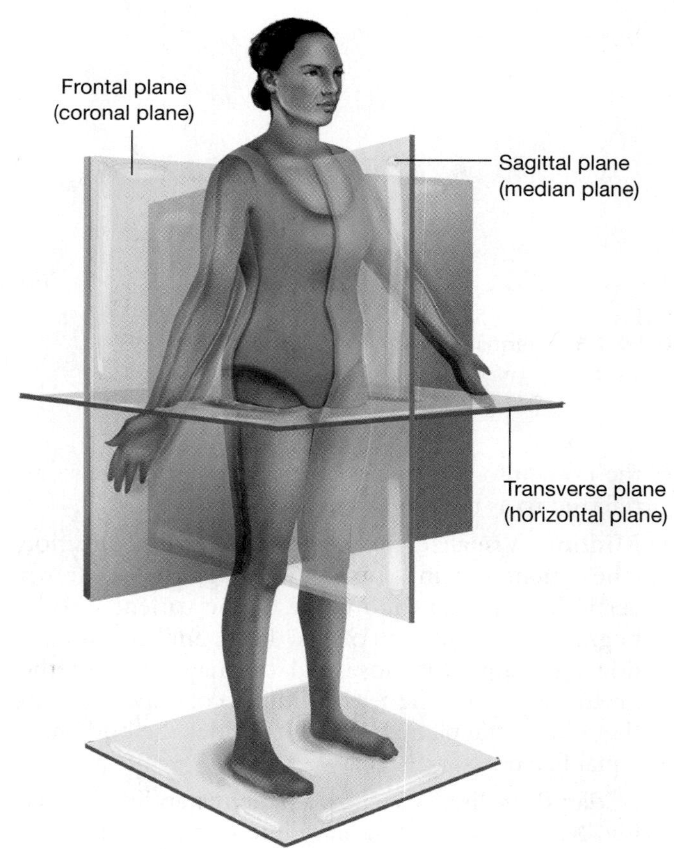

FIGURE 7-2 * Anatomical planes.

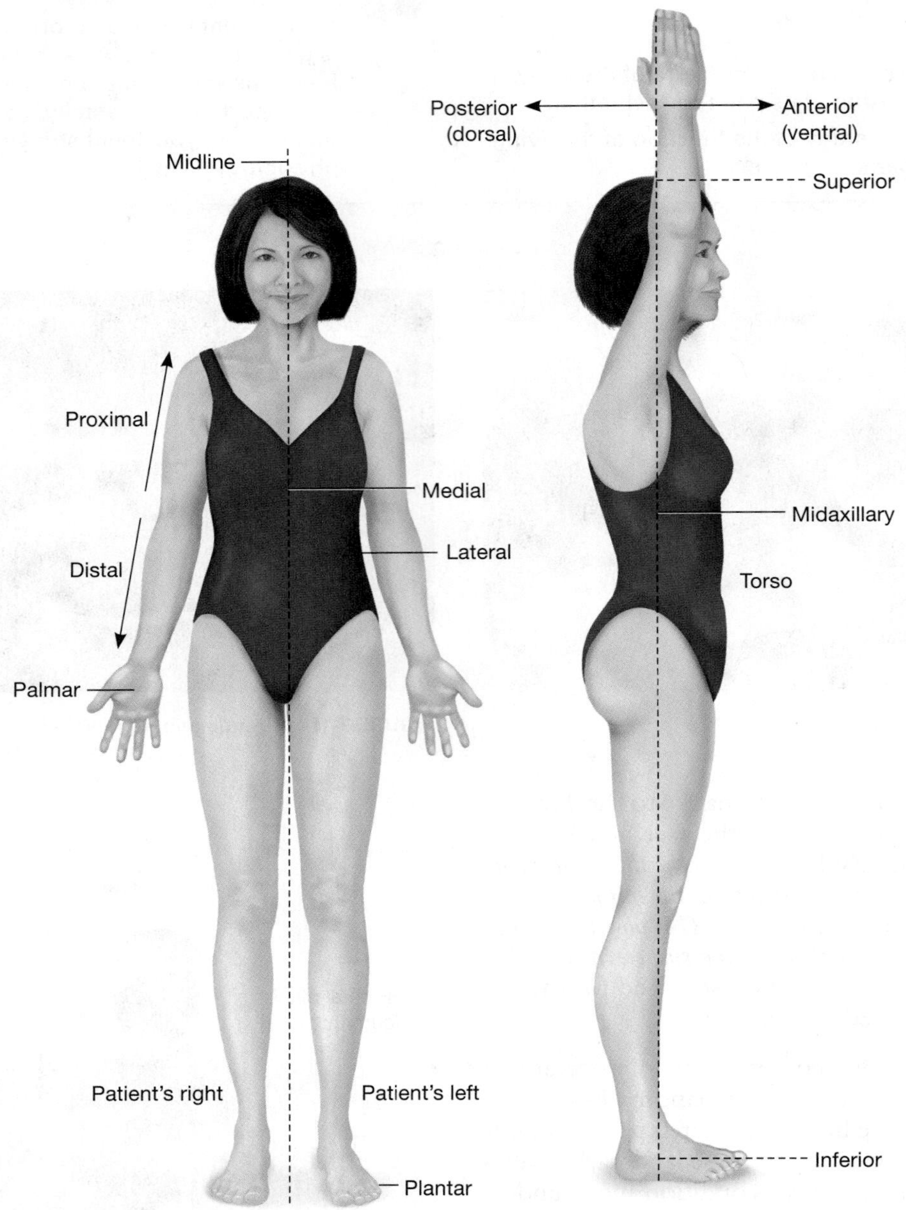

FIGURE 7-3 * Terms of direction.

the body into upper and lower halves. It may also be referred to as the axial plane.

- **Midline**. Visualize the normal anatomical position (the patient is facing you). Now imagine a line drawn vertically through the middle of the patient's body, beginning at the top of the head and continuing down through the nose and the navel and to the ground between the legs. Midline corresponds with the midsagittal plane because it divides the body into equal halves.
- **Midaxillary line**. Visualize a patient standing in profile. Now draw an imaginary line vertically from the middle of the patient's armpit down to the ankle. This is the midaxillary line. A vertical line drawn side to side through the body from the midaxillary line on one side to the midaxillary line on the opposite side forms the frontal plane and divides the body into the **anterior plane** (the patient's front) and the **posterior plane** (the patient's back).
- **Transverse line**. Visualize the normal anatomical position. Draw an imaginary line horizontally through the patient's waist. This is the transverse line. A horizontal line drawn through the body, front to back, at the waist forms the transverse plane and divides the body into the **superior plane** (above the waist) and the **inferior plane** (below the waist).

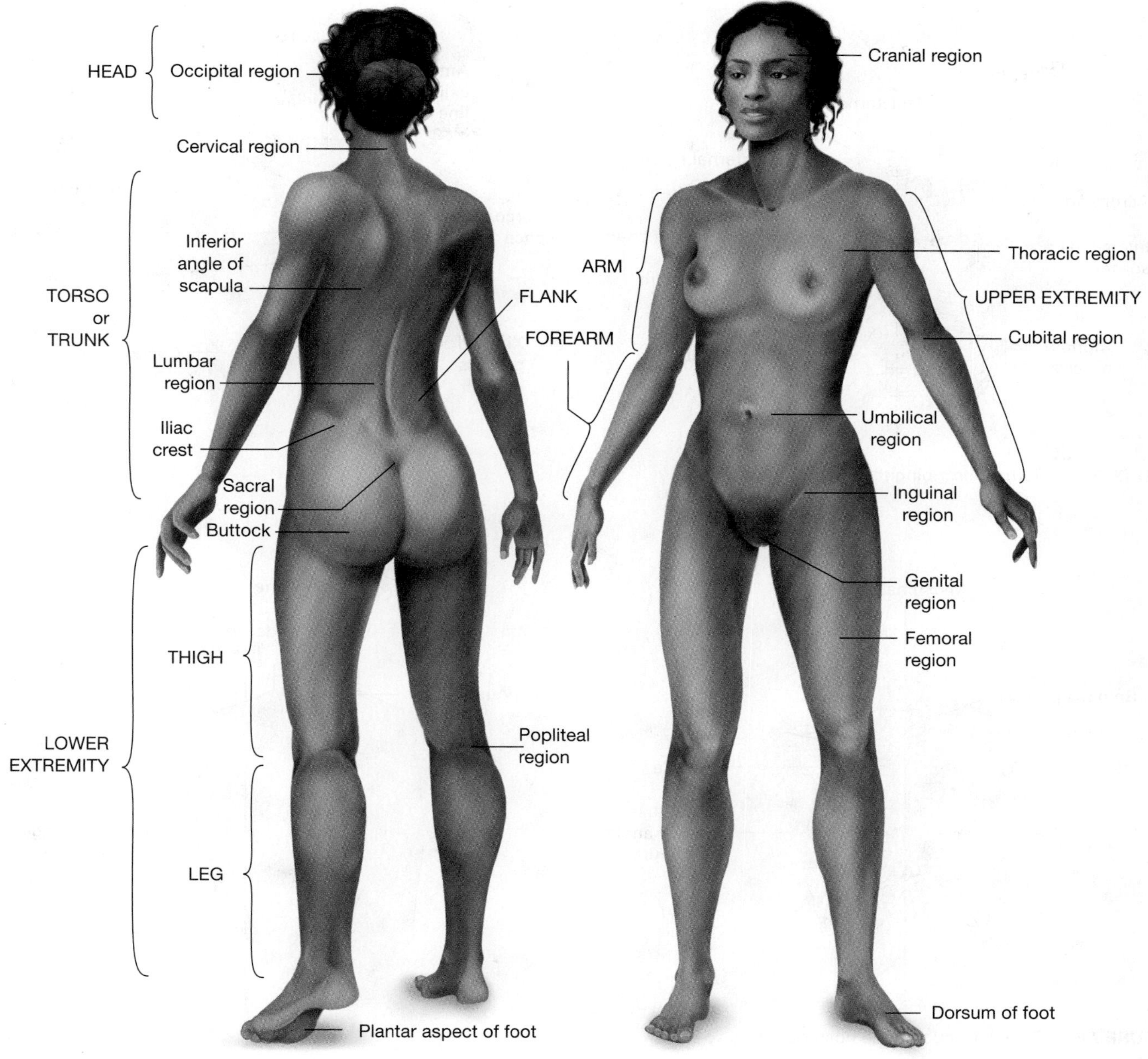

FIGURE 7-4 ✱ Regions of the body.

Other descriptive terms include (Figure 7-3):

- **Anterior** and **posterior**. *Anterior* is toward the front. *Posterior* is toward the back.
- **Superior** and **inferior**. *Superior* means toward the head or above the point of reference. *Inferior* means toward the feet or below the point of reference.
- **Dorsal** and **ventral**. *Dorsal* means toward the back or backbone (spine). *Ventral* means toward the front or belly (abdomen).
- **Medial** and **lateral**. *Medial* means toward the midline or center of the body. *Lateral* refers to the left or right of the midline, or away from the midline of the body. Note that **bilateral** refers to both left and right, meaning "on both sides." *Unilateral* refers to one side. *Ipsilateral* refers to the same side, *contralateral* to the opposite side.
- **Proximal** and **distal**. *Proximal* means near the point of reference. *Distal* is distant, or far from the point of reference.
- **Right** and **left**. Always the patient's right and left.
- **Midclavicular** and **midaxillary**. *Midclavicular* refers to the center of each of the collarbones (clavicle). The midclavicular line (Figure 7-5✱) extends from the center of either collarbone down the anterior thorax.

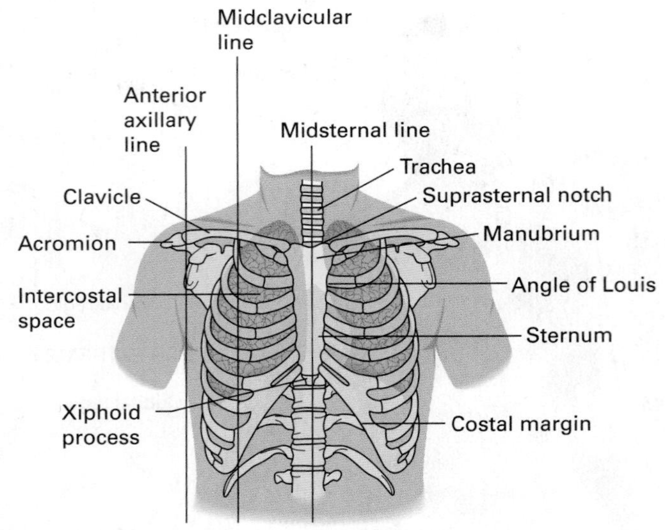

FIGURE 7-5 ✻ Terms describing the anterior chest.

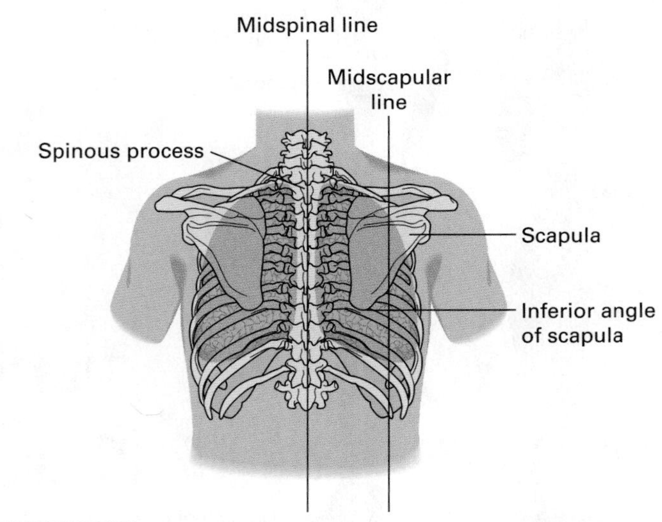

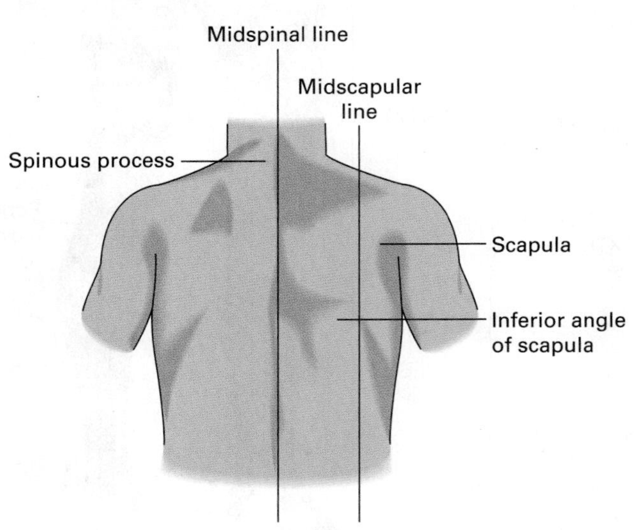

FIGURE 7-6 ✻ Terms describing the posterior chest.

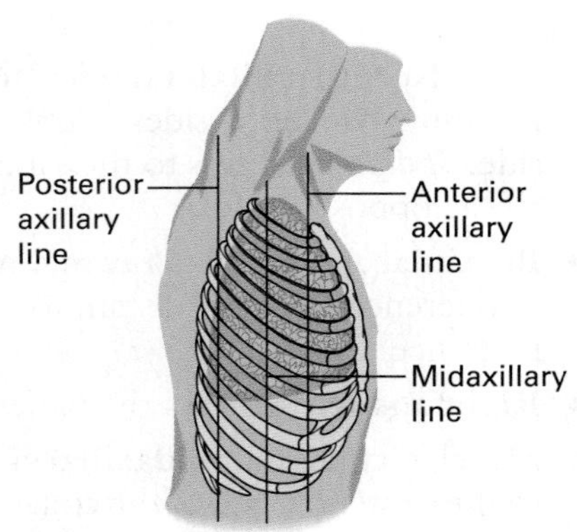

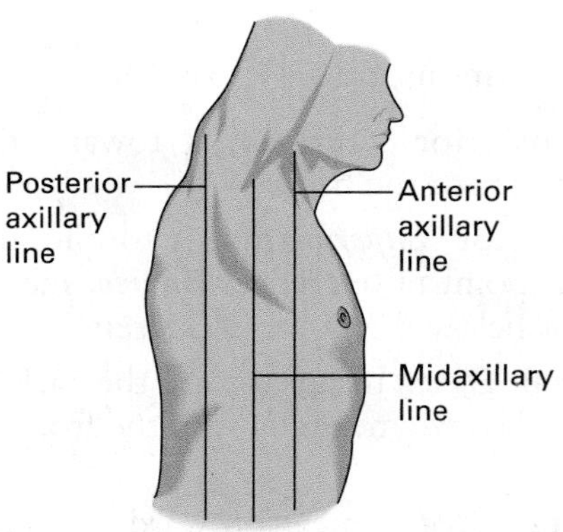

FIGURE 7-7 ✻ Terms describing the lateral chest.

Key Terms

musculoskeletal system the system of bones and muscle plus connective tissue that provides support and protection to the body and permits motion.

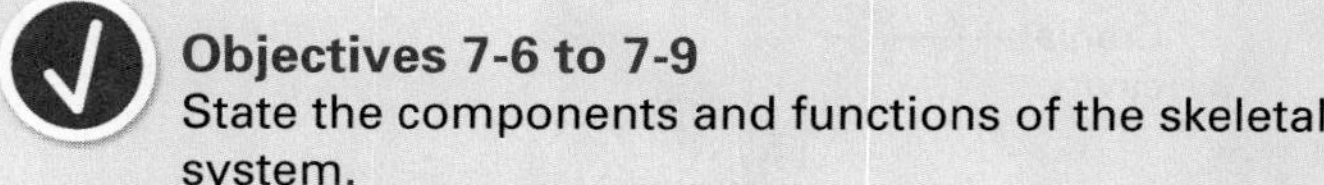

Objectives 7-6 to 7-9

State the components and functions of the skeletal system.

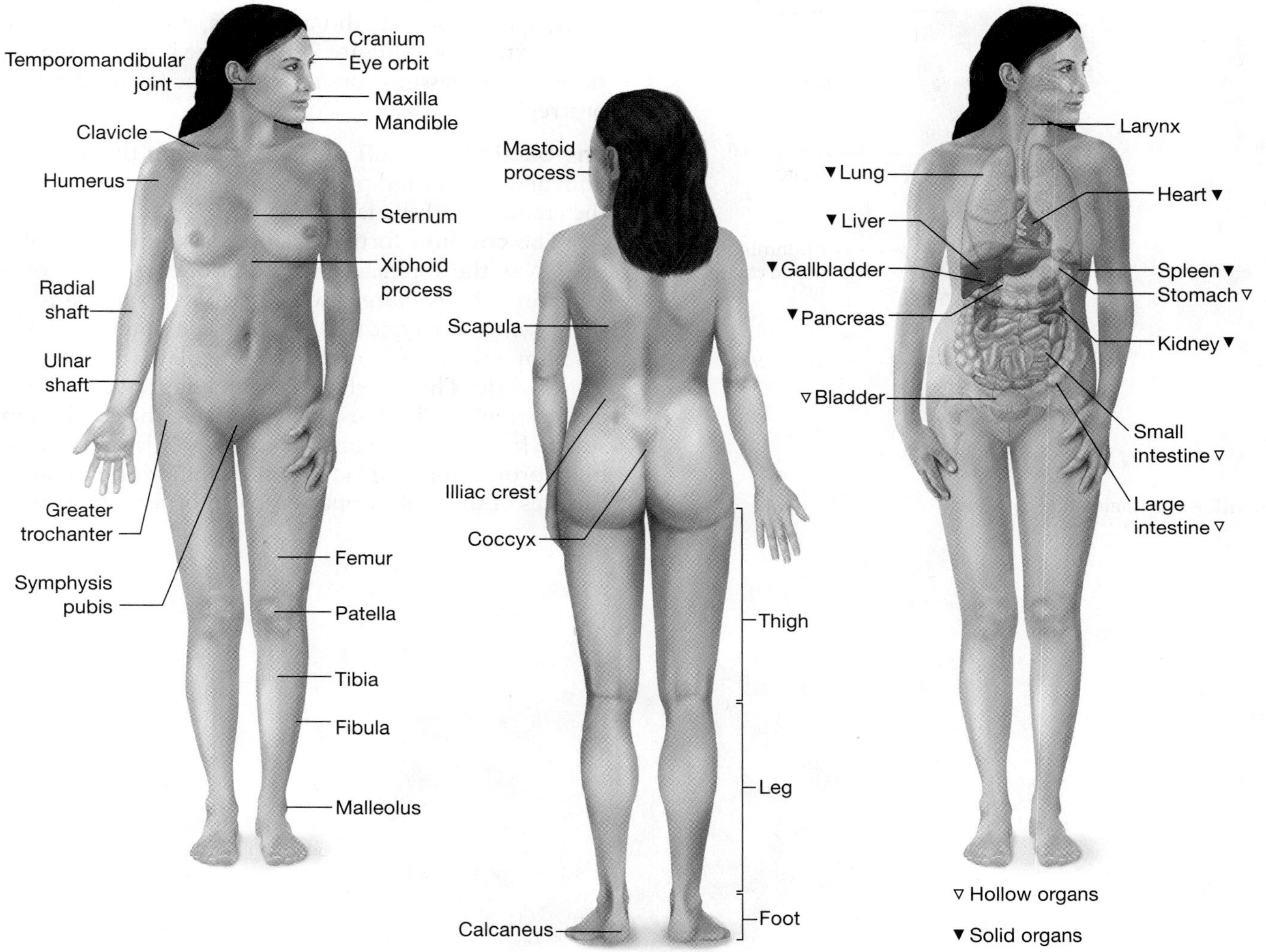

FIGURE 7-8 ∗ Topographic anatomy.

Midaxillary refers to the center of the armpit (axilla). The midaxillary line (Figure 7-7∗) extends from the middle of the armpit to the ankle.

- **Plantar** and **palmar**. *Plantar* refers to the sole of the foot. *Palmar* refers to the palm of the hand.

The abdomen may be referred to as if it were divided by horizontal and vertical lines drawn through the umbilicus (navel). The four parts, or **abdominal quadrants** (Figure 7-10∗), are the right upper quadrant (RUQ), right lower quadrant (RLQ), left upper quadrant (LUQ), and left lower quadrant (LLQ).

Body Systems

The Musculoskeletal System

The **musculoskeletal system** of the human body consists of a bony framework, or skeleton, held together by *ligaments* that connect bone to bone, layers of muscles, *tendons* that connect muscles to bones, and various other connective tissues. The system must be strong to provide support and protection, jointed to permit motion, and flexible to withstand stress.

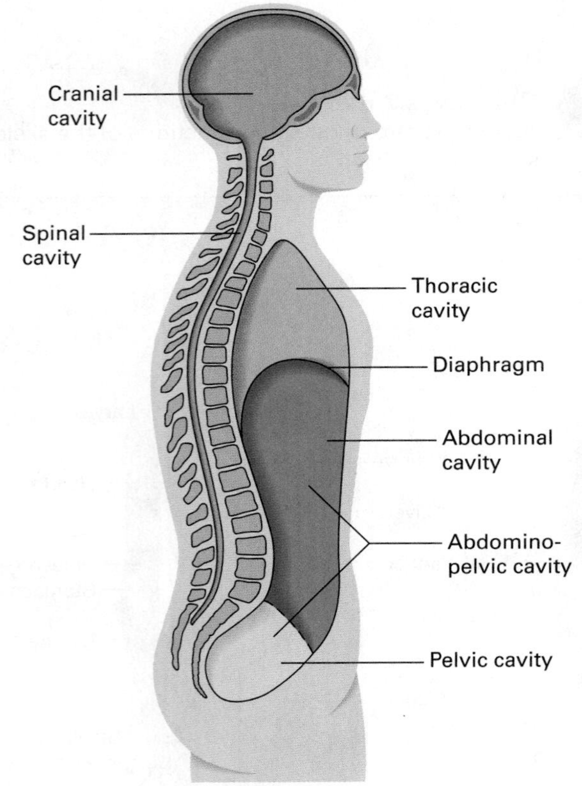

FIGURE 7-9 * Main body cavities.

The Skeletal System

The skeletal system serves four functions:

- Giving the body its shape
- Protecting the vital internal organs
- Allowing for movement
- Storing minerals and producing blood cells

The skeletal system has six basic components: the skull, spinal column, thorax, pelvis, and the upper and lower extremities (Figure 7-11*). The bones of the adult skeleton are classified by size and shape (long, short, flat, or irregular).

The Skull The **skull** rests at the top of the spinal column and houses and protects the brain. It has two parts: the cranium and the face.

The **cranium** forms the top, back, and sides of the skull plus the forehead. The interlocking bones of the cranium—the *occipital,* two *parietal,* two *temporal,* and the *frontal*—are typical flat bones. The outer layer of the cranium is thick and tough. The inner layer is thinner and more brittle. Though this arrangement provides for maximum strength, lightness, and elasticity, the cranium may still be fractured. The brain is commonly lacerated by the bony projections and ridges on the anterior and inferior surfaces of the skull. Impact also can bruise the brain and

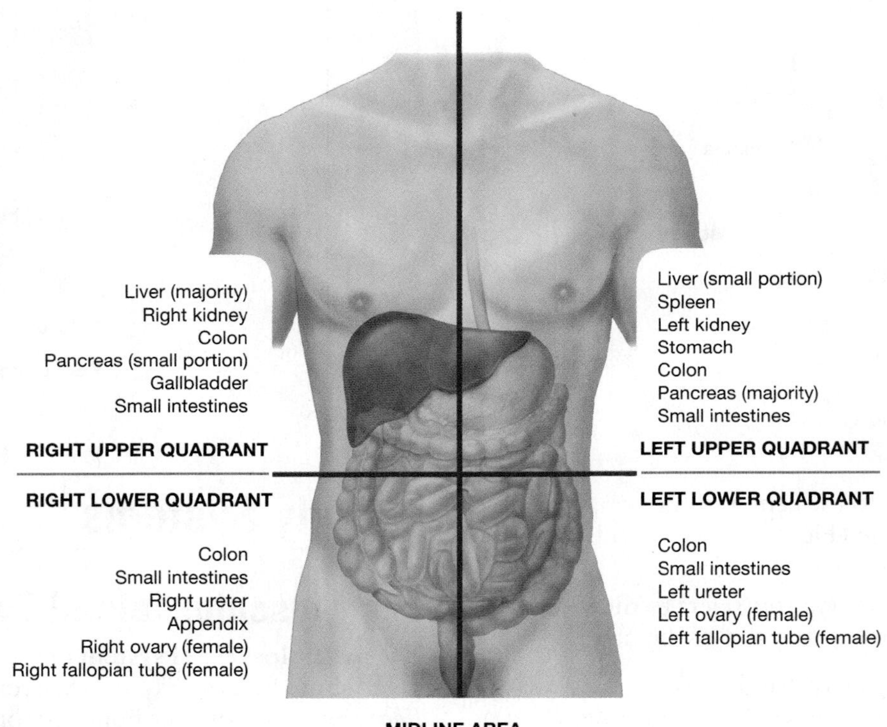

FIGURE 7-10 * The abdominal cavity.

Skeletal System

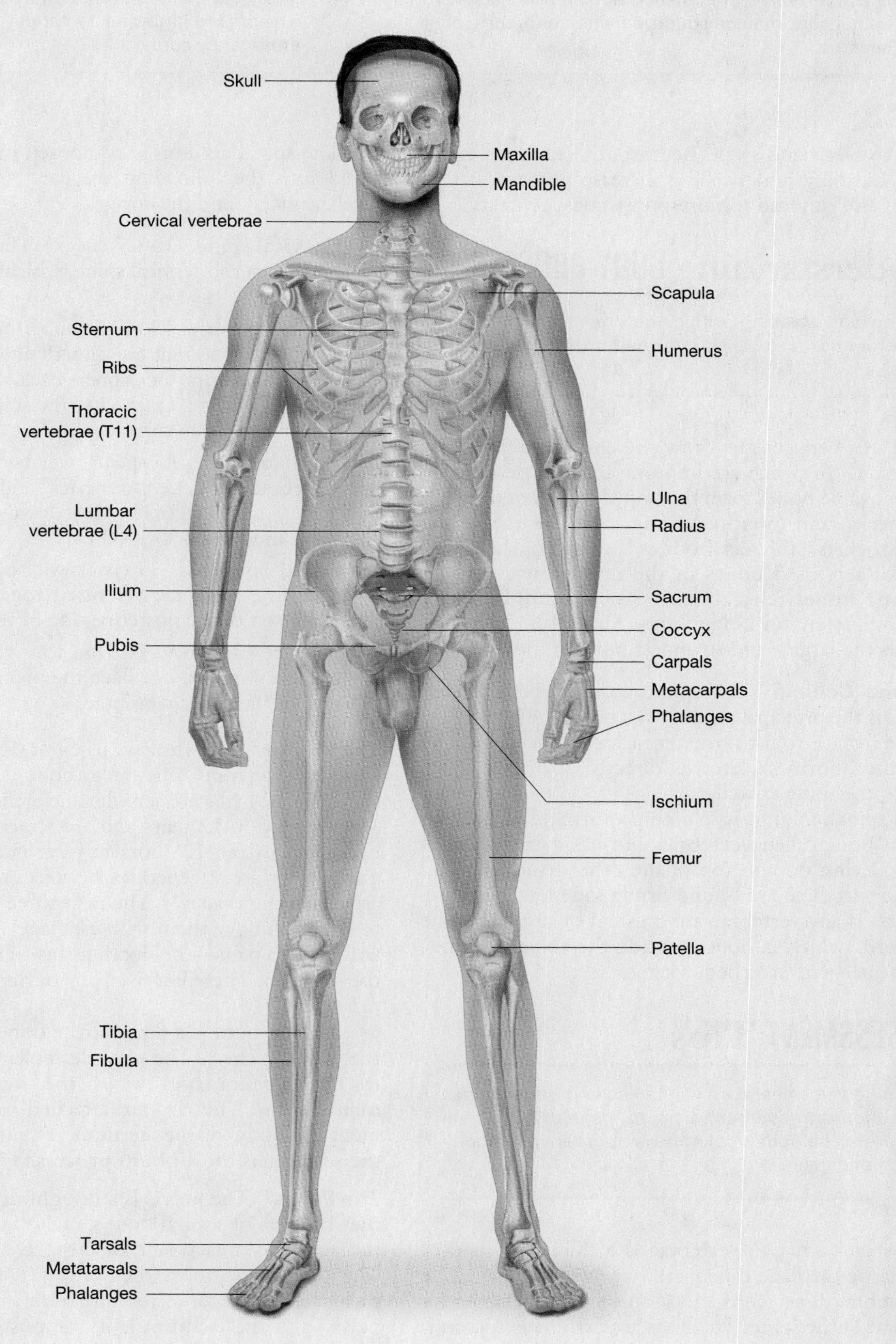

FIGURE 7-11 ✱ The skeletal system.

Key Points
If any vertebrae are crushed or displaced, the spinal cord may be squeezed, stretched, torn, or severed.

Key Points
Knowledge of the human body and its systems is essential to high-quality patient assessment and emergency care.

cause it to bleed and swell. Because the cranium cannot expand, bleeding and swelling increase pressure within the brain and can lead to unresponsiveness or death.

Understanding BODY PROCESSES

Bleeding and swelling within the cranium may compress brain tissue, causing it to malfunction and possibly die. ■

The area between the brow and chin—the **face**—has 14 bones, 13 of which are immovable and interlocking. The immovable bones form the bony settings of the eyes, nose, cheeks, and mouth. Among them are the **orbits** (the eye sockets), the **nasal bones** (the bed of the nose), the **maxillae** (fused bones of the upper jaw), and the **zygomatic bones** (cheekbones). The **mandible** (lower jaw) moves freely on hinge joints. Shaped like a horseshoe, it is the largest and strongest bone of the face.

The Spinal Column The **spinal column**, or **vertebral column**, is the principal support system of the body. Ribs originate from it to form the thoracic (chest) cavity. The rest of the human skeleton is directly or indirectly attached to the spine as well.

The spinal column is made up of irregularly shaped blocks of bone called **vertebrae** and has a great deal of mobility. Lying one on top of the other to form a column, the vertebrae are bound firmly together by strong ligaments. If any vertebrae are crushed or displaced, the spinal cord (which is housed inside the spinal column) may be squeezed, stretched, torn, or severed.

ASSESSMENT Tips

Damage to the spinal cord will typically produce a loss of sensation or movement distal to the injury, whereas an injury to the spinal column (vertebrae) will usually produce only pain. ■

Between each two vertebrae is a fluid-filled pad of tough elastic cartilage called the *intervertebral disk*. The intervertebral disks act as shock absorbers and allow for movement of the spine. The disks are extremely susceptible to injury from twisting, grinding, or improper lifting of heavy objects.

The spinal column is composed of 33 vertebrae divided into the following five parts: cervical, thoracic, lumbar, sacral, and the coccyx.

- **Cervical spine**, C1–C7 (neck). The first seven vertebrae form the cervical spine, which is the most prone to injury.
- **Thoracic spine**, T1–T12 (upper back). The 12 thoracic vertebrae that are directly inferior to the cervical spine form the upper back. The 12 pairs of thoracic ribs are attached to the spine posteriorly and help support the vertebrae.
- **Lumbar spine**, L1–L5 (lower back). The next five vertebrae form the lower back, and are the least mobile of the vertebrae. Most lower-back injuries involve muscles, not vertebrae.
- **Sacral spine**, S1–S5 (back wall of the pelvis). The next five vertebrae are fused together to form the rigid part of the posterior side of the pelvis.
- **Coccyx** (tailbone). The last four vertebrae are fused together and do not have the protrusions characteristic of the other vertebrae.

The Thorax The **thorax**, or chest, is composed of the ribs, the **sternum** (the breastbone), and the thoracic spine. The 24 ribs are semiflexible arches of bone, which are arranged in 12 pairs and are attached posteriorly by ligaments to the 12 thoracic vertebrae. The first seven pairs of ribs are attached to the sternum by cartilage and are called the *true ribs*. The next three pairs are attached to the ribs above them with cartilage. The front ends of the last two pairs—the floating ribs—are not attached to the sternum. These last five pairs of ribs are referred to as *false ribs*.

The sternum is a flat, narrow bone in the middle of the anterior chest. The **clavicle** (collarbone) is attached to the superior portion of the sternum called the **manubrium**. The ribs are attached to the middle segment, or body, of the sternum. The inferior portion of the sternum is the **xiphoid process**.

The Pelvis The **pelvis** is a doughnut-shaped structure that consists of several bones, including the sacrum and the coccyx. At each side of the pelvis is an **iliac crest**. The iliac crests form the "wings" of the pelvis. The **pubis** is in the anterior and inferior portion of the pelvis, and the **ischium** is in the posterior and inferior portion. The pelvis forms the floor of the abdominal cavity. The pelvic cavity supports the intestines and houses the bladder, rectum, and internal reproductive organs.

The Lower Extremities The limbs of the body, the arms and legs, are known as the **extremities**. The legs from the hip to the toes are called the *lower extremities.* On the lateral aspect of each hip is the hip joint. The joint is made up of the pelvic socket, called the **acetabulum**, into which fits the rounded top, or head, of the **femur** (thighbone).

The bottom of the femur is flat with two projections that help to form the hinged knee joint, which like the elbow allows angular movement only. The knee joint is protected and stabilized in front by the **patella** (kneecap), a small, triangular-shaped bone. Because the patella usually receives the force of falls or blows to the knee, it is often bruised and can be fractured.

The two bones of the lower leg are the **tibia** (shin) and the **fibula**. The tibia is the weight-bearing bone located at the anterior and medial side of the leg. Its broad upper surface receives the rounded end of the distal femur to form the knee joint. The much smaller distal end of the tibia forms the medial malleolus of the ankle. The fibula is attached to the tibia at the top and is located at the lateral side of the leg parallel to the tibia.

The bony prominences at the ends of the tibia and fibula form the ankle joint socket. The medial and lateral **malleolus** are the knobby surface landmarks of the ankle joint. A group of bones, including the **calcaneus** (heel bone), are called the **tarsals** and make up the proximal portion of the foot. Five **metatarsals** form the substance of the foot, and 14 **phalanges** on each foot form the toes (two in the big toe and three in each other toe).

The Upper Extremities The upper limbs, including the shoulders, arms, forearms, wrists, and hands, are called the *upper extremities.* Each clavicle (collarbone) and **scapula** (shoulder blade) form a shoulder girdle, the tip of which is called the **acromion**. The powerful muscles of the shoulder girdle help attach the arms to the trunk and extend from it to the arms, thorax, neck, and head.

The proximal portion of the arm is the **humerus**, the largest bone in the upper extremity. Its shaft is roughly cylindrical, its upper end is round, and its lower end is flat. The round head of the humerus fits into a shallow cup in the shoulder blade, forming a ball-and-socket joint that is the most freely movable and easily dislocated joint in the body.

The hinged elbow joint is made up of the distal end of the humerus plus the proximal ends of the **radius** (the lateral bone of the forearm) and the **ulna** (the medial bone of the forearm). The radius is located on the thumb side and the ulna is found on the little-finger side of the forearm. The **olecranon** is a part of the ulna that forms the bony prominence of the elbow. While the ulna can be felt through the skin with your fingertips, the upper two-thirds of the radius cannot because it is sheathed in muscle tissue. Only the lower third of the radius, which enlarges to form most of the wrist joint, can be felt through the skin.

The wrist consists of eight bones called the **carpals**. The structural strength of the hand comes from the **metacarpals**. The bones that make up the fingers and thumbs are the phalanges (three per finger, two per thumb).

The Joints The place where one bone connects to another is called a **joint**. Some joints are immovable (as in the skull), others are slightly movable (as in the spine), and the remaining joints such as the elbow and knee are movable (Figure 7-12*). Movable joints allow changes of position and motion as follows:

- **Flexion.** Bending toward the body or decreasing the angle between the bones or parts of the body
- **Extension.** Straightening away from the body or increasing the angle between the bones or parts of the body
- **Abduction.** Movement away from the midline
- **Adduction.** Movement toward the midline
- **Circumduction.** A combination of the four preceding motions as is possible with the shoulder joint

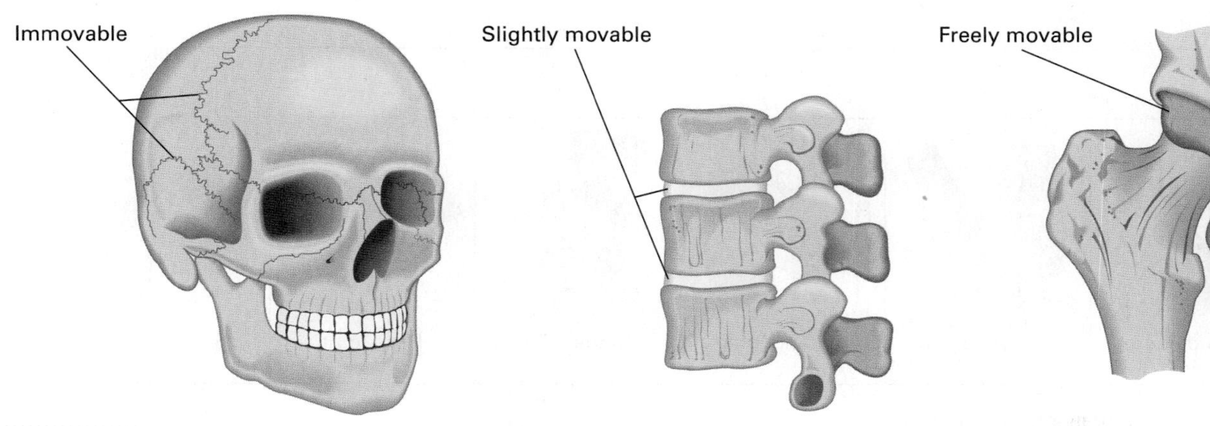

FIGURE 7-12 * Three types of joints.

- **Pronation.** Turning the forearm so the palm of the hand is turned toward the back
- **Supination.** Turning the forearm so the palm of the hand is turned toward the front

The structure of the joint determines the kind of movement that is possible. Types of joints include the following, the most common of which are the ball-and-socket joint and hinged joint (Figure 7-13*):

- **Ball-and-socket joint.** This type of joint permits the widest range of motion—flexion, extension, abduction, adduction, and rotation. Examples: joints at the shoulder and hip.
- **Hinged joint.** Hinged joints (such as those in the elbow, knee, and finger) permit flexion and extension. Elbow joints have forward movement (the anterior bone surfaces approach each other), while knee joints have backward movement (the posterior bone surfaces approach each other).
- **Pivot joint.** This type of joint allows for a turning motion, and includes the joints between the head and neck at the first and second cervical vertebrae and those in the wrist.
- **Gliding joint.** The simplest movement between bones occurs in a gliding joint, where one bone slides across another to the point where surrounding structures restrict the motion. Gliding joints connect the small bones in the hands and the feet.
- **Saddle joint.** This joint is shaped to permit combinations of limited movements along perpendicular planes. For example, the ankle allows the foot to turn inward slightly as it moves up and down.
- **Condyloid joint.** This is a modified ball-and-socket joint that permits limited motion in two directions. In the wrist, for example, it allows the hand to move up and down and side to side, but not to rotate completely.

Bone Injury

A fracture is a loss of continuity in the structure of a bone. When a fracture to a bone occurs, the sharp fragments may injure surrounding tissue, such as nerves, vessels, and connective tissue. However, it is important to note that bones are also living tissue and have a rich blood supply. If a bone is fractured, the vessels within the bone may be torn or ruptured (Figure 7-14*). This sometimes leads to severe bleeding from the bone itself rather than from the surrounding vessels or tissue. A patient can lose from 1,000 to 2,000 mL of blood from a fractured femur. A bleeding pelvic fracture may cause the

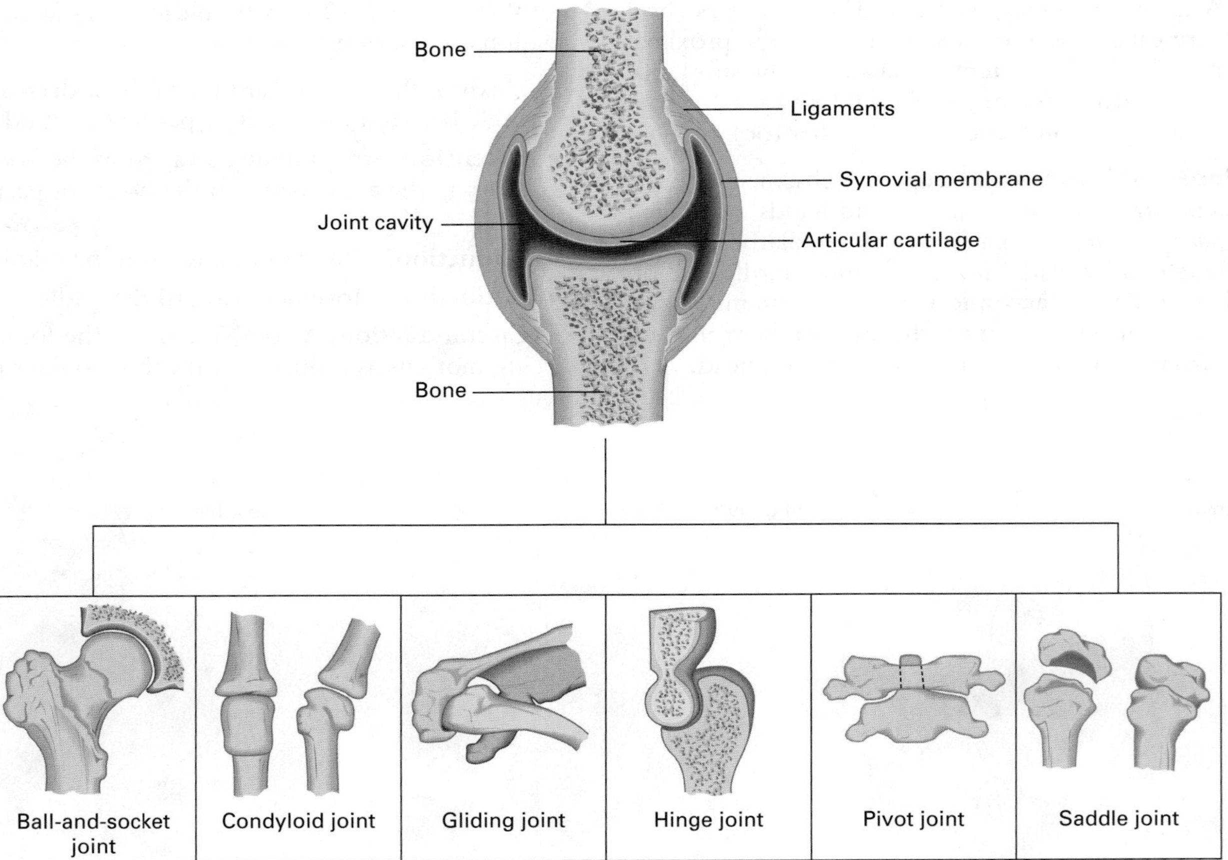

FIGURE 7-13 * Types of freely movable joints.

Key Points
Muscle tissue is enabled to work by its ability to contract when stimulated by a nerve impulse.

Objective 7-10
Differentiate between skeletal (voluntary), smooth (involuntary), and cardiac muscle.

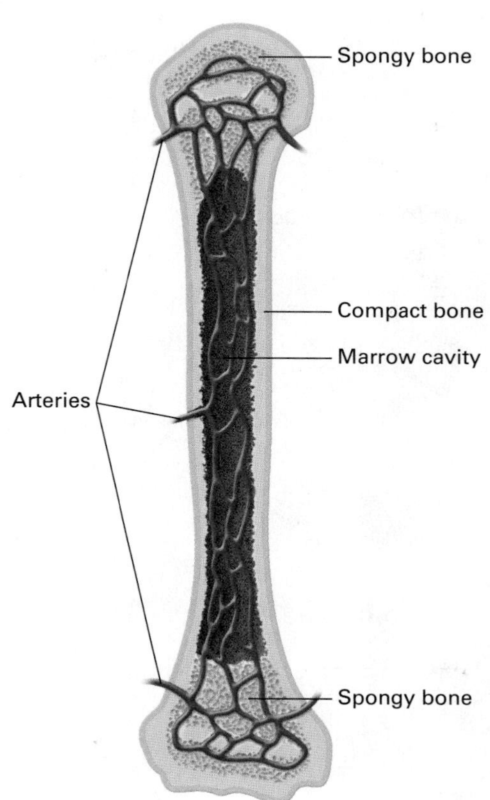

FIGURE 7-14 ✻ Bones have both arteries and veins, though only arteries are shown here. The vessels enter and exit through openings in the compact outer bone layers. They branch and extend throughout the marrow cavity and into the spongy bone at the ends. Because they are so richly supplied with blood vessels, bones can bleed profusely when fractured.

loss of up to 2,000 mL of blood into the pelvic cavity. Thus, when assessing a patient who has suffered a bone fracture, look for signs and symptoms of bleeding at the fracture site. Also, if the bleeding is severe, be aware that it may produce a shock state.

The Muscular System

Movement of the body is due to work performed by the muscles (Figure 7-15✻). What enables muscle tissue to work is its ability to contract (to become shorter and thicker) when stimulated by a nerve impulse. The cells of a muscle are called *fibers,* because they are usually long and threadlike. Each muscle has countless bundles of closely packed, overlapping fibers bound together by connective tissue.

Muscles can be injured in many ways. Overexerting a muscle may tear fibers, and muscles subjected to trauma can be bruised, crushed, cut, torn, or otherwise injured, even if the skin is not broken. Muscles injured in any way tend to become swollen, tender, painful, or weak.

There are three kinds of muscle: skeletal (voluntary), smooth (involuntary), and cardiac muscle (Figure 7-16✻).

Skeletal Muscle Under the control of the brain and nervous system, **skeletal muscle**, or **voluntary muscle**, can be contracted and relaxed by will of the individual. This type of muscle makes possible all deliberate movement, such as walking, chewing, swallowing, smiling, frowning, talking, or moving the eyeballs. It forms the major muscle mass of the body, helps to shape it, and forms its walls.

Skeletal muscle is generally attached at one or both ends to bone by tendons. A few are attached to skin, cartilage, organs (such as the eyeball), or other muscles (such as the tongue). In the trunk, skeletal muscles are broad, flat, and expanded to help form the walls of the cavities they enclose—the abdomen and the chest. In the extremities, the skeletal muscles are long and more rounded, somewhat resembling spindles.

Smooth Muscle **Smooth muscle**, or **involuntary muscle**, is made up of large fibers that carry out the automatic muscular functions of the body through rhythmic, wavelike movements. For example, smooth muscles move blood through the veins, bile from the gallbladder, and food through the digestive tract. The individual has no direct control over this type of muscle, though it responds to stimuli such as stretching, heat, and cold.

Smooth muscle is found in the walls of tubelike organs, ducts, the respiratory tract, and blood vessels and forms much of the walls of the intestines and urinary system. Vasoconstriction, decreasing the diameter of the vessel, and vasodilation, increasing the diameter of the vessel, are controlled by smooth muscle within the vessels (Figure 7-17✻). Vasoconstriction increases the resistance inside the vessel, making it harder for the blood to pass through, and results in an increase in pressure. Conversely, vasodilation results in a decrease in the resistance inside the vessel, making it easier for the blood to flow through, and decreasing the pressure.

Cardiac Muscle Found only in the walls of the heart, **cardiac muscle** is a special kind of involuntary muscle particularly suited for the work of the heart. It has the

Muscular System

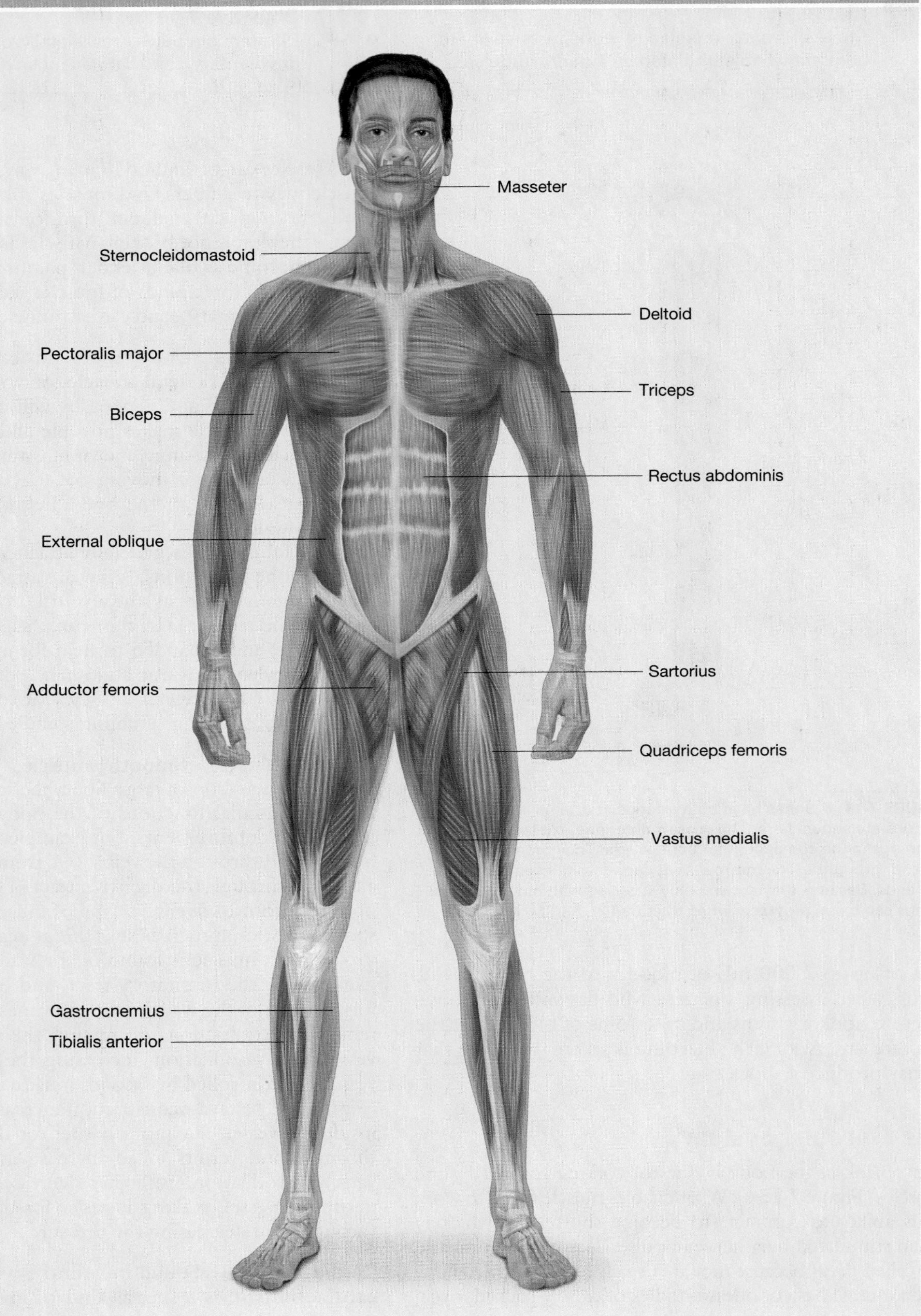

FIGURE 7-15 ✱ The muscular system.

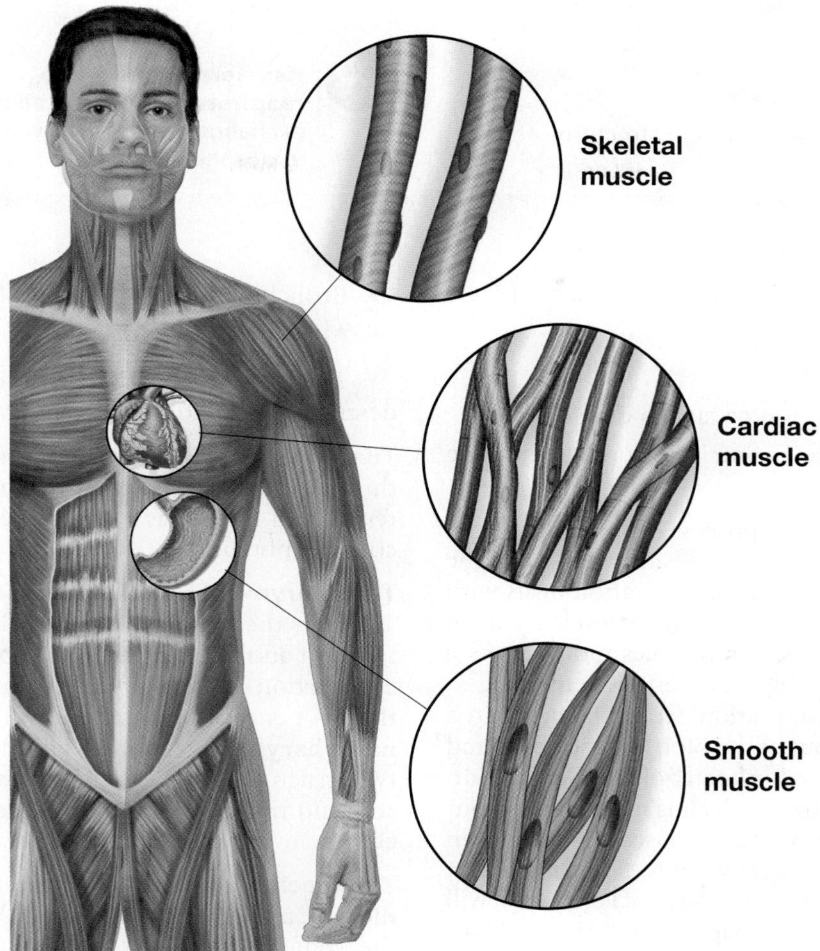

FIGURE 7-16 ✱ Three types of muscle.

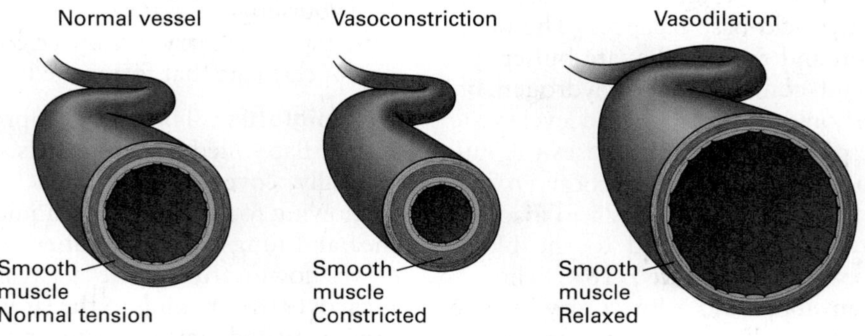

FIGURE 7-17 ✱ Smooth muscle is capable of vasoconstriction or vasodilation.

property of *automaticity*. That is, it has the ability to generate an impulse on its own, even when disconnected from the central nervous system.

Although it is smooth like smooth muscle but striated (stringlike) like skeletal muscle, cardiac muscle is made up of a cellular meshwork that is unlike either smooth or skeletal muscle. It has its own blood supply, furnished by the coronary artery system, and cannot tolerate interruption of the blood supply for even very short periods.

The Respiratory System

Basic Functions and Structures

The body can store food for weeks and water for days, but it can store enough oxygen to last only a few minutes. Simple inhalation normally provides the body with the oxygen it needs. However, if the oxygen supply is cut off, as in a drowning or choking patient, brain cells will ordinarily begin to die in about 5 minutes.

Objectives 7-11 and 7-12
Identify the basic functions and structures of the respiratory system.

Key Terms
respiratory system the organs involved in the exchange of gases between an organism and the atmosphere.

The basic functions of the respiratory system are:

- Respiration
- Ventilation
- Oxygenation and removal of carbon dioxide
- Serving as a buffer to maintain a normal acid-base balance

Respiration refers to the process of moving oxygen and carbon dioxide across membranes, in and out of the alveoli, capillaries, and cells. Thus, respiration deals with the actual gas exchange process. **Oxygenation** is the form of respiration in which oxygen molecules move across a membrane from an area of high oxygen concentration to an area of low oxygen concentration. Cells are oxygenated when the oxygen moves out of the blood in the vessel and into the cell where it is used in metabolism. **Ventilation** is the mechanical process by which air is moved in and out of the lungs. Ventilation is primarily based on changes in pressure inside the chest that cause air to flow into or out of the lungs. The mechanics and control of ventilation will be covered in more detail in Chapter 10, "Airway Management, Artificial Ventilation, and Oxygenation."

The body also relies on the respiratory system to assist in regulating the balance of acid and base elements in the body. Respiration is one of three mechanisms by which the body regulates acid-base balance. (The other two are kidney function and the bicarbonate buffer system, which works through combinations of hydrogen, bicarbonate ions, and carbonic acid.) As the acid level in the body increases, the respiratory system increases the rate and depth of respirations to exhale excess carbon dioxide, which in turn works to decrease the body's acid load.

Oxygen from the air is transported to the blood through the **respiratory system** (Figure 7-18*). The airway is separated into an upper and a lower airway. The upper airway consists of the following structures:

- Nose and mouth
- Pharynx
- Nasopharynx
- Larynx

The upper airway ends at the level of the cricoid cartilage, the ring that forms the most inferior portion of the larynx. The lower airway is composed of the following structures:

- Trachea
- Bronchi
- Bronchioles
- Alveoli

The major components of the respiratory system are described in the following paragraphs.

The Nose and Mouth Air normally enters the body through the nose and mouth. There it is warmed, moistened, and filtered as it flows over the damp, sticky mucous membranes.

The Pharynx From the back of the nose or mouth, the air enters the **pharynx** (throat), the common passageway for food and air. Air from the mouth enters through the oral portion of the pharynx, or the **oropharynx**. Air from the nose enters the nasal portion of the pharynx, or the **nasopharynx**. At its lower end the pharynx divides into two structures—the **esophagus**, which leads to the stomach, and the **trachea**, which leads to the lungs. The trachea is anterior to the esophagus.

The Trachea and Larynx The trachea carries air from the nose and mouth to the lungs. Immediately superior to the trachea is the **larynx**, which houses the vocal cords and is commonly called the "voice box." The "Adam's apple" or **thyroid cartilage** is the anterior cartilage that covers the larynx. The larynx can be easily felt through the skin with your fingertips at the front of the neck. The most inferior part of the larynx is the **cricoid cartilage**, a firm, full ring of cartilage that forms the lower edge of the larynx.

The Epiglottis The trachea is protected by a small, leaf-shaped flap called the **epiglottis**. Usually, this flap automatically covers the entrance of the larynx during swallowing to keep food and liquid from entering the trachea and lungs. When a patient swallows, the epiglottis moves downward and the larynx moves upward, creating a seal over the opening to the larynx. However, during an altered mental status or unresponsiveness, reflexes may not work properly. If liquid, blood, vomit, or another substance is in the mouth of an unresponsive patient, it may be aspirated into the trachea and lungs and cause impaired exchange of oxygen and carbon dioxide.

The Bronchi The distal portion of the trachea branches into two main tubes, or **bronchi**, one branching off to each lung. Each bronchus divides and subdivides into smaller **bronchioles**, somewhat like the branches of a tree. The bronchioles are lined with smooth muscle and have the ability to constrict (bronchoconstriction) or dilate (bronchodilation) to certain stimuli. If bronchoconstriction occurs, the smooth muscle contracts, decreasing the diameter

Respiratory System

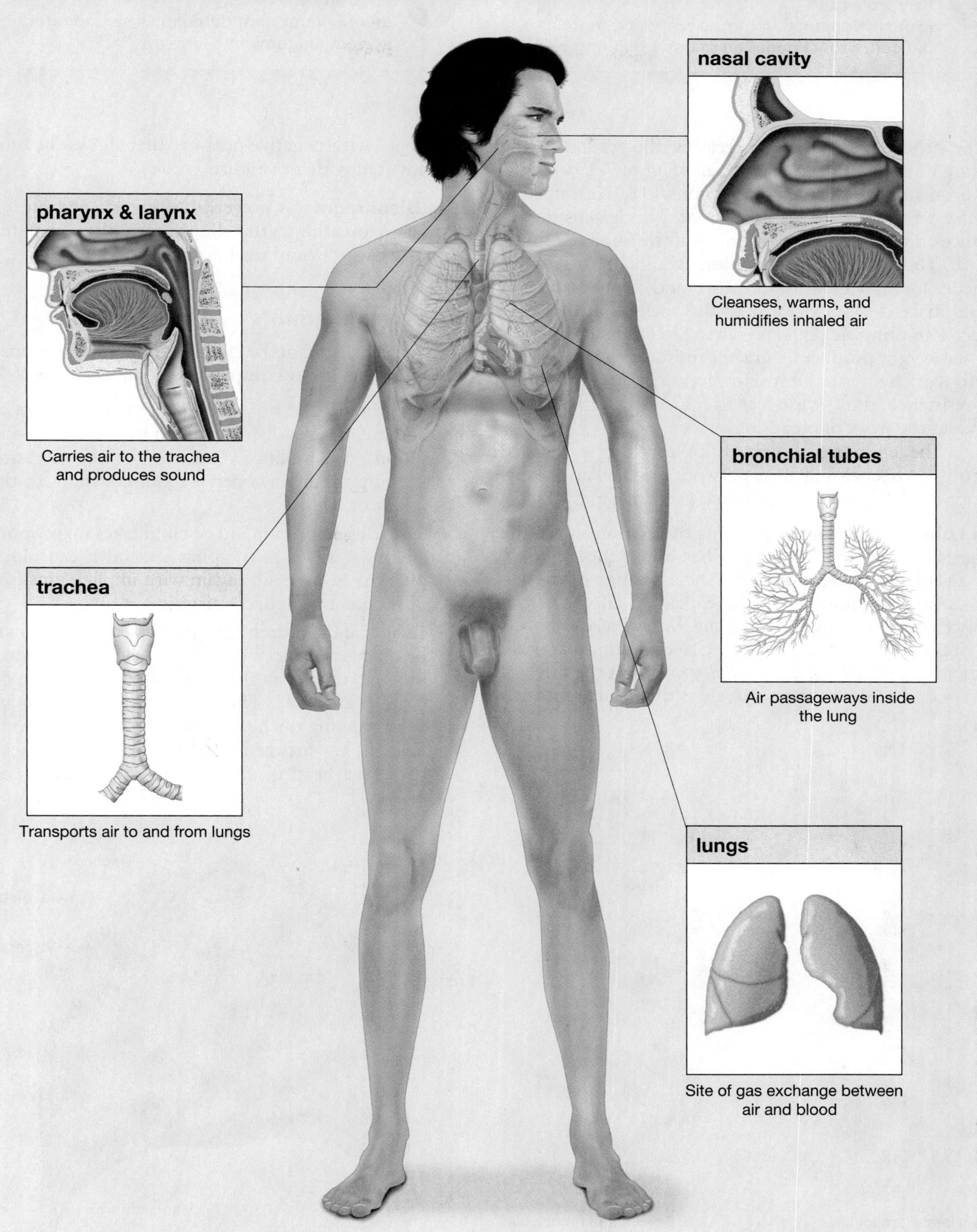

FIGURE 7-18 ✱ The respiratory system.

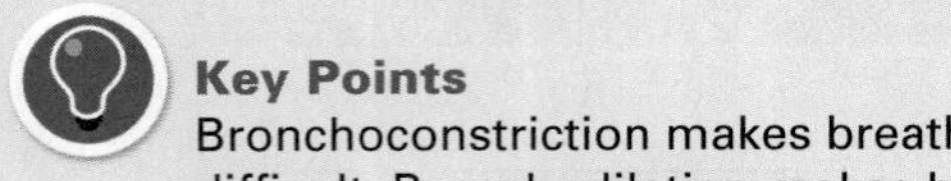

Key Points
Bronchoconstriction makes breathing more difficult. Bronchodilation makes breathing easier.

Objective 7-13
Identify important differences in respiratory system anatomy in children.

of the bronchiole, thereby increasing the resistance and making it more difficult to move air (Figure 7-19∗). During bronchodilation, the smooth muscle relaxes, making the diameter of the bronchiole larger. This lessens the resistance and makes it easier to move air through the bronchiole. Thus, bronchoconstriction would make it more difficult for a patient to breathe, and bronchodilation would make it easier because of the changes in the resistance. This principle could be related to lifting a weight. A heavier weight produces a greater resistance and a muscle has to work harder to lift it. However, a lighter weight has less resistance, thus, it is easier to lift. A greater resistance increases the work of breathing.

At the ends are thousands of tiny air sacs called **alveoli**, each enclosed in a network of capillaries (tiny blood vessels). This is the site of gas exchange in the lungs.

The Lungs The principal organs of respiration are the **lungs**, two large, lobed organs that house thousands of tiny alveolar sacs responsible for the exchange of oxygen and carbon dioxide (as will be explained later). A thin layer of connective tissue called the *visceral pleura* covers the outer surface of the lungs. A layer of thicker, more elastic tissue called the *parietal pleura* covers the internal chest wall. Between the two layers is the *pleural cavity,* a tiny space with negative pressure that allows the lungs to stay inflated with air (Figure 7-20∗).

The Diaphragm A powerful, dome-shaped muscle essential to breathing, the **diaphragm** also separates the thoracic cavity from the abdominal cavity.

Anatomy in Infants and Children

When treating infants or children, remember the anatomical differences in the respiratory system (Figure 7-21∗):

- The mouth and nose are smaller than those of adults and are more easily obstructed by even small objects, blood, or swelling. Therefore, extra attention to keeping the airway open is required when treating an infant or child.
- The tongue of an infant or child takes up proportionally more space in the pharynx and it can block the pharynx more easily, again with implications for care of the infant or child's airway.
- Infants and children have narrower tracheas that may be obstructed more easily by swelling or foreign bodies. The trachea is also softer and more flexible than that of an adult. Therefore, hyperextension of the head (tipping the head back), or flexion (allowing the head to tip forward), can occlude the trachea. Because the head of an infant or young child is quite

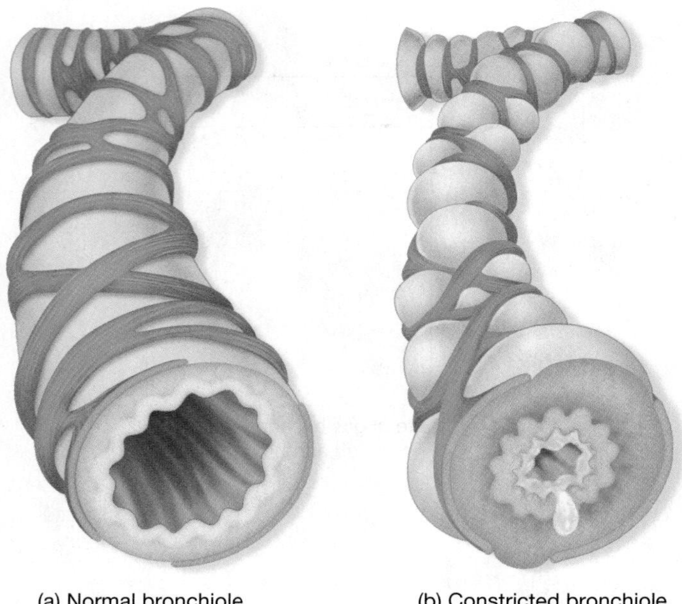

FIGURE 7-19 ∗ **(a)** A normal bronchiole. **(b)** A constricted bronchiole.

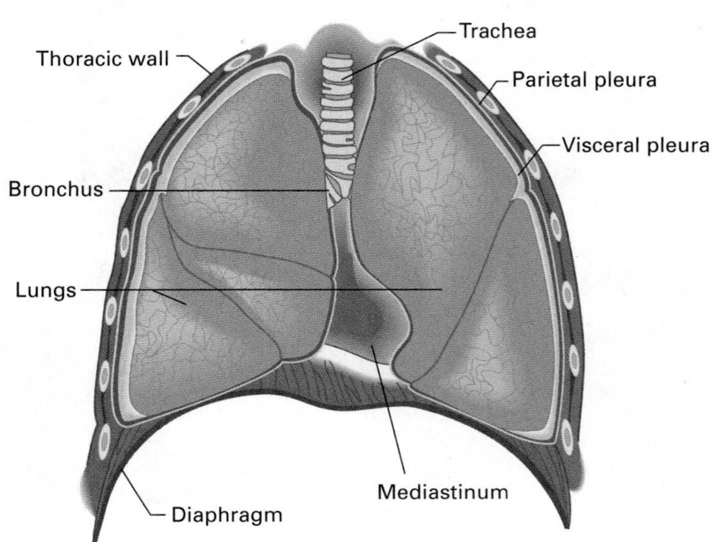

FIGURE 7-20 ∗ The pleural lining of the lung.

Key Points
Children's airway and chest structures are smaller, softer, and less rigid than adults'.

Objective 7-14
Describe the basic mechanics and physiology of normal ventilation, respiration, and oxygenation.

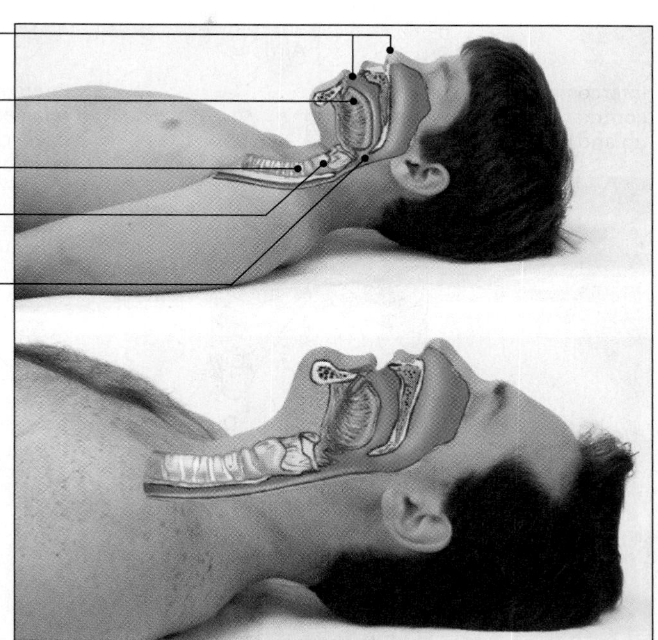

Child has smaller nose and mouth.
In child, more space is taken up by tongue.
Child's trachea is narrower.
Cricoid cartilage is less rigid and less developed.
Airway structures are more easily obstructed.

FIGURE 7-21 ✱ Comparison of child and adult respiratory systems.

large relative to the body, it is necessary to place a folded towel or similar item about one inch thick under the shoulders to keep the trachea aligned and open ("sniffing" position).

- The cricoid cartilage is less developed and much less rigid. Therefore, the maneuver of pressing on the cricoid cartilage to help in placing a tube into the trachea, often used on adults, is not appropriate for an infant or child, since it can depress the soft cartilage and result in obstruction.
- Because the chest wall is softer, infants and children rely more heavily on the diaphragm for breathing. Excessive movement of the diaphragm is a sign of respiratory distress in an infant or child, evidenced by increased movement of the abdominal wall.

ASSESSMENT Tips

The immature respiratory chest muscles of the infant and young child often mean they need to use their abdominal muscles more during breathing; thus, you would expect to see more exaggerated abdominal movement during normal breathing. ■

Mechanics of Ventilation

During inhalation the diaphragm and the **intercostal muscles** (the muscles between the ribs) contract, increasing the size of the thoracic cavity. The diaphragm moves slightly downward, flaring the lower portion of the rib cage, which moves upward and outward. This creates a negative pressure in the chest, which causes air to flow into the lungs. During exhalation the diaphragm and intercostal muscles relax, decreasing the size of the thoracic cavity. The diaphragm moves upward; the ribs move downward and inward, creating a positive pressure within the thorax and causing air to flow out of the lungs (Figure 7-22✱). The diaphragm contributes about 60–70 percent of the effort to breathe, whereas the intercostal muscles contribute the remaining 30–40 percent. Thus, a significant injury that prevents the diaphragm from functioning properly will cause the patient's breathing to become ineffective.

The diaphragm receives its stimulation to contract from the phrenic nerve that exits the spinal cord at the cervical spine between vertebrae C3 and C5. If a spinal cord injury occurs at C3 to C5, the phrenic nerve may be damaged and the diaphragm will not receive a nervous impulse to contract, no longer allowing it to contribute to ventilation. The intercostal muscles will also not work

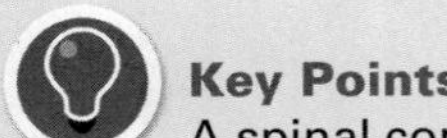

Key Points
A spinal cord injury high in the cervical vertebrae destroys innervation of the muscles of respiration. The patient cannot breathe spontaneously and requires artificial ventilation.

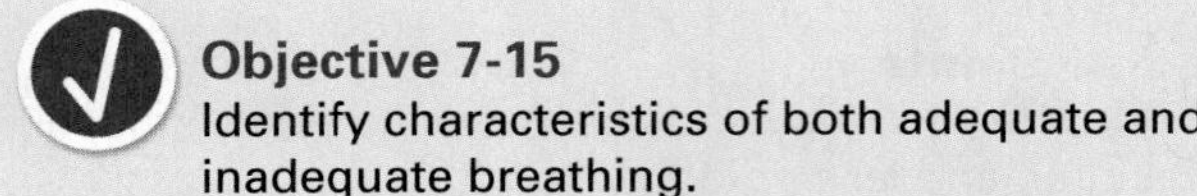

Objective 7-15
Identify characteristics of both adequate and inadequate breathing.

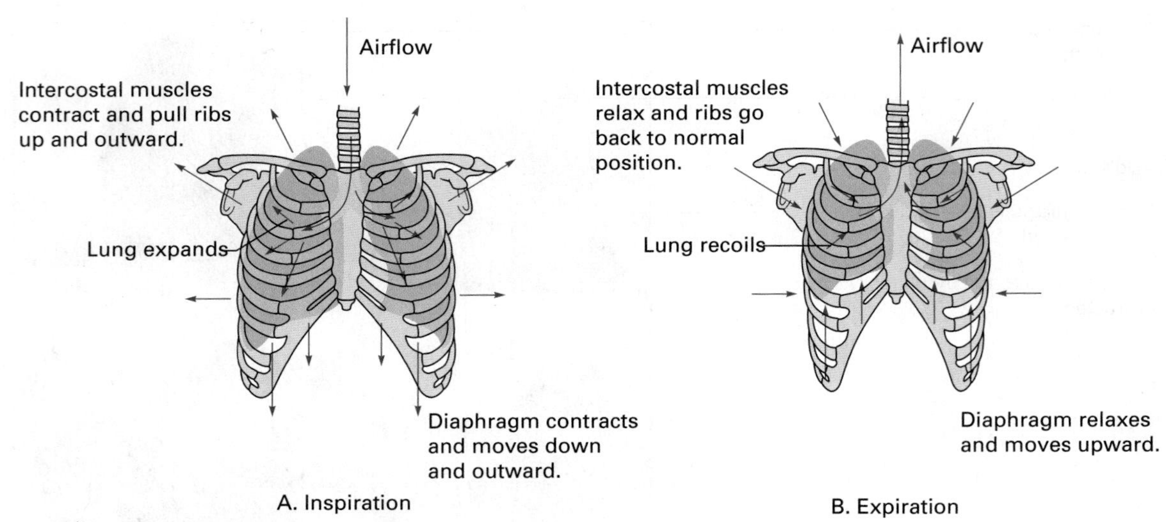

FIGURE 7-22 ✱ Mechanics of respiration.

properly because the nerves that stimulate these muscles exit from the lower thoracic vertebrae. With an injury to the spinal cord high in the cervical vertebrae, the patient would not be able to breathe spontaneously and would require artificial ventilation.

Understanding BODY PROCESSES

The phrenic nerve, which exits the spinal column between the third and fifth cervical vertebrae, transmits the electrical impulses that cause the diaphragm to contract. ■

Physiology of Respiration

In the lungs, oxygen and carbon dioxide are exchanged through the thin walls of the alveoli and the capillaries (Figures 7-23✱ and 7-24✱). In alveolar/capillary exchange, oxygen-rich air enters the alveoli during each inspiration and passes through the capillary walls into the bloodstream. Carbon dioxide and other waste gases move from the blood through the capillary walls into the alveoli and are exhaled. In capillary/cellular exchange throughout the body, carbon dioxide moves from the cells to the capillaries, and oxygen moves from the capillaries to the cells.

Adequate and Inadequate Breathing

Adequate breathing is characterized by an adequate respiratory rate and tidal volume. Respiratory rate is the number of breaths a patient takes in one minute. Tidal volume (V_T) is the amount of air the patient breathes in and out with one regular breath. There is a wide variety of normal ranges of respiratory rates. In adults, the normal range is 8 to 24 breaths per minute, with the average between 12 and 20 breaths per minute. Elderly patients have higher resting respiratory rates that average 20 to 22 per minute. A normal range for children is typically 15 to 30 breaths per minute. Infants typically breathe 25 to 50 breaths per minute. As the infant or child ages, his respiratory rate will decrease. The respirations should be regular in rhythm and free of unusual sounds, such as wheezing. The chest should expand outward and equally with each breath, indicating an adequate depth (tidal volume). The chest wall of an average-sized adult will move outward about 1 inch with each inhalation. Breathing should be virtually effortless (accomplished without the use of accessory muscles of the neck, chest, or abdomen).

Inadequate breathing may be characterized by:

- Rates that are either too slow or too fast as compared to what is normal for the patient
- Irregular pattern of breathing resulting from an illness or injury

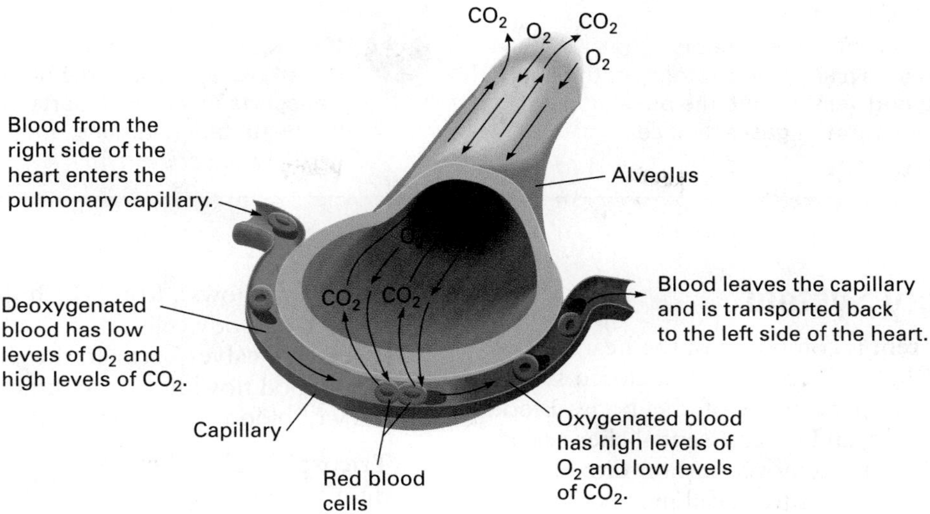

FIGURE 7-23 ✻ Alveolar/capillary gas exchange.

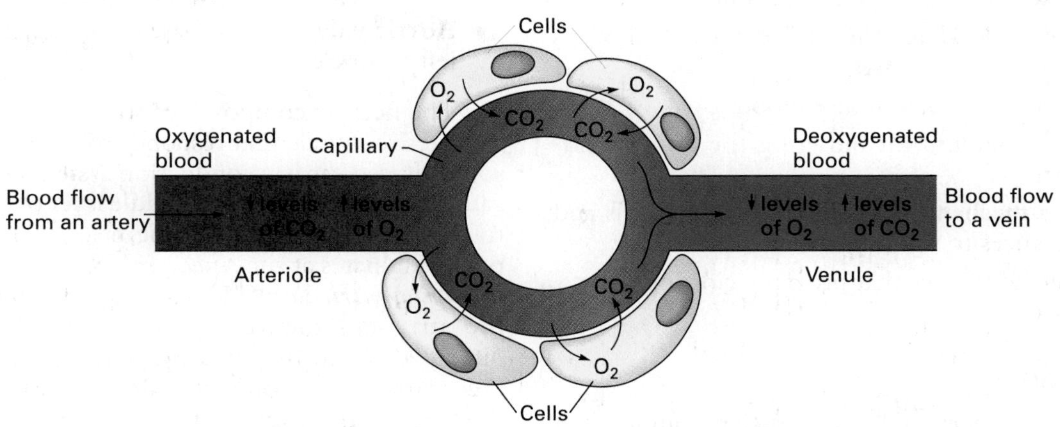

FIGURE 7-24 ✻ Capillary/cell gas exchange.

- Diminished or absent breath sounds, indicating an inadequate volume of air being breathed in and out
- Unequal chest expansion, indicating a chest wall injury that could reduce the tidal volume
- Inadequate chest expansion, indicating a poor volume of air being breathed in (referred to as shallow breathing)
- Pale or bluish mucous membranes or skin that may also be cool and clammy, indicating poor oxygen exchange (respiration and oxygenation)
- Use of accessory muscles, identified by retractions above the clavicles, between the ribs, and below the rib cage and use of the muscles in the neck during breathing, especially among infants and children, indicating an increased work effort to breathe
- Nasal flaring, especially in children, indicating an increased work effort to breathe
- "Seesaw" breathing in infants (the chest and abdomen move in opposite directions)
- Head bobbing, where the head bobs upward on inhalation and downward toward the chest on exhalation, indicating severe respiratory fatigue
- *Agonal respirations* (occasional gasping breaths) that may be seen just before death
- Grunting, especially in newborns, heard at the end of inspiration or the beginning of exhalation

For the breathing to be considered adequate, both rate and tidal volume must be adequate. If *either* rate *or* tidal volume is inadequate, the breathing is considered inadequate, and immediate ventilation is necessary.

Objectives 7-16 to 7-18
List the functions of the circulatory (cardiovascular) system, the anatomy of the heart, blood, and blood vessels, and the physiology of circulation, transport of gases, and cell metabolism.

Key Terms
circulatory system the body system that transports blood to all parts of the body. Includes the heart, blood vessels, and blood. Also called the *cardiovascular system.*

The Circulatory System

The **circulatory system** is composed of the heart, blood vessels, and blood (Figure 7-25a∗). It is a closed system that transports blood to all parts of the body. Blood brings oxygen, nutrients, and other essential chemical elements to tissue cells, and removes carbon dioxide and other waste products resulting from cell metabolism.

The circulatory system has several functions:

- Providing a medium for perfusion of cells with oxygen and other nutrients and removal from the cells of carbon dioxide and other waste products
- Transporting blood to cells and the alveoli for gas exchange
- Serving as a reservoir to house blood
- Serving as a medium for buffering the body's acid-base balance
- Providing a mechanism to deliver immune cells and other substances to fight infection
- Containing substances that promote clotting

Basic Anatomy

The Heart The **heart**, a highly efficient pump, is a chambered muscular organ that lies within the chest in the thoracic cavity between the two lungs. In size and shape, it resembles a closed fist. About two-thirds of its mass is located to the left of the midline of the body. Its lower point, the apex, lies just above the diaphragm.

The *pericardium* is a double-walled sac that encloses the heart, gives support, and prevents friction as the heart moves within this protective sac. The surfaces of the pericardial sac produce a small amount of fluid lubrication needed to facilitate the normal movements of the heart.

The heart has four chambers. (The flow of blood to and from the lungs and the body and through the four chambers is shown in Figure 7-25b∗.) The upper chambers, called the **atria**, receive blood from the veins. The right atrium receives oxygen-depleted blood from the veins of the body. The left atrium receives oxygen-rich blood from the pulmonary veins from the lungs.

The lower chambers are called **ventricles**. They pump blood out to the arteries. The right ventricle pumps oxygen-depleted blood to the pulmonary arteries, which transport the blood to the lungs where it will be oxygenated. The left ventricle pumps oxygen-rich blood to the major artery from the heart, the aorta (see the description that follows), from which the blood is gradually delivered to all body cells.

A series of **valves** between the chambers of the heart keep the blood flowing in one direction and prevent the backflow of blood. The four valves are:

- **Tricuspid valve.** Between the right atrium and the right ventricle
- **Pulmonary valve.** At the base of the pulmonary artery in the right ventricle
- **Mitral valve, also known as the bicuspid valve.** Between the left atrium and the left ventricle
- **Aortic valve.** At the base of the aortic artery in the left ventricle

The heart is composed of specialized contractile and conductive muscle that responds to electrical impulses. A sophisticated cardiac conduction system (Figure 7-25c∗) causes the *myocardium,* or middle layer of muscle, to contract and eject blood from the heart. The electrical impulse originates at the *sinoatrial (SA) node* and travels to the *atrioventricular (AV) node,* which is located between the atria and the ventricles, and finally through the *bundle of His* to the *Purkinje fibers* to the ventricles. As the heart muscle contracts, blood is propelled through the pulmonary arteries and to the lungs and into the aorta. From the aorta, it is eventually circulated throughout the body.

The Arteries An **artery** carries blood away from the heart (Figure 7-26a∗). All arteries except the pulmonary arteries carry oxygen-rich blood. The major arteries include the following:

- **Aorta**—The major artery from the heart, the aorta, lies in front of the spine and passes through the thoracic and abdominal cavities. At about the level of the navel, the aorta divides into the iliac arteries, allowing blood to travel down each leg. The aorta and its branches supply all other arteries with blood.
- **Coronary arteries**—The coronary arteries are the vessels that supply the heart itself with blood (Figure 7-25d∗).
- **Carotid arteries**—The carotid arteries (one on each side of the neck) supply the brain and head with blood. Pulsations of the carotid arteries can be felt on either side of the neck.
- **Femoral arteries**—The femoral artery is the major artery of the thigh and supplies the groin and leg

Cardiovascular System

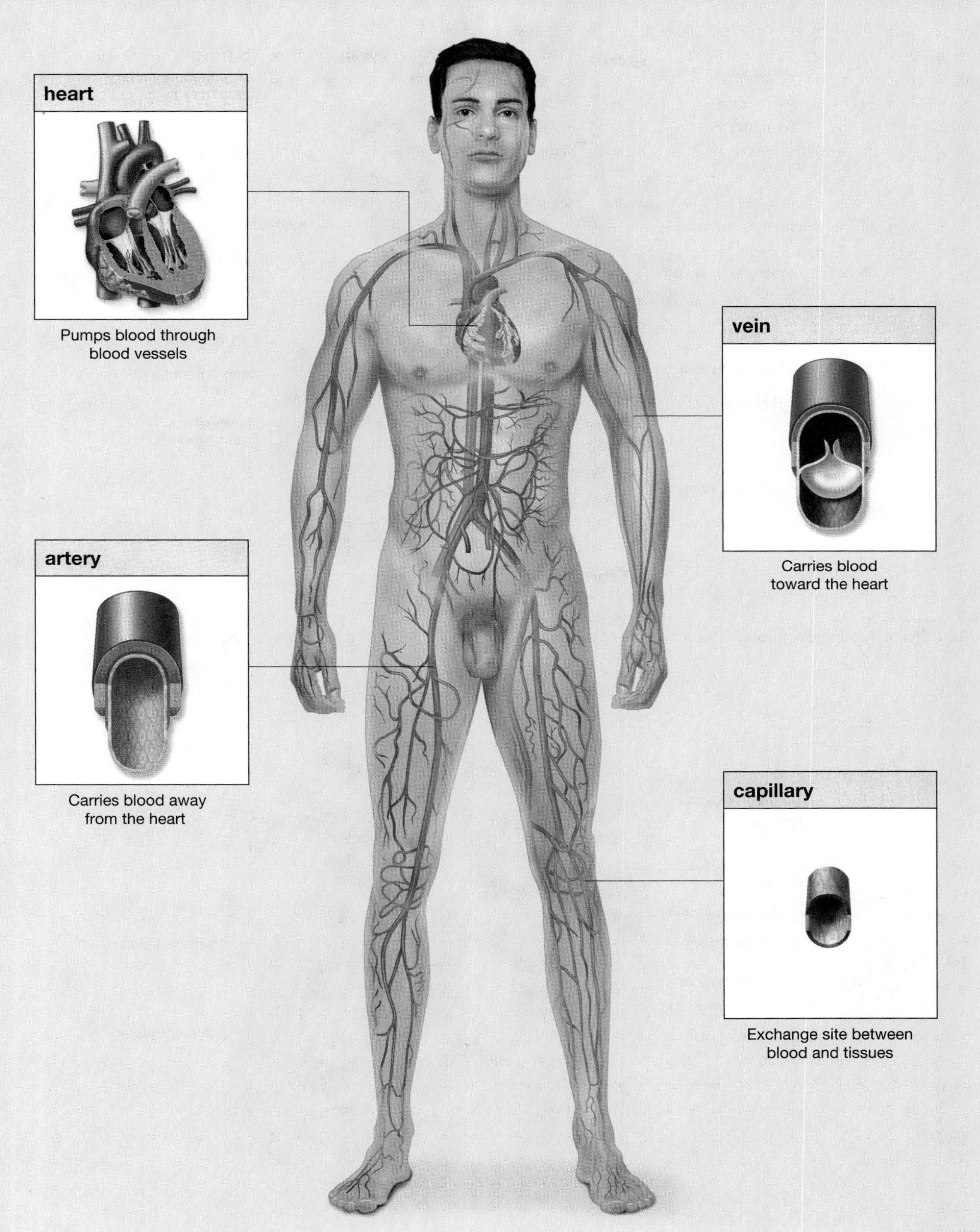

FIGURE 7-25a ✱ The circulatory system. (Red indicates arteries; blue indicates veins.)

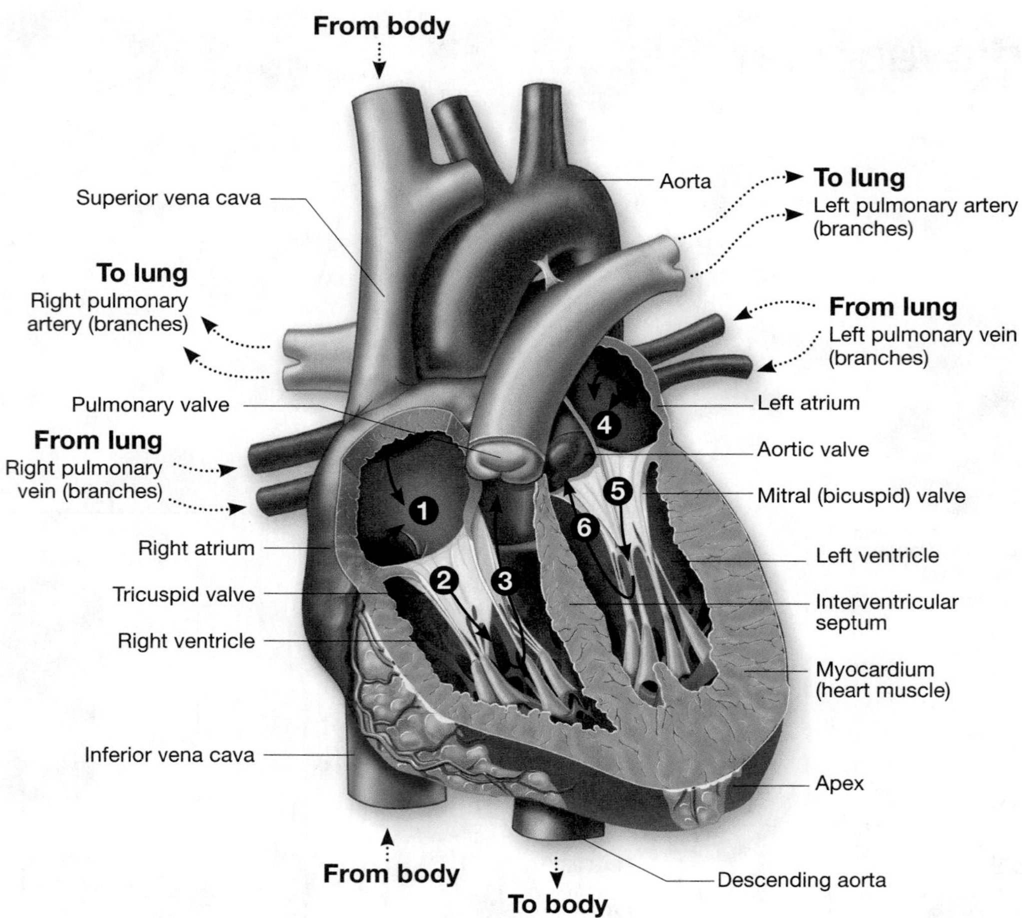

FIGURE 7-25b ✱ Blood flow through the chambers of the heart.

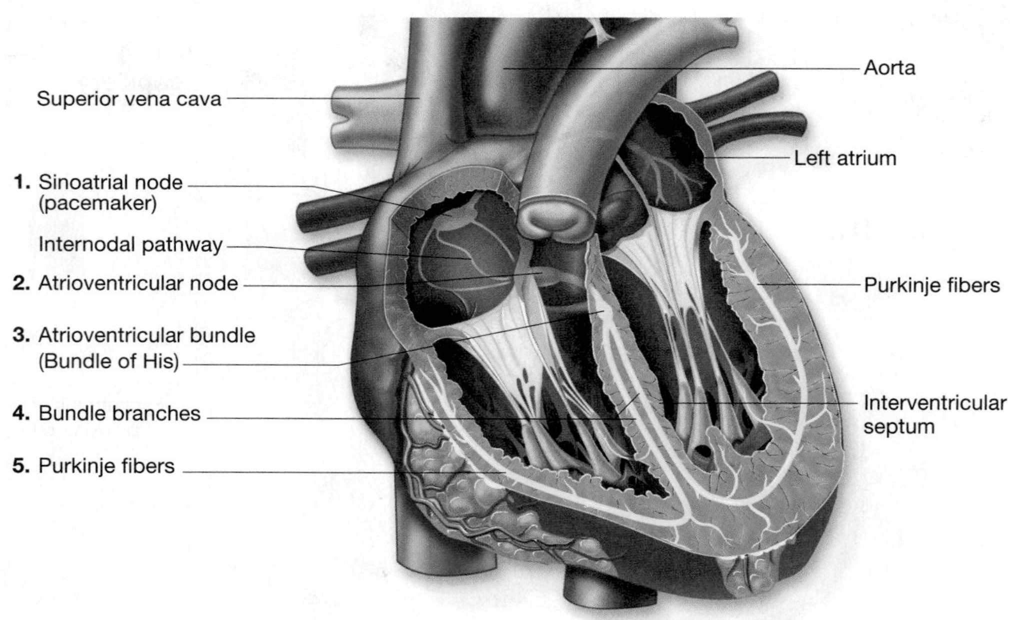

FIGURE 7-25c ✱ The cardiac conduction system.

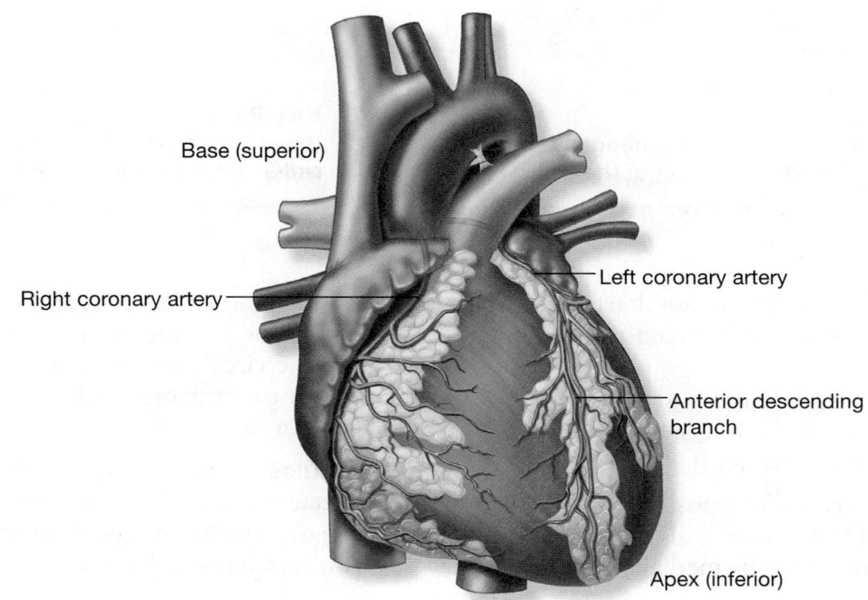

FIGURE 7-25d ✻ The coronary arteries.

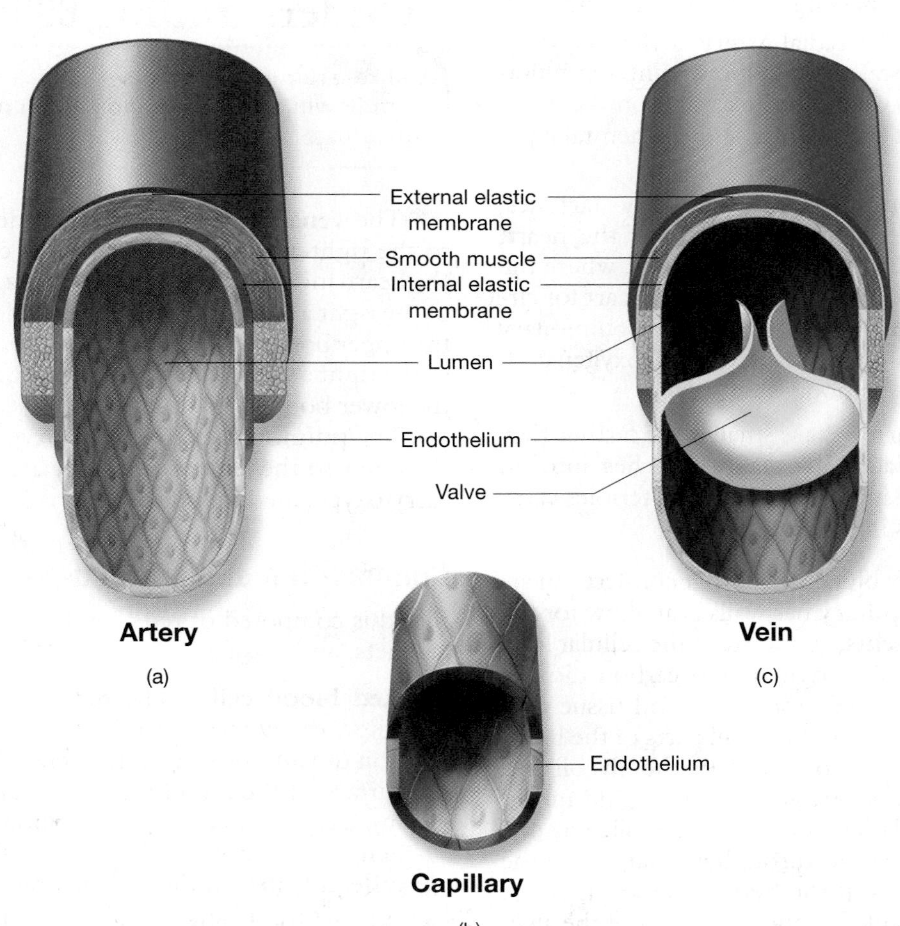

FIGURE 7-26 ✻ Comparative structure of arteries, capillaries, and veins.

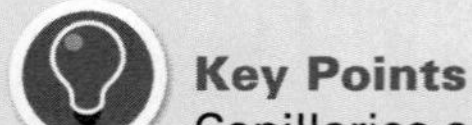

Key Points
Capillaries are the sites for gas exchange at the level of the alveoli and at the level of the cells.

Key Points
Blood is composed of red blood cells, white blood cells, platelets, and plasma.

with blood. Pulsations of the femoral artery can be felt in the groin at the crease between the abdomen and thigh.

- **Dorsalis pedis arteries**—Pulsations of the dorsalis pedis, an artery in the foot, can be felt on the top surface of the foot on the big-toe side.
- **Posterior tibial arteries**—The posterior tibial artery travels from the calf to the foot. Pulsations of this artery can be felt posterior to the medial malleolus (ankle bone).
- **Brachial arteries**—The brachial artery is the major artery of the upper arm. Its pulsations can be felt at the front of the elbow (antecubital region) and on the medial arm midway between the shoulder and elbow. The brachial artery is used when determining blood pressure and when assessing a pulse in an infant.
- **Radial arteries**—The radial artery is the major artery of the arm distal to the elbow joint. Its pulsations can be felt proximal to the thumb on the wrist. It is the artery that is usually assessed when taking a patient's pulse.
- **Pulmonary arteries**—The pulmonary arteries, which originate at the right ventricle of the heart, carry oxygen-depleted blood to the lungs, where the blood is oxygenated and returned to the heart for circulation throughout the body. Note: The pulmonary arteries are the only arteries that carry deoxygenated, or oxygen-depleted, blood.

The Arterioles The arteries are smaller the farther they are from the heart. Each eventually branches into an **arteriole**, the smallest kind of artery. The arterioles carry blood from the arteries into the capillaries.

The Capillaries A tiny blood vessel that connects an arteriole to a venule, a **capillary** has walls that allow for the exchange of gases, nutrients, and waste at the cellular level (Figure 7-26b∗). All fluid, oxygen, and carbon dioxide exchange takes place between the blood and tissue cells through the walls of the capillaries in all parts of the body.

In the lungs, oxygen moves out of the alveoli and into the alveolar capillaries while carbon dioxide moves out of the alveolar capillaries and into the alveoli. The carbon dioxide is then blown off through exhalation. In the tissue capillaries throughout the body, the movement of oxygen and carbon dioxide is opposite to that of the alveolar capillaries. Oxygen moves out of the tissue capillaries and into the cells while carbon dioxide and other wastes move out of the cells and into the tissue capillaries. The carbon dioxide and other wastes are then carried through the circulatory system back to the lungs where the alveolar gas exchange and blowing off of carbon dioxide takes place.

The Venules The smallest branch of the veins, a **venule**, is connected to the distal ends of capillaries. Blood that has been depleted of oxygen flows from the capillaries into the venules, from which it is transported into larger veins.

The Veins A **vein** carries blood back to the heart (Figure 7-26c∗). All veins except the pulmonary veins (see description that follows) carry oxygen-depleted blood. The major veins include the venae cavae and the pulmonary veins.

Understanding BODY PROCESSES

Unlike arteries, veins have valves that keep blood from flowing backward and help in moving the blood forward. ■

The **venae cavae** carry oxygen-depleted blood back to the right atrium, where it begins circulation through the heart and lungs. The *superior vena cava* enters the top of the right atrium, carrying oxygen-depleted blood from the upper body. The *inferior vena cava* enters the bottom of the right atrium, carrying oxygen-depleted blood from the lower body.

The **pulmonary veins** carry oxygen-rich blood from the lungs to the left atrium. They are the only veins that carry oxygenated blood.

Composition of the Blood

Blood is composed of red blood cells, white blood cells, platelets, and plasma.

- **Red blood cells**—The red cells give the blood its color, carry oxygen to the body cells, and carry carbon dioxide away from the cells. Hemoglobin on the surface of the red blood cell is responsible for carrying oxygen molecules and carbon dioxide. The oxygen and carbon dioxide molecules are carried on different sites on the hemoglobin molecule.
- **White blood cells**—The white cells (several types exist) are part of the body's immune system and help to defend against infection.

- **Platelets** and other clotting factors—Platelets and other clotting factors are essential to the formation of blood clots, necessary to stop bleeding.
- **Plasma**—This is the liquid part of the blood, which carries blood cells and transports nutrients to all tissues. The plasma also transports waste products to organs where they can be excreted from the body. A minute amount of oxygen is dissolved in plasma and transported throughout the body. A larger amount of carbon dioxide is carried by the plasma to the lungs for elimination.

Understanding BODY PROCESSES

Plasma contains large molecules of albumin that help keep the water portion of the plasma from leaking outside of the vessel. ■

Physiology of Circulation

Two ways of determining the adequacy of circulation are by assessing the pulse and by assessing the blood pressure.

When the left ventricle contracts, sending a wave of blood through the arteries, the **pulse**, or wave of propelled blood, can be felt at various points called *pulse points*. Simply, the pulse can be felt at the point where an artery passes over a bone near the skin surface. The pulse is a measure of the effectiveness of the left ventricle as a pump and also provides information about the volume of blood being ejected by the left ventricle and being carried in the arteries.

The central pulses are the carotid and femoral—located centrally, closer to the heart. The peripheral pulses are the radial, brachial, posterior tibial, and dorsalis pedis—located on the periphery of the body, farther from the heart. These pulses can be felt at the locations described earlier. An apical pulse is felt on the left side of the chest over the left ventricle. The pulse being felt is from the mechanical contraction of the left ventricle; however, since you are only feeling the mechanical contraction of the heart and not the pressure wave of blood, it does not provide an assessment of the effectiveness of the heart or blood volume. An apical pulse simply indicates that the heart is contracting. If a patient has lost a significant amount of blood, the apical pulse will still be felt since the heart is still producing a mechanical contraction. However, the radial or carotid pulses would feel weak or may even be absent because the amount of blood being ejected by the left ventricle would be reduced.

Blood pressure is the force exerted by the blood on the interior walls of the arteries. The **systolic blood pressure** is exerted against the walls of the arteries when the left ventricle contracts. The **diastolic blood pressure** is exerted against the walls of the arteries when the left ventricle is at rest, or between contractions. The systolic blood pressure measures the effectiveness of the pumping function of the left ventricle. The diastolic blood pressure measures the resistance in the arteries between contractions. The resistance is related to the vessel diameter. As the vessel diameter gets smaller, the resistance in the vessel increases. An increase in resistance will increase the diastolic blood pressure. Likewise, a decrease in resistance will decrease the diastolic blood pressure. If you have a patient whose vessels are dilating (the diameter is getting larger), his diastolic blood pressure would decrease.

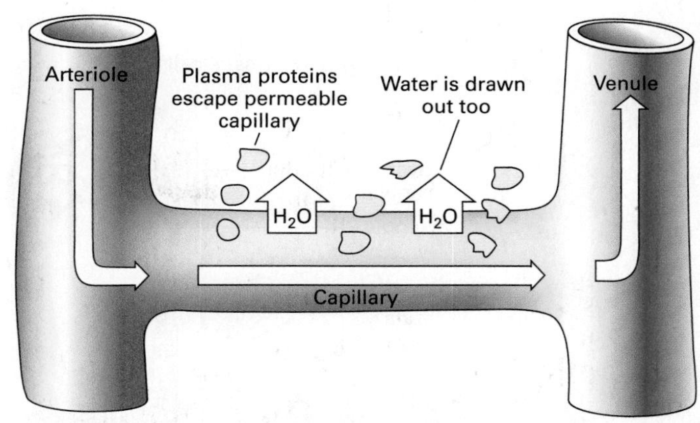

FIGURE 7-27 ✱ The effects of hydrostatic pressure on a vessel.

Another type of pressure found inside the vessel is hydrostatic pressure. **Hydrostatic pressure** is the force exerted on the inside of the vessel walls as a result of the blood pressure and volume (Figure 7-27✱). A significant increase in hydrostatic pressure may cause the blood in the capillaries to force fluid through the capillary wall. Basically, the capillaries begin to leak fluid, which is typically water and not whole blood. This may produce **edema**, which is swelling occurring in the tissues. If the capillaries in the lungs are leaking, the fluid will collect between the alveoli and capillary. This will force the alveoli farther away from the capillary, making gas exchange more difficult and less effective.

Perfusion is the delivery of oxygen, glucose, and other nutrients to the cells of all organ systems, and the elimination of carbon dioxide and other waste products, which results from the constant adequate circulation of blood through the capillaries (Figure 7-28✱).

Shock, or **hypoperfusion**, is the insufficient supply of oxygen and other nutrients to some of the body's cells and the inadequate elimination of carbon dioxide and other wastes that result from inadequate circulation of blood. It is a state of profound depression of the vital processes of the body. (Detailed information will be found in Chapter 15, "Shock and Resuscitation.")

Transport of Gases in the Blood

The two most important gases the EMT is concerned with are oxygen and carbon dioxide. Cells require oxygen to function effectively and survive. Carbon dioxide is a waste product that must be carried away from the cells

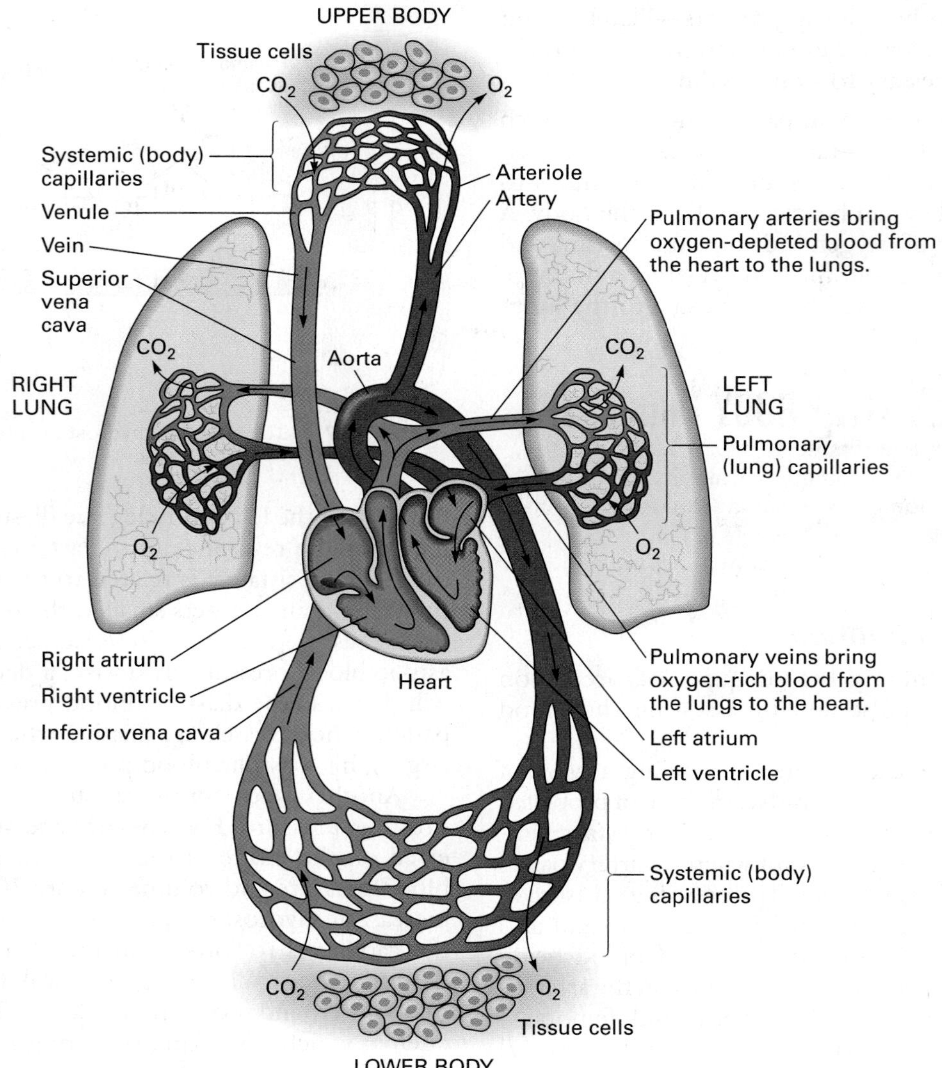

FIGURE 7-28 ✱ The circulatory system and tissue perfusion.

and eliminated by the lungs. An effective transport system must be in place to continuously deliver oxygen to the cells and eliminate carbon dioxide.

Oxygen is carried in the blood in two ways, whereas carbon dioxide is carried in three ways. Oxygen is attached to hemoglobin and dissolved in plasma. About 97 percent of the oxygen carried in the blood is attached to the hemoglobin molecule, which is on the surface of the red blood cell. The remaining 3 percent, not enough to survive on alone, is dissolved in the blood plasma.

Carbon dioxide is transported in the blood as bicarbonate, attached to hemoglobin, and dissolved in plasma. Approximately 70 percent of carbon dioxide is carried in the blood in the form of bicarbonate. The bicarbonate is formed when the carbon dioxide molecule enters the red blood cell and combines with water. The bicarbonate that results leaves the red blood cell and circulates in the blood. When the bicarbonate reaches the lungs, it re-enters the red blood cell, combines with hydrogen, and dissociates into carbon dioxide and water. The carbon dioxide leaves the red blood cell and is blown off by the lungs. Another 23 percent of carbon dioxide attaches to hemoglobin on the surface of the red blood cell. It attaches at a different site than the site where oxygen was attached. Once the blood reaches the lungs, the hemoglobin–carbon dioxide bond is broken and the carbon dioxide enters the alveoli and is exhaled from the lungs. Only 7 percent of carbon dioxide is carried in the blood dissolved in the plasma.

The transport of oxygen and carbon dioxide in the blood can be disrupted in a number of ways, for example a problem in gas exchange in the alveoli or at the level of cells, an inadequate volume of blood, or ineffective pumping by the heart. The disruption could leave cells without an adequate supply of oxygen and/or could result in a dangerous buildup of carbon dioxide.

Cell Metabolism

Cells require energy to survive. The main source of energy is glucose (a simple sugar molecule) that is metabo-

Objectives 7-19 to 7-21
Describe the basic functions of the nervous system, the central and peripheral structural divisions, and the voluntary and involuntary (sympathetic and parasympathetic) functional divisions of the peripheral system.

Key Terms
nervous system the body system including the brain, spinal cord, and nerves that controls the voluntary and involuntary activity of the human body.

lized inside the cell. In the ideal state, glucose metabolism occurs with adequate amounts of oxygen present. The metabolized glucose provides large amounts of energy for the cells to use. The final by-products of glucose metabolism are water and carbon dioxide. The carbon dioxide is transported away from the cell in one of the methods previously discussed and blown off by the lungs. This kind of metabolism is known as **aerobic metabolism**. *Aerobic* means "with oxygen." *Metabolism* refers to chemical and physical changes that take place within the cells.

If oxygen is not available when the cell is metabolizing glucose, very little energy is produced for the cell and the end product is acid. Acid is bad for the body if it accumulates. This process of metabolizing glucose without producing much energy is known as **anaerobic metabolism**; *anaerobic* means "without oxygen." If a patient is losing blood and very little oxygen is being delivered to the cells, very little energy is being produced. This may be seen in the patient who appears quiet and calm at the scene. Because of poor perfusion, he doesn't have enough energy to scream and complain of his injuries. Such patients are those that you should assess first and be more concerned about than the patient who is screaming about his fractured arm with the bone protruding through the skin. The patient who has enough energy to yell and scream is likely getting enough oxygen and glucose to his cells and is producing adequate energy.

The Nervous System

The **nervous system** (Figure 7-29*) controls the voluntary and involuntary activity of the human body. It enables the individual to be aware of and react to the environment. It also coordinates the responses of the body to stimuli and keeps body systems working together. Nerves carry impulses from tissues and organs to the nerve centers, and from nerve centers to other tissues and organs.

The basic functions of the nervous system are:

- Controlling and maintaining a conscious and aware state
- Transmitting sensory stimuli to the brain for interpretation
- Controlling motor function and transmitting motor impulses to muscle for voluntary and involuntary movement
- Controlling body functions through the autonomic nervous system

Structural Divisions of the Nervous System

The nervous system is divided into two main structural divisions: the central nervous system and the peripheral nervous system.

The Central Nervous System The **central nervous system** consists of the brain, which is located within the cranium, and the spinal cord, which is located within the spinal column (Figure 7-30*). The three layers of protective membranes enclosing both the brain and the spinal cord are the meninges. In addition, nature provides a cushion of fluid around and within the brain and spinal cord called *cerebrospinal fluid*. It is formed and circulated constantly, with part perpetually reabsorbed into the brain's venous blood.

The brain, which is the control center of the nervous system, is probably the most highly specialized organ in the body. It weighs about 3 pounds in the average adult, is richly supplied with blood vessels, and requires considerable oxygen to perform effectively. The brain does not store glucose and requires a constant supply. It has three main subdivisions: the cerebrum, the cerebellum, and the brainstem. A smaller subdivision of the brain, the pons, acts as a bridge that connects the three.

- **The cerebrum.** The outermost portion of the brain, the cerebrum occupies nearly all the cranial cavity. It controls specific body functions, such as sensation, thought, and associative memory. It also initiates and manages motions that are under the conscious control of the individual.
- **The cerebellum.** Also called the "small brain," the cerebellum is located in the posterior and inferior aspect of the cranium. It coordinates muscle activity and maintains balance through impulses from the eyes and the ears. Though it cannot initiate a muscle contraction, it can hold muscles in a state of partial contraction.
- **Brainstem.** The brainstem contains the mesencephalon, the pons, and the medulla oblongata. The medulla oblongata consists of three major control centers: the respiratory center, the cardiac center, and the vasomotor center. The *respiratory center* controls the rate and depth of respiration. The *cardiac center* is responsible for regulating the heart rate and force of contraction of the ventricles. The blood pressure is controlled by the *vasomotor center*, which produces dilation (relaxation) and constriction of the blood vessels.

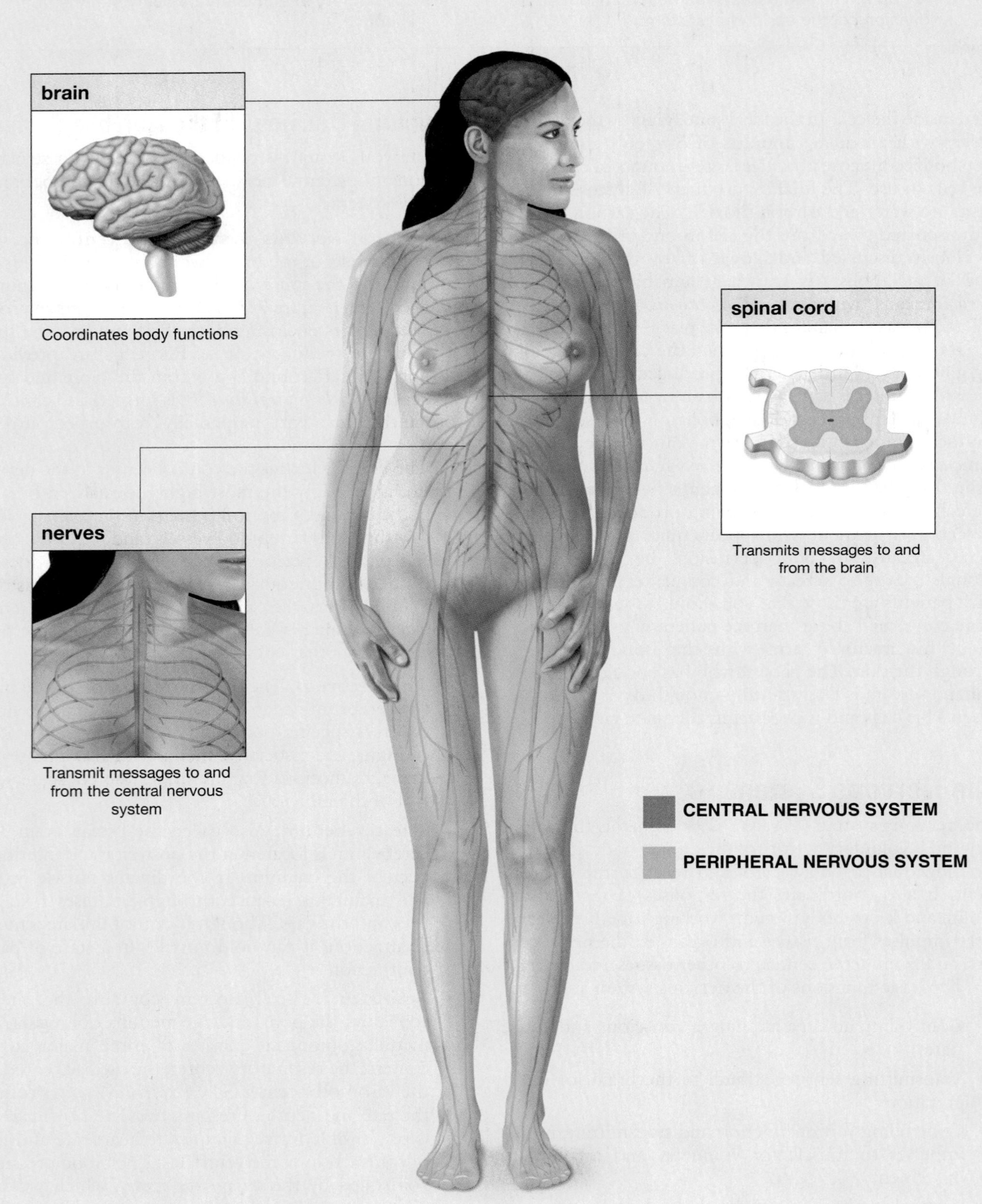

FIGURE 7-29 ✱ The nervous system.

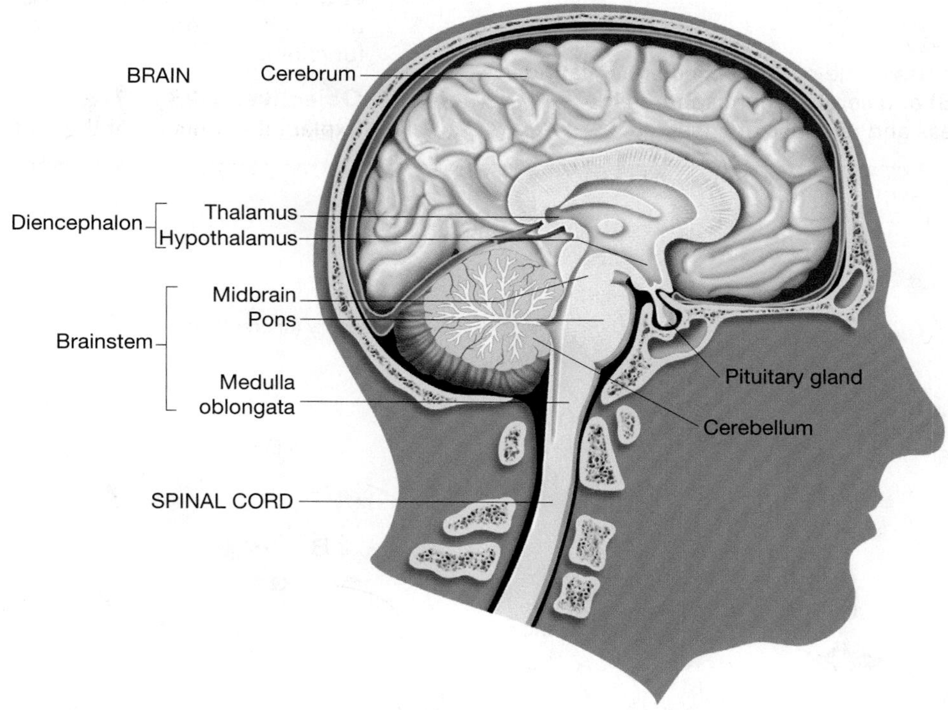

FIGURE 7-30 ✱ The central nervous system.

Understanding BODY PROCESSES

The brain has a specialized network of capillaries called the blood-brain barrier that allows only some substances, such as glucose, to pass through from the blood into the brain. ■

The spinal cord is about 18 inches long and is an extension of the brainstem. The major function of the spinal cord is conduction of nerve impulses. Many nerves enter and leave the spinal cord at different levels. These nerves all connect with nerve centers located in the brain or spinal cord.

The Peripheral Nervous System The **peripheral nervous system** is composed of the nerves located outside the spinal cord and brain. Afferent nerves carry sensory information from the body to the spinal cord and brain. Efferent nerves carry motor information from the brain and spinal cord to the body. Together, they create a complete circuit that permits, for example, the sensation of pain and the reflexive withdrawal from it (Figure 7-31✱).

Functional Divisions of the Nervous System

The functional divisions of the nervous system are the voluntary nervous system and the autonomic nervous system.

The Voluntary Nervous System The voluntary nervous system influences the activity of skeletal (voluntary) muscles and movements.

The Autonomic Nervous System The autonomic nervous system, as its name implies, is automatic. It influences the activities of smooth (involuntary) muscles and glands. It is partly independent of the rest of the nervous system.

The autonomic nervous system is divided into the *sympathetic nervous system* and the *parasympathetic nervous system*. These two systems have opposite effects and act in a delicate balance. The sympathetic nervous system is activated when the body is challenged by stressors: trauma, blood loss, fright, and so on. Its actions are commonly known as the "fight-or-flight" response. The parasympathetic nervous system returns body processes to normal or depresses body function. Figure 7-32✱ illustrates the effects on various organs.

Consciousness and Unconsciousness

Two components of the nervous system that control consciousness are the *cerebral hemispheres* and the *reticular activating system (RAS)*. The cerebral hemispheres are the large right and left sides of the cerebrum of the brain. The RAS is not an actual structure but a group of nerves found in the brainstem. The RAS is often referred to as the "wake and sleep center" or "on/off center" because it determines whether the patient remains awake and aware of his surroundings or not. The RAS is continuously transmitting impulses regarding the patient's surroundings to the brain for constant stimulation and response.

Consciousness In order for the patient to be in a conscious or awake state, the RAS and at least one cerebral hemisphere must be intact and functioning.

Objective 7-22
Describe the basic role of the recticular activating system (RAS) and cerebral hemispheres in consciousness and unconsciousness.

Key Terms
endocrine system a system of ductless glands that produce hormones that regulate body functions.

Objectives 7-23 to 7-25
Explain the function of the endocrine system.

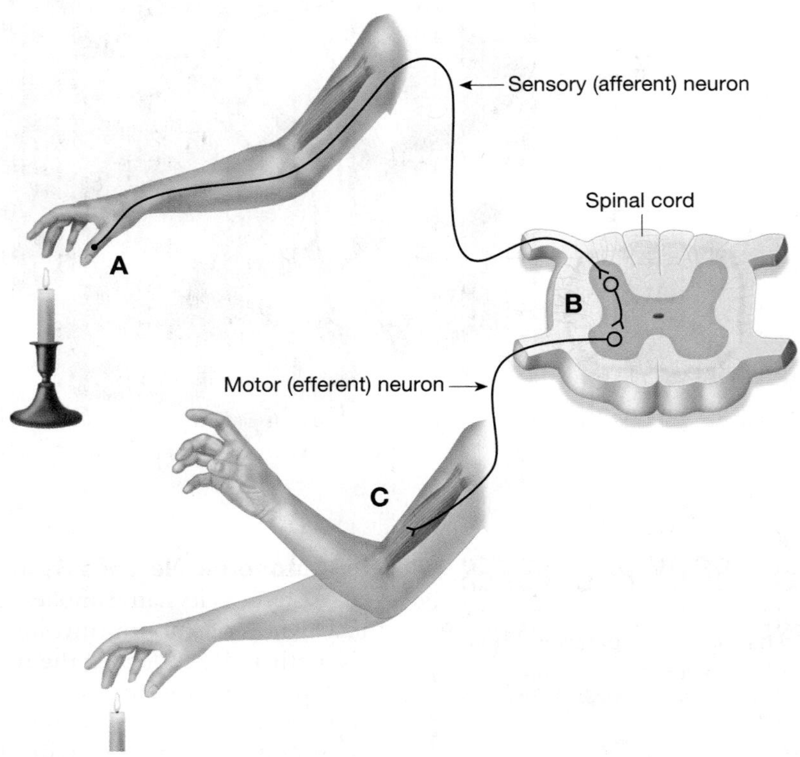

FIGURE 7-31 ✱ Afferent nerves carry sensory information from the body to the spinal cord and brain. Efferent nerves carry motor information from the brain and spinal cord to the body. The resulting circuit permits, for example, quick reflexive withdrawal from pain.

Unconsciousness If either the RAS or both cerebral hemispheres are damaged or not functioning properly, the patient will no longer be in an awake state, or conscious.

Understanding BODY PROCESSES

When a person is injured, the sympathetic nervous system is triggered and provides an immediate response through the nerves. Within minutes, the body also begins to release hormones, such as epinephrine and norepinephrine, to produce a sustained sympathetic nervous system response. ■

The Endocrine System

The **endocrine system** is made up of ductless glands, the body's regulators (Figure 7-33✱). Secretions from these glands are called *hormones,* chemical substances that have effects on the activity of certain organs. Hormones are carried by the bloodstream to all parts of the body, affecting physical strength, mental ability, build, stature, reproduction, hair growth, voice pitch, and behavior. How people think, act, and feel depends largely on these secretions.

The endocrine glands discharge secretions directly into the bloodstream. Good health depends on a well-balanced output of hormones. Endocrine imbalance yields profound changes in growth and serious changes in mental, emotional, physical, and sexual behavior.

The endocrine glands and their functions include the following:

- The *thyroid gland,* which is located in the anterior neck, regulates metabolism, growth and development, and the activity of the nervous system.
- The *parathyroid glands,* behind the thyroid, produce a hormone necessary for the metabolism of calcium and phosphorus in the bones.

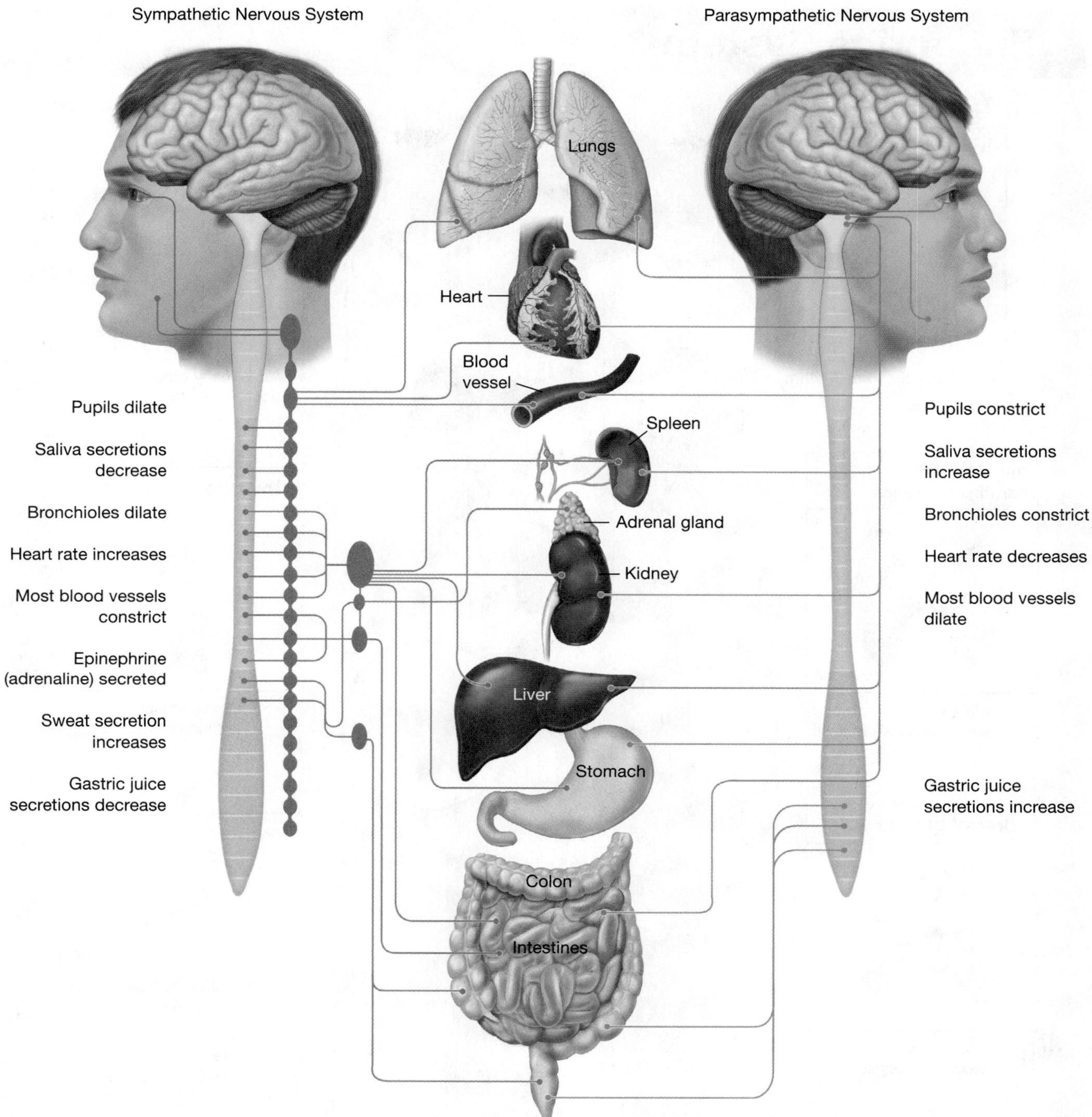

FIGURE 7-32 ✱ The effects of the sympathetic and parasympathetic nervous systems on organs.

- The *adrenal glands,* which sit atop the kidneys, secrete epinephrine (adrenaline) and norepinephrine, postpone muscle fatigue, increase the storage of sugar, control kidney function, and regulate the metabolism of salt and water.
- The *gonads* (ovaries and testes) produce the hormones that govern reproduction and sex characteristics.
- The *islets of Langerhans,* which are in the pancreas, make insulin, which allows glucose (sugar) to enter cells, and also produce glucagon, a hormone that raises the glucose level in the blood.
- The *pituitary gland,* which is at the base of the brain, is considered to be the "master gland." It regulates growth, the thyroid and parathyroid glands, the pancreas, the gonads, metabolism of fatty acids and some basic proteins, blood sugar reactions, and urinary excretion.

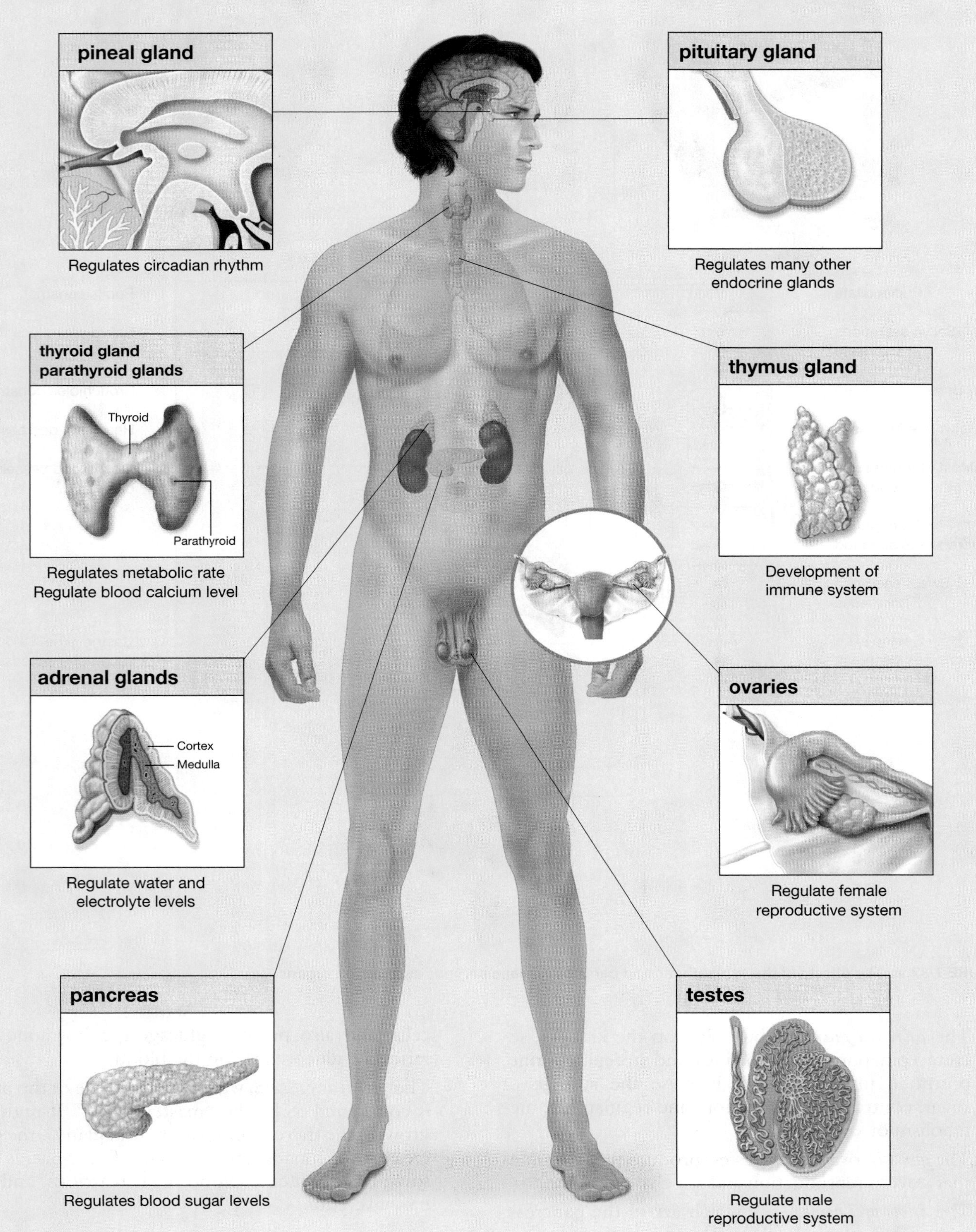
Endocrine System
pineal gland
Regulates circadian rhythm
pituitary gland
Regulates many other endocrine glands
thyroid gland
parathyroid glands
Thyroid
Parathyroid
Regulates metabolic rate
Regulate blood calcium level
thymus gland
Development of immune system
adrenal glands
Cortex
Medulla
Regulate water and electrolyte levels
ovaries
Regulate female reproductive system
pancreas
Regulates blood sugar levels
testes
Regulate male reproductive system

FIGURE 7-33 ✻ The endocrine system.

Key Points
Epinephrine and norepinephrine are the two primary hormones secreted by the sympathetic nervous system.

Key Terms
integumentary system the skin.

Objectives 7-26 and 7-27
List the general functions and structures of the integumentary system.

Epinephrine and Norepinephrine

As just noted, epinephrine, also known as adrenaline, and norepinephrine are two hormones secreted by the adrenal gland. These hormones produce many of the signs and symptoms seen in patients when the sympathetic nervous system is stimulated. In order to understand the signs and symptoms that are produced, you must first understand the basics of the four effects—$alpha_1$, $alpha_2$, $beta_1$, and $beta_2$—activated by these hormones.

- $Alpha_1$ effects cause the vessels to constrict (vasoconstriction). The vessels in the skin are significantly affected by $alpha_1$. When the vessels in the skin constrict, the blood is shunted to the core of the body. The warm red blood is no longer located in great quantities in the skin. This causes the skin to become cool and pale (white looking). $Alpha_1$ stimulation also causes the sweat glands to release sweat. This causes the skin to become moist, or clammy.
- $Alpha_2$ effects are thought to regulate the release of $alpha_1$.
- $Beta_1$ effects all relate to the heart. They increase the heart rate, increase the force of cardiac contraction, and speed up the electrical impulse traveling down the heart's conduction system.
- $Beta_2$ effects cause smooth muscle to dilate, especially in the bronchioles and in some vessels.

Epinephrine and norepinephrine are the two primary hormones secreted by the sympathetic nervous system. The hormone epinephrine has all four properties ($alpha_1$, $alpha_2$, $beta_1$, and $beta_2$). Thus, when it is secreted by the adrenal gland or if it is administered to a patient, you would expect all of the actions just listed to occur and to see the signs related to these actions. Epinephrine is used to treat patients with severe allergic reactions to combat the problems found in the condition, primarily vasodilation and bronchoconstriction.

Norepinephrine causes primarily $alpha_1$ and $alpha_2$ effects plus trace amounts of $beta_1$ and $beta_2$ activity. Thus, the majority of the effects of norepinephrine are seen in the blood vessels and skin (pale, cool, and clammy).

Recognizing these signs and understanding how they are produced may lead you to suspect the presence of some conditions much earlier, affording you the time to provide your patient better care. For example, in a patient who is losing blood, the body will try to compensate by releasing epinephrine and norepinephrine. Being able to recognize the signs and understand why they are occurring may help you to suspect the blood loss much earlier and treat the patient more aggressively. Also, you will be administering or assisting with the administration of drugs containing these properties.

The Integumentary System (Skin)

All the various tissues, organs, and systems that make up the human body are separated from the outside environment by the skin, which is also known as the **integumentary system** (Figure 7-34*). The skin has the following functions:

- Protecting the body from the environment, bacteria, and other foreign organisms
- Regulating the temperature of the body
- Serving as a receptor for heat, cold, touch, pain, and pressure
- Aiding in the regulation of water and electrolytes (sodium and chloride)

The skin has three layers: the epidermis, the dermis, and a subcutaneous layer. The **epidermis**, or outermost layer of skin, is actually composed of four layers of cells. The outer two layers are dying and dead cells that are sloughed off as new cells replace them. The skin's pigmentation—the *melanin*—is located in the deepest layers of the epidermis.

The **dermis**, or second layer of the skin, is much thicker than the epidermis. It contains the vast network of blood vessels that supply the skin as well as the hair follicles, sweat glands, oil glands, and sensory nerves. Composed of dense connective tissue, the dermis gives the skin its elasticity and strength.

Just below the dermis is a layer of fatty tissue called the **subcutaneous layer**, or *subcutaneous connective tissue*. It varies in thickness, depending on what part of the body it covers. Subcutaneous tissue of the eyelids, for example, is extremely thin, but that of the abdomen and buttocks is thick.

The four accessory structures of the skin are the nails, hair, sweat glands, and oil glands.

Objective 7-28
Describe the basic anatomy and physiology of structures of the digestive system.

Key Terms
digestive system the structures and organs that ingest and carry food so that absorption and waste elimination can occur.

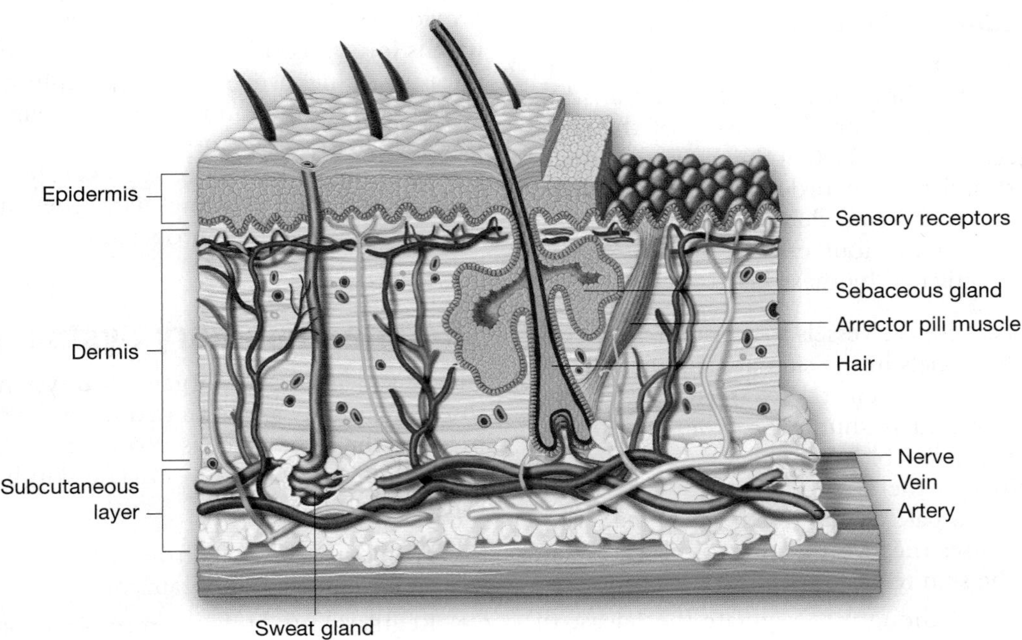

FIGURE 7-34 * Anatomy of the skin.

The Digestive System

Basic Anatomy

The **digestive system** (Figure 7-35*) is composed of the *alimentary tract* (the passage through which food travels) and the *accessory organs* (organs that help prepare food for absorption and use by tissues of the body). The main functions of the digestive system are to ingest and carry food so that absorption can occur and waste can be eliminated.

The abdominal cavity contains all the major organs of the digestive system except for the mouth and the esophagus. The esophagus is a flexible tubelike structure located posterior to the trachea and is responsible for carrying food from the mouth to the stomach.

- *The stomach*, a large, hollow organ, is the main organ of the digestive system. While digestion actually begins in the mouth, where saliva begins to break down foods, the majority of digestion takes place in the stomach, which secretes gastric juices that begin converting ingested foods to a form that can be absorbed and used by the body.
- *The pancreas* is a flat, solid organ that lies just inferior and posterior to the stomach. It secretes *pancreatic juices* that aid in the digestion of fats, starches, and proteins. The islets of Langerhans, located in the pancreas, produce the insulin that regulates the amount of sugar in the bloodstream.
- *The liver*, the largest solid organ in the abdomen, lies immediately beneath the diaphragm in the right upper quadrant of the abdominal cavity. The liver produces bile, which aids in the digestion of fat. It stores sugars until they are needed by the body. It also produces components necessary for immune function, blood clotting, and the production of plasma. Finally, the toxic substances produced by digestion are rendered harmless in the liver.
- *The spleen* is a solid organ located in the left upper quadrant of the abdominal cavity. It helps in the filtration of blood and, because it contains a dense network of blood vessels, serves as a reservoir of blood the body can use in an emergency such as hemorrhage. Although it lies among the digestive organs, the spleen has no digestive function.
- *The gallbladder* is a hollow pouch. Part of the *bile duct* leading from the liver, the gallbladder acts as a reservoir for bile. When food enters the small intestine, contractions are stimulated that empty the

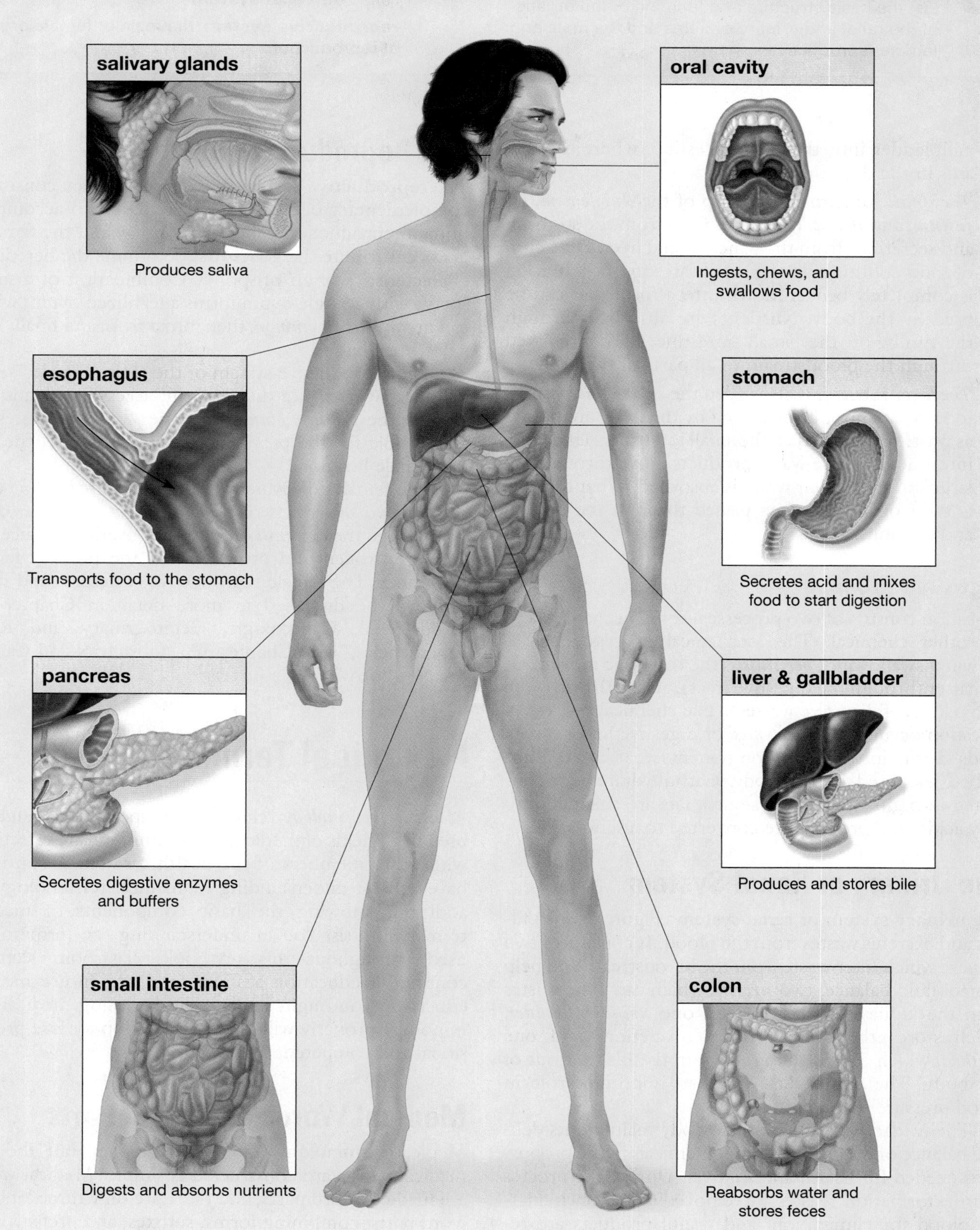
Digestive System
salivary glands
Produces saliva
oral cavity
Ingests, chews, and swallows food
esophagus
Transports food to the stomach
stomach
Secretes acid and mixes food to start digestion
pancreas
Secretes digestive enzymes and buffers
liver & gallbladder
Produces and stores bile
small intestine
Digests and absorbs nutrients
colon
Reabsorbs water and stores feces

FIGURE 7-35 ✱ The digestive system.

Objectives 7-29 and 7-30
List the basic structure and function of the organs of the renal and urinary systems and the male and female reproductive systems.

Key Terms

urinary system the organs and structures that filter and excrete wastes from the blood. Also called the **renal system**.

reproductive system the male or female organs of reproduction.

gallbladder into the small intestine, where the bile aids in the digestion of fats.

- *The small intestine* is made up of the *duodenum, jejunum,* and *ileum*. It receives food from the stomach and secretions from the pancreas and liver. Digestion of food continues in the small intestine, where food is completely broken down into a form that can be used by the body. Nutrients are absorbed through the walls of the small intestine and circulated through the bloodstream to all parts of the body.
- *The large intestine* is also called the *colon*. The parts of food that cannot be absorbed by the body are passed as waste products from the small intestine to the large intestine. As these waste products move through the large intestine, their water is absorbed. What remains is the stool that is then passed through the rectum and the anus.

Digestive Process

Digestion consists of two processes—one mechanical and the other chemical. The mechanical process includes chewing, swallowing, *peristalsis* (the rhythmic movement of matter through the digestive tract), and *defecation* (the elimination of digestive wastes). The chemical process of digestion occurs when *enzymes,* or digestive juices, break foods down into simple components that can be absorbed and used by the body. Carbohydrates are converted into glucose (simple sugar), fats are changed into fatty acids, and proteins are converted to amino acids.

The Urinary or Renal System

The **urinary system** or **renal system** (Figure 7-36*) filters and excretes wastes from the blood. It consists of two *kidneys,* which filter waste from the bloodstream and help control fluid balance; two *ureters,* which carry the wastes from the kidneys to the bladder; one *urinary bladder,* which stores the urine prior to excretion; and one *urethra,* which carries the urine from the bladder out of the body. The kidneys also play an important role in blood pressure regulation.

The urinary system helps the body maintain its delicate balance of water and various chemicals in the proportions needed for health and survival. During the process of urine formation, wastes are removed from the circulating blood for elimination, and useful products are returned to the blood. Kidney function also helps to maintain a normal acid-base balance in the body.

The Reproductive System

The **reproductive system** of women and men consists of complementary organs that can function to accomplish human reproduction. The male's *sperm* and the female's *ovum* contribute the genes that determine the hereditary characteristics of an offspring. Combination of a single sperm with a single ovum forms a fertilized ovum, which can grow into an *embryo,* then into a *fetus,* and finally into a newborn baby.

The reproductive system of the male (Figure 7-37*) includes two *testes,* a duct system, accessory glands (including the *prostate gland*), and the *penis*. The testes are responsible for the production of testosterone, the primary male hormone.

The female reproductive system (Figure 7-38*) consists of two *ovaries,* two *fallopian tubes,* the *uterus,* the *vagina,* and the *external genitals*. The ovaries produce and secrete estrogen and progesterone, the primary female hormones. The female reproductive structures and function will be discussed in more detail in Chapter 23, "Abdominal, Gynecologic, Genitourinary, and Renal Emergencies," and Chapter 37, "Obstetrics and Care of the Newborn."

▶ Medical Terminology

Medical terminology refers to the specialized language used in all fields of medicine. To communicate effectively with other members of the health care team, you must have a basic understanding of medical terminology. In addition, knowing the basic components of medical terms will assist you in understanding the terminology used throughout this textbook, classroom lectures, continuing education sessions, and any future medical education you might pursue. Finally, using medical terminology properly will help you develop a more professional and competent presentation.

Medical Words and Word Parts

Medical terminology may look complex, but the way medical words are constructed is simple. Medical words are made of word parts, and there are only three kinds of word parts: combining forms, suffixes, and prefixes. The ability to break down a medical word into its parts will drastically improve your ability to understand its meaning.

Urinary System

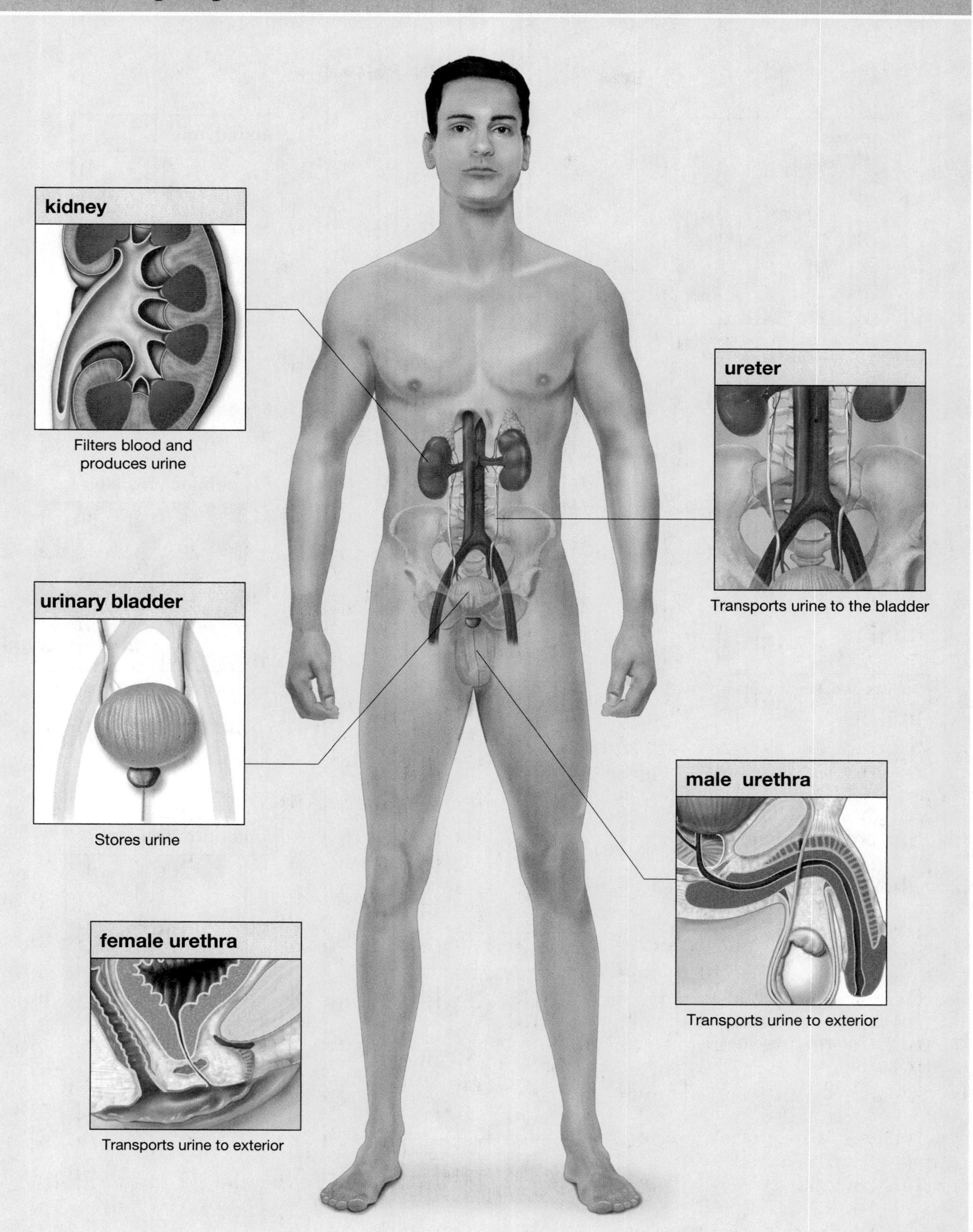

FIGURE 7-36 ✻ The urinary system.

Male Reproductive System

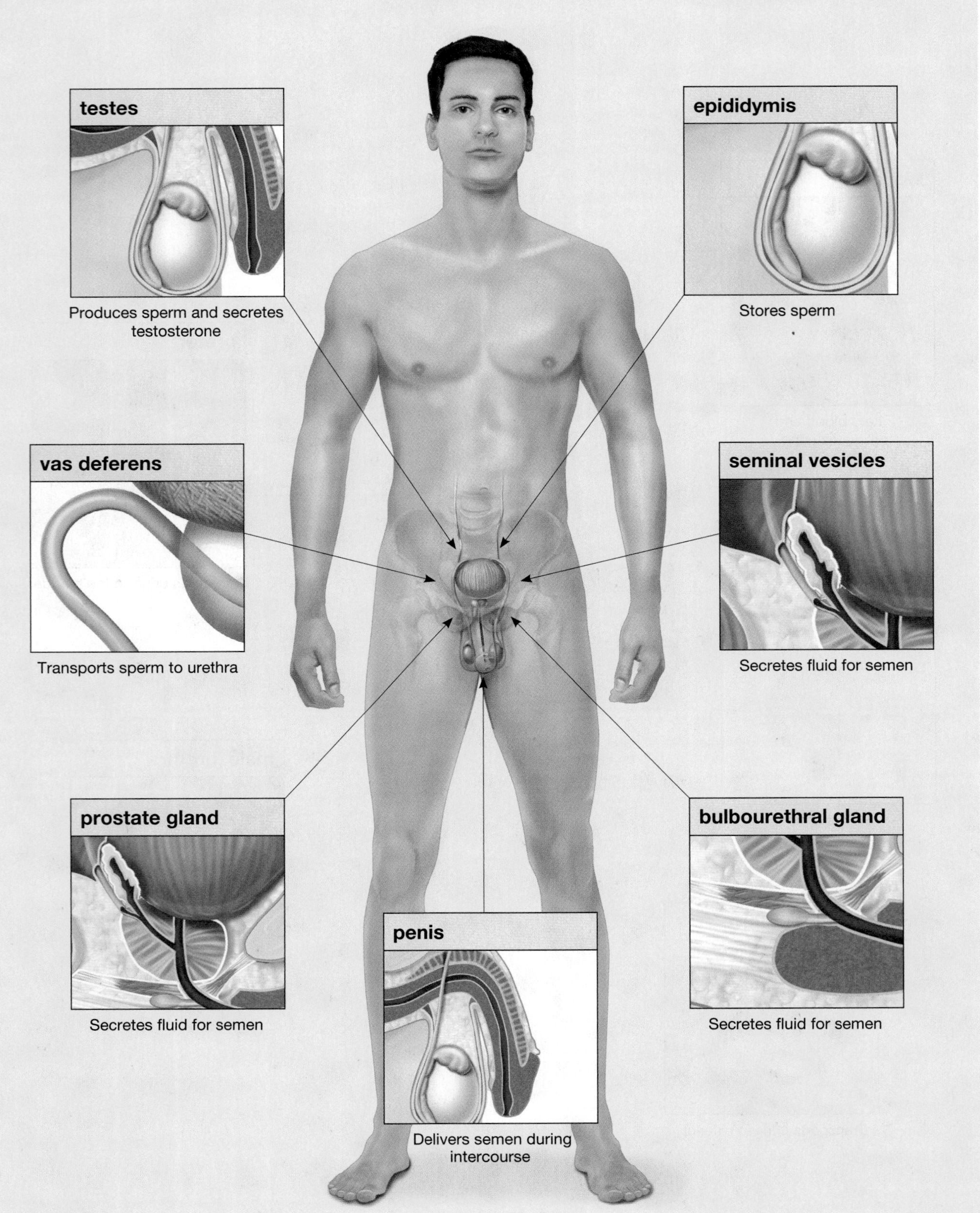

FIGURE 7-37 ✱ The male reproductive system.

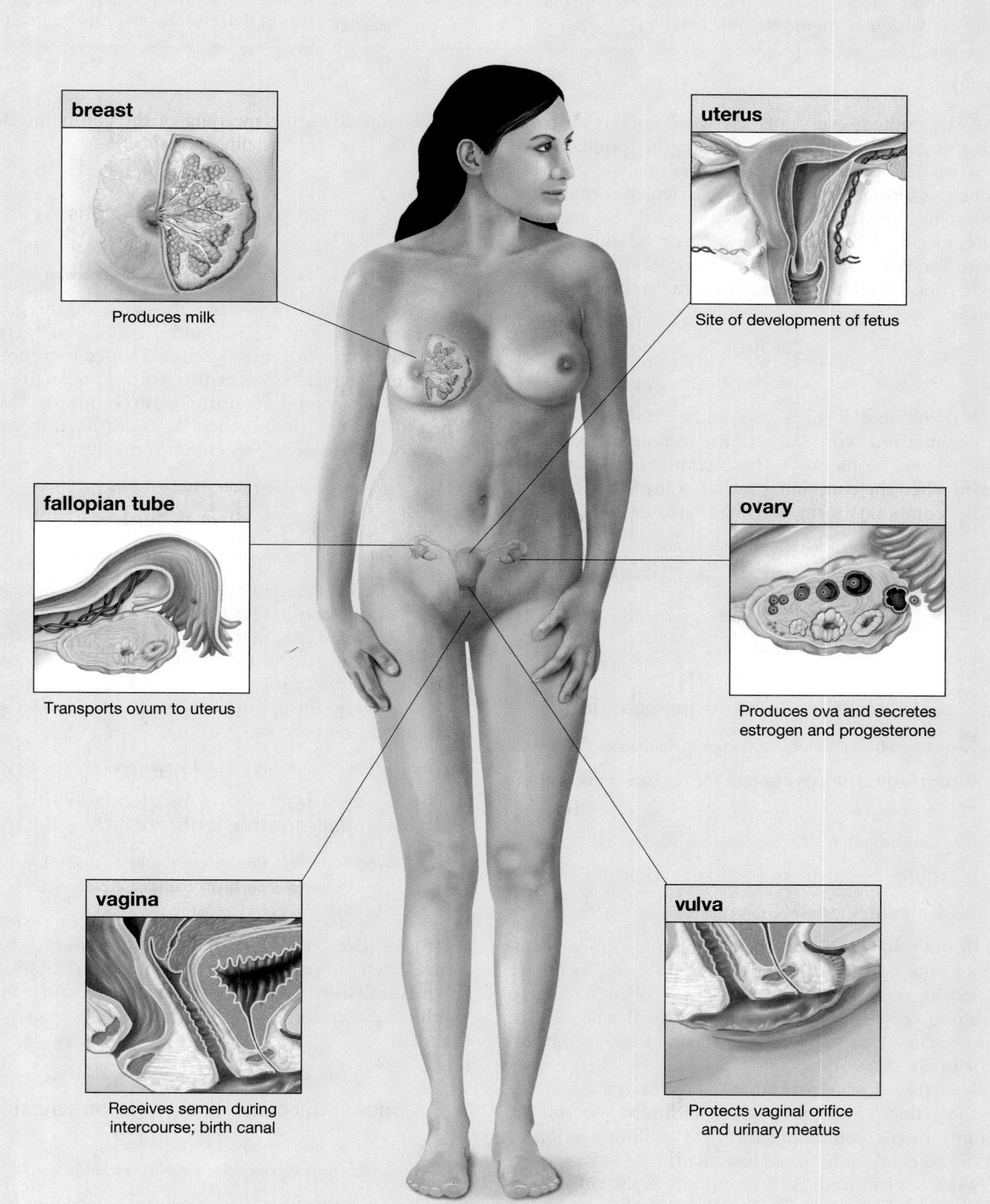

FIGURE 7-38 ✱ The female reproductive system.

Objective 7-31
Explain the importance of knowledge of medical terminology in communicating among health care team members.

Objective 7-32
Apply knowledge of common prefixes, suffixes, and roots to interpret medical terms.

Thinking Critically
Your patient has suffered a possible fracture somewhere between his right hip and knee, the toes of his right foot are numb, and you can't feel a pulse in that ankle or foot. Why would you want to be able to use correct medical terminology when you report these findings to the hospital?

As just noted, every medical word contains a **combining form**. The combining form is the foundation of the word and gives the word its essential meaning. A combining form has two parts: a *root* (which contains the medical meaning) and a *combining vowel.* The combining vowel (usually *o*, but sometimes *a, e,* or *i*) helps join the root to another word part and makes the resulting whole word pronounceable. An example is the combining form *cardi/o-:*

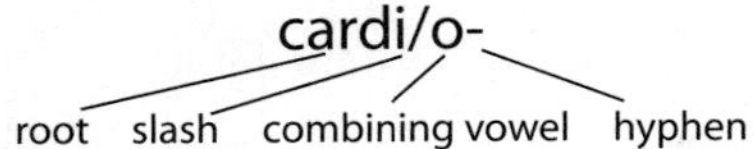

A combining form always ends with a hyphen to show that it is a word part, not a complete word. The hyphen—and sometimes the combining vowel—is deleted when the combining form is joined with a prefix, another combining form, and/or a suffix to make a word.

combining form + suffix = word

cardi/o- + -logy = cardiology

(heart) + (study of) = (study of the heart)

prefix + combining form + suffix = word

peri- + cardi/o- + -um = pericardium

(around) + (heart) + (structure) = (structure that surrounds the heart)

Some medical words contain more than one combining form.

combining form + combining form + suffix = word

my/o- + cardi/o- + -al = myocardial

(muscle) + (heart) + (pertaining to) = (pertaining to heart muscle)

In the prior examples, the combining form *cardi/o-* refers to the heart. Other common combining forms are *pulmon/o-,* referring to the lungs; *angi/o-,* referring to the blood vessels; *bronch/o-,* referring to the bronchi of the lower airway; and *cerebr/o-,* referring to the cerebrum of the brain.

A **suffix** is a word part added to the end of a combining form that modifies or gives additional or specific meaning to the combining form. By adding a suffix to one of the combining forms just mentioned, a new medical word is produced. As an example, if the suffix *-itis,* which means "inflammation," is added to the combining form *bronch/o-,* it becomes the medical word *bronchitis.* By breaking down the meaning of the combining form and suffix, it is easy to define *bronchitis.*

combining form + suffix = word

bronch/o- + -itis = bronchitis

(bronchus) + (inflammation of) =
(inflammation of the bronchi or of the lower airway)

Several suffixes may share the same meaning. The suffixes *-ac, -al, -ary, -eal, -ic,* and *-ous* all mean "pertaining to." When one of these suffixes is added to a combining form, it typically makes the word an adjective. For example, the combining form *hepat/o-* means "liver." When the suffix *-ic* is added to *hepat/o-,* it becomes *hepatic,* which means "pertaining to the liver."

combining form + suffix = word

hepat/o- + -ic = hepatic

(liver) + (pertaining to) = (pertaining to the liver)

As noted earlier, some medical terms may contain more than one combining form. An example is *laryngotracheobronchitis.* At first, you may think this word is confusing and hard to understand, not to mention unpronounceable. However, by breaking the term into the combining forms and suffix, it becomes easy to understand—and even to pronounce.

combining form + combining form + combining form + suffix = word

laryng/o- + trache/o- + bronch/o- + -itis =
laryngotracheobronchitis

(larynx) + (trachea) + (bronchus) + (inflammation of) =
(inflammation of the larynx, trachea, and bronchi)

A **prefix** is a word part that comes before a combining form. The prefix modifies the combining form or forms, often indicating direction, time, or orientation. In the medical word *endotracheal,* the prefix *endo-* means "within." An endotracheal tube is a tube that lies within the trachea.

prefix + combining form + suffix = word

endo- + trache/o- + -al = endotracheal

(within) + (trachea) + (pertaining to) =
(pertaining to something within the trachea)

The easiest way to learn prefixes, combining forms, and suffixes is to memorize them; in fact, memorizing

Key Points

The ability to break down a medical word into its parts will drastically improve your ability to understand its meaning.

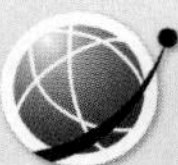

Media Resources

Go to www.bradybooks.com for mykit. Highlights:

- *Animation:* Heart and Major Vessels
- *Animation:* Endocrine System
- *Animation:* Skeletal System

TABLE 7-1 How to Break Down and Understand Medical Terms: Some Examples

Prefix	Combining Form	Suffix	Medical Word	Meaning
hypo- (below normal)	vol/o- (volume)	-emic (pertaining to the blood)	hypovolemic	Pertaining to a below-normal volume of blood
hyper- (above normal)	glyc/o- (glucose, sugar)	-emia (condition of the blood)	hyperglycemia	Condition of an above-normal blood glucose (sugar) level
a- (without, no)	pne/o- (breathing)	-a (condition)	apnea	Condition of no breathing (absence of breathing)
tachy- (fast)	cardi/o- (heart)	-ia (condition)	tachycardia	Condition of a fast heart rate
brady- (slow)	pne/o- (breathing)	-a (condition)	bradypnea	Condition of a slow breathing rate

word parts and their meanings is useful, because they will be encountered in many medical words and always have the same meaning. However, memorizing is not the easiest way to learn whole medical words. Instead, medical words can be easily understood by breaking them down into, and knowing the meanings of, the individual prefixes, combining forms, and suffixes. It is not only impossible to memorize all of the medical words you will need to know, it is not necessary, because you can decode any medical word by separating it into its recognizable parts.

Refer to Table 7-1 for a few medical words that you will encounter when reading this text and an example of how each can be easily broken down and understood.

Refer to Table 7-2 for common combining forms, Table 7-3 for common prefixes, and Table 7-4 for common suffixes. These are not all-inclusive lists. It is strongly recommended that you become familiar with a medical terminology text. You should also acquire a medical dictionary and use it to define medical terms you are not familiar with.

Note: The explanations of medical words and the combining words, prefixes, and suffixes presented in this section and in Tables 7-2, 7-3, and 7-4 are based on the following medical terminology text: Susan Turley. *Medical Language*. Upper Saddle River, NJ: Pearson Prentice Hall, 2007.

TABLE 7-2 Common Combining Forms

Combining Form	Meaning	Combining Form	Meaning
abdomin/o-	abdomen	corpor/o-	body
acous/o-	hearing, sound	cost/o-	rib
acr/o-	extremity, highest part	cry/o-	cold
aden/o-	gland	cubit/o-	elbow
adip/o-	fat	cyan/o-	blue
albin/o-	white	cyst/o-	bladder, cyst
alg/o-	pain	dent/i-	tooth
all/o-	other, strange	derm/a-	skin
andr/o-	male	digit/o-	finger or toe
angi/o-	blood vessel	edem/o-	swelling
aort/o-	aorta	embryon/o-	fetus
arter/o-	artery	enter/o-	intestines
arthr/o-	joint	erythr/o-	red
articul/o-	joint	esthes/o-	sensation
audi/o-	hearing	eti/o-	cause
aur/i-	ear	febr/o-	fever
auscult/o-	listen	fibr/o-	fiber
bi/o-	life	flex/o-	bend
blephar/o-	eyelid	fract/o-	break up
brachi/o-	arm	gastr/o-	stomach
bronch/o-	bronchus	gnos/o-	knowledge
bucc/o-	cheek	gynec/o-	female
burs/o-	pouch or sac, bursa	hem/o-	blood
calcane/o-	heel	hepat/o-	liver
carcin/o-	cancer	heter/o-	other, different
cardi/o-	heart	home/o-	same
carp/o-	wrist	humer/o-	upper arm
caus/o-	burn	lith/o-	stone
cephal/o-	head	medi/o-	middle
cervic/o-	neck, cervix	hydr/o-	water
chol/e-	bile	hyster/o-	womb, uterus
chondr/o-	cartilage	idi/o-	unknown, individual
chrom/o-	color	inguin/o-	groin
cili/o-	hairlike structure	lact/i-	milk
cis/o-	cut	later/o-	side
cleid/o-	collarbone (clavicle)	leuk/o-	white
cochle/o-	cochlea of the inner ear	ligat/o-	tie, bind
cor/o-	pupil	meg/a-	large
coron/o-	encircling structure (like the vessels that encircle and supply the heart)	melan/o-, melen/o-	black

TABLE 7-2 Common Combining Forms *continued*

Combining Form	Meaning
men/o-	monthly
morb/o-	disease
mort/o-	death
myel/o-	bone marrow, spinal cord
my/o-	muscle
nephr/o-	kidney
neur/o-	nerve
noct/o-	night
ocul/o-	eye
odont/o-	tooth
o/o-, ov/i-	egg
ophthalm/o-	eye
orch/o-	testis
osse/o-, oste/o-	bone
ot/o-	ear
palpat/o-	touch, feel
par/o-	birth
pariet/o-	wall of a cavity
path/o-	disease
ped/o-	child
percuss/o-	strike, tap
phag/o-	eat, swallow
phot/o-	light
placent/o-	placenta
pleur/o-	pleura (lung membrane)
pne/o-	breathe
pneum/o-	lung, air
pod/o-	foot
psych/o-	mind
purul/o-, pyl/o-	pus
pyel/o-	pelvis (including pelvis of the kidney)
pyret/o-	fever
ren/o-	kidney
reticul/o-	network
retin/o-	retina of the eye
rhin/o-	nose
rub/o-	red
salping/o-	fallopian tube
sang/o-	blood
scler/o-	hard
seb/o-	sebum (oil)
sect/o-	cut
sept/o-	wall
ser/o-	serum
sinus/o-	cavity or hollow, sinus
somat/o-	body
sphincter/o-	sphincter muscle
spir/o-	coil, breathe
stern/o-	sternum
steth/o-	chest
sthen/o-	strength
stom/o-	opening, mouth
tact/o-	touch
tars/o-	ankle
tele/o-	distance
tempor/o-	time, temple of the head
tendon/o-	tendon
tetr/a-	four
tom/o-	cut
toxic/o-	poison
trache/o-	trachea
trich/o-	hair
urin/o-	urine
vagin/o-	female genital canal
vertebr/o-	vertebra
viscer/o-	viscera (internal organs)
vol/o-	volume
viscos/o-	thick
xen/o-	foreign
xer/o-	dry

TABLE 7-3 Common Prefixes

Prefix	Meaning	Example
a-, an-	without, lack of	apnea (without breath), asthenia (lack of strength, weakness), anemia (lack of blood)
ab-	away from	abnormal (away from the normal)
acr-	pertaining to extremity	acromegaly (enlargement of the bones of the distal parts)
ad-	to, toward	adhesion (something stuck to)
ante-	before, forward	antenatal (occurring or formed before birth)
anti-	against, opposed to	antipyretic (against fever)
auto-	self	autointoxication (poisoning by a toxin generated within the body)
bi-	two	bilateral (two-sided)
brady-	slow	bradycardia (slow heartbeat)
circum-	around, about	circumflex (winding around)
contra-	against, opposite	contralateral (on the opposite side)
di-	twice, double	diplopia (double vision)
dia-	through, completely	diagnosis (knowing completely)
dys-	with pain or difficulty	dyspnea (difficulty breathing)
e-, ex-	from, out of	excise (to cut out or remove completely or surgically)
ecto-	out from	ectopic (out of place)
em-	in	empyema (pus in the chest)
endo-	within	endometrium (within the uterus)
epi-	upon, on	epidermis (outer layer of skin)
eu-	normal, good	eupnea (normal breathing)
exo-	outside	exogenous (produced outside the body)
extra-	outside, in addition	extrasystole (premature contraction of the heart)
hemi-	half	hemiplegia (paralysis of one side of the body)
hyper-	excessive, above normal	hyperplasia (excessive formation)
hypo-	deficient, below normal	hypotension (low blood pressure)
in-	not	inferior (beneath or lower)
infra-	below	infrascapular (below the scapula)
inter-	between	intercostal (between the ribs)
iso-	equal	isotonic (having equal tension)
para-	by the side of	parathyroid (beside the thyroid)
per-	through	percutaneous (through the skin)
peri-	around	pericardium (fibroserous sac surrounding the heart)
poly-	many	polycystic (containing many cysts)
post-	after, behind	postpartum (after childbirth)
pro-	before	prognosis (forecast of the outcome of a disease)
quadri-	four	quadrant (quarter of an area)
retro-	backward	retroflexion (bending backward)
semi-	half	semiflexion (partial flexion)
sub-	below, less than	subacute (moderately sharp)
supra-	above	supraclavicular (above the clavicles)
sym-	with, together	symphysis (growing together)
tachy-	fast	tachycardia (fast heartbeat)
trans-	across	transfusion (pouring across)
tri-	three	tricuspid (have three cusps)
uni-	one	unilateral (one-sided)

TABLE 7-4 Common Suffixes

Suffix	Meaning	Example
-a	condition of	dyspnea (condition of difficulty in breathing)
-ac	pertaining to	insomniac (pertaining to insomnia, or lack of sleep)
-al	pertaining to	carpal (pertaining to the wrist)
-algia	pertaining to pain	neuralgia (pain along a nerve)
-ary	pertaining to	coronary (pertaining to the blood vessels that supply the heart muscle)
-blast	germ of immature cell	myeloblast (bone marrow cell)
-cele	tumor, hernia	enterocele (hernia of the intestine)
-centesis	puncturing	thoracentesis (puncture and draining of the pleural space)
-cyte	cell	leukocyte (white cell)
-eal	pertaining to	tracheal (pertaining to the trachea)
-ectomy	a cutting out	tonsillectomy (excision of the tonsils)
-emia	condition of the blood	hypoxemia (condition of low blood oxygen)
-emic	pertaining to the blood	hyperglycemic (pertaining to high blood sugar)
-gram	record or picture	electrocardiogram (electronic picture of heart activity)
-ic	pertaining to	psychic (pertaining to the mind)
-itis	inflammation	bursitis (inflammation of the bursae)
-logy	study of	ophthalmology (study of the eye)
-lysis	destruction or loosening	glycogenolysis (breakdown of glycogen to form glucose)
-meter	measuring instrument	oximeter (instrument that measures blood oxygen saturation)
-ostomy	creation of an opening	tracheostomy (artificial opening into the trachea)
-oma	tumor, swelling	neuroma (tumor of a nerve)
-osis	condition of	psychosis (a mental disorder)
-ous	pertaining to	fibrous (pertaining to fiber)
-pathy	disease	neuropathy (disease of the nervous system)
-plasty	surgical repair of, tying of	nephroplasty (suturing of a kidney)
-ptosis	falling, drooping	enteroptosis (falling of the intestine)
-rrhagia	excessive flow, bursting forth	hemorrhage (heavy flowing of blood)
-rrhea	flowing or discharge	rhinorrhea (runny nose)
-scope	instrument for examination	laryngoscope (instrument for visualization of the larynx)
-scopy	examination with an instrument	colonoscopy (instrumental examination of the colon)
-stasis	standing still	homeostasis (remaining the same)
-taxia	order, coordination	ataxia (failure of muscle coordination)

CHAPTER REVIEW

SUMMARY

It is essential to develop a foundation of knowledge of basic anatomy and physiology in order to better understand signs and symptoms patients will present with and the reasons for and effects of certain treatments you will administer. This basic understanding will assist you in determining what body systems are affected by an injury or illness and whether there are any potential life threats to that system. Also, knowing how the systems are interrelated will assist you in determining what areas of the body to assess when a patient has a particular complaint or injury.

Anatomical terms, planes, and lines will help you to better describe patient positioning and injuries to the body. Along with medical terminology, it will increase your ability to communicate effectively and professionally with other health care providers.

There are several body systems of which you must have a basic understanding: musculoskeletal, respiratory, circulatory, nervous, endocrine, integumentary (skin), digestive, urinary, and reproductive systems.

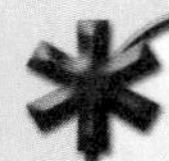

CASE STUDY FOLLOW-UP

SCENE SIZE-UP

You have been dispatched to the scene of a 38-year-old woman who was burned when the fuel for a model airplane ignited. By the time you arrive, the fire has been extinguished and the fuel and airplane no longer pose a threat.

PATIENT ASSESSMENT

Your general impression is that the patient is experiencing extreme pain from burns to her right arm and the right side of her head. When you question the patient, she responds appropriately with her name—Sherry Washington—and is able to describe what happened. Her airway and breathing are adequate. You assess circulation and start oxygen therapy before proceeding with the secondary assessment and care.

Upon examining the injury sites, you find that the entire right arm from the elbow to the fingertips has been severely charred from the burning fuel. The burns to the head are minor but fairly extensive, involving the right side of Ms. Washington's face and singeing to the hair, and you notice some swelling of the mucous membranes in the mouth and singeing of the nasal hair. Since burns to the mouth and nose can have serious effects on the airway and breathing, you are particularly careful to assess burns to her mouth and upper airway.

Pupils are equal and reactive to light. There are no other injuries noted to the head or neck. Breath sounds are equal bilaterally and the patient denies shortness of breath. You inspect the entire body for evidence of other burns. You find present pulses to all extremities, and the patient is able to move her extremities well.

While performing the physical exam, you also ask questions to gather the patient's history. The information you elicit is consistent with the burn injury. There is no other significant medical history.

Your partner readies the wheeled stretcher while you record the patient's vital signs. You find that blood pressure and heart rate are both slightly high while rate and depth of breathing are normal.

You gently place sterile burn sheets on the injury sites and try to help the patient relax as you and your partner prepare her for transport. You place her on the cot in a Fowler position, which she finds is comfortable and helps her to breathe more easily.

En route to the hospital you reassess the patient's mental status, airway, respiration, and circulation, and ensure that the burn sheets are properly protecting the burned skin. Ms. Washington remains alert. You reassess vital signs and record your findings.

COMMUNICATION AND DOCUMENTATION

You notify the hospital en route, describing the types and locations of the burns. You tell the staff that there is a full-thickness burn (through all layers of the skin) originating at the right elbow joint, which extends inferiorly and circumferentially to the distal fingers. The burn to the skull appears to be a superficial burn that involves the right cranium and face. The facial burn involves the lateral aspect of the right mandible, maxilla, and zygomatic arch. The emergency physician reminds you to stay alert to possible airway compromise from upper airway swelling as a result of the burns to the face.

When you arrive at the hospital, Ms. Washington is still alert and suffering severe pain but in no severe respiratory distress. You give a verbal report to the emergency department staff and help transfer the patient to a hospital bed. You and your partner then complete the prehospital care report, restock the ambulance, and prepare for another call.

Reflecting on this call, you are able to take pride in your ability to communicate clearly with the emergency department staff, and to document Ms. Washington's injuries in your prehospital care report, using correct anatomical terminology.

IN REVIEW

1. Describe the following six positions: normal anatomical position, supine, prone, lateral recumbent, Fowler, and Trendelenburg.
2. Define the following five descriptive terms: midline, midclavicular line, midaxillary line, plantar, and palmar. Also define the following five terms and name and define the opposite of each term: anterior, superior, dorsal, lateral, and distal.
3. Briefly describe the anatomy and physiology of the musculoskeletal system.
4. Briefly describe the anatomy and physiology of the respiratory system.
5. Briefly describe the anatomy and physiology of the circulatory system.
6. Identify the central and peripheral pulse points and their locations.
7. Define shock (hypoperfusion).
8. Briefly describe the anatomy and physiology of the nervous system.
9. Briefly describe the anatomy and physiology of the endocrine system.
10. Briefly describe the anatomy and physiology of the skin.
11. Briefly describe the anatomy and physiology of the digestive system.
12. Briefly describe the anatomy and physiology of the urinary or renal system.
13. Briefly describe the anatomy and physiology of the reproductive system for both the male and female.

CRITICAL THINKING

You arrive on the scene and find a 23-year-old male patient who has several stab wounds to the neck, the front of the chest on the right side, and the abdomen. He is screaming in pain. His breathing is 28 per minute and his radial pulse is weak and rapid. His skin is pale, cool, and clammy. His BP is 88/68 mmHg.

1. What body systems do you suspect could be injured by the knife wounds?
2. Pick a knife wound location on this patient's body and provide a brief description of the injury using medical terminology and anatomical terms as you would use them in your written EMS report.
3. What is causing the elevated heart rate?
4. What is causing the skin to be pale, cool, and clammy?
5. What is the significance of the systolic and diastolic blood pressure?

PEARSON

EXPLORE mybradykit™

Please go to **www.bradybooks.com** to access mykit for this text. You will find quizzes, critical thinking scenarios, weblinks, animations, and videos related to this chapter—and much more. Look for online information on identifying body systems as well as animations on the heart, endocrine system, and skeletal system.

Register your access code from the front of your book by going to **www.bradybooks.com** and selecting the mykit links.

PART 3

STANDARD

Pathophysiology

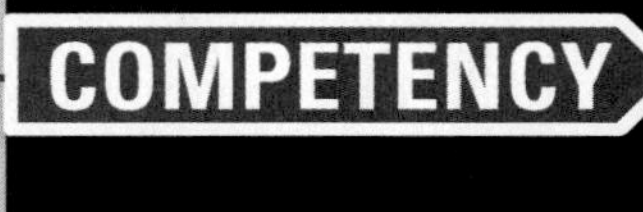

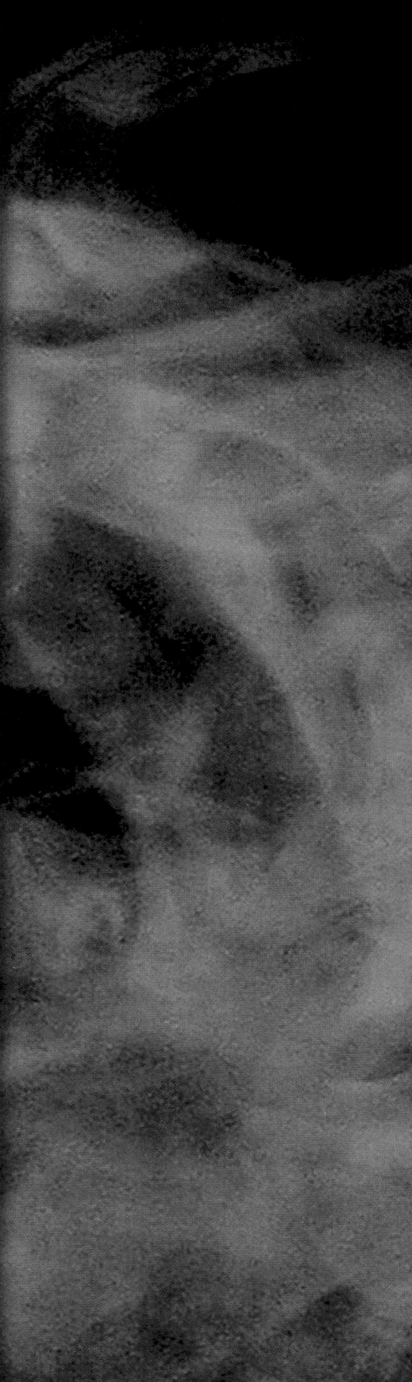

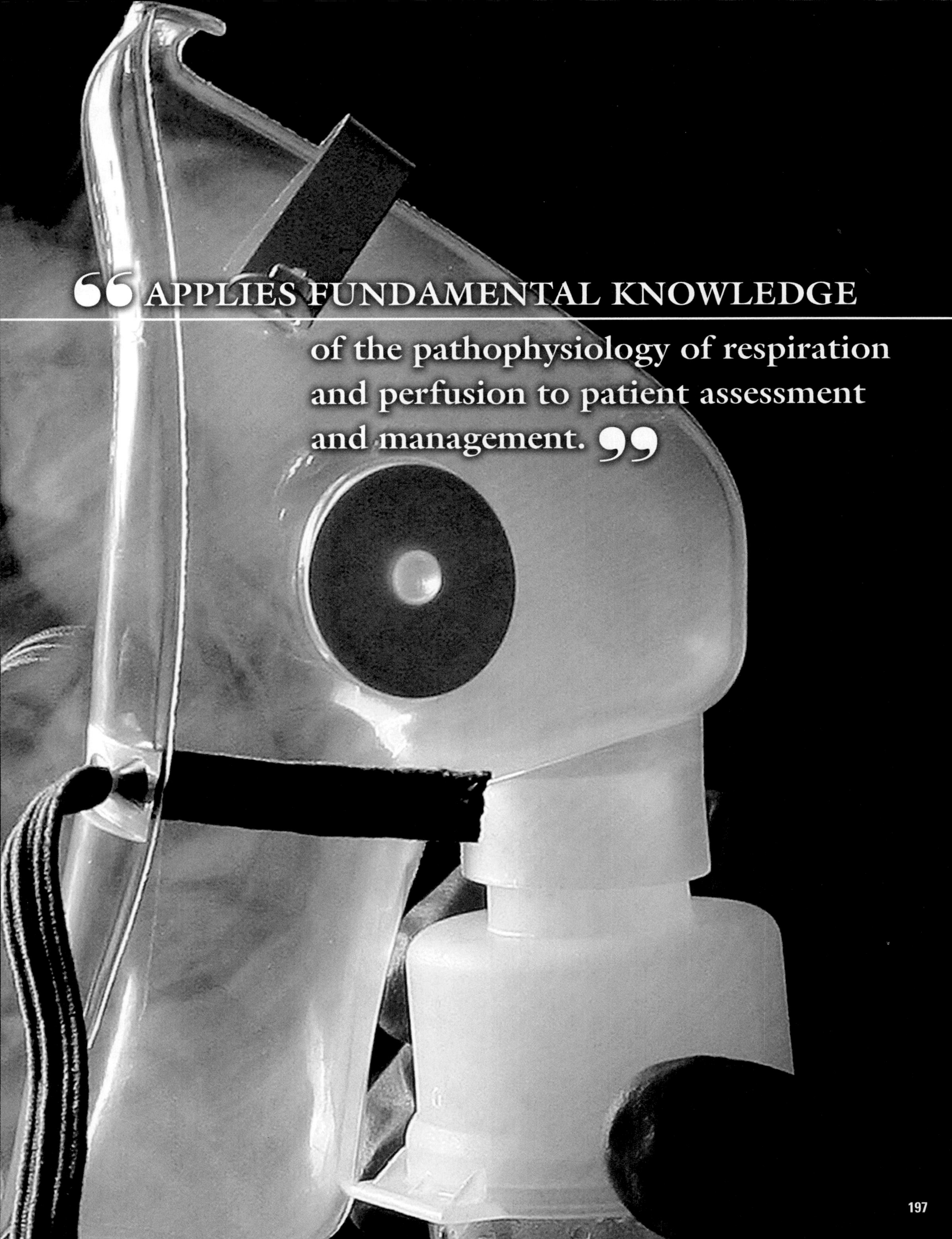
"APPLIES FUNDAMENTAL KNOWLEDGE
of the pathophysiology of respiration
and perfusion to patient assessment
and management."

CHAPTER 8

Pathophysiology

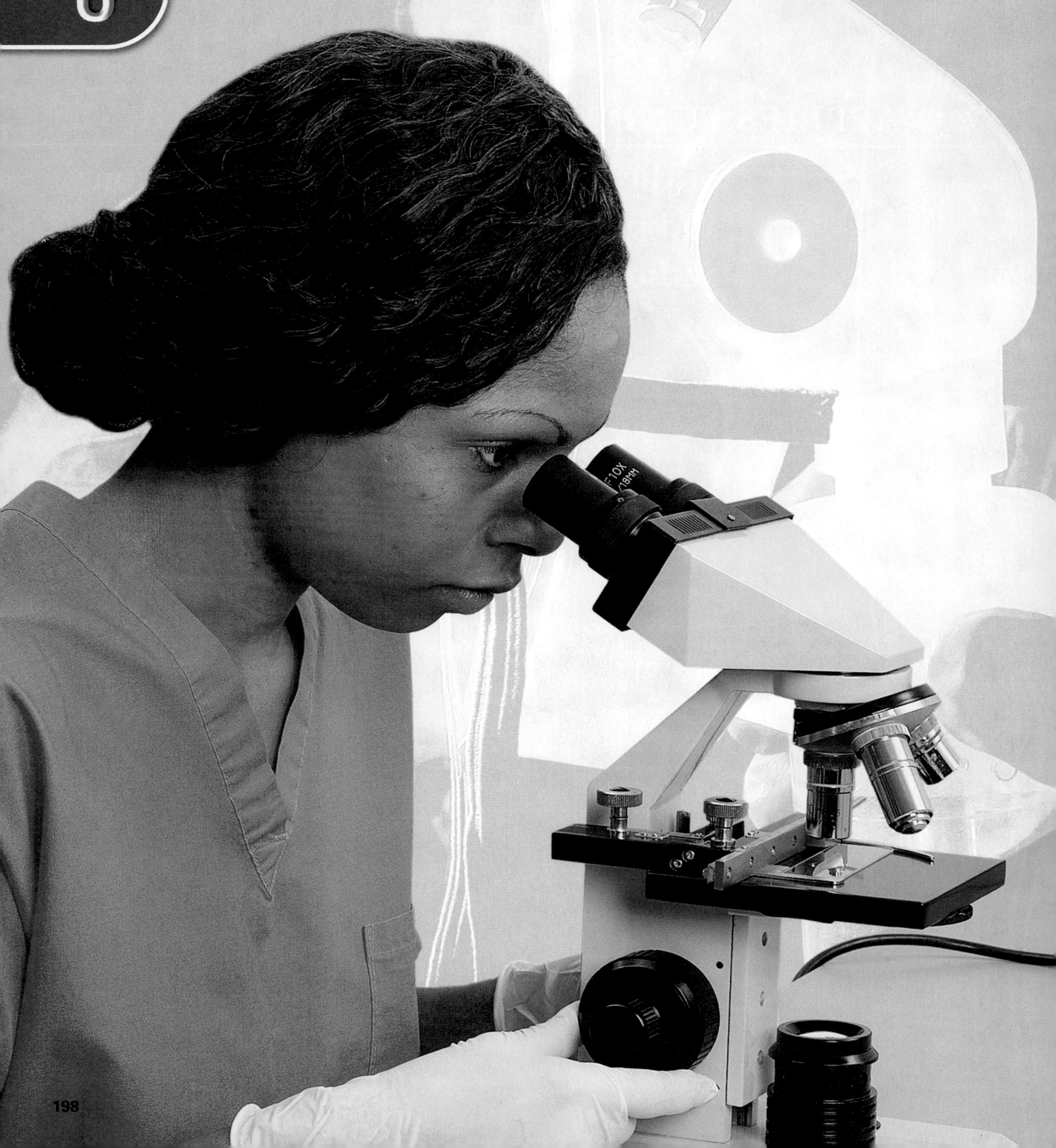

Navigation Guide

The following items provide an overview to the purpose and content of this chapter. The Standard and Competency are from the new National EMS Education Standards.

STANDARD **Pathophysiology**

COMPETENCY Applies fundamental knowledge of the pathophysiology of respiration and perfusion to patient assessment and management.

OBJECTIVES: After reading this chapter, you should be able to:

8-1. Define key terms introduced in this chapter.
8-2. Explain the importance of understanding basic pathophysiology.
8-3. Differentiate between the processes of aerobic and anaerobic cellular metabolism, including explanations of:
  a. The amount of ATP produced
  b. Removal of by-products of metabolism
8-4. Describe the consequences of failure of the cellular sodium/potassium pump.
8-5. Explain the concept of perfusion, including the physical and physiological components necessary to maintain perfusion.
8-6. Describe the composition of ambient air.
8-7. Apply the Boyle law to ventilation.
8-8. Explain how changes in compliance of the lungs and chest wall and changes in airway resistance affect ventilation.
8-9. Describe the consequences of loss of contact between the parietal and visceral pleura.
8-10. Explain the concept of minute ventilation.
8-11. Differentiate between minute ventilation and alveolar ventilation.
8-12. Describe the roles of chemoreceptors, lung receptors, and the nervous system in the control of ventilation.
8-13. Explain the concept of the ventilation/perfusion (VQ) ratio.
8-14. Describe the transport of oxygen and carbon dioxide in the blood.
8-15. Explain the exchange of gases across the alveolar/capillary membrane and the exchange of gases between capillaries and cells.
8-16. Describe the composition of blood, including the function of plasma and the formed elements.
8-17. Explain the effects of changes in hydrostatic pressure and plasma oncotic pressure on the movement of fluid between the circulatory system and interstitial spaces.
8-18. Discuss factors that affect cardiac output, including heart rate, stroke volume, myocardial contractility, preload, and afterload.
8-19. Describe the concept of systemic vascular resistance and its relationship to blood pressure and pulse pressure.
8-20. Summarize the local, neural, and hormonal factors that regulate blood flow through the capillaries.
8-21. Explain the regulation of blood pressure by baroreceptors and chemoreceptors.
8-22. Explain the relationship between ventilation, perfusion, and cellular metabolism.

KEY TERMS: Page references indicate first major use in this chapter. For complete definitions, see the Glossary at the back of the book.

aerobic metabolism p. 200
afterload p. 220
airway resistance p. 207
alveolar ventilation p. 208
anaerobic metabolism p. 201
apneustic center p. 212
baroreceptors p. 224
Boyle law p. 206
cardiac output p. 219
central chemoreceptors p. 210
chemoreceptors p. 210
compliance p. 207
dead air space (V_D) p. 208
deoxyhemoglobin p. 216
dorsal respiratory group (DRG) p. 212
Frank-Starling law of the heart p. 219
frequency of ventilation (f) p. 208
glycolysis p. 200
hydrostatic pressure p. 217
irritant receptors p. 211
J-receptors p. 211
laryngeal spasm p. 205
microcirculation p. 222
minute ventilation p. 208
minute volume p. 208
oxyhemoglobin p. 216
peripheral chemoreceptors p. 210
plasma oncotic pressure p. 218
pneumotaxic center p. 212
preload p. 219
respiratory control centers p. 212
stretch receptors p. 211
stroke volume p. 219
systemic vascular resistance p. 220
tidal volume (V_T) p. 208
ventilation/perfusion (V/Q) ratio p. 212
ventral respiratory group (VRG) p. 212

continued

Navigation Guide *continued*

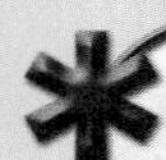

MEDIA RESOURCES: Please go to www.bradybooks.com to access mykit for this text. You will find quizzes, critical thinking scenarios, weblinks, animations, and videos related to this chapter—and much more. Look for online information on cardiac output and blood pressure. You will also find animations on Starling's law and the process of gas exchange.

CASE STUDY

The Dispatch

EMS Unit 204—respond to 143 Clovermeade Avenue—you have a 50-year-old male patient who has been stabbed by his wife —time out 2136 hours.

Upon Arrival

As you turn onto Clovermeade Avenue, you look for signs of the police and quickly note two police cars in the driveway of number 143. A police officer standing in the yard tells you that the victim's wife is in custody and the scene is safe to enter. As you get out of the ambulance, the daughter frantically yells to you, "My father was stabbed in the belly and he doesn't look good." She leads you to the enclosed back porch where you find the patient lying on his left side with blood soaking through his shirt in the area of his abdomen.

How Would You Proceed to Assess and Care for This Patient?

During this chapter, you will read a brief overview of the physiological function of the human body. Later, we will return to the case study and put in context some of the information you learned.

Introduction

One of the most fundamental purposes of emergency care is maintaining adequate perfusion of the body cells to ensure continuous delivery of oxygen and glucose and removal of waste by-products. These basic molecules—oxygen and glucose—are necessary for normal cell metabolism and function. Many illnesses and injuries can disturb the delivery of oxygen and glucose and removal of waste by-products. Understanding these disturbances will allow you to better recognize and explain why certain signs and symptoms occur and to comprehend the emergency care you will need to provide to the patient.

Cellular Metabolism

Cellular metabolism, also known as cellular respiration, is the process in which, normally, the body cells break down molecules of glucose to produce energy for the body. There are two types of cellular metabolism, aerobic and anaerobic, which will be discussed in the following sections. Which of these two types of cellular metabolism occurs is based on whether there is an effective and continuous delivery of oxygen and energy sources, or fuel. Glucose is the primary fuel, and oxygen is the primary catalyst for metabolism within the cell.

Aerobic Metabolism

Aerobic metabolism is the breakdown of molecules such as glucose through a series of reactions that produce energy within the cells *in the presence of oxygen*. (The term *aerobic* means "with oxygen.") When glucose crosses the cell membrane, it is broken down into pyruvic acid molecules. This process, known as **glycolysis**, occurs in the fluid portion of the cell (cytosol) and does not require oxygen. However, glycolysis releases only a small amount of adenosine triphosphate (ATP). ATP is an energy source that is required by the cell to release more energy and a necessity for cells to carry out certain functions, such as contraction of muscles. When oxygen is available, the reaction continues inside the mitochondria of the cell where the process releases a much larger amount of energy (ATP). This large amount of energy is necessary for normal cell function (Figure 8-1a✱).

Other by-products of aerobic metabolism include heat, carbon dioxide, and water. The heat produced is used to maintain a normal body core temperature. As you would expect, an increased metabolism results in in-

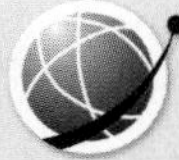

Media Resources

Go to www.bradybooks.com for mykit. Highlights:

- *Web Resource:* Frank Starling's Law and Heart Failure
- *Web Resource:* Blood Composition

Objective 8-2

Explain the importance of understanding basic pathophysiology.

Objective 8-3

Differentiate between the processes of aerobic and anaerobic cellular metabolism.

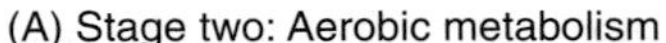

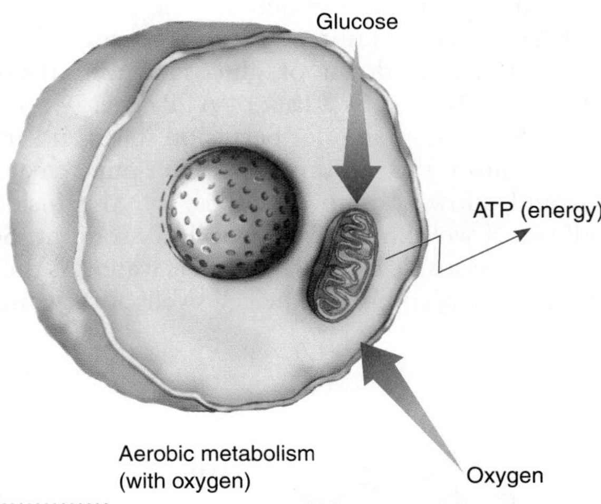

FIGURE 8-1a ✱ Aerobic metabolism. Glucose broken down in the presence of oxygen produces a large amount of energy (ATP).

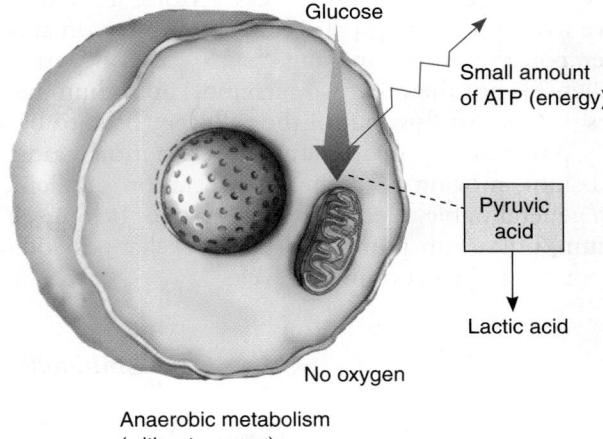

FIGURE 8-1b ✱ Anaerobic metabolism. Glucose broken down without the presence of oxygen produces pyruvic acid that converts to lactic acid and only a small amount of energy (ATP).

creased body core temperature. The carbon dioxide produced by metabolism is transported in the blood and blown off in the exhalation phase of normal respiration. An increase in metabolism results in an increase in the respiratory rate to eliminate the extra carbon dioxide. The water produced by metabolism is reabsorbed and used within the body or excreted. Thus, all of the products of aerobic metabolism are either used by the body or eliminated without causing any harm to the cells or to the patient, and a high amount of energy is made available to allow for normal body functions.

Anaerobic Metabolism

Anaerobic metabolism is the breakdown of molecules in the cells *without the presence of oxygen*. (The term *anaerobic* means "without oxygen.") Just as with aerobic metabolism, glucose crosses the cell membrane and normal glycolysis occurs with the production of pyruvic acid and the release of a small amount of ATP. Without the availability of oxygen, however, the pyruvic acid is not able to enter the next phase of metabolism and is converted to lactic acid. So the by-products of anaerobic metabolism are lactic acid and a small amount of ATP (Figure 8-1b✱).

If the acid is allowed to accumulate, it produces an acidic environment which may disturb its function and stability. High acid levels inactivate enzyme function, disrupt cell membranes, and ultimately lead to cell death. In addition, the cell has very little energy to perform its normal functions. Thus, an inadequate delivery of oxygen and glucose to cells will result in very little energy production, reduced cellular function, and the possibility of cellular damage.

Sodium/Potassium Pump Failure

One detrimental effect of anaerobic metabolism or the lack of glucose delivery to cells is related to the function of the sodium/potassium pump. Sodium and potassium are ions, that is, electrically charged molecules. Sodium (chemical symbol Na^+) is a positively charged ion that is found primarily in the fluid outside the cell, although some sodium is also found inside the cell. It is considered the primary extracellular ion. Potassium (chemical symbol K^+) is also positively charged and is considered the primary intracellular ion. That is, it is found primarily in the fluid on the inside of the cell but also exists outside the cell. Most body cells, to perform their special functions such as muscle contraction and nerve impulse transmission, require an alternating movement of sodium out of the cells and potassium into the cells, with these in-and-out cycles occurring continuously.

Key Terms

aerobic metabolism the breakdown of a molecule of glucose in the cell in the presence of oxygen to produce energy.

glycolysis the breakdown of glucose into pyruvic acid in the cells.

Key Terms

anaerobic metabolism lack of oxygen during the breakdown of a molecule of glucose in the cell, producing lactic acid and very little energy.

Objective 8-4

Describe the consequences of failure of the cellular sodium/potassium pump.

Sodium that is inside a cell wants to stay inside the cell where its concentration is less. (Molecules naturally move from an area of greater concentration to an area of lesser concentration—moving "*with* the concentration gradient"—not the other way around.) So sodium molecules do not just flow out of the cell; they have to be actively pumped out *against* the concentration gradient. Potassium, moving with the concentration gradient, is then generally able to enter the cell where it belongs. The sodium/potassium pump constantly exchanges sodium for potassium in a continuous cycle.

For the sodium/potassium pump to work, as with any other pump, energy is required. The energy is in the form of ATP which, as noted earlier, is released through glycolysis, the breakdown of glucose within the cells (Figure 8-2∗). If there is a lack of ATP/energy production by cells, as found in poor perfusion states and anaerobic metabolism, the sodium/potassium pump may fail. This would allow sodium to collect on the inside of the cell. As is well known, water follows sodium. So as sodium collects inside the cell, it attracts water. As the water continues to accumulate, the cell swells and eventually

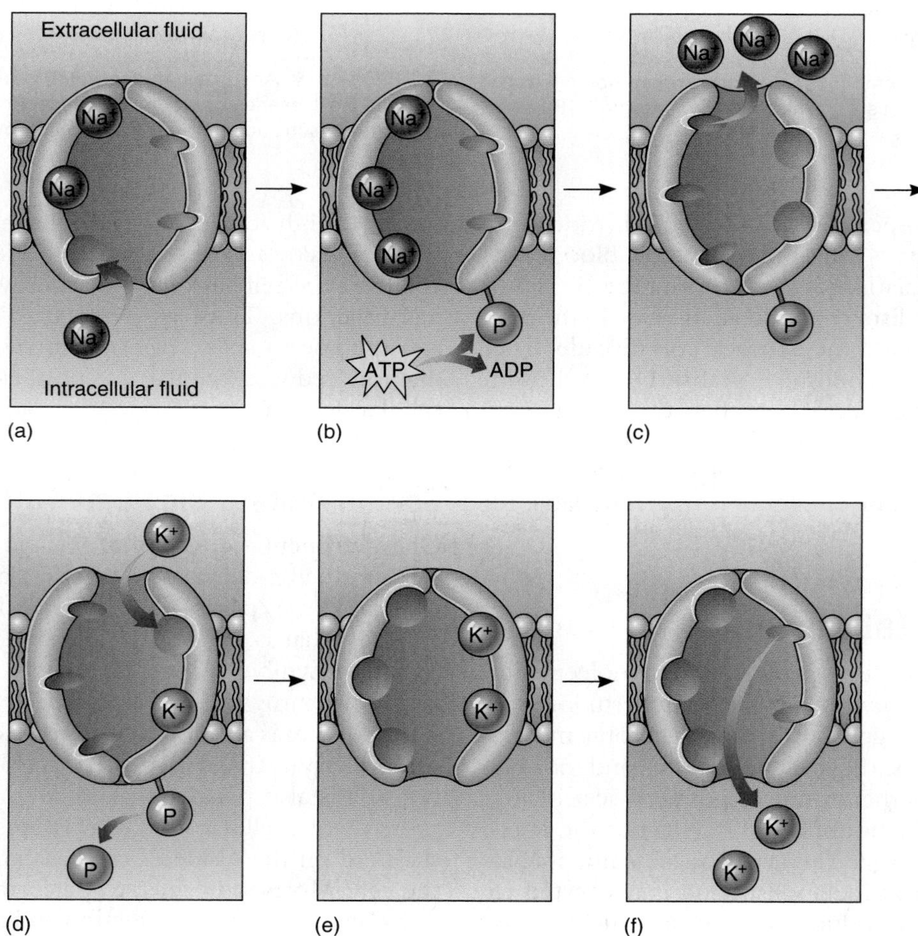

FIGURE 8-2 ∗ The sodium/potassium pump. Energy (ATP) is required to pump sodium molecules out of the cell against the concentration gradient. Potassium then moves with the gradient to flow into the cell. Sodium and potassium are exchanged in a continuous cycle that is necessary for proper cell function. The cycle continues as long as the cells produce energy through aerobic metabolism. When insufficient energy is produced, through anaerobic metabolism, the sodium/potassium pump will fail and cells will die.

Key Points

Poor perfusion has a chain of consequences: insufficient oxygen delivered to the cells→ anaerobic metabolism→insufficient ATP/energy production→sodium/potassium pump failure→ sodium accumulation inside cells→swelling of cells→rupture of cells→cell death.

Objective 8-5

Explain the concept of perfusion, including the physical and physiological components necessary to maintain perfusion.

Objective 8-6

Describe the composition of ambient air.

ruptures and dies. Thus the end result of a lack of energy to run the pump is cell death.

The effect on the cell of failure of the sodium/ potassium pump is an example of how a lack of adequate delivery of oxygen and glucose to cells can lead to cell death and organ failure. It is also an example of why maintaining delivery of oxygen and glucose to the cells and elimination of waste products from the cells is a fundamental purpose of emergency care for any patient.

Components Necessary for Adequate Perfusion

Perfusion can be described as the delivery of oxygen, glucose, and other substances to the cells and the elimination of waste products from the cells. In order to maintain adequate perfusion, the components of the delivery and removal system must work properly. These components (each of which will be discussed in the following sections) are:

- Composition of ambient air
- Patent airway
- Mechanics of ventilation
- Regulation of ventilation
- Ventilation/perfusion ratio
- Transport of oxygen and carbon dioxide by the blood
- Blood volume
- Pump function of the myocardium
- Systemic vascular resistance
- Microcirculation
- Blood pressure

An alteration in any one of these components may lead to poor cellular perfusion with an inadequate delivery of oxygen or glucose to the cell or inadequate elimination of carbon dioxide and other waste products. Inadequate perfusion can shift cells from aerobic to anaerobic metabolism, reduce the production of energy needed for normal cell function, produce harmful by-products, and allow waste products to accumulate. Therefore, your emergency care will focus on establishing and maintaining each of these components to ensure continuous adequate cellular perfusion and aerobic metabolism.

As an example, establishing and maintaining a patent (open) airway will allow adequate amounts of oxygen-rich air to enter the alveoli of the lungs. If the airway is not patent, the amount of oxygen-rich air available in the alveoli will be reduced. Blood passing through the adjoining capillaries will pick up less oxygen and will then deliver less oxygen to the cells. If the amount of oxygen is reduced significantly, the cells will shift from aerobic to anaerobic metabolism. Anaerobic metabolism will reduce the amount of ATP (energy) produced for normal cell function and will begin to produce lactic acid as a by-product, both of which will adversely affect normal cell and organ function and may eventually lead to cell and organ death.

Composition of Ambient Air

The concentration of oxygen in the ambient air will determine the proportion of oxygen molecules that end up in the alveoli to be available for gas exchange with the blood. A lesser proportion of oxygen in the blood means less oxygen for cells to use for metabolism.

Ambient air at sea level contains approximately 79 percent nitrogen, 21 percent oxygen, 0.9 percent argon, and 0.03 percent carbon dioxide. There are trace amounts of other gases. The partial pressures of these gases are found in Table 8-1. The partial pressures of the gases will be discussed later in the chapter.

If the patient is in an environment low in oxygen, such as an enclosed space with toxic gases, the reduced oxygen concentration will result in cellular hypoxia. It is important to ensure that the concentration of oxygen the patient is breathing is at least 21 percent.

Increasing the concentration of oxygen in breathed air will increase the number of oxygen molecules in the alveoli, the blood, and the cells. Thus, one way to improve cellular oxygenation is by increasing the concentration of

TABLE 8-1 Partial Pressure of Gases in Ambient Atmosphere at Sea Level

Gas	%	Partial Pressure
Oxygen	21	159 mmHg
Nitrogen	79	597 mmHg
Argon	0.9	7 mmHg
Carbon Dioxide	0.03	0.3 mmHg

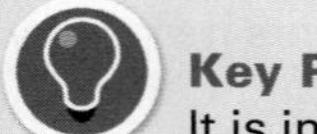

Key Points
It is important to ensure that the concentration of oxygen the patient is breathing is at least 21 percent.

Key Points
One of the most basic and important aspects of any emergency care is to establish and maintain a patent airway.

oxygen in the air breathed in by the patient. This can be achieved by increasing the FiO_2, which is the fraction of inspired oxygen. An FiO_2 is expressed as a fraction or decimal and not a percentage. A patient breathing ambient air that contains 21 percent oxygen would have an FiO_2 of 0.21. A nonrebreather mask can deliver an FiO_2 of approximately 0.95, which is an oxygen concentration of approximately 95 percent. An FiO_2 of 1.0 would be equal to inspiration of a 100 percent oxygen concentration.

An FDO_2 is a fraction of delivered oxygen. The difference between an FiO_2 and an FDO_2 is that the FiO_2 is administered to a patient who is breathing spontaneously and inhaling the air on his own effort; whereas the FDO_2 is delivered by a ventilation device to a patient who is not able to breathe adequately on his own. The concept is the same, though, and FiO_2 is typically used in place of FDO_2. FDO_2 is rarely used. If you are ventilating the patient with a bag-valve-mask device connected to a reservoir with oxygen flowing at 15 lpm, you are likely delivering an oxygen concentration of approximately 95 to 98 percent, or an FDO_2 of 0.95 to 0.98. Both FiO_2 and FDO_2 are numbers you are most likely to encounter when transporting patients from one medical facility to another who are either on a ventilator or require manual ventilation or supplemental oxygen during the transport.

Some toxic gases displace the amount of oxygen in the air and basically suffocate the patient. Other gases, such as carbon monoxide, disrupt the ability of the blood to carry adequate amounts of oxygen to the cells. In either condition, the cells end up hypoxic.

Some toxic gases may not severely reduce the concentration of oxygen in the air or disrupt the ability of the blood to carry oxygen but may interfere with its use by the cell. One example is cyanide poisoning. The patient may be breathing in an adequate percentage of oxygen, and the oxygen is adequately transported to the cells, but the cyanide prevents the oxygen from being used effectively by the cells. In this case, the alveoli and blood have adequate amounts of oxygen; nevertheless, the cells become severely hypoxic.

Patency of the Airway

One of the most basic and important aspects of any emergency care provided is to establish and maintain a patent airway. A patent airway is one that is open and not obstructed by blood, secretions, vomitus, tissue, bone, teeth, or any other substance. Establishing an open airway is typically one of the first steps in emergency care. In some cases, it may be the only care necessary to treat the patient in the prehospital setting. Failure to recognize, establish, or maintain a patent airway—as already noted—will lead to reduced oxygen concentration breathed in, cellular hypoxia, and eventual patient death.

An airway obstruction can occur at several anatomical levels in both the upper and the lower airway including the nasopharynx, oropharynx, posterior pharynx, epiglottis, larynx, trachea, and bronchi (Figure 8-3*).

Nasopharynx

An obstruction may occur to the nasopharynx by blood, secretions, vomitus, tissue swelling, bone fragments, or other substances. This usually does not pose a major airway problem if the oropharynx remains clear. However, the nasopharynx opens into the pharynx, which leads to the larynx, the trachea, and eventually the lungs. Blood, vomitus, or other substances that occlude the nasopharynx may drain into the pharynx and lead to aspiration or occlusion. Thus, it is important to keep the nasopharynx clear to prevent potential aspiration. In addition, if you are unable to gain access to the oropharynx because of a fractured mandible or clenched teeth, the nasopharynx can be used as an alternative location to establish an airway. Infants are obligate nose breathers; thus it is imperative to keep the nasopharynx clear in these patients.

Oropharynx and Pharynx

The oropharynx and pharynx can be obstructed by the tongue, foreign bodies, tissue swelling, hematomas, blood, vomitus, and other substances. Any obstruction must be removed immediately. Liquid substances such as blood or vomitus can easily be aspirated (breathed into the lungs) from the oropharynx and pharynx. Aspirated substances like vomitus may damage the lung tissue or fill the alveoli and interfere with gas exchange. Blockage of airflow in the oropharynx and pharynx or aspiration of liquid substances will lead to a decreased alveolar oxygenation and a reduced delivery of oxygen to cells, leading to cellular hypoxia.

Epiglottis

The epiglottis is a flap of cartilaginous tissue that covers the opening of the larynx, known as the glottic opening, during swallowing. If the epiglottis is injured and swells

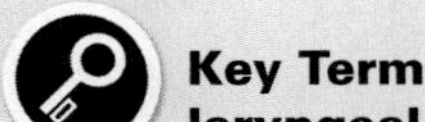

Key Terms
laryngeal spasm a contraction of the vocal cords that causes them to close and prevents air from passing through into the trachea.

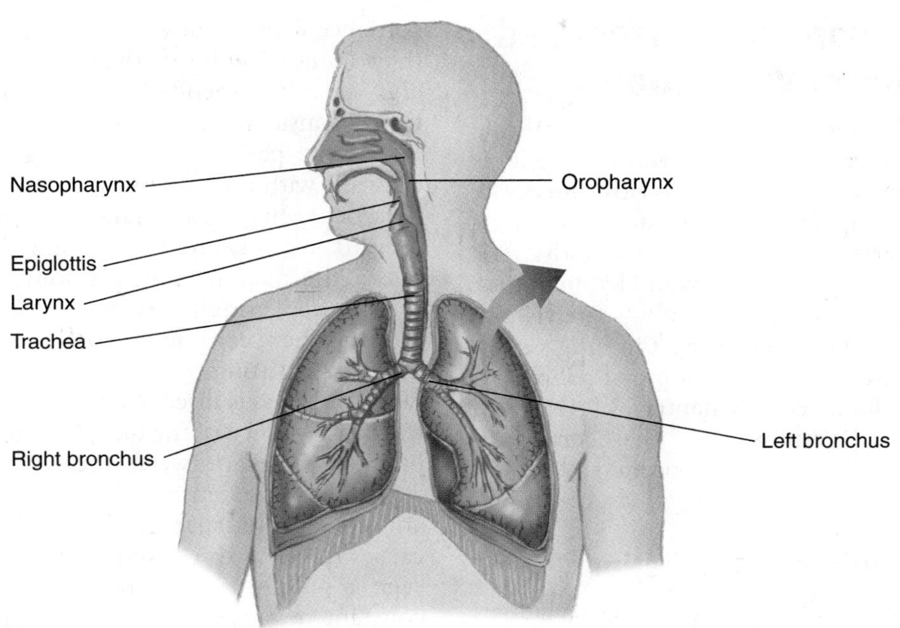

FIGURE 8-3 ✱ Airway obstruction can occur at several levels of the upper and lower airway, including the nasopharynx, oropharynx, posterior pharynx, epiglottis, larynx, trachea, and bronchi.

or becomes inflamed from infection, it can occlude the airway at the level of the larynx. The epiglottis is flexible tissue; thus, it may fall over the glottic opening when the muscles controlling the tongue relax and become flaccid. A jaw-thrust or chin-lift maneuver is designed to lift the epiglottis clear of the glottic opening. If there is obstruction from swelling or inflammation, advanced airway management may be required to establish a patent airway.

Larynx

The larynx is the structure that contains the vocal cords. The anterior portion is composed of the thyroid cartilage, which is the prominent "Adam's apple" often seen in males. The most inferior portion is the cricoid cartilage, a completely circumferential cartilaginous ring. The adult has a cylindrical airway, and the narrowest portion of the upper airway in the adult is at the level of the vocal cords. A child less than 8 years of age, however, has a cone-shaped airway with the narrowest portion at the cricoid ring.

The larynx can be obstructed by **laryngeal spasm**, also called *laryngospasm*, where the vocal cords spasm and close together, which prevents any air from passing through into the trachea. This may result from injury, insertion of mechanical airways, or administration of some medications. A fracture to the larynx may cause the laryngeal structures to lose stability and be drawn inward, creating an obstruction. Any obstruction at the level of the larynx will prevent airflow into the trachea and lungs, leading to a reduced amount of oxygen in the alveoli, which results in poor oxygen levels in the blood and cellular hypoxia.

Trachea and Bronchi

The larynx opens into the trachea, which extends downward and bifurcates at the carina. The carina is located at the second intercostal space (angle of Louis) anteriorly or the fourth thoracic vertebra posteriorly. The trachea is composed of anterior cartilaginous rings that are C-shaped with a soft, flexible muscle on the posterior aspect. The trachea bifurcates into the right mainstem bronchus and left mainstem bronchus. Obstruction of the trachea and bronchi by secretions, blood, vomitus, food particles, objects, tissue, swelling, bone, or other substances blocks airflow to the bronchioles, which supply the alveoli with oxygenated air. This reduces the concentration of oxygen in the alveoli, which in turn reduces gas exchange and the amount of oxygen transported by the blood to the cells, leading to cellular hypoxia.

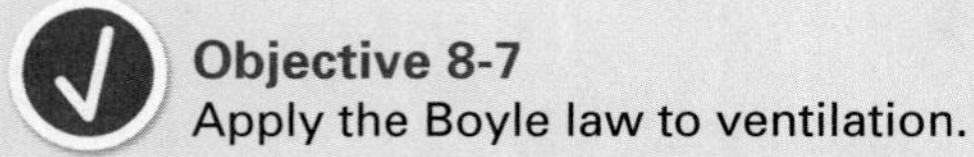
Objective 8-7
Apply the Boyle law to ventilation.

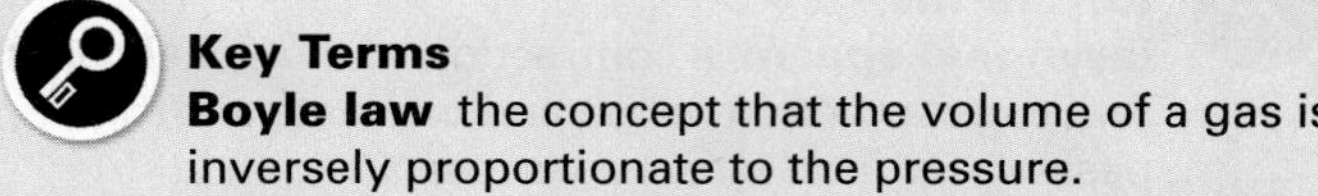
Key Terms
Boyle law the concept that the volume of a gas is inversely proportionate to the pressure.

Respiratory Compromise Associated with Mechanics of Ventilation

The integrity of the thoracic cavity plays an integral role in maintaining normal ventilation. The thoracic cavity is formed by the neck muscles and first two ribs superiorly; diaphragm inferiorly; muscles, ribs, and sternum anteriorly; and muscles, vertebrae, and ribs posteriorly. It is divided by the mediastinum into a right and left hemithorax. The lungs are covered by a pleural lining. The visceral pleura is the innermost lining covering the lung tissue; the parietal pleura is the outermost lining that adheres to the thoracic wall. As discussed in Chapter 7, "Anatomy, Physiology, and Medical Terminology," these structures are necessary for normal ventilation to occur.

The Boyle Law Applied to Ventilation

Ventilation is a mechanical process that relies on changes in pressure inside the thorax to move air in and out of the lungs. The alterations in pressure occur as a result of changes to the size of the thorax. Ventilation conforms to the **Boyle law,** which states that the volume of gas is inversely proportionate to the pressure. It can be quickly summarized as follows:

An increase in pressure (more positive) will decrease the volume of gas.

A decrease in pressure (more negative) will increase the volume of gas.

Increasing the size of a closed container will decrease the internal pressure (create a negative pressure) by creating a partial vacuum. The vacuum may be thought of as "sucking air into the container." More accurately, it is the higher pressure outside that pushes air into the container, increasing the volume of gas. Conversely, decreasing the size of a container will increase the internal pressure (create a positive pressure) and force air out, decreasing the volume of gas.

By contracting the diaphragm (the muscle that provides approximately 60 to 70 percent of the effort of inhalation) and the external intercostal muscles, the diaphragm moves slightly downward while the ribs are lifted upward and outward. This causes the thorax to increase in size, creating a negative pressure. Normal atmospheric pressure is 760 mmHg at sea level. With the expansion of the thorax immediately prior to inhalation, the pressure inside the chest drops to 758 mmHg. In accordance with the Boyle law, this negative pressure causes the volume of air inside the chest to increase. Because energy must be expended to contract the muscles, inhalation is considered an active process.

As the parietal pleural lining is pulled upward and outward with the expansion of the chest wall, the serous fluid between the two linings also pulls the visceral lining upward and outward. (This pulling by the serous fluid between the pleural linings is sometimes called a "water glass" effect, similar to the surface tension created by moisture between the bottom of a glass and the surface the glass is sitting on, which will tend to lift the surface when the glass is lifted.) The visceral lining is attached to the outer surface of the lung; therefore, when the visceral lining is pulled outward, the lung is forced to expand. The natural tendency of the lung, however, is to recoil and collapse because of the elasticity of its tissue. This causes the lung to constantly pull inward as the thoracic cage is pulling it outward. This opposite pull creates a constant negative pressure, or a vacuum, in the pleural space (the space between the pleura).

After inhalation, the diaphragm and external intercostal muscles relax, allowing the chest wall to move inward and downward and, assisted by the inward pull of the elastic lung tissue, decrease the size of the thoracic cavity. As the size of the thorax decreases, the pressure inside increases to about 761 mmHg at sea level, which causes air to be forced out of the lungs. Because this process is brought about by the relaxation of muscles, with no energy expenditure, exhalation is considered a passive process.

Accessory Muscles

Use of accessory muscles (in addition to the diaphragm and intercostal muscles that are normally used for inhalation) may be required either to help increase the chest size to draw more air into the chest and lungs, or to help decrease the chest size to force air out of the lungs and chest. (The accessory muscles of inhalation are listed in Table 8-2.) Contracting the accessory muscles uses more energy than normal. Keep in mind that adequate amounts of oxygen must be constantly delivered to the cells to produce energy. A patient who needs to use accessory muscles to inhale may already be experiencing a lack of oxygen delivery and energy production. If the patient lacks the energy needed to contract both regular and accessory muscles of inhalation, the respiratory muscles will begin to fail. This will result in inadequate ventilation,

Key Terms

compliance the measure of the ability of the chest wall and lungs to stretch, distend, and expand.

airway resistance the restriction of airflow that is related to the diameter of the airways.

Objective 8-8
Explain how changes in compliance of the lungs and chest wall and changes in airway resistance affect ventilation.

Objective 8-9
Describe the consequences of loss of contact between the parietal and visceral pleura.

TABLE 8-2 Accessory Muscles

Accessory Muscles of Inhalation

The following accessory muscles of inhalation are used to increase the size of the thoracic cavity and generate a greater negative pressure, increasing the flow of air into the lungs.

- *Sternocleidomastoid muscles* lift the sternum upward.
- *Scalene muscles* elevate ribs 1 and 2.
- *Pectoralis minor* muscles elevate ribs 3 to 5.

Accessory Muscles of Exhalation

The following accessory muscles of exhalation are used to decrease the size of the thoracic cavity and to create a more positive pressure, forcing air out of the lungs.

- *Abdominal muscles* contract and increase the pressure inside the abdominal cavity, forcing the diaphragm to move higher against the lungs.
- *Internal intercostal muscles* contract and pull the sternum and ribs downward.

which will compound the patient's problems with a further decrease in oxygen delivery to cells.

Accessory Muscles of Exhalation Exhalation is normally a passive process, requiring no expenditure of energy. However, if the patient is struggling to expel air from the lungs, the accessory muscles of exhalation may be used to create more positive pressure in the chest. (The accessory muscles of exhalation are listed in Table 8-2.) If the accessory muscles are used, exhalation becomes an active process, requiring energy. If the patient is also using accessory muscles and additional energy to inhale, the extra energy needed for exhalation may cause the respiratory muscles to fatigue, leading to respiratory failure.

A bellows is a device that pushes air out through a narrow opening when its sides are squeezed together and draws air in when its sides are pulled apart. The movement of air during ventilation relies on what is often called a bellows action of the chest. An injury or illness that interferes with that bellows action will impede the ability of the chest to create the pressure changes necessary to draw air into the lungs and force air out of the lungs. An injury that keeps the chest from expanding properly, such as compression, multiple rib fractures, or severe chest wall injury, will lead to a reduced creation of negative pressure inside the chest, reduced air volume drawn in to the lungs, and less oxygen made available for gas exchange. This will eventually lead to cellular hypoxia.

Compliance and Airway Resistance

Two conditions that may require the use of accessory muscles to generate a greater force to fill and empty the lungs are higher airway resistance and poor compliance. **Compliance** is a measure of the ability of the chest wall and lungs to stretch, distend, and expand. A condition that would cause the lungs or chest wall to become stiff would decrease compliance. A decrease in compliance would make it more difficult for the patient to move air in and out of the lungs. This also would make it more difficult for you to ventilate the patient artificially. Conditions such as pneumonia and pulmonary edema (discussed in Chapter 16, "Respiratory Emergencies") decrease compliance within the lungs. Structural problems with the chest wall can also lead to poor compliance, for example a flail segment where two or more ribs are fractured in more than one place (discussed in detail in Chapter 34, "Chest Trauma") or neuromuscular diseases affecting the ability of the chest muscles to contract.

Airway resistance is related to the ease of airflow down the conduit of airway structures leading to the alveoli. A higher airway resistance makes it more difficult to move air through the conducting airways; a lower airway resistance makes it easier to move air. Higher airway resistance requires the patient to work harder to breathe, expending more energy and possibly using accessory muscles, which may accelerate respiratory muscle fatigue and failure. The most common cause of increased airway resistance is edema (swelling) within the airway structure. Mucus and constriction of the bronchioles will also decrease the radius of the airway and increase resistance.

Poor compliance and higher airway resistance may lead to less air available in the alveoli for gas exchange. This will result in less oxygen in the blood that is delivered to the cells, potentially resulting in cellular hypoxia.

Pleural Space

The potential space between the pleura maintains a negative pressure. If a break occurs in the continuity of either the parietal pleura from an open wound to the thorax or to the visceral pleura from an injury to the lung tissue, the negative pressure will draw air into the pleural space. With each

Key Terms
minute ventilation the amount of air moved in and out of the lungs in one minute. Also called **minute volume.**

tidal volume (V_T) the volume of air breathed in with each breath.

Key Terms
frequency of ventilation (f) the number of ventilations in one minute.

Objectives 8-10 and 8-11
Explain and differentiate between minute ventilation and alveolar ventilation.

inhalation, the thorax increases its size and the pleural pressure becomes more negative. This draws even more air into the pleural space, increasing its volume and collapsing the lung. Lung collapse severely interferes with the ability of the alveoli to fill with air and to create an interface with the pulmonary capillaries, which reduces gas exchange with the blood and leads to hypoxia. This is why occluding any open wound to the chest is done very early in the primary assessment of a patient, as you will learn later.

Minute Ventilation

Minute ventilation, also known as **minute volume**, is the amount of air moved in and out of the lungs in one minute. It is determined by multiplying the tidal volume by the frequency of ventilation in one minute. The **tidal volume (V_T)** is the volume of air breathed in with each individual breath. The **frequency of ventilation (f)** is generally calculated as the number of ventilations in one minute. The formula is:

$$\textbf{Minute ventilation} = \textbf{tidal volume } (\mathbf{V_T}) \times \textbf{frequency of ventilation (f/minute)}$$

An average-sized adult has a tidal volume of approximately 500 mL and breathes approximately 12 times per minute at rest. Thus, the minute ventilation for an average-sized adult would be calculated as:

$$\textbf{Minute ventilation} = \textbf{500 mL} \times \textbf{12/minute}$$
$$\textbf{Minute ventilation} = \textbf{6,000 mL or 6 L/minute}$$

An average-sized adult moves approximately 6,000 mL or 6 L of air in and out of the lungs in one minute. You will not be expected to measure or calculate the minute ventilation in the prehospital environment. The importance of understanding the calculation of minute ventilation is summarized in the following points:

- A decrease in tidal volume will decrease the minute ventilation.
- A decrease in frequency of ventilation will decrease the minute ventilation.
- A decrease in minute ventilation will reduce the amount of air available for gas exchange in the alveoli.
- A decrease in minute ventilation can lead to cellular hypoxia.
- To ensure adequate ventilation, the patient must have *both* an adequate tidal volume *and* an adequate rate of ventilation.

A patient may increase his frequency of ventilation to compensate for a decrease in tidal volume in order to maintain an adequate minute ventilation. As an example, an average-sized person is hypoventilating as a result of a low tidal volume of only 200 mL. If the patient maintains a ventilatory rate of 12/minute, the minute ventilation would be:

$$\textbf{Minute ventilation} = \textbf{200 mL} \times \textbf{12/minute}$$
$$\textbf{Minute ventilation} = \textbf{2,400 mL or 2.4 L/minute}$$

A minute ventilation of 2,400 mL or 2.4 liters/minute for this average-sized adult is 3,600 mL (6,000 mL – 2,400 mL = 3,600 mL) or 3.6 liters/minute less than normal, resulting in a significantly decreased amount of air moved during one minute of ventilation. This would most likely lead to a reduced amount of air in the alveoli, decreased gas exchange, and cellular hypoxia.

One way to compensate for a decreased minute ventilation is to increase the ventilatory rate. If the patient just described increases his ventilatory rate to 28 breaths/minute, the minute ventilation would be:

$$\textbf{Minute ventilation} = \textbf{200 mL} \times \textbf{28/minute}$$
$$\textbf{Minute ventilation} = \textbf{5,600 mL or 5.6 L/minute}$$

With a tidal volume of 200 mL and a ventilatory rate of 28/minute, it appears as if the minute ventilation is near the normal of 6,000 mL or 6 liters/minute. However, even though the minute ventilation appears to be near normal in this patient example, severe hypoxia may still occur as a result of a small amount of air actually getting to the alveoli for gas exchange. Increasing the frequency of ventilation may improve the amount of air moved in and out of the respiratory tract in one minute; however, if the tidal volume is too low, an adequate amount of air may never make it completely down to the alveoli for gas exchange but will instead remain in the trachea and major bronchi.

Alveolar Ventilation

Alveolar ventilation is the amount of air moved in and out of the alveoli in one minute. The key in this definition is specifically the amount of air moving in and out of the *alveoli*—unlike minute ventilation where the calculation is concerned only with air movement in and out of the respiratory tract and lungs.

Alveolar ventilation is related to the concept of anatomical dead air space. **Dead air space (V_D)** consists

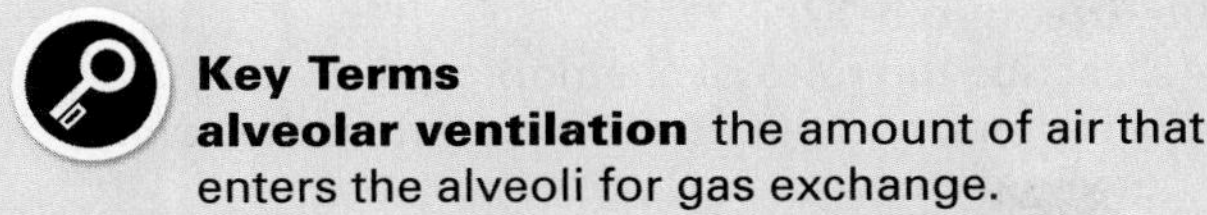

Key Terms
alveolar ventilation the amount of air that enters the alveoli for gas exchange.

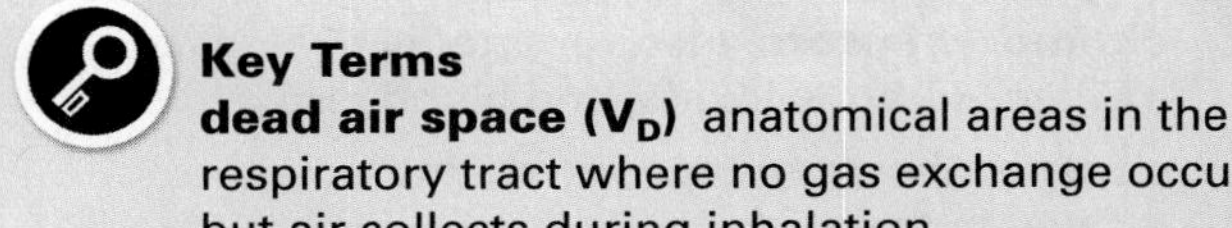

Key Terms
dead air space (V_D) anatomical areas in the respiratory tract where no gas exchange occurs but air collects during inhalation.

of anatomical areas in the respiratory tract where air collects during inhalation—areas where, however, no gas exchange occurs. Thus, the air that moves in and out of these areas is not involved in gas exchange and is wasted. In the average-sized adult, approximately 150 mL of the tidal volume is lost in the dead air space. Thus, of the 500 mL of air breathed in, only 350 mL reaches the alveoli for gas exchange. The equation is:

Alveolar ventilation = (tidal volume − dead air space) × frequency of ventilation/minute

Alveolar ventilation = ($V_T - V_D$) × f/minute

The alveolar ventilation for an average-sized adult with a tidal volume of 500 mL breathing at a rate of 12/minute would be calculated as follows:

Alveolar ventilation = (500 mL − 150 mL) × 12/minute

Alveolar ventilation = 4,200 mL or 4.2 L/minute

This calculation reveals that of the 6,000 mL or 6 liters/minute breathed in and out (minute ventilation), only 4,200 mL or 4.2 liters/minute reach the alveoli for gas exchange. Approximately 1,800 mL or 1.8 liters/minute of air fills the dead air space and is not used in gas exchange. This explains why exhaled air contains an oxygen concentration of 17 to 18 percent when the person is breathing in 21 percent oxygen. The oxygen in air that reaches the alveoli passes into the bloodstream and is replaced with waste carbon dioxide that passes from the blood into the alveoli. The question, therefore, is why there is any oxygen at all in exhaled air. The answer is that the air initially exhaled was not involved in gas exchanges because it was housed in the dead air spaces and still contains the higher concentrations of oxygen. This also explains how mouth-to-mouth ventilation provides an adequate amount of oxygen from the exhalation of the person providing the ventilation.

With alveolar ventilation, just as was true with minute ventilation, tidal volume and frequency of ventilation affect the amount of air from each ventilation that ends up in the alveoli. A reduction in tidal volume may dramatically reduce the alveolar ventilation, even when the patient increases the frequency of ventilation in order to compensate. Using the earlier example, it was found that if the patient began to hypoventilate with a tidal volume of 200 mL per breath but increased his rate of ventilation to 28/minute, his minute ventilation was near normal; however, he was very prone to hypoxia. Consider his alveolar ventilation in the following equation:

Alveolar ventilation = (200 mL − 150 mL) × 28/minute

Alveolar ventilation = 1,400 mL or 1.4 L/minute

Recall that his average normal alveolar ventilation was 4,200 mL or 4.2 liters/minute. Although he more than doubled his ventilatory rate, he is only getting 1,400 mL or 1.4 liters/minute of air into his alveoli for gas exchange. This occurs because the dead air space fills first, regardless of the volume breathed in with each ventilation. This leaves very little volume of air to reach the alveoli where gas exchange occurs, causing a dramatic reduction in the amount of oxygen in the blood and resulting in cellular hypoxia. This patient requires positive pressure ventilation so that more air can be forced into his alveoli to improve gas exchange. If you were to put this patient on supplemental oxygen only, you would not increase the amount of air getting into the alveoli. The air in the dead air space would be enriched with oxygen, but it might be exhaled from the lungs without ever reaching the alveoli.

The key points to consider with alveolar ventilation are:

- The patient may begin to breathe faster to move more air in and out of the thorax; however, that does not mean he is getting more oxygen into his alveoli for gas exchange.
- The dead air spaces will fill first regardless of the volume of air breathed in and the amount made available to the alveoli.
- To improve gas exchange in the patient with an inadequate tidal volume, you must provide positive pressure ventilation to move more air into the alveoli.
- By simply placing a patient with an inadequate tidal volume on oxygen, you will not improve ventilation or reverse the cellular hypoxia.
- Assessing the tidal volume is as important as assessing the ventilatory rate.

Understanding minute ventilation and alveolar ventilation should help you understand the relationship between the tidal volume and ventilatory rate. Inadequate ventilation and cellular hypoxia can occur from:

- A low tidal volume
- A ventilatory rate that is too slow
- A ventilatory rate that is too fast

Key Terms

chemoreceptors monitor arterial content of oxygen, carbon dioxide, and blood pH.

central chemoreceptors chemoreceptors located in the medulla.

Key Terms

peripheral chemoreceptors chemoreceptors located in the aortic arch and the carotid bodies.

Objective 8-12

Describe the roles of chemoreceptors, lung receptors, and the nervous system in the control of ventilation.

A low tidal volume will decrease the alveolar ventilation by not putting enough air into the alveoli with each breath. A ventilatory rate that is too slow will not provide enough air in the alveoli for adequate gas exchange. A ventilatory rate that is too fast can cause two problems: (1) the rate is so fast that it doesn't allow the lungs adequate time between breaths to fill, reducing the tidal volume; and (2) a very fast rate requires a large amount of energy and muscular workload that may not be able to be sustained, setting the patient up for respiratory failure. Ventilatory rates of 40/minute or greater in the adult patient and greater than 60/minute in the pediatric patient are too fast to be sustainable or to allow adequate time for a normal tidal volume.

Regulation of Ventilation

Breathing is mostly an involuntary process that is controlled by the autonomic nervous system to maintain normal gas exchange. Receptors within the body constantly measure the amount of oxygen (O_2), carbon dioxide (CO_2), and hydrogen ions (pH) and send signals to the brain to adjust the rate and depth of respiration (Figure 8-4*). You do have some voluntary control over your breathing that allows you to hold your breath and alter your breathing pattern during talking, laughing, and singing. Primary involuntary control is through the respiratory center located in the brain stem, which sends out stimulatory impulses to the respiratory muscles.

Chemoreceptors

Chemoreceptors are specialized receptors that monitor the pH, carbon dioxide, and oxygen levels in arterial blood. There are two groups of chemoreceptors: central and peripheral.

Central Chemoreceptors The **central chemoreceptors** are located near the respiratory center in the medulla. These receptors are most sensitive to carbon dioxide and changes in the pH of the cerebrospinal fluid (CSF). The pH is a measurement of hydrogen ion concentration. (The abbreviation *pH stands for "potential of hydrogen."*) The pH in CSF is a direct reflection of the carbon dioxide level of the arterial blood. The carbon dioxide is able to cross over the blood-brain barrier and into the CSF. Once it is in the CSF, it combines with water (H_2O) to form carbonic acid. Thus, you can consider the following association between CO_2 and acid:

The greater the amount of CO_2 in the blood, the greater the amount of acid.

The lesser the amount of CO_2 in the blood, the lesser the amount of acid.

A molecule of carbonic acid consists of carbon, oxygen, and hydrogen atoms from the CO_2 and H_2O that combined to create the acid. The hydrogen ions dissociate from the carbonic acid and stimulate the central chemoreceptors. The central chemoreceptors are very sensitive to changes in the pH (hydrogen ion content) of CSF. Even small changes will stimulate a response in the rate and depth of breathing. Faster, deeper breathing blows off more CO_2 during exhalation. Slower, shallower breathing blows off less CO_2. The response of ventilation to stimulation by the central chemoreceptors from changes in CO_2 can be summarized as follows:

An increase in arterial CO_2 will increase the number of hydrogen ions in the CSF, stimulating an increase in the rate and depth of respiration to blow off more CO_2.

A decrease in arterial CO_2 will decrease the number of hydrogen ions in the CSF, causing a decrease in the rate and depth of respiration to blow off less CO_2.

Peripheral Chemoreceptors The **peripheral chemoreceptors** are located in the aortic arch and the carotid bodies in the neck. These chemoreceptors are also somewhat sensitive to CO_2 and pH but are most sensitive to the level of oxygen in the arterial blood. As the level of oxygen in the blood decreases, the peripheral chemoreceptors signal the respiratory center in the brain stem to increase the rate and depth of respiration. It takes a significant decrease in the arterial oxygen content to trigger the peripheral chemoreceptors to stimulate the respiratory center. The activity of the peripheral chemoreceptors can be summarized this way:

A significant decrease in the arterial oxygen content will cause an increase in the rate and depth of respiration to increase the content of oxygen in the blood.

Stimulation by the central chemoreceptors and the peripheral chemoreceptors together has a greater influence on the rate and depth of ventilation than stimulation from either one by itself.

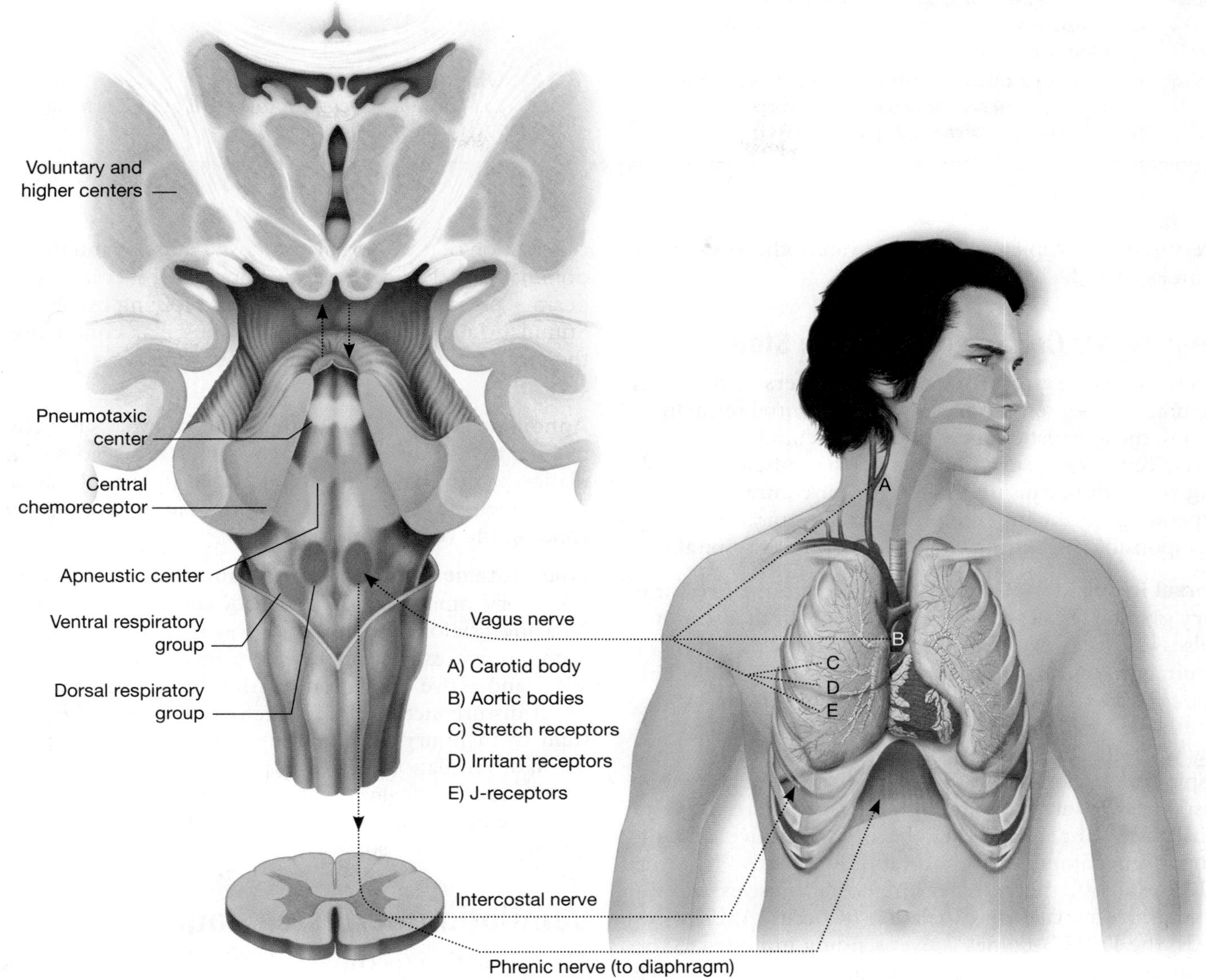

FIGURE 8-4 ✱ Respiration is controlled by the autonomic nervous system. Receptors within the body measure oxygen, carbon dioxide, and hydrogen ions and send signals to the brain to adjust the rate and depth of respiration.

Hypoxic Drive Normally, a person's rate and depth of breathing are regulated primarily by the amount of carbon dioxide in the blood. This is referred to as a *hypercapnic* or *hypercarbic drive.*

The situation is different for patients with chronic obstructive pulmonary disease (COPD), such as emphysema. These patients have a tendency to retain carbon dioxide in arterial blood as a result of their poor gas exchange. When the arterial CO_2 level is chronically elevated, the central chemoreceptors become insensitive to the small changes that typically stimulate ventilation. The peripheral chemoreceptors then become the primary stimulus for ventilation; instead of a small increase in carbon dioxide level being a strong stimulus for ventilation, the peripheral chemoreceptors rely on a decrease in the oxygen level to stimulate ventilation. Hypoxia becomes the stimulus for ventilation in place of hypercarbia. This is known as *hypoxic drive.*

Lung Receptors

There are three types of receptors within the lungs that provide impulses to regulate respiration. These are irritant receptors, stretch receptors, and J-receptors.

Irritant Receptors **Irritant receptors** are found in the airways and are sensitive to irritating gases, aerosols, and particles. Irritant receptors will stimulate a cough, bronchoconstriction, and an increased ventilatory rate.

Stretch Receptors **Stretch receptors** are found in the smooth muscle of the airways and measure the size and volume of the lungs. These receptors stimulate a decrease in the rate and volume of ventilation when stretched by high tidal volumes to protect against lung overinflation.

J-Receptors **J-receptors** are found in the capillaries surrounding the alveoli and are sensitive to increases in

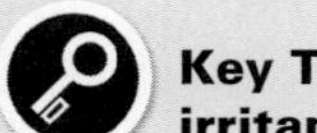

Key Terms
irritant receptors, stretch receptors, J-receptors receptors in the lungs that help to regulate respiration.

respiratory control centers in the brainstem include the **dorsal respiratory group (DRG)** and the **ventral respiratory group (VRG)**.

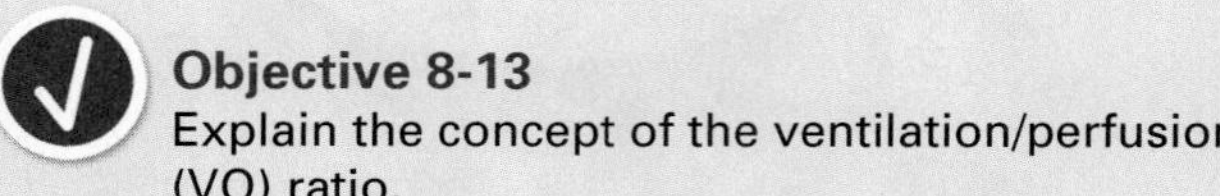

Objective 8-13
Explain the concept of the ventilation/perfusion (VQ) ratio.

pressure in the capillary. When activated, the J-receptors stimulate rapid, shallow ventilation.

Respiratory Centers in the Brain Stem

There are four **respiratory control centers** in the brain stem: the dorsal respiratory group, the ventral respiratory group, the apneustic center, and the pneumotaxic center. These centers transmit impulses to the muscles controlling ventilation, causing them to either contract or relax, depending on the impulse. The dorsal respiratory group is responsible for setting the basic rhythm of respiration.

Dorsal Respiratory Group (DRG) The **dorsal respiratory group (DRG)** has inspiratory neurons that send impulses to the external intercostal muscles and the diaphragm, causing them to contract, which results in inhalation. The DRG functions in every respiratory cycle, whether during quiet breathing or during forced breathing with the accessory muscles involved. In a typical respiratory cycle, the DRG stimulates the external intercostal muscles and diaphragm for 2 seconds, resulting in inhalation. The DRG then becomes inactive and no longer sends impulses for a total of 3 seconds. With the DRG shut off, the external intercostal muscles and diaphragm relax, causing exhalation to occur. After 3 seconds, the DRG becomes active, sending impulses to the respiratory muscles that cause inhalation to occur once again. The process continues to repeat itself.

Ventral Respiratory Group (VRG) The **ventral respiratory group (VRG)** has both inspiratory and expiratory neurons and is basically inactive during regular quiet ventilation. The VRG becomes active when an increase in ventilatory effort is necessary. The VRG inspiratory (VRG_I) neurons control the accessory muscles, such as the scalene, pectoralis minor, and sternocleidomastoid muscles that are involved in maximal inhalation. The VRG expiratory (VRG_E) neurons stimulate muscles involved in forced or active exhalation, such as the internal intercostal and abdominal muscles.

In forced inhalation, the DRG stimulates the external intercostal muscles and diaphragm to contract to their maximal level and the VRG_I stimulates the accessory muscles to contract to further increase the size of the thorax and the inspiratory effort. At the end of inhalation, both the DRG and VRG_I stop sending impulses to the muscles. The respiratory muscles relax and exhalation occurs.

In forced exhalation, as the DRG and VRG_I cease stimulation, the VRG_E becomes active and stimulates contraction of the internal intercostal muscles and the abdominal muscles, decreasing thorax size, increasing the positive pressure inside the chest, and forcing exhalation. Stimulation by the VRG_E causes muscular contraction; therefore, exhalation becomes an active process under its control.

Apneustic Center The **apneustic center** does not control the rhythm of ventilation; however, it provides stimulation to the DRG and VRG_I to intensify the inhalation. The apneustic center may prolong the inspiration, increasing the ventilation volume.

Pneumotaxic Center The **pneumotaxic center** sends inhibitory impulses to the apneustic center to turn off the inhalation before the lungs are too full. It can promote both passive exhalation by shutting off the DRG and VRG_I and active exhalation by stimulating the VRG_E.

A disturbance to the respiratory centers in the brain stem from injury or illness may alter the pattern and depth of ventilation. This may produce inadequate ventilation and abnormal ventilatory patterns that may impede adequate gas exchange and promote cellular hypoxia, requiring ventilatory support.

Ventilation/Perfusion Ratio

The **ventilation/perfusion (V/Q) ratio** describes the dynamic relationship between the amount of ventilation the alveoli receive and the amount of perfusion through the capillaries surrounding the alveoli. This relationship determines the quality of gas exchange across the alveolar-capillary membrane, which influences the amount of oxygen entering the blood and the amount of carbon dioxide exiting the blood. The dynamic relationship between ventilation and perfusion in the lungs can be used to explain the etiology (causes) of hypoxemia, or inadequate oxygen concentrations in the blood (Figure 8-5∗).

In the ideal lung, each alveolus would receive an adequate amount of ventilation and a matching amount of blood flow through the surrounding capillary, resulting in a V/Q ratio that is equal. This ideal condition never exists because of the effects of gravity on blood flow, the structure of the lungs, and shunting of blood.

With an individual in a standing position, gravity pulls the lungs downward toward the diaphragm, compressing the lower lobes. As the lower lobes are compressed and blood is pulled down to the bases of the lungs, air travels upward to the apexes (tops) of the lungs and increases the residual volume. Interestingly, the alveoli in the apexes of

Key Terms

apneustic center the respiratory center in the brain stem that intensifies and prolongs inhalation.

pneumotaxic center located in the brain stem, it sends inhibitory impulses to the apneustic center to turn off the inhalation before the lungs are too full.

Key Terms

ventilation/perfusion (V/Q) ratio the dynamic relationship between the amount of ventilation the alveoli receive and the amount of perfusion through the capillary surrounding the alveoli.

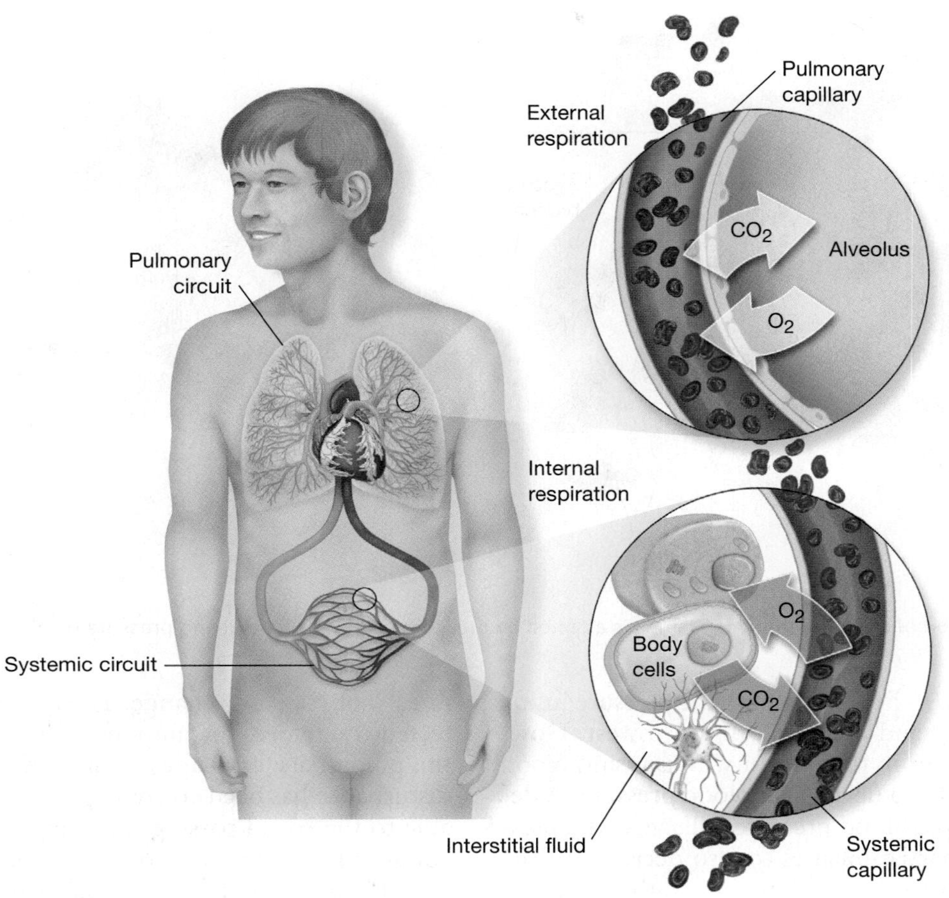

FIGURE 8-5 ✱ Overview of ventilation and perfusion.

the lungs have a greater residual volume of air, are larger, and have a higher surface tension, but they are fewer in number as compared to other areas of the lungs. These larger alveoli in the apexes have a higher surface tension, which makes them less compliant and harder to inflate during ventilation. Thus, the tidal volume is shifted to the lower lobes where the lung is more compliant and there is less surface tension. Because gravity pulls the blood downward, less pressure is required to perfuse the lower lobes of the lungs as compared to the apexes. As a result, the bases of the lungs receive a greater amount of blood and are much better perfused than the apexes. This is a desirable condition, since the greatest amount of ventilation also exists in the base of the lungs.

The ventilation/perfusion ratio is never at an ideal state in any zones of the lungs. In the apexes, the amount of available ventilation in the alveoli exceeds the amount of perfusion through the pulmonary capillaries; that is, there is more oxygen available in the alveoli than the supply of blood is able to pick up and transport. This is considered to be wasted ventilation. In the bases, the amount of perfusion exceeds the amount of ventilation; this means there is more blood moving through the pulmonary capillaries than there is alveolar oxygen available for it to pick up. This is considered to be wasted perfusion. Overall, under normal conditions, perfusion exceeds the amount of available ventilation.

Pressure Imbalances

The perfusion of blood through the pulmonary capillaries is affected by the amount of air and pressure inside the alveoli and the pressure of the blood flowing through the capillary bed (Figure 8-6✱). If the pressure in an alveolus exceeds the blood pressure in the capillary bed, blood flow through the capillary stops. This is most likely to

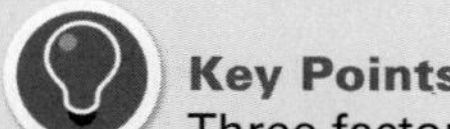

Key Points
Three factors can upset the ideal ventilation/perfusion ratio: pressure imbalances, ventilatory disturbances, and perfusion disturbances.

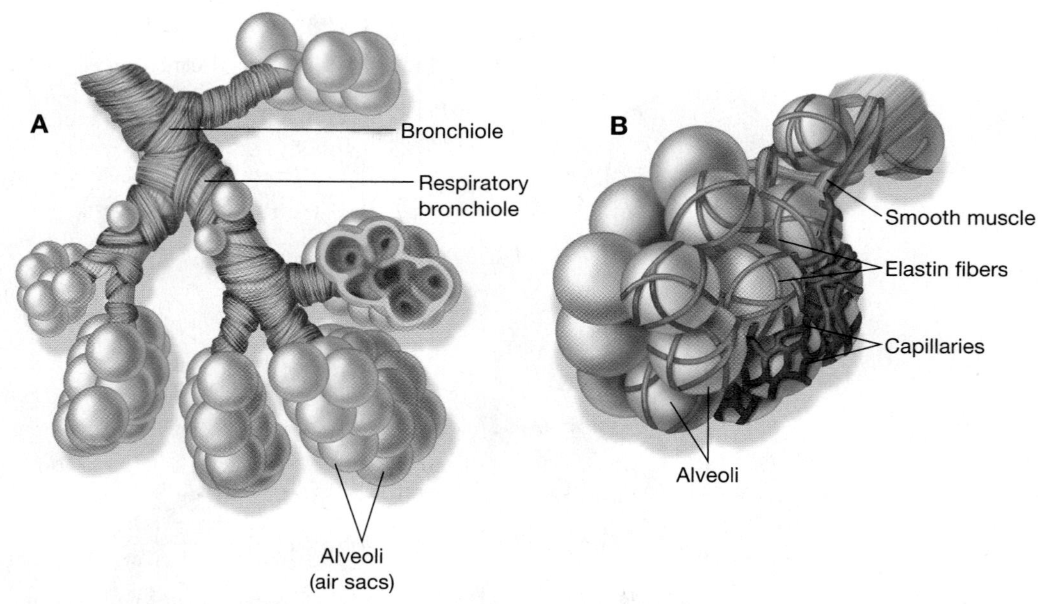

FIGURE 8-6 ✱ Perfusion of the pulmonary capillaries is affected by pressure within the alveoli and pressure within the capillaries.

occur in the apexes of the lungs where the pressure inside the alveoli is highest and the blood flow is lowest. However, it may also occur in the patient who is losing blood from an injury and has a decreasing blood pressure. A decrease in the systemic blood pressure will cause the pressure in the pulmonary capillaries to also decrease. If the patient does not have a chest or lung injury, the lungs will continue to receive adequate volumes of air, creating adequate pressure in the alveoli. However, the reduction in blood pressure may allow the alveolar pressure to exceed the pulmonary capillary pressure and impede blood flow. This will result in poor pulmonary perfusion, hypoxemia (reduced oxygen concentrations in the blood), and cellular hypoxia (oxygen deficiency in the cells).

Ventilatory Disturbances

A disturbance on the ventilation side of the ventilation/perfusion ratio can lead to hypoxia. If a condition or injury causes less oxygenated air to be available in the alveoli for the amount of blood flowing through the pulmonary capillaries, the end result will be less oxygen saturating the blood and less oxygen delivered to the cells, creating hypoxemia and cellular hypoxia. As an example, if a patient is having an asthma attack and the bronchioles are inflamed and constricted, the restricted airways reduce airflow and provide less oxygenated air to the alveoli for gas exchange. The blood pressure is not affected; therefore, the amount of blood passing through the pulmonary capillaries remains normal. A ventilation disturbance has been created by making less oxygen available to the blood passing through the capillaries. In this condition, there is wasted perfusion, since the blood is available but there is an inadequate amount of oxygen to be picked up. This disturbance in ventilation leads to hypoxemia and cellular hypoxia.

In the situation just described in which an asthma attack has caused a ventilatory disturbance, you must improve the ventilation side of the ventilation/perfusion ratio by relieving the bronchiole airway restriction and increasing the amount of oxygenated air entering the alveoli. An EMT would achieve this by placing the patient on oxygen and administering a medication to dilate the bronchioles to improve airflow. This treatment would not only increase the amount of air in the alveoli, it would also increase the concentration of oxygen in the alveolar air, making more oxygen available for the blood moving through the pulmonary capillaries. This would reduce or eliminate the hypoxemia and cellular hypoxia.

Perfusion Disturbances

A perfusion disturbance may also lead to severe cellular hypoxia. Consider a patient you encounter who has cut

Key Points
Managing hypoxia from a ventilatory disturbance should focus on improving ventilation and oxygenation. Managing hypoxia from a disturbance in perfusion must focus on increasing blood flow, hemoglobin availability, and delivery of oxygen to the cells.

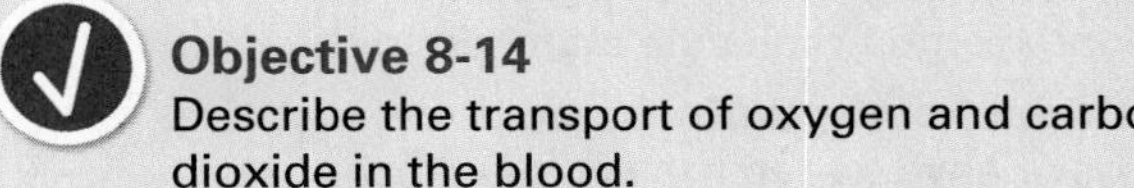

his radial artery on a saw and suffered severe blood loss. The patient has no chest or lung injury and has an increased rate and depth of ventilation. His minute ventilation and alveolar ventilation are increased; however, his cells are becoming hypoxic. Although he is moving more oxygenated air into the alveoli, his blood loss has significantly reduced the amount of blood flow through the pulmonary capillaries. This represents a perfusion disturbance, because there is not enough blood to pick up the oxygen available in the alveoli. This would create a state of wasted ventilation, hypoxemia, and cellular hypoxia. By placing the patient on oxygen, you might reduce some of the cellular hypoxia; however, it will not be eliminated until the perfusion disturbance is fixed. The bleeding must be stopped, and this patient needs to receive fluid and blood to increase the flow and pressure in the pulmonary capillaries so there is enough hemoglobin available for oxygen in the alveoli to attach to and be transported to the cells.

Hypoxia generally results from a ventilation or perfusion disturbance. A myriad of conditions can cause one of these disturbances to occur. The management of hypoxia resulting from a ventilatory disturbance should focus on improving ventilation and oxygenation. Managing a disturbance in perfusion must focus on increasing blood flow through the pulmonary capillaries, the availability of hemoglobin, and delivery of oxygen to the cells.

Transport of Oxygen and Carbon Dioxide in the Blood

Oxygen must be continuously delivered by the blood to the cells in order for normal cellular metabolism to occur. Carbon dioxide, a by-product of aerobic metabolism, must be carried back to the lungs to be blown off in exhalation. A disturbance in the transport system may lead both to cellular hypoxia, a lack of oxygen available to the cells, and to hypercarbia, a buildup of carbon dioxide in the blood. Both hypoxia and hypercarbia pose problems for normal cellular function and stability.

Both oxygen and carbon dioxide are transported by the blood, but in different ways (Figure 8-7∗). It is important to remember that oxygen and carbon dioxide move from areas of higher concentration to areas of lower concentration. This helps explain the movement of gas molecules between alveoli and capillaries and between capillaries and cells.

Oxygen Transport

Approximately 1,000 mL of oxygen is delivered to the cells every minute. Oxygen is transported by the blood in two ways: dissolved in plasma and attached to hemoglobin. A small amount, only 1.5 to 3 percent, is dissolved in plasma. The majority of oxygen, approximately 97 to 98.5 percent, is attached to hemoglobin molecules.

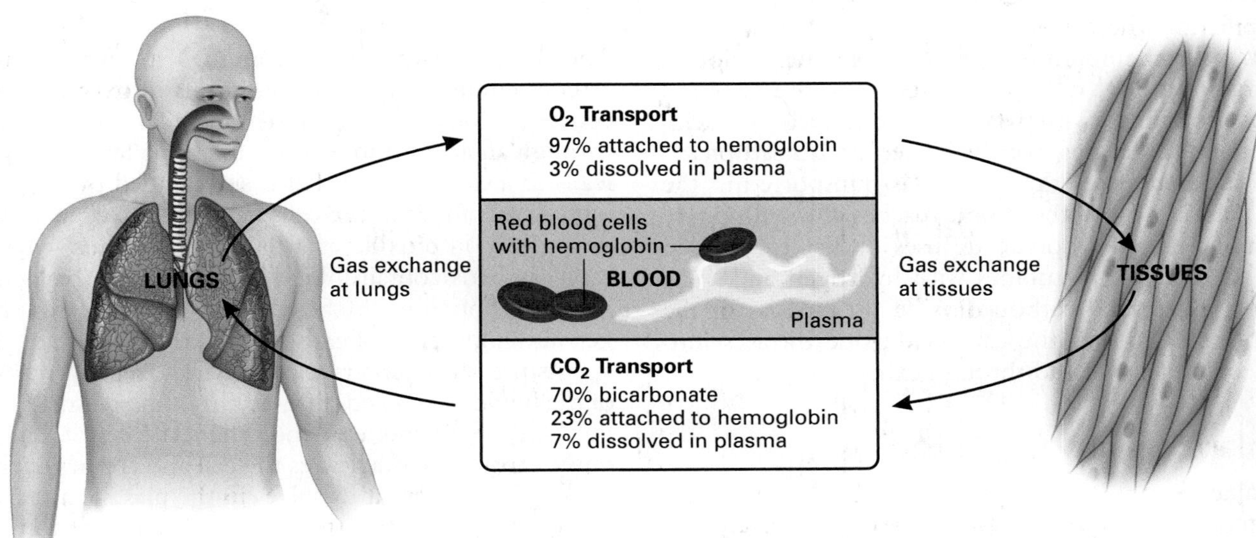

FIGURE 8-7 ∗ Oxygen is transported in the blood two ways: attached to hemoglobin and dissolved in plasma. Carbon dioxide is transported in the blood three ways: as bicarbonate, attached to hemoglobin, and dissolved in plasma.

Key Terms

oxyhemoglobin hemoglobin that has at least one oxygen molecule attached to it.

deoxyhemoglobin hemoglobin that does not have any oxygen molecules attached to it.

Objective 8-15

Explain the exchange of gases across the alveolar/capillary membrane and the exchange of gases between capillaries and cells.

Hemoglobin is a protein molecule that has four iron sites for oxygen to bind to. Thus, one hemoglobin molecule could carry up to four oxygen molecules. If one oxygen molecule is attached to the hemoglobin molecule, it is considered to have 25 percent saturation. Attachment of two oxygen molecules would be considered 50 percent saturation, three molecules 75 percent saturation, and four molecules 100 percent saturation. The attachment of one oxygen molecule to a hemoglobin iron binding site will increase the affinity for the other sites to also bind with oxygen.

Once an oxygen molecule binds with hemoglobin, it is referred to as **oxyhemoglobin**. A hemoglobin molecule that has no oxygen attached is referred to as **deoxyhemoglobin**. Without hemoglobin, the negligible amount of oxygen that can be transported by plasma would not be enough to sustain normal cellular function or life. A loss of hemoglobin, which commonly occurs as a result of bleeding, can easily lead to severe cellular hypoxia, even though an adequate amount of oxygen is available in the alveoli.

Carbon Dioxide Transport

Carbon dioxide is transported in the blood in three ways: Approximately 7 percent is dissolved in plasma, 23 percent is attached to hemoglobin, and 70 percent is in the form of bicarbonate.

As carbon dioxide leaves the cells, it crosses over into the capillaries where a small amount dissolves into the plasma. A larger amount of CO_2 attaches to hemoglobin. The largest amount of CO_2 diffuses into the red blood cell and combines with water to form carbonic acid, which then dissociates into hydrogen and bicarbonate. The bicarbonate exits the cell and is transported in the blood plasma. When the blood reaches the pulmonary circulation, the bicarbonate diffuses back into the red blood cell where it combines with hydrogen and splits back into water and carbon dioxide. Regardless of the transport mechanism, the carbon dioxide diffuses into the alveoli and is released through exhalation.

Alveolar/Capillary Gas Exchange

After inhalation, the alveoli are filled with oxygen-rich air that contains very little carbon dioxide. Conversely, the venous blood that flows through the capillaries surrounding the alveoli contains low levels of oxygen and higher amounts of carbon dioxide.

Since gas molecules naturally move from an area of high concentration to an area of low concentration, the high oxygen content in the alveoli moves across the membranes and into the capillaries where the oxygen content is very low. (Review Figure 8-5, top inset.) There, as described earlier, a small amount of oxygen dissolves in the plasma and a larger amount attaches to the hemoglobin. Simultaneously, carbon dioxide moves in the opposite direction, from the high levels contained in the capillaries into the alveoli where the CO_2 content is low. It happens this way: The bicarbonate ions in the blood convert to water and CO_2. Additional CO_2 diffuses out of the plasma and from the hemoglobin. All of this CO_2 crosses from the capillaries into the alveoli.

After these exchanges—from alveoli to capillaries and from capillaries to alveoli—the alveoli contain low levels of oxygen and high levels of carbon dioxide, while the blood in the capillaries contains high levels of oxygen and low levels of carbon dioxide. Basically, the gases have switched concentrations. The carbon-dioxide-rich air in the alveoli is exhaled from the lungs. The oxygen-rich blood in the capillaries is transported from the pulmonary circulation to the left atrium and then to the left ventricle of the heart, from which it is ejected into the aorta and to the arteries throughout the body. This blood that is circulating throughout the body will be used in the cell/capillary gas exchange described next.

Cell/Capillary Gas Exchange

The blood that was ejected from the left ventricle into the arteries contains high concentrations of oxygen and low concentrations of carbon dioxide. This blood travels through an artery and then enters a smaller arteriole that leads to a capillary bed that is surrounded by cells. During cell metabolism, the cells have used oxygen and produced carbon dioxide as a by-product. Thus, while the capillary beds contain blood that is high in oxygen and low in carbon dioxide, the cells contain low levels of oxygen and high levels of carbon dioxide.

As the blood enters the capillary, oxygen breaks free of the hemoglobin and diffuses out of the plasma, crosses the capillary membrane, and enters the cell. Simultaneously, carbon dioxide leaves the cell and crosses over into the capillary where it dissolves in the plasma, attaches to hemoglobin, or enters the red blood cell to be converted to bicarbonate. (Review Figure 8-5, bottom inset.) As the blood leaves the capillary, it enters a small venule from which it is eventually dumped into a larger vein. The

Key Terms
hydrostatic pressure the force inside the vessel or capillary bed generated by the contraction of the heart and the blood pressure that exerts a "push" effect that forces fluid out of the vessel.

Objective 8-16
Describe the composition of blood, including the function of plasma and the formed elements.

blood in the venules and veins contains low concentrations of oxygen and high concentrations of carbon dioxide. This carbon-dioxide-carrying blood is transported to the right atrium of the heart, from which it enters the right ventricle and is pumped to the lungs. There the blood enters the pulmonary capillaries to give off carbon dioxide and pick up oxygen in the alveolar/capillary gas exchange that was previously described.

For the cells to receive an adequate amount of oxygen and eliminate carbon dioxide, both the alveolar/capillary gas exchange and cell/capillary gas exchange must be functioning properly. A disturbance in either will result in inadequate amounts of oxygen being delivered to the cells or will result in the accumulation of carbon dioxide.

Blood Volume

One of the determinants of an adequate blood pressure and perfusion is blood volume. An adult has approximately 70 mL of blood for every kilogram (2.2 lb) of body weight. Thus, a patient who weighs 154 lb or 70 kg would have approximately 4,900 mL or 4.9 liters of blood volume. Blood volume correlates with body mass; therefore, a larger patient would normally have a greater blood volume. The loss of 1 liter of blood in a 100-lb patient would be much more significant than in a 200-lb patient.

Composition of Blood

Blood is composed of formed elements and plasma. The formed elements, which are cells and proteins, make up approximately 45 percent of blood composition. Plasma is the fluid component that accounts for the remaining 55 percent. The primary function of plasma is to suspend and carry the formed elements. Plasma is made up primarily of water and plasma proteins. Water comprises 91 percent of plasma. The plasma proteins consist of albumin, antibodies, and clotting factors. Albumin is a large molecule that does not pass easily through a capillary; it plays a major role in maintaining the fluid balance in the blood, as will be explained later in the section on plasma oncotic pressure. Antibodies are produced by the lymphatic system and are responsible for the defense against infectious organisms. The clotting factors are key in coagulation of blood from damaged vessels. Fibrinogen is the most plentiful clotting factor and is the precursor to the fibrin clot.

The formed elements in the blood are red blood cells, white blood cells, and platelets. Red blood cells (erythrocytes) make up approximately 48 percent of the blood cell volume in men and 42 percent in women. The red blood cells, which contain hemoglobin, are primarily responsible for carrying oxygen and delivering it to cells for metabolism. The white blood cells (leukocytes) protect the body against infection and eliminate dead and injured cells and other debris. The platelets (thrombocytes) are not actual cells but fragments that play a major role in blood clotting and the control of bleeding.

Distribution of Blood

Blood is distributed throughout the cardiovascular system (Table 8-3). The majority of blood is housed within the venous system, which is also known as a reservoir or capacitance system. The venous system is capable of enlarging or reducing its capacity to respond to increases or decreases in the blood volume. As a patient bleeds, the venous volume is continuously reduced regardless of whether the bleeding is from a vein, an artery, or a capillary.

The venous system is responsible for supplying the right side of the heart with an adequate volume of blood. If the volume entering the right side of the heart is decreased, the amount ejected from the left ventricle, through the arteries, and to the cells, is also reduced. Thus, the venous volume plays a major role in maintaining blood pressure and adequate perfusion of the cells. This will be discussed in more detail later in the chapter. The capillary network is the site of gas exchange occurring with the alveoli or cells.

Hydrostatic Pressure

Hydrostatic pressure is the force inside the vessel or capillary bed generated by the contraction of the heart and

TABLE 8-3 Distribution of Blood in the Cardiovascular System

Blood is distributed in the various components of the cardiovascular system as follows.

Venous	64%
Arterial	13%
Pulmonary vessels	9%
Capillaries	7%
Heart	7%

Key Terms

plasma oncotic pressure the force responsible for keeping fluid inside a vessel by exerting a "pull" effect.

Objective 8-17

Explain the effects of changes in hydrostatic pressure and plasma oncotic pressure on the movement of fluid between the circulatory system and interstitial spaces.

the blood pressure. Hydrostatic pressure exerts a "push" inside the vessel or capillary. That is, it wants to push fluid out of the vessel or capillary, through the vessel wall, and into the interstitial space. A high hydrostatic pressure would force more fluid out of the vessel or capillary and promote edema—swelling from excess fluid outside the vessels (Figure 8-8∗).

As an example, if a patient has a left ventricle that is failing and unable to pump blood effectively, the volume and pressure in the left atrium, pulmonary vein, and pulmonary capillaries rise. This occurs because the pulmonary capillaries, pulmonary vein, and left atrium are the pathways by which blood enters the left ventricle. When the left ventricle fails to empty effectively, blood backs up into the left atrium and pulmonary vessels, which increases the pressure within them. The increased hydrostatic pressure inside the pulmonary capillaries forces fluid out of them. The extruded fluid has a tendency to collect in the spaces between the alveoli and capillaries and around the alveoli, which reduces the ability of oxygen and carbon dioxide to be exchanged across the alveolar/capillary membrane. This disturbance reduces the blood oxygen content, leading to cellular hypoxia, and also causes the blood to retain carbon dioxide. The fluid will eventually begin to collapse and fill the alveoli, further diminishing gas exchange. This condition is known as pulmonary edema.

Plasma Oncotic Pressure

Plasma oncotic pressure, also known as colloid oncotic pressure or oncotic pressure, is responsible for keeping fluid inside the vessels. A force is generated inside vessels by large plasma proteins, especially albumin, that attract water and other fluids. Opposite to hydrostatic pressure, oncotic pressure exerts a "pull" inside the vessel. A high oncotic pressure would pull fluid from outside the vessel, through the vessel wall, and into the vessel. (Review Figure 8-8.)

A balance between hydrostatic pressure and plasma oncotic pressure must be maintained for equilibrium of fluid balance. The effects of high and low hydrostatic and oncotic pressures are summarized as follows:

- A high hydrostatic pressure will push fluid out of a capillary and promote edema.
- A low hydrostatic pressure will push less fluid out of the vessel.
- A high oncotic pressure will draw excessive amounts of fluid into the vessel or capillary and promote blood volume overload.
- A low oncotic pressure will not exert an adequate pull effect to counteract the push of hydrostatic pressure and will therefore promote loss of vascular volume and promote edema.

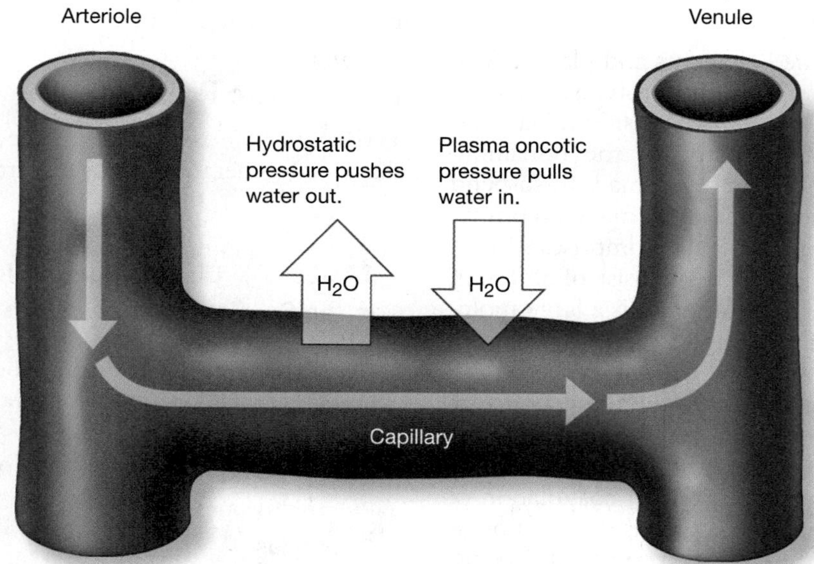

FIGURE 8-8 ∗ Hydrostatic pressure pushes water out of the capillary. Plasma oncotic pressure pulls water into the capillary.

Key Terms

cardiac output the volume of blood ejected from the left ventricle in one minute.

stroke volume the volume of blood ejected by the ventricle with each contraction.

Key Terms

preload the pressure generated in the left ventricle at the end of diastole (resting phase).

Objective 8-18

Discuss factors that affect cardiac output, including heart rate, stroke volume, myocardial contractility, preload, and afterload.

Pump Function of the Myocardium

In order to have an adequate blood pressure and perfusion, the myocardium must work effectively as a pump. The heart is capable of varying its output to meet a wide range of physiological demands. It can drastically increase its pump function, up to sixfold. The pump function is typically expressed as the cardiac output. **Cardiac output** is defined as the amount of blood ejected by the left ventricle in one minute. The cardiac output has a major influence on blood pressure and perfusion, as will be discussed later in the chapter.

Cardiac Output

A normal cardiac output for an adult at rest is 5 liters/minute. That means the ventricles will pump the entire blood volume through the vascular system in one minute. If a drop of blood left the left ventricle, in one minute it should be back at the left ventricle. The cardiac output is determined by the heart rate and the stroke volume. Cardiac output is expressed by the following equation:

Cardiac output = heart rate × stroke volume

Heart Rate

The heart rate is defined as the number of times the heart contracts in one minute. The heart has the property of automaticity, meaning it can generate its own impulse. This is achieved through the conduction system with the sinoatrial (SA) node being the primary pacemaker. The heart rate can also be influenced to increase or decrease its rate of firing by several factors outside of the heart. The primary factors are hormones and the autonomic nervous system, composed of the sympathetic and parasympathetic systems. The influence of the autonomic nervous system on the heart rate is summarized as follows:

An increase in stimulation by the sympathetic nervous system increases the heart rate.

A decrease in stimulation by the sympathetic nervous system decreases the heart rate.

An increase in stimulation by the parasympathetic nervous system decreases the heart rate.

A decrease in stimulation by the parasympathetic nervous system increases the heart rate.

The sympathetic and parasympathetic nervous systems exert control over the heart rate through the cardiovascular control center located in the brain stem. The cardiovascular control center is composed of the cardioexcitatory center and the cardioinhibitory center. The cardioexcitatory center increases the heart rate by increasing sympathetic stimulation and decreasing parasympathetic stimulation. The cardioinhibitory center decreases the heart rate by decreasing sympathetic stimulation and increasing parasympathetic stimulation.

Direct neural stimulation provides an immediate response in the heart rate and force of ventricular contraction. In addition, stimulation of the sympathetic nervous system may cause the release of epinephrine and norepinephrine from the adrenal gland located on top of the kidney. The release of these hormones may take a few minutes; however, the response will be sustained as long as the hormones are continuously released and circulating. As discussed in Chapter 7, "Anatomy, Physiology, and Medical Terminology," the $beta_1$ properties in the epinephrine will cause an increase in the heart rate and force of contraction.

Stroke Volume

Stroke volume is defined as the volume of blood ejected by the left ventricle with each contraction. Stroke volume is determined by preload, myocardial contractility, and afterload.

Preload is the pressure generated in the left ventricle at the end of diastole (the resting phase of the cardiac cycle). Preload pressure is created by the blood volume in the left ventricle at the end of diastole. The available venous volume, which determines the volume of blood in the ventricle, consequently plays a major role in determining preload. An increase in preload generally increases stroke volume, which in turn increases the cardiac output. Preload determines the force necessary to eject the blood out of the ventricle.

As blood fills the left ventricle, the muscle fibers stretch to house the blood. The stretch of the muscle fiber at the end of diastole determines the force available to eject the blood from the ventricle. This is known as the **Frank-Starling law of the heart**. As the blood volume increases in the left ventricle, the increased stretch in the muscle fibers generates a commensurate contraction force. In short, the volume of blood in the ventricle automatically generates a contraction forceful enough to eject it. There is a limit, however, to applicability of the Frank Starling law—a limit to the effectiveness of fiber

Key Terms
Frank-Starling law of the heart the stretch of the muscle fiber in the left ventricle at the end of diastole determines the force necessary to eject the blood contained within it.

Key Terms
afterload the force of contraction that the left ventricle has to generate to overcome the resistance in the aorta to eject the blood.

stretch. In the case of a severely dilated ventricle where the fibers are overstretched, the heart will no longer be able to produce contractions strong enough to eject blood from the ventricle adequately.

In order to have an adequate stroke volume, the left ventricle must be able to generate enough force to effectively eject its blood volume. An increase in myocardial contractility will increase the stroke volume and improve cardiac output. Conversely, a decrease in myocardial contractility will lead to a decrease in stroke volume and a resulting decrease in cardiac output. For example, a patient with congestive heart failure will have a decrease in contractile force of the left ventricle that is likely to result in a diminished cardiac output. A patient who has suffered a heart attack will have a deadened portion of cardiac muscle that will no longer contribute to the contractile force. If the area of necrosis is large, the contractile force will be significantly reduced with a proportional decrease in stroke volume and cardiac output.

Afterload is the resistance in the aorta that must be overcome by contraction of the left ventricle to eject the blood. The force generated by the left ventricle must overcome the pressure in the aorta to move the blood forward. A high afterload places an increased workload on the left ventricle. A chronically elevated diastolic blood pressure will create a high afterload, generating an increased myocardial workload that could lead to left ventricular failure over a period of time.

In general, a decrease in either the heart rate or stroke volume will decrease the cardiac output:

A ↓ in heart rate = ↓ in cardiac output

A ↓ in stroke volume = ↓ in cardiac output

The effects of heart rate, blood volume, myocardial contractility, autonomic nervous system stimulation, hormone release, and diastolic blood pressure on cardiac output are these:

- A decrease in heart rate will decrease cardiac output.
- An increase in heart rate, if not excessive, will increase cardiac output.
- A decrease in blood volume will decrease preload, stroke volume, and cardiac output.
- An increase in blood volume will increase preload, stroke volume, and cardiac output.
- A decrease in myocardial contractility will decrease stroke volume and cardiac output.
- An increase in myocardial contractility will increase stroke volume and cardiac output.
- Neural stimulation from the sympathetic nervous system will increase heart rate, myocardial contractility, and cardiac output.
- Neural stimulation from the parasympathetic nervous system will decrease heart rate, myocardial contractility, and cardiac output.
- $Beta_1$ stimulation from epinephrine will increase heart rate, myocardial contractility, and cardiac output.
- $Beta_1$ blockade (patient on beta blocker) will block $beta_1$ stimulation, decrease heart rate, decrease myocardial contractility, and decrease cardiac output.
- An extremely high diastolic blood pressure will increase the pressure in the aorta, requiring a more forceful contraction to overcome the aortic pressure and a higher myocardial workload, and may weaken the heart and decrease the cardiac output over time.
- A reduction in the diastolic blood pressure will decrease the pressure in the aorta, require a less forceful contraction to overcome the aortic pressure, and reduce the myocardial workload, which may improve the cardiac output in a weakened heart.

A faster heart rate may increase cardiac output; however, if the rate is extremely fast the cardiac output may actually decrease. With excessively fast heart rates, usually >160 bpm in the adult patient, the time between beats is so short that there is not an adequate amount of time for the ventricles to fill. This reduces the preload, which in turn reduces the cardiac output.

Systemic Vascular Resistance

Systemic vascular resistance is the resistance that is offered to blood flow through a vessel. As a vessel constricts (decreases its diameter), resistance inside the vessel increases, which typically increases pressure inside the vessel. Conversely, as a vessel dilates (increases its diameter), resistance inside the vessel decreases, which typically decreases pressure inside the vessel. *Vasoconstriction* is the term for a decrease in vessel diameter. *Vasodilation* is the term for an increase in vessel diameter. Vessel size influences blood pressure. Vasoconstriction decreases vessel size, increases resistance, and increases blood pressure. Vasodilation increases vessel diameter, decreases resistance, and decreases blood pressure.

Objective 8-19
Describe the concept of systemic vascular resistance and its relationship to blood pressure and pulse pressure.

Key Terms
systemic vascular resistance the resistance of blood flow through a vessel based on the diameter of the vessel.

Key Points
One determinant of an adequate blood pressure and perfusion is blood volume.

Pressure within the vessels is greatest during cardiac contraction (systole) and least during cardiac relaxation (diastole). The basic measure of systemic vascular resistance is the diastolic blood pressure because it is assessed during the relaxation phase, indicating the resting pressure within the vessels. Systolic blood pressure, created by the wave of blood ejected from the left ventricle during contraction, increases the pressure within the vessels beyond their resting pressure.

An abnormally high diastolic blood pressure is not a desirable condition. The diastolic blood pressure is the pressure inside the arteries and the aortic root immediately prior to contraction of the left ventricle. The higher the diastolic blood pressure, the greater the resistance to blood being ejected from the left ventricle. That means the left ventricle has to work harder to pump the blood out against a higher diastolic pressure. If the diastolic blood pressure is chronically elevated, it will eventually cause the heart to fail. It is all related to resistance of flow and harder workloads.

As an example, a person is given two weights to lift simultaneously. The weight in the right hand weighs only 1 lb, whereas the weight in the left hand weighs 10 lb. Which extremity and muscle would become fatigued and fail first if the person were asked to continuously lift the weights? Obviously the left arm lifting the 10-lb weight would fatigue and fail first. Why? The muscle is working against a greater resistance. Relate this example to the heart of a patient with a chronically elevated diastolic blood pressure. The high resistance to blood flow causes the left ventricle to work harder to pump the blood out. If the left ventricle has to contract against the high resistance chronically, it eventually weakens and fails. This condition is known as left ventricular failure or congestive heart failure.

The autonomic nervous system influences the systemic vascular resistance. Direct neural stimulation from the sympathetic nervous system causes the vessels to constrict, increasing vessel resistance and pressure. Parasympathetic nervous system stimulation causes the vessels to dilate, reducing resistance and pressure. Additionally, epinephrine and norepinephrine that are released by the adrenal gland in response to sympathetic stimulation have alpha properties. Alpha$_1$ receptor stimulation causes the vessels to constrict, increasing the vessels' resistance and pressure.

If the volume of blood inside a vessel decreases, one way to maintain the pressure is to decrease vessel size and increase resistance. When blood is being lost and overall volume is decreasing, vessels will usually compensate for this loss by continuing to constrict to raise resistance and pressure. Blood pressure may thus be maintained at a normal level, making it appear as if no volume has been lost. That is why it is so important not only to evaluate the vital signs in a patient with blood loss but also to look for signs of poor perfusion.

Think back to the beginning of the chapter and the discussion of cellular metabolism. As vessels decrease in size to maintain blood pressure, they do so at the expense of cellular perfusion. As the vessels constrict, less blood flows through them and less oxygen is delivered to the cells. As oxygen delivery decreases, the cells change from aerobic to anaerobic metabolism. The loss in energy is often noted in the patient's general appearance at the scene. The patient with poor perfusion is typically quiet, reserved, and may actually appear sleepy. The patient who is screaming and yelling and constantly moving about has to have lots of energy in order to do so. There has to be an adequate delivery of oxygen and glucose to the cells to produce this amount of energy. Be careful not to mistake this high level of patient energy with the agitation and aggression experienced by patients whose brain cells are hypoxic.

The effects of the autonomic nervous system on the systemic vascular resistance are summarized as follows:

- Sympathetic stimulation causes vasoconstriction, which decreases vessel diameter and increases systemic vascular resistance.
- Parasympathetic stimulation causes vasodilation, which increases vessel diameter and decreases systemic vascular resistance.
- The alpha$_1$ properties in epinephrine and norepinephrine, released in response to sympathetic stimulation, cause vasoconstriction, which decreases vessel diameter and increases systemic vascular resistance.

Systemic Vascular Resistance Effect on Pulse Pressure

The systolic blood pressure is a relative indicator of the cardiac output, whereas the diastolic blood pressure measures the systemic vascular resistance. If the systolic blood pressure is decreasing, it is an indication of a diminishing cardiac output. The following describes the effect of the systemic vascular resistance on diastolic blood pressure:

- An increase in the systemic vascular resistance will increase the diastolic blood pressure.

Key Terms
microcirculation the flow of blood through the arterioles, capillaries, and venules that is the site of exchange of gases, nutrients, and waste products with the cells.

Key Points
Cardiac output is determined by heart rate and stroke volume.

Objective 8-20
Summarize the local, neural, and hormonal factors that regulate blood flow through the capillaries.

- A decrease in the systemic vascular resistance will decrease the diastolic blood pressure.

The *pulse pressure* is the difference between the systolic and the diastolic blood pressure readings. If the patient has a blood pressure of 132/74 mmHg, the pulse pressure would be derived by subtracting the diastolic from the systolic. In this case, the pulse pressure would be 58 mmHg (132 − 74 = 58). A narrow pulse pressure is defined as being less than 25 percent of the systolic blood pressure reading. In this case, a narrow pulse pressure would be less than 33 mmHg (132 × 25% = 33 mmHg).

In the patient with blood or fluid loss, a narrow pulse pressure is a significant sign. As a patient loses blood, the following occurs:

Blood loss ↓ venous volume which ↓ preload which ↓ stroke volume which ↓ cardiac output.

The systolic blood pressure begins to decrease from the drop in cardiac output. One way the body attempts to compensate for the decrease in blood pressure is by increasing the systemic vascular resistance. You will see the following in the blood pressure reading:

↓ Systolic blood pressure
Narrow Pulse Pressure =
↑ Diastolic blood pressure

Although the blood pressure may appear to be within normal limits, the narrow pulse pressure may warn you of a dropping cardiac output from blood or fluid loss and a rising systemic vascular resistance as an attempt to compensate for the decreasing pressure.

As an example, a patient with suspected bleeding in his abdomen presents with a blood pressure of 108/88 mmHg. Based on normal blood pressure ranges that you will learn in Chapter 11, "Baseline Vital Signs, Monitoring Devices, and History Taking," this blood pressure falls well within a normal range and may not alarm you. However, if you look at the pulse pressure, it is only 20 mmHg (108 − 88 = 20 mmHg). A normal pulse pressure would be greater than 25 percent of the systolic blood pressure. In this case, a normal pulse pressure would be 27 mmHg or greater (108 × 25% = 27 mmHg). Thus, this patient has a narrow pulse pressure, which may be an indication of a dropping cardiac output from a decrease in venous volume and preload and an increasing systemic vascular resistance to compensate for the decrease in pressure. By just looking at the patient's blood pressure, you could easily say it is normal. When considering the pulse pressure, as well as other signs of perfusion, such as skin color, temperature, condition, and mental status, you might reclassify it as abnormal.

Microcirculation

Microcirculation is the flow of blood through the smallest blood vessels—the arterioles, capillaries, and venules (Figure 8-9*). As mentioned previously, the veins and venules primarily serve a capacitance function by pooling blood as needed and supplying it to the heart as necessary to maintain cardiac output. Arteries branch into arterioles, which are at the terminal ends of the arteries. The arterioles, which are made up of almost all smooth muscle, control the movement of blood into the capillaries. Vasoconstriction reduces the flow into the capillaries, and vasodilation increases the capillary blood flow.

The true capillaries are the sites of exchange of nutrients, oxygen, carbon dioxide, glucose, waste products, and metabolic substances between the blood and the cells. Metarterioles are described often as thoroughfares or channels that connect the arterioles and venules. True capillaries branch from the metarterioles. Precapillary sphincters control the movement of blood through the true capillaries. If the precapillary sphincter is relaxed, blood moves through the capillary. If the precapillary sphincter is contracted, the blood is shunted away from the true capillary. The precapillary sphincters help to maintain arterial pressure and control the movement of blood through the capillary beds.

Three regulatory influences control blood flow through the capillaries: local factors, neural factors, and hormonal factors. Local factors are found in the immediate environment around or within the capillary structure, for example, temperature, hypoxia, acidosis, and histamine. A cold temperature would cause the peripheral arterioles to constrict and precapillary sphincters to close, shunting blood away from the capillaries in an attempt to reduce the blood exposure to the cold environment. The opposite would be true in a warm environment where the arterioles would dilate and the precapillary sphincters would open to shunt the blood to the periphery where it can cool.

Neural factors are associated with the influence of the sympathetic and parasympathetic nervous systems on the arterioles and precapillary sphincters. Sympathetic nervous stimulation would cause the arterioles to constrict and precapillary sphincters to close. Parasympathetic stimulation would cause the arterioles to dilate and the precapillary sphincters to open.

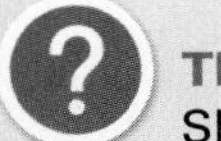

Thinking Critically

Shock results from inadequate perfusion of the body cells. Poor perfusion is usually caused by (1) inadequate blood volume and/or (2) inadequate pumping of the heart and/or (3) inadequate blood vessel tone (systemic vascular resistance). Based on what you have learned in this chapter, explain how each of these three factors would affect perfusion.

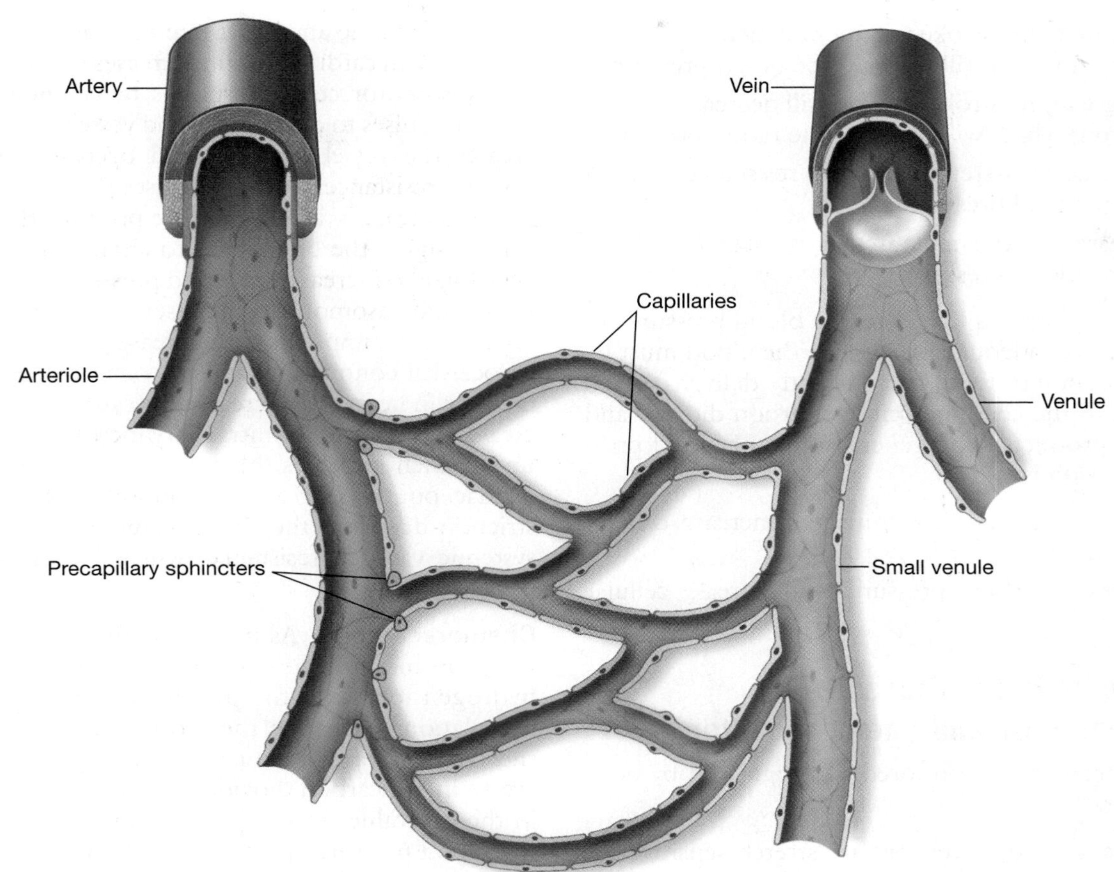

FIGURE 8-9 ✱ Microcirculation is the flow of blood through the smallest blood vessels: arterioles, capillaries, and venules. Precapillary sphincters control the flow of blood through the capillaries.

Hormones may also control the movement of blood through the capillaries. As an example, the $alpha_1$ stimulation from epinephrine causes the arterioles to constrict and the precapillary sphincters to close.

In a resting state, the local factors predominantly control blood flow through the capillaries. When adaptation is necessary, the neural factors will change the capillary blood flow. Hormones are usually responsible for a sustained effect on the arterioles and capillaries.

Blood Pressure

As previously noted, the systolic blood pressure is a measure of cardiac output. The diastolic blood pressure is a measure of systemic vascular resistance. The body's compensation mechanisms are geared toward maintaining pressure inside the vessel and perfusion of the cells.

The blood pressure is derived by multiplying two major factors: cardiac output and systemic vascular resistance:

Blood pressure (BP) = cardiac output (CO) × systemic vascular resistance (SVR)

Both the cardiac output and systemic vascular resistance have a direct effect on the blood pressure, which is summarized as follows:

- An increase in cardiac output will increase the blood pressure.
- A decrease in cardiac output will decrease the blood pressure.
- An increase in the heart rate will increase the cardiac output which will increase the blood pressure.
- A decrease in the heart rate will decrease the cardiac output which will decrease the blood pressure.

Key Terms
baroreceptors stretch-sensitive receptors located in the aortic arch and carotid bodies that constantly measure the blood pressure.

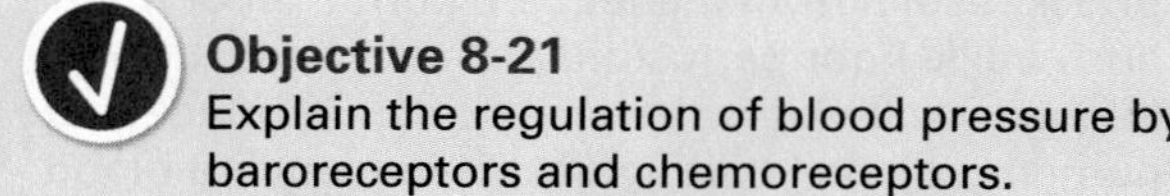

Objective 8-21
Explain the regulation of blood pressure by baroreceptors and chemoreceptors.

- An increase in the stroke volume will increase the cardiac output which will increase the blood pressure.
- A decrease in the stroke volume will decrease the cardiac output which will decrease the blood pressure.
- An increase in systemic vascular resistance will increase the blood pressure.
- A decrease in systemic vascular resistance will decrease the blood pressure.

Perfusion of cells is linked to the blood pressure. In order to maintain adequate perfusion, the blood must be pushed with enough force to constantly deliver oxygen and glucose to the cells and remove carbon dioxide and other waste products. The general effect of blood pressure on perfusion is:

- An increase in blood pressure will increase cellular perfusion.
- A decrease in blood pressure will decrease cellular perfusion.

Regulation of Blood Pressure by Baroreceptors and Chemoreceptors

The blood pressure is monitored and regulated by both baroreceptors and chemoreceptors.

Baroreceptors **Baroreceptors** are stretch-sensitive receptors, located in the aortic arch and carotid sinuses, that detect changes in blood pressure. As the pressure inside the vessels changes, it decreases or increases the stretch of the fibers of the baroreceptors. The baroreceptors, having thus detected the change in blood pressure, send impulses to the cardioregulatory and vasomotor centers in the brain stem to make compensatory alterations in the blood pressure. The cardioregulatory center consists of the cardioexcitatory (cardioacceleratory) center and the cardioinhibitory center that control heart rate and force of cardiac contraction. The vasomotor center controls the vessel size and resistance through vasoconstriction and vasodilation.

An increase in blood pressure prompts the baroreceptors to signal the brain stem to alter heart function and vessel size to decrease the blood pressure. The cardioinhibitory center responds by sending parasympathetic nervous system impulses that cause the heart to decrease heart rate and myocardial contractility. A decrease in myocardial contractility decreases stroke volume. A decrease in stroke volume and heart rate decreases cardiac output. A decrease in cardiac output decreases the blood pressure. The vasomotor center responds by sending parasympathetic impulses to dilate the blood vessels. Vasodilation increases the vessel diameter and decreases the systemic vascular resistance, which decreases the blood pressure.

A decrease in blood pressure prompts the baroreceptors to signal the brain stem to alter heart function and vessel size to increase the blood pressure. The cardioexcitatory and vasomotor centers send out sympathetic nervous system impulses to increase the heart rate and myocardial contractility and to constrict the vessels. The increase in heart rate increases the cardiac output. The increase in myocardial contractility increases the stroke volume, which increases the cardiac output. An increase in cardiac output increases the blood pressure. Vasoconstriction decreases the vessel diameter and increases the systemic vascular resistance, which increases the blood pressure.

Chemoreceptors As previously discussed, the chemoreceptors monitor the content of oxygen, carbon dioxide, hydrogen ions, and the pH of the blood. The greatest stimulation to change the blood pressure occurs when the oxygen content in arterial blood decreases. An increase in the carbon dioxide level, resulting in a decrease in the pH value (more acid) has a much lesser effect on the blood pressure. When the oxygen content in the arterial blood falls, carbon dioxide level increases, or pH decreases (more acid in the blood), the brain stem triggers the sympathetic nervous system through the cardioexcitatory center and vasomotor centers to increase the blood pressure by increasing the heart rate, myocardial contractility, and vasoconstriction. The increase in blood pressure is intended to improve the delivery of oxygen to the brain cells and to remove more carbon dioxide. These changes account for the signs you may observe as an EMT. Hypoxia may produce pale, cool skin and an increase in heart rate. The pale, cool skin is from vasoconstriction, and the increase in heart rate is from sympathetic stimulation of the SA node.

A decrease in blood pressure and oxygen content in the blood will also trigger the release of a whole cascade of hormones from different endocrine organs in the body. This will be discussed in greater detail in Chapter 15, "Shock and Resuscitation."

Maintaining aerobic metabolism is essential for the cells, the organs, and the patient to survive. To summa-

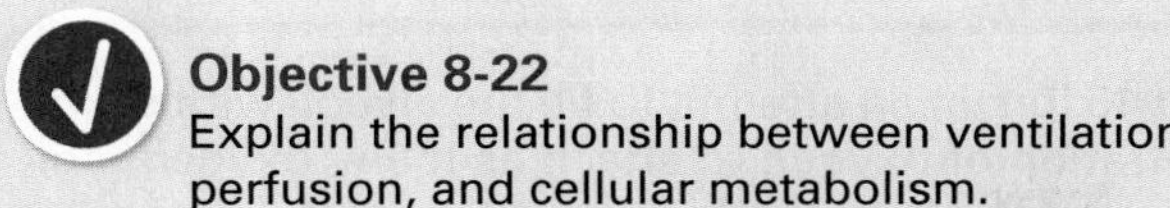

Objective 8-22
Explain the relationship between ventilation, perfusion, and cellular metabolism.

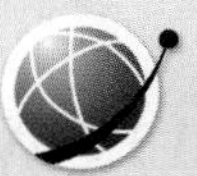

Media Resources
Go to www.bradybooks.com for mykit. Highlights:

- *Web Resource:* Cardiac Output and Blood Pressure
- *Animation:* Transport of Carbon Dioxide

rize, in order to maintain aerobic metabolism of cells, the following must be adequate:

- Oxygen content in ambient air
- Patency of the airway
- Minute ventilation
  - Ventilatory rate
  - Tidal volume
- Alveolar ventilation
  - Ventilatory rate
  - Tidal volume
- Perfusion in the pulmonary capillaries
  - Venous volume
  - Right ventricular pump function
- Gas exchange between the capillaries and the alveoli
- Content of blood
  - Red blood cells
  - Hemoglobin
  - Plasma
- Cardiac output
  - Heart rate
  - Preload
  - Stroke volume
  - Myocardial contractility
  - Afterload
- Systemic vascular resistance
  - Sympathetic nervous system stimulation
  - Parasympathetic nervous system stimulation
- Gas exchange between the capillaries and the cells

CHAPTER REVIEW

SUMMARY

The most fundamental purpose of your emergency care is to restore or sustain perfusion of cells with oxygen and glucose. With adequate delivery of oxygen and glucose, the cells can maintain aerobic metabolism resulting in the production of water, carbon dioxide, and ATP for energy. With adequate perfusion and ventilation, carbon dioxide can be effectively eliminated through exhalation. A shift to anaerobic metabolism occurs when oxygen is not made available to cells during metabolism, which results in the production of lactic acid as the primary by-product. Acid can have a detrimental effect on cell structure and function.

The key to constant delivery of an adequate supply of oxygen and glucose to cells and the elimination of carbon dioxide and other waste products of metabolism is to establish and maintain an adequate and effective airway, ventilation, oxygenation, gas exchange at both the alveoli and cells, transportation of gases in the blood, blood volume, cardiac function, and blood pressure. An alteration in any one of these components can result in poor perfusion and cellular hypoxia.

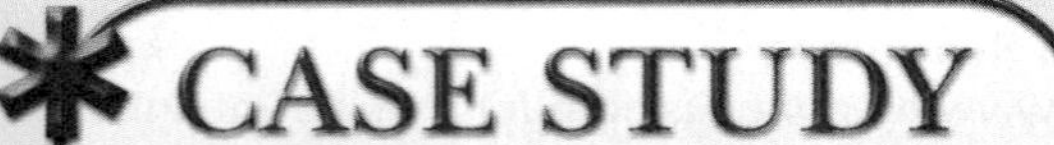

CASE STUDY FOLLOW-UP

SCENE SIZE-UP

You have been dispatched for a 50-year-old male patient who has been stabbed by his wife. The wife is in police custody and the scene is safe to enter. The daughter leads you to an enclosed back porch where you find the patient lying on his side in a pool of blood. Suddenly, a dog rushes from the house and begins barking ferociously. The daughter yells, "Winston! Go back inside the house!" You ask the daughter to take Winston into the house and place him in a room and close the door to secure him.

PATIENT ASSESSMENT

The patient is moaning in pain and clutching his abdomen. You ask the patient his name to determine the level of responsiveness. He states, "Paul—my name is Paul. I can't believe she stabbed me. I just wanted to watch the football game in peace." From his response, you gather that he is alert, oriented to his name, has an open airway, and is breathing adequately.

You note that the patient is breathing at a rate of 24/minute and slightly shallow. You think that his minute ventilation appears to be slightly increased because of an increased ventilatory rate; however, you want to be sure that his alveolar ventilation is also adequate. His chest is rising and falling adequately with each breath; thus, he appears to be moving enough tidal volume to sustain the alveolar ventilation. His radial pulse is barely palpable and his skin is pale, cool, and clammy. You expect that the skin is pale, cool, and clammy as a result of vasoconstriction occurring from sympathetic nervous system stimulation and circulating epinephrine and norepinephrine to maintain the blood pressure. The weak pulse is likely due to a loss of volume, a decreased preload, and a decreased cardiac output and intense peripheral vasoconstriction. His heart rate is 122 bpm. You think that the heart rate is elevated as an attempt to raise the cardiac output and to increase or maintain the blood pressure. Your partner places him on a nonrebreather mask at 15 lpm in an attempt to fill the alveoli with a high concentration of oxygen to attach as many oxygen molecules as possible to the binding sites on the hemoglobin in the blood.

You expose the patient and perform a quick examination of his body from head to toe, looking for other injuries and signs. During the assessment, he complains, "My belly hurts really bad." The abdomen is rigid and tender when you palpate it. You suspect this is from blood loss in the abdominal cavity. Your partner assesses the vital signs: BP 102/88 mmHg, heart rate 122 bpm, respirations 24/minute, and skin pale, cool, and clammy.

The pulse pressure appears to be narrow. You do a quick mental calculation and determine that 25 percent of 100 is 25; thus, the pulse pressure should be around 25 mmHg or greater. You quickly subtract the diastolic blood pressure from the systolic and determine that the pulse pressure is 14 mmHg. You suspect the narrow pulse pressure is correlated with blood volume loss from the stab wound to the abdomen, causing a drop in preload and a decrease in stroke volume and cardiac output, causing the systolic blood pressure to decrease. The baroreceptors sensed the decrease in pressure inside the aortic arch and carotid sinuses and sent impulses to the brain stem to trigger the sympathetic nervous system to raise the blood pressure. Based on the formula $BP = CO \times SVR$, you suspect the increased heart rate is an attempt to raise the cardiac output, and the pale, cool, clammy skin is a sign of vasoconstriction in an attempt to increase the systemic vascular resistance. The decrease in cardiac output and increase in systemic vascular resistance are creating the narrow pulse pressure.

You cover the stab wounds to the abdomen and prepare the patient for transport. En route you continue to reassess the patient, contact the receiving medical facility, and provide a radio report. Once at the medical facility, you provide an oral report to the physician and complete your transfer of care. You clean up the ambulance and prepare for your next call.

IN REVIEW

1. Describe the difference between aerobic metabolism and anaerobic metabolism.
2. Define FiO_2 and FDO_2.
3. Describe how the content of gases in the ambient air affects the oxygenation status of the patient.
4. Describe possible causes of airway obstruction at the nasopharynx, oropharynx, pharynx, and larynx.
5. Describe the mechanical process of inhalation and exhalation.
6. Describe how the Boyle law affects ventilation.
7. List and describe the role of the respiratory centers located in the brain stem.
8. List, identify the location, and describe the role of the two different types of chemoreceptors.
9. Describe the ventilation/perfusion ratio and its relationship to cellular hypoxia.
10. Describe the transport of oxygen in the blood.
11. Describe the transport of carbon dioxide in the blood.
12. List the components of the blood and describe the function of each component.

13. Define hydrostatic pressure and plasma oncotic pressure.
14. List, define, and describe the factors that determine the cardiac output, systemic vascular resistance, and blood pressure.
15. Describe the influence of the sympathetic nervous system and parasympathetic nervous system on the cardiac output and blood pressure.
16. Define microcirculation and describe how it affects blood pressure and perfusion.
17. Identify the location and describe the role of the baroreceptors.
18. Discuss how the chemoreceptors influence changes in blood pressure.

CRITICAL THINKING

You arrive on the scene and find a 28-year-old construction worker who has sustained a large, gaping laceration to his left upper leg. Blood is spurting from the wound. The patient only responds with moans when you yell his name. His respiratory rate is 26/minute. His radial pulse is absent. His skin is extremely pale, cool, and clammy. His blood pressure is 98/76 mmHg and heart rate is 134/minute.

1. In order to determine if his ventilation is adequate, what else must you assess?
2. Based on the ventilation/perfusion ratio, why would the cells in the patient become and remain hypoxic?
3. Why is the patient responding so poorly?
4. How is the spurting blood affecting the perfusion of the cells?
5. What is causing a decrease in the systolic blood pressure?
6. Is the pulse pressure narrow? If so, describe why.
7. Why is the skin pale, cool, and clammy?
8. Why is the heart rate 134 bpm?
9. Are the cells of this patient likely undergoing aerobic or anaerobic metabolism? Why?
10. Why does the patient have such a lack of energy?

EXPLORE PEARSON **mybradykit**™

Please go to **www.bradybooks.com** to access mykit for this text. You will find quizzes, critical thinking scenarios, weblinks, animations, and videos related to this chapter—and much more. Look for information on cardiac output and blood pressure as well as animations on Starling's law and the process of gas exchange.

Register your access code from the front of your book by going to **www.bradybooks.com** and selecting the mykit links.

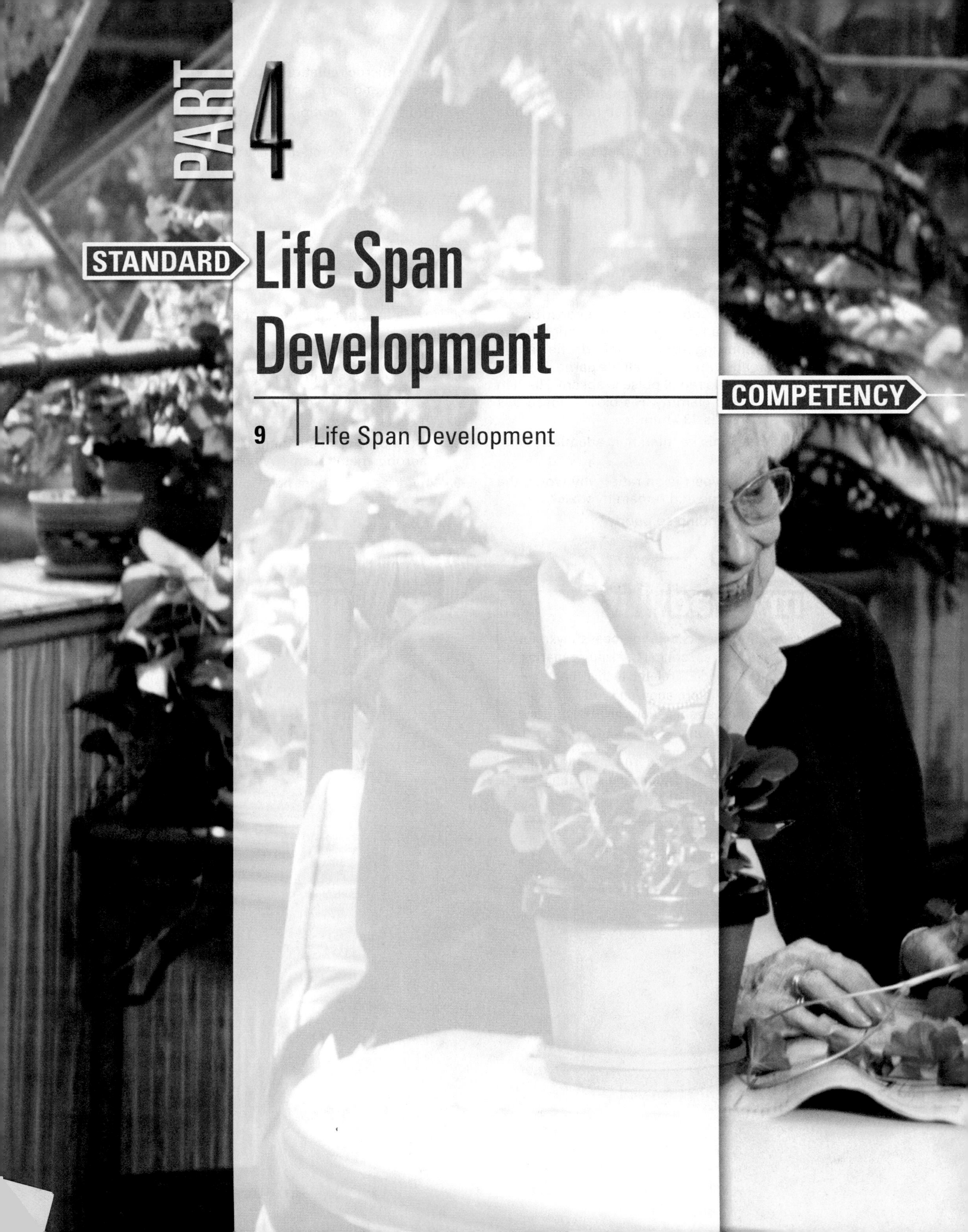

PART 4

STANDARD

Life Span Development

COMPETENCY

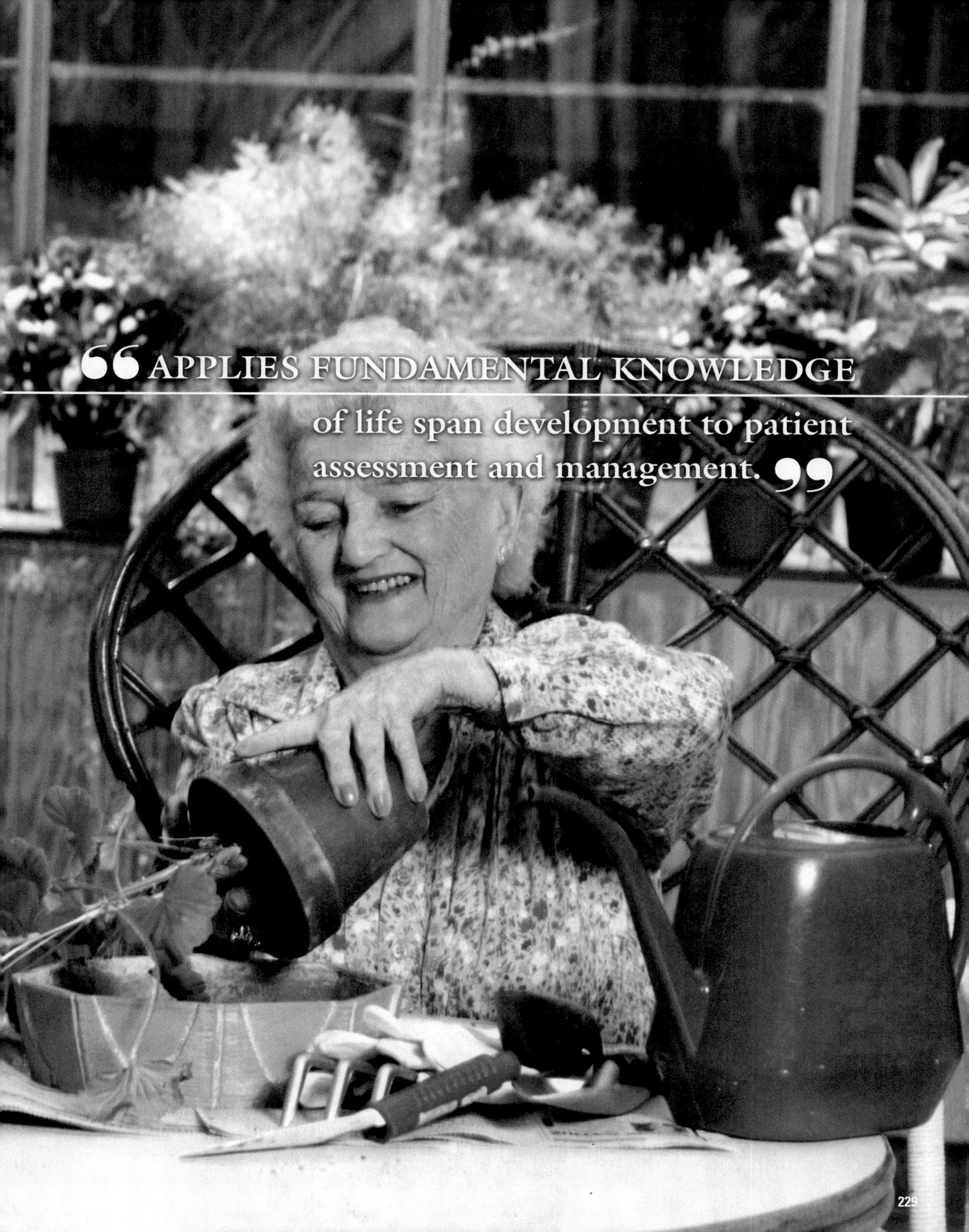
APPLIES FUNDAMENTAL KNOWLEDGE
of life span development to patient
assessment and management.

CHAPTER 9

Life Span Development

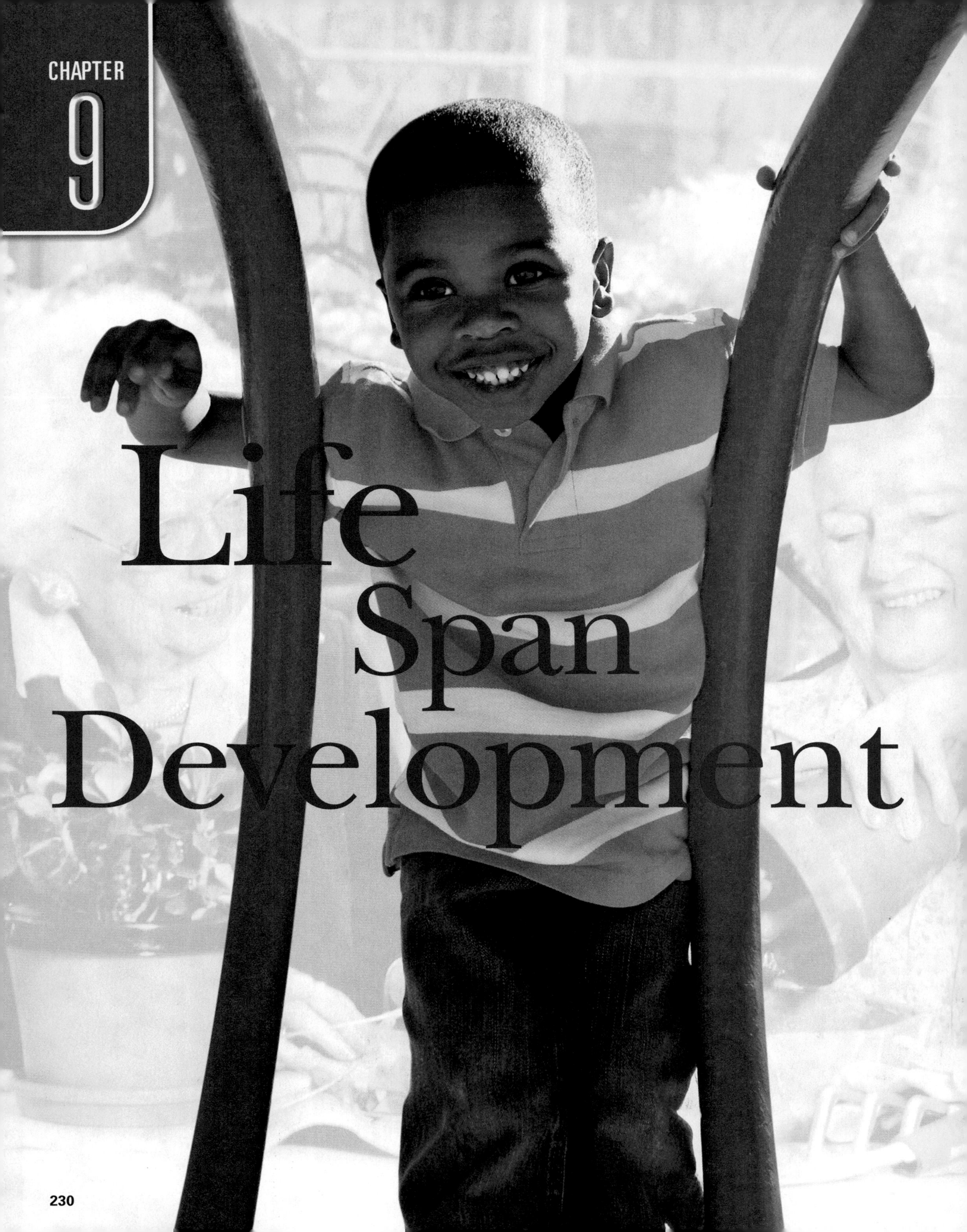

Navigation Guide

The following items provide an overview to the purpose and content of this chapter. The Standard and Competency are from the new National EMS Education Standards.

STANDARD **Life Span Development**

COMPETENCY Applies fundamental knowledge of life span development to patient assessment and management.

OBJECTIVES: After reading this chapter, you should be able to:

9-1. Define key terms introduced in this chapter.
9-2. Identify the age ranges associated with each of the following terms:
  a. Neonate
  b. Infant
  c. Toddler
  d. Preschooler
  e. School age
  f. Adolescent
  g. Early adulthood
  h. Middle adulthood
  i. Late adulthood
9-3. Describe the physiological changes that occur immediately after birth.
9-4. Discuss the key physical and psychosocial characteristics of individuals in each of the following age groups:
  a. Neonates and infants
  b. Toddlers
  c. Preschool-age children
  d. School-age children
  e. Adolescents
  f. Early adulthood
  g. Middle adulthood
  h. Late adulthood

KEY TERMS: Page references indicate first major use in this chapter. For complete definitions, see the Glossary at the back of the book.

adolescent p. 237
fontanelles p. 234
infant p. 232
life expectancy p. 240
maximum life span p. 240
menopause p. 240
neonate p. 232
nocturnal enuresis p. 237
preschooler p. 235
puberty p. 238
reflex p. 233
school age p. 236
toddler p. 235

MEDIA RESOURCES: Please go to www.bradybooks.com to access mykit for this text. You will find quizzes, critical thinking scenarios, weblinks, animations, and videos related to this chapter—and much more. Look for online information on the process of aging. You will also find a video clip on pediatric growth and development.

CASE STUDY

The Dispatch

EMS Unit 112—respond to 408 Windsor Avenue—you have a 16-year-old male patient who is complaining of difficulty urinating. Time out is 1345 hours.

Upon Arrival

Upon your arrival, a 37-year-old woman answers the door. She states that her son has complained that it hurts when he urinates and that she wants him checked out. As you enter the back bedroom, you find an alert and oriented 16-year-old male text-messaging on his cell phone. He yells at his mother and asks why she called the ambulance. She yells back and tells him that he is going to go to the hospital.

How Would You Proceed to Assess and Care for This Patient?

During this chapter, you will learn about the stages of life span development and how to apply this knowledge to your assessment and emergency care for a patient. Later, we will return to the case and apply the knowledge learned.

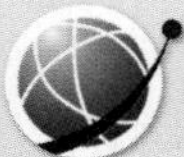

Media Resources
Go to www.bradybooks.com for mykit. Highlights:

- *Web Resource:* Lifespan Development
- *Web Resource:* Pediatric Stages of Development

Objective 9-2
Identify the age ranges associated with the terms neonate, infant, toddler, preschooler, school age, adolescent, early adulthood, middle adulthood, and late adulthood.

Introduction

Throughout the course of a lifetime, people experience changes, both physical and psychosocial. Although each individual matures at a different rate, most changes normally occur within a specific period of life. As an EMT, you will assess and treat patients who are in various life stages. You will need to incorporate your knowledge of what is expected for each stage into your patient assessment and management. Life span development begins at conception; however, prenatal development will be discussed later in Chapter 37, "Obstetrics and Care of the Newborn."

Life Span Development

The life stages discussed in this chapter are infants, toddlers and preschool-age children, school-age children, adolescents, and adults at early adulthood, middle adulthood, and late adulthood. For each group, normal vital signs are discussed. Normal vital signs for the various age groups are summarized in Table 9-1.

Neonates and Infants

The term **neonate** refers to the child from birth to 1 month of age (Figure 9-1a∗), while the term **infant** refers to the child from 1 month to 1 year of age (Figure 9-1b∗). During this period, a child undergoes some of the most rapid growth and development.

Vital Signs

At birth, the neonate has a respiratory rate of 40–60 breaths per minute and a tidal volume of only 6–8 mL/kg. His respiratory rate will drop to 30–40 breaths per minute after a few minutes of life. By the age of 1 year, his respiratory rate will be 20–30 breaths per minute and the tidal volume will increase to 10–15 mL/kg. At birth a neonate's heart rate is normally 140–160 beats per minute. Within the first 30 minutes after birth, the baby's heart rate decreases to 100–160 beats per minute. Then the heart rate will normally settle to around 120 beats per minute and remain that way or will slightly decrease throughout infancy. The average systolic blood pressure of an infant increases from 70 mmHg at birth to 90 mmHg by 1 year of age. An infant's temperature is normally 98°F–100°F, which is the thermoneutral range.

TABLE 9-1 Normal Vital Signs Throughout a Life Span

Stage of Development	Respirations (average in breaths per minute)	Pulse (average in beats per minute)	Blood Pressure (average in mmHg)	Temperature (degrees Fahrenheit)
Infancy: At birth	40–60	140–160	70 systolic	98–100
Infancy: Neonate	30–40	100–160	70–90 systolic	98–100
Infancy: At one year	20–30	100–120	90 systolic	98–100
Toddlers	20–30	80–130	70–100 systolic	98.6–99.6
Preschoolers	20–30	80–120	80–110 systolic	98.6–99.6
School age	20–30	70–110	80–120 systolic	98.6
Adolescents	12–20	55–105	100–120 systolic	98.6
Early adulthood	16–20	70	120/80	98.6
Middle adulthood	16–20	70	120/80	98.6
Late adulthood	Depends on patient's physical and health status	Depends on patient's physical and health status	Depends on patient's physical and health status	98.6

Objectives 9-3 and 9-4
Describe the physiological changes that occur immediately after birth and the key characteristics of neonates and infants, toddlers, preschool-age children, school-age children, and early, middle, and late adulthood.

Key Terms

neonate a child from birth to 1 month of age.

infant a child from 1 month to 1 year of age.

reflex an instantaneous and involuntary movement resulting from a stimulus.

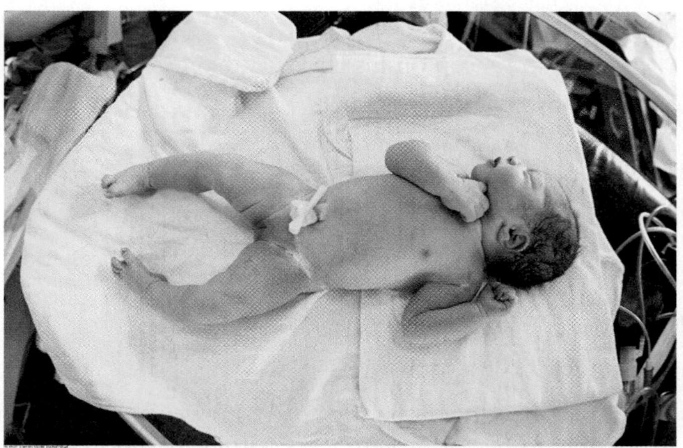

FIGURE 9-1a ✻ A newborn infant (neonate).
(© Rommel/Masterfile)

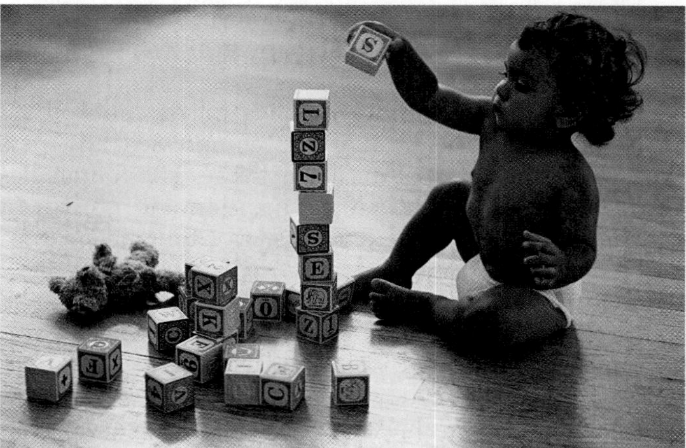

FIGURE 9-1b ✻ A 12-month-old infant.
(© Raoul Minsart/Masterfile)

In general, as an infant ages his heart rate and respiratory rate become lower and his systolic blood pressure becomes higher.

Physiological Changes

At birth the neonate normally weighs 3.0–3.5 kg and the head accounts for 25 percent of the total body weight. The initial birth weight of the neonate normally drops 5–10 percent in the first 2 weeks of life, but the lost weight is normally regained shortly thereafter. The baby's weight will continue to increase throughout infancy with proper nutrition. Infants require breast milk or formula to meet their nutritional needs. As his first year progresses, the infant will be able to consume other soft foods without yet having teeth. During infancy, the primary teeth will begin to emerge, and the baby will be slowly introduced to solid foods.

A baby's pulmonary system also undergoes changes throughout infancy. An infant's airways are shorter, narrower, less stable, and more easily obstructed than those of an adult. This can make him more easily susceptible to airway obstructions. Until 4 weeks of age, infants are primarily nose breathers. They have fewer alveoli with decreased collateral ventilation. Their lung tissue is also fragile and is prone to trauma from pressure. It is important for the EMT to be mindful of this when manually ventilating an infant. Infants also have immature accessory muscles. This makes them easily susceptible to early fatigue from labored breathing. The infant's less rigid chest wall and more horizontally placed ribs promote diaphragmatic breathing. Therefore the EMT should examine both the chest and the abdomen when assessing an infant's respiration. If an infant's respiratory rate is rapid, it can lead to rapid heat and fluid loss. The EMT can help to prevent some of the heat loss by keeping the baby warm and dry.

The infant's immune system is also immature. Most of the neonate's immunity is based on antibodies that he received through the placenta from his mother during pregnancy. This is called passive immunity and is normally retained through the first 6 months of life. Babies who are breast-fed may also receive antibodies from their mother's breast milk and will thus retain immunity as long as breast-feeding continues. Because infants are more susceptible to infections and diseases, it is important for them to be immunized early. Childhood immunizations normally begin after birth and should continue to be provided at various times throughout the child's development.

The infant's nervous system allows him to have normal movement and sensation. Infants also have special **reflexes**, or instantaneous and involuntary movements, that result from a stimulus at birth. These reflexes include blinking, startling, rooting, sucking, swallowing, stepping, gagging, and grasping reflexes. Their very strong and coordinated sucking and gag reflexes help them survive. They also have well-flexed extremities that move equally when the infant is stimulated. An EMT should look for symmetrical movement when assessing an infant. Infants are able to sense pain and touch. Although they are not capable of localizing pain, it is

Key Terms
fontanelles soft spots on a baby's skull that allow the head to pass through the birth canal during delivery and to expand during development.

Key Points
Crying is how infants communicate with the world around them.

important to consider that an infant may be experiencing pain if he is crying. As the baby grows, his response to pain will become more specific.

Babies are born with **fontanelles**, or soft spots on the skull that allow the head to be compressed and pass through the birth canal during delivery. The fontanelles also allow room for the rapid expansion and growth of the brain during infancy. The posterior fontanelle closes at 3 months and the anterior fontanelle closes between 9 and 18 months. The EMT should never press on the fontanelles. The fontanelles may provide the EMT with an indirect estimate of hydration. Normally, the fontanelles will be level to the skull. If the child is dehydrated, the fontanelles may appear depressed or sunken in relation to the rest of the skull.

The bones in the baby's musculoskeletal system will grow throughout infancy. As the infant grows, he will be able to perform more activities. The EMT should know what activities are normally present at various stages of infancy.

By 2 months, an infant will be able to do the following:

- Track objects with his eyes
- Focus on objects 8–12 inches away
- Recognize familiar faces
- Display primary emotions and facial expressions
- Hear and recognize some familiar sounds and voices
- Move in response to stimuli

By 6 months, the infant should be able to do the following:

- Sit upright in a high chair
- Make one-syllable sounds (e.g., ma, mu, da, di)
- Raise and support his upper body when he is on his stomach
- Grasp and shake hand toys
- Push down on his legs and feet when held over a firm surface
- Follow moving objects with his eyes
- Recognize familiar objects at a distance
- Begin to babble and try to imitate familiar sounds

By 12 months, the infant should be able to do the following:

- Walk with help
- Know his own name
- Sit without assistance
- Crawl and creep on his hands and knees
- Put objects into containers
- Poke objects with fingers
- Respond to simple requests and "no"
- Say "mama" or "dada"
- Imitate some words, gestures, and facial expressions
- Begin to use objects like brushes, cups, or phones correctly
- Finger feed himself

Every child develops at his own pace. However, if an infant is not able to perform these tasks within the normal time frame, the infant should be evaluated by a physician. EMTs should know what types of movements and activities are expected during each of these periods so they can better assess the pediatric patient and understand his responses.

Psychosocial Changes

Just as the infant experiences many physical changes, he will also develop psychosocially throughout infancy. The relationships built during this period most often revolve around the infant's parents and primary caregivers. The parents are responsible not only for meeting the infant's physical needs but also for providing a stable home filled with love and affection. Children who lack fulfillment of any of their physical, emotional, or psychological needs are less likely to become healthy self-reliant adults. Infants bond with the people who meet their needs.

As an EMT you may encounter different responses when you attempt to take an infant away from his parent. In most cases, the infant will protest and act as if in despair and withdrawal when separated from his caregiver. To him, you are not his caregiver and he will tend to be afraid of you. Crying and restlessness may persist even after the child is returned to the parent. If the infant does not seem anxious or upset when separated from his parent, the EMT should consider underlying causes that may be affecting the infant's response.

Crying is how infants communicate with the world around them. Although the EMT may not recognize a difference in an infant's cry, the parent or caregiver should be able to. An infant normally cries in response to a basic need, anger, or pain. The basic cry normally indicates that the child is hungry, wet, or tired. Once this need is met, the infant normally does not continue to cry. An infant may also

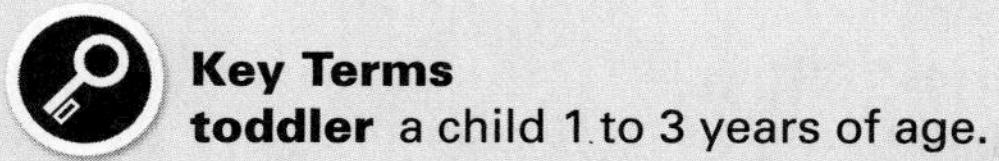

Key Terms
toddler a child 1 to 3 years of age.

Key Terms
preschooler a child 3 to 6 years of age.

cry as a result of being angry. This type of cry can usually be noted by the EMT who separates the infant from his parent. This type of crying can be avoided if you allow the parent to hold the infant during your assessment. The child may also cry as a response to pain. If the cry persists for a long period of time and all the other needs of the child have been met, the EMT should suspect that something else, such as pain, is contributing to the infant's response.

By the end of infancy, the baby will have developed relationships with his parents and family. He should be able to recognize his favorite things and people. Some infants may have a favorite toy or other item they can hold that may provide some comfort while you perform your assessment. However, never allow an infant to have anything that could possibly cause an airway obstruction. Smile and speak in a calm voice when assessing a patient in this age group. Try to keep the parents calm, too. Although the infant may not be able to understand what is occurring, he is able to identify changes in emotion and gestures, especially from his parents. If the parent is upset and scared, the infant usually will respond in the same way.

Toddlers and Preschool-Age Children

The term **toddler** refers to a child who is 1 to 3 years of age. A **preschooler** is a child who is 3 to 6 years of age (Figures 9-2a and 9-2b*). The children in these stages continue to grow physically and psychosocially.

Vital Signs

As children age, their heart and respiratory rates tend to decrease while their systolic blood pressure increases. Typically, a toddler will have a normal heart rate of 80–130 beats per minute. He will have a normal respiratory rate of 20–30 breaths per minute. The toddler's normal systolic blood pressure will range from 70–100 mmHg. The child's temperature will range from 98.6°F–99.6°F.

Preschoolers typically have a normal heart rate of 80–120 beats per minute. Their respiratory rate is normally 20–30 breaths per minute. The normal systolic blood pressure for a preschooler ranges from 80–110 mmHg. The body temperature of a preschooler will range from 98.6°F–99.6°F.

Physiological Changes

As children get older, they experience more physiological changes. The bones in the musculoskeletal system continue to grow and increase in density. By the end of this period, children will have all of their primary teeth. Toddlers and preschoolers continue to increase their muscle mass, but their weight gain slows down. They normally shed extra fat and become leaner.

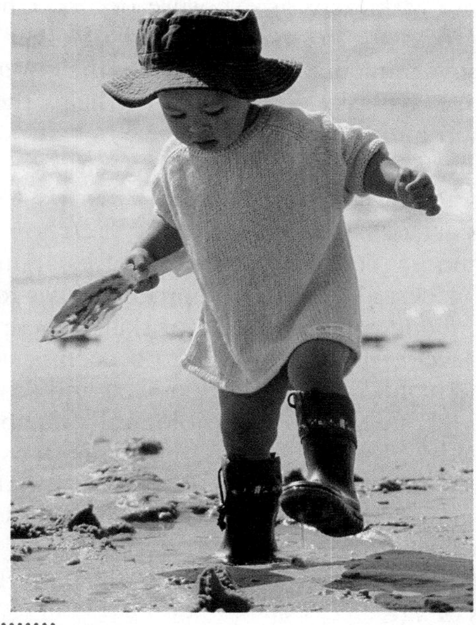

FIGURE 9-2a * A toddler. (© Pierre Arsenault/Masterfile)

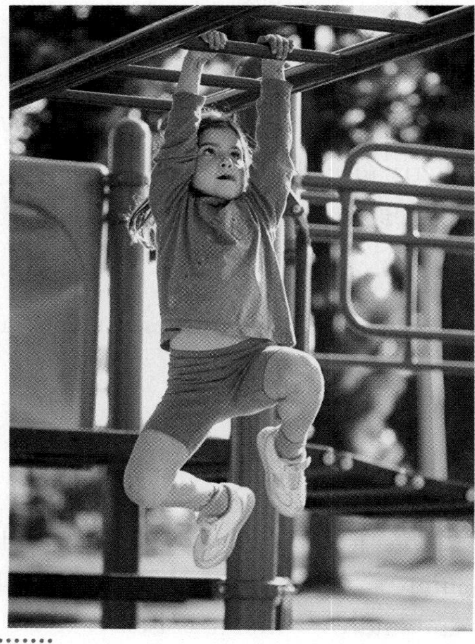

FIGURE 9-2b * A preschooler. (© WireImageStock/Masterfile)

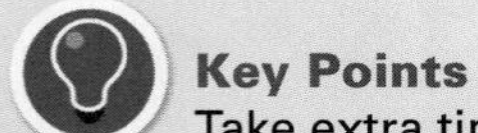

Key Points
Take extra time to communicate with a toddler or preschooler on a level he understands.

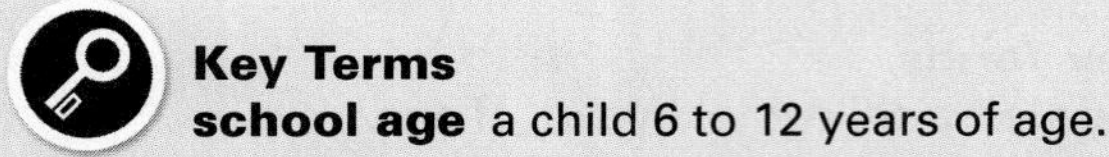

Key Terms
school age a child 6 to 12 years of age.

In the pulmonary system, the terminal airways continue to branch and the alveoli continue to grow in number. Passive immunity from the mother is lost, which makes the child more susceptible to minor respiratory and gastrointestinal infections. However, the child begins to develop his own immunity, known as active immunity, to common pathogens as exposure occurs. Children in this age group are normally exposed to other children and new environments, which increases the number of infections they typically contract, but it helps them build their own immunities.

The nervous system of toddlers and preschoolers continues to develop quickly. The brain is the fastest growing part of their body, and by preschool age the child's brain has reached 90 percent of its adult weight. During this period, their development allows for effortless walking and other basic motor skills. These children begin to develop fine motor skills, too, such as using their fingers and hands to manipulate objects and scribble.

Although children are physiologically capable of toilet training by 12 to 15 months, most are not psychologically ready until they reach 18 to 30 months. The average age for toilet training completion is 28 months. Although they are toilet trained, most children will continue to experience bed-wetting at night until they are 6 or 7 years of age.

It is important for the EMT to recognize what activities toddlers and preschoolers are capable of performing. This information may help in identifying what is normal for a child in this age group.

By the age of 3, the child should be able to:

- Walk alone and begin to run
- Pull or carry several toys when walking
- Climb up and down furniture or stairs with minimal support
- Scribble and play with toys
- Recognize names, faces, voices, objects, and body parts
- Find hidden objects
- Sort objects by shape or color

By the age of 5, children should be able to:

- Stand on one foot for more than 10 seconds
- Hop, jump, swing, climb, and do somersaults
- Dress and undress without assistance
- Use forks, spoons, and sometimes knives appropriately
- Count ten or more objects
- Trace and draw pictures

Psychosocial Changes

Toddlers and preschoolers experience many psychosocial and cognitive changes. Language takes the place of crying as the sole form of communication. The basics of language are usually mastered by approximately 36 months, and the child can say single words and make simple phrases and sentences. As the child grows, his language will continue to expand and be refined. By 18 to 24 months, a child can understand cause and effect. Most children develop separation anxiety at approximately 18 months of age. This reaction normally includes the child clinging to the parent or caregiver and crying when the person leaves. By age 5, a preschooler can say his name and address. He can also recall and tell stories using sentences.

Children use play in a variety of ways. They explore new ideas and objects, identify and resolve simple problems, and learn from engaging in different activities. During this period, children are able to play simple games and follow basic rules. Play time also serves as a social outlet and encourages the children to learn and improve their social skills. Many children attend preschool or day care and begin to develop friendships outside their immediate families. Children in this group begin to display competitiveness. Toddlers and preschoolers may express feelings and frustrations they can't express through play.

When assessing a toddler or preschooler, the EMT should take extra time to communicate with the patient on a level he understands. Children take language literally, so phrases like "take your blood pressure" should be replaced with a phrase that can be interpreted literally, such as "measure your blood pressure." It also helps if you allow the child to touch the equipment before you use it and demonstrate on a parent how the equipment will be used. Techniques like these will help decrease the child's anxiety and increase the trust he will have in you. Never lie to a child, because you will not regain his trust during the short period you will see him. Allow the parent to stay with the child during the assessment if possible. This will also help alleviate some of the child's fears and provide you with more information pertinent to the situation.

School-Age Children

The term **school age** refers to a child between 6 and 12 years of age (Figure 9-3*).

Key Points
Most school-age children identify EMTs, firefighters, and law enforcement officers as people who can help them in a crisis.

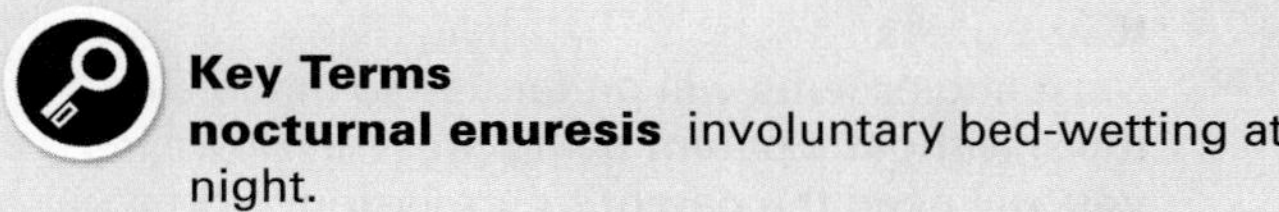

Key Terms
nocturnal enuresis involuntary bed-wetting at night.

Key Terms
adolescent a child 12 to 18 years of age.

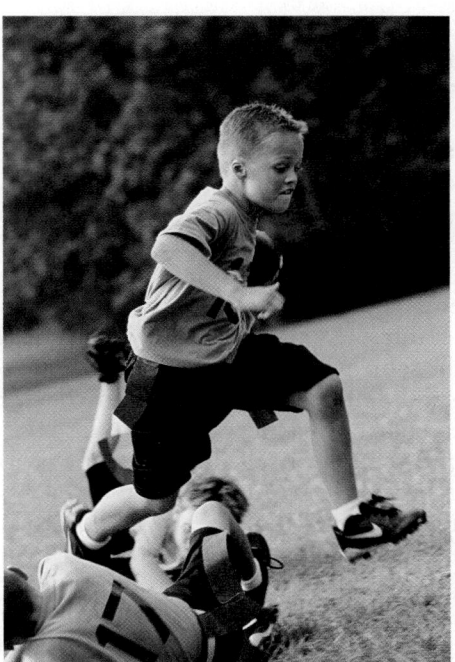

FIGURE 9-3 * A school-age child. (© Kevin Dodge/Masterfile)

Vital Signs

School-age children have normal heart rates ranging from 70–110 beats per minute. Their respiratory rates range from 20–30 breaths per minute. They typically have a systolic blood pressure of 80–120 mmHg. A school-age child's temperature is normally 98.6°F.

Physiological Changes

As school-age children get older, they continue to grow and change. The bones in the musculoskeletal system continue to increase in density and grow larger. Most children experience some discomfort when this occurs. School-age children lose their primary teeth and replace them with permanent teeth. Their brain function increases in both hemispheres. Children in this age group are normally able to read and write. Although school-age children are able to control their bodily functions better, some still struggle with **nocturnal enuresis**, or involuntary bed-wetting at night, after the age of 10.

Psychosocial Changes

Most children in this age group attend school and develop relationships outside of the home. Because of this, they interact more with adults and other children. Friendships are formed, especially with the same sex, and become more important during this period. Most children in this age group participate in a variety of social activities and develop problem-solving skills. They are capable of fundamental reasoning and problem solving, but have not developed the insight to do so in all situations.

School-age children develop their own self-concept, that is, a personal concept of who they are. These children compare themselves with others to help determine their own values and to seek the approval of others. School-age children also begin to develop a sense of self-esteem and morals. They understand how to obey rules and avoid punishment. School-age children understand concepts associated with pain, illness, death, and loss, but most are still uneasy or scared when those situations occur. They will usually turn to a parent or other adult or to a trusted friend to help them cope with their fears.

Most school-age children identify EMTs, firefighters, and law enforcement officers as people who can help them in a crisis. They may actually have unrealistic expectations about what you are able to do, but assure them that you are doing everything you can to help them or their family member. Make sure you communicate at a level they can understand.

Adolescence

An **adolescent** is a child between 12 and 18 years of age (Figure 9-4*). Although most adolescents want to feel and be treated as adults, they are not adults and are continuing to experience physiological and psychosocial changes throughout this period.

Vital Signs

Adolescents have normal heart rates ranging from 55–105 beats per minute. Their normal respiratory rate ranges from 12–20 breaths per minute. They typically have a systolic blood pressure of 100–120 mmHg. An adolescent's temperature is normally 98.6°F.

Physiological Changes

Most adolescents will experience a rapid 2- to 3-year growth spurt. Their muscle mass and bone growth and development are nearly complete by the end of this period. The adolescent's growth spurt begins distally with the enlargement of the feet and hands and progresses

Key Terms
puberty the period in which the sexual organs mature during adolescence.

Key Points
Most adolescents will prefer you to interview them without a parent being present. However, you will need the parent's permission to do so.

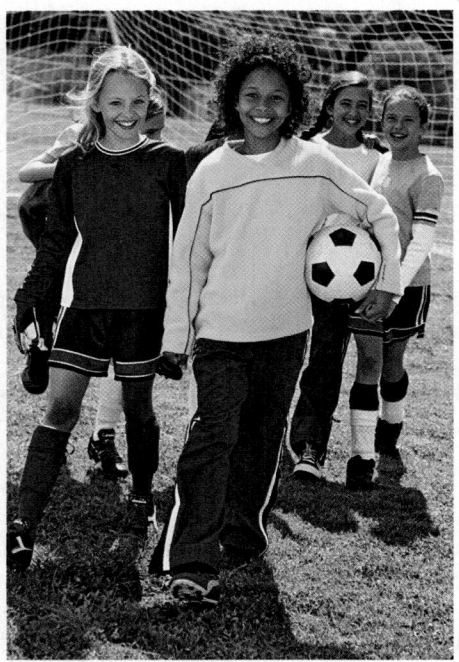

FIGURE 9-4 * Adolescents. (© JJ/Getty Images)

along the extremities. In the final stages of adolescence, the chest and trunk enlarge. Girls are mostly done growing by age 16, while boys are mostly done by age 18.

During this period, adolescents go through **puberty**, the period in which the sexual organs mature and reproductive maturity is reached. Girls usually begin puberty around age 10, which is about 2 years before most boys. Primary and secondary sexual development occurs. Endocrine changes occur and specific hormones are released into the adolescent's bloodstream. During this period, males grow facial, pubic, and axillary hair. They also develop a deeper voice. Their shoulders broaden and their muscles become larger. The adolescent male's penis and testes also increase in size and the adolescent has erections that result in the ejaculation of semen. Females begin menstruation and their breasts enlarge. They also grow pubic and axillary hair. Their hips normally widen and the waist gets smaller.

Psychosocial Changes

The many biological, social, and emotional changes that occur during adolescence can cause family conflicts. Most of these conflicts revolve around the adolescent and his parents. Adolescents become more argumentative and more aware of the shortcomings of others. They also believe that they are the focus of others' attention and that they are invulnerable. As a result, many participate in risky behaviors.

Adolescents desire to be treated as adults although most are not capable of making their own medical decisions. (See Chapter 3, "Medical, Legal, and Ethical Issues.") Adolescents want privacy, and most will prefer if their parents are not present during the patient interview. If possible, interview the adolescent in private. Interview them in the same way you would an adult, but remember that you should obtain the parent's consent before doing so. Adolescents may be more willing to disclose pertinent medical information or self-destructive behaviors if their parents are not present.

During this time, adolescents develop their identity. They often try to imitate others and experiment with alternative identities in an attempt to find their own. Peer pressure increases during this stage. Self-consciousness increases and adolescents desire more independence and responsibility. They begin to make decisions that will influence their careers and their futures.

Adolescents understand that there are consequences to their actions and are capable of discerning what is right and socially acceptable and what is wrong. Antisocial behavior peaks around eighth or ninth grade. Some adolescents begin to participate in self-destructive behaviors such as tobacco, alcohol, and/or illicit drug use. These types of behaviors can cause both physical and psychosocial problems for the adolescent. Depression and suicide are more common in this age group than in any other.

Adolescents are also very concerned with body image. How they look and feel about themselves has a profound impact on their sense of identity and self-esteem. They make continual comparisons between themselves and their peers and often look to outside sources for what a "perfect body" should be like. Because of this, eating disorders within this age group are common. Bulimia (eating and deliberately throwing up) and anorexia nervosa (not eating enough to meet nutritional needs) in order to control weight are more frequently identified in females; however, these disorders are also becoming more common among males. These eating disorders can cause both psychological and physical problems and occasionally become severe enough to be life threatening.

During adolescence, both males and females experience an increased interest in the opposite sex and begin dating and/or participating in sexual activity. Because their bodies and sex cells have matured, they are capable of reproduction. Some adolescents choose to abstain from sexual activity during this period. Many adolescents who engage in sexual activity do not use condoms or otherwise practice safe sex. Some may feel they are invulnerable to the risks, while others may be embarrassed to ask for their partner's sexual history or simply get too carried away to be pragmatic. Participation in unprotected sexual activities increases the risk of acquiring sexually transmitted diseases as well as the risk of pregnancy.

Early Adulthood

Early adulthood is defined as the stage of development when a person is 20 to 40 years of age (Figure 9-5*).

Vital Signs

The average heart rate for a person in early adulthood is 70 beats per minute. Average respiratory rate is 16–20 breaths per minute. Average blood pressure is 120/80 mmHg. Normal temperature is 98.6°F.

Physiological Changes

During early adulthood, all body systems are operating at optimal levels. Most people reach peak physical condition between 19 and 26 years of age. Because of their excellent physical condition, they are capable of risky activity, and hence accidents are the leading cause of death in this age group. Once young adults reach their peak, however, their physical condition begins to slow down. They gain weight, store fat, and experience decreased muscle tone. Their spinal disks settle. During this period, adults also develop lifelong habits and routines that will impact the quality of their health and life.

Psychosocial Changes

Upon entering early adulthood, people generally take on more responsibility and become more independent. Many young adults choose to leave their parents' homes and make homes of their own. During this period, most people develop both romantic and affectionate relationships. Many young adults marry and begin new families. Childbirth is most common in this age group. Their new families provide new challenges and stress for the early adults. It is also during this time that many adults finish school and find a career. They experience the highest levels of job stress during this period. Early adults are more capable of coping with their stress than when they were younger. This period is less associated with psychological problems related to well-being than other age groups.

Middle Adulthood

Middle adulthood is the stage of development when a person is 41 to 60 years of age (Figure 9-6*).

Vital Signs

The average heart rate for a person in middle adulthood is 70 beats per minute. Their average respiratory rate is 16–20 breaths per minute. They have an average blood pressure of 120/80 mmHg, and their temperature is normally 98.6°F. There are no significant changes in normal levels from early adulthood.

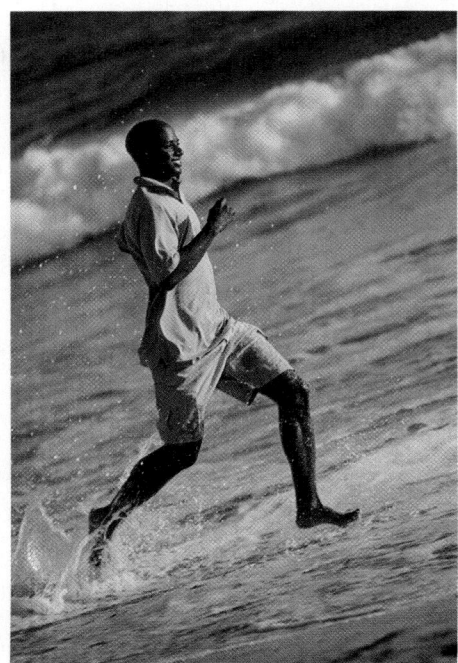

FIGURE 9-5 * A young adult. (© Ty Milford/Masterfile)

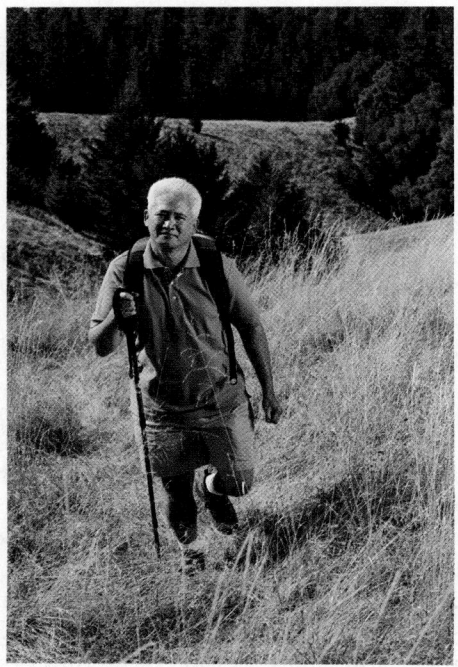

FIGURE 9-6 * A middle-aged adult. (© Masterfile)

Key Terms

menopause the permanent end of menstruation and fertility, which usually occurs in a woman's late 40s or 50s.

Thinking Critically

What expectations should you have when called to an emergency for an older adult that are different from those for a younger patient? How should you adjust your communication with this patient? the physical exam? preparations for transport?

Physiological Changes

During middle adulthood, the body is still functioning at a high level but with varying degrees of degradation. Body systems are beginning to experience more changes as a result of disease and lifestyle decisions. Adults in this stage are more susceptible to chronic illnesses and diseases like diabetes and arthritis.

It is usually during middle adulthood when cardiovascular health becomes a concern. Cardiac output decreases throughout this period. Cholesterol levels increase. This makes people more susceptible to cardiovascular diseases. Cancer is also a concern and strikes this age group frequently. Screenings for various types of cancers are recommended to those in this age group.

Middle-aged adults continue to gain weight easily, while controlling weight becomes more difficult. Many individuals have vision changes and require corrective lenses to see properly. Because of environmental and physical changes, most do not hear as well as they did during early adulthood.

Normally, women in their late 40s and 50s will go through **menopause**, or the permanent end of menstruation and fertility. Many women during this period are prone to a decrease in height as a result of osteoporosis.

Psychosocial Changes

During middle adulthood, people tend to approach problems more as challenges than as threats. This is the period when many individuals reach their goals and try to find ways to help younger generations. Some adults experience a period of self-questioning if they have not been able to accomplish their goals. These adults have experienced many different problems within previous stages of life, and have developed coping strategies that can be useful throughout the remainder of adulthood. This age group is aware of the limits of time, and many formulate new goals for the remainder of their lives.

Many adults focus on others rather than themselves during this stage. Because of this, some may delay seeking help for health issues. Many of these adults are burdened by financial commitments both for elderly parents and for young adult children. Transitions in parenting also occur during this period. As the children leave the home, some adults experience a feeling of loss known as empty nest syndrome; others embrace the extra time they didn't have before. Sometimes, grown-up children return home because of economic or social reasons. This can be both positive and negative for the families. It is also during this period that many adults become grandparents.

Late Adulthood

Late adulthood is the stage of development when a person is 61 years of age and older (Figure 9-7*).

Vital Signs

The heart rate, respiratory rate, and blood pressure in late adulthood depend on the person's physical and health status. Underlying diseases, poor physical conditioning, and some medications can alter the vital signs for these patients. Normal temperature in late adulthood is 98.6°F.

Physiological Changes

The **maximum life span**, which is the theoretically longest period of time for an organism to live, is 120 years for a human being. However, an individual's **life expectancy** is the average years of life remaining based on the individual's year of birth. Almost all individuals will

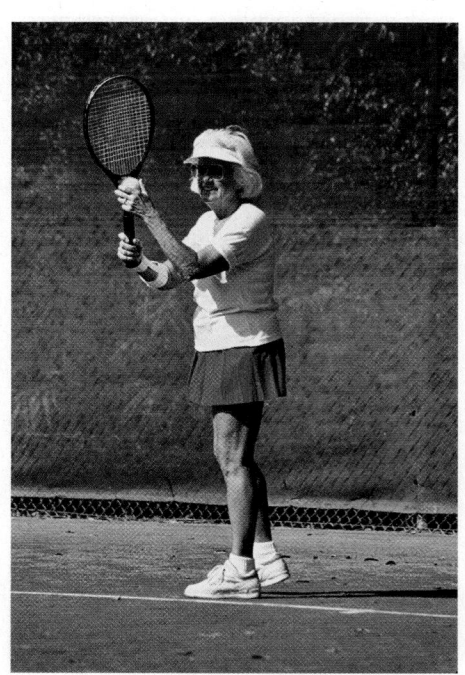

FIGURE 9-7 * An older adult. (© Dion Ogust/The Image Works)

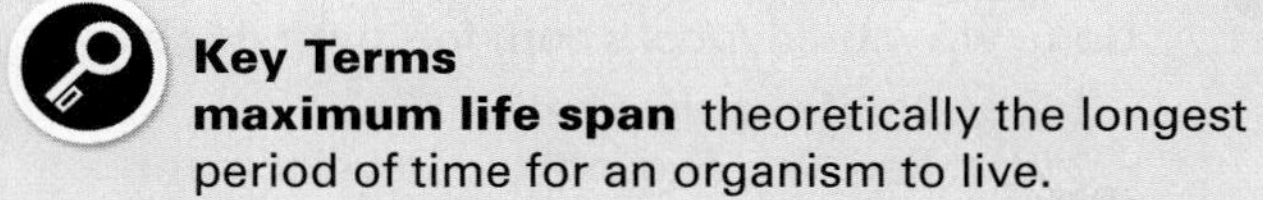
Key Terms
maximum life span theoretically the longest period of time for an organism to live.

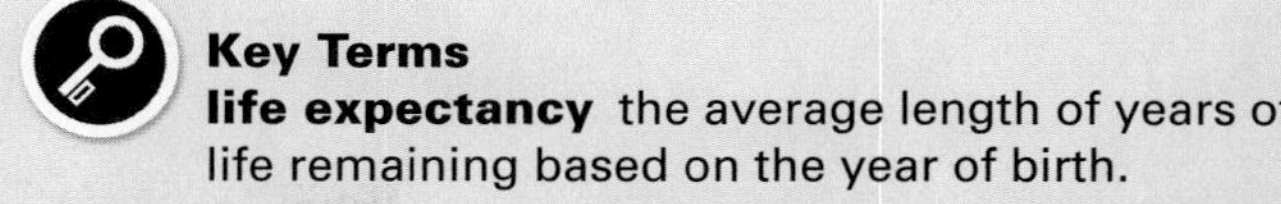
Key Terms
life expectancy the average length of years of life remaining based on the year of birth.

die from diseases or accidents before reaching the maximum life span. The incidence of diseases and illnesses continues to increase with age. During late adulthood, most body systems continue to become less efficient.

The cardiovascular system undergoes several changes in late adulthood. The efficiency of circulation decreases. The blood vessels within the cardiovascular system thicken, which results in increased peripheral resistance, which in turn reduces blood flow to the organs. The workload and size of the heart increase, which puts additional demands on the myocardium. Many older adults have heart problems and diseases that contribute to the additional workload on the heart. The myocardium is less able to respond to exercise, and tachycardia is not well tolerated in this age group. The functional blood volume is also decreased in late adulthood.

The respiratory system also develops changes in the mouth, nose, and lungs during late adulthood. The chest wall and bone structure weaken and make coughing ineffective. The elasticity of the diaphragm and the lung capacity of these adults are diminished. Metabolic changes and lifelong exposure to pollutants have diminished the lung capacity and diffusion of the gases through the alveoli.

The nervous system also changes during late adulthood. The brain gets smaller and these adults lose neurons, which causes problems with memory, balance, and movement. The sleep cycle may be disrupted, and many older adults experience sleep problems. Reaction time to various stimuli is decreased, and it takes longer to respond than before. This makes older adults more prone to falls or injury.

These adults experience many sensory changes. They lose taste buds, which results in a diminished sense of taste. Their olfactory senses are also diminished. They experience diminished pain perception and diminished kinesthetic sense. Adults in this period also experience hearing loss and their visual acuity is decreased. Many adults need corrective lenses and hearing aids to help compensate for these sensory losses.

The endocrine, reproductive, and renal systems are also affected in late adulthood. These adults have decreased metabolism and insulin production. Some adults in late adulthood may have underlying problems resulting from diabetes. The reproductive organs atrophy in women during this developmental stage. There is a 50 percent nephron loss within the kidneys, and the amount of abnormal glomeruli increase during this period. Adults in late adulthood have a decreased elimination of urine from the renal system. Problems with hydration are common in this age group.

Older adults experience changes to the mouth, teeth, and saliva during this period. Many adults lose permanent teeth and must use dentures. This can lead to changes in diet that could result in vitamin and mineral deficiencies. Their ability to chew their food can be impaired and may result in possible airway obstructions. Dentures, or the loss of teeth without them, may influence speech and communication. The gastrointestinal system functions less efficiently and gastrointestinal secretions are decreased. The rate of absorption of minerals, foods, and medications also changes, and many adults suffer from constipation during this period.

Because of the nature of EMS, many older patients that you are called to treat will be experiencing not only the current emergency but one or more chronic illnesses as well. However, there is a wider variation of health status in this age group than in any other. While some at this time of life have serious mental or physical problems, many others maintain good mental and physical health and lead active lives throughout their 60s, 70s, 80s, and even their 90s. When dealing with an older adult, be aware of the possibility of underlying ill health, but do not assume that every older patient has chronic physical or mental deficits.

Psychosocial Changes

During late adulthood, people face new challenges that may not have been present throughout the previous stages. In some cultures, wisdom is attributed to age. The experiences and behaviors developed throughout their lifetime have influenced who they have become. These adults tend to reflect on their lives and generally are either satisfied with the outcome or have regrets that may lead to depression or despair.

Some adults have families and friends who can provide support during this period, while many others do not. Even those who have support networks may feel alone and isolated at this stage.

Although many adults have lived in their homes for a great portion of their lives, many during late adulthood must make decisions about moving. Many older adults live in assisted-living communities that can help provide social, emotional, and physical support to their residents. However, these communities are expensive and many individuals must sell their homes and possessions in order to reside there, while many others cannot afford them at all. Some remain at home or may move in to a family

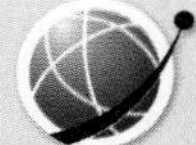

Media Resources
Go to www.bradybooks.com for mykit. Highlights:

- *Video:* Notifying the Family
- *Video:* Pediatric Growth and Development

member's home. Sometimes the decision to move is based on the financial burdens associated with living alone and no longer working. Many adults during this period live on fixed incomes and must make difficult decisions about how to manage their finances.

Because older adults have been independent and self-reliant for most of their lives, some may feel ashamed or otherwise reluctant to give up their independence and ask for assistance. Combined with many of the physical changes and illnesses they may have, this can lead to a decline in the older adult's well-being and sense of self-worth. Many find themselves not capable of performing activities that they once performed easily. Many of these adults also experience the death or dying of their spouses or companions. This may leave them feeling more alone and isolated than before and may cause them to think more about their own death.

However, while there are many psychosocial challenges associated with aging, the majority of older adults are able to remain in their own homes and lead rewarding lives. Most do not need to go to a nursing home, to an assisted-living facility, or to live with relatives until very advanced age or at all.

CHAPTER REVIEW

SUMMARY

People develop and change continuously throughout their life span. These changes are both physical and psychosocial in nature. It is important to understand the different stages of life and to know what is normal for each stage. It is also important to understand what changes and challenges your patients may be experiencing during each stage of development. Such understanding can help you identify your patient's needs and appropriately modify your assessment and management approach. The stages an EMT should be knowledgeable about are infancy, toddlerhood, preschool age, school age, adolescence, early adulthood, middle adulthood, and late adulthood.

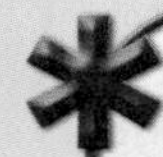

CASE STUDY FOLLOW-UP

SCENE SIZE-UP

You have been dispatched to a 16-year-old male patient complaining of difficulty urinating. As you arrive on the scene, you are greeted by a 37-year-old woman who answers the front door. She states that her name is Linda Shively and that her 16-year-old son, Jeremiah, has been complaining that it hurts when he urinates. She states that she wants him checked out and taken to the local emergency department. She leads you into the back bedroom of a neat and orderly residence. As you enter the back bedroom, you see a young man on his bed.

PATIENT ASSESSMENT

The patient, a 16-year-old male who is dressed in jeans and a T-shirt, is actively text-messaging on his cell phone as you approach him. As you say "Hello," he begins to yell at his mother and asks her, "Why did you call the ambulance?" His mother yells back that he is going to go to the hospital. Because you know conflict between adolescents and their parents is normal, you ask your partner to take Mrs. Shively into another room to gather the patient's medical history.

The teenager identifies himself as Jeremiah Shively and states that he really doesn't want to go to the ED. He is alert and oriented. His airway is open and he is breathing adequately at 12 breaths per minute. His pulse is 60 beats per minute and his skin is warm and dry. His blood pressure is 110/74 mmHg. His vitals appear within normal ranges for his age.

You begin your patient interview by introducing yourself and explaining that you are there to help him. You know that adolescents want to be treated as adults. You also understand that Jeremiah will be more likely to disclose information to you in private than with his mother in the room. You ask him if he is having any problems. He continues to text-message and says, "No." You state his mother called and said he was having pain when he urinates. He then replies, "That's just what I told her."

You attempt to develop a good rapport with Jeremiah. You ask him again if he is having any problems either urinating or in general. This time he states that he is not having much pain when he urinates, but that he does have itching and redness around his genitals. Because you are aware that many adolescents are sexually active, you know that you will need to ask more personal questions that may potentially embarrass the teen. As you proceed to obtain a history from him, he confides in you that he has been sexually active. You ask him directly about his sexual history, and he states that he has had unprotected sex with several partners. You know this type of behavior puts him at risk for sexually transmitted diseases.

You ask Jeremiah if you may examine him, and he agrees. You perform a complete physical assessment, noting nothing out of the ordinary for Jeremiah's age except in the genital area, as he stated. You explain that his mother wants him to be evaluated at the local hospital and that he should be assessed and treated by a physician. You also explain the consequences of not seeking medical treatment for his current condition. Knowing that adolescents are capable of reasoning and understanding the consequences of their actions, you ask him if he will go with you to the hospital. Although he is a minor and cannot provide you with full consent—or refusal—for treatment, it is important that you make him feel that he has an active role in his care. You understand that if you address Jeremiah as you would an adult, he will most likely cooperate and agree to go; however, if he doesn't agree you will need to explain how his mother's request for treatment and transport must be honored. Fortunately, Jeremiah acknowledges that he should seek medical attention and agrees to go with you to the emergency department.

TRANSPORT AND TRANSFER OF CARE

As you prepare Jeremiah for transport, his mother enters the room with your partner. Your partner provides you with the information he has received from Mrs. Shively. In order to help maintain patient rapport and avoid other potential conflicts between the mother and son, you inform Mrs. Shivley that you have talked to Jeremiah and he has agreed to go with you to the ED and to be seen by a physician as she asked. You ask her if she would like to accompany your partner in the front of the ambulance or if she would prefer to meet you at the receiving facility. Mrs. Shively elects to meet you at the receiving facility and leaves the scene after you have. You assure her that you will provide proper care and treatment for her child en route to the receiving facility.

En route you continue to reassess Jeremiah. You also call the receiving facility and give a verbal report to the triage nurse on duty. Upon arrival at the emergency department, Mrs. Shively meets you at the door. As she proceeds to go in and register Jeremiah, you transfer care to the ED physician and provide him with a complete report about the call, your assessment findings, and your management. You then place Jeremiah in the hospital cubicle he has been assigned to. You again suggest to Jeremiah that he speak to the physician about his risky sexual behaviors.

When Mrs. Shively comes into the cubicle, you finish your documentation and ask her to sign your patient care report. You wish them both the best as you leave the cubicle. As you depart the ED, you make sure to leave a copy of your documentation with the staff.

IN REVIEW

1. Describe each stage of development with regard to vital signs, physiological changes, and psychosocial changes.
2. List the normal vital signs for infants, toddlers, preschoolers, school-age children, adolescents, and adults.
3. List activities that a child should be capable of performing at 1, 3, and 5 years of age.
4. Explain how the physical changes a patient experiences can affect him psychosocially.

CRITICAL THINKING

You arrive on the scene and find a 2-year-old child in her father's arms. The father is crying and obviously very upset. He states that he thinks his daughter may have eaten some food that was left out overnight. He explains that he was washing the dishes a couple of minutes ago when he saw her drink from her old cup and he noticed some of the food was missing that had been left on her plate from supper the evening before. The patient is alert and watching your every move. As you approach her, she clings to her father and begins to cry. She has a foul odor on her breath and her dress is wet. Her respirations are 26 per minute with good chest rise. Her radial pulse is regular at a rate of 110 beats per minute. Her skin is warm and dry.

1. Was the young girl's reaction toward you normal for her age?
2. What can you do to help build a good rapport with the patient?
3. Based on her developmental stage, what vital signs did you expect this patient to have?
4. How will you adjust your assessment techniques to meet this patient's needs?
5. What would you say to the father in this scenario?

EXPLORE PEARSON **mybradykit**™

Please go to **www.bradybooks.com** to access mykit for this text. You will find quizzes, critical thinking scenarios, weblinks, animations, and videos related to this chapter—and much more. Look for information on the process of aging as well as a video clip on pediatric growth and development.

Register your access code from the front of your book by going to **www.bradybooks.com** and selecting the mykit links.

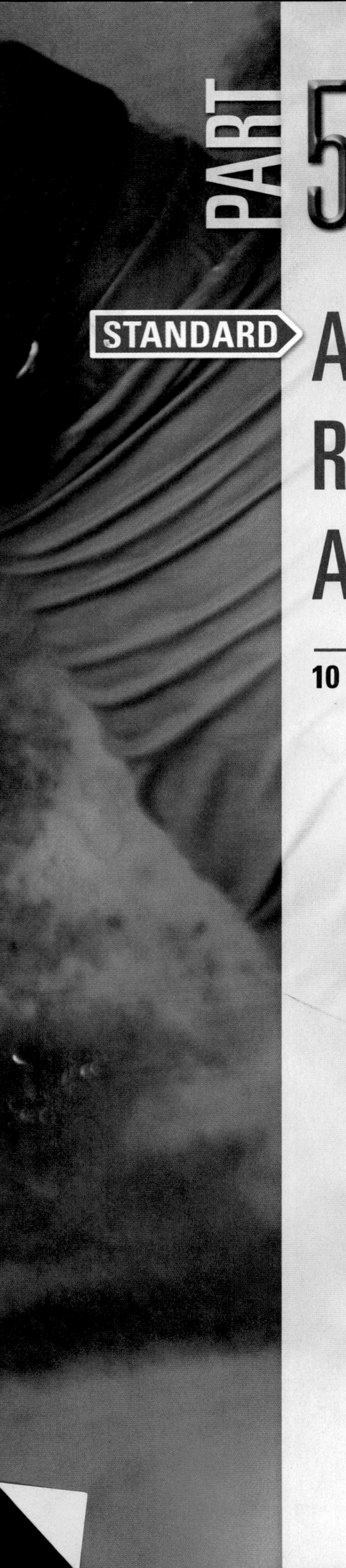

PART 5

STANDARD

Airway Management, Respiration, and Artificial Ventilation

COMPETENCY

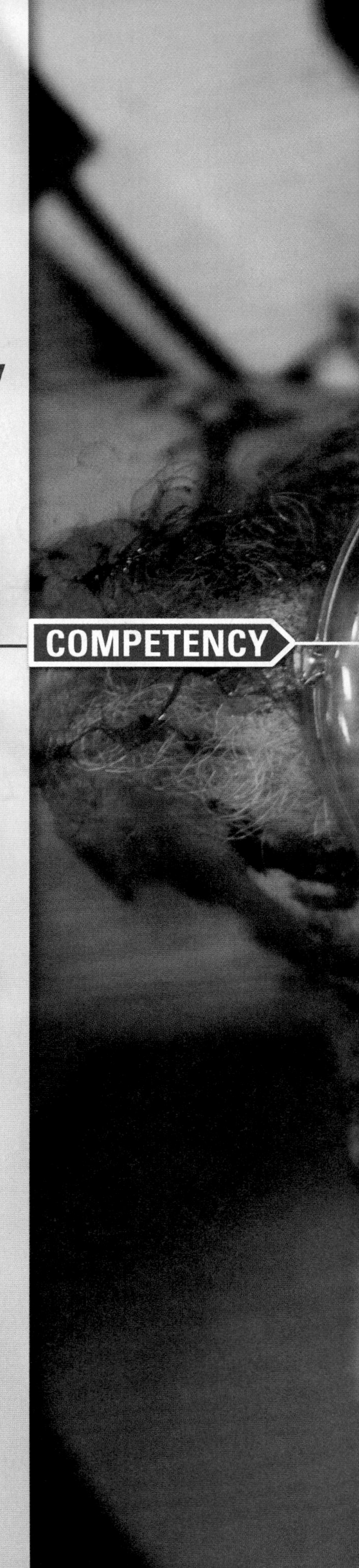

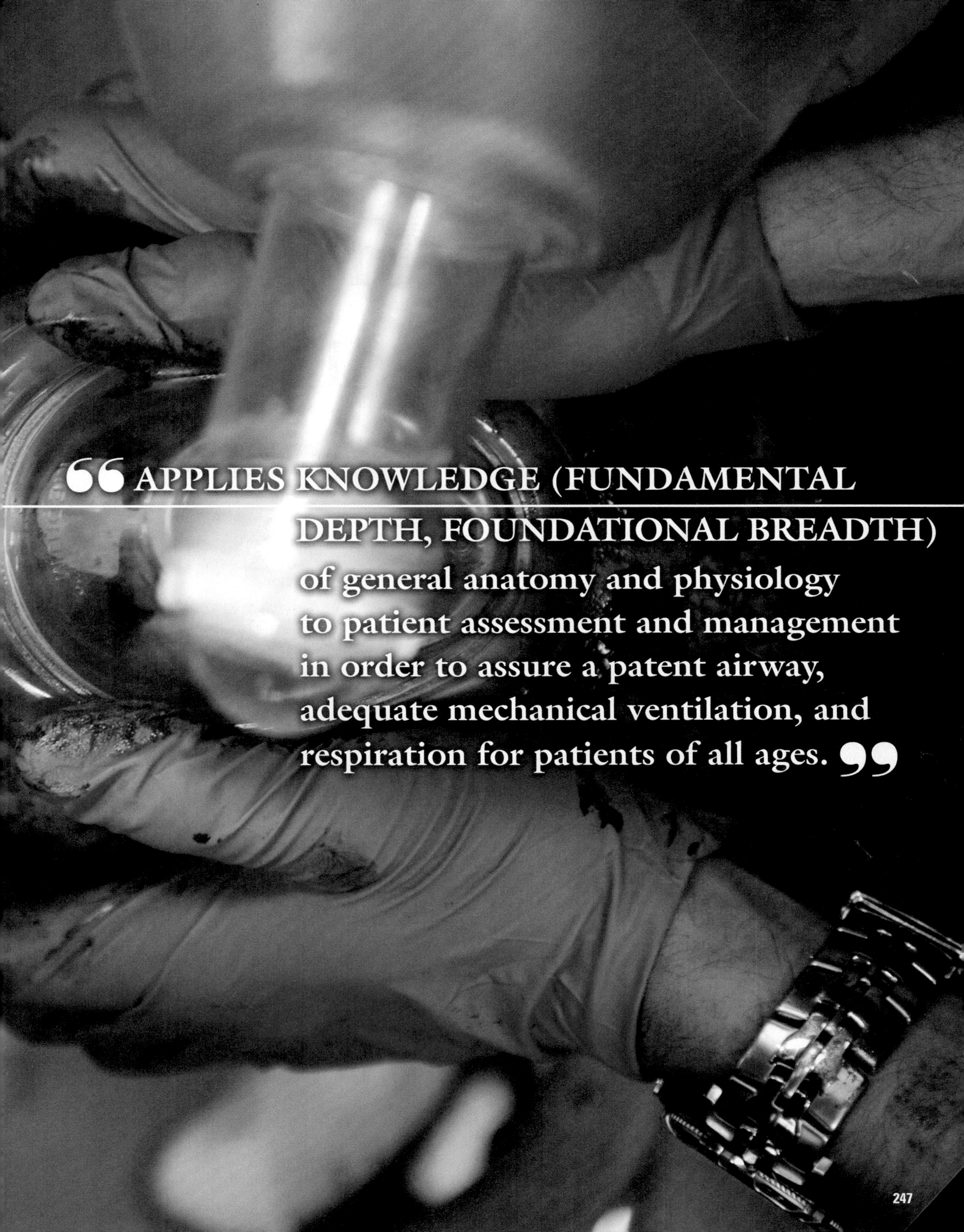

“APPLIES KNOWLEDGE (FUNDAMENTAL DEPTH, FOUNDATIONAL BREADTH) of general anatomy and physiology to patient assessment and management in order to assure a patent airway, adequate mechanical ventilation, and respiration for patients of all ages.”

CHAPTER 10

Airway Management, Artificial Ventilation, and Oxygenation

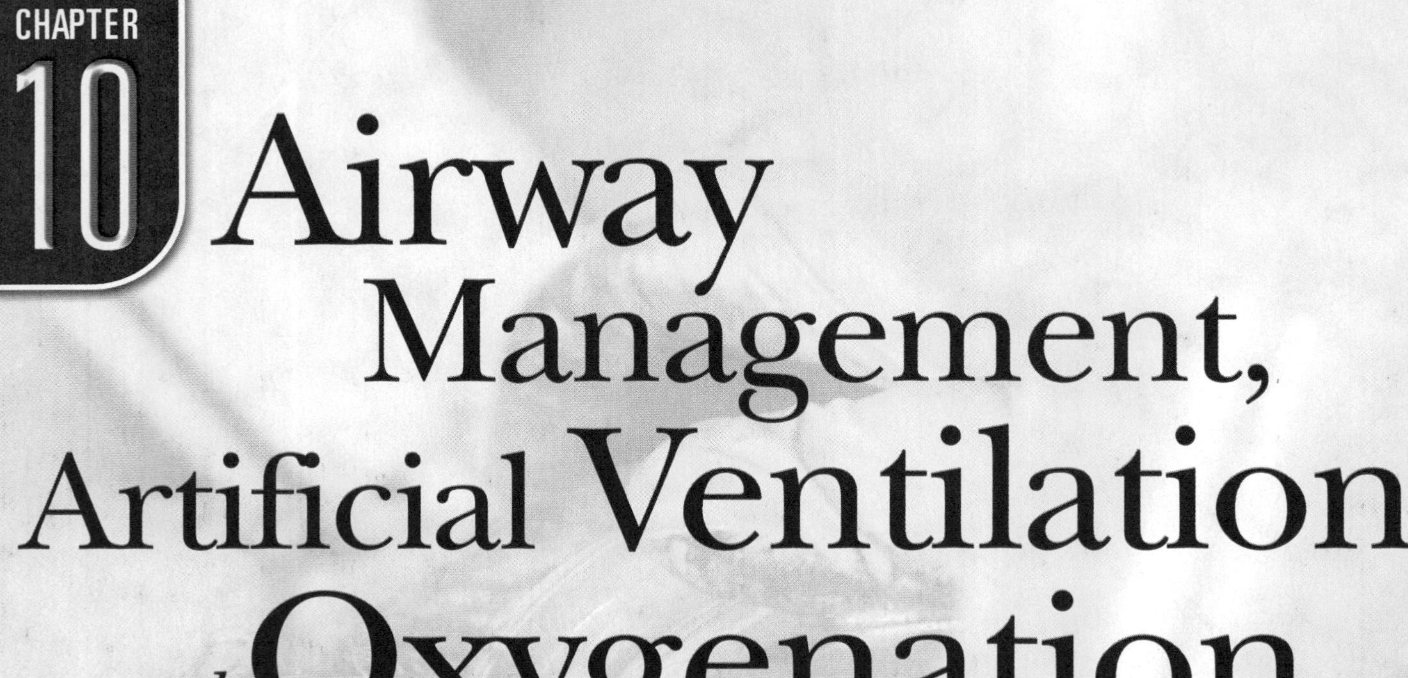

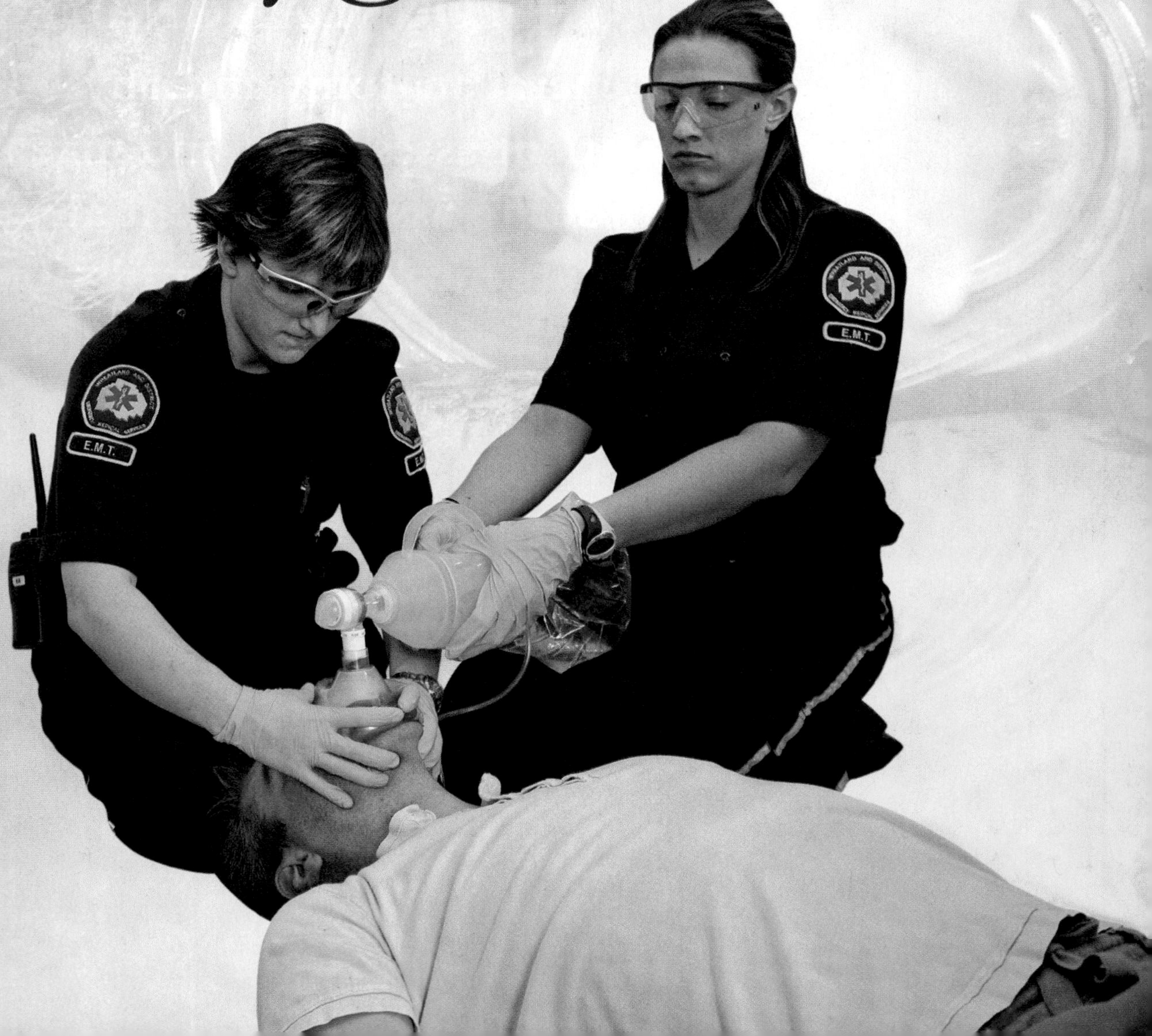

Navigation Guide

The following items provide an overview to the purpose and content of this chapter. The Standard and Competency are from the new National EMS Education Standards.

STANDARD **Airway Management, Respiration, and Artificial Ventilation** (Content Areas: Airway Management; Respiration; Artificial Ventilation)

COMPETENCY Applies knowledge (fundamental depth, foundational breadth) of general anatomy and physiology to patient assessment and management in order to assure a patent airway, adequate mechanical ventilation, and respiration for patients of all ages.

OBJECTIVES: After reading this chapter, you should be able to:

10-1. Define key terms introduced in this chapter.
10-2. Distinguish between the terms *respiration, ventilation, pulmonary ventilation, external respiration, internal respiration*, and *cellular ventilation.*
10-3. Relate the anatomy and physiology of the respiratory system to ventilation and respiration.
10-4. Recognize signs of mild to moderate and severe hypoxia.
10-5. Explain differences between adults and children in the signs of hypoxia.
10-6. Describe the relationship between airway status and mental status.
10-7. Give examples of conditions that can lead to impaired ventilation and respiration.
10-8. Describe how partial or complete obstruction of the airway leads to hypoxia.
10-9. Describe differences between adults and children in the anatomy and physiology of the respiratory system.
10-10. Explain the causes of each of the following abnormal upper airway sounds:
- **a.** Snoring
- **b.** Crowing
- **c.** Gurgling
- **d.** Stridor

10-11. Demonstrate each of the following procedures necessary for airway assessment and correction:
- **a.** Opening the mouth of an unresponsive patient
- **b.** Suctioning the mouth
- **c.** Head-tilt, chin-lift maneuver
- **d.** Jaw-thrust maneuver
- **e.** Insertion of an oropharyngeal airway
- **f.** Insertion of a nasopharyngeal airway
- **g.** Positioning a patient for control of the airway

10-12. Describe the performance requirements for fixed suction devices.
10-13. Compare the function of fixed and portable suction devices.
10-14. Compare the use of rigid and soft suction catheters.
10-15. Explain special considerations to be kept in mind when suctioning patients, including signs of hypoxia and patients with copious amounts of vomit that cannot be quickly suctioned.
10-16. Describe the indications, advantages, disadvantages, precautions, uses, and limitations of oropharyngeal and nasopharyngeal airways.
10-17. Distinguish between patients with adequate and inadequate breathing by considering the following:
- **a.** Minute ventilation
- **b.** Alveolar ventilation
- **c.** Inspection of the chest
- **d.** Patient's general appearance
- **e.** Regularity of breathing
- **f.** Flaring of the nostrils
- **g.** Patient's ability to speak
- **h.** Airflow
- **i.** Breath sounds

10-18. Identify patients with indications for supplemental oxygen and positive pressure ventilation.
10-19. Describe the physiological differences between spontaneous and positive pressure ventilation.
10-20. Distinguish between adequate and inadequate positive pressure ventilation.
10-21. Demonstrate each of the following procedures for artificial ventilation:
- **a.** Mouth-to-mouth and mouth-to-mask ventilation
- **b.** Delivery of positive pressure ventilations with a bag-valve-mask device (one-person and two-person), with a flow-restricted, oxygen-powered ventilation device, and with an automatic transport ventilator

10-22. Differentiate between the duration and volume of ventilation for patients with and without pulses.
10-23. Explain the significance of avoiding gastric inflation when administering positive pressure ventilation.
10-24. Describe indications and methods for administering positive pressure ventilations to a patient who is breathing spontaneously.
10-25. Discuss the indications, contraindications, and methods for administering continuous positive airway pressure (CPAP) or bilevel positive airway pressure (BiPAP).
10-26. Discuss the hazards of overventilation.

continued

Navigation Guide *continued*

10-27. Discuss special considerations of airway management and ventilation for the following:
- **a.** Patients with stomas or tracheostomy tubes
- **b.** Infants and children
- **c.** Patients with facial injuries
- **d.** Patients with foreign body airway obstructions
- **e.** Patients with dental appliances

10-28. Describe the properties of oxygen.

10-29. Differentiate between the various sizes of oxygen cylinders available.

10-30. Describe the hazards associated with oxygen use and safety precautions to be observed when using oxygen or handling oxygen cylinders.

10-31. Describe the regulation of oxygen pressures, including the uses of high-pressure and therapy regulators.

10-32. Discuss the use of oxygen humidifiers.

10-33. Discuss the administration of oxygen by nonrebreather mask, nasal cannula, simple face mask, partial rebreather mask, Venturi mask, and tracheostomy mask.

KEY TERMS: Page references indicate first major use in this chapter. For complete definitions, see the Glossary at the back of the book.

alveolar ventilation p. 271
bradypnea p. 275
cricoid pressure p. 281
cyanosis p. 257
dead air space p. 272
external respiration p. 251
gastric distention p. 281
hypoperfusion p. 256
hypoxia p. 256
internal respiration p. 251
minute volume p. 271
oxygenation p. 256
positive pressure ventilation (PPV) p. 278
residual volume p. 268
respiration p. 251
respiratory arrest p. 275
respiratory distress p. 274
respiratory failure p. 275
tachypnea p. 275
tidal volume p. 271
ventilation p. 255

MEDIA RESOURCES: Please go to www.bradybooks.com to access mykit for this text. You will find quizzes, critical thinking scenarios, weblinks, animations, and videos related to this chapter—and much more. Look for online information on effective BVM ventilations. You will also find a video clip on the two-person BVM technique.

CASE STUDY

The Dispatch

EMS Unit 108—respond to the Twilight Bar, 59 South Market Street—You have an unresponsive male patient—time out 1703 hours.

Upon Arrival

As your ambulance draws up to the bar, you and your partner recognize it as one you've been sent to several times in the past to handle injuries caused in fights. "They must have changed the name of the bar," you say to your partner. She contacts dispatch and inquires, "Is this patient's unresponsiveness a result of a fight or other violent act?"

Dispatch responds, "EMS Unit 108, be advised the bartender states the patient was drinking heavily this afternoon. He was found unresponsive in the bathroom by another patron."

You cautiously approach the scene and enter the bar. It is quite dark and a typical "bar smell" fills the air. You are directed to the men's bathroom at the end of a short hallway. You enter and find a man approximately 30 years of age lying prone on the bathroom floor. Vomitus surrounds the patient's face.

How Would You Proceed to Assess and Care for This Patient?

During this chapter, you will learn special considerations of assessment and management of the airway and breathing status and techniques of oxygen administration. Later we will return to the case and apply the procedures learned.

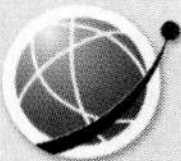

Media Resources

Go to www.bradybooks.com for mykit. Highlights:

- *Web Resource:* Effective BVM Ventilations
- *Video:* OPA Insertion

Objective 10-2

Distinguish between the terms *respiration, ventilation, pulmonary ventilation, external respiration, internal respiration*, and *cellular ventilation.*

Objective 10-3

Relate the anatomy and physiology of the respiratory system to ventilation and respiration.

Introduction

Without an open and clear airway, adequate ventilation, or sufficient oxygenation, all other emergency care is futile since the patient will rapidly deteriorate and die. Therefore, these components are part of the primary assessment that is conducted on every patient regardless of the injuries or illness. By understanding the mechanical and physiological processes of respiration and ventilation and the various ways to assist patients with artificial ventilation, you will be able to quickly initiate and maintain an adequate airway and oxygenation in cases of emergency.

Respiration

Respiration is also commonly referred to as *ventilation* or *breathing*. These terms are often used synonymously. However, there are true physiological differences between ventilation or breathing and the various types of respiration.

Respiration can be broken down into four distinct components: pulmonary ventilation, external respiration, internal respiration, and cellular respiration and metabolism. Physiologically, the term *respiration* refers to the gas exchange process that occurs between the alveoli or cells and the capillaries, or to the utilization of glucose and oxygen during normal metabolism within the cells. The following is a brief summary of the components associated with respiration. More detail regarding each component will be provided later in the chapter. You can also review Chapter 8, "Pathophysiology," for more detail on ventilation and gas exchange.

- *Pulmonary ventilation*, or simply ventilation or breathing, is the mechanical process of moving air in and out of the lungs. It is related to minute ventilation and alveolar ventilation.
- *External respiration* is the gas exchange process that occurs between the alveoli and the surrounding pulmonary capillaries. **External respiration,** also referred to as alveoli/capillary gas exchange, serves to oxygenate the blood and eliminate carbon dioxide in the lungs.
- *Internal respiration* is the gas exchange process that occurs between the cells and the systemic capillaries. **Internal respiration,** also known as cell/capillary gas exchange, is responsible for delivering oxygen to the cells and removing carbon dioxide from the cell.
- *Cellular respiration and metabolism,* also known as aerobic metabolism, occurs in the cell. The process breaks down glucose in the presence of oxygen, produces high amounts of energy in the form of ATP, and releases carbon dioxide and water as a by-product.

Respiratory System Review

To ensure that you can establish and maintain an open airway and properly ventilate a patient, you should understand some basics of the anatomy and physiology of the respiratory system. What follows is a brief review of that system. You may also wish to review the material on the respiratory system in Chapter 7, "Anatomy, Physiology, and Medical Terminology," and in Chapter 8, "Pathophysiology."

Anatomy of the Respiratory System

The respiratory system takes oxygen from air that is breathed in, transports it to the alveoli where the oxygen crosses over into the capillary, and attaches the oxygen to the hemoglobin on the red blood cell or dissolves it in the plasma of the blood. The blood then transports the oxygen to body cells through the arteries and capillaries of the circulatory system. At the capillary/cell interface, the oxygen leaves the blood in the capillary and crosses over into the cell. If the oxygen supply is decreased by an obstructed airway, inadequate breathing, ineffective oxygen exchange in the lungs, or an inadequate delivery system to the cells, the body cells will become hypoxic (low in oxygen) and eventually die. The respiratory system is also responsible for eliminating carbon dioxide, the major waste product of cellular metabolism, when carbon dioxide crosses out of the cells into the capillaries and is carried by the venous system back to the lungs to be exhaled.

The respiratory system is divided anatomically into the upper airway and the lower airway. Often, conditions are described as affecting the upper or lower airway.

The Upper Airway

The **upper airway** extends from the nose and mouth to the cricoid cartilage, the most inferior portion of the larynx (Figure 10-1*).

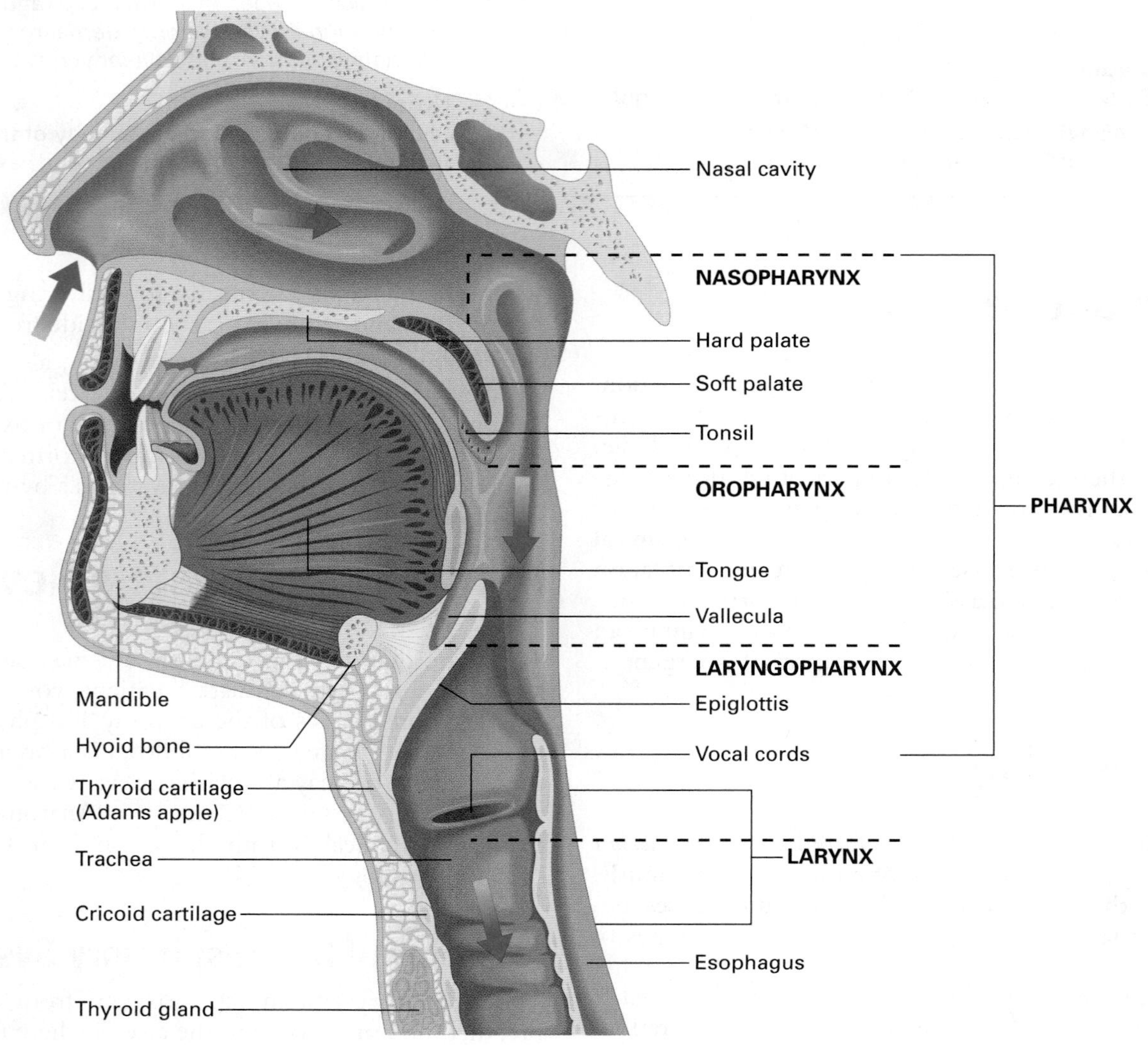

FIGURE 10-1 * Anatomy of the upper airway.

Nose and Mouth Air normally enters the body through the nostrils. It is warmed, moistened, and filtered as it flows over the damp, sticky **mucous membrane** lining the nose. Air also enters through the mouth; however, there is less filtration and warming by that route than through the nostrils. The tongue is a common cause of airway obstruction in the patient with an altered mental status. This occurs when the muscles controlling the tongue (the submandibular muscles) relax. This causes the tongue to fall back and occlude (block) the airway.

Pharynx Air entering the body through the mouth and nostrils travels into the **pharynx** (throat). Air from the nasal passages enters through what is referred to as the **nasopharynx.** Air entering through the mouth travels through the **oropharynx.** Both the oropharynx and nasopharynx enter into the pharynx at the back of the throat. The pharynx must be kept clear because obstructions in it can prevent air from traveling into the lower airways, or the substance may be aspirated into the lungs, thus interfering with oxygen and carbon dioxide exchange in the alveoli.

Two passageways are found at the lower end of the pharynx—the **trachea** and the **esophagus.** The trachea is the passageway for air traveling into the lungs. Food and water are routed to the esophagus, which leads to the stomach.

Epiglottis The trachea is protected by a small, leaf-shaped flap of cartilaginous tissue called the **epiglottis.** This acts as a valve that closes over the opening to the larynx while food and drink are being swallowed. At other times, the epiglottis is pulled away from the opening to the larynx, which permits breathing. This controlled diversion usually works automatically to keep food and drink out of the trachea and air from going into the esophagus.

At times, the epiglottis may fail to close, and food or liquids can enter the larynx and the upper portion of the trachea, causing a patient to choke. If a patient is unresponsive, the protective reflexes may not work during swallowing, so that foreign objects, blood, secretions, and vomitus can enter the trachea and cause an airway obstruction or lung infection.

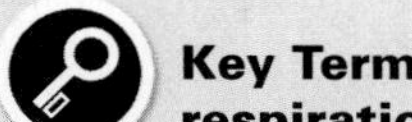

Key Terms
respiration the exchange of oxygen and carbon dioxide that takes place during inhalation and exhalation.

external respiration the gas exchange process that occurs between the alveoli and the pulmonary capillaries.

Key Terms
internal respiration the gas exchange process that occurs between the cells and the capillaries.

When the muscles controlling the tongue relax in a patient with an altered mental status, the muscles controlling the epiglottis also relax and may cause the epiglottis to fall over the opening of the larynx (glottic opening). This will block the only opening to the trachea and cause an airway obstruction at the level of the larynx that cannot be directly seen by the EMT. The best method to relieve this type of obstruction is to perform a head-tilt, chin-lift maneuver or jaw-thrust maneuver (described later), which will pull the epiglottis up away from the opening of the larynx.

Larynx Just superior to (above) the trachea and just inferior to (below) the epiglottis is the **larynx,** or voice box, which contains the vocal cords (Figure 10-2*). The vocal cords are thin muscles that produce speech and also protect the lower airway. The anterior portion of the larynx is composed of the large bulky **thyroid cartilage,** commonly known as the **Adam's apple,** which can be felt at the front of the throat. The **cricoid cartilage,** which forms the most inferior portion of the larynx and is the only completely circular cartilaginous ring of the upper airway, is found at the lower portion of the larynx just below the thyroid cartilage. Pressure applied to the cricoid ring, a technique that will be discussed later, is often used in airway management to help prevent air from filling the stomach and to help prevent regurgitation of stomach contents. The larynx is a common site of airway obstruction in adults, infants, and children.

The Lower Airway

The **lower airway** extends from the cricoid cartilage at the lower edge of the larynx to the alveoli of the lungs (Figure 10-3*).

Trachea The trachea, commonly known as the windpipe, is the passageway for air entering the lungs. It extends from the larynx to the **carina,** the point at which the trachea splits into the right and left mainstem bronchi. The anterior portion of the trachea is composed of strong C-shaped cartilaginous rings that provide support and structure. The posterior wall of the trachea is made up of muscle and therefore is not a rigid structure.

Bronchi and Bronchioles The right and left mainstem **bronchi,** which are the two major branches of the trachea, extend from the carina into the lungs, where they continue to divide into smaller sections or branches known as **bronchioles.** The bronchi are larger airways and contain cartilage. The bronchioles, which become increasingly smaller as they continue to branch, are lined with smooth muscle and mucous membranes. The smooth muscle can contract and the mucous lining can become inflamed and swollen, severely narrowing the diameter of the bronchiole and causing lower airway obstruction, as is seen in asthma. This narrowing causes an increase in airway resistance inside the bronchiole, which makes it more difficult for the patient to move air into and out of the alveoli and the lower airway passages. An increase in airway resistance causes the patient to work

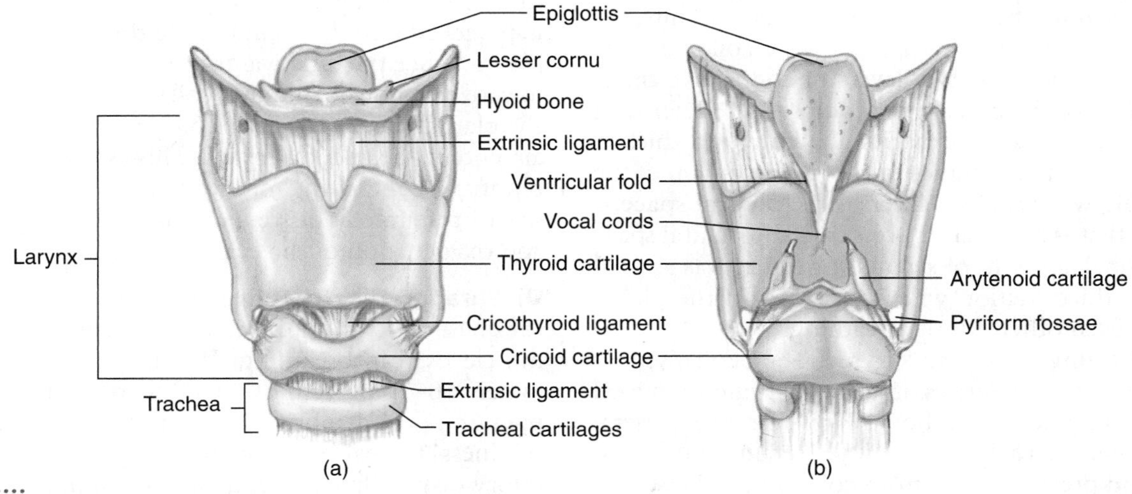

FIGURE 10-2 * The larynx. **(a)** Anterior view. **(b)** Posterior view.

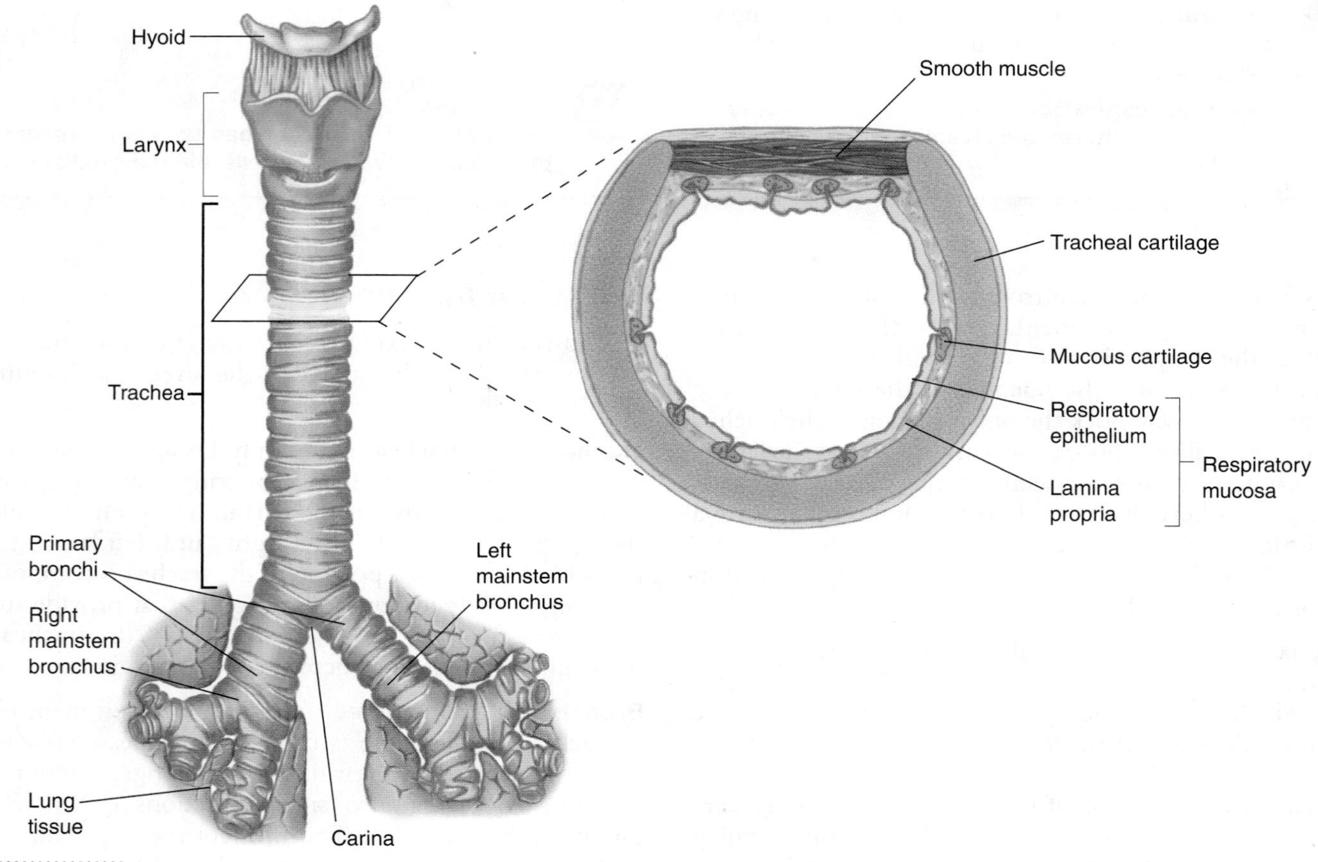

FIGURE 10-3 * Anatomy of the lower airway.

harder to breathe, which may lead to fatigue and failure of the respiratory muscles. This would produce ineffective and inadequate ventilation and oxygenation, leading to cell hypoxia.

Lungs The bronchioles terminate in thousands of tiny air sacs in the lungs. These are called the **alveoli.** Each air sac is wrapped in a web of thin-walled capillaries referred to as the pulmonary capillaries. This is the site for gas exchange between the alveoli and the blood in the capillaries.

The lungs are made of elastic tissue. This elastic tissue causes the lungs to react like a rubber band; thus, the lungs' natural tendency is to recoil and collapse. The lungs are surrounded by two layers of connective tissue called the **pleura.** The **visceral pleura** is the innermost covering of the lung. The **parietal pleura** is a thicker, more elastic layer that adheres to the inner portion of the chest wall. Between the two layers is the **pleural space,** a small space that is at negative pressure. The pleural space contains a small amount of **serous fluid** that acts as a lubricant to reduce friction when the layers of the pleura rub against each other during breathing.

Since the lung tissue wants to recoil and collapse, because of its elastic properties, it is always tugging inward toward the midline of the body. However, the parietal pleura, connected to the chest wall, retains the lungs' structure and prevents them from collapsing. The serous fluid between the attached parietal pleura and the visceral pleura, which is always tugging inward, creates a "water glass" effect. If a water glass is placed open end down on a flat surface covered with water, then pulled straight upward, a vacuum is created between the flat surface and the glass. The water creates a seal. If the seal is broken, air is sucked inward and allows the glass to be moved off the flat surface. To apply this principle, think of the patient who has an open wound to the chest with a tear in the parietal or visceral pleura. The visceral pleural pull is continuously creating a vacuum, so air from outside the chest gets sucked into the pleural space through the hole in the pleura. Since the lung wants to recoil, it continues to pull inward toward the midline, collapsing the lung as air fills the pleural space. The lung continues to collapse as more air enters the pleural space. This is frequently seen in blunt and penetrating injuries to the chest and can lead to severe respiratory distress and inadequate gas exchange and oxygenation of the cells.

Diaphragm The **diaphragm** is a muscle that separates the chest cavity from the abdominal cavity. It is the major muscle used in breathing. It is responsible for approximately 60–70 percent of the effort of ventilation. If contraction of the diaphragm is ineffective because of trauma or illness, the patient may show signs of significant respiratory distress from inadequate breathing.

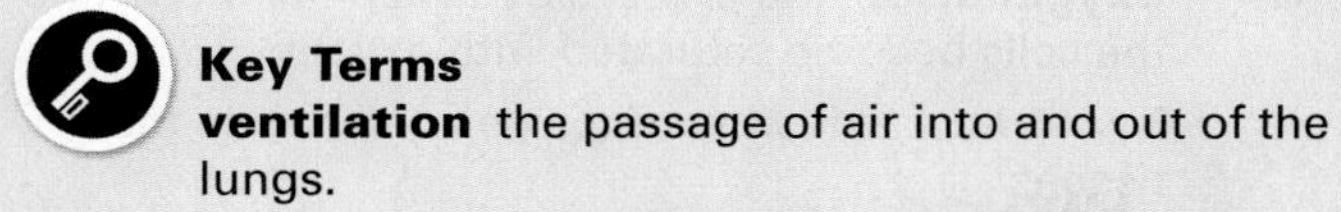

Key Terms
ventilation the passage of air into and out of the lungs.

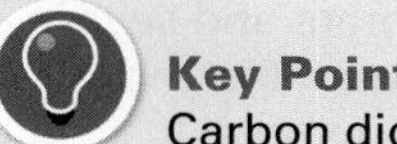

Key Points
Carbon dioxide levels in arterial blood provide the constant stimulation and regulation of respiration in the normal person.

Mechanics of Ventilation (Pulmonary Ventilation) Review

The passage of air into and out of the lungs is called **ventilation.** It is also often referred to as breathing, pulmonary ventilation, or respiration. Ventilation is a mechanical process that creates pressure changes in the lungs to draw air in and force air out. **Inhalation** or **inspiration** is the process of breathing air in, and **exhalation** or **expiration** is the process of breathing air out.

Inhalation

During inhalation, the diaphragm and the **intercostal muscles,** or muscles between the ribs, contract. The diaphragm moves slightly downward and flares the lower portion of the rib cage outward. The intercostal muscles pull the ribs and sternum upward and outward. These actions increase the size of the chest cavity, creating negative pressure inside the chest cavity. This draws air by way of the nose, mouth, trachea, and bronchi into the lungs until the pressure inside the lungs is equal to the atmospheric pressure outside the body. Inhalation is an active process because it requires energy to contract the muscles.

Exhalation

During exhalation, the diaphragm and intercostal muscles relax, moving the diaphragm upward and the ribs and sternum downward and inward back to their normal resting positions. The size of the chest cavity is reduced, the elastic lung tissue recoils to its normal position, and the pressure in the chest cavity becomes positive. This forces a volume of air out of the lungs. Because this process involves relaxation of muscles and little energy is expended, it is considered to be passive.

In some respiratory diseases affecting the lower airway, such as asthma, the patient has a difficult time moving air out of the lungs because of an increased resistance in the airways or diseased lung tissue. There is a loss of the elastic recoil of the chest wall and lungs because air is trapped in the alveoli. Therefore, the patient has to contract muscles, not only to draw air into the lungs but also to force air out of the lungs. As a consequence, both inhalation and exhalation become active, requiring energy. Such patients have a tendency to become exhausted very quickly because of the amount of energy it takes to breathe. They are prone to a rapid deterioration from fatigue of the respiratory muscles.

Control of Respiration

Unlike the heart, which can generate contractions from within the heart's own muscle and conductive system, the respiratory organs do not have the ability to control their function from within the respiratory system. Respirations are controlled by the nervous system in a variety of ways. The dorsal respiratory group (DRG), ventral respiratory group (VRG), apneustic center, and pneumotaxic center in the brain stem are respiratory rhythm centers that control the impulses being sent to the respiratory muscles. The **chemoreceptors** continuously monitor levels of oxygen, carbon dioxide, and pH (hydrogen) in the arterial blood and stimulate an increase or decrease in impulses from the respiratory rhythm centers to control the rate and depth of ventilation.

Understanding BODY PROCESSES

The central chemoreceptors located in the medulla are most sensitive to changes in the blood pH and carbon dioxide, whereas the peripheral chemoreceptors located in the carotid arteries and aortic arch are more sensitive to changes in arterial oxygen. ■

The respiratory system responds primarily to changes in the carbon dioxide levels. If the carbon dioxide level in arterial blood increases, the chemoreceptors sense the increase and the brain stem sends impulses to the respiratory muscles to increase the rate and depth of respiration. The increase in respirations results in the increased elimination of carbon dioxide. Thus healthy people breathe on a *hypercarbic* (high carbon dioxide) *drive.* When the carbon dioxide level decreases in the blood, the chemoreceptors sense this and send signals to the respiratory muscles to slow down the **respiratory rate** and depth and the respirations return to normal. Oxygen is much less of a stimulus for breathing in healthy people.

In patients with a category of conditions known as chronic obstructive pulmonary disease (COPD), which includes emphysema and chronic bronchitis, the carbon dioxide level in arterial blood is typically chronically elevated as a result of the disease process. Because of the constant high carbon dioxide levels, the chemoreceptors

Objectives 10-4 to 10-6
Recognize signs of mild to moderate and severe hypoxia, the differences between adults and children in the signs of hypoxia, and the relationship between airway status and mental status.

Key Terms

oxygenation the process by which the blood and the cells become saturated with oxygen.

hypoxia a reduction of oxygen delivery to the tissues.

become relatively insensitive to changes in carbon dioxide. Instead, the chemoreceptors of COPD patients tend to rely on oxygen levels in the blood to regulate their breathing. These patients breathe on a *hypoxic* (low oxygen) *drive,* since they breathe to increase their oxygen levels and not to reduce their carbon dioxide levels. This could affect your management of the patient when considering oxygen therapy.

In some cases, if oxygen is provided at high concentrations to a patient with COPD over a long period of time, the oxygen levels in the arterial blood will rise beyond a normal level for that patient. The chemoreceptors will sense this rise and may send signals to the respiratory muscles to slow down or even stop respirations, because the oxygen levels are more than adequate in the blood and no more oxygen is needed at that time. The result can be respiratory failure or respiratory arrest, although this rarely happens in the short period of time when a patient is receiving prehospital care. Even though this could be a complication in the COPD patient, oxygen should never be withheld from a patient if he needs it, whether he has COPD or not. If it should occur, ventilate the patient artificially, just as with any patient who suffers respiratory failure or arrest.

Respiratory Physiology Review

Oxygenation is the process by which the blood and the cells become saturated with oxygen. This happens as a result of *internal respiration* and *external respiration*, the processes in which fresh oxygen replaces waste carbon dioxide, a gas exchange that takes place between the alveoli and the capillaries in the lungs, and also between the capillaries and the cells throughout the body. As noted earlier, *ventilation* is the mechanical process of moving air in and out of the lungs, and *respiration* is the physiological process of gas exchange.

Hypoxia

Hypoxia is an inadequate amount of oxygen being delivered to the cells. Hypoxia can result from a large number of causes including an occluded airway, inadequate breathing, inadequate delivery of oxygen to the cells by the blood (**hypoperfusion** or **shock**), inhalation of toxic gases (e.g., carbon monoxide), lung and airway diseases (e.g., asthma, emphysema), drug overdose that suppresses the respiratory center in the brain (e.g., morphine, heroin, and other narcotics), stroke, injury to the chest or respiratory structures, and head injury. There are many more conditions or injuries that may create a blockage to the airway or produce inadequate breathing by depressing the respiratory centers in the brain, interfering with gas exchange at the level of the alveoli, or restricting the movement of the chest wall.

The signs of hypoxia may be subtle. It is extremely important to continuously assess the patient for hypoxia and to recognize the subtle signs and symptoms. The following are signs of hypoxia:

Signs of Mild to Moderate Hypoxia

Tachypnea (increased respiratory rate)

Dyspnea (shortness of breath)

Pale, cool, clammy skin (early)

Tachycardia (increase in heart rate)

Elevation in blood pressure

Restlessness and agitation

Disorientation and confusion (from high carbon dioxide levels in the blood)

Headache

Signs of Severe Hypoxia

Tachypnea

Dyspnea

Cyanosis (bluish gray color to skin, mucous membranes, and nail beds)

Tachycardia that may lead to dysrhythmias (irregular heart rhythms) and eventually bradycardia (slow heart rate)

Confusion

Loss of coordination

Sleepy appearance

Head bobbing (head bobs upward with inhalation and downward with exhalation, as if falling asleep while sitting upright) with droopy eyelids

Slow reaction time

Altered mental status

In a newborn, bradycardia (slow heart rate) may be an early sign of hypoxia. Infants and young children normally have higher heart rates than adults. As an example, a heart rate of 80 bpm, which would be normal in an adult, may be an indication of hypoxia in a week-old infant where a

Key Terms
hypoperfusion the insufficient supply of oxygen and other nutrients to some of the body's cells that results from inadequate circulation of blood. Also called **shock.**

Key Terms
cyanosis a bluish color of the skin and mucous membranes that indicates poor oxygenation of tissue.

heart rate of 120–150 bpm would be normal. It is important in the assessment of newborns to suspect hypoxia as a cause of a slower-than-expected heart rate, since this is a primary cause of bradycardia in this group. In infants, children, and adults, bradycardia is a sign of severe hypoxia and impending respiratory and cardiac arrest.

It is important to assess for the early signs of hypoxia. The skin will become pale, cool, and clammy early. You may also find tachypnea (rapid breathing) and tachycardia (rapid heartbeat). Early changes in the mental status may occur in the form of restlessness or agitation and confusion. Hypoxia causes restlessness and agitation in the patient, whereas the buildup of carbon dioxide in the blood will cause the patient to become confused. These most often occur together; therefore, your patient will likely appear both agitated and confused. If a patient presents with agitation and confusion, it is extremely important that you suspect and assess for evidence of inadequate ventilation and oxygenation in the patient.

ASSESSMENT Tips

An early sign of hypoxia is an alteration in the patient's mental status. ■

Cyanosis, a bluish gray color, is a late sign of hypoxia and may be found in and around several areas of the body, including the lips, mouth, nose, fingernail beds, conjunctiva (the normally red area between the bottom eyelid and the eyeball), and oral mucosa (between the lips and gums, and the tongue) (Figure 10-4*). In a dark-skinned patient, the fingernail beds may appear more pale than cyanotic. In dark-skinned patients, be sure to check the oral mucosa or conjunctiva for cyanosis. In summary, it is important in your assessment of the patient to look at these various areas to determine if cyanosis exists.

Understanding BODY PROCESSES

Cyanosis occurs when adequate amounts of oxygen are no longer attached to the hemoglobin molecules. However, hemoglobin must be present in the blood to change its color. Thus, a patient with severe bleeding who is hypoxic may not exhibit extreme cyanosis, since there may not be large enough amounts of hemoglobin in the blood to produce the bluish color of cyanosis. ■

If the patient is displaying any signs of hypoxia, immediately assess the airway and adequacy of breathing. If the airway is open and the patient is breathing adequately (adequate rate and volume), apply a nonrebreather mask and administer a high concentration of oxygen. If the patient's airway is not open, immediately open it and assess the breathing status. If the breathing status is inadequate (either an inadequate rate or an inadequate volume), immediately begin positive pressure ventilation. These oxygen administration and ventilation techniques will be discussed in greater detail later in the chapter.

Alveolar/Capillary Exchange (External Respiration)

Oxygen-rich air enters the alveoli during each inspiration. Surrounding the alveoli are capillaries that deliver blood to the alveoli. The blood moving into the capillaries is **deoxygenated,** that is, with low oxygen concentration, but is high in carbon dioxide. The alveoli contain

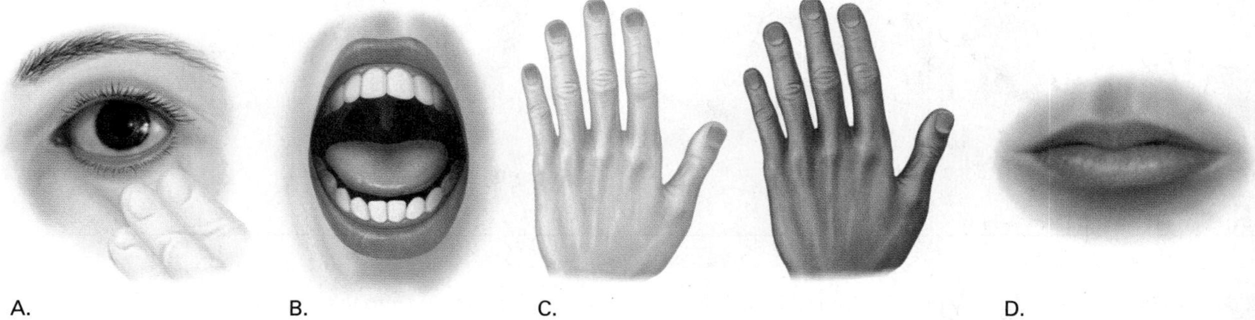

FIGURE 10-4 * Cyanosis at the **(a)** conjunctiva, **(b)** mucosa, **(c)** fingernail beds, **(d)** circumoral area.

an enriched supply of oxygen and very little carbon dioxide. Because both gases move from areas of high concentration to areas of low concentration, the oxygen diffuses (moves) from the alveoli into the capillaries, and the carbon dioxide diffuses (moves) from the capillaries into the alveoli (Figure 10-5a∗).

From this point, the blood in the capillaries is **oxygenated,** that is, with high oxygen concentration and low carbon dioxide. **Hemoglobin,** found on the surface of red blood cells, is responsible for picking up the majority of oxygen in the blood, approximately 97 percent, and carrying it through the arterial system to the capillaries throughout the body. The carbon dioxide is exhaled from the alveoli and out of the lungs. Oxygenation is required; however, it does not ensure adequate internal respiration and aerobic metabolism. Although the blood may be saturated with oxygen from the alveolar capillaries, a disturbance in the delivery or the off-loading of the oxygen from the hemoglobin would result in a decrease in internal respiration and, consequently, in cellular hypoxia.

Capillary/Cellular Exchange (Internal Respiration)

The blood entering the capillaries surrounding the body's cells has a high oxygen content and a low carbon dioxide content. The cells have high levels of carbon dioxide and low levels of oxygen from normal metabolism. Again, because oxygen and carbon dioxide move from areas of high concentration to those of low concentration, the oxygen moves out of the capillaries and into the cells and the carbon dioxide moves out of the cells and into the capillaries (Figure 10-5b∗). The blood, now low in oxygen and high in carbon dioxide, moves out of the capillaries and into the venous system where it is transported back to the lungs for gas exchange.

Pathophysiology of Pulmonary Ventilation and External and Internal Respiration

A disturbance in pulmonary ventilation, oxygenation, external respiration, internal respiration, or circulation can lead to cellular hypoxia and the conversion from aerobic to anaerobic metabolism. Anaerobic metabolism is associated with insufficient energy production and the buildup of lactic acid, which can affect cellular function and integrity. A severe alteration in perfusion can also cause a decrease in glucose delivery to the cells. Without a fuel source, the cells will fail to produce energy and will eventually die.

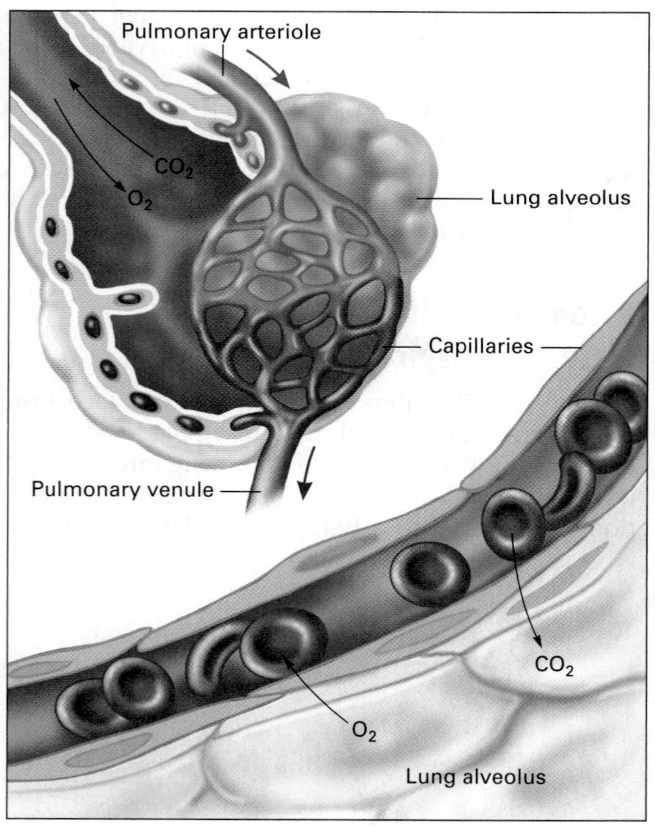

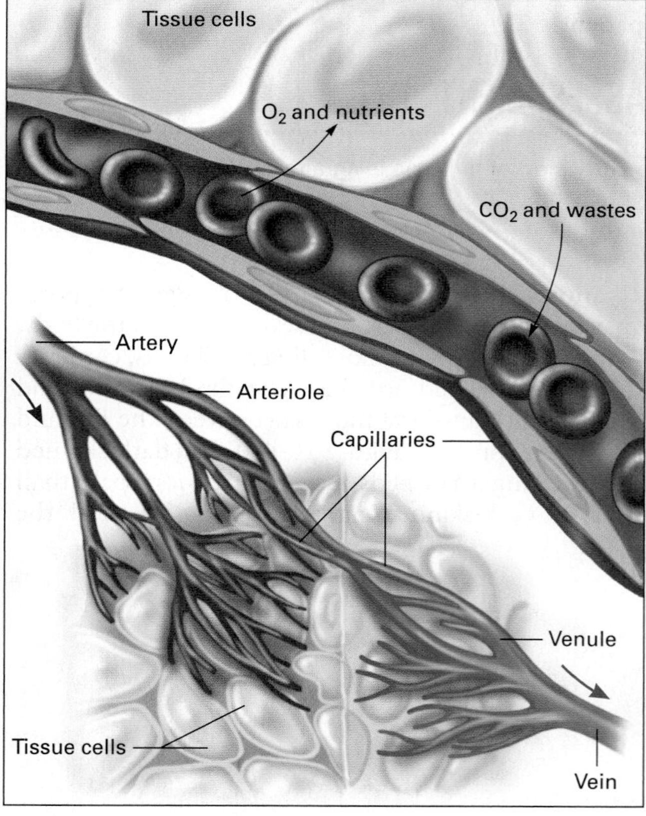

FIGURE 10-5 ∗ **(a)** Alveolar/capillary gas exchange. Oxygen moves from the lung alveolus into the capillary. Carbon dioxide moves from the capillary into the lung. **(b)** Capillary/cell gas exchange. Oxygen and nutrients move from the capillary into the cell. Carbon dioxide and other wastes move from the cell into the capillary.

Objectives 10-7 and 10-8
Give examples of conditions that can lead to impaired ventilation and respiration and describe how partial or complete airway obstruction leads to hypoxia.

Objective 10-9
Describe differences between adults and children in the anatomy and physiology of the respiratory system.

A disruption in the mechanical process of pulmonary ventilation may occur from one of the following:

- Interruption of the nervous system's control and stimulation of the diaphragm or of the external intercostal muscles may result from a brain injury, from drugs that depress the central nervous system, or from neuromuscular diseases such as muscular dystrophy.
- Structural damage to the thorax may interfere with the bellows action of the chest. This will impede the ability of the thorax to generate pressure changes necessary to draw air into the lungs for inhalation and to allow airflow out of the lungs during exhalation. Pain associated with chest injury, flail chest (two or more ribs fractured in two or more places), rupture or injury to the diaphragm, or compression of the chest wall can reduce the effective bellows action of the chest.
- Increased airway resistance will reduce airflow through the respiratory tract and reduce the amount of air in the alveoli. This will make less oxygen available for gas exchange. An increase in airway resistance may occur from bronchoconstriction or from inflammation inside the vessel.
- Disruption of airway patency can occur from swelling caused by infection, allergic reaction, or burns; from trauma; from foreign body obstruction; or from loss of muscle tone associated with an altered mental status or unresponsiveness. Reduction or loss of airway patency will reduce the tidal volume, minute ventilation, alveolar ventilation, and volume of gas in the lungs for gas exchange.

A reduction in the oxygen content of the ambient atmosphere will decrease the available oxygen for gas exchange in the alveoli and at the cells, leading to cellular hypoxia. The oxygen content may be reduced by toxic gases, an enclosed space without adequate ventilation, or a high altitude.

Certain conditions or diseases can obstruct or disrupt the exchange of gas between the alveoli and capillaries. Pneumonia, pulmonary edema, and drowning cause fluid to fill the alveoli, collapse the alveoli, or increase the space between the alveoli and the capillaries, all of which hinder the movement of oxygen from the alveoli into the capillaries and the movement of carbon dioxide from the capillaries into the alveoli. Other diseases, such as emphysema, distort the structure of the alveoli and change the surface area for effective gas exchange. Some toxic gases, such as cyanide and carbon monoxide, interfere with oxygen use by the cell once it has been delivered. These conditions lead to a disruption in both internal and external respiration.

Another cause of cellular hypoxia is poor perfusion or a decreased ability of the blood to carry oxygen. Conditions that obstruct forward movement of blood flow, such as a pulmonary embolism, tension pneumothorax, heart failure, and cardiac tamponade, reduce the delivery of oxygenated blood to the cells. They also reduce perfusion in the pulmonary capillaries, making less blood available to pick up oxygen. Other conditions such as anemia or hypovolemia reduce the concentration of red blood cells and hemoglobin in the blood, making oxygen transport less effective.

Airway Anatomy in Infants and Children

The causes of airway obstruction and inadequate breathing in infants and children are usually similar to those in adults. However, there are several anatomical features in infants and children that may cause them to deteriorate more rapidly than adults (Figure 10-6*).

Mouth and Nose

The noses and mouths of infants and children are smaller than those of adults. Thus, they are more easily obstructed by foreign bodies, swelling, blood, mucus, and secretions. Infants are obligate nose breathers, meaning that they want to breathe through the nose and not the mouth; thus it is especially important to keep the nose clear of obstructions.

Pharynx

Because the tongue of an infant or a child is relatively large in proportion to the size of the mouth, it takes up more room. Therefore, an infant or a child is more prone to airway obstruction by posterior displacement of the tongue at the level of the pharynx. Also, the epiglottis is more U-shaped and can protrude into the pharynx, contributing to obstruction.

Trachea and Lower Airway

The trachea and lower airway passages of infants and children are narrower, softer, and more flexible than those of adults. Thus, airway obstructions occur more easily from

Key Points
Because of the young child's larger head, padding must be placed under the shoulders to keep the airway aligned.

Key Points
Cardiac arrest in infants and children is commonly due to an airway compromise or to ineffective ventilation or oxygenation.

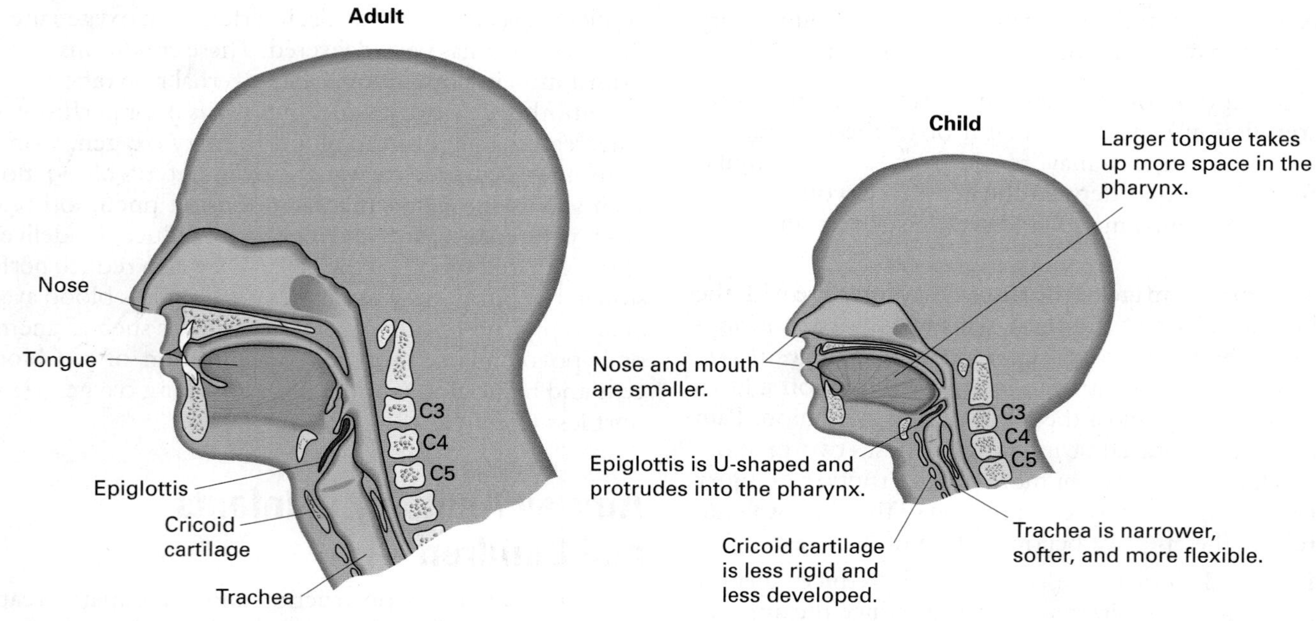

FIGURE 10-6 ✱ Comparison of airways of adult and infant or child.

mucus, pus, blood, secretions, swelling (edema), constriction, and kinking of the trachea with flexion or extension. Very small reductions in the diameter of the lower airway result in significant airway obstruction and high resistance to airflow, reducing effective breathing and oxygenation. Because the young child's head is larger in proportion to his body, the head tends to tilt forward, flexing the neck and potentially collapsing the trachea, when the child is placed on his back for oxygenation or ventilation. Padding under the child's shoulders is necessary to keep the airway aligned and the trachea open (Figure 10-7✱).

Cricoid Cartilage

The cricoid cartilage, like other cartilage in infants and children, is less developed and less rigid. Also, in infants and children less than 10 years of age, the cricoid cartilage is typically the narrowest portion of the upper airway.

Chest Wall and Diaphragm

The chest wall in an infant or a child is softer and more pliable than in an adult. This leads to a much greater compliance (elasticity, response to pressure) or movement during ventilation. Infants and children rely more on the diaphragm for breathing. The intercostal muscles contribute less in normal breathing and act more like accessory muscles. That is why retractions are seen more prominently in infants and young children as compared to adults. When you perform artificial ventilation on an infant or child, the chest should expand and rise easily. If the chest does not rise, you should assume that the airway is not adequately open or is occluded by an obstruction, or the ventilation volume is inadequate. Because the chest expands so easily, it is much easier for the EMT to overinflate the lungs and cause possible lung injury.

Oxygen Reserves

Infants and children are smaller and have more limited oxygen reserves than adults. Therefore, they have less oxygen in the lungs available during periods of inadequate breathing or apnea (complete cessation of breathing). Also, they have twice the metabolic rate of adults, causing them to use oxygen at a much faster rate. Their smaller reserve of oxygen and greater metabolic rate will cause infants and children to become hypoxic more rapidly than adult patients. Hypoxia is the most common cause of cardiac arrest in children.

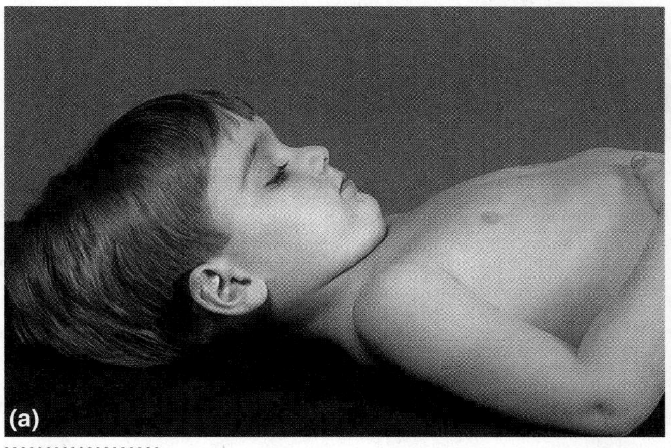

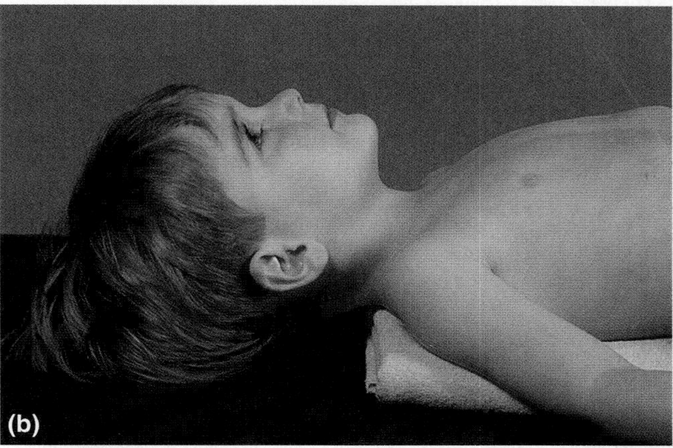

FIGURE 10-7 * **(a)** In the supine position, an infant's or child's larger head tips forward, causing airway obstruction. **(b)** Placing padding under the patient's back and shoulders will bring the airway to a neutral alignment.

Airway Assessment

An open airway is necessary for adequate breathing and oxygenation. Therefore, assessment of the airway is the first component in the primary assessment of the patient. An open airway is commonly referred to as a **patent airway.**

Airway Functions and Considerations

The following are general functions and considerations regarding the airway:

- The airway and respiratory tract is the conduit that allows air to move from the atmosphere and into the alveoli for gas exchange.
- No matter what the patient's condition, the airway must remain patent at all times.
- Any obstruction (food, blood, swelling, vomit) of the airway will result in less air movement, which will lead to some degree of poor gas exchange and potential hypoxia.
- The degree of the obstruction will directly affect the amount of air available for gas exchange. The tongue may create only a partial airway obstruction, whereas a piece of food may completely stop airflow.

The mental status of a patient typically correlates well with the status of his airway. An alert, responsive patient who is talking to you in a normal voice has an open airway. It takes an open and clear airway, along with adequate breathing, to enable a patient to communicate easily. Table 10-1 lists signs of an open airway.

A patient who has an altered mental status or is completely unresponsive cannot adequately protect his own airway and has the potential for airway occlusion, or obstruction. The tongue relaxes and falls back, blocking the pharynx. The epiglottis can also relax and obstruct the airway at the level of the larynx. The patient may lose his gag or cough reflex, making him susceptible to aspiration. Efforts by the patient to breathe will create a negative pressure; this may draw the tongue, epiglottis, or both into the airway to block airflow into the trachea and lungs. The airway may also be obstructed from injuries such as burns and soft tissue trauma to the face and upper airway (Figure 10-8*).

TABLE 10-1 Signs of an Open Airway

- Air can be felt and heard moving in and out of the mouth and nose.
- The patient is speaking in full sentences or with little difficulty.
- The sound of the voice is normal for the patient.

ASSESSMENT Tips

A patient who has an altered mental status but continues to maintain a gag or cough reflex could still aspirate blood, secretions, vomitus, or other substances. ■

Abnormal Upper Airway Sounds

When assessing the airway in the patient with a severely altered mental status, it is necessary to open the mouth manually, perform a manual airway maneuver, inspect inside the mouth, and listen for any abnormal sounds. The following are sounds that may indicate airway obstruction:

- **Snoring** (sonorous sounds) occurs when the upper airway is partially obstructed by the tongue or by relaxed tissues in the pharynx. The snoring and obstruction can be corrected by performing a head-tilt, chin-lift maneuver. This lifts the base of the tongue from the back of the pharynx (throat). In a patient with a suspected spinal injury, a jaw-thrust maneuver should be used.

Objective 10-10
Explain the causes of these upper airway sounds: snoring, crowing, gurgling, and stridor.

Objective 10-11
Demonstrate the procedures necessary for airway assessment and correction.

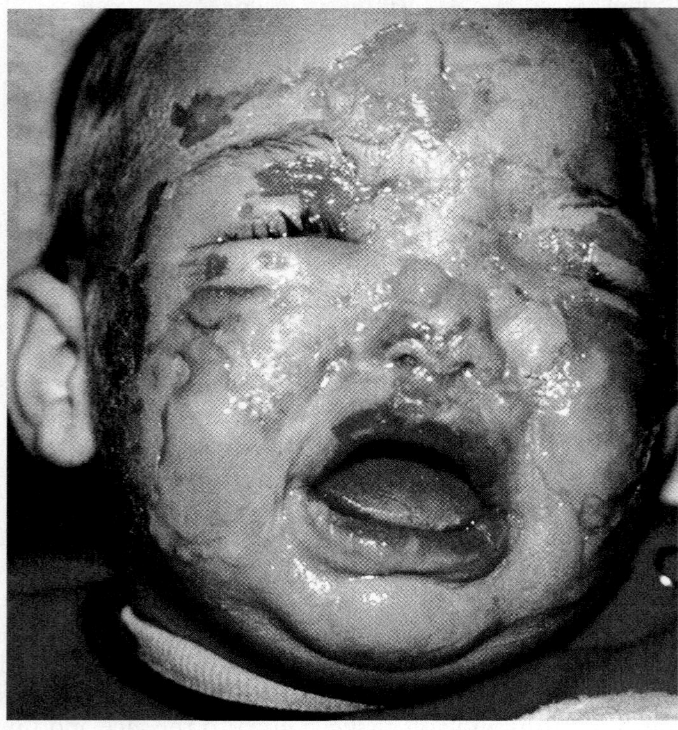

(a)

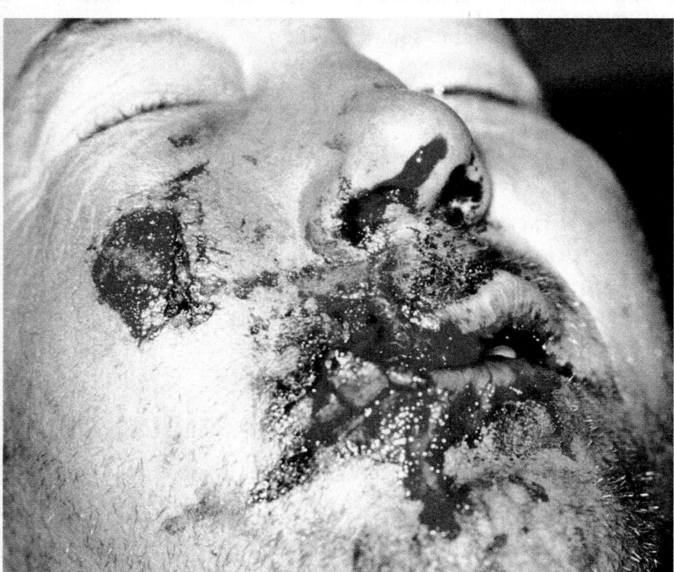

(b)

FIGURE 10-8 ∗ The airway can be blocked by injuries such as **(a)** burns or **(b)** soft tissue trauma.

- **Crowing** is a sound like a crow cawing that occurs when the muscles around the larynx spasm and narrow the opening into the trachea. Air rushing through the restricted passage causes the sound.
- **Gurgling,** a sound like gargling, usually indicates the presence of blood, vomitus, secretions, or other liquid in the airway. Immediately suction the substance from the airway.
- **Stridor** is a harsh, high-pitched sound heard during inspiration. It is characteristic of a significant upper airway obstruction from swelling in the larynx. Stridor may also be heard if a mechanical obstruction by food or other objects is present.

Signs of a blocked or inadequate airway are found in Table 10-2.

TABLE 10-2 Signs of a Blocked or Inadequate Airway

- Abnormal upper airway sound (stridor, snoring, crowing, or gurgling)
- An awake patient who is unable to speak
- Evidence of a foreign body airway obstruction (tongue, food, vomit, blood, or teeth in the upper airway, mouth, or nose)
- Swelling to the mouth, tongue, or oropharynx

Opening the Mouth

It is necessary to open the mouth of an unresponsive patient or a patient with an altered mental status to adequately assess the airway. This is done by using the **crossed-finger technique** (Figure 10-9∗):

1. Kneel above and behind the patient.
2. Cross the thumb and forefinger of one hand.
3. Place the thumb on the patient's lower incisors and your forefinger on the upper incisors.
4. Use a scissors motion or finger-snapping motion to open the mouth.

Inspect inside the mouth for vomitus, blood, secretions, broken teeth, or foreign bodies that can obstruct

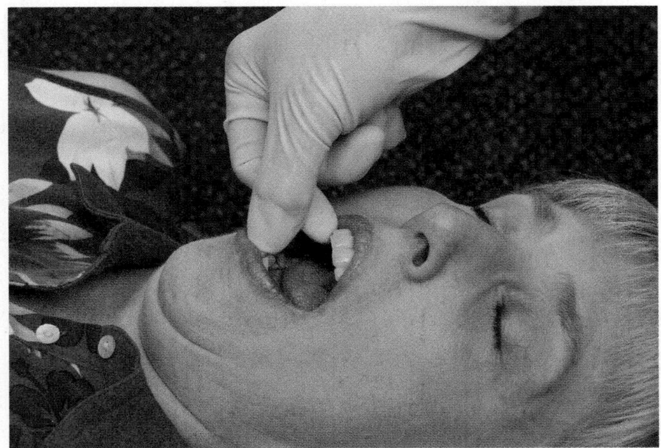

FIGURE 10-9 * Open the mouth using a crossed-finger technique.

the airway. Suction any foreign substance from the mouth. If suction equipment is not immediately available, turn the patient on his side (only perform this move if *no* spinal injury is suspected) and wipe the fluids away with your index and middle fingers wrapped in a cloth or gauze pad. If you can see foreign objects, such as food, broken teeth, or dentures, sweep the mouth with your index finger and remove them. Do this quickly. Be extremely cautious because the patient could bite down on your fingers, gag, or vomit.

Opening the Airway

Before a patient who is breathing inadequately can receive positive pressure ventilation, or breathing assistance in which air is forced into his lungs, he must have an open airway. The following are techniques that are used to open and maintain a patent airway.

- Manual airway maneuvers
  1. Head-tilt, chin-lift maneuver
  2. Jaw-thrust maneuver
- Suction
- Mechanical airways
  1. Oropharyngeal airway (oral airway)
  2. Nasopharyngeal airway (nasal airway)

If obvious blood, vomitus, secretions, or other substances are found in the mouth when you come in contact with the patient, immediately suction the substance from the oropharynx and nasopharynx prior to initiating a manual airway maneuver. It may be necessary to turn the patient on his side to remove heavy vomitus or large amounts of blood, fluid, or other secretions. Turning the patient on his side can only be done when you do not suspect a spine injury. Open the airway manually by using either the head-tilt, chin-lift maneuver or the jaw-thrust maneuver. Generally, the head-tilt, chin-lift maneuver is used. *However, if you suspect that a patient may have suffered a spinal injury, then use the jaw-thrust maneuver in conjunction with manual in-line spinal stabilization.*

Head-Tilt, Chin-Lift Maneuver

The **head-tilt, chin-lift maneuver** should be used for opening the airway in a patient who has no suspected spinal injury. This is only a temporary maneuver and must be supplemented with a mechanical airway device if the airway can't be adequately maintained with the head-tilt, chin-lift maneuver alone, or if ventilation of the patient is necessary. The head-tilt, chin-lift maneuver is illustrated in Figures 10-10a to 10-10d* and summarized here:

1. Place one hand on the patient's forehead, and apply firm, backward pressure with the palm of the hand to tilt the head back. Place the tips of the fingers of the other hand underneath the bony part of the lower jaw.
2. With the head tilted backward, lift the jaw upward to bring the patient's chin forward. Do not compress the soft tissues underneath the chin; they might obstruct the airway.
3. Continue to press the other hand on the patient's forehead to keep the head tilted backward.
4. Lift the chin and jaw so that the teeth are brought nearly together. (If necessary, you can use your thumb to depress or retract the lower lip; this will keep the patient's mouth slightly open.)
5. If the patient has loose dentures, hold them in position, making obstruction by the lips less likely. A seal is easier to form when the dentures are in place. If the dentures cannot be managed, remove them.

Examples of patients who require a head-tilt, chin-lift maneuver are:

- An unresponsive patient with no suspicion of spinal trauma
- A patient with cardiac arrest not due to trauma
- An apneic (not breathing) patient with no signs of trauma

Head-Tilt, Chin-Lift Maneuver in Infants and Children

The preferred method of opening the airway in infants and children without suspected spinal injury is the head-tilt, chin-lift maneuver (Figure 10-11*).

The hand positions and procedures for performing the head-tilt, chin-lift maneuver with infants and children are the same as with adults except for a variation in head positioning. With an infant, the head should be tilted back gently into a "sniffing" or neutral position. As noted earlier, because of the large size of the head, it may be necessary to place a pad behind the shoulders to keep the airway open, until about the age of 4 years. Because of the underdeveloped airway structures in the infant, care must be taken not to overextend the infant's head; this could lead to an obstruction of the trachea. With a child, the head is tilted only slightly back from the neutral position. Only the index finger of one hand lifts the chin and jaw.

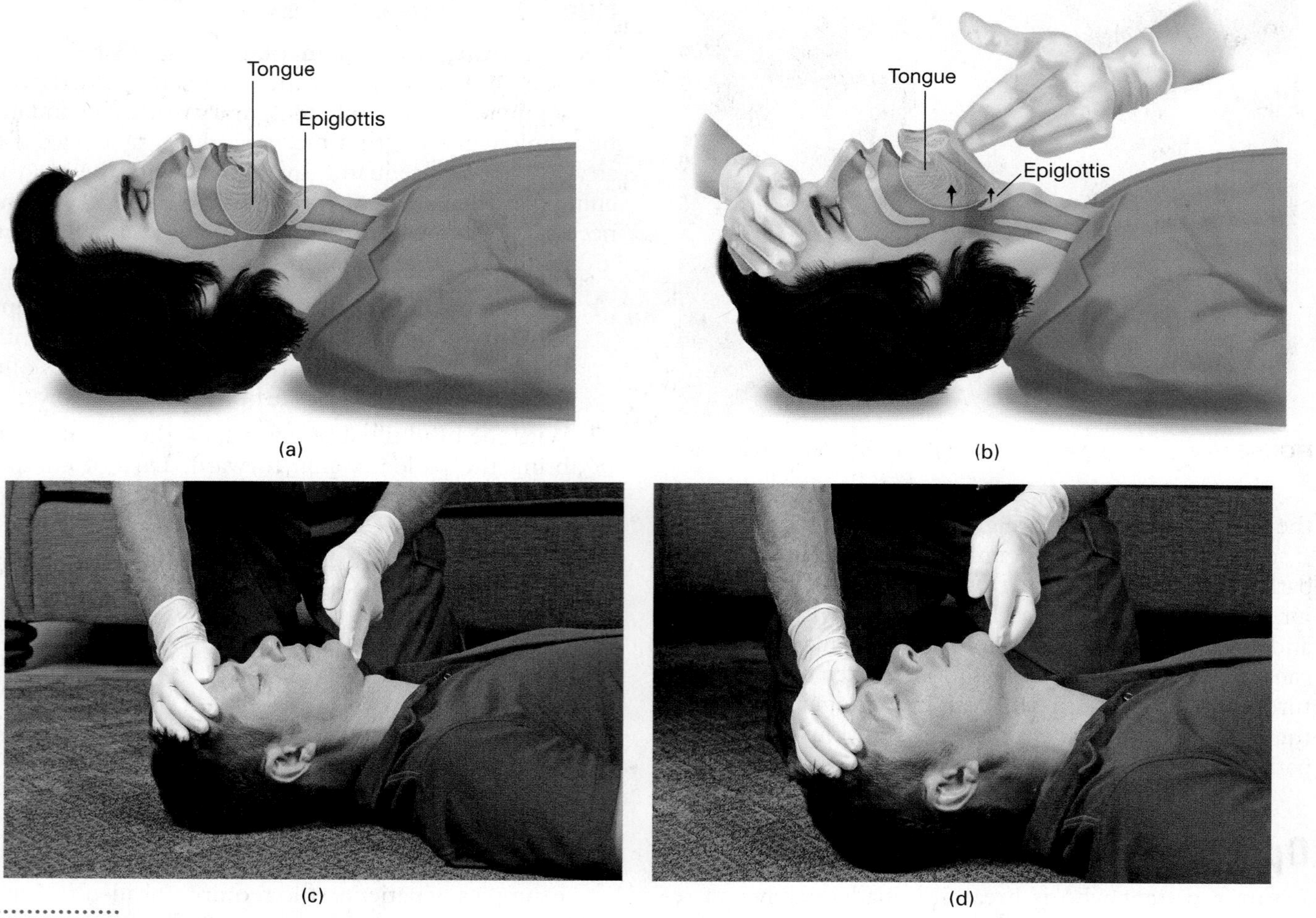

Tongue
Epiglottis

(a)

Tongue
Epiglottis

(b)

(c)

(d)

FIGURE 10-10 ✱ **(a)** The supine adult. **(b)** The head-tilt, chin-lift maneuver in the adult. **(c)** Head-tilt, chin-lift maneuver in the adult: neutral starting position. **(d)** Head-tilt, chin-lift maneuver in the adult: final tilted position.

Be careful not to press on the soft tissue beneath the chin, which may cause an airway obstruction.

Jaw-Thrust Maneuver

If a spinal injury is suspected, the patient's head and neck must be brought into and maintained in a neutral, in-line position. This means that the head is not turned to the side, tilted forward (flexed), or tilted backward (extended). The **jaw-thrust maneuver** is used to open the airway in such a patient because the head and neck are not tilted back during this maneuver. The jaw (mandible) is displaced forward by the EMT's fingers; this causes the patient's tongue to be pulled forward, away from the back

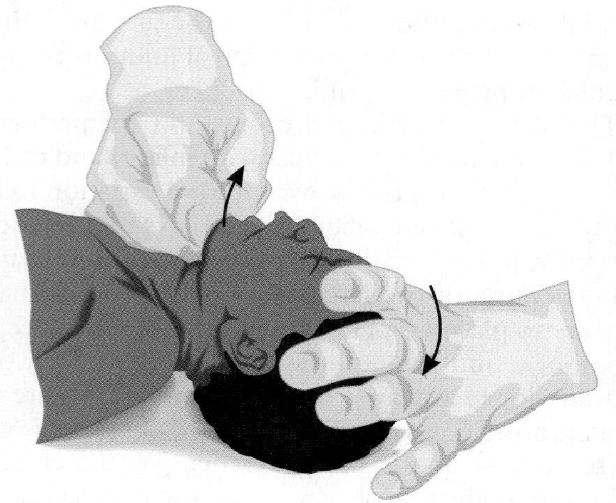

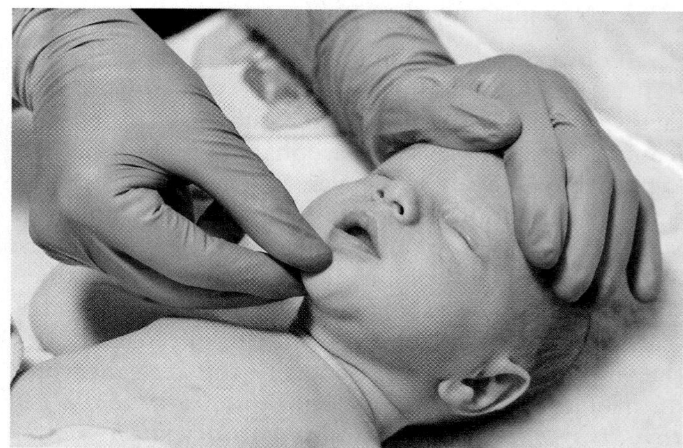

FIGURE 10-11 ✱ Head-tilt, chin-lift maneuver in the infant. Be sure to avoid overextension.

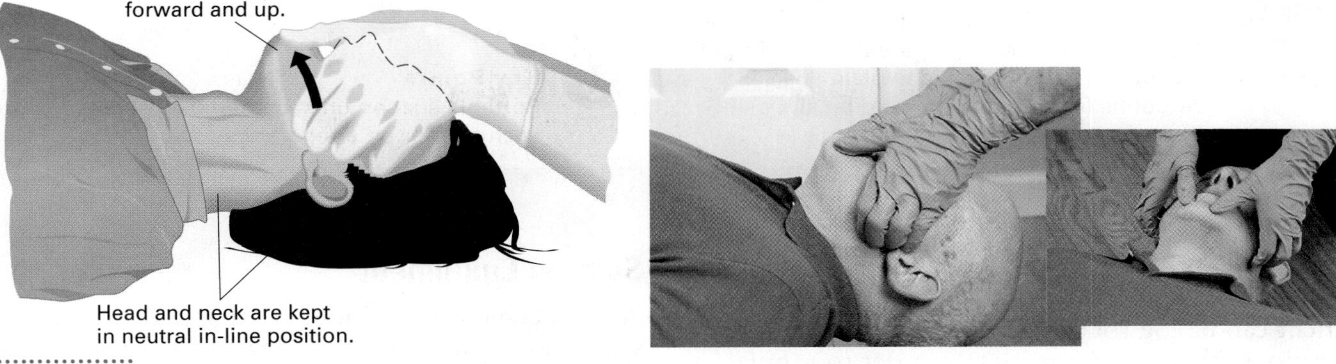
Mandible is moved forward and up.
Head and neck are kept in neutral in-line position.

FIGURE 10-12 ✱ The jaw-thrust maneuver is used to open the airway in patients with suspected spinal injury.

of the airway. If the head-tilt, chin-lift maneuver is unsuccessful in opening the airway of the non-spine-injured patient, perform the jaw-thrust maneuver. This is only a temporary maneuver and must be supplemented with a mechanical airway device if the airway can't be adequately maintained with the jaw thrust alone, or if continued ventilation of the patient is necessary. The procedure for the jaw thrust is illustrated in Figure 10-12✱. It involves the following steps:

1. Kneel at the top of the patient's head. Place your elbows on the surface on which the patient is lying, putting your hands at the side of the patient's head.
2. Grasp the angles of the patient's lower jaw on both sides. Move the jaw forward with both hands. This will move the tongue forward, away from the airway. If no spinal injury is suspected, the head could be tilted backward.
3. Retract the lower lip with your thumb if the lips close.

If the jaw thrust does not establish an open airway, reposition the jaw. If repositioning is not effective, insert an oral or nasal airway adjunct, as explained later in this chapter. The EMT holding the in-line stabilization can also establish and maintain the jaw thrust. The jaw thrust would be used in unresponsive patients with suspected spinal injury or trauma patients in need of a manual maneuver to open the airway.

Jaw-Thrust Maneuver in Infants and Children

Follow the basic procedure just described for adults when performing the jaw-thrust maneuver in infants and children (Figure 10-13✱). Place two or three fingers of each hand at the angle of the jaw to lift it up and forward while the other fingers guide the movement. Insert an airway adjunct if the jaw thrust does not open the airway.

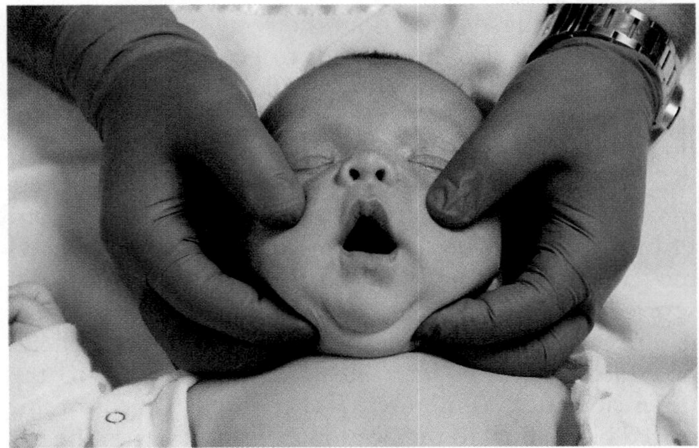

FIGURE 10-13 ✱ Jaw-thrust maneuver in an infant.

Positioning the Patient for Airway Control

If the patient has an altered mental status and may be at risk of aspirating blood, secretions, or vomitus, place the patient in a modified lateral (recovery) position (Figure 10-14✱). This is also known as the coma or recovery position. Place the patient's arm that is closest to you flat on the ground at a right angle to the body. Log roll the patient onto his side. Place the hand of the opposite arm (now on top) under his lateral face and cheek. Bend the leg at the hip and knee to stabilize the body in this position. This positioning is only used in patients who do not have a suspected spinal injury and in patients who are not in need of positive pressure ventilation. If a spinal injury is suspected, the patient must remain supine with manual in-line stabilization

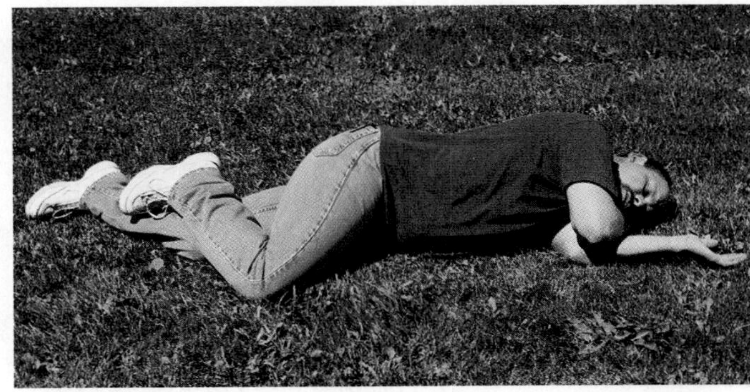

FIGURE 10-14 ✱ The modified lateral (recovery) position is used to help prevent aspiration in patients who do not have suspected spinal injury.

Objectives 10-12 to 10-15
Describe the performance requirements for fixed suction devices; compare the function of fixed and portable suction devices; compare the use of rigid and soft suction catheters; and explain special considerations for suctioning including signs of hypoxia and patients with copious vomit.

Key Points
Portable suction units should be inspected before each shift or on a regular basis.

maintained until the patient is completely immobilized to a backboard. At that point, the entire board-with-patient can be log rolled to assist with the drainage of secretions, blood, and vomitus. In order to ventilate a patient effectively when no advanced airway device is in place, the patient must be in a supine position.

When using this position, the body should be as lateral as possible. The head needs to be placed so that the secretions, blood, or vomitus will flow out of the mouth freely. Any pressure on the chest that might interfere with breathing must be avoided. A prone position (face down) will drain secretions; however, it may reduce effectiveness of ventilation by pushing the abdominal contents upward toward the head and against the diaphragm, limiting its movement. This may lead to inadequate ventilation and severe hypoxia. Therefore, never use a prone position. If it is necessary to leave the patient in the modified lateral position for greater than 30 minutes, turn him to the other side after 30 minutes. If there are any signs of impaired blood flow to the bottom extremities, turn the patient to the opposite side.

Suctioning

It is necessary to remove any blood, vomitus, secretions, and any other liquids, food particles, or objects from the mouth and airway since they can cause obstruction. Such substances are best removed through the use of suction devices. If a gurgling sound is heard when you are assessing the airway or during artificial ventilation, immediately apply suction to remove the liquid from the airway. Failure to do so will force the liquid substance farther down the airway and possibly into the lungs.

Some suction equipment is not very effective in removing thick vomitus or solid objects, such as teeth, foreign bodies, or food, from the airway. In such situations, it may be necessary to place the patient on his side and perform a finger sweep to remove the material.

Standard Precautions During Suctioning

Because suctioning involves removal of body fluids and the potential for coughing and spatters, you must take appropriate Standard Precautions. Protective eyewear, a mask, and gloves should be used. If a patient is known to have tuberculosis or displays signs and symptoms consistent with tuberculosis, an N-95 or high-efficiency particulate air (HEPA) respirator should be worn at all times in addition to eyewear and gloves.

Suction Equipment

Suction equipment includes the device that creates the suction as well as the catheters that are inserted in the airway. Various types of fixed and portable suction devices and catheters are available.

Mounted Suction Devices Fixed or installed units should be part of the required on-board ambulance equipment (Figure 10-15*). They should be powerful enough to provide an airflow of $>$ 40 lpm at the end of the delivery tube and create a vacuum of more than –300 mmHg on the gauge when the tubing is clamped or kinked. The device should be adjustable to allow for a reduced vacuum when suctioning infants and children. Such fixed systems are powered by an electric vacuum pump or by the vacuum produced by the ambulance engine manifold.

Portable Suction Devices A portable unit must produce a vacuum adequate to suction substances from the pharynx. Portable suction units can be electric-, oxygen- or air-, or hand-powered (Figure 10-16*). These suction units should be inspected before each shift or on a regular basis.

Electric suction devices must have fully charged batteries to function effectively. A low battery charge will reduce the effective vacuum and the length of time the unit can be used. Some units allow for constant charging so that the batteries are always fully charged when needed.

Oxygen-powered devices function only as long as a source of oxygen is available. Once the oxygen source has run out, the vacuum is lost and suction becomes ineffective.

Hand-powered suction devices (Figure 10-17*) do not require any energy source other than an EMT to cre-

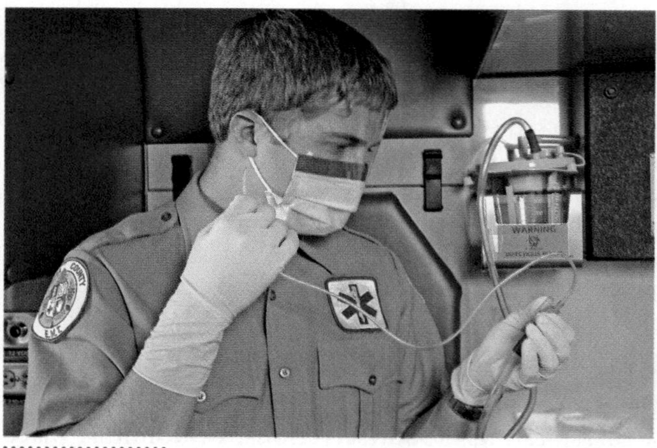

FIGURE 10-15 * On-board suction unit.

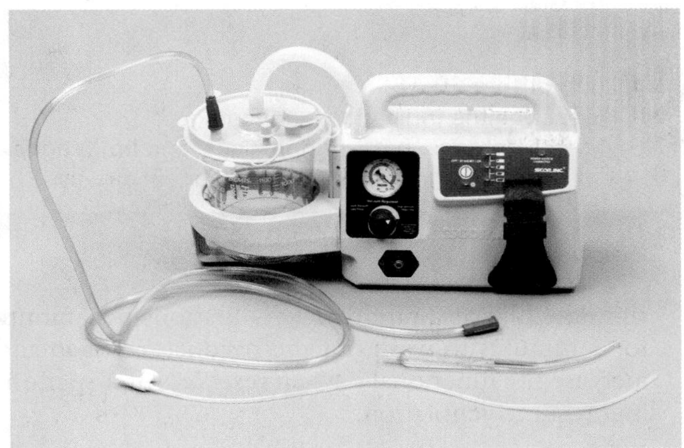

FIGURE 10-16 * A portable suction unit.

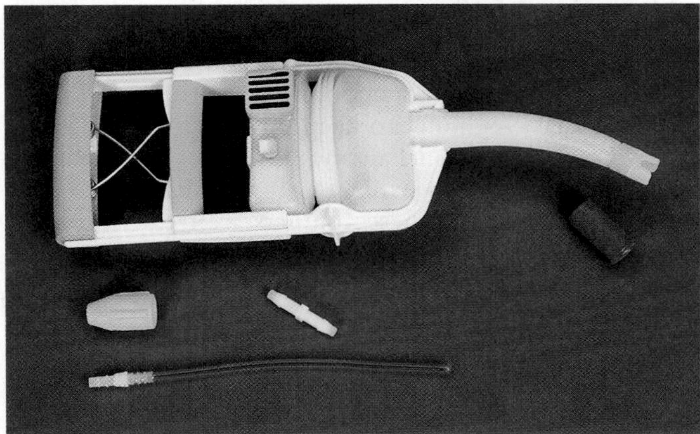

FIGURE 10-17 * A hand-powered suction device.

ate the vacuum. Therefore, these devices lack some typical problems associated with electric- or oxygen-powered devices. Also, hand-powered units can more effectively suction heavier substances, such as thick vomitus.

Any type of portable suction device must have the following:

- Wide-bore, thick-walled, nonkinking tubing that fits standard rigid or soft suction catheters
- An unbreakable collection bottle or container and a supply of water for rinsing and clearing the tubes and catheters
- Enough vacuum pressure and flow to suction substances from the pharynx effectively

Suction Catheters Suction catheters must be disposable and capable of being connected to the suction unit's tubing. Two different types of suction catheters are available:

- **Hard or rigid catheter**—This type of catheter is a rigid plastic tube. It is called a Yankauer catheter and is commonly referred to as a **"tonsil tip"** or **"tonsil sucker."** It is used to suction the mouth and oropharynx of an unresponsive patient. It is more effective for particulate matter than a soft catheter. The catheter should be inserted only as far as you can see, typically not farther than the base of the tongue. The tip of the suction catheter may stimulate a gag reflex and cause vomiting if it touches the back of the oropharynx. Also, the vagus nerve may be stimulated, causing the patient to become bradycardic. If you are using a hard catheter on an infant or child, be careful when applying suction, because doing so might cause soft tissue trauma and may also stimulate bradycardia. In infants and children, never touch the back of the airway.

ASSESSMENT Tips

Prior to suctioning—to avoid inserting the catheter too far into the oropharynx—the hard suction catheter can be measured with the tip placed at the angle of the jaw and a landmark established at the corner of the mouth. ■

- **Soft catheter**—The soft suction catheter consists of flexible tubing. It is also called a **"French" catheter.** It is used in suctioning the nose and nasopharynx and in other situations where the rigid catheter cannot be used. The length of catheter should be determined by measuring from the tip of the patient's nose to the tip of his ear if it is being inserted in the nasopharynx or from the corner of his mouth to the tip of his ear if it is being inserted in the mouth and oropharynx. The soft suction catheter should not be inserted beyond the base of the tongue.

Technique of Suctioning

There are many suctioning techniques. They vary depending on the device and type of catheter used. One technique is described here (EMT Skills 10-1):

1. Position yourself at the patient's head. If this is not possible, take a position in which you can observe the airway.
2. Turn on the suction unit.
3. Select the appropriate type of catheter. Use a rigid catheter when suctioning the mouth or oropharynx. If the nasal passages need to be suctioned, select a soft (French) catheter and use low to medium suction (80–120 mmHg). A bulb syringe may be used if a soft catheter is not available.
4. Measure the catheter and insert it into the oral cavity without suction, if possible. Insert it no farther down than the base of the tongue.
5. Apply suction only on the way out of the airway. Begin suction after the tip has been positioned, moving the catheter tip from side to side to clear material from the mouth as the catheter is being removed. If possible, suction for no more than 15 seconds at a time in the adult; in infants and children, suction in

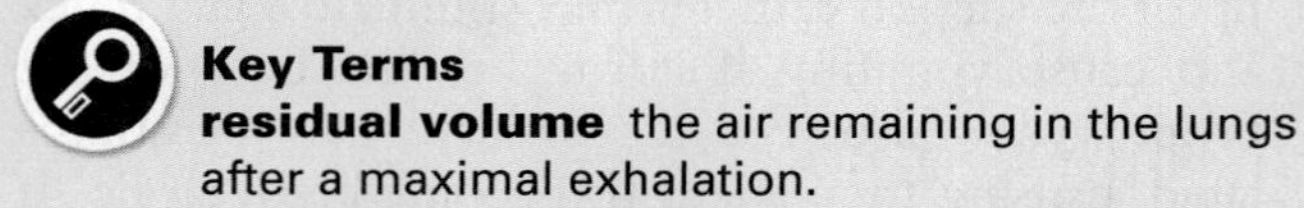

Key Terms
residual volume the air remaining in the lungs after a maximal exhalation.

Objective 10-16
Describe the indications, advantages, disadvantages, precautions, uses, and limitations of oropharyngeal and nasopharyngeal airways.

shorter periods, approximately 5 seconds. Suction until the substance is clear from the airway to prevent aspiration from spontaneous or artificial ventilation.

6. If necessary, rinse the catheter with water to prevent obstruction of the tubing from dried or thick material. Do this by keeping a bottle of water available and applying suction to the water as necessary to clear the tubing.

Special Considerations When Suctioning

The following are special considerations when suctioning the airway:

- If the patient has secretions or vomitus that cannot be removed quickly and easily by suctioning, the patient should be log rolled onto his side and the oropharynx cleared by finger sweeping the foreign material from the mouth.
- If the patient in need of artificial ventilation is producing frothy secretions as rapidly as suctioning can remove them, apply suction for 15 seconds, provide positive pressure ventilation with supplemental oxygen for 2 minutes, then apply suction for another 15 seconds. Repeat this sequence until the airway is cleared. Consult medical direction in such a situation.
- During suctioning, the **residual volume** of air in the lungs between respirations is removed. Residual volume is defined as the air remaining in the lungs after a maximal exhalation. This will cause a quick decrease in blood oxygen levels. Therefore, monitor the patient's pulse, heart rate, and pulse oximeter reading while suctioning. If the heart rate drops during suctioning, especially in infants and children, immediately remove the catheter, administer oxygen, and be prepared to begin positive pressure ventilation with supplemental oxygen.

  In the adult patient, a rapid heart rate (tachycardia), slow heart rate (bradycardia), or an irregular heart rate may be seen during suctioning. These can occur from stimulation of the airway by the suction catheter or may be an indication that the oxygen level in the blood is getting dangerously low. Stop the suction procedure and resume positive pressure ventilation for at least 30 seconds if the patient is being artificially ventilated.
- Before suctioning mucus and small amounts of secretions in a patient who is being artificially ventilated, ventilate him at a rate of 12 ventilations per minute for 5 minutes to wash out the residual nitrogen and increase the functional oxygen reserve. After suctioning, resume ventilation.

Airway Adjuncts

Once the airway is opened by the head-tilt, chin-lift maneuver or the jaw-thrust maneuver, and all foreign substances are removed by suctioning, it may be necessary to insert an airway adjunct to keep the airway open. There are two types of artificial airways: the oropharyngeal and nasopharyngeal. Both extend near to, but do not pass through, the larynx. These adjuncts are frequently used during artificial ventilation. When using these devices, keep the following points in mind:

- The adjunct must be clean and clear of obstructions.
- The proper size airway adjunct must be selected to avoid complications and ineffectiveness.
- The airway adjuncts do not protect the airway from aspiration of secretions, blood, vomitus, or other foreign substances into the lungs.
- The mental status of the patient will determine whether an adjunct can be used. The patient's mental status must be continually and carefully monitored. If the patient becomes more responsive or gags, remove the airway adjunct.
- A head-tilt, chin-lift or jaw-thrust maneuver must still be maintained, even when an airway adjunct is in place and properly positioned.

Oropharyngeal (Oral) Airway

The **oropharyngeal airway,** also known as the **oral airway,** is a semicircular device of hard plastic or rubber that holds the tongue away from the back of the airway (Figure 10-18*). The device also allows for suctioning of secretions. There are two common types of oropharyngeal airway: One is tubular and the other has a channeled side. Both are disposable and come in a variety of adult, child, and infant sizes.

The patient must be completely unresponsive and must have no gag or cough reflex. *Do not use this device on a patient who is responsive or has a gag or cough reflex.* If inserted in such a patient, it may cause vomiting or spasm of the vocal cords. This will further compromise the airway.

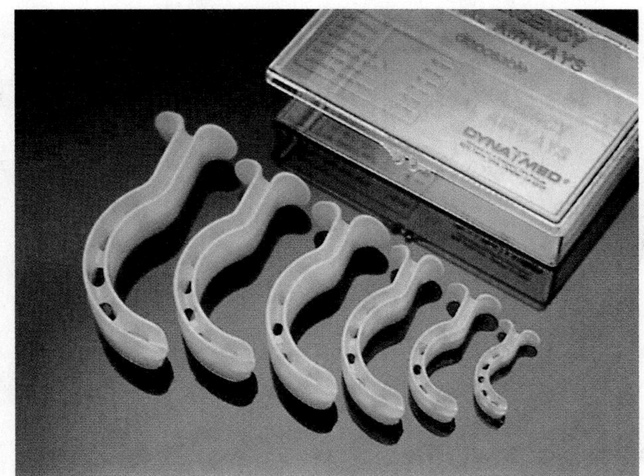
FIGURE 10-18 * Oropharyngeal (oral) airways.

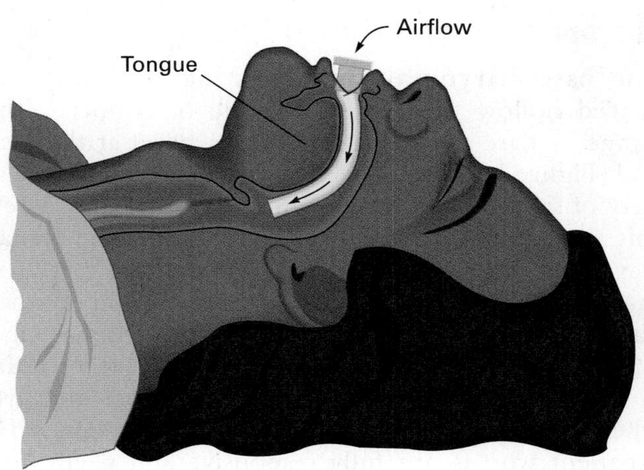

FIGURE 10-19 * Oropharyngeal airway that is properly placed. The tongue is kept from falling back to occlude the patient's airway.

Use of an improperly sized airway adjunct can result in major complications. If the device is too long, it can push the epiglottis over the opening to the larynx, obstructing airflow to the trachea and causing a complete obstruction of the airway. Also, if not inserted properly it may push the tongue back into the airway, causing complete or partial obstruction.

Even with the adjunct properly inserted, it is often necessary to maintain the position of the patient's head with the head-tilt, chin-lift or jaw-thrust maneuver to ensure an open airway. Airway management improves significantly with placement of the adjunct.

Inserting the Oropharyngeal Airway The procedure for inserting an oropharyngeal airway is illustrated in EMT Skills 10-2. When inserting such a device, follow these steps:

1. Select the proper size airway. Measure the airway by holding it next to the patient's face. A properly sized airway should extend the distance from the level of the front teeth to the angle of the jaw. Thus, the flange will be at the level of the teeth while the distal portion of the airway will be at the level of the angle of the jaw.
2. Open the patient's mouth using the crossed-finger technique. In adults, insert the airway upside down, tip pointing to the roof of the mouth.
3. When the airway comes in contact with the soft palate at the back of the roof of the mouth, gently rotate it 180° while continuing to advance it until the flat flange at the top of the airway rests on the patient's front teeth. The airway follows the natural curve of the tongue and the oropharynx (Figure 10-19*). Following this procedure will reduce the chances of the tongue being pushed back and obstructing the airway. The airway can also be inserted sideways in the corner of the mouth and rotated 90° while it is being advanced into position.

An alternative method of inserting the oropharyngeal airway involves the use of a tongue depressor (blade). The tongue depressor is inserted in the mouth until its tip is at the base of the tongue. The tongue is then pressed down toward the mandible and forward with the tongue depressor. The airway is inserted in its normal anatomical position until the flange is seated on the teeth (Figure 10-20*). This is the preferred method of airway insertion in infants and children.

If a patient at any time gags during the insertion, remove the oropharyngeal airway. It may then be necessary to use a nasopharyngeal airway or no adjunct at all. If a patient tries to dislodge the device after it has been inserted, remove it by gently pulling it out and down. Because this airway adjunct commonly causes the patient to gag, be prepared for vomiting.

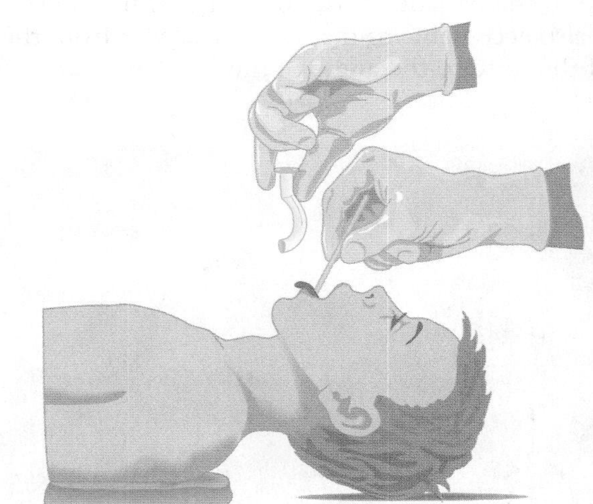
FIGURE 10-20 * The preferred method of inserting the oropharyngeal airway in the infant or child is to use a tongue blade to hold the tongue forward and down toward the mandible as the airway is inserted.

Nasopharyngeal (Nasal) Airway

The **nasopharyngeal airway,** or **nasal airway,** is a curved hollow tube of soft plastic or rubber with a flange or flare at the top end and a bevel at the distal end (Figure 10-21*). This airway adjunct comes in a variety of sizes based on the diameter of the tube. Use of this airway is indicated in patients in whom the oral airway cannot be inserted because of clenched teeth, biting, or injuries to the maxilla or face, and in those patients who are unable to tolerate an oropharyngeal airway. The nasopharyngeal airway is less likely to stimulate vomiting because the soft tube moves and gives when the patient swallows. Therefore, it can be used on a patient who is not fully responsive and needs assistance in maintaining an open airway but who still has a minimally intact gag reflex.

Be careful to select an airway of proper length. Avoid use of the nasal airway in patients with a suspected fracture to the base of the skull or severe facial trauma.

Insertion and use of this device may still cause gagging, vomiting, and spasming of the vocal cords. Also, like the oropharyngeal airway, it does not protect the trachea and lungs from aspiration of blood, vomitus, secretions, or other foreign substances. Even though the tube is lubricated, insertion is painful and may cause injury to the nasal mucosa, causing the nose to bleed and allowing blood to enter the airway, resulting in possible obstruction or aspiration. It is still necessary to maintain a head-tilt, chin-lift or jaw-thrust maneuver once the airway is inserted.

Inserting the Nasopharyngeal Airway The procedure for inserting the nasopharyngeal airway is illustrated in EMT Skills 10-3. When inserting such a device, follow these steps:

1. Measure the airway by placing it next to the patient's face. A properly sized airway should extend from the tip of the patient's nose to the tip of the earlobe. It is also acceptable to measure the airway from the tip of the nose to the angle of the jaw. The diameter of the airway must be such that it can fit inside the patient's nostril without blanching the skin of the nose.
2. Lubricate the outside of the airway well with a sterile, water-soluble lubricant. This will ease the insertion and lessen the chance of trauma to the nasal mucous lining.
3. Insert the device in the larger or more open nostril. The bevel should be facing the septum (wall between the nostrils) or floor of the nostril. The device is inserted close to the midline, along the floor of the nostril, and straight back into the nasopharynx. If you meet resistance, rotate the device gently from side to side as you continue to insert it. If you still meet resistance, remove the airway and try the other nostril. When the device is properly inserted, the flange should lie against the flare of the nostril (Figure 10-22*).
4. Check to be sure that air is flowing through the airway during inhalation and exhalation. If the patient is spontaneously breathing and no air movement is felt through the tube, remove it and attempt reinsertion in the other nostril.

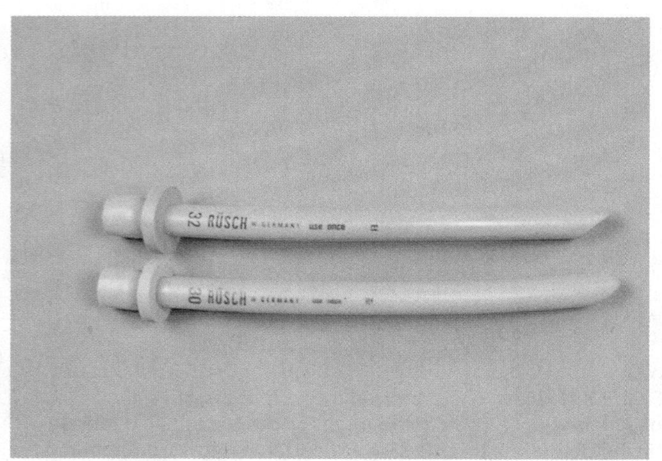

FIGURE 10-21 * Nasopharyngeal (nasal) airways.

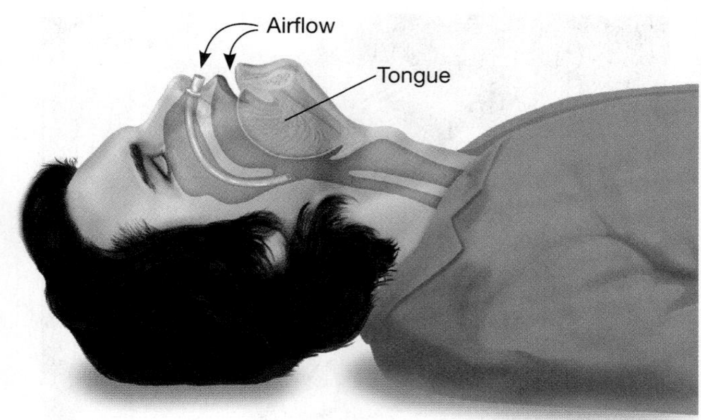

FIGURE 10-22 * A nasopharyngeal airway properly placed.

Nasopharyngeal airways come in a variety of pediatric sizes. In very young patients, the nasopharyngeal airway is so small that it is easily obstructed by secretions and other upper airway substances. Children may have large adenoids, which will make insertion of the nasopharyngeal airway very difficult. This may also lead to injury and bleeding. Even if insertion is possible, the large adenoids may compress the nasopharyngeal airway and increase the resistance in the airway. This may make the use of a nasopharyngeal airway in the very young ineffective.

Assessment of Breathing

After establishing a patent airway, it is necessary to assess the adequacy of the patient's breathing. Inadequate breathing leads to both poor gas exchange in the alveoli and ineffective delivery of oxygen to the cells. To deter-

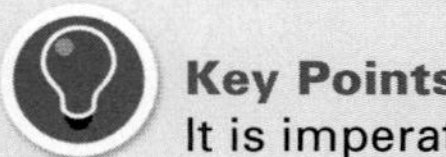

Key Points
It is imperative to assess both volume and rate to determine if a patient's breathing is adequate or not.

Key Terms

minute volume the amount of air breathed in and out in one minute. Also called *minute ventilation*.

tidal volume the amount of air breathed in and out in one normal respiration.

alveolar ventilation the amount of inspired air that reaches the alveoli of the lungs.

mine whether the breathing is adequate, you must focus on both the rate at which the patient is breathing and the volume of each of his breaths.

Relationship of Tidal Volume and Respiratory Rate in Assessment of Breathing

It is imperative to assess the relationship between the volume, or amount of air taken in with each breath, and the rate at which the patient is breathing when determining whether the patient's breathing is adequate or not. This is a key decision-making process that the EMT must accomplish quickly and accurately on every patient. The wrong decision about breathing status can have serious consequences, the most serious being death of the patient. Thus, understanding the basic relationship between the volume of air the patient breathes in, the respiratory rate, and the volume of air that actually reaches the alveoli for gas exchange is critical in determining whether the patient is breathing adequately and, if not, recognizing the need for immediate intervention with ventilation.

Minute Volume

Both adequate and inadequate breathing depend on two specific variables: the rate at which the patient is breathing and the depth of each breath. Because **minute volume** deals with both depth and rate, it typically correlates with how adequately the patient is breathing. A decrease in either the **tidal volume** or the respiratory rate may lead to a decrease in minute volume so severe that the patient is no longer moving an adequate amount of air per minute in and out of the lungs. The consequence will be a decrease in gas exchange at the level of the alveoli which, in turn, can cause the cells to become hypoxic.

It is not important for the EMT to determine the actual minute volume value; however, it is imperative to assess both respiratory rate and volume when determining whether the breathing is adequate, since a change in either of these could lead to inadequate breathing. If you arrive on the scene and ask your partner if the adult patient you are treating is breathing adequately and he answers that the respiratory rate is 14 per minute, you have only half the information necessary to determine whether the patient is breathing adequately or not. A respiratory rate of 14 per minute for an adult patient is well within the normal respiratory range. However, if that patient is moving only a very small volume into the lungs with each of the 14 breaths, he would have an inadequate breathing status and would need to be ventilated. On the other hand, if your partner were to tell you that a different adult patient is breathing full and deep, you can't make a decision about the breathing status without also knowing the respiratory rate. If the respiratory rate is only six per minute in this patient, even though the volume with the six breaths is full and deep, the breathing would be considered inadequate and the patient would need to be ventilated. These examples reinforce the principle that you must know both variables, respiratory rate and tidal volume, before you can make any decision about the adequacy of breathing.

Typically, an increase in either the respiratory rate or the depth (tidal volume) would increase the respiratory minute ventilation. If a patient starts breathing at a faster rate, your assumption might be that he is moving more air in and out of the lungs in 1 minute, which would increase the minute volume and gas exchange in the alveoli of the lungs, thereby providing more oxygen to the cells. For example, if a patient has increased his respiratory rate from 12/minute to 20/minute, you might believe that the patient now has a greater minute volume because he is moving more air in and out of his lungs per minute. However, that would be true only if the tidal volume (depth of each breath) has remained at or near a normal level or has increased. A decrease in the tidal volume, even though the rate has increased, may have a profound negative effect on the volume of air reaching the alveoli and how much air is therefore available for gas exchange, as explained in the next section.

ASSESSMENT Tips

The best method to assess for tidal volume is to look for adequate chest rise and to feel and listen for air movement from the nose and mouth. ■

Alveolar Ventilation

It is important to understand how the two variables just discussed, respiratory rate and tidal volume, determine the amount of air that actually reaches the alveoli, which is the site of gas exchange, as well as how they impact ventilatory management and oxygen therapy.

Alveolar ventilation is the amount of air breathed in that reaches the alveoli. Only the air that reaches the alveoli can be used for gas exchange (oxygenation of the

Key Terms
dead air space inspired air that fills the respiratory tract but never reaches the alveoli of the lungs.

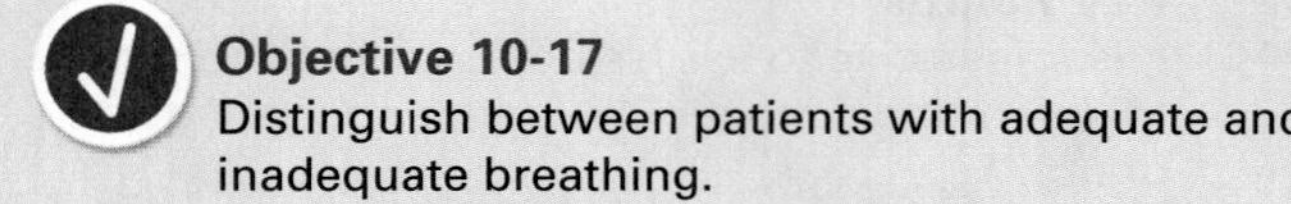

Objective 10-17
Distinguish between patients with adequate and inadequate breathing.

blood and removal of carbon dioxide) since the trachea and bronchi do not participate in gas exchange.

Because of the effect of **dead air space** on ventilation, decreases in tidal volume can dramatically reduce the amount of air reaching the alveoli for gas exchange. As an example, take the average-sized adult who is breathing at 12 times per minute; however, because of a condition that depresses the respiratory system, he is only breathing in 200 mL of air (tidal volume) with each breath. The minute ventilation would be calculated as follows:

Minute volume = 200 mL × 12 per minute
Minute volume = 2,400 mL

Of the 200 mL of air taken in with each breath, 150 mL will fill the dead air space, leaving only 50 mL to reach the alveoli for gas exchange (200 mL of tidal volume – 150 mL of dead air space = 50 mL). Although the patient is still breathing at 12 times per minute, which is well within the normal range of breathing, the amount of air reaching the alveoli for gas exchange is thoroughly inadequate. If left untreated, the patient will become severely hypoxic. This patient needs to be immediately ventilated to increase the tidal volume so that the amount of air reaching the alveoli is increased to an adequate level. One might ask, if the patient is already breathing at 12 times per minute, how would that be done? When the patient begins to take in his own breath, the ventilation is delivered. The delivered volume of your ventilation will supplement and increase the tidal volume of each of the patient's breaths to an adequate level, restoring the adequate alveolar ventilation.

A high respiratory rate can also lead to a decrease in alveolar ventilation. A very fast respiratory rate allows less time for the lungs to fill fully. If the patient is breathing at a very fast rate, the time for inhalation is decreased and the breaths become shallow, thereby reducing tidal volume. Typically, an adult patient with a respiratory rate of 40 breaths per minute or greater will have a significant reduction in tidal volume. Even though the respiratory rate is excessively elevated, the severely decreased tidal volume leads to a decrease in alveolar ventilation and poor gas exchange. Consider the following as an example in a patient breathing at 42 times per minute, but breathing in only 200 mL with each breath:

Minute volume = 42 breaths per minute × 200 mL
Minute volume = 8,400 mL

This appears to be much better minute ventilation than the average-sized adult breathing at 12 times per minute (6,000 mL). However, when you consider the volume of each breath, you can see how the ventilation is severely inadequate and the gas exchange is dramatically reduced.

Alveolar ventilation = (200 mL of tidal volume – 150 mL of dead air space) × 42 breaths per minute
Alveolar ventilation = 2,100 mL

Even though this patient is breathing 3½ times as fast as the patient breathing at 12 times per minute, he is getting less volume to his alveoli, creating a significantly inadequate breathing status.

As these examples have shown, it is necessary to carefully assess the tidal volume of the patient in addition to the respiratory rate, because a reduction in tidal volume affects the alveolar ventilation more drastically and leads to poor gas exchange sooner than rate disturbances. It is not your intent to determine an actual number value, but you must determine if the tidal volume is adequate. Also, as you can see by the example just given, an increased respiratory rate will not necessarily compensate for lower tidal volumes.

Remember that the dead space is filled with each breath regardless of the volume breathed in. If the average-sized patient is breathing in a tidal volume of only 200 mL with each breath, only 50 mL of air will reach the alveoli. This leads to severely inadequate breathing. A patient with an inadequate respiratory rate—or a poor tidal volume regardless of the respiratory rate—needs ventilation.

Assessing for Adequate Breathing

The rate, rhythm, quality, and depth of respirations should be assessed. This is done by looking, listening, feeling, and auscultating (listening with a stethoscope).

- **Look (inspect).** Inspection includes the following:
  1. *Inspect the chest.* Observe for adequate expansion by watching the chest wall rise and fall. Look for **retractions,** or pulling inward, of the intercostal muscles of the chest as well as excessive use of the neck muscles during inspiration. In the unresponsive patient, you should place your ear near the patient's mouth or nose while looking at the chest. You will simultaneously look, listen, and

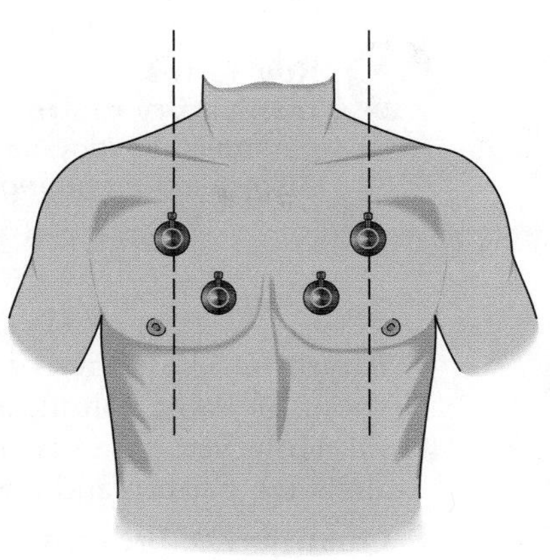
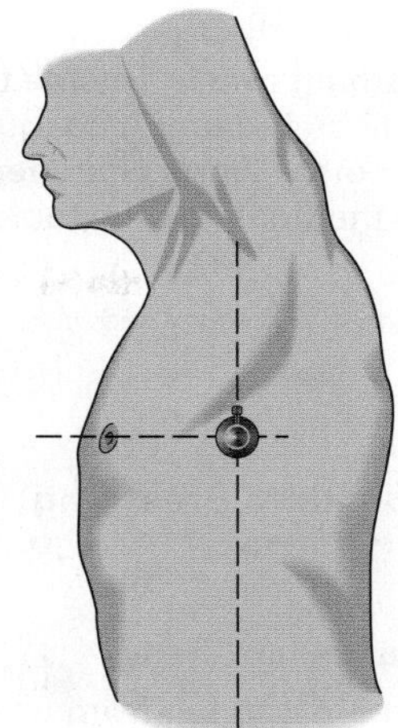

FIGURE 10-23 ✱ Auscultation landmarks on the anterior and lateral chest.

feel for air movement. If the chest does not rise adequately or appears to have a shallow rise, the tidal volume with each breath is inadequate. This patient needs to be ventilated.

2. *Observe the patient's general appearance.* Does he appear to be anxious, uncomfortable, or in distress? Is the patient lying down or sitting erect? (Typically, a patient who has difficulty in breathing is sitting up, leaning forward.) Does it appear that the patient is straining to breathe? Look for use or straining of the large muscle in the neck. This is often associated with a patient having a difficult time moving an adequate amount of air on inhalation.
3. *Decide if the breathing pattern is regular or irregular.* Injuries to the brain commonly produce irregular breathing patterns that are ineffective.
4. *Look at the nostrils* to see if they open wide during inhalation. Such flaring indicates difficulty in breathing.

- **Listen.** How does the patient speak to you? Does he speak only a few words at a time, then have to catch his breath? If the patient has an altered mental status or is unresponsive, place your ear next to the patient's nose and mouth and listen and feel for air escaping during exhalation. The sound or movement of air will indicate that the patient is breathing. If you do not hear an adequate volume of air being exhaled with each breath, the tidal volume would be considered inadequate. If the tidal volume is inadequate, you must ventilate the patient.
- **Feel.** With your ear next to the patient's nose and mouth, feel the volume of air escaping during exhalation. Feeling the air against your ear and cheek will provide you with a sense of the volume that the patient is breathing. If you do not feel an adequate volume of air being exhaled with each breath, the tidal volume would be considered inadequate. If the tidal volume is inadequate, you must ventilate the patient.
- **Auscultate.** Place your stethoscope at the second intercostal space, about 2 inches below the clavicle, at the midclavicular line. You can also auscultate at the fourth or fifth intercostal space on the anterior or midaxillary line, or at the fifth intercostal space next to the sternum on the anterior chest (Figure 10-23✱). Listen to one full inhalation and exhalation and determine if the breath sounds are present and equal **bilaterally** (on both sides). An adequate volume of air being inspired will produce full breath sounds that are equal on both sides. Breath sounds that are diminished or absent indicate inadequate breathing. Breath sounds are not the primary method to check for breathing status. You must first look at the chest for rise and listen for air movement with the naked ear. Checking breath sounds will be done later in the assessment to provide more information about the breathing status of the patient.

The rate, rhythm, quality, and depth of the breathing must be checked during assessment. The rate is checked by counting the number of respirations in 1 minute (one inhalation + one exhalation = one respiration). The rhythm is checked by looking at the pattern of respirations (regular or irregular). The quality of breathing refers to assessment of tidal volume. It is assessed by inspecting for adequate chest rise with each inhalation. Also inspect for use of accessory muscles. Later in the assessment, the breath sounds will be assessed for presence or absence of breath sounds or abnormal noises.

Adequate Breathing

The patient whose breathing is adequate will exhibit the following characteristics (see Table 10-3):

- **Rate.** The respiratory rate falls within a range of 8–24 respirations per minute for an adult, 15–30 per minute for a child, and 25–50 per minute for an infant. Elderly adults have resting respiratory rates of

Key Points

A patient whose breathing rate is outside the normal range may still be breathing adequately. Assess the patient for other signs of inadequate breathing, especially the tidal volume, before intervening.

Key Terms

respiratory distress a condition in which a person is working harder than normally to breathe. Also called *breathing difficulty.*

TABLE 10-3 Signs of Adequate Breathing

- Normal respiratory rate
- Clear and equal breath sounds bilaterally
- Adequate air movement heard and felt from nose and mouth (tidal volume)
- Good chest rise and fall with each ventilation (tidal volume)

approximately 20 per minute. If the respiratory rates are too low, even though the tidal volume may be adequate, the patient will not move enough air into the lungs and alveoli to meet the oxygen demands of the cells of the body. The cells will become hypoxic and may eventually die. If the respiratory rate is too high, the fast rate may not allow the lungs to inflate fully with each breath, causing a decrease in the tidal volume with each breath. This will lead to a decrease in the volume of air getting to the alveoli for gas exchange, causing cells to become hypoxic.

Even though a range of 8–24 breaths per minute is listed as the normal range for the adult patient, it is important that you assess the whole patient when considering rates as being outside a normal range. For example, in situations where the patient is frightened or nervous, the respiratory rate will typically be elevated. This does not automatically mean that the patient's breathing status is inadequate. Assess the patient for other signs of inadequate breathing, especially low or poor tidal volume, before intervening. As an example, you arrive on the scene and find a 22-year-old patient who just crashed his new car. He is alert and visibly upset. He is breathing at a rate of 28 times per minute. His speech is clear and appropriate, and he is completely oriented. He displays no other evidence of inadequate breathing. You would not decide to ventilate this patient based on the respiratory rate, even though it is outside the normal range. It is important that you consider the respiratory rates in relation to the whole patient. Typically, if the adult is breathing greater than 40 times per minute, the rate is so fast that the tidal volume will fall and the patient will need to be ventilated. Again, look for signs of inadequate tidal volume in the patient and do not ventilate purely based on the excessive rate.

- **Rhythm.** The pattern is regular. Each breath is of about the same volume and comes at a regular interval. However, it is normal for a patient to sigh, which alters the pattern and makes it slightly irregular.
- **Quality.** The breath sounds are equal and full bilaterally, indicating good expansion of each lung. The chest rises and falls adequately and equally with each breath. No excessive accessory muscle use is seen with inhalation and exhalation. It is normal for infants and children to use the abdominal muscles more than adults do in breathing; therefore, expect greater movement of the abdomen with these patients.
- **Depth (tidal volume).** The chest will rise fully with each inhalation. The volume of air felt and heard by placing your ear next to the patient's mouth and nose will be full and adequate with each breath.

A patient who is breathing adequately may, nevertheless, be in respiratory distress. **Respiratory distress** is a condition where the patient is working harder to breathe. The difficulty breathing may be from the patient working harder to move air into the lungs, out of the lungs, or both. The key to respiratory distress is that, even though the patient is working harder to breathe, the respiratory rate and tidal volume are still adequate. Because both are adequate, the patient does not need to be ventilated; however, he does need supplemental oxygen. Keep in mind that if, at any time, either the respiratory rate or tidal volume becomes inadequate, the patient needs to be ventilated.

ASSESSMENT Tips

For the patient to have adequate breathing he must have both an adequate tidal volume and an adequate respiratory rate. ■

Inadequate Breathing

Inadequate breathing leads to both inadequate oxygen exchange at the level of the alveoli and inadequate delivery of oxygen to the cells. It also causes inadequate elimination of carbon dioxide from the body. If the breathing remains inadequate, the cells become hypoxic and begin to die. The brain, heart, and liver are the organs most sensitive to hypoxia. The brain will begin to die in about 4 to 6 minutes without an adequate oxygen supply.

Key Terms

respiratory failure insufficient respiratory rate and/or tidal volume.

respiratory arrest complete stoppage of breathing. Also called *apnea.*

Key Terms

tachypnea a breathing rate that is faster than the normal rate.

bradypnea a breathing rate that is slower than the normal rate.

Inadequate breathing may be categorized as respiratory failure or respiratory arrest. **Respiratory failure** occurs when the respiratory rate and/or tidal volume (amount of air breathed in and out) is insufficient. This results in hypoxia to the cells and organs. **Respiratory arrest,** also called *apnea*, occurs when the patient completely stops breathing. There is no movement of air; therefore, there is no rate or tidal volume. The patient quickly becomes hypoxic. Conditions that commonly cause respiratory arrest are:

Common Causes of Respiratory Arrest

Stroke
Myocardial infarction (heart attack)
Drug overdose
Toxic inhalation (e.g., carbon monoxide poisoning)
Electrocution and lightning strike
Suffocation
Traumatic injuries to the head, spine, chest, or abdomen
Infection to the epiglottis
Airway obstruction by a foreign body

ASSESSMENT Tips

A patient who exhibits signs of respiratory failure or respiratory arrest requires immediate intervention with positive pressure ventilation. ■

A type of respiratory pattern that is completely inadequate and may be seen in witnessed cardiac arrest or in some other conditions is called agonal breathing or **agonal respirations.** Agonal respirations are gasping-type breaths. If seen in the cardiac arrest patient, they usually appear soon after the person goes into cardiac arrest. These are totally ineffective respirations. A patient with agonal respirations must be provided positive pressure ventilation. When agonal respirations are found in a patient who does not yet seem to be in cardiac arrest, immediately check the patient's pulse, since these respirations are often found early in cardiac arrest.

It is important to recognize the signs of inadequate breathing and to immediately begin positive pressure (artificial) ventilation when they are present. Some of the signs are subtle and require careful evaluation (Figure 10-24∗). If you are uncertain as to whether a patient requires breathing assistance, it is better to err on the side of safety and provide ventilation. Any time ventilation is administered, oxygen must be connected and delivered with each ventilation.

Signs of Inadequate Breathing

Figure 10-24 and Table 10-4 summarize the signs of inadequate breathing. Note how the rate, rhythm, quality, and depth differ from those of adequate breathing.

- **Rate.** The respiratory rate is either too fast or too slow—outside the normal rate ranges that were listed under "Adequate Breathing." **Tachypnea** is an excessively rapid breathing rate and may indicate inadequate oxygenation and breathing, especially in an adult. **Bradypnea** is an abnormally slow breathing rate and an ominous sign of inadequate breathing and

TABLE 10-4 Signs of Inadequate Breathing

- Abnormal work of breathing
  - retractions
  - nasal flaring
  - abdominal breathing
  - diaphoresis
- Abnormal breath sounds
  - stridor
  - wheezing
  - crackles
  - silent chest (no breath sounds heard)
  - unequal breath sounds (trauma, infection, pneumothorax)
- Reduced minute ventilation
  - decreased tidal volume
  - inadequate respiratory rate
- Inadequate chest wall movement or chest wall injury
  - paradoxical chest wall movement
  - splinting of the chest wall
  - asymmetrical chest wall movement
- Irregular respiratory pattern (head injury, stroke, metabolic derangement, toxic inhalation)
- Rapid respiratory rate without clinical improvement in the patient's condition

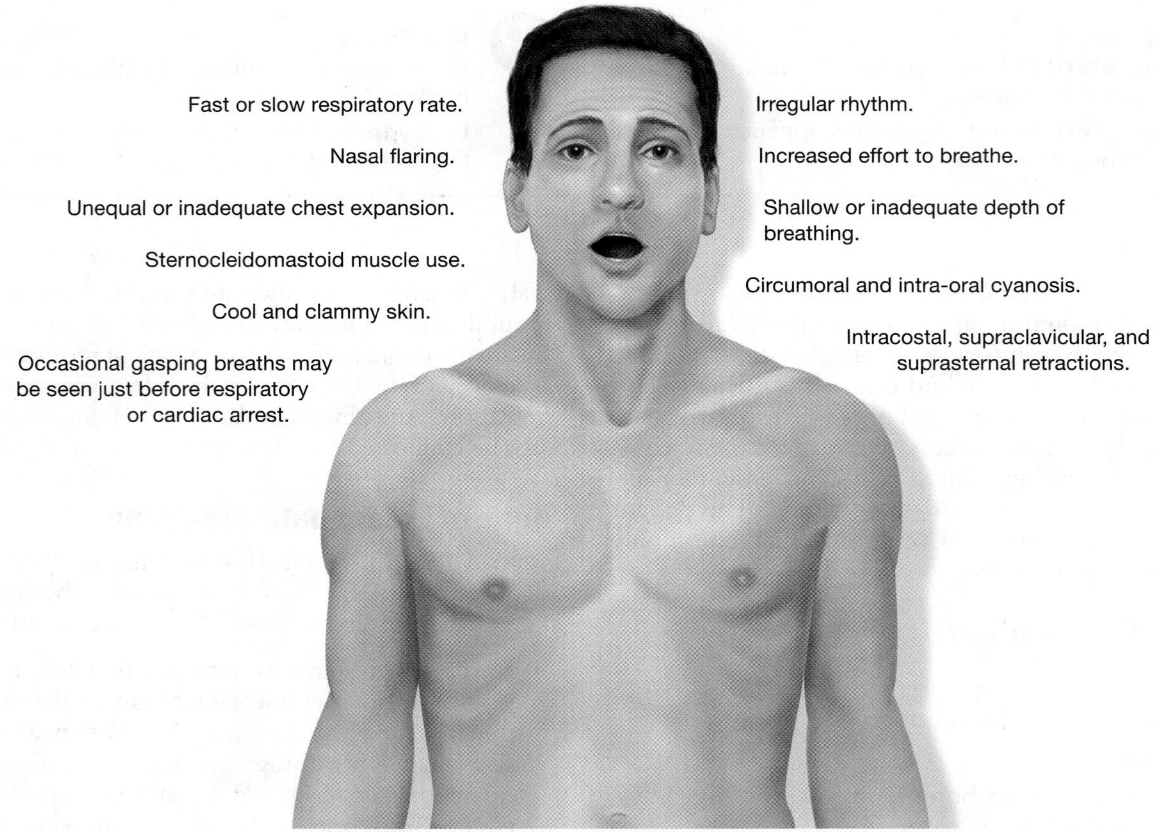
Fast or slow respiratory rate.
Nasal flaring.
Unequal or inadequate chest expansion.
Sternocleidomastoid muscle use.
Cool and clammy skin.
Occasional gasping breaths may be seen just before respiratory or cardiac arrest.
Irregular rhythm.
Increased effort to breathe.
Shallow or inadequate depth of breathing.
Circumoral and intra-oral cyanosis.
Intracostal, supraclavicular, and suprasternal retractions.

FIGURE 10-24 ✱ Signs of inadequate breathing and severe respiratory distress.

oxygenation in infants and children. Bradypnea may also be seen in adult patients, particularly those with central nervous system depression, drug, or alcohol emergencies. Again, it is important to assess the patient for other signs of inadequate breathing, such as altered mental status; however, keep in mind that rate could be the single cause of inadequate breathing.

- **Rhythm.** An irregular breathing pattern may indicate a severe brain injury or medical illness. Most irregular breathing patterns also produce an inadequate rate, depth, and quality.
- **Quality.** Breath sounds that are decreased or absent indicate an inadequate volume of air moving in and out of the lungs with each breath. If the chest wall is not rising and falling adequately with each breath, or if the sides of the chest rise and fall unequally, the breathing is inadequate.
  - Inadequate breathing can lead to excessive use of the neck muscles and intercostal muscles during breathing in an attempt to increase the size of the chest, creating greater negative pressure and drawing in more air. This can produce retractions, or depressions between the ribs, above the clavicles, around the muscles of the neck, and below the rib cage with inspiration. These retractions are seen more often in infants and children.
  - The abdomen may also move excessively in a patient breathing inadequately. Such a patient is using the abdomen to push up on the diaphragm in an effort to force air out of the lungs. Remember, however, that infants and children normally use their abdominal muscles in breathing.
  - Infants may display a "seesaw" breathing motion in which the abdomen and chest move in opposite directions during breathing.
  - The nostrils may flare during inspirations, an indication that a patient is working hard to breathe. Flaring is seen most often in children.
- **Depth.** The depth of breathing (tidal volume) is shallow and inadequate. The chest wall movement is minimal and does not rise adequately with inhalation. This is referred to as shallow breathing. Shallow breathing implies an inadequate tidal volume and requires assisted ventilation.

Not all of the signs of inadequate breathing will be present at the same time. *Any of these signs—a breathing rate that is too low or too high, a shallow depth, a poor quality, or an inadequate tidal volume—is by itself a reason to artificially ventilate a patient without delay. Waiting for additional signs to appear would only risk further compromise in the patient's condition.*

Objective 10-18
Identify patients with indications for supplemental oxygen and positive pressure ventilation.

Thinking Critically
In one week, you encounter four unresponsive patients who are breathing spontaneously. Patient #1 is taking deep full breaths at 7 per minute; patient #2 deep full breaths at 18 per minute; patient # 3 shallow breaths at 12 per minute; patient # 4 shallow breaths at 28 per minute. Which patient(s) require positive pressure ventilation? Which need oxygen by nonrebreather? What is your reasoning in each case?

Making the Decision to Ventilate or Not

A difficult decision that the EMT must make is whether the patient needs to be ventilated or if oxygen alone will be sufficient (EMT Skills 10-4). If the patient needs to be ventilated and you make the decision to simply place the patient on oxygen, it may mean the difference in whether the patient survives or dies. Recall from the previous discussion of alveolar ventilation that only the air getting to the alveoli is used in gas exchange. If a patient's tidal volume is inadequate and only oxygen is placed on the patient, the tidal volume he is breathing may only be filling the dead air space and none or very little air is actually reaching the alveoli. The oxygen on the patient will be of very little use since the oxygen will stay within the dead air space and not reach the alveoli. Thus, placing oxygen on a patient with inadequate breathing is ineffective and will not prevent deterioration of the patient. It is necessary to get the air and oxygen to the alveoli. The only way that can be done is by ensuring that both the rate and the tidal volume of each breath are adequate to move oxygenated air into the alveoli for gas exchange.

Remember that neither rate nor depth by itself is enough to ensure that the breathing is adequate. You may, for example, determine that an adult patient is breathing at a rate of 16 respirations per minute, which falls within the normal limits. If you also note, however, that his chest shows only a slight rise and fall, that you hear and feel very little air being expelled, and that his breath sounds are diminished bilaterally, the patient's breathing is inadequate. On the other hand, you might find a patient who has very good tidal volume but who is only breathing at 6 respirations per minute. Based on the rate, this patient's breathing is also inadequate.

In order to have adequate breathing, the rate of respiration and the tidal volume must *both* be within adequate limits. If *either* is inadequate, the patient must be provided with positive pressure ventilation (artificial ventilation). This requires you to pay close attention to the chest wall activity during the assessment. If the chest wall is moving minimally, and very little air movement is heard or felt, you must immediately intervene and provide positive pressure ventilation to the patient. To reemphasize: Applying oxygen alone in this patient will be totally ineffective. It is necessary for you to closely monitor the respiratory rate and the chest wall movement continuously.

The need for ventilation is determined as follows:

Adequate respiratory rate *and* an adequate tidal volume with each breath = Adequate breathing

Thus, *two* adequates, rate and tidal volume, are necessary to have adequate breathing. When *both* adequates exist, there is no need for positive pressure ventilation. Adequate volumes of air are getting into the alveoli. This patient can be placed on an oxygen mask.

Inadequate respiratory rate and an adequate tidal volume = Inadequate breathing

Even though the patient may have an adequate tidal volume with each breath, the respiratory rate is not sufficient to maintain adequate breathing. This patient needs to be ventilated to move an adequate amount of air into the alveoli for gas exchange.

Adequate respiratory rate and an inadequate tidal volume = Inadequate breathing

This patient is breathing at an adequate rate; however, he is not moving enough volume with each breath to overcome the dead air space and place adequate amounts of oxygenated air into the alveoli for gas exchange. This patient needs to be ventilated.

To sum up how to determine the need for ventilation, remember the following (Table 10-5):

- Two adequates must be present to have adequate breathing: adequate respiratory rate **and** adequate tidal volume. (No need for ventilation. Supplemental oxygen can be applied if necessary.) ***Thus, it takes two adequates to produce adequate breathing!***
- Only one inadequate needs to be present to have inadequate breathing: **either** inadequate respiratory rate **or** an inadequate tidal volume. This patient needs to be ventilated. Placing an oxygen mask on the patient will not move the necessary volume into the alveoli for gas exchange. The patient will become hypoxic and will deteriorate. ***Thus, it only takes one inadequate (rate or tidal volume) to produce inadequate breathing and the need for ventilation.***

Key Points
It only takes *one* "inadequate" (rate or tidal volume) to produce inadequate breathing and the need for ventilation. However, assess the whole patient for signs of inadequate breathing before intervening, especially if the rate is abnormal but tidal volume is normal.

Key Terms
positive pressure ventilation (PPV) method of aiding a patient whose breathing is inadequate by forcing air into his lungs.

Objective 10-19
Describe the physiological differences between spontaneous and positive pressure ventilation.

TABLE 10-5 Making a Decision: Should I Ventilate the Patient or Apply Oxygen?

Assessment: **Adequate** respiratory rate + **adequate** tidal volume
Conclusion: **Adequate** breathing
Emergency Care: Apply oxygen if necessary by nonrebreather mask

Assessment: **Inadequate** respiratory rate + adequate tidal volume
Conclusion: **Inadequate** breathing
Emergency Care: Immediately begin ventilation of the patient

Assessment: Adequate respiratory rate + **inadequate** tidal volume
Conclusion: **Inadequate** breathing
Emergency Care: Immediately begin ventilation of the patient

Techniques of Artificial Ventilation

The EMT can use several methods to artificially ventilate, or force air into, the patient who is breathing inadequately or not breathing at all. Because air is being forced into the patient's lungs, the technique is referred to as **positive pressure ventilation (PPV).** The methods for providing positive pressure ventilation vary and require different levels of skill and different types of equipment. Each method has different advantages and disadvantages; the method you select should be based on the characteristics of the situation and the resources available.

Differences Between Normal Spontaneous Ventilation and Positive Pressure Ventilation

There are significant physiological differences in the patient who is breathing spontaneously (on his own) and one who is receiving positive pressure ventilation. These differences may affect other body systems or require other management techniques:

- **Air movement.** In normal spontaneous ventilation, the negative pressure created by increasing the size of the thorax draws air into the lungs. Positive pressure ventilation is just that—you are delivering ventilation through positive pressure. You are forcing air into the lungs regardless of the pressure changes in the thorax. If a patient has a condition or injury that does not allow the thorax to expand adequately, such as a flail segment, enough negative pressure is not generated to draw a sufficient amount of air into the lungs. Positive pressure ventilation does not rely on negative pressure; thus, it becomes the treatment of choice to force air into the lungs and the alveoli.
- **Airway wall pressure.** Airway wall pressure is not affected during normal ventilation. However, during positive pressure ventilation the airway walls are pushed outward creating a larger space. This requires higher volumes to fill the larger space and ventilate the patient effectively.
- **Esophageal opening pressure.** The esophagus is a soft, flexible structure. During normal ventilation, the esophagus remains collapsed and no air moves into it. Positive pressure ventilation can overcome the esophageal opening pressure, allowing air to enter the esophagus and filling the stomach with air during ventilation. This leads to gastric distention and the possibility of regurgitation, which increases the risk of compromising the airway and aspiration of gastric contents. Cricoid pressure is used during positive pressure ventilation to reduce the incidence of air passage into the stomach and regurgitation of vomitus. Cricoid pressure will be discussed later in the chapter.
- **Cardiac output.** Normal spontaneous ventilation does not adversely affect the cardiac output or blood pressure. Actually, the negative pressure generated in the thorax prior to inhalation acts like a vacuum and sucks the venous blood into the inferior vena cava from the body below the level of the diaphragm. This provides an adequate amount of venous blood volume to the right side of the heart. Preload is dependent on the venous volume and amount of blood ejected from the right ventricle. An adequate preload contributes to an adequate stroke volume, cardiac output, and blood pressure. This is known as the cardiothoracic pump effect. During positive pressure ventilation, the thorax becomes positive during the inhalation phase as air is forced into the lungs. With the loss of the negative pressure generated during

Key Points
There is a high risk of coming into contact with secretions, blood, or vomitus while ventilating a patient, so be sure to take Standard Precautions.

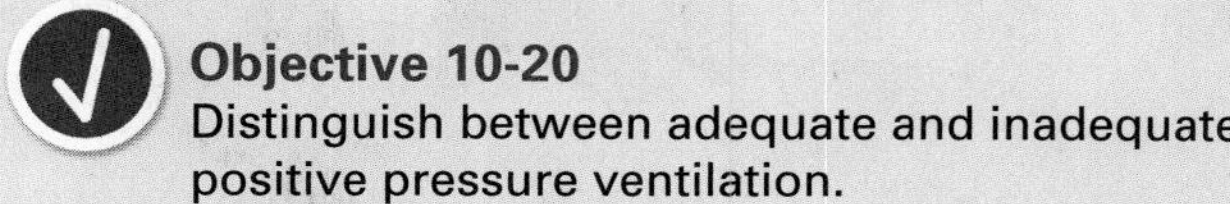

Objective 10-20
Distinguish between adequate and inadequate positive pressure ventilation.

normal ventilation, the vacuum effect is diminished and the venous return decreases. This then decreases the preload, which in turn reduces the stroke volume, cardiac output, blood pressure, and perfusion. In a patient with no pulse who is in cardiac arrest or has a condition where air is already trapped in the lungs, creating a more positive environment, such as with a severe asthma attack or tension pneumothorax, this effect can be significant and lead to poor perfusion of the brain, heart, and body.

Basic Considerations

The methods that the EMT can use to artificially ventilate the patient are as follows (Figure 10-25*):

Methods of Artificial Ventilation

- Mouth to mask
- Bag-valve mask (BVM) operated by two people
- Flow-restricted, oxygen-powered ventilation device (manually triggered ventilation device)
- Bag-valve mask (BVM) operated by one person

There are three major considerations when using a device for artificial ventilation:

1. You must be able to maintain a good mask seal and not allow excessive air leakage from between the mask and the patient's face. An inadequate mask seal will lead to an insufficient volume of air being delivered.
2. The device must be able to deliver an adequate volume of air to sufficiently inflate the lungs.
3. There must be a connection to allow for simultaneous oxygen delivery while artificially ventilating.

Standard Precautions

As with any technique in which there is a risk of coming in contact with body fluids, it is necessary to take Standard Precautions when performing artificial ventilation. The risks of coming in contact with secretions, blood, or vomitus while ventilating are relatively high; therefore, the EMT must, at minimum, use gloves and eyewear. If large amounts of blood or secretions are present, use a face mask. If tuberculosis is suspected, use a HEPA or N-95 respirator during the entire patient contact.

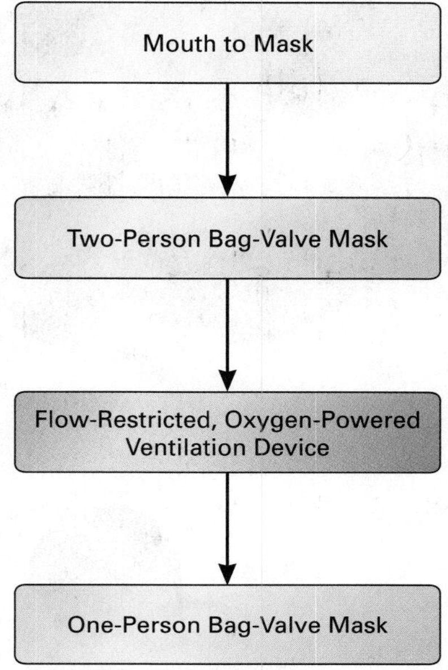

FIGURE 10-25 * Methods of ventilation in a patient.

Adequate Ventilation

When performing artificial ventilation, regardless of the device being used, it is necessary to monitor the patient continuously to ensure that the ventilation is adequate. Inadequate ventilation may occur because of problems with the patient's upper or lower airway or because of improper use of a ventilation device. You must be completely familiar with any device you use to ventilate a patient. Keep in mind that ventilation must not be interrupted for greater than 30 seconds.

Indications that the patient is being adequately ventilated (Figure 10-26a*) include the following:

Indications of Adequate Ventilation

- *The rate of ventilation is sufficient.* Infants and children must be ventilated at a rate of 12–20 times per minute, once every 3 seconds (20 times per minute) to 5 seconds (12 times per minute) *if a pulse is present.* The rate for adults *with a pulse* is 10–12 times per minute, once every 6 seconds (10 times per minute) or once every 5 seconds (12 times per minute). Each ventilation should be delivered over 1 second. If the patient *has no pulse,* the ventilations are performed in conjunction with chest compressions at a ratio of 30 compressions to 2 ventilations in adults, children, and infants (excluding newborns).

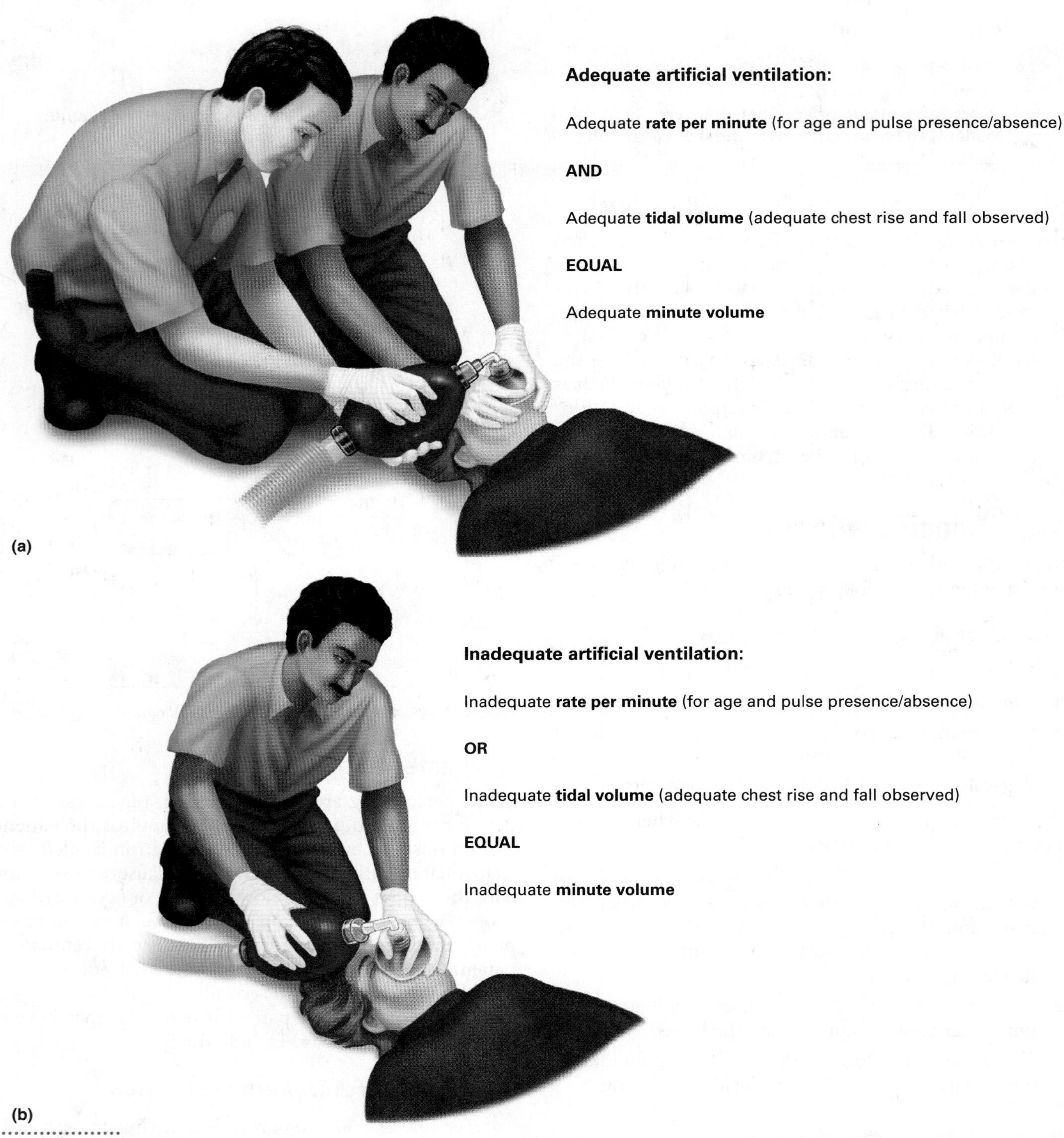

Adequate artificial ventilation:
Adequate rate per minute (for age and pulse presence/absence)
AND
Adequate tidal volume (adequate chest rise and fall observed)
EQUAL
Adequate minute volume
(a)
Inadequate artificial ventilation:
Inadequate rate per minute (for age and pulse presence/absence)
OR
Inadequate tidal volume (adequate chest rise and fall observed)
EQUAL
Inadequate minute volume
(b)

FIGURE 10-26 ✱ **(a)** Adequate artificial ventilation with good alveolar ventilation. **(b)** Inadequate artificial ventilation with poor alveolar ventilation.

The rate of ventilation for a newborn infant *with a pulse* is 40–60 ventilations per minute. In the newborn *with no pulse,* the ratio of chest compressions to ventilations is 3:1 or 90 compressions to 30 ventilations.

- *The tidal volume must be consistent; it must also be sufficient to cause the chest to rise during each ventilation.* Inspect the chest with each ventilation to ensure adequate rise.
- *The patient's heart rate returns to normal.* (Other underlying conditions may prevent return of a normal heart rate even when ventilations are adequately performed.)
- *Color improves.* The pale, gray, or cyanotic color begins to lessen and disappear.

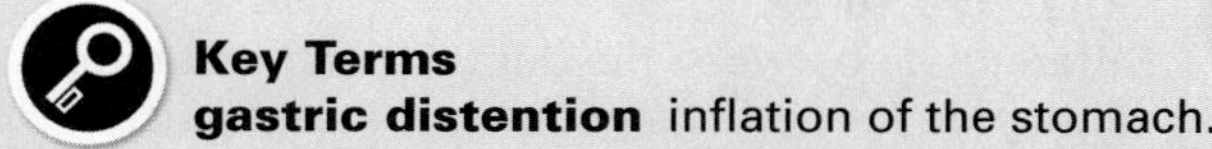

Key Terms
gastric distention inflation of the stomach.

Key Terms
cricoid pressure pressure applied to the cricoid cartilage to compress the esophagus. Also called *Sellick maneuver.*

Inadequate Ventilation

Indications of inadequate artificial ventilation (Figure 10-26b✱) include the following:

Indications of Inadequate Ventilation

- *The ventilation rate is too fast or too slow.* Ventilating a patient too rapidly does not allow for adequate exhalation and can also cause **gastric distention.** Too slow a rate of ventilation will not provide an adequate amount of oxygen. Other dangers associated with overventilating patients will be discussed later in the chapter.
- *The chest does not rise and fall with artificial ventilation.* This is an indication that the volume being delivered is not adequate. This may be due to a failure to use the ventilation device properly or to an airway obstruction. A common cause of ineffective ventilation is a poor mask seal that allows a portion of the ventilation to escape. If the patient's chest does not fall, it may be a sign that the airway is not properly opened or that the ventilation device or the upper or lower airway is obstructed, preventing adequate exhalation.
- *The heart rate does not return to normal with artificial ventilation.* (Remember, however, to consider other sources of heart rate disturbance, such as blood loss, anxiety, or heart problems.)
- *Color does not improve.* The skin color remains extremely pale, cyanotic, or gray.

ASSESSMENT Tips

An already rapid heart rate that continues to increase may be an indication of worsening hypoxia from inadequate ventilation. Conversely, a rapid heart rate that begins to decrease may indicate an improvement in the oxygenation and ventilation status; however, if the decrease in rate continues to bradycardia, it may be an indication of inadequate ventilation and oxygenation and worsening hypoxia. ■

Cricoid Pressure

Cricoid pressure (*Sellick maneuver*) (Figure 10-27a and 10-27b✱) was once thought to reduce complications associated with positive pressure ventilation when the unresponsive patient's airway is not protected by an advanced airway device. The technique was intended to reduce the incidence of gastric inflation, regurgitation, and aspiration of gastric contents.

According to the American Heart Association guidelines of 2010, cricoid pressure is not recommended for routine use but can be used to facilitate insertion of an endotracheal tube in an adult. In the pediatric patient, cricoid pressure can be considered only if an extra EMT is available to apply the pressure without compromising the airway or effective ventilation and to guard against collapse of the trachea from excessive pressure.

Cricothyroid membrane
Thyroid cartilage
Trachea
Esophagus
Cricoid cartilage occluding esophagus
(a)

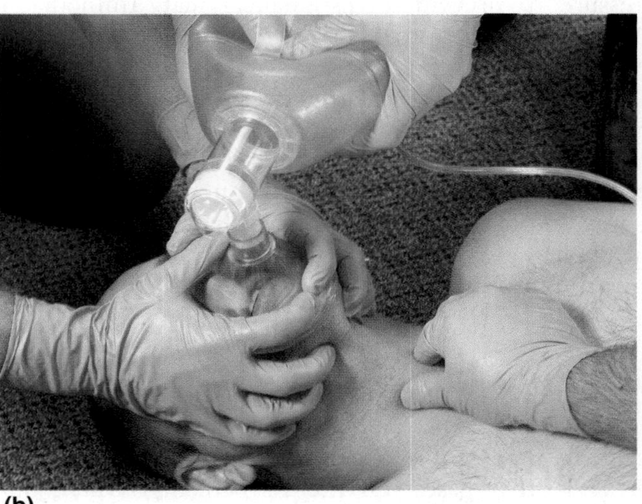
(b)

FIGURE 10-27 ✱ **(a)** and **(b)** Cricoid pressure.

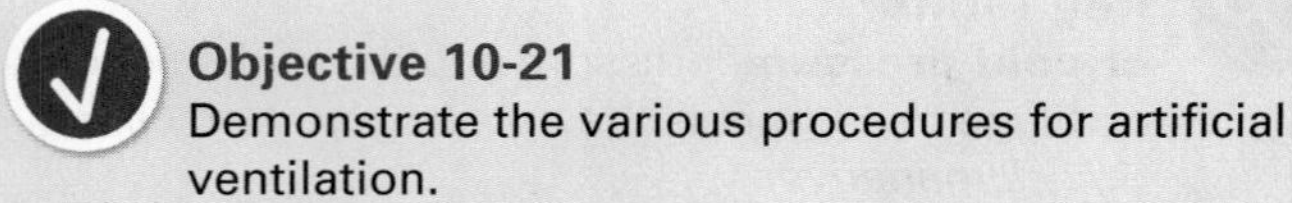
Objective 10-21
Demonstrate the various procedures for artificial ventilation.

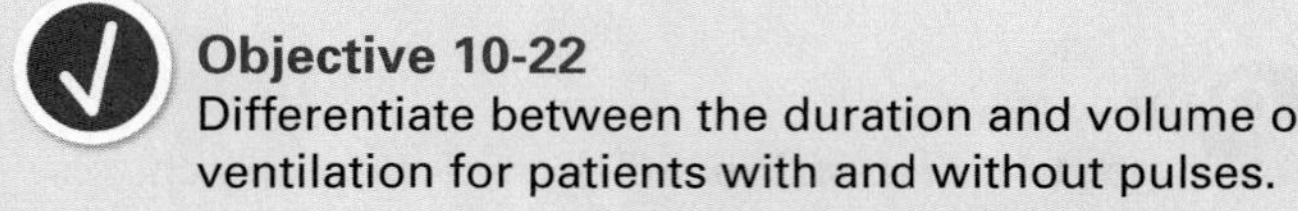
Objective 10-22
Differentiate between the duration and volume of ventilation for patients with and without pulses.

Cricoid pressure may facilitate visualization of the glottic opening, the laryngeal opening that leads to the trachea, where an endotracheal tube is inserted during intubation (laryngoscopy). The backward pressure displaces the larynx posteriorly, allowing the intubator a better view of the opening. A paramedic or other advanced practitioner may ask you to apply cricoid pressure during laryngoscopy. Once the tube is in place, the cricoid pressure is released.

The technique to perform cricoid pressure is:

1. Locate the thyroid cartilage (Adam's apple) by sliding index and middle fingers slowly down from the chin until you feel an obvious cartilage prominence.
2. Continue downward until you feel the base of the thyroid cartilage and, below it, a small, soft midline indentation, the cricothyroid membrane. Immediately below that membrane is the bulky cricoid cartilage.
3. Place your index finger on one side of the cricoid cartilage, your thumb on the other side, and apply firm backward pressure.

The cricoid cartilage is the only complete cartilaginous ring (review Figure 10-2). When forced backward, it may collapse the esophagus behind it against the cervical vertebrae, preventing air from traveling down to inflate the stomach and stomach contents from moving up. In this way, cricoid pressure protects the airway from regurgitation and consequent aspiration of stomach contents and also protects against gastric inflation. If the patient starts to regurgitate, release the cricoid pressure to prevent an esophageal tear. Immediately turn the patient onto his side, if possible, and suction the airway until clear.

Slow, sustained ventilation over 1 second with a controlled tidal volume is the best method to prevent gastric inflation. Also, proper positioning of the airway with the head-tilt, chin-lift maneuver will reduce resistance in the airway and allow more of the ventilation to flow down the trachea and into the lungs instead of down the esophagus and into the stomach.

Mouth-to-Mouth Ventilation

The air we breathe contains approximately 21 percent oxygen, 78 percent nitrogen, and 1 percent carbon dioxide and other gases. Of the 21 percent oxygen, only 5 percent is used by the body; the remaining 16 percent is exhaled. Dead air space, volume that was not used in gas exchange, makes the greatest contribution to maintaining a high oxygen content in the exhaled air. Because the exhaled breath contains about 16 percent oxygen, a patient can be oxygenated with the rescuer's exhaled breath. This is the principle behind mouth-to-mouth ventilation taught in many first-aid and CPR courses.

However, the risk of contracting infectious diseases makes this technique too dangerous for regular use by EMTs.

Mouth-to-Mouth and Mouth-to-Nose Technique

The EMT forms a seal with his mouth around the patient's mouth or nose and uses his exhaled air to ventilate. The nose is pinched during mouth-to-mouth ventilation, and the mouth is closed during mouth-to-nose ventilation. This technique provides adequate volumes of air for ventilating a patient. Its major limitations are the inability to deliver high concentrations of oxygen while ventilating and the risk posed to the EMT by contact with the patient's body fluids. To reduce risks, a barrier device must be used.

Use mouth-to-nose ventilation when the patient's mouth cannot be opened, when severe soft tissue or bone injury has occurred to the mouth or around it, in infants, or when you cannot achieve a tight mouth-to-mouth seal.

Mouth-to-Mask and Bag-Valve Ventilation: General Considerations

The next sections describe mouth-to-mask and bag-valve-mask ventilation. As you read about these techniques, keep in mind the general considerations regarding ventilation volumes, duration of ventilation, and gastric inflation.

Ventilation Volumes and Duration of Ventilation

When ventilating a patient by mouth-to-mask or bag-valve-mask technique, it is necessary to adjust the volume and rate of ventilation based on whether the patient has a pulse (Table 10-6). If the patient has a pulse (perfusing rhythm), the amount of air volume (tidal volume) delivered to the patient should be approximately 10 mL/kg (700–1,000 mL), enough to make the chest rise adequately and effectively with each ventilation. The ventilation rate in the adult patient *with a pulse* is 10–12 breaths

TABLE 10-6 Ventilation Rates

Ventilation Rates for the Patient with a Pulse

Patient	Age	Rate of Ventilation	Frequency of Ventilation
Adult	Adolescent and older	10–12 ventilations per minute	One ventilation every 5–6 seconds
Child	1 year of age to adolescent	12–20 ventilations per minute	One ventilation every 3–5 seconds
Infant	Up to 1 year of age	12–20 ventilations per minute	One ventilation every 3–5 seconds
Newborn	Birth to 30 days	40–60 ventilations per minute	One ventilation every 1–1.5 seconds

Ventilation Rates for the Patient Without a Pulse

Patient	Age	Ratio of Compression to Ventilation (one-person CPR)	Ratio of Compression to Ventilation (two-person CPR)
Adult	Adolescent and older	30 compressions to 2 ventilations	30 compressions to 2 ventilations
Child	1 year of age to adolescent	30 compressions to 2 ventilations	15 compressions to 2 ventilations
Infant	Up to 1 year of age	30 compressions to 2 ventilations	15 compressions to 2 ventilations
Newborn	Birth to 30 days	3 compressions to 1 ventilation	3 compressions to 1 ventilation

Ventilation Rates for the Patient Without a Pulse with an Advanced Airway in Place

Patient	Age	Compression Rate	Ventilation Rate	Ventilation Frequency
Adult	Adolescent and older	100 per minute with no pause for ventilation	8–10 per minute	One ventilation every 6–7.5 seconds
Child	1 year of age to adolescent	100 per minute with no pause for ventilation	8–10 per minute	One ventilation every 6–7.5 seconds
Infant	Up to 1 year of age	100 per minute with no pause for ventilation	8–10 per minute	One ventilation every 6–7.5 seconds
Neonate	Birth to 30 days	3 compressions to 1 ventilation	30 per minute	One ventilation after every third compression

per minute (one breath every 6 to 5 seconds, respectively). The pediatric patient, from 1 year of age to 12–14 years of age (adolescent), is ventilated at 12–20 times per minute (5 to 3 seconds, respectively) *when a pulse is present.* The infant who is less than 1 year of age is ventilated at 12–20 times per minute (5 to 3 seconds, respectively) *when a pulse is present.* In every patient, the ventilation is delivered over a 1-second period. The rate of ventilation for a newborn infant *with a pulse* is 40–60 ventilations per minute.

If the patient is pulseless (no perfusing rhythm), the ventilation rates are reduced and are performed in conjunction with chest compressions. The compression-to-ventilation ratio in the adult patient for both one- and two-person CPR is 30 compressions to 2 ventilations. For the infant and child, when one-person CPR is performed, the ratio remains at 30 compressions to 2 ventilations; however, in the infant and child, the ratio changes to 15 compressions to 2 ventilations when two-person CPR is performed. In the newborn *with no pulse,* the ventilation rate is approximately 30 per minute being performed in conjunction with chest compressions. This is done at a ratio of 3 compressions to 1 ventilation. Each ventilation in the pulseless patient, regardless of age, should be delivered over 1 second. The volume of air delivered should be enough to make the chest visibly rise with each ventilation.

At any time a patient is being ventilated, an airway adjunct must be inserted to facilitate maintenance of the airway and to ensure delivery of good ventilation volumes. Also, supplemental oxygen must be connected to the ventilation device and delivered at the highest possible concentration.

Ventilating a Pulseless Patient with an Advanced Airway in Place If the patient has an advanced airway in place, such as an endotracheal tube, esophageal–tracheal

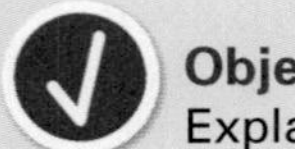

Objective 10-23
Explain the significance of avoiding gastric inflation when administering positive pressure ventilation.

Combitube, or Laryngeal Mask Airway (LMA), the ventilation in the patient *without* a pulse is reduced to 8–10 ventilations per minute. One EMT provides continuous chest compressions at a rate of 100 compressions per minute *without* pausing for any ventilation. The ventilations should be delivered at a rate of 8–10 per minute, which is every 7.5 to 6 seconds, respectively. It is extremely important *not* to overventilate the patient by providing either too fast a rate or too great a volume. Even though you may assume that more ventilation is better than less, overventilating may cause the blood flow to the brain and heart to be reduced.

Gastric Inflation

Decreasing the ventilation volume is aimed at reducing the incidence of gastric distention and the potential regurgitation and aspiration that can occur during mouth-to-mask or bag-valve-mask ventilation. The smaller tidal volume reduces airway pressure and avoids causing the lower sphincter in the esophagus to open.

When higher tidal volumes are used, the increased air pressure can force the esophageal sphincter to open, allowing the stomach to become inflated with air and causing gastric inflation. When this happens, several complications may occur. The air-filled stomach may cause stomach contents to enter the esophagus, leading to regurgitation and possibly aspiration. Aspiration of gastric contents may interfere with gas exchange and cause pneumonia. Also, an inflated stomach places pressure on the diaphragm, which can elevate the diaphragm and restrict its movement. This can lead to difficult and ineffective ventilation, particularly in children.

When supplemental oxygen is connected, adequate oxygen saturation can be maintained with smaller tidal volumes. Supplemental oxygen should be connected to the pocket mask or BVM at a liter flow of 15 lpm as early as possible when ventilating a patient.

Mouth-to-Mask Ventilation

The mouth-to-mask technique, like the mouth-to-mouth or mouth-to-nose technique, uses the exhaled breath of the EMT to ventilate the patient. But with this technique, a plastic pocket mask is used to form a seal around the patient's nose and mouth (Figure 10-28∗). The EMT then blows into a port at the top of the mask to deliver the ventilation.

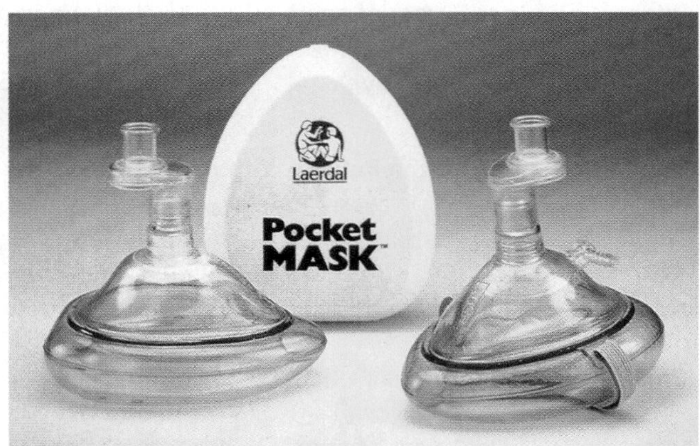

FIGURE 10-28 ∗ Pocket mask with one-way valve and oxygen connection. (© Laerdal Medical Corporation)

Mouth-to-mask ventilation is the preferred method to use when performing artificial ventilation because of the following advantages:

- One EMT can ventilate using the two-handed mask seal technique, achieving a better mask seal.
- The mask eliminates direct contact with the patient's nose, mouth, and secretions.
- Use of a one-way valve at the ventilation port prevents exposure to the patient's exhaled air.
- The method can provide adequate tidal volumes and possibly greater tidal volumes than bag-valve-mask ventilation.
- Supplemental oxygen can be administered through the oxygen inlet that most pocket masks have in addition to the ventilation port.

Disadvantages of mouth-to-mask include the following:

- The mask is perceived by some EMTs as having an increased risk of infection.
- The EMT providing the ventilation may fatigue after a period of time.
- The device doesn't allow for the highest possible concentration of oxygen to be delivered with each ventilation.

The mask used to ventilate the patient must have the following characteristics:

- It should be of a transparent material to permit the detection of vomitus, secretions, blood, or other substances in the patient's mouth.

- It must be able to fit tightly on the patient's face and form a good seal.
- It must have an oxygen inlet to allow for high-concentration oxygen delivery at 15 liters per minute (lpm).
- It should be available in one average adult size and additional sizes for infants and children.
- It must have or be connectable to a one-way valve at the ventilation port.

Mouth-to-Mask Technique—No Suspected Spine Injury

Mouth-to-mask ventilation is illustrated in Figure 10-29*. The procedure is described as follows:

1. Connect a one-way valve to the ventilation port of the mask and connect tubing that is attached to an oxygen supply to the oxygen inlet. Set the oxygen flow for 15 lpm.
2. Position yourself, if possible, at the top of the patient's head. This is referred to as a *cephalic technique*. It is easier to monitor the patient's chest rise and fall in this position. However, if you are performing one-person CPR, it is better to position yourself to one side of the patient's head. This is called a *lateral technique*. It is the preferred technique when performing one-person CPR because it allows easier movement from the chest to the airway to provide both chest compressions and ventilations.
3. Place the mask on the patient's face. The narrow top portion of the mask should be seated on the bridge of the nose, and the broader portion should be seated in the cleft above the chin. Hold the mask with a "C-E" technique. Place your thumbs on the top and lateral edges of the mask, the thumb sides of your palms along the sides of the mask, and your index fingers over the bottom of the mask over the cleft above the chin. In this way, your thumbs and index fingers form "Cs" around the mask chimney. With your middle, ring, and little fingers, grasp under the mandible just in front of the earlobes, forming "Es" with those fingers. Pull upward on these fingers, using the "Es" to lift the mandible upward and lift the chin. Be careful to keep the patient's mouth open if no oropharyngeal or nasopharyngeal airway is in place. While lifting the mandible upward, tilt the head backward, performing a head tilt while achieving a chin lift by lifting the mandible to the mask. Squeeze the mask tightly to achieve an airtight seal between the mask and the patient's face.
4. Place your mouth around the one-way valve and blow into the ventilation port of the mask. Give a breath over a 1-second period. When the chest rises adequately, stop the ventilation to allow for exhalation. If you cannot ventilate, or if the chest does not rise adequately, reposition the patient's head and try again. Improper head position is the most common cause of difficulty with ventilation. If the second try also fails, assume the airway is blocked by a foreign object and follow the guidelines for removing a foreign body airway obstruction found in Appendix 1.

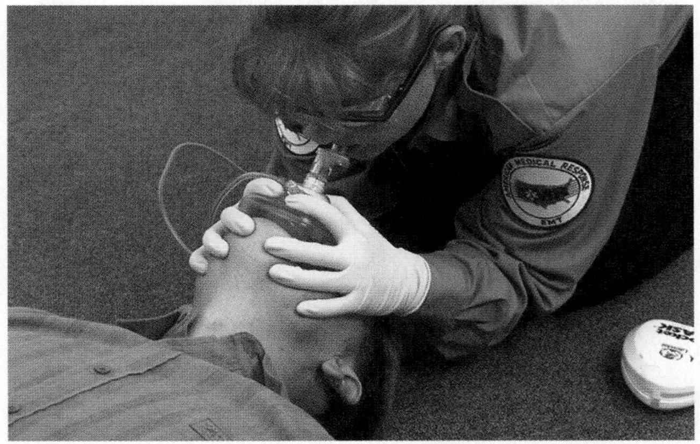

FIGURE 10-29 * Mouth-to-mask ventilation. The mask should be connected to oxygen at a flow of 15 liters per minute (lpm).

Mouth-to-Mask Technique—Suspected Spine Injury

If the patient has a suspected spine injury, you will ventilate the patient with the mouth-to-mask technique, taking care not to manipulate the head and neck during the procedure. Mouth-to-mask ventilation in the patient with a suspected spine injury would be performed as follows:

1. Connect a one-way valve to the ventilation port of the mask and connect tubing that is attached to an oxygen supply to the oxygen inlet. Set the oxygen flow for 15 lpm.
2. Position yourself, if possible, at the top of the patient's head or at the side.
3. Place the mask on the patient's face. The narrow top portion of the mask should be seated on the bridge of the nose, and the broader portion should be seated in the cleft above the chin. Hold the mask with a "C-E" technique. With your middle, ring, and little fingers, grasp under the angle of the mandible just in front of the earlobes. Pull upward on the angle of the jaw to lift the mandible upward and to lift the chin forward *without* tilting the head backward and while keeping the head and neck in a neutral position (jaw-thrust maneuver). Squeeze the mask tightly to achieve an airtight seal between the mask and the patient's face.
4. Deliver the ventilation as you would in the non-spine-injured patient.

If the patient is in cardiac arrest (pulseless) and an open airway cannot be established or the patient cannot be adequately ventilated by using the jaw-thrust maneuver, it may be necessary to perform a head-tilt, chin-lift maneuver to gain an adequate airway and ventilation of the patient. This can be done by continuing to slightly lift the patient's head backward until the airway is achieved. As soon as the airway is achieved, stop, maintain spinal stabilization, and begin to ventilate the patient. It may be necessary to reposition the airway several times while chest compressions are being performed.

Ineffective Ventilation

If the ventilations are ineffective and are not producing adequate chest rise and fall, it is necessary to immediately identify and correct the problem. Ineffective ventilation may be due to several possible causes. If the chest does not rise adequately during ventilation with any ventilation device, perform the following sequence to identify and correct possible causes of the problem:

1. *Reposition the head and neck* to ensure the airway is open. In a suspected spine injury, reposition the jaw thrust while keeping the head in a neutral position. If the jaw thrust is ineffective in opening or maintaining an airway, use the head-tilt, chin-lift maneuver to ventilate the patient, even if the potential for a spine injury exists. Opening the airway and providing adequate ventilation is a priority in patients in cardiac arrest and takes precedence over other procedures, even with suspected spine injury.
2. *Change from a head-tilt, chin-lift to a jaw-thrust maneuver or from a jaw-thrust to a head-tilt, chin-lift maneuver if the patient is in cardiac arrest.*
3. *Readjust the face mask* and make sure there are no seal leaks between the face and the mask.
4. *Administer a greater tidal volume.* The tidal volume may be insufficient to ventilate the patient adequately, especially in patients with a history of airway and lung disease, or if the patient's condition is related to an airway problem (such as an acute asthma attack or allergic reaction), chest injury (such as a collapsed lung), or lung condition (such as pneumonia).
5. *Insert an oropharyngeal or nasopharyngeal airway* to assist in maintaining an open airway.

ASSESSMENT Tips

When using a jaw-thrust maneuver in a patient with suspected spinal injury, if you are unable to ventilate the patient after several attempts, you can slightly extend the head until a decrease in airflow resistance is felt and the chest rises adequately with each ventilation. ■

Bag-Valve-Mask Ventilation

A **bag-valve-mask (BVM) device** (Figures 10-30a and 10-30b*) is a manual resuscitator used to provide positive pressure ventilation. The bag-valve mask consists of a self-inflating bag, a one-way nonrebreather valve, a face mask, an intake/oxygen reservoir valve, and an oxygen reservoir. Most adult-sized BVM devices have a volume of approximately 1,600 milliliters. It is important to use a bag that can deliver between 1 and 2 liters in the adult. Bag-valve-mask devices used for ventilation of full-term newborns, infants, and children should have a minimum volume of 450–500 mL. In children 8 years of age or greater, use an adult BVM device.

Regardless of the size of the BVM, be sure to use only enough volume to cause the chest to rise. When used without an oxygen source, the device will only deliver

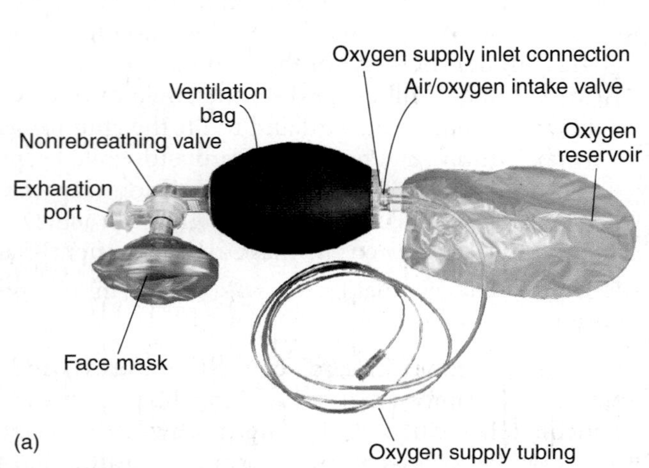

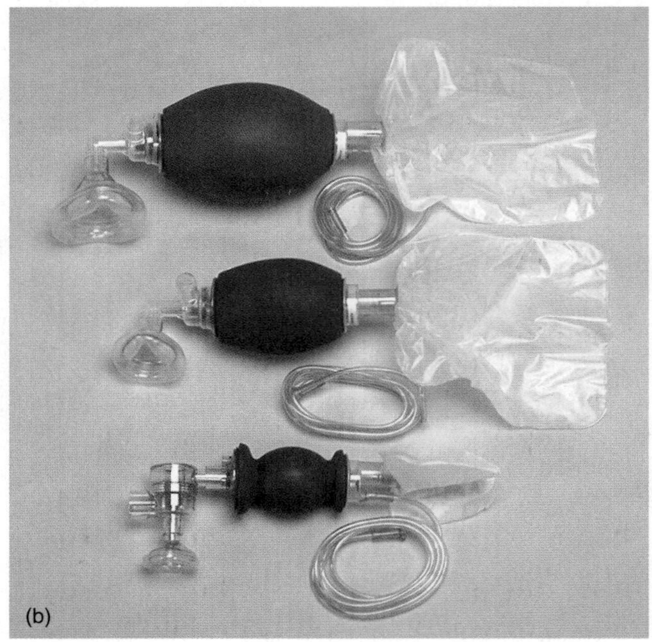

FIGURE 10-30 * **(a)** Bag-valve-mask unit with oxygen bag reservoir. Tubing-type reservoirs are also available. **(b)** Adult, child, and infant bag-valve-mask units.

Key Points
Mouth-to-mask ventilation can provide more consistent tidal volumes than are likely with one-person bag-valve-mask ventilation.

Key Points
Two-person bag-valve-mask ventilation provides a better mask seal and greater ventilation volumes and is the preferred method when using a BVM.

21 percent oxygen, the amount found in room air. By adding oxygen and a reservoir, you can deliver close to 100 percent oxygen to the patient, a major advantage of using the device.

The principal advantages of the BVM device over mouth-to-mask ventilation are its convenience for the EMT and its ability to deliver enriched oxygen mixtures. Also, if two EMTs are performing the procedure, one EMT achieves and maintains the mask seal with two hands, while the second EMT squeezes the bag to deliver the ventilation. However, the bag-valve mask may not consistently generate the tidal volumes that are possible with mouth-to-mask ventilation during one-EMT bag-valve-mask use. Thus, a disadvantage of the BVM device is the need for two EMTs to perform a two-handed mask seal to typically achieve the best ventilation results.

The BVM device is harder to use than it looks and is fatiguing to the operator when performing a one-person technique. The EMT must simultaneously provide a tight mask seal, maintain an open airway by properly positioning the patient's head and chin, and squeeze the bag to deliver the ventilation. It takes frequent practice to maintain the skills needed to deliver adequate ventilation with the device. Because of the difficulty in working the bag-valve mask, use of the device by two persons is highly recommended but not always possible. A single-operator mask such as the pocket mask has few of these disadvantages, takes less skill and maintenance, and is much easier to use by all practitioners, experienced or inexperienced.

A bag-valve mask should have these features:

- A self-refilling bag that is disposable or easy to clean and sterilize.
- A nonjamming valve system that allows a maximum oxygen inlet flow of 30 lpm.
- Either no pop-off valve or a pop-off valve that can be manually disabled. A pop-off valve that is not disabled may lead to inadequate ventilation.
- Standard 15/22 couplings for masks, endotracheal tubes, tracheostomy tubes, laryngeal mask airways, and Combitubes.
- An oxygen inlet and a reservoir that can be connected with an oxygen source to deliver high concentrations of oxygen during ventilation. An oxygen reservoir should be used when ventilating all patients.
- A true nonrebreather valve that vents the patient's exhalations and does not allow him to rebreathe any exhaled gas and cannot be obstructed by foreign material.
- Adaptability to all environmental conditions and temperature extremes.
- A variety of infant-, child-, and adult-sized masks. A properly sized mask will fit snugly over the bridge of the nose and into the cleft above the chin.
- Transparent masks to permit detection of vomitus, blood, or secretions during ventilation.

Note that oropharyngeal or nasopharyngeal airway adjuncts can help in maintaining an open airway and should be used any time the BVM device is used.

Bag-Valve-Mask Technique—No Suspected Spine Injury

A bag-valve-mask device can be used by one or two EMTs. For reasons already cited, use of the device by two EMTs is preferred. One EMT holds a tight mask seal with both hands while the second EMT uses both hands to squeeze the bag to deliver the full volume of oxygenated air inside it (Figure 10-31*). This technique is considerably more effective than one-person use of the device and should always be employed unless the number of personnel or the circumstances of the run, such as an extremely cramped working area, do not allow it.

Two-Person BVM Technique Procedures for two-person use of the bag-valve mask are as follows:

1. If possible, position yourself at the top of the patient's head. If you do not suspect a spinal injury, open the airway using the head-tilt, chin-lift maneuver. Raise the patient's head slightly with a towel or

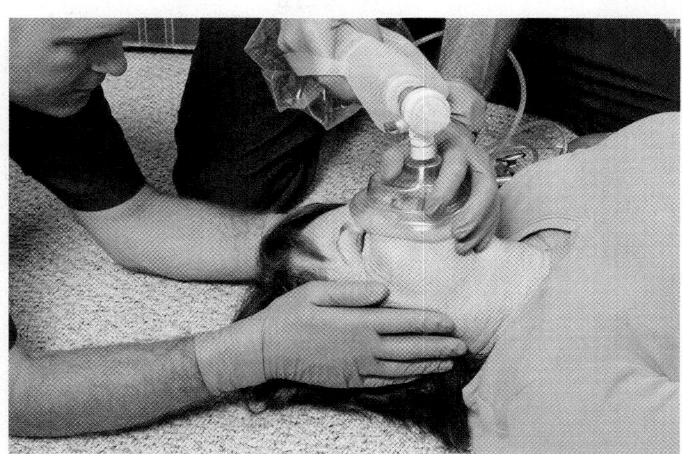

FIGURE 10-31 * Two-person bag-valve-mask method.

pillow to achieve a better sniffing position. If a spinal injury is suspected, follow procedures described later under "Bag-Valve-Mask Technique—Patient with Suspected Spinal Injury."

2. Select the correct size mask and bag-valve device. If the patient is unresponsive, an oropharyngeal or nasopharyngeal airway should be inserted to help maintain a patent airway.
3. Place the upper, narrower part of the mask over the bridge of the nose and lower it over the mouth and into the cleft above the chin. If the mask has a large round cuff surrounding the ventilation port, center the port over the mouth (Figure 10-32∗).
4. Position your thumbs over the top half of the mask and your index fingers over the bottom portion of the mask. Use your ring and little fingers to bring the patient's jaw up to the mask. The middle fingers, depending on the size of the EMT's hands, may be placed either under the mandible or over the mask. The thumb-side edges of the palms are placed over both sides of the mask to hold it in place and form an airtight seal. This forms the "E-C" hand position, as previously described.
5. Have another EMT connect the bag valve to the mask, if it is not already attached.
6. Begin ventilation as soon as possible. The other EMT or qualified person will squeeze the bag with two hands and deliver the ventilation steadily over 1 second while watching for adequate chest rise. Oxygen must be connected to the reservoir of the BVM and flowing at 15 lpm as quickly as possible. If you cannot ventilate or if the chest does not rise adequately, take the measures that will be described under "Bag-Valve-Mask Problems."
7. An adult with a pulse should be ventilated once every 6 to 5 seconds (10–12 breaths/minute) and infants and children once every 5 to 3 seconds (12–20 breaths/minute). Review Table 10-6 for ventilation rates in the pulseless patient. The chest should be monitored continuously for adequate rise and fall.

One-Person BVM Technique When you must operate the bag-valve mask alone, apply the mask to the patient's face with one hand. Your thumb should be placed over the part of the mask covering the bridge of the nose, and your index finger is placed over the part covering the cleft above the chin. Seal the mask firmly on the face by pushing down with the thumb and index finger while pulling up on the mandible with the other fingers to maintain a head-tilt, chin-lift. The "E-C" hand position technique will be performed with only one hand. Squeeze the bag with the other hand while observing the chest rise to make certain the lungs are being inflated effectively (Figure 10-33∗). The bag may alternatively be compressed against your body or forearm to deliver a greater tidal volume to the patient. If you are performing one-person BVM, ventilate the patient for approximately 1 minute and then connect the oxygen to the BVM. Be sure that you do not interrupt ventilation for more than 30 seconds when doing so.

Bag-Valve-Mask Problems If you are ventilating with a bag-valve mask and the patient's chest does not rise and fall, re-evaluate the BVM device and the patient's airway, considering these possible problems and remedies:

1. *Check the position of the head and chin.* Reposition the airway and repeat your attempt at ventilation.
2. *Check the mask seal* to ensure that an excessive amount of air is not escaping from around the mask. Reposition your fingers and the mask to attain a tight seal.
3. *Assess for an obstruction.* If the airway is repositioned, the seal is adequate, and you are still unable to ventilate effectively, consider an airway obstruction. Inspect inside the mouth for evidence of an obstruction. If one is found, remove it with a finger sweep. If none is found, begin the foreign body airway obstruction maneuver described in Appendix 1 until you are able to effectively ventilate.
4. *Check the bag-valve-mask system* to ensure that all the parts are properly connected and operational. Some systems with a bag-type oxygen reservoir will refill extremely slowly if the oxygen flow rate is inade-

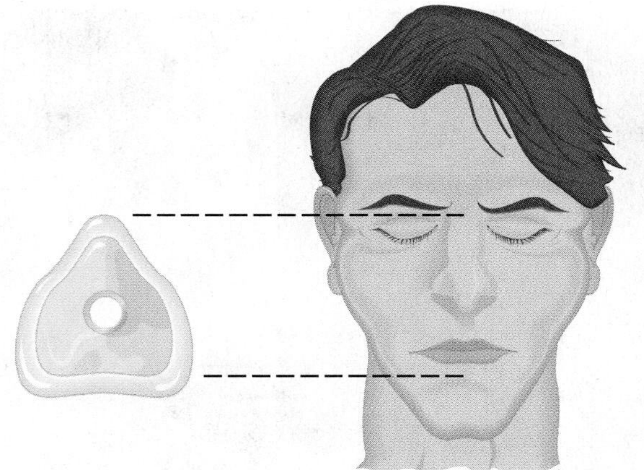

FIGURE 10-32 ∗ Always use the proper size mask. It should fit securely over the bridge of the nose and in the cleft above the chin.

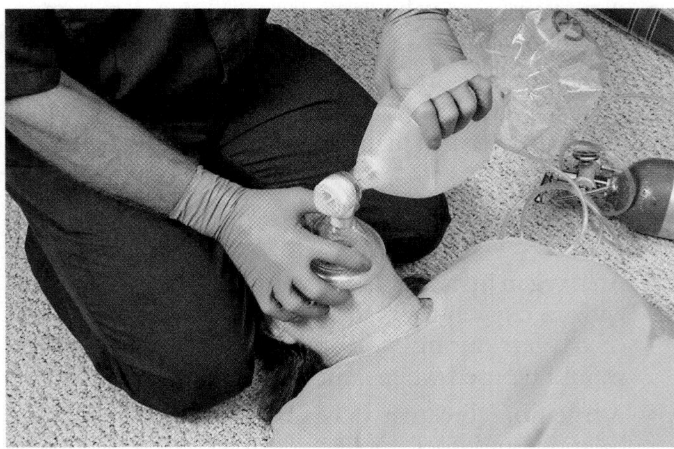

FIGURE 10-33 ∗ One-person bag-valve-mask method.

quate. This causes a reduction in the tidal volume delivered to the patient and subsequently produces minimal chest rise and fall and leads to hypoxia.

5. *If the chest still does not rise and fall, use an alternative method* for positive pressure ventilation, for example, a pocket mask or a flow-restricted, oxygen-powered ventilation device.
6. *If you are having difficulty maintaining an open airway, insert an oropharyngeal or nasopharyngeal airway.* Either device will help keep the tongue from falling back to block the airway.
7. *If the patient's abdomen rises with each ventilation or it appears to be distended,* it may be an indication of one of the following:
   - *The head-tilt, chin-lift maneuver is not being performed properly* and is allowing an excessive amount of air into the esophagus and stomach. Reposition the head and neck and resume ventilation.
   - *The patient is being ventilated too rapidly or with too great a tidal volume.* Such excessive ventilation increases the pressure in the esophagus and allows air to enter the stomach. Squeeze the bag slowly to deliver the volume over a 1-second period and allow for adequate exhalation after each ventilation. Ensure that an excessive tidal volume is not being delivered and causing the stomach to fill with air.

Bag-Valve-Mask Technique—Patient with Suspected Spinal Injury

If you suspect a patient has a spinal injury, you must establish and maintain in-line spinal stabilization as a priority. The airway maneuvers and use of the bag-valve-mask technique must be performed with special care to avoid movement of the head or spine while maintaining in-line spinal stabilization until the patient is fully immobilized to a backboard. The procedures for using a bag-valve mask with a patient with suspected spinal injury are illustrated in EMT Skills 10-5 and are described here:

1. While following procedures for manual in-line stabilization of the head and neck (see Chapter 32, "Spinal Column and Spinal Cord Trauma"), open the airway using a jaw-thrust maneuver.
2. Have another EMT or a trained assistant maintain the in-line stabilization of the head and neck while you select the correct size mask. If no other personnel are available, you can kneel at the patient's head and hold his head between your thighs and knees to prevent movement.
3. Position your thumb over the top portion of the mask and your index finger over the bottom portion of the mask. Use your ring and little fingers to bring the patient's jaw up to the mask. The middle finger, depending on the size of your hands, may be placed either under the mandible or over the mask. Place the top of the mask over the bridge of the nose. Lower the mask over the mouth until the bottom half of the mask fits snugly in the cleft above the chin. Place the thumb-side edge of your palm over the side of the mask to hold it in place and form an airtight seal. This forms the "E-C" hand position, as previously described.
4. Place the mask to the face and bring the jaw up to the mask without tilting the head back or moving the neck.
5. Have another EMT connect the bag-valve device to the mask, if this has not already been done. Hold a mask seal with your thumbs at the bridge of the nose and the index fingers over the bottom half of the mask. The edges of the palms on the thumb side should hold the mask down on the face. The middle, ring, and little fingers are used to maintain the jaw thrust. EMTs with smaller hands may be able to form the "E-C" position with the thumb, index, and middle fingers and grasp the mandible only with the ring and little fingers.
6. Begin ventilation as soon as possible. Have the other EMT or trained assistant squeeze the bag with two hands to deliver the volume over a 1-second period.
7. An adult with a pulse should be ventilated once every 6 to 5 seconds (10–12 breaths/minute) and infants and children once every 5 to 3 seconds (12–20 breaths/minute). Review Table 10-6 for ventilation rates in the pulseless patient. The chest should be monitored continuously for adequate rise and fall.
8. If the bag-valve mask has not already been connected to the oxygen supply, the patient should receive positive pressure ventilation for 1 minute. At that point the other EMT should make the connection, set the flow at 15 lpm, attach a reservoir, and resume ventilation. *Ventilation should not be interrupted for more than 30 seconds at any time.*
9. In-line manual stabilization must be maintained until the patient is completely immobilized to the backboard.
10. Once the patient is fully immobilized, follow the standard two-person bag-valve-mask technique, using the jaw-thrust maneuver to maintain a patent airway. If the patient is in cardiac arrest and the airway cannot be established with a jaw-thrust maneuver, it may be necessary to tilt the head until the airway can be established. The priority in the cardiac arrest patient is airway management and effective ventilation.

If only two EMTs are at a scene, it may be necessary for one to hold the in-line stabilization with his thighs and knees, while performing all the additional steps of the one-person bag-valve-mask technique. This is the most ineffective method for providing bag-valve-mask ventilation and should be replaced with the two-person technique as soon as possible. Also apply cricoid pressure, if enough personnel are available, to reduce the risk of gastric inflation, regurgitation, and aspiration.

Flow-Restricted, Oxygen-Powered Ventilation Device (FROPVD)

Another method of providing positive pressure ventilation is through the flow-restricted, oxygen-powered ventilation device (FROPVD), also known as a manually triggered ventilation device. The device is powered by oxygen and, with a proper mask seal, will deliver 100 percent oxygen to the patient. In the spontaneously breathing patient, the valve is opened automatically by the negative pressure created by the patient's inspiration. Oxygen flow ceases automatically when the inhalation ends. The major advantages of the device are that it delivers 100 percent oxygen during ventilation and that it can be used by one EMT to deliver ventilation using a two-handed mask seal.

A major disadvantage of this device is that it is designed to be used *only on adult patients.* Because it delivers oxygen at high pressure and at a high flow rate, it cannot be used on infants or children. Also, the EMT is unable to feel the compliance of air being delivered during the ventilation.

According to the American Heart Association guidelines of 2010, the FROPVD is an aid in ventilating a patient in cardiac arrest when used in the manual mode, which requires the EMT to trigger the device to deliver a ventilation. Avoid the automatic mode in cardiac arrest, because it may cause an increase in positive end-expiratory pressure (air remains in the terminal bronchioles and alveoli), which may lead to a decrease in blood return to the heart and subsequent reduction in perfusion of the cerebral and coronary arteries.

The FROPVD should have the following features:

- Peak flow rate under 40 lpm of 100 percent oxygen
- Inspiratory pressure relief valve that opens at about 60 centimeters of water pressure and vents remaining volume to the atmosphere or ceases gas flow
- Alarm that sounds when relief valve pressure is exceeded
- Adaptability to a variety of environmental conditions and extremes of temperature
- Activating trigger or on/off button placed so the EMT can keep both hands on the mask to hold a seal
- Standard 15/22 mm couplings for masks, endotracheal tubes, tracheostomy tubes, laryngeal mask airways, and Combitubes
- Rugged, compact design, easy to hold and operate
- Can be used with advanced alternative airways

FROPVD Techniques

Follow the steps described next when using a flow-restricted, oxygen-powered ventilation device:

1. Check the unit to ensure it is properly functioning. Also, check the oxygen source to ensure there is an adequate supply to operate the unit effectively.
2. Open the airway using a head-tilt, chin-lift maneuver if no spinal injury is suspected (Figure 10-34a*). If a spinal injury is suspected (Figure 10-34b*), use the same technique of establishing a mask seal with a jaw thrust as described in the bag-valve mask section. In-

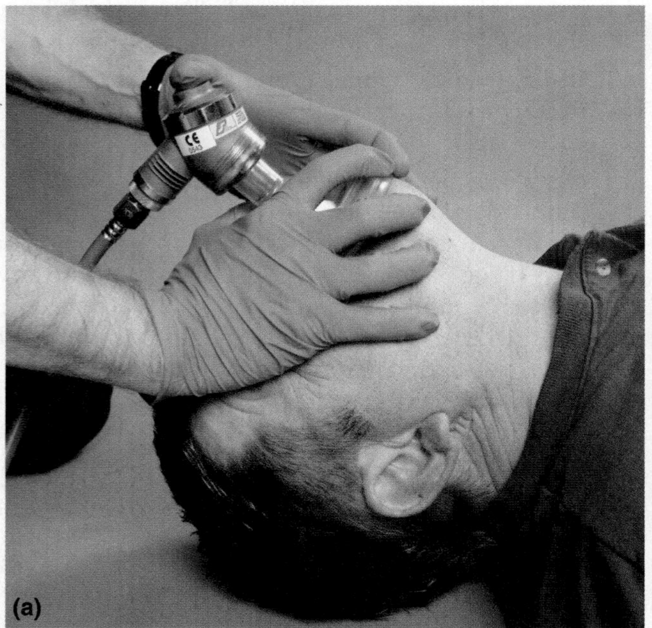

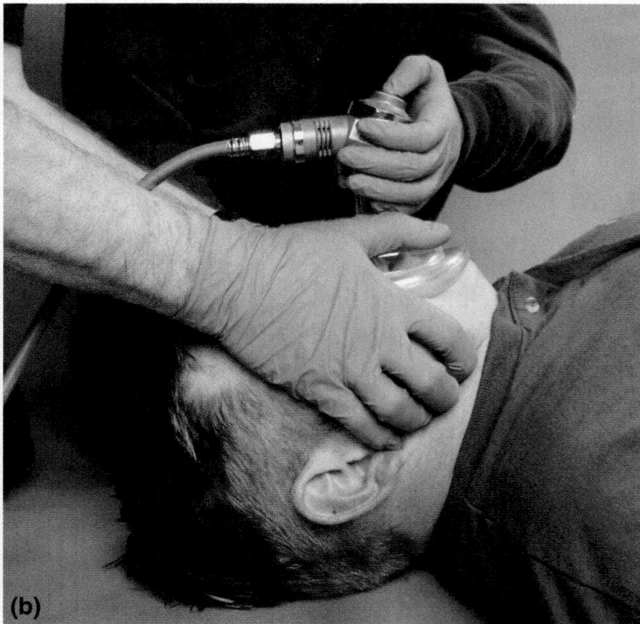

FIGURE 10-34 * **(a)** A flow-restricted, oxygen-powered ventilation device on a patient *with no* suspected spine injury. **(b)** A flow-restricted, oxygen-powered ventilation device on a patient *with* a suspected spine injury.

sert an oropharyngeal or nasopharyngeal airway. Apply the adult mask to the patient's face in the same manner as for the bag-valve mask.

3. Connect the flow-restricted, oxygen-powered ventilation device to the mask if not already done.
4. Activate the valve by depressing the trigger or button on the valve. As soon as the chest begins to rise, deactivate the valve by releasing the trigger or button. The oxygen flow ceases and the patient's exhaled gas is released through a one-way valve. The device is driven by 100 percent oxygen, thus, there is no need to attach any supplemental oxygen source once ventilation has begun.
5. An adult with a pulse should be ventilated once every 6 to 5 seconds (10–12 breaths/minute). The adult patient in cardiac arrest will be ventilated twice after every 30 compressions. The chest should be monitored continuously for adequate rise and fall.

If you suspect that a patient has a spinal injury and two EMTs are available, one can perform the in-line stabilization while the other holds a mask seal and triggers the device. If only one EMT is available, he can hold in-line stabilization of the head and neck with his thighs and knees while holding a mask seal and triggering the device.

FROPVD Problems If a patient's chest does not rise adequately during use of the flow-restricted, oxygen-powered ventilation device, re-evaluate the position of the head and chin and the mask seal. If the chest does not rise after repositioning and the mask seal proves adequate, an airway obstruction is a possibility; follow the procedure for adult foreign body airway obstruction in Appendix 1.

If the oxygen source that powers the device runs out or the user cannot effectively use the device, it is necessary to use an alternative means to ventilate the patient, such as pocket mask or bag-valve-mask device.

Automatic Transport Ventilator (ATV)

Another device used for positive pressure ventilation is the **automatic transport ventilator (ATV)** (Figure 10-35*). Several different devices are available. They have been shown to be excellent at providing and maintaining a constant rate and tidal volume during ventilation, and maintaining adequate oxygenation of arterial blood. In addition, most ATVs use oxygen as their power source, thereby delivering 100 percent oxygen during ventilation.

The ATV can deliver oxygen at lower inspiratory flow rates and for longer inspiratory times. Therefore, the devices have a lesser likelihood of causing gastric distention compared with other methods of positive pressure ventilation, including mouth-to-mask and bag-valve mask ventilation. However, as with any ventilation device, gastric distention can occur if the patient's head and neck are improperly positioned.

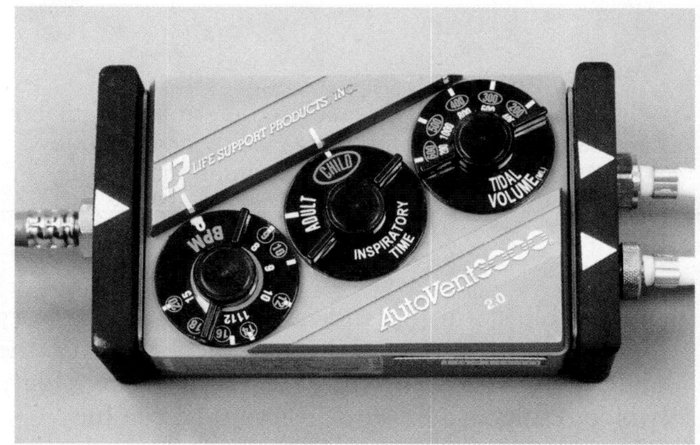

FIGURE 10-35 * An automatic transport ventilator.

Among other advantages of the ATV are the following:

- The EMT is free to use both hands to hold the mask and maintain the airway position as the device delivers the ventilation automatically.
- The device can be set to provide a specific tidal volume, respiratory rate, and minute ventilation.
- Alarms indicate low pressure in the oxygen tank as well as accidental disconnection of the ventilator.
- One EMT can hold in-line stabilization with his thighs and knees and hold the mask seal with two hands while the ventilation is delivered.
- While holding the mask seal with one hand, the EMT can apply cricoid pressure with the other hand.

There are a few disadvantages associated with the ATV:

- Because the ATV is usually oxygen powered (although one type of ATV does use electric power), once the oxygen supply is depleted, the device cannot be used. A pocket mask or bag-valve-mask device must always be available when using an ATV in case of failure or oxygen depletion.
- Some ATVs cannot be used in children less than 5 years of age.
- When using the ATV device, it is not possible to feel an increase in airway resistance or a decrease in the compliance in the lungs.

ATV Recommended Features

ATVs used for prehospital care should have the following features:

- A device that is simple and time- or volume-cycled (pressure-cycled devices should be avoided)
- A standard lightweight 15/22 mm connector
- Lightweight (less than or equal to 4 kg) and rugged in design that can function in temperature extremes
- A default peak inspiratory pressure limit of 60 cm H_2O that is adjustable from 20 to 80 cm H_2O and easily accessible to the EMT

Key Points
Consult medical direction to determine ventilator settings when using the ATV, and always follow the manufacturer's recommendations.

Objective 10-24
Describe indications and methods for administering positive pressure ventilations to a patient who is breathing spontaneously.

- An audible alarm that indicates the peak inspiratory pressure is generated and alerts the EMT that the lung compliance is low or the airway pressure is high, which results in a lower delivered tidal volume
- Ability to deliver 50–100 percent oxygen
- An inspiratory time of 1 second
- An adjustable inspiratory flow of 30 lpm for the adult and 15 lpm for the child
- A rate of 10 breaths per minute for adults and 20 breaths per minute for children

Some ATVs have a demand valve built in, in the event that the patient begins to breathe spontaneously. The valve should be able to deliver a peak inspiratory flow rate of 120 lpm. Also, it is necessary that the ATV have an appropriate inspiration-to-exhalation ratio of 1:2 seconds. Some ATVs have alarms that indicate low oxygen levels, disconnection from the mask, or a low battery. The ATV may also have the ability to provide positive end-expiratory pressure (PEEP) or continuous positive airway pressure (CPAP). Those using an ATV must be specially trained and well aware of the device and its specific features.

ATV Techniques

It is necessary to consult with medical direction to determine the ventilator settings when using the ATV. Always follow the manufacturer's recommendations. The following are general guidelines for the operation of an ATV:

1. Check the ATV to ensure it is properly functioning.
2. Attach the ATV to a mask. Seal the mask on the face by using the same technique described earlier in the bag-valve mask section.
3. Select the appropriate tidal volume and rate to be delivered. On some models the tidal volume and rate are preset. Turn the unit on.
4. Observe the chest for adequate rise and fall. Adjust the tidal volume until adequate rise of the chest is achieved.
5. Continuously monitor both the device for proper functioning and the rise of the patient's chest for adequate ventilation. If a failure of the device is detected or suspected, immediately discontinue use of the ATV and begin ventilation with a pocket mask or a bag-valve-mask device.

Ventilation of the Patient Who Is Breathing Spontaneously

If the patient presents with either an inadequate respiratory rate or an inadequate tidal volume, even though he is still breathing, it is necessary to ventilate the patient and provide supplementary oxygen to ensure that he is receiving an adequate alveolar ventilation volume. The most important step is to assess accurately and recognize the need for ventilation of the patient who is breathing, but breathing inadequately. Signs of inadequate breathing include an altered mental status, inadequate respiratory rate, poor chest rise and fall, and fatigue from an increased work of breathing.

Complications that you may encounter when ventilating a spontaneously breathing patient include combativeness in the hypoxic patient who does not cooperate, an inadequate mask seal, overventilation leading to lung injury, and risk of regurgitation and aspiration.

Explain the procedure to any patient with spontaneous ventilation who requires positive pressure ventilation. Coach the patient to work with you during the ventilation. You may not know if the patient can understand; regardless, it is necessary to explain what you are doing in case he can understand but is unable to respond appropriately.

The following breathing patients would need ventilation:

- *The patient who has a reduced minute volume due either to an inadequate respiratory rate or to an inadequate tidal volume.* This is termed *hypoventilation.* The adult patient would need to be ventilated at a rate of 10–12, the infant or child with tidal volumes adequate to make the chest rise with each ventilation.
- *The patient with an adequate respiratory rate but an inadequate tidal volume (shallow breathing).* This is termed *hypopnea* (low volume of breathing). The rate is adequate; however, the tidal volume is inadequate. Because the ventilation rate is adequate, you would assist the ventilation at the rate at which the patient is already breathing. When the patient begins to inhale, you would deliver your ventilation, ensuring an adequate tidal volume with each ventilation. Be sure to connect supplemental oxygen, and watch for chest rise with each ventilation.
- *The patient who has an adequate tidal volume but has a respiratory rate that is too slow.* This is termed *bradypnea* (slow breathing). Even though the tidal

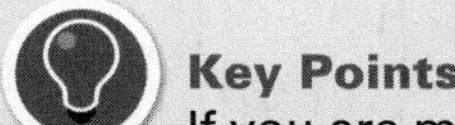

Key Points
If you are meeting resistance with ventilation in the breathing patient, be sure to coordinate your ventilation with the patient's spontaneous breaths.

Key Points
Continuous positive airway pressure (CPAP) is a form of noninvasive positive pressure ventilation used in the awake and spontaneously breathing patient who needs ventilatory support.

volume of each breath may be adequate, the rate is not fast enough to maintain adequate oxygenation of the tissues. In the patient with bradypnea, you would need to supplement ventilation to bring the rate to 10–12 in the adult and 12–20 in the infant or child. For example, if the adult patient was breathing only six times per minute, you would need to deliver another six breaths in 1 minute to achieve an adequate minute volume. Begin by ventilating with each of the patient's inhalations and then, over the next 5–10 ventilations, increase the rate to once every 5–6 seconds. Be sure that each breath the patient takes on his own has an adequate tidal volume. If not, as the patient begins to inhale, deliver a ventilation and then deliver another ventilation within 5–6 seconds to achieve an adequate ventilation rate.

- *The patient who has a respiratory rate that is too fast (tachypnea) that leads to an inadequate tidal volume (hypopnea).* You must deliver ventilations at a rate of 10–12 per minute with an adequate tidal volume with each ventilation. As an example, if the adult patient is breathing at a rate of 42 per minute and the tidal volume is shallow, you would initially assist the ventilations at the patient's rate by delivering a ventilation with each breath. Over the next 5–10 ventilations, slowly adjust the rate so that you are ventilating every 5–6 seconds with one of the patient's breaths.

If you are meeting resistance with ventilation in the breathing patient, be sure to first coordinate your ventilation with the patient's spontaneous breaths. Increase or decrease the ventilation rate from that point. Once you have control over the ventilation, the patient may relax and allow you to ventilate with greater ease.

Continuous Positive Airway Pressure (CPAP)

Continuous positive airway pressure (CPAP) is a form of noninvasive positive pressure ventilation used in the awake and spontaneously breathing patient who needs ventilatory support. CPAP is applied typically to patients with a respiratory disease or cardiac failure with pulmonary involvement who are in severe respiratory distress or respiratory failure. CPAP applied by the EMT would be delivered via a tight-fitting mask and a specialized CPAP device designed to deliver a continuous flow of air under pressure (Figure 10-36*).

CPAP is often used to avoid the need to place an endotracheal tube or other advanced airway to artificially ventilate the patient. As already noted, it is delivered via a tightly fitted mask and a device that generates a continuous flow of air through the airways under positive pressure that is higher than normal air pressure. Oxygen is typically delivered with the positive pressure.

The continuous delivery of air under positive pressure is intended to inflate collapsed alveoli, improve oxygenation, and reduce the patient's work of breathing. It takes a great deal of work and energy to reinflate the alveoli with each breath. By keeping the alveoli open with CPAP, less work is required and less energy is used. This typically averts complete respiratory failure or arrest and allows the patient to continue to breathe on his own.

Left ventricular failure increases hydrostatic pressure inside the pulmonary capillaries, forcing fluid out of the capillaries and into the adjoining alveoli, displacing the air in the alveoli and inhibiting gas exchange. The continuous pressure created in the alveoli by CPAP prevents further fluid leakage into the alveoli and actually forces fluid that may already have accumulated out of the alveoli and back into the interstitial space and the capillaries. CPAP improves the heart rate and blood pressure and reduces the sympathetic tone by improving gas exchange and oxygenation. This also decreases afterload and reduces the myocardial workload in an already failing heart.

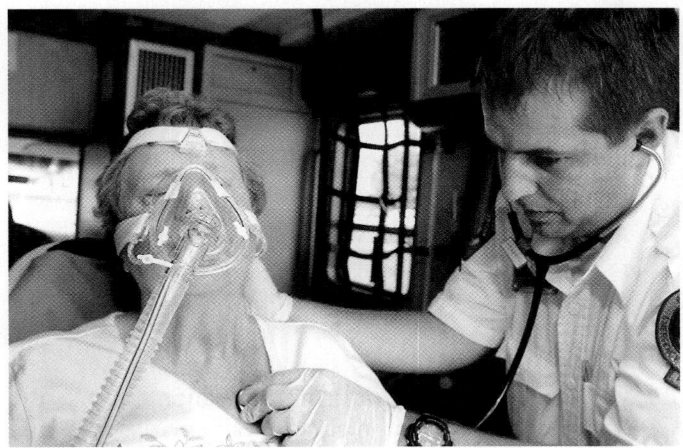

FIGURE 10-36 * CPAP is a form of noninvasive positive pressure ventilation used in the awake and spontaneously breathing patient who needs ventilatory support. (© Ken Kerr)

Objective 10-25
Discuss the indications, contraindications, and methods for administering continuous positive airway pressure (CPAP) or bilevel positive airway pressure (BiPAP).

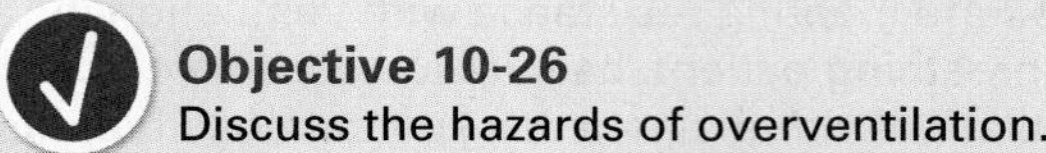

Objective 10-26
Discuss the hazards of overventilation.

Indications for CPAP

CPAP is used to support ventilations and not as a device to provide artificial ventilation. Patient criteria for CPAP include:

- Awake and alert enough to obey commands
- Able to maintain his own airway
- Able to breathe on his own

The indications for CPAP for the patient in severe respiratory distress or failure, but who is alert and awake enough to obey commands, maintain his own airway, and continue to breathe on his own, include:

- Congestive heart failure
- Pulmonary edema (fluid around and in the alveoli from a high hydrostatic pressure in the pulmonary capillaries)
- Chronic obstructive pulmonary disease (COPD)
- Asthma

Contraindications for CPAP

CPAP is contraindicated in patients with:

- Apnea
- Inability to understand or obey commands
- Inability to maintain their own airway
- Unresponsiveness
- Responsiveness only to verbal or painful stimuli
- Cardiac arrest
- Need for frequent suctioning

Relative contraindications include patients with:

- Pulmonary trauma
- Increased intracranial pressure
- Abdominal distention with a risk for vomiting
- Hypotension

Administering CPAP

Be sure to completely inform the patient about the CPAP device, how it will feel, and its benefits. It is vital that you continuously coach the patient in order to lessen his anxiety and fear. This is a very difficult procedure for most patients who are struggling to breathe, even though it will improve their condition. Increasing their anxiety will increase their sympathetic nervous system response, increase breathing workload, increase oxygen demand, increase myocardial workload, and worsen their condition. It is imperative that you work into the CPAP quickly, yet slowly enough to allow the patient to become comfortable with the procedure. It may take only 5 to 10 minutes before the patient begins to show improvement.

BiPAP

BiPAP (bilevel positive airway pressure) is similar to CPAP but allows for different airway pressures to be set for inspiration and expiration. The effectiveness of BiPAP in the prehospital setting has not been adequately studied; therefore, its use in prehospital care is not recommended.

Hazards of Overventilation

Performing ventilation on patients has many risks. It is often thought that providing more ventilation than what is necessary might be helpful to the patient. On the contrary, scientific evidence has found that overventilating a patient can lead to serious complications, especially in the cardiac arrest patient and those with increased pressures in the chest from injury or illnesses.

In the cardiac arrest patient, hyperventilation and prolonged positive pressure ventilation can lead to a decrease in the cardiac output, blood pressure, and perfusion. In one study, it was speculated that higher ventilation rates and volumes increased the pressure inside the chest, not allowing for the development of negative pressure between compressions. The negative pressure between compressions is necessary to draw blood into the chest cavity and increases the blood flow to the right side of the heart. With the pressure in the chest remaining higher than it should be, the amount of blood entering the left side of the heart to be ejected out to the body is severely diminished. This leads to a decrease in the perfusion of both the coronary vessels in the heart and the cerebral vessels in the brain.

When a spontaneously breathing patient is overventilated, where the rate and volume delivered with the ventilation is in excess of the recommended rate and volume, large amounts of air may become trapped in the alveoli, causing the pressure in the chest to remain higher than it

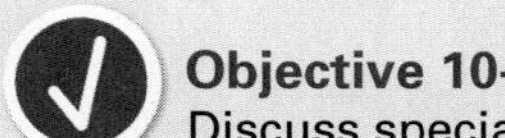

Objective 10-27
Discuss special considerations of airway management and ventilation for infants and children and for patients with stomas/tracheostomy tubes, facial injuries, foreign body airway obstructions, or dental appliances.

should during inhalation and exhalation. The overinflated alveoli may cause the capillaries in the lungs to become compressed and obstruct blood flow to the left atrium. Also, the constant high pressure in the chest would reduce the negative pressure that is able to be generated, thereby reducing the vacuum effect that sucks blood into the right side of the heart with each breath. This would reduce the blood volume that is available to the left ventricle, causing a reduction in cardiac output. This can reduce the blood pressure and perfusion of essential organs such as the brain, heart, lungs, liver, and kidneys.

It is essential to adhere to the recommended ventilation rates and volumes when ventilating a patient, especially the cardiac arrest patient. More ventilation is *not* good for the patient. What *is* good for the patient is establishing and maintaining a patent airway, providing good ventilations at the right rate and tidal volume, and providing supplemental oxygen with ventilations.

Special Considerations in Airway Management and Ventilation

You will sometimes encounter patients or emergency situations that will require you to alter or adjust your technique when controlling the airway or providing artificial ventilation. It is necessary for you to recognize these special situations and to be prepared to provide the appropriate intervention to ensure adequate airway control, ventilation, and oxygenation.

A Patient with a Stoma or Tracheostomy Tube

A **stoma** is a surgical opening in the front of the neck that may be permanent or temporary. One reason for the presence of a stoma in the patient's neck is that a **tracheostomy** has been performed. During a tracheostomy, a stoma is created by cutting through the skin and into the trachea to relieve an obstruction higher in the trachea or to serve in place of an endotracheal tube (a tube through the mouth and into the trachea) that has been in place for a number of hours or days. Often, a **tracheostomy tube**—a curved hollow tube made of rubber, plastic, or metal—is inserted into the stoma to help hold it open. The patient may be breathing completely through the stoma and tube or may still be getting some air through the mouth and nose, around whatever blockage exists in the trachea. A tracheostomy is usually temporary and will eventually be closed and allowed to heal.

Another reason for the presence of a stoma is a **laryngectomy.** In a laryngectomy, typically because of cancer, all or part of the patient's larynx has been removed. In a *total laryngectomy,* there is no longer any connection of the trachea to the mouth and nose. The trachea is disconnected from the pharynx, brought forward, and connected to the stoma in the neck. This alters the airway so that the patient breathes completely through the stoma. In a *partial laryngectomy,* some of the tracheal connection to the mouth and nose remains so that the patient may be getting some air through the stoma and some through the mouth and nose (Figure 10-37∗). With a laryngectomy, the stoma is permanent.

When you encounter a patient with a stoma (with or without a tube in the stoma), it will probably not be immediately obvious whether the patient is able to take in any air through the mouth and nose or can get air only through the stoma, unless a family member is able to tell you. The procedures described next take this into account.

Bag-Valve-Mask-to-Tracheostomy-Tube Ventilation

The bag-valve device is designed so that it can connect directly to the tracheostomy tube to provide positive pressure ventilation (Figure 10-38∗). When ventilating through the tracheostomy tube, it may be necessary to seal the patient's mouth and nose to prevent air from escaping. If this is not done, ineffective ventilation may result, with inadequate tidal volumes delivered to the patient.

If you are unable to ventilate through the tube, first suction it using a soft suction catheter. If you are still unable to ventilate, attempt to ventilate through the mouth and nose while sealing the stoma; this may improve the ability to ventilate or may clear the obstruction preventing ventilation through the tracheostomy tube.

Bag-Valve-Mask-to-Stoma Ventilation

The permanent stoma of a laryngectomy patient is usually at the base of the neck with no tube inserted.

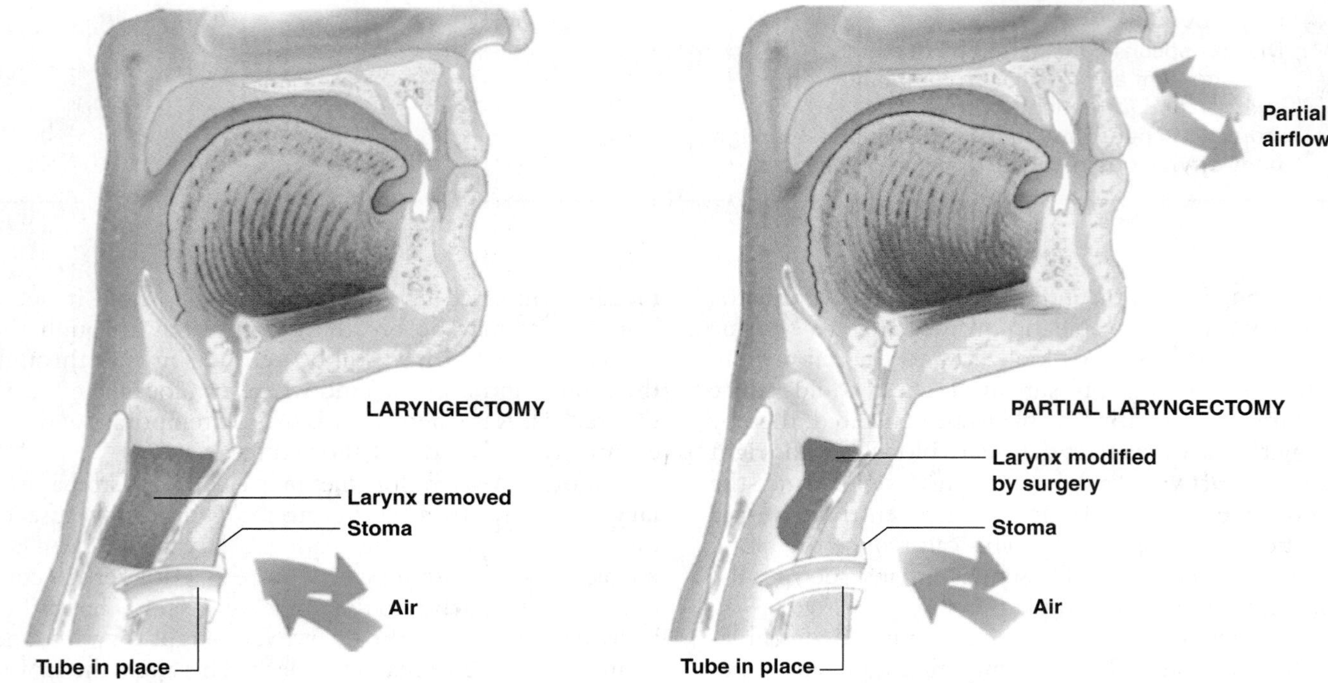

FIGURE 10-37 ✱ The neck breather's airway has been changed by surgery.

Remember that a total laryngectomy patient has no airflow from the mouth and nose, but a partial laryngectomy patient may still have some airflow from the mouth and nose. To perform artificial ventilation with a bag-valve mask to the stoma, follow these guidelines:

1. Remove all coverings (e.g., scarves and ties) from the area of the stoma.
2. Clear the stoma of any foreign matter. Suction the stoma by passing a sterile soft suction catheter through the stoma and into the trachea no more than 3–5 inches. Suction enough to partially open the airway.
3. *You will not need to perform a head-tilt, chin-lift or jaw-thrust maneuver on a patient with a stoma.* Keep the patient's head straight and the shoulders slightly elevated.
4. Select a mask, most often a child or infant mask, that fits securely over the stoma and can be sealed against the neck. Hold the mask seal with your hand and squeeze the bag delivering the ventilation over a 2-second period. Watch for adequate chest rise and fall. Feel to be sure that the air is escaping back through the stoma during exhalation.
5. If the chest does not rise, suspect a partial laryngectomy. Seal the nose and mouth with one hand so that air will not leak out of the mouth and nose. Pinch off the nose between the third and fourth fingers; seal the lips with the palm of the hand. Place the thumb under the chin, and press upward and backward. Repeat the ventilation process.

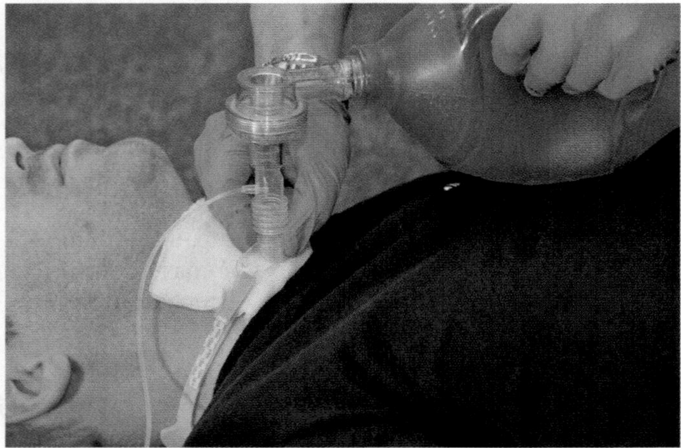

FIGURE 10-38 ✱ Artificial ventilation can be accomplished in the patient with a tracheostomy tube by attaching the bag-valve-mask device directly to the tube.

Mouth-to-Stoma Ventilation

Mouth-to-stoma ventilation is not recommended because it exposes the EMT to respiratory secretions and droplets, causing possible contamination with infectious disease. It is preferable to use a bag-valve-mask device with an infant- or child-sized mask to form a seal over the stoma. Follow the same procedure as for adult ventilation with a bag-valve mask with the exception of forming the mask seal over the stoma instead of over the mouth. If a BVM is not present and you have no other option, you must use a barrier device over the stoma before you perform mouth-to-stoma ventilation.

Infants and Children

Keep the following special considerations in mind when establishing and controlling the airway and providing artificial ventilation in infants and children:

- When establishing an airway by head-tilt, chin-lift maneuver, place the infant's head in a neutral position without hyperextension. The child's head should be placed in a neutral position and then only slightly extended. Because of immature development of the airways, hyperextension may actually produce an airway obstruction. Because of the large size of the head, it may be necessary to elevate the upper chest of an infant or small child by placing padding under the shoulders to achieve an adequate airway.
- When providing positive pressure ventilation, regardless of the device or technique used, it is necessary to avoid excessive ventilation volumes and pressures. Excesses in these areas will lead to gastric distention, a common problem while ventilating infants and children. Gastric distention can impede lung inflation, reducing the ventilation volume being delivered, or it can cause the patient to vomit and possibly aspirate the vomitus. Also, excessive volumes can cause lung rupture and injury. The smallest volume that causes the chest to visibly rise is adequate.
- Use a bag-valve-mask device with a minimum volume of 450–500 mL without a pop-off valve. If a pop-off valve is present, disable it by placing it in a closed or off position. Because of the smaller airways and higher resistance in infants and children, a pop-off valve may unnecessarily vent air and lead to ineffective ventilation.
- Insert an oropharyngeal or nasopharyngeal airway if the airway cannot be maintained with a head-tilt, chin-lift or jaw-thrust maneuver alone or if prolonged ventilation is necessary.
- The ventilation rate for infants and children is 12–20 per minute or one ventilation delivered every 5 to 3 seconds. Be sure the chest rises with each ventilation.

Patients with Facial Injuries

The blood supply to the face is extremely rich; this can lead to two major complications with facial injuries:

1. Blunt injury can cause excessive swelling that may partially or completely occlude the airway. It may be necessary to insert an airway adjunct to establish and maintain the airway. Avoid the use of a nasopharyngeal airway with mid-face trauma. Also, positive pressure ventilation may be needed to force ventilation past the swollen airway.
2. Bleeding into the pharynx may be severe and can cause problems with airway management. Frequent or constant suctioning may be necessary.

Foreign Body Airway Obstruction

You may encounter a responsive or unresponsive patient with a known upper airway foreign body obstruction. It is also possible that an unresponsive patient may have a foreign body obstruction that is only detected after unsuccessful attempts at positive pressure ventilation. In these events, follow the procedure for foreign body airway obstruction to establish a patent airway. Refer to Appendix 1 to review the techniques of managing a foreign body airway obstruction.

If the patient is responsive and choking but is effectively moving air when inhaling and exhaling, instruct him to cough. Do not perform abdominal thrusts or other foreign body airway obstruction maneuvers. Place the patient on high-concentration oxygen and begin transport. If the breathing becomes weak and ineffective, indicating poor air exchange and severe obstruction, immediately manage the patient as a complete foreign body obstruction. Perform abdominal thrusts in the adult or child, or chest thrusts and back blows (slaps) in the infant. Signs of a severe partial airway obstruction with poor air exchange are:

- Cough that becomes silent
- Stridor heard on inhalation
- Increase in labored breathing

If the patient is 1 year of age or older, perform abdominal thrusts as you would for an adult patient. In an infant who is less than 1 year of age, perform back blows (slaps) and chest thrusts in an attempt to relieve the obstruction.

If the airway is completely occluded and there is no air movement, perform three cycles of the foreign body airway obstruction maneuver. If the obstruction is not relieved, transport the patient expeditiously and continue with the foreign body airway obstruction cycles en route to the hospital until the obstruction is relieved.

Once the obstruction is relieved, closely assess the patient's breathing status and pulse. If the breathing is inadequate or absent, begin positive pressure ventilation with supplemental oxygen. If no pulse is present, apply the automated external defibrillator (AED) (see Chapter 15, "Shock and Resuscitation) or, if the AED is not available, begin CPR.

Dental Appliances

If the patient has dentures that are secure in the mouth, leave them in place. It is much easier to establish a tight mask seal with the dentures in place. If the dentures are extremely loose, remove them so they do not dislodge and occlude the airway. Partial dentures (plates) may also become dislodged and occlude the airway. If the partial plate is loose, remove it. Reassess the mouth frequently in patients who have dentures or partial dentures to ensure that these appliances have not come loose.

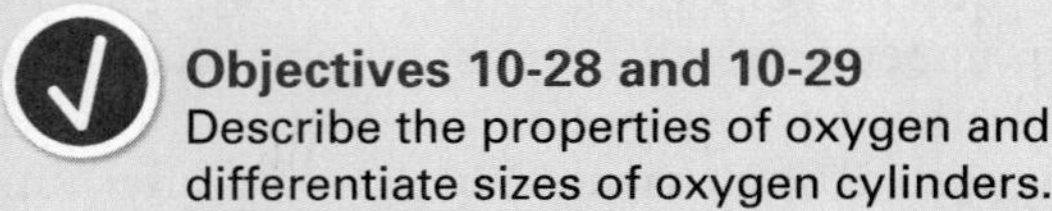

Objectives 10-28 and 10-29
Describe the properties of oxygen and differentiate sizes of oxygen cylinders.

▶ Oxygen Therapy

Oxygen is a colorless, odorless gas normally present in the atmosphere in a concentration of approximately 21 percent. Pure, or 100 percent oxygen is obtained commercially by fractional distillation, a process by which air is liquefied and the gases other than oxygen, primarily nitrogen, are boiled off. Liquid oxygen is then converted under high pressure to a gas and stored in steel or aluminum cylinders under a pressure of about 2,000 pounds per square inch (psi) (Figure 10-39∗).

Oxygen Cylinders

A number of different types of oxygen cylinders are available. They vary in size and in the volume of oxygen contained. Even though the volume of oxygen may vary, all of the cylinders when full are at the same pressure, about 2,000 psi. The cylinders are given letter designations according to their size. The following are sizes and related volumes of oxygen cylinders used in emergency medical care:

- D cylinder—350 liters
- E cylinder—625 liters
- M cylinder—3,000 liters
- G cylinder—5,300 liters
- H cylinder—6,900 liters

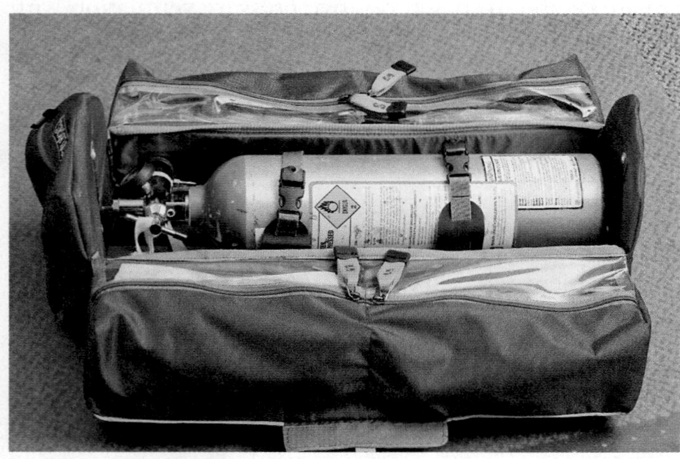

FIGURE 10-39 ∗ A basic portable resuscitator.

Duration of Flow

The only way to truly determine the amount of oxygen in the tank is to apply the gauge and identify the psi of pressure remaining in the tank. The pressure remains constant; however, the volume varies based on the size of the tank. Thus, if a D tank had 1,000 psi it would have approximately 175 liters of oxygen remaining (350 ÷ 2 = 175), whereas an M cylinder with 1,000 psi would have approximately 1,500 liters remaining in the tank (3,000 ÷ 2 = 1,500). The M cylinder would allow a much longer oxygen administration period as compared to the D cylinder.

One method to determine the oxygen duration of a tank is to apply some basic numbers to a simple formula (Table 10-7). This is necessary when a patient must be transported for a long period of time while on high-concentration oxygen and you need to determine if the oxygen content of the tank will last the entire time. A nonrebreather mask at 15 lpm uses a significant amount of oxygen. The higher the flow rate, the faster the oxygen is depleted from the tank.

TABLE 10-7 Oxygen Duration

Formula to Calculate Oxygen Tank Duration

Take the tank pressure measured by the gauge in psi minus the safe residual pressure that is always set at 200 psi times the constant (see the tank constant listed below) divided by the flow rate expected to be delivered or being delivered to the patient in liters per minute. This will provide you with how long the oxygen will last at a desired flow rate for the specified tank (E tank, for example).

Cylinder Constant

D = 0.16	G = 2.41
E = 0.28	H = 3.14
M = 1.56	K = 3.14

As an example, to determine how long the full (2,000 psi) E cylinder will last with a patient on a nonrebreather mask at 15 lpm, you would calculate the following:

$$\frac{(2{,}000 - 200) \times 0.28}{15} = \frac{504}{15} = 33.6 \text{ minutes}$$

The oxygen tank will provide oxygen at 15 lpm to the patient for a period of 33.6 minutes.

Key Points
An oxygen tank can cause serious injury or death to the EMS crew and the patient if not properly handled.

Objectives 10-30
Describe the hazards associated with oxygen use and safety precautions to be observed.

Objectives 10-31 and 10-32
Describe the regulation of oxygen pressures and the use of oxygen humidifiers.

Safety Precautions

Because oxygen is a gas that acts as an accelerant for combustion and oxygen cylinders are under high pressure, they must be handled very carefully. Observe the following safety precautions:

- Never allow combustible materials such as oil or grease to touch the cylinder, regulator, fittings, valves, or hoses. Oil and oxygen under pressure will explode if they come into contact. This includes petroleum-based adhesive (adhesive tape) or lubricants such as petroleum jelly.
- Never smoke or allow others to smoke in any area where oxygen cylinders are in use or on standby. Because oxygen makes fires burn more rapidly, it greatly increases the risk of fire, not only from the tank but in towels, sheets, and clothing with which oxygen has come in contact.
- Store the cylinders below 125°F.
- Never use an oxygen cylinder without a safe, properly fitting regulator valve. Never use a valve that has been modified from another gas.
- Keep all valves closed when the oxygen cylinder is not in use, even if the tank is empty.
- Keep oxygen cylinders secured to prevent their toppling over. In transit, they should be in a carrier rack or secured to the stretcher. An oxygen tank should never be left unsecured anywhere in the patient or driver compartment.
- When you are working with an oxygen cylinder, never place any part of your body over the cylinder valve. A full cylinder is at 2,000 psi. If the tank is punctured or if a valve breaks off, an oxygen cylinder can accelerate with enough force to penetrate concrete walls. A loosely fitting regulator can be blown off the cylinder with sufficient force to decapitate a head, penetrate the body, or demolish any object in its path. Never stand an oxygen tank upright or in any position in which it may fall and possibly break off its valve. Lay the oxygen tank down next to the patient.

Pressure Regulators

Gas flow from an oxygen cylinder is controlled by a regulator that reduces the high pressure in the cylinder to a safe range, from 30 to 70 psi, and controls the flow of oxygen from 1 to 15 lpm. These regulators attach to the cylinder by a yoke, a series of pins configured to fit cylinders holding only one type of gas. The yoke prevents a regulator from being attached accidentally or purposefully to another type of gas. In addition, all gas cylinders are color-coded according to their contents. Oxygen cylinders in the United States are generally steel green or aluminum gray.

Two types of regulators may be attached to an oxygen cylinder: high-pressure regulators and therapy regulators. The **high-pressure regulator** can provide 50 psi to power a flow-restricted, oxygen-powered ventilation device. It has only one gauge, which registers the cylinder contents, and a threaded outlet. It cannot be used interchangeably with the therapy regulator because it has no mechanism for controlling and adjusting the flow rate. To use the high-pressure regulator, attach the equipment supply line to the threaded outlet and open the cylinder valve fully; then turn it back one-half turn for safety.

The **therapy regulator** can administer oxygen from 0.5 lpm up to 25 lpm. It typically has two gauges, one indicating the pressure in the tank and the other indicating the measured flow of oxygen being delivered to the patient. Some therapy regulators have only one gauge and a dial. The gauge shows the tank pressure. The dial, which has lpm markings, is used to select the flow of oxygen to be delivered to the patient. The various oxygen delivery devices require different flow rates.

The pressure in the tank, about 2,000 psi when full, decreases proportionately as the volume of oxygen in the tank decreases. Therefore, a pressure reading of 1,000 psi would indicate that the tank is half full. The pressure in the tank will vary with changes in ambient temperature. An increase in ambient temperature would cause the pressure in the tank to increase, whereas a decrease in ambient temperature would cause a decrease in tank pressure.

Oxygen Humidifiers

Oxygen exits the tank in a dry gaseous form. The dryness can be irritating to a patient's respiratory tract if used over a long period of time. It is possible to add moisture to the oxygen by attaching an **oxygen humidifier** (Figure 10-40*) to the regulator. The humidifier, which consists of a container that is filled with sterile water, is connected directly to the regulator. The oxygen device tubing is attached directly to the humidifier. The

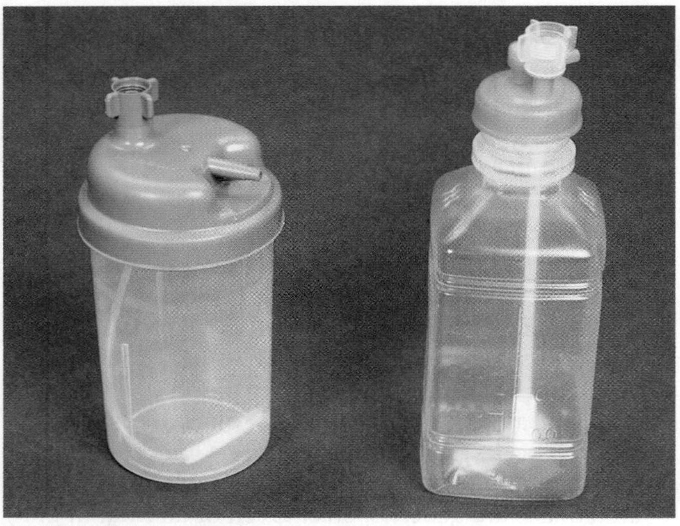

FIGURE 10-40 ✻ An oxygen humidifier.

oxygen leaving the regulator is forced through the water in the humidifier, picking up moisture before exiting and being delivered to the patient. Disposable humidifiers are available for one-time use.

For short periods, it is not harmful to deliver dry oxygen to the patient. Generally, a humidifier is not needed for prehospital administration of oxygen. If oxygen is to be delivered over a long period, as in a transport of an hour or more, a humidifier should be considered. Humidified oxygen is recommended in asthma patients.

Indications for Oxygen Use

Oxygen is actually a drug. Like other drugs, there are recognized indications for its use:

- Any patient in cardiac arrest or respiratory arrest (100 percent oxygen, or as close to 100 percent as possible, attached to a ventilation device)
- Any patient who is being ventilated via positive pressure ventilation
- Any signs of hypoxia in a patient with an adequate respiratory rate and an adequate tidal volume (amount of air breathed in and out)
- Any patient with an SpO_2 reading less than 94 to 95%, depending on the condition.
- Medical conditions that may cause hypoxia to cells or organs, such as stroke, heart attack, drug overdose, toxic inhalation, suffocation, foreign body airway obstruction, drowning, asthma attack, allergic reaction, seizures, poisoning, and environmental emergencies where the patient is exhibiting signs and symptoms of hypoxia, shock or heart failure, or complains of dyspnea.
- Any patient with an altered mental status or who is unresponsive
- Injuries to any body cavity or central nervous system component, including head, spine, chest, abdomen, and pelvis
- Multiple fractures and multiple soft tissue injuries
- Severe bleeding that is either external or internal
- Any evidence of hypoperfusion (shock)
- Exposure to toxins e.g., carbon monoxide, cyanide

If there is any doubt, it is better to err on the side of benefiting the patient and deliver the oxygen. Never withhold oxygen from a patient who you think may need it.

Should the oxygen be supplied via a mask or nasal cannula, relying on the patient's own breathing effort to take the oxygen into the body—or should the oxygen be supplied in conjunction with positive pressure ventilation to force the oxygen into the patient's lungs? *Be sure to carefully assess the patient to determine the breathing status prior to making this decision.* It is necessary to determine *both* that the respiratory rate is adequate *and* that the tidal volume (amount of air breathed in with each inhalation) is adequate in order to apply oxygen by mask or cannula. If *either* the respiratory rate *or* the tidal volume is inadequate, immediately begin positive pressure ventilation with oxygen flowing at 15 lpm to the ventilation device.

To assess tidal volume, look at chest rise and fall and listen and feel for air movement from the nose and mouth. If the chest does not appear to be rising and falling adequately or the air movement from the nose and mouth is minimal (shallow breathing), immediately begin positive pressure ventilation. Administration of oxygen by mask or nasal cannula will not provide the tidal volume necessary to get the oxygen to the alveoli for gas exchange. The patient will remain hypoxic and become more hypoxic. Likewise, if the respiratory rate is inadequate, oxygen administration by nasal cannula or mask will not provide an adequate tidal volume nor rate per minute that will reverse or prevent hypoxia. This patient will also need to be ventilated.

Determining whether to ventilate or apply oxygen by a mask or nasal cannula is a critical decision that could alter the outcome for the patient. Always closely assess the patient and be aggressive in management of the airway and ventilation status. Do not withhold ventilation from a patient with inadequate breathing, thinking that the oxygen flowing from an oxygen mask will provide an equal benefit. In many cases, the oxygen provided by mask or cannula will have no benefit, and the patient will continue to deteriorate.

Always err to benefit the patient.

Hazards of Oxygen Administration

Oxygen administration is clearly indicated in a large number of patients you will be called upon to treat. However, oxygen therapy also carries hazards or risks. As mentioned earlier, oxygen is a drug. The following are hazards of oxygen administration:

- Oxygen toxicity is a rare event in the prehospital environment. However, if you are called to transport a patient to another facility, it may be necessary to use a low-concentration delivery device for a patient who has been on oxygen for a long period of time. Oxygen toxicity may cause the alveoli in the lungs to collapse, reducing the function of the lungs, and may lead to seizures.

- Damage to the retina of the eye through scar tissue formation may occur in premature newborns with excessive oxygen administration. This is not usually a major consideration in the prehospital environment, and oxygen must never be withheld from an infant with any signs of hypoxia or inadequate breathing. However, if you are on a team transporting a premature newborn to another facility, calling for a longer period of oxygen administration, potential oxygen toxicity may be a consideration.
- Respiratory depression or respiratory arrest in patients with COPD (emphysema and chronic bronchitis) may occur from administration of high-concentration oxygen. In COPD patients, the body responds to low oxygen levels in the blood as a stimulus to breathe. It was originally thought that raising the oxygen level considerably in such a patient would lead to a quick depression of the respiratory status. (This is unlike a typical person, whose body uses the level of carbon dioxide in the blood, rather than the level of oxygen, to regulate respiration.)

    However, it has been discovered that it takes a longer period of time on high-concentration oxygen to "knock out" the COPD patient's low oxygen drive, known as hypoxic drive, than is normally encountered in the prehospital environment. Thus, never withhold oxygen from a COPD patient who is displaying any signs of hypoxia or who is suffering from respiratory failure or arrest. Again, this may be a consideration in a transport of a patient with a history of COPD from a facility where the patient has been on oxygen for a long period of time. It is usually necessary to deliver lower concentrations of oxygen to this patient, based on the physician's advice. Monitor the patient closely and be prepared to assist ventilations.

Oxygen Administration Procedures

To administer oxygen to a patient, it is necessary to prepare the oxygen tank and regulator. The oxygen system should be full and ready for patient use. However, in some situations, the tank must be changed and the regulator reattached. Follow the guidelines listed next when initiating oxygen administration (EMT Skills 10-6). Before administering oxygen, explain to the patient why the oxygen is needed, how it is to be administered, and how the oxygen delivery device will fit on the patient.

1. Check the cylinder to be sure it contains oxygen. Remove the protective seal on the tank valve.
2. Quickly open, then shut, the cylinder valve for 1 second to remove any dust or debris from the valve assembly.
3. Place the yoke of the therapy regulator over the valve and align the pins. Be sure the regulator washer is present and in the proper place. Hand-tighten the T-screw on the regulator.
4. Slowly open the main cylinder valve about one-half turn to charge the regulator. Check the pressure gauge to be sure an adequate amount of oxygen is available.
5. Attach the oxygen mask or nasal cannula tubing to the nipple of the regulator.
6. Open the flowmeter control. Set the oxygen flow rate at the desired liters per minute.
7. With the oxygen flowing, apply the oxygen mask or nasal cannula to the patient.

Terminating Oxygen Therapy

Follow these steps to terminate oxygen administration:

1. Remove the mask or cannula from the patient.
2. Turn off the oxygen regulator flowmeter control, then turn off the cylinder valve.
3. Open the regulator valve to allow the oxygen trapped in the regulator to escape until the pressure gauge reads zero. Turn the regulator flowmeter control completely off.

Transferring the Oxygen Source: Portable to On-Board

When switching over from a portable oxygen tank to the on-board oxygen source, do not disconnect the oxygen tubing from the regulator while the mask is still on the patient's face. Instead, remove the mask from the patient's face before attempting to switch over. The oxygen tubing can easily become caught in sheets, blankets, straps, or other equipment and may require a few minutes to untangle. During this time, if no oxygen is flowing to the mask, the patient's tidal volume and blood oxygen content will be drastically reduced. Do not inadvertently cause the patient to become hypoxic while switching oxygen sources. Once the oxygen has been reconnected and is flowing, reapply the mask to the patient's face.

Oxygen Delivery Equipment

A variety of oxygen delivery devices can be used to deliver supplemental oxygen to the patient. The two primary devices used in the prehospital setting are the nonrebreather mask and the nasal cannula. Other devices that you may encounter or use are the simple face mask, partial rebreather mask, Venturi mask, and tracheostomy mask.

Nonrebreather Mask

The preferred method for delivering oxygen in the prehospital setting when a high concentration is desirable is with

Objective 10-33
Discuss the administration of oxygen by nonrebreather mask, nasal cannula, simple face mask, partial rebreather mask, Venturi mask, and tracheostomy mask.

Thinking Critically
Your patient is a teenager with a possible rib fracture. The pain is forcing her to breathe shallowly. You approach her with a nonrebreather mask and she freaks out, saying it will "smother me." How would you proceed?

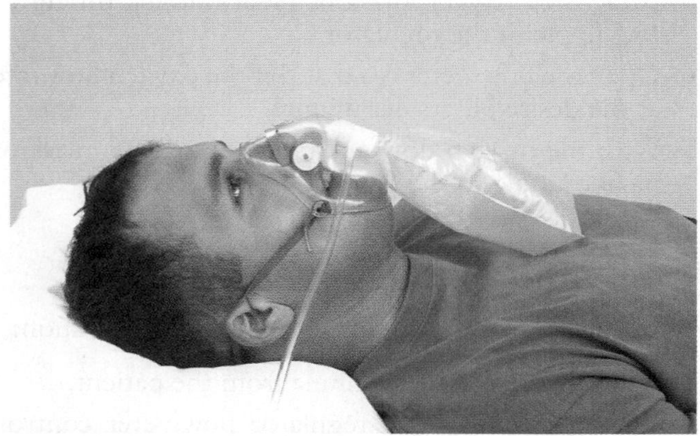

FIGURE 10-41a * Nonrebreather mask.

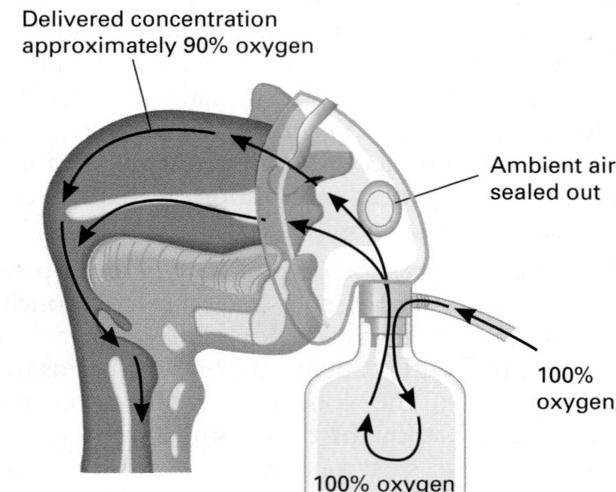

FIGURE 10-41b * Cutaway view of nonrebreather mask.

a **nonrebreather mask** (Figures 10-41a and 10-41b*). This device has an oxygen reservoir bag attached to the mask with a one-way valve between them that prevents the patient's exhaled air from mixing with the oxygen in the reservoir. The mask also has rubber washers that cover the exhalation ports. This allows air to escape on exhalation but restricts air to flow in the exhalation ports during inhalation. With each inhalation, the patient draws in the contents of the reservoir bag, which is 100 percent oxygen. Because some ambient air is inhaled from around the edges of the mask, the oxygen concentration actually delivered is usually around 90 percent.

The flow from the oxygen cylinder should be set at a rate that prevents the reservoir bag from collapsing when the patient inhales. Most typically, this is 15 lpm. Inflate the reservoir bag completely before applying it to the patient.

ASSESSMENT Tips

A poorly inflated nonrebreather mask reservoir may cause a decrease in the patient's tidal volume and worsen the patient's ventilation and oxygenation status. ■

Various size nonrebreather masks are available for infants, children, and adults. Select the correct size mask to ensure that maximum oxygen concentration is being delivered.

Most adult patients tolerate the nonrebreather mask well. However, it is restrictive and not tolerated well by infants, children, and some adults. Some patients feel as if they cannot breathe adequately with the device on. You may need to coach the patient to breathe at a normal rate and depth and provide reassurance that he is getting a sufficient amount of oxygen and air. If an infant or small child does not tolerate the mask, either you, a parent, or someone else familiar with the child can hold the mask close to his face, enriching the air he inspires.

Applying the Nonrebreather Mask To apply the nonrebreather mask:

1. Explain to the patient that you are going to apply oxygen through a mask. Reassure him that he will be getting an increased amount of oxygen and instruct him to breathe normally.
2. Select the appropriate-sized mask. Prepare the oxygen tank and set the regulator at 15 lpm. Connect the nonrebreather tubing to the regulator. Fill the reservoir bag completely. You may need to press down on the rubber valve gasket found covering the one-way valve between the mask and the reservoir. This will cause the reservoir bag to fill much faster.
3. Once the reservoir is completely inflated, fit the mask to the patient's face. Bring the elastic strap around the back of the head and secure it. Form the soft metal piece at the top of the mask to conform with the nose.
4. Constantly monitor the reservoir bag to ensure that it remains filled during inhalation.

Nasal Cannula

An alternative oxygen delivery device is a **nasal cannula.** It provides a very limited oxygen concentration ranging from approximately 24 to 44 percent. The main indication for its use is a patient who is not able to tolerate a nonrebreather mask, despite coaching and reassurance from the EMT, and a patient who requires a low concentration of supplemental oxygen.

The nasal cannula consists of two soft plastic tips, commonly referred to as nasal prongs, that are connected by thin tubing to the main oxygen source (Figures 10-42a and 10-42b*). The nasal prongs are inserted a short distance into the nostrils. The nasal cannula is a "low-flow" system that does not supply enough oxygen to provide the entire tidal volume during inspiration. Therefore, a large portion of the patient's inhalation consists of ambient air that is mixed with the oxygen supplied by the nasal cannula. This significantly reduces the concentration of oxygen delivered by the device. As a general rule, for every liter per minute of flow delivered, the oxygen concentration the patient inhales increases by 4 percent. *The liter flow for the nasal cannula should be set at no less than 1 lpm and no greater than 6 lpm.* Thus, the delivered oxygen concentration ranges from 24 to 44 percent.

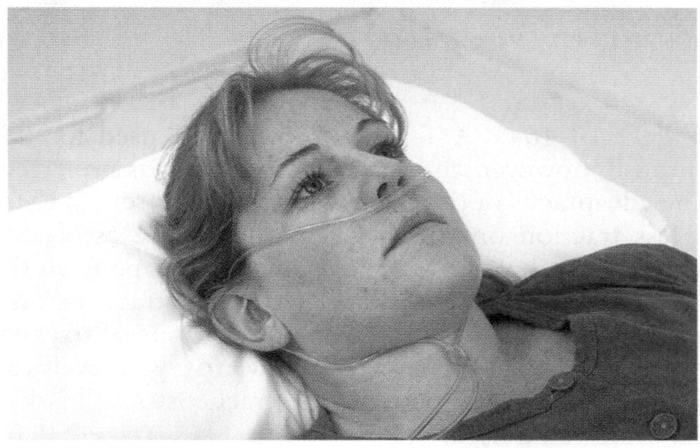

FIGURE 10-42a * Nasal cannula.

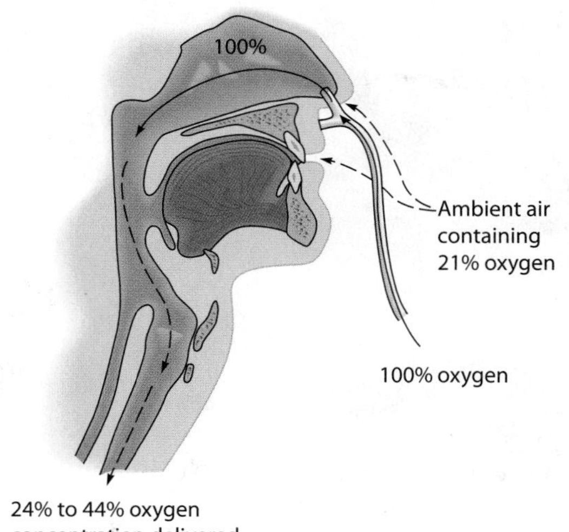

FIGURE 10-42b * Cutaway view of nasal cannula.

Applying the Nasal Cannula Follow these procedures when using the nasal cannula:

1. Explain to the patient that the oxygen will be delivered through the prongs that will fit in each nostril. Instruct the patient to breathe normally while the prongs are in place.
2. Prepare the oxygen tank and regulator. Connect the nasal cannula tubing to the regulator and set the liter flow between 4 and 6 lpm or according to your local protocol or medical direction.
3. Insert the two prongs of the cannula into the patient's nostrils with the tab facing down. Make sure that the prongs curve downward.
4. Position the tubing over and behind each ear. Gently secure it by sliding the adjuster underneath the chin. Do not make the tubing too tight. If an elastic strap is used, adjust it so it is secure and comfortable.
5. Check the cannula position periodically to ensure that it has not dislodged.

Other Oxygen Delivery Devices

The following devices are also used to deliver oxygen to the patient.

Simple Face Mask A simple face mask has no reservoir and can deliver up to 60 percent oxygen, depending on the patient's tidal volume and the oxygen flow rate (Figure 10-43*). Exhaled air exits through the holes on each side of the mask. Air is drawn in through the holes in the side of the mask, diluting the oxygen concentration being delivered. The oxygen flow rate is usually set at 10 lpm but must not be set at less than 6 lpm. Because it

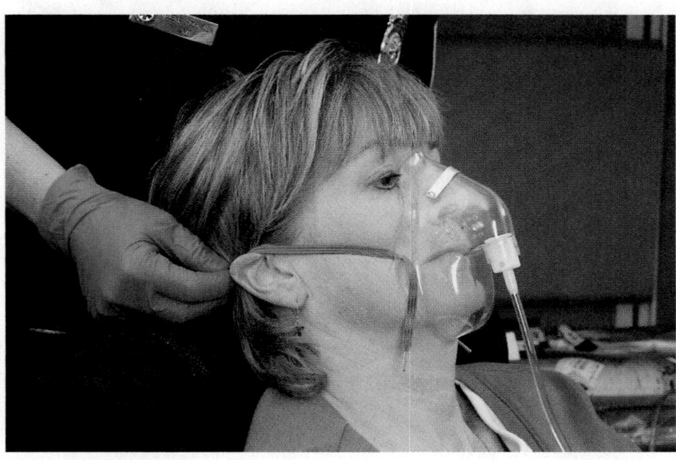

FIGURE 10-43 * Simple face mask.

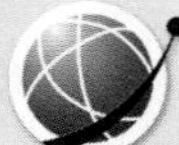

Media Resources
Go to www.bradybooks.com for mykit. Highlights:

- *Video:* Two-person BVM Technique
- *Video:* Oxygen Delivery Devices
- *Video:* Pulse Oximetry

does not deliver as high a concentration of oxygen as the nonrebreather mask, it is not recommended for prehospital use.

Partial Rebreather Mask The partial rebreather mask looks very similar to the nonrebreather mask but is equipped with a two-way valve that allows the patient to rebreathe about one-third of his exhaled air (Figure 10-44*). Since the initial portion of exhaled air is principally from the patient's dead space, areas of the respiratory system where gas exchange does not occur, it contains mostly oxygen-enriched air from the previous inhalation. The flow rate is typically set at 10 lpm but should be no less than 6 lpm. Partial rebreather masks can provide oxygen concentrations of between 35 and 60 percent.

Venturi Mask The Venturi mask is a low-flow oxygen system that provides precise concentrations of oxygen through an entrainment valve connected to the face mask (Figure 10-45*). The entrainment valve can be changed to deliver precise oxygen concentrations at preset flow rates. This mask is commonly used for a patient with a history of COPD because of its ability to deliver a precise concentration of oxygen.

Tracheostomy Mask The tracheostomy mask is used to deliver aerosolized medication, bland aerosol therapy, or oxygen to a patient with a tracheostomy tube (Figure 10-46*). A T-tube is commonly used for this purpose; however, the tracheostomy mask is preferred. The advantages of the tracheostomy mask are: (1) there is less traction on the airway from pulling associated with the T-tube, and (2) secretions can escape from the tube. The main disadvantage is that the tracheostomy mask will deliver only lower concentrations of oxygen, typically less than 50 percent. If lower oxygen levels can be tolerated by the patient, the tracheostomy mask is the preferred device.

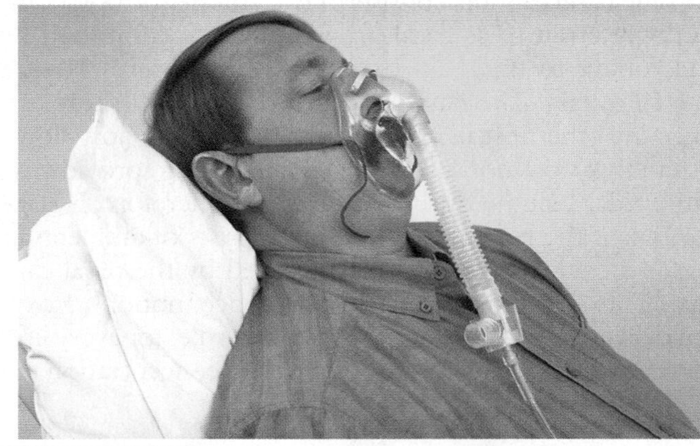

FIGURE 10-45 * Venturi mask.

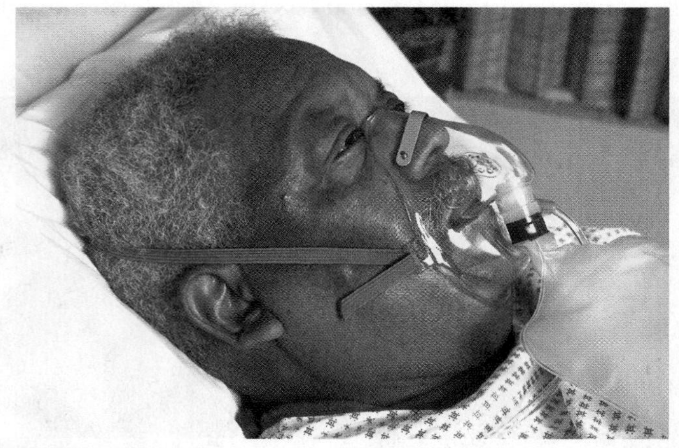

FIGURE 10-44 * Partial rebreather mask.

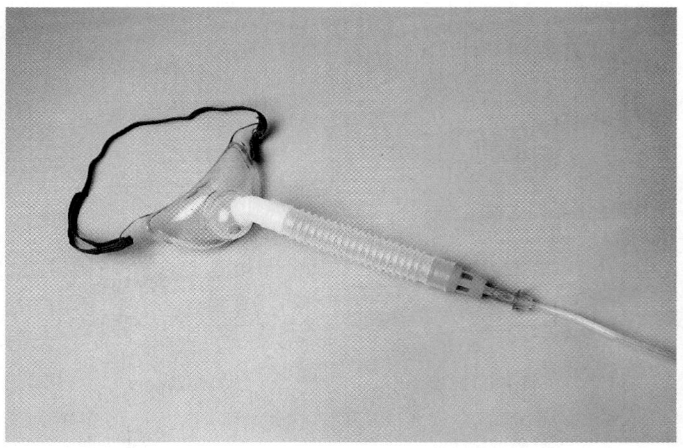

FIGURE 10-46 * Tracheostomy mask. (© Carl Leet)

EMT skills 10-1 Suctioning Technique

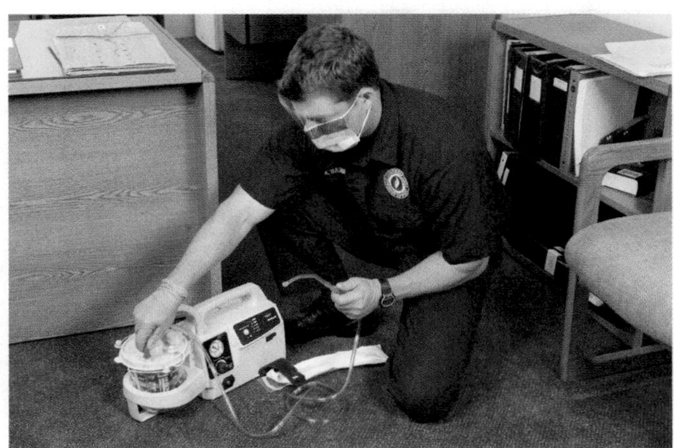
10-1A * Make sure the suction unit is properly assembled.

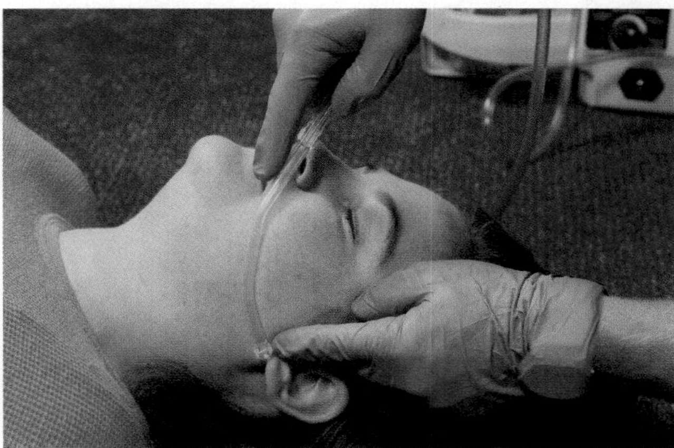
10-1B * Measure the catheter from the corner of the mouth to the earlobe.

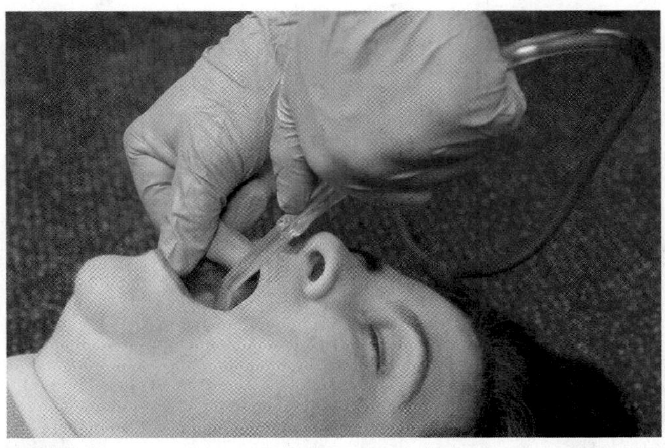
10-1C * Open the patient's mouth and insert the catheter.

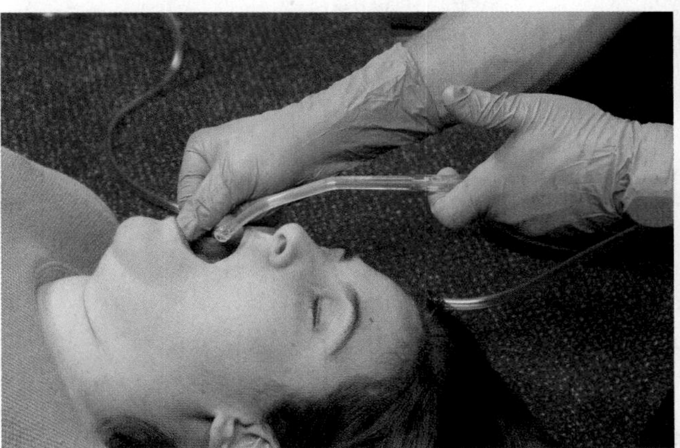
10-1D * Apply suction as you withdraw the catheter.

EMT skills 10-2 Inserting an Oropharyngeal Airway

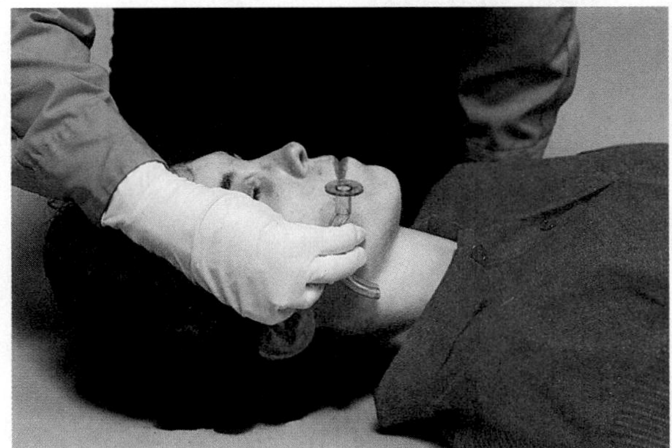
10-2A * Measure to ensure correct size.

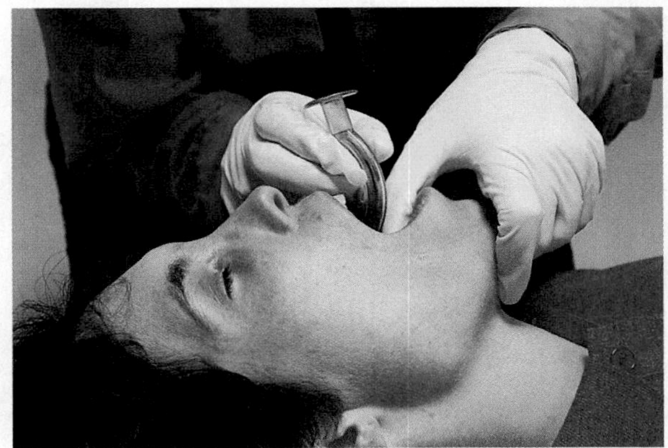
10-2B * Insert with tip pointing up toward roof of mouth.

continued

EMT skills 10-2 Inserting an Oropharyngeal Airway *continued*

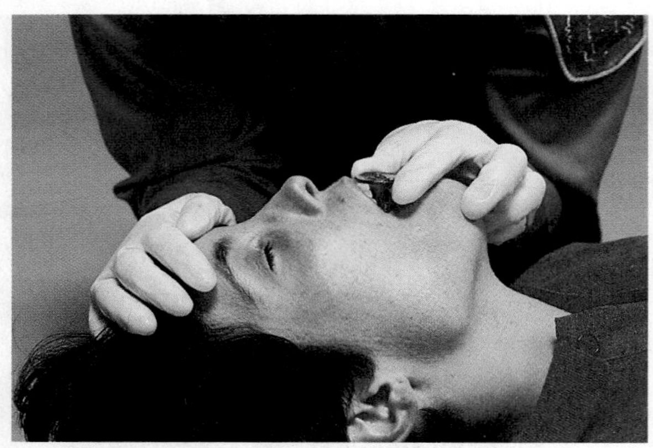

10-2C ✱ Advance while rotating 180°.

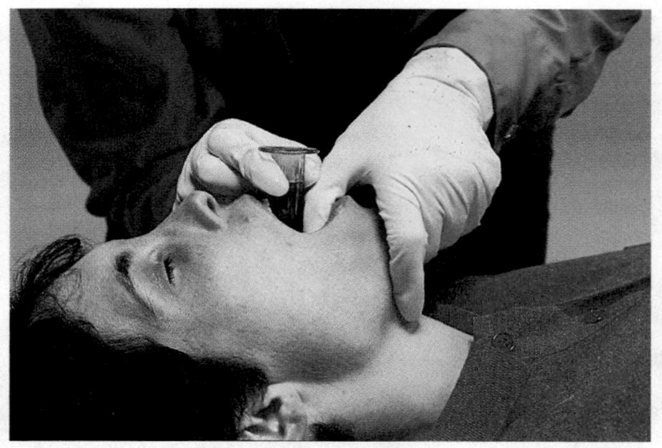

10-2D ✱ Continue until flange rests on the teeth.

EMT skills 10-3 Inserting a Nasopharyngeal Airway

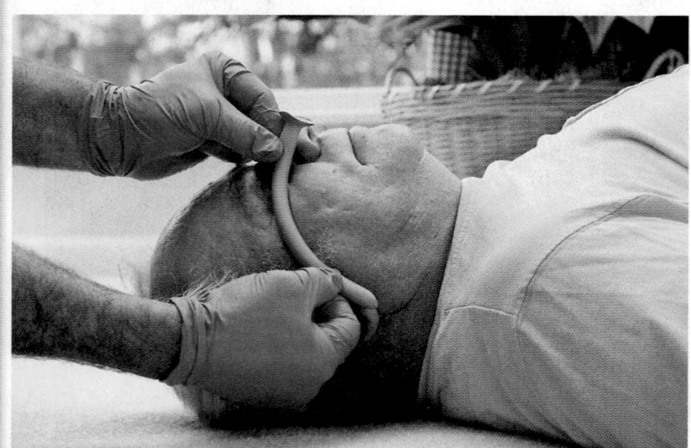

10-3A ✱ Measuring the nasopharyngeal airway.

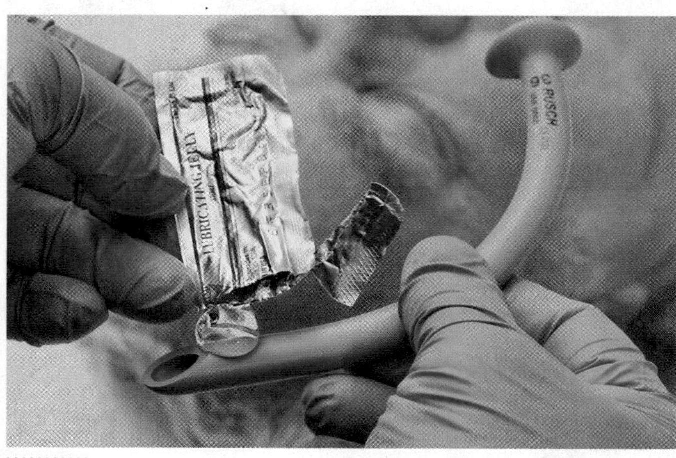

10-3B ✱ Lubricate it with water-soluble lubricant.

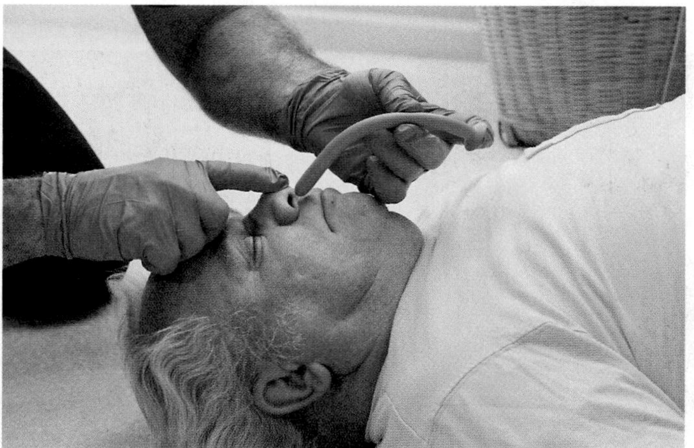

10-3C ✱ Insert with the bevel toward the septum or base of the tonsil.

EMT skills 10-4 Patient Has Breathing Difficulty: When and How to Intervene

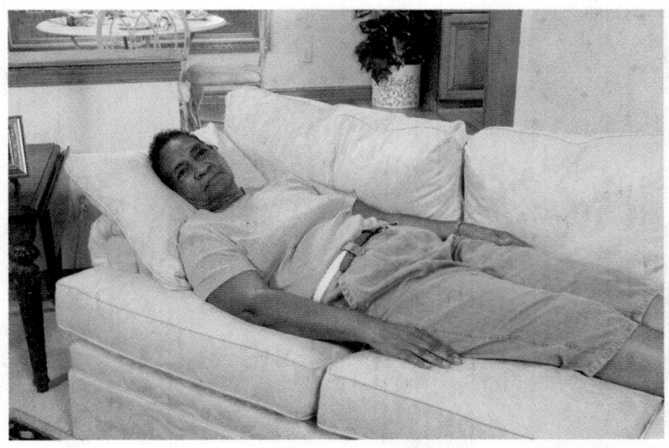

10-4A ✱ The patient is breathing normally but has an underlying condition that requires oxygen.

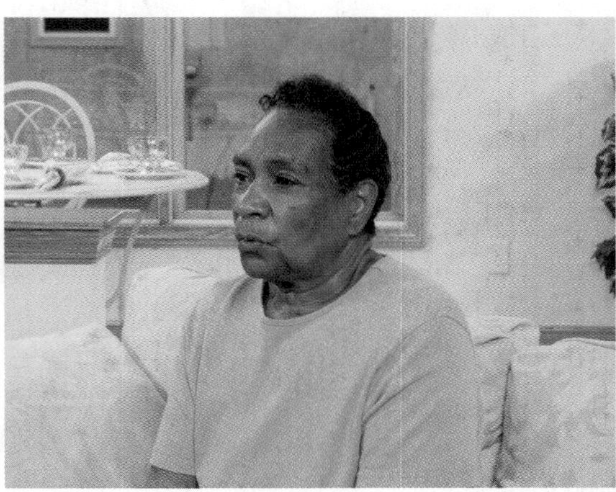

10-4B ✱ The patient is suffering mild respiratory distress but still breathing with an adequate rate and tidal volume.

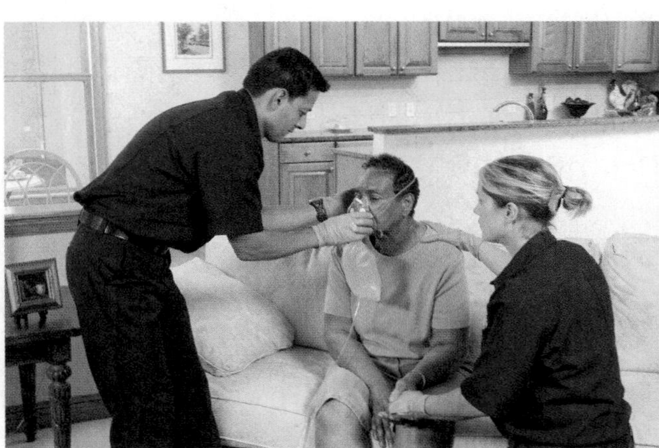

10-4C ✱ The EMT places a nonrebreather mask on the patient and administers high-concentration oxygen.

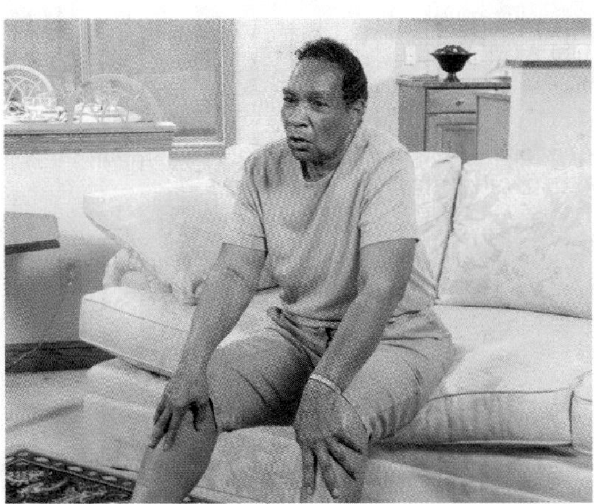

10-4D ✱ The patient is suffering respiratory failure with rapid ventilations and inadequate tidal volume.

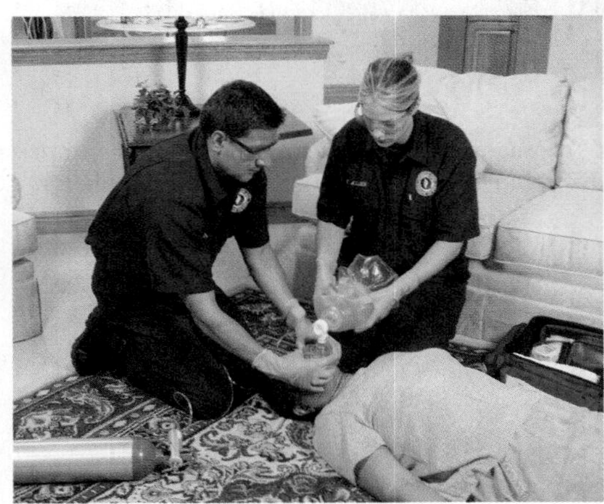

10-4E ✱ The EMTs administer positive pressure ventilation.

continued

EMT skills 10-4 Patient Has Breathing Difficulty: When and How to Intervene *continued*

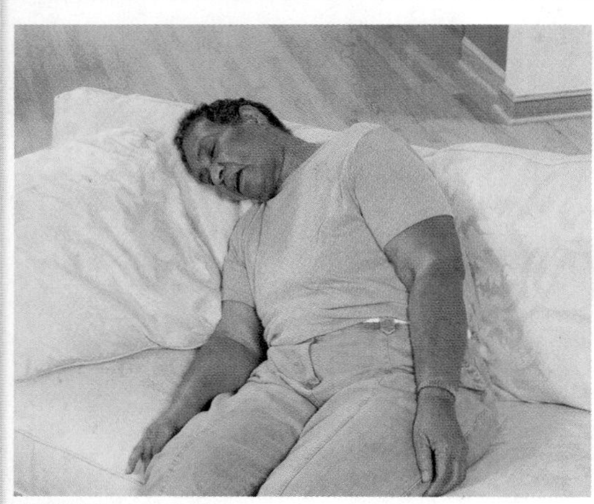

10-4F * The patient is in severe respiratory failure with completely inadequate respirations.

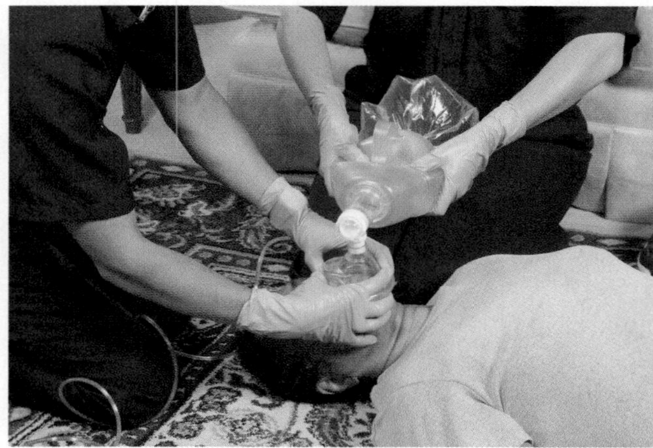

10-4G * The EMTs administer positive pressure ventilation.

EMT skills 10-5 In-Line Stabilization During Bag-Valve Ventilation

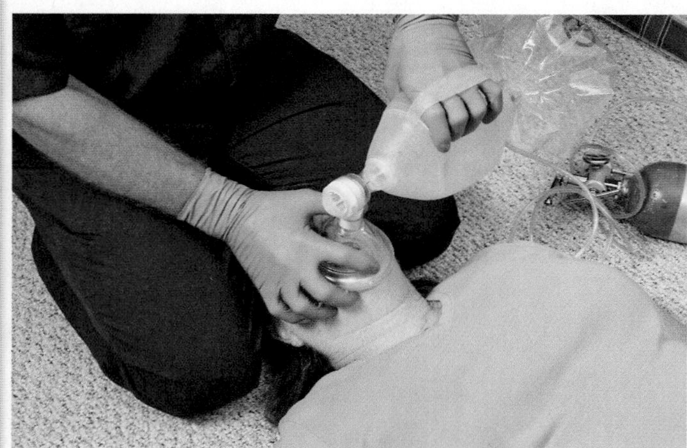

10-5A * Technique for one EMT to maintain in-line stabilization while performing one-person bag-valve-mask ventilation.

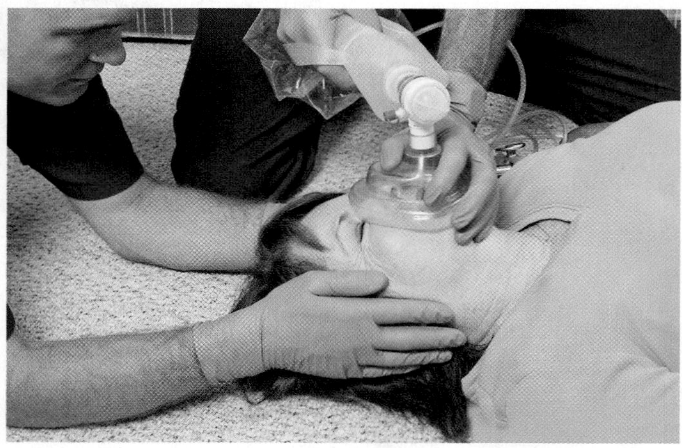

10-5B * Technique for two EMTs to maintain in-line stabilization while performing bag-valve-mask ventilation.

EMT skills 10-5 In-Line Stabilization During Bag-Valve Ventilation *continued*

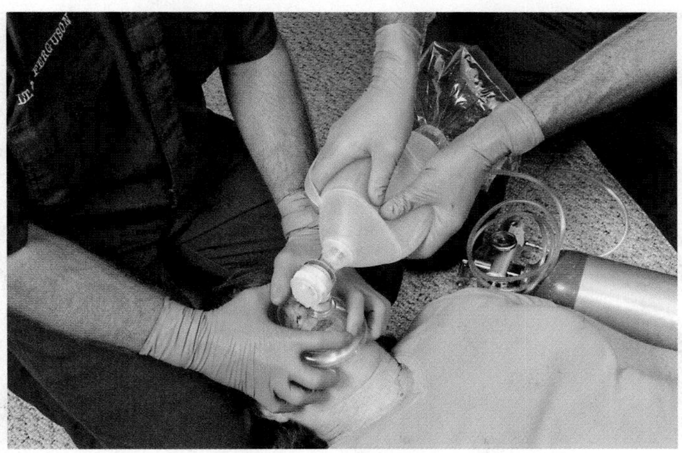

10-5C ✱ Alternative technique for two EMTs to maintain in-line stabilization while performing bag-valve-mask ventilation.

EMT skills 10-6 Initiating Oxygen Administration

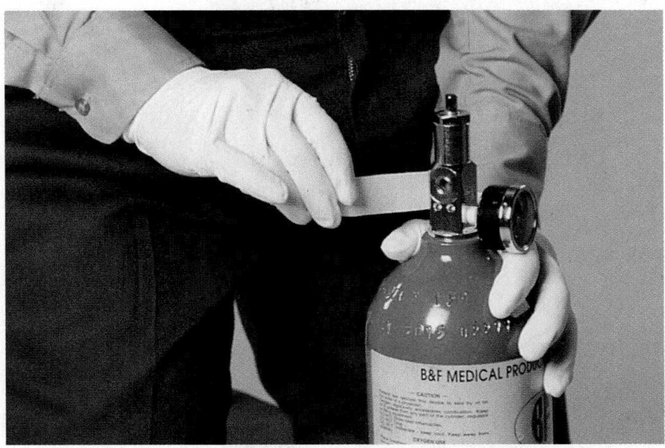

10-6A ✱ Identify the cylinder as oxygen and remove the protective seal.

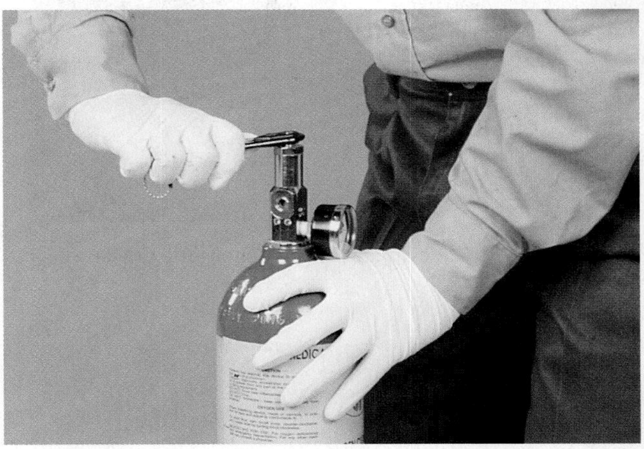

10-6B ✱ Crack the main cylinder for 1 second to remove dust and debris.

continued

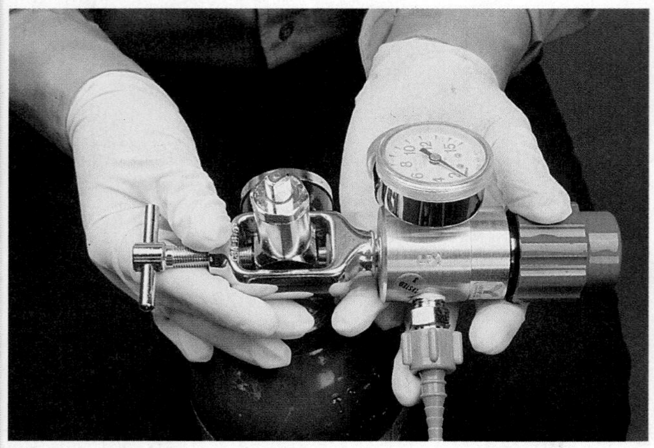

10-6C ✱ Place the yoke of the regulator over the cylinder valve and align the pins.

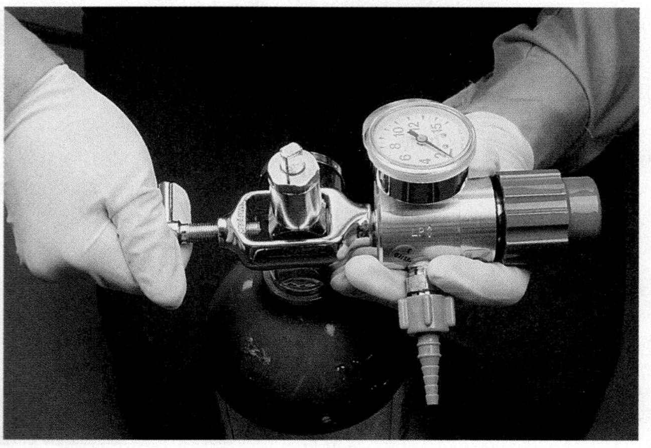

10-6D ✱ Hand-tighten the T-screw on the regulator.

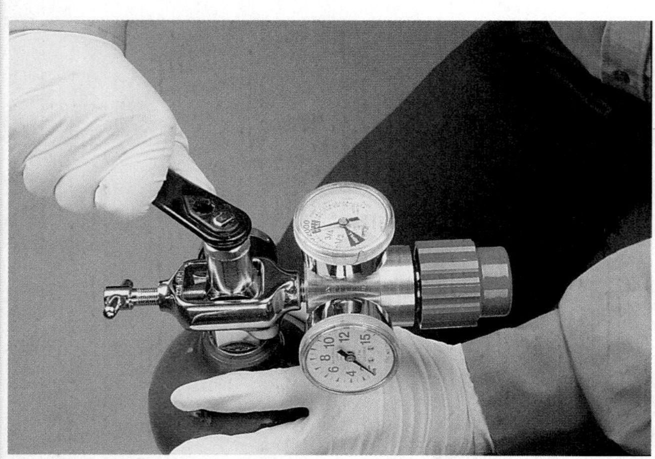

10-6E ✱ Open the main cylinder valve to check the pressure.

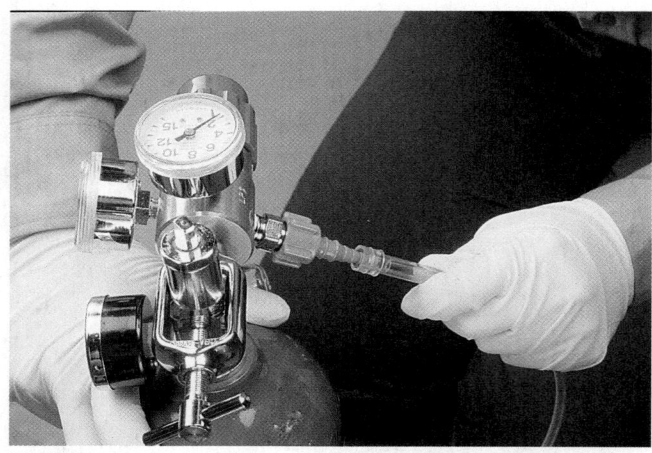

10-6F ✱ Attach the oxygen delivery device to the regulator.

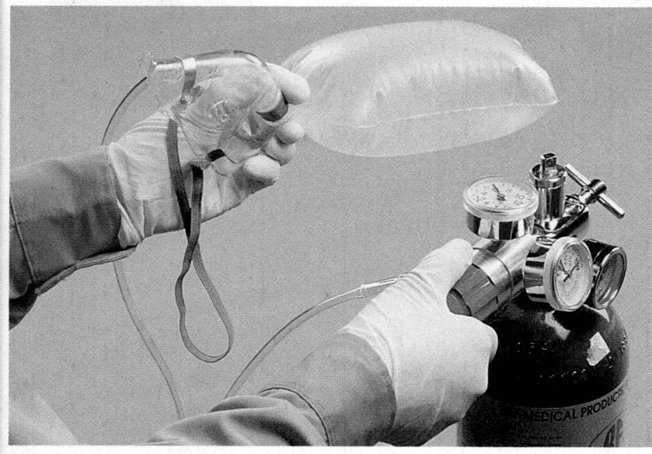

10-6G ✱ Adjust the flowmeter to the appropriate liter flow.

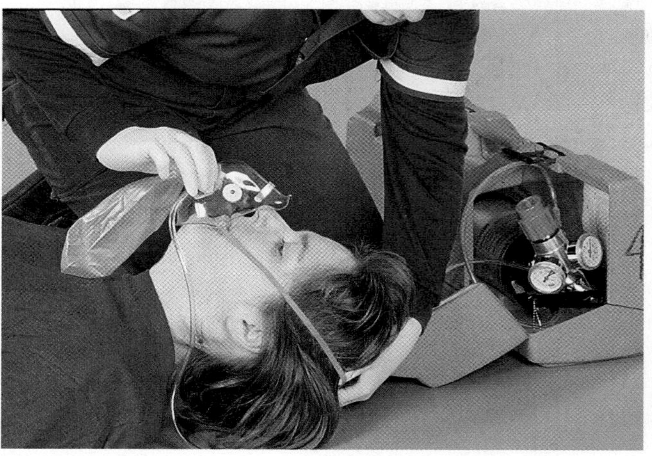

10-6H ✱ Apply an oxygen device to the patient.

CHAPTER REVIEW

SUMMARY

Without an adequate airway, oxygenation, or ventilation, all other emergency care provided to the patient will be futile. The most basic and fundamental care provided to all patients focuses on establishing and maintaining a patent airway and providing adequate ventilation and oxygenation. A foundation of knowledge of airway and respiratory anatomy and physiology will help you achieve a better understanding of the signs and symptoms and the emergency care related to these systems.

Assessment of the airway, oxygenation, and ventilation status occurs very early in your patient contact. Each of these is a separate and distinct component. Assessing or managing one component—airway, oxygenation, or ventilation—does not necessarily mean that the other components will be assessed or managed effectively. As an example, a patient can have an open airway but ineffective ventilation, or adequate ventilation but ineffective oxygenation. Thus, it is imperative to become highly efficient in the assessment of all three components and remain vigilant of any changes in their status.

A closed airway is opened using either the head-tilt, chin-lift maneuver or the jaw-thrust maneuver. The head-tilt, chin-lift maneuver is performed on patients who do not have any suspected spinal injury, whereas the jaw-thrust maneuver is used to open the airway in a patient who has a suspected spinal injury while maintaining manual in-line spinal stabilization. Airway adjuncts can be used to assist in establishing and maintaining an airway. The oropharyngeal airway can be inserted only in patients who have no gag reflex. The nasopharyngeal airway can be used in patients who still have a slight gag reflex. Suctioning may be needed to clear an airway of blood, vomitus, secretions, or other obstructions.

Once the airway is established, the ventilation status is assessed. If the patient has inadequate breathing, he must be immediately ventilated using a pocket mask, bag-valve-mask device, or flow-restricted, oxygen-powered ventilation device. Some systems use automatic transport ventilators once the need for prolonged ventilation has been established.

Oxygen therapy is used to reduce, eliminate, or prevent hypoxia from occurring in the patient. The oxygen status is often assessed through the use of a pulse oximeter. Oxygen may be delivered through the ventilation device or by a nonrebreather mask or nasal cannula. The nonrebreather mask delivers the highest concentration of oxygen, and thus it is the preferred device for EMTs in the prehospital setting.

When assessing and managing the airway, ventilation, and oxygenation, you must also be aware of special circumstances or patient conditions that may provide challenges, such as a patient with a stoma or tracheostomy tube, infants and children, facial injuries, foreign body obstruction, and dental appliances.

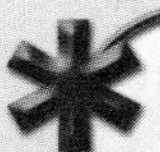

CASE STUDY FOLLOW-UP

SCENE SIZE-UP

You and your partner have been dispatched to the Twilight Bar for an unresponsive male patient. Because the bar is frequently the site of fights, stabbings, and shootings, you approach the scene cautiously. You contact dispatch to inquire as to whether the unresponsive patient was involved in some type of altercation. Dispatch informs you that the patient is thought to be unresponsive because of drinking heavily.

As you enter the bar, it is dark and hard to see. You turn on your flashlight and weave your way around the patrons, tables, and bar stools. You continuously scan the scene for any indication of hazards to you and your partner. You finally make your way to the bar and ask the bartender, "Where is the unresponsive patient?" The bartender says, "Oh, he's in the john." You ask what happened. He replies, "This kid was in here drinking all morning and afternoon. He stumbled to the bathroom. One of the other guys found him passed out in there."

You proceed to the bathroom and cautiously open the door, continuously scanning the scene for any signs of a hazard. You find a male patient about 30 years of age on the floor lying in a puddle of vomit. The scene does not reveal any overt signs of a mechanism of injury, but you are still unsure why the patient is unresponsive. No one at the scene knows his name or has ever seen him before.

PATIENT ASSESSMENT

You instruct your partner to take in-line stabilization. You quickly inspect and palpate the back, and on the count of three, you log roll the patient into a supine position on a backboard. You immediately suction the remaining vomitus out of the mouth and then perform a jaw-thrust maneuver. The patient is not responsive, even to a painful pinch, and has no gag reflex, so you are able to insert an oropharyngeal airway without incident.

The breathing rate is approximately 6 per minute with minimal chest rise on inspiration. The breathing rate and tidal volume is inadequate, so you begin positive pressure ventilation with a bag-valve mask and supplemental oxygen at a rate of 10 ventilations per minute by delivering a ventilation every 6 seconds. There are only two of you to work on the patient, so your partner holds in-line stabilization with her knees and thighs, maintains the jaw thrust and seals the mask to the patient's face with one hand, and squeezes the bag against her side with the other. While she is doing this, you call for a backup and continue with the primary assessment, which reveals a radial pulse that is slow and weak at a rate of about 55 per minute. The skin is pale, cool, and cyanotic. Because the patient is unresponsive and has no gag reflex, he is considered a priority for transport.

Your partner maintains in-line stabilization and continues to ventilate the patient. You quickly begin a physical exam to check the patient's body, starting at the head, for any evidence of injury. There are no signs of trauma to the head or neck. You palpate the posterior cervical region and apply a cervical spinal immobilization collar. You continue by checking the chest, abdomen, pelvis, and extremities (having checked the posterior body) and find no signs of trauma. You obtain a set of baseline vital signs.

Since the patient is unresponsive and there were no witnesses, except the bartender who reported his prolonged drinking, there is no way to get any additional history on the patient.

As you are completing the vital signs, your backup crew arrives, bringing in the stretcher. You completely immobilize the patient to the backboard. One newly arrived EMT establishes a seal on the bag-valve mask and your partner begins two-handed ventilation. You move the patient into the ambulance and begin transport.

En route to the hospital, you pinch the patient's hand and there is still no response. You interrupt ventilation for about 2 seconds to ensure that the airway is clear of vomitus and secretions. Ventilation is continued and the oxygen source is switched over to the on-board tank. You take another set of vital signs and continue with ventilation, monitoring the airway and breathing.

The patient begins to vomit, and you immediately begin to suction as your partner and the other EMT tilt the board, with the patient firmly secured to it, up on its side to help drain the vomitus from the mouth. Once the vomitus is cleared, you continue ventilation. You record the vitals and contact the hospital.

Upon arrival at the hospital, you help transfer the patient to the hospital bed. You report your assessment findings and emergency care to the physician. Once your prehospital care report is completed and the unit is cleaned and restocked, you clear and mark back into service.

IN REVIEW

1. Describe the two manual methods used to open an airway, and explain the circumstances in which each should be used.
2. Name the two airway adjuncts that can be inserted to assist in establishing and maintaining an open airway, and explain the circumstances in which each should be used.
3. Outline the assessment techniques you would use to determine if the patient's breathing is adequate or inadequate.
4. Name the signs of adequate breathing.
5. Name the signs of inadequate breathing.
6. Name the recommended methods that the EMT can use to artificially ventilate the patient.
7. Explain the difference in the technique for ventilation of a patient with and without a suspected spinal injury.
8. List the indications that the patient is being ventilated adequately.
9. Describe the appropriate procedure for initiating oxygen administration.
10. Describe the appropriate procedure for terminating oxygen administration.

CRITICAL THINKING

You arrive on the scene and find a 67-year-old male patient lying supine on the couch in the living room. The family states the patient began complaining of a sudden onset of an extremely severe headache, and then he appeared to be confused and losing consciousness. They laid him on the couch to prevent further injury. The patient is not alert and exhibits flexion posturing when a trapezius pinch is applied. You hear snoring sounds with inhalation and exhalation. His chest is moving minimally with each breath and his respirations are approximately 5–6 per minute. His radial pulse is strong. His heart rate is approximately 50 per minute. His skin is normal color, warm, and dry. Your partner applied a pulse oximeter and it reads 79%.

1. What is the status of the patient's airway?
2. How would you manage the airway in this particular patient?
3. What is the status of his ventilation?
4. What emergency care would you provide to manage the ventilation?
5. What is the oxygenation status of the patient?
6. What intervention would you provide to manage the oxygenation status?

EXPLORE PEARSON **mybradykit**™

Please go to **www.bradybooks.com** to access mykit for this text. You will find quizzes, critical thinking scenarios, weblinks, animations, and videos related to this chapter—and much more. Look for information on effective BVM ventilation as well as a video clip on the two-person BVM technique.

Register your access code from the front of your book by going to **www.bradybooks.com** and selecting the mykit links.

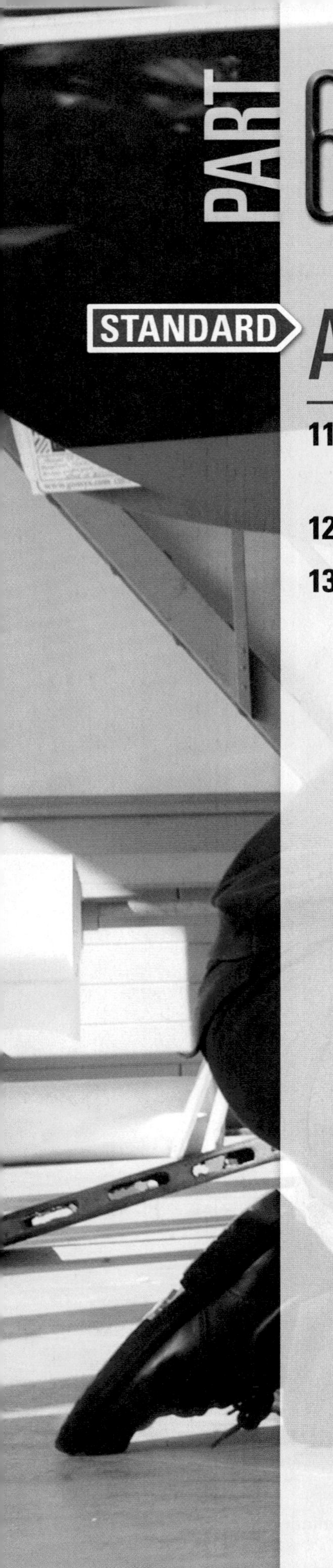

PART 6

STANDARD

Assessment

COMPETENCY

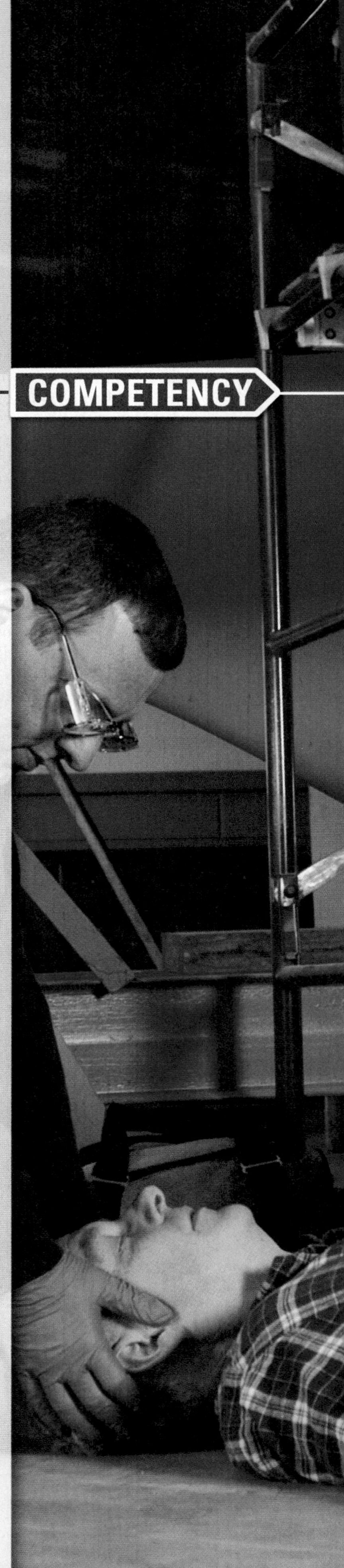

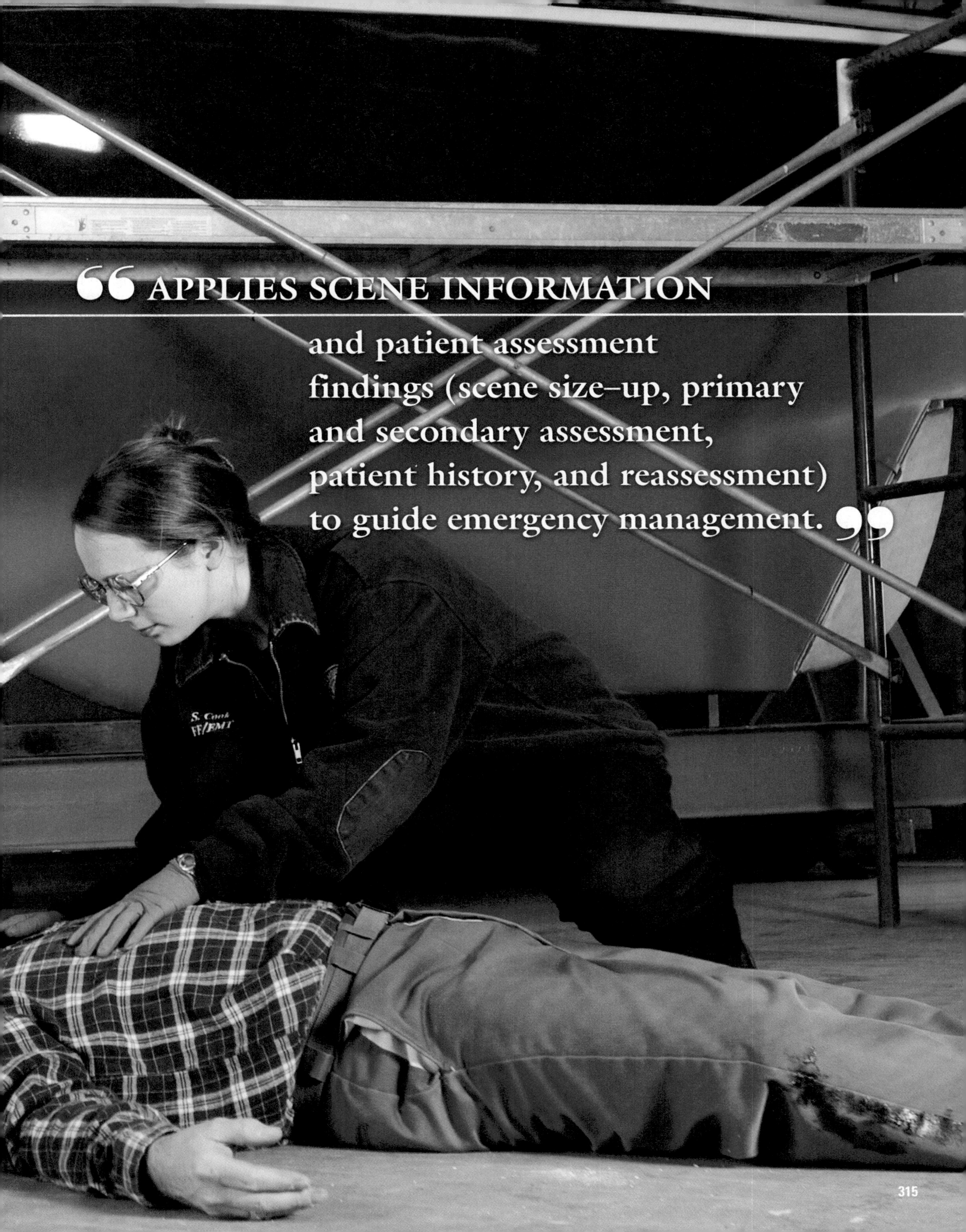
“APPLIES SCENE INFORMATION
and patient assessment
findings (scene size–up, primary
and secondary assessment,
patient history, and reassessment)
to guide emergency management.”
S. Cook
FF/EMT

▶ Components of the Patient Assessment: An Overview

During an emergency call, you will perform certain procedures, known as ***patient assessment***, to find out what is wrong with the patient to help you decide what emergency medical care should be provided and how quickly the patient needs to be transported to a medical facility. As the EMT at the scene, you also become the eyes and ears of all emergency care personnel, since you will have access to the home or other emergency scene and to family and bystanders who will not be available to other health care providers, especially those at the hospital emergency department to whom you will transfer the care of your patient.

Components of Patient Assessment

- Scene size-up
- Primary assessment
- Secondary assessment
- Reassessment

The purposes of patient assessment are described below with, in brackets, the step(s) when each would primarily be accomplished.

- *To determine whether the patient is injured or has a medical illness* [scene size-up; primary assessment]
- *To identify and manage immediately life-threatening injuries or conditions* [primary assessment; as appropriate during secondary assessment]
- *To determine priorities for further assessment and care on the scene vs. immediate transport with assessment and care continuing en route* [primary assessment; as appropriate, throughout the assessment]
- *To further examine the patient and gather a patient history* [secondary assessment]
- *To provide further emergency care based on additional findings* [secondary assessment]
- *To monitor the patient's condition, assessing the effectiveness of the care that has been provided and adjusting care as needed* [reassessment, until the patient is transferred to the receiving facility]

Always remember that each patient's condition is unique—even though the patient may have the same signs and symptoms as another patient you treated previously. It is easy to develop tunnel vision and focus on the patient's chief complaint (the reason that EMS was called), especially if the complaint is dramatic, while failing to determine the entire extent of the patient's condition.

For example, if you find an elderly man lying on the living room floor complaining of excruciating pain to his hip with obvious deformity, you would quickly conclude that the patient must have fallen and injured his hip. Immediate immobilization of the hip, followed by transport to the hospital, might then seem to be the most appropriate care for this patient.

However, it is vital that you question the patient to determine the cause of the fall. If the patient says he fell after tripping on the rug, the apparent hip injury is your primary concern. But suppose the patient tells you he fell because, while crossing the room, he began to suffer severe chest pain and dizziness. You realize that the patient's fall was probably caused by a medical condition, possibly a heart attack. Now your focus has changed. You will deal first with the medical condition, which is potentially more serious than the hip injury. The hip injury, though significant, becomes a secondary priority.

So, you can see that it is necessary to perform a complete assessment on every patient. Immediately focusing in on whatever is obvious or dramatic will often cause the EMT to miss injuries or conditions that are important, even potentially life threatening. No matter how significant—or insignificant—the most obvious complaint or injury may seem, you must be suspicious that other injuries or medical conditions exist that you have not yet found.

Throughout the patient assessment, respect the patient's feelings. Protect his dignity and modesty, explain what you are doing, and—without being dishonest—reassure him that everything is being done to help him.

For a detailed overview of the components of patient assessment and how they apply to different kinds of patients, see the flowchart on the next page. Return to this chart as you read through this module to track the steps of patient assessment you are learning about.

Patient Assessment Flowchart

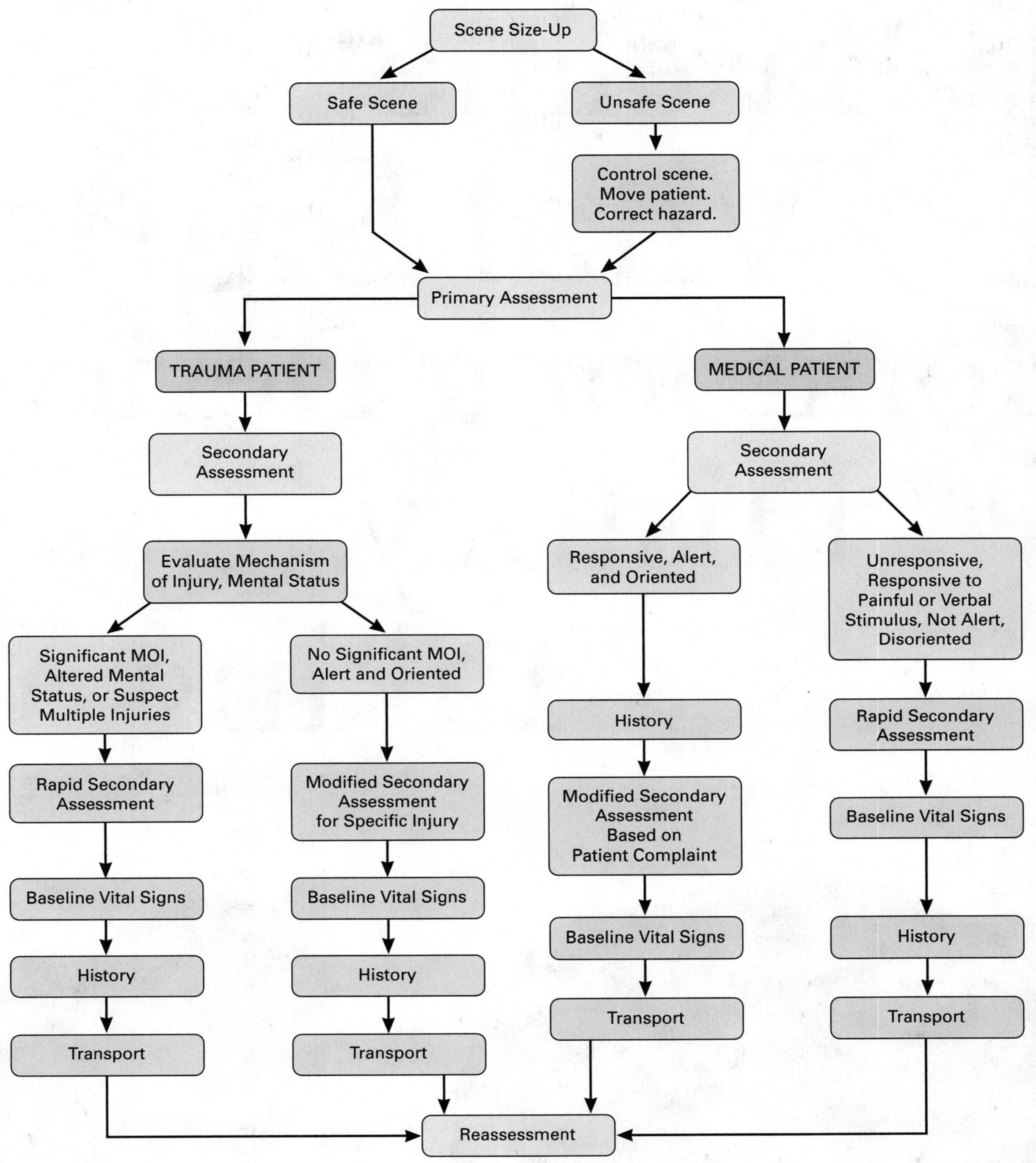

CHAPTER 11

Baseline Vital Signs, Monitoring Devices, and History Taking

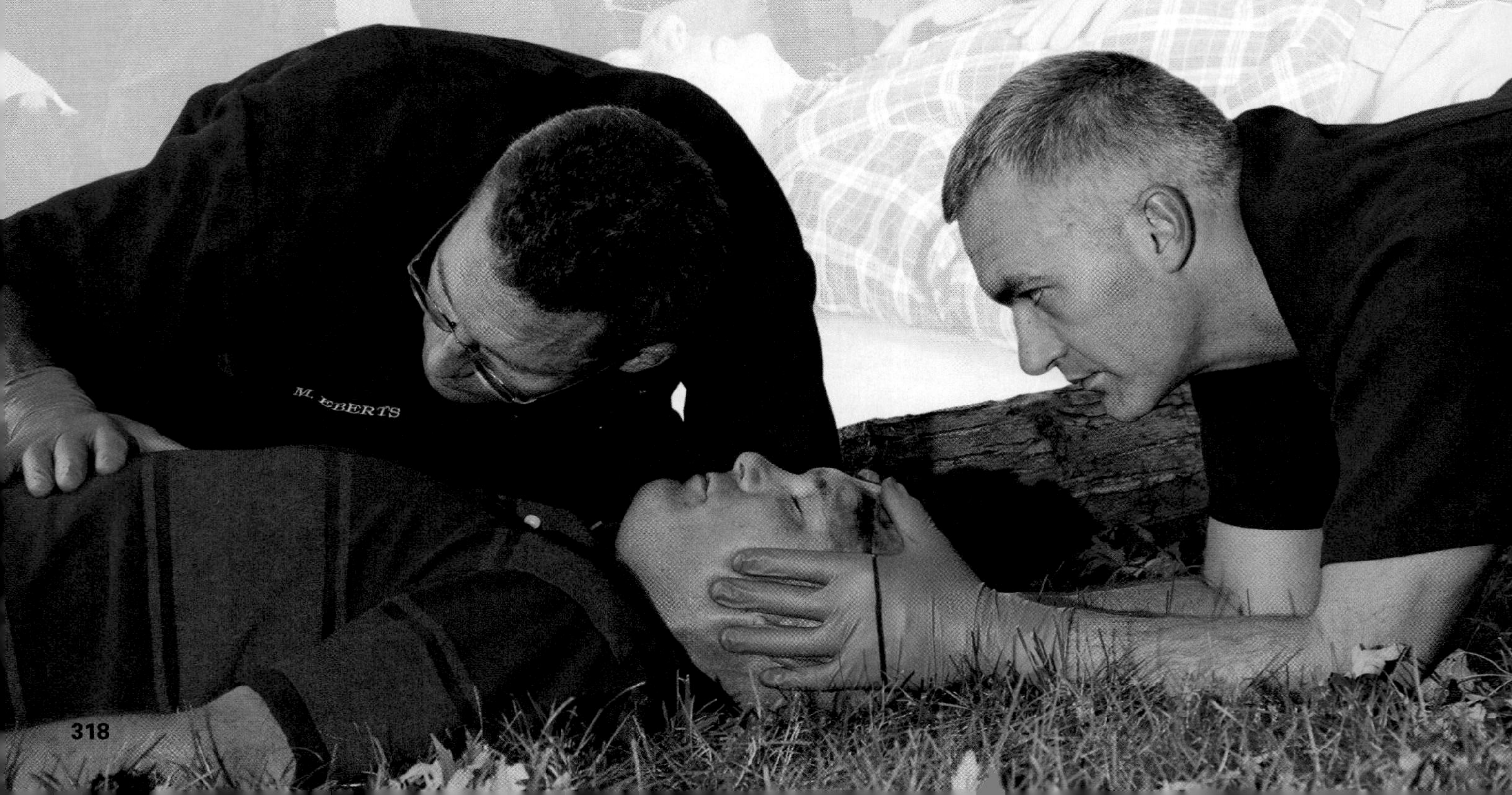

Navigation Guide

The following items provide an overview to the purpose and content of this chapter. The Standard and Competency are from the new National EMS Education Standards.

STANDARD **Assessment** (Content Areas: Secondary Assessment; Monitoring Devices; History Taking)

COMPETENCY Applies scene information and patient assessment findings (scene size-up, primary and secondary assessment, patient history, and reassessment) to guide emergency management.

OBJECTIVES: After reading this chapter, you should be able to:

11-1. Define key terms introduced in this chapter.
11-2. Explain the importance of taking and recording a patient's vital signs over a period of time to identify problems and changes in the patient's condition and of accurately documenting the vital signs and patient history.
11-3. Perform the steps required to assess the patient's breathing, pulse, skin, pupils, blood pressure, and oxygen saturation and consider the patient's overall presentation when interpreting the meaning of vital sign findings.
11-4. Differentiate between normal and abnormal findings when assessing a patient's breathing, to include the respiratory rate, quality of respirations, rhythm of respirations, and signs that may indicate respiratory distress or respiratory failure.
11-5. Differentiate between normal respiratory rates for adults, children, infants, and newborns and evaluate the need to administer treatment based on assessment of a patient's breathing.
11-6. Auscultate breath sounds to determine the presence of breath sounds, equality of breath sounds, and the presence and likely underlying causes of abnormal breath sounds.
11-7. Assess the pulse at various pulse points and consider the patient's age and level of responsiveness when selecting a site to palpate the pulse.
11-8. Differentiate between normal and abnormal findings when assessing a patient's pulse, to include the pulse rate, quality of the pulse, and rhythm of the pulse.
11-9. Associate pulse abnormalities with possible underlying causes and describe the changes in the pulse associated with pulsus paradoxus.
11-10. Recognize normal and abnormal findings in the assessment of skin color, temperature, condition, capillary refill, and color of the mucous membranes and associate abnormal skin findings with potential underlying causes.
11-11. Explain factors that can affect capillary refill findings.
11-12. When assessing the pupils, recognize dilation, constriction, inequality, and abnormal reacitivty and associate abnormal findings with potential underlying causes.
11-13. In relation to blood pressure measurement, explain systolic and diastolic blood pressure, consider normal values for age and gender, find the pulse pressure, and identify potential causes of abnormal findings or changes.
11-14. Compare palpation and auscultation of blood pressure as to processes, useful findings, and documentation and discuss how technique and selection of equipment can affect the accuracy of readings.
11-15. Demonstrate assessment of orthostatic vital signs.
11-16. Given a patient scenario, determine the frequency with which vital signs should be reassessed.
11-17. Explain what pulse oximetry measures, use pulse oximetry to help determine the need for supplemental oxygen, and describe factors and limitations in interpreting pulse oximetry findings.
11-18. Describe the correct procedure for noninvasive blood pressure monitoring.
11-19. Describe the processes for controlling the scene, achieving a smooth transition of care, and reducing the patient's anxiety.
11-20. Determine a patient's chief complaint.
11-21. Given a scenario, efficiently elicit an adequate patient history using closed-ended and open-ended questions and active listening techniques.
11-22. Use the mnemonics SAMPLE and OPQRST to ensure a complete prehospital patient history.
11-23. React appropriately when asking questions about sensitive topics or when caring for patients who present special challenges to history-taking and assessment.

continued

Navigation Guide *continued*

KEY TERMS: Page references indicate first major use in this chapter. For complete definitions, see the Glossary at the back of the book.

auscultation p. 332
bradycardia p. 325
capillary refill p. 328
constricted p. 329
diastolic blood pressure p. 330
dilated p. 329
orthostatic vital signs p. 333
palpation p. 332
pulse oximetry p. 334
pulse pressure p. 331
pulsus paradoxus p. 326
systolic blood pressure p. 330
tachycardia p. 325
vital signs p. 321

MEDIA RESOURCES: Please go to www.bradybooks.com to access mykit for this text. You will find quizzes, critical thinking scenarios, weblinks, animations, and videos related to this chapter—and much more. Look for online information on taking a pulse. You will also find a video clip on vital sign assessment.

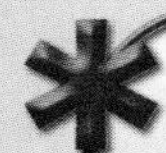

CASE STUDY

The Dispatch

EMS Unit 114—proceed to 1895 East State Street for an unknown medical emergency called in by a family member—time out 1748 hours.

Upon Arrival

Upon arrival a woman approaches you. She says she is the patient's daughter, Ms. Kennedy. She adds that she had been trying to reach her father, Mr. Li, by phone all day, but he had not answered. After driving to her father's house, she says, she broke in and found her father lying on the floor in the kitchen. The daughter adds that Mr. Li seems pretty weak and in pain.

How Would You Proceed to Assess and Care for This Patient?

During this chapter, you will learn about taking vital signs, monitoring devices, and gathering a patient history. Later, we will return to the case and put in context some of the information you learned.

Introduction

Accurate measurement and recording of vital signs over a period of time may reveal critical trends in the patient's condition. The patient history is just as important. It can guide your pace, shine a light on underlying problems, and—if the patient loses consciousness—can be the only source of information important for hospital personnel to know.

As an EMT, you will perform a variety of skills necessary to manage a patient's injuries or illness. There is one skill, however, that you will perform on every patient—one skill that is the basis for all the emergency care you will provide. That skill is patient assessment. Like putting together the pieces of a puzzle, the EMT uses each detail revealed by the assessment to help build a picture of the patient's condition and to make informed decisions on emergency care.

Among the fundamental pieces of information you will gather during your assessment of each patient are the patient's vital signs and the patient's history. Monitoring equipment will be used to gather additional assessment information not obtainable in the traditional physical exam, such as the amount of glucose in the blood or amount of hemoglobin saturated with oxygen.

Gathering Patient Information

When you arrive at the scene of an emergency call, you will need to find out all you can about the patient's condition: What's wrong with the patient right now? What led up to the problem? and so on. The process of finding out is called assessment. Most of your EMT course and

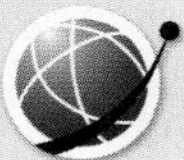

Media Resources

Go to www.bradybooks.com for mykit. Highlights:

- *Web Resource:* Blood Pressure
- *Web Resource:* Taking a Pulse

Objective 11-2

Explain the importance of taking and recording a patient's vital signs over a period of time.

Key Terms

vital signs assessments related to breathing, pulse, skin, pupils, and blood pressure.

most of the chapters of this text are devoted to teaching you how to assess, as well as how to care for, a patient in the prehospital setting.

Much of the information you gain during assessment is readily obvious or available. An open bottle of bleach may provide the clue to a poisoning. The patient or a family member may tell you the chief complaint—for example, "I can't catch my breath," or "I hurt my leg when I fell." The fact that the patient is answering questions clearly may tell you that he is alert, has an open airway, is breathing adequately, and has a pulse. As you conduct a physical exam, you may spot swelling, cuts, bruises, or other signs of injury.

Other indications of the patient's condition require a bit of "detective work"—some special skills for finding out more than what is readily obvious. These skills include measuring the patient's vital signs and asking questions to obtain the patient's history.

Always be aware of the feelings, such as anxiety or embarrassment, that a patient may experience during assessment. Continually reassure the patient and respect his dignity.

Baseline Vital Signs

You can't get inside the patient's body to see what is going on, but you can measure the **vital signs.** These are the "signs of life"—outward signs that give clues to what is happening inside the body. The vital signs that you will measure are:

- Breathing (respiration)
- Pulse
- Skin
- Pupils
- Blood pressure

Pulse oximetry is often considered to be the sixth vital sign. The pulse oximeter is one of the monitoring devices that will be discussed later in the chapter.

Correctly reading and interpreting the vital signs significantly affects the success of prehospital emergency care as well as providing critical information for the hospital staff. Taking two or more sets of vital signs and comparing them will reveal changes in the patient's condition and may indicate how effectively you are managing the patient's injury or illness, or if the patient is deteriorating. The first set of measurements you take are known as the **baseline vital signs,** to which subsequent measurements can be compared. It is important to look for trends in the vital sign readings. As an example, a blood pressure that continues to decrease and a heart rate that continues to increase would be significant findings in a patient who is losing blood.

Although you can monitor most of the vital signs with your senses (looking, listening, feeling), it is necessary that you use and routinely carry the following equipment:

- A **sphygmomanometer** (blood pressure cuff) in adult and pediatric sizes to measure blood pressure
- A stethoscope to take blood pressure and listen to lung sounds
- A wristwatch that counts seconds to measure pulse and respiratory rates
- A penlight to examine pupils
- A pair of EMT shears for cutting away clothing
- A pen and pocket notebook for recording vital signs and other findings
- Your personal protective equipment for Standard Precautions, such as protective gloves, eyewear, and face mask
- Pulse oximeter to establish and monitor the oxygen saturation in the blood

Breathing (Respiration)

Breathing (Respiratory) Rate

The breathing (respiratory) rate is assessed by observing the patient's chest rise and fall (Figure 11-1∗). The normal respiratory rate range for an adult patient at rest is 8 to 24 per minute. On average, the range falls between 12 and 20 breaths per minute. Typically, respiratory rates that are less than 8 or greater than 24 are of concern. First, however, look at the patient and determine if he looks to be in respiratory distress; second, assess his mental status and pay attention to his speech pattern. For example, if you encounter a patient with a respiratory rate of 8 who is alert, oriented, and able to answer your questions without gasping for a breath or showing a struggle to breathe, 8 may be his normal respiratory rate, and no intervention is necessary. On the other hand, if the patient has his eyes closed, needs to be aroused with verbal

Objective 11-3

Perform the steps required to assess the patient's breathing, pulse, skin, pupils, blood pressure, and oxygen saturation and consider the patient's overall presentation when interpreting the meaning of vital sign findings.

Objective 11-4

Differentiate between normal and abnormal findings when assessing a patient's breathing, to include the respiratory rate, quality of respirations, rhythm of respirations, and signs that may indicate respiratory distress or respiratory failure.

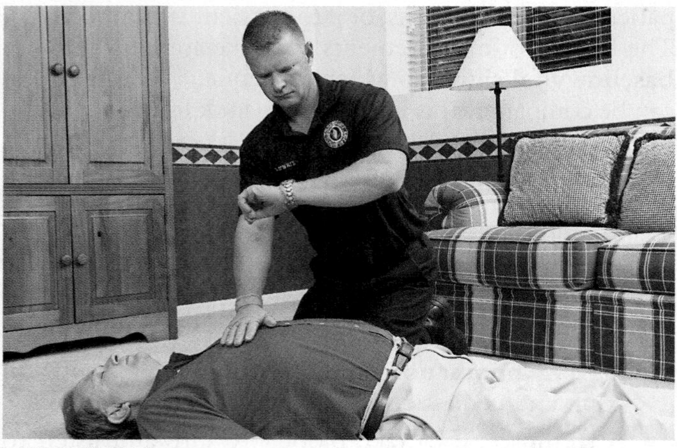

FIGURE 11-1 * Assess the breathing (respiratory) rate, quality, and rhythm.

stimuli, appears fatigued, appears to be struggling to breathe, or speaks only a couple of words before gasping for a breath, you would consider ventilating the patient.

Look at the respiratory rate in relation to the presentation of the patient. Do not be misled by a respiratory rate that falls within the normal limit and consider it "normal" when the patient's clinical signs tell you otherwise. Base your determination of "normal" on the patient's presentation and not on a predetermined "normal" range. What may be normal for one patient may be abnormal for another.

Keep in mind that the resting respiratory rate of the elderly is typically higher, with an average of 20 breaths per minute. Elderly patients have a decreased tidal volume. As a consequence, they must make up the deficit in the volume they breathe by increasing the respiratory rate. A respiratory rate of 22 in an 18-year-old may be alarming, but the same rate of 22 in an elderly person may be considered normal.

Any adult patient breathing at a rate greater than 40 per minute should be ventilated for two reasons: (1) The patient will not be able to sustain that rate for a long period because of the increase in workload to breathe and the respiratory muscle fatigue that will follow, and (2) the rate is so fast the lungs don't have time to fill adequately, leading to a drastic reduction in tidal volume. General ranges for respirations per minute are (see also Table 11-1):

- Adults—8–24 per minute
- Adolescents—12–20 per minute
- Children—15–30 per minute
- Infants—20–40 per minute
- Newborns—30–60 per minute

TABLE 11-1 Normal Breathing Rates

Patient	Normal Breathing Rate per Minute
Adult	8–24
Adolescent 11–16 years	12–20
School-age child 6–10 years	15–30
Preschooler 3–5 years	20–30
Toddler 1–3 years	20–30
Infant 6 months–1 year	20–30
Infant 30 days–5 months	25–40
Newborn–30 days	30–60

Breathing, or respiratory, rate—the number of respirations per minute—is usually determined by counting the number of breaths in a 30-second period and multiplying by 2. (One breath = one inhalation + one exhalation.) If the patient knows you are counting, it can influence the rate. Instead, you can pretend you are checking the radial pulse and cross the patient's arm over the lower chest while actually counting respirations.

Understanding BODY PROCESSES

Pain will trigger the sympathetic nervous system, causing an increase in the respiratory rate. As the pain is reduced, the respiratory rate will decrease. ■

Breathing (Respiratory) Quality

Determining quality of breathing, or respiration, is as important as determining rate. It will tell you the volume of air moving in and out of the lungs with each breath, the volume per minute, and how well it is moving. The quality of breathing is an assessment of tidal volume. If <u>either</u> the respiratory rate <u>or</u> the tidal volume is found to be inadequate, then the patient's respiratory status is inadequate and positive pressure ventilation must be initiated. The quality of breathing may be normal or abnormal. A

Objective 11-5
Differentiate between normal respiratory rates for adults, children, infants, and newborns and evaluate the need to administer treatment based on assessment of a patient's breathing.

Objective 11-6
Auscultate breath sounds to determine the presence of breath sounds, equality of breath sounds, and the presence and likely underlying causes of abnormal breath sounds.

normal quality correlates with an ***adequate*** tidal volume, whereas an ***abnormal*** quality is usually an indication of an ***inadequate*** tidal volume. An abnormal quality of breathing may be shallow, labored, or noisy. You can assess the quality of breathing while you are counting the rate.

- ***Normal breathing*** involves average chest wall motion, which is at least one inch of expansion in an outward direction. The patient does not use the accessory muscles of the chest, neck, or abdomen while breathing. Rate is normal, and inhalations are neither prolonged nor excessively short. Exhalation is typically twice as long as inhalation. Normal breathing is quiet; it does not produce abnormal sounds or noises.
- ***Shallow breathing*** is indicated by only slight chest or abdominal wall expansion upon inhalation. This typically indicates an inadequate tidal volume and requires positive pressure ventilation.
- ***Labored breathing,*** where the patient is working hard to breathe, is indicated by an abnormal sound of breathing that may include grunting or **stridor** (a harsh, high-pitched sound); the use of accessory muscles in the neck, chest, or abdomen to breathe; nasal flaring; and sometimes gasping. In infants and children, there may be retraction of the skin, muscles, and other tissues around the clavicle and between the ribs. The use of accessory muscles in the neck and chest usually indicates that the patient is struggling to inhale, whereas excessive abdominal muscle use is usually an indication of trouble exhaling. The use of accessory muscles requires an increase in the amount of energy expended to breathe. This may lead to respiratory muscle fatigue and a failure in the ability of the patient to breathe adequately.
- ***Noisy breathing,*** or an abnormal sound of breathing (Table 11-2), may include snoring, wheezing, gurgling, crowing, or stridor. Auscultate the chest with a stethoscope to determine if breath sounds are present on both sides and to identify any noisy breathing sounds not audible to the ear alone. In the trauma patient you will auscultate the lungs primarily to determine if breath sounds are present or absent, whereas in the medical patient you are more focused on abnormal breath sounds. Sounds heard during auscultation may include wheezing, rhonchi, and crackles (rales).

Remember to record your observations.

TABLE 11-2 Noisy Breathing

Sounds Audible Without a Stethoscope	Potential Cause
Snoring	Tongue partially blocking the upper airway at the level of the pharynx
Gurgling	Fluid in the upper airway
Stridor or crowing	Partial obstruction of the upper airway at the level of the larynx
Sounds Audible with a Stethoscope	**Potential Cause**
Wheezing	Constriction (narrowing) and inflammation reducing the internal diameter of the bronchioles in the lungs
Rales	Fluid surrounding and filling the alveoli
Rhonchi	Mucus blocking the larger bronchioles

Breathing (Respiratory) Rhythm

The breathing, or respiratory, rhythm—the regularity or irregularity of respirations—can be easily affected by speech, activity, emotions, and other factors in the conscious and alert patient. However, an abnormal respiratory rhythm—that is, an irregular pattern of respiration—in the patient with an altered mental status is a serious concern. It may indicate a medical illness, a chemical imbalance, or brain injury. It is important to assess for adequacy of breathing by assessing the rate and tidal volume when faced with an irregular breathing pattern. Intervene by ventilating, if necessary, and document and report your findings.

Pulse

Location of Pulses

As mentioned in Chapter 7, the pulse is the pressure wave generated by the contraction of the left ventricle. The pulse directly reflects the rhythm, rate, and relative strength of the contraction of the heart as well as the volume of blood being pumped out of the heart, and it can be felt at any point where an artery crosses over a bone near the surface

Objective 11-7
Assess the pulse at various pulse points and consider the patient's age and level of responsiveness when selecting a site to palpate the pulse.

Key Points
When assessing the carotid pulse, do not press too hard and never assess the carotid on both sides at the same time—to avoid impeding circulation to the brain.

of the skin. Central pulses (carotid and femoral) and peripheral pulses (radial, brachial, posterior tibial, and dorsalis pedis) can be felt at the following locations:

- ***Carotid artery,*** on either side of the neck in the groove between the trachea and the muscle mass
- ***Femoral artery,*** in the crease between the lower abdomen and the upper thigh (groin)
- ***Radial artery,*** proximal to the thumb on the palmar surface of the wrist
- ***Brachial artery,*** on the medial aspect of the arm, midway between the shoulder and the elbow between the biceps and triceps muscles
- ***Popliteal artery,*** in the crease behind the knee
- ***Posterior tibial artery,*** behind the medial malleolus (ankle bone)
- ***Dorsalis pedis artery,*** on the top of the foot on the great-toe side

A radial pulse should be assessed in all patients 1 year or older (Figure 11-2∗). In patients younger than 1 year the neck is short and stubby, making it difficult to locate the carotid pulse; thus, assess a brachial pulse (Figures 11-3a and 11-3b∗). When a peripheral pulse cannot be obtained in patients older than 1 year of age, assess the carotid pulse (Figures 11-4a and 11-4b∗). When palpating the carotid pulse, take care not to compress too hard, which may impede circulation to the brain. Never assess the carotid pulse on both sides at the same time, and avoid excessive pressure in elderly patients.

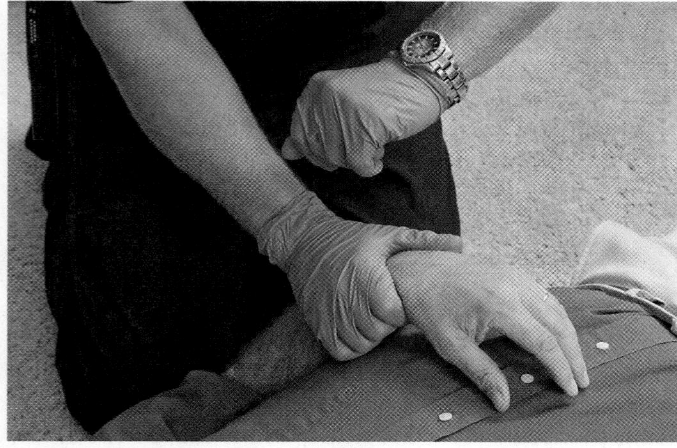

FIGURE 11-2 ∗ Assess the pulse rate, quality, and rhythm. The radial pulse is assessed in patients older than 1 year of age.

ASSESSMENT Tips

If the patient is unresponsive, assess the carotid (central) and the radial (peripheral) pulse at the same time so that there is no delay in determining if a pulse is truly present. This also provides a quick assessment of the patient's perfusion status. ■

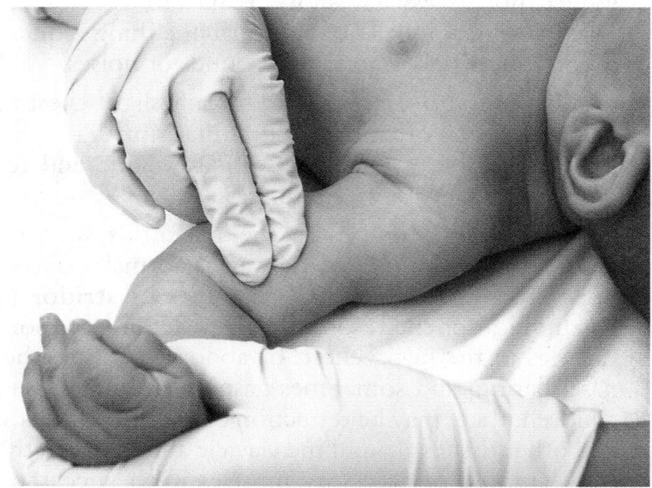

FIGURE 11-3a ∗ Assess the brachial pulse in patients who are less than 1 year of age.

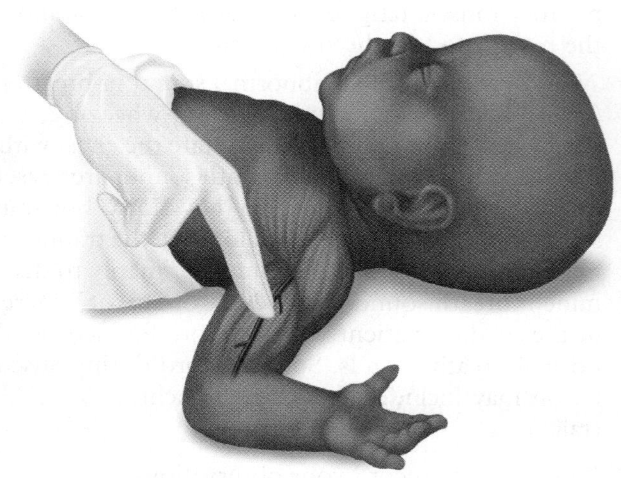

FIGURE 11-3b ∗ Taking a brachial pulse.

Objective 11-8
Differentiate between normal and abnormal findings when assessing a patient's pulse, to include the pulse rate, quality of the pulse, and rhythm of the pulse.

Key Terms
tachycardia a heart rate greater than 100 beats per minute.
bradycardia a heart rate less than 60 beats per minute.

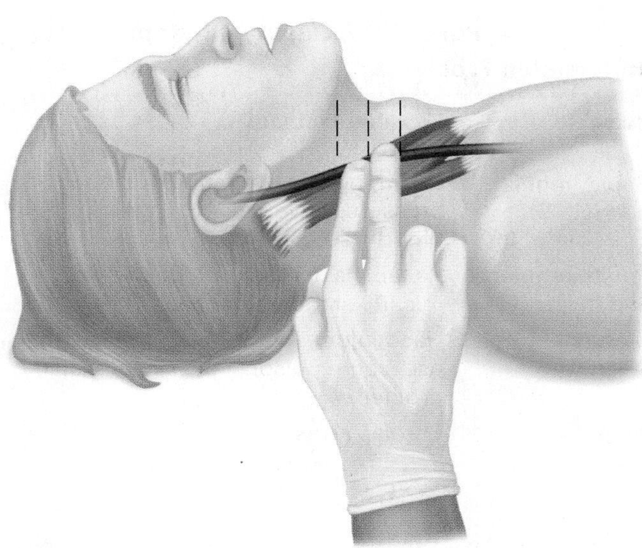

FIGURE 11-4a ✻ Locate the carotid pulse.

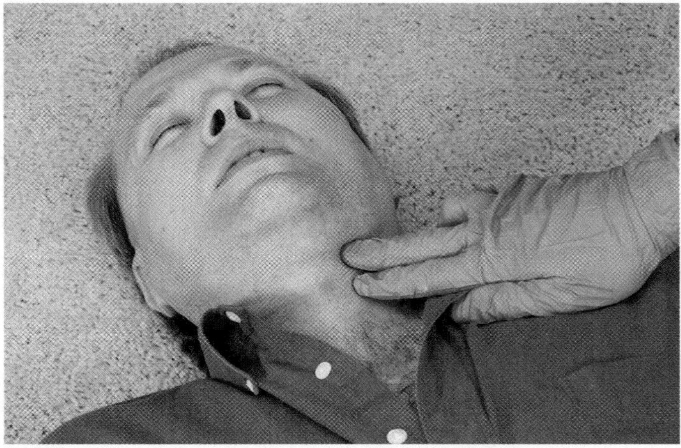

FIGURE 11-4b ✻ Assess the carotid pulse.

Pulse Rate

A pulse rate (Table 11-3) should be taken as soon as possible and frequently. The average resting rate range is 60–80 beats per minute (bpm) for an adult, 60–105 for an adolescent, 60–120 for a school-age child, 80–150 for a preschooler, 120–150 for an infant, and 100–180 for a newborn. In the adult patient, a heart rate greater than 100 bpm is termed **tachycardia** and a heart rate less than 60 bpm is called **bradycardia.**

TABLE 11-3 Normal and Abnormal Pulse Rates

Patient	Pulse Rate (approx. per minute at rest)	Description
Elderly (over 75 years)	90	Normal
Adult	60–80	Normal
	100+	Rapid (tachycardia)
	Below 60	Slow (bradycardia)
Adolescent	60–105	Normal
	Above 105	Rapid
	Below 50	Slow
Child (5–12 years)	60–120	Normal
	Above 120	Rapid
	Below 60	Slow
Child (1–5 years)	80–150	Normal
	Above 150	Rapid
	Below 80	Slow
Infant	120–150	Normal
	Above 150	Rapid
	Below 120	Slow
Newborn	100–180	Normal

Like respirations, the heart rate must be considered in relation to the patient's presentation and assessment findings. A heart rate that falls within the limits of 60 to 100 bpm could be considered abnormal for some patients, whereas a heart rate falling outside of these limits could be considered normal. As an example, a resting heart rate of 42 bpm is obtained for a 34-year-old male patient who injured his ankle. The patient appears to be physically fit and presents as being alert, oriented, and showing no signs of poor perfusion. Although the heart rate is only 42 bpm and would be reported as bradycardic, it would not be cause for alarm based on the patient presentation. On the other hand, a heart rate of 42 bpm in a 56-year-old male patient who must be aroused with verbal stimuli and has pale, cool, and clammy skin is very concerning. As another example, a heart rate of 92 bpm in an elderly patient at rest would be considered normal; however, a heart rate of 92 bpm in a

Objective 11-9
Associate pulse abnormalities with possible underlying causes and describe the changes in the pulse associated with pulsus paradoxus.

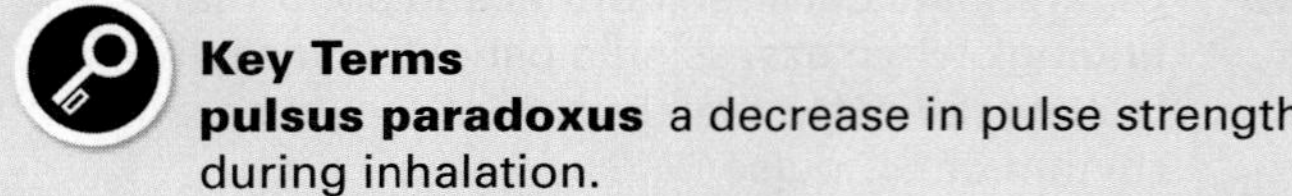

Key Terms
pulsus paradoxus a decrease in pulse strength during inhalation.

20-year-old at rest may be a cause for concern, even though it falls within the definition of a normal range and is not tachycardic. In an elderly patient (greater than 75 years of age), the resting heart rate is normally around 90 bpm. It is not typical for a 20-year-old to have a resting heart rate of 92 bpm; thus, you would consider that heart rate to be potentially abnormal and look for possible causes.

To take the pulse rate:

1. Position the patient. He should be sitting or lying down.
2. Using the tips of two or three fingers, palpate the artery (feel it gently). Avoid using your thumb, because it has a prominent pulse of its own.
3. Count the number of beats in a 30-second period. Then multiply by 2. An irregular pulse should be taken for a full minute.

The pulse can help you gauge the patient's condition. For example, a rapid pulse may indicate shock (hypoperfusion). Absence of a pulse indicates that the heart has stopped beating, the blood pressure is extremely low, or the artery has been blocked or injured. Absence of a pulse in a single extremity may indicate obstruction to the artery in that extremity and may be associated with bone or joint injuries. If so, the patient may complain of numbness, weakness, and tingling, and the skin may gradually turn mottled, blue, and cold.

Pulse Quality and Rhythm

The quality of the pulse can be characterized as strong or weak, the rhythm regular or irregular (Table 11-4):

- ***Strong pulse*** usually refers to a pulse that is both full and normally strong. A "bounding" pulse is one that is abnormally strong.
- ***Weak pulse*** is one that doesn't feel full or may be difficult to find and palpate. A weak pulse may also be quite rapid. The general term for a weak, rapid pulse is "thready."
- ***Regular pulse*** is usually a normal pulse that occurs at regular intervals with a smooth rhythm.
- ***Irregular pulse*** is one that occurs at irregular intervals, which may indicate a cardiac disease. An irregular pulse can be regularly irregular or irregularly irregular. A regularly irregular pulse is one in which the irregular beat occurs at a regular interval and has a pattern. An example would be an abnormal beat that occurs early after each fourth regular beat. An irregularly irregular pulse has no predictable pattern and presents as a chaotic rhythm.

Remember to record the pulse quality.

TABLE 11-4 Pulse Rate, Quality, Rhythm, and Related Problems

Pulse	Possible Problem
Rapid, regular, and full	Exertion, fright, fever, high blood pressure, or very early stage of blood loss
Rapid, regular, and thready	Reliable sign of shock, often evident in early stage of blood loss
Slow	Head injury, barbiturate or narcotic use, some poisons, possible cardiac problem
No pulse	Cardiac arrest

Understanding BODY PROCESSES

A weak pulse typically indicates that not enough blood is being ejected from the left ventricle, as associated with volume loss, or that the blood is not being ejected from the left ventricle with enough force, as seen in heart failure. ■

When assessing a pulse, you may note that it decreases in strength or can't be felt for a short period of time and then returns. If this occurs, look at the patient's respiratory pattern when taking the pulse. If the pulse weakens or disappears during inhalation, be sure to note it and provide the information in your oral report to the advanced life support unit or medical facility. This could be a sign of pulsus paradoxus. **Pulsus paradoxus** is a decrease in the strength of the pulse during the inspiratory phase of the patient. This may be an indication of a severe cardiac or respiratory injury or illness, or significant blood loss. Another method for determining pulsus paradoxus is upon blood pressure measurement. This will be discussed in the blood pressure section.

Objective 11-10
Recognize normal and abnormal findings in the assessment of skin color, temperature, condition, capillary refill, and color of the mucous membranes and associate abnormal skin findings with potential underlying causes.

Key Points
In dark-skinned people, assess skin color on the palms of the hands and soles of the feet.

Skin

The appearance and condition of the skin (Table 11-5) is another important indicator of the body's perfusion status. In assessing the skin, you should check color, temperature, condition, and capillary refill.

Skin Color

Skin color indicates how well the blood is being oxygenated and circulated to the skin and, therefore, how well the lungs and heart (respiratory and circulatory system) are functioning. In all patients, check the color of the nail beds, oral mucosa (mucous membranes of the mouth), and **conjunctiva** (mucous membranes that line the eyelid). They all should be pink. In infants and children and dark-skinned people, check the palms of the hands and the soles of the feet. They should be pink, too.

Abnormal skin colors include the following:

- ***Paleness,*** or **pallor,** may be a sign of extreme vasoconstriction, blood loss, or both. It may indicate shock (hypoperfusion), heart attack, fright, anemia, fainting, or emotional distress. Pale, cool, and clammy skin may be an early skin sign of inadequate oxygenation.
- ***Blue-gray color,*** or **cyanosis,** indicates inadequate oxygenation or poor perfusion. It often appears first in the fingertips and around the mouth, which is referred to as circumoral cyanosis. It can indicate conditions such as suffocation, inadequate respirations, lack of oxygen, heart attack, or poisoning. Cyanosis always indicates a serious problem but often is seen very late.
- ***Red color,*** or **flushing,** may be a sign of heat exposure, vessel dilation, or very late finding in carbon monoxide poisoning.
- ***Yellow color,*** or **jaundice,** may indicate liver disease.
- **Mottling** is a discoloration similar to cyanosis; however, it occurs as a blotchy pattern. Mottled skin may be seen in some shock patients or patients with blood pooling in the extremities for a long period of time.

Skin Temperature

The most common measurement of temperature in the field is relative skin temperature (Figure 11-5∗). This can be assessed by placing the back of your hand against the patient's skin. Relative skin temperature is not a precise measurement but is a good indicator of abnormally low or high temperatures.

Normal skin feels warm to the touch. Abnormal skin temperatures include the following:

- ***Hot,*** which indicates a fever or exposure to heat
- ***Cool,*** which may be a sign of inadequate circulation, shock, or exposure to cold
- ***Cold,*** which indicates extreme exposure to cold

TABLE 11-5 Skin Color, Temperature, and Condition

Color	**Possible Problem**
Pallor (white)	Vasoconstriction, blood loss, shock, heart attack, fright, anemia, fainting, emotional distress
Cyanosis (blue-gray)	Inadequate oxygenation or perfusion (shock), inadequate respiration, heart attack
Flushing (red)	Heat exposure, carbon monoxide poisoning (late)
Jaundice (yellow)	Liver disease
Temperature	**Possible Problem**
Hot	Fever, heat exposure
Cool	Inadequate circulation (shock), cold exposure
Cold	Extreme cold exposure
Condition	**Possible Problem**
Wet or moist	Shock, heat emergency, diabetic emergency
Abnormally dry	Spinal injury, dehydration, heat stroke, poisoning

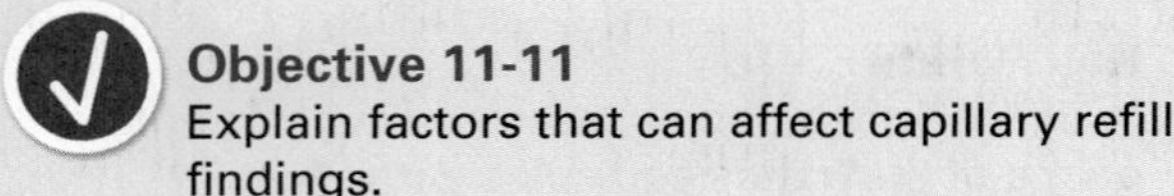

Objective 11-11
Explain factors that can affect capillary refill findings.

Key Terms
capillary refill the amount of time it takes for capillaries that have been compressed to refill with blood.

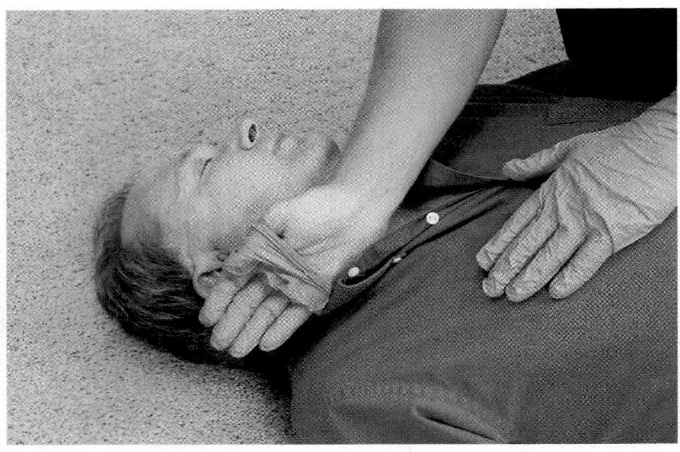

FIGURE 11-5 * Assess relative skin temperature.

Changes in skin temperature over a period of time, or different temperatures in various parts of the body, can be significant. For example, circulatory problems can result in a cold foot, while an isolated "hot" area may indicate a localized infection.

Skin Condition

Normally, skin is dry. Wet or moist skin (often referred to as clammy skin) may indicate shock (hypoperfusion); poisoning; a heat-related, cardiac, or diabetic emergency; or many other conditions. Skin that is both cool and moist is often described as **clammy.** *Diaphoresis* is the term used to describe profuse sweating. Skin that is abnormally dry may be a sign of spinal injury or severe dehydration.

Understanding BODY PROCESSES

Direct sympathetic nervous stimulation and circulating epinephrine and norepinephrine will cause the vessels in the skin to constrict, shunting the warm, red blood away from the skin, which causes the skin to become cool and pale. The nerves and alpha properties will trigger the sweat glands, making the skin clammy (moist) or making the patient diaphoretic. ■

Capillary Refill

The time it takes for compressed capillaries to fill up again with blood is called **capillary refill** time. It is a more reliable sign in infants and younger children than in older children or adults, since younger children usually have very little existing disease that might affect the perfusion in the capillaries. It is acceptable to assess the capillary refill in the older child or adult patient; however, be aware of the influence a cold environment, pre-existing conditions of poor circulation, and certain medications could have on the capillary refill. Keep in mind that capillary refill is only one measure, only a part of the overall picture.

To measure capillary refill, press firmly on the skin or nail bed (Figure 11-6a*). When you remove your finger, the compressed area will be white (Figure 11-6b*). Count the time it takes to return to the original color. Normally capillary refill times vary based on the patient's

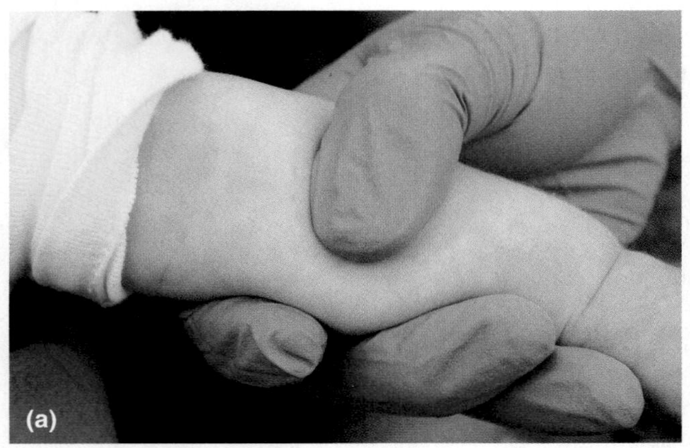

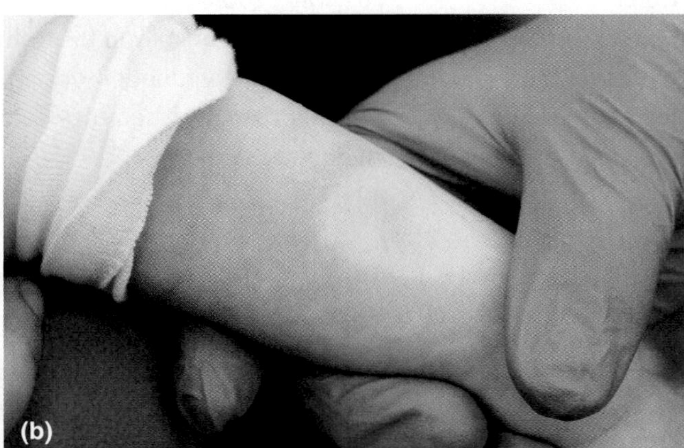

FIGURE 11-6 * Assess capillary refill in infants and children. **(a)** Press on the nail or skin. **(b)** Release the pressure and count the number of seconds that elapse before color returns to the blanched (whitened) area. (Both photos: © Daniel Limmer)

Objective 11-12
When assessing the pupils, recognize dilation, constriction, inequality, and abnormal reacitivty and associate abnormal findings with potential underlying causes.

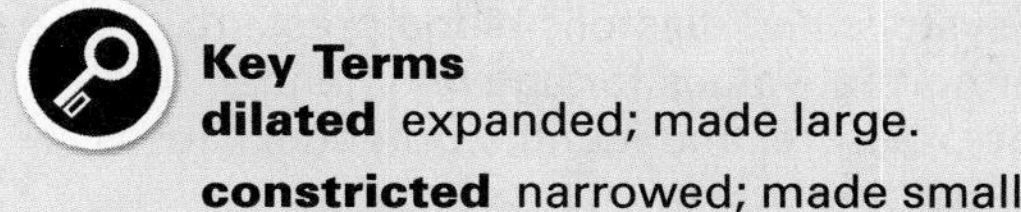

Key Terms
dilated expanded; made large.
constricted narrowed; made small.

age, current disease states, and temperature of the environment. When assessed at room temperature, the upper limits of normal capillary refill times are 2 seconds for infants, children, and male adults; 3 seconds for females; and 4 seconds in the elderly. When it takes longer, the circulation of blood through the capillaries may be inadequate, indicating that the patient is suffering from shock (hypoperfusion).

Capillary refill alone does not provide enough information to determine shock. You need to look at the entire patient and other signs and symptoms. Also look at the color of the mucous membranes inside the mouth, especially in an adult, as a reliable indicator of perfusion status.

Pupils

To assess the pupils, briefly shine a penlight into the patient's eyes (Table 11-6 and Figure 11-7✱).

- **Size.** Pupils that are **dilated** (large) may indicate cardiac arrest or the use of certain drugs, including LSD, amphetamines, atropine, and cocaine. Pupils that are **constricted** (small) may indicate a central nervous system disorder, the use of narcotics, glaucoma medications, or a brightly lit environment.
- **Equality.** Pupils of unequal size may indicate a stroke, head injury, an artificial eye, disease of the eye, use of certain eye drops, or injury to the eye or nerve that controls the pupil. Some people normally have unequal pupils; if it is a normal condition, however, the pupils remain reactive to light and the size difference is not great (< 2 mm). This condition is termed anisocoria. It is usually due to a congenital defect or an ophthalmic injury.
- **Reactivity.** *Reactivity* refers to the pupil changing in size in response to light shined in the eye. The pupils, which are normally midsize, will constrict when light is shined in them. The pupils will dilate when shaded or in a dark environment. Both pupils will have the same response, even when the light is shined in only one eye. This is called a consensual reflex. For example, you shine a light in the right eye and the right and left pupil constrict simultaneously. Pupils that remain midsize may indicate cranial nerve damage.

It is important to assess how briskly the pupils respond to light. Sluggish pupils may indicate a poor oxygen state

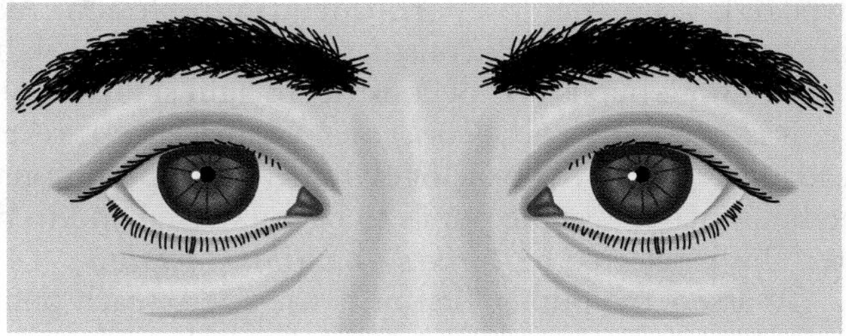

Constricted pupils

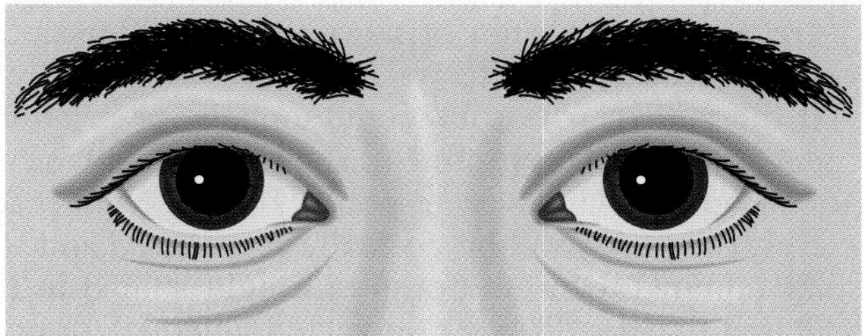

Dilated pupils

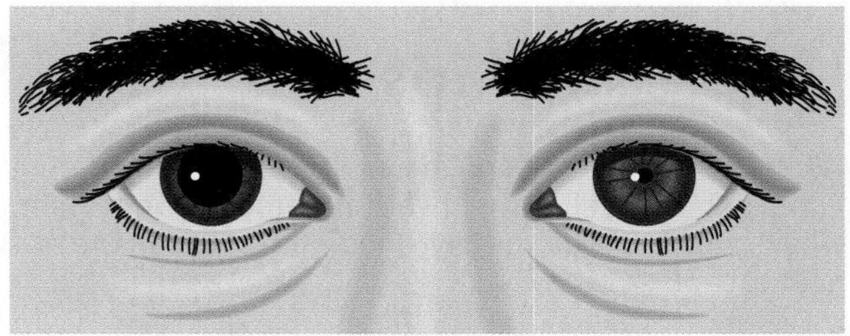

Unequal pupils

FIGURE 11-7 ✱ Assess pupils for size, equality, and reactivity.

TABLE 11-6 Pupil Size, Equality, and Reactivity

Factor	Possible Problem
Dilated	Cardiac arrest, drug use such as LSD, amphetamines, cocaine
Constricted	Central nervous system disorder, narcotics use
Unequal	Stroke, head injury, artificial eye (occasionally a normal finding), eye drops
Nonreactive	Cardiac arrest, brain injury, drug intoxication or overdose

Objective 11-13
In relation to blood pressure measurement, explain systolic and diastolic blood pressure, consider normal values for age and gender, find the pulse pressure, and identify potential causes of abnormal findings or changes.

Key Terms
systolic blood pressure the amount of pressure exerted against the walls of the arteries when the left ventricle of the heart contracts and ejects blood.

diastolic blood pressure the pressure exerted against the walls of the arteries while the left ventricle of the heart is at rest.

(hypoxia), drug overdose, or inadequate perfusion. Also note whether both pupils constrict in response to the light. If one or both pupils do not constrict to light shined in one eye, it is referred to as a *fixed pupil.* Cardiac arrest, severe head injury, severe hypoxia, or extremely poor perfusion to the brain may cause the pupils to become fixed and to dilate. This is referred to as *fixed and dilated pupils.*

To assess the pupils, first note the size of each pupil. Then shine the light in one eye and watch the response of both pupils. Note if the pupil constricts and how brisk the response is. Remove the light and note if the pupil returns to its resting state and how briskly it responds. Repeat the procedure on the opposite eye.

If the patient is out in bright sunlight or in an extremely brightly lit environment, shade the patient's eyes before testing the pupillary response. If you do not shade the eyes, the pupils will be normally constricted and will display minimal to no response to a light shined in the eye. Pupils that are dilated, constricted, unequal, or nonreactive may indicate a variety of conditions, as noted in Table 11-6.

ASSESSMENT Tips

When assessing for pupillary reaction, use only a penlight, not a flashlight with an extremely bright light, which would be extremely uncomfortable for the patient to look at. ■

Blood Pressure

When the left ventricle of the heart contracts, it ejects blood into the aorta and throughout the arteries of the body. The pressure that is exerted on the walls of the arteries by the blood flowing through them is referred to as the **blood pressure.** The blood pressure normally includes two readings: the systolic blood pressure and the diastolic blood pressure.

The top number is always the **systolic blood pressure,** which is the amount of pressure exerted on the walls of the arteries during the contraction and ejection of blood from the left ventricle. The systolic blood pressure correlates with the wave of blood that creates the pulse. Therefore, the pulse is an assessment of the systolic blood pressure. If the systolic blood pressure is low, the pulse will be weak or absent. If the systolic blood pressure is high, the pulse will be bounding (feel very strong). The systolic blood pressure is identified by the first distinct sound (Korotkoff sound) heard when measuring the blood pressure by auscultation (listening with a stethoscope while using a sphygmomanometer, or blood pressure cuff).

The bottom number is always the **diastolic blood pressure,** which is the amount of pressure on the artery walls while the ventricle is at rest and *not* contracting. The diastolic blood pressure is related to both the amount of blood in the artery and the diameter of the artery. If the artery is constricted (diameter is made smaller), the diastolic blood pressure will increase. During auscultation, the diastolic blood pressure is recorded when the systolic (Korotkoff) sound disappears or changes drastically.

In a patient who has a reported blood pressure of 128/68 mmHg, 128 is the systolic blood pressure and 68 is the diastolic blood pressure. The systolic and diastolic readings are expressed in millimeters of mercury (mmHg), units that correspond to the marks on the sphygmomanometer gauge.

The blood pressure reading taken with a sphygmomanometer is always expressed as an even number. If the reading falls between two even numbers, the reading is rounded up to the nearest even number. For example, if the systolic sound is heard between 110 and 112, you would not express the reading as 111. You would round the systolic reading up to 112. Electronic blood pressure measurement equipment expresses readings in both even and odd numbers. It is acceptable to report the blood pressure using the numbers provided from the device, but be sure to record on your prehospital care report that the blood pressure was taken by an electronic device. These devices are referred to as noninvasive blood pressure monitors and will be discussed in more detail later in the chapter under "Monitoring Equipment."

Blood pressures vary widely for different patients (Table 11-7). A normal systolic blood pressure in an adult is considered to be less than 140 mmHg. A normal diastolic blood pressure is less than 85. You often hear 120/80 mmHg expressed as being the "normal blood pressure." Actually, 120/80 represents an average, rather than a "normal," blood pressure for an adult patient. Quick guidelines to determine if the systolic blood pressure falls within a normal range are as follows:

- **Adult male.** In the adult male patient at rest who is less than 40 years of age, add the patient's age to 100. As an example, a 32-year-old male patient would have an estimated normal systolic blood pressure of

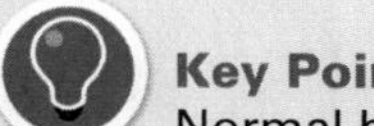

Key Points
Normal blood pressures can vary widely. In addition to blood pressure, always use other assessments of perfusion, such as skin temperature and color and mental status.

Key Terms
pulse pressure the difference between the systolic blood pressure and the diastolic blood pressure.

TABLE 11-7 Normal Blood Pressures in Adults, Children, and Infants

Patient	Systolic	Diastolic
Adult male	100 + age in years to age 40	60–85 mmHg
Adult female	90 + age in years to age 40	60–85 mmHg
Adolescent	90 mmHg (lower limit of normal)	2/3 of systolic pressure
Child 1–10 years	90 + (2 age in years) (upper limit of normal)	2/3 of systolic pressure
	80 + (2 age in years) (middle range of normal)	
	70 + (2 age in years) (lower limit of normal)	
Infant 1–12 months	70 mmHg (lower limit of normal)	2/3 of systolic pressure

132 mmHg (100 + 32 years = 132 mmHg). A systolic blood pressure greater than 140 mmHg would be considered a mild form of hypertension (high blood pressure). The normal range for the diastolic blood pressure is between 60 and 85 mmHg. Any diastolic blood pressure greater than 90 mmHg is referred to as diastolic hypertension.

- **Adult female.** Since an adult female's blood pressure is typically 8 to 10 mmHg lower than in an adult male, you would take the patient's age in years plus 90 mmHg to estimate the normal blood pressure of an adult female at rest. As an example, a 28-year-old female would have an estimated systolic blood pressure of 118 mmHg (90 + 28 = 118 mmHg). The adult female's diastolic blood pressure is normally 60–85 mmHg. Any pressure greater than 90 mmHg is considered to be diastolic hypertension.
- **Child age 1–10 years.** In children between 1 and 10 years of age, the normal expected systolic blood pressure is calculated by taking the child's age times 2 and then adding it to 80 mmHg. As an example, the normal expected blood pressure for a 6-year-old child is 92 mmHg (80 + (2 × 6 years) = 92 mmHg). The upper limit of a normal systolic blood pressure would be calculated by taking 90 + (2 × years in age). Thus, the 6-year-old would have an expected upper limit systolic blood pressure of 102 mmHg (90 + (2 × 6 years) = 102). The lower limit of a normal systolic blood pressure would be calculated by taking 70 + (2 × years in age). The lower limit of a normal systolic blood pressure in the 6-year-old would be 82 mmHg (70 + (2 × 6 years) = 82). The lower limit of normal of a systolic blood pressure in an infant from birth to 1 month of age is 60 mmHg, and from 1 month to 1 year is 70 mmHg. This provides you with a quick reference when estimating blood pressures in children.

  The diastolic blood pressure is normally two-thirds the systolic blood pressure. As an example, a child with a systolic blood pressure of 90 mmHg would have an expected diastolic blood pressure of 60 mmHg.
- **Child or adolescent greater than age 10 years.** Children greater than 10 years of age would have a minimum systolic blood pressure of 90 mmHg. A blood pressure less than the minimum expected blood pressure would be a possible indication of shock.

It is important to use the blood pressure as only one indicator of shock or hypoperfusion. Assess the entire patient while looking for other indicators of shock or hypoperfusion. Normal blood pressure could vary widely. Be sure to use many different assessments of perfusion, such as skin temperature and color and mental status. Always treat the patient and not the blood pressure.

The difference between the systolic blood pressure and the diastolic blood pressure is called the **pulse pressure.** As an example, if the patient's blood pressure is 124/80, the pulse pressure would be 44 mmHg (124 – 80 = 44 mmHg). If the pulse pressure is less than 25 percent of the systolic blood pressure, it would be considered a narrow pulse pressure. If the pulse pressure is greater than 50 percent of the systolic blood pressure, it would be considered a widened pulse pressure. Using the example just given, a narrow pulse pressure would be less than 31 mmHg (124 × .25 = 31 mmHg) and a widened pulse pressure would be greater than 62 mmHg (124 × .50 = 62 mmHg).

Objective 11-14
Compare palpation and auscultation of blood pressure as to processes, useful findings, and documentation and discuss how technique and selection of equipment can affect the accuracy of readings.

Key Terms
auscultation listening for sounds within the body with a stethoscope.

palpation feeling, as for a pulse.

Normally, the two blood pressures rise and fall together. However, there are conditions in which the systolic and diastolic readings become closer together than normal (narrow pulse pressure) or become much further apart (widened pulse pressure). These are important indicators of possible conditions or injuries that a patient may be suffering. For example, a patient with a head injury may suffer a widened pulse pressure where the systolic blood pressure sharply rises but the diastolic does not rise or even falls. Shock, cardiac tamponade (sac around the heart that is filled with blood and compressing the heart), and tension pneumothorax (one lung is injured and collapses, compressing the heart and uninjured lung) cause a narrow pulse pressure where the systolic blood pressure is falling and the diastolic blood pressure is rising.

Understanding BODY PROCESSES

A narrow pulse pressure is usually a result of less blood being ejected from the left ventricle because of either volume loss or left ventricular failure, which causes the systolic blood pressure to decrease while peripheral vasoconstriction causes the diastolic blood pressure to remain stable or increase. ■

As an EMT, you should note and record any abnormalities in the pulse pressure so that the emergency department can determine trends that may be occurring with the blood pressure. This could lead to suspicion and diagnosis of life-threatening conditions.

A low blood pressure indicates that there is not enough pressure in the arteries to keep the organs supplied with an adequate amount of blood. In an adult patient, a systolic blood pressure of less than 90 mmHg is typically considered to be low, although this is somewhat variable. This can cause an inadequate oxygen delivery to the cells and organs, which in turn can lead to cell and organ damage and death. This condition of inadequate delivery of oxygen and nutrients to the cells and tissues is known as shock or hypoperfusion.

The blood pressure can decrease as a result of blood or fluid loss, cardiac pump failure, or blood vessel dilation (the vessel diameter increases in size). Conditions that may cause shock or hypoperfusion include severe bleeding, heart attack, heart failure, or spinal injury. A low blood pressure may be an indication of these conditions. High blood pressure, also known as hypertension, can result from a variety of causes. The abnormally high blood pressure can cause damage to the heart and blood vessels, leading to heart damage and failure, stroke, ruptured blood vessels, and kidney disease.

It is difficult to assess blood pressure in infants and children less than 3 years of age. Therefore, the EMT should measure blood pressures only in patients greater than 3 years of age. In a child less than 3 years of age, you will rely on the skin temperature, color, and condition; the patient's mental status; and quality and location of pulses to determine the perfusion status.

Methods of Measuring Blood Pressure

There are two methods of measuring blood pressure with a sphygmomanometer: by **auscultation,** or listening for the systolic and diastolic sounds through a stethoscope, and by **palpation,** or feeling for the return of the pulse as the cuff is deflated.

To assess blood pressure by auscultation (EMT Skills 11-1):

1. *Choose the proper size sphygmomanometer cuff.* It should completely encircle the patient's bare arm about one inch above the antecubital space (at the front of the elbow) without overlapping. The cuff should cover two-thirds of the upper arm. Its bladder should be centered over the brachial artery, and cover half the arm's circumference. Properly fitted, the cuff should fit snugly, but you should still be able to place one finger easily under its bottom edge. An improperly sized blood pressure cuff will provide an inaccurate reading. A cuff that is too small will provide a reading that is higher than it should be; a cuff that is too large will provide a reading that is lower than it should be.
2. *Position the arm.* If the patient is seated, position the arm so that the brachial artery at the antecubital fossa is at the level of the heart. If the arm is allowed to dangle, the increase in blood flow due to gravity may provide a false high reading. If the arm is too high above the heart, it may provide a false low reading. If the patient is standing, position the arm at the midchest level. Regardless if standing or sitting, do not allow the patient to support his own arm by holding it up. The strain on the arm may change the blood pressure reading.
3. *Palpate the radial pulse.* Inflate the cuff rapidly to 70 mmHg and then increase by 10-mmHg incre-

Thinking Critically

While taking a patient's blood pressure you notice that the pressure drops suddenly by more than 10 mmHg when the patient inhales. This is a sign of what condition? Why is it important to report this sign in both your oral and your written report?

Objective 11-15

Demonstrate assessment of orthostatic vital signs.

Key Terms

orthostatic vital signs a comparison of blood pressure and heart rate readings while a patient is supine and while sitting upright or standing.

ments until the radial pulse is no longer felt. Note the number on the dial and deflate the cuff.

4. *Place the stethoscope in your ears with the earpieces facing forward.* Locate the brachial artery on the medial (inner) aspect of the antecubital fossa (front of the elbow). Position the head of the stethoscope over the brachial artery. Be careful not to place the stethoscope under the cuff, which will distort the sounds when listening through the stethoscope.
5. *Close the thumb valve and squeeze the bulb to inflate the cuff.* Inflate the cuff to 30 mmHg above the level noted in step 3.
6. *Slowly turn the thumb valve counterclockwise or press the release mechanism to release air.* Deflate the cuff at approximately 2 mmHg per second, watching the pressure gauge as it slowly decreases.
7. *As soon as you hear the first sound* (clear but dull tapping or swooshing sound), *record the pressure.* This is the systolic pressure.
8. *Continue releasing air from the bulb.* At the point where you hear the last sound, record the diastolic pressure. Continue to deflate slowly for at least 10 mmHg. With children and some adults, you may hear sounds all the way to zero. In those cases, record the pressure when the sound changes from a clear tapping to a soft, muffled tapping.
9. *After you have recorded the blood pressure, leave the cuff deflated but in place* so you can take more blood pressure readings during treatment and transport. Carefully record the blood pressure each time you take it. Changes can be significant.

To measure the blood pressure by palpation (EMT Skills 11-2):

1. *Inflate the cuff rapidly* with the rubber bulb while palpating the radial pulse until you can no longer feel it. (Make a mental note of that reading.) Without stopping, continue to inflate the cuff to 30 mmHg above the level where the radial pulse could no longer be felt.
2. *Slowly deflate the cuff.* Make a note of the pressure at which the radial pulse returns. This is the systolic pressure as measured by palpation. In a noisy situation where you cannot hear well enough to measure the blood pressure by auscultation, this will be the only blood pressure measurement you can make. You will not be able to measure the diastolic pressure by palpation. Record the palpated blood pressure as, for example, 120/P.

A palpated systolic blood pressure is approximately 7 mmHg lower than a systolic blood pressure taken by auscultation.

It was previously thought that the location of a palpable pulse would provide an estimation of the systolic blood pressure. For example, if a radial pulse was felt, the systolic blood pressure would have to be higher than if only the carotid pulse was felt. This was based only on a guess. Research has shown that a radial pulse may be present with a systolic blood pressure as low as 60 mmHg in some patients. Therefore, this method of estimating systolic blood pressure is inaccurate. However, the research did find that it is necessary to have a systolic blood pressure of at least 60 mmHg to produce a carotid, femoral, or radial pulse. Once the systolic blood pressure falls below 60 mmHg, a severe condition of hypotension (low blood pressure), no pulses will be palpable.

Blood pressure should be measured in all patients older than 3 years of age. In infants or young children, however, the general appearance, physical assessment, and quality of pulse are more valuable than the blood pressure.

If, when taking the blood pressure, you note a sudden drop of greater than 10 mmHg, continue with the process. Take another blood pressure and watch for the drop. If the drop is greater than 10 mmHg and is noted during the patient's inspiration, this is another sign of pulsus paradoxus (as described earlier in the chapter). Note this in your written report and in your oral report to the advanced life support crew or receiving medical facility. Pulsus paradoxus could indicate a serious cardiac or lung illness or injury, or severe bleeding.

In the patient experiencing chest pain, it is important to assess the blood pressure in both upper extremities. If a difference of greater than 20 mmHg is noted between the systolic readings in the two upper extremities, report this finding to the advanced life support crew or the receiving medical facility. This finding may indicate an evolving problem with the aorta in the patient's chest.

Testing Orthostatic Vital Signs

In a patient with suspected volume loss, you may be asked to obtain a set of **orthostatic vital signs.** This is done by placing the patient in a supine position and measuring his blood pressure and heart rate, then standing the patient

Objective 11-17
Explain and demonstrate the use and interpretation of pulse oximetry readings.

Objective 11-16
Given a patient scenario, determine the frequency with which vital signs should be reassessed.

Key Terms
pulse oximetry measurement of blood oxygen saturation level.

up and, after 2 minutes, reassessing the blood pressure and heart rate. If, while the patient is standing, the heart rate increases by greater than 10–20 bpm and the systolic blood pressure decreases by 10–20 mmHg as compared to the readings taken while the patient was supine, it is considered to be a positive orthostatic test, which typically indicates a significant loss of blood or fluid volume (EMT Skills 11-3). The orthostatic vital signs test is also commonly known as the **tilt test.**

ASSESSMENT Tips

When you take orthostatic vital signs, moving the patient from a supine to a standing position provides the best results. A supine-to-seated position will provide orthostatic vital signs if they are present but is not as accurate. ■

You must be careful when using the systolic blood pressure reading as conclusive in this test, because a large percentage of patients, especially the elderly, experience a normal drop in systolic blood pressure when rising from a supine position even if they have not lost any blood volume. One study indicated that 25 percent of patients over 65 years of age will falsely test positive when an orthostatic tilt test uses a drop in the systolic blood pressure of 10–20 mmHg as the clinical indicator. An increase in the heart rate is a much more sensitive indicator of blood loss when checking orthostatic vital signs. However, bear in mind that some medications, such as beta blockers, may prevent the heart rate from increasing significantly.

If the patient can't be placed in a standing position, you can move him from a supine to a seated position. Wait the 2 minutes, then reassess heart rate and blood pressure. You will look for the same findings as in the standing patient. However, performing the orthostatic tilt test with a patient in the seated position will not provide the same sensitivity as with the patient in a standing position.

Do not perform this test on patients who you suspect may have a possible spinal injury. It would be imprudent to place this patient in a standing or seated position. When moving a patient from a supine to a standing position, be sure that you assist him and have a good grasp on his body. If the patient has a significant volume loss, he may pass out when moving to a standing position. This would, of course, be a significant indication of volume loss.

Vital Sign Reassessment

If the patient is stable, vital signs should be taken and recorded at least every 15 minutes and as often as necessary to ensure proper care. Take and record vital signs every 5 minutes if the patient is unstable. Reassess vital signs immediately following every medical intervention, regardless of how soon it follows your previous assessment of vital signs.

▶ Monitoring Equipment

Specialized equipment may be used to monitor certain aspects of the patient's status. Two common monitoring devices used by EMTs in the prehospital environment are the pulse oximeter and the noninvasive blood pressure monitor. Many EMTs also use glucometers, or glucose meters, to determine the amount of glucose (sugar) in the patient's blood. Unlike the pulse oximeter and noninvasive blood pressure monitor, the glucometer does not provide continuous monitoring. It will be covered in detail in Chapter 20, "Acute Diabetic Emergencies."

Pulse Oximeter: Oxygen Saturation Assessment

Pulse oximetry is a method of detecting hypoxia in patients by measuring oxygen saturation levels in the blood. The device used to measure the level of hemoglobin saturated with oxygen is a **pulse oximeter** (EMT Skills 11-4). The pulse oximeter probe is clipped, somewhat like a clothespin, or attached by adhesive-backed sensors, onto a patient's finger, toe, earlobe, or across the bridge of the nose. (Since the pulse oximeter measures arterial blood oxygen saturation, the probe must be placed in an area where the light from the oximeter shines through arterial blood flow. The most common placement in the adult patient is the finger.) One side of the pulse oximeter probe sends out a red light and infrared light. The light shines through the tissue to a photosensor on the opposite side. The light detects the amount of hemoglobin in the blood that is saturated with oxygen and the amount of hemoglobin that is not saturated with oxygen.

The pulse oximeter provides a reading as a percent of hemoglobin saturated with oxygen. This is recorded as % SpO_2, which indicates the reading was measured by a

Key Points
The pulse oximeter is just one tool. It must be used in conjunction with other assessment findings to determine hypoxia.

Key Points
A pulse oximeter reading is commonly called the "sixth vital sign," indicating that it should be a standard measure in all patients.

pulse oximeter. A normal pulse oximeter reading for a person breathing room air is in the high 90s, typically 97–100% SpO_2. A pulse oximeter reading in a compromised patient that is less than 95% may indicate hypoxia. Therefore, any SpO_2 reading of less than 95% in a patient must be investigated and oxygen must be applied to the patient. An SpO_2 reading of 90% or less is an indication of severe hypoxia. Assess your patient carefully, paying close attention to his respiratory rate and tidal volume. He may need to be ventilated if either the rate or tidal volume is found to be inadequate. Whether the patient requires assisted ventilation or not, apply oxygen to the patient. Be aggressive in your management of the patient, bearing in mind that the result of severe and prolonged hypoxia is cell death.

The pulse oximeter is just one tool used in assessment of the patient. It is not the only tool to detect hypoxia. The pulse oximeter reading must be used in conjunction with other assessment findings to make a determination of whether the patient is hypoxic. Treat the patient and not the pulse oximeter reading. However, keep in mind that the pulse oximeter is a sensitive device that may detect hypoxia long before overt signs and symptoms are present.

In addition to indicating hypoxia, the pulse oximeter is a good tool for monitoring the effectiveness of airway management and oxygen therapy and to detect if the patient is deteriorating or improving. If possible, apply the pulse oximeter prior to administration of oxygen so you can measure trends. However, do not delay administration of oxygen to apply the pulse oximeter in a suspected hypoxic patient.

As an example of the pulse oximeter's effectiveness as a monitoring tool, consider a patient with obvious respiratory distress in whom you apply the pulse oximeter as your partner prepares to administer oxygen by a nonrebreather mask. You obtain an SpO_2 reading of 92%, indicating obvious hypoxia. Following application of the nonrebreather mask at 15 lpm, the pulse oximeter reading begins to increase. After 10 minutes on the oxygen mask, the patient's SpO_2 reaches 99%. The pulse oximeter readings have shown a dramatic improvement in the patient's status. On the other hand, if the patient's SpO_2 reading is 93% on a nonrebreather mask and continues to fall, it is an indication that the patient is deteriorating and may need positive pressure ventilation to maintain or increase the level of oxygenation.

One consideration: If the patient is on a nonrebreather at 15 lpm for a period of time and the pulse oximeter reading is near or slightly less than 95%, it may still be an indication that the patient is hypoxic. If the nonrebreather were removed, it is likely that the SpO_2 reading would decrease rapidly.

Understanding BODY PROCESSES

A patient with a small amount of hemoglobin from blood loss but a large amount of oxygen attached to the remaining hemoglobin may have a high SpO_2 reading, even though his cells are truly hypoxic. When carbon monoxide attaches to hemoglobin, it will cause abnormal absorption at one of the emitted light frequencies the hemoglobin to become red. The pulse oximeter will falsely read this color and interpret it as a high level of oxygen attached to hemoglobin, although the cells are severely hypoxic. ■

Indications for Pulse Oximetry

The pulse oximeter should be applied in any situation where the patient's oxygen status is a concern or when hypoxia may be even remotely suspected. In many systems, the pulse oximeter is applied and used routinely on all emergency call patients. The pulse oximeter reading is referred to commonly as the "sixth vital sign," indicating that it should be a standard measure in patients along with respirations, pulse, skin, pupils, and blood pressure.

Limitations of the Pulse Oximeter

The pulse oximeter needs pulsatile arterial blood flow to determine an accurate reading. Any condition that interferes with the blood flowing to the area where the probe is attached may produce an erroneous reading. The pulse oximeter must be used appropriately, because erroneous readings provide false information and may adversely affect your treatment. As an example, it would be inappropriate to gauge the oxygenation of a cardiac arrest patient by using a pulse oximeter. The perfusion status is too poor for the pulse oximeter to provide accurate or reliable information. Another limitation is that the pulse oximeter does not provide a direct measurement of the blood oxygen content. There is a lag time from when the patient initially becomes hypoxic to when the pulse oximeter reading indicates it, because it relies on an indirect measure of the oxygen content in the blood. Also, it does not indicate the amount of oxygen being off-loaded to cells, the oxygenation status of the cells, or the ability of

Thinking Critically
Your patient is a victim of carbon monoxide poisoning. After she has been removed from the toxic environment, can you assess her SpO_2 level? If so, how? If not, why not?

Objective 11-18
Describe the correct procedure for noninvasive blood pressure monitoring.

the cells to use the oxygen. The following are conditions in which the pulse oximeter would produce no reading or an inaccurate reading:

- Shock or hypoperfusion states associated with blood loss or poor perfusion will lead to inaccurate readings.
- Hypothermia or cold injury to the extremities will reduce peripheral perfusion and limit the blood available in the capillaries to be read by the probe.
- Excessive movement of the patient (for example, during some types of seizures) will lead to inaccurate readings.
- Nail polish on the finger the probe is attached to will produce an inaccurate reading. Clean the fingernail with an acetone wipe before applying the finger probe.
- Carbon monoxide will give an abnormally high reading although the cells are actually becoming severely hypoxic. Carbon monoxide binds with the hemoglobin in the blood and absorbs light at the emitted frequencies, creating a red tone. The pulse oximeter erroneously reads the absorbed light of hemoglobin attached to carbon monoxide molecules, providing a false high reading.
- Cigarette smokers may have falsely high SpO_2 readings, because carbon monoxide is a by-product of the smoke. Up to 15 percent of the hemoglobin may be bonded with carbon monoxide, not oxygen, giving a false high reading.
- Anemia may produce abnormally high readings. The hemoglobin may be saturated with oxygen, but the anemic patient has decreased levels of hemoglobin. The hemoglobin is saturated with oxygen, but the combined hemoglobin-oxygen content of the blood is inadequate.

Most pulse oximeters display a pulse rate along with the SpO_2 reading. If the pulse rate shown on the pulse oximeter does not correspond with the patient's actual pulse rate, there is a good chance that the pulse oximeter is also not accurately reading the blood flow and oxygen saturation.

To elaborate on the point just listed about carbon monoxide: In a carbon monoxide poisoning patient, the pulse oximeter reading will be excessively high, but totally inaccurate. This patient may be severely hypoxic and still have an SpO_2 reading of 100%. This occurs because the pulse oximeter measures the percentage of hemoglobin that is saturated. The pulse oximeter cannot distinguish between hemoglobin saturated with oxygen and hemoglobin saturated with carbon monoxide. With carbon monoxide having an affinity for hemoglobin that is 200–300 times greater than oxygen, a large amount of the hemoglobin is saturated with carbon monoxide and not oxygen. This creates a deadly hypoxic state. Yet, the SpO_2 provides an extremely high reading. There are portable devices available to measure the carbon monoxide level in the blood. These devices distinguish between hemoglobin saturated with carbon monoxide and hemoglobin saturated with oxygen.

Again, remember to assess the patient as a whole. The SpO_2 reading is just one tool in that assessment.

Procedure for Determining the SpO_2 Reading

To determine the patient's SpO_2 level:

1. Connect the sensor to the SpO_2 monitor device.
2. Attach the probe to the fingertip. In an infant, the toe or distal foot can be used.
3. Turn on the device and wait for a few seconds for the reading to appear. Match the pulse reading on the SpO_2 monitor with the patient's. If the heart rate is different, it is likely the SpO_2 reading is inaccurate.
4. If a poor signal is detected or an "error" reading is indicated, check the probe to be sure it is on properly. Check for nail polish on the fingernails. Remove the nail polish or change the probe to another fingertip.
5. Once an accurate reading is provided, reassess and document the SpO_2 reading every 5 minutes in the unstable patient, every 15 minutes in the stable patient.

Noninvasive Blood Pressure Monitor

A noninvasive blood pressure monitor is a device that automatically measures a blood pressure and provides an electronic readout (Figure 11-8*). The monitor can be set to reassess the blood pressure at selected intervals, such as every 5 or 15 minutes, or it can be activated manually. Alarms can be set to signal pressures that exceed or fall below set upper and lower limits. It is important that you become completely familiar with the manufacturer's instructions for the device you are using and follow your local protocol. Currently, finger- and

Objective 11-19
Describe the processes for controlling the scene, achieving a smooth transition of care, and reducing the patient's anxiety.

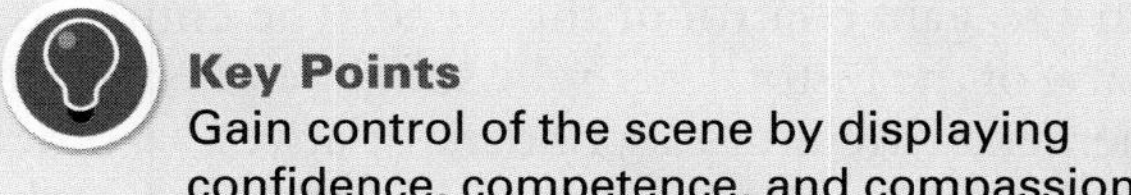

Key Points
Gain control of the scene by displaying confidence, competence, and compassion.

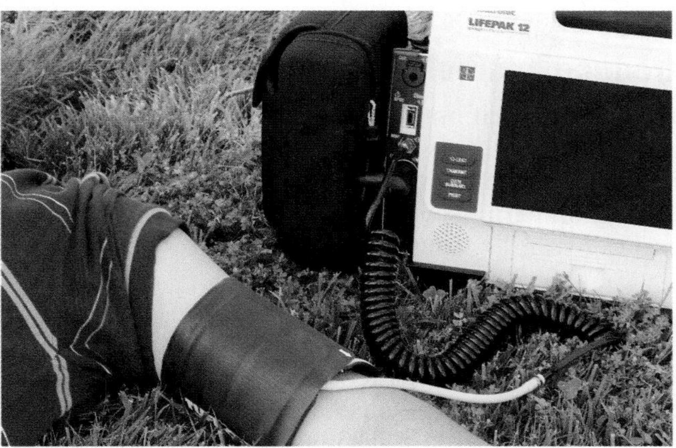

FIGURE 11-8 ✱ A noninvasive blood pressure device.

wrist-automated blood pressure monitors have not been found to be accurate and should not be used in the prehospital environment.

Procedure for Noninvasive Blood Pressure Monitoring

1. Always obtain the first blood pressure reading by the auscultation method, using a stethoscope and a sphygmomanometer. Once this reading has been documented, proceed with applying the noninvasive blood pressure monitor (Figures 11-9a and 11-9b✱).
2. Apply and position the cuff. Be sure the cuff is the appropriate size to avoid erroneous readings. The cuff is measured and applied in the same manner as for an auscultated blood pressure.
3. Activate the device. If in a manual mode, you typically depress a button to begin the measurement process. The cuff inflates. You may need to prepare the patient prior to activating the device by describing what he will feel and instruct the patient not to move the arm during the measurement.
4. Obtain the reading. After the cuff deflates, a systolic and diastolic blood pressure reading will be displayed on the device. Be sure to record the reading. If the reading is unobtainable, the device will so indicate.

▶ Preparing to Take the History

Gain Control of the Scene

When arriving on the scene, you will frequently encounter patients and family members who are frightened, injured, anxious, or in shock. In addition, you may find an angry or hostile crowd and law enforcement or fire department personnel anxiously awaiting your arrival. You must display competence, confidence, and compassion—through your personal appearance and professional manner—in order to obtain cooperation not only from

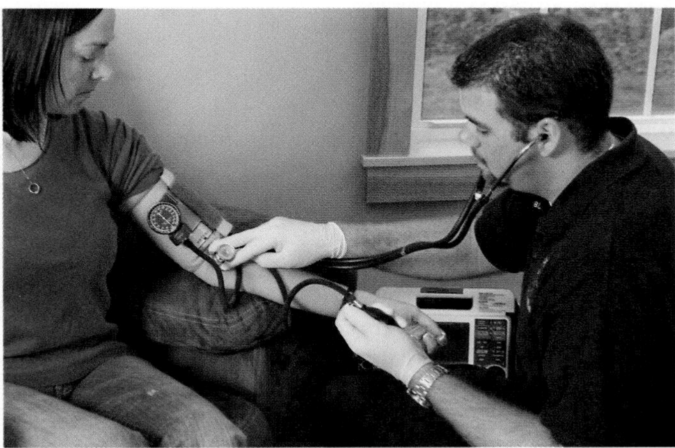

FIGURE 11-9a ✱ Always obtain at least one blood pressure by auscultation prior to applying the noninvasive blood pressure monitor.

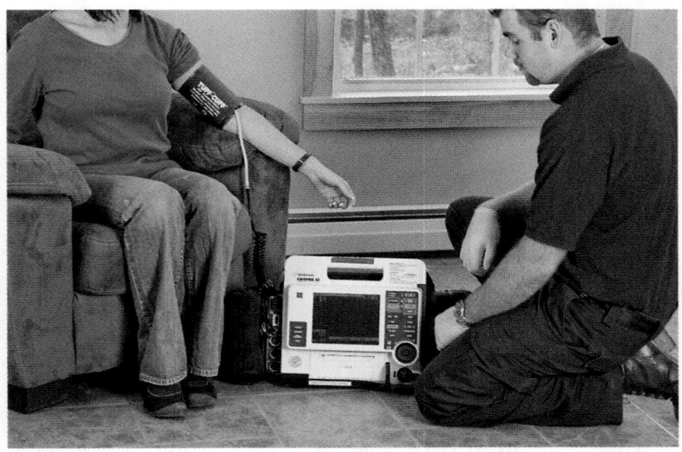

FIGURE 11-9b ✱ Apply the noninvasive blood pressure monitoring device to obtain regular blood pressure readings.

the patient but also from others at the scene. Prior to obtaining a history or performing a physical examination it is necessary to gain control of the scene. The entire history or parts of the history might be sought and obtained from Emergency Medical Responders, relatives, or other caregivers at the scene. By using the following techniques, you should be more successful in taking the history and obtaining the necessary information.

Achieve a Smooth Transition of Care

When you arrive on the scene, it is important to achieve a smooth transition of care from an Emergency Medical Responder, police officer, or other individual who is providing first aid. Announce your arrival by stating, for example, "I'm John Brady and this is Susan Kechlow. We are emergency medical technicians. Can you tell us what has happened and what care has been given?"

If the patient appears to be alert and responsive, you will have time to quickly gain information from the Emergency Medical Responders before you make actual patient contact. This should take less than 1 minute. Do not carry on a conversation that is irrelevant to the patient, as this tends to ruin your presentation of confidence, competence, and compassion. An unresponsive or obviously injured patient needs your immediate attention. In this situation, proceed directly to the patient and obtain information from others at the scene as you begin to perform your primary assessment.

Reduce the Patient's Anxiety

Once you make contact with the patient, attempt to reduce his anxiety and that of others at the scene. You can do this by employing the following simple techniques:

1. Bring order to the environment.
2. Introduce yourself.
3. Gain patient consent.
4. Position yourself.
5. Use communication skills.
6. Be courteous.
7. Use touch when appropriate.

Bring Order to the Environment

As quickly as possible, bring order to the environment by asking that televisions or radios be turned down, dogs removed from the area in which you are working, and children supervised by a family member, police officer, or Emergency Medical Responder. Do not walk up to a television and simply turn it off while someone is watching it. No matter how serious the situation or patient appears, there are people who become extremely agitated when treated in this manner. You would be setting yourself up for a possible violent confrontation. You must explain, for example, "It is extremely important that you turn the television off so that we can hear and focus on caring for your mother." If the person refuses, ask for the sound to be turned down or remove the patient as quickly as possible from the scene.

Remember, not everyone at the scene is happy to see you. Some people will become agitated and resist your simple requests. You must remain calm and nonconfrontational and continue to focus on patient care.

Introduce Yourself

Introduce yourself and ask for the patient's name. Address older individuals formally as "Mr. Jones" or "Mrs. Smith" to avoid any implication of disrespect. If time or the situation permits, you can ask, "What would you like me to call you?"

Gain Patient Consent

Gain consent from the patient. This step is necessary before you may legally provide emergency care. You can do it simply by asking, "Is it all right for me to help you?" If the patient has an altered mental status, is unresponsive, or is unable to make a rational decision, provide emergency care based on implied consent.

If the patient refuses your assistance, do not immediately pack up your equipment and pull out the refusal form, ready for the patient's signature. Many times the patient initially refuses care out of denial (a normal, and usually temporary, psychological response in which the patient cannot accept that he is ill or injured) or because he is frightened or confused. Keep talking with the patient to establish a rapport and help the patient accept the need for you to assess and treat him. If necessary, enlist the aid of a family member in convincing the patient. If the patient continues to refuse, contact medical direction for advice on how to proceed. Refer to Chapter 3, "Medical, Legal, and Ethical Issues," for further discussions on the legal implications of patient consent and refusal of emergency care.

Position Yourself

Your body position and posture are forms of nonverbal communication. Position yourself at a comfortable level in relation to the patient. If the eye levels are equal, so is the authority. If you are standing over the patient, you are in a dominant position of authority and control. This may be uncomfortable for the patient and may set the wrong tone for the scene. (At some scenes, when you need to establish control, this position is warranted.)

In the general American culture, intimate space generally starts at about 18 inches from the body. Unless you are intentionally touching your patient (see the next section), the patient is likely to be most comfortable if you maintain at least this distance from him during history taking or other conversation.

Thinking Critically
A family is yelling at you to "do something" for your chest pain patient. They rudely refuse your requests to turn down the TV and get the dog out of the room. You'd like to yell back but know it's important to be courteous. Why?

Standing with your arms crossed over your chest is a closed communication posture, conveying hostility or disinterest. Instead, you want to display an openness and willingness to help.

Use Communication Skills

As much as possible, maintain eye contact when talking with the patient to help establish rapport and to convey your sincere concern.

Speak calmly and deliberately to allow the patient to process the information. Raise your voice only if the patient appears to be hearing impaired. An elderly patient is not necessarily hard of hearing. Speak slowly, clearly, and directly to elderly patients. Give them additional time to respond to each question. Also speak in a calm and confident manner when you are communicating to your partner or others at the scene. Yelling or screaming while directing the scene and giving orders will only increase the anxiety of the patient and bystanders and exhibits a loss of control on your part.

Your body movements should be purposeful, displaying competence and confidence, and not hasty or jerky.

Actively listen to what the patient is telling you. This avoids having to unnecessarily, and annoyingly, ask the same question several times. Make sure that the patient realizes you are listening by leaning forward, maintaining eye contact, and not allowing your attention to wander while the patient is talking to you.

Be Courteous

The scene of an emergency is very stressful. As a result, the patient, family members, and bystanders may not be at their best. They may often seem quarrelsome, petty, rude, or hostile. As a professional, you must resist yielding to the same stresses. Try to understand why people behave as they do, and maintain a courteous manner throughout the call.

Use Touch When Appropriate

Touching the patient is a powerful comfort measure when dealing with most people. Use eye contact to avoid the patient's perception of the touching as encroachment. Hold a hand, pat a shoulder, or lay your hand on a forearm. In order for touch to be effective, you must be sincere in your gestures, not using them as a gimmick.

Maintain Control

It is difficult to conduct an assessment, gather information from the patient, and provide emergency care at a scene that is not controlled. The greater the distractions at the scene, the higher the anxiety level of the patient, family, and bystanders. Use the scene control measures described earlier to lessen confusion, reduce anxiety, and convey a professional attitude that the patient is in the care of capable EMTs.

It is important to recognize when a scene cannot be adequately controlled. It may be impossible to gain scene control when the crowd is extremely hostile, the family is emotionally charged or upset, threats are being made toward you, or the scene is unstable because of the risk of fire, explosion, or other hazards. You must consider your own safety when working in an uncontrolled environment. If the scene remains uncontrolled, it is best to move as rapidly as possible to remove yourself and the patient from the scene and/or to call for additional resources as needed.

Taking the History

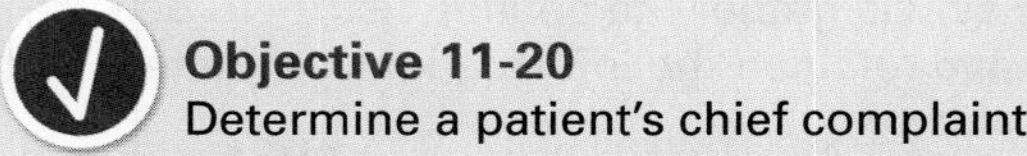

Objective 11-20
Determine a patient's chief complaint.

Information gained in the history is as important in most medical cases as the information determined through the physical examination. The history typically begins with determining the **chief complaint.** The chief complaint is the reason why the EMS crew was called to the scene. You will continue with obtaining information about the present illness, significant past medical history, and the current health status of the patient. The information gathered may provide direction for the physical examination. Often, the history and physical examination are conducted concurrently depending on the resources at the scene and the condition of the patient. Although a structured approach to history taking will be presented, the process must remain dynamic to allow you to pursue pieces of information provided by the patient or other persons as they are presented.

The best source to gather the history from is the patient. If that is not possible, you can attempt to obtain history information from the family, friends, bystanders, other emergency responders, medication containers, medical identification tags, and any other source possible. When using sources other than the patient, the accuracy of the information may be questionable.

Once the chief complaint is obtained, you will proceed with a history of the present illness. This is a more

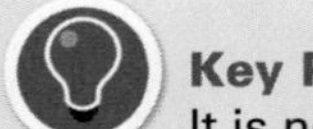

Key Points
It is not only acceptable, it is necessary to take notes as you gather the patient history to be sure you have retained the information completely and accurately.

Objective 11-21
Given a scenario, efficiently elicit an adequate patient history using closed-ended and open-ended questions and active listening techniques.

detailed evaluation of the chief complaint and associated signs and symptoms. Other components include demographic information, current health status, and past medical history. You may need to ask questions about sensitive topics such as alcohol or drug use or sexual history. You will build your history-taking technique and become comfortable through practice and experience.

Statistical and Demographic Information

Certain data will be collected for statistical, record keeping, and demographic purposes. These data include the following:

- **Date.** Be sure to document the correct current date and dates of information provided by the patient regarding complaints, signs, treatments, illnesses, hospitalizations, and any other pertinent information.
- **Time.** Document the time of events accurately.
- **Identifying data.** Record the patient's age, sex, and race.

Current Health Status

Determine the current health status of the patient relevant to the chief complaint and medical illness or injury. The current health status focuses on the patient's present state of health. Take into consideration environmental and individual factors. Environmental conditions may include what the patient is exposed to at work, in the home, or in recreational activities. Individual factors to consider are:

- Current medications, including prescription and over-the-counter medications
- Allergies to medications or other substances
- Tobacco use, including type of tobacco and how much
- Alcohol, drugs, and related substances
- Diet, including daily food and drink intake
- Screening tests that may have been done recently
- Immunization against certain diseases
- Environmental hazards the patient is exposed to
- Use of safety equipment such as seat belts and bike helmets
- Family history, especially for disease with a hereditary link

Techniques for Taking a Patient History

Certain techniques that can be used to better facilitate the history-taking and information-gathering process are described next.

Note Taking

Document the information the patient provides as accurately as possible. It is typically impossible to remember all the information the patient provides, especially when you are doing multiple calls back-to-back. The information seems to meld together and it is sometimes difficult to recall the history of the current patient and not confuse it with information gained from previous patients in the day. Thus, it is not only acceptable but also necessary to take notes to present the most accurate information as possible.

Types of Questions

There are basically two types of questions used by EMTs to gather a history: open-ended questions and closed-ended questions. An **open-ended question** requires the patient to respond with a descriptive or more detailed answer. "How are you feeling today?" and "Can you describe the discomfort?" are examples of open-ended questions. The patient is unable to provide a "yes" or "no" answer to open-ended questions.

A **closed-ended question** is often a rapid-fire-type question that requires only a "yes" or "no" answer. "Are you having pain in your chest?" and "Do you feel lightheaded?" are examples of closed-ended questions. Often, both types of questions are used throughout the history. A multiple-choice question that uses a mix of both formats may also be used. "When are you more short of breath: when you lie flat or when you sit up?" is an example of a multiple-choice question.

The patient's condition may require that you use more of one type of question than the other. If a patient is struggling to breathe because of an acute asthma attack, you don't want him expending lots of energy trying to provide long answers to your open-ended questions. Thus, you would use rapid-fire, closed-ended questions to gather a great amount of information in a short time with less effort on the patient's part. Be careful, however, since it is easy to lead the patient with closed-ended questions. You might find a patient answering "yes" to all the questions, even the ones that contradict each other.

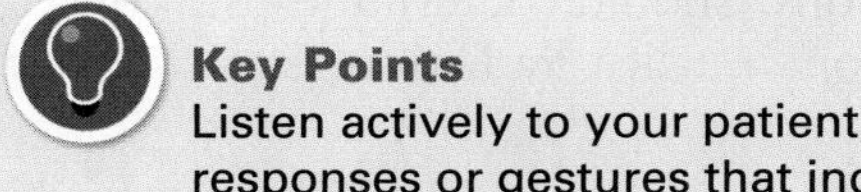

Key Points
Listen actively to your patient, providing responses or gestures that indicate you understand.

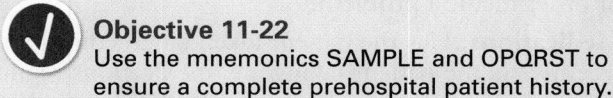

Objective 11-22
Use the mnemonics SAMPLE and OPQRST to ensure a complete prehospital patient history.

To determine the chief complaint, use an open-ended question. "Why did you call EMS?" or "What seems to be the problem today?" are often used to elicit a chief complaint. Be aware that the chief complaint is not always the primary problem. For example, the patient states "My belly hurts" when asked why he called EMS. However, as you pursue the history you find that he has had the belly pain for 3 weeks and called EMS today because he had bloody diarrhea.

Be sure to use plain English and not medical terminology when asking any of the questions.

Active Listening Techniques

Listen actively to your patient and provide responses or gestures that indicate you understand. The following are active listening techniques.

- **Facilitation.** Maintain eye contact with the patient in a sincere manner. Use posture, actions, words, facial expressions, or cues while listening to help your patient feel comfortable, open up, and provide more information. Phrases such as "I'm listening" or "Go on" may be used.
- **Reflection.** Repeating the patient's words will encourage him to provide additional responses. Avoid interrupting the patient's train of thought while practicing reflection. This may encourage the patient to reveal information you might not otherwise have discovered. The patient states, "My belly hurts" as a response to your open-ended question to gather the chief complaint. "Your belly hurts?" is your response. The patient then states, "Yes, it has hurt ever since I haven't had a bowel movement for this past week." Your response is, "You haven't had a bowel movement for a week?" The patient then responds with, "No, it has been more than a week and my belly began hurting a few days ago." As you can see, the chief complaint has changed its focus from abdominal pain to a possible bowel obstruction.
- **Clarification.** Clarification is used to clarify ambiguous statements, responses, symptoms, or words. The patient states, "I feel bad all over." You then clarify by asking, "Can you describe what the bad feeling feels like?" The patient responds with, "It feels like pins and needles in my arms and legs." The clarification technique provided a much more descriptive symptom.
- **Empathetic Response.** Show empathy through verbal responses and gestures. "I understand" or "I see how that would be difficult" are some verbal responses that show empathy.
- **Confrontation.** Sometimes patients will not provide the entire truth or will try to downplay symptoms. You may need to confront them to determine the accurate information. "You said you have never been to the doctor, but there is a prescription for Glucophage in your name on the table" is an example of confrontation.
- **Interpretation.** Interpretation takes confrontation to the next level. You may need to make an inference based on your observations. As an example, "You say you have never been to the doctor, yet you have a prescription medication in your name. Are you afraid your current medical condition is worsening and you might have to be admitted to the hospital?"

Standardized Approach to History Taking

The SAMPLE History

The **SAMPLE history** is a medical history of the patient that you gather by asking questions of the patient, family, and bystanders. *SAMPLE* is a mnemonic (memory aid) used to help you remember the information that must be included in a patient history. It spells out the first letters of the following categories:

- **Signs and symptoms. Signs** are any objective physical evidence of medical or trauma conditions that you can see, hear, feel, or smell. For example, you can hear stridor, you can see bleeding, and you can feel skin temperature. **Symptoms** are conditions that cannot be observed and must be described by the patient, such as pain in the abdomen or numbness in the legs. When you begin to question the patient, ask: "What are you feeling? When and where did the first symptoms occur? What were you doing at the time?" Another mnemonic used to evaluate the patient's symptoms is OPQRST (onset, provocation/palliation, quality, radiation, severity, and time).
- **Allergies.** Determine whether the patient has any allergies to medications, food, or environmental agents such as pollen, grass, ragweed, or molds. Ask about the type of reaction to the allergen, such as a rash or wheezing. If you have not already done so during the

physical exam, check for a medical alert tag, necklace, anklet, or bracelet, which can alert you to an allergy or other medical problem.

- **Medications.** Has the patient taken any medications recently? Is the patient taking any medications regularly? It is important to determine if the patient takes (1) prescription medications, (2) nonprescription or over-the-counter medications, (3) birth control pills, (4) illicit drugs, (5) herbal medications, (6) erectile dysfunction drugs, (7) another person's prescription medication, or (8) vitamins. If you suspect illegal drug use, you might say something like, "I'm an EMT, not a police officer. I need all the information you can give me so I can provide the proper care. Let's work on helping you right now." As with allergies, look for a medical alert tag if the patient is unresponsive.
- **Pertinent past history.** Find out about underlying medical problems like seizures, heart disease, diabetes, kidney disease, or emphysema. Ask if there have been past surgical procedures or trauma, and whether the patient is currently under a doctor's care. Again, look for a medical alert tag if the patient is unresponsive.
- **Last oral intake.** Find out when the patient last ingested a solid or liquid. Find out what it was, when it was consumed, and the quantity that was consumed. Ask: "When did you last eat or drink anything?"
- **Events leading to the injury or illness.** What occurred before the patient became ill or had the accident? Were there any unusual circumstances? What was the patient doing? Did the patient have any peculiar feelings or experiences?

ASSESSMENT Tips

When patients are asked about their last meal, they often interpret this as breakfast, lunch, or dinner, which may have been several hours from the time of the call, and not provide information about snacks between meals, which may have occurred very close to the time of the call. That is why you ask about last oral intake and not the last meal. ■

As you conduct a SAMPLE history, try to get more detailed information about the conditions that are directly related to or that could adversely affect the present problem. If you are caring for a burn victim, for example, it would be important to learn if there are underlying cardiac or respiratory problems that might impair breathing. It would not be relevant to learn that the patient had a hernia surgery 5 years ago or had measles as a child.

Assessing Patient Complaints: OPQRST

OPQRST is a mnemonic for remembering the questions to ask when assessing the patient's chief complaint or major symptoms, such as pain, that the patient can tell you about. Your questions should determine the onset, provocation/palliation, quality, radiation, severity, and time of the complaint.

- **Onset.** *When and how did the symptom begin?* Ask the patient if the onset was sudden or gradual. Also determine if the onset was associated with a particular activity. For example, you arrive on the scene and find a patient complaining of chest pain. The patient states the onset of the chest pain was sudden. You then ask, "What were you doing when the chest pain started?" The patient replies, "I was playing tennis at the time." Based on this response, you would document the onset of chest pain as being associated with strenuous activity.

ASSESSMENT Tips

It is crucial to determine the exact time of onset of the first sign of weakness, slurred speech, numbness, paralysis, facial droop, or other signs of stroke and report it to the emergency department or receiving medical facility. You may be the only person who can collect this vital information at the scene from relatives, friends, or bystanders. It may make a critical difference in stroke and cardiac treatment once at the hospital. ■

- **Provocation/palliation/position.** *What makes the symptom worse? What makes it better? In what position is the patient found?* A patient complaining of chest pain may tell you that walking up the steps made the pain much worse, or a patient complaining of dyspnea states, "When I lie flat in bed, I can't breathe." Determine if the patient has taken any medication to attempt to relieve the symptoms. A patient complaining of abdominal pain may have taken an antacid. If something was taken, determine if the symptoms were relieved, made worse, or remained the same. Also, pay attention to the position the patient was found in since it can provide clues to the condition. As an example, if the patient is found in a fetal position with his legs drawn up and does not want to move, you would assume the patient is having severe abdominal pain. A patient in a tripod position is likely having difficulty breathing. You will need to consider whether the patient should be allowed to remain in that position or if it is necessary to reposition the patient to conduct the physical exam or to prepare to transport.
- **Quality.** *How would you describe the pain?* Quality is most often associated with a complaint of pain. Ask the patient to describe the pain. Most often, pain is described as crushing, aching, dull, stabbing, knifelike, crampy, gnawing, burning, or tearing. Do not lead the patient by asking, "Is the pain sharp or dull?" Ask an open-ended question such as, "What does the pain feel like?"

Key Points
To obtain the most effective information, ask open-ended questions when you can.

Objective 11-23
React appropriately when asking questions about sensitive topics or when caring for patients who present special challenges to history-taking and assessment.

The quality of pain, with other signs and symptoms, usually helps to determine what organ system is involved. For example, dull, aching, tight, pressure-type chest pain is usually associated with a cardiac problem; conditions involving the lung or chest wall muscles or nerves usually produce a sharper, knifelike pain.

- **Radiation.** *Where do you feel the pain? Where does the pain go?* Prior to asking about radiation, it is necessary to determine the exact location of the pain. Ask the patient to point to the pain with one finger. The pain is localized if he can isolate it to one area. Generalized pain cannot be localized and is spread over a general area. From the point of the initial pain, ask if the pain extends, moves, or radiates. Commonly, pain associated with the heart radiates to the arms, neck, and back. Pain associated with an aortic aneurysm (a weakened and ballooned segment of the wall of the aorta) commonly radiates to the back in the lumbar region or to the groin. Kidney stones commonly produce pain in the flank area (side) that radiates down along the groin.
- **Severity.** *How bad is the symptom?* Ask the patient to rate the pain on a scale of 1 to 10 with 10 being the most severe. Have the patient compare the pain with a previous condition he may have suffered that involved pain. The patient's appearance should give you some indication as to the severity of the pain. Is the patient squirming about in pain or easily distracted from the pain?
- **Time.** *How long have you had the symptom?* Determine if the symptom has been present for minutes, hours, days, weeks, months, or years. If you get called to the scene and find a patient complaining of a symptom that has been present for more than a day, ask the patient, without appearing to be judgmental, "Why did you call us today?" If the symptoms have been present for a few hours or more, ask the patient, "Was there any change in the symptoms that caused you to call?" Most times the patient will call EMS when the pain gets worse, changes in quality, or if other associated signs or symptoms occur. Do not assume that a patient suffering pain or some other symptom accesses EMS immediately. Document the length of time the symptoms have been present.

To gather the most effective information, ask open-ended questions when you can—ones that cannot be answered merely "yes" or "no" but require a fuller response or description from the patient. Then wait for the patient's response. Whenever trauma is involved, try to identify the mechanism of injury (the manner by which the injury occurred) through observation or questioning. Pertinent negatives, things the patient denies, are also important to note. For example, if you ask a patient with chest pain if he is short of breath and he says no, you would document "Patient denies having shortness of breath." Finally, remember to write all pertinent findings from the SAMPLE history on the prehospital care report.

Sensitive Topics or Special Challenges

Sensitive Topics

It may be necessary to ask questions in the history that you might consider to be sensitive in nature, such as alcohol or drug use, physical or sexual abuse, or sexual history. When asking questions that may be sensitive, remain nonjudgmental and only ask questions that pertain directly to the medical history and are necessary to gain answers that are pertinent to your assessment and emergency care. Respect the patient's privacy and ask questions of a sensitive nature at the appropriate time and in an appropriate location. You are not a mental health professional and are not trained in counseling; thus, your interaction with the patient on sensitive topics must remain within the scope of your practice.

Special Challenges

Some patients create special challenges to gathering a history. Typically, as you become more experienced and build a solid technique for history taking, the challenges become easier to manage. Some of the challenges are:

- **Silence.** Silence can be uncomfortable for both you and the patient. Attempt to determine why the patient has become silent. It may be due to several factors. The patient may have suffered a medical condition such as a stroke or brain injury that renders him unable to speak. The patient may just need time to respond to your question. This is often true in the elderly. The patient may be overwhelmed with the situation or you may have asked too many questions and he is trying to sort his thoughts. Provide the patient adequate time to respond. Watch his body language for nonverbal clues such as crying; facial expressions of anger, confusion, or depression; a closed body posture; and signs of being tense. Try to determine the cause for the silence, rectify it if possible, and proceed with the history.

- **Overly talkative patient.** Some patients will continue to talk and not allow you enough time to ask questions. Give your patient a free rein for a period of time to talk and express himself. You can interrupt him and summarize his statements frequently. You can also proceed to closed-ended questions in an attempt to control the history. Maintain patience and gather as much information as possible.
- **Patient with multiple symptoms.** Some patients will present a multitude of complaints. The challenge is attempting to determine the true chief complaint. You will need to use clarification to bring the patient to a primary chief complaint. Asking "But why did you call today?"or "What was the primary reason for calling us today?" may assist you in determining the actual chief complaint.
- **Anxious patient.** Many patients experience anxiety in an acute emergency. The patient may exhibit many nonverbal clues such as sweating, nervousness, trembling, and tachycardia. Encourage the patient to freely express his feeling of anxiousness or anxiety. The best approach you can take is to provide reassurance.
- **Angry and hostile patient.** Anger and hostility are a natural part of illness and injury. Because you are likely to be the first medical person to provide care for the patient, it may be you that the patient or family directs the anger toward. They are not really angry at you, even though it may appear that way. Remain calm, confident, professional, and competent. Accept the patient and family members' feelings. Do not become frustrated, angry, or defensive.
- **Intoxicated patient.** The most significant concern with an intoxicated patient is your own safety. An intoxicated patient may suddenly change his behavior and become violent. Always remain vigilant when dealing with an intoxicated patient. The easiest way to deal with this patient is not to challenge but to accept him. Do not ask the patient to lower his voice or stop pacing. Listen to what the patient is saying through the loud voice, shouting, or cursing. Avoid trapping the intoxicated patient in a small area as well as any other behavior that may appear threatening to the patient. Remain nonjudgmental and attempt to provide assistance to the patient. In some cases it may be necessary to involve law enforcement to protect yourself, the patient, or bystanders.
- **Crying patient.** Crying is a nonverbal clue to the patient's emotions. Be patient, empathetic, and supportive. It is okay to allow the patient to cry. Provide reassurance and remain supportive.
- **Depressed patient.** Look for signs of depression such as weight loss, flat affect, poor eye contact, insomnia, loss of appetite, fatigue, or complaints of aches or pains. Listen carefully to the patient and remain nonjudgmental. If there are signs of serious depression, such as thoughts of suicide, be sure to get the patient the assistance and care that he needs.
- **Confusing behavior or history.** A patient who presents with a confusing history or bizarre or unusual behavior may be suffering from a mental illness, dementia, or delirium. Dementia is associated with a gradual decline in the mental status of the patient due to some type of neurological disease. Delirium is an acute alteration in the mental function of the patient that is usually due to a reversible cause such as intoxication or drug use. Do not spend an excessive amount of time trying to collect a history in these patients.
- **Patient with limited intelligence.** The patient will often be able to provide you with adequate history information. Be alert to possible omissions of information. If the patient has a severe cognitive impairment, obtain the history from the family or caregivers.
- **Language barrier.** If the patient speaks a language that you are not fluent in, try to find an interpreter such as a family member. Realize that some history information may be confused or lost in the translation. If a translator is not available, contact a telephone translation service or transport the patient and notify the hospital of the need for a translator.
- **Hearing impairment.** Hearing impairment offers many of the same challenges as a language barrier. The advantage in this situation, however, is that you can revert to writing to ask questions and obtain information. When speaking to a hearing-impaired person, face the patient and look at him when you speak. Such patients often read lips. Use a person who can sign as your translator if available.
- **Visual impairment.** Remember to tell the visually impaired patient everything you are doing. These patients cannot see your movements or hand gestures. You may increase their anxiety significantly if they are not continuously made aware of what is happening at the scene. Constantly communicate with the patient.

Key Points
A child 4 years or older should be the primary source of his history.

Key Points
Do not assume dementia in an elderly patient. If mental impairment presents, ask family or friends if this is normal for the patient.

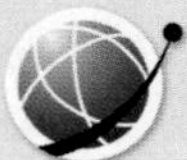

Media Resources
Go to www.bradybooks.com for mykit. Highlights:

- *Web Resource:* Pulse Oximetry
- *Video:* Vital Sign Assessment

- **Talking with friends and family.** Some patients will only be able to provide limited information. You may need to rely on family members or friends to fill in the gaps or provide the entire history. Family or friends may be very useful in providing information about the events leading up to the emergency.
- **Pediatric patient.** The pediatric patient may present with special challenges based on ability to understand the questions you are asking. A child may not have the ability to respond appropriately. Once the child reaches 4 years of age, he should become the primary source of the history. Use the parent or caregiver to fill in the gaps.
- **Elderly patient.** The elderly patient may have physical limitations such as impaired sight or hearing that make history gathering a challenge. Do not assume that an elderly patient suffers from dementia. If mental impairment seems evident, ask family or friends if this is the patient's normal presentation or if it may be a result of the current medical condition or emergency. Normally, the elderly patient should be the primary source for the information. Be patient and, if necessary, allow extra time for responses to your questions.

EMT skills 11-1 Taking Blood Pressure by Auscultation

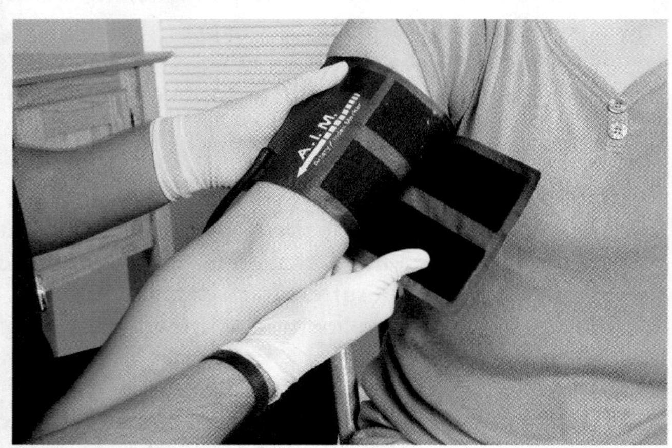

11-1A * Apply the cuff.

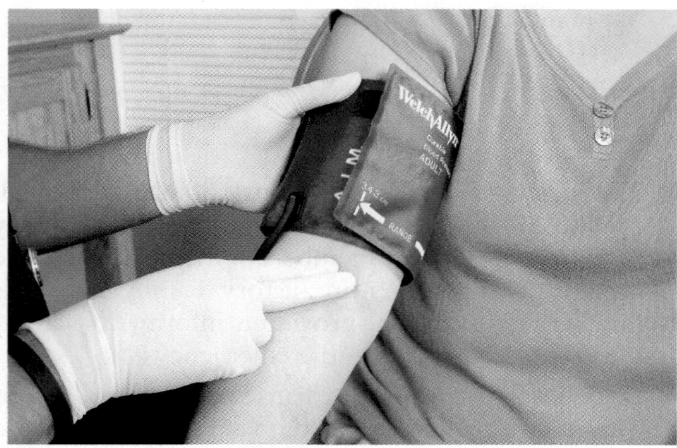

11-1B * Palpate the brachial artery.

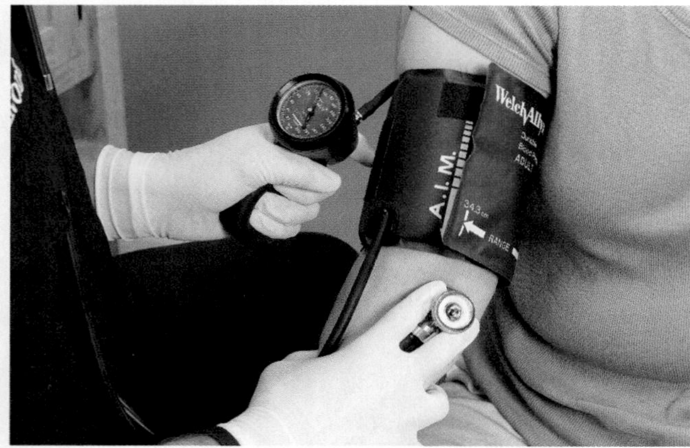

11-1C * Close the valve and pump until the radial pulse is no longer felt. Note the number and deflate the cuff. Position the stethoscope over the brachial artery and inflate the cuff to 30 mmHg above the level where you previously stopped feeling the radial pulse.

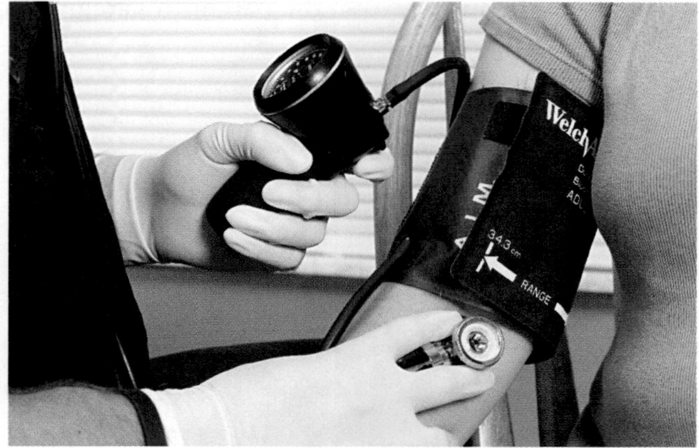

11-1D * Deflate the cuff at about 2 mmHg per second. When you hear the first sound, record the pressure (systolic). Continue releasing air. When you hear the last sound, record the pressure (diastolic).

EMT skills 11-2 Taking Blood Pressure by Palpation

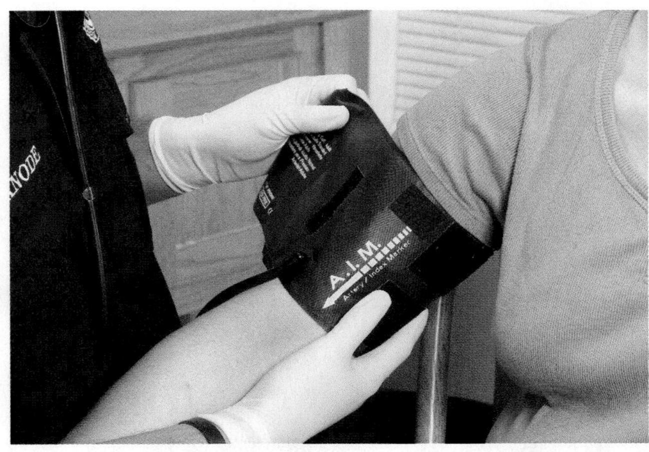

11-2A * Apply the cuff and inflate rapidly to 30 mmHg above the level where you can no longer feel the radial pulse.

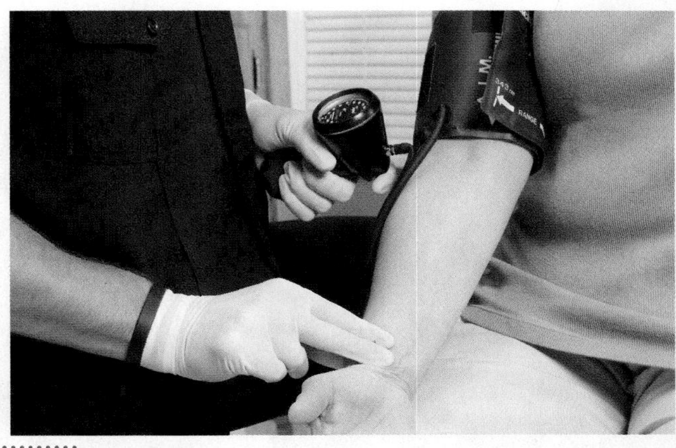

11-2B * Slowly deflate the cuff. Note the pressure at which the radial pulse returns (systolic). You will not be able to measure the diastolic pressure by palpation.

EMT skills 11-3 Taking Orthostatic Vital Signs

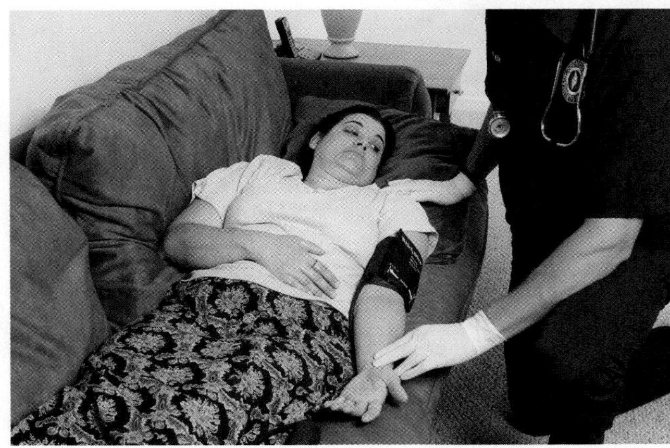

11-3A * Place the patient supine and measure heart rate and blood pressure.

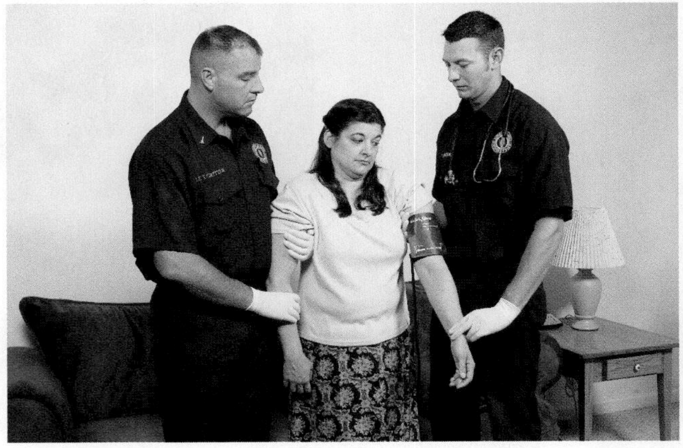

11-3B * Help the patient to a standing position, wait 2 minutes, then measure heart rate and blood pressure. Compare the readings to those taken while the patient was supine. An increase in heart rate more than 10–20 bpm and a decrease in blood pressure by 10–20 mmHg is considered a positive orthostatic test, indicating inadequate blood volume.

EMT skills 11-4 Pulse Oximetry

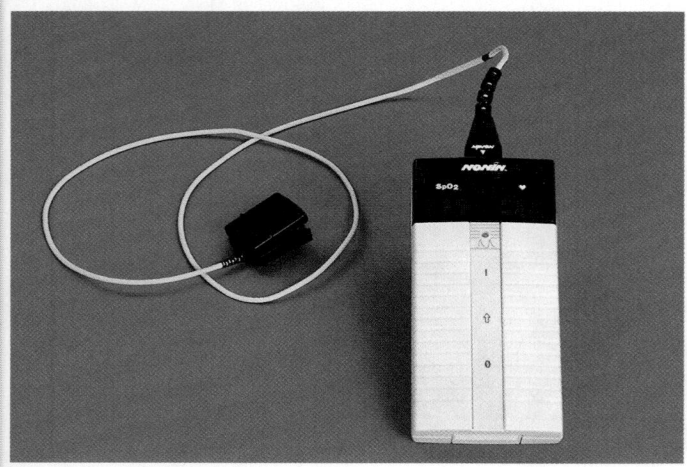

11-4A ✱ A pulse oximeter.

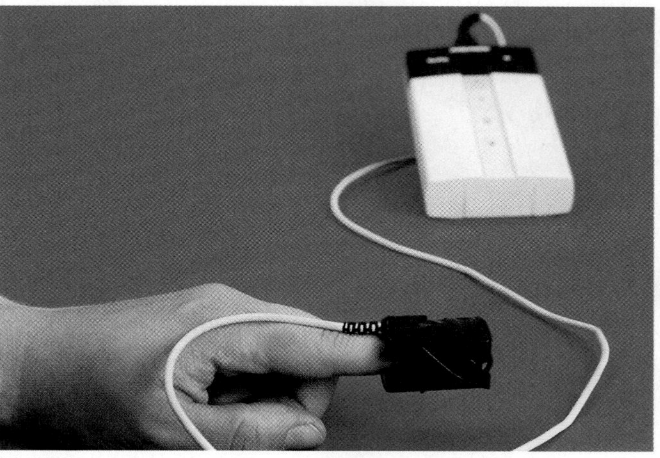

11-4B ✱ A pulse oximeter placed on the patient's finger.

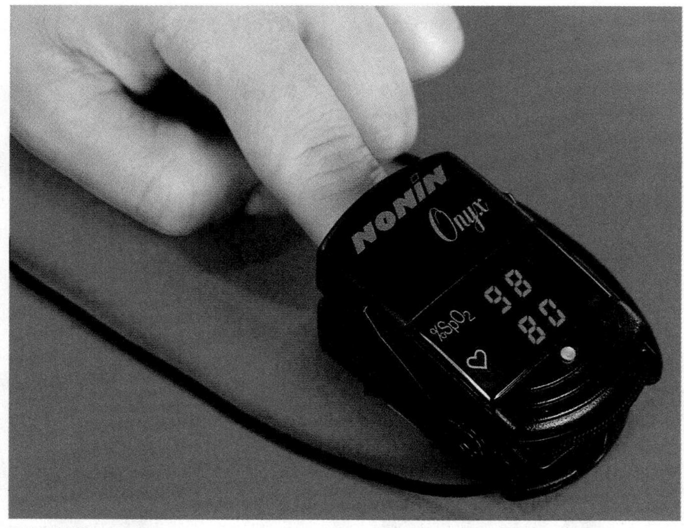

11-4C ✱ A mini "finger-size" pulse oximeter.

CHAPTER REVIEW

SUMMARY

Assessing vital signs is an important EMT function. You will take vital signs on every patient you encounter. These vital signs are typically the first ones taken in the emergency situation and are often used as the baseline from which the medical team gauges changes in the patient's condition. You will often take several sets of vital signs on each patient in an attempt to identify trends in the patient's condition, that is, whether he is improving or deteriorating. The vital signs cannot be used as the sole indicator of the patient's condition but, instead, must be viewed in the context of the whole patient along with other indicators, such as signs and symptoms.

The six vital signs that you will assess are breathing (respirations), pulse, skin, pupils, blood pressure, and pulse oximetry. In a stable patient the vital signs are assessed every 15 minutes, whereas they are assessed every 5 minutes in the unstable patient.

Obtaining a history is important in determining the condition of the patient and what emergency care is necessary, especially in the medical patient. You will often use closed-ended questions in the trauma patient where history is less important and in those who are having trouble responding. Open-ended questions are used in the medical patient and generally provide more information. You must be prepared for many challenges in history taking.

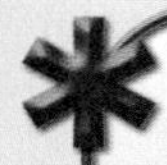

CASE STUDY FOLLOW-UP

SCENE SIZE-UP

You have been dispatched to the scene of an 86-year-old male who lives alone. His daughter, who found him, reports that the patient, Mr. Li, fell early this morning and was unable to get up. As you and your partner enter the home, you note no safety hazards.

Upon entering the kitchen, you see Mr. Li supine on the floor, eyes closed, with a blanket covering him from shoulders to feet. The kitchen is very tidy and clean. The daughter, Ms. Kennedy, says she thinks he fell off a chair he had been standing on to reach the top of a cupboard.

PATIENT ASSESSMENT

You crouch next to Mr. Li as your partner provides manual stabilization of his head and neck and ask, "Are you okay?" He opens his eyes and responds, "I think so." You check for life-threatening problems with the airway, breathing, and circulation and find none. You conduct a more thorough exam before you transport Mr. Li to the hospital.

You administer oxygen, conduct a head-to-toe physical exam (during which you discover that Mr. Li is wearing a bracelet identifying him as a diabetic), and apply a spinal cervical immobilization collar. Then you obtain a set of baseline vital signs. Your findings are: respirations 18 and normal; pulse 78 and regular; skin pink, warm, and dry; pupils normal, equal, and reactive; blood pressure 168/82 mmHg; and SpO_2 is 98%.

Finally, you gather a SAMPLE history. By questioning Mr. Li and his daughter, you learn that Mr. Li's main symptom is the pain in his left hip, which he says was brought on by the fall several hours ago. In answer to your questions, he says the pain is especially severe when he tries to move his left leg, describes the pain as sharp, and says it does not radiate to any other location. Mr. Li also states that he is allergic to penicillin to which he develops a rash. Questioned about his medications, he says he takes insulin daily to help control blood sugar. When you ask about pertinent past history, the daughter confirms that Mr. Li has a history of diabetes and tells you that he had both hip joints replaced in 1989. You inquire about last oral intake—what Mr. Li last ate or drank—and Mr. Li says he has not eaten a meal since dinner last night. Ms. Kennedy adds that while they were waiting for the ambulance, she gave her father a glass of water. The patient describes the events that led to the injury by explaining that he slipped and fell from the chair at about 11:00 A.M.

You prepare your patient for transport by applying a splint to the left leg and hip, immobilizing him to a long spine board, securing him to your wheeled stretcher, and placing him in the ambulance.

En route to the hospital, you reassess Mr. Li's airway, breathing, and circulation and find no abnormalities. You frequently check that he is comfortable; that he is properly secured to the splint, spine board, and stretcher; and that the oxygen mask is secure and oxygen flowing properly. Because Mr. Li's condition is considered stable, you repeat and record his vital signs every 15 minutes before reaching the hospital without finding any significant changes. Transport is uneventful, and you transfer Mr. Li to the emergency department personnel. After completing a prehospital care report, you and your partner prepare the ambulance for the next call.

IN REVIEW

1. Identify the components of vital signs, and state how often they should be taken.
2. Explain how to assess a patient's breathing rate and quality of breathing. Also state the normal ranges of respirations per minute for the adult, child, and infant.
3. Describe what you would observe when a patient is breathing normally and when a patient is breathing abnormally.
4. State the general circumstances under which you would choose to take a radial pulse, a brachial pulse, or a carotid pulse.
5. Explain how to take a pulse. Also identify normal resting pulse rates in an adult, adolescent, school-age child, preschool child, and infant. Define the terms that you would use to describe pulse quality.
6. List the places on the body to check for skin color. Also identify normal and abnormal skin colors.
7. Explain how to assess a patient's pupils, and describe normal and abnormal findings.
8. Explain how to take a blood pressure by palpation and by auscultation. Also identify the normal ranges of systolic and diastolic blood pressure for an adult male and an adult female.
9. Explain the indications for and limitations of pulse oximetry. Explain how to take an SpO_2 reading.
10. Name the categories of information you need to obtain through a SAMPLE history.
11. List the information collected by using the OPQRST mnemonic.
12. Describe special challenges to history taking and methods of how you would overcome each challenge.

CRITICAL THINKING

You are called to a residence for a patient who has fallen. A neighbor has made the call to 911. Upon your arrival, you find a 56-year-old male patient who has fallen from the roof of his house onto the concrete driveway. As you approach the patient, he is not alert and has severe trauma to the head. It appears he has fallen head first. He has a large amount of blood coming from his mouth, nose, and ears. You hear gurgling sounds with each respiration. His respirations are rapid at approximately 45 per minute with minimal chest movement. His radial pulse is slow at a rate of 48 per minute, but strong. His BP is 198/72 mmHg. The SpO_2 reading is 76% on room air. His skin is cyanotic, warm, and dry. His wife arrives home while you are on the scene and begins to scream frantically.

1. What is the significance of the gurgling sound?
2. How would you document the pulse rate?
3. What does the pulse oximeter reading indicate?
4. What do the skin signs indicate?
5. What other vital signs would be important to assess in this patient?
6. When would you attempt to gather a SAMPLE history?
7. How would you gather the SAMPLE history?
8. What information would you be able to gather using the OPQRST mnemonic?

PEARSON

EXPLORE mybradykit™

Please go to **www.bradybooks.com** to access mykit for this text. You will find quizzes, critical thinking scenarios, weblinks, animations, and videos related to this chapter—and much more. Look for online information on taking a pulse. You will also find a video clip on vital sign assessment.

Register your access code from the front of your book by going to **www.bradybooks.com** and selecting the mykit links.

CHAPTER 12 Scene Size-Up

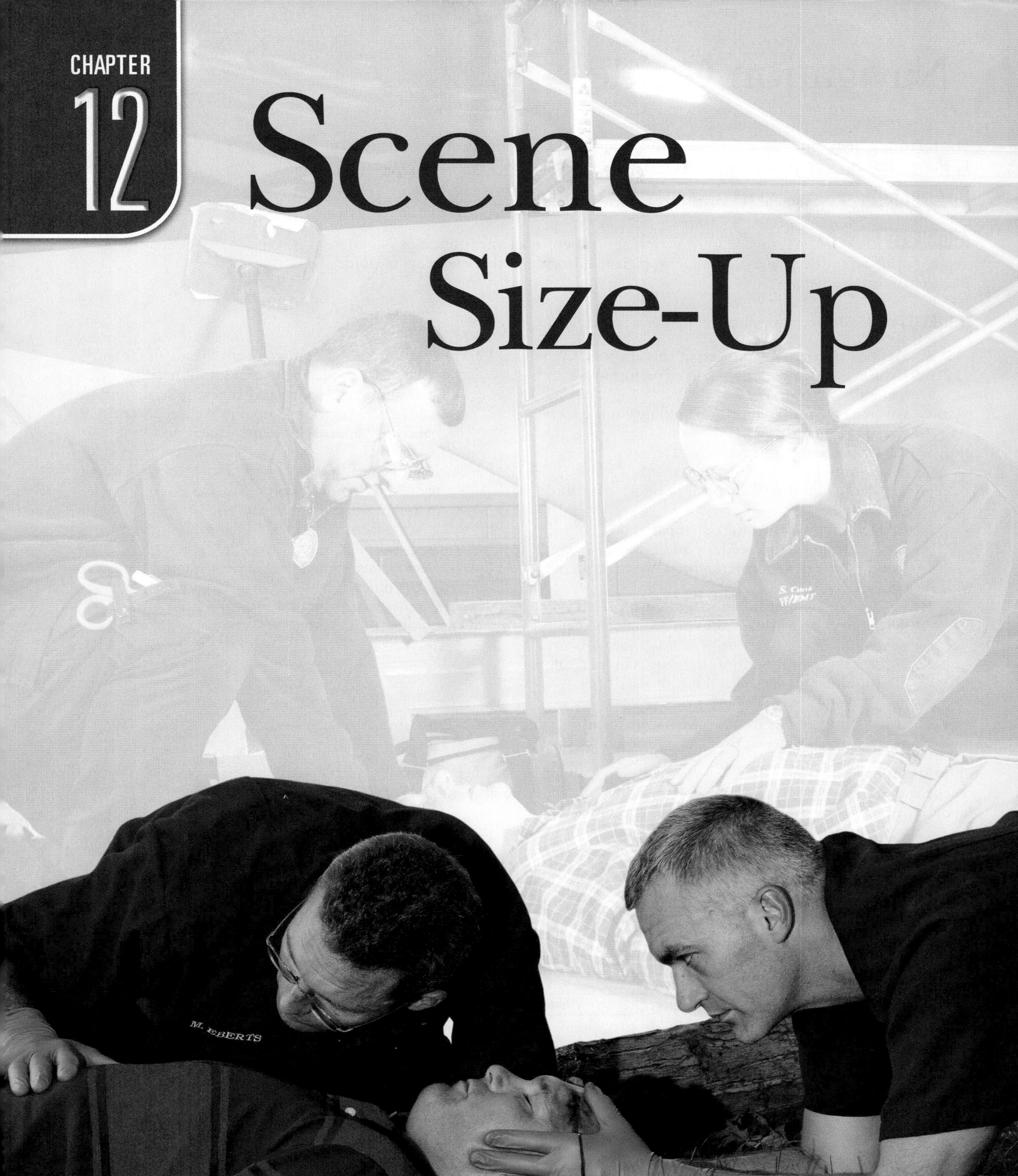

Navigation Guide

The following items provide an overview to the purpose and content of this chapter. The Standard and Competency are from the new National EMS Education Standards.

STANDARD **Assessment** (Content Area: Scene Size-Up)

COMPETENCY Applies scene information and patient assessment findings (scene size-up, primary and secondary assessment, patient history, and reassessment) to guide emergency management.

OBJECTIVES: After reading this chapter, you should be able to:

12-1. Define key terms introduced in this chapter.

12-2. Explain the purposes and goals of performing a scene size-up on every EMS call.

12-3. Given a scenario, identify key findings in the scene size-up related to:

- **a.** Taking Standard Precautions
- **b.** Identifying possible scene hazards
- **c.** Identifying the mechanism of injury or nature of illness
- **d.** Determining the number of patients
- **e.** Determining the need for additional resources

12-4. Describe the dynamic nature of scenes and scene size-up.

12-5. Utilize dispatch information and information determined on arrival at the scene to assess scene safety.

12-6. Discuss types of situations that may require a call for additional or specialized resources.

12-7. Describe scenes you are likely to encounter and points to consider before entering such scenes, including crash scenes, other rescue scenes, crime scenes, and barroom scenes as well as potential hazards in approaching any vehicle and its passengers.

12-8. Discuss measures necessary to protect the patient, protect bystanders, control the scene, and maintain situation awareness.

12-9. Discuss factors involved in determining a mechanism of injury.

12-10. Discuss factors involved in determining the nature of the illness.

12-11. Discuss factors involved in determining the number of patients.

KEY TERMS: Page references indicate first major use in this chapter. For complete definitions, see the Glossary at the back of the book.

index of suspicion p. 365
mechanism of injury (MOI) p. 365
medical p. 365
nature of the illness (NOI) p. 367
personal protective equipment (PPE) p. 354
scene safety p. 355
scene size-up p. 353
trauma p. 365

MEDIA RESOURCES: Please go to www.bradybooks.com to access mykit for this text. You will find quizzes, critical thinking scenarios, weblinks, animations, and videos related to this chapter—and much more. Look for online information on ice hazards and power line safety.

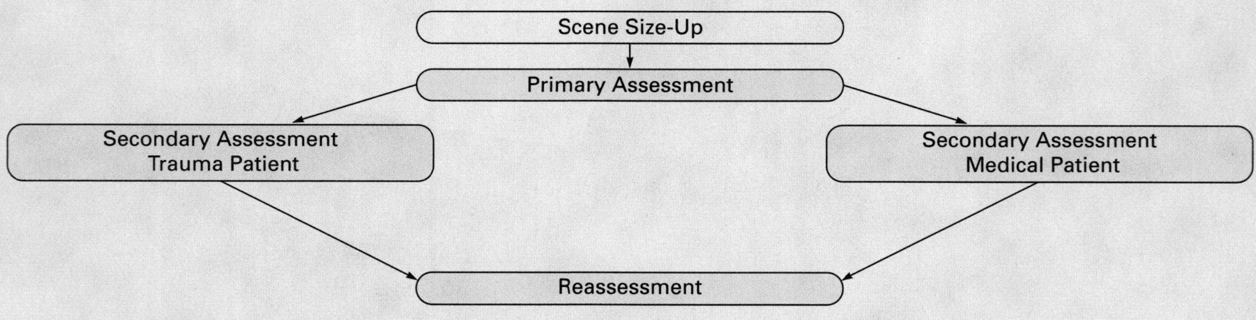

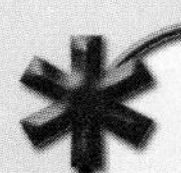

CASE STUDY

The Dispatch
EMS Unit 104—respond to an emergency at 68 Chicago Avenue—unknown problem—time out 2316 hours.

Upon Arrival
As you approach the street, you shut off the siren and the emergency lights to reduce the attention that you will draw. Your partner, EMT McKeown, is identifying the addresses out loud, "56, 58, 64, 66." As she shines a spotlight on a run-down house with a front door standing open, you can barely see the number 68. Your partner calls out, "Hey, where are the lights? The whole house is pitch black."

How Would You Proceed at This Scene?
During this chapter, you will learn about the special considerations of scene size-up. Later, we will return to this case and apply the procedures you have studied.

Introduction

The prehospital setting is an uncontrolled environment. An EMT who does not pay close attention to the characteristics of the scene, who fails to follow basic guidelines before entering a scene, and who fails to follow his intuition when things do not seem right runs the risk of serious injury. Many subtle hazards confront EMTs at the scenes of calls. With good sense developed through experience and study, it becomes easier to recognize such hazards. But experience should never lead you to become complacent and let down your guard. The costs of failing to recognize the hazards of an unstable scene can be high for yourself, your partners, and your patients. It is imperative that you identify and pay close attention to the scene size-up characteristics on every call, not just the ones that sound bad. Doing so can save your life.

The **scene size-up** is the EMT's initial evaluation of a scene to which he has been called. You have three basic goals during scene size-up:

1. Identify possible hazards at the scene and ensure the safety of yourself and other members of your EMS crew, the patient, and the bystanders.
2. Identify what led to your being called to the scene—either an injury or a medical problem. This identification will determine the steps you follow in patient assessment and emergency care.
3. Determine whether any factors, such as the number of patients or unusual characteristics of the scene, might require a call for additional assistance.

With these goals in mind, you will proceed with the scene size-up by evaluating the following components in a stepwise manner:

1. Take the necessary Standard Precautions (body substance isolation) to protect yourself against contact with blood and other body fluids, and put on any other necessary personal protective equipment:
   - Gloves
   - Eye protection
   - Surgical mask
   - High-efficiency particulate air (HEPA) or N-95 mask
   - Gown
   - Helmet
   - Turnout gear
2. Evaluate the scene for safety hazards (environmental, hazardous materials, violence, roadway traffic, power lines):
   - If the scene is not safe, do not enter until it is made safe.
   - Protect yourself, your crew, the patient, and bystanders.
   - Retreat if necessary if the scene becomes unsafe.
3. Determine the mechanism of injury or the nature of the illness:
   - Is the patient injured (a trauma patient)? ill (a medical patient)? both injured and ill?
   - Determine the mechanism of injury (MOI) for a trauma patient.
   - Determine the nature of the illness (NOI) for a medical patient.

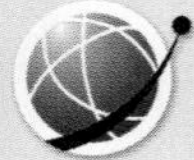

Media Resources

Go to www.bradybooks.com for mykit. Highlights:

- *Web Resource:* Ice Hazards

Objective 12-2

Explain the purposes and goals of performing a scene size-up on every EMS call.

Key Terms

scene size-up an assessment of the scene for safety hazards and to determine the nature of the patient's problem and the number of patients.

personal protective equipment (PPE) items that protect against injury and disease.

- Is the MOI or NOI unknown at this time and unable to be determined until further assessment is done?

4. Determine the number of patients at the scene.
5. Determine the need for additional resources to effectively manage the scene or the patient:
   - Additional EMS units
   - Law enforcement
   - Fire department
   - Hazardous materials team for chemical and biological threats
   - Special rescue teams (swift water, high altitude)
   - Specialized search and extrication teams (structural collapse)
   - Power or utility company

Always remember that the scene size-up is a dynamic and ongoing process that continues throughout the call. Scene size-up does not end once you make contact with the patient. Also, only those who are specifically trained should wear the specialized equipment and attempt a specialized rescue.

Take the Necessary Standard Precautions and Other Personal Protection Precautions

The first goal of the scene size-up is to ensure the safety of the responding EMTs. As you learned in Chapter 2, "Workforce Safety and Wellness of the EMT," you must consider contact with all body fluids to be a true safety hazard. Appropriate Standard Precautions will definitely reduce your risk of contracting an infectious disease in the prehospital setting. What follows are some key points to remember as you prepare for and perform the scene size-up.

Because the prehospital setting is so uncontrolled, unexpected exposures to blood and body fluids may often occur. *Gloves must be considered standard protective equipment.* Wear examination gloves for every patient where you suspect there is any chance of coming into contact with blood, other body fluids, mucous membranes, a break in the continuity of the skin, or other potential exposure to transmissible diseases. The extent of Standard Precautions used and application of other personal protective equipment will vary according to the suspected pathogen and anticipated exposure to blood or other body fluids.

The call from dispatch can help you begin to plan your Standard Precautions. A report of a laceration with active bleeding should indicate a high probability of exposure to blood and body fluids. In such circumstances, in addition to gloves you might need protective eyewear. If the dispatch information alerts you to a patient with tuberculosis, or to a patient in an institutional setting such as a nursing home where such infections are common, you should wear gloves, eyewear, and an N-95 or HEPA respirator.

Dispatch information can be incomplete or inaccurate. You will have to make your own assessment of the scene and of the need for additional protection.

Prior to arriving on the scene, you must anticipate what Standard Precautions and other personal protection is necessary. Any type of equipment that you put on to reduce your risk of personal injury or illness is referred to as **personal protective equipment (PPE).** This may range from simple examination gloves to complex breathing apparatus and suits used in a toxic environment. In addition to Standard Precautions, it is necessary for all EMTs to recognize the need for additional PPE, such as a helmet, puncture-proof or leather gloves, steel-toe boots, turnout gear or other heat-resistant outerwear, high-angle rescue gear, or specialized breathing apparatus, depending on the situation. You should not use any PPE for which you have not been specially trained in its use. As an example, you should not use a self-contained breathing apparatus (SCBA) to enter a confined space with a low-oxygen environment unless you have been specifically trained in the use of the SCBA and have been approved to use it on scene.

As a general rule, the EMT should use the same level of personal protection that is required of other personnel on the scene and in the immediate environment. For instance, if you respond to a factory and every factory worker is required to wear eye protection and a hard hat, you should not enter the scene without eye protection and a helmet. Recognize, however, that some personal protective equipment that is needed in the hazardous zone may not be necessary outside of that area. As an example, a firefighter will wear full protective equipment to enter the burning structure to rescue a patient. The firefighter, still wearing full protective equipment, may deliver that patient to you in a staged area well away from any danger from the structure fire. Since you are working

Objective 12-3
Given a scenario, identify key findings in the scene size-up.

Objective 12-4
Describe the dynamic nature of scenes and scene size-up.

Objective 12-5
Utilize dispatch information and information on arrival at the scene to assess scene safety.

Key Terms

scene safety steps taken to ensure the safety and well-being of the EMT, his partners, patients, and bystanders.

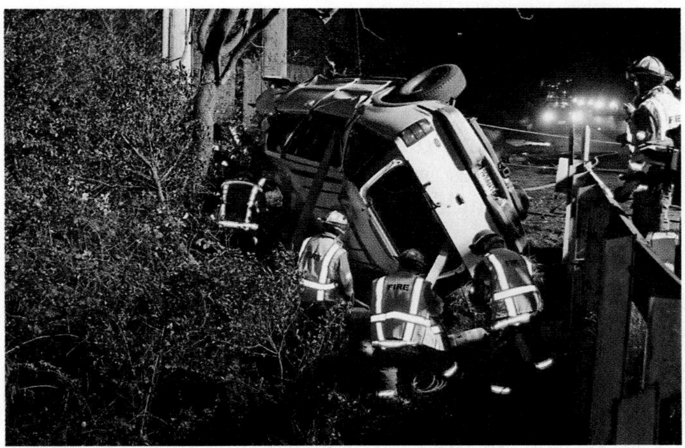

FIGURE 12-1 ✱ Firefighters wearing full protective gear at the scene of a motor vehicle crash. Source: (© Joshua Menzies)

in a safe and protected area, not in the immediate hazard zone, it is not necessary to wear the same full protective equipment as the firefighter.

Consider a different situation, where firefighters or those responsible for extrication at the scene of a crashed vehicle with exposed jagged metal and glass are wearing personal protective equipment to protect against personal injury, which may include turnout gear, helmet, heavy gloves, reflective vest, and eye protection (Figure 12-1✱). Prior to entering the crashed vehicle to assess and manage a patient, you must consider what level of personal protection is needed to protect yourself against the same personal injury. Your PPE should be at the same level of the other rescuers on scene, because you are in the same immediate hazard zone and exposed to the same hazards.

It is unfortunate that some EMTs do not have the proper protective equipment available to them or do not practice proper personal protection beyond Standard Precautions and may be injured unnecessarily at a scene.

Determine Scene Safety

Once standard and PPE precautions have been taken, the primary goal of EMTs upon arrival at a scene to which they have been dispatched is **scene safety.** This means assessment of a scene to ensure the well-being of the EMTs, their patient or patients, and any bystanders.

The process of ensuring scene safety is dynamic and ongoing. It is not done quickly upon arrival at the scene and then forgotten. The EMT must adjust his actions and precautions as additional information becomes available. Information gained from assessment of the scene is applied throughout the response—through the encounter with the patient, treatment, transportation, and, ultimately, delivery of the patient to the hospital. You must think scene safety on every call, whether the scene is a street corner riot or the bedroom of an elderly patient who has fallen. Be alert at all times.

Scene safety requires that the EMT exercise leadership and take control of the scene. If he fails to do so, the scene will control the EMT. Someone has to be in charge. That "someone" might become the patient, a family member, or a crowd of bystanders if the EMT fails to take charge.

Sleeplessness, preoccupation with other problems, apathy, and overconfidence can lead an EMT to shortcut or ignore the principles of scene safety. Don't let this happen to you. The consequences can be costly for the patient, your partners, and you.

Consider Dispatch Information

The process of ensuring scene safety should begin well before the EMTs arrive at the actual scene. It should start upon receipt of the call notification from the dispatcher. The dispatch information can help you anticipate what Standard Precautions and other personal protection equipment you will need at the scene.

However, the dispatch information is only a starting point. It is critical to remember that dispatchers may not have complete and accurate information to work with. The person calling to report an accident may have hung up before giving details. The person calling may fail to recognize a medical condition that would require increased precautions.

Be aware, too, that callers at times may deliberately give inaccurate information. For example, a caller may report chest pains when the problem actually is a stabbing or a gunshot wound. If the caller had reported the facts, it is likely that law enforcement personnel as well as EMTs would have been dispatched, something the caller wished to avoid.

Dispatch information can have other, unintended effects on EMTs. Consider the following sets of calls:

Unit 102, respond to a call at 223 Garfield Street, reports of shots fired, man down in the street.

Unit 107, caller now reports wires down and arcing at the accident scene. Fire and power companies en route. Use caution.

Objective 12-6
Describe points to consider regarding crash and other rescue scenes, crime scenes, barroom scenes, and potential hazards in approaching a vehicle and its passengers.

Objective 12-7
Discuss types of situations that may require a call for additional or specialized resources.

Unit 101, proceed to I-80 at the scales. State Patrol reports accident with multiple injuries involving tanker truck. Be advised, tanker is leaking unknown product.

Calls of this nature automatically alert the EMT to be cautious. They highlight an obvious risk that must be dealt with. With such calls, EMTs—from those on their first run to seasoned veterans—automatically begin to think of their safety at the scene. Such calls indicate that assistance from police, fire, power company, additional medical personnel, or other resources will be necessary. The reaction to the following calls, however, may be different:

Unit 105, respond to 6776 Quail Hollow Drive for a 67-year-old male with chest pain.

Unit 101, you have an unknown problem at Dr. Smith's office, 2225 Greenbriar Drive.

Calls such as these appear to be routine. The voice of the dispatcher lacks the urgency that might be displayed in the earlier types of calls. The routine nature of these calls may also lull the responding EMTs into a lesser state of readiness. Ironically, these "routine" calls may present a greater threat than the "major" incidents first discussed. The patient may have been involved in a domestic dispute. Or family members may become hostile during the call. Or the patient may have an infectious disease that can be transmitted to the EMTs. Or the patient may have inhaled toxic fumes that are still present and dangerous at the scene. Or, as noted earlier, the "chest pain" patient may actually have a stabbing or a gunshot wound. If the EMTs don't consider scene safety on the way to a call, they will expose themselves to increased danger and possible injury.

Remember, use the dispatch information to prepare for the scene, but remain alert to the possibility of very different circumstances upon your arrival.

Consider the Need for Additional or Specialized Resources

At any time during the scene size-up it may be necessary to recognize your own limitations and call for additional resources or specially trained personnel for situations or rescues that are beyond your training. As an example, it may be necessary to request a hazardous materials team to respond to a scene involving a chemical exposure. The team may wear encapsulated suits and use specialized equipment and procedures to rescue and decontaminate the patient. Not doing so may put you, your partner, and other personnel at the scene at considerable risk of exposure. Other examples of rescues that may require specialized equipment and personnel include difficult or complicated extrication, high-altitude emergencies, deep diving emergencies, structural collapse, swift water rescues, and high-angle rescues.

Consider Scene Characteristics

Personal protection of the EMT is of primary importance. An injured or helpless EMT cannot provide emergency care to a patient. In addition, attention and resources may be diverted from the patient to the injured EMT, risking further compromise to the patient.

You must study the scene carefully and determine if it is safe to approach the patient. This determination must be made on all responses, but different scenes will present different characteristics to consider (EMT Skills 12-1). Your final determination must be tailored to the specific scene, keeping these overriding principles in mind:

- Do not enter unstable crash scenes.
- Managing patients at crash scenes or on roadways and highways places the EMT at extreme risk of being struck by moving traffic.
- Take extra precautions at crime scenes, suspected crime scenes, and scenes involving volatile crowd situations; wait for the arrival of police or, if a scene turns threatening, retreat and wait for the police.
- Be sure to bring your portable radio with you when you leave the ambulance so you can contact dispatch or medical direction from the scene for needed resources or advice.
- Call for help from the appropriate agencies—police, fire department, rescue squad, utility company, water rescue squad, hazmat team, or other—if a scene is outside your area of training or expertise.
- Remove yourself if a scene turns hazardous.

Scenes you are likely to encounter and points to consider before entering those scenes are discussed next.

Crash Scenes

At a crash scene, the EMT's attention is drawn naturally and immediately to the patient or patients. This may put the EMT at considerable risk if the crash scene is not

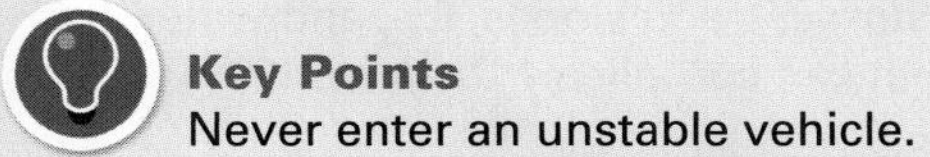

Key Points
Never enter an unstable vehicle.

Key Points
Take as many precautions as necessary to reduce your risk of being struck by moving traffic.

properly controlled and safety precautions have not been taken to protect emergency medical and other personnel—not only from hazards that exist because of the crash itself but also from vehicle traffic around the crash scene.

Before exiting the ambulance and approaching the scene or patients, the EMT must assess the total crash scene. This includes the areas to the left, right, front, back, top, and bottom of the vehicles involved. The boundaries of the accident scene can be limited to a single vehicle or can extend for hundreds of feet in multiple-vehicle or high-speed crashes. When assessing a crash scene, pay particular attention to the points in the following list. For more detailed information on crash scenes, see Chapter 42, "Gaining Access and Patient Extrication."

- Is the vehicle stable?
- If not, can you safely make it stable or are additional personnel and equipment necessary?
- Are power lines involved (Figure 12-2*)?
  - *Consider all power lines to be energized until a power company representative tells you they are not.*
  - Power lines can be on the car, under the car, or touching a guardrail or wire fence that the car is in contact with.
  - The lines may be lying on wet ground and energizing a large area.
- Does jagged metal or broken glass pose a threat?
  - Can such material be avoided, covered, or otherwise isolated to minimize the threat?
- Are there air bags that have not deployed in the crash?

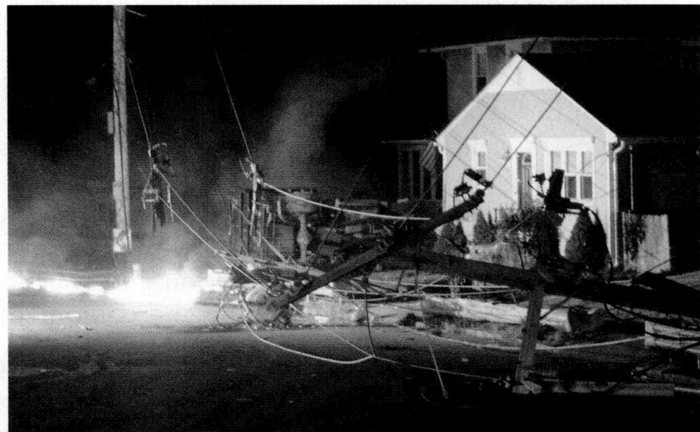

FIGURE 12-2 * Downed electrical wires pose a threat to the EMT. Source: (© Mark C. Ide)

- Is there fuel leaking and, if so, is there an ignition source nearby?
- Is there fire?
  - If so, has the fire department been called?
  - If rescue is possible, do not approach a burning vehicle directly from the front or the rear, where fire or explosion hazards are greatest, but from the side.
- Are there hazardous materials involved?

Protecting Yourself and Others at the Crash Scene from Being Struck by Traffic Another serious threat to emergency medical and other rescue personnel at a crash scene is moving traffic. There are many well-documented incidents of EMTs being killed or severely injured by vehicles crashing into emergency personnel and emergency vehicles at a crash scene on a highway or roadway. You must always remain alert and take as many precautions as necessary to reduce your risk of being struck by moving traffic.

Guidelines for working in or near traffic will be discussed in more detail in Chapter 41, "Ambulance Operations and Air Medical Response." Some general rules to reduce the incidence of being struck are:

- Limit your time on scene to reduce your exposure to traffic.
- Shut down traffic on the roadway if necessary to ensure your safety.
- Place flares or cones far enough from the crash scene to give oncoming traffic plenty of warning of the crash scene.
- Place apparatus and vehicles strategically so they protect the scene.
- Wear bright safety reflective clothing or a vest at the crash scene to make yourself highly visible both day and night.
- Do as much work as possible away from and out of the traffic flow.
- Don't turn your back to moving traffic.
- Don't jump highway dividers to provide emergency care while leaving yourself extremely exposed to moving traffic.
- Reduce any unnecessary scene lighting that may distract or impair visibility of oncoming traffic.
- Turn the wheels of the parked emergency vehicles so they are pointed away from the scene.
- Avoid stopping and standing between vehicles.

Key Points
If you can't make the scene safe without risk to yourself, retreat and call for appropriate assistance to make the scene safe for you.

Key Points
Unstable surfaces and slopes, ice, and water are hazards that can complicate treatment and transport.

Other Rescue Scenes

Some rescue scenes require specialized training and equipment. The EMT must be prepared to call upon additional specialized resources to ensure not only his own well-being but also the successful rescue of the patient. *It is the EMT's duty to ensure that adequate numbers of appropriately trained and equipped personnel are summoned if necessary to handle special rescues.* Examples of rescue scenes where specialized training and equipment must be considered include the following:

- Chemical, biological, and nuclear weapons of mass destruction
- Heights (rooftops, trees, catwalks, construction areas)
- Natural disasters (e.g., tornadoes, hurricanes, floods) (Figure 12-3*)
- Underground areas (caves, manholes, trenches, excavations)
- Collapses/cave-ins (buildings, construction sites, excavations)
- Storage tanks/vats (regardless of contents)
- Silos/bins (suffocation hazards, regardless of contents)
- Farm equipment (This might include equipment such as combines, corn pickers, or augers. See Appendix 4, "Agricultural and Industrial Emergencies.")

Some special situations that EMTs might frequently encounter include those described next.

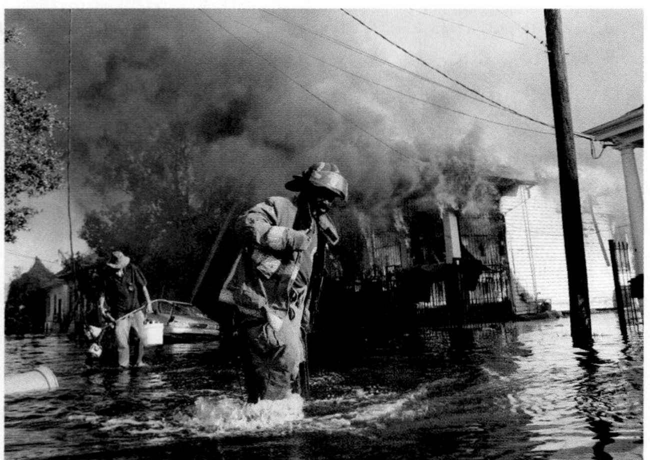

FIGURE 12-3 * A firefighter helps a man out of floodwaters as a home burns in New Orleans after Hurricane Katrina in 2005. Source: (© Shannon Stapleton/Reuters/Corbis)

Unstable Surfaces and Slopes Victims of injury or illness may be encountered on unstable surfaces or slopes. Such surfaces create additional difficulties and hazards and can greatly complicate treatment and transport of the patient. Access to patients in such circumstances may require the use of ropes. If you are not trained in the proper use of ropes in such situations, summon or wait for a trained rescue crew. If you have been properly trained, keep the following points in mind:

- Remember to secure the patient to the hillside to prevent him from sliding downslope during assessment, treatment, and stabilization.
- Be sure that vehicles that have gone over embankments have been secured to prevent them from sliding and carrying occupants and EMS personnel away.
- Beware of loose rocks and stones that may be knocked down to your position by rescuers working above.

Ice The presence of ice can complicate any scene, making what would normally be a simple rescue hazardous. Keep the following points in mind:

- Apply sand, salt, or gravel to walks, steps, and roadways where you will be working or over which you will be moving a patient.
- Avoid walking onto frozen ponds, lakes, or other bodies of water if the safety and thickness of the ice is unknown. In these cases, notify rescue teams who are trained and equipped for ice rescue.
- If the ice surface is known to be safe, a tarp, rug, or other portable nonskid surface should be brought to the patient's side to provide a safe surface from which to stabilize, treat, and prepare the patient for transport.

Water Drownings are common reasons for the dispatch of an EMT team. But water can also be a factor in other types of calls. Always proceed with caution in situations where water is a factor. See Chapter 25, "Submersion Incidents: Drowning and Diving Emergencies," for more details. If you are faced with a situation beyond your capacity to handle, summon and wait for backup from those with proper training and equipment.

- **Swimming pools**—The comparatively controlled environment of a swimming pool presents a major challenge for rescue of a patient. The patient will be visible but, to the EMT who is untrained in water rescue, retrieving the patient will be very difficult and

Key Points
Force of the current is an additional complication to rescues in moving water.

Key Points
Entry into a confined space should be made with SCBA. Such spaces may be very low in oxygen or high in toxic fumes.

should never be attempted alone. The EMT's partner should be close at hand to lend assistance, preferably from the pool's edge. A personal flotation device (life jacket) and a line or pole to assist the rescuer and patient to the pool's edge should be used.

- **Open water**—Rescue in open water is a specialized technique that requires training and equipment. The EMT must ensure that adequate resources are summoned to open-water scenes where people have been reported as drowned or missing. If the EMT goes out into the water, he must wear a personal flotation device. Under no circumstances should an EMT wear boots or heavy clothing that can pull him under if he goes into the water.
- **Moving water**—Rescue in moving water such as rivers, streams, or creeks presents all the problems of open-water rescue further complicated by the force of the current. Often, the current will make swimming difficult if not impossible. Patients and rescuers alike can easily be swept away, even in shallow water, if the current is strong enough. Never wade or walk into moving water in an attempt to effect a rescue without adequate training and equipment. Flooded streams, creeks, and drainage ditches as well as rivers have swept many well-meaning but untrained rescuers to their deaths. Whitewater or moving-water rescues involve specialized techniques and equipment and extensive training (Figure 12-4*). The EMT must ensure that adequate resources are summoned to reports of a drowning or of a person caught in moving water.

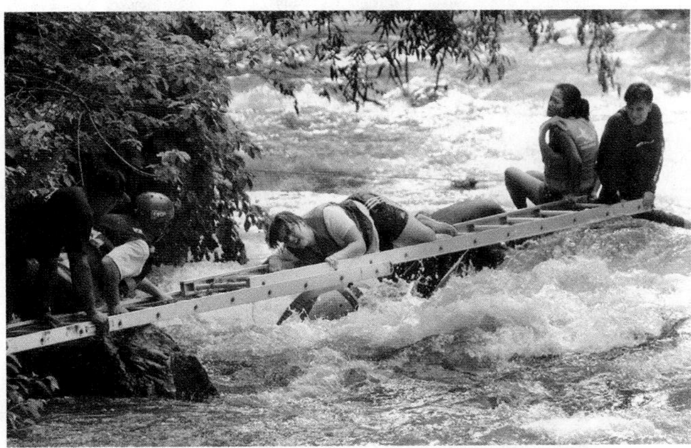

FIGURE 12-4 * Moving-water rescues require specialized techniques and equipment. (© AP Photo/Standard Examiner, Brian Nicholson)

Toxic Substances and Low-Oxygen Areas The EMT must be alert to the possible presence of toxic substances or areas of low oxygen during the scene size-up. Some scenes, such as an accident involving a tanker truck, will present obvious hazards. At other scenes, the hazard may not be as obvious. For example, a call to aid someone who fell in his kitchen might present a toxic hazard if, during the fall, the person knocked over and spilled bleach and ammonia. The combination of the two creates chloramine gas, a lung irritant.

Often, the caller requesting assistance will be unaware that a toxic environment exists. It is your responsibility during the initial scene size-up to determine if the environment is safe. Suspect the presence of toxic substances or an oxygen-depleted atmosphere in the following circumstances:

- **A spill, leak, or fire**—Scenes that involve highly visible incidents such as tanker spills, pipeline ruptures, and heavy smoke conditions should automatically alert you to call upon specialized assistance to control the situation.
- **A confined space**—Caves, wells, tankers, vats, manholes, sewers, culverts, underground utility vaults, silos, closed garages, and other confined spaces are areas where the EMT must exercise extreme caution. Such areas may be very low in oxygen and/or high in toxic substances such as methane. Entry into a confined space to effect a rescue should be made with appropriate SCBA in place. Many well-meaning rescuers have failed to recognize the risk of confined-space entry and have themselves become victims along with the patients they planned to rescue.
- **Multiple patients with similar symptoms**—A toxic environment will generally cause all people within it to suffer from similar symptoms. Therefore, the EMT called to a residence in which all occupants, including pets, exhibit similar signs and symptoms must assume that the environment is toxic until it is proven not to be. Faulty furnaces cause such problems every winter. The EMT encountering this situation during the winter months should be prepared to consider the possibility of carbon monoxide poisoning. A blocked flue on a gas hot-water tank can produce the same problem in a closed, air-conditioned residence at the peak of summer.

The EMT must be alert to the possibility of encountering such situations on every call. If the EMT is not trained to make the environment safe in such situations, he must contact specialized rescue or fire units who can.

You will learn more about the dangers of these situations and how to cope with them in Chapter 22, "Toxicologic Emergencies"; Chapter 43, "Hazardous Materials"; and Appendix 4, "Agricultural and Industrial Emergencies."

Crime Scenes

Chances are good that, as an EMT, you will respond to crime scenes almost as frequently as you will to motor vehicle crashes. Firearms are second only to motor vehicle crashes as a cause of death by trauma. Crime scenes require special attention to ensure the personal protection of the EMT. Review material about crime scenes in Chapter 2, "Workforce Safety and Wellness of the EMT," for additional information.

Remember that ensuring your own safety is the first step in scene size-up. If you are sent to the scene of a crime, wait for the police to arrive and secure the scene before you attempt to enter. As a general rule, *do not enter a known crime scene unless it has been secured by police.*

However, there will be times when you are sent to scenes at which no crime has been reported but where you suspect that a crime might be involved. A report of an injury at a bar late at night might be one such circumstance. A call to an area with a high crime rate might be another. Be alert to the possibility of danger on such calls. A dispatcher may not know that the scene to which he is directing you is, in fact, a crime scene. While you are en route to such a scene, check to see if police have also been called. If they have not, request their support. *If you arrive at such a scene and feel uneasy or suspect that a threat might exist, do not enter the scene. Wait for police backup.*

On calls to known or possible crime scenes, take the precautions that follow.

Arriving at the Scene While still several blocks from the scene, turn off the siren and emergency lights. By arriving discreetly, you will draw less attention to the scene and minimize the chances of drawing a crowd. This will give you better conditions in which to perform the scene size-up. If the scene appears too hostile or threatening, do not stop but drive on and await police backup in a secure area.

It is a prudent practice to anticipate the address and to park two to three houses away from the scene. This affords you an additional opportunity to study the scene before becoming involved in it.

At crime scenes in which guns might be involved, parking in such a position will usually put you outside the killing zone. This is defined as the area controlled by hostile fire. If someone inside the house has a gun, an area about 120° in front of the house is at least partially exposed to hostile fire. This area can be much larger depending on the location of the house—for example, one on a corner lot—and on the mobility of the person with the gun. The killing zone is not static and is always subject to change.

Studying the Crowd If a crowd has gathered before your arrival, assess the crowd. Be aware that the size of the crowd is less important than its mood. Is the scene chaotic? If so, do not allow yourself to be pulled into the chaos. Is the scene hysterical? Again, do not be pulled in. Does the crowd seem hostile to your presence? If it does, your options include retreating until appropriate backup arrives or taking the patient and leaving.

Approaching the Scene When you have completed your initial evaluation and see no immediate danger, leave the ambulance to approach the scene. Be alert, however, to the possibility that the scene could suddenly turn dangerous. Be prepared to retreat if it does. When approaching the scene, follow these procedures:

- Walk on the grass, not the sidewalk, for a quieter, less obvious approach.
- If you are using a flashlight, hold it beside, not in front of, your body—so that you don't make your body a possible target (Figure 12-5∗).
- If you are walking with a partner, walk single file. The last person in line should carry the jump kit (Figure 12-6∗). This will leave the person or persons at the front of the line unencumbered and better able to react to any problems that may be encountered.
- Only the first person in line should carry a flashlight, because anyone with a flashlight behind the first person will backlight those in front.
- As you approach the scene, make a mental map of possible places of concealment (objects, such as

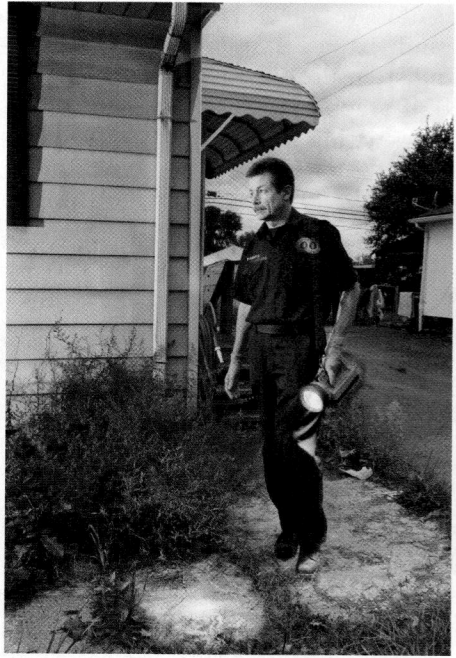

FIGURE 12-5 ∗ Hold a flashlight out and to the side of your body.

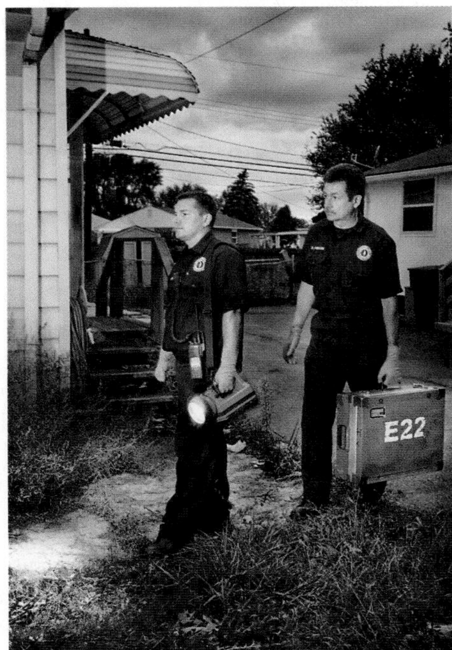

FIGURE 12-6 ✱ Walk single file to a potentially unstable scene.

shrubbery, that will hide you) and cover (objects, such as trees, that will both hide you and stop bullets). Keep illuminating or scanning dark or shadowed areas for movement as you approach a house.

- Take a moment to look at windows and corners. If you need to take a longer look, change positions to make it harder for a hostile person to get a fix on you.
- Stand to the side of a door when you knock on it; never in front of it—to avoid being a target for someone shooting, springing out, or reaching to grab at you through the door (Figure 12-7✱). Standing to the knob side prevents a door that opens outward from blocking you. If the door opens inward, the person opening it will most likely be looking toward the hinge side, letting you see him before he sees you.

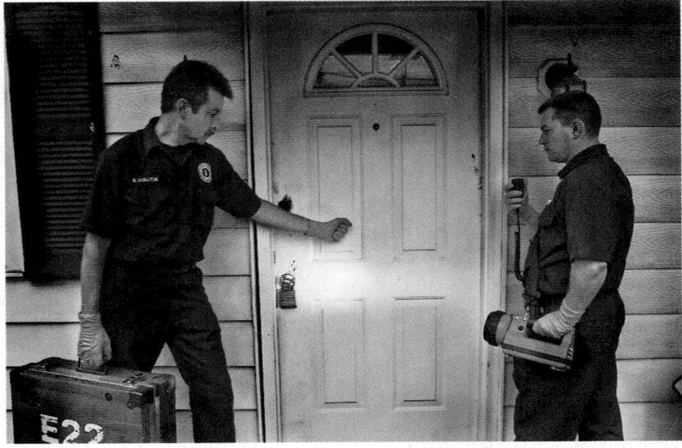

FIGURE 12-7 ✱ Stand to the side of the door when knocking. Do not stand directly in front of a door or window.

- As soon as the door is open, assess the situation before you decide whether to retreat and call for reinforcement or to have your partner move the ambulance up to the front of the building. As you enter, leave doors open behind you to ensure an escape route. Likewise, never appear to block the patient's route of escape.

At the Patient's Side Once you are at the patient's side, your first priority remains protecting yourself and your partner. The next priority is to protect and treat the patient. If you reach a patient and discover that a crime is, in fact, involved in the situation, be aware that a perpetrator may still be on the scene and police intervention will be necessary. Ensure that the police have been called and follow local protocols. Be ready to retreat.

When you are assisting a patient at a properly secured crime scene, follow these procedures:

- Limit the number of responders at a possible crime scene to the number required to care for the patient.
- Do not allow bystanders to touch or disturb the patient or his immediate surroundings.
- Introduce yourself to the patient carefully and say that you are there to help him. Crime victims are often confused and fearful of contact with strangers.
- Be alert to the possibility that the patient at the crime scene may be not simply a victim but also a perpetrator. Always keep track of the patient's hands in a hostile situation. Be prepared for the possibility that such a patient may suddenly reach for a weapon.
- If possible, have one EMT keep a constant watch on the bystanders and the surrounding area while you work on the patient—to alert you if a scene begins to turn dangerous.
- *Remember as you work on the patient that your task is to render medical assistance and to save his life, not to aid in solving a crime. Be as considerate of police requests as possible, but keep your primary task in mind.*
- Where appropriate, assist police in collecting and recording anything on the patient, such as blood, hair, seminal fluid, gunpowder residue, or clothing fibers. Follow local protocol.
- Take extreme care not to disturb any evidence that is not directly on the patient's body (footprints, soil, broken glass, tire tracks, and so on).
- Never touch or move suspected weapons unless it is absolutely necessary for treating the patient's injuries. Many guns found are loaded and extremely dangerous to handle because of the possibility of accidental discharge. Such a gun in the hands of an untrained person could pose an extreme hazard to you, your partner, the patient, and bystanders. If you do touch a weapon, do not disturb any fingerprints that may be on it. Pick up a gun by the edge of the grip, and use gauze pads to pick up a knife at the very edge of the blade.

- Wear gloves the entire time on the scene to avoid leaving your fingerprints at the crime scene.
- If you need to tear or cut away clothing to expose a wound, make sure you do not cut through a bullet hole or knife slash in the clothing. Keep the clothing and submit it as evidence to the police.
- If the patient was strangled or tied with a rope or other material, cut at a point away from the knot instead of untying it—the knot can be used as evidence and may help identify the perpetrator.
- If the patient is responsive, do not burden him with questions about the crime. Treat his injuries and transport him.
- Realize that the patient will probably show extremes of emotion and be prepared to handle them.
- Document who is at the crime scene when you arrive.
- If a patient is obviously dead when you arrive, do nothing and disturb nothing. Summon the police, if they have not already been called, and wait for their arrival. However, remember that you must provide basic life support and other appropriate care, as you would for any patient, unless injuries are so extreme or the patient has obviously been dead for so long that resuscitation is out of the question. Follow your local protocol and standard operating policies and procedures.

Barroom Scenes

Barrooms can quickly become places of danger for EMTs responding to a call. The presence of people consuming alcohol makes any situation volatile and unpredictable. Scenes in which the patient or bystanders are prone to sudden changes in behavior put the emergency medical personnel at risk for violence and personal injury. The problems are compounded in a barroom, where patrons often know each other and their actions may be affected by long-standing friendships or feuds about which you have no knowledge. In such circumstances, violence can easily erupt, even in what appears to be a routine situation.

Simply entering a barroom can present a special challenge to the EMT. Barrooms are often dark places. If you receive a call to one during daylight hours, your eyes can require several minutes to adjust from bright sunlight to low-light vision. By wearing sunglasses while outside, you can shorten the time of adjustment considerably. You might also keep one eye closed while still outside; this will give the closed eye a marked head start on accommodating to the low light inside the bar.

You will sometimes respond to barroom calls where none of the patrons will be able to tell you what happened to an injured person; often, however, some of them will offer advice on medical treatment. Be patient in such situations. It is critical that you do not antagonize the patrons. A routine question or comment can easily be misunderstood by an inebriated patient or bystander and lead to a violent confrontation.

While working at a barroom call, have your partner stand and survey the patrons at all times. Do not turn your back on the people in the bar. Don't reply to verbal threats, but never ignore them, either. It only takes an instant for verbal abuse to turn into a physical assault. If the situation becomes threatening, retreat temporarily and call for police support.

Car Passengers

Approaching people in vehicles is another seemingly routine situation that can hold unexpected danger for the EMT. The EMT's uniform or the emergency lights on the ambulance may be misinterpreted as the police by the occupants of a vehicle, who may be intoxicated on alcohol and/or drugs. You should plan the approach to a parked vehicle carefully, following these steps:

- Park the ambulance at least one car-length behind the vehicle. Park with your wheels turned slightly to the left, so that if you have to back up you will not go any deeper into the shoulder of the road.
- Align your headlights in the middle of the trunk of the vehicle, and turn them to high beam. Try to reflect your beams off the rearview mirror, illuminating the car's interior and also making your approach more difficult for the occupants of the car to see.
- While still in the ambulance, write down the license number of the vehicle and leave it at the radio.
- Note how many people are in the vehicle, their positions, and the driver's apparent condition. Be wary around tinted windows.
- As you approach the vehicle, be alert to the possibility of other unseen occupants. Check to see if the trunk is locked, and look on the rear seat and the floor as you pass.
- Have your partner open the passenger door a split second before you open the driver's door; if you are alone, wait for help to arrive.
- Keep behind the center post. Carry an object, such as a report book or bag, that you can throw at the occupant's face if he becomes violent.
- If you have to retreat, immediately get into your vehicle and back up rapidly. Move 100 to 150 yards to clear the killing zone.

Protect the Patient

Ensuring the safety of the patient is an important part of the scene size-up. Accidents and sudden medical emergencies frequently occur in public places or outdoors, away from the patient's home. Such emergencies expose the patient to a wide range of environmental factors that can cause him discomfort and also contribute to the deterioration of his condition (see Chapter 24, "Environmental Emergencies"). Emergencies can also expose a

Objective 12-8
Discuss measures necessary to protect the patient and bystanders, control the scene, and maintain situation awareness.

Key Points
Your attention must be directed toward the patient, but you must also make sure bystanders are safe.

patient to the curiosity of the public, a situation some may find highly stressful (Figure 12-8*). The EMT must have a keen awareness of how such factors affect the patient and be prepared to do what is necessary to change them in order to ensure the patient's safety and comfort. If you are unable to control the scene to make it safe for the patient, move the patient quickly to a safer environment, such as in the back of the ambulance.

A victim of a fall onto a sidewalk on a hot, sunny day, for example, can experience extreme discomfort, even burns, from the hot sidewalk. By placing the patient on a backboard as quickly as possible, you can make the patient much more comfortable and may prevent additional injury.

Conversely, the victim of a fall in a wet, slushy parking lot in midwinter faces the risk of hypothermia. This is a potentially life-threatening condition in which the body temperature falls below normal. Providing such a patient with just a blanket is not enough. Major heat loss will occur through the patient's wet clothing and through the cold, wet surface on which he is lying. Placing such a patient on a backboard as soon as possible will slow heat loss and make him more comfortable. Also, with the patient on a backboard, he may be loaded into the ambulance for the balance of assessment and treatment, minimizing exposure to the elements.

Shade a patient's face from either the sun or precipitation. This will make him more comfortable and allow you to complete the assessment more easily.

You can protect a patient from the public's gaze in a way that will also assist you in crowd control. Ask several bystanders to turn their backs to the patient while holding up unfolded bed sheets at shoulder level. The patient appreciates the privacy provided. The bystanders also become involved in the patient's care and thus become easier to manage. Such a technique is usually far more effective than sternly telling the crowd to "step back."

Protect Bystanders

Emergencies do draw crowds. Your attention as an EMT must be directed toward the patient. However, the crowd is part of the scene and making sure the bystanders are safe is one of your responsibilities during scene size-up. If hazards to the bystanders cannot be minimized or eliminated, remove the bystanders from the scene.

Keeping the crowd out of the way can be as big a challenge as treating the patient (Figure 12-9*). In cases of spills, leaks, fires, or heavy smoke, bystanders must be kept back through the use of roadblocks, detours, police lines, and public address systems advising bystanders of the risk. In such situations, bystanders who do not disperse should be dealt with by the police.

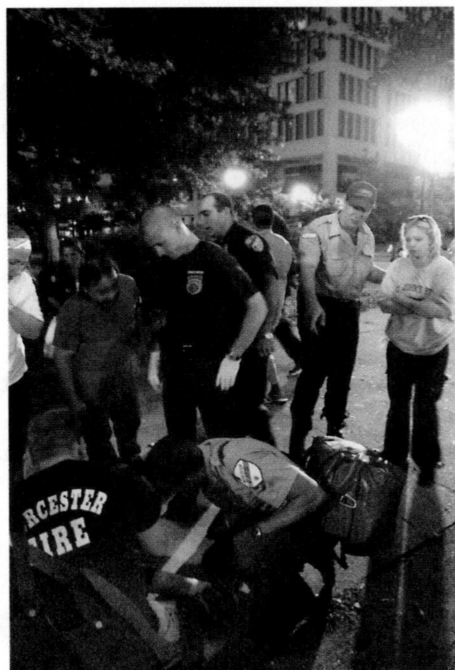

FIGURE 12-8 * The stares of curious bystanders will be highly stressful to some patients. (© Mark C. Ide)

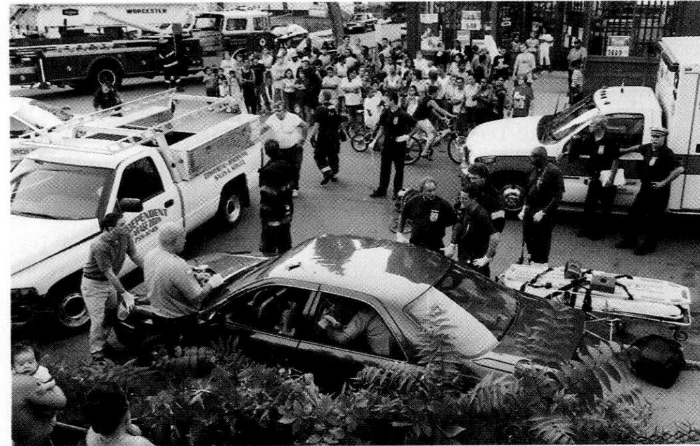

FIGURE 12-9 * For their own safety, bystanders must be kept back in cases of possible spills, leaks, fire, or other emergency scene hazards. (© Mark C. Ide)

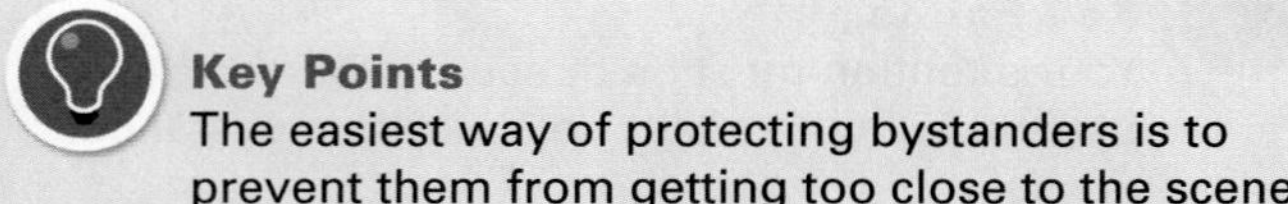

Key Points
The easiest way of protecting bystanders is to prevent them from getting too close to the scene.

Thinking Critically
What is meant by the statement "scene size-up is a dynamic process"? How should you apply this idea to your thoughts and actions at the scene?

The hazards to the bystanders in smaller-scale emergencies are less dramatic but equally important. A one-car crash can down potentially deadly electrical wires. It can also scatter sharp glass and metal that can cut unwary bystanders. The easiest way of protecting bystanders is to prevent them from getting too close to the scene.

Control the Scene

At a scene, it is the responsibility of the EMT to provide for the safety of himself and his partners, his patient, and any bystanders. To carry out these responsibilities, the EMT must sometimes take action to create a workable environment. This can be done through a variety of measures that range from providing more light, to eliminating noise, to moving the patient.

The EMT may need to improve the environment subtly, avoiding a disruption of the scene. For example, a television set may be a source of noise, but turning it off may also eliminate the only source of light in a room. Therefore, if the television's noise is the interfering factor, turn it down rather than off, or ask that it be turned down. Following is a list of basic measures that you might consider adopting to improve working conditions at a scene:

- *Provide light.* Make it a point to have a good flashlight and keep it handy day and night.
- *Consider moving furniture* that interferes with access to the patient. This should be done after advising the patient or the bystanders of your intentions. In a residence, you must remember that, in spite of the emergency, you are a guest in the home and should demonstrate a proper level of respect toward the owners or occupants. If furniture is moved, it should be moved carefully to avoid any impression of ransacking the room. If possible, attempt to return furniture to its original position before leaving the scene.
- *Consider moving the patient* to an area more conducive to patient care. Attempting to resuscitate a patient in a cramped bathroom would generally make little sense when, by moving the patient 5 feet to the bedroom, you would have plenty of space in which to work. However, whenever an injury is suspected, the patient must be properly immobilized to a backboard before any movement is attempted. Always adapt your actions to the prevailing circumstances.
- *Maintain an escape route* and keep it open when a scene is tense or danger exists. If operating outdoors, try to position the ambulance in such a way that the crowd will not get between you and the patient and the ambulance. When working indoors, consider asking bystanders to keep all doors along the route to the ambulance open. Do not allow yourself to be cornered. If all else fails, remember that windows may be a good emergency escape route.
- *Pay attention to bystanders.* If the mood of a crowd turns ugly, you, your partners, and your patient may be in danger. Remember that a concerned crowd poses far less of a threat than an unruly crowd. Consider involving bystanders in crowd control. If the bystanders are parents or relatives of the patient, a continuing explanation of the measures you are taking will be appropriate.
- *Control the scene* or the scene will control you. Stay in control and anticipate things that will happen before they occur. Initiate action rather than respond to the actions of others at the scene.
- *Stay calm.* Other team members, the patient, and the bystanders will respond more positively.
- *Use tact and diplomacy.* A compassionate, understanding tone may produce more positive results than a harsh, demanding one.
- *Be flexible.* Have a Plan A to deal with the situation you are facing, but remain ready to shift to Plans B, C, or D if conditions indicate that Plan A won't work.
- *Be open-minded* about the situations, circumstances, and conditions you encounter on the job. Prehospital care involves working with people of a variety of ages, races, religions, and backgrounds. Many people have ways of life quite different from yours; some of them are ways that you would not choose to follow. Remember that you have been called to assess, treat, and transport patients, not to judge them.
- *Be alert* to yourself, your partners, your patient, and your surroundings.
- *Be compassionate* toward the people you have been called upon to serve. Treat all people the way you would wish to have your loved ones treated in their time of need; someday you, too, may be in need.

Maintain Situation Awareness

Scene size-up is a dynamic process. EMS personnel must continuously assess the emergency scene for unusual characteristics such as sounds, smells, or things that look odd.

Key Terms
trauma concerning injury.
medical concerning illness.

Objective 12-9
Discuss factors involved in determining a mechanism of injury.

Key Terms
mechanism of injury (MOI) the factors and forces that cause traumatic injury.
index of suspicion an anticipation that certain types of accidents and mechanisms will produce specific types of injuries.

For example, as you are treating a patient who claims to be home all alone, the door of the bedroom opens slightly. That should immediately draw your attention to a potential hazard. It could be the family dog, it might be an open window that blew the door open, or it could be someone who does not want to be recognized behind the door. Whatever it may be, you need to investigate and not leave it to chance that it might be the wind. If the patient is alert and responding appropriately, ask immediately what or who is behind the door. If you are extremely uncomfortable with the situation, you may choose to load the patient immediately and move him to the ambulance. The key to remaining safe is to remain vigilant at all times.

One mistake commonly made by EMS personnel is that once they have performed the initial scene survey for safety hazards, they focus completely on the patient. In essence, they switch from a "scene awareness" to a "patient awareness." Such a complete transfer of attention to the patient without any recognition of what is happening around you may cause you to be injured or even killed. When at the scene, always maintain a situation awareness. You need to shift your attention to patient assessment and management once you have entered the scene and deemed it safe; however, you still need to be aware of all aspects of the scene around you. To re-emphasize the point, you must maintain a situation awareness.

Determine the Nature of the Problem

Once scene safety has been ensured, the next step in the scene size-up is determining the nature of the patient's problem that brought you to the scene. There are two basic categories of problems: **trauma** and **medical**. Which category a patient falls into will determine how you proceed with your continuing assessment and treatment of the patient.

Trauma is a physical injury or wound caused by external force or violence. Injuries caused by blunt, penetrating, or blast forces are examples of trauma, as are burns. Such injuries are typically to the skin, muscle, bone, ligaments, tendons, vessels, or organs.

A *medical condition* is brought on by illness or by substances or by environmental factors that affect the function of the body. A heart attack, a drug overdose, and a case of heat stroke are three examples of medical conditions that you may have to confront.

In prehospital care, the EMT first looks for evidence of an injury. If the possibility of injury is ruled out, the EMT may assume that the patient has a medical condition.

The dispatch information that starts you out on a call will often provide information that can be helpful in categorizing a patient. But, as you have seen, that information can be incomplete or inaccurate. You will have to be alert during the scene size-up for physical clues or other information that will help you understand the nature of the problem.

As always, you should remain open-minded and flexible as you try to determine the nature of the problem. Sometimes a patient will not fit neatly into one category or the other. For example, you may encounter a diabetic suffering from an altered mental status from taking too much insulin who, as a result, has fallen down a flight of stairs. This patient is suffering from both trauma and a medical condition. When in doubt, treat the patient as a trauma patient as this will mandate attention to possible spinal injury.

Determine the Mechanism of Injury

When arriving on the scene of a suspected trauma, you will be looking for the **mechanism of injury (MOI)**. Mechanism of injury refers to how the patient was injured. It includes the strength, direction, and nature of the forces that caused the injury. The mechanism of injury is the basis for your index of suspicion. The **index of suspicion** is the degree of your anticipation that the patient has been injured, or has been injured in a specific way, based on your knowledge that certain mechanisms usually produce certain types of injuries.

The mechanism of injury only provides a degree of suspicion of the types of injuries. It does not, however, provide any indication of the actual injuries or condition. At some point in your career, you will arrive on the scene of a motor vehicle crash where you suspect the driver did not survive or is severely injured based on the condition of the vehicle, only to find the minimally or noninjured driver outside walking around the scene, smoking a cigarette. On the contrary, you will also arrive on the scene of what appears to be a "fender bender" and find a patient who is critically injured inside the passenger compartment. It is extremely important to use physical examination findings to determine the actual patient injuries and the severity of the condition. Findings such as an altered mental status, elevated heart rate, increased respiratory rate, and pale, cool, and clammy skin are much more important indicators of the patient's condition and severity than the mechanism of injury.

Identification of the mechanism of injury in a trauma patient may begin with the dispatch information. Dispatch to an automobile crash, a shooting, a fall, or a stabbing will provide some preliminary information as to the mechanism of injury. Once you arrive at the scene, however, it is necessary to take a much closer look at such scene characteristics as damage to the automobile, the use of restraint devices, the distance the patient fell, the type of surface the patient fell on (e.g., grass, carpet, concrete), the position in which the patient landed, the object that struck the patient, or the caliber of the gun the patient was shot with. Such characteristics provide clues to what forces were applied to the body and the possible patterns of injury that may have resulted from them.

Common situations that should create a high index of suspicion for trauma injuries include the following:

- Falls
- Motor vehicle crashes
- Motorcycle crashes
- Recreational vehicle crashes (snowmobile, all-terrain vehicle)
- Contact sports involving intentional or unintentional collision
- Recreational sports (e.g., skiing, diving, basketball)
- Pedestrian collision with a car, bus, truck, bike, or other force
- Blast injuries from an explosion
- Stabbings
- Shootings
- Burns

Chapter 27, "Trauma Overview: The Trauma Patient and the Trauma System," will provide more details about the nature of injuries resulting from a variety of mechanisms. The following information concerns characteristics you should look for during scene size-up in a number of common situations.

Falls

Look for evidence of a fall when arriving on a scene. Fallen ladders, collapsed scaffolding, ropes in a tree or on buildings, trees in the immediate proximity of the patient, stairs, balconies, roofs, and windows are all common places to fall from or indicators that a fall may have occurred. When inspecting the scene of a suspected fall, you will develop a clearer idea of the types of injury the patient may have suffered if you determine the following information:

- Distance the patient fell
- Surface the patient landed on
- Body part that impacted first

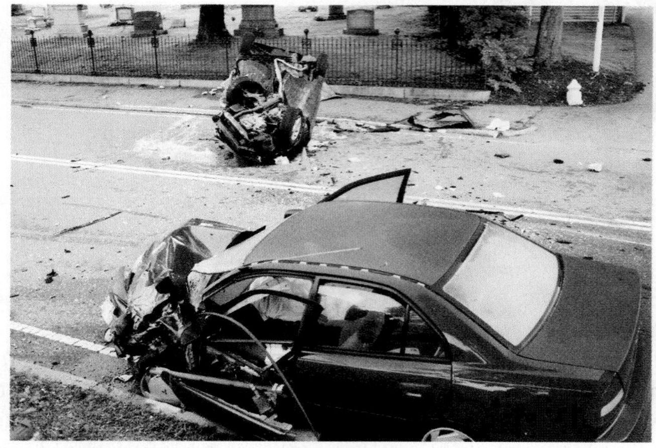

FIGURE 12-10 * Motor vehicle crashes produce some of the most lethal mechanisms of injury. (© Mark C. Ide)

Motor Vehicle Crashes

Motor vehicle crashes produce some of the most lethal mechanisms of injury (Figure 12-10*). Blunt forces applied to the body produce widespread injury to organs, bones, muscles, nerves, and blood vessels. The type of collision or point of impact to the vehicle commonly dictate the types of injuries to expect. Study the vehicle carefully, if possible, to identify this information. Common types of crashes include the following:

- Head-on or frontal collision
- Rear-end collision
- Side or lateral-impact collision
- Rotational impact collision
- Rollover

When approaching the scene of a motor vehicle crash, look for evidence of both external impact to the vehicle from an outside force and internal impact to the vehicle caused by a patient's body. One EMT should quickly walk around all sides of the vehicle to identify the points of impact. That EMT should also conduct a close inspection of the passenger compartment for signs of impact that correlate with specific types of injury.

The following are significant external signs of vehicle impact to look for and document:

- Deformity to the vehicle greater than 20 inches
- Intrusion into the passenger compartment
- Displacement of a vehicle axle
- Rollover

The following are significant signs of patient impact in the passenger compartment to look for and document:

- Impact marks on the windshield caused by the patient's head
- Missing rearview mirror
- Collapsed steering wheel

- Broken seat
- Side-door damage
- Cracked or smashed dashboard
- Deformed pedals
- Use of restraint devices and deployment of air bags

Deployment of driver and front seat passenger air bags may produce an impact mark that resembles what would be made by the patient's head contacting the windshield. In this case, determine if the safety belt restraint system was used and examine the head for evidence of trauma. A restrained patient with no evidence of trauma to the head likely did not impact the windshield.

Ejection from the vehicle usually produces significant blunt or penetrating trauma. Patients often die not from the ejection itself, but from the car rolling on top of them.

The death or significant injury of one passenger should cause you to suspect significant injury to other passengers.

Motorcycle Crashes

Try to determine and document the type of impact involved in the crash of a motorcycle. The following types of impacts are common:

- Head-on—The rider is propelled forward off the motorcycle.
- Angular impact—The rider strikes an object.
- Ejection—The rider is thrown from the motorcycle and impacts the ground, the object involved in the collision, or both.
- "Laying the bike down"—The rider purposefully lays the bike down on its side to avoid another, potentially more serious impact.

It is important to determine and document whether the patient was wearing a helmet. The use of a helmet may prevent or reduce the severity of head injury.

Recreational Vehicle Crashes

Snowmobiles, also known as snow machines, and all-terrain vehicles (ATVs) are commonly operated on uneven terrain, a factor that contributes to rollovers. Crush-type injuries are common. Snowmobiles can travel at high speed, producing severe impact upon collision with trees, rocks, or other vehicles.

With these vehicles be especially alert for "clothesline"-type injuries. In these injuries, a rider is pulled off the vehicle by a low branch, wire, rope, or other low-hanging object. Severe trauma to the neck and airway is common with this type of crash.

Penetrating Trauma

Whenever you receive reports of a shooting or stabbing at the scene of a call, it is necessary to expose and assess the patient's body to confirm or rule out a stabbing or a gunshot wound (Figure 12-11*). With an unresponsive patient, completely expose him and look for a penetrating injury, whether or not blood is visible at the scene or around the body. Be sure to log roll the patient to inspect the posterior body for open wounds. Heavy coats, dark clothing, poor lighting, dark environments, or dark hair hide blood very well. You must inspect the body carefully for open wounds. Open wounds to the chest may not produce much bleeding but can be lethal if not immediately identified and managed.

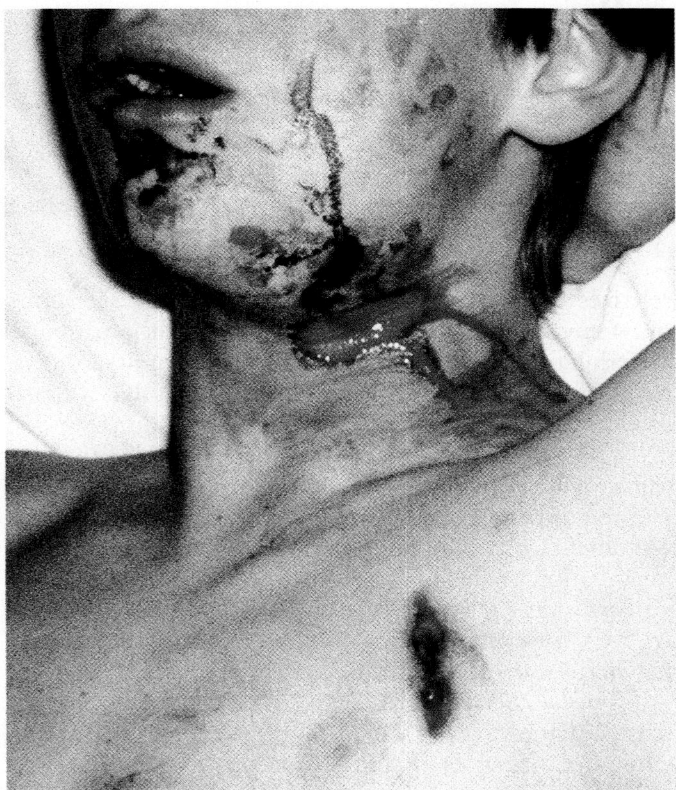

FIGURE 12-11 * Expose the patient's body to confirm or rule out a stabbing or gunshot wound.

Blast Injuries

Explosions are another source of trauma. Gasoline, fireworks, natural gas, propane, acetylene, grain dust in grain elevators, and criminal intent are common causes of explosion. Look for injuries caused by the pressure wave associated with the blast, by flying debris, and by the collision that results when a patient propelled by the blast comes into contact with the ground or with other objects. Note also that burns are common at blast scenes.

Determine the Nature of the Illness

In a patient who is not injured but is suffering from a medical condition, you will begin to determine the **nature of the illness (NOI)** during scene size-up. The patient,

Key Terms
nature of illness (NOI) the type of medical condition or complaint a patient is suffering from.

Objective 12-10
Discuss factors involved in determining the nature of the illness.

Objective 12-11
Discuss factors involved in determining the number of patients.

relatives, bystanders, or physical evidence at the scene may provide you with clues to determine what the patient is suffering from. You are not attempting to diagnose the patient's illness. You are gathering information that will narrow down the nature of the patient's complaint.

The initial information provided by the dispatcher can provide you with some preliminary clues. For example, the dispatcher may transmit, "Respond to a 77-year-old female complaining of chest pain." You can use such information to help you focus your questioning when you arrive at the scene. As usual, be alert to the possibility that information given to and relayed by the dispatcher is incomplete or inaccurate.

Once you arrive at the scene, you must determine the reason that you were called. Simply asking the patient, family members, or bystanders an open-ended question like, "What seems to be the problem today?" could provide you with the exact nature of the illness. Even if that does not happen, you might obtain at least some information that will help determine the nature of the illness.

Be aware, though, that the patient or his family may try to mislead you or to cloud the real nature of the illness. For example, use of drugs such as heroin or cocaine is illegal. Therefore, the family of a drug-overdose patient may claim they do not know why the patient is unresponsive. They may deny any drug use by the patient if directly asked. They may or may not eventually tell the truth regarding the real reason for the unresponsiveness.

Inspect the scene for clues about the illness. Look for prescription and nonprescription medications, drugs, drug paraphernalia, alcohol, and other pertinent clues. Home oxygen equipment may indicate a pre-existing respiratory disease or cardiac condition; thus, you would likely suspect complaints of chest pain or difficulty breathing associated with either condition.

The physical position and condition of the patient may provide information about the illness. A tripod position—sitting up and leaning forward—may indicate respiratory distress or cardiac compromise. Patients with respiratory distress rarely lie flat unless they are completely exhausted. A patient lying very still with his legs drawn up to his chest is likely suffering from severe abdominal pain. A fruity odor emanating from the patient may indicate a diabetic condition. Look for loss of bowel or bladder control, which may have resulted from a seizure or stroke.

Environmental conditions may provide clues to the nature of the illness. Extreme cold, wet and cold clothing, or a patient found outdoors in cool weather should suggest the possibility of hypothermia (low body temperature). A hot and humid environment, especially if the patient was playing a sport or performing some other strenuous activity, should suggest a possible heat emergency. Wooded areas may make you suspect snakebites or spider bites. Bites and stings from marine life are a real possibility if the patient is found at the beach. Scuba equipment should heighten your suspicion that the patient may be suffering a condition brought on while diving. If more than one person complains of similar symptoms in a home, consider the possibility of poisoning from carbon monoxide or some other gas.

The key to this phase of scene size-up is to study both the scene and the patient carefully as you look for clues that increase your suspicion of a particular nature of illness. Remember to write down your findings. Your report will provide emergency department personnel with valuable information that might not be otherwise available, especially if the patient is unresponsive.

Determine the Number of Patients

The last major element of the scene size-up is determining the total number of patients. Sometimes this may be simple, as in the case of a single, responsive patient who has called for help because of chest pain. At other times, as in the case of a multiple-vehicle accident during a nighttime snowstorm or a suspected carbon monoxide poisoning in a multifamily dwelling, it may be more complicated.

If you discover that conditions at a scene are beyond your ability to handle, call for additional resources. Such resources may include law enforcement, fire, rescue, or utility company personnel; a hazardous materials team; or an additional basic life support unit or advanced life support team.

Key Points
Call for additional resources before you make patient contact and get too busy to make the call. It is better to overestimate the resources you will need than to underestimate.

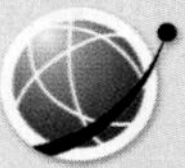

Media Resources
Go to www.bradybooks.com for mykit. Highlights:
- *Web Resource:* Power Line Safety

If, after studying the scene, you determine that there are more patients than your unit can effectively handle, initiate your local multiple-casualty plan. Follow local protocols in doing so. Such incidents will be covered in Chapter 44, "Multiple-Casualty Incidents and Incident Management."

Try to make any call for additional assistance before making contact with patients. Once you have made patient contact, you are likely to be completely focused on patient needs and not call for additional help.

If the number of patients surpasses your resources, begin triage and prioritization of patients. If you and your partner can manage the scene and the patients, consider spinal precautions based on the mechanism of injury, proceed with the assessment, and provide emergency care.

It is important to recognize when a scene cannot be adequately controlled. It may be impossible to gain scene control when the crowd is extremely hostile, the family is emotionally charged or upset, threats are being made toward you, or the scene is unstable because of the risk of fire, explosion, or other hazards. You must consider your own safety when working in an uncontrolled environment. If the scene remains uncontrolled, it is best to move as rapidly as possible to remove yourself and the patient from the scene and/or to call for additional resources as needed.

EMT skills 12-1 Scene Characteristics

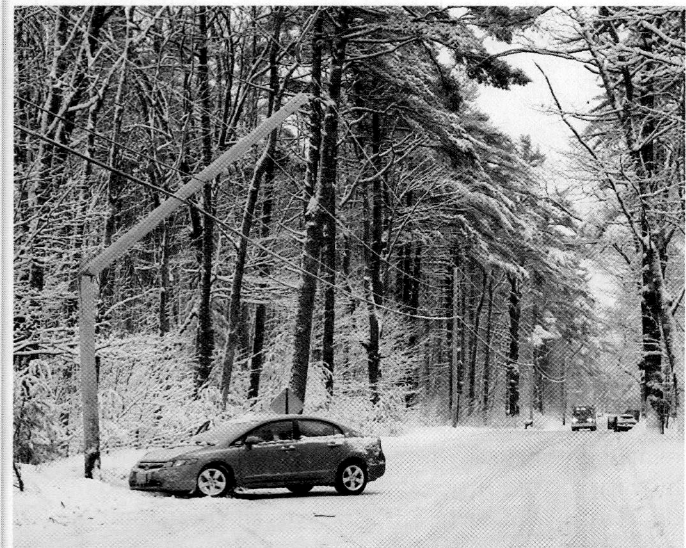

12-1A * Motor vehicle strikes utility pole. (© Daniel Limmer)

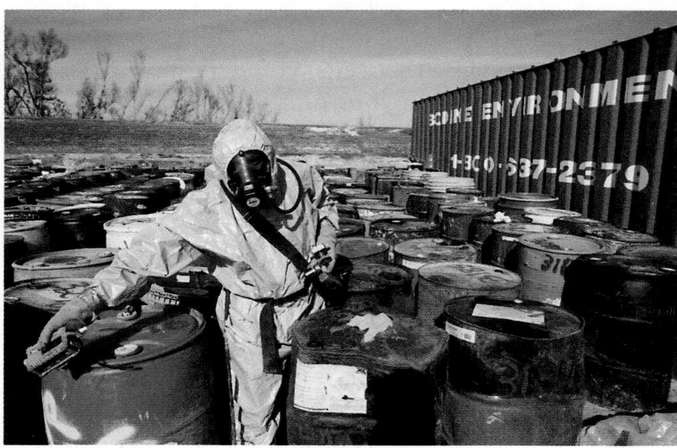

12-1B * Hazardous materials. (© Ed Kashi/Corbis)

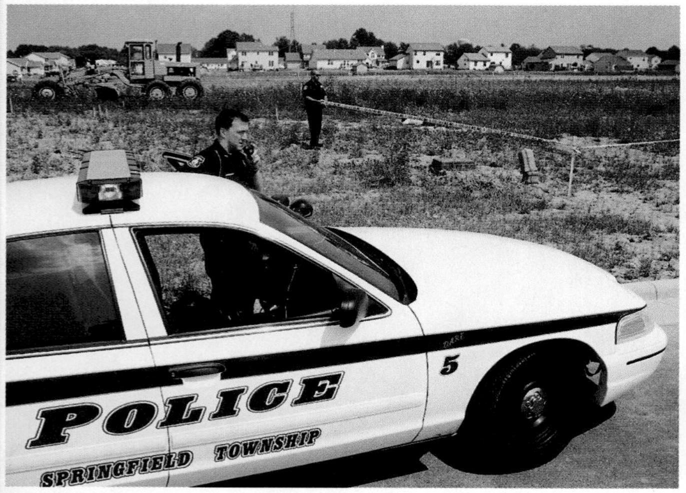

12-1C * Crime scene.

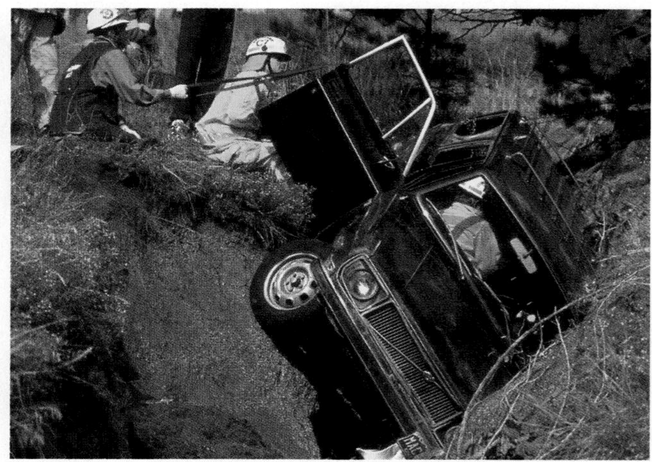

12-1D * Motor vehicle in ditch. (© Howard M. Paul/Emergency! Stock)

CHAPTER REVIEW

SUMMARY

Scene size-up involves an initial evaluation of the scene. This is considered the first component of the patient assessment because the scene size-up can provide evidence as to whether the patient is injured or ill. If injured, the scene size-up may provide clues as to the mechanism and the potential severity of the injury. This information will dictate what type of assessment is performed and may lead to changes in the initial emergency care provided to the patient.

The goals of the scene size-up are to ensure the safety of those at the scene, to use the characteristics of the scene to determine whether the patient is a trauma patient or medical patient, and to request additional resources as early as possible. The components of the scene size-up are to take the necessary personal protection precautions to include Standard Precautions and other personal protective equipment (PPE), to evaluate the scene for safety hazards, to determine the mechanism of injury or nature of the illness, to establish the number of patients at the scene, and to ascertain and request additional resources to effectively manage the scene or patient(s).

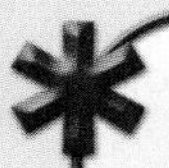

CASE STUDY FOLLOW-UP

SCENE SIZE-UP

You have been dispatched to an unknown problem. As you approach the street, you shut off the siren and the emergency lights. Pulling up to the house, you notice that 68 Chicago is completely dark. No lights are noted outside or inside of the house. Your partner instructs you to proceed past the scene and park two houses up the street.

Because the house is completely dark and there appears to be no activity in it or around it, you contact dispatch and inquire if they have a call-back number. Dispatch responds, "EMS Unit 104, be advised, the call came from 71 Chicago. The patient at 68 Chicago has no phone." You look out and see that 71 Chicago is well lit. You then request, "Dispatch, can you call back the number for 71 Chicago and verify that this is a legitimate call?" A short time later dispatch contacts you, indicating that the woman at 71 Chicago said the man from 68 Chicago came to her house, said he had an emergency, and asked her to call 911. You contact dispatch and advise, "We are going to approach the scene. Please give us a radio check-up in 2 minutes."

Before leaving the ambulance, you turn on all the scene lights and focus the floodlight on the front door. You and your partner, EMT McKeown, exit the ambulance after agreeing that you will carry the flashlight while she brings the equipment from the ambulance. You take the lead and approach the house, holding your flashlight out in front of you and to the side. McKeown follows about 8 feet behind with the jump kit. You walk up the front steps and approach the door. McKeown stays at the bottom of the steps watching the rest of the house and your back. You stand to the knob side of the door and knock. An older man opens the door and says nothing, but motions you in. You enter the house cautiously, on the alert for threats or hazards. After you are inside, McKeown enters, taking care to leave the door open behind her.

The man tells you he is Mr. Ziegler. He leads you to the living room where you find an elderly woman lying on the couch. He says, "My wife isn't feeling well," and sits in an armchair. You contact dispatch on your portable radio and indicate that you are okay and on the scene.

The room seems neat but sparsely furnished. The only light comes from a small television set. The rest of the house is completely dark. McKeown reaches for the light on the end table and Mr. Ziegler advises her, "The fuses blew. Nothing works but the TV. It's on batteries." McKeown walks over to the TV set and you tell her, "Just turn the volume down and leave the TV on. We need the light."

As you approach the patient, you notice a bottle of the medication Diabenase, used in treating diabetes, on a table next to the couch. Mrs. Ziegler looks up at you and says, "My legs are swollen. They've been like this all week."

McKeown is watching your back and the rest of the room. The scene seems secure. You note no mechanism of injury. Mrs. Ziegler appears to be suffering from a medical condition. There are no other patients to worry about at the scene. You can now begin to assess and provide treatment to the patient.

PATIENT ASSESSMENT

Having determined during scene size-up that Mrs. Ziegler is a medical patient with no signs of trauma, you proceed with the steps of patient assessment care as appropriate for a medical patient. You check for life-threatening conditions and find none. Her mental status, airway, breathing, and circulation are all normal. When you ask, "Why did you call the ambulance today?" Mrs. Ziegler states that she figured the emergency department wouldn't be busy on a Monday night. As you continue to ask questions to get her medical history, she confirms that she has diabetes controlled by Diabenase. The physical exam confirms that her legs are swollen but reveals no other problems. Her vital signs are normal.

You prepare Mrs. Ziegler for transport, positioning her on the stretcher in a sitting position, which she finds comfortable. En route to the hospital you continue to check on her condition and speak with her reassuringly. Mr. Ziegler rides along up front beside EMT McKeown, who is driving.

You contact the emergency department and give a brief report. You transfer Mrs. Ziegler's care to the nurse in the emergency department following an oral report. You write your prehospital report and prepare the ambulance for the next call. You contact dispatch and mark back in service.

Upon return to the emergency department on another call 3 hours later, you inquire about Mrs. Ziegler. The nurse states she was okay and released about an hour ago. The next-door neighbor came to pick up Mr. and Mrs. Ziegler and take them home.

IN REVIEW

1. Define and list three goals of the scene size-up.
2. List basic guidelines an EMT should follow at potentially dangerous or unstable scenes.
3. List guidelines to follow to protect the EMT from moving traffic at a crash scene or while managing patients on a highway or roadway.
4. Explain the special problems an EMT is likely to encounter in confined areas like a cave, well, or sewer.
5. Explain how EMTs should approach a house that they feel may be the scene of a crime.
6. Explain the chief determination about the nature of the patient's problem an EMT should make during the scene size-up.
7. Define mechanism of injury.
8. List clues to mechanism of injury that the EMT should be alert to at an automobile crash.
9. List clues at a scene that might indicate the nature of a patient's illness.
10. Explain why the EMT must determine the total number of patients at a call during the scene size-up.

CRITICAL THINKING

You are dispatched for a possible shooting at a residence. The communications officer informs you, once you are en route, that a 26-year-old female patient has been shot in the abdomen. As you respond to the scene, you begin to formulate your scene size-up plan.

1. What Standard Precautions do you anticipate?
2. What indicators will you look for to determine if the scene is safe to enter?
3. What criteria will you use to categorize the patient as trauma or medical?
4. How will you determine if more than one patient is present on the scene?
5. What other resources may be needed at the scene?
6. When will you call for the additional resources if they are needed?

PEARSON

EXPLORE mybradykit™

Please go to **www.bradybooks.com** to access mykit for this text. You will find quizzes, critical thinking scenarios, weblinks, animations, and videos related to this chapter—and much more. Look for online information on ice hazards and power line safety.

Register your access code from the front of your book by going to **www.bradybooks.com** and selecting the mykit links.

CHAPTER 13

Patient Assessment

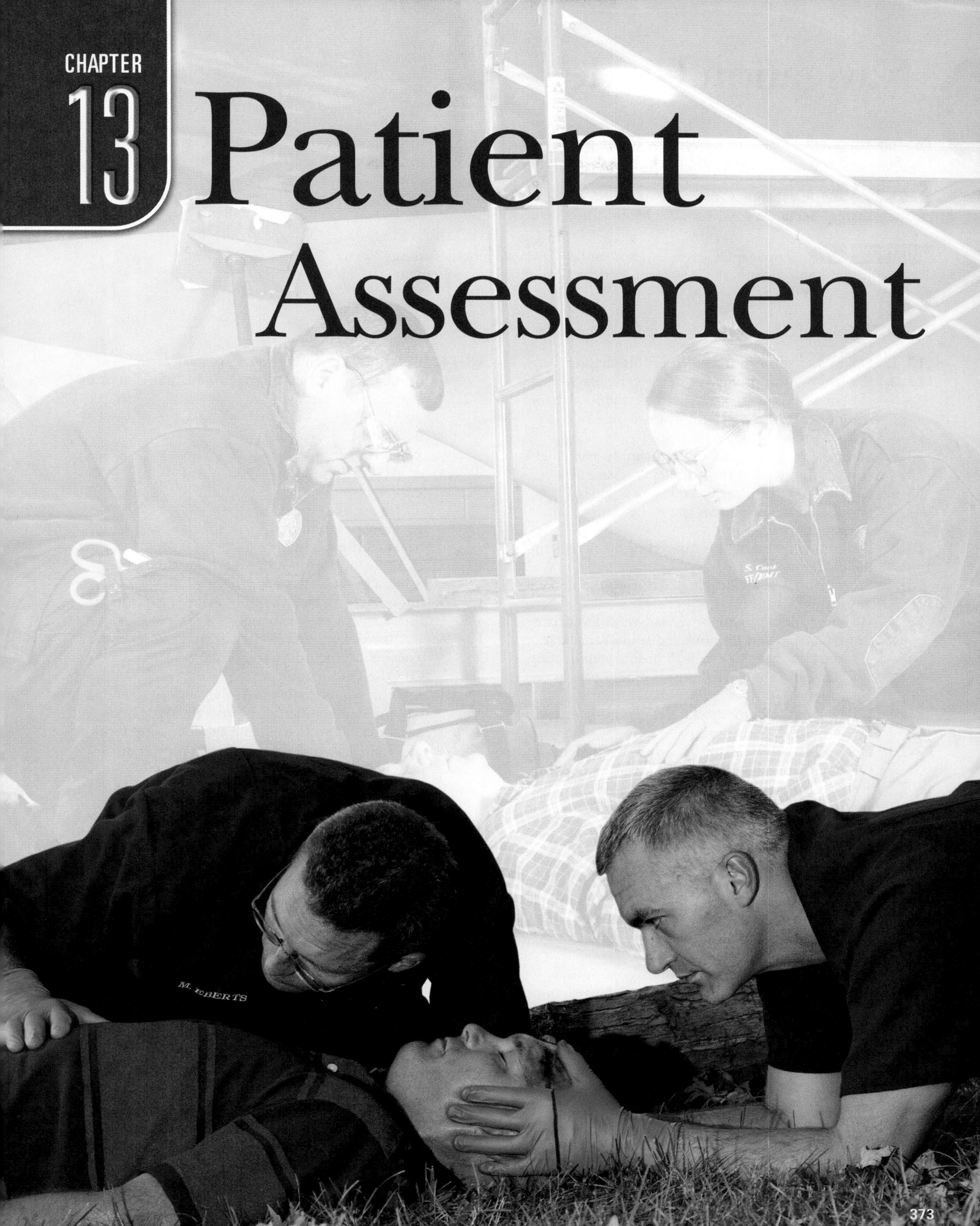

Navigation Guide

The following items provide an overview to the purpose and content of this chapter. The Standard and Competency are from the new National EMS Education Standards.

STANDARD **Assessment** (Content Areas: Scene Size-Up; Primary Assessment; History Taking; Secondary Assessment; Monitoring Devices; Reassessment)

COMPETENCY Applies scene information and patient assessment findings (scene size-up, primary and secondary assessment, patient history, and reassessment) to guide emergency management.

OBJECTIVES: After reading this chapter, you should be able to:

13-1. Define key terms introduced in this chapter.
13-2. Explain the importance of developing a systematic patient assessment routine and list the four main components of the patient assessment.
13-3. List the steps of the scene size-up.
13-4. State the main purpose of the primary assessment and list the steps of the primary assessment.
13-5. Explain how forming and revising a general impression of the patient spans the entire patient assessment process.
13-6. Determine if a patient is injured or ill and obtain the chief complaint.
13-7. Identify immediate life threats during the general impression.
13-8. Given a variety of patient scenarios, differentiate those who do and do not need spinal stabilization, demonstrate how to establish in-line stabilization, and demonstrate patient positioning for assessment.
13-9. Using the AVPU method, assess and document the level of responsiveness.
13-10. Determine airway status in responsive patients and those with an altered mental status, demonstrate methods of establishing and maintaining an open airway, and recognize indications of partial airway occlusion.
13-11. Assess the rate and quality of breathing; determine if the patient has absent, inadequate or adequate breathing; provide positive pressure ventilation in the patient with absent or inadequate breathing; and provide oxygenation as determined by the SpO_2 level in the patient who is breathing adequately.
13-12. Assess the circulation to include assessing the pulse, identifying and controlling major bleeding, and assessing perfusion through skin color, temperature, and condition and capillary refill, and recognize and begin treatment for shock.
13-13. Discuss establishing patient priorities by evaluating critical findings to the airway, breathing, or circulation to determine if a patient is unstable and a candidate for rapid secondary assessment and immediate transport to the hospital.
13-14. Describe performing the secondary assessment using an anatomical approach, including steps for assessing the following:
- **a.** Head
- **b.** Neck
- **c.** Chest
- **d.** Abdomen
- **e.** Pelvis
- **f.** Lower extremities
- **g.** Upper extremities
- **h.** Posterior body

13-15. Describe performing the secondary assessment using a body systems approach.
13-16. Summarize assessment of the vital signs during the secondary assessment.
13-17. Discuss obtaining a history during the secondary assessment, including use of the SAMPLE and OPQRST mnemonics.
13-18. List the sequence in which the steps of the secondary assessment are generally performed for a trauma patient and define the following types of physical exam that can be chosen for a trauma patient:
- **a.** Rapid secondary assessment for a trauma patient
- **b.** Modified secondary assessment for a trauma patient

13-19. List the mechanisms of injury that have a high incidence of producing critical trauma and the special considerations for infants and children.
13-20. For the trauma patient with a significant mechanism of injury, discuss how to continue spinal stabilization, reasons to consider requesting advanced life support, and reasons to reconsider transport decisions.
13-21. Explain how to use the Glasgow Coma Scale (GCS) to rank the patient's level of consciousness and how to interpret the resulting GCS score.
13-22. Discuss how to conduct a rapid secondary assessment for a trauma patient with significant mechanism of injury, altered mental status, multiple injuries, or critical finding (unstable patient).

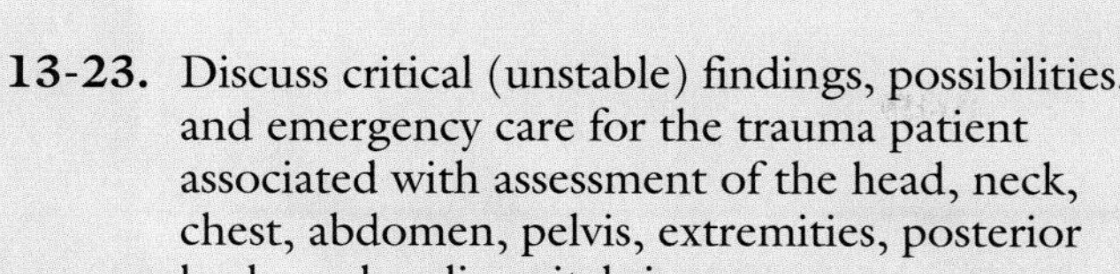

Navigation Guide *continued*

13-23. Discuss critical (unstable) findings, possibilities, and emergency care for the trauma patient associated with assessment of the head, neck, chest, abdomen, pelvis, extremities, posterior body, or baseline vital signs.

13-24. Explain the purpose and elements of the trauma score.

13-25. Discuss how to conduct a modified secondary assessment for a trauma patient with no significant mechanism of injury, altered mental status, multiple injuries, or critical finding (stable patient).

13-26. Explain circumstances when you should perform a complete, rather than a modified, secondary assessment on a trauma patient with no significant mechanism of injury.

13-27. Name the key differences in the secondary assessment for the responsive medical patient versus the unresponsive medical patient with regard to:

  a. Sequence of steps
  b. Appropriate type of physical exam (modified or rapid)

13-28. Explain how to conduct a secondary assessment for a medical patient who is not alert or is disoriented, is responding only to verbal or painful stimuli, or is unresponsive.

13-29. Discuss critical (unstable) findings, possibilities, and emergency care for the medical patient with an altered mental status associated with assessment of the head, neck, chest, or pelvic region.

13-30. Explain how to conduct a secondary assessment for a medical patient who is alert and oriented.

13-31. Explain the purposes of reassessment.

13-32. Explain how to conduct and to complete the reassessment.

KEY TERMS: Page references indicate first major use in this chapter. For complete definitions, see the Glossary at the back of the book.

MEDIA RESOURCES: Please go to www.bradybooks.com to access mykit for this text. You will find quizzes, critical thinking scenarios, weblinks, animations, and videos related to this chapter—and much more. Look for online information on simulated patient assessments.

OVERVIEW: This chapter on patient assessment is divided into four parts. The chapter parts begin on the pages listed here.

continued

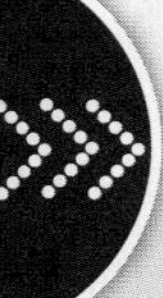

CASE STUDY

During your shift as an EMT, you are called to two different kinds of cases. The first call is to a patient who has been injured—a trauma patient. The second is to a patient who is suffering from a medical problem.

CALL ONE—A TRAUMA PATIENT

The Dispatch

EMS Unit 74—respond to Newton Drive, Greenway Apartments, Building 24. Unresponsive patient with an unknown problem. Be advised police are at the scene. Time out is 1512 hours.

Upon Arrival

Upon arrival, you find an adult male patient lying supine at the bottom of a two-story fire-escape ladder. The police are on the scene and indicate that they were called for a domestic incident and the neighbors heard fighting and gunshots.

How would you proceed with the assessment of this patient?

CALL TWO—A MEDICAL PATIENT

The Dispatch

EMS Unit 74—respond to 33 East Sassafras Street. Patient with an unknown problem. Patient's daughter made the call. Time out is 1623 hours.

Upon Arrival

You arrive at the address, a well-kept home in a quiet neighborhood. A middle-aged woman hurries out into the driveway as you pull up.

"It's my mother," she says. "She can't seem to catch her breath."

How Would You Proceed with the Assessment of This Patient?

In this chapter, you will learn about the patient assessment procedures you will perform as an EMT for trauma and medical patients in a variety of situations. Later, we will return to these two cases and apply the procedures learned.

Introduction

An EMT's most important functions are assessing the patient plus providing emergency care and transport to a medical facility. Of these functions, performing an accurate and reliable assessment is the most important, because all of your decisions about care and transport will be based on it.

It is very important that you develop a systematic assessment routine. This will ensure that you assess every patient consistently and appropriately, based on the nature of that patient's illness or injury. This systematic approach to patient assessment will become second nature as you apply it to each patient, whether that patient's condition is minor or critical. Without this systematic approach, you are far more likely to become distracted or to develop tunnel vision. For example, the horror of a gory abdominal evisceration might tempt you to immediately begin treating the wound and cause you to delay more critical tasks such as ensuring an open airway or providing needed assisted ventilations.

In this chapter, you will learn about the components of the patient assessment—scene size-up, primary assessment, secondary assessment, and reassessment—that you will perform on every patient you encounter as an EMT.

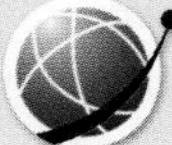

Media Resources

Go to www.bradybooks.com for mykit. Highlights:

- *Video:* Initial Assessment
- *Video:* Abdominal Assessment Techniques
- *Video:* Assessment of Pain

Objective 13-2

Explain the importance of developing a systematic patient assessment routine and list the four main components of the patient assessment.

Objective 13-3

List the steps of the scene size-up.

Part 1: Scene Size-Up

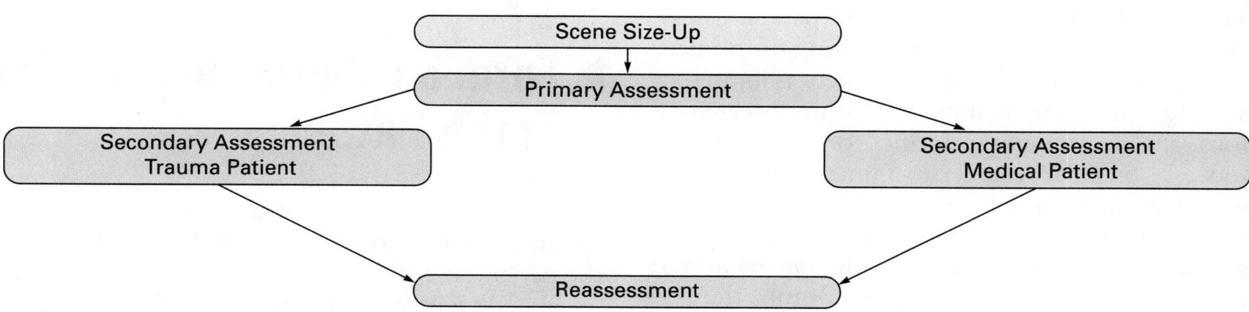

The first component of patient assessment is the scene size-up. The scene size-up is a dynamic process that continues throughout the entire call. Much of the scene size-up is operational, such as ensuring scene safety and ascertaining the need for additional resources. However, determining the mechanism of injury or nature of the illness and determining the number of patients actually constitute the beginning of the patient assessment process. As you learned in Chapter 12, the phases of the scene size-up are as listed here:

Steps of the Scene Size-Up

1. Take necessary Standard Precautions.
2. Evaluate scene hazards and ensure scene safety.
    - Personal protection
    - Protection of the patient
    - Protection of bystanders
3. Determine the mechanism of injury or the nature of the illness.
    - Trauma patient
    - Medical patient
4. Establish the number of patients.
5. Ascertain the need for additional resources to manage the scene or the patient(s).

Part 2: Primary Assessment

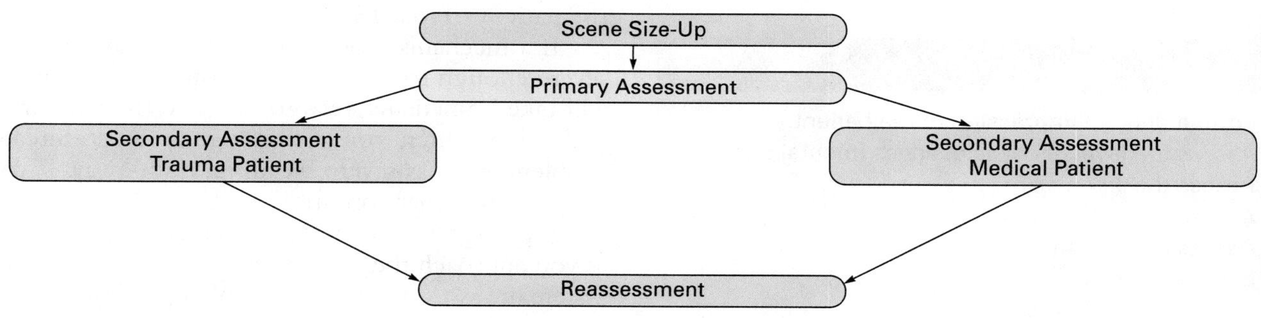

Key Terms

primary assessment assessment following scene size-up to discover and treat immediately life-threatening conditions.

Objective 13-4

State the main purpose of the primary assessment and list the steps of the primary assessment.

Key Points

A life threat must be treated immediately after being found.

Objective 13-5

Explain how forming and revising a general impression of the patient spans the entire patient assessment process.

Once you have ensured that the scene is safe and has been controlled, you are prepared to begin the **primary assessment**. A primary assessment is conducted on every patient regardless of the mechanism of injury or nature of the illness.

A number of the overall purposes of patient assessment are served—in whole or in part—during the primary assessment: determining whether the patient is injured or ill, identifying and managing immediately life-threatening conditions, and determining priorities for further assessment and care on the scene versus immediate transport with assessment and care to continue en route.

The main purpose of the primary assessment is to identify and manage immediately life-threatening conditions to the airway, breathing, or circulation. During the primary assessment, you will quickly form a general impression of the patient and assess the patient's level of consciousness (mental status), airway, breathing, and circulation. *Any life-threatening condition that is identified must be treated immediately as found—before moving on to the next portion of the primary assessment.* As a result of the primary assessment, you will make decisions about priorities for further assessment, care, and transport.

The steps of the primary assessment allow a systematic approach to assessment for, and control of, life threats. It is vital that you progress through the steps in this exact sequence, and do not allow dramatic but non-life-threatening injuries or conditions to cloud your priorities. For example, a fractured humerus that is protruding through the skin is a dramatic injury. However, the fracture will not immediately cause the death of the patient unless it is associated with major bleeding. By contrast, a patient with clotted blood in the mouth causing the airway to be blocked is in immediate danger. The blood in the mouth is not as dramatic and could easily be missed by an EMT who is not systematically performing the primary assessment. Systematically following the steps of the primary assessment will keep you focused and allow you to identify and correct immediately life-threatening injuries or conditions.

The steps of primary assessment are conducted in the following sequence:

Steps of the Primary Assessment

1. Form a general impression of the patient.
2. Assess the level of consciousness (mental status).
3. Assess the airway.
4. Assess breathing.
5. Assess circulation.
6. Establish patient priorities.

You should be able to conduct this survey (shown in more detail in Figure 13-1*) in about 60 seconds, unless confronted with life-threatening problems that must be treated immediately as found.

Form a General Impression of the Patient

Primary assessment begins as soon as you approach the patient, allowing you to gain your firsthand impression of the patient.

As you gain experience as an EMT, you will become more adept at gaining valuable information about your patient from your first impressions. For example, if this information has not already been provided to you by dispatch, Emergency Medical Responders, or bystanders, you will immediately observe the patient's general age (for example, child, adult, elderly) and sex, which may have a bearing on the patient's condition or care.

You will often be able to gain a quick impression, just from the patient's general appearance, as to whether the patient seems well or ill, is possibly stable or unstable, or appears to have been injured. A patient who greets you at the door, talks in full sentences, and does not appear to be in much distress would provide a quick initial impression of being stable; whereas, the patient who is alert but appears to be in distress may be potentially unstable (Figures 13-2a and 13-2b*). A patient who is bleeding excessively and appears to have a decreased mental status or is extremely pale, or one who appears to be unconscious upon your arrival would cause you to immediately consider him unstable (Figures 13-2c and 13-2d*).What the patient tells you about what is wrong with him (the chief complaint) and the items or conditions you notice in the patient's immediate environment are additional elements of the general impression you form as you approach and make your first contact with the patient (Table 13-1).

If a mechanism of injury that you have identified is severe enough to cause you to suspect spinal injury, you will take immediate steps to stabilize the patient's head and spine. Often you will recognize a life-threatening problem, such as severe bleeding, right away. If you do, you will treat that condition immediately.

Although you form your general impression quickly as you approach the patient, even before you can begin a systematic assessment, the general impression can provide

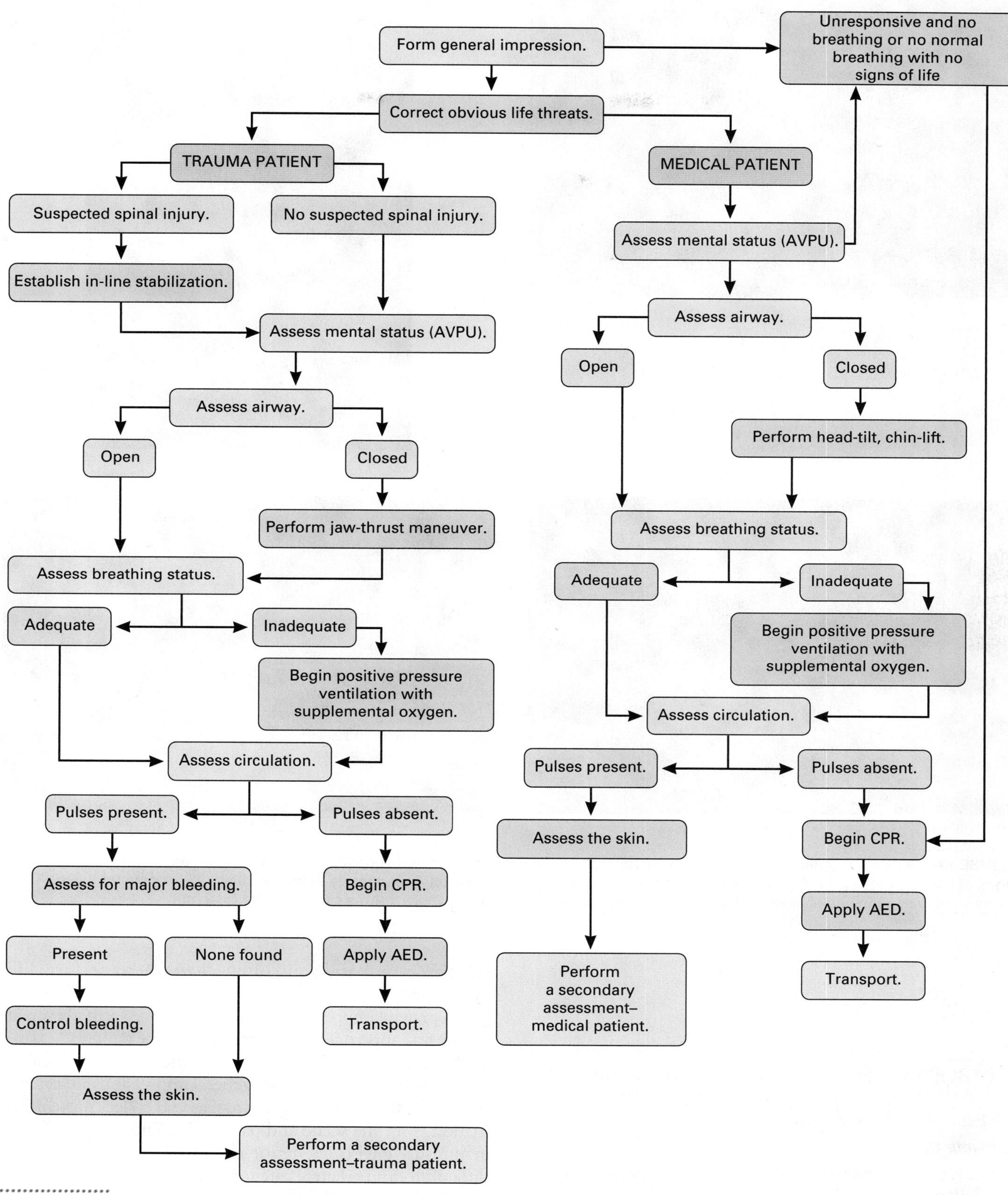

FIGURE 13-1 ✱ Steps of the primary assessment.

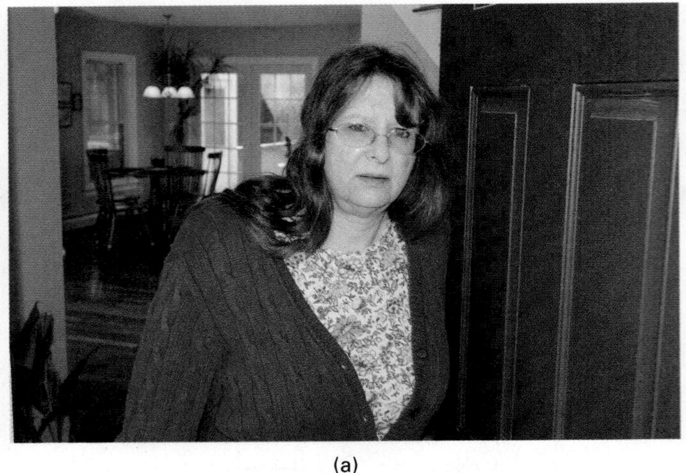

(a)

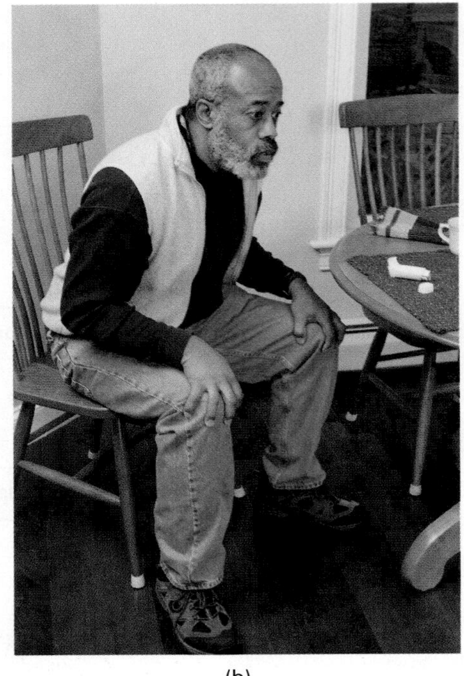

(b)

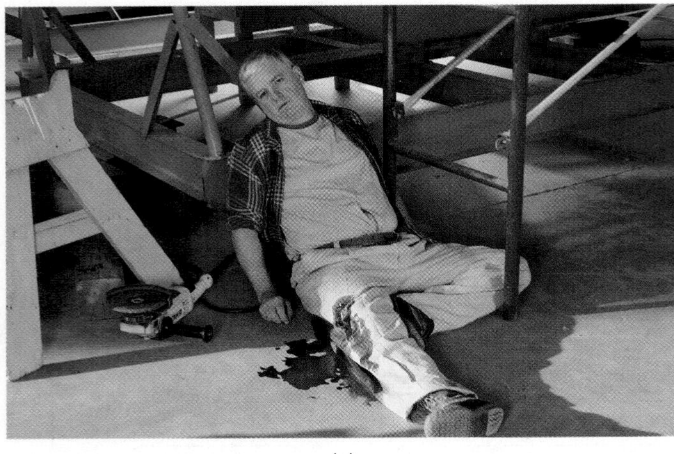

(c)

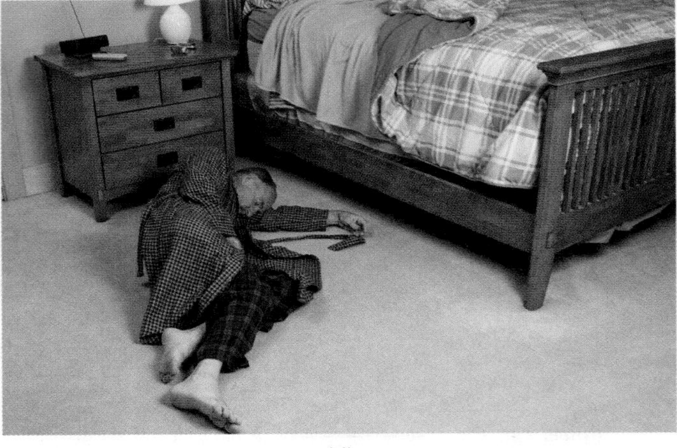

(d)

FIGURE 13-2 ✱ Form a general impression as you approach the patient. Shown in this photo group: **(a)** An alert patient with no obvious signs of illness or injury. **(b)** A patient exhibiting signs of respiratory distress. **(c)** A responsive patient with an obvious leg injury. **(d)** An unresponsive patient who is likely suffering from a medical condition but for whom trauma cannot yet be ruled out.

valuable information and often allow you to perform lifesaving procedures without delay.

A general impression can continue to be formed even after the first approach to the patient. In some patients, it is difficult to immediately determine if they are a medical or trauma patient or both. Your general impression and categorization of the patient may change as you collect more information from the scene and patient. Patients who are found in unusual environments or circumstances are sometimes difficult to immediately categorize as medical or trauma, especially those who are intoxicated, are under the influence of drugs, or have psychiatric disorders (Figure 13-3✱). Be alert for general clues to the patient's condition or history throughout the assessment (Figure 13-4✱).

TABLE 13-1 Forming a General Impression

- Estimate the patient's age.
- Note the patient's sex.
- Determine if the patient is a trauma or medical patient.
- Obtain the patient's chief complaint.
- Identify (and manage) immediate life threats.

Objective 13-6
Determine if a patient is injured or ill and obtain the chief complaint.

Key Terms
penetrating trauma a force that pierces the skin and body tissues, for example, a knife or gunshot wound.

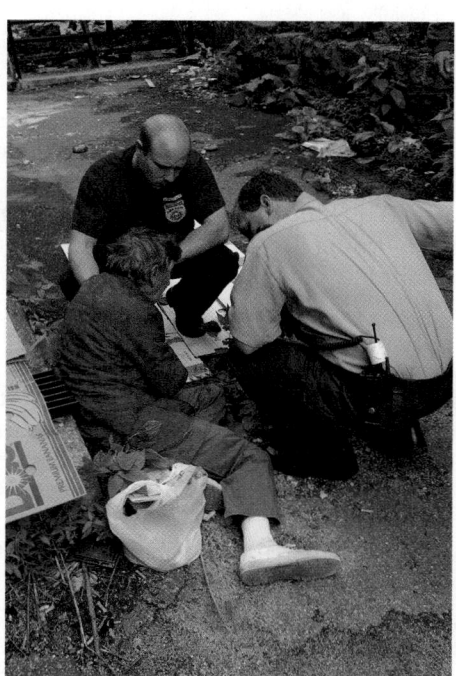

FIGURE 13-3 * Patients found in unusual environments or circumstances are sometimes difficult to immediately categorize as medical or trauma. (© Mark C. Ide)

Determine If the Patient Is Injured or Ill

As you form your general impression at the beginning of the primary assessment, categorize the patient as injured (a trauma patient) or ill (a medical patient) (Figure 13-5*). You will often confirm information already gathered from the dispatcher, scene size-up, First Responders, and bystanders. This determination is important in the next step of assessment.

There are two types of trauma: penetrating and blunt-force. **Penetrating trauma** is a force that pierces the skin and body tissues, often from gunshots and knives but also sometimes from screwdrivers, ice picks, handlebars, broken glass, metal, wood, or any other sharp object.

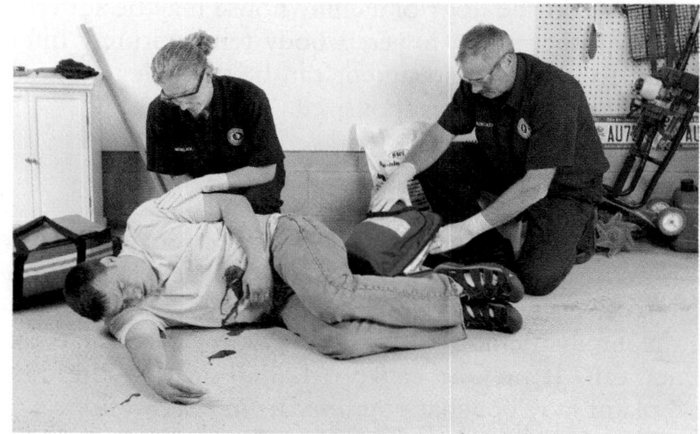

(a)

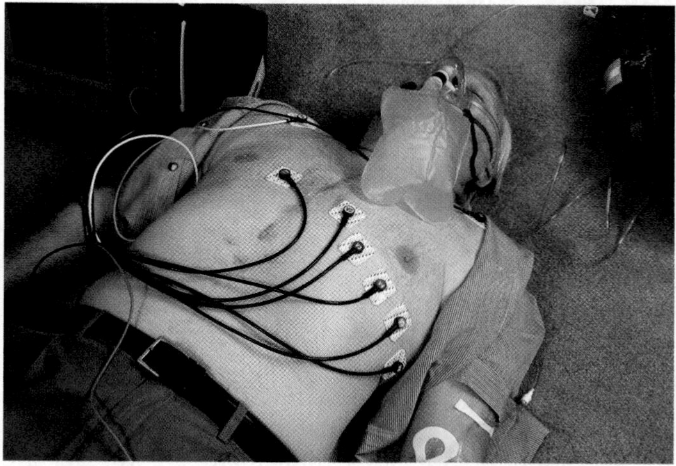

FIGURE 13-4 * Be alert for clues to the patient's condition or history throughout the assessment. When this patient's chest was exposed for a 12-lead ECG, obvious scars from prior bypass surgery were visible.

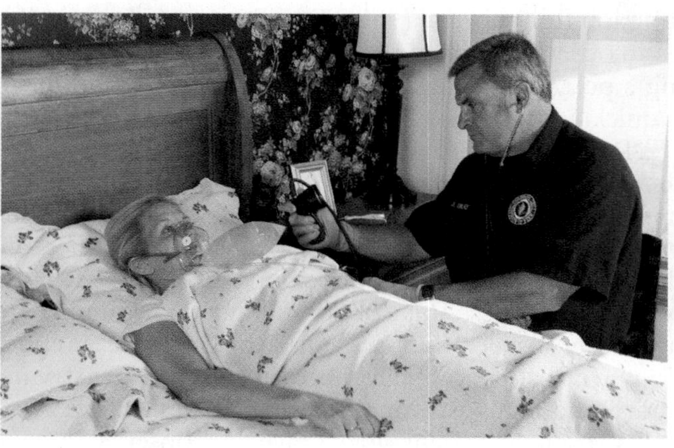

(b)

FIGURE 13-5 * As you form your general impression, categorize the patient as being **(a)** injured—a trauma patient or **(b)** ill—a medical patient.

Key Terms

blunt trauma a force that impacts or is applied to the body but is not sharp enough to penetrate it, such as a blow or a crushing injury.

chief complaint the patient's answer to the question "Why did you call the ambulance?"

Thinking Critically

As you approach the patient's home you immediately see an overturned ladder, a gutter hanging from the second story, and the patient on the ground bleeding copiously. What interventions should you perform before you complete the primary assessment—if any?

Blunt trauma is caused by a force that impacts or is applied to the body but is not sharp enough to penetrate it. Blunt trauma usually results from blows (as in vehicle crashes, falls, and fights) or from crushing (as in a building collapse or when an extremity gets caught in machinery). Clues to the mechanism of injury may be present in the patient's immediate environment, for example, a dent in the dashboard, the presence of a bloody knife, or a heavy object that appears to have fallen on the patient.

On the other hand, the environment may offer clues that the patient is suffering not from trauma but from a medical problem. For example, a bottle of nitroglycerin pills may indicate he was having chest pain prior to your arrival. A patient in bed in pajamas at 2:00 in the afternoon may have been sick all day. A pail next to the bed may make you suspect the patient has been vomiting. An elderly patient lying on the floor of a chilly house may be suffering from hypothermia (a lowered body temperature). Information from the environment can be valuable, especially when the patient is unresponsive.

Obtain the Chief Complaint

The **chief complaint** is the patient's answer to the question "Why did you call EMS today?" If the patient is unable to answer, the chief complaint may be the response of the family member or bystander who placed the emergency call. If no one can provide an answer, the chief complaint may be what you infer from observation.

The chief complaint may regard pain ("My stomach hurts"), abnormal function (slurred speech), a change in function from normal ("She doesn't seem to be herself"), or an observation made by you (bizarre behavior indicating a possible psychiatric problem). The chief complaint is quickly ascertained during the general impression.

Do not always assume that the original complaint is the true chief complaint. In a patient who is injured, you may think the chief complaint is obvious. You might suspect the pain associated with an obviously crushed and deformed leg to be the chief complaint. However, if the patient also states, "My chest is killing me," you must immediately suspect a possible chest injury or heart condition, which are potentially more serious than an extremity injury, and focus assessment on the patient's chest.

A trauma patient may have an observable chief complaint—for example, a wound. Medical conditions, rarely offer such obvious signs. So obtaining the chief complaint from a medical patient is extremely important.

Ask additional questions that refine a broad chief complaint, such as generalized abdominal pain. Suppose through further questioning you determine that the patient has been complaining of the same pain for the past 2 years. You must then ask, "Why did you call EMS *today?*" This will tend to focus the patient on what has changed to make him more concerned. He may now state, "This morning I vomited bright red blood." The chief complaint has changed and has set the tone for further assessment and emergency care.

In unresponsive patients, the chief complaint may need to be established through family, friends, or bystanders at the scene or from the environment itself. Ask, "Can you tell me what happened?" and "Was the patient complaining of anything before he became unconscious?" Do not assume that the bystander at the scene understands what unconsciousness truly means. You may need to ask, "Did the patient respond in any way when you were talking to him?"

If there is a possible life threat, the chief complaint, along with scene size-up, will help determine priorities for further assessment, care, and transport. You would opt for immediate transport following the primary and secondary assessments, with further assessment continuing en route. For a less serious complaints, you would proceed with assessment and emergency care on scene before transporting the patient.

Identify Immediate Life Threats During the General Impression

If you identify an obvious life-threatening condition during the general impression phase as you begin to assess the patient, you must immediately treat it. For example, you arrive at the scene of an injury incurred during a domestic dispute. After ensuring that the scene is safe, you enter. From the doorway, you spot a stab wound to the patient's left lateral chest. Since an open wound to the chest is an immediate life threat, you immediately place your gloved hand over the wound until your partner can prepare and apply the appropriate dressing. Only then do you continue with the primary assessment, watching especially for other injuries related to the stabbing. Obvious immediate life threats are those that you identify as you approach the patient—without having to look or feel for the problem. There are few obvious life threats that you would stop the

Objective 13-7
Identify immediate life threats during the general impression.

Objective 13-8
Discuss and demonstrate spinal stabilization and patient positioning for assessment.

Key Terms
in-line stabilization bringing the patient's head into a neutral position in which the nose is lined up with the navel and holding it there manually.

primary assessment to manage. Life threats that require immediate management if found during the general impression are listed in Table 13-2.

The American Heart Association guidelines of 2010 emphasize the need to quickly recognize cardiac arrest and immediately begin chest compressions. Thus, the intervention sequence in the cardiac arrest patient has changed from ABC to CAB: immediate initiation of chest compressions followed by opening the airway and providing ventilation, along with AED application. It is also recognized that many of the interventions can be accomplished simultaneously with enough EMTs or emergency medical personnel on the scene. It is extremely important to reinforce that upon recognition of cardiac arrest the resuscitation must begin immediately with chest compressions. During the resuscitation, the EMT must ensure minimal interruption of chest compressions while providing other interventions or assessments.

If the patient appears to be unresponsive, with no breathing or no normal breathing (gasping or agonal breaths), quickly assess the carotid pulse in the adult and child, brachial pulse in the infant (no more than 10 seconds). If no signs of life are present, immediately begin chest compressions. Apply the AED as soon as it is available without interruption to chest compressions until the AED indicates a "stand clear" or analysis of the rhythm. Follow the AED prompts. Also, delay ventilation until after the first set of compressions is delivered.

Establish In-Line Stabilization

If you determine or suspect that the patient has been injured, ask yourself if the mechanism of injury could have been significant enough to injure the spine. (Do not automatically rule out possible spinal injury in patients who are ill. Consider a diabetic patient who is found unconscious at the bottom of a stairway.)

If you suspect a possible spinal injury based solely on the mechanism of injury, you must manually stabilize the patient's spine before other assessment or care. Take manual **in-line stabilization** by bringing the patient's head into a neutral in-line position and holding it there. The procedure (Figure 13-6*) is:

1. Place one hand on each side of the patient's head.
2. Gently bring the head into a position in which the nose is in line with the patient's navel.
3. Position the head neutrally so the head is not extended (tipped backward) or flexed (tipped forward).

It is possible to have a stable injury of the vertebrae in which the spinal cord has not been damaged. If immediate and proper manual in-line stabilization is not accomplished, however, the vertebral injury may become unstable as a result of the patient moving or being moved. For example, you and your partner grasp the patient by the armpits and knees to move him onto the stretcher, causing permanent spinal cord damage, paralysis, or death.

TABLE 13-2 Immediate Life Threats That May Be Obvious During the General Impression

The following are life threats that require immediate management if found during formation of the general impression:

- An airway that is compromised by blood, vomitus, secretions, the tongue, bone, teeth, or other substances or objects
- Obvious open wounds to the chest
- Paradoxical movement of a segment of the chest (inward movement on inhalation and outward movement on exhalation)
- Major bleeding (steady flow or spurting)
- Unresponsive with no breathing or no normal breathing (agonal or gasping breaths)

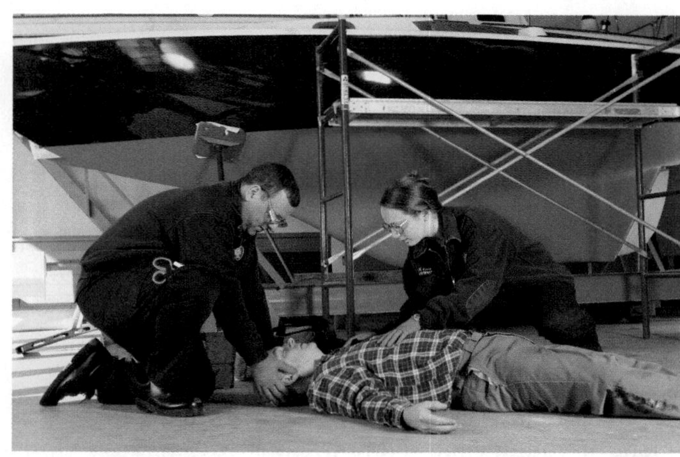

FIGURE 13-6 * Establish manual in-line stabilization if spinal injury is suspected.

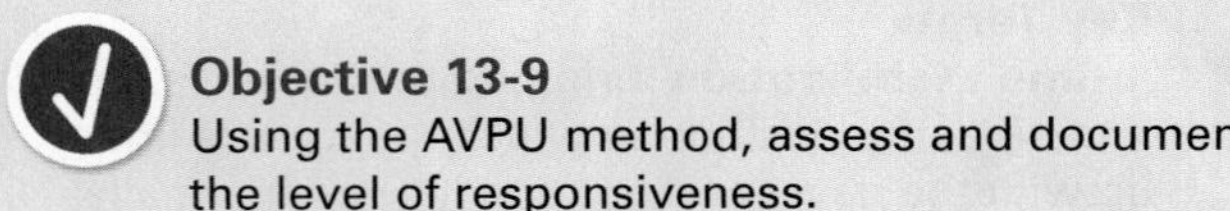

Objective 13-9
Using the AVPU method, assess and document the level of responsiveness.

Key Terms
AVPU a mnemonic for alert, responds to verbal stimulus, responds to painful stimulus, unresponsive, to characterize levels of responsiveness.

Thus, having a high index of suspicion and recognizing the need for proper spinal stabilization is extremely important prior to and during the primary assessment.

Once manual in-line stabilization is established, it must be maintained, even after a cervical spinal immobilization collar (CSIC) is applied, until the patient is completely immobilized to a backboard with backboard straps and a head immobilization device. Complete spinal immobilization will be discussed in Chapter 32.

Position the Patient for Assessment

If you find the patient prone (face down), it is necessary to quickly log roll him into a supine position (face up) (EMT Skills 13-1). It is not possible to properly assess the airway and breathing with the patient prone. Prior to log rolling the patient, quickly assess the posterior thorax and lumbar regions, the vertebral column, buttocks, and posterior aspects of the lower extremities by inspecting and palpating for any major bleeding, deformities, open wounds, bruises, burns, tenderness, or swelling. If an open wound to the posterior thorax is present, quickly occlude the wound with a nonporous or occlusive dressing prior to log rolling the patient into a supine position. If spinal injury is possible, establish in-line stabilization before log rolling.

Assess Level of Consciousness (Mental Status)

Indicate to the patient that you are an emergency medical technician and you are there to help. In the trauma patient, do this only after taking manual in-line stabilization to avoid any unnecessary movements by the patient. Quickly determine if the patient is awake, if he responds to a stimulus, or if he is unresponsive.

Assess the Level of Responsiveness

The patient's level of responsiveness can be rapidly assessed by using the **AVPU** mnemonic (Table 13-3).

Make adjustments in gauging the mental status of an infant or young child. Note whether the child is following movements with his eyes. Crying may replace speech as a response. For response to verbal stimulus, watch and listen for the child's reaction to a shout. The response to painful stimulus should be similar to an adult's.

TABLE 13-3 AVPU: Mnemonic for Assessment of Mental Status

A	Alert
V	Responds to Verbal Stimulus
P	Responds to Painful Stimulus
U	Unresponsive

Alertness and Orientation

If the patient's eyes are open and he is able to speak as you approach him, you would assume that the patient is alert. However, a patient can be alert but agitated, confused, or disoriented. If the patient is not alert, proceed to check his response to verbal stimulus.

Understanding BODY PROCESSES

Low oxygen levels (hypoxia) cause a patient to be agitated and anxious. High carbon dioxide levels (hypercapnia) cause the patient to become confused and sleepy. ■

Responsiveness to Verbal Stimulus

If the patient opens his eyes and responds or makes an attempt to respond only when you speak to him, he is responsive to verbal stimulus. If the patient does not speak, quickly check to determine if he will obey your commands. Instruct the patient to "squeeze my fingers" or "wiggle your toes." If the patient obeys the commands, you can assume he has a higher level of responsiveness than the patient who stares off, talks inappropriately, mumbles incomprehensibly, or does nothing at all.

Responsiveness to Painful Stimulus

If there is no response when you speak to the patient, you should try a painful stimulus. Painful stimulus is just that: applying pain to the patient to determine if and how he responds. Painful stimuli can be applied either centrally or peripherally. A central painful stimulus is applied to the core of the body. The following are methods of applying central painful stimuli (Figures 13-7a to 13-7d*):

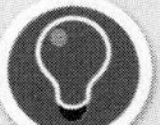

Key Points
To determine if the patient is responding to a painful stimulus, watch his face as well as his body.

- **Trapezius pinch.** Pinch the trapezius muscle that extends from along the base of the neck to the shoulder. Grasp 1 to 2 inches of the trapezius muscle and squeeze the muscle. Be sure that you have the muscle and not just the skin.
- **Supraorbital pressure.** Slide your finger under the upper ridge of the eye socket and apply upward pressure. Be careful not to produce any damage to the eyelid or globe during this procedure.
- **Sternal rub.** Apply hard downward pressure to the center of the sternum with the knuckles of your hand.
- **Earlobe pinch.** Pinch the soft tissue portion of the earlobe.
- **Armpit pinch.** Pinch the skin and underlying tissue along the margin of the armpit.

Peripheral painful stimuli can be applied; however, you must use caution in interpreting the results of the test. Common peripheral painful stimuli include:

- **Nail bed pressure.** Apply point pressure to the cuticle portion of the nail bed.
- **Pinch to the web between thumb and index finger**
- **Pinch to the finger, toe, hand, or foot**

To determine if the patient is responding to the painful stimulus, watch his face as well as his body. Look for a facial grimace or any other body movement.

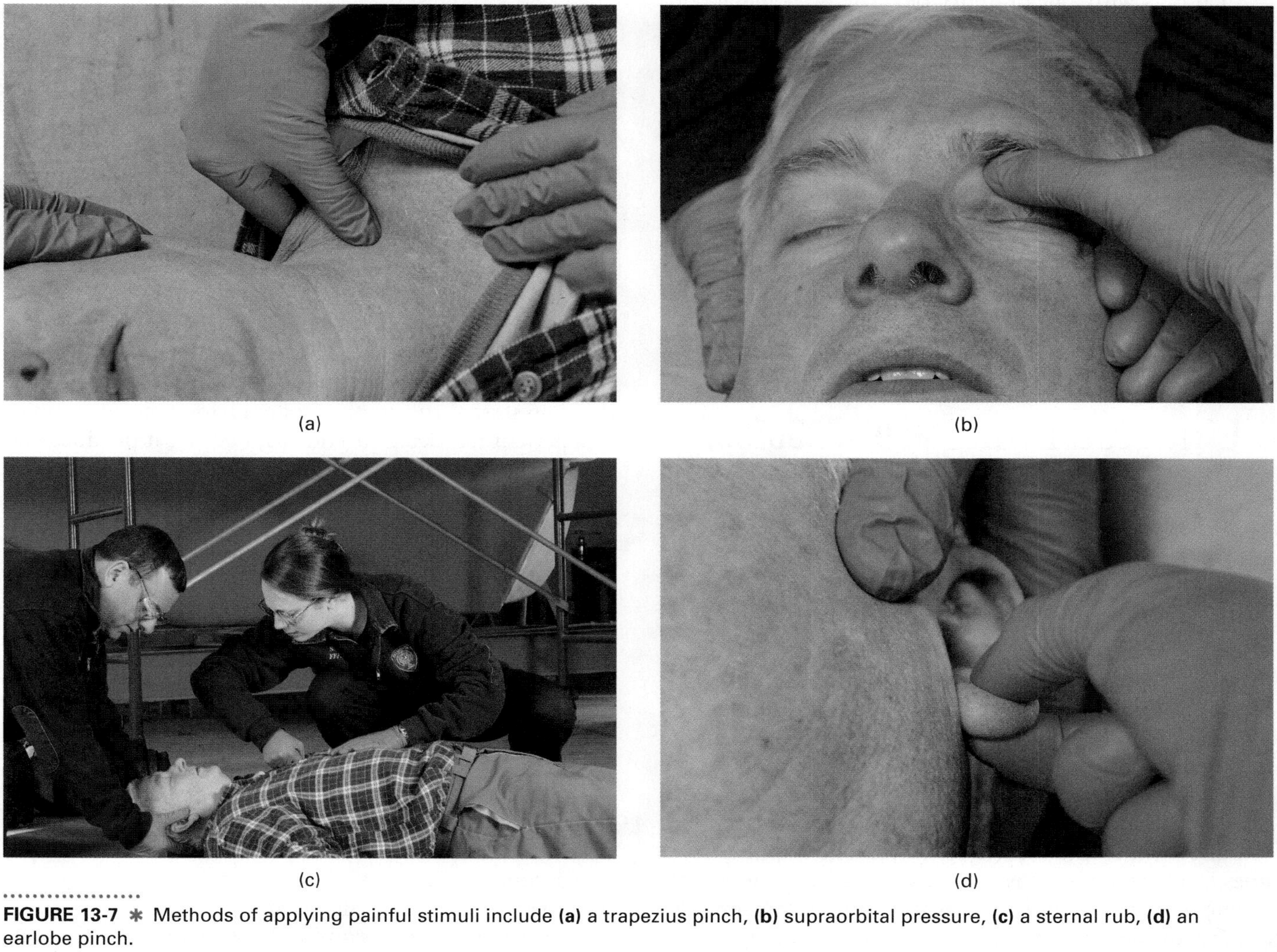

(a)

(b)

(c)

(d)

FIGURE 13-7 ✱ Methods of applying painful stimuli include **(a)** a trapezius pinch, **(b)** supraorbital pressure, **(c)** a sternal rub, **(d)** an earlobe pinch.

Key Terms

flexion posturing back arched, arms flexed inward toward the chest. Also called *decorticate posturing.*

extension posturing back arched, arms extended straight out parallel to the body. Also called *decerebrate posturing.*

Thinking Critically

Why is pinching the patient's fingernail not a reliable painful stimulus to assess severity of brain injury? What kind of painful stimulus would produce more reliable results? Why?

The patient who responds to a painful stimulus typically responds with either purposeful or nonpurposeful movements. The purposeful movements are attempts made by the patient to remove the stimulus or avoid the pain. This could be as significant as the patient grabbing your hand or as insignificant as a small movement away from the pain or a slight upward sweeping motion of the hand. If the patient lifts his arm and makes a purposeful movement toward the painful stimulus as if to push it away, or if he moves his body away from the painful stimulus, you would document this as "withdraws the stimulus" or "withdraws from pain." If the patient reaches up and grabs your hand, you can be sure the movement is purposeful and that he has a higher level of brain function than the patient who just moves his arm toward the pain.

Patients with a head injury or those with spinal cord injuries may respond to a painful stimulus but may not respond appropriately or normally. The patient with a spinal cord injury may only respond to pain applied above the site of the injury or to pain on only one side of the body. Two nonpurposeful movements—that is, having no purpose relative to the painful stimulus—are flexion posturing and extension posturing (Figures 13-8a and 13-8b*). In **flexion posturing**, also known as *decorticate posturing,* the patient arches the back and flexes the arms inward toward the chest. In **extension posturing**, also known as *decerebrate posturing,* the patient arches the back and extends the arms straight out parallel to the body. Both are signs of serious head injury.

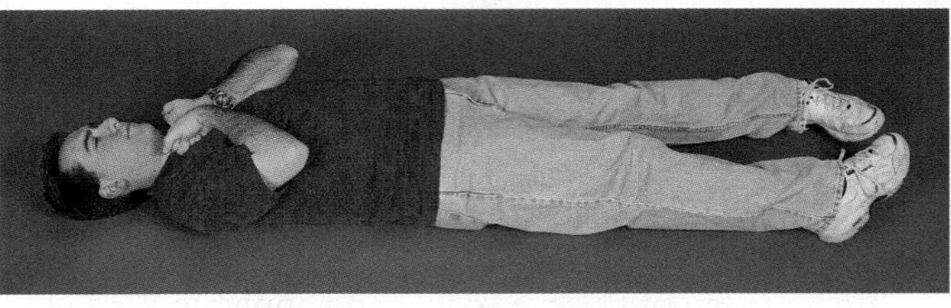

(a)

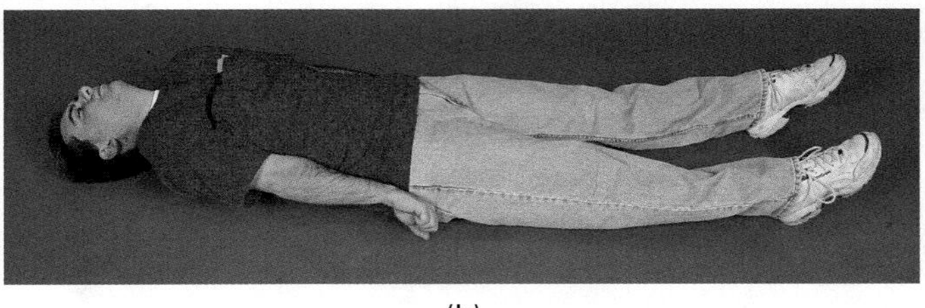

(b)

FIGURE 13-8 * Nonpurposeful movements: **(a)** flexion (decorticate) posturing, and **(b)** extension (decerebrate) posturing.

Understanding BODY PROCESSES

Flexion (decorticate) posturing is associated with compression of the brain at the upper portion of the brain stem. Extension (decerebrate) posturing is produced when the lower portion of the brain stem is being compressed. These are signs of serious head injury. ■

Problems with Some Types of Painful Stimuli It is important to always assess a central painful stimulus in a patient who is not responding to verbal stimuli. When the nail bed is pinched (a peripheral painful stimulus), the pain impulse travels to the spinal cord. The spinal cord may turn the impulse immediately around and send an impulse back to the muscle to move. The impulse never goes to the brain, so it is not the brain telling the muscle to move but the spinal cord just turning the impulse around and sending it back out again. If you pinch a nail bed on the right hand and the patient moves the right hand, you would want to interpret this as purposeful movement generated by the brain to withdraw from the painful stimulus. However, since this is a peripheral stimulus, the brain may never have received the stimulus. So interpreting this as purposeful movement would be a false assessment finding and might make you believe the patient's brain is responding more appropriately than it is. Thus, always be sure to assess a central painful stimulus, which will be transmitted to the brain.

The sternal rub method of applying painful stimulus to a patient has been questioned, because it produces results that may be less specific than the trapezius pinch and supraorbital pressure. When the sternal rub is applied, the patient may move his arm upward. This may be nonpurposeful movement; however, it appears as if the patient is making a movement to withdraw the stimulus, which can be incorrectly interpreted as purposeful. Also, some anecdotal evidence suggests that hard downward sternal pressure must be applied for 30 seconds to get an accurate response from a sternal rub. This may produce bruising and damage to the tissue over the sternum.

Unresponsiveness

A patient who does not respond to verbal or painful stimuli is considered to be unresponsive. Unresponsive patients commonly lose their gag and cough reflexes and the ability to control the tongue and epiglottis, often leading to airway compromise. Because unresponsiveness

Key Terms

occluded closed or blocked; not patent, as an occluded airway.

patent open; not blocked, as a patent airway.

Objective 13-10

Determine airway status in responsive patients and those with an altered mental status, demonstrate methods of establishing and maintaining an open airway, and recognize indications of partial airway occlusion.

is a significant finding, the unresponsive patient is considered a priority for emergency care and transport.

The patient who is not alert but responds to either verbal or painful stimulus is considered to have an altered mental status. This patient is not completely unresponsive but, like the unresponsive patient, may be prone to airway compromise.

Document the Level of Responsiveness

It is important to document the exact response to the stimulus, for example, "The patient groaned and flexed his left arm" or "The patient made a facial grimace and grasped my hand." A patient who grabs your hand when you apply a painful stimulus versus a patient who has flexion posturing indicates two significantly different levels of cerebral function. Obviously, the patient with the ability to grasp your hand has a much better level of neurological function than the flexion-postured patient; however, both could be placed generally into the category of responding to painful stimulus. The more specific you are regarding how the patient responds, the easier it is for others to assess for a deteriorating mental status at a later point in time.

Assessment of the patient's mental status should take you no longer than a few seconds to accomplish. Do not waste time performing an extensive neurological exam during the primary assessment. The AVPU check is to quickly establish a baseline for mental status. A much more detailed neurological exam will be performed later in the assessment process.

Assess the Airway

Once you have assessed the patient's level of responsiveness, you must immediately progress to assessment of the airway (Figure 13-9*). A closed or blocked or **occluded** airway is an immediately life-threatening condition. Your patient will not survive without a **patent** (open) airway, no matter how diligent your emergency care. You must closely assess the airway and, if it is not patent, immediately open it, using manual techniques and mechanical devices if necessary.

Determine Airway Status

The AVPU check of the patient's level of responsiveness can be used to quickly rule out a possible airway problem. A patient who is alert, responsive, and talking without signs of distress can be assumed to have a patent airway. Thus, the mental status check is a helpful tool for simultaneously gathering information about airway status.

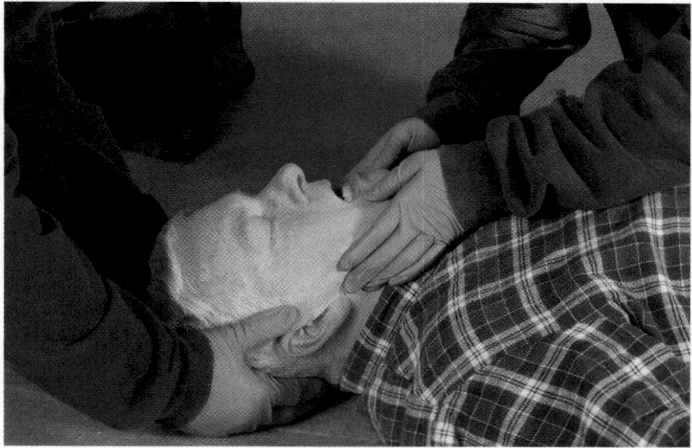

FIGURE 13-9 * Assess the airway. To open the airway, use the jaw-thrust maneuver for a trauma patient. Use the head-tilt, chin-lift maneuver for a medical patient.

In the Responsive Patient

If the patient is alert and talking without difficulty, or if the infant or child is crying, you can assume the airway is patent and move on to the assessment of breathing. However, an alert patient who has stridor on inspiration or exhalation or who is having difficulty in speaking, gasping between words, using extremely short sentences, or not talking at all should be examined closely for a blocked or partially blocked airway or for other causes of respiratory distress. If you have any doubt that the airway is open, you should immediately take the necessary steps to open it (as will be described).

In the Unresponsive or Severely Altered Mental Status Patient

Unresponsive patients or patients with a severely altered mental status, such as those only responding to painful stimuli with flexion or extension, have a high incidence of airway occlusion resulting from relaxation of the muscles in the upper airway. The muscle relaxation allows the tongue and epiglottis to fall back and partially block the lower part of the pharynx and the opening to the trachea. In this situation, use the techniques described next to open or to maintain an open airway.

Open the Airway

If the patient is not talking or responding normally, has a severely altered mental status, or is unresponsive, assume that the airway is or may become closed. You must immediately open the airway and take measures to maintain the airway's patency.

The airway is opened and maintained by using, as needed, any or all of the following techniques:

- Manual airway maneuvers to prevent the tongue and epiglottis from blocking the airway: the head-tilt, chin-lift maneuver or the jaw-thrust maneuver. The head-tilt, chin-lift maneuver is used for medical patients in whom you do not suspect the possibility of a spinal injury. The jaw-thrust maneuver is used for trauma patients in whom you suspect a possible spinal injury.
- Suction and/or finger sweeps to remove blood, vomitus, food, secretions, or foreign objects.
- Airway adjuncts to maintain a patent airway: the oropharyngeal airway or the nasopharyngeal airway.
- Manual thrusts to the abdomen (Heimlich maneuver), or a combination of chest thrusts and back blows for infants, to force bursts of air from the lungs—used to relieve a blockage of the airway by a foreign body that cannot be relieved by any of the techniques already listed.
- Positioning of the medical patient who has no suspected spinal injury in a modified lateral position (recovery or coma position) to allow secretions, blood, or vomitus to flow out of the mouth instead of into the airway. If the medical patient requires ventilation, he must be maintained in a supine position. It is not possible to effectively ventilate the patient while he is on his side. The patient can be quickly turned on his side if he vomits or has a large amount of secretions and then placed supine again to resume ventilation. Always have suction available in the patient who is unresponsive or who has an altered mental status.

The head-tilt, chin-lift and jaw-thrust maneuvers, suctioning techniques, and the use of airway adjuncts were taught in Chapter 10, "Airway Management, Artificial Ventilation, and Oxygenation."

Indications of Partial Airway Occlusion

When you approach the patient, you may hear abnormal sounds from the upper airway. These sounds are an indication that the airway may be partially blocked. Sounds that frequently indicate partial airway occlusion are listed in Table 13-4 and discussed next.

TABLE 13-4 Sounds That May Indicate Partial Airway Obstruction

- *Snoring (sonorous)*—a rough, snoring-type sound on inspiration and/or exhalation
- *Gurgling*—a sound similar to air rushing through water on inspiration and/or exhalation
- *Crowing*—a sound like a cawing crow on inspiration
- *Stridor*—harsh, high-pitched sound on inspiration

Snoring

If a snoring (sonorous) sound is heard, it is an indication that the tongue and likely the epiglottis are partially blocking the airway. Use the head-tilt, chin-lift maneuver (if there is no suspicion of spinal injury) or the jaw-thrust maneuver (if spinal injury is possible) to relieve any obstruction of the airway by the tongue. If this does not correct the snoring, insert an oropharyngeal airway (for an unresponsive patient without a gag reflex). If the patient gags when you insert an oropharyngeal airway, remove it immediately, be prepared to suction, and consider insertion of a nasopharyngeal airway.

Gurgling

A gurgling sound is an indication that a liquid substance is in the airway. Immediately open the mouth and suction out the contents. If the contents are too thick to be suctioned, turn the patient on his side and sweep the mouth out with your fingers, a tongue blade, or the suction catheter itself. A patient with possible spinal injury must be log rolled onto his side while manual in-line stabilization is maintained. Be cautious when placing your fingers in a patient's mouth, even if he is unresponsive. The patient can very easily, and unintentionally, bite down and injure you significantly. Place a bite stick between the teeth if necessary to avoid a patient bite.

Do not waste time when clearing the airway. The key is to be prepared and use whatever device or technique is most readily available that clears the contents so they are not aspirated into the airway, respiratory tract, or lungs.

Crowing and Stridor

Crowing and stridor are both high-pitched sounds produced on inspiration. Both are most commonly associated with the swelling or muscle spasms that result from conditions such as airway infections, allergic reactions, or burns to the upper airway. These conditions typically cannot be relieved by manual maneuvers, suctioning, or insertion of an airway adjunct.

Inserting anything such as an airway adjunct, suction tip, tongue blade, or fingers into the mouth or throat of a pediatric patient with a suspected upper airway infection can cause extremely dangerous spasm and a complete airway obstruction. (Such a patient may complain of a sore or hoarse throat and typically will be leaning forward with the neck jutted out or drooling. A patient with these signs

Objective 13-11
Assess the rate and quality of breathing; determine if the patient has absent, inadequate or adequate breathing; provide positive pressure ventilation in the patient with absent or inadequate breathing; and provide oxygenation as determined by the SpO_2 level in the patient who is breathing adequately.

Key Points
Both too slow and too fast respiratory rates can lead to hypoxia.

and symptoms should be suspected of having an upper airway infection.) Instead, in these cases, it may be necessary to begin ventilation with a bag-valve-mask device with supplemental oxygen immediately to ensure adequate movement of air past the swollen tissues. For more details on assessing respiratory illnesses, see Chapter 16, "Respiratory Emergencies."

Assess Breathing

As soon as you secure an open airway, assess the patient's breathing status (Figure 13-10∗). Assess to:

- Determine if breathing is adequate or inadequate (Table 13-5).
- Determine the need for early oxygen therapy if breathing is adequate.
- Provide positive pressure ventilation with supplemental oxygen for inadequate breathing.

Assess Rate and Quality of Breathing

The best method to assess breathing is by *looking, listening,* and *feeling.* When doing so, assess both the amount of air breathed in and out (tidal volume) and the approximate respiratory rate. Remember that one respiration consists of one inhalation and one exhalation.

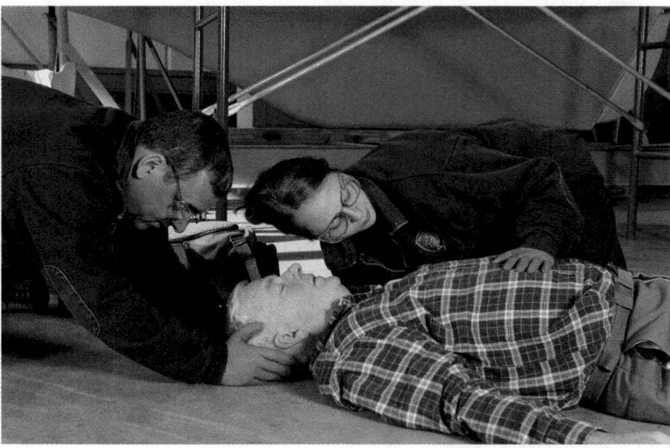

FIGURE 13-10 ∗ Assess breathing. If breathing is adequate and the patient requires oxygen, administer oxygen at 15 lpm via nonrebreather mask. If breathing is inadequate, begin positive pressure ventilation with supplemental oxygen.

TABLE 13-5 Inadequate Breathing Versus Adequate Breathing

Inadequate Breathing	Adequate Breathing
Inadequate *rate* **or** inadequate *tidal volume* = inadequate breathing	Adequate *rate* **and** adequate *tidal volume* = adequate breathing

Look

Get down and place your ear and face close to the patient's nose and mouth while looking at the chest. Look for the following:

- **Inadequate tidal volume.** Poor movement (rise) of the chest wall, indicating that an inadequate amount of air is being breathed in with each respiration. This is typically described as shallow respiration.
- **Abnormal respiratory rate.** Breathing that is either too fast or too slow (outside the ranges of 8–24 per minute for an adult, 15–30 per minute for a child, 25–50 per minute for an infant).
- **Bradypnea.** A respiratory rate that is too slow, called bradypnea, may cause the minute volume (amount of air breathed into the lungs in 1 minute) to be inadequate. Thus, the slow rate will lead to hypoxia (inadequate oxygen delivery to the tissues). The amount of air taken in with each breath may be adequate, but there are not enough breaths to maintain an adequate supply of oxygen to the cells. The breathing rate that would be defined as bradypnea varies with the type of patient. Obviously, adults breathe at slower rates than infants and young children; therefore, a rate that is considered bradypnea in an adult is much slower than a rate that is considered bradypnea in an infant or child. As an example, a respiratory rate of 16 per minute is more than adequate in an adult or older child; however, it may be too slow in an infant.

  You must consider the rate with the whole assessment of the patient. Consider the mental status and other signs when determining if the rate is adequate or inadequate. For instance, if a patient has a respiratory rate of 8 per minute and an altered mental status with signs of respiratory insufficiency (retractions, poor air exchange) and hypoxia (agitation, restlessness, cyanosis), you would consider the rate inadequate and begin positive pressure ventilation. Thus, the rate is not considered inadequate unless there are other signs of respiratory insufficiency present.

ASSESSMENT Tips

Because brain cells require a constant supply of oxygen, an altered mental status may be an early sign of hypoxia (low oxygen levels). ■

The following conditions may cause bradypnea (abnormally slow respiratory rates): hypoxia (especially in young children and infants), drug overdose on depressant drugs, head injury, stroke, hypothermia (cold emergency), and toxic inhalation.

- **Tachypnea.** A respiratory rate that is too fast, called tachypnea, may not always result in better breathing status for the patient. When the rate becomes excessive, the lungs do not have enough time between breaths to fill adequately; therefore, the minute volume (volume of air the patient is breathing in 1 minute) becomes inadequate. The result is inadequate breathing, leading to hypoxia. Keep in mind that a rate that is too fast in an adult may be normal in a young child or infant. As an example, a respiratory rate of 40 per minute in an adult is excessive and may lead to inadequate breathing, whereas a rate of 40 per minute in an infant is considered normal.

Understanding BODY PROCESSES

When the respiratory rate is greater than 40 per minute in the adult, the time for the lungs to fill is so short that the tidal volume will become inadequate and the patient will likely become hypoxic. ■

ASSESSMENT Tips

A rapid respiratory rate should alert you to the possibility that the patient is hypoxic. However, be aware that elderly patients typically have higher resting respiratory rates than younger patients: an average of 20 per minute. ■

Again, you must view the respiratory rate as one part of the whole patient assessment. If the patient is talking and alert, without distress, the breathing is adequate. However, if the patient has signs and symptoms of inadequate breathing, the rate or depth would be considered ineffective and intervention with positive pressure ventilation would be necessary.

Conditions that may lead to tachypnea (abnormally fast respiratory rates) are hypoxia, fever, pain, drug overdose, stimulant drug use, shock, head injury, chest injury, stroke, and other medical conditions.

Understanding BODY PROCESSES

Chemoreceptors constantly measure the amount of carbon dioxide and oxygen in the arterial blood. Carbon dioxide is a strong stimulus to breathe. As its level in the blood increases, the respiratory rate increases in an attempt to eliminate the excess carbon dioxide from the body. ■

Look for the following additional signs of inadequate breathing:

- *Retractions*—identified by a sunken-in appearance of tissues that are pulled inward on inhalation at any of these locations:
  - the suprasternal notch (above the sternum)
  - intercostal spaces (between the ribs)
  - supraclavicular spaces (above the clavicles)
- *Use of the neck muscles* on inhalation
- *Nasal flaring*—the nostrils flaring out as the patient inhales
- *Excessive abdominal muscle use*
- *Tracheal tugging*—pendulum motions of the trachea in the anterior neck during inhalation
- *Pale, cool, clammy skin*—a sign of poor perfusion to and oxygenation of the cells and tissues
- *Cyanosis*—a bluish or blue-gray tone of the skin seen early around the lips, nose, and fingernail beds indicating inadequate oxygenation
- *A pulse oximeter (SpO_2) reading of less than 95%*

ASSESSMENT Tips

Pale, cool, and clammy (moist) skin is an early sign of hypoxia. Cyanosis is a late sign. ■

Also, quickly observe the patient's respiratory pattern. Look for:

- *Asymmetrical movement of the chest wall*—The chest wall should move symmetrically (both sides moving together) and smoothly. Unequal movement—for example, one side moving up and outward as the other moves down and inward—is an indication of a significant chest injury.

Listen and Feel

Listen for air movement and feel for escape of warm humidified air. Very little air movement is an indication of inadequate tidal volume and inadequate breathing.

Key Terms

apnea absence of breathing; respiratory arrest.

dyspnea shortness of breath or perceived difficulty in breathing.

Key Points

A patient with an insufficient or ineffective breathing rate that is too slow or too fast requires positive pressure ventilation with supplemental oxygen.

Absent or Inadequate Breathing

Not all of the breathing difficulties that you may observe, or that the patient may tell you about, are immediately life threatening. A patient may be experiencing some difficulty in breathing, yet be breathing adequately to support life, at least for the time being.

During the primary assessment, you are observing for signs of absent or inadequate breathing—conditions that are immediately life threatening and that must be treated at once. Life-threatening breathing problems are:

- **Absence of breathing (apnea**). Identified by no chest wall movement and no sensation or sound of air moving in and out of the nose or mouth
- **Inadequate breathing.** Identified by:
  - An insufficient or ineffective respiratory rate
  - Signs of an inadequate tidal volume such as poor chest rise and little air movement from the nose and mouth
  - Signs of inadequate oxygenation, such as deteriorating mental status; pale, cool, clammy skin; or cyanosis
  - Signs of serious respiratory distress, including difficulty in breathing (**dyspnea**), poor chest wall movement, retractions, nasal flaring, use of neck muscles during inhalation, and/or poor air exchange from the nose and mouth

Understanding BODY PROCESSES

Dyspnea, the uncomfortable sensation of breathing difficulty, is produced when the oxygen demands of the cells are not being met by the respiratory or circulatory system. ■

If the patient is apneic (not breathing) or is breathing inadequately, you must immediately begin positive pressure ventilation with supplemental oxygen. Any delay in treatment could lead to brain death and cardiac arrest.

As you learned in Chapter 10, "Airway Management, Artificial Ventilation, and Oxygenation," positive pressure ventilation is any method that forces air and oxygen into the patient's lungs when the patient is unable to breathe adequately, or at all, on his own. It can be achieved by mouth-to-mask, bag-valve-mask device, or a flow-restricted, oxygen-powered ventilation device. Whenever you perform positive pressure ventilation, you need to attach and deliver supplemental oxygen within the first few minutes after beginning ventilation. To ensure a patent airway so that the ventilations reach the patient's lungs, you should insert an oropharyngeal or nasopharyngeal airway prior to beginning ventilation.

A patient with an insufficient or ineffective breathing rate that is too slow or too fast requires positive pressure ventilation with supplemental oxygen. If an ill or injured patient with a breathing rate greater than 24 per minute is responsive and has an adequate tidal volume, administer oxygen and continually reassess the patient for signs of inadequate breathing.

Adequate Breathing

If the chest is rising and falling adequately, you hear and feel good air exchange, the respiratory rate is adequate, and no evidence of serious respiratory distress is present, assume that the patient's breathing is adequate.

If the patient with adequate breathing is responsive, but is ill or injured, consider administering oxygen.

Oxygen Therapy in the Patient with Adequate Breathing

In the patient who is breathing adequately, oxygen administration is based on the patient's condition; on signs and symptoms of hypoxia, poor perfusion, or respiratory distress; and on the SpO_2 reading. As an example, if an alert patient is complaining of abdominal pain and has no signs of hypoxia, poor perfusion, or respiratory distress, and the SpO_2 reading is 96% on room air—you can elect to place the patient on a nasal cannula at 2 to 4 lpm or not to administer any oxygen at all. If at any time the patient's mental status deteriorates; the patient becomes anxious, confused, sleepy, or disoriented; the patient exhibits other signs or symptoms of hypoxia, poor perfusion, or respiratory distress; or the patient complains of chest discomfort or shortness of breath—immediately place the patient on a nonrebreather mask at 15 lpm. If the patient with adequate breathing has an altered mental status or is unresponsive—administer oxygen at 15 lpm by nonrebreather mask.

Always err to benefit the patient, and never withhold oxygen if it is needed. If you have any doubt about whether to administer oxygen, administer it. If you have any doubt about whether the patient should be placed on a nonrebreather mask or on a simple face mask or a nasal cannula, place the patient on the nonrebreather mask. Most patients will benefit from—or at least not be

Objective 13-12
Assess the circulation to include assessing the pulse, identifying and controlling major bleeding, and assessing perfusion through skin color, temperature, and condition and capillary refill, and recognize and begin treatment for shock.

Key Points
In the unresponsive patient, check the pulse. If you cannot feel a radial pulse, immediately check for a carotid pulse.

harmed by—oxygen. Always follow your local protocol and do what is right for the patient. As you become more experienced, it will become easier to make clinical decisions regarding the extent of oxygen therapy to provide for the patient.

Adequate Oxygenation Based on the SpO_2 Reading

A pulse oximeter (SpO_2) reading of 95% or greater on room air is an indicator of adequate oxygenation. A patient who is on a nonrebreather mask for a period of time and has an SpO_2 reading of only 95% is a concern. The patient is breathing a high concentration of oxygen; thus, he should have an SpO_2 reading that reflects the high oxygen saturation in the blood (> 95%). You would assume that if you removed the oxygen from the patient, his SpO_2 would fall well below 95%, indicating hypoxemia.

ASSESSMENT Tips

The patient with an SpO_2 reading of 95% or 96% who has been receiving oxygen by nonrebreather mask at 15 lpm for a period of time will likely become hypoxemic upon removal of the oxygen. ■

Once you have assessed and controlled any immediate life threats associated with breathing, and have begun positive pressure ventilation with supplemental oxygen or have considered oxygen therapy, you must quickly progress to assessment of the circulation.

Assess Circulation

An assessment of the circulation includes checking the following (Table 13-6):

- Pulse
- Possible major bleeding
- Skin color, temperature, and condition
- Capillary refill

During the primary assessment, the main purposes for checking circulation are to determine whether the heart is beating, whether there is any severe bleeding, and whether blood is circulating adequately (the patient may be suffering from a perfusion problem or shock). A problem in any of these areas is life threatening and must be treated immediately.

TABLE 13-6 Primary Assessment of Circulation

Assessment of circulation during the primary assessment should occur in this sequence:

- Assess for presence or absence of *pulse.*
- Assess for possible major *bleeding.*
- Assess *skin* color, temperature, and condition.
- Assess *capillary refill.*

Assess the Pulse

You learned about pulses and how to assess them in Chapter 11, "Baseline Vital Signs, Monitoring Devices, and History Taking." During the primary assessment, you will not attempt to make a precise reading of heart rate. This will happen later, when you take the vital signs during the secondary assessment. For now, if the patient is unresponsive you first want to ascertain whether the heart is beating. In the adult patient, if you cannot feel a radial pulse (at the wrist), immediately assess for a carotid pulse (in the neck) (Figure 13-11∗). The carotid pulse is

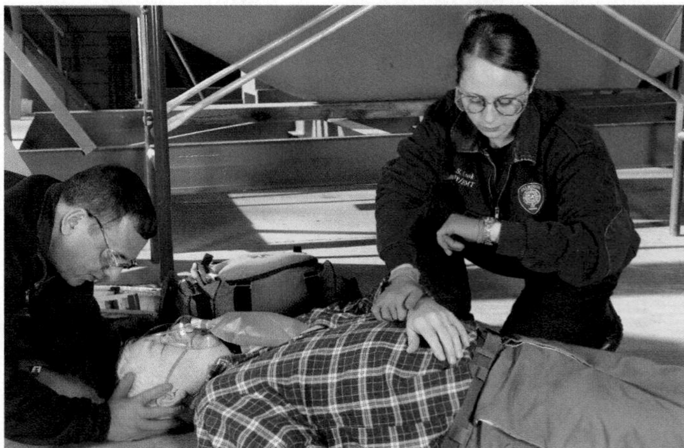

FIGURE 13-11 ∗ Assess pulses. If there is no radial pulse, palpate the carotid pulse. If the patient is pulseless or is unresponsive and has no breathing or no normal breathing, immediately begin chest compressions followed by airway and ventilation and apply the automated external defibrillator according to your local protocol.

typically the most prominent pulse and is the last to be lost in the patient. A pulse that is growing faint usually can be felt in the carotid artery even when it can no longer be felt in a peripheral artery.

To assess for a carotid pulse, locate the thyroid cartilage (Adam's apple) and slide your fingers down the neck laterally on the same side on which you are positioned until you feel the groove between the larynx and the bulk of muscles in the neck. The carotid artery is located there and should be felt with the index and middle fingers.

Maintain in-line stabilization when assessing for pulses in a trauma patient. The EMT who is at the patient's head holding in-line stabilization can assess the carotid pulse by sliding the index and middle fingers of one hand down the neck to the correct landmark until feeling the pulse. Do not assess or compress the carotid pulses on both sides of the neck simultaneously as this may reduce circulation to and oxygenation of the brain.

As you learned in Chapter 11, in a patient who is 1 year old or less, it is necessary to palpate a brachial pulse, which is found on the lateral aspect of the upper section of the arm between the biceps and triceps muscles (Figure 13-12*).

When palpating the pulses, quickly determine:

- If the pulse is present or not
- The approximate heart rate (beats per minute)
- The regularity and strength

ASSESSMENT Tips

Elderly patients commonly have "irregularly irregular" heart rhythms (that is, an irregular, or abnormal, rhythm that has no regular pattern). In many elderly patients, this kind of abnormality *is* their normal rhythm; however, it is important to report and document this finding since it may be related to their current condition. ■

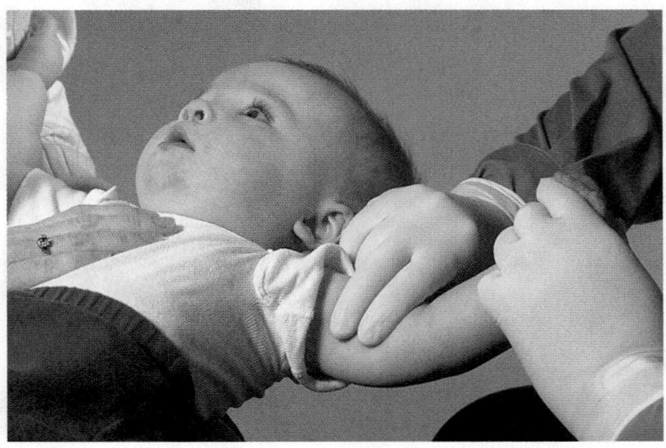

FIGURE 13-12 * Assess the brachial pulse in an infant less than 1 year old.

When determining approximate heart rate, remember that a more accurate heart rate will be determined later in the patient assessment. During the primary assessment, it is most appropriate to estimate the heart rate as fast, normal, or slow.

Note heart rates that are less than 60 per minute or greater than 100 per minute. Bradycardia, a heart rate less than 60 per minute, may indicate severe hypoxia (oxygen starvation), head injury, drug overdose, heart attack, or some other medical condition. (It is important to remember, however, that athletes and other well-conditioned individuals commonly have heart rates less than 60 bpm at rest.) Bradycardia is an ominous sign of hypoxia in infants and children. Tachycardia, a heart rate greater than 100 per minute, may indicate anxiety, blood loss, shock, abnormal heart rhythms, heart attack, drug overdose, early hypoxia, fever, and other medical or traumatic conditions.

It was once thought that the pulse location could provide an estimate of the systolic blood pressure; however, this method of estimating the systolic pressure has not been supported by the scientific literature. One thing that has been established is that, in order for a pulse to be palpated, the systolic pressure must be at least 60 mmHg. A peripheral (radial, brachial, or femoral) or central (carotid) pulse will likely not be felt with a systolic blood pressure less than 60 mmHg. It is important to determine the quality of the pulse in relation to its location. Peripheral pulses may be weaker and less prominent or absent in hypoperfusion states.

If the carotid pulse is absent, immediately begin chest compressions followed by positive pressure ventilation with supplemental oxygen and application of the automated external defibrillator (AED). If the cardiac arrest was witnessed, immediately begin chest compressions, apply the AED during chest compressions, and begin rhythm analysis as soon as the AED is ready. If the cardiac arrest was not witnessed, immediately begin chest compressions and perform five cycles (approximately 2 minutes) of 30 compressions followed by 2 ventilations (a 15-compression-and-2-ventilation ratio may be used in two-rescuer CPR in infants and children). During the CPR, apply the AED and begin the rhythm analysis immediately following the fifth set of compressions. Cardiac arrest resulting from traumatic injuries requires CPR and quick transport. Consult medical direction regarding use of the AED in a traumatic cardiac arrest. (The AED will be covered in detail in Chapter 15, "Shock and Resuscitation.")

Identify Major Bleeding

Scan the body looking for any indication of major bleeding. If you notice large pools of blood or completely blood-soaked clothing, immediately expose the area by cutting away clothing with your scissors (Figures 13-13a and 13-13b*). Major bleeding is typically identified as bright red, spurting bleeding (arterial) or dark red, steady, rapid bleeding (venous). If either of these types of major

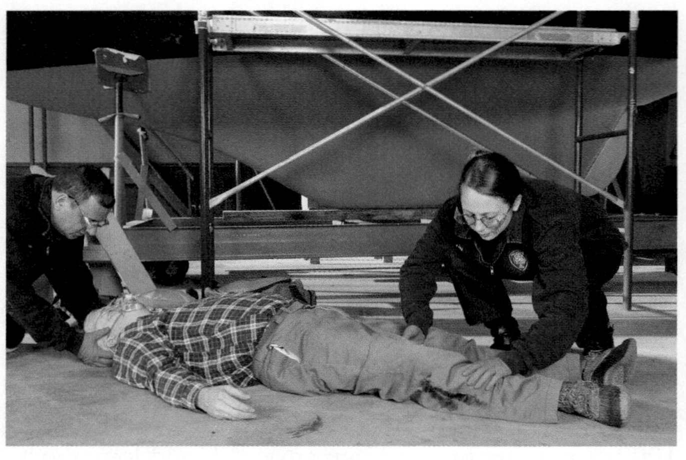

(a)

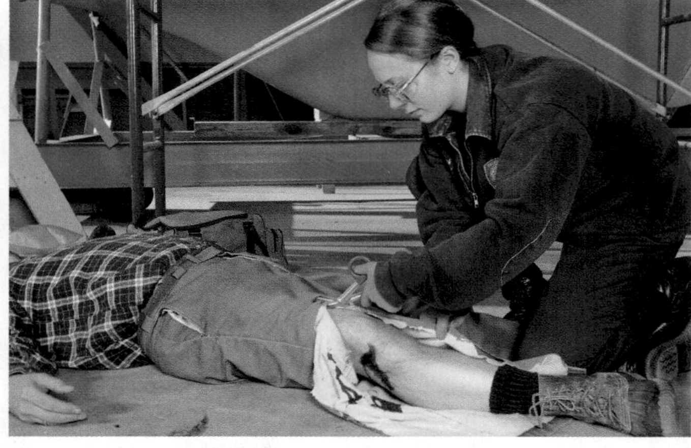

(b)

FIGURE 13-13 ∗ **(a)** Check for major bleeding. **(b)** Cut away blood-soaked clothing to expose potentially life-threatening bleeding. Control bleeding with direct pressure, then a pressure dressing.

bleeding is present, immediately place gloved fingers or a gloved hand on the wound and apply direct pressure to control the bleeding. Apply a pressure dressing once the bleeding has been controlled. During the primary assessment, do not waste time dealing with slow, oozing capillary bleeding or other wounds that do not present with major bleeding, no matter how dramatic they may appear. The control of bleeding will be covered in detail in Chapter 28, "Bleeding and Soft-Tissue Trauma."

ASSESSMENT Tips

If the patient has lost a significant amount of blood, the arterial bleeding may not be spurting by the time you reach the scene. The loss of blood volume will reduce the pressure to the point that it is no longer great enough to make the blood spurt. Instead, the bleeding will be a steady flow. ■

Assess Perfusion

The patient's perfusion (the sufficient supply of oxygen to the body's cells that results from adequate circulation of blood through the capillaries) can be assessed by checking the skin's color, temperature, and condition (Figure 13-14∗). Capillary refill is typically a more reliable indicator of perfusion status in infants and children. The assessment of skin was discussed in detail in Chapter 11, "Baseline Vital Signs, Monitoring Devices, and History Taking."

ASSESSMENT Tips

Capillary refill alone cannot provide an accurate assessment of perfusion in infants, children, or adults. You must also assess the mental status, heart rate, peripheral and central pulses, skin signs, and blood pressure to determine the perfusion status of the patient. ■

Skin Color

The skin is normally referred to as pink, even though it doesn't have a pink color tone. In all patients, including dark-skinned patients, the color can be observed at the mucous membranes of the mouth (including the lips), at the mucous membranes that line the eyelids, under the tongue, and at the nail beds. The nail bed is the least desirable place to check color because cold temperatures, some chronic medical illnesses, smoking, and other conditions may reduce or restrict blood flow to the hands and feet.

Because the skin plays a major role in body temperature regulation, it is important to realize the effects of the environment on the skin. You would expect a patient in a cold temperature to present with cooler and more pale-looking skin. A patient in a hot environment would typically have flushed (red), warm skin. With these exceptions, the skin colors listed next are considered to be abnormal.

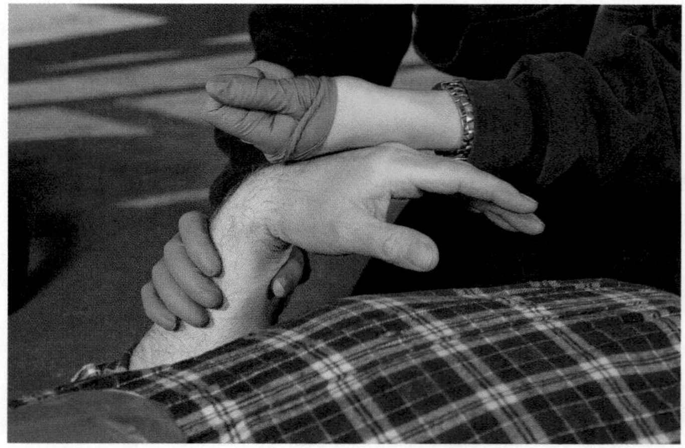

FIGURE 13-14 ∗ Assess perfusion by assessing color, temperature, and condition of the skin. Assess capillary refill.

Understanding BODY PROCESSES

In a cold environment, the vessels in the skin constrict, causing the blood to be shunted to the core of the body to preserve the heat at the core. Because the warm, red blood has been shunted away from the skin, the skin takes on a pale appearance and becomes cool. In a hot environment, the vessels in the skin dilate (increase the diameter) to increase the flow of blood to the skin. This allows the hotter blood to flow to the skin where it can be distributed over a large surface area and cooled by the air and through evaporation of sweat. The flow of hotter blood to the skin may cause the skin to appear flushed and feel warm. ■

- **Pale or mottled.** Skin that is pale or mottled typically indicates a decrease in perfusion and the onset of shock (hypoperfusion). If the patient's skin is pale or mottled, suspect that the patient is losing blood internally or externally or suffering another cause of shock.

Understanding BODY PROCESSES

The alpha receptor properties of epinephrine (adrenaline) that circulates in response to shock will cause the vessels in the skin to constrict, shunting the blood away from the vessels in the skin and to the core of the body. Because the warm red blood is no longer in the skin, it will take on a pale appearance and feel cool. ■

- **Cyanotic.** Cyanotic, or blue-gray, skin may indicate reduced oxygenation from chest injuries, blood loss, or conditions like pneumonia or pulmonary edema that disrupt gas exchange in the lungs. It is a late sign of poor perfusion.

Understanding BODY PROCESSES

The hemoglobin in the red blood cells changes color when starved of oxygen, thus giving the skin of a hypoxic patient its bluish (cyanotic) tint. ■

ASSESSMENT Tips

A patient with anemia, who has a low number of red blood cells or low hemoglobin content to start with, may take longer to become cyanotic when hypoxic. ■

- **Red.** A flushed, or red, color usually indicates an increase in the amount of blood circulating in the blood vessels in the skin. This could indicate anaphylactic or vasogenic shock, poisonings, overdose, or some diabetic or other medical conditions. Alcohol ingestion, local inflammation, cold exposure, or a severe heat emergency (heat stroke) may also turn the skin red.
- **Yellow.** Liver dysfunction usually produces a yellow skin color termed *jaundice*. This is common in patients suffering from some form of liver disease, chronic alcoholism, or endocrine disturbance caused by increased bilirubin, a product of hemoglobin breakdown that is normally eliminated by the liver.

During the primary assessment, you are most concerned with the pale or cyanotic (blue) colors that indicate possible shock (hypoperfusion) or inadequate oxygen intake.

Skin Temperature

The skin temperature is best assessed by partially taking off your gloves and placing the back of your hand or fingers on the patient's abdomen, face, or neck. The skin is normally warm to the touch but may instead be hot, cool, or cold:

- **Hot skin.** This may result from a hot environment or extremely elevated body core temperatures.
- **Cool skin.** Decreased perfusion as seen in shock, as well as exposure to cold temperatures, fright, anxiety, drug overdose, or other medical conditions that interfere with the body's ability to regulate temperature, may result in cool skin.
- **Cold skin.** A patient with frostbite, significant cold exposure, immersion in cold water, or severe hypothermia (general cooling resulting from cold exposure) will have cold skin. The skin may appear to be firm or stiff. This is a significant sign of frostbite or a cold-induced injury.
- **Cool and clammy skin.** Cool skin that is moist is referred to as cool and clammy. It may be related to blood loss, fright, nervousness, anxiety, pain, or other medical conditions. It is the most common sign of shock (hypoperfusion).

Skin Condition

Skin condition refers to the amount of moisture found on the skin surface. This can be checked during palpation of the skin for temperature. The skin is usually either dry or moist:

- **Dry skin.** A patient who is dehydrated or suffering from severe heat exposure (heat stroke) or from some medical emergencies may have dry skin.
- **Moist skin.** Skin that is moist or wet to the touch may indicate sweating in a hot environment, exercise or exertion, or fever. Moist skin may also be associated with heart attack, hypoglycemia, shock (hypoperfusion), or many other conditions.

Thinking Critically
Capillary refill alone cannot determine perfusion status. What other assessments should you use to evaluate perfusion?

Objective 13-13
Discuss establishing patient priorities by evaluating critical findings to the airway, breathing, or circulation to determine if a patient is unstable and a candidate for rapid secondary assessment and immediate transport to the hospital.

Understanding BODY PROCESSES

Moist, or clammy, skin associated with medical or trauma conditions is typically produced from circulating epinephrine. The alpha stimulant property in the epinephrine stimulates the sweat glands. ■

Skin temperature, color, and condition will be discussed in more detail in the chapters dealing with specific medical conditions and injuries.

Capillary Refill

Capillary refill is a quick method to check peripheral perfusion. It is more reliable in infants and children than in adult patients, in whom other influences may provide an inaccurate reading. In adults, depress the nail bed, the fleshy part of the palm along the ulnar margin, the forehead, or the cheeks and release. In children and infants, depress the forearm or over the kneecap (EMT Skills 13-2).

Capillary refill is most reliable when assessed at room temperature. Cold exposure causes a delay in the refill and causes refill time to increase. If the refill of capillaries (a return of the pink color) takes longer than 2 seconds in the infant, child, or adult male at room temperature, tissue perfusion may be inadequate. The upper limit for adult females is 3 seconds and for the elderly is 4 seconds. Thus a capillary refill time at room temperature of greater than 3 seconds in adult females or greater than 4 seconds in the elderly would be considered a "delayed" capillary refill. Once again, capillary refill is only one indicator of many that must be assessed to determine the perfusion status of the patient. Capillary refill alone will not provide an accurate determination of the perfusion status.

Shock (Hypoperfusion)

Shock (hypoperfusion) is a life-threatening condition. If your primary assessment reveals pale, cool, and clammy skin, especially if there is a significant mechanism of injury, an altered mental status, or severe bleeding, assume that the patient is in shock.

Treatment for shock needs to begin during the primary assessment and continue until the patient is transferred to the medical facility staff. Control any serious bleeding. If possible, splint any bone or joint injuries, but only if it does not delay transport. Provide positive pressure ventilation with supplemental oxygen, if needed, or oxygen at 15 lpm by nonrebreather mask; keep the patient warm; and consider immediate transport with assessment.

▸ Establish Patient Priorities

In the course of the primary assessment, you should have identified and managed any immediately life-threatening conditions related to the status of the airway, breathing, and circulation. Any critical finding to the airway, breathing, or circulation makes the patient unstable (Table 13-7). During the primary assessment, the airway must be opened. High-concentration oxygen should be administered for any unresponsive patient or for a responsive patient based on the patient's condition; signs and symptoms of hypoxia, poor perfusion, or respiratory distress; and a low SpO_2 reading. Inadequate breathing must be managed by positive pressure ventilation with supplemental oxygen. Any major bleeding must be controlled. If the patient is unresponsive, with no breathing (apneic) or no normal breathing, immediately initiate CPR, beginning with chest compressions, and apply the automated external defibrillator (AED) when appropriate. Treatment for shock (hypoperfusion) must be undertaken if the patient displays signs of shock.

At this point in the primary assessment—based on your general impression and your assessment of the patient's mental status, airway, breathing, and circulation—it is necessary to decide if the patient is unstable and a priority for a rapid secondary assessment and immediate transport or if, instead, the patient is stable and you will continue with the secondary assessment on the scene. For example, the trauma patient who is critically injured and categorized as unstable requires a rapid secondary assessment and immediate transport to the emergency department with continued assessment and treatment provided in the ambulance, whereas the injured patient who appears stable should be further assessed and treated at the scene prior to transport. The medical patient could fall into either category—rapid secondary assessment and transport or continued on-scene assessment and stabilization—depending on the conditions found during the primary assessment. Consider the factors listed in Table 13-8 when determining the need for a rapid secondary and immediate transport.

If your priority decision is for immediate transport, you will first conduct a rapid secondary assessment to identify any additional signs of injury or illness, and to be

TABLE 13-7 Critical Findings Indicating an Unstable Patient in the Primary Assessment and Emergency Care

Primary Assessment Step	Critical Finding Making the Patient Unstable	Emergency Care
General impression	Obvious blood, vomitus, secretions, or other obstructions to the airway	Immediately suction or clear the obstruction from the airway.
General impression	Obvious open wound to the anterior, lateral, or posterior chest	Immediately cover the open wound with a nonporous or occlusive dressing.
General impression	Paradoxical movement of the chest	Stabilize the segment with your hand, or provide bag-valve-mask ventilation, if necessary for inadequate breathing
General impression	Major bleeding that is spurting or flowing steadily	Apply direct pressure to the site of bleeding.
General impression	Mechanism of injury that might produce spinal injury	Establish and hold manual in-line stabilization of the head and neck.
Mental status assessment (AVPU)	Altered mental status to include a patient who is confused, responds only to verbal or painful stimuli, or one who does not respond	Closely assess airway and breathing status and administer high-concentration oxygen.
Airway	Blood, secretions, vomitus, or other substance in mouth and airway (gurgling, stridor, or crowing sounds)	Immediately suction the airway and clear any other obstructions.
Airway	Occluded from the tongue (sonorous sounds)	Immediately perform a head-tilt, chin-lift or jaw–thrust maneuver if a spine injury is suspected.
Breathing	Inadequate respiratory rate (too slow or too fast, with other signs of inadequate breathing)	Immediately begin positive pressure ventilation with supplemental oxygen connected to the ventilation device.
Breathing	Inadequate tidal volume (shallow breathing or poor chest rise)	Immediately begin positive pressure ventilation with supplemental oxygen connected to the ventilation device.
Circulation	Rapid and weak pulses	Apply a nonrebreather mask at 15 lpm.
Circulation	Carotid pulse present, but absent peripheral pulses	Apply a nonrebreather mask at 15 lpm.
Circulation	Pale, cool, clammy skin	Apply a nonrebreather mask at 15 lpm.
Circulation	Capillary refill greater than 2 seconds with other signs of poor perfusion	Apply a nonrebreather mask at 15 lpm.
Circulation	Major bleeding that is spurting or flowing steadily	Immediately stop the bleeding by applying direct pressure.
Circulation	Absent carotid pulse in the adult or child; absent brachial pulse in the infant	Immediately initiate CPR, beginning with chest compressions, and apply AED.

sure that nothing significant has been overlooked, before the patient is fully immobilized and/or secured to the stretcher. The rapid secondary assessment for trauma or the rapid secondary assessment for the medical patient will be explained in detail later in the chapter.

The rapid secondary assessment can typically be accomplished in no more than 60 to 90 seconds (hence the name "rapid"). One partner can conduct the rapid secondary assessment while the other sets up the immobilization equipment or the stretcher, so there should be no needless delay in loading the patient into the ambulance and getting transport under way.

If you have made a priority decision for rapid secondary assessment and immediate transport, consider requesting ALS (advanced life support; paramedic) intercept en route.

A decision for rapid secondary assessment and immediate transport does not mean that a full secondary assessment and appropriate emergency care are not conducted. However, the priority decision you make at the conclusion of the primary assessment will dictate when and where the remainder of the assessment and treatment will occur, whether at the scene or en route to the hospital. Thus, the primary assessment sets the pace for the entire patient encounter.

TABLE 13-8 Criteria for Which Rapid Transport Is Required

- A poor general impression (The patient looks ill or is severely injured. Look for cyanosis, pale skin, significant blood loss, and multiple wounds or injuries to the head, chest, abdomen, pelvis, posterior thorax, or multiple extremities.)
- An unresponsive patient or patient with an altered mental status who lacks a gag or cough reflex (This is significant because the patient cannot protect his own airway.)
- A responsive patient who is not obeying commands
- Inability to establish or maintain a patent airway
- A patient experiencing difficulty in breathing or who exhibits signs of respiratory distress
- Absent or inadequate breathing for which the patient requires continuous positive pressure ventilation
- A pulseless patient
- Uncontrolled hemorrhage or severe blood loss
- A patient with pale, cool, clammy skin who you suspect is in shock (hypoperfusion)
- A patient with an open wound to the chest or a flail segment
- Severe chest pain with a systolic blood pressure of less than 100 mmHg
- Severe pain anywhere
- Complicated childbirth
- Extremely high body temperature—above 104°F
- Signs of generalized hypothermia
- Severe allergic reaction
- Poisoning or overdose of unknown substance

Part 3: Secondary Assessment

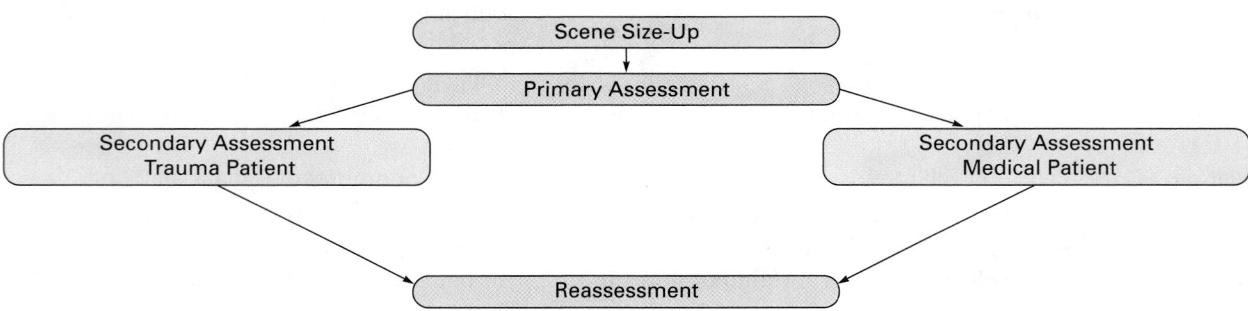

Once you have conducted the scene size-up and the primary assessment to identify and manage immediately life-threatening conditions involving the airway, breathing, and circulation, your next step is to conduct the **secondary assessment** to identify any additional injuries or conditions that may also be life threatening.

Further emergency care will be based on the information you gain from the history and physical exam. There are three major steps to the secondary assessment.

Components of the Secondary Assessment

- Conduct a physical exam.
- Take baseline vital signs.
- Obtain a history.

The way these steps are carried out will vary according to the condition of the patient: trauma or medical, responsive or unresponsive, with a serious or a minor complaint.

For example, a patient who has lacerated his shin while operating a weed cutter does not necessarily need a complete head-to-toe exam if you are certain that the injury was isolated to that one anatomical region and involves no underlying organs or body systems. Your physical exam and history will deal primarily with the leg injury. This type of focused exam deals only with isolated injuries where the patient is completely alert, oriented, and has not experienced any mechanism that might result in organ damage or multiple injuries.

Likewise, a medical patient does not need to have his entire body inspected and palpated; however, it is

Key Terms

secondary assessment the portion of patient assessment conducted after the primary assessment, for the purpose of identifying additional serious or potentially life-threatening injuries or conditions and as a basis for further emergency care.

Key Points

The physical exam is conducted in the trauma patient to identify evidence of injury, in the medical patient to identify the severity of the condition.

important that you examine all body systems that are potentially related to the medical condition. As an example, a medical patient with no mechanism of injury who is complaining of shortness of breath does not need to have his pelvis and symphysis pubis inspected or palpated. However, it would be important to examine the central nervous system, cardiovascular system, and respiratory system. This would involve examination of the head, neck, chest, abdomen, upper and lower extremities, and posterior body for signs associated with the complaint. Examining only the thorax in this case would cause you to possibly miss a number of other signs and the potential cause of the patient complaint or severity of the condition.

You must tailor your assessment to the needs of the patient and the suspected condition or injury. However, if you have any doubt as to the significance of the mechanism of injury or the illness, or if the potential exists that the patient may have suffered multiple injuries, or if the mental status is altered, err on the side of benefit to the patient and perform a complete secondary assessment from head to toe.

The sequence of the steps of the secondary assessment will depend on whether the patient has suspected injuries or a medical problem and whether the patient is responsive or unresponsive. For example, history taking precedes the physical exam and vital signs for a responsive medical patient for two reasons: (1) the most significant information about a medical condition will usually be obtained from what the patient tells you, and (2) if the patient loses responsiveness, you will have lost the opportunity to get the history, whereas you can conduct the physical exam and obtain vital signs whether the patient is responsive or not.

For a trauma patient, the physical exam and vital signs are done before the history, because the most significant information about injuries will usually come from the physical exam. (When EMT partners are working together, these steps can often be done almost simultaneously, for example, with one partner obtaining the history and taking vital signs while the other does the physical exam.)

Although the physical exam for a trauma patient and for a medical patient are similar, the type of information that you are assessing for may differ. In the trauma patient, the physical exam is conducted to identify evidence of injury. In the medical patient, the physical exam is often conducted to determine the severity of the condition. For example, you will assess the lower extremities for both the trauma patient and the medical patient in most cases, including assessment of distal pulses and motor and sensory function. However, in the trauma patient you are primarily looking for tenderness (pain in response to palpation), swelling, and deformities—in addition to weak or absent pulses or poor motor or sensory function—as an indication of injury. In the medical patient, you may be looking more for signs of an inadequate pumping function of the heart, as in a heart attack or congestive heart failure—for example, discoloration of the lower extremities or swelling to the ankles plus poor pulses—or for poor or absent motor and sensory function as a sign of the status of the brain in a suspected stroke patient.

If you are unable to categorize the patient as a trauma or a medical patient by the time you complete the primary assessment, you should continue with a complete head-to-toe secondary assessment to gain additional information to appropriately categorize the patient.

Suppose you are called to the scene for a "man down." When you arrive on the scene, you find a patient supine on the side of the street. Only one bystander is present who states that she found the patient lying in the street. You have no immediate clues from the dispatcher, scene, or bystander as to the emergency problem. Your general impression and primary assessment of the airway, breathing, and circulation do not provide any clear indications as to whether the patient's condition has resulted from trauma or a medical cause.

You must suspect that the patient has been hit by a car, shot, assaulted, stabbed, fallen and hit his head, or suffered from some other mechanism of injury. However, you must also suspect that the patient could have had a heart attack or a stroke, has a low blood sugar level, or is suffering from some other medical condition. You would conduct a rapid secondary assessment from head to toe and continue to look for indications of both trauma and medical problems while you continue your emergency care.

EMS runs of this nature require a high index of suspicion on your part and the application of judgment and common sense to the sequence and manner in which you conduct the secondary assessment.

In most cases, you will have determined whether the patient is suffering from trauma or from a medical condition by the time the primary assessment has been completed. For a patient who has been injured, you will continue with a *secondary assessment for a trauma patient.* A patient who is suffering from a medical condition requires a *secondary assessment for a medical*

Thinking Critically
Inspection, palpation, and auscultation are used in the secondary assessment. What might you be looking for with each of these techniques?

Objective 13-14
Describe performing the secondary assessment using an anatomical approach.

patient. These two variations of the secondary assessment (for a trauma patient and for a medical patient) will be discussed later in the chapter. In order to perform a secondary assessment on either the trauma or the medical patient, it is important to first learn the components and techniques of the complete secondary assessment. From that foundational information and technique, you will be able to alter the secondary assessment to meet the needs of any particular patient, complaint, condition, or situation.

Overview of Secondary Assessment: Anatomical and Body Systems Approaches, Baseline Vital Signs, and History

Use the techniques of inspection, palpation, and auscultation to identify additional signs, symptoms, and complaints of the patient. Any potential immediate life threats should be managed as found. For example, if an open wound is found on inspection of the chest, it must be immediately managed by placing your gloved hand over the wound and then occluding it with a nonporous or occlusive dressing. Non-life-threatening injuries in the noncritical or stable patient will be noted and treated after the examination, or en route in the critical or unstable patient, if time and the patient's condition permit.

When conducting the secondary assessment in a stable, noncritical trauma patient, the injuries can be managed as found. If you note swelling and deformity to the lower portion of the left arm, you will closely assess the area, immobilize it, and continue with the assessment. Bone injuries and soft tissue injuries, such as lacerations, abrasions, and punctures, are managed as found during the physical exam in the stable, noncritical trauma patient.

Any clothing that interferes with your ability to properly examine the trauma patient should be cut on the anterior part and allowed to fall away, if this was not already done during the primary assessment. Take modesty into consideration and cover the patient with a sheet.

If any doubt exists as to how extensively to assess the patient, complete the entire secondary assessment. In the critical or unstable patient, conduct a rapid secondary assessment so that you do not divert attention that is required for the ongoing care of life-threatening injuries or medical conditions.

Performing the Secondary Assessment: An Anatomical Approach

The secondary assessment should be conducted systematically, starting at the head moving to the feet (EMT Skills 13-3). A *rapid* secondary assessment would be conducted to identify life-threatening injuries or conditions in the unstable or critically injured trauma patient or in the unstable or critically ill medical patient. The rapid secondary assessment uses the same techniques as those for the complete secondary assessment illustrated in EMT Skills 13-3 and discussed in this section, but the approach is abbreviated to focus on rapidly finding potential life threats. Thus, the rapid secondary assessment may not use all of the techniques discussed in this section. The rapid assessment for the trauma and medical patient will be discussed later in the chapter.

The trauma patient who has suffered a significant mechanism of injury or who potentially has multiple injuries must be completely exposed at the end of the primary assessment prior to beginning the secondary assessment (Figure 13-15*). If the patient is not exposed, you

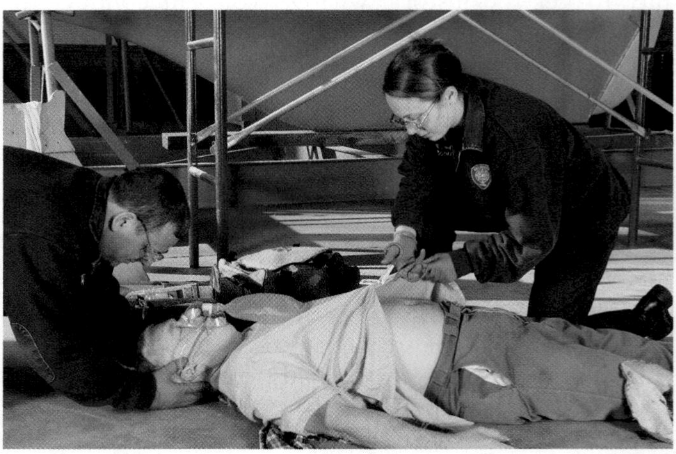

FIGURE 13-15 * Completely expose the trauma patient who has suffered a significant mechanism of injury or who has potential multiple injuries.

Key Terms
cerebrospinal fluid (CSF) a clear fluid that surrounds and cushions the brain and the spinal cord.

Thinking Critically
The "halo test" is no longer considered reliable for identifying CSF. Why?

are at a high risk of missing potentially life-threatening injuries. Keep patient modesty and environmental concerns in mind when exposing the patient.

Assess the Head

Inspect the head and scalp for any deformities, contusions, abrasions, punctures, burns, lacerations, or swelling (EMT Skills 13-3A). If conducted at the scene on the trauma patient with a spinal injury, maintain spinal stabilization as applied during the primary assessment. If adequate resources are available and the patient has critical findings or is unstable, the patient may be immobilized to the backboard prior to the secondary assessment. Depending on the type of device used and whether the patient is immobilized or not, your access to the head may be limited. Do not remove any immobilization device to further examine the head.

Palpate the entire head. Start at the parietal region (top of the head) and work your way down to the occipital region (back of the head). Palpate the temporal (side) and frontal regions of the skull. Do not poke your fingers into the scalp or skull. Cup your hands together and palpate with the palms of the hands. This will reduce the possibility of damage to the brain from inadvertently pushing in bone ends during palpation. Note any crepitation, depressions, deformities, or protrusions. Also note any tenderness to the head or scalp. Look at your gloved hands for evidence of blood when palpating. This is useful in patients with dark hair or at night when blood is difficult to see.

Ears Inspect the ears for trauma to the external auditory canal. Look for deformities, contusions, abrasions, punctures, burns, lacerations, or swelling. Move into a position to allow you to look inside the ear with a penlight for blood or other fluid (EMT Skills 13-3B). A clear fluid flowing from the ear is most likely **cerebrospinal fluid (CSF)**, a clear fluid that surrounds and cushions the brain and the spinal cord. Leakage of CSF usually indicates a skull fracture. If bleeding is occurring from the ear, place a loose dressing over the ear to catch the blood. Do not pack the ears or restrict the bleeding.

Look behind the ears for discoloration over the bony prominence known as the mastoid process (EMT Skills 13-3C). Ecchymosis (black-and-blue discoloration) to the mastoid area is known as the Battle sign. This is a late sign of possible skull or head injury that may not appear until hours after the injury.

ASSESSMENT Tips

A "halo test" has frequently been taught to be performed on blood and fluid leaking from the ears, nose, or mouth to determine if it contains cerebrospinal fluid. It was done by dropping blood onto a piece of cotton, such as a gauze pad, a pillowcase, or a sheet. If a yellow circle or "halo" formed around the blood, it was thought to be CSF. Research has found, however, that nasal secretions, saline, and other substances when mixed with blood will create the same effect. Therefore, this test is not reliable for identifying CSF leakage. ■

Understanding BODY PROCESSES

If time permits and you want to test to see if a clear fluid leaking from the ears, nose, or mouth is cerebrospinal fluid, place a drop of the clear fluid on a glucose test strip and test it in the glucometer. CSF contains sugar, whereas nasal secretions and other fluids do not. The sugar level in CSF is much lower than that found in blood. If the fluid is mixed with blood, this will not work since the blood itself contains sugar. *Do not delay transport to perform this test.* ■

Face Inspect the entire facial region to include the eyes, nose, and mouth. Look for deformities, contusions, abrasions, punctures, burns, lacerations, or swelling. Palpate for deformity, swelling, and tenderness (EMT Skills 13-3D). Injuries to the face are typically dramatic and potentially life threatening. Bleeding or displacement of bone or tissue into the airway may cause an obstruction. Clear the airway with suction and insert an oropharyngeal airway if necessary and appropriate. Avoid the use of a nasopharyngeal airway. Palpate the facial bones for deformity, instability, and crepitation. If you note any trauma, continue to closely monitor the airway for bleeding and excessive swelling. Inspect and palpate the maxilla (upper jawbone) and mandible (lower jawbone) for any deformity or instability. The patient should be able to move the mandible without excessive pain. If the patient is unable to close his mouth, or if the teeth do not align well, the mandible is likely to be fractured or dislocated. With an injury to the maxilla or mandible, your major concern is maintaining a patent airway.

Inspect the face for singed or burnt eyebrows, nasal hair, beard, or hairline. Burns to the face should make you suspicious that the patient may be suffering from an

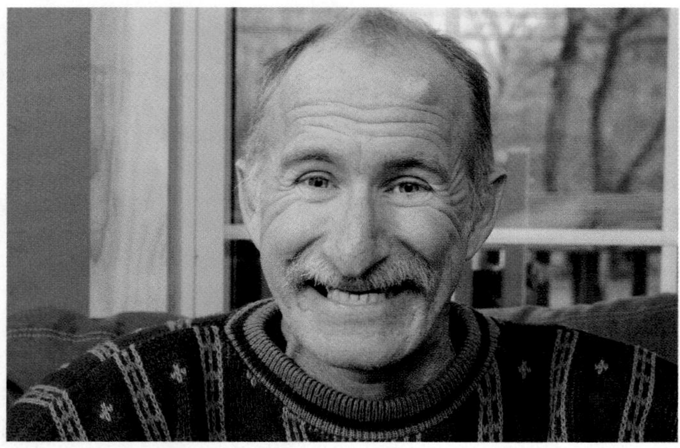

FIGURE 13-16 ✱ Have the patient grin to check facial symmetry.

upper airway burn. Upper airway burns frequently result in severe swelling and airway closure at the level of the larynx. If stridor (high-pitched sounds on inspiration) is noted, consider positive pressure ventilation with supplemental oxygen, immediate transport, and advanced life support intervention for advanced airway management.

In the medical patient, have the patient make a big smile and show his teeth while doing so to check for facial asymmetry (Figure 13-16✱). If the facial muscles are paralyzed you will note a droop to one side of the face. It is likely that you will miss the asymmetry if you examine the face without having him exaggerate a smile.

Eyes Inspect for deformities, contusions, abrasions, punctures, burns, lacerations, or swelling. Look especially for lacerations or trauma to the eyelids and eyeballs. Do not attempt to remove foreign bodies embedded in the eye. If the patient has burns, lacerations, or any other injuries to the eyelids, assume that the eye is also damaged. Do not force the eyelid open. Do not apply any pressure to the eye.

If the patient is unresponsive and is wearing hard contact lenses that are not properly positioned over the pupil, remove the lenses. Place them in a container with a small amount of saline, marking the container for the left and right contact. Be sure to transport the lenses with the patient. If the patient has a chemical burn to the eye, remove the contact lens to allow for adequate flushing. If the contact lens is left in place during flushing, the chemical trapped under the lens will continue to burn the eye.

Check for pupillary response (EMT Skills 13-3E). In a dark environment, shine a light in the eye of the patient. In a bright environment, shade the eye with your hand. Both pupils should react simultaneously and equally to light being shined in either eye. This is referred to as a *consensual reflex.* While shining a light into one eye, watch the pupillary reaction of the other eye. Then shine the light a second time in the first eye and watch the pupillary reaction of that eye. Thus, the light is shined in each eye twice, first to check the response of the opposite pupil to the light, and then to check the reaction of the pupil in the eye to which the light is applied. Observe whether pupil response is brisk or sluggish. Under normal conditions, the pupils should respond briskly. Poor perfusion to the brain, high levels of carbon dioxide, or brain injuries may cause the pupils to respond sluggishly.

Note the size of the pupils. Unequal pupils usually indicate a head injury or stroke. A pupil that is large in size and not responding to light is referred to as being *fixed and dilated.* In cardiac arrest or severe injury to the brain, both pupils may be fixed and dilated. Pupils that are pinpoint, or extremely constricted, and unresponsive usually indicate an injury to the brain stem or a patient under the influence of a narcotic substance. Also assess pupil shape. A teardrop-shaped pupil may indicate severe trauma.

A small portion of the population normally have unequal pupils. However, there is usually less than 1 mm difference, and their pupils remain reactive to light. It is extremely important to consider the patient's level of responsiveness when determining the seriousness of the pupillary size. If the patient has unequal pupils but is completely alert and oriented, consider direct trauma to the eye, a localized nerve injury, or that the patient has used eye drops such as atropine or pilocarpine. Rely heavily on the level of responsiveness to confirm the findings of the pupils.

Check *visual acuity* (clarity of vision) by having the patient tell you how many fingers you are holding up or by having him read your name tag. Hold your finger in front of the patient and have him follow it up, down, left, right, and in a circular pattern (EMT Skills 13-3F). This checks the extraocular muscle movements. The eyes should move together (*conjugate movement*) and smoothly. Jerky eye movements (*nystagmus*) usually result from drugs or central nervous system effects. A single eye that is fixed or has a gaze in one direction (*dysconjugate gaze*) usually indicates injury to the orbit, ocular muscles, or nerves (Figure 13-17✱).

Inspect the white portion of the eye, termed the *sclera,* for a redness or a yellow color. Yellow sclerae,

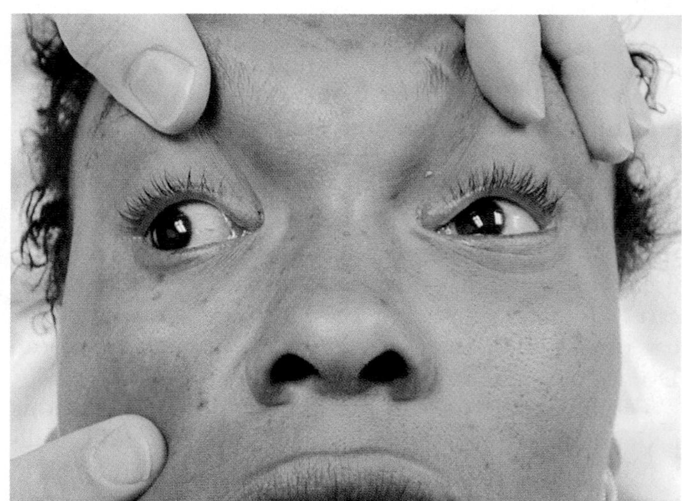

FIGURE 13-17 ✱ Dysconjugate gaze. (© Charles Stewart, MD, and Associates)

known as *icterus*, is an indication of possible liver damage or failure. Pull the bottom part of the eye down and check the conjunctiva (EMT Skills 13-3G). Poor perfusion, as in shock, causes the conjunctiva to appear pale. Extremely red conjunctivae with reddened sclerae is typically caused by eye irritation.

Blood in the anterior eye is a sign that the eye or the head has received a forceful blow. Inspect the eye by shining a light from the side to detect a reddish discoloration over the iris (the colored portion around the pupil). This blood will typically form a straight fluid line across the cornea.

Nose Inspect the nose for deformities, contusions, abrasions, punctures, burns, lacerations, or swelling (EMT Skills 13-3H). Look for fluid or blood drainage, nasal flaring, and singed nasal hair. Bleeding from the anterior nose is usually easily controlled by pinching the nostrils together. However, some patients, especially the elderly with a history of high blood pressure, experience severe posterior nosebleeds in which the bleeding is difficult to control. Many times, the patient swallows large amounts of blood, becomes nauseated, and vomits. The vomitus contains blood and may be incorrectly assessed as internal bleeding in the stomach. The patient could lose a large volume of blood from the nosebleed.

Leakage of cerebrospinal fluid indicates a skull fracture, which may have an associated brain injury. Singed nasal hair should increase your suspicion that the patient has been involved in a fire and possibly has an upper airway burn.

Nasal flaring, which is identified by the nares (nostrils) opening wide during inspiration, is a sign of respiratory distress. Reassess the patient closely for other evidence of airway or breathing problems.

Palpate the nose for deformity, swelling, or instability. Your major concern with an injury to the nose is possible bleeding into the airway. Be prepared to suction the airway.

Mouth Open the mouth and inspect for deformities, contusions, abrasions, punctures, burns, lacerations, or swelling (EMT Skills 13-3I). Look for loose or missing teeth, loose or missing dentures, and discoloration of the mucosa (lining). Loose dentures should be removed in unresponsive patients so they do not fall back into the throat and become an airway obstruction. Remove any objects by suction or, if too large to suction, with your fingers. Inspect the tongue for lacerations and swelling, a possible sign that the patient has had a seizure (biting the tongue is common during seizures). Look for discoloration. Cyanosis (bluish color) of the mucosa indicates inadequate oxygenation. A pale tongue may indicate poor perfusion and shock. Any burns or extremely white areas may be caused by ingestion of a chemical poison.

Smell for any unusual odors. An alcoholic beverage odor may make you suspect alcohol intoxication as a reason for an altered mental status. It is always necessary to be suspicious that the patient's condition is from some cause other than alcohol. Look for other evidence of trauma or medical illness. A fruity odor on the breath may indicate a diabetic patient with an abnormally high blood sugar level. Smell for other unusual odors like rubbing alcohol, cologne, cleaners, and solvents. A desperate alcoholic may drink cologne or cough syrup because of the alcohol content. Children may accidentally ingest cleaners or solvents. Antifreeze may be ingested by teenagers as a means to get drunk, which can be lethal.

Look for black sputum and burns inside the mouth if the patient was involved in a fire. Suspect upper airway burns and be prepared to aggressively manage the airway and breathing if burning to the mouth or face is noted.

The mouth may provide some signs as to the oxygenation, breathing, or perfusion status. However, your chief concern is to ensure that the mouth is clear of potential airway obstructions.

Assess the Neck

Inspect the neck much more closely than you did during the rapid assessment (EMT Skills 13-3J). Look for deformities, contusions, abrasions, punctures, burns, lacerations, or swelling. Large lacerations of the neck must be covered with an occlusive dressing to prevent air being sucked into a large vein, causing an air embolus. With any trauma to the neck, you should suspect possible cervical spinal injury and provide in-line spinal stabilization, if it has not already been applied. If a cervical spinal immobilization collar is in place, you typically will not remove it to inspect or palpate the neck. Most devices are manufactured with a large hole on the anterior surface to permit reassessment of the neck for jugular vein distention (JVD), blood collecting under the skin, or tracheal deviation.

The neck may appear large or swollen. This may be due to blood collection in or around the tissues or air trapped under the skin. Because of the large vessels, bleeding in the neck could be severe. A *hematoma* (collection of blood) could compress the airway or trachea and cause obstruction. Air trapped under the skin may be better palpated than seen. If you palpate an unusual sensation of air under the skin, and feel or hear crepitation (crackling), it is a sign of subcutaneous emphysema. *Subcutaneous emphysema* (which means, simply, air under the skin) is a sign of trauma to the airway, respiratory tract, lung, or esophagus. You should closely reassess the chest for evidence of chest injury and closely monitor the breathing status.

Reassess the jugular veins for distention. The jugular veins slightly distend normally in the supine patient with a normal blood volume. If possible, the jugular veins should be assessed with the patient sitting at a 45° angle. If two-thirds of the jugular vein is filled or engorged from the base of the neck up toward the angle of the jaw, then JVD is present. Do not have the trauma patient with suspected spinal injuries sit up to check the neck veins. JVD is a sign of a possible *tension pneumothorax* (air trapped in the chest cavity as a result of chest or lung injury), *pericardial tamponade* (blood filling the sac around the heart), or congestive heart failure. It is vital to reassess the effectiveness of the breathing status, pulses, perfusion, and blood pressure if JVD is noted.

Check the trachea to ensure it is midline. A shifted or deviated trachea is a late sign of tension pneumothorax. It may be easier to palpate the location of the trachea than to see it. Start at the suprasternal notch (the indention where the right and left clavicle come together at the top of the sternum) and palpate with your thumb and index finger to feel the position of the trachea. It should be midline all the way up to the larynx.

Since a tension pneumothorax is a life-threatening condition, whenever tracheal deviation is noted you must immediately reassess the breathing and perfusion status. If the trachea tugs or moves to one side during inhalation, there may be an airway obstruction in the bronchi. Reassess for adequate breathing.

Another sign to look for is excessive neck muscle use. These muscles become very prominent when a patient is having difficulty with inspiration. Check for other signs of respiratory distress and inadequate breathing and provide positive pressure ventilation with supplemental oxygen, if necessary.

If a cervical spinal immobilization collar was applied, the neck would have been quickly palpated for any deformities during the rapid assessment. If a collar is not in place, palpate the anterior neck and posterior neck for deformities or spasms.

Assess the Chest

In the trauma patient, if not already done, expose the chest completely. Inspect the chest (EMT Skills 13-3K) for evidence of trauma including open wounds, deformities, contusions, abrasions, burns, lacerations, or swelling. If an open wound is found, immediately occlude it with a gloved hand and apply a nonporous or an occlusive dressing taped on three sides or a commercial occlusive device. Watch for retractions (the muscles between the ribs pulling inward during inspiration), a sign of respiratory distress. Retractions are seen more often in infants and children than in adults.

Determine if the chest is rising and falling symmetrically (evenly on both sides) or if one side of the chest appears to remain elevated during exhalation. Asymmetrical (uneven) chest wall movement is a sign of a significant chest injury.

Look for any segments of the chest that are moving inward during inspiration and outward during exhalation, opposite to the direction of the rest of the chest. This is referred to as **paradoxical movement** and is a sign of a flail segment. A flail segment is an immediately life-threatening injury that should be managed as discovered. Immediately following the blunt chest injury in which a flail segment has occurred, the muscles between the ribs will commonly spasm and keep the free rib section stabilized. Therefore, you may not see exaggerated movement of the flail segment and may not detect it during the earlier assessments. Later during the call, it may become apparent that the chest wall is moving paradoxically. Stabilization of the segment is necessary. Usually, palpation will more easily identify an unstable section. Closely palpate the sides of the chest since the most common site of a flail segment is to the lateral chest wall.

Feel the chest to confirm the findings of the inspection. Check for symmetry of respirations by placing each hand with the thumbs pointed inward toward the sternum (breastbone) over the right and left lower portion of the rib cage. Both hands should move an equal distance with each breath. Also palpate for any tenderness, instability, and crepitation (crackling or crunching sounds beneath the skin), signs of subcutaneous emphysema. Apply light pressure with both hands downward and inward, slightly compressing the rib cage. If there is any rib or muscular injury, the patient will complain of pain. If the patient is already complaining of chest pain from an injury, do not compress the chest. If you suspect possible rib fractures or chest wall injury, reassess the breathing status. Because of the pain, the patient may be purposely breathing extremely shallowly and rapidly, decreasing the adequacy of breathing.

ASSESSMENT Tips

A patient with a simple rib fracture may breathe very shallowly and rapidly because of the pain associated with deeper breathing. By intentionally breathing shallowly, the patient is lowering his tidal volume and making his ventilation inadequate. This can lead to hypoxia in the patient with a rib fracture, particularly in the elderly and those with underlying lung disease. ■

Palpate the sternum by pushing down gently with the ulnar edge of one or both hands. A pain response may indicate rib or sternum injury.

Children's rib cages are extremely pliable and flexible. Significant blunt or compression injury may not cause any fractures to occur; however, significant injury to the internal organs may be present. Look at the mechanism of injury and have a high index of suspicion if the mechanism of injury has been significant. Continuously monitor the patient for signs and symptoms of poor perfusion, respiratory distress, and shock.

Inspect and palpate the shoulder girdle (articulation of the clavicle and shoulder), the clavicles (collarbones), and scapulae (shoulder blades) for deformity, crepitation, and tenderness. Palpate the clavicles with the pads of your fingers beginning at the sternum and moving toward the shoulder. Gently slide your hand under the back on each side to palpate each scapula. Cup your hand around the shoulder girdle and compress lightly.

Key Terms

paradoxical movement a section of the chest that moves in the opposite direction to the rest of the chest during the phases of respiration. Typically seen with a flail segment.

Thinking Critically

Six-year-old Megan was hit by a softball her brother batted in their backyard. The skin over her ribs is reddened but the ribs seem to be intact. Should you conclude that she is not badly injured? Why or why not?

If the patient is not immobilized or secured to a backboard and does not have a suspected spinal injury, roll the patient or sit the patient forward to assess the posterior thorax, looking for signs of trauma. Prior to being immobilized to the backboard, the posterior thorax must be inspected and palpated for injury.

Inspect and palpate the entire anterior and lateral chest. Injuries could easily be missed if you do not look at the patient's sides and in the axillary region (under the armpit).

Auscultation Listen to the chest with your stethoscope to determine if the breath sounds are present or absent, equal or unequal, normal or abnormal (EMT Skills 13-3L). Place your stethoscope just below the second rib at the midclavicular line to listen to the apices of the lungs and just below the fourth rib at the midaxillary line for breath sounds in the bases. Compare the sounds of the lobes on both sides of the chest. Absent or diminished breath sounds are a sign of air, blood, or fluid in the chest cavity or obstruction of a bronchus. Typically only one side has diminished or absent breath sounds, indicating which lung is injured.

In the medical patient, breath sounds are important to auscultate if the patient is complaining of dyspnea (shortness of breath or difficult breathing), has hives and itching, or has a history of allergies, anaphylactic (severe allergic) reaction, asthma, emphysema, or chronic bronchitis.

Wheezes are prolonged, high-pitched sounds most often heard on exhalation. Wheezes indicate narrowing of the airways at the level of the bronchiole. Note whether the wheezing is diffuse (throughout the lung fields) or isolated to one section of the lung. Diffuse wheezing heard in all the lung fields is usually due to narrowing or spasm of the airways associated with asthma, anaphylaxis, emphysema, or chronic bronchitis. Isolated wheezing heard in only one area is a sign of localized lung infection, obstruction, or a foreign body.

Fluid collection in the lungs produces crackles, a sound sometimes called rales. A harsher snoring sound heard upon auscultation, called rhonchi, is from mucus in the larger airways within the lung.

Stridor, a high-pitched sound, is from partial obstruction of the upper airway at the level of the larynx. It is usually caused by a foreign body or swelling. Closely monitor the airway and provide positive pressure ventilation with supplemental oxygen if inadequate breathing is found.

Coughing is a response to bronchial irritation. Smoke, chemicals, or other inhaled gases may cause the patient to cough. If you suspect the patient has inhaled a toxic substance such as smoke, place the patient on a nonrebreather mask at 15 lpm. If mucus is produced with the cough, which is referred to as a *productive cough,* note the color, consistency, amount, and odor. Mucus is normally white and clear. Yellow or green mucus is a sign of possible infection. Also note any blood-tinged sputum (substance produced by coughing). This may indicate lung injury, airway trauma, or a cardiac or pulmonary disease. Be sure to inspect inside the mouth for lacerations if blood is found in the sputum.

Assess the Abdomen

It is best to examine the abdomen with the patient lying flat (EMT Skills 13-3M). Notice the posture of the patient. A patient lying extremely still with his knees drawn up toward the chest and with breathing that is fast and shallow is most likely suffering from significant abdominal pain. Expose the abdomen and inspect all four anterior quadrants and the lateral aspects for obvious signs of injury such as deformities, contusions, abrasions, punctures, burns, or lacerations. Look for impaled objects or open wounds with protruding organs.

ASSESSMENT Tips

A patient with severe abdominal pain will often lie extremely still, draw his knees up toward the chest, and breathe fast and shallowly to reduce the movement of the diaphragm. The condition usually involves irritation of the peritoneum (lining of the abdomen). A patient who is complaining of pain but feels better if he is up and walking may be suffering from a bowel obstruction. ■

Look at the abdomen for signs of swelling or distention. The abdomen could be distended from air, fluid, or blood. If the abdomen appears to be distended, look for signs of poor perfusion and shock. A significant amount of blood must be lost in the abdomen before it distends. (Two liters of blood in the abdomen may distend the girth of the abdomen by only 1 inch.) Note any discoloration around the navel or in the flank areas. Bleeding in the abdomen may cause discoloration to these areas; however, this is a very late sign that takes several hours to develop.

The patient may have a colostomy or ileostomy. This is a surgical opening in the abdominal wall with a bag to hold excretions from the digestive tract. Leave the bag in place and be careful not to displace or cut it. Keep the bag covered from view to save the patient from possible embarrassment.

Ask if the patient is having any abdominal pain prior to palpating. Palpate all four quadrants of the abdomen separately using the pads of your fingers with one hand on top of the other. Roll the hands across the quadrant assessing for rigidity or stiffness, tenderness or pain, and distention. (A soft abdomen is normal.) If the patient is complaining of pain, have him point to the pain with one finger. If the patient can localize the pain in this manner, start your palpation at the point farthest away from the pain and move inward. Palpate the painful quadrant last. When palpating, listen to the patient's response. In the unresponsive patient, watch the patient's face and body movement for an indication of a painful response to palpation.

A pulsating mass in the abdomen may indicate that the abdominal aorta is weakened and bulging. If noted, stop any further palpation, rapidly complete the remainder of the secondary assessment, and begin immediate transport to a medical facility.

The patient may reflexively guard his abdomen by tightening the muscles. Voluntary guarding (guarding the patient is able to control) is common when you begin to assess the abdomen. Attempt to distract the patient with conversation to stop the guarding. If the abdomen remains rigid, it is a sign of *peritonitis* (inflammation or irritation of the lining of the abdomen) from blood, gastric contents, bacteria, or other substances. Taking a deep breath usually produces pain, so the patient typically breathes shallowly and fast.

A better test to perform is the Markle test, also called the heel drop test. If the patient is able to stand, have him stand up and get up on the balls of his feet, then suddenly drop down onto his heels (Figures 13-18a and 13-18b✱). Don't tell the patient what you are testing for. Watch the patient's face for a grimace, or note if he complains of pain to the abdomen. If the medical patient has pain to the abdomen, this is a positive for rebound tenderness, an indication of peritonitis or other inflammation within the abdomen, such as appendicitis. Perform a heel jar test if the patient is supine or unable to stand when you are assessing the lower extremities. Make a fist and strike the bottom of the heel forcefully enough to jar the abdomen (Figure 13-19✱). Again, don't tell the patient what you are testing for and watch his face for a grimace. If he complains of pain, ask where. If it is to the abdomen, this is positive for rebound tenderness and probable peritonitis or other intra-abdominal inflammation.

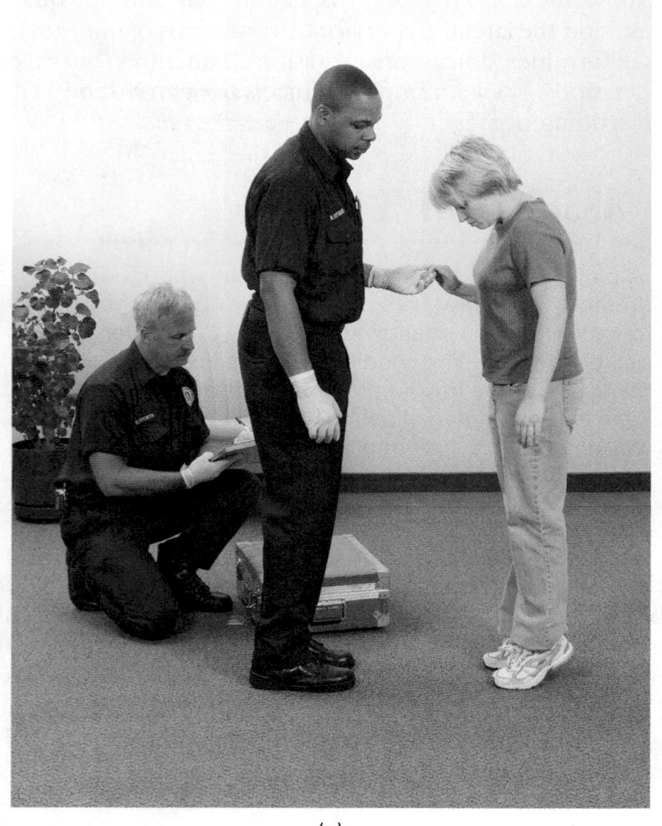

(a)

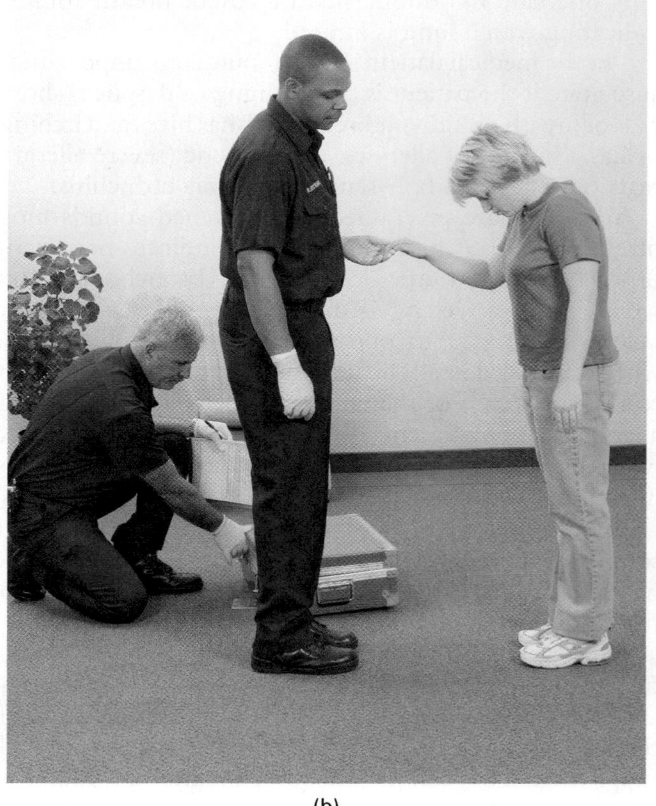

(b)

FIGURE 13-18 ✱ A heel drop test is performed by **(a)** having the patient stand on the balls of her feet, then **(b)** dropping suddenly onto her heels.

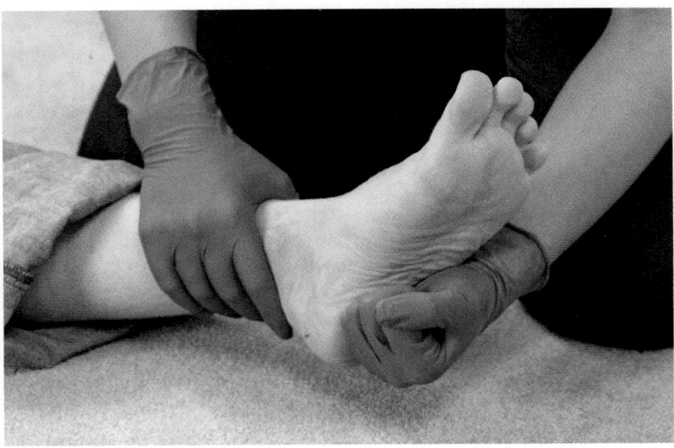

FIGURE 13-19 * A heel jar test is performed by striking the bottom of the heel forcefully with a fist.

Understanding BODY PROCESSES

Acids and other chemicals leaking into the abdominal cavity will usually produce pain immediately on contact with the peritoneal lining. The pain is typically sharp, constant, and severe. By contrast, bacteria leaking from the large intestine may take several hours to produce pain. ■

Do not palpate over obvious injuries or areas of severe pain. Do not poke the abdomen. If an impaled object is present, do not remove it. Stabilize the object in place. An evisceration is when organs, most commonly the small intestines, are protruding from an open abdominal wound. Do not attempt to put the organs back into the abdominal cavity. Cover them with a moist sterile dressing and seal with a large occlusive dressing.

Assess the Pelvis

Look for injury to the pelvis during the secondary assessment because of the potential seriousness of associated bleeding. If the patient does not complain of pain or is unresponsive, gently flex and compress the pelvis to determine instability (EMT Skills 13-3N). Pelvic injuries are considered to be critical. If you identify a painful or unstable pelvis during the exam, rapidly complete the secondary assessment and consider immediate transport.

Expose the pelvic area and inspect for deformities, contusions, abrasions, punctures, burns, lacerations, or swelling. Do not palpate if there is obvious injury or the patient is complaining of pain to the pelvis. Note any loss of bladder control, bleeding, or priapism. *Priapism* is a persistent erection of the penis in a male patient that is a sign of a possible spinal cord injury.

If the patient has no pain in the pelvic region or is unresponsive, place each hand on the anterior lateral wings of the pelvis and gently compress inward and downward. Do not rock the pelvis or apply unnecessary pressure. Assess for instability, tenderness, and crepitation. Place the base of your hand on the symphysis pubis (pubic bone), located immediately above the genitalia, and apply gentle pressure backward, checking for tenderness, crepitation, and instability.

ASSESSMENT Tips

If the scrotum is swollen and red in a male patient with trauma to the pelvis, suspect a possible pelvic fracture with internal bleeding. ■

If serious trauma to the area of the genitalia is suspected—for example, penetrating trauma or major bleeding—expose and inspect the area. The male genitalia are relatively vascular (having many blood vessels); therefore, injury could result in significant blood loss. The female genitalia are most susceptible to penetrating trauma. Control bleeding to the external genitalia with direct pressure. If the female patient complains of vaginal bleeding, assess for signs and symptoms of shock. To assess the amount of bleeding, ask the patient how many tampons or sanitary pads she has used since the onset of bleeding.

Respect the patient's feelings of modesty or embarrassment. Explain what you are doing and why and protect the patient's dignity and privacy by shielding the patient from the view of others during examination.

Assess the Lower Extremities

If any injury is suspected, cut the clothing away from the patient. Inspect the lower extremities, one at a time, from the hip to the toes (EMT Skills 13-3O). Look for deformities (e.g., angulation), contusions, abrasions, punctures, burns, lacerations, or swelling. Watch for abnormal positioning. Injuries to the hip or femur may cause the leg to shorten or rotate inward or outward.

In the medical patient, look for excessive swelling around the ankles (peripheral edema). This may be an indication of possible cardiac failure, especially to the right ventricle.

Palpate the extremity by placing a hand on each side of the leg with the thumbs anteriorly and touching, if possible, and the little fingers to the posterior. Begin at the level of the groin and palpate down to the feet. The hands should never lose contact with the leg. Feel for any deformities, angulation, crepitation, or depressions. Determine if the patient feels pain, tenderness, numbness, or tingling. In the medical patient, check for pain in the calf during dorsiflexion (pull his foot back and point his toes toward his head; Figure 13-20a*) and plantar flexion (push his foot downward and point his toes away from the head). Also, palpate the calf for tenderness, swelling, or redness (Figure 13-20b*). This may be an indication of a deep vein thrombosis and is a significant sign in a patient complaining of shortness of breath or fainting.

If an injury is suspected, remove the shoes or boots. It may be necessary to cut the laces to avoid any

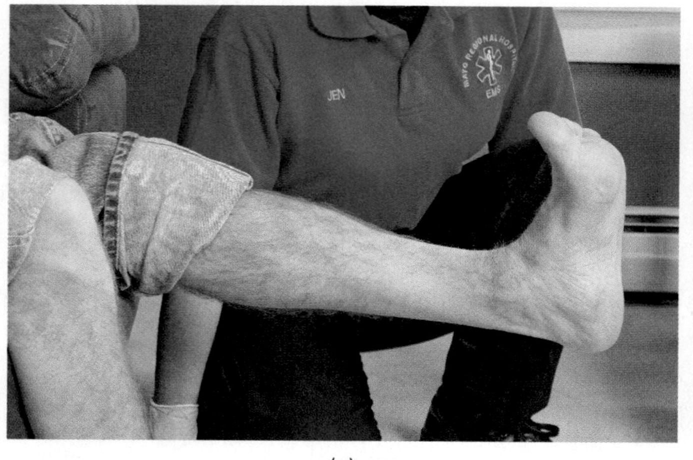

(a)

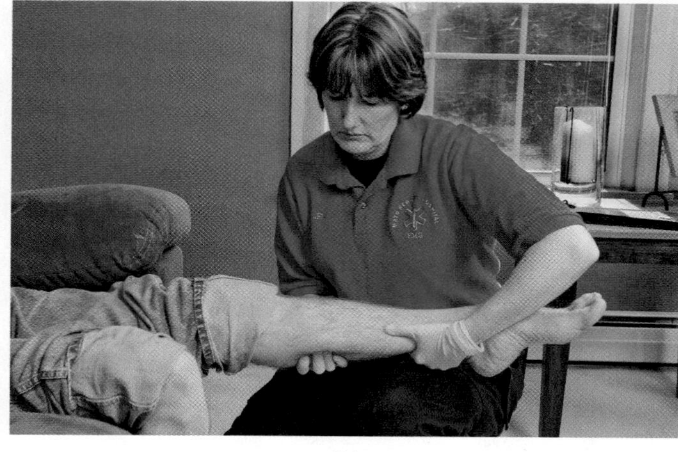

(b)

FIGURE 13-20 ✱ In the medical patient, **(a)** check for pain in the calf during dorsiflexion and plantar flexion. **(b)** Also palpate the calf for tenderness, swelling, or redness, possible indications of deep vein thrombosis.

unnecessary manipulation of the foot or leg during removal. If injury to the ankle or foot is suspected, cut the sock away. Ski boots should not be removed unless you are specially trained to do so.

Assess the distal pulses, motor function, and sensation. Loss of these functions is a sign of possible brain, spinal cord, or extremity injury.

Pulses Assess the dorsalis pedis pulse on the top surface of the foot or the posterior tibial pulse located behind the medial malleolus (inner ankle bone) (EMT Skills 13-3P). Compare the equality of the pulses in the two lower extremities. While feeling the pulse, check the skin color, temperature, and condition. If the pulse is absent and the skin is pale or cyanotic and cool, expect a possible blocked artery in that lower extremity. A blocked vein causes the extremity to become flushed, warm, swollen, and painful. Pedal and tibial pulses are frequently absent in patients suffering from severe blood loss and shock.

Motor Function Have the patient move his toes. Check for equality of strength in the lower extremities by placing your hands on the soles of both feet and having the patient push down against your hands (EMT Skills 13-3Q). Then place your hands on the dorsal surface of the feet and have the patient pull up against your hands. Note any inequality in strength. Do not check equality of strength if any obvious bone or joint injury is found in the lower extremity. Any unnecessary movement should be avoided. Unequal strength may be a sign of head, spinal, or extremity injury.

ASSESSMENT Tips

If the foot or ankle is injured, you can still check motor function in the distal extremity by having the patient push against your finger and pull back against your finger with his great (big) toe. This should give you the same results as if the foot were tested. ■

Paralysis, in which the patient is unable to move the extremity, may result from head or spinal injury or a stroke. Spinal injuries usually result in *paraplegia* (paralysis involving both legs only) or *quadriplegia* (paralysis involving both arms and both legs). A stroke or head injury commonly produces *hemiplegia* (paralysis of an arm and leg on one side of the body). A special exam for stroke will be discussed in Chapter 18, "Altered Mental Status, Stroke, and Headache."

Sensation Begin by lightly touching the toe on one foot and asking the patient to identify which toe you are touching (EMT Skills 13-3R). Then pinch the foot to elicit a pain response. Repeat the same procedure for the opposite foot. It is important to test both light touch and pain, since each stimulus is carried by a different spinal cord nerve tract. Record if the patient responds appropriately to both light touch and painful stimulus. Make sure the patient is unable to see which foot you are touching or pinching. The patient may provide the right response because he is able to see which toe you are touching instead of feeling it.

In the unresponsive patient, pinch the extremity while looking at the patient's facial expression. A facial grimace usually indicates that the patient feels the pain. Also note any movement of the extremity, especially if it is withdrawal away from the source of pain. Clearly document the response to pain in your prehospital care report.

Assess the Upper Extremities

Inspect the upper extremities from the shoulder to the fingertip (EMT Skills 13-3S). Look for deformities (e.g., angulation), contusions, abrasions, punctures, burns, lacerations, or swelling.

Palpate the entire extremity by placing a hand on each side of the arm with the thumbs touching on the anterior surface. Start at the most proximal portion of the arm and move down to the fingertips. Feel for any deformity, crepitation, or swelling. Note any pain or tenderness the patient experiences. In the unresponsive patient, watch the patient's face for grimacing and extremity movement (e.g., withdrawing the arm from the pain) when applying a painful stimulus.

Assess the distal pulses, motor function, and sensation in both upper extremities.

Pulses Assess the radial pulse, which is located at the base of the hand at the wrist on the thumb side (EMT Skills 13-3T). Assess the color, temperature, and condition of the hand. Radial pulses may not be felt when there is severe blood loss. It is important to evaluate the mechanism of injury, mental status, and skin if radial pulses are not present.

Motor Function Have the patient move his fingers. Check the equality of strength in both extremities simultaneously by having the patient grip your fingers and squeeze (EMT Skills 13-3U). Head, spinal, or extremity injuries may cause the grip strength to be unequal. Do not check grip strength in an extremity with obvious injury as this will cause unnecessary movement.

In the medical patient, have the patient close both eyes and hold his arms straight out in front of him for 10 seconds while seated or standing to assess for arm drift (Figure 13-21*). Check for the following: (1) an arm that drifts downward; (2) the patient can't lift one arm to the same level as the other, or the patient can't lift the arm at all.

Sensation Lightly touch the finger of one hand and ask the patient to identify which finger you are touching, making sure the patient cannot see what you are doing. Pinch the hand and note the response. In an unresponsive patient, pinch the hand in an attempt to elicit a response. Watch the face for a grimace and movement of the extremity that may indicate a response to the pain. Repeat the process for the other hand. Clearly document the type of response and the type of painful stimulus in your prehospital care report.

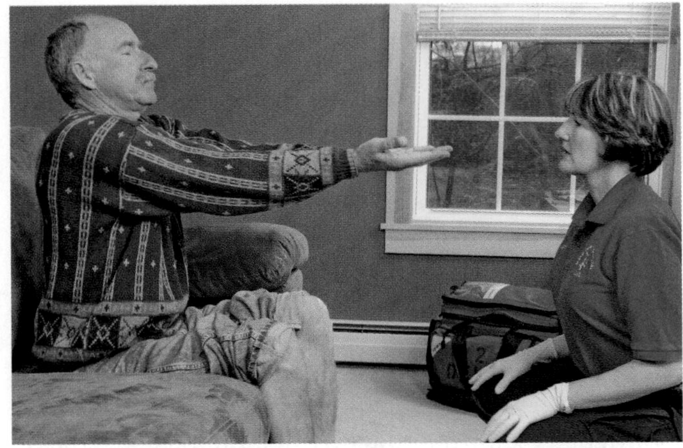

FIGURE 13-21 * Have the patient close both eyes and hold his arms straight out to check for arm drift.

ASSESSMENT Tips

On one side of the body, a patient may be able to move and feel light touch but can feel no pain. On the opposite side, he may be able to feel pain but is unable to feel light touch, or perhaps he can't move on that side. These findings are consistent with a spinal cord injury that is incomplete, where some nerve tracts are intact and others are not. ■

Assess the Posterior Body

If the patient is not already secured to the backboard, roll the supine patient onto his side. If a spinal injury is suspected, manual in-line spinal stabilization must be maintained at all times until the patient is completely immobilized to the backboard. Inspect the posterior thorax, lumbar area, buttocks, and lower extremities for any deformities, contusions, abrasions, punctures, burns, lacerations, or swelling.

Palpate the posterior body for deformities and tenderness. If pain or tenderness is noted around any of the vertebrae, note the location and do not palpate the area. Palpating may cause further damage. If no pain is noted, lightly palpate along the vertebrae for deformities or tenderness. Muscle spasm, tenderness, deformity, or pain to or around the vertebrae is a sign of vertebral injury. Be extremely cautious in handling the patient. Ensure proper in-line spinal stabilization and avoid any excessive or unnecessary movements.

Understanding BODY PROCESSES

While assessing the patient's back, you may note muscle spasms along the vertebral column. These spasms may occur as a protective reflex to keep the injured or fractured vertebrae stable and in line following an injury. ■

If the patient is already immobilized to the backboard, do not roll him to assess the posterior body. Simply place your hand at the flank area and slide it as far under the patient as possible. Check for any obvious deformity or pain.

Performing the Secondary Assessment: A Body Systems Approach

An anatomical head-to-toe approach, as described in the prior sections, provides a systematic method in performing the secondary assessment. This systematic approach allows the EMT to perform the assessment in an organized manner, even when there is a great deal of distraction at the scene. Not performing the systematic head-to-toe

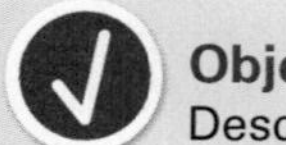

Objective 13-15
Describe performing the secondary assessment using a body systems approach.

Thinking Critically
Why is the body systems approach to assessment not enough by itself? Why is the body systems assessment also important?

approach leaves you vulnerable to missing injuries or signs of conditions that could be life threatening. Thus it is highly recommended you practice this type of approach throughout your career as an EMT.

Once an injury or condition has been identified, however, it is important not to focus on just that one particular anatomical region but rather to consider all other body systems that might also be affected. As an example, if the patient has a penetrating wound to the chest, it may have caused damage to the respiratory system and cardiovascular system which could lead to poor perfusion and cellular hypoxia. In this case, you must assess the respiratory, cardiovascular, and neurological systems to determine the extent of the injury. It is important to link the body systems together to establish the severity of the condition. In this case, you would perform a rapid secondary assessment from head to toe for two reasons: (1) to identify and manage additional penetrating or other life-threatening injuries, and (2) to determine the severity of the penetrating injury to the chest on perfusion and oxygenation.

The following is an example of the linkage of body system findings during the secondary assessment of the penetrating-chest-injury patient. The complete head-to-toe exam will be performed. Additionally, however, the body systems approach will help you to link findings from the complete head-to-toe exam that will provide information about the extent of the specific injury and its effects on other body systems. Linked findings from the head-to-toe exam of the penetrating-chest-trauma patient might include the following:

- Pupils that are dilated and sluggish may indicate hypoxia.
- Conjunctiva that is cyanotic may indicate hypoxia, and pale may indicate hemorrhage.
- Cyanotic oral mucosa indicate possible hypoxia.
- Distended jugular veins indicate possible backup of venous blood caused by impedance on the cardiac output from a tension pneumothorax or pericardial tamponade, leading to poor perfusion.
- Subcutaneous emphysema indicates a possible air leak from an injury to the lung or respiratory structure, which may lead to poor gas exchange and hypoxia.
- An open wound to the chest could interfere with lung expansion, leading to poor gas exchange and hypoxia.
- Decreased or absent breath sounds indicate a partially or completely collapsed lung that would cause a ventilation disturbance, poor gas exchange, and hypoxia.
- Extremities that are pale, cool, and clammy, with absent or weak peripheral pulses indicate vasoconstriction likely associated with blood loss leading to poor perfusion. Pale, cool skin and cyanosis indicate hypoxia.
- Decreased mental status indicates poor cerebral perfusion and cerebral hypoxia.

The major body systems assessment includes the respiratory (pulmonary), cardiovascular, neurological, and musculoskeletal. systems. The body systems approach is integrated into the head-to-toe anatomical assessment. While conducting the head-to-toe exam, you must identify the findings that are related to the body systems and make the links. Body systems assessment should include, but not be limited to, the following:

Respiratory (Pulmonary) System

- Chest shape and symmetry
- Accessory muscle use (retractions)
- Auscultation (normal and abnormal breath sounds)

Cardiovascular System

- Peripheral and central pulse (rate, rhythm, strength, location)
- Blood pressure (systolic, diastolic, pulse pressure)

Neurological System

- Mental status (AVPU, orientation)
- Posture and motor activity (appropriateness of posture and movement, arm drift) (Review Figure 13-21.)
- Facial expression (anxiety, depression, anger, fear, sadness, pain, facial asymmetry or droop) (Review Figure 13-16.)
- Speech and language (slurred, garbled, aphasia)
- Mood (nature, intensity, suicidal ideation)
- Thought and perceptions
  - Thought process (logic, organization)
  - Thought content (unusual, unpleasant)
  - Perceptions (unusual, auditory hallucinations, visual hallucinations)
- Memory and attention (orientation to person, place, time, purpose)

Objective 13-16
Summarize assessment of the vital signs during the secondary assessment.

Objective 13-17
Discuss obtaining a history during the secondary assessment, including use of the SAMPLE and OPQRST mnemonics.

Musculoskeletal System

- Pelvic region (symmetry, tenderness)
- Lower extremities (symmetry, superficial findings, range of motion, sensory, motor function)
- Upper extremities (symmetry, superficial findings, range of motion, sensory, motor function, arm drift)
- Peripheral vascular system (tenderness, temperature, distal pulses)
- Perfusion (distal pulses, skin color, temperature, condition)
- Posterior body (symmetry, contour, superficial findings, flank tenderness, spinal column tenderness)

Assess Baseline Vital Signs

The assessment of vital signs will occur at different times depending on if you are dealing with a trauma or medical patient, if the patient is responsive or unresponsive, and if the patient is stable or unstable. Remember, however, that if you have enough assistance and can be sure that in-line stabilization is being maintained by a trained person, these steps may overlap. For example, one EMT may be able to get vital sign measurements while the other is conducting the physical exam, or vital signs and history may be taken at the same time.

The methods for assessing the vital signs were discussed in Chapter 11, "Baseline Vital Signs, Monitoring Devices, and History Taking." The following vital signs must be assessed during the secondary assessment and reassessed throughout the entire call:

- *Breathing* (rate and tidal volume)
- *Pulse* (location, rate, strength, regularity)
- *Skin* (temperature, color, condition)
- *Capillary refill*
- *Blood pressure* (both systolic and diastolic)
- *Pupils* (equality, size, rate of reactivity)
- SpO_2

The vital signs with specific findings will be discussed further in the trauma assessment and medical assessment sections.

Obtain a History

The history was covered in detail in Chapter 11, "Baseline Vital Signs, Monitoring Devices, and History Taking." For a systematic approach the EMT commonly uses the SAMPLE and OPQRST mnemonics in the history-taking process. You can use whatever approach or technique works for you as long as you collect all of the necessary information. The mnemonics have a tendency to keep the EMT from doing a shotgun approach to history taking and allow him to collect all of the necessary information.

Components of the SAMPLE history are:

- **S**igns and **S**ymptoms
- **A**llergies
- **M**edications
- **P**ast medical history
- **L**ast oral intake
- **E**vents prior to the incident

The OPQRST mnemonic is used to further evaluate the chief complaint and other complaints of the patient. As an example, if a patient complains of chest discomfort, shortness of breath, and nausea, the OPQRST mnemonic (onset, provocation/palliation, quality, radiation, severity, and time of the complaint) will be used to further investigate each of the complaints.

The history is conducted at different times in the secondary assessment depending on whether the patient is categorized as trauma or medical, responsive or unresponsive, and stable or unstable. The history is a much more important component of the secondary assessment of the medical patient than it is for the trauma patient. This will be discussed further in the section on assessment of the medical patient later in the chapter.

Objective 13-18
List the sequence in which the steps of the secondary assessment are generally performed for a trauma patient and differentiate between the rapid secondary assessment and the modified secondary assessment for a trauma patient.

Key Terms
rapid secondary assessment a head-to-toe physical exam that is swiftly conducted on a trauma patient who has an altered mental status or a significant mechanism of injury or on a medical patient who has an altered mental status.

Secondary Assessment: Trauma Patient

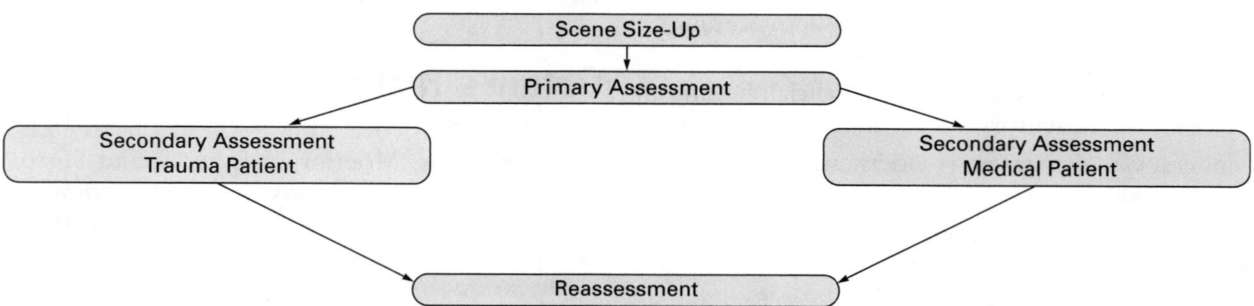

For the patient who has an injury or injuries rather than a medical condition, perform the secondary assessment for a trauma patient, which is generally performed in the following sequence:

1. Physical exam
2. Baseline vital signs
3. History

As mentioned earlier, you can often reduce the time before transport by performing some of these steps simultaneously. For example, while an Emergency Medical Responder maintains in-line stabilization, your partner might be taking vital signs and a history while you conduct the physical exam. Over a period of time, you and your partner can develop ways of accomplishing several things at the same time.

One of two kinds of physical exam can be chosen for a trauma patient: a **rapid secondary assessment** (a rapid head-to-toe exam) or a **modified secondary assessment** (an exam focused on a specific injury site), which will be described on the following pages. Your first decision during the focused history and physical exam will be which kind of exam is most appropriate for this patient:

- *A rapid secondary assessment* followed by prompt transport, or on-scene emergency care, or
- *A modified secondary assessment* followed by on-scene emergency care

The kind of physical exam you will conduct is based on the mechanism of injury—the force that caused the injury—and findings in your primary assessment. (Mechanism of injury was introduced in Chapter 12 and will be further discussed in Chapter 27.) You must determine whether the mechanism of injury is significant enough to have caused critical injury, if multiple injuries exist, if the patient has an altered mental status, or if any other critical finding identified in the primary assessment makes the patient unstable. If so, choose the rapid secondary assessment (the rapid head-to-toe exam) followed by prompt emergency care and transport. If the mechanism of injury is not significant enough to produce critical injuries, but you suspect the patient could be suffering from multiple or serious injuries anywhere on the body, or if the patient has an altered mental status, conduct a rapid secondary assessment as a basis for further on-scene emergency care. If the patient is suffering from an isolated injury that is not critical, the mechanism of injury is minor, there is no evidence of multiple injuries, and the patient is alert and oriented, conduct a modified secondary assessment of the injury site, followed by appropriate on-scene emergency care.

The following chart compares the two approaches.

Secondary Assessment for a Trauma Patient Who Has . . .

A Significant Mechanism of Injury, Multiple Injuries, Altered Mental Status, or Critical Findings in Primary Assessment (or for Whom Unknown Injuries Are Suspected)

1. Rapid secondary assessment (head to toe)
2. Baseline vital signs
3. SAMPLE history

Isolated Injury with No Significant Mechanism of Injury, No Multiple Injuries, Alert and Oriented Mental Status, and No Critical Finding in Primary Assessment

1. Modified secondary assessment (focused on the injury site)
2. Baseline vital signs
3. SAMPLE history

Key Terms

modified secondary assessment a physical exam that is focused on a specific injury site on a responsive trauma patient with no significant mechanism of injury or critical injuries or on a medical patient who is alert, oriented, and stable.

Objective 13-19

List the mechanisms of injury that have a high incidence of producing critical trauma and the special considerations for infants and children.

Reevaluate the Mechanism of Injury

Your first step in the secondary assessment (Figure 13-22*) is to re-evaluate the mechanism of injury. Remember, the mechanism of injury is directly related to the potential for critical injuries. The more significant or severe the mechanism of injury, the greater the chance that the patient is critically injured. You must ask yourself, "Was this mechanism of injury significant enough to cause critical or multiple injuries?"

The emergency care you provide is frequently based on the findings of the scene size-up and a high index of suspicion. Most often, spinal immobilization is performed based solely on your suspicion that the patient might have suffered an injury to the spinal column. You provide the necessary emergency care for a spinal injury even though you detect no signs or symptoms of such an injury.

When there is a significant mechanism of injury—as soon as you have completed the primary assessment and management of immediately life-threatening conditions—you should proceed with a rapid secondary assessment to identify any additional serious or potentially life-threatening injuries.

Significant Mechanisms of Injury

Mechanisms of injury that have a high incidence of producing critical trauma are:

- Ejection (partial or complete) of the patient from a vehicle in an automobile crash
- A crash that causes death to a person in the same passenger compartment in which the patient is found
- A fall of greater than 20 feet
- Rollover of the vehicle the patient was in (Figure 13-23a*)
- A vehicle collision that has occurred at a high speed
- An intrusion of greater than 12 inches into the passenger compartment or greater than 18 inches at any site on the vehicle (Figure 13-23b*)
- A pedestrian/bicyclist struck by a vehicle
- A motorcycle crash at greater than 20 mph with separation of rider from motorcycle
- Blunt or penetrating trauma that results in an altered mental status, from confusion to unresponsiveness

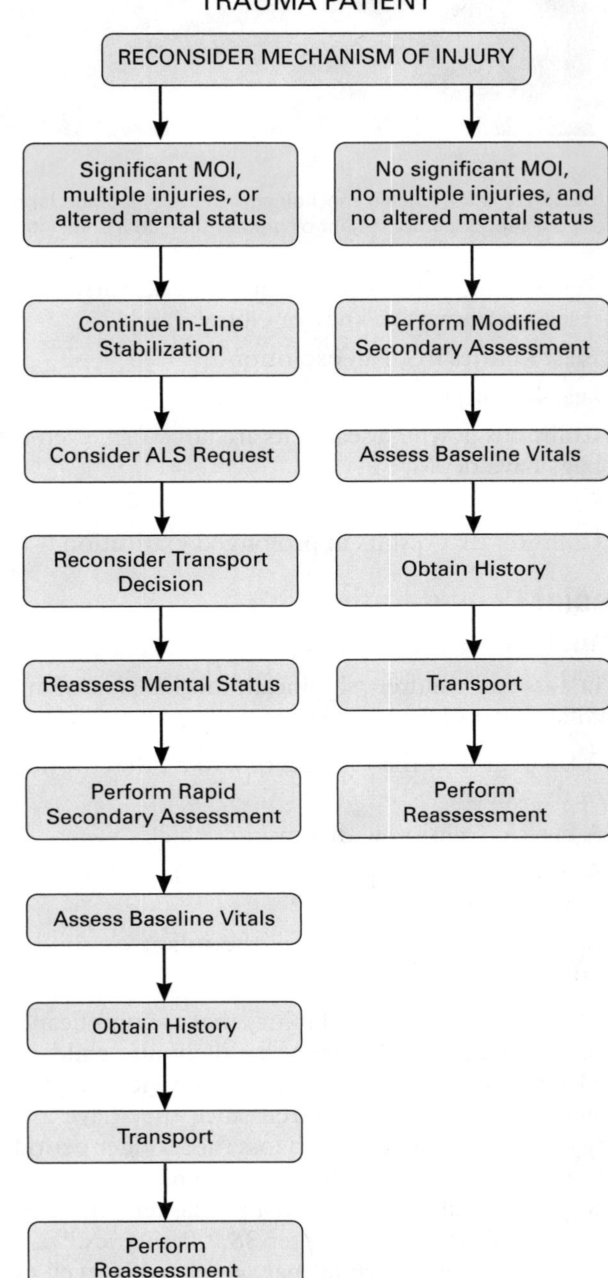

FIGURE 13-22 * Steps of the secondary assessment for a trauma patient.

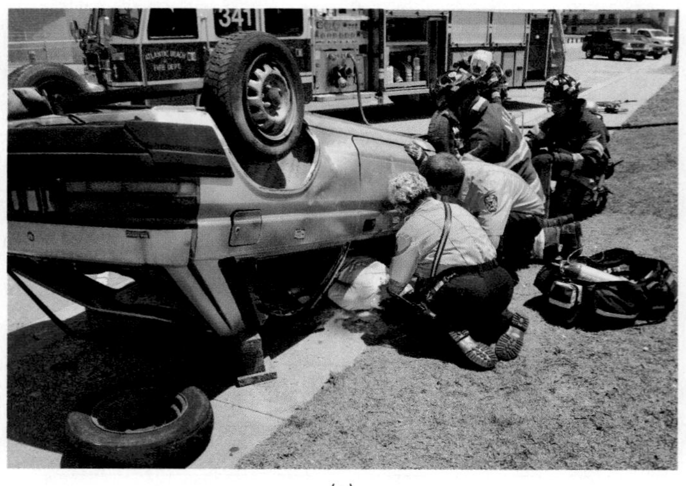
(a)

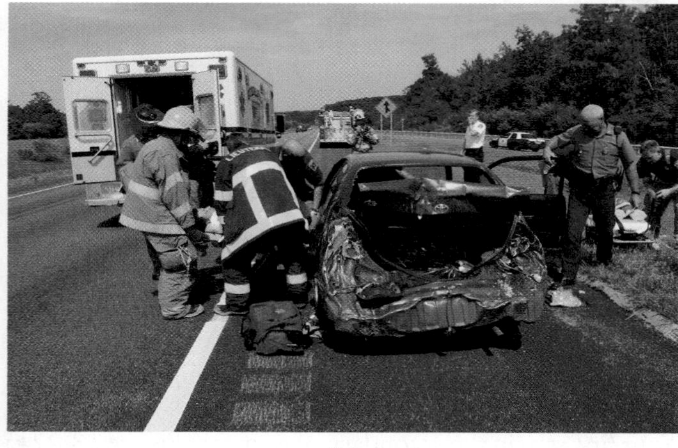
(b)

FIGURE 13-23 * Significant mechanisms of injury include **(a)** rollover of a vehicle a patient was in; **(b)** intrusion of greater than 12 inches into the passenger compartment or greater than 18 inches into any site on the vehicle. (Photo b: © Mark C. Ide)

- Penetrating injuries to the head, neck, torso, or extremities above the knee or elbow
- Blast injuries from an explosion
- Seat-belt injuries
- Collisions in which seat belts are not worn, even if air bags have deployed
- Impact causing deformity to the steering wheel
- Collision that results in prolonged extrication

Special Considerations for Infants and Children

For infants and children, significant mechanisms of injury would also include:

- A fall of greater than 10 feet or 2 to 3 times the height of the child
- A bicycle collision with a motor vehicle
- A pedestrian occupant in a vehicle collision at a medium speed
- Any vehicle collision where the infant or child was unrestrained

All other mechanisms of injury that are significant for the adult are also significant in the infant and child.

Mechanism of injury is a vital component in the assessment of infants and children since they have a tendency to compensate for blood loss for a longer period of time compared to adults, then decompensate faster. (This phenomenon will be explained in Chapter 15, "Shock and Resuscitation," and Chapter 38, "Pediatrics.") Consequently, an infant or child may appear to be well even though injured as severely as an adult who displays all the signs of shock. When that infant or child does deteriorate, it will happen very rapidly and perhaps too late for emergency care to save the child's life. So for the infant or child, even more than for an adult, you must rely on the mechanism of injury in your assessment. If there is a significant mechanism of injury, you must assume that the child is critically injured and in shock, even if the child looks all right, and provide treatment accordingly.

ASSESSMENT Tips

If the patient—adult or child—has not suffered a significant mechanism of injury (MOI) but is exhibiting signs and symptoms of shock or a severe injury, assume the patient is injured and provide immediate emergency care based on the clinical findings and not the MOI. ■

Rapid Secondary Assessment: Trauma Patient with Significant Mechanism of Injury, Altered Mental Status, Multiple Injuries, or Critical Finding (*Unstable*)

If any of the significant mechanisms of injury listed earlier are encountered at the scene, if the patient has an altered mental status, if you are unsure of the extent of injury to the patient, if you cannot clearly identify the mechanism of injury, if multiple injuries exist or are suspected, or if critical findings were identified in the primary assessment, you should proceed with a rapid secondary assessment to quickly identify other life threats and prepare the patient for rapid transport.

The rapid secondary assessment is a head-to-toe physical exam that is swiftly conducted on a patient who has suffered or may have suffered severe injuries. If the patient is responsive, he can be questioned as to symptoms and

Objective 13-20
For the trauma patient with a significant mechanism of injury, discuss how to continue spinal stabilization, reasons to consider requesting advanced life support, and reasons to reconsider transport decisions.

Objective 13-21
Explain how to use the Glasgow Coma Scale (GCS) to rank the patient's level of consciousness and how to interpret the resulting GCS score.

history while the exam is in progress. This will aid in identifying injuries and related problems the patient may be suffering from, such as breathing difficulty. If the patient is unresponsive, the rapid secondary assessment alone can identify a majority of the injuries.

Prior to performing the rapid secondary assessment, make sure that spinal stabilization—established during the primary assessment—is continued. Consider requesting ALS backup, reconsider your transport decision, and reassess the patient's mental status. These steps are described in further detail in the next sections.

Continue Spinal Stabilization

Maintain in-line spinal stabilization until the patient is completely immobilized to a backboard. While one EMT performs the rapid secondary assessment, another EMT or assistant should continue to hold the head and neck in a neutral in-line position until a cervical spinal immobilization collar is applied, the patient is placed on the backboard and strapped in place, and a head immobilization device is applied. Once manual spinal stabilization is established, it should never be released until immobilization is completed. Typically, complete immobilization of the patient will not be performed until the rapid assessment is completed.

Consider an Advanced Life Support Request

Some trauma patients may benefit from advanced life support at the scene or while en route to the hospital. Airway trauma, an occluded airway, or any indication that air from an injured lung is trapped in the chest cavity, causing the uninjured lung and the heart to be compressed (tension pneumothorax), may be reason to consider calling for advanced life support. These are life-threatening problems in which advanced airway maneuvers or chest decompression could be life saving. These decisions should not delay transport to an appropriate facility. Follow local protocols and consult medical direction.

Reconsider the Transport Decision

Normally, if a decision for immediate transport has not been reached at the end of the primary assessment, transport will take place after the rapid secondary assessment, assessment of baseline vital signs, gathering of the SAMPLE history, and completion of appropriate emergency care based on these assessments. Throughout the exam, however, keep in mind the possibility of immediate transport if evidence of critical injury or deterioration is discovered.

Reassess Mental Status

Any deterioration in the patient's condition can have an adverse effect on functioning of the brain and a consequent deterioration in mental status. Therefore, continuous reassessment of the patient's mental status is necessary to provide you with valuable information regarding the deterioration or improvement of the patient's condition. This is often referred to as "trending."

Common causes of decreased mental status in trauma patients are compromised airways, inadequate breathing, hypoxia, blood loss, poor perfusion, poor oxygenation, and brain injuries. These commonly result from:

- Bleeding or trauma to the face, mouth, or neck
- Head injuries
- Chest injuries
- Abdominal injuries
- Bone injuries associated with blood loss

Critical Findings: Unstable Trauma Patient

Critical Finding:	Already altered or deteriorating mental status
Possibilities:	Hypoxia and high carbon dioxide levels (head injury, chest injury, spinal cord injury, blood loss, inadequate airway or breathing, shock, toxins)
Emergency Care:	Establish an airway, begin positive pressure ventilation if respiratory rate or tidal volume is inadequate, and administer oxygen.

ASSESSMENT Tips

The mental status of a patient with a brain injury will continue to deteriorate or will not improve if it is already altered. ■

Key Points
Once manual in-line spinal stabilization is established, do not release it until the patient is completely immobilized to a backboard or if you determine there is no possibility of spinal injury.

Thinking Critically
Your patient has a mental status that is altered and deteriorating. You immediately administer oxygen, but the mental status continues to deteriorate. Why might oxygen not improve mental status in a given patient?

A patient who is already unresponsive upon your arrival at the scene should be considered seriously injured. If a responsive patient's mental status shows signs of deteriorating, you should move rapidly through the assessment, looking for the potential cause of the unresponsiveness or deterioration of the mental status, and take steps to immediately correct the problem. To assess mental status, use the AVPU method (alert, responds to verbal stimulus, responds to painful stimulus, unresponsive) that was described in Part 2 of this chapter.

In an alert patient, assess the level of orientation. This is accomplished by asking the following questions about the time, place, and person/self:

- Do you know what year, month, and day it is?
- Can you tell me where you are right now?
- Who is this person with you?
- What is your full name?

Determine if the patient can provide you with the year, month, day, and approximate time of day. Orientation to place is assessed by asking the patient if he can identify where he is. If he is at home, he should be able to provide you with his address. If he is in an automobile crash, he should be able to tell you where he was coming from and where he is going. If he is at the mall or a store, he should be able to give the name of the mall or the store he is in. If another person is at the scene who is a friend or relative of the patient, have the patient identify him or her. If no other person is with the patient at the scene, it is somewhat difficult to assess for orientation to person. Finally, ask the patient his own full name.

If the patient correctly answers all of the questions, he is noted to be alert and oriented to time, place, and person/self. Commonly, this is documented as "alert and oriented × 3."

Orientation to time is usually the first to be lost in a deteriorating mental status. As the patient continues to progressively deteriorate, he will lose orientation to place, then person, and finally to his own self. At this point, he would not be able to identify himself or anyone else at the scene.

If the patient is not alert, determine what type of stimulus is needed to arouse the patient. As described in Part 2 of this chapter, first attempt verbal stimulus. If the patient does not respond to verbal stimulus, attempt painful stimulus.

The patient may respond in the following ways to a verbal stimulus:

- Responds to verbal stimulus with inappropriate words
- Responds to verbal stimulus with incomprehensible sounds, such as mumbling
- Responds with eye opening or obeying a command
- No response to verbal stimulus

The patient may respond to a painful stimulus with:

- Purposeful movements aimed at attempting to remove the stimulus, such as grabbing your hand or making a pushing-away gesture
- Nonpurposeful movements noted by flexion or extension posturing (back arched, arms pulled upward toward the chest or extended parallel to the body) that is not an attempt to remove the stimulus
- No response

Document precisely the alert patient's orientation or the nonalert patient's response to verbal or painful stimulus. Examples: "The patient is alert and oriented to person and self but not time or place," or "The patient responds to painful stimulus with upward movement of the left arm only." This information provides other emergency personnel with criteria to use later to determine if the patient's mental status has improved or deteriorated. The Glasgow Coma Scale (GCS) (Tables 13-9 and 13-10) is used to rank the patient's level of consciousness by assigning a numeric score from 3 to 15. This scoring tool is used in emergency medical services to identify trends of improvement or deterioration in the mental status of the patient. The GCS score is widely accepted, is reproducible, and can be reported and recorded as evidence of the mental status trending. A GCS score of 8 or less indicates a severe alteration in brain function. A GCS score of 13 or less is an indication for limited on-scene time (less than 10 minutes) and rapid transport.

If bystanders, relatives, or friends are present at the scene, it is important to determine from them if the patient suffered an altered mental status, lost orientation, or became unresponsive at any time prior to your arrival. If the patient is unresponsive, determine if the patient was responding and oriented at any time after the incident but prior to your arrival. Also note if the patient lost responsiveness, awoke for a period of time, and then became unresponsive again. Most of these are reliable indicators of possible head injury. Patients with these patterns of responsiveness and loss of responsiveness need very close monitoring.

Objective 13-22
Discuss how to conduct a rapid secondary assessment for a trauma patient with significant mechanism of injury, altered mental status, multiple injuries, or critical finding (unstable patient).

Key Points
You must expose the multiple-trauma patient completely to look for any and all evidence of injury.

TABLE 13-9 Glasgow Coma Scale

Eye Opening	
Spontaneous	4
To verbal command	3
To pain	2
No response	1
Verbal Response	
Oriented and converses	5
Disoriented and converses	4
Inappropriate words	3
Incomprehensible sounds	2
No response	1
Motor Response	
Obeys verbal commands	6
Localizes pain	5
Withdraws from pain (flexion)	4
Abnormal flexion in response to pain (decorticate rigidity)	3
Extension in response to pain (decerebrate rigidity)	2
No response	1

Perform a Rapid Secondary Assessment

When performing the rapid secondary assessment, you will inspect and palpate the patient to identify signs and symptoms of potential injuries. Also, auscultation could reveal a collapsed lung and potential life-threatening chest injuries.

During the rapid secondary assessment of each major body area, inspect and palpate for evidence of trauma. Common signs of trauma include deformities, contusions, abrasions, punctures and penetrations, burns, tenderness, lacerations, and swelling (EMT Skills 13-4). This is not an all-inclusive list; many other signs and symptoms should be assessed for as evidence of trauma:

- *Inspect (look) for* deformities, contusions (bruises), abrasions, punctures, penetrating wounds, burns, lacerations, swelling, unusual chest wall movements, angulated extremities, bleeding, discoloration, open wounds, and significant bleeding.
- *Palpate (feel) for* tenderness, deformities, swelling, masses, muscle spasms, skin temperature, and pulsations. When palpating for tenderness (pain on palpation) in the unresponsive patient, watch the patient's face for grimacing. This provides a good indication that tenderness is present without the patient being able to tell you.
- *Auscultate (listen with a stethoscope) for* presence and equality of breath sounds.
- *Listen for* sucking sounds, gurgling, stridor (high-pitched sound of the upper airway), and crepitation (grating sound heard when broken bone ends rub against each other, or a crackling sound caused by air under the skin).
- *Use your sense of smell* to detect any unusual odors on the patient's breath, body, or clothing, such as alcohol, feces, or urine.

As you conduct the rapid secondary assessment, talk calmly to the patient, even if he appears to be unresponsive. Don't distress the patient by describing wounds and injuries, but rather indicate what areas you are going to assess. In the responsive patient and if the condition permits, ask any relevant questions about the area to be assessed prior to examining it. If you assess the area and then ask questions, the patient will suspect that you have found something wrong.

In the rapid secondary assessment, be most concerned with identifying potentially life-threatening injuries. If you find any injuries that are potentially life threatening, you must manage them immediately to avoid further deterioration of the patient. Each situation is different and will dictate how you proceed.

Be careful not to move the patient unnecessarily to avoid aggravating any neck or spinal injury that might exist. Do not manipulate the patient to attempt to remove clothing. If necessary, expose the areas to be examined by cutting the clothing off the patient. In patients with a significant mechanism of injury or for whom serious trauma is a possibility, it is important to completely expose the patient to look for additional injuries.

ASSESSMENT Tips

A distracting injury, such as an extremity fracture, may cause the patient to not complain of other, more significant or critical injuries, such as a knife wound to the chest. If a patient has a distracting injury, expose him completely to assess for other, more potentially life-threatening injuries that he may not be complaining of. ■

Thinking Critically
Why is it important to completely expose the body of a patient with a significant mechanism of injury or possible major trauma?

Objective 13-23
Discuss critical (unstable) findings, possibilities, and emergency care for the trauma patient associated with assessment of the head, neck, chest, abdomen, pelvis, extremities, and posterior body.

TABLE 13-10 Pediatric Glasgow Coma Scale

		> 1 Year	**< 1 Year**	
Eye Opening	4	Spontaneous	Spontaneous	
	3	To verbal command	To shout	
	2	To pain	To pain	
	1	No response	No response	
		> 1 Year	**< 1 Year**	
Best Motor Response	6	Obeys		
	5	Localizes pain	Localizes pain	
	4	Flexion-withdrawal	Flexion-withdrawal	
	3	Flexion-abnormal (decorticate rigidity)	Flexion-abnormal (decorticate rigidity)	
	2	Extension (decerebrate rigidity)	Extension (decerebrate rigidity)	
	1	No response	No response	
		> 5 Years	**2–5 Years**	**0–23 Months**
Best Verbal Response	5	Oriented and converses	Appropriate words and phrases	Smiles, coos, cries appropriately
	4	Disoriented and converses	Inappropriate words	Cries
	3	Inappropriate words	Cries and/or screams	Inappropriate crying and/or screaming
	2	Incomprehensible sounds	Grunts	Grunts
	1	No response	No response	No response

Suppose that you arrive on the scene of a shooting and find a patient with a gunshot wound to the left upper thigh. It appears the bullet fractured the femur. Because the femur fracture is so painful, the patient is only complaining of that injury. You focus in on the femur fracture and neglect to expose the patient to look for any other injuries. It is winter and the patient has a heavy coat on. It is nighttime, and the patient is wearing dark clothing. Therefore, it is difficult to see blood. The patient was shot with a .22 caliber gun, which is very small. En route to the hospital, the patient begins to complain of severe breathing difficulty. You finally become suspicious and expose the chest to find a gunshot wound of the anterior chest. You missed a life-threatening injury in this patient. If you had quickly exposed the chest during your assessment, you would have found the injury.

When exposing the patient, keep modesty and environmental conditions in mind. Do not completely expose the patient in front of a crowd or television camera. Cover the patient with a sheet to protect the modesty of any patient, male or female, young or old. Also, do not inadvertently induce hypothermia by exposing the patient to the cold. Consider moving into the ambulance before completely exposing the patient.

As described in the following sections, the rapid secondary assessment is performed in a systematic sequence to ensure that all major body areas are inspected and palpated (EMT Skills 13-5).

Assess the Head

When examining the head, it is necessary to quickly examine the skull, scalp, face, ears, pupils, nose, and mouth. *The exam is not detailed unless an injury is found or suspected in that particular area. A more detailed exam of each area can be conducted at a later time.* You are prima-

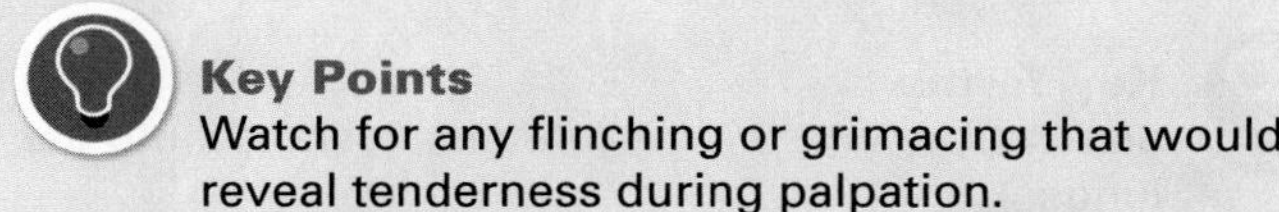

Key Points
Watch for any flinching or grimacing that would reveal tenderness during palpation.

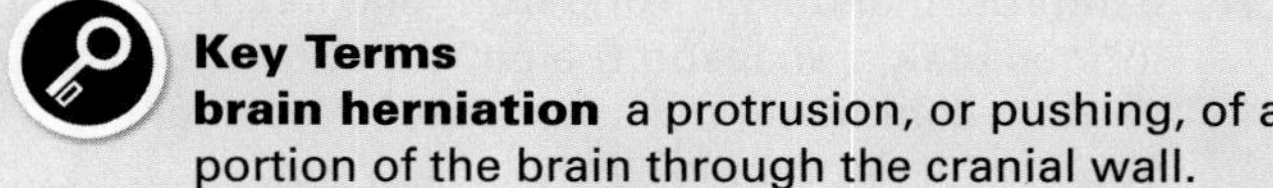

Key Terms
brain herniation a protrusion, or pushing, of a portion of the brain through the cranial wall.

rily concerned with identifying a possible head injury by examining the scalp, skull, pupils, and ears. Also, you must quickly reassess the nose and mouth for potential obstructions of the airway.

Scalp and Skull Inspect the scalp and skull (EMT Skills 13-5A) for any obvious deformities, contusions, abrasions, punctures, burns, lacerations, swelling, depressions, protrusions, impaled objects, or bleeding. Palpate for any crepitation (grating sound or feeling resulting from fractured bone ends rubbing together), depressions, protrusions, swelling, bloody areas, instability, or lack of symmetry. Listen for any sounds the patient makes and look for flinching or grimacing that reveals any tenderness the patient experiences when you are palpating. If you discover burns or the patient's hair is singed, suspect that the patient was involved in a fire and pay particular attention to the airway, breathing, and oxygenation status.

Critical (Unstable) Findings: The Head	
Critical Finding:	Trauma to the head or face with altered mental status Unequal pupils Fixed pupils Cerebrospinal fluid leaking from ears, nose, or mouth
Possibility:	Head injury
Emergency Care:	Establish an airway, begin positive pressure ventilation if respiratory rate or tidal volume is inadequate, and administer oxygen.
Critical Finding:	Blood, secretions, vomitus, teeth, bones, or other debris in the mouth
Possibility:	Airway obstruction
Emergency Care:	Suction the mouth and nose. If necessary, log roll the patient onto his side to clear the airway if heavy vomitus or clotted blood is present.

Palpate the scalp and skull by cupping your hands and moving from the frontal region to the back of the skull. Do not poke with your fingers, since you may aggravate a depressed skull fracture by pushing the bony ends into the brain. Be careful not to move the head or neck when palpating in the patient with a suspected spine injury.

In a dark environment, it is difficult to see blood in the hair. Thus, when assessing the head, periodically look at your gloves for evidence of blood. Also, pay attention to areas that feel warm during the exam as this usually indicates leakage of blood or cerebrospinal fluid. Leakage of cerebrospinal fluid is evidence of a skull fracture.

Avoid unnecessary pressure to any areas of the skull that appear unstable, depressed, or deformed. Refrain from palpating the depressed or deformed area to avoid further injury. If an impaled object is found in the skull, stabilize it in place with bulky dressings. Do not remove or move the object. (Management of impaled objects will be discussed in detail in Chapter 28, "Bleeding and Soft-Tissue Trauma," and Chapter 33, "Eye, Face, and Neck Trauma.") Abnormalities to the skull, especially with an altered mental status, are a clear indication of a critical head injury that requires prompt attention and transport.

A severe and detrimental condition that may occur in a head injury is called **brain herniation**. This occurs when a significant amount of swelling and/or bleeding to or around the brain creates excessive pressure within the skull and causes the brain to be compressed and pushed downward toward the brain stem at the base of the skull. Herniation results when a portion of the brain is pushed out, usually through the foramen magnum, the opening through which the spinal cord exits from the brain, or through the fibrous tentorium, which divides the upper and lower brain. Compressed brain tissue does not function properly. If the medulla in the brain stem is compressed, the respiratory center, cardiac center, and vasomotor center (which controls blood pressure) will not function. This will quickly lead to death.

Assess for signs of brain herniation and treat the patient aggressively. Signs of brain herniation include a severely altered mental status, abnormal posturing (flexion or extension), fixed pupils, or unequal pupils. If the patient has a suspected head injury and is displaying signs of herniation and is breathing inadequately, an airway must be established and the patient artificially ventilated. Hyperventilation may be considered; however, this emergency care is controversial and may not be recommended in your local protocol. Always follow your local protocol. Hyperventilation is achieved by positive pressure ventilation

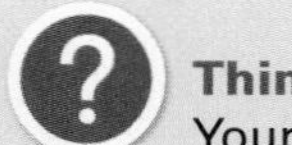

Thinking Critically
Your patient displays signs of severe head injury, including bradycardia, unequal pupils, and cerebrospinal fluid leaking from one ear. You immediately transpsort the patient to the hospital without continuing the secondary assessment. Did you do the right thing? Why or why not?

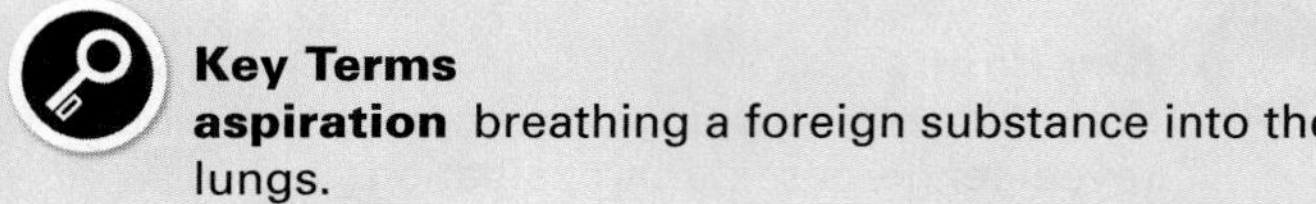

Key Terms
aspiration breathing a foreign substance into the lungs.

initiated and maintained at a rate of 20 ventilations per minute in the adult patient. If there are no signs of brain herniation but the patient is not breathing adequately, establish an airway and provide positive pressure ventilation at a rate of 10–12 ventilations per minute. If the patient is breathing adequately (i.e., both rate and tidal volume are adequate), apply a nonrebreather mask at 15 lpm. (Head injuries will be discussed in detail in Chapter 31, "Head Trauma.")

ASSESSMENT Tips

Bradycardia (a slow heart rate) in a patient with a suspected head injury is a very serious sign of brain injury. ■

Even though prompt transport is key in treatment of the patient with a head injury, it is vital to continue with the exam to identify any other potential injuries that need immediate attention. For example, the patient could die from an open wound to the chest that you missed because of failure to continue with the exam.

If the patient is wearing a hairpiece or a wig, do not attempt to remove it. It may be held in place with permanent adhesive or tape or may be sewn into the scalp. Feel gently through the netting to assess for bleeding, swelling, or deformity. Do not reach under the wig.

Face Inspect the face (EMT Skills 13-5B), looking for any evidence of trauma and bleeding that may be obstructing the airway. Look for deformities, contusions, abrasions, penetrating wounds, lacerations, swelling, or other evidence of trauma. Palpate for deformities, instability, and swelling.

Of particular concern is trauma to the midface region. This is a common injury from blunt forces being applied to the area between the lower lip and the bridge of the nose. A patient who strikes his face on the dashboard in an automobile crash commonly suffers trauma to the midface. Also, blows to the face from punches, kicks, baseball bats, or other objects will cause significant trauma.

If trauma to the face is found, carefully assess the airway for possible occlusion. Many times the bones of the face are pushed posteriorly into the airway, causing a blockage. Bleeding, which is common with injuries to the face, may occlude the airway or increase the risk of **aspiration** of the blood (the patient breathing the blood into the lungs). Insertion of an oropharyngeal airway and constant suction may be necessary to maintain a patent airway. Do not use a nasopharyngeal airway when injuries to the midface are present. The airway may be improperly placed, with the risk of the airway entering the skull, because of a fracture to the nasal structures.

When inspecting the face, in addition to looking for burns to the skin, look for singed or burned nasal hair, eyebrows, and facial hair. This would indicate that the patient has potentially suffered an upper airway burn. Reassess the airway for stridor and adequate air movement. If stridor is present, begin positive pressure ventilation with supplemental oxygen.

ASSESSMENT Tips

You may meet more resistance when ventilating a patient with stridor because of the increase in resistance to airflow through the swollen larynx. If you feel resistance, however, make sure it is not from a poorly established head-tilt, chin-lift maneuver or jaw-thrust maneuver. ■

Ears Quickly look inside the ears with a flashlight. Inspect for leakage of blood, cerebrospinal fluid, or other fluid, which are signs of a possible head injury (Figure 13-24∗).

Pupils Assess the patient's pupils by opening the eyes and shining a penlight into each eye, checking for equality of pupil size and reactivity. The pupils are normally equal in size and constrict briskly to light. Unequal pupils (Figure 13-25∗) or pupils that do not respond to light (fixed pupils) usually indicate a severe head injury. Poor tissue perfusion and hypoxia (inadequate oxygen supply) will cause the pupils to respond sluggishly.

If a patient has unequal pupils but is alert and oriented, the unequal pupils are probably not from a head injury. You need to suspect a possible eye injury, effect of eye medications, or some other condition. Approximately 6 to 10 percent of the population normally have unequal pupils. This is termed *anisocoria*.

ASSESSMENT Tips

Some patients take medicated eye drops that cause the pupils to dilate. Also, patients who have had their eyes examined that day may have dilated pupils. The pupils will continue to respond to light changes, but very slightly. ■

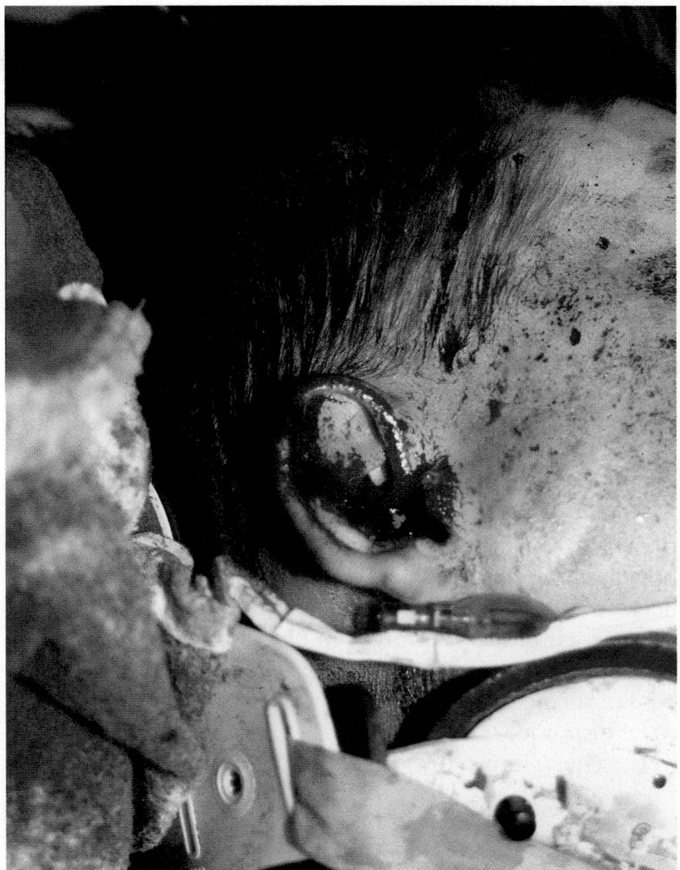

FIGURE 13-24 ✱ Blood and cerebrospinal fluid draining from a patient's ear. (© Edward T. Dickinson, MD)

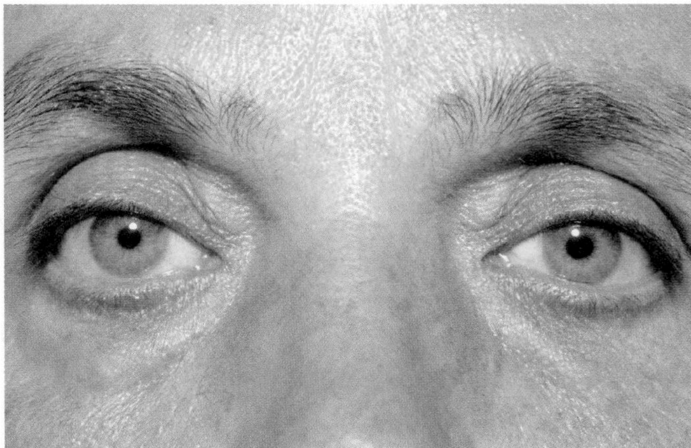

FIGURE 13-25 ✱ Unequal pupils. (© Medscan/Corbis)

Nose Inspect the nose for evidence of bleeding and leakage of cerebrospinal fluid. Suction the nose clear of blood if it is draining posteriorly into the nasopharynx. Your major concern with the nose is bleeding into the airway, causing occlusion or possible aspiration. Check the nose for burned nasal hair or carbonaceous (charcoal black) discharge. This indicates likely inhalation of smoke and a possible upper airway burn.

Mouth Your major concern when inspecting the inside of the mouth is to reassess the patency of the airway. Inspect for any bleeding, bone fragments, or dislodged teeth that may need to be suctioned or removed by finger sweeps. Also, inspect for swelling, lacerations to the tongue, and tissue damage that may cause possible obstruction.

When inspecting inside the mouth, look at the color of the mucous membranes. The mucous membranes are normally pink. Cyanotic membranes indicate hypoxia and pale membranes indicate poor tissue perfusion, possibly from long-term blood loss.

If the patient is being ventilated, quickly inspect the inside of the mouth in between ventilations. Never interrupt ventilation for more than 30 seconds.

Assess the Neck

Inspect the anterior neck (EMT Skills 13-5C) for deformities, contusions, abrasions, punctures, burns, lacerations, swelling, and any other evidence of trauma. A large collection of blood under the skin in the neck might actually occlude the airway by compressing the posterior portion of the trachea. Any large puncture wound or laceration to the neck must be immediately covered with an occlusive dressing (one that will not allow air through) and taped on all four sides. This is to prevent the possibility of air being sucked into a large vein and causing an air embolus. (Neck injuries will be discussed in detail in Chapter 33, "Eye, Face, and Neck Trauma.")

Critical (Unstable) Findings: The Neck	
Critical Finding:	Jugular venous distention (JVD) with a patient at a 45° angle or excessively engorged jugular veins
Possibility:	Injury to heart (pericardial tamponade) or lungs (tension pneumothorax) or poor heart function
Emergency Care:	Rapid transport upon recognition. Consider ALS intercept. Establish an airway, begin positive pressure ventilation (PPV) if respiratory rate or tidal volume is inadequate, and administer oxygen. *Caution:* Aggressive PPV may worsen a lung injury.
Critical Finding:	Tracheal deviation
Possibility:	Lung injury with excessive buildup of pressure in the pleural space (tension pneumothorax)

continued

Key Points

Subcutaneous emphysema indicates that there is an air leak somewhere in the respiratory tract, lungs, or esophagus. It indicates a significant neck or chest injury.

Thinking Critically

In one supine trauma patient, the jugular veins are flat. In another trauma patient who is sitting up, the jugular veins are distended. What are some possible causes of these abnormal presentations?

Critical (Unstable) Findings: The Neck *continued*

Emergency Care:	Rapid transport upon recognition. Consider ALS intercept. Establish an airway, begin positive pressure ventilation if respiratory rate or tidal volume is inadequate, and administer oxygen. *Caution:* Aggressive PPV may worsen a lung injury.
Critical Finding:	Tracheal tugging
Possibility:	Blockage of the airway, usually at the level of the bronchi
Emergency Care:	Rapid transport upon recognition. Consider ALS intercept. Establish an airway, begin positive pressure ventilation if respiratory rate or tidal volume is inadequate, and administer oxygen.

Understanding BODY PROCESSES

Veins in the neck drain downward toward the heart. A laceration to a large vein in the neck may cause air to be sucked into the vein as it is draining toward the heart. If the air bubble (embolus) is large enough, it will likely be caught up in the circulation in the lungs, blocking blood flow and causing hypoxia. ■

Inspect the neck for evidence of subcutaneous emphysema. Subcutaneous emphysema is air trapped under the lower layer of the skin. It appears as if the skin is bloated or inflated. Air leaking from the trachea, bronchus, bronchiole, lung, or esophagus will commonly collect in the neck. Thus, subcutaneous emphysema is a good indicator of a significant chest or neck injury. It may be easier to find subcutaneous emphysema when palpating. It feels like bubble package wrap. Crepitation (a crackling sound) when palpating is an indication of air trapped under the skin.

Look at the trachea to determine if it is midline. A trachea shifted to one side is a late indication of a significant amount of air trapped in the pleural space of the chest cavity, the result of a severe lung or chest injury. The trachea will deviate away from the injured side. This condition is a tension pneumothorax. Also, look for a pendulum motion of the trachea called tracheal tugging. This usually indicates an airway obstruction on the side the trachea moves toward.

Assess the jugular veins for distention (Figure 13-26*). Normally, the jugular veins are slightly engorged in a patient who is lying supine. With the patient at a 45° angle, however, the neck veins should be flat. If the patient has neck veins that are flat in a supine position, it may indicate a decreased blood volume from bleeding. If the neck veins are engorged more than two-thirds the distance from the base of the neck to the angle of the jaw, they are considered to be distended. In trauma, JVD is a sign of a serious injury to the chest, lungs, or heart.

Understanding BODY PROCESSES

The jugular veins drain downward into the superior vena cava and into the right side of the heart. If the right side of the heart is not able to off-load the blood effectively, if the heart is being compressed and not able to fill completely, or if the superior vena cava is kinked or compressed, the pressure and volume of blood inside the jugular vein will increase and produce the distended appearance. ■

ASSESSMENT Tips

If the patient exhibits the signs and symptoms of shock or hypoperfusion and you find jugular vein distention on inspection of the neck, look for a cause of poor perfusion other than blood loss. ■

ASSESSMENT Tips

If jugular vein distention is present, the veins in the hand will likely be engorged with blood and distended. ■

Inspect the posterior portion of the neck (EMT Skills 13-5D) for evidence of trauma. Look for deformity, contusions, and swelling. If in-line stabilization is being maintained, do not have it released to inspect or

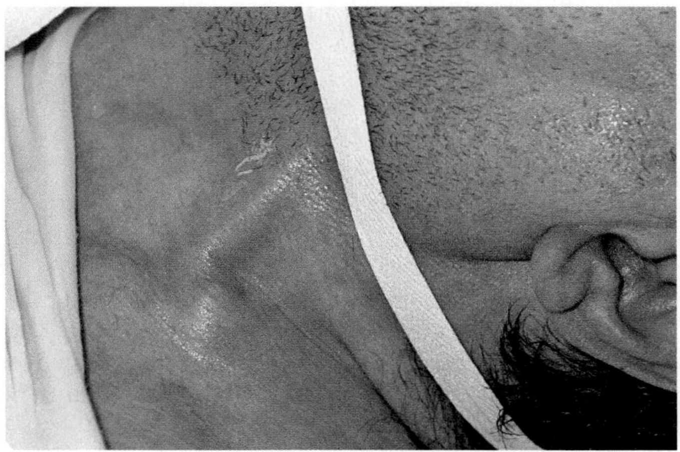

FIGURE 13-26 ✱ Jugular vein distention. (© David Effron, MD)

palpate. Inspection is difficult to accomplish with in-line stabilization. You may only be able to gently palpate the posterior cervical region for any deformities, tenderness, or muscle spasms. Do not move the head or neck to palpate. It is better to skip the inspection than to jeopardize the in-line stabilization and cause further injury.

Note any muscle spasms in the posterior cervical region. Muscle spasms occur in cervical injuries as a protective reflex, in an attempt to maintain support. Thus, a patient complaining of muscle spasms anywhere along the vertebral (spinal) column who has a mechanism of injury consistent with vertebral injury needs spinal immobilization.

Inspect the larynx for evidence of deformity and swelling. Injuries to the larynx from steering wheels, clothesline injuries, kicks, punches, and other blunt trauma could cause serious airway occlusion. With larynx injuries, the patient is typically hoarse or cannot speak, shows signs of respiratory distress, and may cough up blood. Oropharyngeal or nasopharyngeal airways are of no use in an isolated laryngeal injury because they do not reach to the depth of the injury. If the patient is unable to breathe adequately, you must provide positive pressure ventilation with supplemental oxygen. If the patient is able to breathe adequately, apply oxygen via a nonrebreather mask at 15 lpm.

ASSESSMENT Tips

A patient who is hoarse or cannot speak and who has evidence of trauma to the neck may have an injury to the larynx. ■

The patient may have a stoma, which is a surgical opening at the base of the throat. The stoma usually has a plastic or metal tube in the opening. The patient breathes through this opening. Therefore, make sure the tube is not occluded by blood, mucus, or other secretions.

Apply a Cervical Spinal Immobilization Collar

If the patient is suspected of having a possible spinal injury, a cervical spinal immobilization collar (CSIC) must be applied as soon as assessment of the neck is completed (EMT Skills 13-5E). The person who is maintaining manual in-line spinal stabilization continues to do so while the CSIC is sized and applied. It is very important not to move or manipulate the head or neck while applying the CSIC. At no time should in-line spinal stabilization be let go before, during, or after application of the CSIC. Even after the CSIC is properly applied, in-line spinal stabilization must be maintained until the patient is completely immobilized to a backboard with straps and a cervical spinal immobilization device. See Chapter 32, "Spinal Column and Spinal Cord Trauma," for the proper techniques of measuring and applying the CSIC and providing immobilization.

If the cervical spinal immobilization collar has been applied prior to your arrival by Emergency Medical Responders or by additional EMTs during the primary assessment, do not remove the cervical collar to assess the neck. Inspect and palpate for evidence of trauma as best you can through the large opening in the front of the collar.

Assess the Chest

In order for the chest to be properly examined, it is necessary to expose it (EMT Skills 13-5F). Cut the clothing from the patient. Inspect the chest anteriorly, laterally, and in the axillary regions (armpits) for open wounds (Figure 13-27a✱). Any open wound to the chest must be immediately covered with your gloved hand. Then apply an occlusive dressing taped on three sides over the wound. The dressing will prevent air from entering the thorax (pleural space) and worsening the chest injury. The loose side will possibly allow air to escape during exhalation, relieving the possible buildup of air in the chest.

Inspect the chest for evidence of deformities, contusions, abrasions (Figure 13-27b✱), burns, lacerations, swelling, lack of symmetry, and any other evidence of trauma. Look for segments of the chest that are moving in a paradoxical movement. Paradoxical movement occurs when a section of the chest sinks inward upon inhalation while the rest of the chest is moving outward, and upon exhalation bulges outward while the rest of the chest is moving inward.

This type of motion may be seen when two or more adjacent ribs are fractured in two or more places. This is termed a *flail segment*. A flail segment interferes with the effectiveness of chest wall movement, altering the negative pressure in the chest, thus reducing the adequacy of breathing and oxygenation. Since this is a life-threatening injury, you must immediately place your hand over the section to stabilize it in an inward position. Then place the patient's arm, a pillow, or bulky dressings or towels

Thinking Critically

A flail segment is usually accompanied by a severe contusion to the lung. What are the possible consequences of this injury? What treatment may be required?

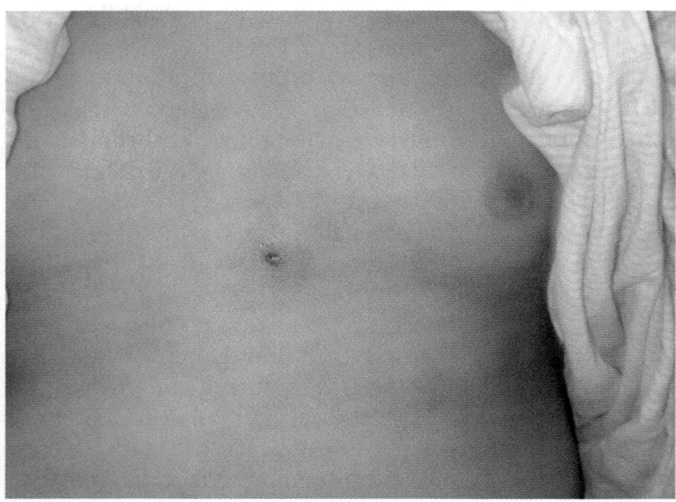

(a)

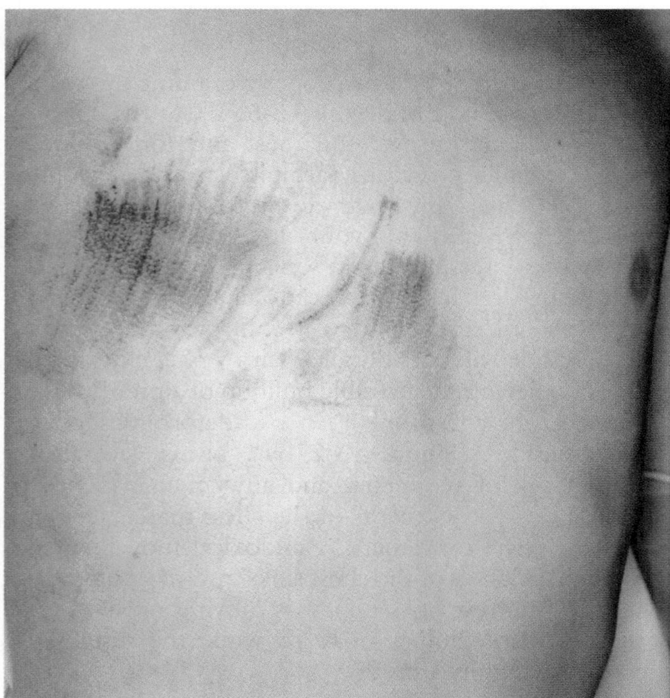

(b)

FIGURE 13-27 ✱ Expose the chest to inspect for injuries such as these: **(a)** Pellet wound to the chest. **(b)** Abrasions to the chest wall. (Both photos: © Charles Stewart, MD, and Associates)

taped in position over the site of injury. A flail segment is usually accompanied by a severe contusion (bruise) to the lung, causing hypoxia. Closely monitor the patient's breathing status. If the patient's breathing is inadequate, you must initiate positive pressure ventilation with supplemental oxygen.

Critical (Unstable) Findings: The Chest

Critical Finding:	Open wound to the chest
Possibility:	Sucking chest wound (air sucked into pleural space, causing the lung to collapse [pneumothorax])
Emergency Care:	Occlude the open wound immediately with a gloved hand and then with a nonporous dressing or occlusive dressing taped on three sides. Rapid transport upon recognition. Consider ALS intercept. Establish an airway, begin positive pressure ventilation if respiratory rate or tidal volume is inadequate, and administer oxygen. *Caution:* PPV may worsen the lung injury.
Critical Finding:	Paradoxical movement of the chest
Possibility:	Fracture of two or more adjacent ribs in two or more places (flail segment) Lung bruise (pulmonary contusion) may occur with injury Severe hypoxia can result from either condition
Emergency Care:	Stabilize flail segment in inward position. Rapid transport upon recognition. Consider ALS intercept. Establish an airway, begin positive pressure ventilation if respiratory rate or tidal volume is inadequate, and administer oxygen.
Critical Finding:	Absent or severely decreased breath sounds

Critical (Unstable) Findings: The Chest *continued*

Possibility:	Lung injury with excessive buildup of pressure in the pleural space (possible tension pneumothorax)
Emergency Care:	Begin positive pressure ventilation with supplemental oxygen if respiratory rate or tidal volume is inadequate. Look for deviated trachea or jugular vein distention, signs of air in the chest cavity. If you suspect this condition, consider rapid transport, requesting an ALS intercept. If an occlusive dressing is in place over an open chest wound, lift it off the wound for a few seconds during exhalation to allow any trapped air to escape, then reseal it. *Caution:* PPV may worsen the lung injury.
Critical Finding:	Poor chest wall movement with inhalation
Possibility:	Lung injury with excessive buildup of pressure in the pleural space (tension pneumothorax) Complete collapse of one or both lungs (pneumothorax) Severe chest wall pain from injury causing the patient to breathe shallowly Head or spinal cord injury Injury to the diaphragm (rupture or laceration) from trauma to chest or abdomen
Emergency Care:	Rapid transport upon recognition. Consider ALS intercept. Establish an airway, begin positive pressure ventilation if respiratory rate or tidal volume is inadequate, and administer oxygen. *Caution:* PPV may worsen the lung injury.

Understanding BODY PROCESSES

A flail segment may interfere with the ability of the thorax to produce the pressure changes necessary to effectively move air in and out of the lungs. This can be easily overcome by the EMT who provides positive pressure ventilation so that the thorax no longer needs to generate pressure changes to draw in air. ■

ASSESSMENT Tips

A flail segment may initially be stabilized by contraction of the muscles between the ribs (intercostal muscles). This will suppress paradoxical movement that would otherwise alert you to the presence of a flail segment. As the intercostal muscles fatigue, however, the stabilization is lost and the paradoxical movement becomes much more obvious. It is important to palpate for a flail segment early in your assessment, even though paradoxical movement may not yet be obvious. ■

Determine if the patient is in respiratory distress by inspecting the intercostal muscles (the muscles between the ribs) and the muscles above the suprasternal notch (the notch where the clavicles come together above the sternum). If the muscles are retracted inward during inhalation, it is likely that the patient is having a difficult time breathing. Look for flaring at the nostrils, use of the neck muscles, and excessive use of the abdominal muscles. If you suspect the patient is in respiratory failure, begin positive pressure ventilation with supplemental oxygen.

Quickly palpate the chest to confirm the findings of inspection. Check for symmetry of chest movement by placing the tips of your thumbs on the xiphoid process (the lower tip of the sternum) and spreading your hands over the lower rib cage. Both hands should move an equal distance with each breath. Apply slight pressure downward and inward on the rib cage. It may be easier to palpate for paradoxical movement in the chest wall rather than to see it on inspection, since muscle spasms usually keep the segment from moving dramatically. Also palpate for tenderness, subcutaneous emphysema, crepitation, and instability.

Use a stethoscope to auscultate for breath sounds (EMT Skills 13-5G). Listen to the breath sounds in the apices (top portions) and bases (bottom portions) of the lungs, comparing the left to the right side at each level. To assess each apex of the lung, place the stethoscope at the second intercostal space at the midclavicular line. Listen to each base at the fourth or fifth intercostal space in the midaxillary line. Listen during both inspiration and exhalation.

When listening to breath sounds, determine if the sounds are present and equal on both sides. Absent or diminished breath sounds on one side may indicate a serious lung or chest injury or bronchial obstruction.

If the breath sounds are absent or severely diminished on one side, quickly reassess the heart rate and quality, reassess respiratory rate and quality, assess for evidence of severe respiratory distress and hypoxia, and assess for jugular venous distention and tracheal deviation. Suspect a tension pneumothorax if the breath sounds are absent or severely diminished and the heart rate is increasing (tachycardia), the pulse is becoming weaker, the respiratory rate is increasing (tachypnea), ventilations are becoming more shallow, signs of respiratory distress are worsening, and signs of hypoxia are present.

A tension pneumothorax (a life-threatening condition) occurs when the injured lung is completely collapsed from air trapped in the pleural space. The pleural space continues to take in air and creates a high pressure, reducing the volume of the lung on the injured side. This pressure begins to shift over to the uninjured lung, compressing the heart, kinking the vena cava, and compressing the uninjured lung. This causes the signs and symptoms previously described. If the pressure is not released, the patient will rapidly deteriorate and become severely hypoxic.

Understanding BODY PROCESSES

Because of gravity, blood moves toward the feet and air travels toward the head. If the patient has suffered a pneumothorax (air trapped in the pleural space) and is standing or seated, the air will tend to collect in the top portion of the lungs (apex) near the clavicles. Thus the patient with a pneumothorax will likely have diminished breath sounds to the apex of the lungs early, whereas if the lung collapse is due to the presence of blood in the pleural space, breath sounds at the lower lobes of the lungs may be diminished early. ■

Prompt transport and calling for an ALS intercept is very important. ALS providers can provide lifesaving decompression of the pleural space and reverse the condition. If a nonporous or occlusive dressing is covering an open wound to the chest on the injured side, lift the dressing off the chest for a few seconds during exhalation to allow any trapped air to escape, then replace it.

During your examination of the chest, reassess the patient's adequacy of breathing by looking at the depth of rise and fall of the chest wall, listening and feeling for air movement, auscultating for adequate and full breath sounds, and assessing the rate. If the breathing appears to be inadequate at any time, begin positive pressure ventilation with supplemental oxygen.

All of the findings listed under "Critical (Unstable) Findings: The Chest" require immediate intervention and prompt transport to the emergency department.

Assess the Abdomen

Inspect the abdomen for evidence of deformities, contusions, abrasions, penetrations, burns, lacerations, and any other evidence of trauma. These signs could indicate trauma to the abdomen, the possibility of underlying abdominal organ injury, and life-threatening bleeding into the abdominal cavity.

While inspecting the abdomen, look for discoloration around the umbilicus (navel) and in the flank areas (sides). This is a sign that blood has collected in the abdomen. Usually this is not seen until several hours after the injury. It takes an extremely large amount of blood in the abdomen to produce abdominal distention, in which the abdomen appears to be abnormally large or swollen. By the time this is seen in the patient, it is an indication that a significant amount of blood has been lost in the abdominal cavity.

Critical (Unstable) Findings: The Abdomen	
Critical Finding:	Severe abdominal pain Abdominal tenderness on palpation Discoloration of the abdomen, especially in the flank areas or around the navel Abdominal rigidity (contracted abdominal muscles) Distended abdomen
Possibility:	Bleeding within the abdominal cavity, obstruction of the gastrointestinal tract Irritation of the lining of the abdomen (peritonitis)
Emergency Care:	Rapid transport upon recognition. Establish an airway, begin positive pressure ventilation if respiratory rate or tidal volume is inadequate, and administer oxygen.
Critical Finding:	Organs protruding from an abdominal laceration
Possibility:	Abdominal evisceration
Emergency Care:	Do not replace the organs. Rinse with sterile water or saline. Apply a wet sterile dressing. Cover that dressing with a large occlusive dressing. Rapid transport.
Establish an Airway:	Administer oxygen. Begin positive pressure ventilation if respiratory rate or tidal volume is inadequate.

Palpate each of the four quadrants of the abdomen with the pads of your fingers by placing one hand on top of the other and rolling the hands across the quadrant (EMT Skills 13-5H). Each quadrant should be quickly palpated once for tenderness, guarding (spasm of the abdominal muscles), and rigidity (hardness or stiffness from the contraction of the abdominal muscles). To get the most reliable exam, first palpate areas farthest from the pain.

Understanding BODY PROCESSES

Different signs and symptoms are produced by internal bleeding and by the spilled contents of ruptured organs. Blood in the abdominal cavity is not very irritating and will not produce serious pain, but it will cause the abdomen to become rigid or stiff. However, the peritoneum (abdominal lining) has a large number of sensory nerves that typically respond quickly and severely to irritating substances leaking from organs. Bleeding can occur behind the lining of the abdomen (retroperitoneal space). Since there are not many nerves located in this area, the bleeding and injury can be easily missed. ■

Tenderness is a pain response elicited when the abdomen is palpated. If the patient is unresponsive, watch his face for a grimace while palpating. This would indicate pain on palpation. Also when palpating, feel if the abdomen is firm or soft. A firm or rigid abdomen is due to guarding. This is an indication of organ injury or irritation of the abdominal lining. A soft abdomen is a normal finding.

The Markle test, or heel jar test, is another way to assess for rebound tenderness and possible internal injury to abdominal organs. With the patient supine, strike the bottom of the heel sharply with your clenched fist, using enough force to shake and jar the abdomen (review Figure 13-19). If there is an existing irritation of the peritoneum (abdominal lining), for example by contents spilled from an injured or ruptured organ, the result of the heel strike will be a sharp pain to the abdomen. The responsive patient will report the pain; the patient who is responsive to pain will likely grimace.

Assess the Pelvis

Inspect the pelvis (EMT Skills 13-5I) for any evidence of trauma: deformities, contusions, abrasions, penetrations, burns, lacerations, or swelling. If the patient complains of pain or has obvious deformity to the pelvic region, you should suspect a pelvic injury. Do not palpate the pelvis if an injury is suspected.

Critical (Unstable) Findings: The Pelvis	
Critical Finding:	Pain to the pelvis without palpation Tenderness or instability on palpation of iliac crest or symphysis pubis
Possibility:	Pelvic fracture
Emergency Care:	Rapid transport. Administer oxygen. Establish an airway and begin positive pressure ventilation if respiratory rate or tidal volume is inadequate. Stabilize the pelvis.

If the patient is not complaining of any pain in the pelvic region, or no deformities are noted, place each hand on the iliac crest and gently compress the pelvis inward and downward. Also compress the symphysis pubis for any tenderness, facial grimace, or instability. Note any instability, crepitation, tenderness, or deformity.

ASSESSMENT Tips

A pelvic fracture can be associated with severe bleeding. Be prepared to treat hemorrhagic shock in a patient with a pelvic fracture. ■

Assess the Extremities

Assess first the lower, then the upper, extremities (EMT Skills 13-5J to 13-5N). Inspect and palpate the extremities for deformities, contusions, abrasions, penetrations, burns, tenderness, lacerations, swelling, and any other evidence of trauma. Trauma to the extremities rarely produces life-threatening injuries. Major bleeding will be your major concern. Like the pelvis, a fractured femur may lead to profuse bleeding from the bone and surrounding blood vessels. Since bone and joint injuries are usually not life threatening, splinting in the critical patient must be conducted en route to the hospital and not at the scene. Too much time is lost when splints are applied at the scene of an incident.

Following inspection and palpation, check for "PMS"—distal pulses, motor function, and sensation:

- **Pulses.** Check distal pulses in all extremities. In the lower extremities, check the dorsalis pedis pulse. This is the pulse that is located on the top of the foot approximately midway between the toes and the ankle on the big toe side. Another distal pulse that could be assessed in the lower extremities is the posterior tibial pulse. This pulse is located behind the medial malleolus, the knob at the inner side of the ankle.

  When assessing for either pulse, bare the area where the pulse is to be felt. In the upper extremities, assess for a radial pulse. The radial pulse is located on the thumb side near the anterior base of the wrist.

  Determine if pulses are present in each extremity. Compare the strength of the pulses of each extremity. Absent or weak pulses could indicate poor perfusion from shock, a pinched or damaged artery from a bone injury, or a blood clot blocking circulation. When feeling for the pulse, also note the patient's skin color, temperature, and condition in each extremity as an indication of perfusion.
- **Motor Function.** If the patient is able to obey commands, ask the patient to wiggle his toes and squeeze your fingers. Simply determine if the patient can move his fingers and toes.
- **Sensation.** In a responsive patient, touch a finger on one hand and ask the patient to identify what finger

Critical (Unstable) Findings: The Extremities	
Critical Finding:	Open wound with spurting or steadily flowing blood loss
Possibility:	Lacerated artery or vein
Emergency Care:	Apply direct pressure to the wound. Apply pressure dressing. If not controlled with direct pressure, apply a tourniquet. Rapid transport. Administer oxygen.
Critical Finding:	Pain, swelling, discoloration, and deformity to thigh
Possibility:	Femur fracture
Emergency Care:	Application of a traction splint. Rapid transport. Administer oxygen.

you are touching. Then pinch the hand and ask the patient to identify the extremity with pain. (Test both light touch and pain, since each of these stimuli is carried by a different nerve tract in the spinal cord.) Repeat this procedure on the other hand and then each foot, using the toes.

Understanding BODY PROCESSES

The sensation of light touch and the sensation of pain are carried by different nerve tracts within the spinal cord. It is possible that a patient who can feel light touch in an extremity may be unable to feel pain in that same extremity because of an incomplete injury of the spinal cord. ■

If the patient is unresponsive, pinch the hand or foot and watch the response. It is important in the unresponsive patient to note the motor response associated with the painful stimulus applied to the extremity. Be careful when interpreting the response to pain applied to an extremity, since it may be the spinal cord returning the impulse and not the brain.

Understanding BODY PROCESSES

When a painful stimulus is applied to an extremity, it may travel to the spinal cord and be returned immediately by the spinal cord through a reflex arc. The result will be movement in the pinched extremity, without the impulse ever having been transmitted to the brain. This could provide a false finding in a patient who you think is responding to a painful stimulus when he is actually unresponsive. ■

Injury to the femur is an exception to the rule that extremity injuries are not life threatening. Injury to the femur could result in severe bleeding within the bone and around the muscle and tissue in the leg. Therefore, injury to the femur is considered critical. If the thigh is discovered to be painful, swollen, or deformed and a femur fracture is suspected, immobilize the patient on a backboard and initiate prompt transport.

Assess the Posterior Body

With in-line spinal stabilization being maintained, roll the patient to inspect and palpate the posterior aspect of the body (EMT Skills 13-5O). With the patient positioned on his side, quickly inspect the posterior thorax, lumbar region, buttocks, and backs of the legs. Look for deformities, contusions, abrasions, punctures, burns, lacerations, swelling, or any other evidence of injury. Any open wound to the posterior thorax must be covered with an occlusive dressing.

If the patient is not complaining of pain along the vertebrae, lightly and gently palpate the vertebral column for any deformity and tenderness. Be extremely careful not to move the patient or cause excessive pain when palpating. This may jeopardize the in-line stabilization. If the patient is complaining of pain, assume that a spinal injury exists. Provide complete spinal immobilization.

With the patient on his side, place a backboard alongside him and roll him back down onto the backboard. Continue manual in-line stabilization until the patient is completely secured to the backboard.

Critical (Unstable) Findings: The Posterior Body	
Critical Finding:	Open wound to the posterior thorax
Possibility:	Sucking chest wound Lung injury (pneumothorax)
Emergency Care:	Occlude the open wound immediately with a gloved hand and then with a nonporous dressing or occlusive dressing taped on three sides. Rapid transport upon recognition. Consider ALS intercept. Establish an airway, begin positive pressure ventilation if respiratory rate or tidal volume is inadequate, and administer oxygen. *Caution:* Aggressive PPV may worsen a lung injury.
Critical Finding:	Open wound with spurting or steadily flowing blood loss

Key Points
In the rapid secondary assessment for the trauma patient, the vital sign assessment follows the physical exam and precedes the SAMPLE history. However, if enough trained personnel are present, these steps may overlap.

Key Points
Any SpO_2 less than 95% should heighten suspicion of hypoxia. Look for other evidence and a cause for the hypoxia and take steps to ensure adequate respiration and oxygenation.

Critical (Unstable) Findings: The Posterior Body *continued*

Possibility:	Lacerated artery or vein
Emergency Care:	Apply direct pressure to the wound. Apply pressure dressing if possible. Rapid transport. Administer oxygen.

Assess Baseline Vital Signs

In the rapid secondary assessment for the trauma patient, vital sign assessment follows the physical exam and precedes the SAMPLE history. However, if you have enough assistance and can be sure that in-line stabilization is being maintained by a trained person, these steps may overlap. For example, one EMT may be able to get vital sign measurements while the other conducts the physical exam, or vital signs and history may be taken at the same time.

The methods for assessing the vital signs were discussed in Chapter 11, "Baseline Vital Signs, Monitoring Devices, and History Taking." The vital signs are reviewed briefly here with notes about vital sign assessment for the trauma patient:

- **Breathing.** Assess the rate, tidal volume, and quality of breathing. Determine the quality of breathing as normal, shallow, labored, deep, or noisy. (See Table 13-5 regarding adequate and inadequate breathing.)
- **Pulse.** Assess the radial pulse in the adult and child patient and the brachial pulse in an infant less than 1 year of age. If the radial pulse is not present, assess the carotid pulse. If there is a carotid pulse (central pulse) but no radial pulse (peripheral pulse), or if the radial pulse is weak and rapid, the patient is likely to be suffering from shock (hypoperfusion).

ASSESSMENT Tips

A pulse that becomes very weak or disappears only when the patient inhales may indicate shock from blood loss, a tension pneumothorax, or pericardial tamponade. ■

- **Skin.** The skin is assessed to determine the perfusion status of the patient. Inspect for pale or cyanotic nail beds and pale skin, oral mucosa, and conjunctiva. Feel the skin with the back of the hand for the temperature and condition. Pale, cool, clammy skin is a strong indication of poor tissue perfusion. A trauma patient with tachycardia (rapid pulse) and pale, cool, clammy skin should be assumed to be in shock.

  Assess for capillary refill. A delayed capillary refill may indicate poor tissue perfusion and shock. However, cold exposure and other conditions may lengthen the capillary refill time, making it a less reliable sign of shock. Capillary refill alone cannot identify a shock patient. You must look at several different assessment findings to determine a shock state.
- **Pupil.** Quickly assess the pupils for size and reactivity by shining a light into the patient's eyes. Poor perfusion could cause the pupils to dilate and respond sluggishly to light, so this sign may be considered along with other indicators of shock. Head injury may cause the pupils to become unequal and unresponsive to light.
- **Blood pressure.** Take the blood pressure by auscultation. Determine the systolic and diastolic pressure. Two signs of serious blood loss and shock are narrow pulse pressure (the difference between the systolic and diastolic pressures) and hypotension (low blood pressure). If the blood pressure cannot be auscultated because of excessive noise at the scene, use the palpation method. Since palpation provides only the systolic pressure, pulse pressure cannot be determined by this method.
- **Pulse oximeter.** The pulse oximeter (Figure 13-28✱) can be applied to determine the level of oxygenation. Any SpO_2 reading less than 95% should heighten your suspicion that the patient is hypoxic. You must look for other evidence and a cause for the hypoxia. Closely assess the respiratory status, to include rate and tidal volume, to be sure that both are adequate. Be aggressive with airway management, positive pressure ventilation, and oxygen therapy. Be careful when using the pulse oximeter in patients with suspected hypoperfusion or shock. You may not get a reading on the pulse oximeter or the reading may be erroneous because of the poor perfusion status and blood loss.

Critical (Unstable) Findings: Baseline Vital Signs

Critical Finding:	Inadequate respiratory rate Inadequate tidal volume (poor air movement)
Possibility:	Lung injury with excessive buildup of pressure in the pleural space (tension pneumothorax) Complete collapse of one or both lungs (pneumothorax) Severe chest wall pain from injury that causes the patient to breathe shallowly Head or spinal cord injury Injury to the diaphragm (rupture or laceration) from trauma to the chest or abdomen
Emergency Care:	Rapid transport upon recognition. Consider ALS intercept. Establish an airway, begin positive pressure ventilation if respiratory rate or tidal volume is inadequate, and administer oxygen. *Caution:* Aggressive PPV may worsen a lung injury.
Critical Finding:	Absent carotid pulse in the adult or child greater than 1 year of age Absent brachial pulse in an infant less than 1 year of age No movement, breathing, or other signs of life
Possibility:	Cardiac arrest
Emergency Care:	Immediately initiate CPR, beginning with chest compressions, and apply the automated external defibrillator (AED) according to your AED protocol. In a cardiac arrest patient who has suffered traumatic injuries immediately initiate CPR, beginning with chest compressions, manage the traumatic injuries, and follow your local protocol regarding application of the AED. Call for ALS intercept.
Critical Finding:	Cool, clammy skin, weak pulses, rapid heart rate (tachycardia), decreasing systolic blood pressure, narrow pulse pressure, delayed capillary refill
Possibility:	Hypoperfusion (shock)
Emergency Care:	Stop any bleeding. Administer oxygen. Rapid transport. Splint fractures.
Critical Finding:	Unequal pupils Fixed pupil
Possibility:	Head injury
Emergency Care:	Establish an airway, begin positive pressure ventilation if respiratory rate or tidal volume is inadequate, and administer oxygen.
Critical Finding:	SpO_2 reading of less than 95%
Possibility:	Hypoxia associated with an injury, occluded airway, or inadequate respiration
Emergency Care:	If the breathing is adequate, administer oxygen. If the breathing is inadequate, establish an airway and begin positive pressure ventilation with supplemental oxygen connected to the ventilation device.

Blood Glucose Test

The blood glucose level (BGL) is not considered one of the vital signs; however, any patient who presents with an altered mental status may be suffering from a low BGL (a low blood sugar level). This condition is referred to as hypoglycemia (low blood glucose). A test can be performed using a drop of the patient's blood and an electronic glucometer (Figure 13-29*) to determine the blood glucose level. This may guide your treatment of the patient and provide you with an indication of whether to administer glucose to the patient or not. Refer to Chapter 11, "Baseline Vital Signs, Monitoring Devices, and History Taking," to review blood glucose measurement. Hypoglycemia will be discussed in Chapter 20, "Acute Diabetic Emergencies."

The vital signs should be reassessed and recorded every 5 minutes in the unstable patient. In the stable patient, the vitals should be reassessed and recorded a minimum of every 15 minutes. Consider any trauma patient with a significant mechanism of injury to be unstable and assess vital signs every 5 minutes.

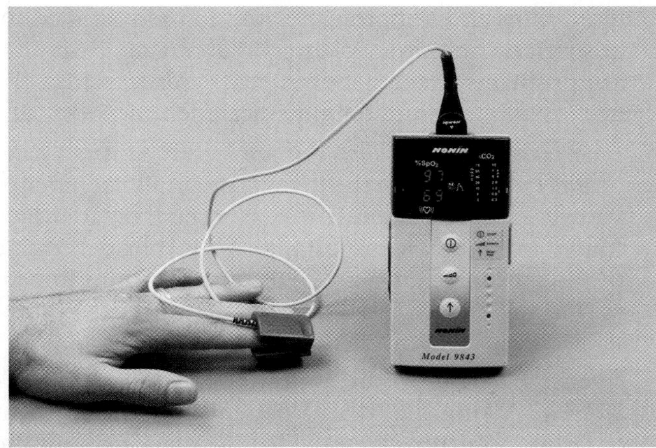

FIGURE 13-28 ✻ Apply a pulse oximeter to measure the arterial blood oxygen level.

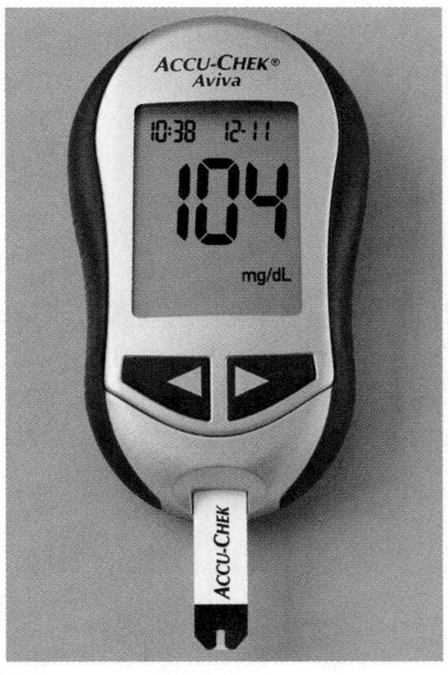

FIGURE 13-29 ✻ Use an electronic glucometer, such as this Roche Accu-Chek Aviva, to measure the blood glucose level. (© Roche Diagnostics Corporation, Indianapolis, Indiana)

Understanding BODY PROCESSES

A narrowing pulse pressure (where the systolic and diastolic pressure readings get closer together) typically occurs when the amount of blood being ejected from the left ventricle decreases (systolic blood pressure measure) while the vessels constrict, decreasing their diameter and increasing resistance (diastolic blood pressure measure), in an attempt to increase the blood pressure. ■

ASSESSMENT Tips

A palpated systolic blood pressure is an average of 7 mmHg lower than an auscultated systolic blood pressure. ■

ASSESSMENT Tips

A systolic blood pressure that suddenly drops more than 10 mmHg only when the patient inhales may indicate shock from blood loss, a tension pneumothorax, or pericardial tamponade. ■

Understanding BODY PROCESSES

If a patient is bleeding, there are fewer red blood cells available to become oxygenated. This may produce a false high SpO_2 reading, since the remaining smaller number of red blood cells are oxygenated. However, there are not enough red blood cells carrying oxygen to the cells, and so the cells remain hypoxic. ■

ASSESSMENT Tips

A normal blood glucose level in a nondiabetic patient who has had nothing to eat or has had no drink containing sugar or other carbohydrates for 8–12 hours is, on average, 80–90 mg/dL. It may range from 70–100 mg/dL. Shortly after a meal and for an hour or so, the nondiabetic BGL is usually 120–140 mg/dL. ■

Obtain a SAMPLE History

For a trauma patient, the SAMPLE history follows the physical exam and vital signs measurements. With two EMTs working together, the SAMPLE history can be conducted while the physical exam and vital signs are being assessed, or—if the patient is responsive—the SAMPLE history can be taken en route to the hospital. If the patient is unresponsive, you must attempt to get as much of the history as possible from family members or bystanders prior to leaving the scene.

History taking and questioning should not interfere with any assessment or treatment of life threats or delay transport of a critically injured patient.

Methods of obtaining a SAMPLE history were covered in Chapter 11, "Baseline Vital Signs, Monitoring Devices, and History Taking." The elements of the SAMPLE history are reviewed briefly here with notes about their relevance for the trauma patient with a significant mechanism of injury:

- **Signs.** *During your assessment, you are continuously inspecting for signs of trauma.* Deformities, contusions, abrasions, punctures, burns, lacerations, swelling, and indication of pain on palpation (tenderness) are all signs of blunt or penetrating trauma. It is important to correlate the sign with the mechanism of injury to focus your index of suspicion on specific possible injuries.
- **Symptoms.** *How do you feel? Do you hurt anywhere? What symptoms are you experiencing? (If the patient is*

unresponsive, ask bystanders if he complained of pain or any other symptoms before losing consciousness.) The patient may complain of pain, light-headedness, weakness, dizziness, dyspnea, numbness, tingling, nausea, or many other symptoms associated with trauma. Any complaints of dyspnea, severe headache, chest pain, or abdominal pain should cause you to closely examine the related area for life-threatening injuries. For example, a patient who is complaining of dyspnea should be examined closely for possible life-threatening chest injuries such as a flail segment, open chest wound, or air in the chest cavity. Symptoms are gathered throughout assessment. Signs, symptoms, and mechanism of injury are the basis for emergency care provided to trauma patients.

- **Allergies.** *Do you have any allergies? Are you allergic to any medications?* For the trauma patient, gather information on allergies to medications that may be important for the medical facility staff to know about. Look for a medical tag that may identify an allergy.
- **Medications.** *Are you currently taking any medications?* In the trauma patient, it is not extremely important to gather extensive information regarding the prescription or over-the-counter medications the patient is currently taking. However, this information may help to provide a medical history in the unresponsive trauma patient, and some medications may alter the signs and symptoms expected in some conditions or may cause the patient to decompensate (succumb to shock) faster. For example, beta blocker drugs are frequently taken to control hypertension and heart rhythms. A beta blocker will slow the heart rate. A patient who is on a beta blocker and is in shock may not have the classic signs of shock, such as tachycardia or clammy skin. Also, this patient will not compensate well and will deteriorate more quickly.

ASSESSMENT Tips

If the patient is taking a beta blocker or calcium channel blocker drug, the heart rate may remain slower than expected in some conditions, such as shock. Therefore, the one significant sign of shock that might **not** be seen in this patient is tachycardia, because of the effects of the drugs. ■

Gather whatever information about medications you can, but do not expend any extra time at the scene to determine the patient's medications. This information is not vital for the trauma patient.

- **Pertinent Past Medical History.** *Have you had any recent illnesses? Have you been seeing a doctor for any condition?* Quickly determine the medical history from the patient or, if the patient is unresponsive, from a family member. A patient with an existing medical condition may decompensate faster and exhibit altered signs and symptoms related to the past medical or surgical condition. Ask quickly about any past medical problems, trauma, or surgeries. Also, inspect the neck and extremities for a medical identification tag.
- **Last Oral Intake.** *When did you last eat or drink anything?* Find out from the patient or family member or knowledgeable bystander the last time the patient ate solid food or drank any liquids. If possible, determine the approximate amount. This information is important to the hospital staff if the patient needs anesthesia for surgery.
- **Events Leading to the Injury.** *How did the incident happen?* Asking the trauma patient how the accident or injury occurred can provide information about the mechanism of injury. Information from the patient or bystanders may shed additional light on the mechanism of injury, for example the height from which the patient fell. It is also important to determine why an accident occurred. Did the patient get dizzy and swerve off the road? Was the patient having chest pain that caused him to fall down the stairs? Did the patient lose consciousness before wrecking the car? A patient in an automobile crash who tells you that he was driving 90 mph because he was shot in the abdomen and was trying to get to the hospital has a clear mechanism of injury that provides you with suspicions of other injuries. Knowing what events led up to the accident or incident could also be helpful in determining if an illness exists in addition to the trauma.

Prepare the Patient for Transport

Normally, the critical trauma patient is prepared for transport simultaneously as the rapid secondary assessment is being conducted. Other EMTs and First Responder personnel should be preparing the backboard, head immobilization device, and stretcher. Following or simultaneously with assessment of the vital signs, the patient is secured to the backboard with straps. The head is immobilized with a head immobilization device or blanket rolls and tape (Figure 13-30*). The patient should then be transported to the cot and into the ambulance. (The SAMPLE history can be taken during this process or delayed to be taken in the ambulance.) Techniques for immobilization and transfer of the patient to the ambulance are covered in detail in Chapter 32, "Spinal Column and Spinal Cord Trauma," and Chapter 6, "Lifting and Moving Patients."

Once the patient is completely immobilized, transport should not be delayed. If any critical findings are present and the trauma patient is unstable, on-scene time should be limited to 10 minutes or less. See Table 13-11 for factors to consider as part of a decision for prompt transport. Bear in mind that prompt transport is key in survival of the critically injured patient.

To ensure the best chance of survival in certain situations, the trauma patient must be transported to an

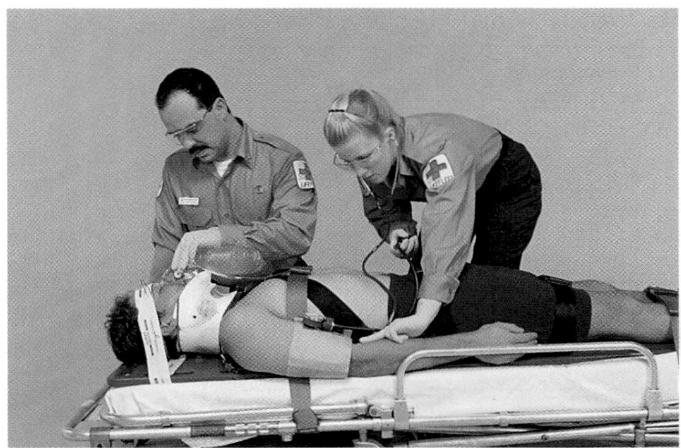

FIGURE 13-30 ✱ Prepare the patient for transport.

TABLE 13-11 Indications for a 10-Minutes-or-Less On-Scene Time and Rapid Transport

- Airway occlusion or difficulty in maintaining a patent airway
- Respiratory rate < 10/minute or > 29/minute
- Inadequate tidal volume
- Hypoxia (SpO_2 < 95%)
- Respiratory distress, failure, or arrest
- Open wound to chest
- Flail chest
- Suspected pneumothorax
- Uncontrolled external hemorrhage
- Suspected internal hemorrhage
- Signs and symptoms of shock
- Significant external blood loss with controlled hemorrhage
- GCS 13 or less
- Altered mental status
- Seizure activity
- Sensory or motor deficit
- Any penetrating trauma to the head, neck, anterior or posterior chest and abdomen, and above the elbow or knee
- Amputation of an extremity proximal to the finger
- Trauma in a patient with significant medical history (MI, COPD, CHF), > 55 years of age, hypothermia, burns, and pregnancy

appropriate trauma center. The decision should be based on physiological criteria, such as blood pressure, respiratory rate, and Glasgow Coma Scale score; anatomical criteria, such as where the patient was injured; mechanism of injury; and special considerations, such as age and medical history. The Centers for Disease Control has developed the *Field Triage Decision Scheme: The National Trauma Triage Protocol* to assist EMS providers with making a decision regarding destination of transport. This protocol (Figure 13-31✱) provides objective criteria and recommendations for rapid transport to a trauma center.

Provide Emergency Care

In addition to the interventions that have been mentioned for each critical finding listed in this section, the information that follows provides overall advice about emergency care based on the rapid secondary assessment.

The entire rapid secondary assessment is typically conducted in a period of about 2–2½ minutes. This includes the head-to-toe assessment, baseline vital signs, and SAMPLE history. For this kind of patient, who is likely to be in critical condition, the head-to-toe assessment should identify any immediately life-threatening injuries and conditions, as well as any other less severe injuries or problems the patient may have.

A decision to rapidly transport the patient is made based on the findings of the rapid secondary assessment. Any of the critical findings summarized in Table 13-11 is an indication for prompt transport, with further treatment and continued assessment to take place en route to the hospital. *However, life-threatening injuries and conditions must be appropriately managed as found at the scene prior to transport.* In critical patients, splinting for suspected bone or joint injuries is not done at the scene because these injuries are not life threatening, with the exception of a suspected fracture to the pelvis or femur if adequate resources are available and transport is not delayed to apply the splint.

During transport, the life threats are reassessed while further evaluating the patient and providing care, as possible, for additional conditions or injuries that are not immediately life threatening.

If the patient's condition is stable, emergency treatment for non-life-threatening conditions or injuries may be completed at the scene before transport. However, in a trauma patient with a significant mechanism of injury or a critical finding, a decision to transport rapidly is likely.

En route to the hospital, your priority is to continuously reassess the components of the primary assessment—mental status, airway, breathing, and circulation—plus vital signs and components of the rapid secondary assessment focused on the patient's injuries. You will also reassess the effectiveness of your interventions. This is known as a reassessment and is described in Part 4 of this chapter.

You must set priorities for management of critical injuries and conditions both at the scene and throughout the transport to the hospital. If a patient has suffered blunt trauma to the face with significant bleeding in the upper airway, the EMT caring for the patient in the back of the ambulance is most concerned with maintaining a patent airway. This can only be done with continuous suction. In addition, the EMT must reassess the breathing and perfusion status and reassess vital signs.

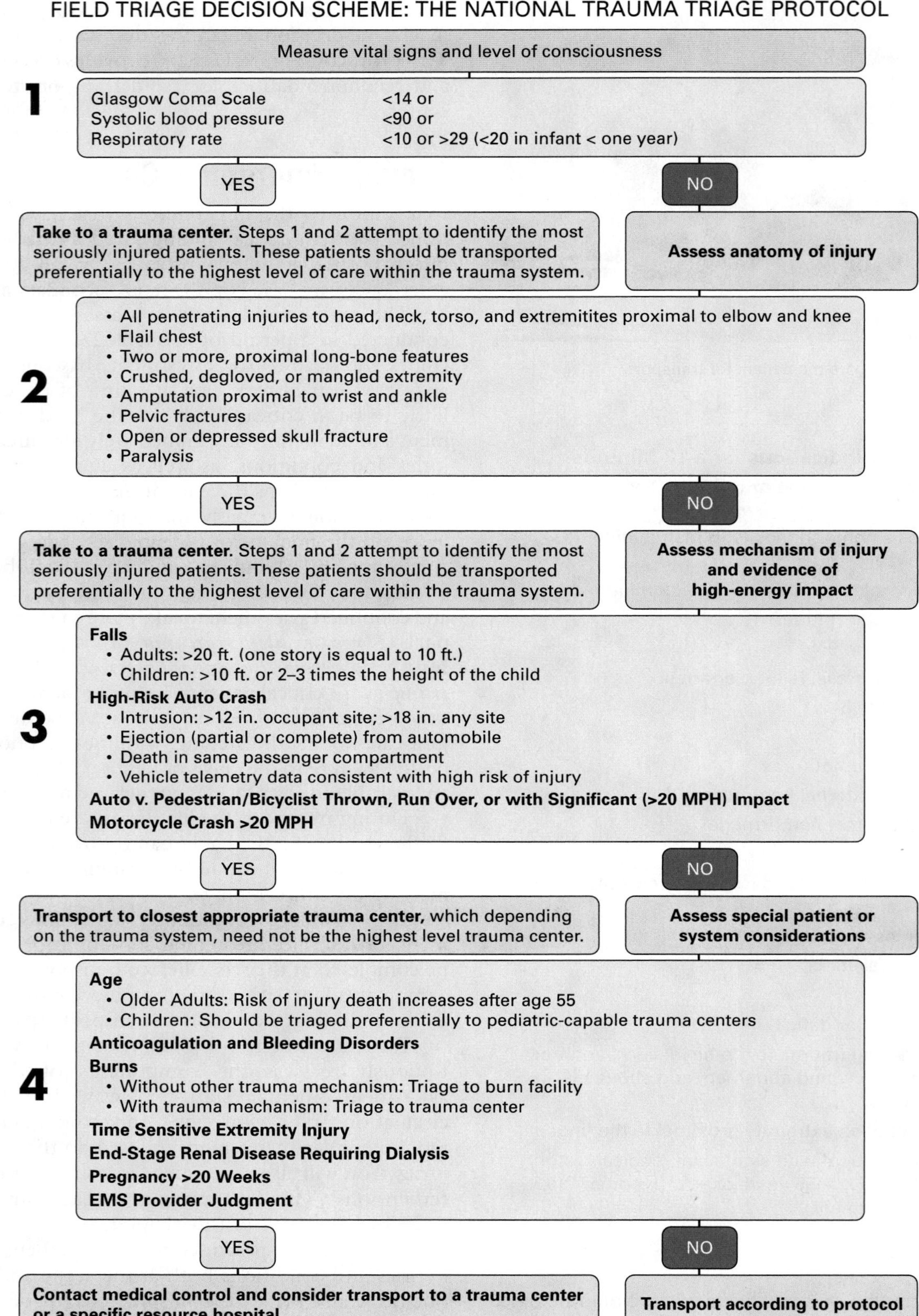

FIGURE 13-31 ✱ Field Triage Decision Scheme: The National Trauma Triage Protocol.

Objective 13-24
Explain the purpose and elements of the trauma score.

Objective 13-25
Discuss how to conduct a modified secondary assessment for a trauma patient with no significant mechanism of injury, altered mental status, multiple injuries, or critical finding (stable patient).Using the AVPU method, assess and document the level of responsiveness.

Management of the airway takes precedence over any other condition and over any additional assessment.

Trauma Score

A trauma score is a numerical way to identify the severity of trauma. Many EMS systems use the scoring system as a means to communicate the severity of the patient to the receiving facility. You should be familiar with the trauma scoring system used in your region and be familiar with the elements of that scoring system.

The Revised Trauma Score (Table 13-12), which includes the Glasgow Coma Scale, is one type of scoring system used. A number is assigned to each parameter being assessed. The numbers from each subset are totaled and a score is derived for that particular patient. The lower the score, the more severe the patient's condition.

The major components of the trauma score are:

- Respiratory rate
- Systolic blood pressure
- Glasgow Coma Scale (GCS) score

Report and document the findings of the Revised Trauma Score. This information is extremely useful to the receiving facility for purposes of reassessment.

Modified Secondary Assessment: Trauma Patient with *NO* Significant Mechanism of Injury, Altered Mental Status, Multiple Injuries, or Critical Finding (*Stable*)

On the prior pages, we discussed how to conduct the secondary assessment when you have determined that the patient has a significant mechanism of injury, altered mental status, multiple injuries, or a critical finding. Here we will discuss the trauma patient whose mechanism of injury is not significant, who is alert and oriented, who does not have multiple injuries, and for whom no critical findings are present. If you are ever in doubt as to what assessment to perform, err to benefit the patient and perform the rapid secondary assessment to avoid missing injuries.

Perform a Modified Secondary Assessment

Consider a patient whose injury is a laceration to one finger that resulted from a slip of the knife while cutting a tomato. The finger may be bleeding profusely, but the mechanism of injury is not significant—that is, it is a mechanism that does not lead you to suspect additional injuries or problems, the patient is alert, and no critical findings are present.

For this patient, a complete head-to-toe rapid secondary assessment is not necessary or appropriate. Instead, you conduct a modified secondary assessment—an exam that focuses primarily on the injury site, in this case the injured finger. You use the same techniques as in a secondary assessment—inspecting and palpating for deformities, contusions, abrasions, punctures, burns, tenderness, lacerations, and swelling—but you assess just the specific localized site of the injury. For the patient with the cut finger, you have already controlled the bleeding as part of the primary assessment, and now you conduct the modified secondary assessment to ensure that there is no further injury to the patient's hand or arm, such as a burn or a bone or joint injury.

Another example is a suspected bone or joint injury. Earlier, it was stated that injuries to the extremities are seldom life threatening, and that complete assessment and treatment of such injuries for a critical trauma patient would not take place at the scene. Instead, treatment would be carried out in the ambulance en route to the hospital if time and care of the patient's more serious problems permit. However, for the patient who has no significant mechanism of injury, is alert and oriented, has no multiple injuries, and has no critical findings, but presents with indications of a possible fracture or other injury to a bone or joint, full assessment and splinting of the injured extremity would be carried out at the scene before transport to the hospital.

For instance, a high school student is playing volleyball and jumps up for the ball. She lands on the lateral aspect of her right ankle with her leg in a twisted position. You are called to the scene. The patient is complaining of severe pain to her ankle. You perform a scene size-up and brief primary assessment and determine that no significant

TABLE 13-12 The Revised Trauma Score with Glasgow Coma Scale

Brief Neurological Evaluation

A—**Alert**

V—Responds to **Verbal** stimuli

P—Responds to **Painful** stimuli

U—**Unresponsive**

Revised Trauma Index

TRAUMA SCORE

Operational Definitions

Respiratory Rate

Number of respirations in 15 seconds; multiply by 4

Systolic Blood Pressure

Systolic cuff pressure, either arm—auscultate or palpate

No pulse—no carotid pulse

Best Verbal Response

Arouse patient with voice or painful stimulus

Best Motor Response

Response to command or painful stimulus

Projected estimate of survival for each value of the Trauma Score based on results from 1,509 patients with blunt or penetrating injury[2]

Trauma Score	Percentage Survival
12	99
11	97
10	88
9	77
8	67
7	64
6	63
5	46
4	33
3	33
2	29
1	25
0	4

REVISED TRAUMA SCORE

The Trauma Score is a numerical grading system for estimating the severity of injury.[1] The score is composed of the Glasgow Coma Scale (reduced to approximately one-third total value) and measurements of cardiopulmonary function. Each parameter is given a number (high for normal and low for impaired function). Severity of injury is estimated by summing the numbers. The lowest score is 0 and the highest score is 12.

Respiratory Rate	10–29/min	4
	> 29/min	3
	6–9/min	2
	1–5/min	1
	None (0/min)	0
Systolic Blood Pressure	> 89 mmHg	4
	76–89 mmHg	3
	50–75 mmHg	2
	1–49 mmHg	1
	No Pulse or 0 SBP (Systolic Blood Pressure)	0
Trauma Scale Total		

GLASGOW COMA SCALE

			Total Glasgow Coma Scale Points
Eye Opening	Spontaneous	4	
	To verbal command	3	
	To pain	2	
	No response	1	
Verbal Response	Oriented and converses	5	
	Disoriented and converses	4	13 – 15 = 4
	Inappropriate words	3	9 – 12 = 3
	Incomprehensible sounds	2	6 – 8 = 2
	No response	1	4 – 5 = 1
Motor Response	Obeys verbal commands	6	< 4 = 0
	Localizes pain	5	
	Withdraws from pain (flexion)	4	
	Abnormal flexion in response to pain (decorticate rigidity)	3	
	Extension in response to pain (decerebrate rigidity)	2	
	No response	1	
Glasgow Coma Scale Total			
Total Trauma Score (Trauma Scale + GCS)			0–12

Source: A Revision of the Trauma Score. (1989). *Journal of Trauma, 29*(5), 623–629.

[1]Champion, H. R., Sacco, W. J., Carnazzo, A. J., et al. (1981). Trauma Score. *Critical Care Medicine, 9*(9), 672–676.

[2]Endorsed by the American Trauma Society.

Key Points

If there is any doubt about whether you should perform a complete rapid trauma assessment or a modified trauma assessment focused on the injury, always err to benefit the patient and perform a complete rapid trauma assessment.

Objective 13-26

Explain circumstances when you should perform a complete, rather than a modified, secondary assessment on a trauma patient with no significant mechanism of injury.

mechanism of injury has occurred, the patient is alert and oriented, and no multiple or critical injuries exist. You would immediately focus in on the ankle injury and inspect and palpate the entire extremity. Then you would immobilize the ankle while still at the scene.

To assess an upper or lower extremity when a bone or joint injury is suspected, inspect for deformity (such as angulation to a bone where no joint exists), contusions, and swelling. Palpate by placing your hands around the entire extremity so that the thumbs come together on the anterior surface and the little fingers are on the posterior surface. Your thumbs and fingers should never lose contact with the extremity during the palpation. Begin at the most proximal point (closest to the heart) and palpate to the most distal point (farthest from the heart), noting any deformity, swelling, tenderness, or crepitation.

Following inspection and palpation, check the distal pulses, motor function, and sensation. Always assess distal pulses, motor function, and sensation both before the injury is splinted (to detect any impairment of function caused by the injury) and after the injury is splinted (to detect any improvement or deterioration of function resulting from the intervention). Be sure to document this assessment on the prehospital care report.

Obtain Baseline Vital Signs and SAMPLE History

Once the modified secondary assessment is completed, assess the baseline vital signs and obtain the SAMPLE history. Then provide emergency care for the injuries found and prepare the patient for transport. While en route to the hospital, reassess the airway, breathing, and perfusion; reassess vital signs; and check the effectiveness of the emergency care provided.

Perform a Rapid Secondary Assessment If Indicated

Although the modified secondary assessment is usually appropriate for a trauma patient with no significant mechanism of injury, no altered mental status, no evidence of multiple injuries, and no critical finding, occasionally it is wise to conduct a full head-to-toe secondary assessment.

One such instance would be when you undertake a modified secondary assessment in a patient with no significant mechanism of injury but you develop a suspicion that more injuries may exist than what the patient is complaining of, or the patient begins to deteriorate. In this case, immediately conduct a complete secondary assessment.

Another instance would be when you are conducting a modified secondary assessment on a patient and you make a critical finding. Immediately perform a secondary assessment and consider prompt transport. For example, you arrive on the scene and find a patient lying on the kitchen floor complaining of pain to his left hip. He says that he slipped on some water and fell. The mechanism of injury is not significant, and the primary assessment does not reveal any critical findings. Therefore, you decide to perform a modified secondary assessment on the left hip area, extending to the pelvis and both lower extremities. When you begin to palpate the pelvis, the patient complains of severe pain and you feel instability and crepitation. A pelvic injury is considered a critical finding, so you quickly conduct a secondary assessment, assess baseline vitals, and prepare the patient for immediate transport. En route, you reassess airway, breathing, and perfusion; reassess vital signs; complete the SAMPLE history; and reassess the abdomen, pelvis, and lower extremities.

Another kind of patient with no significant mechanism of injury and no critical findings, who nevertheless must have a complete secondary assessment, is the patient suffering from multiple injuries each of which, by itself, would not be considered critical. The patient may have multiple minor soft tissue injuries. Or the patient may have suspected multiple fractures to the extremities. In either situation, the multiple injuries may indicate a more significant mechanism of injury than was first suspected. The multiple injuries may also, cumulatively, be causing significant internal or external blood loss and shock. For this patient, perform a head-to-toe assessment and, if these are critical findings, consider prompt transport.

Remember: If there is any question in your mind as to what assessment to perform on a patient—the limited modified secondary assessment versus the complete secondary assessment—err to benefit the patient and conduct the complete secondary assessment.

Objective 13-27
Name the key differences in the secondary assessment for the responsive medical patient versus the unresponsive medical patient with regard to the sequence of steps and the appropriate type of physical exam (modified or rapid).

Key Points
A medical patient is one who has not suffered any type of injury or trauma but instead is experiencing signs and symptoms related to a disease or condition affecting the body's organs or systems.

Secondary Assessment: Medical Patient

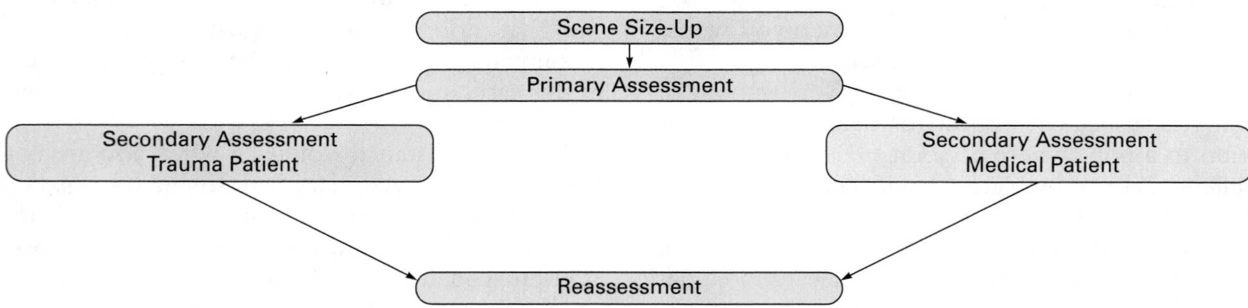

A medical patient has not suffered from any type of injury or trauma, but instead is experiencing signs and symptoms related to a disease process or condition affecting the body's organs or systems.

As was true for the trauma patient, you will perform the secondary assessment on the medical patient (Figure 13-32∗) immediately following the primary assessment. Life-threatening conditions of the airway, breathing, and circulation will have already been managed as part of the primary assessment. Further emergency care will be based on your findings from the secondary assessment.

First, you will categorize the medical patient in one of three ways: as alert, oriented, and responsive; or as not alert, disoriented, and responsive to only verbal or painful stimuli; or as unresponsive. For ease of categorization, the alert, oriented, and responsive patient will be referred to as "responsive" and the patient who is not alert, is disoriented, is responsive to verbal or painful stimuli, or is unresponsive will be referred to as "unresponsive."

ASSESSMENT Tips

A responsive medical patient is one who not only responds to your questions and commands but responds appropriately. If the patient responds, but not appropriately, consider the patient's responses to be unreliable and conduct a rapid secondary assessment. ■

There are two key differences in the way you will conduct the secondary assessment for the responsive medical patient versus the unresponsive medical patient.

The first difference is in the sequence of steps. For the responsive medical patient, you will gather the history from the patient first, then conduct the physical exam and obtain the vital signs. The history comes first for the responsive medical patient for two reasons: (1) the most valuable information on a medical condition in the prehospital setting usually comes from what the patient can tell you about how he feels; and (2) it is important to get information from the patient before he, possibly, becomes unresponsive. For the patient who is already unresponsive when you arrive on the scene, the physical exam and vital signs will come before the history, which will need to be gathered, to the extent possible, from family members or bystanders.

The second difference is in the kind of physical exam you will conduct. For the responsive medical patient, you will conduct a *modified secondary assessment*—an exam that is focused on the patient's chief complaint, signs, and symptoms. For the unresponsive medical patient, you will conduct a *rapid secondary assessment*—the quick head-to-toe assessment that is similar to the rapid secondary assessment conducted on the trauma patient. You will look for signs relating to the patient's medical condition as well as any signs of possible trauma that may have been missed earlier.

As the next chart reveals, the secondary assessment for an unresponsive medical patient is similar to the secondary assessment for a trauma patient with significant mechanism of injury because, in both instances, you first need to examine the whole body for information the patient cannot tell you. The modified secondary assessment for a responsive medical patient (the majority of your medical calls) begins with the history, followed by a physical exam focused on the patient's chief complaint, signs, and symptoms.

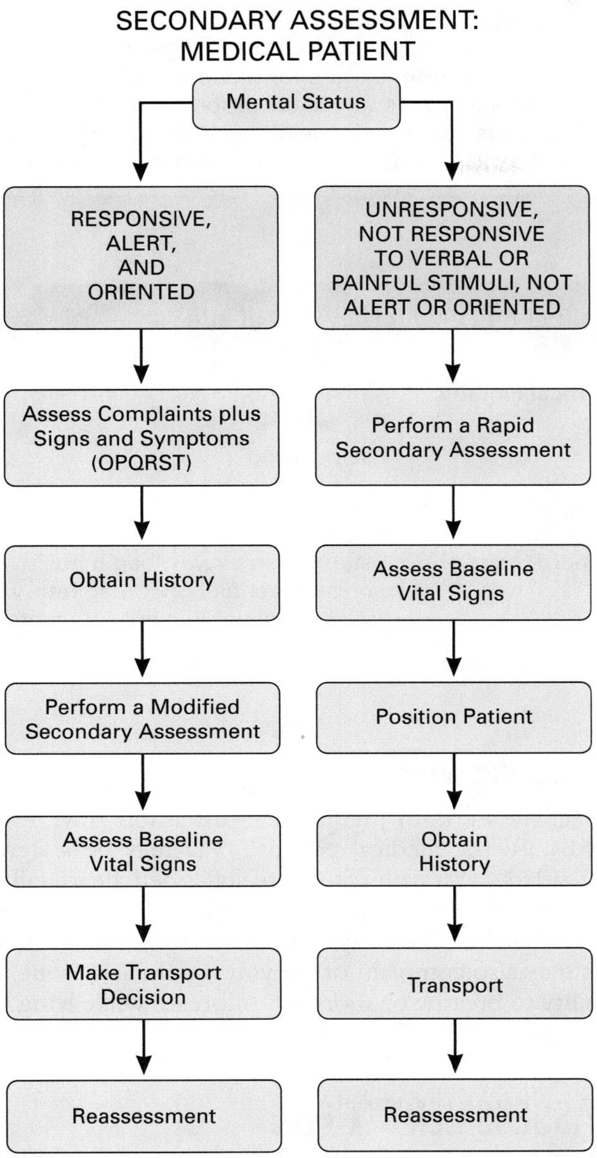

SECONDARY ASSESSMENT: MEDICAL PATIENT

RESPONSIVE, ALERT, AND ORIENTED	UNRESPONSIVE, NOT RESPONSIVE TO VERBAL OR PAINFUL STIMULI, NOT ALERT OR ORIENTED
Assess Complaints plus Signs and Symptoms (OPQRST)	Perform a Rapid Secondary Assessment
Obtain History	Assess Baseline Vital Signs
Perform a Modified Secondary Assessment	Position Patient
Assess Baseline Vital Signs	Obtain History
Make Transport Decision	Transport
Reassessment	Reassessment

Mental Status → (left) RESPONSIVE, ALERT, AND ORIENTED → Assess Complaints plus Signs and Symptoms (OPQRST) → Obtain History → Perform a Modified Secondary Assessment → Assess Baseline Vital Signs → Make Transport Decision → Reassessment; (right) UNRESPONSIVE, NOT RESPONSIVE TO VERBAL OR PAINFUL STIMULI, NOT ALERT OR ORIENTED → Perform a Rapid Secondary Assessment → Assess Baseline Vital Signs → Position Patient → Obtain History → Transport → Reassessment

FIGURE 13-32 ✱ Steps of the secondary assessment for a medical patient.

Secondary Assessment for a Medical Patient Who Is . . .

Unresponsive (Not Alert, Disoriented, Responsive to Verbal or Painful Stimuli, or Unresponsive)

1. Rapid secondary assessment (head to toe)
2. Baseline vital signs
3. SAMPLE history

Responsive (Alert and Oriented)

1. SAMPLE history
2. Modified secondary assessment (focused on the chief complaint, signs, and symptoms)
3. Baseline vital signs

Medical Patient Who Is Not Alert or Is Disoriented, Is Responding Only to Verbal or Painful Stimuli, or Is Unresponsive

An altered mental status in a medical patient should be considered critical. You must perform a rapid secondary assessment, followed by prompt transport, continued assessment, and emergency care en route to the hospital.

Attempt to gain as much information from the scene as possible. Note the patient's medications, both prescribed and over-the-counter; any evidence of drugs or alcohol; signs that the patient may have been sick for a period of time; and the condition of the place in which the patient was found. Look at how the patient is dressed, where he was found, and what he may have been doing prior to the emergency. If you walk into the scene and find an oxygen tank or concentrator in the living room, you are likely to suspect that the patient has a history of emphysema, chronic bronchitis, or some other type of respiratory condition. A patient in a hospital-type bed usually has a chronic illness or severe debilitating disease.

Critical (Unstable) Findings: Medical Patient	
Critical Finding:	Unresponsive or altered mental status
Possibility:	Stroke Severe hypoxia Drug overdose Cardiac compromise Blood loss Seizure Diabetic emergency
Emergency Care:	Establish an airway, begin positive pressure ventilation if respiratory rate or tidal volume is inadequate, and administer oxygen.

Make use of other sources of information. Question bystanders, family members, or other relatives or friends. The patient may have been complaining of symptoms prior to the altered mental state or unresponsiveness. Look for a medical identification tag on the patient as evidence of a chronic illness.

Objective 13-28
Explain how to conduct a secondary assessment for a medical patient who is not alert or is disoriented, is responding only to verbal or painful stimuli, or is unresponsive.

Objective 13-29
Discuss critical (unstable) findings, possibilities, and emergency care for the medical patient with an altered mental status associated with assessment of the head, neck, chest, abdomen, pelvic region, extremities, and posterior body.

Perform a Rapid Secondary Assessment for the Medical Patient

Perform a rapid medical assessment on the unresponsive patient to determine the possible nature of the medical illness. The patient's airway, breathing, and perfusion status will have been assessed and managed during the primary assessment. As you perform the rapid secondary assessment, reassess the airway, breathing, and circulation status and manage these or any additional life-threatening problems immediately.

Like the rapid secondary assessment for the trauma patient, the rapid secondary assessment for the medical patient should be conducted systematically, beginning at the head and covering all major portions of the body (EMT Skills 13-6). The techniques of inspection, palpation, and auscultation are used to search for any signs of abnormality or dysfunction.

Assess the Head

Inspect the head for any evidence of trauma (EMT Skills 13-6A). You may not initially expect to find trauma, because of a lack of mechanism of injury; however, the patient may have fallen several hours, days, or even weeks prior to the onset of the signs, symptoms, or unresponsiveness. Inspect for contusions, lacerations, depressions, abrasions, punctures, and any other evidence of trauma. Palpate the head for any deformities.

Quickly inspect inside the mouth for pale mucosa, bleeding, secretions, or vomitus. Reassess the airway and ensure that it is patent. Inspect the nose and ears for fluid discharge or blood. Quickly inspect the pupils for equality, size, and reactivity. Unequal pupils may indicate a stroke or possible head injury. Pupil size and reactivity may provide evidence of drug overdose, poisoning, hypoxia, or adverse environmental conditions. Inspect for a droop to one side of the face.

ASSESSMENT Tips

A pale oral mucosa (inside the mouth) may indicate that the medical patient has been losing blood over a long period of time. ■

Critical (Unstable) Findings: The Head	
Critical Finding:	Unequal pupils with an altered mental status Facial droop
Possibility:	Stroke
Emergency Care:	Establish an airway, begin positive pressure ventilation if respiratory rate or tidal volume is inadequate, and administer oxygen.

Assess the Neck

Inspect the neck for jugular vein distention (EMT Skills 13-6B). In the medical patient, JVD may be a sign of right-sided heart failure or late left-sided heart failure. You might find JVD associated with complaints of chest pain, dyspnea, or severe fatigue and weakness. The patient may also complain of (or you should ask about) the inability to breathe or shortness of breath while lying flat, which is termed **orthopnea**.

ASSESSMENT Tips

If you see jugular vein distention, also inspect the veins in the hands. They will be engorged from an increase in the venous blood volume and pressure. ■

Inspect the neck for excessive accessory muscle use. If the muscles in the neck bulge and become very prominent during inhalation, respiratory distress should be suspected. Reassess the adequacy of breathing.

Understanding BODY PROCESSES

In labored breathing, the neck muscle that is used as an accessory muscle for breathing lifts the sternum higher than normal. By doing so, it is attempting to increase the thorax to a greater-than-normal size, thus increasing the negative pressure inside and allowing more air to flow into the lungs. ■

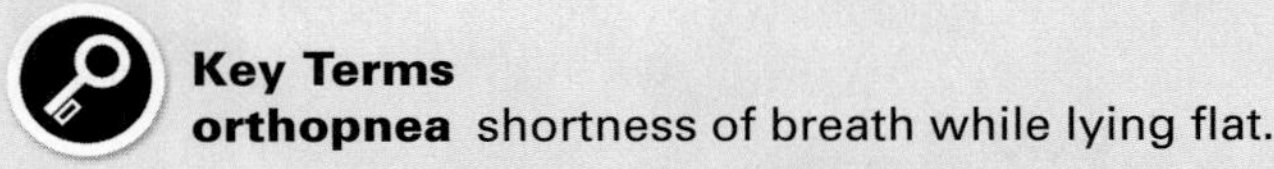

Key Terms

orthopnea shortness of breath while lying flat.

Key Points

Noisy breath sounds heard on auscultation indicate an abnormal condition such as congestive heart failure or pneumonia (crackles), asthma, allergic reaction, or emphysema (wheezing).

While inspecting the neck, look for a medical identification necklace with pertinent information about the patient inscribed on the back (or the medical ID tag may, instead, be worn as a bracelet) (EMT Skills 13-6C). The information on the tag may provide you with an indication of the patient's condition.

Check for a tracheostomy tube at the base of the neck. Because the patient breathes through this tube, secretions and mucus could block the tube, causing an airway obstruction.

Critical (Unstable) Findings: The Neck

Critical Finding:	Jugular venous distention
Possibility:	Right- or late left-sided heart failure
Emergency Care:	Establish an airway, begin positive pressure ventilation if respiratory rate or tidal volume is inadequate, and administer oxygen.
Critical Finding:	Tracheal tugging
Possibility:	Obstruction in the bronchi
Emergency Care:	Establish an airway, begin positive pressure ventilation if respiratory rate or tidal volume is inadequate, and administer oxygen.

Assess the Chest

Inspect the chest for adequate rise and fall, retraction of the intercostal muscles, and symmetrical movement (EMT Skills 13-6D). An inward pulling of the muscles between the ribs during inhalation indicates respiratory distress. In a patient who is unresponsive or has a deteriorating mental status, begin positive pressure ventilation with supplemental oxygen if retractions are noted and the respiratory rate or tidal volume is inadequate.

Look for scars and evidence of implanted cardiac devices such as a pacemaker or automated internal cardiac defibrillator (Figure 13-33*). These will provide a history of cardiac disease even if the patient is unable to respond to your history questions.

Quickly auscultate the breath sounds at the second intercostal space at the midclavicular line and at the fourth or fifth intercostal space at the midaxillary line.

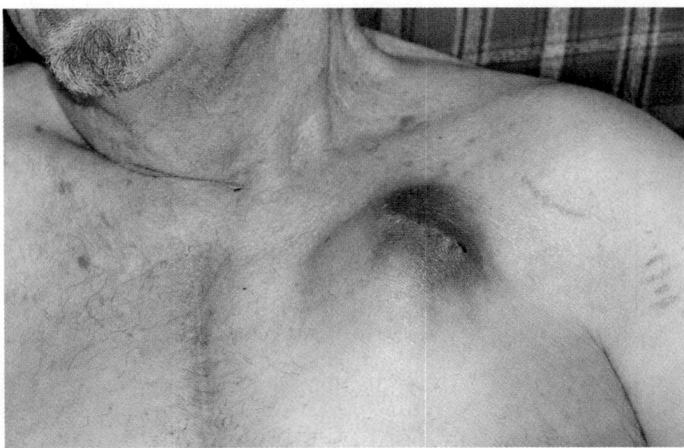

FIGURE 13-33 * An implanted pacemaker. (© Michal Heron)

Compare the breath sounds from side to side. Determine if the breath sounds are present or absent, equal or unequal, clear or noisy.

Noisy breath sounds are not normally heard in the lungs upon auscultation. These sounds are a possible indication of a condition the patient may be suffering. The sounds that you may hear are:

- **Crackles.** Also known as rales, these are a fine crackling sound on inhalation similar to hair being rubbed together close to your ear. This is an indication of fluid in and around the alveoli and the terminal end of the bronchiole. Crackles are also heard as the alveoli "pop" open to allow air to pass through. Patients whose left ventricle is failing and who are in congestive heart failure may experience an increase in the pressure in the pulmonary vessels in the lungs. This increase may force fluid out of the capillaries and force the fluid around or into the alveoli. Another condition in which crackles may be heard is pneumonia, when puslike fluid collects in the alveoli.

Understanding BODY PROCESSES

The pressure inside the pulmonary capillaries (capillaries in the lungs) is very low. An increase in pressure inside the pulmonary capillaries may force the plasma portion (primarily water) of the blood out of the capillary and into the space between the capillary and the alveolus as well as into the alveolar sac. This may interfere with gas exchange and lead to hypoxia. It will also produce the crackle sound heard on auscultation. ■

Critical (Unstable) Findings: The Chest

Critical Finding:	Retractions Accessory muscle use (neck muscles) Diminished breath sounds on both sides of the chest
Possibility:	Inadequate breathing due to a respiratory condition (asthma, emphysema, pneumonia, allergic reaction, pulmonary embolus, pulmonary edema)
Emergency Care:	Establish an airway, begin positive pressure ventilation if respiratory rate or tidal volume is inadequate, and administer oxygen.
Critical Finding:	Crackles upon auscultation
Possibility:	Congestive heart failure Pneumonia
Emergency Care:	Establish an airway, begin positive pressure ventilation if respiratory rate or tidal volume is inadequate, and administer oxygen.
Critical Finding:	Wheezing upon auscultation
Possibility:	Asthma attack Allergic reaction Emphysema Congestive heart failure
Emergency Care:	Establish an airway, begin positive pressure ventilation if respiratory rate or tidal volume is inadequate, and administer oxygen. Patient medications may be administered (epinephrine, metered dose inhaler).

- **Wheezing.** Wheezing is heard as a musical-type sound on inhalation and exhalation. It is an indication that there is a higher resistance in the bronchioles with restricted airflow. The higher resistance may be caused by constriction of the smooth muscle surrounding the bronchiole and swelling and inflammation within the bronchiole. This commonly occurs in asthma, allergic reactions, and emphysema.

Assess the Abdomen

Inspect the abdomen for any abnormal distention or discoloration (EMT Skills 13-6E). Look for evidence of scars from previous surgeries. Palpate for tenderness, distention (Figure 13-34∗), rigidity, or pulsating masses. A rigid, distended, or tender abdomen is a sign of possible internal bleeding, perforation of an organ, or infection. An aortic aneurysm, which is a weakened area of the abdominal aorta, may produce a palpable pulsating mass in the midline of the abdomen.

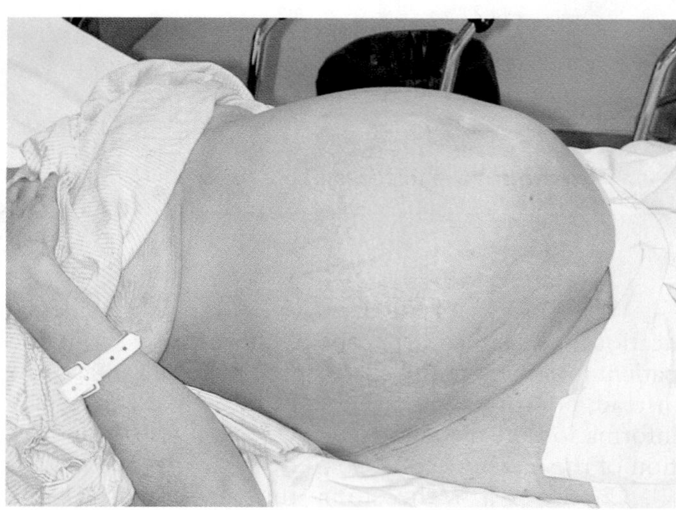

FIGURE 13-34 ∗ Ascites (fluid accumulation in the abdomen) from ovarian cancer. (© Charles Stewart, MD, and Associates)

Understanding BODY PROCESSES

Wheezing is produced from turbulent air moving through higher resistance in the lower respiratory tract, which is caused by constriction of smooth muscle and inflammation of the mucous lining inside the bronchioles. Thus, when wheezing is heard you must suspect the patient has an increase in lower airway resistance. ■

ASSESSMENT Tips

An extremely distended abdomen in the medical patient may be the result of a large amount of fluid, not blood, in the abdomen. This could still lead to hypoperfusion from fluid loss and respiratory compromise from upward pressure to the diaphragm. ■

You can also assess for rebound tenderness, which indicates the lining of the abdomen, the peritoneum, is irritated. The irritation may result from leakage of a substance from a ruptured organ or from an infection of the peritoneum. This is referred to as peritonitis. To assess for rebound tenderness, you can press down firmly on the abdomen and then suddenly release your hand. If the patient complains of pain or grimaces, you could assume the patient has rebound tenderness and peritonitis.

Critical (Unstable) Findings: The Abdomen	
Critical Finding:	Severe abdominal pain Abdominal tenderness on palpation Discoloration of the abdomen, especially in the flank areas or around the navel Abdominal rigidity (contracted abdominal muscles) Distended abdomen
Possibility:	Bleeding within the abdominal cavity, obstruction of hollow organ Irritation of the lining of the abdomen (peritonitis)
Emergency Care:	Rapid transport upon recognition. Establish an airway, begin positive pressure ventilation if respiratory rate or tidal volume is inadequate, and administer oxygen.

Since many patients will complain of pain before you even press down, the test may not provide much information about the abdomen. Perform the Markle test if the patient is able to stand or the heel jar test if the patient is unable to stand (review Figures 13-18 and 13-19).

Assess the Pelvic Region

Look for signs of incontinence. Inspect and palpate for distention or tenderness (EMT Skills 13-6F). This is most significant in the female patient of childbearing age who could have an ectopic pregnancy. If a female patient complains of abdominal pain, usually isolated to the lower quadrants, has a history of a missed menstrual period, and exhibits signs and symptoms of poor perfusion, suspect an ectopic pregnancy—a surgical emergency requiring prompt transport. Note that the history of a missed period may be unreliable.

Assess the Extremities

Note any excessive peripheral edema (swelling around the hands, feet, and ankles). Excessive edema could indicate congestive heart failure, fluid overload, or a clot blocking a vein in that extremity (EMT Skills 13-6G). Also assess the extremities for pulses, motor function, and sensation (EMT Skills 13-6H and 13-6I). Assess the radial and dorsalis pedis pulses. Check motor function and sensation by pinching the hands and feet. Note the patient's response. Look for a medical identification tag around the wrist or ankle.

Critical (Unstable) Findings: The Pelvic Region	
Critical Finding:	Lower quadrant abdominal pain in the pelvic region Tenderness on palpation Female patient in childbearing years with history of missed period (patient may present with vaginal bleeding)
Possibility:	Ectopic pregnancy with bleeding within the abdominal cavity
Emergency Care:	Rapid transport upon recognition. Establish an airway, begin positive pressure ventilation if respiratory rate or tidal volume is inadequate, and administer oxygen.

ASSESSMENT Tips

In a medical patient who complains of a sudden onset of shortness of breath, assess the lower extremities for pain, redness, or swelling to one calf. The patient may also have pain in his calf when pulling his foot backward toward his head. This may be an indication of a blood clot in a deep vein of the lower leg that has broken off and traveled to the lungs. ■

Assess the Posterior Body

Inspect and palpate the back for discoloration, edema, and tenderness. Edema to the sacral region may be from fluid collection associated with congestive heart failure.

ASSESSMENT Tips

Assess for edema (collection of fluid in the tissues under the skin) to the sacral region, called sacral edema, in patients who are bedridden and have their legs level with the heart. Excess fluid in patients who are mostly in a seated position and dangle their legs, or those who are moving about, will collect in the hands, ankles, and feet rather than in the sacral region. ■

Assess Baseline Vital Signs

In the secondary assessment for a medical patient who is not alert, is disoriented, is responding to verbal or painful stimuli, or is unresponsive, vital sign assessment follows the physical exam and precedes the SAMPLE history. Remember, however, that with EMT partners working together, some of these steps can be done simultaneously.

The methods for assessing the vital signs were discussed in Chapter 11, "Baseline Vital Signs, Monitoring Devices, and History Taking." The vital signs are reviewed briefly here, with notes about vital sign assessment for the medical patient who is not alert, is disoriented, is responding only to verbal or painful stimuli, or is unresponsive.

- **Breathing.** Tachypnea (rapid breathing) may indicate a central nervous system disorder, respiratory distress, cardiac problem, anxiety, poisoning, overdose, high blood sugar level, abdominal disorder, or a pulmonary problem. Abnormal respiratory patterns may be seen in patients with central nervous system disorders like stroke, poisoning, overdose, and diabetic emergencies.

ASSESSMENT Tips

Abnormal respiratory patterns typically do not allow for adequate breathing. Assess the patient carefully to ensure the respiratory rate and tidal volume are adequate. ■

- **Pulse**
- **Skin**
- **Pupils.** Pupillary signs are important to document in the unresponsive patient. Note the size, equality, and reactivity to light.
- **Blood pressure**
- **Pulse oximeter.** The pulse oximeter can be applied to determine the level of oxygenation. In many systems, the pulse oximeter reading is used as a sixth vital sign, and the pulse oximeter is applied to virtually all patients being transported to the emergency department. A normal room air reading is typically 95–99%. Any SpO_2 reading less than 95% should heighten your suspicion that the patient is hypoxic. You must look for other evidence and a cause for the hypoxia. Closely assess the respiratory status to include rate and tidal volume to be sure that both are adequate. Be aggressive with airway management, positive pressure ventilation, and oxygen therapy. Be careful when using the pulse oximeter in patients with suspected hypoperfusion or shock, cold environments, or toxic inhalation of carbon monoxide. You may not get a reading on the pulse oximeter or the reading may be erroneous. Patients with carbon monoxide poisoning who are truly hypoxic will display an abnormally high SpO_2 reading due to the carbon monoxide molecules attached to the hemoglobin on the red blood cell.

The vital signs should be reassessed and recorded every 5 minutes in the unresponsive medical patient.

Understanding BODY PROCESSES

When oxygen attaches to hemoglobin on the red blood cell, it turns the molecule red. The pulse oximeter measures oxygen saturation by reading the redness of hemoglobin. Carbon monoxide (CO) attached to the hemoglobin also turns it red. Thus, the SpO_2 reading will be inaccurately high in a patient with carbon monoxide poisoning, even though that patient's cells are truly hypoxic. ■

Blood Glucose Test

Any patient who presents with an altered mental status may be suffering from a low blood glucose (sugar) level, referred to as hypoglycemia. As noted earlier, a test can be performed using a drop of the patient's blood and an electronic glucometer to determine the blood glucose level. This may guide your treatment of the patient and provide an indication of whether to administer glucose to the patient. Hypoglycemia will be discussed in more detail in Chapter 20, "Acute Diabetic Emergencies."

ASSESSMENT Tips

It is important to determine the true last oral intake when testing the blood glucose level, because it will determine whether the reading is normal or not. Shortly after a meal or carbohydrate intake, the blood glucose level in the *nondiabetic* patient will be 120–140 mg/dL. A fasting (8 to 12 hours without food) blood glucose in the *diabetic* patient may be 120–140 mg/dL. ■

Position the Patient

A patient with a severely altered mental status or who is unresponsive most typically cannot protect his own airway. Secretions, mucus, blood, or vomitus can easily be aspirated into the lungs. To avoid the potential for aspiration, place the patient in the *recovery position*, also known as the *coma position*—a modified left lateral recumbent position—as you prepare the patient for transport (Figure 13-35*). In this position, the secretions, blood, mucus, or vomitus will flow out of the mouth and not into the patient's lungs. You must still have a suction device available to assist with clearing the airway, if necessary. If the patient needs to be ventilated, keep him in a supine position. It is very difficult to ventilate a patient on his side with a bag-valve mask or pocket mask.

Obtain a SAMPLE History

Methods of obtaining a SAMPLE history were covered in Chapter 11, "Baseline Vital Signs, Monitoring Devices, and History Taking." For the disoriented, severely

Critical (Unstable) Findings: Baseline Vital Signs

Critical Finding:	Inadequate breathing rate
Possibility:	Stroke Drug overdose Toxic inhalation Respiratory emergency (asthma, pneumonia, allergic reaction) Cold emergency (hypothermia) Heat emergency (heatstroke)
Emergency Care:	Establish an airway, begin positive pressure ventilation if respiratory rate or tidal volume is inadequate, and administer oxygen. Consider ALS intercept.
Critical Finding:	Absent carotid pulse in the adult or child greater than 1 year of age Absent brachial pulse in the infant less than 1 year of age No movement, breathing, or other signs of life
Possibility:	Cardiac arrest
Emergency Care:	Immediately initiate CPR, beginning with chest compressions, and apply the automated external defibrillator (AED) according to your protocol. Consider ALS intercept.
Critical Finding:	Cool, clammy skin, weak pulses, rapid heart rate (tachycardia), decreasing systolic blood pressure, narrow pulse pressure, delayed capillary refill
Possibility:	Hypoperfusion (shock) Possible internal bleeding, infection, other fluid loss
Emergency Care:	Administer oxygen. Rapid transport.
Critical Finding:	Unequal pupils Fixed pupil
Possibility:	Stroke
Emergency Care:	Establish an airway, begin positive pressure ventilation if respiratory rate or tidal volume is inadequate, administer oxygen, and consider hyperventilation if signs of brain herniation are present (abnormal posturing, fixed or unequal pupils).
Critical Finding:	SpO_2 reading of less than 95%
Possibility:	Hypoxia associated with an occluded airway or inadequate respiration
Emergency Care:	Administer oxygen by nonrebreather mask at 15 lpm if breathing is adequate. If breathing is inadequate, establish an airway, begin positive pressure ventilation, and administer a high concentration of oxygen through the ventilation device.

altered mental status, or unresponsive patient, it is necessary to gain as much information as possible from any family members, friends, and bystanders at the scene (Figure 13-36✱). The SAMPLE history is a quick method for obtaining limited but extremely important information. Because the patient has an altered mental status, a more detailed history that goes beyond the SAMPLE is not pursued. The following is a review of the SAMPLE history for the unresponsive medical patient:

- **Signs.** *Signs will be revealed in the physical exam and vital signs assessment.* As you conduct your rapid medical assessment and find specific signs, it may be necessary to ask the people at the scene relevant questions regarding the complaints of the patient. For example, if you find unequal pupils, it would be appropriate to ask those at the scene: Was the patient complaining of a headache, weakness, numbness, or paralysis in the extremities?
- **Symptoms.** *Was the patient complaining of any symptoms prior to becoming unresponsive?* Was the patient complaining of:
  - Shortness of breath?
  - Chest pain or any other type of pain?
  - Severe headache?
  - Light-headedness, dizziness, or faintness?
  - Severe itching?
  - Feeling excessively cold or hot?
  - Abdominal pain or pain in the lumbar region?

  If the patient was complaining of a particular symptom, try to determine from those at the scene:
  - Was the onset sudden or gradual?
  - Did anything provoke the symptom?

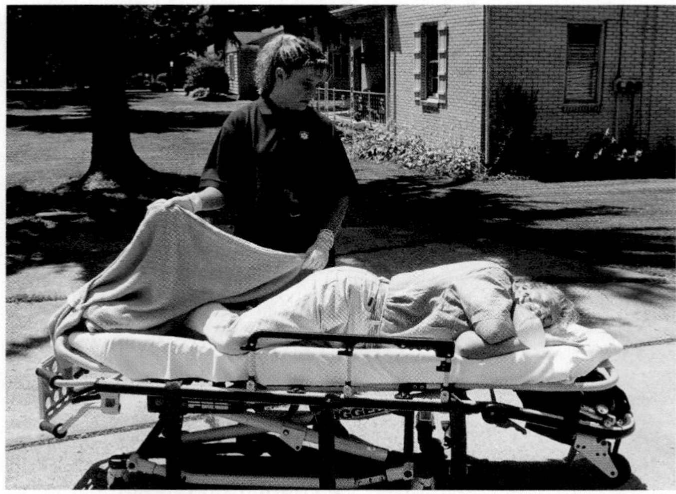

FIGURE 13-35 ✱ Position the unresponsive medical patient in the recovery position to protect the airway and prevent aspiration of secretions, blood, or vomitus.

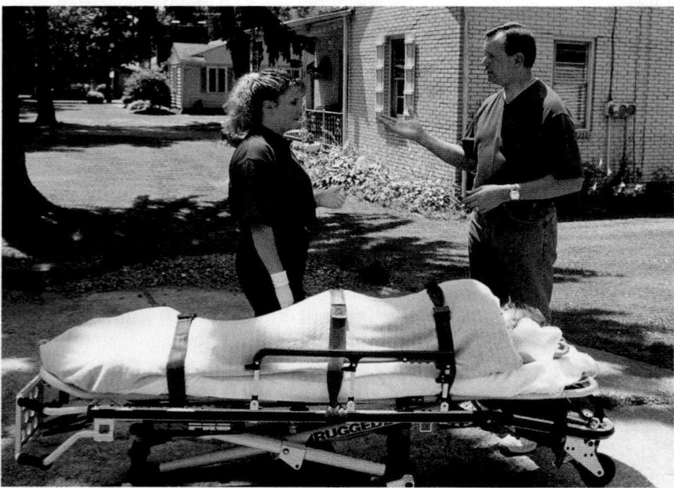

FIGURE 13-36 ✱ Prepare the patient for transport. Obtain a SAMPLE history from any bystanders, family, or friends of the unresponsive patient.

- How severe was the symptom?
- How long was the patient complaining of the symptom?
- Where exactly was the symptom felt?
- Was anything done or taken to relieve the symptom?

ASSESSMENT Tips

Pain is typically produced by ischemia (tissue that is hypoxic), inflammation, infection, or obstruction. ■

- **Allergies.** *Does the patient have any known allergies?* The patient may have a medical identification tag that identifies his allergies.

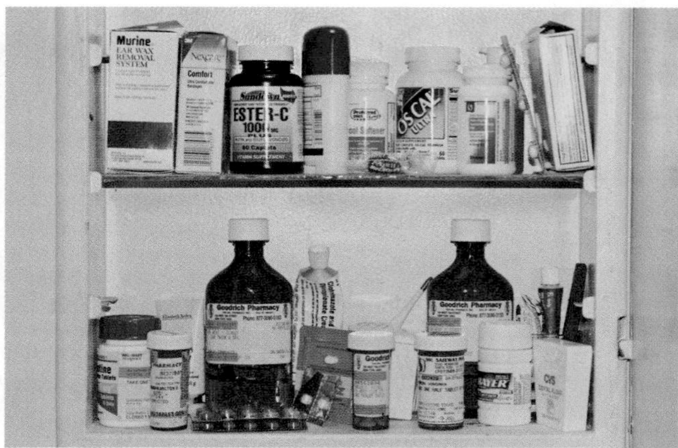

FIGURE 13-37 ✱ Check the patient's medications. Look for both prescription and over-the-counter medications. Check the refrigerator for insulin if the patient is unresponsive with an unknown medical history. (© Michal Heron)

- **Medications.** *What medications has the patient been taking?* Have someone gather the medications the patient takes. These will provide information about the patient's past medical history. If no family members are at the scene, have your partner look around the kitchen, bathroom, and bedroom for medications, both prescription and over-the-counter medications (Figure 13-37✱). If the patient is suspected of being a diabetic, look in the refrigerator for insulin.
- **Pertinent past medical history.** *Does the patient have any pre-existing medical condition?* Ask if the patient has ever been hospitalized or is seeing a physician. If so, for what condition? If the patient was hospitalized for the condition, ask how recently and for how long. This should provide some indication of the severity of the illness and may provide an indication as to why the patient is unresponsive.
- **Last oral intake.** *When did the patient last eat or drink anything?* It is of extreme importance to determine when the diabetic patient most recently had a meal or last had anything to eat or drink. Attempt to determine how long after the meal the signs and symptoms occurred. Gastrointestinal disorders, anaphylaxis, and diabetic emergencies are often associated with eating. Also, if the patient will require surgery, the anesthetist will need this information.
- **Events leading to the present illness.** *What was the patient doing prior to the onset of the unresponsiveness? What were his signs or symptoms?* This is useful in trying to rule out trauma as the cause for the unresponsiveness.

Provide Emergency Care

Following the secondary assessment, you will provide emergency care based on the signs, symptoms, and history gathered. All medical patients with an altered mental

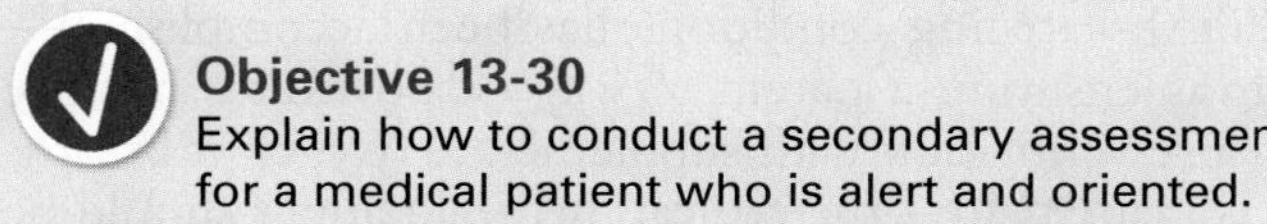

Objective 13-30
Explain how to conduct a secondary assessment for a medical patient who is alert and oriented.

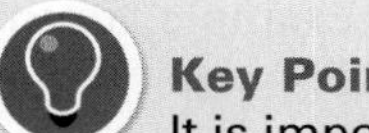

Key Points
It is important to assess all body systems related to the patient's chief complaint, not just the one most immediately associated with it.

status or who are unresponsive must receive oxygen via a nonrebreather mask at 15 lpm or positive pressure ventilation with supplemental oxygen, if needed.

Make a Transport Decision

Altered mental status in a medical patient is considered to be a critical finding. Transport should be prompt. However, life-threatening injuries and conditions must be appropriately managed at the scene prior to transport.

During transport, closely monitor the airway, breathing, and circulation status. Reassess vital signs every 5 minutes. Following any intervention that you provide, check for a change in the patient's condition. If at any time the patient regains responsiveness, perform a secondary assessment and reevaluate the history.

Responsive Medical Patient Who Is Alert and Oriented

In the responsive medical patient who is alert and oriented, closely assess the history of the present illness. You do this mainly by asking the patient a series of questions. In the medical patient, the SAMPLE history should be the baseline for gathering information. It is often desirable to collect additional information from the history (refer to Chapter 11, "Baseline Vital Signs, Monitoring Devices, and History Taking"). With the responsive medical patient, you can add the OPQRST questions to the SAMPLE history to gain as complete a picture as possible of the illness the patient is experiencing. The manner in which you conduct the modified secondary assessment and provide emergency care will be based on the information you gather from the OPQRST, SAMPLE, and other history questions.

Assess Patient Complaints: OPQRST

OPQRST was discussed in detail in Chapter 11, "Baseline Vital Signs, Monitoring Devices, and History Taking." It is a mnemonic for the questions you should ask when assessing the patient's chief complaint or major symptoms like pain, as follows:

- **Onset.** *When and how did the symptom begin?*
- **Provocation/palliation.** *What makes the symptom worse? What makes it better?*
- **Quality.** *How would you describe the pain?*
- **Radiation.** *Where do you feel the pain? Where does the pain go?*
- **Severity.** *How bad is the symptom?*
- **Time.** *How long have you had the symptom?*

ASSESSMENT Tips

It is crucial to determine the exact time of onset of the first sign of weakness, slurred speech, numbness, paralysis, facial droop, or other signs of stroke and report it to the emergency department or receiving medical facility. You may be the only person who can collect this vital information at the scene from relatives, friends, or bystanders. It may make a critical difference in stroke and cardiac treatment once at the hospital. ■

Complete the SAMPLE History

You will have gained information about the patient's symptoms in response to the OPQRST questions. Information about the patient's signs will be gained during the physical exam and vital signs measurements. To complete the SAMPLE history, determine the patient's allergies, medications, pertinent past medical history, last oral intake, and events leading to the present illness, as described in detail in Chapter 11 and earlier in this chapter for the unresponsive medical patient. Consider obtaining additional information in the history that might be helpful in determining the patient's condition and in the continuum of care once at the medical facility.

Perform a Modified Secondary Assessment

For the responsive medical patient who is alert and oriented, the physical exam comes after the SAMPLE history. The physical exam may be more focused, or it may be a complete head-to-toe secondary assessment, depending on the patient complaint and suspected body systems involved. For example, if a patient is complaining of nontraumatic chest pain, possibly related to a heart problem, you would focus the exam on the pupils, conjunctiva, oral mucosa, neck, chest, abdomen, posterior body, and extremities. You would palpate the patient's head, inspect inside the ears and nose, and palpate the pelvis and symphysis pubis. However, if the patient's signs and symptoms are not specific enough to make a decision about what areas to focus on—for example, a complaint such as "I just don't feel well"—you should perform a complete head-to-toe secondary assessment.

Assess Baseline Vital Signs

Obtain the breathing rate and quality; pulse rate and quality; skin temperature, color, and condition; capillary refill; pupil size and reactivity; blood pressure; and SpO_2 reading.

Critical findings and interventions would be the same as those that were listed for the medical patient who is not alert, is disoriented, responds only to verbal or painful stimuli, or is unresponsive.

Provide Emergency Care

Emergency care provided to the patient will be based on the information gathered from the medical assessment and in consultation with medical direction. General care involves maintaining a patent airway, administering oxygen, and assisting ventilation, if necessary.

Make a Transport Decision

For a patient whose condition is not critical, the patient can be prepared for transport following the secondary assessment and provision of any required emergency care at the scene. If the patient's condition is critical, this procedure can be expedited by having one EMT partner begin preparing the patient for transport while the other is completing the assessment. Once on-scene management of life-threatening conditions has been accomplished—such as ensuring a patent airway or providing positive pressure ventilation with supplemental oxygen if breathing is inadequate—the critical medical patient should be transported promptly with additional assessment and emergency care provided en route. Review Table 13-8 for the criteria for immediate transport. Prompt transport is the key to survival of the critical patient.

During transport, reassess the airway, breathing, and pulses. Take the vital signs every 5 minutes in the critical patient or unstable patient and every 15 minutes in the noncritical or stable patient. On every patient, assess the effectiveness of the interventions provided. For example, make sure that a nonrebreather mask is securely placed and that oxygen is flowing adequately. You should develop a pattern:

1. Assess
2. Intervene
3. Reassess

In the medical patient, you must rely heavily on the complaints of the patient and the signs and symptoms found during the secondary assessment to proceed with emergency care. You are not required to diagnose a medical condition or disease process but rather to recognize significant signs and symptoms and, based on these findings, provide care to manage life threats. Whenever you are in doubt or whenever local protocols require it, consult with medical direction prior to providing care.

Part 4: Reassessment

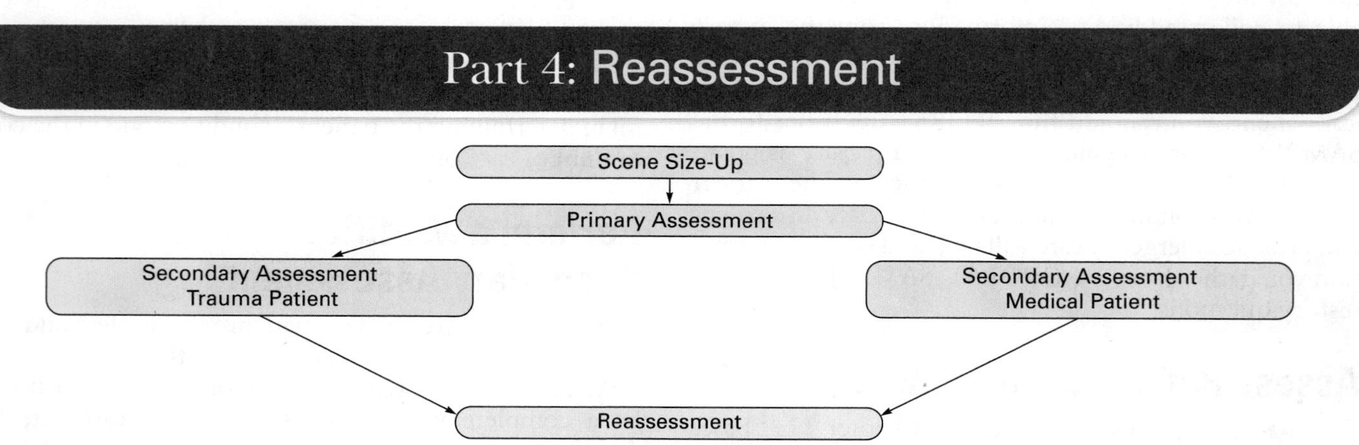

The **reassessment** (Figures 13-38∗ and 13-39∗) is conducted following the secondary assessment. Reassessment is most often performed in the ambulance, continuously, until care of the patient is transferred to hospital personnel (EMT Skills 13-7). If there is a delay in arrival of an ambulance to transport the patient—for example, when the EMT is performing a first-response function or emergency care when off duty, when multiple patients require dispatch of additional ambulances, or when the patient is entrapped or requires extrication—reassessment may begin at the scene and continue in the ambulance.

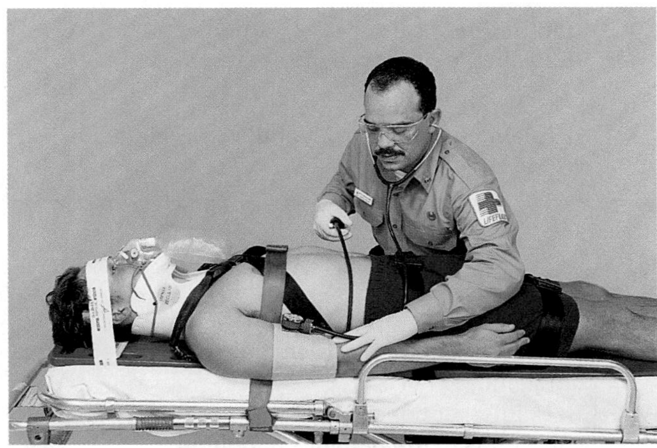

FIGURE 13-38 * Reassess the vital signs.

Purposes of the Reassessment

The purposes of the reassessment are to determine any changes in the patient's condition and to assess the effectiveness of your emergency care. It should be performed on both the trauma and the medical patient, whether the patient is responsive or unresponsive, stable or unstable. If during the reassessment you identify a critical patient condition, you should provide immediate care to correct the problem. For example, as you perform the assessment you note that the patient's breathing depth and quality have become inadequate. You would intervene immediately to begin positive pressure ventilation with supplemental oxygen.

If this is a trauma patient, you would repeat the rapid secondary assessment looking for the possible cause of the deterioration of the patient. Does the patient have signs of pneumothorax (air in the chest cavity, possibly from a damaged lung)? Did the occlusive dressing over an open chest wound become clotted, not allowing air to escape? Does the patient have a possible head injury? The rapid assessment should identify any signs and symptoms that may identify the possible cause of the patient's condition.

The main objective is to intervene and provide the necessary emergency care for the life-threatening injuries or conditions, followed by reassessment. Remember that your routine should be as follows:

1. Assess
2. Intervene
3. Reassess

The reassessment must be performed on all patients. The three basic reasons for performing a reassessment are:

1. To detect any change in the patient's condition
2. To identify any missed injuries or conditions, especially those that are life threatening
3. To adjust the emergency care as needed

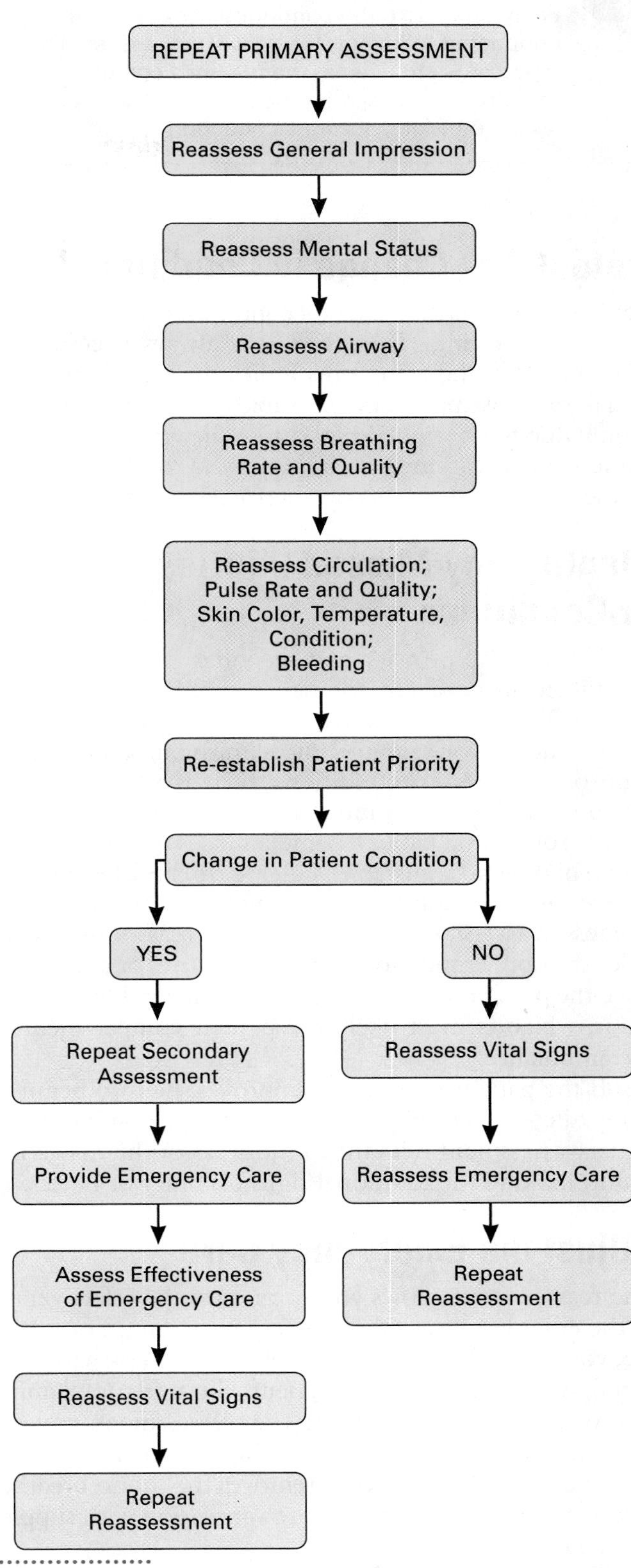

FIGURE 13-39 * Steps of the reassessment.

Key Terms

reassessment the continuous assessment that is conducted following the secondary assessment to detect any changes in the patient's condition, to identify any missed injuries or conditions, and to adjust emergency care as needed.

Objective 13-31
Explain the purposes of reassessment.

Objective 13-32
Explain how to conduct and to complete the reassessment.

Detect Any Change in Condition

Rapid changes in the patient's condition can occur in the prehospital setting. Therefore, it is always necessary to look for signs and symptoms indicating deterioration as well as signs of improvement. Rapid deterioration is commonly due to continued blood loss, airway compromise, inadequate breathing, poor perfusion, or brain injury. These areas are the focus of the reassessment.

Identify Any Missed Injuries or Conditions

Many times the primary and secondary assessments are conducted in poor environmental conditions that limit the EMT's ability to assess adequately. Extremely dark environments, for example, may limit your ability to see signs of injury. Noisy conditions, such as a hostile crowd or a busy highway, may interfere with your ability to hear breath sounds or patient complaints. Rain, bright sunshine, high winds, unstable vehicles, threats of explosion, smoke, or other conditions commonly reduce the effectiveness of assessment at the scene. The reassessment provides the opportunity to reassess for injuries or conditions once the patient is in a more stable and favorable environment, which is most likely the patient compartment of the ambulance.

If the patient's condition improves, he may begin to complain of other symptoms. You can then conduct a secondary assessment relevant to the areas of the new complaint, looking for additional signs of injury or illness.

Adjust the Emergency Care

The reassessment allows you to reassess the effectiveness of the emergency care that you are providing. For example, you may have placed a nonrebreather mask with oxygen flowing at 15 lpm on a patient who was complaining of shortness of breath. During the reassessment, you determine that the patient's breathing depth has become extremely shallow, so you remove the nonrebreather mask and begin positive pressure ventilation with supplemental oxygen.

The steps of the reassessment are as follows:

Steps of the Reassessment

1. Repeat the primary assessment.
2. Reassess and record vital signs.
3. Repeat the secondary assessment for other complaints, injuries, or a change in the chief complaint.
4. Check interventions.
5. Note trends in the patient's condition.

Repeat and record the assessment findings—particularly the components of the primary assessment and the vital signs—at least every 5 minutes in the unstable patient with critical injuries and every 15 minutes in a stable patient.

Repeat the Primary Assessment

Since the main objective of the primary assessment was to identify and manage life-threatening injuries, repetition of the primary assessment is also a key component of the reassessment. It is necessary to assess the same parameters that were initially assessed.

Reassess Mental Status

If the patient continues to talk to you throughout the entire call, reassess for any change in the speech pattern and appropriateness of his responses. A patient with a head injury may continue to talk to you, but his speech pattern may become garbled and his responses inappropriate. This is a sign of continued bleeding or swelling within the skull. Also assess the patient's ability to obey commands appropriately. Repeat the Glasgow Coma Scale and obtain another score and compare it to the others.

If the patient is not alert or loses alertness, reassess the response based on the AVPU mnemonic. Record any change in the patient's mental status, whether it is improved or worsened.

Reassess the Airway

If the patient is talking to you and in no distress, assume the airway is patent. In the unresponsive patient, open the mouth and look inside for any evidence of blood, secretions, or vomitus. Suction the mouth, if necessary. Listen for snoring sounds, gurgling, or stridor. Reassess the position of the nasopharyngeal or oropharyngeal airway if one has been inserted. Check to make sure either airway is not clogged with secretions, blood, or vomitus. If the patient is being ventilated, ask the EMT who is ventilating if any unusual resistance is felt. This may indicate an airway obstruction.

If the patient's condition improves and he can no longer tolerate an airway adjunct and begins to gag, remove it. Have suction available and position the patient on his side, if possible, before removing the airway. Loss of a gag or cough reflex, on the other hand, may require insertion of an airway.

Reassess Breathing

Look, listen, and feel for adequate breathing. If the breathing is determined to be inadequate because of poor quality or rate, begin positive pressure ventilation with supplemental oxygen. If the patient is already being ventilated, reassess effectiveness of the ventilation by looking at the rise and fall of the chest and watching for improvement in the patient's color and mental status. Ask the EMT who is ventilating if any unusual resistance is felt when squeezing the bag. If so, reevaluate the airway, the chest, the device being used for ventilation, the seal of the face mask, or the manner in which ventilation is being provided.

ASSESSMENT Tips

Increasing resistance during ventilation can mean that the airway is not being maintained effectively, that the stomach is filling with air and pushing up on the diaphragm, or that the patient with a chest injury may be developing a tension pneumothorax. Immediately reassess the airway and breath sounds. ■

Apply oxygen to any patient who becomes unresponsive, has an alteration in mental status, becomes anxious or agitated, suddenly becomes sleepy, or exhibits a decrease in the SpO_2 reading. Once oxygen is applied, continue to provide it, even if the patient's condition improves. The pulse oximeter is a good tool to monitor the effectiveness of oxygen therapy and positive pressure ventilation.

Reassess Circulation

Reassess Pulse

Reassess and record the patient's pulse rate and quality. An increasing rate with poor quality may be a sign of continued bleeding. A decreasing pulse with poor quality may indicate a head injury or severe hypoxia (oxygen starvation). An increasing pulse in a patient who initially had a low rate may indicate an improvement in breathing and oxygenation. If a patient initially had an elevated pulse associated with bleeding, a decrease may indicate a reduction in the bleeding and an improvement in the patient's condition. Evaluate the pulse rate in relationship to the initial findings and the injuries or medical condition.

Reassess Bleeding

Check the site of any major bleeding for blood seeping through the dressing and bandage, indicating the need to recontrol bleeding through direct pressure. If the bleeding is severe and cannot be controlled with direct pressure, apply a tourniquet. If you detect any signs of increasing or continued blood loss, such as a decrease in perfusion or elevated pulse with poor quality, conduct a rapid assessment to detect the site of any external blood loss that you can control. Continue to treat for shock.

Reassess Skin

Look for skin color changes. Feel for changes in skin temperature and condition. Reassess capillary refill. Improvements in oxygenation typically improve the color of the skin. Likewise, poor oxygenation from airway or breathing compromise will cause the skin to become cyanotic or blue-gray. As a patient continues to lose blood, the skin becomes more pale, cool, and clammy. Capillary refill may be delayed. Continue to treat for shock.

Return of normal skin color, temperature, and condition are obvious indications of improvement.

Re-establish Patient Priorities

If reassessment is undertaken at the scene and deterioration of the patient's condition is noted, it may be necessary to reconsider your emergency care and transport decision. If the patient becomes a priority patient because of the injuries or conditions found, begin prompt transport and continue to provide emergency care while en route to the hospital. If the patient's condition deteriorates, reassess and adjust interventions as needed.

▶ Complete the Reassessment

Reassess and Record Vital Signs

During the reassessment, reassess the breathing rate and quality, pulse rate and quality, perfusion status, pupils, blood pressure, and SpO_2. Record the vital signs and the time that they were taken.

Repeat Components of the Secondary Assessment for Other Complaints

If the patient begins to complain of a symptom that was not initially identified or a change in the original symptom, complete the relevant components of the secondary

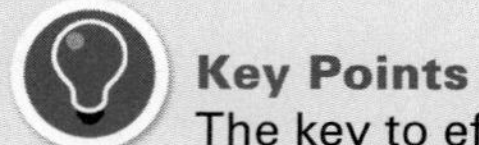

Key Points
The key to effective management of the patient is to assess-intervene-reassess.

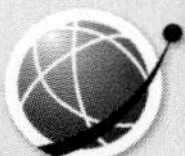

Media Resources
Go to www.bradybooks.com for mykit. Highlights:

- *Video:* Detailed Physical Exam
- *Video:* Ongoing Assessment

assessment related to the area of the complaint and other relevant body systems. Obtain additional history information, if necessary. The patient may have been initially unresponsive and unable to identify any complaints. However, as a result of effective care and improvement in his condition, the patient begins to complain of symptoms of injury or medical illness. Repeat components of the physical assessment as necessary to focus on those areas or symptoms. For example, during the reassessment a patient begins to complain of abdominal pain. You must reinspect and palpate the abdomen, looking for any additional signs of injury or abnormality.

Check Interventions

Determine if your emergency care is adequate and your interventions are effective for the patient's condition. Ensure adequacy of oxygen delivery, positive pressure ventilation, bleeding control, CPR or AED, and immobilization.

Ask yourself the following questions when considering adequacy of intervention:

- Have the patient's vital signs improved, or deteriorated?
- Is the patient's airway still patent?
- Is the oxygen mask and liter flow adequate? Is oxygen connected and flowing to the bag-valve-mask device?
- Has the patient's color improved with oxygen or should I consider positive pressure ventilation?
- Is the patient's chest rising and falling adequately with the ventilations?
- Are the chest compressions producing pulses? Is the rate and depth of compression adequate?
- Has a cardiac arrest patient whose heartbeat has been restored lapsed into arrest again?
- Is the AED indicating that a shock is needed (or not needed)?
- Is the pressure dressing adequately controlling the bleeding? Has the bleeding stopped or do I need to proceed to the next step in bleeding control?
- Is the patient's spine completely immobilized?
- Are bone or joint injuries adequately immobilized?

If an intervention is not effective, it may be necessary to reassess the patient's condition, look for signs of other injuries or illness, check the equipment, ensure that the equipment is being used properly, and/or select alternative methods for emergency care.

Assessment, intervention, and reassessment of the patient is the key to all emergency care provided in the prehospital environment.

Note Trends in Patient Condition

The changes for the better or worse in the patient's condition will be the basis for interventions or changes in intervention and reassessment that you will perform en route to the hospital. It is also important to document and report to the staff of the receiving facility any changes in the patient's condition. For both the EMTs and the hospital staff, it is not only the patient's condition, but the trends in the patient's condition, indicating improvement or deterioration, that are important.

EMT skills 13-1 Log Rolling from a Prone to a Supine Position When Spinal Injury Is Suspected

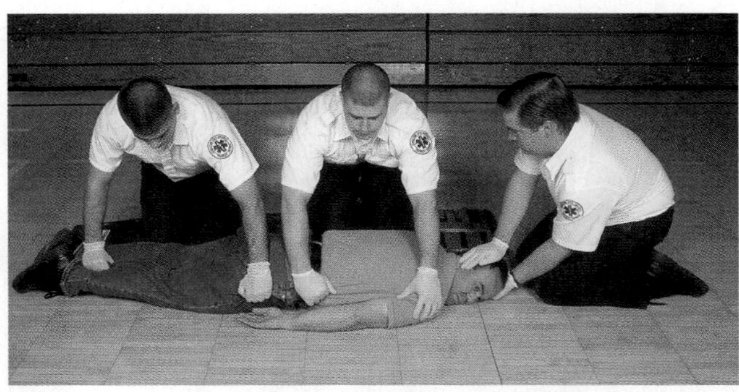

13-1A ✻ A rescuer at the patient's head establishes and maintains manual in-line spinal stabilization. A backboard is placed alongside the patient, and two other rescuers kneel on it. One grasps the patient's shoulder and hip. The other grasps the patient's thigh and ankle.

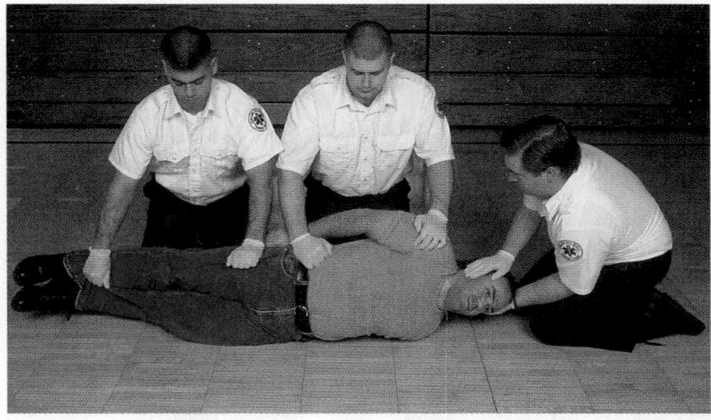

13-1B ✻ On the command of the rescuer at the head, the patient is rolled up against the thighs of the kneeling rescuers. The rescuer who is grasping the patient's thigh and ankle makes sure that the legs are slightly raised off the floor to keep them aligned with the spine as the patient is turned.

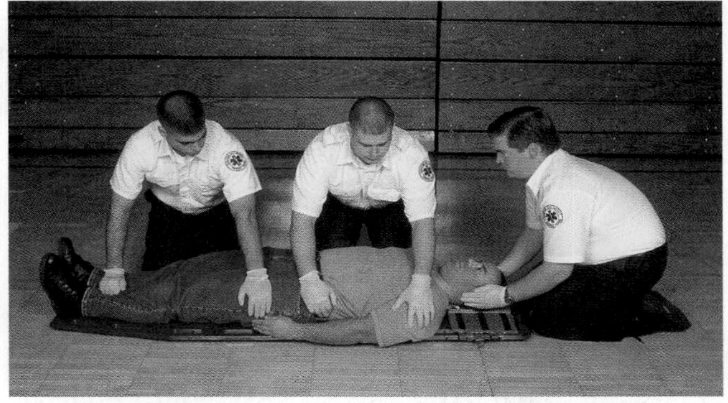

13-1C ✻ The patient is then rolled into the supine position on the backboard. In-line spinal stabilization is maintained by the rescuer at the head.

EMT skills 13-2 Assessing Capillary Refill in Children and Infants

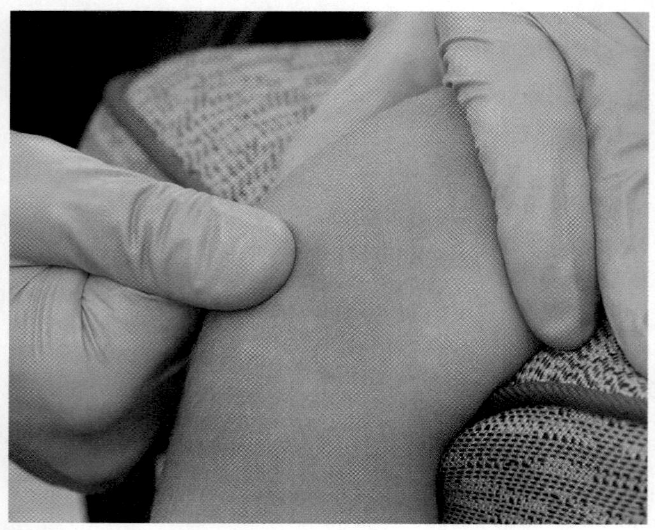

13-2A ✱ To assess capillary refill, press your thumb down on the child's kneecap for several seconds.

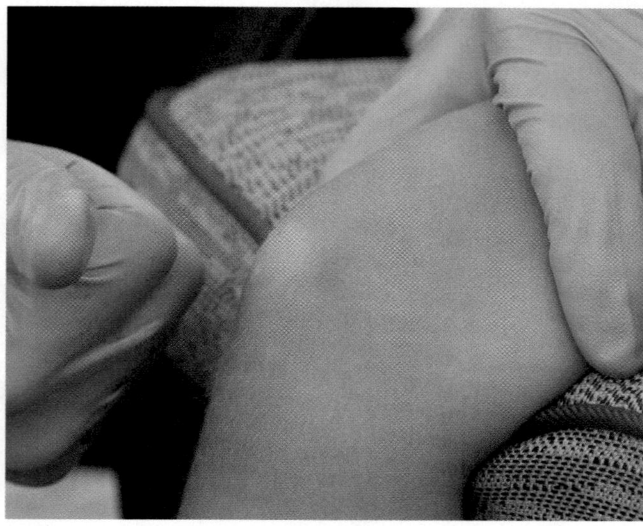

13-2B ✱ Release your thumb and observe the whitened (blanched) area where you had been pressing. Count the number of seconds it takes for the color to return to normal. Normal color should return to the area in 2 seconds or less. If it takes longer, capillary refill is said to be delayed. This is only one sign of inadequate circulation. You must assess for other signs of poor perfusion.

EMT skills 13-3 The Secondary Assessment: Anatomical Approach

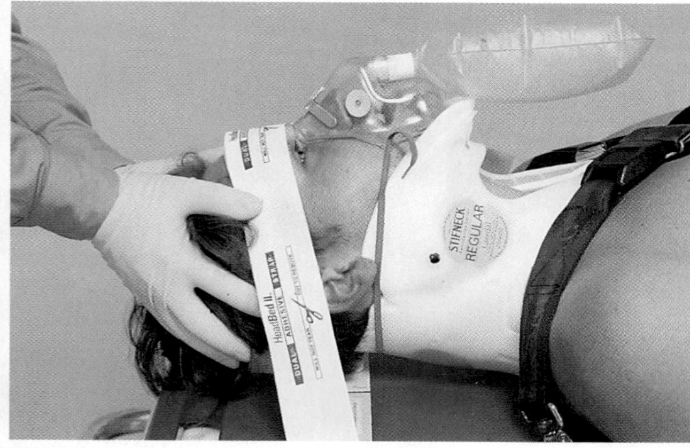

13-3A ✱ Inspect the head for signs of trauma. Carefully palpate the skull for abnormalities.

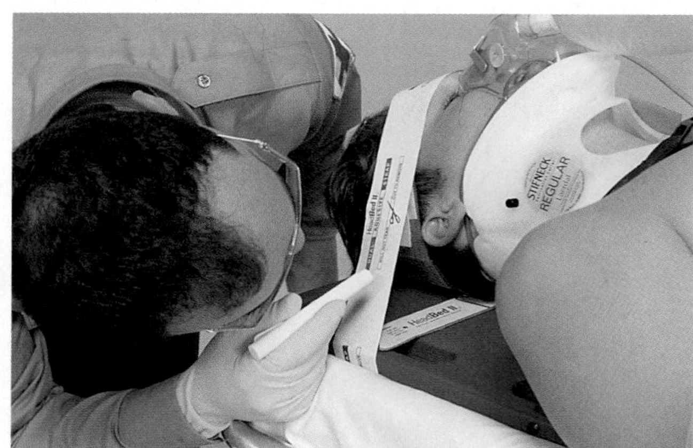

13-3B ✱ Inspect and palpate the ear. Note any leakage of blood or fluid.

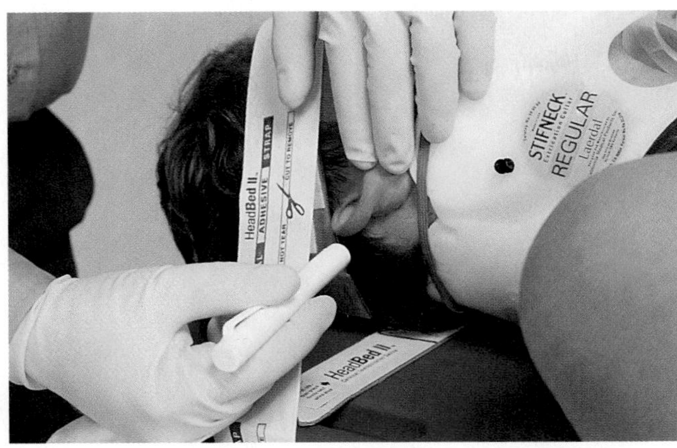

13-3C ✱ Inspect behind the ears for any injury or discoloration.

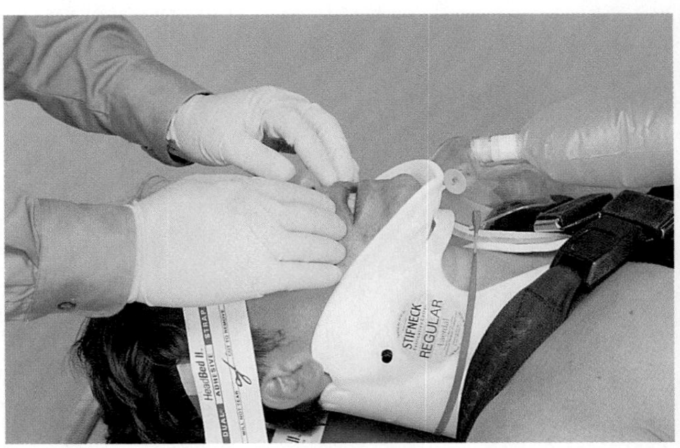

13-3D ✱ Inspect and palpate the face. Note any deformity, instability, burns, or swelling.

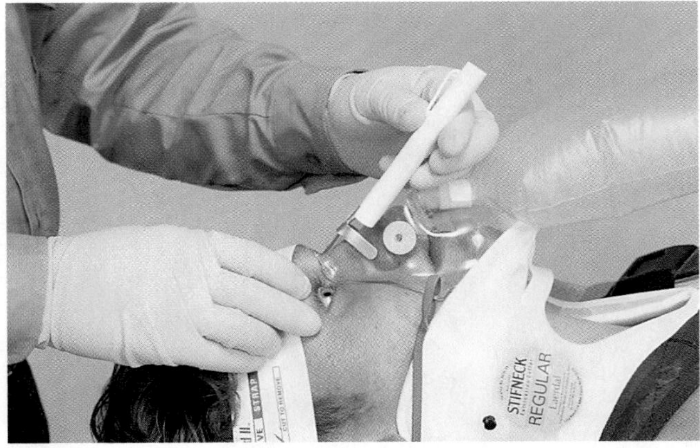

13-3E ✱ Assess both pupils for equality of size and reactivity to light. Inspect the color of the sclerae.

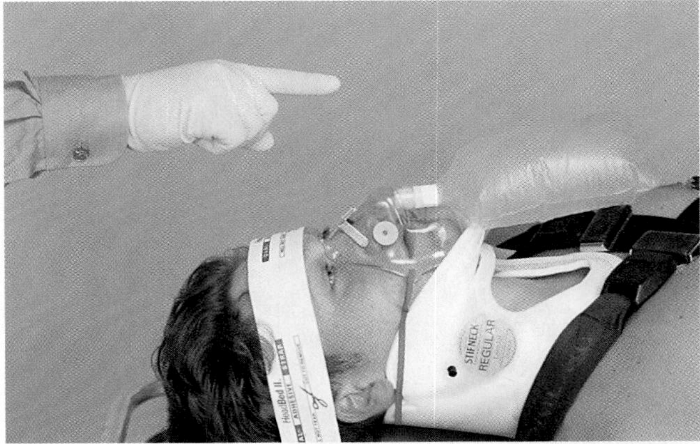

13-3F ✱ Check eye movement by having the patient follow your finger. Note any gazes in one direction or jerky eye movements.

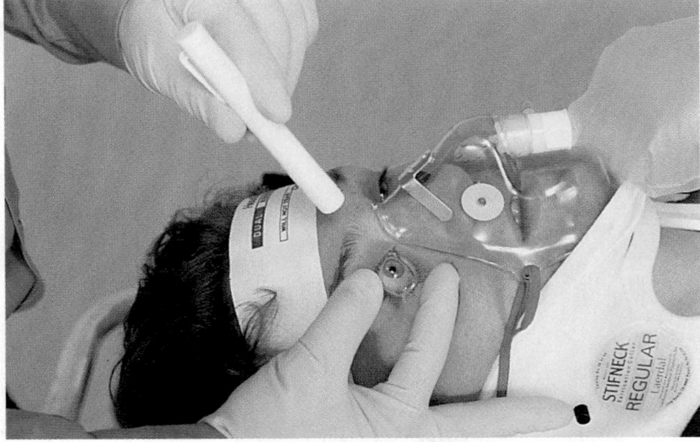

13-3G ✱ Inspect the conjunctiva by pulling the lower eyelid down.

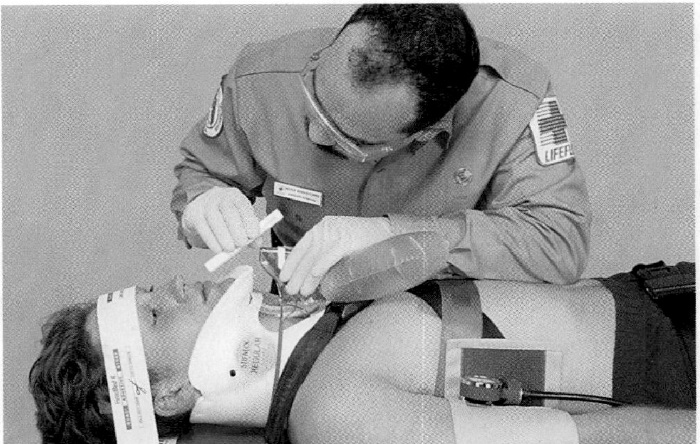

13-3H ✱ Inspect and palpate the nose for any signs of trauma, burns, bleeding, or fluid leakage.

continued

The Secondary Assessment: Anatomical Approach *continued*

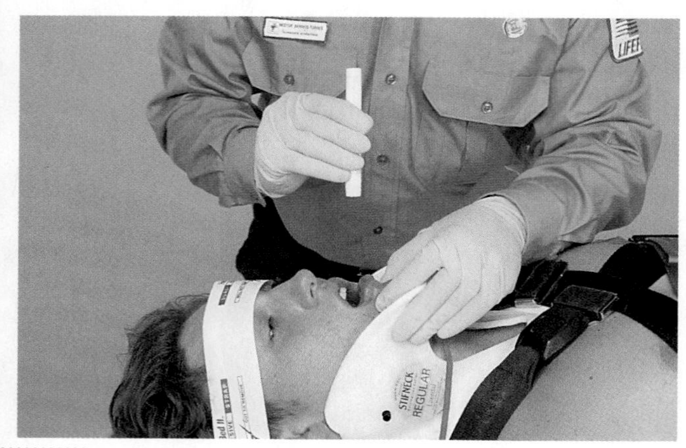

13-3I ✱ Inspect the inside of the mouth for signs of trauma, burns, and discoloration. Note the color of the mucous membranes. Smell the breath for any unusual odor.

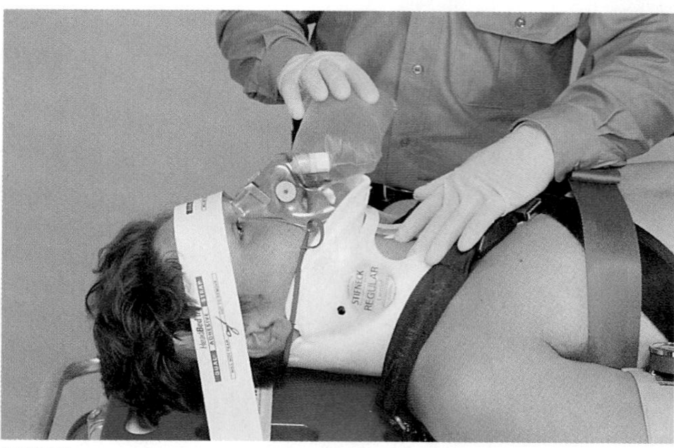

13-3J ✱ Assess the neck for jugular vein distention, tracheal deviation, accessory muscle use, and subcutaneous emphysema.

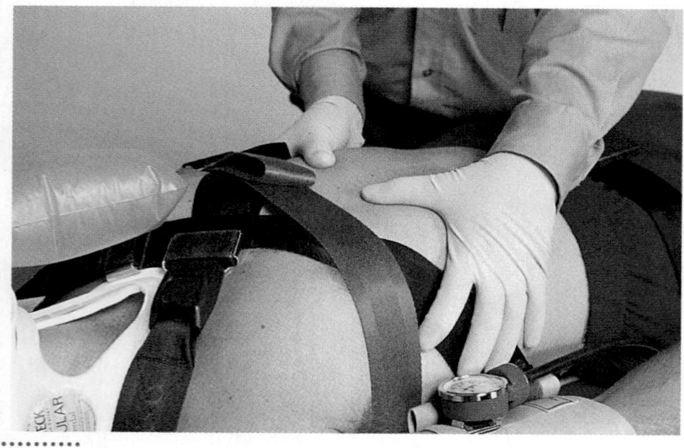

13-3K ✱ Inspect and palpate the entire chest. Check for symmetry of chest wall movement. Palpate the sternum, clavicles, and shoulders.

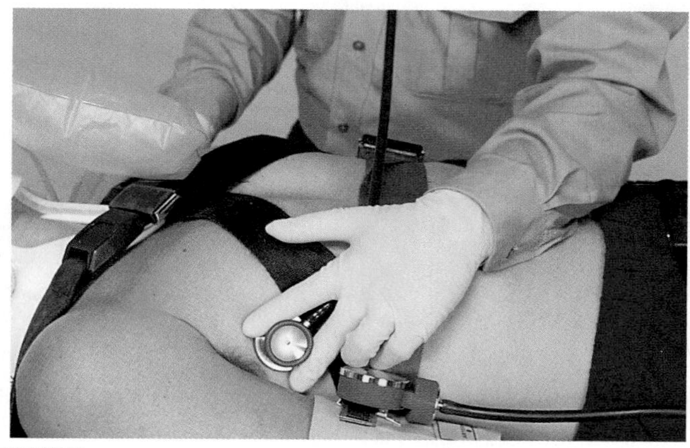

13-3L ✱ Auscultate breath sounds, comparing one side to the other.

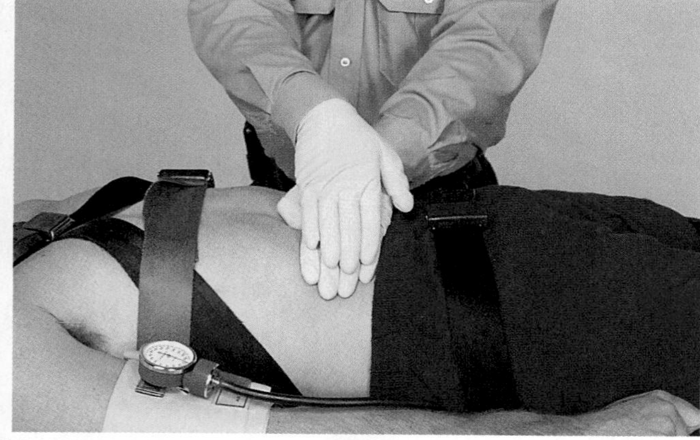

13-3M ✱ Inspect and palpate each quadrant of the abdomen. Note any guarding, tenderness, or rigidity.

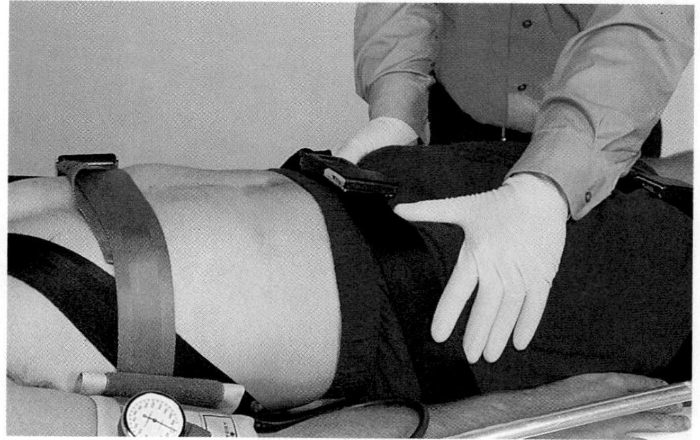

13-3N ✱ Assess the stability of the pelvis in a patient who is unresponsive or who has no noted pain in that area.

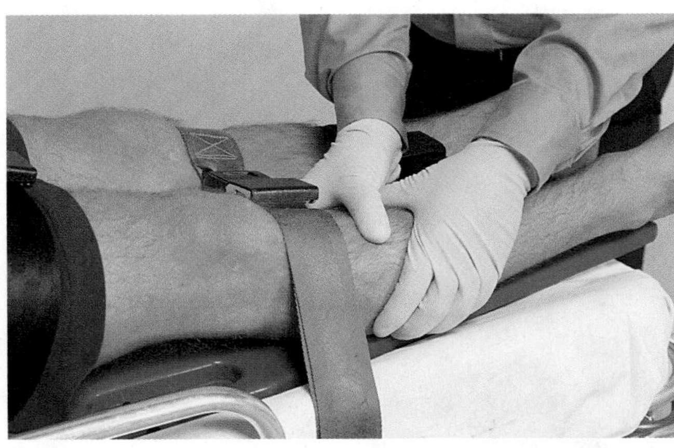

13-3O ✱ Inspect and palpate each lower extremity. Look for signs of wounds, bleeding, deformity, swelling, and discoloration.

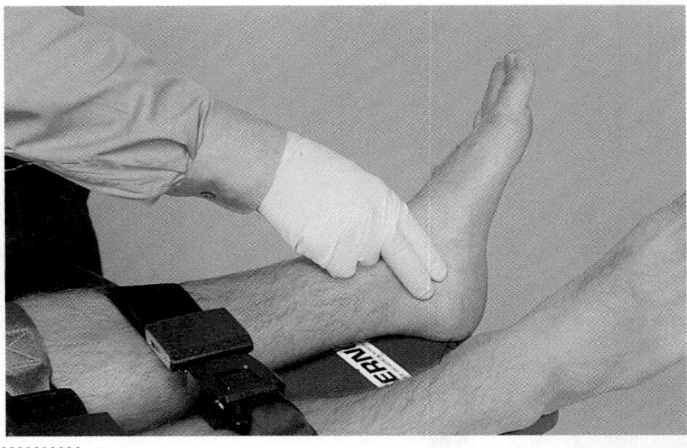

13-3P ✱ Assess distal pulses in each lower extremity. Also note skin color, temperature, and condition.

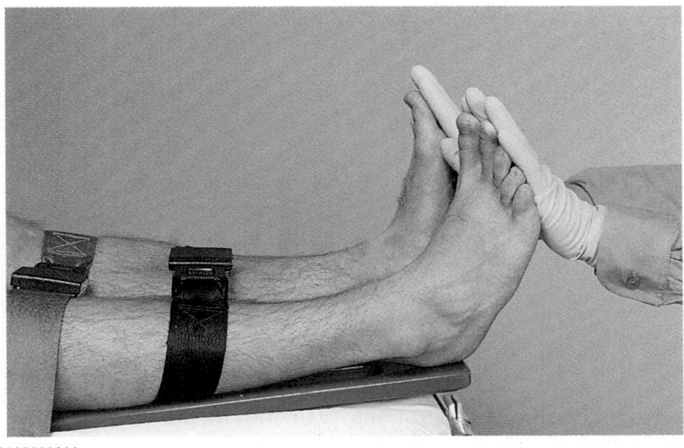

13-3Q ✱ Check motor response of both lower extremities by having the patient push both feet against your hands. Compare and note the equality of strength.

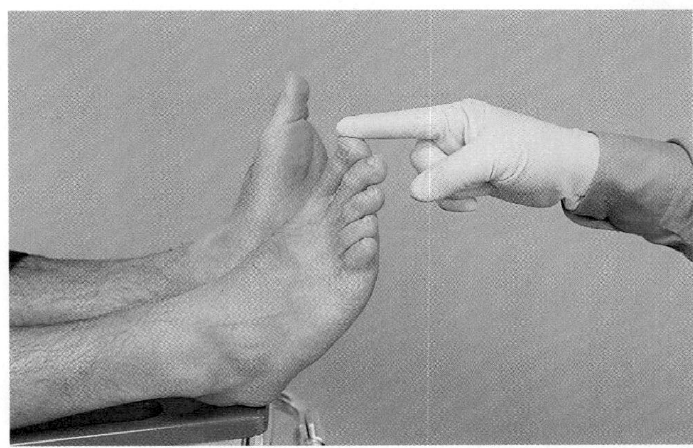

13-3R ✱ Assess sensation by first lightly touching a toe and asking the patient to identify which toe you are touching and then pinching the foot to check for pain response. If the patient is unresponsive, pinch the foot and note the patient's reaction.

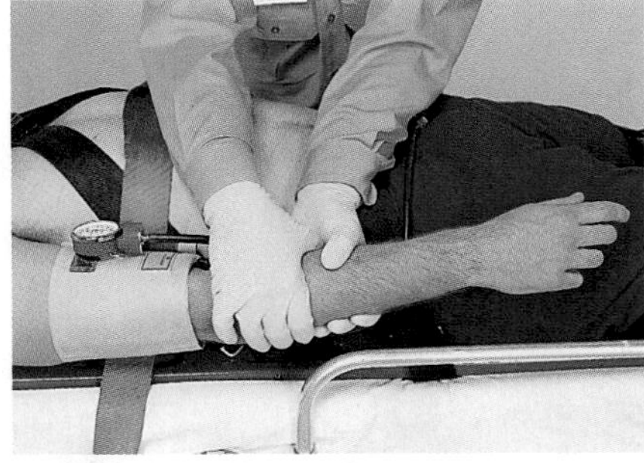

13-3S ✱ Inspect and palpate each upper extremity.

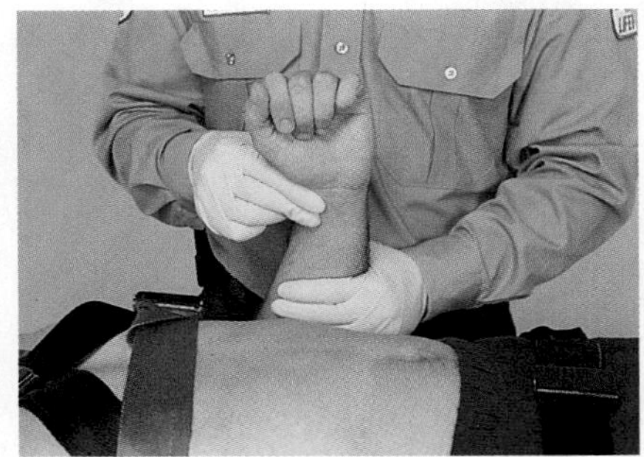

13-3T ✱ Assess the radial pulse on each upper extremity. Note skin color, temperature, and condition.

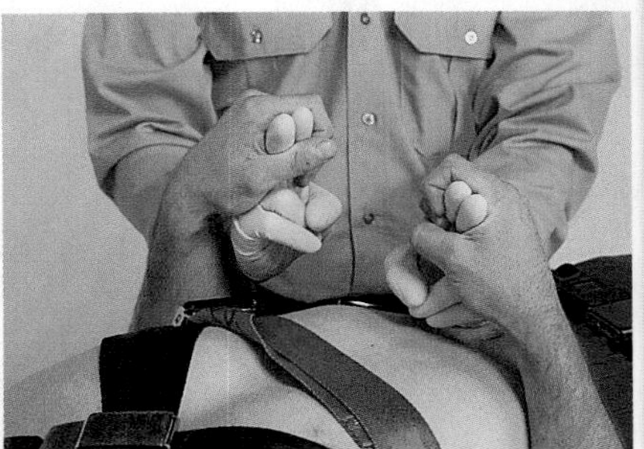

13-3U ✱ Assess motor function by having the patient grip the fingers of both your hands simultaneously. Note equality of strength. Assess sensory function by asking the patient to identify which finger you are touching. Then pinch the hand and ask the patient to identify the hand where he feels pain. If the patient is unresponsive, pinch the hand and note the patient's reaction.

EMT skills 13-4 Common Signs of Trauma

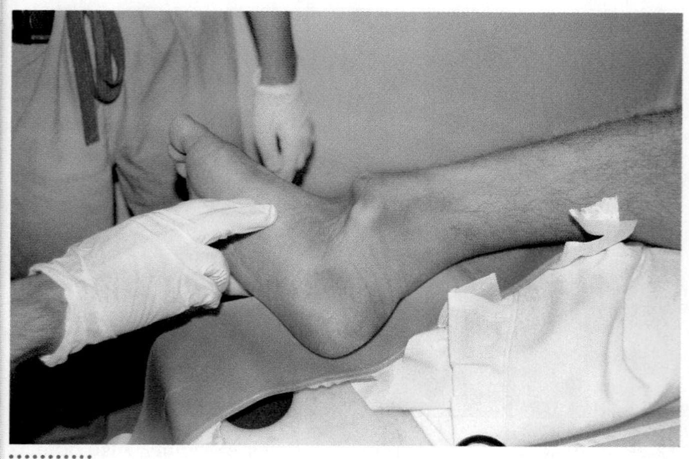

13-4A * Deformities. (© Edward T. Dickinson, MD)

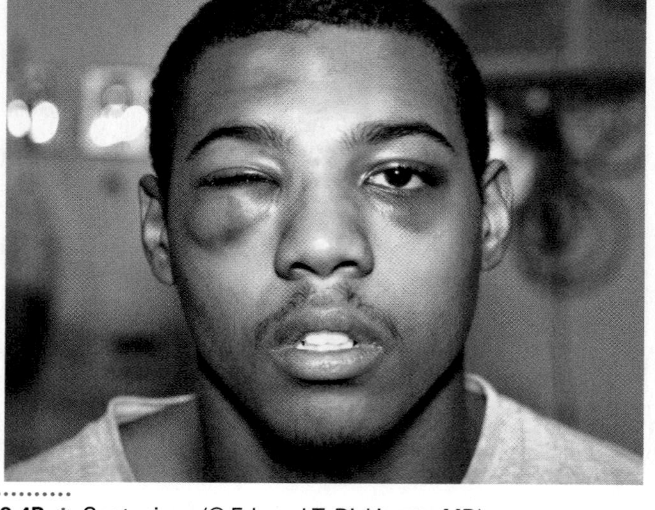

13-4B * Contusions (© Edward T. Dickinson, MD).

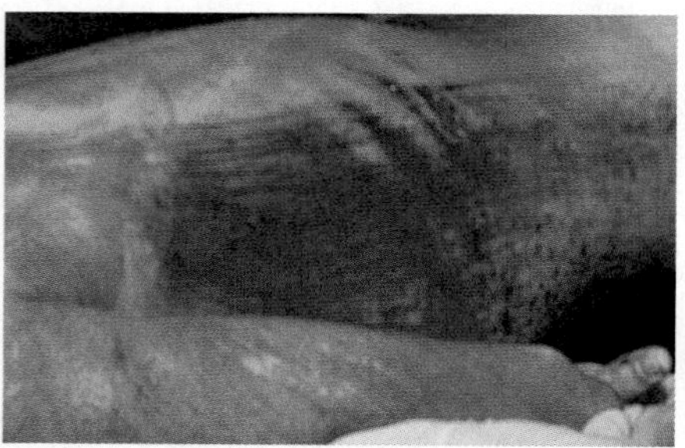

13-4C * Abrasions.

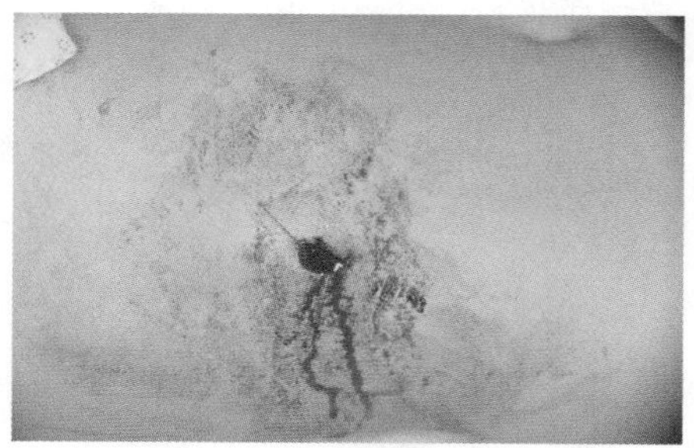

13-4D * Punctures/penetrations (© Charles M. Stewart, MD, and Associates).

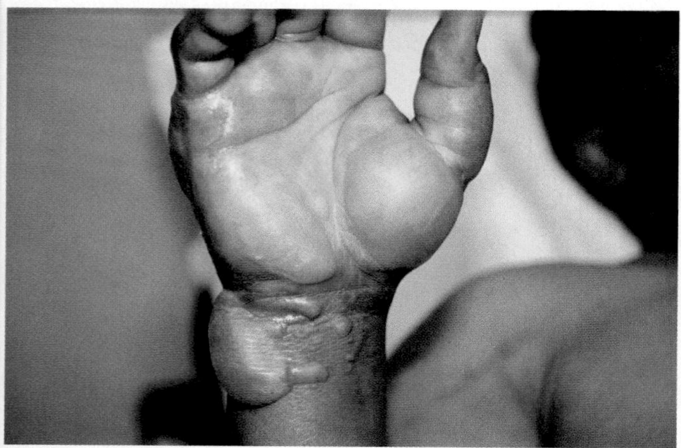

13-4E * Burns. (© Edward T. Dickinson, MD)

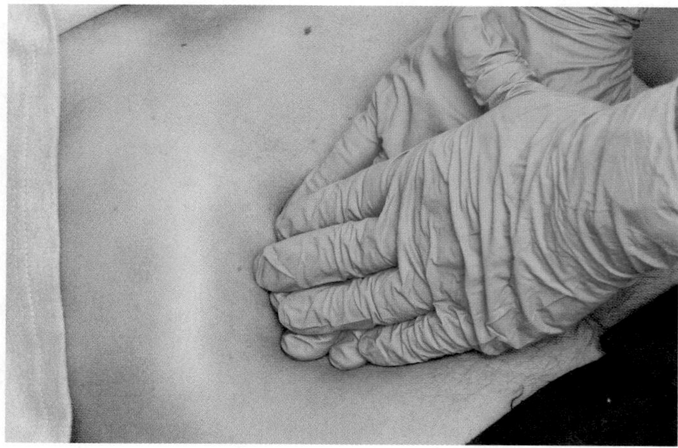

13-4F * Tenderness.

EMT skills 13-4 Common Signs of Trauma *continued*

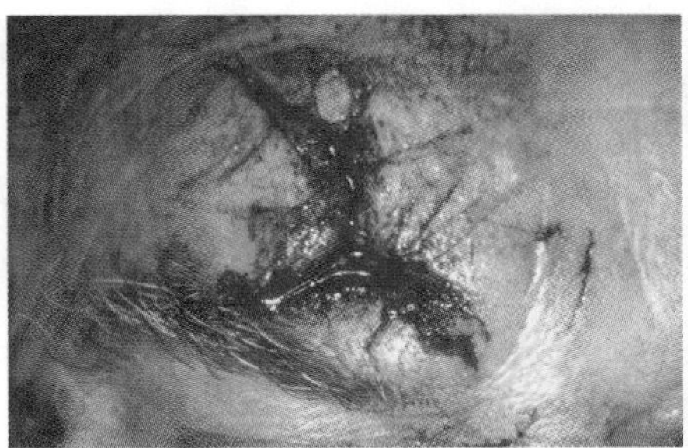

13-4G ✱ Lacerations.

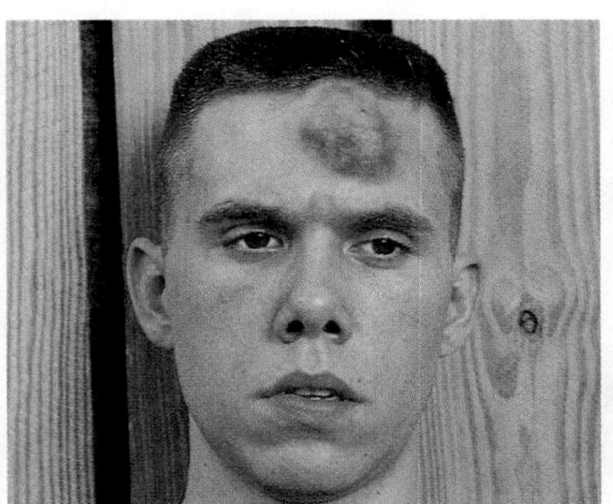

13-4H ✱ Swelling.

EMT skills 13-5 The Rapid Secondary Assessment for the Trauma Patient

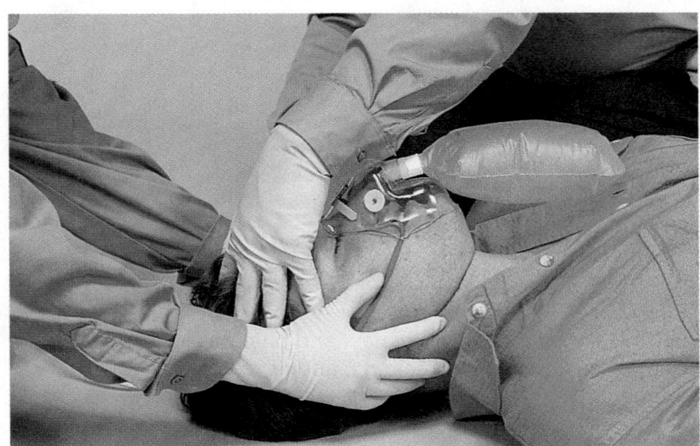

13-5A ✱ Inspect and palpate the scalp and skull.

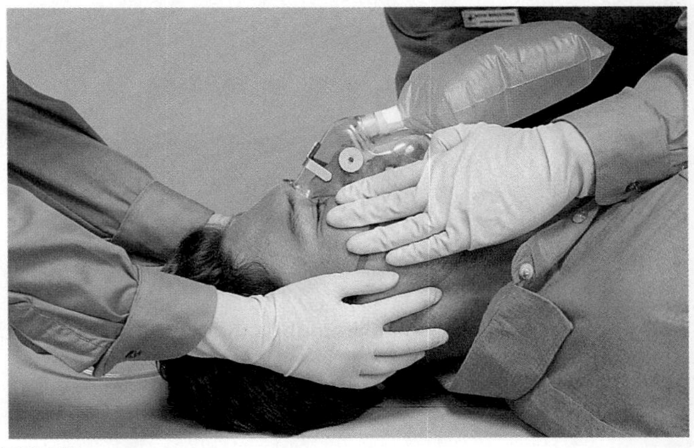

13-5B ✱ Inspect and palpate the face, including ears, pupils, nose, and mouth. Pay particular attention to injuries that could block the airway with blood, bone, teeth, or tissue.

continued

The Rapid Secondary Assessment for the Trauma Patient *continued*

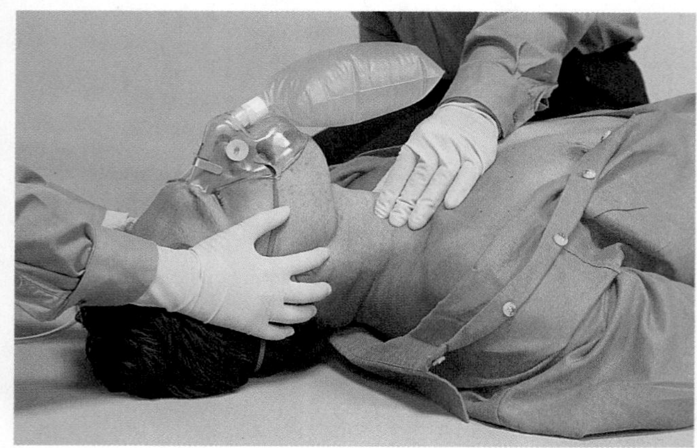

13-5C ✱ Inspect the neck for tracheal deviation, tracheal tugging, jugular vein distention, subcutaneous emphysema, and large lacerations or punctures.

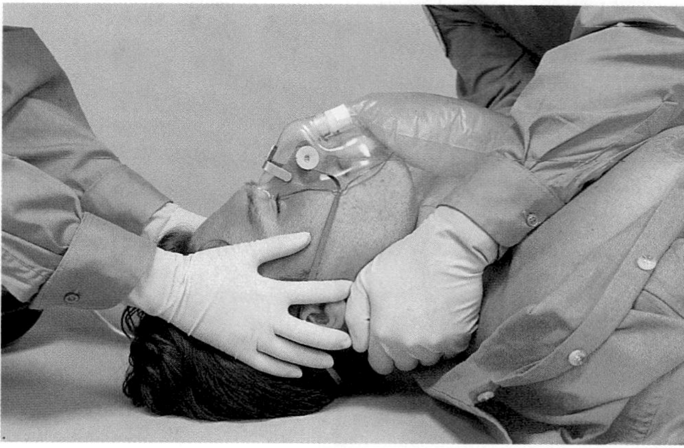

13-5D ✱ Palpate both the anterior and posterior aspects of the neck. Note posterior muscle spasms that may indicate injury to the cervical spine.

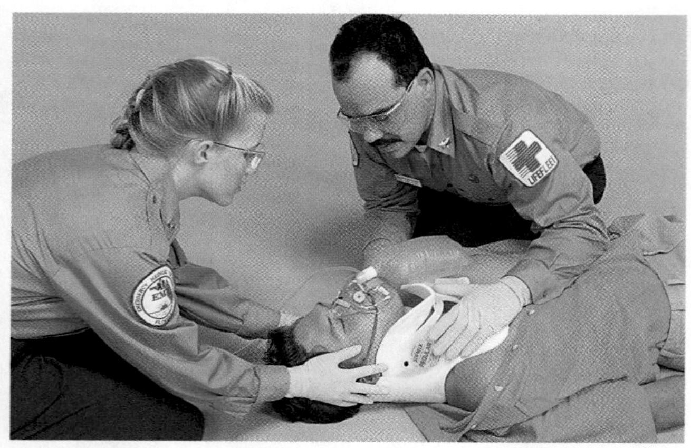

13-5E ✱ Apply a cervical spinal immobilization collar (CSIC) if not already done during or after the primary assessment.

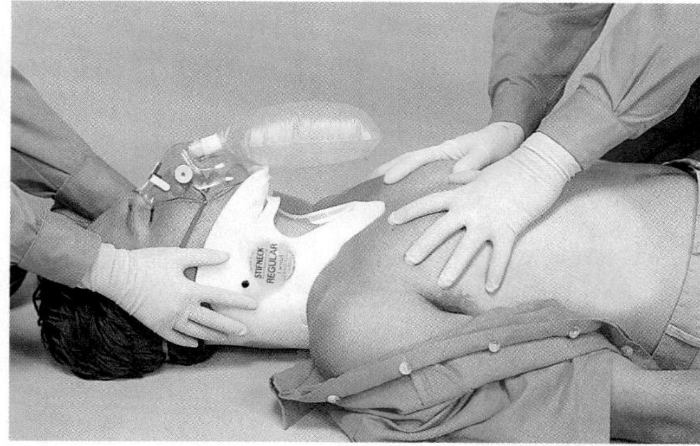

13-5F ✱ Expose the chest. Inspect and palpate for open wounds, flail segments, muscle retractions, and asymmetrical chest movement.

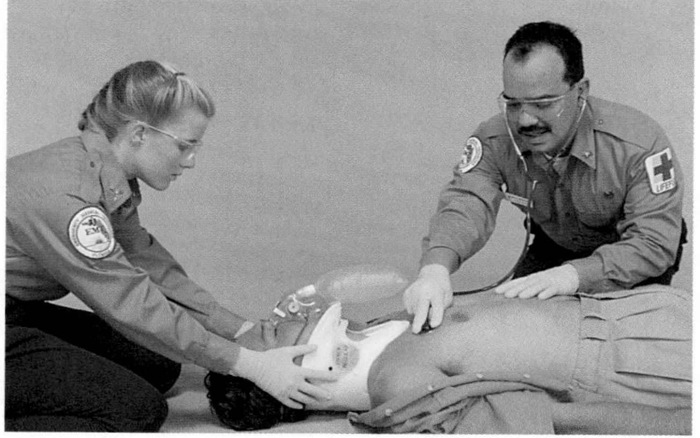

13-5G ✱ Perform a quick four-point auscultation of the chest to listen for the presence and equality of breath sounds.

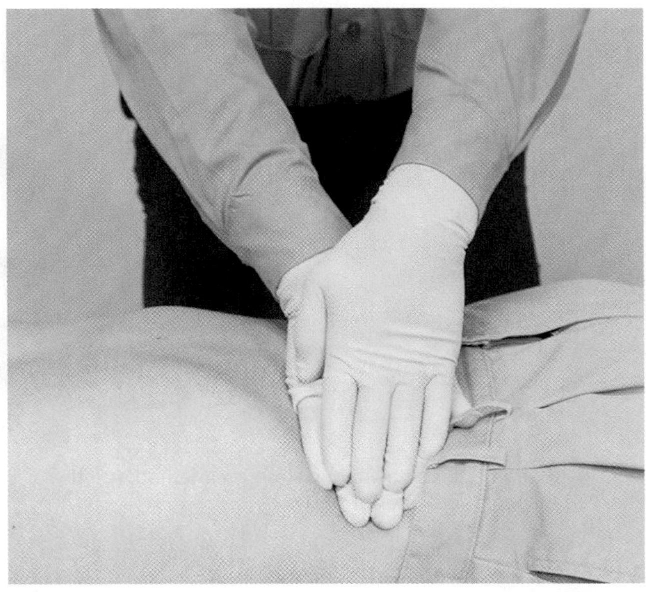

13-5H ✱ Inspect the abdomen for any evidence of trauma or distention. Palpate for tenderness and rigidity.

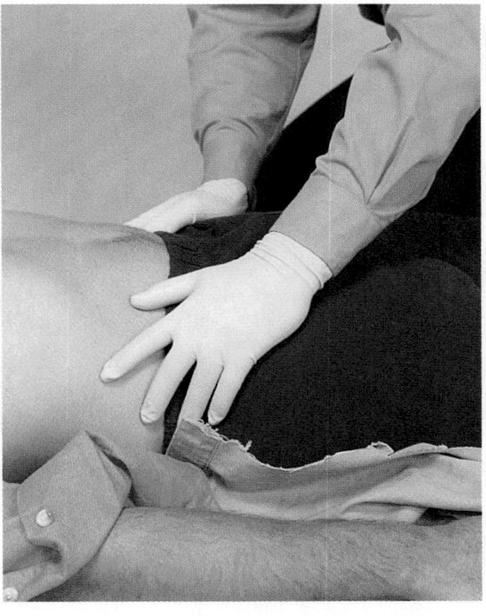

13-5I ✱ Inspect the pelvis for evidence of trauma. If the patient complains of pain or there is obvious deformity, do not palpate.

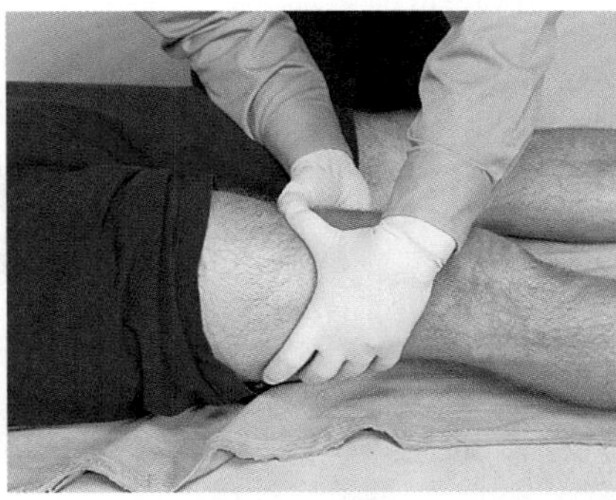

13-5J ✱ Inspect and palpate each lower extremity.

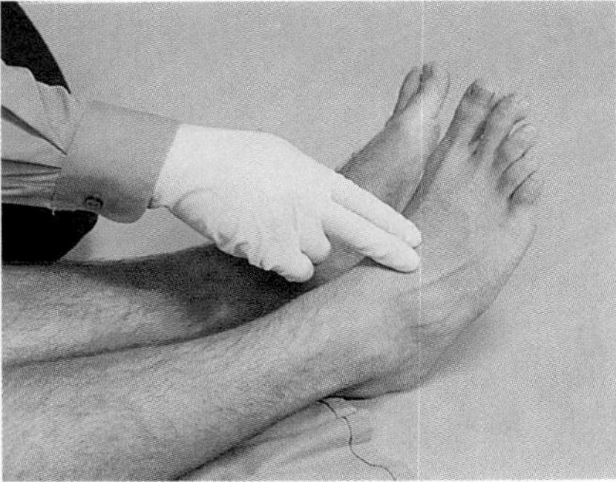

13-5K ✱ Assess pedal pulses.

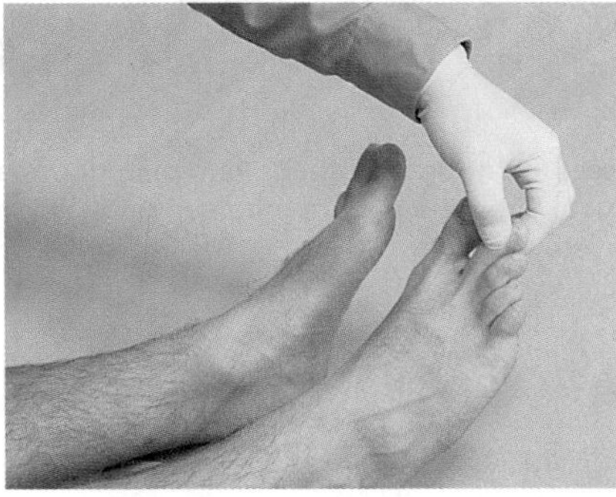

13-5L ✱ Assess motor and sensory function in each foot.

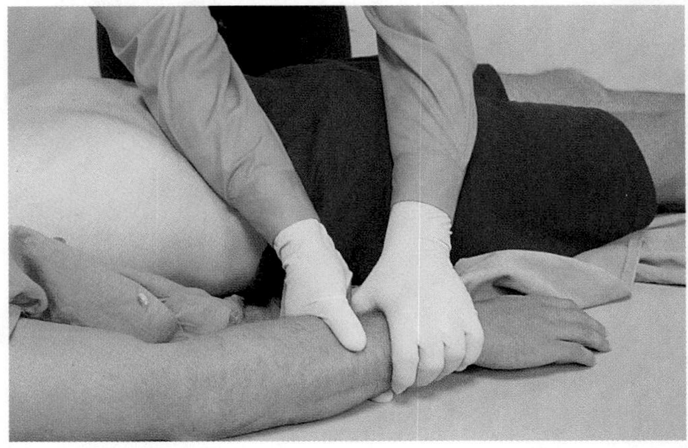

13-5M ✱ Assess and palpate each upper extremity.

continued

EMT skills 13-5 The Rapid Secondary Assessment for the Trauma Patient *continued*

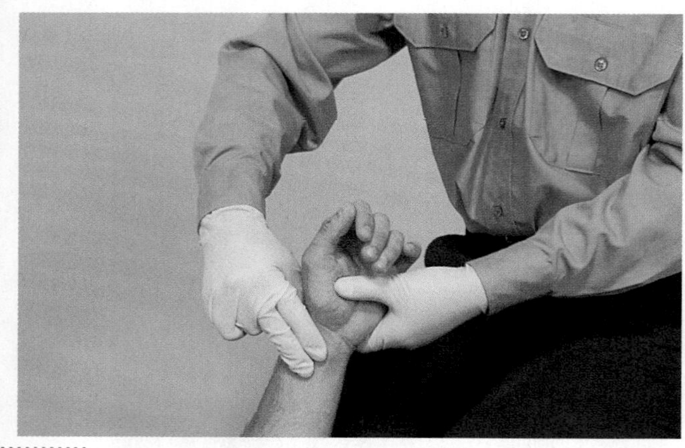

13-5N ✱ Assess distal pulse, motor, and sensory function in each upper extremity.

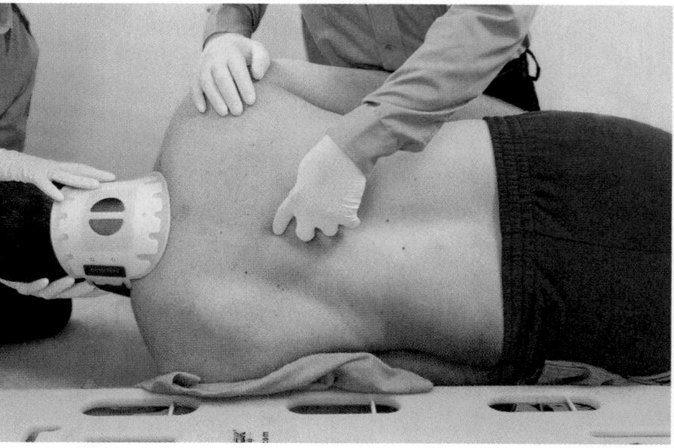

13-5O ✱ With in-line spinal stabilization maintained, roll the patient to inspect the posterior body.

EMT skills 13-6 The Rapid Secondary Assessment for the Medical Patient

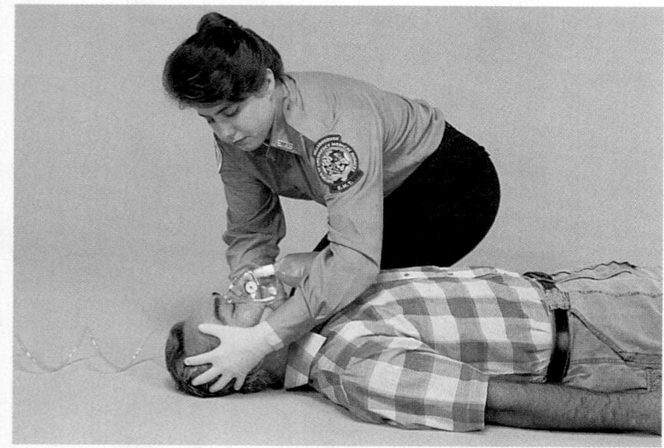

13-6A ✱ Inspect and palpate the head.

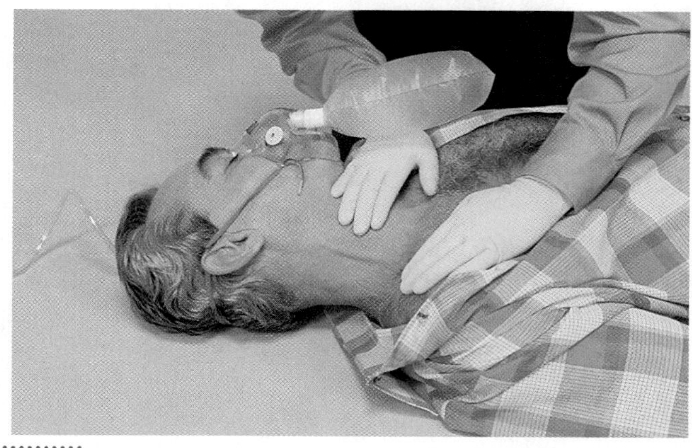

13-6B ✱ Inspect the neck for jugular vein distention, excessive neck muscle use when the patient inhales, medical identification tag, or tracheostomy tube.

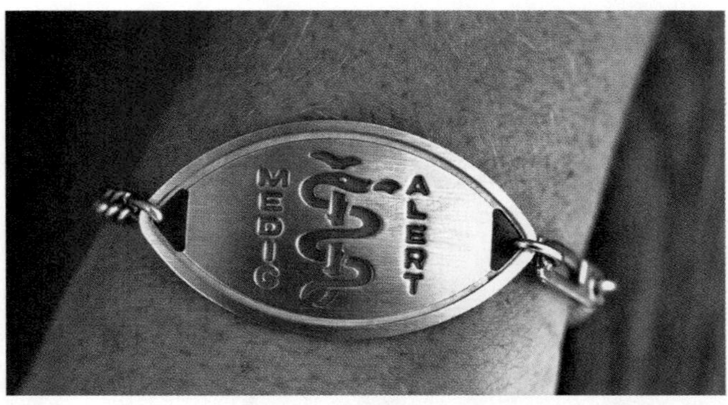

13-6C * A medical identification tag, usually worn around the neck or the wrist, will provide medical information about the patient.

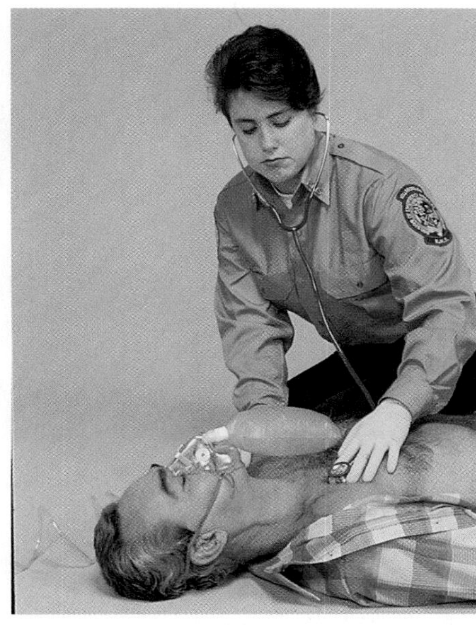

13-6D * Inspect the chest for adequate rise and fall, muscle retractions, and symmetry. Auscultate the breath sounds.

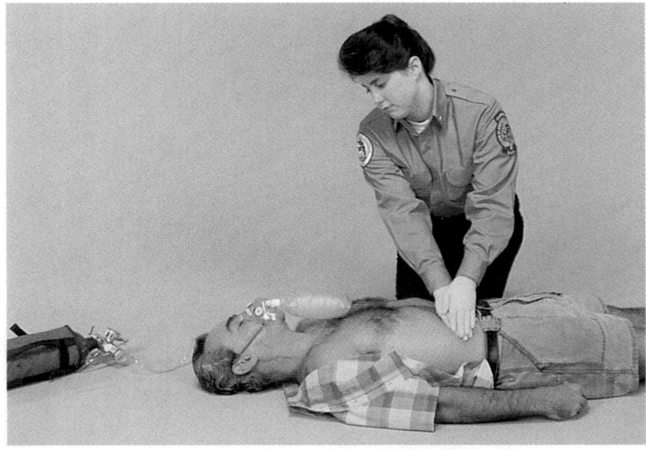

13-6E * Inspect the abdomen for scars, discoloration, or distention. Palpate for tenderness, rigidity, distention, and pulsating masses.

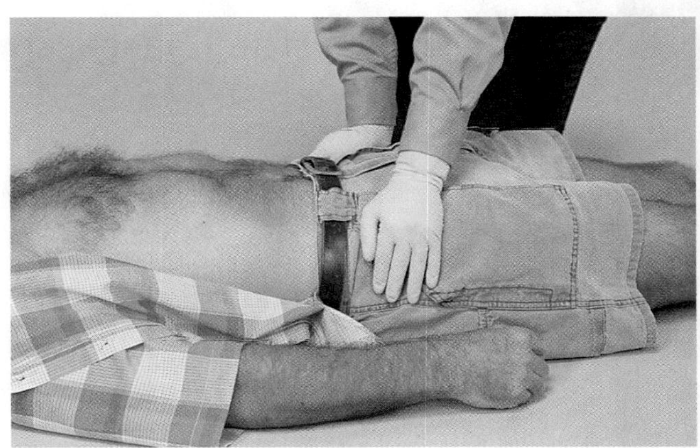

13-6F * Inspect and palpate the pelvic region.

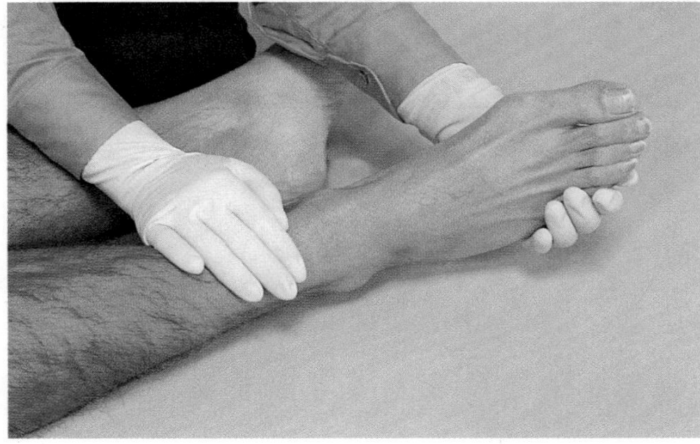

13-6G * Assess the upper and lower extremities for swelling and discoloration. Look for a medical identification tag around the wrist or ankle.

continued

EMT skills 13-6 The Rapid Secondary Assessment for the Medical Patient *continued*

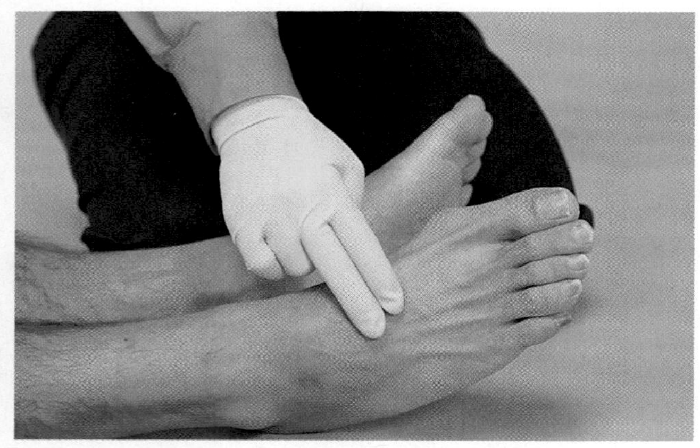

13-6H ✱ Assess pulses in all four extremities.

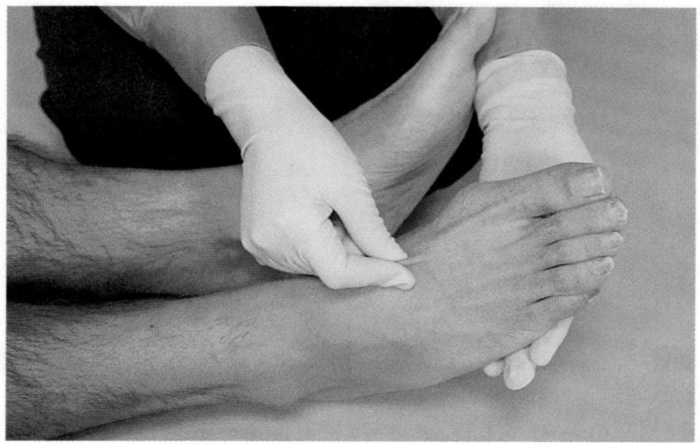

13-6I ✱ Assess motor and sensory function in all four extremities.

Conclude the rapid secondary assessment for the medical patient by inspecting and palpating the posterior body.

EMT skills 13-7 The Reassessment

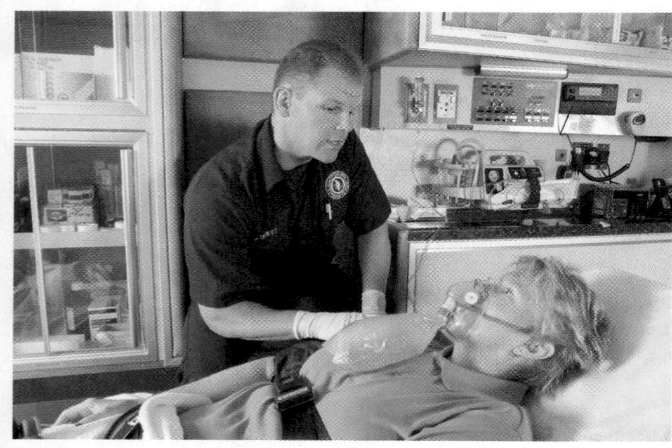

13-7A ✱ Reassure the patient as you begin to repeat the primary assessment.

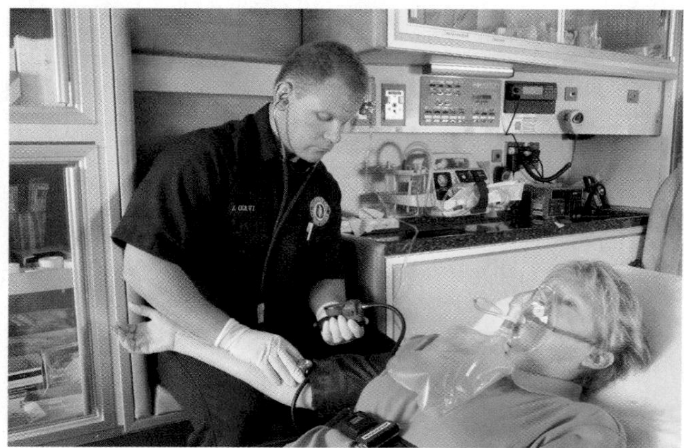

13-7B ✱ Reassess vital signs.

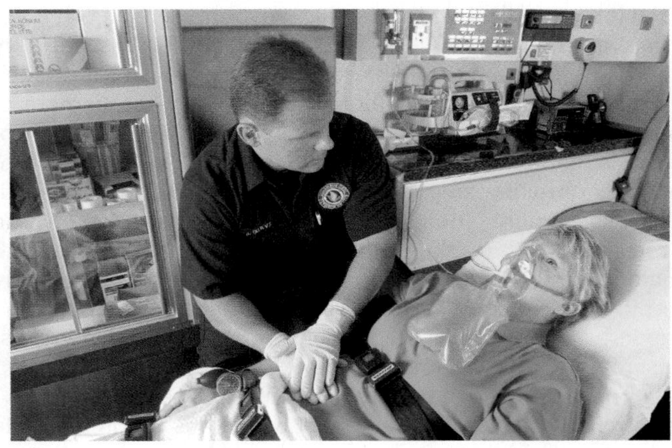

13-7C * Repeat appropriate elements of the physical exam.

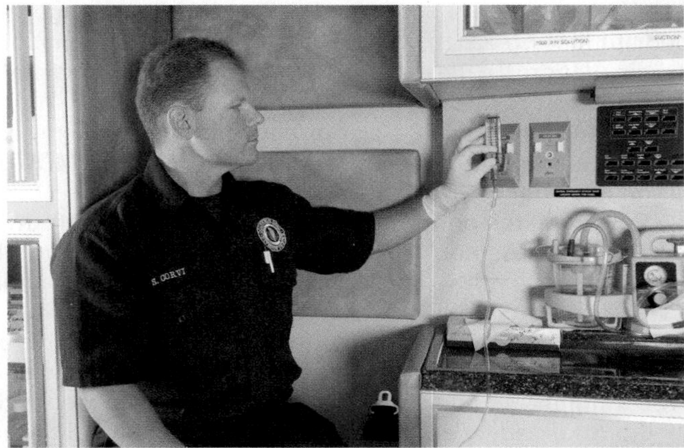

13-7D * Check and adjust interventions as necessary.

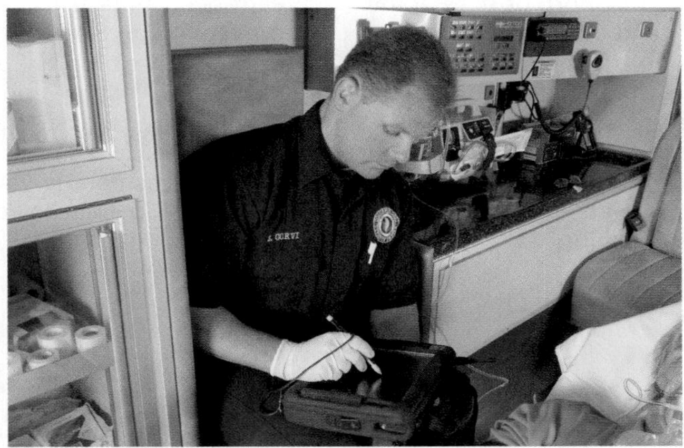

13-7E * Record trends in the patient's condition.

CHAPTER REVIEW

SUMMARY

The patient assessment is one of the most important functions you will perform as an EMT. The assessment determines your emergency care of the patient. If the assessment is not performed accurately or thoroughly, your emergency care may not be adequate, because injuries and conditions may have been overlooked.

Every patient assessment begins with the scene size-up. This was covered in detail in Chapter 12. The scene characteristics may provide clues as to whether the patient is injured or ill. In addition, it may provide information on the mechanism of injury (how the patient was injured) that may lead you to a higher index of suspicion for certain injuries.

The scene size-up will also determine the approach to your secondary assessment, whether it will be for a trauma or a medical patient.

The actual physical examination begins with the primary assessment, which is performed to identify and manage immediate life threats to the airway, breathing, oxygenation, and circulation. If a life threat is found, you must immediately intervene to provide the necessary emergency care. A primary assessment will be performed on every patient, regardless of his complaint, his mechanism of injury (MOI) or nature of the illness (NOI), or his mental status.

Following the primary assessment, you must perform a secondary assessment. A trauma assessment is performed on any patient with an MOI. There are two types of trauma assessment: the rapid secondary assessment and the modified secondary assessment. If the patient is unresponsive or has an altered mental status, has multiple injuries, has suffered a significant MOI, or is unstable, you will proceed with the rapid secondary assessment. This is a rapid head-to-toe assessment that is done to identify and manage all other life threats (other than those already managed during the primary assessment). You are assessing for critical injuries that require rapid intervention or rapid transport, or both. If the patient has only an isolated injury and there is no evidence of an altered mental status, no abnormal finding in the primary assessment, and no suspicion of multiple injuries, you will conduct a modified secondary assessment, a physical exam that focuses on the specific injury or body systems. If there is any doubt as to which assessment to perform (the rapid head-to-toe secondary assessment or the modified secondary assessment on the specific injury), always err on the side of benefiting the patient and do a rapid secondary assessment.

In the medical patient, more information can be gathered from the history than from the physical exam. Therefore, if the medical patient is alert, responsive, and oriented, you will first conduct a SAMPLE history, then a secondary assessment of anatomical areas and body systems associated with the chief complaint, and finally an assessment of baseline vital signs. However, if the medical patient is not alert, is disoriented, is responding to verbal or painful stimuli, or is unresponsive, you will first conduct a rapid secondary assessment (head-to-toe physical exam), then the assessment of baseline vital signs, and finally a SAMPLE history (which you will gather as best you can from family or other witnesses). The rapid secondary assessment for the medical patient is almost identical to the rapid secondary assessment for the trauma patient.

The last phase of the assessment is the reassessment. A reassessment is performed every 5 minutes in the unstable patient and every 15 minutes in the stable patient. It is conducted to reassess the primary assessment, baseline vital signs, any other complaints, and the interventions that have already been done. It also allows you to monitor trends—any improvement or deterioration—in the patient's condition.

You will perform the following three parts of the assessment on every patient you encounter in the prehospital setting: a primary assessment, a secondary assessment, and a reassessment.

The assessment is your tool to gather critical information about the patient so you can provide efficient and effective emergency care.

CASE STUDY FOLLOW-UPS

During your shift as an EMT, you are called to two different kinds of cases. The first call is to a trauma patient. The second is to a patient who is suffering from a medical problem.

CALL ONE—A TRAUMA PATIENT

SCENE SIZE-UP

You have been dispatched to an unresponsive patient with an unknown problem. Upon arrival, you see an adult male supine at the bottom of a two-story fire-escape ladder. A police officer approaches the ambulance and tells you that they have been called for a reported domestic incident and gunshots. The officer motions you to park a safe distance away until the scene is secured. Moments later you see police leading a suspect from the building. The officer motions you forward and tells you the scene is safe. Anticipating that the patient may be bleeding, you already have on gloves, mask, and eyewear with side shields as you jump from the ambulance and approach the patient.

PRIMARY ASSESSMENT

As you approach the patient, you notice that the shirt front and left pants leg are soaked in blood, the skin is extremely pale, and the right lower leg is severely deformed. This is obviously a trauma patient with a significant mechanism of injury—a probable fall from the fire escape and a possible gunshot wound.

Your partner immediately establishes in-line stabilization of the head and neck and performs a jaw thrust to open the airway. The patient does not respond to verbal commands; however, he moans and makes a facial grimace as you pinch the trapezius muscle.

You assess the breathing status and determine that the patient's chest is barely rising and falling and only minimal air movement can be felt or heard. You immediately instruct your partner to insert an oropharyngeal airway and begin bag-valve-mask ventilation with supplemental oxygen while maintaining in-line stabilization. A radial pulse is not palpable and the carotid pulse is extremely weak, fast, and thready. The skin is pale, cool, and clammy.

As you continue with your assessment, you quickly cut the shirt off and find a gunshot wound to the left anterior chest. You immediately place your gloved hand over the wound. You then tape the plastic package from an oxygen mask over the wound on three sides and continue to scan the anterior and lateral aspects of the chest for any other wounds.

Next, you expose the area around the left thigh and find a wound with dark red bleeding at a steady flow. You apply direct pressure to control the bleeding and then immediately apply a pressure dressing.

You indicate to your partner that this is going to be a rapid patient transport.

SECONDARY ASSESSMENT

Now that immediate life threats are under control, you begin the rapid secondary assessment. You quickly assess the head and neck and apply a cervical spinal immobilization collar. Your partner continues in-line stabilization.

As you continue with your assessment, you find decreased breath sounds on the left side of the chest. You find no abnormalities in the abdominal or pelvic region, but the right lower extremity is swollen and deformed and the patient moans when you palpate the angulated area. With assistance from police First Responders, spinal stabilization is maintained as the patient is log rolled and the posterior thorax and lumbar region and buttocks are exposed. No additional injuries are revealed.

While the patient is still on his side, a police First Responder slides the backboard next to the patient and the patient is rolled onto it and secured with straps. A head immobilization device is applied. The right lower extremity is also carefully secured to the board for stabilization.

The blood pressure is measured at a low 70/50 mmHg; skin remains pale, cool, and clammy; pupils are normal in size, equal, and sluggish to respond to light; the heart rate is rapid at 136 per minute; and the spontaneous respiratory rate is only 6 per minute. You continue positive pressure ventilation with supplemental oxygen at a rate of 10 per minute.

No one at the scene knows the patient, so the only portion of the SAMPLE history you are able to gather is information about events leading to the injury. A neighbor reports hearing gunshots, seeing the patient stagger out onto the second-story fire escape clutching his chest, then watching in horror as the patient pitched over the railing and fell to the pavement.

The patient is promptly loaded into the ambulance for transport with lights and siren.

En route to the hospital, you apply a vacuum splint to the right lower leg for better immobilization.

You apply a sterile dressing and bandage to a small laceration at the left temporal region of the patient's head.

REASSESSMENT

Because this is a patient with critical injuries, you continuously reassess the mental status, airway, breathing, and circulation, and you take and record vital signs every 5 minutes while en route to the emergency department. You reassess the patient's injuries and check the effectiveness of interventions, making sure that positive pressure ventilation is adequate, the dressing on the chest wound is permitting escape of air on the unsecured side, the bleeding at the chest and thigh is under control, and the immobilization to the backboard and splints is secure. You radio the hospital emergency department to report patient information and to alert them to your estimated time of arrival. No change in the patient's condition has occurred and you arrive at the hospital without further incident.

You give the hospital staff your oral report on the patient, complete the written documentation, and prepare the ambulance for the next call.

CALL TWO—A MEDICAL PATIENT

SCENE SIZE-UP

Shortly after the call to the man injured in the domestic dispute, you are again dispatched to a patient with an unknown problem. This time, you arrive at a well-kept home in a quiet neighborhood and are met by a middle-aged woman who says she called EMS for her mother, who cannot catch her breath. The woman, Mrs. Conlon, leads you into the house. As you enter the living room, you see an elderly woman sitting up in a chair and an oxygen tank in the corner. You conclude that your patient likely is suffering from a medical problem rather than trauma.

PRIMARY ASSESSMENT

Mrs. Conlon introduces you to her mother, Mrs. Ortega, and tells you that her mother is 72 years old. Mrs. Ortega is sitting up in a chair, leaning forward, with her hand on her chest. She says, "I'm glad—you came. I feel like—I can't breathe." Her remarks assure you that her mental status is alert and her airway is open. You observe that she is breathing in fast, short puffs, but with adequate rise and fall of the chest. You apply a nonrebreather mask connected to oxygen flowing at 15 lpm, explaining that this will help relieve her distress. Because she has a home supply of oxygen that she has occasionally used, she understands and welcomes the oxygen therapy. You are able to palpate a somewhat rapid radial pulse, and you note that her skin is warm, pink, and dry. You instruct your partner to apply the pulse oximeter.

SECONDARY ASSESSMENT

You sit down on a chair next to Mrs. Ortega and begin to take the history, starting with an elaboration of the chief complaint. She is not experiencing pain, so most of the OPQRST questions do not apply, but she does tell you that the onset of her symptoms was gradual over this morning and afternoon and that she has been suffering from the breathing difficulty for several hours. You determine that she chronically has a difficult time breathing, but this episode was slightly worse than usual—a 5 on a scale of 1 to 10. You continue with the assessment using the SAMPLE mnemonic as the foundation for asking questions. She has no allergies that she knows of. The medications she takes, including oxygen, are related to her history of emphysema, a serious lung disease. Her last oral intake was lunch at around noon. There were no unusual events leading to the onset of the symptom.

Meanwhile, your partner has been taking and recording Mrs. Ortega's baseline vital signs. Her respirations are puffy, somewhat labored, and at a rate of 28 per minute with adequate chest rise. Her pulse is rapid at 100 per minute and irregular. Her skin color, temperature, and condition remain normal. Pupils are normal, equal, and reactive. Her blood pressure is 120/90 mmHg. The pulse oximeter reading is 88% while on the nonrebreather mask.

The physical exam you conduct is focused on Mrs. Ortega's complaint and related body systems. You assess her pupils and find that they are midsize and sluggish to respond. Her oral mucosa and conjunctiva are slightly cyanotic. Her neck veins are flat. You quickly inspect the chest by lifting her shirt to look for any potential evidence of trauma. You auscultate her chest with your stethoscope and detect wheezing noises that, in fact, you can hear even without the stethoscope. The breathing sounds are present and equal on both sides. Her abdomen is nontender and no distention is noted. You inspect the lower extremities for redness and swelling, especially to one calf. You quickly palpate trying to elicit a tenderness response. You ask Mrs. Ortega to "Point your toes back toward your head" checking for tenderness in either calf region. You then ask her to "Point your toes" again checking for any tenderness. You inspect the ankles and feet for edema.

You place Mrs. Ortega on the wheeled stretcher and transfer her to the ambulance. You raise the head of the stretcher so that she can ride to the hospital in a sitting position, which she finds is more comfortable and helps her to breathe.

REASSESSMENT

You perform a reassessment by reassessing her mental status, airway, breathing, oxygenation, and circulation, and reassessing and recording her vital signs. You repeat an assessment focused on her breathing problem by using your stethoscope to auscultate her chest and reconfirm that breath sounds are present and equal with wheezing sounds on both sides. You check to be sure that the nonrebreather mask is correctly placed and that the oxygen continues to flow at 15 lpm. Because Mrs. Ortega is a stable patient, you repeat the reassessment every 15 minutes en route. You radio the hospital emergency department with patient information and your estimated time of arrival.

You arrive at the hospital with no further incident, give your oral report to the receiving staff, complete the transfer of care, finish the prehospital care report, and prepare the ambulance for the next call.

IN REVIEW

1. Briefly state the purposes of patient assessment by the EMT.
2. List the main components of patient assessment.
3. List the three steps of the scene size-up.
4. List the steps of the primary assessment.
5. Contrast the order of the three steps of the secondary assessment for a responsive medical patient with the order of the steps for an unresponsive medical patient or trauma patient. Explain why the order of the steps differs.
6. Describe the kinds of patients for whom the physical exam should be a rapid head-to-toe assessment (rapid secondary assessment). Describe the kinds of patients for whom the physical exam should be focused on a specific site or area of complaint (modified secondary assessment).
7. Name the five categories of measurements that are included in the vital signs.
8. Name the categories of information sought during history taking that the letters in OPQRST and SAMPLE represent.
9. State how often, at a minimum, during the reassessment, the components of the primary assessment and the vital signs should be reassessed for the following: (a) a critical or unstable patient and (b) a stable patient.

CRITICAL THINKING

SCENARIO 1

You are called to the scene for a 23-year-old male who fell approximately 20 feet from a balcony at a concert. The patient is not alert as you approach him. He has blood coming from his mouth and ears. His left arm is angulated and obviously fractured. A bystander states he was talking and moaning right after he fell, but now he won't respond.

1. What would be your first immediate action when you arrive at the patient?
2. What assessment should you conduct first?
3. What are the components of that assessment and in what order would you perform them?
4. What life threats are you assessing for and how would you manage them?
5. What injuries should you suspect in this patient?
6. What baseline vital signs would you assess?
7. Would you perform a rapid secondary assessment or a modified secondary assessment?
8. What does the change in his mental status indicate?
9. When would you transport?
10. How would you prepare the patient for transport?
11. What would you do while en route to the medical facility?

SCENARIO 2

You are called to the scene for a 78-year-old female complaining of shortness of breath. As you arrive on the scene, her daughter lets you into the house and directs you to her mother. The patient is lying supine on the couch and appears to be extremely pale and cyanotic. You hear snoring sounds when she breathes. The daughter states that her mother has a heart condition and hasn't been feeling well for 2 days. She thought her mother was napping on the couch, but when she went to wake her, her mother did not respond.

1. Do you suspect she is a trauma or medical patient?
2. What would be your first immediate action when you arrive at the patient?
3. What assessment should you conduct first?
4. What are the components of that assessment and in what order would you perform them?
5. What life threats are you assessing for and how would you manage them?
6. Would you collect a SAMPLE history first or do a medical assessment?
7. Would you perform a rapid secondary assessment or a modified secondary assessment?
8. How would you collect a SAMPLE history?
9. What does the mental status possibly indicate?
10. What would you expect the SpO_2 reading to be?
11. When would you transport?
12. How would you prepare the patient for transport?
13. What would you do while en route to the medical facility?

PEARSON

EXPLORE mybradykit™

Please go to **www.bradybooks.com** to access mykit for this text. You will find quizzes, critical thinking scenarios, weblinks, animations, and videos related to this chapter—and much more. Look for online information on simulated patient assessments.

Register your access code from the front of your book by going to **www.bradybooks.com** and selecting the mykit links.

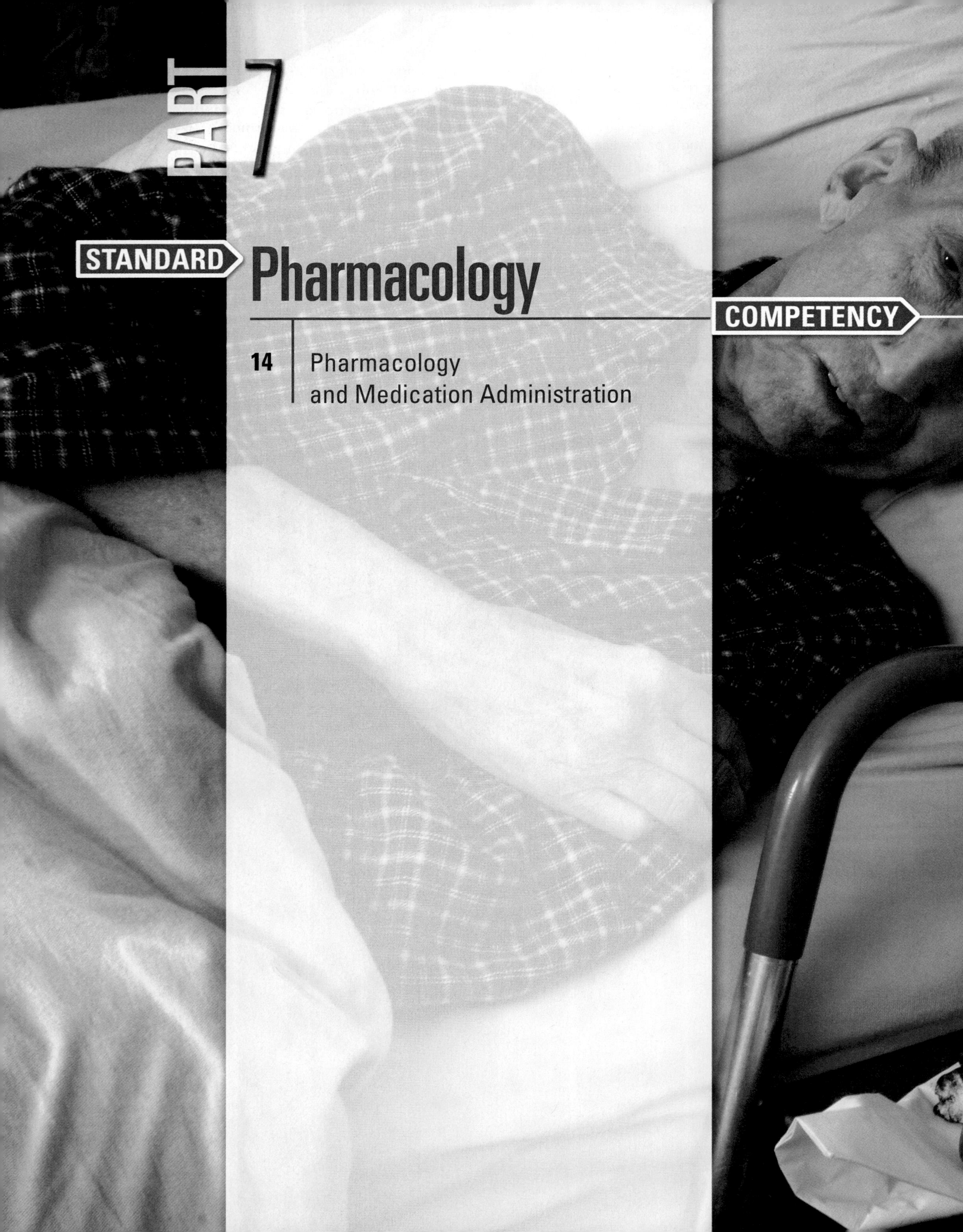

PART 7

STANDARD

Pharmacology

COMPETENCY

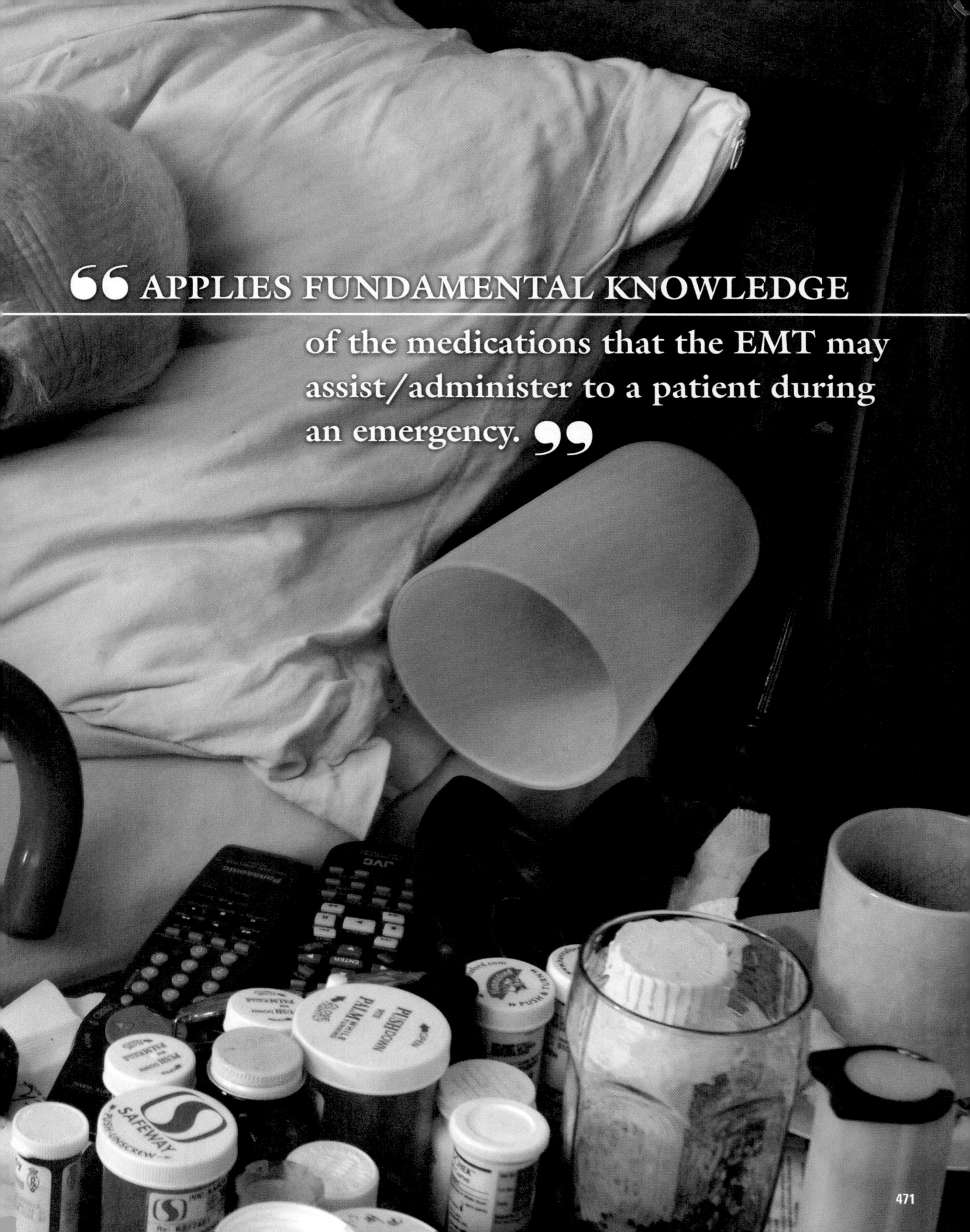

"APPLIES FUNDAMENTAL KNOWLEDGE of the medications that the EMT may assist/administer to a patient during an emergency."

CHAPTER 14

Pharmacology *and* Medication Administration

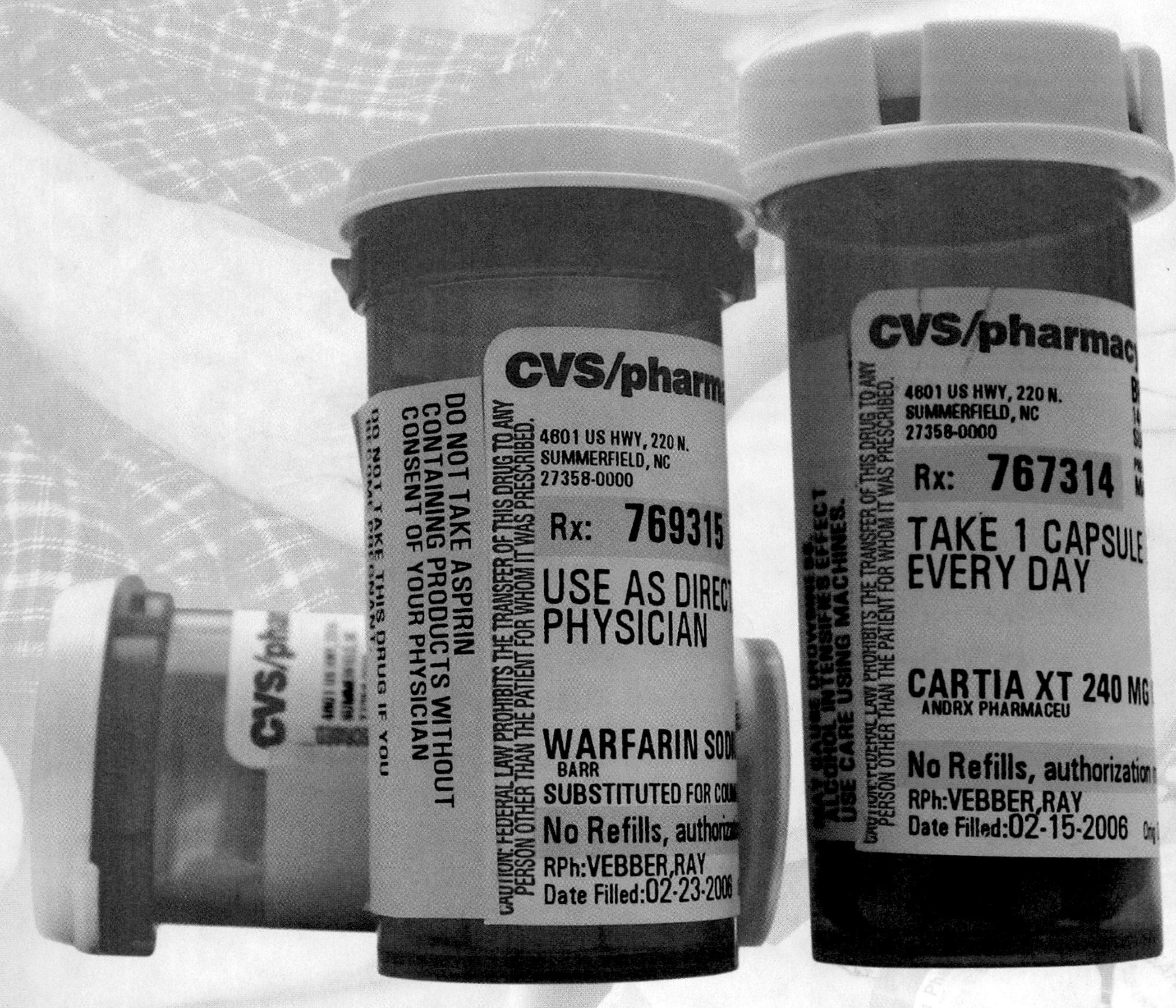
DO NOT TAKE ASPIRIN
CONTAINING PRODUCTS WITHOUT
CONSENT OF YOUR PHYSICIAN
CAUTION: FEDERAL LAW PROHIBITS THE TRANSFER OF THIS DRUG TO ANY
PERSON OTHER THAN THE PATIENT FOR WHOM IT WAS PRESCRIBED.
4601 US HWY, 220 N.
SUMMERFIELD, NC
27358-0000
Rx: 769315
PHYSICIAN
BARR
RPh:VEBBER,RAY
MAY CAUSE DROWSINESS.
ALCOHOL INTENSIFIES EFFECT
USE CARE USING MACHINES.
Rx: 767314
EVERY DAY
ANDRX PHARMACEU
RPh:VEBBER,RAY
Date Filled:02-15-2006

Navigation Guide

The following items provide an overview to the purpose and content of this chapter. The Standard and Competency are from the new National EMS Education Standards.

STANDARD **Pharmacology** (Content Areas: Principles of Pharmacology; Medication Administration; Emergency Medications)

COMPETENCY Applies fundamental knowledge of the medications that the EMT may assist/administer to a patient during an emergency.

OBJECTIVES: After reading this chapter, you should be able to:

14-1. Define key terms introduced in this chapter.
14-2. Describe the roles and responsibilities associated with administering and assisting patients with administration of medications.
14-3. Differentiate between administration of medication and assisting a patient in taking his own medications.
14-4. List the medications in the EMT's scope of practice.
14-5. Differentiate between a drug's chemical, official, generic, and trade names.
14-6. Demonstrate the proper administration of drugs by each of the following routes:
- **a.** Sublingual
- **b.** Oral
- **c.** Inhalation
- **d.** Intramuscular (epinephrine auto-injector only)

14-7. Differentiate between the following medication forms:
- **a.** Tablet
- **b.** Liquid for injection
- **c.** Gel
- **d.** Suspension
- **e.** Fine powder for inhalation
- **f.** Gas
- **g.** Liquid for spray or aerosolization

14-8. Explain the roles of off-line and on-line medical direction with regard to medication administration.
14-9. Adhere to the following key steps of medication administration:
- **a.** Obtain an order.
- **b.** Verify on-line orders.
- **c.** Select the proper medication.
- **d.** Verify the patient's prescription.
- **e.** Check the expiration date.
- **f.** Check for impurities and discoloration.
- **g.** Verify the form, route, and dose.
- **h.** Ensure that the "five rights" of medication administration are followed.

14-10. Document required information regarding medication administration.
14-11. Describe the reassessment of a patient after you have administered or assisted the patient in taking a medication.

KEY TERMS: Page references indicate first major use in this chapter. For complete definitions, see the Glossary at the back of the book.

action p. 482
administration p. 482
contraindications p. 482
dose p. 482
drug p. 474
form p. 479
indications p. 482
medication p. 474
metered-dose inhaler (MDI) p. 476
pharmacology p. 474
route p. 478
side effects p. 482
small-volume nebulizer p. 476

MEDIA RESOURCES: Please go to www.bradybooks.com to access mykit for this text. You will find quizzes, critical thinking scenarios, weblinks, animations, and videos related to this chapter—and much more. Look for online information on medications that can be administered by an EMT. You will also find video clips on the administration of activated charcoal, oral glucose, and nitroglycerin.

continued

CASE STUDY

The Dispatch
EMS Unit 202—respond to 1934 Lincoln Avenue—you have a 76-year-old male patient complaining of severe chest pain. Time out is 2136 hours.

Upon Arrival
The house is unlit and the surrounding area dark. You and your partner approach the house from the side, walk up onto the front porch, and stand on either side of the door. You ring the doorbell and hear a voice say, "Please help me. . . . The door is open," and then, between gasps, "I'm having bad chest pain." With flashlights in hand, you and your partner decide to enter the scene very cautiously. Upon entry, you find an elderly man sitting on the hallway floor against the wall. You immediately turn on the hall light. A scan of the scene does not reveal any potential hazards. The patient is clutching his chest, complaining of severe, crushing pain.

How Would You Proceed to Assess and Care for This Patient—Including the Administration of Medication?
During this chapter, you will learn about assessment and emergency care for a patient whose condition may require administration of a medication. Later, we will return to the case and apply the procedures learned.

Introduction

As an EMT you will be responsible for administering or assisting the patient with the administration of certain medications. Unlike a mathematician, you cannot erase your mistakes and start over. Once a medication has been administered, you cannot extract it or prevent its effects. Improper use of a medication may have dangerous consequences for the patient. Therefore, it is vital that you be completely familiar with the medications and the proper procedures for administration.

Only certain patients who have specific chief complaints or signs and symptoms will require medication. Either the medication will be carried on the EMS unit or it will be prescribed to the patient. Regardless of the source of the medication, you must attain medical direction's permission, whether as an off-line standing order found in your written protocols or as an on-line order you receive by direct communication with medical direction, before you administer or assist the patient with administering a medication.

Administering Medications

A **medication** is generally defined as a drug or other substance that is used as a remedy for illness. A **drug** is a chemical substance that is used to treat or prevent a disease or condition. The terms *drug* and *medication* are often used interchangeably by EMTs. The study of drugs is referred to as **pharmacology**.

The EMT must take seriously the responsibility of administering medications. Medications have specific physiological effects on the cells, organs, or body systems. When the correct dose is administered appropriately, the patient's condition may improve significantly and uncomfortable symptoms may be relieved. If administered inappropriately, some drugs can cause serious side effects and deterioration in the patient's condition.

As an EMT, you will be administering medications under the direct order of a licensed physician. Without this order, you cannot administer any type of medication. Also, the EMT is only able to administer the medications identified in the local protocol, which may include all or some of the medications covered in this chapter.

Remember that you may not administer or assist with administration of any medication other than the medications that are identified in local protocols. For example, if you arrive on the scene and find a patient experiencing excruciating pain associated with a dislocated shoulder, and you find the patient's prescription of Percodan at his side, it would be inappropriate for you to suggest, administer, or assist with the administration of the medication. Even though Percodan is a pain reliever, and it might seem to "make sense" to use it to make the patient more comfortable, it is not an acceptable medication to be administered by an EMT. An EMT can only administer medications within his scope of practice.

Some systems clearly distinguish between the EMT administering and assisting the patient with the adminis-

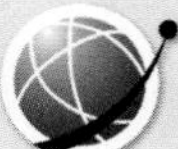

Media Resources
Go to www.bradybooks.com for mykit. Highlights:

- *Web Resource:* Six Rights of Med. Admin.
- *Web Resource:* Medications That Can Be Administered by an EMT
- *Video:* Epi-pen Actions and Use
- *Video:* MDI Administration

Key Terms

medication a drug or other substance that is used as a remedy for illness.

drug a chemical substance that is used to treat or prevent a disease or condition.

pharmacology the study of drugs.

tration of a medication. *Administration* of a medication implies that the EMT will actually take all of the steps necessary to give the patient the medication via an oral, injection, or inhalation route. The patient simply takes the direction from the EMT while receiving the medication. If the orders clearly state that the EMT will *assist* with the administration of the medication, the EMT will prepare the medication and then hand it over to the patient who will then proceed with taking the medication. As an example, if the orders state that the EMT can *administer* aspirin to the patient, the EMT will obtain the aspirin, instruct the patient to chew the aspirin, and place it in his mouth. If the orders only allow the EMT to assist with administration of the aspirin, the EMT will obtain the aspirin, instruct the patient to chew the aspirin, hand the patient an aspirin tablet, and have the patient place it into his mouth.

Medications Commonly Administered by the EMT

Medications administered by the EMT are either carried on the EMS unit or are prescribed for the patient. The prescription medications may be found on the patient or at the scene. General steps for properly administering all of the medications mentioned in this section are detailed at the end of this chapter.

Medications Carried on the EMS Unit

The following medications may be carried on the EMS unit. Even though the EMT controls the administration of these medications and they are ready at hand on the ambulance, an off-line or on-line order from medical direction is still necessary.

Oxygen

Oxygen is an odorless, tasteless, colorless gas that is found in the ambient atmosphere at a concentration of approximately 21 percent. When it is used for medical purposes, it is administered as a 100 percent compressed gas concentration. Oxygen is indicated in any patient who is experiencing a medical or trauma condition and who may be hypoxic or may become hypoxic (without sufficient oxygen in the body cells). By increasing the oxygen concentration breathed in by the patient, you are attempting to put a higher concentration of oxygen into the alveoli of the lungs. By doing so, you will increase the amount of oxygen crossing over from the alveoli and into the pulmonary capillary. This will allow more oxygen molecules to be available to attach to the hemoglobin on the surface of the red blood cell. By increasing the number of oxygen molecules attached to the hemoglobin, more oxygen will circulate in the blood and be delivered to the hypoxic or potentially hypoxic cells. Oxygen was covered in detail in Chapter 10, "Airway Management, Artificial Ventilation, and Oxygenation."

Oral Glucose

Glucose is a simple sugar that is found in the blood. It is the primary energy source for the body cells. Most cells throughout the body are capable of using other energy sources if they can't get enough glucose. Brain cells, however, can use only glucose for energy. When the brain cells do not get an adequate amount of glucose, they begin to function improperly, and the patient will exhibit an altered mental status. The signs and symptoms of a low blood glucose level will appear very rapidly. If the level drops too low for a long period of time, the brain cells can actually die.

Oral glucose is administered to the patient with a history of diabetes who is suspected of having a low blood glucose level. The oral glucose is absorbed in the mouth and through the intestines and eventually into the blood, where it will raise the blood glucose level, making more glucose available to the starving brain cells. The brain cells will once again begin to function normally. This will be seen as an improvement in the mental status. Oral glucose will be covered in detail in Chapter 20, "Acute Diabetic Emergencies."

Activated Charcoal

Activated charcoal is a fine black powder that is designed to adsorb, or bind, an ingested poison to the charcoal. Once this occurs, the poison will be carried by the charcoal through the digestive tract and then eliminated in a bowel movement. The efficacy of activated charcoal has been questioned. Activated charcoal has been removed from many protocols. Activated charcoal will be covered in detail in Chapter 22, "Toxicologic Emergencies."

Objectives 14-2 and 14-3
Describe the roles and responsibilities associated with, and differentiate between, administering and assisting a patient in taking his own medications.

Objective 14-4
List the medications in the EMT's scope of practice.

Key Terms

metered-dose inhaler (MDI) device consisting of a plastic container and a canister of medication used to inhale an aerosolized medication.

small-volume nebulizer (SVN) device used to create a fine vapor or mist containing a beta$_2$-specific medication for inhalation.

Aspirin

Aspirin is administered to a patient who is having chest discomfort or pain that is related to the lack of oxygen getting to the heart. The administration of aspirin may keep the vessels that deliver blood to the heart (the coronary arteries) from completely closing shut. Aspirin will be covered in detail in Chapter 17, "Cardiovascular Emergencies."

Understanding BODY PROCESSES

Aspirin keeps the platelets in the blood from sticking together. This prevents the platelets from forming a clot and completely closing off a coronary blood vessel in the heart, thereby maintaining some blood flow to that portion of the heart muscle. ■

Medications Prescribed for the Patient

Some of the medications that the EMT may administer or assist the patient with administering are not carried on the EMS unit. Instead, they are medications prescribed for the patient. Through good history taking, you should identify any medications the patient is currently taking.

The patient typically will have the medication in his possession; however, it may be necessary for you to locate it at the scene. For example, you arrive on the scene and find a patient who is experiencing severe chest pain. During your assessment, you determine that the patient has a prescription for nitroglycerin tablets. The patient states that the tablets are upstairs next to the bed. You must remain with the patient while your partner, a family member, or a First Responder retrieves the medication. Do not let the patient attempt to get the medication, since the activity may increase the discomfort and aggravate the medical condition.

Whether the EMT actually administers the medication or assists the patient in administering the medication is up to medical direction and local protocol.

The following are prescribed medications that EMTs may administer or assist in administering.

Inhaled Bronchodilator

Medications that cause the bronchioles to dilate are delivered via two different routes: metered-dose inhaler or small-volume nebulizer.

Metered-Dose Inhaler A **metered-dose inhaler (MDI)** is used by a patient who has some type of respiratory disease. Most often, you will find MDIs prescribed to patients with a history of asthma, emphysema, and chronic bronchitis. These patients will have episodes of bronchoconstriction in which the bronchioles in the respiratory tract will constrict, increasing the resistance to air flowing into the lungs and down into the alveoli. The patient will experience shortness of breath and signs and symptoms of respiratory difficulty from the increased effort to breathe and from the decreased flow of oxygen to the alveoli. The only MDI that you are able to administer or assist the patient with is one that contains a beta$_2$-agonist drug. A beta$_2$-agonist drug will cause the bronchioles to dilate (open; increase in diameter), decreasing the airway resistance and increasing the airflow through the respiratory tract and into the alveoli. Metered-dose inhaler medications (albuterol, levalbuterol) will be covered in detail in Chapter 16, "Respiratory Emergencies."

Small-Volume Nebulizer The beta$_2$-specific medication administered via a metered-dose inhaler can also be delivered through a **small-volume nebulizer (SVN).** The indications, actions, side effects, and contraindications of the medication are the same; only the route of delivery is different.

To nebulize a medication, you place it into a specialized chamber and pass oxygen or compressed air through it to create a fine vapor. The fine vapor is expelled through a T-tube and into a mouthpiece or mask. The patient then inhales the vapor through the mouthpiece or mask over a period of several minutes and until the medication is completely gone from the chamber. Note that an MDI is designed to deliver the medication with one inhalation, whereas the nebulizer is designed to create a continuous flow of vapor that contains the medication. With each inhalation, the patient breathes in the beta$_2$-specific medication, which is then topically deposited in the bronchioles and at the site of bronchoconstriction.

Some EMTs carry nebulizer equipment and beta$_2$-specific drugs for nebulization on the ambulance. Others are allowed to administer or assist the patient with administration of the beta$_2$ by using the patient's home nebulizer.

Nitroglycerin

Nitroglycerin is a medication that is used to treat cardiac patients with diseases of the coronary arteries that deliver

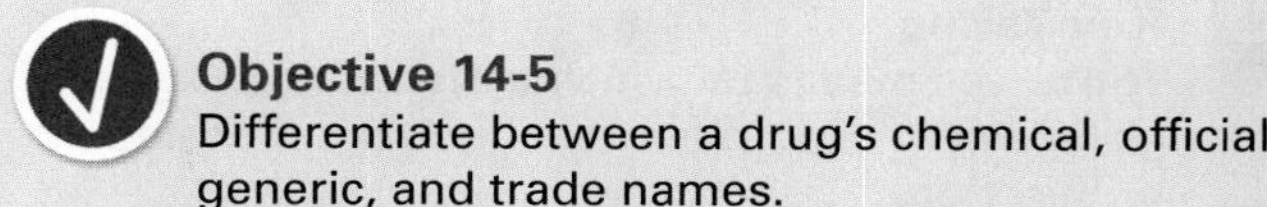

Objective 14-5
Differentiate between a drug's chemical, official, generic, and trade names.

blood to the heart. The medication is commonly referred to as "nitro." Nitroglycerin is a vasodilator; that is, it dilates the blood vessels in the body. By doing so, it reduces the workload of the heart, thereby decreasing the demand for oxygen by the heart muscle. In addition, it dilates the coronary arteries themselves, which increases the supply of oxygenated blood to the heart muscle.

Because it is a vasodilator, the major side effect of the drug is hypotension (low blood pressure). It is extremely important to measure the blood pressure prior to and after administration of nitroglycerin. Nitroglycerin must not be administered (that is, it is contraindicated) to patients taking medications for erectile dysfunction, which themselves lower blood pressure. In particular, patients who have taken tadalafil (Cialis), vardenafil (Levitra), or sildenafil (Viagra) should never be given nitroglycerin. The combined blood-pressure-lowering effects of the nitroglycerin and the erectile dysfunction medication may cause serious drops in blood pressure and perfusion and can lead to death. Nitroglycerin will be covered in detail in Chapter 17, "Cardiovascular Emergencies."

ASSESSMENT Tips

Nitroglycerin should not be administered to a patient with a systolic blood pressure of less than 90 mmHg or a systolic blood pressure that drops greater than 30 mmHg from the baseline blood pressure. ■

Epinephrine

Epinephrine is a drug used to treat patients suffering from severe allergic reactions known as anaphylaxis. An anaphylactic reaction usually occurs when the patient ingests, injects, inhales, or absorbs a substance that the body views as foreign. The body then reacts with a misdirected and exaggerated immune response that can easily lead to death. The patient's blood vessels dilate (vasodilation), decreasing the blood pressure and perfusion; the bronchioles constrict (bronchoconstriction), increasing the airway resistance and making it difficult to move air into the alveoli; and the capillaries leak fluid out (from increased capillary permeability), causing the blood volume to decrease. These all can produce serious signs and symptoms in the patient and lead to failure of the respiratory and cardiovascular systems.

Many patients with a history of anaphylactic reaction will carry an epinephrine auto-injector. This is a prefilled single-dose or multidose spring-loaded device that delivers a specific dose of epinephrine when activated. The epinephrine constricts the vessels, increasing the blood pressure; dilates the bronchioles, allowing the patient to move more air into the alveoli; and decreases capillary permeability, reducing the leakage of fluid. Epinephrine will be covered in detail in Chapter 21, "Anaphylactic Reactions."

ASSESSMENT Tips

Epinephrine stimulates four receptors: $alpha_1$, $alpha_2$, $beta_1$, and $beta_2$. These properties make up the sympathetic nervous system function. Following the administration of epinephrine, the patient may experience an increase in the heart rate due to the $beta_1$ properties of the epinephrine. ■

Medication Names

A medication, or drug, can have up to four different names: chemical, generic, trade (brand), and official. These names are assigned during the development of the drug and are used interchangeably. The EMT must be most familiar with the generic and trade names. Table 14-1 lists generic and trade names and common uses for the medications the EMT may be allowed to administer or assist the patient with administering.

A description of the four drug names is as follows:

- **Chemical name.** The chemical name describes the drug's chemical structure. It is usually the first name associated with the drug.
- **Generic name.** Also referred to as the nonproprietary name, the generic name still reflects the chemical characteristic of the drug, but in a shorter form than the full chemical name. It is the name assigned to the drug before it is officially listed and is independent of the manufacturer. The generic name is listed in the U.S. Pharmacopoeia, a publication listing all drugs officially approved by the U.S. Food and Drug Administration.
- **Trade name.** The trade name, also referred to as the brand name, is assigned when the drug is released for

Key Terms
route the means by which a medication is given or taken; for example, sublingual, oral, inhalation, or injection.

Objective 14-6
Demonstrate the proper administration of drugs by the sublingual, oral, inhalation, and intramuscular routes.

TABLE 14-1 Common Generic and Trade Medication Names

Generic Name	Trade Name(s)	Used for
Oxygen	none	A wide range of medical emergencies, traumatic emergencies, and obstetric and gynecologic emergencies
Glucose, oral	Glutose, Insta-Glucose	Altered mental status associated with diabetic history
Activated charcoal	SuperChar, InstaChar, Actidose, LiquiChar	Poisoning and overdose emergencies
Nitroglycerin	Nitrostat	Chest pain
Nitroglycerin spray	Nitrolingual Spray	Chest pain
Epinephrine	Adrenalin	Allergic reactions
Albuterol	Proventil, Ventolin	Breathing difficulty associated with respiratory conditions
Metaproterenol	Alupent, Metaprel	Breathing difficulty associated with respiratory conditions
Isoetharine	Bronkosol	Breathing difficulty associated with respiratory conditions
Bitolterol	Tornalate	Breathing difficulty associated with respiratory conditions
Levalbuterol	Xopenex	Breathing difficulty associated with respiratory conditions
Pirbuterol	Maxair	Breathing difficulty associated with respiratory conditions
Terbutaline	Brethaire, Brethine	Breathing difficulty associated with respiratory conditions
Salmeterol xinafoate	Serevent	Breathing difficulty associated with respiratory conditions
Ipratropium	Atrovent	Breathing difficulty associated with respiratory conditions
Aspirin	Bayer aspirin, Easprin, Ecotrin, Empirin, Ascriptin, Bufferin, Buffex	Patient experiencing chest pain or chest discomfort suggestive of an acute coronary syndrome

commercial distribution. The name is usually short and easy to recall, and may be based on the chemical name or the type of problem it is used to treat. This is the name the manufacturer uses to market the drug.

- **Official name.** Drugs meeting the requirements of the U.S. Pharmacopoeia or National Formulary are given an official name. It is commonly the generic name followed by the initials U.S.P. or N.F.

An example of the four drug names for the common nitroglycerin tablet taken by many patients with chronic chest pain is as follows:

Chemical Name:	1,2,3-propanetriol trinitrate
Generic Name:	nitroglycerin tablets
Official Name:	nitroglycerin tablets, U.S.P.
Trade Name:	Nitrostat

Routes of Administration

The **route** describes how the medication is actually given to or taken by the patient. The route that is chosen controls how fast the medication is absorbed by the body and its effect. Each medication administered by the EMT is prepared in a form that allows for the quickest and safest absorption into the body.

The following are common routes of administration of medications given by the EMT:

- **Sublingual.** The medication is placed under the patient's tongue. The patient does not swallow the medication. It is dissolved and absorbed across the mucous membrane in the mouth. The drug usually has a relatively quick absorption rate into the blood. The patient must be alert in order for you to administer the medication in this manner. (Medication

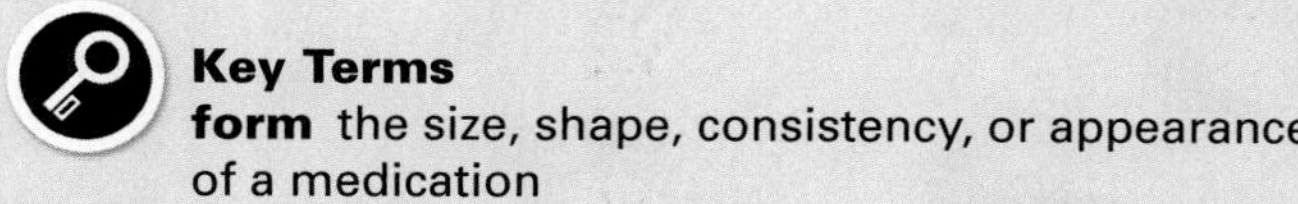

Key Terms
form the size, shape, consistency, or appearance of a medication

Objective 14-7
Differentiate between the following medication forms: tablet, liquid for injection, gel, suspension, fine powder for inhalation, gas, and liquid for spray or aerosolization.

placed into the mouth of a patient who is not alert or who is unresponsive can become lodged in the airway or aspirated into the lungs.) Only a very limited number of medications are able to be given by the sublingual route. Medications administered by the EMT by the sublingual route are:
- Nitroglycerin tablets
- Nitroglycerin spray

- **Oral.** The drug is swallowed. Except for activated charcoal, it is absorbed from the stomach or intestinal tract. The patient must be responsive and able to swallow. The patient may refuse to swallow the drug if it is unpleasant, or may vomit it. Aspirin is first chewed, so that the medication absorption can begin immediately through the oral mucosa, and is then swallowed. Medications administered by the EMT by the oral route are:
  - Aspirin
  - Oral glucose
  - Activated charcoal

Understanding BODY PROCESSES

Enteric-coated aspirin is designed to dissolve more slowly and be absorbed in the small intestine. Because of the increased time it takes to dissolve and get into the blood, this type of aspirin should not be used for patients complaining of chest discomfort. ■

- **Inhalation.** The medication is prepared as a gas or aerosol and is inhaled by the patient. This method typically deposits the medication directly to the target site where the effect is needed most. The patient must be spontaneously breathing for this route to be effective. With some medications, the patient must be responsive and breathing deeply enough to move air into the lower portions of the respiratory tract in order for the drug to be properly deposited. Medications administered by the EMT by the inhalation route are:
  - Oxygen
  - Metered-dose inhaler
  - Small-volume nebulizer
- **Intramuscular injection.** The drug is injected into a muscle mass. The absorption is relatively rapid. This requires the use of a needle; therefore, it poses the danger of a needlestick injury to the EMT. Some discomfort is felt by the patient. Serious side effects might occur if the drug is accidentally injected into a vein. The medication can only be injected in specific muscle groups. Medication administered by the EMT by the intramuscular injection route is:
  - Epinephrine with the use of an auto-injector

Medication Forms

Medications come in several different forms. The **form** usually limits administration to one specific route. This ensures the proper administration of the medication, its correct controlled release, and also the appropriate effect on the target organ or body system. The medication form also determines the effects of the drug. Some drugs have a more local effect on specific cells or organs, whereas other drugs have a much broader, or systemic, effect on the entire body.

Common forms of medications administered by the EMT are:

- **Compressed powder or tablet.** A compressed powder that is shaped into a small disk or elongated shape. Nitroglycerin tablets and aspirin tablets are examples of this type of medication form (Figure 14-1∗).
- **Liquid for injection.** A liquid substance with no particulate matter. Because epinephrine is injected into the muscle, it is in a liquid form (Figure 14-2∗).
- **Gel.** A viscous (thick, sticky) substance that the patient swallows. Oral glucose is a gel (Figure 14-3∗).
- **Suspension.** Drug particles that are mixed in a suitable liquid. These mixtures do not remain mixed for long periods of time and have a tendency to separate. Suspensions must be shaken well prior to administration. Activated charcoal is administered as a suspension (Figure 14-4∗).
- **Fine powder for inhalation.** This form is actually a crystalline solid that is mixed with liquid to form a suspension. A prescribed metered-dose inhaler carried by the patient for inhalation has medication in this form (Figure 14-5a∗). Because it is a suspension, it is necessary to shake the canister vigorously prior to administration. The medication appears as a mist or aerosol. Each spray delivers a precise measured amount of drug to the patient.

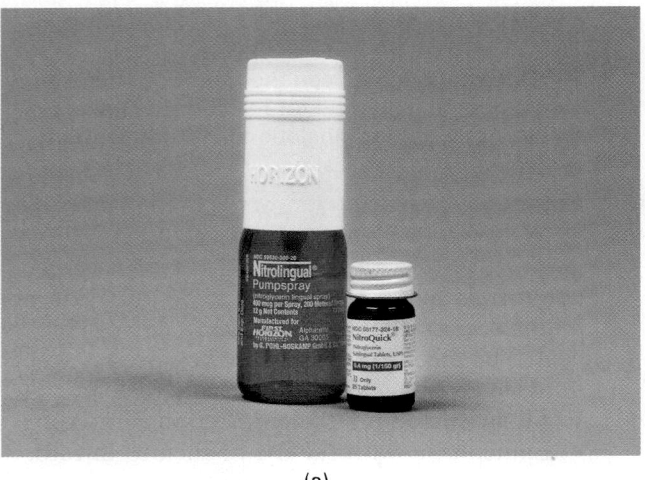

(a)

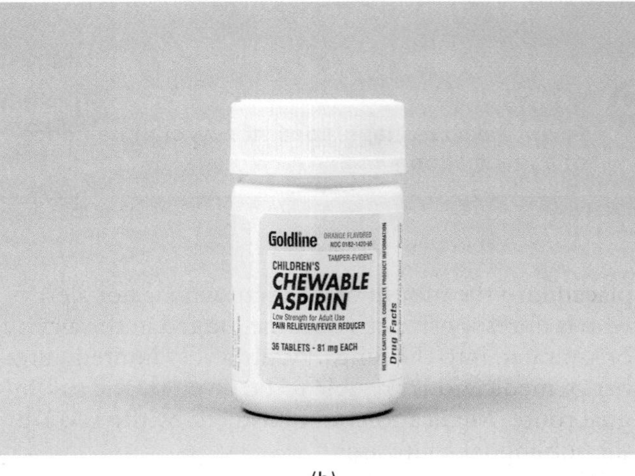

(b)

FIGURE 14-1 ✱ **(a)** The EMT may assist the patient with administration of nitroglycerin prescribed for chest pain. Two common forms are tablet and spray. **(b)** Aspirin, in pill form, may be administered for chest pain when a heart attack is suspected.

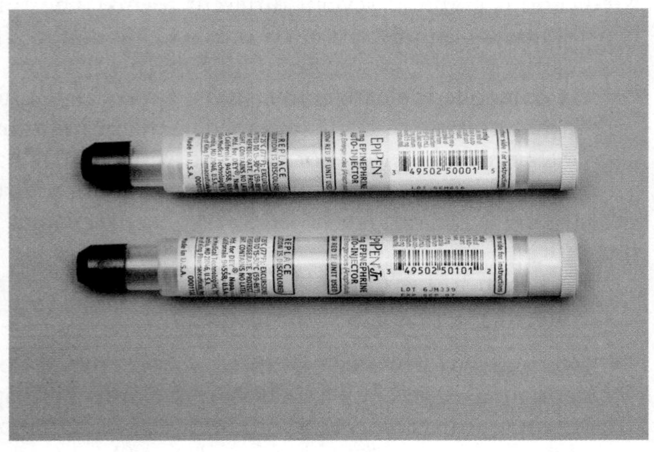

(a)

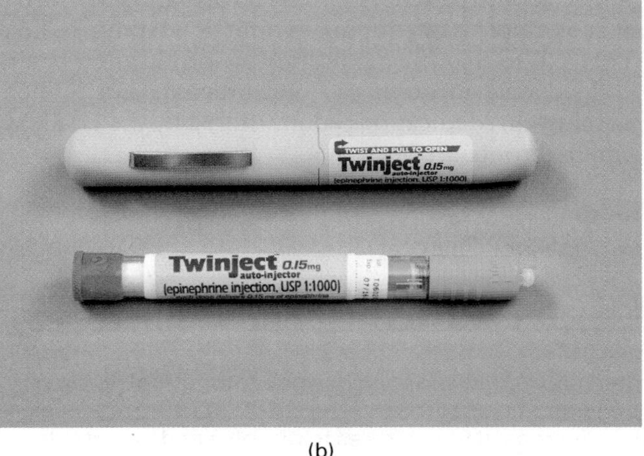

(b)

FIGURE 14-2 ✱ The epinephrine auto-injector may be prescribed for patients with a history of severe allergic or anaphylactic reaction. **(a)** The EpiPen and **(b)** the Twinject are two brands of epinephrine auto-injector.

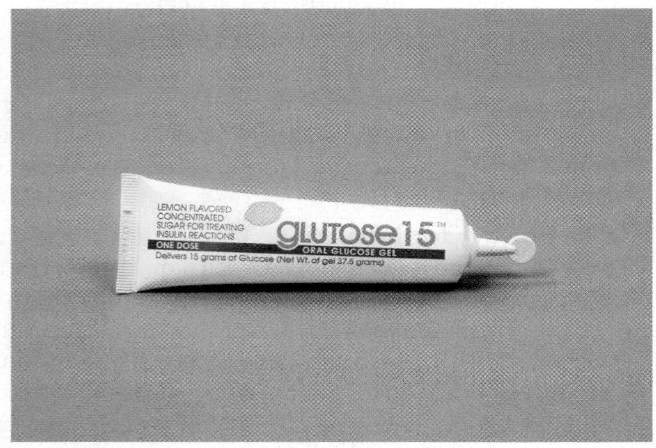

FIGURE 14-3 ✱ Oral glucose is a viscous gel used in acute diabetic emergencies. It is carried on the EMS unit.

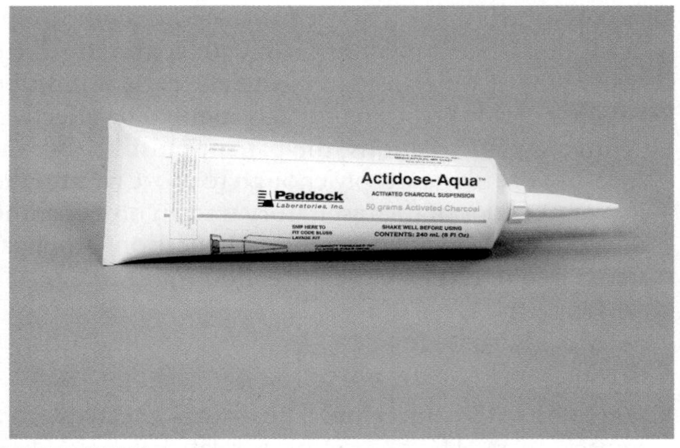

FIGURE 14-4 ✱ Activated charcoal is administered in suspension form and is carried on some EMS units. It may be used in poisoning and overdose emergencies.

Key Points
It is essential to understand the indications, contraindications, dose, administration, actions, and side effects of any medication to be administered.

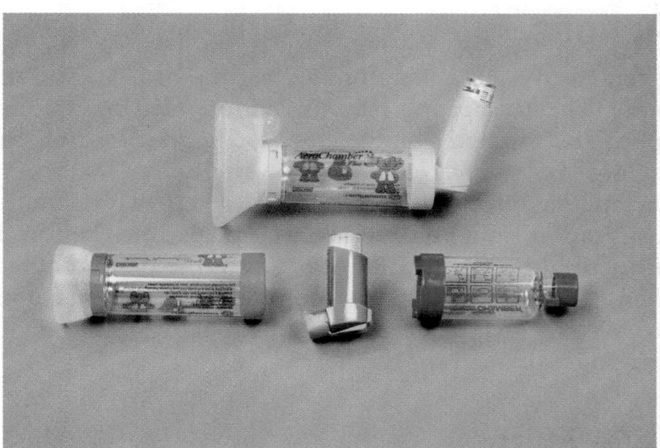

(a)

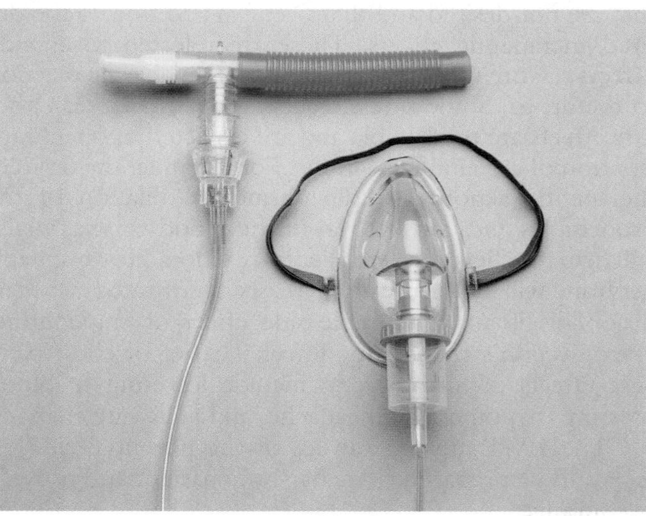

(b)

FIGURE 14-5 ✱ **(a)** A metered-dose inhaler or a metered-dose inhaler with a spacer may be prescribed for respiratory conditions. **(b)** Nebulized medications may be administered by a small-volume nebulizer, through either a mouthpiece or a face mask. (Photo b: © Carl Leet, YSU)

- **Small-volume nebulizer.** A nebulizer is a device that uses a compressed gas, typically oxygen, that is forced into a chamber containing medication. The gas mixes with the liquid medication and forms an aerosol. The aerosol is inhaled by the patient—either through a mouthpiece or through a face mask (Figure 14-5b✱)—and the medication is directly deposited on the mucosal lining deep in the respiratory tract. By depositing the medication at the desired site, the effect is more immediate and direct than when given by other routes, and fewer systemic side effects are usually noted. The medication comes packaged in a premeasured and premixed fixed-dose container or inhaler.

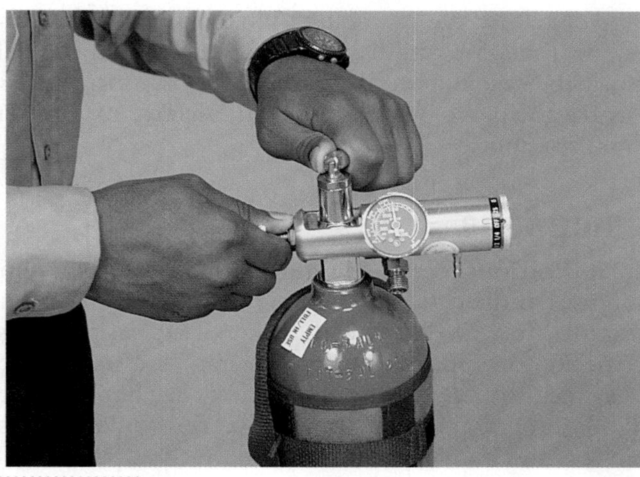

FIGURE 14-6 ✱ The gas oxygen is considered a medication. It is the most commonly used medication in EMS and is carried on the EMS unit.

- **Gas.** Oxygen is the medication most commonly administered by EMTs. It is inhaled and has systemic effects on the cells and organs (Figure 14-6✱).
- **Spray.** Spray droplets may be deposited under the tongue. Nitroglycerin, often in tablet form, may instead be in the form of a spray. Nitroglycerin spray is an aerosol that contains nitroglycerin in a propellant. Each spray delivers a precise metered dose.

Essential Medication Information

It is important that the EMT understand the following terminology associated with the medications to be administered:

- Indications
- Contraindications
- Dose
- Administration
- Actions
- Side effects

Key Terms
indications the common reasons for using a medication to treat a specific condition.

contraindications situations in which a medication should not be used.

dose the amount of a medication that is given to a patient at one time.

Key Terms
administration the route and form by which a drug is given.

action the effect a drug has on the body.

side effects the undesired effects of a medication.

We will use the example of nitroglycerin so you can see how the information applies to a medication you will actually be called upon to administer. This information is essential to ensure proper, safe, and effective medication administration.

Indications

The **indications** for a medication include the most common uses of the drug in treating a specific condition. Indications are geared toward the relief of signs, symptoms, or specific conditions—a direct therapeutic benefit derived from the administration of the drug. For example, an indication for the use of nitroglycerin would be chest pain (because nitroglycerin may relieve chest pain).

Contraindications

Contraindications are situations in which the drug should not be administered because of the potential harm that could be caused to the patient. In some cases, the drug may not have any benefit to the patient in improving his condition; therefore, the drug should not be given. Low blood pressure is a contraindication for the use of nitroglycerin (because nitroglycerin will lower the blood pressure, possibly causing an already-low blood pressure to become dangerously low).

Dose

The **dose** indicates how much of the drug should be given to the patient. It is important to distinguish between adult dosages and dosages for infants and children so that the correct dose is administered. Too much of the drug could cause serious side effects, whereas an inadequate amount of the drug may have little or no effect. For nitroglycerin, EMTs are advised to administer one dose (one tablet or one spray) and repeat it in 3–5 minutes if there is no relief, to a maximum of three doses (including any doses the patient may already have taken before the ambulance arrived).

Administration

Administration refers to the route and form in which the drug is given. The EMT will administer medications sublingually, orally, by inhalation, or by injection. Nitroglycerin, for instance, is administered sublingually in tablet or spray form.

Actions

The **action** is, in general, the effect the drug has on the body. The *therapeutic effect* is the intended positive response by the body. The *mechanism of action* is how the drug works to create its effect on the body. The action, therapeutic effect, and mechanism of action provide the justification for administering a particular medication. If the action described will not produce the desired effect, then the drug should not be administered. Actions of nitroglycerin include relaxation of blood vessels and decreasing workload for the heart.

Side Effects

Even when given appropriately, drugs often have actions that are not desired and that occur in addition to the desired therapeutic effects. These are referred to as **side effects**. (Note that a side effect is not an allergic reaction to the drug.) Some side effects are unpredictable. Other side effects are predictable and are expected upon administration of certain medications. For example, the desired, therapeutic actions of epinephrine are dilation of the bronchioles and constriction of the blood vessels, which will help to relieve a severe allergic reaction. However, epinephrine will also cause an increased heart rate (tachycardia). This is an undesirable side effect of epinephrine. Nitroglycerin's therapeutic effect is relief of chest pain. Side effects of nitroglycerin include lowering of blood pressure (hypotension), headache, and pulse rate changes.

The EMT must be aware of the potential side effects and be prepared to manage the patient and provide reassurance.

▶ Key Steps in Administering Medications

The following are key steps that must be followed when administering a medication to the patient.

Obtain an Order from Medical Direction

Every medication the EMT administers, or assists the patient with, requires an order from medical direction (Figure 14-7*). The medication order may be obtained

Objective 14-9
Adhere to the key steps of medication administration regarding obtaining, verifying, checking for, or ensuring the following: orders, proper medication, prescription, expiration date, impurities/discoloration, form, route, dose, and the "five rights."

Objective 14-8
Explain the roles of off-line and on-line medical direction with regard to medication administration.

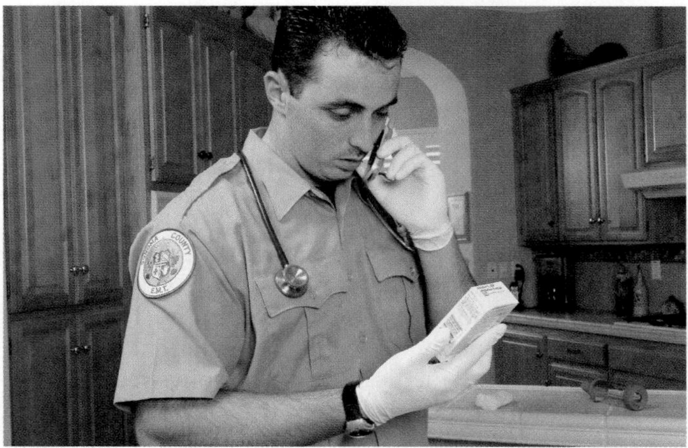

FIGURE 14-7 * You must obtain an order from medical direction to administer medication or to assist the patient with administration of medication. Be sure the prescription is for the patient you are treating, and check the expiration date of the medication.

either on-line by direct communication with medical direction by phone or radio, or off-line through protocols or standing orders. It is important to know and understand your local protocols prior to responding to any emergency call.

If you receive an on-line order from medical direction, you must verify it by restating the drug to be administered, the dose, and the route. This reduces the chances that an improper medication is inadvertently administered, the wrong dose is given, or an inappropriate route is used.

It may be necessary for the EMT to make a judgment as to whether the patient can tolerate the administration of the medication. For example, you may have received an on-line order for the administration of oral glucose. The patient was talking incoherently when you called medical direction for the order; however, his mental status has deteriorated, and now he is only responding to painful stimuli. Obviously, administration of oral glucose may lead to aspiration in this patient. Even though the medication order exists, it is now inappropriate to administer the oral glucose to this patient. You should contact medical direction and report the deterioration in the patient's condition. At the same time, it will be appropriate to seek further orders for emergency care from medical direction.

Select the Proper Medication

Once the medication order has been received, it is the EMT's responsibility to ensure that the proper medication has been selected. You must carefully read the medication label, especially in medications that are prescribed to the patient, to determine that the medication is consistent with the order. Many medications have several trade names. This may be confusing, since many trade names are very similar. (The various trade names of drugs relevant to emergency care will be identified in later chapters that discuss each particular medication.)

Verify the Patient's Prescription

When the medication to be given is not carried on the EMS unit and must be obtained from the patient, it is extremely important to verify that the medication is actually prescribed for the patient and not some other individual such as a spouse, relative, or friend. Some patients may take medications that are not specifically prescribed for them. They believe that if the signs and symptoms are similar to those of someone who is taking the medication, then it is appropriate for them to take it also.

For example, you arrive on the scene of a 55-year-old female patient complaining of chest pain. Through your history, you determine that the patient has taken nitroglycerin in the past for similar bouts of chest pain. Your assumption is that the patient must have a prescription for nitroglycerin. However, upon inspection of the name on the prescription label, and following further questioning, you determine that the medication is actually prescribed for her husband. The patient has been taking the medication, not based on a physician's order, but because she recognized signs and symptoms similar to her husband's.

As you can see, it may be somewhat misleading when a patient states that he has been taking a medication for a condition or symptom. To avoid medication administration errors, it is vital to check the prescription label and verify the patient's name. *The EMT should never administer medication that is not prescribed for the patient unless ordered to do so by medical direction.* For instance, in the case of the patient just mentioned, the EMT would not assist the patient with administration of nitroglycerin unless medical direction issued orders to administer the husband's nitroglycerin. (For a medication carried on the EMS unit—such as oxygen, oral glucose, or activated charcoal—prescription information is not relevant.)

Some medication labels are not affixed to the medication container itself but are placed on or inside the box or other outer packaging. Nitroglycerin, epinephrine autoinjectors, and metered-dose inhalers are packaged this way. If your patient has one of these medications, you will not

Thinking Critically

A patient with chest pain has no prescribed medication, but a friend at the scene has nitroglycerin spray with him and says, "Here. Give him this." Should you? Why or why not?

Key Points

Before helping to administer any prescribed medication, always check the "five rights": right patient, right medication, right route, right dose, right date.

be able to tell by looking at the container if the medication has been prescribed for this patient. If the outer packaging cannot be found, you must determine through careful questioning if the prescription truly belongs to the patient.

Check the Expiration Date

Check the medication's expiration date. Dependent on the type of package and the medication, the expiration date is either printed on the container itself or on the prescription label.

Do not administer expired medication. Properly dispose of the medications according to your state drug or pharmacy guidelines.

Check for Discoloration or Impurities

Epinephrine, or any other medication that comes in liquid form, should be inspected for any discoloration or cloudiness prior to administration. If the medication appears to be cloudy or discolored, or if any particulate material is found in the container, do not use it. Discard the medication.

Verify the Form, Route, and Dose

Be sure the proper drug form is used for the route selected. Verify that the dose to be administered is correct. Check the medication label to ensure it matches the drug order received from medical direction. Some drug packages are similar but contain different doses. For example, the epinephrine auto-injector comes in adult and pediatric sizes. The packages look very similar. Without close inspection it would be easy to mistake one for the other. Administering an adult dose to a child could have detrimental effects, whereas administering a pediatric dose to an adult may have no or little effect.

The drugs are in a form that corresponds to a specific route of administration. Attempting to administer the medication by some other route may lead to ineffective action or potentially harmful side effects.

Medication Administration: The Five "Rights"

Medication administration is a serious role performed by the EMT. As easily as one of the drugs may improve the condition of a patient, the administration of the wrong medication, the wrong route, or the wrong dose may lead to unwarranted effects and possible serious patient deterioration. An easy way to remember what needs to be checked prior to administration of a medication is to use the principle of the "five rights" of medication administration, as follows:

- **Right patient.** You must be sure that the medication you are administering is prescribed for that specific patient. Do not administer medications that are prescribed for anyone other than the patient unless ordered by the medical direction physician. If the medication to be administered is one that is carried on the EMS unit, the EMT must make the judgment whether this medication is right for this particular patient.
- **Right medication.** Once you have determined what medication is appropriate to administer to the patient, it is vital to be sure that the medication being administered is actually the medication that is intended to be administered. Many patients put several different types of medications into one prescription bottle. Be sure that you have selected the correct medication before administering it to the patient.
- **Right route.** After determining you have the right drug for the right patient, be sure to administer the medication by the right route. The route may be oral, sublingual, inhalation, or intramuscular injection. Administering the drug by the wrong route may have deleterious effects or no effect on the patient. For example, having the patient swallow a nitroglycerin tablet will end with no substantial clinical effect on the patient.
- **Right dose.** When administering a medication, you must know the appropriate dose for the patient. Be sure to understand differences in doses for adults and children. By not knowing the proper dose of the medication, you may underdose the patient, resulting in the medication having little effect, or you may overdose the patient by administering too much of the drug. The overdose may cause serious harm. Once the drug is "on board," there is no way to retract it if too much is administered. You must wait out the period and hope the patient does not suffer serious consequences from your action.
- **Right date (time).** Always check the expiration date of the medication. Do not administer drugs that are

Objective 14-10
Document medication administration.

Objective 14-11
Describe the reassessment of a patient after administration or assistance in taking a medication.

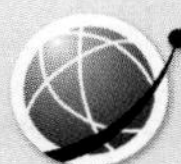

Media Resources
Go to www.bradybooks.com for mykit. Highlights:
- *Video:* Activiated Charcoal Administration
- *Video:* Epi-pen Administration
- *Video:* Oral Glucose Administration
- *Video:* Nitro Administration

expired. The drug expires on the first day of the month listed unless otherwise specified. Once the drug is expired, it does not typically change its composition but weakens in strength and its effectiveness in achieving the desired action.

The "five rights" will help you remember what must be checked prior to medication administration. *Take your role very seriously when administering any type of medication.*

Documentation

Once you administer the medication, you must document the drug, dose, route, and time the medication was administered. Report any changes in the patient's condition, and report whether the signs or symptoms have been relieved. Also report any deterioration in the patient's condition or if side effects associated with the drug have occurred.

Reassessment Following Administration

ASSESSMENT Tips

Once a medication has been administered, it is important to reassess the patient to determine if there is any change in the condition. Aspirin and activated charcoal may not produce obvious changes in the patient's condition. ■

Following the administration of a medication, it is necessary to perform a reassessment. During the reassessment, repeat measurement of vital signs and assess for any changes in the patient's condition.

Assess the following and document changes after drug administration:

- Mental status
- Patency of the airway
- Breathing rate and quality
- Pulse rate and quality
- Skin color, temperature, and condition
- Blood pressure
- Change or relief of the patient's complaints
- Relief of signs and symptoms associated with the patient's complaints
- Medication side effects
- Improvement or deterioration in the patient's condition following medication administration

During the reassessment, be sure to check the adequacy of oxygen administration, whether it is being delivered by a nasal cannula, simple face mask, nonrebreather mask, or in conjunction with positive pressure ventilation. In addition to the medication that was administered, assess the adequacy of any other care that has been administered to manage the patient's condition. Based on the care provided, determine if improvement or deterioration in the patient's condition has occurred. Document any improvement or deterioration.

Sources of Medication Information

The following are sources you can use to gather more information about specific medications. These sources may also provide valuable information relevant to the patient's prescription medications:

- American Hospital Formulary Service, published by the American Society of Hospital Pharmacists
- AMA Drug Evaluation, published by the American Medical Association Department of Drugs
- Physicians' Desk Reference (PDR), published yearly by the Medical Economics Data Production Company
- Package inserts—information that is packaged with the particular drug
- Poison control centers
- EMS pocket drug reference guide
- ePocrates for the PDA
- Other on-line sources approved by your medical director

CHAPTER REVIEW

SUMMARY

Administration of medication is a very serious part of the EMT's responsibility. As much as a medication might help a patient and relieve pain and suffering or potentially relieve a condition, it can be harmful or fatal if administered to the wrong patient or for the wrong condition. The medications that the EMT will carry on the ambulance are oxygen, oral glucose, activated charcoal, and aspirin. The patient-prescribed medications that the EMT may assist the patient with taking are a beta$_2$ agonist by metered-dose inhaler or small-volume nebulizer, nitroglycerin, and epinephrine.

Medications can be administered via various routes, including sublingual, oral, inhalation, and injection. Injection provides the most rapid absorption into the body. The medication itself may come in the form of a compressed powder or tablet, liquid for injection, gel, suspension, fine powder for inhalation, gas, spray, or vaporized liquid in a fixed-dose nebulizer.

Before administering any medication, you must understand the indications, contraindications, dose, administration route and form, actions, and side effects. Be sure to obtain the appropriate order from medical direction, whether off-line or on-line, depending on your protocol. Follow the "five rights" of medication administration: right patient, right medication, right route, right dose, and right date (time). Following the administration of any medication, perform a reassessment to determine if there is any change in the patient's condition.

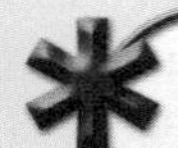

CASE STUDY FOLLOW-UP

SCENE SIZE-UP

You have been dispatched to the scene of an elderly male complaining of chest pain. You and your partner enter the darkened scene cautiously and find the patient sitting against the wall on the floor of the hallway. The phone is off the hook and lying next to the patient. You turn on the hallway lights and scan the scene. The scene appears to be safe. You notice a prescription bottle of nitroglycerin on the table next to the patient. He complains, "I have this crushing pain in my chest. I've never experienced pain like this before." You ask, "What is your name, sir?" He responds, "Jack Brookline."

PRIMARY ASSESSMENT

Your general impression is that of an elderly male patient in severe distress from chest pain. His skin is pale, sweaty, and cool to the touch. His airway is open, breathing is approximately 20 per minute and full, and the radial pulse is 80 per minute and strong. You immediately apply a nonrebreather mask to supply oxygen at 15 liters per minute.

SECONDARY ASSESSMENT

The history reveals chest pain that occurred suddenly as the patient was sleeping on the couch. Mr. Brookline was tired and was taking a nap when the pain started. It woke him from his sleep. He got up to get his nitroglycerin off the table in the hallway, but the short walk greatly intensified the pain and caused him to collapse to the floor. He describes the pain as "crushing, like I've never experienced before." The pain does not radiate and is described as 10 on a scale of 1 to 10, with 10 being the worst. The pain began about 10 minutes prior to his call to 911.

Mr. Brookline denies having any allergies and has a prescription of nitroglycerin related to his past medical history of angina, or recurring chest pain. He states that he had a cup of coffee and a sandwich at about 6:00 P.M. He denies doing anything unusual today or prior to the onset of the chest pain.

You obtain a set of baseline vital signs. The blood pressure is 140/100 mmHg; the radial pulse is 104 per minute and regular; the skin is pale, moist, and cool; the breathing is 20 per minute with good volume; the SpO_2 is 95% on room air.

You ask, "Mr. Brookline, did you take any nitroglycerin before we arrived?" He states, "No, once I sat down in the hallway, I couldn't reach it."

After having the patient chew 160 mg of aspirin, you contact medical direction by radio for permission to administer the nitroglycerin to Mr. Brookline. You report the physical findings, history, and baseline vital signs. Medical direction orders, "Administer one tablet sublingually, recheck the blood pressure within 2 minutes, and re-evaluate the intensity of the chest pain. If the chest pain does not subside after 5 minutes and the systolic blood pressure remains greater than 90 mmHg, administer a second tablet and reassess the blood pressure and the chest pain intensity." You repeat the order to medical direction and sign off.

You inspect the medication container, checking the medication name to make sure it is really nitroglycerin, the patient's name to make sure it is prescribed to Jack Brookline, and the expiration date to be sure the prescription is current.

You instruct, "Mr. Brookline, I need you to open your mouth and lift your tongue. I am going to place a nitroglycerin tablet under your tongue. Do not swallow the tablet and be sure to keep your mouth closed until it is completely dissolved. It may burn slightly and you may get a headache." With a gloved hand you place a nitroglycerin tablet under his tongue. You record the medication administered, dose, route, and time.

REASSESSMENT

After 2 minutes, Mr. Brookline's blood pressure is 110/60 mmHg—slightly lower than before, but still in the normal range. Mr. Brookline indicates that the pain has subsided greatly. On a scale of 1 to 10, the pain is now a 2 or a 3. His radial pulse remains strong at 82/minute, and his breathing is normal at 18/minute and of good volume. His skin is now slightly warmer, less moist, and more normal in color. You check the oxygen to ensure that it is flowing adequately. His SpO_2 is now 99% while on the nonrebreather mask.

You place Mr. Brookline on the stretcher and move him to the ambulance for transport, making sure to transport the medication along with him. You reassess the vital signs and determine that the chest pain is almost completely gone. You record the vital signs, contact the receiving medical facility, and give a report.

Upon arrival at the hospital, Mr. Brookline is transferred without incident. He now appears to be resting comfortably and in better spirits, even managing to say a hearty, "Thanks, guys, for helping me out." You complete the necessary EMS report and prepare the unit for another call.

IN REVIEW

1. Name the medications that are carried on the EMS unit.
2. Name the medications an EMT may administer or assist in administering if prescribed for the patient.
3. Name four routes by which medications may be administered by the EMT.
4. Name several common forms of medications that may be administered by the EMT.
5. Define the following six terms related to medications:
   - indications
   - dose
   - actions
   - contraindications
   - administration
   - side effects
6. Describe the key steps to follow in administering a medication to a patient.
7. Describe proper reassessment following administration of a medication.

CRITICAL THINKING

You arrive on the scene and find a 46-year-old male patient who is complaining of shortness of breath and chest discomfort after exercising on the treadmill at the gym. The patient is alert and oriented. His respirations are 22 per minute with a good tidal volume. His radial pulse is 102 bpm and the skin is pale, cool, and clammy. He states that the pain started about 15 minutes prior to the end of his workout. It got so bad he had to stop working out. He felt light-headed and nauseated. He has had no relief in the pain and he reports that it continues to worsen. He describes the pain as a "tightening" feeling in the middle of his chest. He states he also feels an aching-type pain down the medial aspect of both arms. The pain is an 8 on a 1-to-10 scale, with 10 being the worst. It has now been approximately 30 minutes since the onset of the pain. His blood pressure is 138/92 mmHg, and his SpO_2 is 96% on room air. He has no previous significant medical history and takes no medication. He denies any allergies. He had a sports drink about 45 minutes prior to your arrival.

1. What medications might you consider administering in this patient?
2. What medication would the patient possibly have on his person?
3. What are the forms of the medications that you would possibly administer to this patient?
4. Why are those forms of medications used?
5. What information must you understand about the medication prior to administering it?
6. What are the possible ways to obtain an order for the medication from medical direction?
7. What are the five "rights" you would check prior to administering the medication?

EXPLORE PEARSON **mybradykit**™

Please go to **www.bradybooks.com** to access mykit for this text. You will find quizzes, critical thinking scenarios, weblinks, animations, and videos related to this chapter—and much more. Look for online information on medications that can be administered by an EMT as well as video clips on administration of activated charcoal, oral glucose, and nitroglycerin.

Register your access code from the front of your book by going to **www.bradybooks.com** and selecting the mykit links.

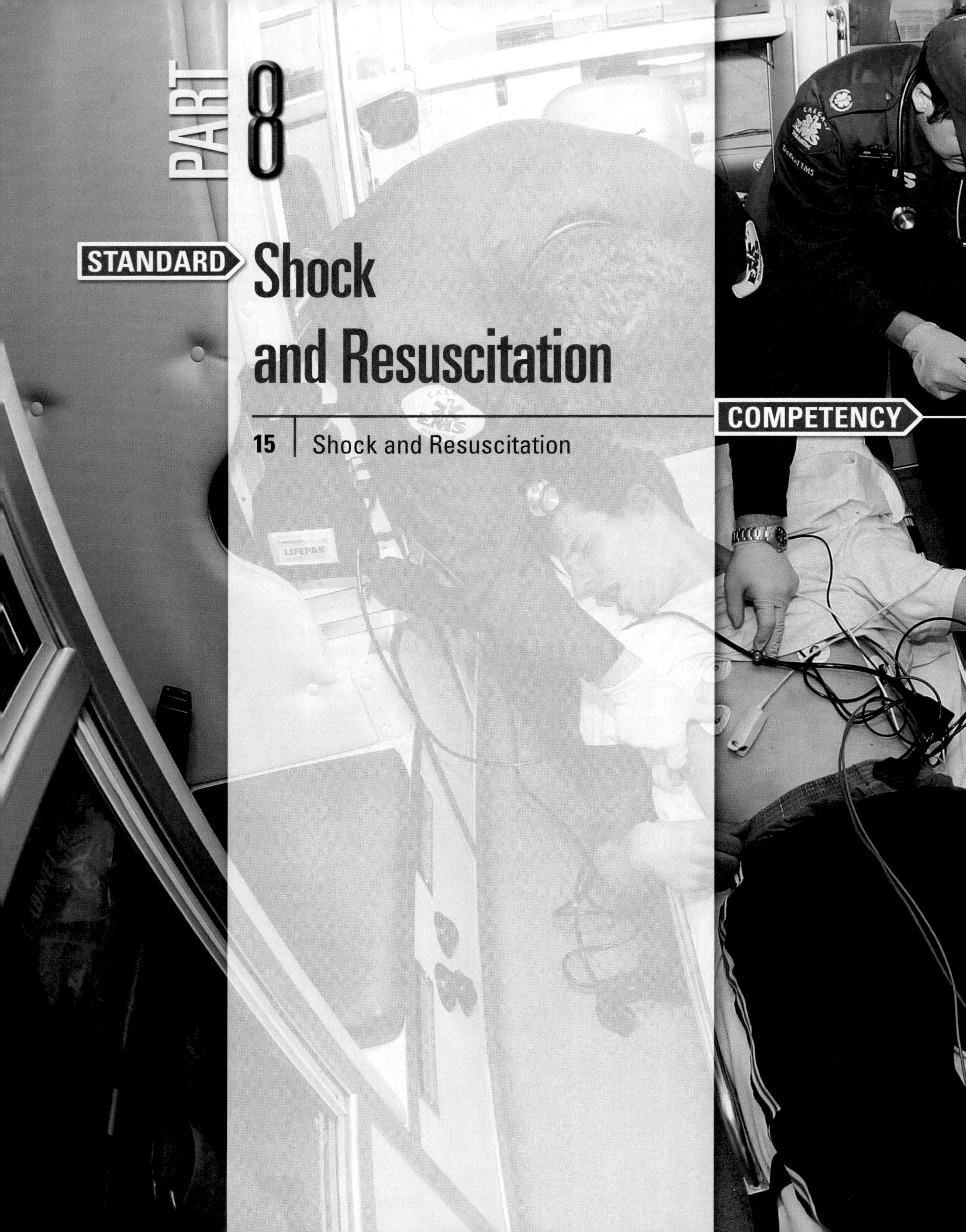

PART 8

STANDARD

Shock and Resuscitation

COMPETENCY

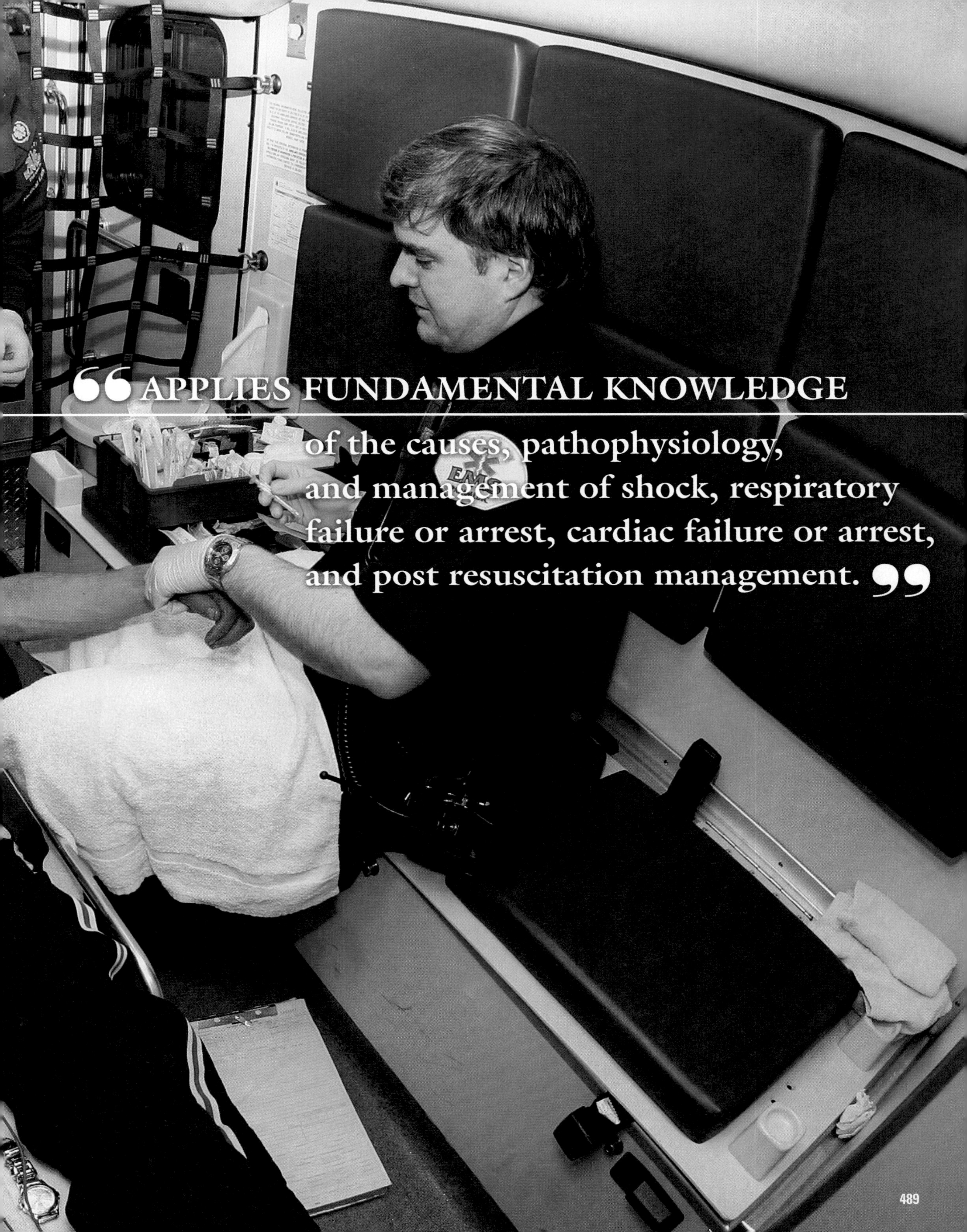
“APPLIES FUNDAMENTAL KNOWLEDGE
of the causes, pathophysiology, and management of shock, respiratory failure or arrest, cardiac failure or arrest, and post resuscitation management.”

CHAPTER 15

Shock *and* Resuscitation

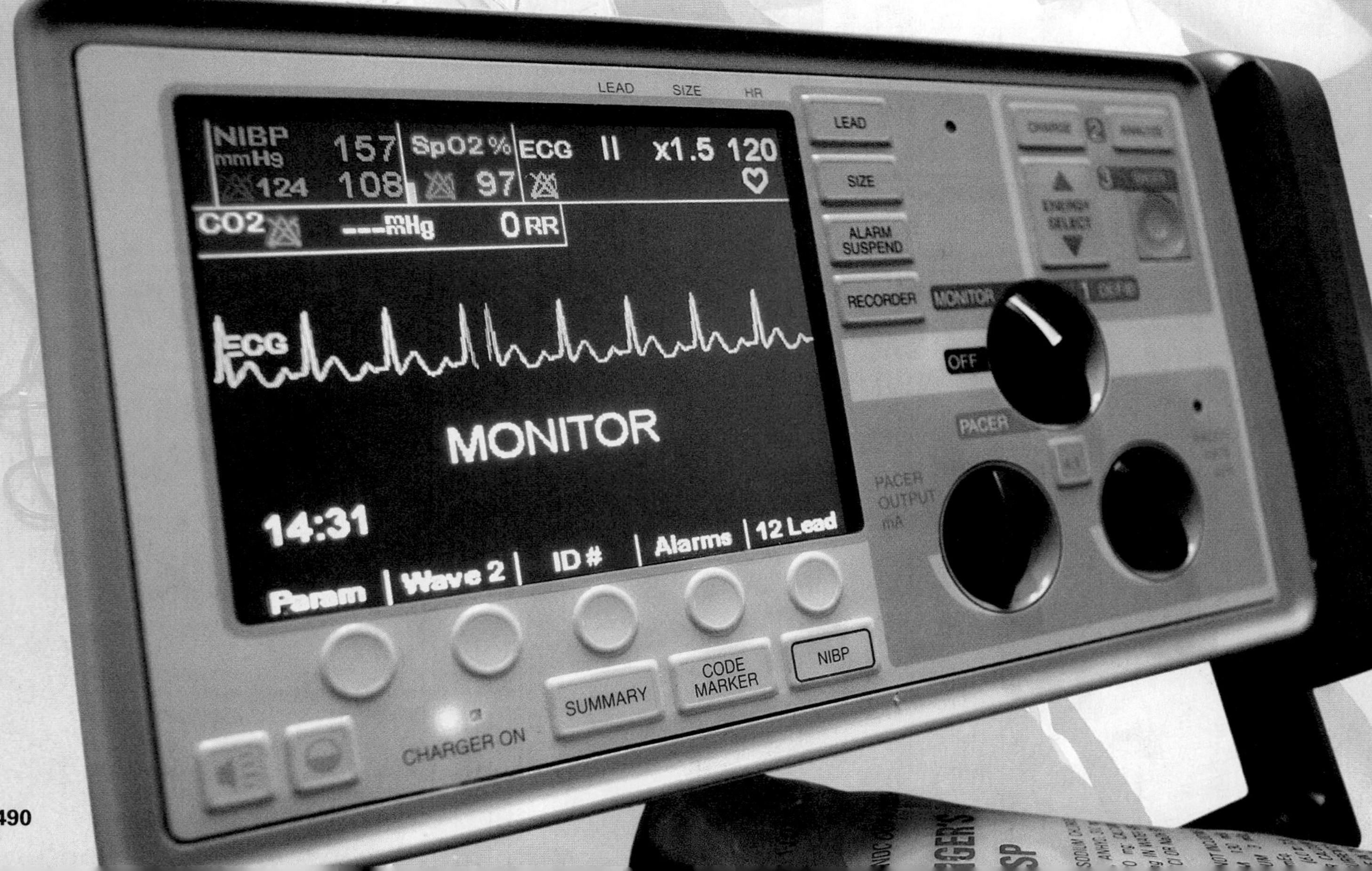

Navigation Guide

The following items provide an overview to the purpose and content of this chapter. The Standard and Competency are from the new National EMS Education Standards.

STANDARD **Shock and Resuscitation**

COMPETENCY Applies fundamental knowledge of the causes, pathophysiology, and management of shock, respiratory failure or arrest, cardiac failure or arrest, and postresuscitation management.

OBJECTIVES: After reading this chapter, you should be able to:

15-1. Define key terms introduced in this chapter.

15-2. Explain the pathophysiology of shock (hypoperfusion), including the consequences of cellular hypoxia and death.

15-3. Describe the physiology of maintaining adequate perfusion.

15-4. Describe how inadequate vascular volume, inadequate heart function, and decreased peripheral vascular resistance can lead to shock.

15-5. Give examples of conditions that can lead to:
- **a.** Loss of vascular volume
- **b.** Inadequate heart function
- **c.** Decreased peripheral vascular resistance

15-6. Explain the mechanisms and pathophysiology of each of the following categories and types of shock:
- **a.** Hypovolemic (hemorrhagic and nonhemorrhagic)
- **b.** Distributive (anaphylactic, septic, neurogenic)
- **c.** Cardiogenic
- **d.** Obstructive
- **e.** Metabolic or respiratory

15-7. Explain how compensatory mechanisms to shock are maintained through:
- **a.** Direct nerve stimulation
- **b.** Release of hormones

15-8. Explain the body's compensatory responses to hypoperfusion and how they manifest in the early signs and symptoms of shock.

15-9. Differentiate between early (compensatory) and late (decompensatory/irreversible) signs of shock.

15-10. Describe the progression of shock through the compensatory, decompensatory (progressive), and irreversible stages.

15-11. Explain how to identify the patient who is in a shock state and demonstrate the assessment of patients to identify shock.

15-12. Explain the influence of age on the assessment and management of patients with shock.

15-13. Discuss the goals of prehospital management of patients with shock.

15-14. Describe the pathophysiology of cardiac arrest.

15-15. Differentiate between the electrical, circulatory, and metabolic phases of cardiac arrest.

15-16. Identify situations in which resuscitative attempts should be withheld.

15-17. Explain each of the links in the Chain of Survival of cardiac arrest.

15-18. Explain the importance of early defibrillation in cardiac arrest.

15-19. Explain the rationale for the "push hard and push fast" approach to cardiopulmonary resuscitation (CPR).

15-20. Describe the features, functions, advantages, disadvantages, use, and precautions in the use of automated external defibrillators (AEDs).

15-21. Compare and contrast ventricular fibrillation, ventricular tachycardia, asystole, and pulseless electrical activity.

15-22. Given a series of cardiac arrest scenarios involving infants, children, and adults, demonstrate appropriate assessment and resuscitative techniques, including the integrated use of AEDs (automated and semiautomated), ventilation, and CPR, and explain the purpose and procedure for reassessment of the cardiac arrest patient.

15-23. Demonstrate assessment and management of a post cardiac-arrest patient with return of spontaneous circulation.

15-24. Given a cardiac arrest scenario, make decisions regarding obtaining advanced cardiac life support (ACLS).

15-25. Describe the safety precautions to be taken to protect yourself, other EMS providers, the patient, and bystanders in resuscitation situations.

15-26. Explain the importance of AED maintenance, EMT training and skills maintenance, and medical direction in the Chain of Survival of cardiac arrest.

15-27. Discuss special considerations in the use of an AED in patients with cardiac pacemakers and automatic implanted cardioverter-defibrillators.

15-28. List the advantages and disadvantages of automated chest compression devices, impedance threshold devices, and other circulation-enhancing devices.

continued

Navigation Guide *continued*

KEY TERMS: Page references indicate first major use in this chapter. For complete definitions, see the Glossary at the back of the book.

anaphylactic shock p. 501
asystole p. 514
automated external defibrillator (AED) p. 511
burn shock p. 501
cardiac arrest p. 508
cardiogenic shock p. 498
Chain of Survival p. 509
compensatory shock p. 503
decompensatory shock p. 505
defibrillation p. 510
distributive shock p. 497
downtime p. 509
hemorrhagic hypovolemic shock p. 500
hypoperfusion p. 493
hypovolemic shock p. 496
irreversible shock p. 505
neurogenic shock p. 501
nonhemorrhagic hypovolemic shock p. 500
obstructive shock p. 498
pulseless electrical activity (PEA) p. 514
resuscitation p. 508
return of spontaneous circulation (ROSC) p. 509
septic shock p. 501
shock p. 493
sudden death p. 508
survival p. 509
total downtime p. 509
ventricular fibrillation (VF or V-Fib) p. 513
ventricular tachycardia (VT or V-Tach) p. 513

MEDIA RESOURCES: Please go to www.bradybooks.com to access mykit for this text. You will find quizzes, critical thinking scenarios, weblinks, animations, and videos related to this chapter—and much more. Look for online information on toxic shock syndrome. You will also find a video clip on bleeding control/shock management.

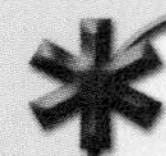

CASE STUDY

The Dispatch
EMS Unit 102—respond to 46 Hillman Street. You have a 26-year-old male patient who has been stabbed in the leg and is bleeding profusely. Law enforcement is en route. Time out is 2102 hours.

Upon Arrival
You and your partner arrive at the scene and are directed into the house by a police officer. He leads you into the basement where you find the patient lying supine on the floor with a large pool of blood around his right thigh. His pant leg is completely soaked in blood. The patient is not alert and doesn't respond when you call out to him. He appears to be extremely pale.

How Would You Proceed to Assess and Care for This Patient?
During this chapter, you will learn about assessment and emergency care for a patient suffering from shock and those needing resuscitation. Later, we will return to the case and apply the procedures learned.

▶ Introduction

Shock is a critical condition that results in the inadequate perfusion of cells, tissue, and organs. It carries a high morbidity and mortality if it is allowed to progress. If shock is not managed effectively, it will eventually lead to cell injury, organ dysfunction, multisystem organ failure, and patient death. Every cell, tissue, organ, and organ system can be affected by shock. In a shock state, the body attempts to restore homeostasis through a response of the nervous system and release of hormones, which cause many of the signs and symptoms seen in the shock patient. There are many different etiologies and types of shock. Determining the underlying cause is important to providing effective emergency care.

Resuscitation is the emergency care process that attempts to restore lost vital functions. It focuses on managing the airway, oxygenation, ventilation, and circulation. Resuscitation is most often associated with cardiac arrest; however, it is also performed in cases of respiratory failure, respiratory arrest, shock, and many other conditions.

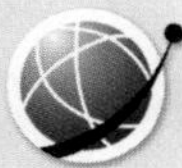

Media Resources
Go to www.bradybooks.com for mykit. Highlights:

- *Web Resource:* Toxic Shock Syndrome
- *Web Resource:* Stages of Shock

Objectives 15-2 and 15-3
Explain the pathophysiology of shock and the physiology of maintaining adequate perfusion.

Key Terms
shock insufficient supply of oxygen and other nutrients to body cells resulting from inadequate circulation of blood. Also called **hypoperfusion**.

Shock

Shock is defined as inadequate tissue perfusion. It is also often referred to as **hypoperfusion**. During a shock state, inadequate amounts of oxygen and glucose are delivered to cells. The inadequacy is defined as an amount of oxygen delivered to the cells that is less than the amount required for normal metabolism. In addition, an impaired elimination of carbon dioxide and other waste products occurs.

As discussed in Chapter 8, "Pathophysiology," a lack of oxygen in the cell causes a shift from aerobic to anaerobic metabolism. Aerobic metabolism takes a glucose molecule and breaks it down in the presence of oxygen, yielding the large amount of adenosine triphosphate (ATP) that is necessary for energy production along with water and carbon dioxide as by-products. The waste carbon dioxide is transported in the venous blood back to the heart and lungs, where it is eliminated during exhalation. When there is a lack of available oxygen, anaerobic metabolism takes place that results in a drastically lower production of ATP and the creation of lactic acid as a by-product.

Energy is needed to maintain the function of the cell's sodium/potassium pump. If the pump fails, the sodium is no longer removed from the cell in exchange for potassium. Potassium and lactic acid leave the cell and begin to collect in the interstitial fluid and eventually enter the blood. The sodium collects inside the cell and attracts water. As a result, the cell swells and eventually ruptures and dies. The acid that has been liberated causes the failure of enzyme systems and the release of lysozymes. The lysozymes begin to autodigest the cell, leading to cell death and eventual organ death.

Restoring perfusion (oxygen and glucose delivery) will restore production of the larger amounts of energy required, reverse the lactic acid buildup, and re-establish the function of the sodium/potassium pump.

In order to maintain cellular perfusion, several components must be functioning adequately. One of the most important is the ability of the body to deliver an adequate amount of oxygen to the cells. For this to happen, the following components associated with oxygen delivery and perfusion must be intact:

- The patient must be breathing an adequate concentration of oxygen (FiO_2) with each breath. If the oxygen content of the ambient air that is being inhaled is diminished, the amount of oxygen in the alveoli available for gas exchange will also be decreased. By increasing the oxygen concentration of inhaled air through oxygen therapy, more oxygen will be made available in the alveoli for gas exchange.
- The oxygen in the alveoli must diffuse across the alveolar/capillary membrane to enter the capillary and be transported to the cells. If there is a disturbance in the ability of the oxygen to diffuse into the capillary, the blood oxygen content would be diminished.
- Once the oxygen diffuses across the capillary, it has to be transported to the cells. Only a small amount (1.5 to 3 percent) of oxygen dissolves into the plasma. The majority of oxygen must bind with hemoglobin in the red blood cells. If there is an inadequate number of red blood cells with hemoglobin, the oxygen-carrying capacity of the blood will be decreased. This will result in a decrease in the delivery of oxygen to the cells.
- Once the oxygen has effectively bonded with hemoglobin, there must be an adequate volume of blood and pressure to move the blood forward through the systemic circulation, enabling it to be delivered to the cells.
- When the oxygen-saturated hemoglobin reaches the cell, the oxygen must break its bond, be released from the hemoglobin, and diffuse across the capillary and into the cell. If a condition exists that causes the oxygen to remain bound to the hemoglobin, the blood will appear to be well oxygenated but the cells will become severely hypoxic.

Most of the emergency care of the patient in shock is geared toward maintaining or restoring oxygen and glucose delivery to the cells. As you can gather from the aforementioned list of necessary components, some of the disturbances of oxygen delivery are not effectively managed in the prehospital setting—for example, increasing the amount of red blood cells and hemoglobin to restore or improve the blood's oxygen-carrying capability. This requires the administration of red blood cells and hemoglobin, which is generally not a prehospital function. Thus, a patient who presents in shock must be categorized as critical and unstable and considered for expeditious transport following the primary assessment and initial emergency care.

Objective 15-4
Describe how inadequate vascular volume, inadequate heart function, and decreased peripheral vascular resistance can lead to shock.

Objective 15-5
Give examples of conditions that can lead to loss of vascular volume, inadequate heart function, and decreased peripheral vascular resistance.

Etiologies of Shock

Three basic etiologies of shock will be described in this section. These etiologies are the basis for the categories and types of shock that will be defined later. The etiologies also provide a foundation for the general emergency care necessary to manage a shock patient as well as an understanding that not all shock treatment is the same.

Poor tissue perfusion (shock) is typically due to one or more of the following basic etiologies:

- **Inadequate volume.** A patient who has a decreased blood volume will have a decrease in preload which, in turn, will cause the stroke volume and cardiac output to fall. A decrease in cardiac output will cause a drop in the systolic blood pressure. As you recall, the systolic blood pressure is responsible for transporting the oxygenated blood throughout the systemic circulation. Therefore, a decrease in systolic blood pressure can result in inadequate tissue perfusion.

  A decrease in blood volume may result from the loss of whole blood, which includes the formed elements (red blood cells, white blood cells, and platelets) and plasma (Figure 15-1∗), or from loss of plasma volume alone. Bleeding causes whole blood loss, whereas diarrhea, burns, excessive urination, increased capillary leakage, and excessive vomiting are examples of conditions that cause loss of plasma volume alone.

  The patient who is in shock from inadequate volume obviously needs an increase in blood volume to restore adequate perfusion. However, if the patient lost whole blood from hemorrhage, there has been a loss of oxygen-carrying capability of the blood in addition to the decrease in pressure and perfusion. This patient would benefit most from administration of whole blood with fluids, which would increase the oxygen-carrying capability of the blood as well as improving pressure and perfusion. If only fluid is administered, the pressure and perfusion may be improved, but the cells may remain hypoxic because there still are not enough red blood cells and hemoglobin to carry the needed amount of oxygen.

  On the other hand, consider a patient who is in shock from fluid depletion resulting from excessive diarrhea. No red blood cells were lost in the diarrhea, only large amounts of water and some electrolytes. The patient has enough red blood cells and hemoglobin available to carry oxygen; however, his depleted fluid volume has decreased the blood pressure and ability of the blood to deliver the oxygen to the cells. This patient does not need whole blood, but does need to have the fluid or water portion of his blood restored. This is also typical in the burn patient who has lost plasma from the burned areas but still has adequate red blood cells and hemoglobin. This patient, too, needs fluid but does not need whole blood.

- **Inadequate pump function.** The heart is the pump responsible for generating the force necessary to move the blood throughout the body. If the pump fails, regardless of the blood volume, the delivery of oxygen and glucose to cells will be decreased (Figure 15-2∗). Pump function failure may result from an injury to the heart that reduces its ability to generate contractions strong enough to push the blood forward throughout the body. For example, a heart attack (myocardial infarction) deadens a portion of the heart muscle. Like any other muscle, a portion that is dead doesn't contribute to the force of contraction. If the heart attack has affected a large enough area of heart muscle, the pump will fail and lead to a shock state. A heart attack

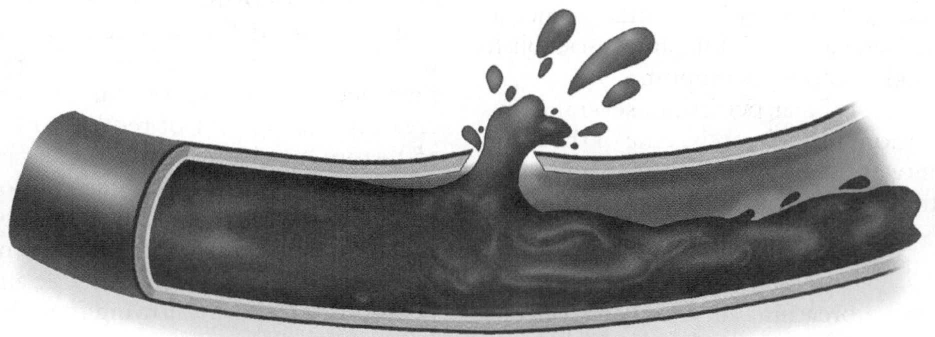

FIGURE 15-1 ∗ Etiology of shock: volume loss.

Key Points
Loss of blood volume results in decreased preload, stroke volume, and cardiac output.

Key Points
If the pump fails, regardless of blood volume, delivery of oxygen and glucose to cells will be decreased.

Key Points
In order to have adequate blood pressure, vessel tone must be maintained.

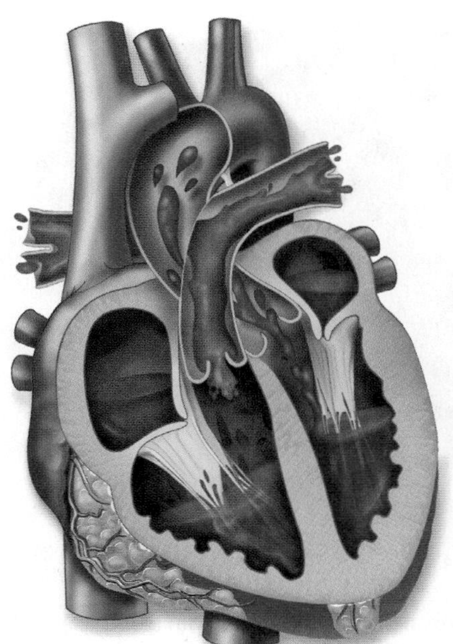

FIGURE 15-2 ✱ Etiology of shock: pump failure.

is not the only condition that can cause pump failure. The heart may be weakened over time from disease, old age, or injury and fail to adequately pump the blood. This is often seen in congestive heart failure patients, resulting in an inadequate delivery of oxygen and glucose to the cells.

Mechanical obstruction of the movement of blood into the heart may also contribute to pump failure. For example, the heart chambers may be compressed from a collection of blood in the pericardial sac, the fibrous sac that surrounds the heart. If the chambers are compressed, the ventricular filling space is decreased, leading to a decrease in preload. This condition is referred to as pericardial tamponade. Another condition that leads to a decrease in preload from compression and poor filling is a tension pneumothorax. This results from an injury to the lung that permits a large collection of air in the pleural space of one hemithorax. As the air continues to collect in the pleural space, it builds pressure and pushes the mediastinum toward the uninjured lung. This causes the inferior vena cava to kink and the aorta and heart to be compressed, resulting in a decrease in preload. A decrease in preload causes a drop in stroke volume and cardiac output, which in turn reduces blood pressure and perfusion. Pericardial tamponade and tension pneumothorax will be discussed in greater detail in Chapter 34, "Chest Trauma."

As just described, ineffective pump function can result either from damage to the heart or from a mechanical obstruction. In either condition, the patient requires improvement of pump function to eliminate the shock state. Remember, this patient has not lost any blood volume. With pump failure, administering fluids will not improve the condition and may actually make it worse.

- **Inadequate vessel tone.** In order to have an adequate blood pressure, the tone of the vessels must be maintained. The tone is related to the size of the vessel and the resistance created within it and is referred to as the systemic vascular resistance or peripheral vascular resistance. Recall from the pathophysiology chapter that as vessel size decreases, resistance increases. The result is an increase in the blood pressure (BP), which is governed by both cardiac output (CO) and systemic vascular resistance (SVR): (BP = CO × **SVR**). Conversely, if the vessel size increases because of massive vasodilation, the resistance decreases and the blood pressure and perfusion also decrease. In this case, the patient has not lost any blood volume; however, there is no longer enough intravascular blood volume to fill the vascular space because of the increase in vessel size (Figure 15-3✱). The result is a decrease in vascular resistance with a decrease in blood pressure and perfusion. The pumping function of the heart is normal, but the relative reduction in blood volume returning to the left ventricle will reduce preload, reduce cardiac output, and further decrease blood pressure and perfusion.

The sympathetic nervous system provides tone by keeping the vessel size regulated to a certain size to maintain the resistance and pressure. Therefore, inadequate vessel tone may occur if the sympathetic nervous system stimulation of the vessels is lost because of an injury to the spinal cord. Another cause of inadequate vessel tone may be chemical mediators released within the body that cause a systemic dilation of vessels. In either case, the only way to increase the blood pressure and perfusion is either to decrease the size of the vessel through vasoconstriction to restore resistance or to fill the vessel with more volume to increase the internal vessel pressure. Typically, both approaches—vasoconstriction and volume restoration—are used in an emergency care for cases where both blood pressure and perfusion are extremely poor.

Objective 15-6
Explain the mechanisms and pathophysiology of hypovolemic, distributive, cardiogenic, obstructive, and metabolic or respiratory shock.

Key Terms
hypovolemic shock shock caused by the loss of blood or fluid from the intravascular space resulting in a low blood volume.

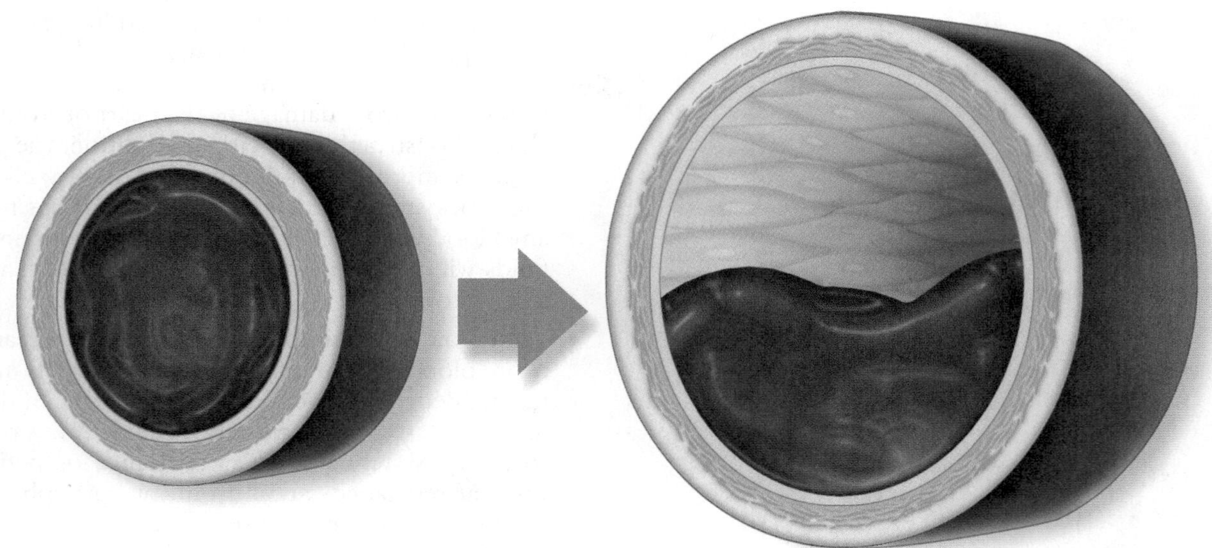

Normal-sized vessel full of blood.

Dilated vessel only partially filled with blood.

FIGURE 15-3 ✱ Etiology of shock: vasodilation.

As you can see, it is not only the cause of shock but also the needed emergency care that may vary, depending on the etiology: inadequate volume, inadequate pump function, or inadequate vessel tone—or a combination of these. A treatment that is effective for low blood pressure and poor perfusion based on one etiology of shock may worsen the condition from another etiology. Many emergency care procedures for shock are beyond the scope of the EMT; however, it is vital that an EMT recognizes a shock state, provides appropriate emergency care, and initiates rapid transport.

In some cases, it may be highly desirable to contact an advanced life support unit that has medications, intravenous fluids, and procedures that can restore the pressure, perfusion, cellular oxygenation, and delivery of glucose to cells. Keep in mind, however, that ALS is also limited in some cases, and delaying or interrupting transport may worsen the patient outcome. This is especially true for patients who are in shock from blood loss. ALS units typically carry only water-based fluids with electrolytes that do not have the capability to transport oxygen. Using these fluids in the patient who continues to bleed may cause the injury to bleed faster from the fluid infusion that is increasing the pressure and making the blood less viscous. In these cases it is critical to get the patient to a medical facility as expeditiously as possible.

Categories of Shock

There are four major categories of shock and a fifth category that some sources list (Figure 15-4✱). These categories are a further classification of the etiology and are somewhat more descriptive. The category of shock provides insight not only into the cause but also into the treatment necessary to reverse the shock state.

Hypovolemic Shock

If you break down the word *hypovolemic* based on what you learned in the medical terminology section of Chapter 7, "Anatomy, Physiology, and Medical Terminology," it clearly defines the cause of the shock. *Hypo-* means low or inadequate, *vol* refers to volume, and *-emic* pertains to blood. Thus, the term **hypovolemic shock** means shock that is caused from a low blood volume. Hypovolemic shock is the most common form of shock. It can be due to blood loss or loss of some other fluid—basically any condition or injury that decreases the blood content or the fluid portion of the blood. The most common cause of hypovolemic shock is hemorrhage (Figure 15-5a✱). Hemorrhage refers specifically to the loss of whole blood. This may be due to an injury, such as a laceration to a vessel or organ, or to a medical illness, such as bleeding from the gastrointestinal tract. Nonhemorrhagic forms of hypo-

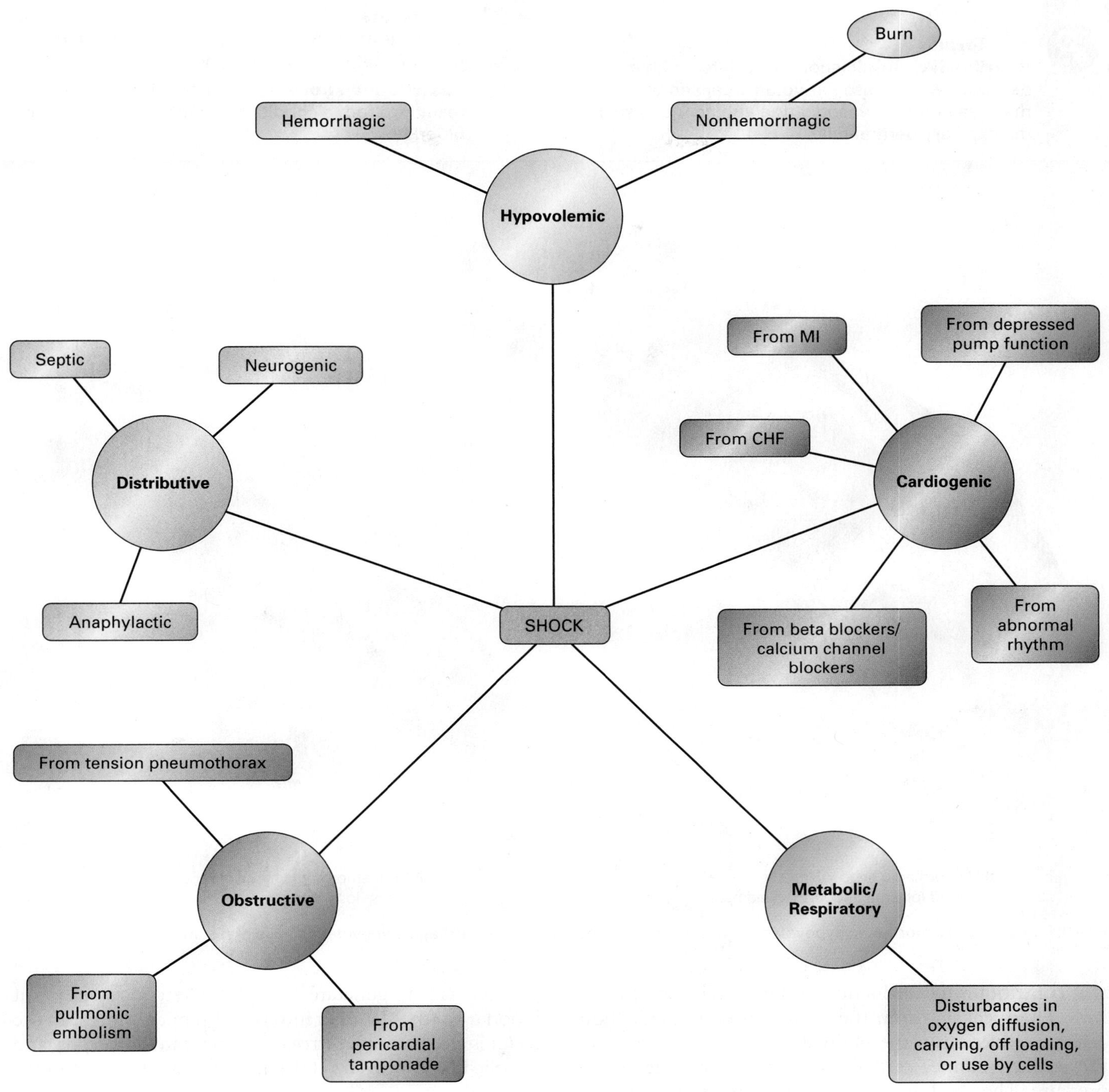

FIGURE 15-4 ✱ Categories and types of shock.

volemia are associated with fluid loss from burns and dehydration (Figure 15-5b✱). Hypovolemic shock will be further discussed later in the chapter.

Distributive Shock

Distributive shock is associated with a decrease in intravascular volume caused by massive systemic vasodilation and an increase in capillary permeability (Figure 15-6✱). In massive systemic vasodilation there is usually no actual loss of fluid or blood from the vessels but rather a *relative* reduction in volume; that is, a volume that has become inadequate to fill the increased size and capacity of the vessels. In some conditions, however, not only will the vessels dilate but also the capillaries will become permeable, which allows fluid to leak out of the capillaries and into the interstitial space. This causes an actual fluid loss, because the fluid is moving out of the vessels and into the spaces between the cells. If treated properly, the fluid will eventually re-enter the vessels.

In distributive shock, the shock state is caused by a reduction in systemic and peripheral vascular resistance

Key Terms

distributive shock shock associated with a decrease in intravascular volume caused by massive systemic vasodilation and an increase in the capillary permeability.

Key Terms

cardiogenic shock poor perfusion resulting from an ineffective pump function of the heart.

obstructive shock a poor perfusion state resulting from a condition that obstructs forward blood flow.

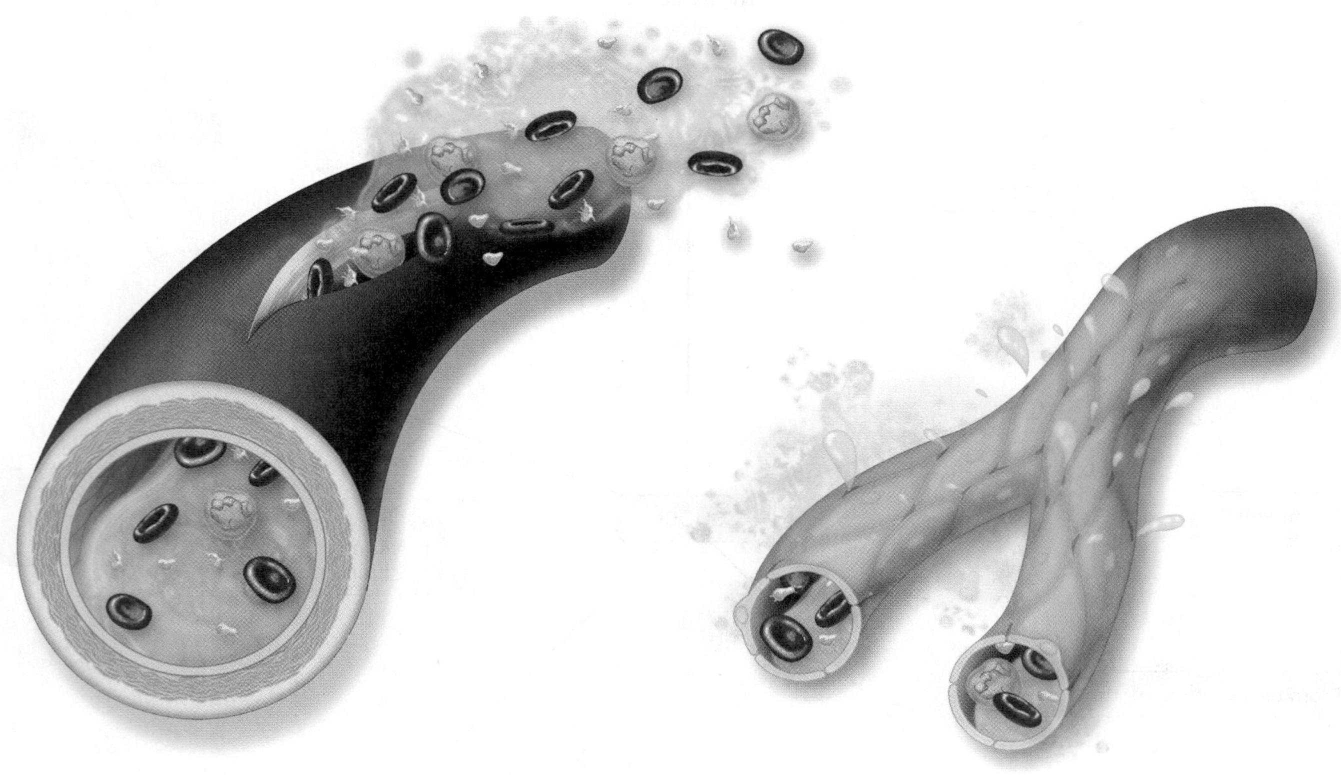

FIGURE 15-5 * **(a)** Hemorrhagic hypovolemia: loss of whole blood; **(b)** Nonhemorrhagic hypovolemia: loss of plasma.

that contributes to a reduction in the systolic blood pressure. Fluid leakage from the capillaries and vasodilation cause a reduction in the preload, which in turn reduces the stroke volume, cardiac output, and systolic blood pressure. The result is a decrease in tissue perfusion.

Cardiogenic Shock

Cardiogenic shock is caused by ineffective pump function of the heart. The patient has an adequate blood volume and vessel tone; however, hypoperfusion results from the inability of the heart to contract effectively. Typically, when more than 40 percent of the left ventricle has been lost, cumulatively, because of damage from a heart attack (Figure 15-7*), congestive heart failure, infection, or abnormal heart rhythms, the patient is prone to cardiogenic shock. The heart muscle that is lost no longer contributes to the force of contraction. When the left ventricle fails to generate enough force to eject sufficient blood from the chamber into the systemic circulation, the result is a reduction in stroke volume, cardiac output, and systolic blood pressure, leading to poor tissue perfusion.

Obstructive Shock

Obstructive shock results from a condition that obstructs forward blood flow. The volume is adequate, the heart is not damaged, and the vessels are of a normal size with adequate resistance. However, an obstruction is not allowing the blood to move forward. For example, a large clot that obstructs blood flow in the lungs (pulmonary embolism) will prevent an adequate amount of blood from getting to the left atrium and, subsequently, the left ventricle (Figure 15-8a*). This will reduce the preload and in turn decrease the stroke volume, cardiac output, systolic blood pressure, and tissue perfusion.

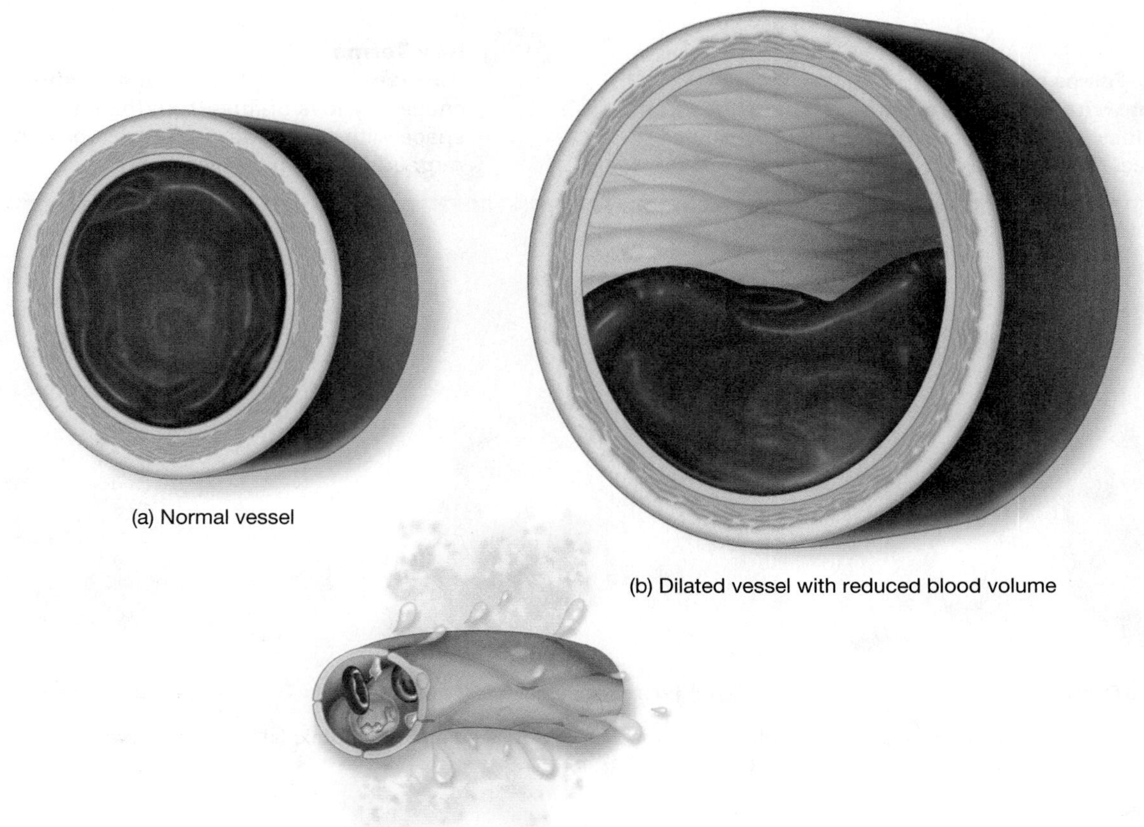
(a) Normal vessel
(b) Dilated vessel with reduced blood volume
(c) Permeable capillaries

FIGURE 15-6 ✱ Causes of distributive shock: **(a and b)** vasodilation; **(c)** capillary permeability.

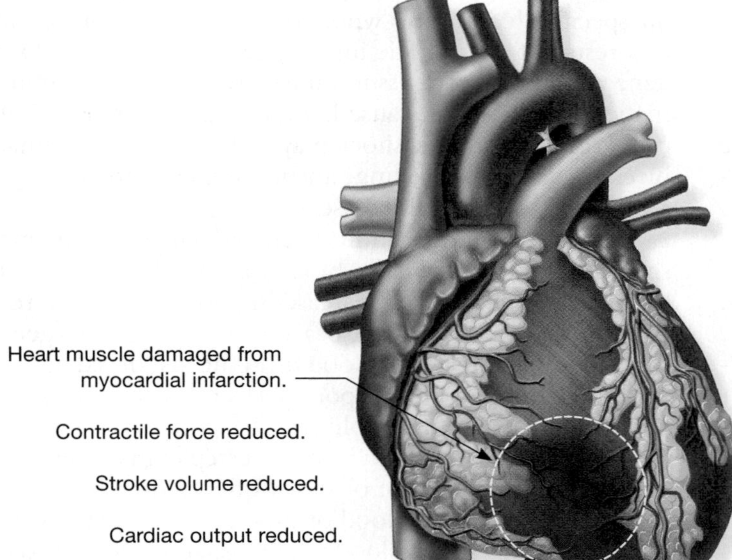
Heart muscle damaged from myocardial infarction.
Contractile force reduced.
Stroke volume reduced.
Cardiac output reduced.

FIGURE 15-7 ✱ Heart attack as a cause of cardiogenic shock: Damaged heart muscle results in reduced force of contractions, reduced stroke volume, and reduced cardiac output.

Two other conditions often associated with injury that can lead to obstructive shock are tension pneumothorax and pericardial tamponade (Figures 15-8b and 15-8c✱). Both of these conditions, as previously described, compress the heart and prevent adequate ventricular filling. This reduces the preload, stroke volume, cardiac output, systolic blood pressure, and tissue perfusion. Once the pressure is relieved, the heart regains its normal function. Although the pump function of the heart is disturbed, once the condition is reversed and the pressure on the heart is relieved, it functions normally.

Key Terms
hemorrhagic hypovolemic shock shock from the loss of whole blood from the intravascular space. Often called just *hemorrhagic shock.*

Key Terms
nonhemorrhagic hypovolemic shock shock caused by loss of fluid from the intravascular space with red blood cells and hemoglobin remaining within the vessels.

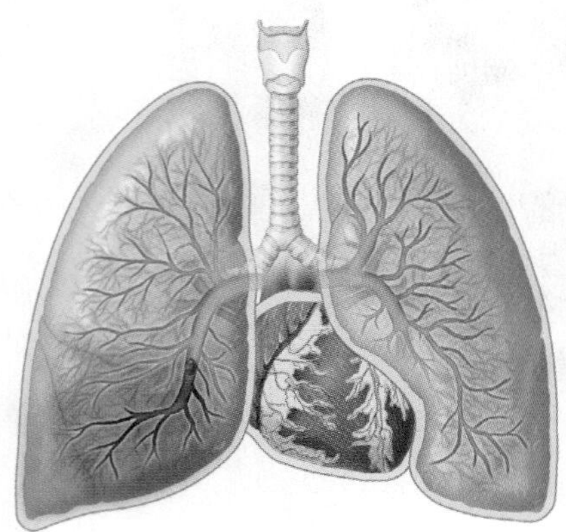

(a) Pulmonary embolism

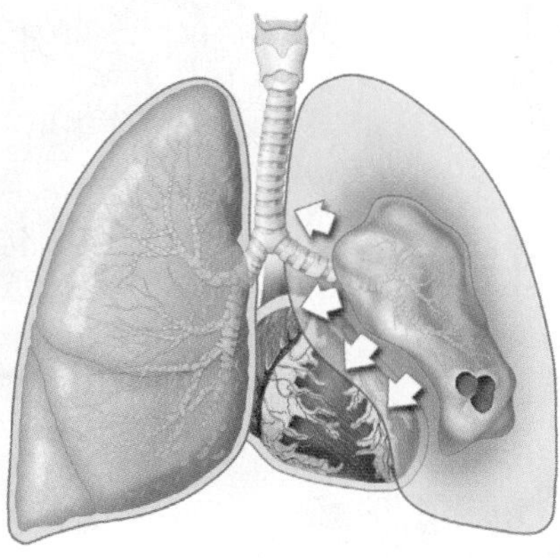

(b) Tension pneumothorax

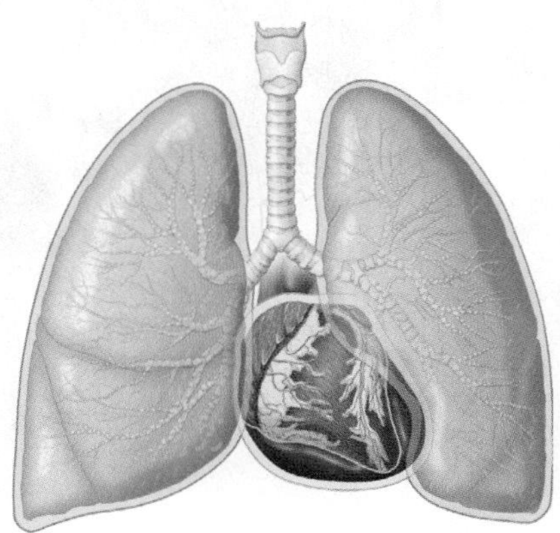

(c) Pericardial tamponade

FIGURE 15-8 * Causes of obstructive shock: **(a)** pulmonary embolism; **(b)** tension pneumothorax; **(c)** pericardial tamponade.

Metabolic or Respiratory Shock

Some sources list *metabolic* or *respiratory shock* as a fifth category of shock—in addition to hypovolemic, distributive, cardiogenic, and obstructive shock. This type of shock is described as a dysfunction in the ability of oxygen to diffuse into the blood, be carried by hemoglobin, off-load at the cell, or be used effectively by the cell for metabolism. Certain poisons, such as cyanide, interfere with the cell's ability to use oxygen. In this case, the blood is carrying an adequate amount of oxygen; however, the cyanide prevents the cell from using it. Carbon monoxide poisoning interferes with the ability of hemoglobin to carry oxygen. Carbon monoxide binds much more readily to the hemoglobin molecule than oxygen, which prevents oxygen from binding. Carbon dioxide cannot be used by the cells, which creates a severe hypoxic state in the blood and in the cells.

Specific Types of Shock

The categories of shock can be further broken down into specific types (review Figure 15-4). The category and etiology primarily describe the immediate reason for the poor perfusion state; whereas, the type of shock indicates the initial cause such as blood loss, spinal cord injury, or allergic reaction. Understanding the specific type of shock will allow you to recognize particular signs and symptoms of the various conditions and provide specialized emergency care in some cases.

Hemorrhagic Hypovolemic Shock

Hemorrhagic hypovolemic shock, often referred to simply as *hemorrhagic shock*, results from the loss of whole blood from the intravascular space. The term *hemorrhagic* specifically indicates whole blood loss that can occur as a result of a traumatic injury or a medical illness. Organ, vessel, and soft tissue injury are examples of traumatic injury that can cause hemorrhagic shock. Medical causes of hemorrhagic shock may include gastrointestinal bleeding, uterine bleeding, aortic disease, ectopic pregnancy, and esophageal disease.

The key to understanding hemorrhagic hypovolemic shock is the loss of whole blood. Once whole blood is lost, there is not only a decrease in perfusion from a reduction in pressure but also a decrease in the oxygen-carrying capability of the blood from the loss of red blood cells and hemoglobin. The poor perfusion state is from an inadequate intravascular volume.

Stopping the bleeding is the first step in management of this patient. This type of shock often requires the administration of whole blood or blood components to replace the intravascular blood volume that was lost. Thus, this patient requires immediate transport.

Nonhemorrhagic Hypovolemic Shock

Nonhemorrhagic hypovolemic shock is caused by the loss of fluid from the intravascular space; however, red blood cells and hemoglobin remain within the vessels. It is primarily water, plasma proteins, and electrolytes that

Key Terms

burn shock a form of nonhemorrhagic hypovolemic shock resulting from a burn injury.

anaphylactic shock distributive shock in which chemical mediators cause massive systemic vasodilation and permeable, leaking capillaries.

Key Terms

septic shock a type of distributive shock caused by an infection that releases bacteria or toxins into the blood.

neurogenic shock a type of distributive shock that results from massive vasodilation. Also called *vasogenic shock.*

are lost in nonhemorrhagic hypovolemic shock. This reduces the blood volume, pressure, and perfusion of cells; however, the oxygen-carrying capability of the remaining blood is preserved. The poor perfusion state is from an inadequate intravascular volume. Examples of nonhemorrhagic causes of shock include severe diarrhea, vomiting, excessive sweating, and excessive urination.

Administration of intravenous fluids may be beneficial in this patient; therefore, you might consider advanced life support backup. Always follow your local protocol.

Burn Shock

Burn shock is a specific form of nonhemorrhagic hypovolemic shock resulting from a burn injury. Burns may interrupt the integrity of the capillaries and vessels and allow them to leak plasma and plasma proteins. Recall from Chapter 8, "Pathophysiology," that hydrostatic pressure exerts a "push" effect and plasma proteins exert a "pull" effect on fluid inside the capillary. When the capillary is damaged from a burn, it becomes permeable. The push from hydrostatic pressure forces fluid outside of the capillary and into the interstitial space. The damaged capillary allows plasma proteins to leak out and collect in the interstitial space. The pull effect of the plasma proteins that are outside the vessel draws fluid out of the capillary and into the interstitial space and does not allow it to return to the inside of the vessel. This collection of fluid causes the edema seen in the burn patient and leads to burn shock. The shock is a direct result of inadequate intravascular volume.

The key emergency care in the burn patient is to establish and maintain an adequate airway, ventilation, and oxygenation. Also, prevent further contamination of the burn injury. Most burn patients die in the prehospital setting from airway obstruction, inadequate ventilation, or toxic exposure. Burn shock takes several hours to occur. Burns and burn management are covered in detail in Chapter 29, "Burns."

Anaphylactic Shock

Anaphylactic shock is a type of distributive shock. Anaphlyactic reactions are covered in detail in Chapter 21, "Anaphylactic Reactions." Chemical mediators that are released in the anaphylactic reaction cause massive and systemic vasodilation. These chemical mediators also cause the capillaries to become very permeable and to leak. The hydrostatic pressure inside the capillary forces (pushes) the fluid out into the interstitial space. The dilated vessels cause a reduction in the systemic vascular resistance, resulting in a decrease in blood pressure and perfusion. The loss of fluid from the capillary further reduces the intravascular volume, causing the preload, stroke volume, cardiac output, systolic blood pressure, and perfusion to decrease, resulting in a shock state.

Epinephrine is the medication of choice in the anaphylactic shock patient. Recall from Chapter 7, "Anatomy, Physiology, and Medical Terminology," that epinephrine contains alpha properties that cause systemic vasoconstriction. The vasoconstriction reduces the vessel size and increases the resistance, which results in an increase in blood pressure and perfusion. In addition, the vasoconstriction tightens the capillaries and lessens the fluid leakage. Airway management, ventilation, and oxygenation are also key components of the emergency care of the anaphylactic reaction patient.

Septic Shock

Septic shock is another type of distributive shock. It results from an infection that releases bacteria or toxins in the blood, causing the vessels throughout the body to dilate and become permeable. Fluid leaks out of the vessels into the interstitial space. The shock state is created by the massive vasodilation, which reduces the systemic vascular resistance, blood pressure, and perfusion. Also, the loss of fluid reduces the intravascular volume and decreases the preload, stroke volume, cardiac output, systolic blood pressure, and perfusion.

As an EMT, you will focus on managing the airway, ventilation, and oxygenation. This patient would benefit from intravenous fluids and medication to constrict the vessels. Thus, consider contacting an advanced life support unit. Always follow your local protocol.

Neurogenic Shock

Neurogenic shock, also commonly referred to as *vasogenic shock*, is another type of distributive shock. Spinal cord injury is a cause of neurogenic shock. A spinal cord injury may damage the sympathetic nerve fibers that control vessel tone below the level of injury. Loss of sympathetic tone causes the vessels to dilate. If the injury is high in the thoracic spinal cord or in the cervical region, enough vessel tone may be lost to cause a drop in systemic vascular resistance, blood pressure, and perfusion.

Objective 15-7
Explain how compensatory mechanism to shock are maintained through direct nerve stimulation and through release of hormones.

Objective 15-8
Explain how the body's compensatory responses to hypoperfusion manifest in the early signs and symptoms of shock.

There is no fluid loss from the intravascular space. The drop in perfusion is solely from widespread vasodilation. Blood will begin to pool in the peripheral vessels, causing a decrease in the preload, stroke volume, cardiac output, and systolic blood pressure, causing a further decrease in perfusion.

Emergency care focuses on spinal immobilization and management of the airway, ventilation, and oxygenation. This patient may also benefit from intravenous fluids to fill the vascular space and medication to constrict the vessels. Consider contacting an advanced life support unit. Again, always follow your local protocol.

Cardiogenic Shock

Cardiogenic shock is both a category and a type of shock. It is most often due to an acute myocardial infarction (heart attack), congestive heart failure, abnormal cardiac rhythm, or overdose on drugs that depress the pumping function of the heart such as beta blockers or calcium channel blockers. The depressed pump function reduces the force of the left ventricular contraction, stroke volume, cardiac output, systolic blood pressure, and perfusion.

Emergency care focuses on management of the airway, ventilation, and oxygenation. The patient may benefit from intervention and medications administered by an advanced life support unit. Follow your local protocol.

The Body's Response to Shock

When shock occurs, the body attempts to compensate for the disturbance and return the perfusion and tissue function to a normal state. Many of the signs and symptoms the patient exhibits while in shock are related to the compensatory mechanisms. The sympathetic nervous system plays a significant role in trying to restore a normal blood pressure and reverse the shock state.

Recall the function of the baroreceptors from Chapter 8, "Pathophysiology." These are stretch-sensitive receptors that continuously measure the pressure inside the aorta and carotid arteries. When there is a reduction in blood volume or pump function, or when there is a massive vasodilation with a redistribution of blood volume away from the core circulation, the cardiac output decreases. This causes a decrease in pressure inside the aorta and carotid arteries, which results in a reduction in stretch or tension in the arterial walls. The baroreceptors sense the reduction in arterial wall tension and trigger compensatory mechanisms.

The compensatory mechanisms associated with shock are initiated and maintained through two major pathways: direct sympathetic nerve stimulation and the release of hormones.

Direct Nerve Stimulation

When shock occurs, the sympathetic nervous system is activated and stimulates primarily the vessels and the heart in an attempt to restore the blood pressure in the arteries. The effects of the sympathetic stimulation, which occur immediately, are:

- Increase in heart rate
- Increase in force of ventricular contraction (stroke volume)
- Vasoconstriction
- Stimulation of the release of epinephrine and norepinephrine from the adrenal gland

The increase in heart rate and force of ventricular contraction, or stroke volume (SV), attempts to increase the cardiac output (CO = <u>**HR**</u> × <u>**SV**</u>). If the cardiac output can be improved and/or vasoconstriction increases the systemic vascular resistance, the systolic blood pressure would increase (BP = <u>**CO**</u> × <u>**SVR**</u>). The adrenal medulla, which is the middle center portion of the adrenal gland that is located on the top of the kidney, is stimulated by the nervous system to release the hormones epinephrine and norepinephrine. The sympathetic nervous system also increases the respiratory rate.

Release of Hormones

While direct nerve stimulation occurs immediately, the hormones epinephrine and norepinephrine are released from the center portion of the kidneys within a few minutes. They exert a sustained sympathetic effect on the organs. Recall from Chapter 7, "Anatomy, Physiology, and Medical Terminology," and Chapter 8, "Pathophysiology," that epinephrine stimulates alpha and beta receptors while norepinephrine mostly stimulates alpha receptors.

Alpha receptors are located primarily in vessel smooth muscle. When stimulated, the smooth muscle contracts, causing vasoconstriction. Thus, alpha stimulation results in vasoconstriction, which attempts to increase systematic vascular resistance and, in turn, blood

Objectives 15-9 and 15-10
Differentiate between early and late signs of shock and describe the progression of shock through the compensatory, decompensatory (progressive), and irreversible stages.

Key Terms
compensatory shock stage of shock in which a cascade of organ and gland stimulation and hormones increases blood pressure, restores arterial wall tension, and maintains a near normal blood pressure and perfusion of vital organs.

TABLE 15-1 Effects of Alpha and Beta Stimulation

Receptor	Stimulatory Effect	Sign or Symptom
Alpha$_1$	Contraction of the muscles controlling the iris	Dilated pupils
	Contraction of vascular smooth muscle causing vasoconstriction	Pale cool skin, narrow pulse pressure
	Stimulation of sweat glands	Localized sweating, clammy skin
Beta$_1$	Increased heart rate	Tachycardia
	Increased speed of impulse through conduction system	Tachycardia
	Increased force of contraction	Pounding heart
Beta$_2$	Bronchial smooth muscle dilation	Decreased resistance in airway
	Skeletal muscle contractility	Tremors

pressure. The beta$_1$ effect stimulates the heart and causes an increase in the heart rate and force of contraction. It also speeds the electrical impulse traveling through the conduction system of the heart, allowing for a faster heart rate. The heart rate and force of contraction are increased in an attempt to increase cardiac output. By increasing the cardiac output, the blood pressure may also be increased. The effects of alpha and beta receptor stimulation are summarized in Table 15-1.

In addition to epinephrine and norepinephrine, the body releases other hormones. Some of these hormones decrease urine output in an attempt to conserve body fluid through the reabsorption of water, while others cause further vasoconstriction, an increase in heart rate and contractility, and an increase in glucose in the blood. See Table 15-2.

Stimulation by the sympathetic nervous system and the release of hormones are geared to reversing the shock state and restoring the pressure in the arteries and perfusion to the cells. Many of the responses of the body to the stimulation or hormones produce the signs and symptoms seen in the shock patient.

Stages of Shock

As just discussed, the body attempts to compensate for disturbances in perfusion through the sympathetic nervous system and the release of hormones. The intention is to bring the dysfunction under control and restore the blood pressure and perfusion of tissues. There are three stages of shock: compensatory, decompensatory, and irreversible (Figure 15-9*).

Compensatory Shock

When the pressure in the aorta and carotid bodies decreases, the arterial wall tension is reduced, which triggers the baroreceptors to send decreased signals to the hypothalamus. This is an indication that the pressure is falling in the large arteries. In response, the hypothalamus activates a whole cascade of organ and gland stimulation and hormone releases in an attempt to increase the blood pressure to restore the arterial wall tension. This process is compensation, also known as **compensatory shock** or *compensated shock*, which is able to maintain a near normal blood pressure and perfusion of the vital organs.

Direct nerve stimulation of the heart by the sympathetic nervous system increases the heart rate and contractility in an attempt to increase cardiac output. This occurs within seconds of the fall in pressure. An increase in cardiac output may increase the blood pressure (BP = **<u>CO</u>** × SVR). Nerves also stimulate vessels to constrict. This increases the systemic vascular resistance and may also increase blood pressure (BP = CO × **<u>SVR</u>**). The respiratory system is stimulated to increase rate and tidal volume.

The sympathetic nerves also stimulate the adrenal medulla gland to release epinephrine and norepinephrine. The release of the hormones takes a few minutes; however, these hormones provide a sustained effect. The primary effects of epinephrine and norepinephrine are an increase in heart rate and contractility as well as vasoconstriction in an attempt to increase the blood pressure and perfusion. Vasoconstriction causes blood to be shunted away from nonessential areas, such as the skin and gastrointestinal tract, and to the core of the body to improve perfusion of the brain, heart, lungs, and other vital organs. An increase

Thinking Critically
An EMT concludes that her patient is not in shock because his blood pressure is normal. What's wrong with this reasoning?

Key Points
The blood pressure may appear to be relatively normal in compensatory shock, however, you might also note a narrow pulse pressure.

TABLE 15-2 Effects of Hormones Released in Shock

Hormone	Effect on Body	Sign or Symptom
Epinephrine	Increased heart rate (beta$_1$)	Tachycardia
	Increased contractility (beta$_1$)	Pounding heart
	Vasoconstriction (alpha$_1$)	Pale cool skin
	Sweat gland stimulation (alpha$_1$)	Clammy skin
	Decreased insulin secretion (alpha$_2$)	Increased blood glucose level
	Conversion of stored glucose in liver to blood glucose	
	Conversion of noncarbohydrates into sugar	
	Iris muscle contraction (alpha$_1$)	Pupillary dilation
Norepinephrine	Vasoconstriction (alpha$_1$)	Pale cool skin
	Sweat gland stimulation (alpha$_1$)	Clammy skin
Antidiuretic Hormone (Vasopressin)	Increased sodium reabsorption in the kidneys	Decreased urine output
	Vasoconstriction	Increased blood pressure
Angiotensin II	Vasoconstriction	Pale cool skin
	Increased heart rate	Tachycardia
	Sodium reabsorption in the kidney	Decreased urine output
Aldosterone	Sodium reabsorption in the kidney	Decreased urine output
Glucagon	Conversion of stored glucose in liver to blood glucose	Increased blood glucose level
	Conversion of noncarbohydrates into sugar	
	Increased heart rate and contractility	Tachycardia

in the respiratory rate and tidal volume provides more oxygen in the alveoli for gas exchange. This coupled with an improvement in circulation is designed to deliver better oxygenated blood to the tissues.

Other hormones cause the kidneys to reabsorb sodium. In Chapter 8, "Pathophysiology," you learned that water follows sodium. Thus, as the kidneys reabsorb sodium, water is also reabsorbed within the body. Body fluid is conserved by decreasing urine output. However, the reduction in urine excretion also causes retention of waste products, which could increase the acidity of the blood.

This stage is referred to as "compensatory" because the body is able to compensate for the decrease in pressure. If the etiology of shock is reversed in this stage, for example, by stopping the hemorrhage, then the compensatory mechanisms will continue to maintain the blood pressure and perfusion and will eventually begin to signal the body to decrease its response as the pressure is restored.

The blood pressure may appear to be relatively normal in compensatory shock. However, you might also note a narrow pulse pressure. Recall that as the systolic blood pressure falls because of a decrease in cardiac output, the vessels constrict. This raises the diastolic blood pressure, which causes the systolic and diastolic values to come closer together.

As an example, if a patient is losing blood from a hemorrhage, as the cardiac output falls the systolic blood pressure reading decreases. The decrease in volume in the vessels causes a reduction in resistance and pressure inside the vessel. To compensate for the lowered pressure, the vessels constrict to increase resistance. By doing so, the pressure increases even though the volume inside the vessel is less. This may provide a deceiving picture of the normal perfusion and blood pressure. However, the narrow pulse pressure is an early sign of shock and provides important additional information about the cardiac output in relation to vasoconstriction.

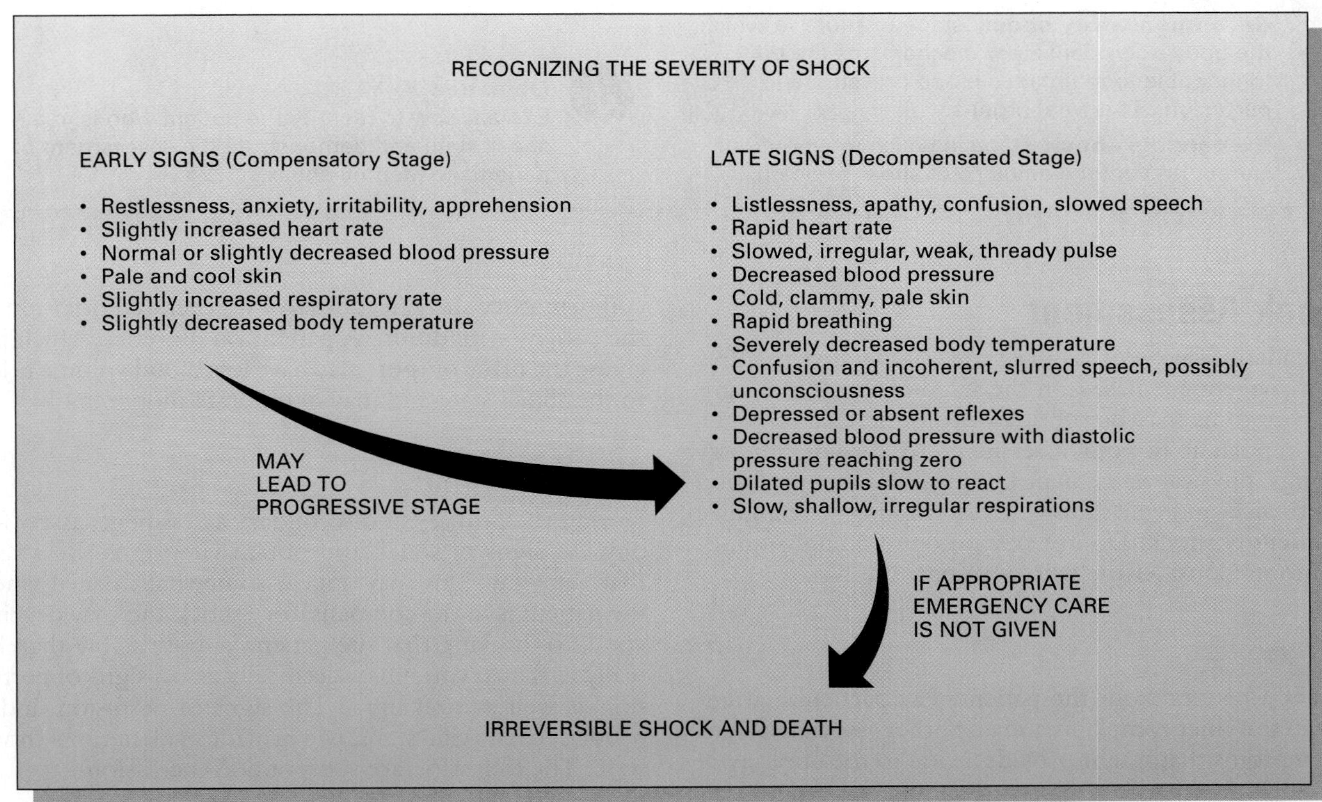

FIGURE 15-9 ✱ Recognizing the severity of shock.

This is an example of why you cannot rely on the presence or absence of only one sign when assessing for shock. You must at least assess mental status, blood pressure, pulse pressure, heart rate, and respiratory rate, as well as skin color, temperature, and condition.

Decompensatory Shock

Decompensatory shock, also commonly referred to as *decompensated shock* or *progressive shock*, is an advanced stage of shock in which the body's compensatory mechanisms are no longer able to maintain a blood pressure and perfusion of the vital organs. If the shock state continues unopposed and is not managed effectively, the compensatory mechanisms become exhausted or overwhelmed, leading to a failure to maintain pressure inside the vessels and perfusion of the vital organs.

Cells, tissues, and organs become ischemic from a lack of perfusion and delivery of oxygen and glucose. Acid begins to build up in the blood from the anaerobic metabolism occurring in the cells. Heart function is depressed from the lack of adequate blood flow through the coronary arteries, leading to myocardial ischemia. Blood in the capillaries begins to sludge and form microemboli (small clots) as the capillaries become permeable from acid accumulation resulting from anaerobic metabolism, hypoxia, and lack of nutrients. The increased capillary permeability allows blood to leak out of the vessels and into the interstitial space, further lowering the vascular volume and pressure. A decrease in brain perfusion leads to cerebral ischemia. When the vasomotor center in the medulla becomes hypoxic it begins to fail, thereby reducing sympathetic nervous system stimulation, which allows vessels to dilate and cause a further drop in pressure and perfusion. This vicious cycle continues to breed more shock. Aggressive shock management may or may not reverse the process in the later stages of decompensation.

Irreversible Shock

Irreversible shock is the stage where, regardless of the intervention, the patient outcome is death. Cell, tissue, and organ failure and damage is so pervasive and severe that no matter what treatment is provided organ death is inevitable and unable to be reversed. Microemboli begin to block capillaries throughout the body, leading to lung failure, kidney failure, and other multiple system organ failure (MSOF). Clotting factors are used in the formation of the microemboli in the blood. The body responds to the clots by releasing substances to attempt to break them up (fibrinolysis). Because the clotting factors were used up in the formation of the microemboli, the substances that are released to break down the clots are unopposed in the body and lead to widespread uncontrolled bleeding from any wound that was previously clotted, intravenous catheter sites, mucous membranes, and the skin.

Key Terms

decompensatory shock stage of shock in which the body's compensatory mechanisms are no longer able to maintain a blood pressure and perfusion of the vital organs.

irreversible shock stage in which interventions cannot prevent the advance of shock to death.

Objective 15-11

Explain how to identify the patient who is in a shock state and demonstrate the assessment of patients to identify shock.

Shock Assessment

Rapid identification of a shock state is imperative to effective management. Based on the stage of shock, the signs and symptoms may be subtle or profound (Table 15-3). It is important in your assessment to consider history findings, physical assessment findings, signs of perfusion disturbance, and vital signs when attempting to recognize and identify shock. Do not rely on one finding, sign, or symptom. Consider the whole patient.

History

Obtain a history from the patient. Pay particular attention to the chief complaint and any other associated signs or symptoms that might provide a clue to the etiology of the shock. Also gather information about the patient's allergies, medications, past medical history, last oral intake, and events prior to the incident.

Pay particular attention to certain medications such as beta blockers and calcium channel blockers. Both of these types of medications keep the heart rate from dramatically increasing, making it appear that the patient is not in a compensatory stage of shock. As an example, a patient on beta blockers or calcium channel blockers may present with a heart rate of only 72 bpm while in a shock state. Without knowledge of the medication, one would consider this to be a normal finding and may be deceived from thinking the patient is in shock.

This is another example of why you should consider all of the assessment findings and not just one individually. In addition to the lowered heart rate, both beta blockers and calcium channel blockers may prevent the cardiac output from effectively responding during the compensatory stage, leading to a quicker deterioration in the patient's condition. A patient on diuretics, which increase the urine output, may have less blood volume prior to the shock state and may deteriorate more rapidly.

Physical Exam

During the primary and secondary assessment, assess for physical signs of shock and obtain vital signs. Be aware that the vital signs may appear somewhat normal when the patient is in the compensatory shock and may deceive you into thinking that the patient is more stable than he really is. Thus, you must specifically assess signs of perfusion as well as vital signs. The signs of perfusion, independent of the vital signs, will provide evidence of a shock state. The following are signs of poor perfusion:

- Altered mental status
- Pale, cool, clammy skin
- Delayed capillary refill
- Decreased urine output
- Weak or absent peripheral pulses

In distributive shock, the skin is warm and flushed (red) from the vasodilation. After a period of time, the blood that has pooled in the extremities begins to deoxygenate and the skin becomes mottled. In cardiogenic shock, the skin appears to be pale, cool, and clammy early but takes on a cyanotic and mottled appearance as the shock state continues and the perfusion worsens.

Vital sign assessment must include the following:

- Blood pressure (both systolic and diastolic)
- Heart rate

TABLE 15-3 Signs and Symptoms of the Stages of Shock

Sign or Symptom	Compensatory Shock	Decompensatory Shock	Irreversible Shock
Mental Status	Normal to anxious	Decreased	Severely decreased or unresponsive
Heart Rate	Increased	Significantly increased	Significantly increased or decreased
Peripheral Pulse Quality	Peripheral pulses slightly weak	Very weak to absent	Absent
Blood Pressure	Normal or slightly decreased	Decreased	Severely decreased to absent
Pulse Pressure	Slightly narrow to narrow	Very narrow	No longer narrow
Skin—Hypovolemic	Slightly pale, cool, clammy	Severely pale, cool, clammy	Cold, cyanotic, mottled
Skin—Distributive	Warm, dry	Cool	Cool, cyanotic, or mottled

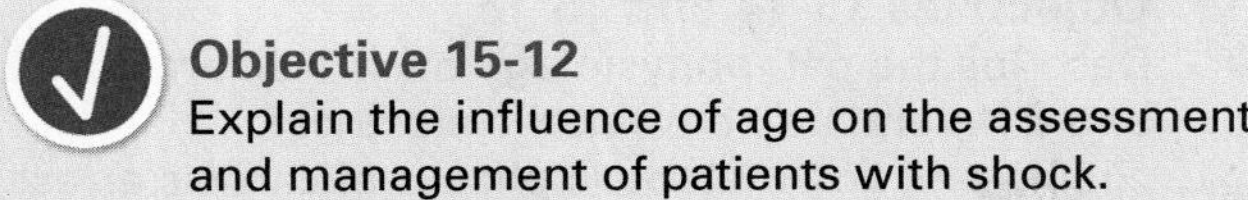
Objective 15-12
Explain the influence of age on the assessment and management of patients with shock.

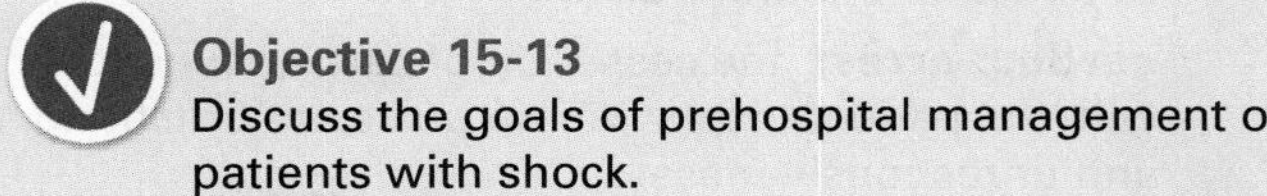
Objective 15-13
Discuss the goals of prehospital management of patients with shock.

- Pulse character
- Respiratory rate and tidal volume
- Skin color, temperature, and condition
- Pulse oximeter reading

The vital signs may vary, depending on the type of shock. Cardiogenic shock may present with an extremely slow heart rate or an irregular rhythm. Distributive shock from a spinal cord injury may present with a normal to slow heart rate and a blood pressure that is not extremely low. Both upper and lower airway compromise may be found in anaphylactic shock. These are only a few examples of variations of vital signs that might be found in the differing shock states.

Age Considerations in Shock

Age may influence the development, presentation, and management of shock, as well as recovery from shock. Shock states specific to pediatrics and geriatrics are discussed in Chapter 38, "Pediatrics," and Chapter 39, "Geriatrics." Briefly, elderly persons and newborns do not compensate well for shock. Thus, they have a tendency to deteriorate rapidly. Children and young adults compensate very well, often exhibiting only minor signs and symptoms for a long period of time and then decompensating suddenly.

Normal vital sign findings vary with age for pediatric patients. For children less than 10 years of age, a systolic blood pressure of 70 mmHg plus two times the age in years is a lower limit of normal. A systolic blood pressure less than the lower limit would be considered hypotensive. Hypotension is a late finding in pediatric patients and often leads to cardiac arrest.

The geriatric patient does not compensate well for shock. In addition, the medications the elderly patient is taking may prevent some signs or symptoms from appearing, such as an elevated heart rate. An altered mental status and tachypnea may be the most profound signs of shock in the elderly.

General Goals of Prehospital Management of Shock

Management of shock is geared to improving oxygenation of the blood and delivery of oxygen and glucose to the cells. The general goals of shock management are:

- Secure and maintain a patent airway.
- Establish and maintain adequate ventilation.
- Establish and maintain adequate oxygenation via a nonrebreather mask at 15 lpm in the patient who is breathing adequately or supplemental oxygen delivered at the highest concentration via the ventilation device for the patient who is not breathing adequately.
- Do not hyperventilate the shock patient. Making the blood alkalotic from hyperventilation will reduce the off-loading of oxygen from the hemoglobin and promote further cellular hypoxia. Increasing the pressure inside the chest in a poor volume and perfusion state may further decrease preload and cardiac output.
- Stop the bleeding as quickly as possible using direct pressure. If direct pressure is not effective, proceed to application of a tourniquet. Consider hemostatic agents to control hemorrhage if permitted by your local protocol.
- Splint fractures to reduce bleeding; however, do not delay transport to perform individual splinting of fractures. Fracture management should be initially achieved with a long backboard and then continued en route if the patient's condition and time allows.
- Do not remove an impaled object.
- Maintain the body temperature by removing wet clothing from water or blood, covering the patient to prevent further heat loss, and warming the patient compartment to 85 degrees for transport.
- Keep the patient in a supine position. Immobilize the patient to a backboard if a spinal cord or column injury is suspected.
- Apply the pneumatic antishock garment (PASG) if a pelvic fracture is suspected and the systolic BP is < 90 mmHg, profound hypotension is present (< 50 to 60 mmHg), intra-abdominal hemorrhage is suspected with severe hypotension, or retroperitoneal hemorrhage is suspected with hypotension. See Chapter 28, "Bleeding and Soft-Tissue Trauma," for more detailed information on the PASG.
- Rapidly transport the patient to the most appropriate medical facility.
- Consider ALS intercept for distributive, cardiogenic, obstructive, and nonhemorrhagic categories of shock. Follow your local protocol.

Key Terms
resuscitation bringing a patient back from a potential or apparent death.
cardiac arrest the cessation of cardiac function with the patient displaying no pulse, no breathing, and unresponsiveness.

Key Terms
sudden death death of a patient within one hour of the onset of signs and symptoms.

Objectives 15-14 and 15-15
Describe the pathophysiology of cardiac arrest and differentiate between the electrical, circulatory, and metabolic phases of cardiac arrest.

Resuscitation in Cardiac Arrest

The term **resuscitation** basically means bringing the patient back from a potential or apparent death. The potential or apparent death may result from many different causes, including trauma and medical conditions. Resuscitation focuses on management of the airway, ventilation, and oxygenation, and restoring adequate circulation.

Cardiac arrest, the worst manifestation of cardiac compromise from an acute coronary event, occurs when the ventricles of the heart, for any of a variety of reasons, are not contracting or when the cardiac output is completely ineffective and no pulses can be felt. The normal electrical impulses are usually absent or disrupted or the mechanical response to the electrical impulse does not occur. Instead of smooth, coordinated contractions, the heart shows a different type of activity, most commonly the uncoordinated twitching known as ventricular fibrillation. Pumping action ceases and the body's cells, without oxygenated blood, begin to die. Brain cells begin to die within 4 to 6 minutes following cardiac arrest. The patient presents as unresponsive and without a detectable pulse or spontaneous respiration.

Cardiac arrest patients are often described as having suffered **sudden death**, which occurs when the patient dies within 1 hour of the onset of the signs and symptoms.

Understanding BODY PROCESSES

Ventricular fibrillation is a chaotic and disorganized cardiac rhythm that causes the ventricles to quiver and does not produce ventricular contraction. No pulse or perfusion occurs during ventricular fibrillation. ■

Pathophysiology of Cardiac Arrest

Time is a critical issue in cardiac arrest. As time passes, the heart continues to deteriorate from a lack of oxygen and glucose and begins to undergo changes that lead to severe myocardial cell ischemia and eventually organ death. Unfortunately, the time is in minutes and begins immediately upon the onset of cardiac arrest. As soon as the patient goes into cardiac arrest, the resuscitation clock is ticking. If it is 5 minutes before someone finds the patient after he collapses and calls 911, and you have a 5-minute response time to get to the patient's side, you are already 10 minutes into the cardiac arrest, which results in a less than favorable condition of the myocardium to begin resuscitative efforts. The brain is the most sensitive organ to cardiac arrest and, as previously noted, undergoes irreversible changes after 4 to 6 minutes.

There are three phases the patient goes through following cardiac arrest that lead to biological death: electrical phase, circulatory phase, and metabolic phase. Each phase is associated with variations in organ function and damage and has implications for emergency care.

Electrical Phase

The electrical phase begins immediately upon cardiac arrest and ends 4 minutes afterward. During this early and initial phase, the heart still has a good supply of oxygen and glucose; therefore, aerobic metabolism is maintained with continued energy production for cell function and prevention of mass production of acid. During this phase, the heart is in a good physiological condition for resuscitation. If CPR is started within these 4 minutes, the circulation of additional oxygen and glucose to the heart improves even further the chance of resuscitation, especially in the latter two phases. The primary issue during this phase in resuscitation is to restore an effective electrical rhythm to generate ventricular contractions that effectively eject blood and create an adequate cardiac output. Thus, during this phase, the heart is prepared for immediate defibrillation and restoration of the cardiac rhythm.

Circulatory Phase

The circulatory phase begins at 4 minutes and lasts through 10 minutes following the cardiac arrest. During this phase, the oxygen stores have been exhausted and the myocardial cells shift from aerobic to anaerobic metabolism. This results in very little energy production for cell function, in addition to the production of acid. The myocardial cells are becoming ischemic and are in need of oxygen and glucose. Because of the lack of oxygen and glucose, the heart is not prepared for defibrillation and is not prone to restarting. CPR will provide oxygen and glucose to the heart and improve the chance of a successful conversion following defibrillation. Thus, if the patient has been in cardiac arrest for 4 to 5 minutes or more and CPR is not being performed on your arrival, it is necessary to provide 2 minutes of CPR to deliver oxygen and glucose to the myocardial cells prior to any defibrillation to increase the chance of conversion to a perfusing rhythm.

Key Terms

downtime the time from cardiac arrest until effective CPR; **total downtime** the time from cardiac arrest until delivery to the emergency department.

return of spontaneous circulation (ROSC) spontaneous pulse return during resuscitation.

Key Terms

survival term applied to a patient who survives cardiac arrest to be discharged from the hospital.

Objective 15-16

Identify situations in which resuscitative attempts should be withheld.

Metabolic Phase

The metabolic phase begins 10 minutes after cardiac arrest. At this point the heart is starved of oxygen and glucose and has a large amount of acid buildup. The tissues are very ischemic and may begin to die. The chances of survival drop dramatically during this phase. Because of the lack of glucose and ATP, the sodium/potassium pump fails, allowing sodium to enter and stay within the cell. The sodium attracts water inside the cell. The cell swells and eventually ruptures and dies. This leads to the beginning of organ death. Resuscitation during this phase does not typically produce favorable results. If the patient is resuscitated, the widespread organ damage often leads to continued deterioration after restoration of the pulse and limited chances of the patient surviving or returning to a near normal level of neurological function.

Terms Related to Resuscitation

There are several terms related specifically to resuscitation of the cardiac arrest patient.

- **Downtime** is from the time the patient goes into cardiac arrest until CPR is effectively being performed.
- **Total downtime** is the total time from when the patient went into cardiac arrest until you delivered the patient to the emergency department.
- **Return of spontaneous circulation (ROSC)** is when the patient regains a spontaneous pulse during the resuscitation effort. The patient may not yet have begun to breathe on his own; however, if the pulse returns spontaneously it is considered a ROSC.
- **Survival** in cardiac arrest is defined as a patient who survives to be discharged from the hospital. If a patient regained ROSC but later died in the hospital, it is not considered a survival.
- **Witnessed cardiac arrest** for the purposes of this chapter and the provision of resuscitation and defibrillation, is when the EMT witnesses the patient become unresponsive, apneic, and pulseless. It does not refer to a layperson watching the patient collapse.
- **Unwitnessed cardiac arrest** for the purposes of this chapter and the provision of resuscitation and defibrillation, is when the EMT arrives on the scene and the patient is already unresponsive, apneic, and pulseless.

Withholding a Resuscitation Attempt

There are some situations in which you will not begin resuscitation on a patient in cardiac arrest. Some of these situations may include a patient with a valid do not resuscitate (DNR) order, physician orders for life-sustaining treatment (POLST), medical orders for life-sustaining treatment (MOLST), a patient with injuries that are not compatible with life such as a decapitation, and obvious death in patients who are in rigor and beyond the point of a resuscitation effort. Be sure to follow your local protocol when considering a decision to withhold resuscitation.

The Chain of Survival

Successfully resuscitating a cardiac arrest patient in the prehospital setting can rarely be done solely with CPR. Success, instead, depends on a sequence of events that the American Heart Association has termed the **chain of survival**. This chain has five links (Figure 15-10*):

- **Immediate recognition and activation.** Time is a critical factor. The quicker someone can recognize a patient in cardiac arrest, begin chest compressions and CPR, and contact EMS the better the chance of survival. The, the two key factors are: (1) recognition that a person who is unresponsive and has no breathing or no normal breathing has suffered a cardiac arrest, and (2) immediate activation of the EMS system. Immediate recognition can be achieved through public education programs, such as CPR courses for the layperson. Immediate activation of EMS is achieved by providing a simple access number, such as 911, to the community. In areas not serviced by 911, people must identify and call a seven- or ten-digit number to access EMS, which usually leads to time delays that may make the difference between successful resuscitation or not.
- **Early CPR.** Cardiopulmonary resuscitation (CPR), by providing coronary perfusion, significantly increases prehospital cardiac arrest survival rates. Research has shown that immediate CPR can double or even triple the chance of survival from ventricular-fibrillation-induced sudden cardiac arrest (VF SCA). This can be achieved through faster response by EMS and First Responders, more lay CPR providers, and EMS communications personnel providing CPR instructions to a person at the scene. Community CPR courses should aim to train as many people as

Objective 15-17
Explain each of the links in the Chain of Survival of cardiac arrest.

Objective 15-18
Explain the importance of early defibrillation in cardiac arrest.

Key Terms
Chain of Survival series of interventions—early access, CPR, defibrillation, and ACLS—that provides the best chance for successful cardiac resuscitation.

defibrillation electrical shock delivered to help the heart restore a normal rhythm.

FIGURE 15-10 ✱ The chain of survival. (Reprinted with permission, 2010 American Heart Assosiation Guidelines for Cardiopulmonary Rresuscitation and Emergency Cardiovascular Care, Part 4: CPR Overview. Circulation, 2010; 122[suppl 3]: S676–S684, © 2010 American Heart Assosiation, Inc.)

possible. Recognition of a cardiac event and the proper access number should be emphasized as heavily as CPR skills. CPR should be initiated, beginning with chest compressions, immediately upon recognition of cardiac arrest. Minimize interruption of chest compressions.

- **Rapid defibrillation.** Defibrillation—but more important, early and rapid defibrillation (shock within minutes)—is another component in determining survival of cardiac arrest. Survival rates of patients in VF SCA decrease with every minute defibrillation is delayed. **Defibrillation**, the procedure of sending an electrical current through the chest, is necessary to convert an abnormal and lethal rhythm with no pulse to an organized rhythm capable of producing a pulse. The time from the onset of cardiac arrest to the time defibrillation is performed is the most essential factor in increasing prehospital cardiac arrest survival rates. Chest compressions should be initiated until the AED is available and applied. Minimize interruption of chest compressions during the AED application.
- **Effective advanced life support.** Advanced life support (ALS) is delivered most often by paramedics who can provide advanced cardiac life support (ACLS). In some systems, Advanced EMTs may be able to provide all or some ALS interventions.
- **Integrated post-cardiac arrest care.** Once the heart is restarted, post-resuscitation care will focus on improving the patient's chance to recover as nearly as possible to a normal neurological condition.

Even though the paramedic is able to perform all the functions of the EMT and also provide other advanced functions such as medication administration, tracheal tube placement, and cardiac pacing, it is important to recognize that *high-quality chest compressions and early defibrillation are the two single most critical factors* to successful resuscitation. Both of these interventions, defibrillation and chest compressions, are well within the scope of practice for the EMT. The role of ALS is to perform certain interventions to increase the possibility of successful defibrillation or to administer medications to keep the patient from going back into cardiac arrest.

A system that has 911 or another easily recognizable public access number, CPR performed within minutes after the arrest by First Responders or laypersons, defibrillation within 4 minutes, and ALS capabilities will have better success rates for prehospital cardiac arrest patients.

Automated External Defibrillation and Cardiopulmonary Resuscitation

Early research from the American Heart Association (AHA) revealed that communities with early defibrillation programs—even those with no prehospital ACLS services—had improved survival rates of patients with cardiac arrest. It also verified that the earlier defibrillation took place, the better the outcome.

Following is the AHA rationale for early defibrillation:

- The most frequent initial rhythm in sudden cardiac arrest is ventricular fibrillation.
- The most effective treatment for terminating ventricular fibrillation is electrical defibrillation.
- The probability of successful defibrillation is directly related to the time from fibrillation to defibrillation. Success decreases as the time to compressions and defibrillation increases.

Key Terms

automated external defibrillator (AED) a device that can analyze the electrical activity or rhythm of a patient's heart and deliver an electrical shock (defibrillation) if appropriate.

Objective 15-19

Explain the rationale for the "push hard and push fast" approach to CPR.

- Successful defibrillation depends on effective chest compressions during CPR. The **automated external defibrillator (AED)** should be readied and applied during chest compressions if more than one rescuer is present. Interruptions in chest compressions for rhythm analysis, defibrillation, and advanced care must be minimized.
- Ventricular fibrillation will, without prompt or appropriate treatment, degenerate into asystole (no cardiac electrical activity). Successful resuscitation from asystole is unlikely.

Research by AHA reinforces the necessity of early defibrillation in the management of VF SCA. However, high-quality CPR focusing on immediate chest compressions with minimal interruption was found to be even more important. Additional research shows that high-quality chest compressions with minimal interruption and early defibrillation are the greatest determinants of successful cardiac arrest management.

The AHA advocates "push hard and push fast" to provide effective chest compressions. Compressions delivered at 100/minute have been shown to provide suitable blood flow to essential organs during cardiac arrest. The AHA advocates a uniform compression-to-ventilation ratio of 30:2 for all patients (other than two-rescuer CPR for infants and children). The 30:2 ratio delivered over 1 minute will result in fewer breaths per minute overall, but in cardiac arrest, the patient's need for oxygen is diminished (thus fewer breaths are needed).

If the cardiac arrest is not witnessed, providers should give five cycles of 30:2 compressions/ventilations (about 2 minutes of CPR) prior to defibrillating. The AED should be readied and applied during CPR to minimize interruption of compressions. CPR prior to defibrillation provides oxygenated blood, glucose, and other metabolic substrates to the myocardium so that defibrillation is more likely to produce conversion from ventricular fibrillation to a perfusing rhythm. If the arrest was witnessed, one EMT should immediately initiate CPR beginning with chest compressions while a second EMT applies the AED. If only one EMT is present, apply the AED as soon as it is available. Follow the AED prompts and defibrillate if advised. Immediately reinitiate chest compressions following defibrillation, minimizing compression interruption.

Pulse checks are not performed immediately after defibrillation because, although successful conversion from ventricular fibrillation occurs with the initial shock more than 85 percent of the time, it then takes several minutes for a perfusing rhythm to return. A pulse check immediately after defibrillation only lengthens the time until chest compressions resume, reducing the effectiveness of CPR and the chance of successful resuscitation. Thus, the most productive intervention following a defibrillation is to immediately resume CPR with chest compressions for 2 minutes, then follow the AED prompts to check the pulse.

The AHA offers this rationale to underscore the importance of current CPR and AED standards:

- "Push hard and push fast" will help avoid delivering compressions that are too slow or too shallow.
- The ratio of 30:2 minimizes interruptions to compressions for pulse checks and ventilations, which have been shown to be detrimental to blood flow, especially to the brain and heart.
- Five cycles of CPR delivered prior to defibrillation in unwitnessed cardiac arrest helps ensure the heart is better perfused, making defibrillation more successful.
- Resuming chest compressions immediately after defibrillation without a pulse check is desirable since rarely will a perfusing rhythm be immediately evident.
- In VF SCA cases, the provision of CPR as just described can double or triple the chance of survival (as opposed to defibrillation alone).
- Avoid excessive ventilation. Excessive ventilation increases pressure inside the thorax and decreases the perfusion pressures generated by chest compressions.

Types of Defibrillators

A defibrillator, as alluded to up to this point, is a device that will deliver an electric shock to convert a fibrillating heart to an organized rhythm with a pulse. External defibrillators used in emergency care are called "external" because they are applied to the outside of the chest.

There are two basic categories of external defibrillators: manual and automated. The use of manual defibrillators requires extensive training, and they are used by qualified ALS providers. The operator uses the machine's monitor to determine the heart's rhythm as

Objective 15-20
Describe the features, functions, advantages, disadvantages, use, and precautions in the use of automated external defibrillators (AEDs).

Key Points
Advantages of the AED over manual defibrillation include ease of use, speed, safety, effective delivery, and efficient monitoring.

displayed on a screen. The operator must analyze the rhythm and decide whether it is appropriate to defibrillate. He must apply the defibrillator pad or gel, hold the paddles firmly against the patient's chest (or attach large defibrillation pads to the chest wall), and administer the shock. Automated external defibrillators are much simpler to operate. This has made possible a broader use of defibrillation.

With AEDs, external adhesive defibrillator pads are attached to the patient's chest. Those pads are connected by cables to the AED. The pads transmit the patient's cardiac rhythm to the AED's circuitry, where the rhythm is analyzed. If the AED determines that an electrical shock (defibrillation) is appropriate, the device delivers the shock through the cables via the pads to the patient.

Advantages of AEDs

With the AED, the device analyzes the rhythm and indicates if a shock is required. The AED operator need only recongnize that the patient is in cardiac arrest and understand the steps in operating the device. Therefore, initial training and continuing education are much simpler with AEDs than with manual defibrillators.

There are several other advantages of the AED:

- **Speed of operation.** The first shock can be delivered to the patient within 1 minute of the AED's application at the patient's side. Clinical trials conducted by the AHA found that operators of AEDs can consistently deliver a first shock more quickly than operators of manual defibrillators.
- **Safer, more effective delivery.** Because it uses adhesive external pads, instead of the paddles that must be held against the chest during manual defibrillation, the AED allows for "hands-free" defibrillation, which is safer for EMS personnel. In addition, the adhesive pads cover a larger surface area than the manual paddles and, therefore, deliver a more effective shock.
- **More efficient monitoring.** AEDs are manufactured with sensors that detect loose leads and false or misleading rhythm readings. The large electrodes make better contact with the patient's body and provide a better ECG tracing, even when the patient is severely diaphoretic (sweaty).

Types of AEDs

In general, there are two types of AEDs:

- **Fully automated AEDs.** The fully automated AED is completely automatic. The operator determines that the patient is in cardiac arrest, attaches the device to the patient, and pushes a button to turn on the power. The device does the rest. The fully automated AED analyzes the heart rhythm and determines whether ventricular fibrillation is present. If ventricular fibrillation is detected, the AED charges automatically and delivers the appropriate electrical shock. Semiautomated AEDs are preferred; however, fully automated models are still available and possibly in use by laypersons and some First Responders.
- **Semiautomated AEDs.** The semiautomated AED requires more involvement by the operator. The operator attaches the AED to the patient in the normal manner, pushes a button to turn on the power, and initiates the heart rhythm analysis. Some models may require the operator to push an analysis button as well. The AED then begins the analysis. When the analysis is complete, a computer voice synthesizer and/or display message indicates to the operator when a shock is advised. The operator must then push another button to deliver the shock. Some devices also provide a display of the heart rhythm as it is being analyzed.

AEDs are often equipped with a variety of features that can provide a record of both the operator's use of the device and the AED's own functions. Such devices include voice and ECG recorders and memory modules.

Some external defibrillators use the older monophasic waveform. Most now use the newer biphasic waveform (Figures 15-11a to 15-11d∗). The monophasic AED delivers the energy at 200, 300, and 360 joules in one direction. The biphasic delivers less energy (typically less than or equal to 150–200 joules) pulses. The lower energy delivered by the biphasic AED is thought to cause less heart cell damage, yet is still more effective at terminating ventricular fibrillation.

Whichever type of AED your service uses, always follow the manufacturer's directions and service recommendations as well as any local protocols for AED use.

Objective 15-21

Compare and contrast ventricular fibrillation, ventricular tachycardia, asystole, and pulseless electrical activity.

Key Terms

ventricular fibrillation (VF or V-Fib) a continuous, uncoordinated, chaotic rhythm that does not produce pulses.

ventricular tachycardia (VT or V-Tach) a rapid heart rhythm that may or may not produce a pulse; usually too fast to adequately perfuse body organs.

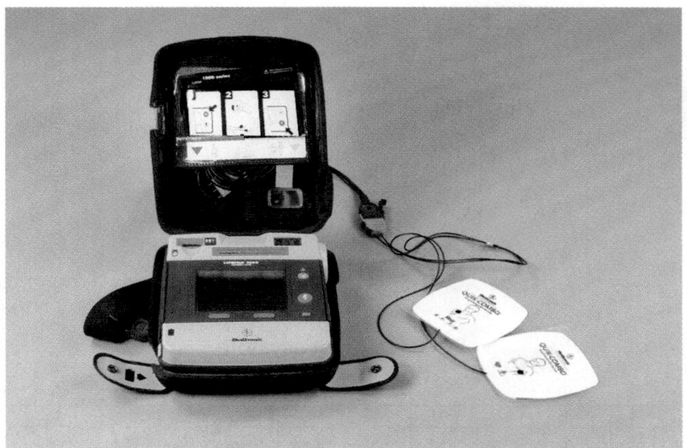

FIGURE 15-11a * Medtronic Lifepak 1000.

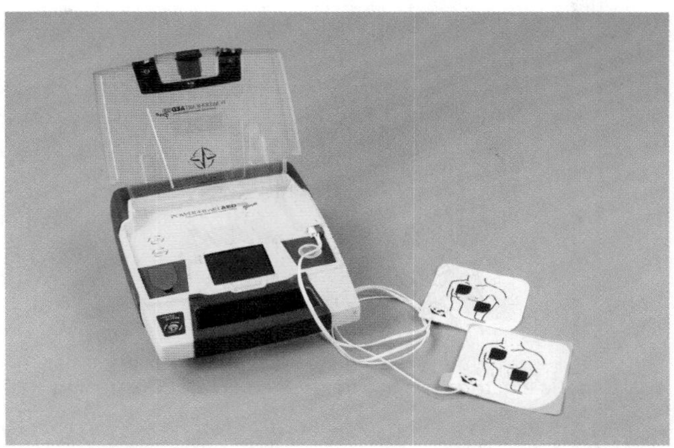

FIGURE 15-11b * Cardiac Science Powerheart AED G3 Pro.

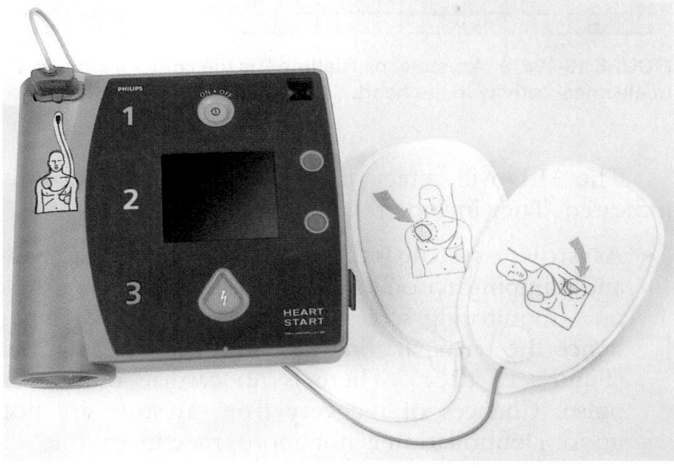

FIGURE 15-11c * HeartStart FR2+. (© Phillips Medical Systems)

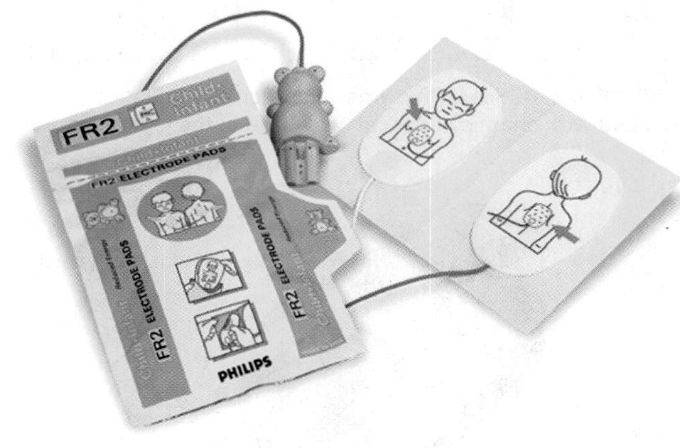

FIGURE 15-11d * Pediatric pads are available for the pediatric version of the HeartStart FR2+. (© Phillips Medical Systems)

Analysis of Cardiac Rhythms

The main component of the AED is the computer microprocessor that records and analyzes whether a heart rhythm should be defibrillated. The rhythms for which defibrillation is appropriate are these:

- **Ventricular fibrillation.** As noted earlier, **ventricular fibrillation (VF or V-Fib)** is a disorganized cardiac rhythm that produces no pulse or cardiac output (Figure 15-12a*). It is commonly associated with advanced coronary artery disease, though it may have other causes. Somewhere between 50 and 60 percent of cardiac arrests will be in ventricular fibrillation during the first 8 minutes after becoming pulseless. V-Fib is most commonly the rhythm that the AED defibrillates.
- **Ventricular tachycardia. Ventricular tachycardia (VT or V-Tach)** is a very fast heart rhythm (Figure 15-12b*) that is generated in the ventricle instead of the sinoatrial node in the atrium. Because the pumping is so rapid, the heart does not refill properly and cardiac output is sharply reduced. This rhythm can easily degenerate into ventricular fibrillation. The AED will respond to V-Tach, usually when the heart rate exceeds 180 beats per minute. However, you should be aware that some V-Tach patients remain responsive;

Key Terms

asystole a heart rhythm indicating absence of any electrical activity in the heart.

Key Terms

pulseless electrical activity (PEA) a condition in which the heart generates relatively normal electrical rhythms but fails to perfuse the body adequately because of a decreased or absent cardiac output from cardiac muscle failure or blood loss.

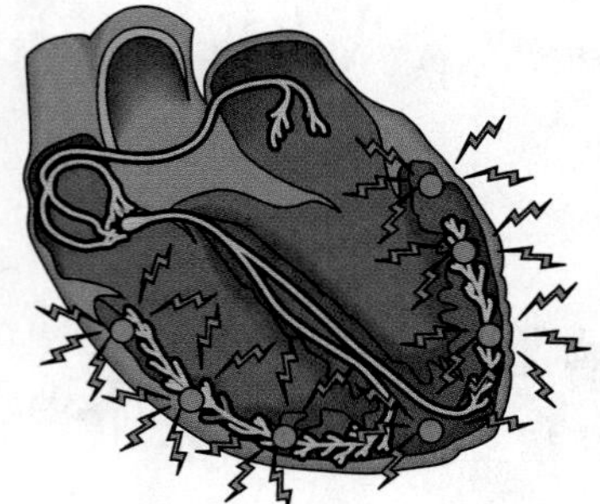

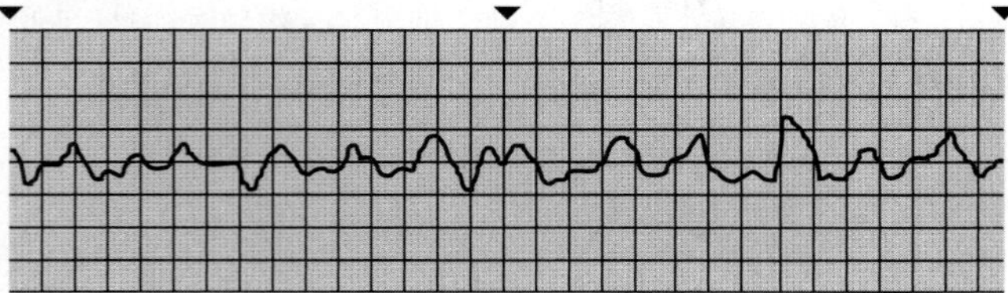

FIGURE 15-12a * Heart Rhythms Ventricular fibrillation is associated with chaotic electrical discharge in the ventricles.

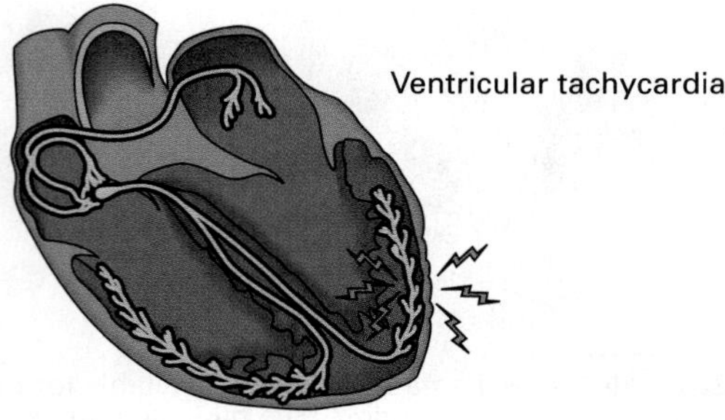

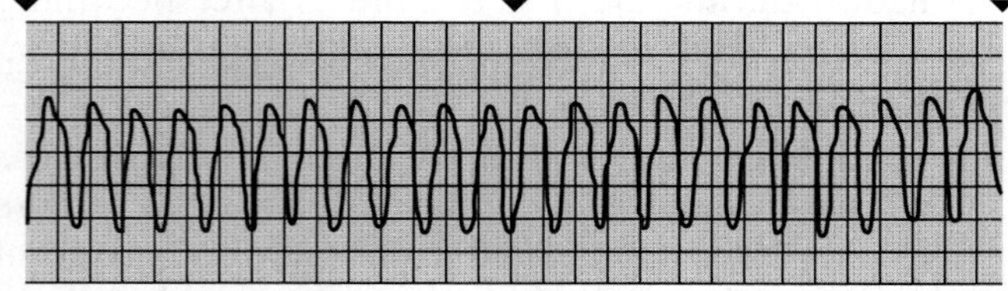

FIGURE 15-12b * Ventricular tachycardia originates in the conduction system of the ventricle.

since they are not pulseless, they are not appropriate candidates for defibrillation. The AED should ONLY be applied to patients who are *pulseless*, not breathing (apneic), and unresponsive.

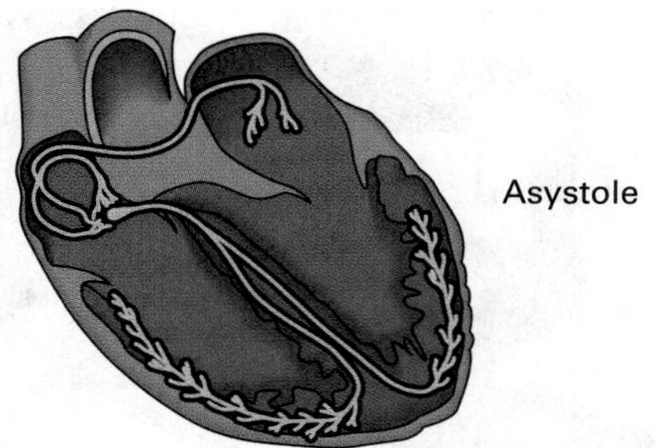

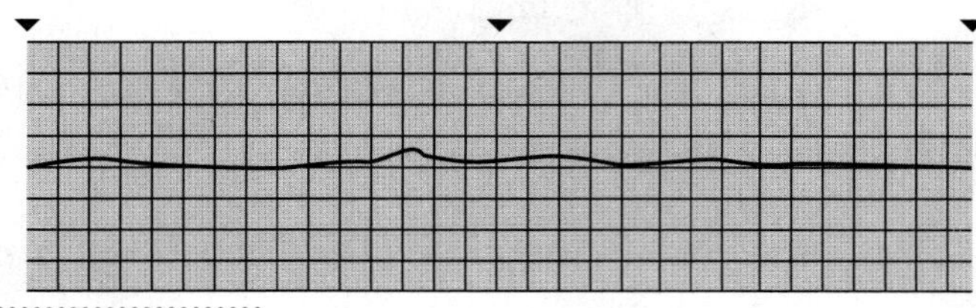

FIGURE 15-12c * Asystole, or "flatline," is the complete absence of electrical activity in the heart.

The AED will detect rhythms for which no shock is indicated. They include the following:

- **Asystole. Asystole** is the absence of electrical activity and pumping action in the heart. This often registers on a monitoring screen as a flat or nearly flat line; hence the term "flatline" is often used for asystole (Figure 15-12c*). There is no cardiac output or pulse. Chances of recovery from asystole are not good. Defibrillation is not appropriate in asystole.
- **Pulseless electrical activity.** In cases of **pulseless electrical activity (PEA)**, the heart has an organized rhythm, but either the heart muscle is so weakened that it fails to pump, or the heart muscle does not respond to the electrical activity, or the circulatory system has lost so much blood that there is nothing to pump. Defibrillation is not appropriate in these rhythms.

Note that the AED is a very sensitive instrument. It can sense spontaneous patient movement, movement of the patient by others, engine vibrations if the patient is in a vehicle, and even some radio transmissions. Such "noise" interferes with the AED's analysis of the patient's heart rhythms.

For these reasons, no one should be touching the patient when the AED is analyzing the rhythm. (Nor should anyone be touching the patient during administration of AED shocks.) Always alert people to move away from the patient by saying "Clear!" in a loud voice before begin-

Objective 15-22
Demonstrate assessment and resuscitative techniques for infants, children, and adults, including the integrated use of AEDs, ventilation, and CPR, and explain the purpose and procedure for reassessment of the cardiac arrest patient.

Thinking Critically
At the scene of a vehicle crash, you find the driver in cardiac arrest. "Give him a shock," begs his wife. Why would you or would you not apply the AED to this patient?

ning the analysis and be sure to look around to verify visually that no one is in contact with the patient.

A properly maintained and operated AED will rarely deliver inappropriate shocks, but mechanical or human error can lead to them. Mechanical error is usually caused by poorly maintained or poorly charged batteries. Human error occurs when an operator misinterprets a patient's condition and uses the AED on someone not in cardiac arrest. Remember, the AED should be used ONLY on pulseless, nonbreathing, unresponsive patients that are older than 1 year of age.

When and When Not to Use the AED

The AED was initially developed for adults. However, the 2010 AHA guidelines indicate it can be used with any age, even those less than 1 year of age. However, manual defibrillation is preferred for patients less than 1 year old to better control the amount of energy delivered. If the patient is between 1 and 8 years of age, an adult AED can be used, preferably with a dose attenuating system to reduce the defibrillation energy being delivered to the child (Figure 15-13*). If no dose-attenuating system is available, proceed with the regular adult pads and defibrillation.

Apply the adult AED without the dose-attenuating system in any patient over 8 years of age. In either group of patients, if the cardiac arrest is witnessed, immediately begin chest compressions and apply the AED as soon as if becomes available. During application of the electrode pads, continue chest compressions until the AED is completely ready for analysis of the patient rhythm. Once applied, proceed with the AED protocol. The goal is to deliver the defibrillation within 3 minutes from the onset of ventricular fibrillation.

If the cardiac arrest was not witnessed, immediately initiate CPR beginning with chest compressions. Ready the AED for use; however, perform five cycles of CPR at a ratio of 30 compressions to 2 ventilations, which takes approximately 2 minutes. Following the five cycles of CPR, immediately initiate rhythm analysis and the AED protocol. Always keep interruption of chest compressions at a minimum.

As mentioned previously, the AED is intended for nontraumatic cardiac arrest patients. These patients must be unresponsive, with no breathing or agonal breathing, no signs of life, and no pulse. The AED is not

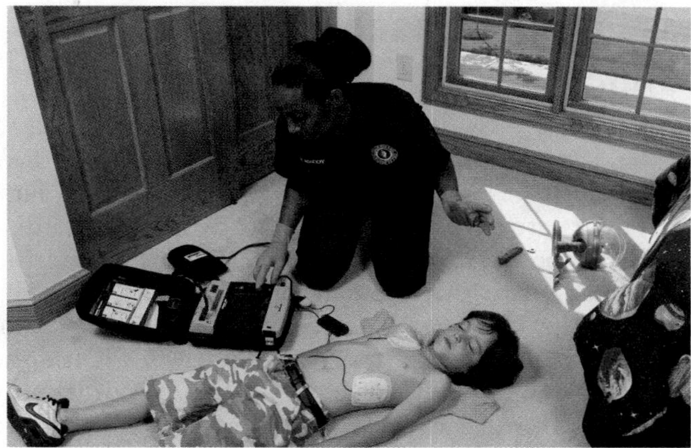

FIGURE 15-13 * AED pads applied to a pediatric patient.

intended for trauma patients. In trauma patients, cardiac arrest is more likely to have resulted from the trauma than from an underlying cardiac cause. If such patients are in cardiac arrest, the condition often is the result of blood loss. Defibrillation usually will not help these patients. Follow local protocols and contact medical direction if in doubt. If a trauma patient is in cardiac arrest, begin CPR and perform bleeding control and spinal immobilization. Contact medical direction to consider use of the AED.

You may come across situations where you cannot tell if the trauma led to cardiac arrest or vice versa. Suppose, for example, that you discover a man in cardiac arrest in a car that has gone off the road and hit a tree. Did the man go into cardiac arrest while driving, then swerve off and hit the tree? Or did he drive off the road for some other reason and go into cardiac arrest only after hitting the tree and sustaining other injuries? In such cases, err to benefit the patient and immediately initiate chest compressions, continue with CPR, and apply the AED. Follow local protocols to determine when use of the AED is appropriate.

Recognizing and Treating Cardiac Arrest

Now that you have reviewed abnormal rhythms, basic information about defibrillation, and the AED, you can learn the procedure for defibrillation.

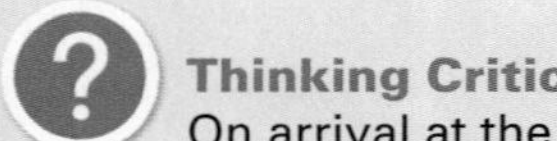

Thinking Critically

On arrival at the scene of a reported cardiac arrest, you find a bystander performing CPR on a patient who is dazed but responsive. "He's having a heart attack," the bystander says while continuing to push on the patient's chest, "so I'm giving him CPR." What should you do?

Key Points

Managing a patient in cardiac arrest is one of the most dynamic situations an EMT can face, calling on almost all of the skills the EMT has learned.

Assessment-Based Approach: Cardiac Arrest

Dispatch may provide information that will lead you to suspect cardiac arrest. Reports that a patient doesn't appear to be breathing, is unresponsive, or that First Responders are performing CPR clearly indicate cardiac arrest. But be alert to the possibility of cardiac arrest in calls to patients with chest pain or discomfort, difficulty in breathing, or seizures. Although not all chest pain patients will go into cardiac arrest and need CPR and the AED, patients with cardiac compromise can rapidly deteriorate to cardiac arrest. Some patients will suffer a brief seizure immediately after going into cardiac arrest. Bring the AED from the ambulance to the patient on such calls.

Scene Size-Up and Primary Assessment

On arrival, take appropriate Standard Precautions. Ensure that the scene is secure. Then proceed rapidly with the primary assessment.

Form a general impression of the patient and his mental status as you approach. If the suspected cardiac patient is responsive, follow the procedures for assessment and care described earlier for cardiac-related emergencies.

In an unresponsive patient who appears to have no signs of life, quickly assess for apnea or agonal ventilations while simultaneously checking a carotid pulse (a brachial pulse in pediatric patients less than 1 year of age). Assess for no longer than 10 seconds. If the patient is unresponsive, is apneic or has agonal ventilations and appears to have no other signs of life, immediately begin CPR using the CAB intervention sequence outlined in the 2010 AHA guidelines. CAB stands for chest compressions, airway, and ventilation. This sequence requires the EMT to immediately initiate CPR beginning with 30 chest compressions followed by opening the airway and 2 ventilations. If multiple EMTs are on the scene, many of the interventions can be accomplished simultaneously, such as preparing the AED, inserting an airway, and readying the bag-valve-mask for ventilation while the first 30 compressions are being performed. The key is to initiate chest compressions as the first intervention and to minimize any interruption in chest compressions during the entire resuscitation. Once you have determined that a patient is in cardiac arrest, proceed with CPR while you prepare to deliver emergency care as described next.

- **Patients under 1 year of age (infants).** For pediatric patients less than 1 year of age, use the CAB intervention approach to CPR and resuscitation. A ratio of 30 compressions:2 ventilations is used when one EMT is performing CPR; however, a ratio of 15 compressions:2 ventilations is used when two EMTs are performing CPR. Chest compressions should be delivered at a rate of 100/minute. The compression depth should be one-third the anterior-posterior chest diameter or approximately 1½ inches or 4 cm. Because most cardiac arrests in this age group occur from an airway, oxygenation, or ventilation issue, ensure you have an open airway, are providing good ventilations, and are adequately oxygenating the patient. Apply the AED after 5 cycles of CPR (approximately 2 minutes). It is preferred that defibrillation be done manually in pediatric patients less than 1 year of age; however, this can only be performed by ALS. If ALS is not on the scene, attach the AED, using a pediatric dose-attenuating system. If manual defibrillation or a pediatric dose-attenuating system is not available, proceed with the use of the adult AED. Follow your local protocol.

  If the heart rate is >60/minute and ventilations are absent or inadequate, immediately begin positive pressure ventilation at 12–20/minute (1 ventilation every 3 to 5 seconds). If the heart rate is <60/minute with signs of poor perfusion (pallor, mottling, cyanosis) after ventilation and oxygenation have been delivered, initiate CPR beginning with chest compressions.
- **Patients 1–8 years of age.** For pediatric patients between 1 and 8 years of age, use the CAB intervention approach to CPR and resuscitation. A ratio of 30 compressions:2 ventilations is used when one EMT is performing CPR; however, a ratio of 15 compressions:2 ventilations is used when two EMTs are performing CPR. Chest compressions should be delivered at a rate of 100/minute. The compression depth should be one-third the anterior-posterior chest diameter or approximately 2 inches or 5 cm. Because most cardiac arrests in this age group occur from an airway, oxygenation, or ventilation issue, ensure you have an open airway, are providing good ventilations, and are adequately oxygenating the patient. Apply the AED after 5 cycles of CPR (approximately 2 minutes) unless cardiac arrest from a rhythm disturbance is suspected, such as the patient suddenly

collapsing at a sporting event. In that case, immediately begin CPR with chest compressions and apply the AED as soon as it is available. It is preferred that defibrillation be done using a pediatric dose-attenuating system. If a pediatric dose-attenuating system is not available, proceed with the use of the adult AED. Follow your local protocol.

If the heart rate is >60/minute and the ventilations are absent or inadequate, immediately begin positive pressure ventilation at 12–20/minute (1 ventilation every 3 to 5 seconds). If the heart rate is <60/minute with signs of poor perfusion (pallor, mottling, cyanosis) after ventilation and oxygenation have been delivered, initiate CPR beginning with chest compressions.

- **Patients over 8 years of age.** Adult interventions are used for patients over 8 years of age. If the cardiac arrest was witnessed, immediately initiate CPR beginning with chest compressions (CAB intervention sequence). As soon as the AED is available, apply it while chest compressions are being performed. When the AED is ready to start the rhythm analysis, stop chest compressions and proceed with the AED protocol. If the cardiac arrest was unwitnessed, immediately initiate CPR beginning with chest compressions (CAB intervention sequence). Apply the AED and initiate rhythm analysis after 5 cycles (approximately 2 minutes) of CPR have been performed. Then proceed with the AED protocol.

  A ratio of 30 compressions:2 ventilations is used when one or two EMTs are performing CPR. Chest compressions should be delivered at a rate of 100/minute. The compression depth should be at least 2 inches or 5 cm.

  When performing CPR on a patient who is obviously pregnant or in her third trimester, use a manual maneuver to displace the uterus laterally while the patient is supine. Use your hand(s) to push the uterus to one side. If not successful, tilt the patient no more than 30 degrees by placing padding under the right side of the backboard.

Secondary Assessment

While CPR is being done and the AED is being set up and applied, an EMT may be able to gather the history from bystanders or relatives.

Signs and Symptoms The signs and symptoms of cardiac arrest are as follows:

- Unresponsive
- No breathing (apnea) or no normal breathing (gasping type agonal ventilations)
- No pulse (should be checked simultaneously with breathing and for less than 10 seconds)
- No other signs of life

Emergency Medical Care

Follow the steps listed under "Performing Defibrillation" to provide emergency medical care with an AED to cardiac arrest patients. Remember to use CPR and defibrillation as appropriate for arrest patients according to their age and estimated downtime. Managing a patient in cardiac arrest is one of the most dynamic situations the EMT will be in, necessitating almost all the skills you acquire during your education.

Reassessment

CPR and, as needed, defibrillation will be performed to restore the patient's pulse and perfusion. Once the pulse is restored, you will continue to perform reassessments en route to the hospital. As will be discussed in the following segment, a patient whose pulse has been restored may revert into cardiac arrest, so the reassessment will be focused especially on monitoring the patient's pulse, breathing, and mental status.

Performing Defibrillation

Ideally, at least two EMTs should be available when the AED is to be used, one to operate the device and provide ventilation and the other to perform good chest compressions with minimal interruption (Figure 15-14*).

Using a Semiautomated AED

The steps that follow are for providing defibrillation with a semiautomated AED, followed by a section on use of the fully automated AED.

Note that the most recent semiautomated AED typically has two buttons. Button number 1 turns on the power and starts analysis of the patient's heart rhythms; button number 2 delivers the defibrillation. Visualize these two buttons as you read the following steps. Some older semiautomated AEDs have three buttons to turn the device on, start the rhythm analysis, and deliver the defibrillation.

Bear in mind, as you read the following steps (see also EMT Skills 15-1A to H), that you should deliver only one shock before intervening with five cycles of CPR, which is approximately 2 minutes in duration.

1. *Take Standard Precautions.* This should normally be done en route to the scene.
2. *Perform a brief primary assessment of the patient* (EMT Skills 15-1A). *If the patient is unresponsive, is apneic or has agonal ventilation, has no pulse (checked simultaneously with ventilation and for no more than 10 seconds), and has no other signs of life, immediately initiate CPR beginning with chest compressions (CAB intervention sequence)*—whether the arrest was witness or unwitnessed. If the cardiac arrest was witnessed, as soon as the AED is available, apply it while

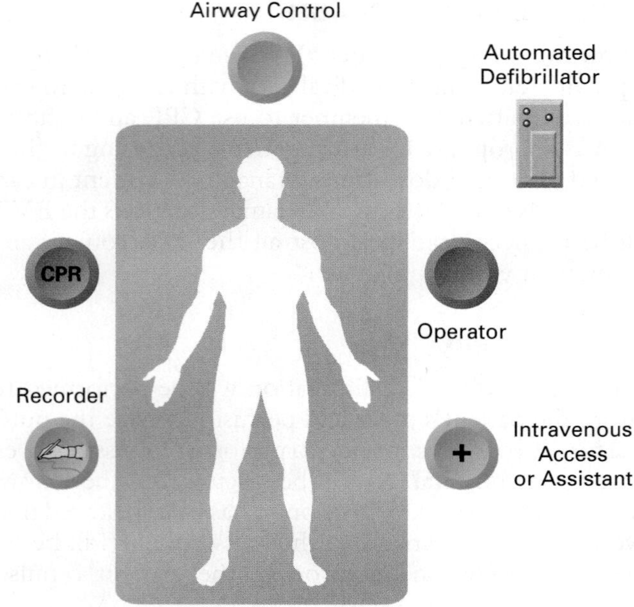

FIGURE 15-14 ✻ This is the preferred layout for automated defibrillation. It may not be possible in all field situations, so alternative arrangements should be tried and practiced.

chest compressions are being performed. When the AED is ready to start the rhythm analysis, stop chest compressions and proceed with the AED protocol. If the cardiac arrest was unwitnessed, apply the AED and initiate rhythm analysis after 5 cycles (approximately 2 minutes) of CPR with chest compressions have been performed. Then proceed with the AED protocol.

If bystanders or First Responders are already performing CPR upon your arrival, instruct them to continue while you prepare application of the AED.

3. *Continue chest compressions while the AED is readied for operation* (EMT Skills 15-1B). If possible, perform AED operations from the patient's side to minimize any interruption in chest compressions.
4. *Turn on power to the AED* (EMT Skills 15-1C).
5. *Attach the adhesive monitoring-defibrillation pads to the chest while chest compressions are being performed* (EMT Skills 15-1D). Minimize any interruption to chest compressions.
6. *Apply the two defibrillation pads to the patient's bared chest* (EMT Skills 15-1D). Follow the AED manufacturer's instructions for applying the pads, turning on power, and pad placement. Please note that the specific location of the (−) and (+) pads is important for the older monophasic AEDs. Biphasic AEDs use the same locations, but the (−) and (+) pads are interchangeable. Follow the anatomic pad placement instructions on the defibrillator pads.

The following are four position options for electrode pad placement:

a. One pad is placed on the right upper border of the sternum; the top edge should be just below the clavicle. The other pad is placed over the left lower ribs at the anterior axillary line (below and to the left of the nipple). This is known as the anterolateral position (Figure 15-15a✻).
b. One pad is placed on either the upper left or right posterior thorax, and the other pad is placed over the left lower ribs at the anterior axillary line (below and to the left of the nipple). This is known as the anterior–posterior position (Figure 15-15b✻).
c. One pad is placed on the left anterior chest, and the other pad is placed below the left scapula. This is known as the anterior-left infrascapular position.
d. One pad is placed on the left anterior chest, and the other pad is placed below the right scapula. This is known as the anterior-right infrascapular position.

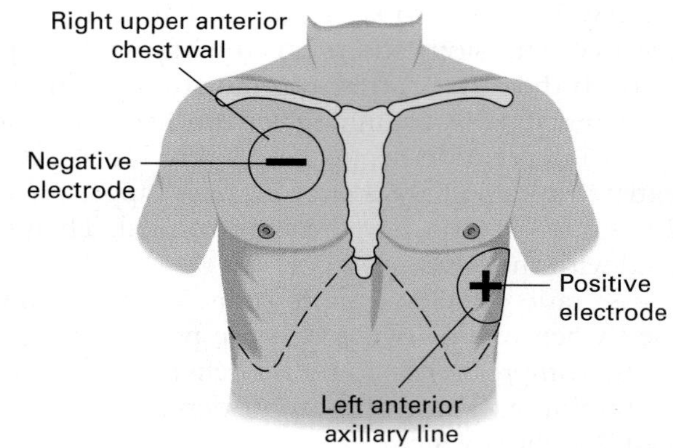

FIGURE 15-15a ✻ Conventional placement of defibrillator electrodes: sternum pad (−) on upper right border of sternum just below the clavicle; apex pad (+) over the left lower ribs at the anterior axillary line.

Alternative Placement of Defibrillator Electrodes

Posterior pad near the center of the back

Anterior pad over the apex of the heart

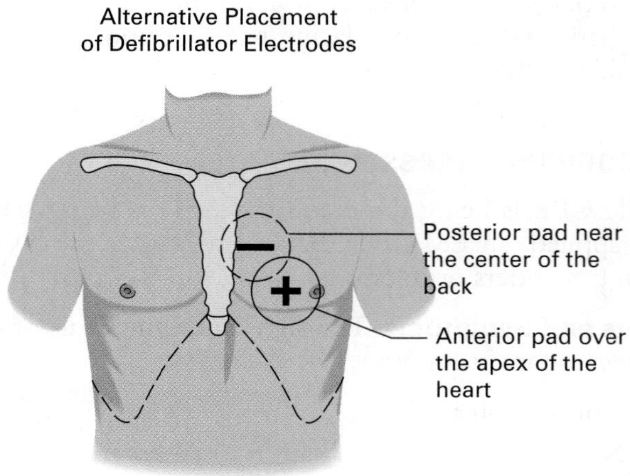

FIGURE 15-15b ✻ An alternative placement of defibrillator electrodes has the anterior electrode (+) placed over the apex of the heart and the posterior electrode (−) placed near the center of the back, 1–2 inches above the anterior pad.

Thinking Critically
What are the differences between resuscitation performed by two EMTs and resuscitation performed by a single EMT?

Objective 15-23
Demonstrate assessment and management of a post cardiac-arrest patient with return of spontaneous circulation.

7. *Begin analysis of the patient's cardiac rhythm* (EMT Skills 15-1E). The AED will automatically monitor and analyze the rhythm and will indicate the start of analysis mode by prompting you to clear the patient, stop any ongoing CPR and say "Clear!" making sure that no one is touching the patient. The AED cannot effectively analyze the cardiac rhythm while CPR is being performed. Also, anyone in contact with the patient during delivery of a shock could be injured. Finally, minimize any interruption of chest compressions each time the AED analyzes and delivers a shock.
8. If the AED's analysis determines a shock is appropriate, it provides a "deliver shock" message. In that case, proceed with defibrillation by depressing the shock or defibrillation button (EMT Skills 15-1F). If the AED's analysis determines a nonshockable rhythm, it gives a "no shock" message. In that case, immediately resume CPR beginning with chest compressions.
9. After a shock has been delivered, immediately resume CPR beginning with chest compressions. Perform CPR for approximately 2 minutes (EMT Skills 15-1G).
10. After 2 minutes, the AED reanalyzes the rhythm. If a shock is indicated, proceed with the defibrillation, then immediately resume CPR beginning with chest compressions. If there is a prompt to check breathing and pulse, quickly assess the patient's breathing and carotid pulse (EMT Skills 15-1H). (Check a brachial pulse in the pediatric patient <1 year of age.)

    The AED may indicate the patient now has a pulse or no longer has a shockable rhythm. If the patient is unresponsive, apneic or has agonal ventilations, and has no pulse, immediately resume CPR beginning with chest compressions. Continue to repeat this sequence. If the patient has a pulse, continue with ventilation at 10 to 12/minute or one ventilation every 5 to 6 seconds in the adult and 12 to 20/minute or one ventilation or one ventilation every 3 to 5 seconds in the pediatric patient (<8 years of age). Continuously reassess the patient.
11. Follow your local protocol regarding when to transport the patient in cardiac arrest.

Use of the AED by a Single EMT

There are times when only a single EMT is initially available to provide emergency care for a cardiac arrest patient. If the EMT has access to an AED and the patient's profile meets the inclusion criteria for AED usage, he should follow this sequence:

1. Verify that the patient is unresponsive, with no breathing and no pulse.
2. Call for additional EMS and get the AED.
3. If the cardiac arrest was witnessed, immediately apply the AED and proceed with the AED protocol. If the cardiac arrest was unwitnessed, immediately initiate CPR beginning with chest compressions (CAB intervention sequence). Apply the AED and initiate rhythm analysis after 5 cycles (approximately 2 minutes) of CPR have been performed. Then proceed with the AED protocol.

Using a Fully Automated AED

Most AEDs used today are semiautomated; however, some older models that are fully automated may still be in use.

Procedures for using the fully automated AED are similar to those for semiautomated AED, already described. The major difference is that the fully automated AED will deliver the shock without operator intervention. Once the machine is connected to the patient and turned on, it also uses a voice synthesizer to give directions such as "Stop CPR," "Stand back," and "Check breathing and pulse" to prompt you through the defibrillation process. This would include delivery of the necessary shock separated by 2 minutes of CPR, or checks of breathing and pulse if the rhythms are inappropriate for shocking. Procedures for the operation of fully automated defibrillators vary, so the manufacturer's instructions should be followed closely.

Because defibrillations are delivered automatically with a fully automated defibrillator, it is important to ensure that all EMTs and bystanders are clear of the patient.

As already noted, most EMS systems use a semiautomatic AED, but fully automated AEDs may be used by some emergency responders or found in public facilities.

Transporting the Cardiac Arrest Patient

If you have followed the emergency medical care procedures and operation of the AED as just described and no ALS backup is responding to the scene, you should transport the patient when any one of the following conditions applies:

- The patient regains a pulse.
- Your local protocol indicates transport.

Key Points

Patients who have been brought out of ventricular fibrillation through use of the AED have a high likelihood of slipping back into that state. Monitor these patients closely.

Objective 15-24

Given a cardiac arrest scenario, make decisions regarding obtaining advanced cardiac life support (ACLS).

The patient you transport after defibrillation will be in one of two conditions: with a pulse or without a pulse.

Transporting a Patient with a Pulse

If a patient's pulse has returned after defibrillation:

1. Check the patient's airway and provide oxygen at 15 lpm by nonrebreather mask if the patient's breathing is adequate, or provide positive pressure ventilation with supplemental oxygen if the patient's breathing is inadequate.
2. Since many cardiac arrest patients vomit, have suction ready for use and clear the airway of any obstructions or fluids.
3. Secure the patient to a stretcher and transfer him to the ambulance. If you regained a pulse while still on scene, the patient should be placed on a backboard so that compressions will be more effective if the cardiac arrest recurs en route to the medical facility.
4. Consider the most efficient way of getting ACLS to the patient. Consult with dispatch and medical direction and consider rendezvousing with an ALS unit en route or awaiting arrival of the ALS unit if that will get the patient advanced care more rapidly.
5. Continue to keep the AED attached to the patient during transport.
6. If you have not already done so, perform the secondary assessment en route.
7. Perform reassessment every 5 minutes.

Patients who have been brought out of ventricular fibrillation through use of the AED have a high likelihood of deteriorating back into that state. Monitor these patients closely. With unresponsive patients, check the pulse every 30 seconds.

If the patient returns to cardiac arrest, follow the AED prompts. If no shock is advised, immediately initiate CPR beginning with chest compressions. If a shock is advised, deliver the shock safely and immediately initiate CPR beginning with chest compressions. Follow the AED protocol.

Transporting a Patient Without a Pulse

If the patient has no pulse, continue to provide CPR and defibrillation and follow local protocol. Use extreme caution and safety precautions when defibrillating a patient in the back of the ambulance to avoid accidental shocks to EMTs. Rendezvous with ALS as early as possible.

Providing for Advanced Cardiac Life Support

As an EMT, you can operate an AED without advanced life support personnel on scene. With cases of cardiac arrest, however, you should keep the AHA's chain of survival in mind. The fourth link of that chain is effective advanced cardiac life support (ACLS).

There are often several options for obtaining ACLS for a patient. Higher-level EMS providers, such as paramedics and some Advanced EMTs, can provide it. If prehospital personnel are not available, other sources for ACLS might be a hospital or clinic.

Whenever you have a cardiac arrest patient, follow your protocol, which may include informing medical direction and requesting ACLS backup as possible. Your system will have protocols about the transport of such patients, but medical direction, or your protocol, depending on the circumstances, may tell you to wait for the arrival of the ALS team, to rendezvous with them en route, or to proceed directly to a hospital or other facility. The goal is to minimize the time from the delivery of CPR and defibrillatory shocks to the arrival of ACLS.

Summary: Assessment and Care

To review assessment findings that may be associated with cardiac arrest and emergency care for cardiac arrest, see Figures 15-16∗ and 15-17∗.

Special Considerations for the AED

Safety Considerations

When you are using an AED, you are operating a device that delivers an electric shock. That shock can save the life of a cardiac arrest patient, but it can injure others who come in contact with it. Such shocks are unlikely to be lethal, but they should be avoided.

Electricity can be conducted, or carried, through a variety of different substances. The human body is one of them. No one should be in contact with the patient during the AED's rhythm analysis or its delivery of defibrillating shocks. Remember to say loudly, "I'm clear, you're

Assessment Summary

CARDIAC ARREST

The following are findings that indicate cardiac arrest. These findings are obtained during the primary assessment:

- Unresponsive
- Apneic (not breathing) or agonal (gasping) ventilation
- Pulseless
- No signs of life

Emergency Care Protocol

CARDIAC ARREST

1. Take Standard Precautions.
2. Perform a brief primary assessment of the patient. If the patient is unresponsive, is apneic or has agonal ventilation, has no pulse (checked simultaneously with ventilation and for no more than 10 seconds), and no other signs of life, immediately initiate CPR beginning with chest compressions.
3. If the cardiac arrest was witnessed, immediately initiate CPR beginning with chest compressions (CAB intervention sequence). As soon as the AED is available, apply it while chest compressions are being performed. When the AED is ready to start the rhythm analysis, stop chest compressions and proceed with the AED protocol. If the cardiac arrest was unwitnessed, immediately initiate CPR beginning with chest compressions (CAB intervention sequence). Apply the AED and initiate rhythm analysis after 5 cycles (approximately 2 minutes) of CPR have been performed. Then proceed with the AED protocol.

   If bystanders or First Responders are already performing CPR when you arrive, instruct them to continue while you prepare application of the AED.
4. Continue with chest compressions while the AED is readied for operation.
5. Turn on power to the AED.
6. Attach the adhesive monitoring-defibrillation pads to the chest while chest compressions are being performed. Minimize any interruption to chest compressions.
7. Begin analysis of the patient's cardiac rhythm.
8. If the AED's analysis indicates a shock, it provides a "deliver shock" message. In that case, proceed with defibrillation by depressing the shock or defibrillation button. If the AED's analysis determines a nonshockable rhythm, it gives a "no shock" message. In that case, immediately resume CPR beginning with chest compressions.
9. After a shock has been delivered, immediately resume CPR beginning with chest compressions. Perform CPR for approximately 2 minutes.
10. After 2 minutes, the AED reanalyzes the rhythm. If a shock is indicated, proceed with the defibrillation, then immediately resume CPR beginning with chest compressions. If the AED gives a prompt to check breathing and pulse, quickly assess the patient's breathing and pulse. The AED may indicate the patient now has a pulse or no longer has a shockable rhythm. If the patient is unresponsive, apneic or has agonal ventilations, and has no pulse, immediately resume CPR beginning with chest compressions. Continue to repeat this sequence. If the patient has a pulse, continue with ventilation. Continuously reassess the patient.
11. Follow your local protocol regarding when to transport the patient in cardiac arrest.

FIGURE 15-16 ✻ **(a)** Assessment summary and **(b)** emergency care protocol: cardiac arrest.

clear, everyone's clear!" and to make sure that everyone is, in fact, clear of the patient before beginning the analysis or defibrillating.

Water is an excellent conductor of electricity. The AED should not be operated if the machine or the patient is lying in water, the chest is covered with water, or the patient is extremely diaphoretic. If the patient is lying in water, it may be necessary to move the patient to a dry and safe area before using the AED. You must also dry the patient's chest if wet or excessively diaphoretic before delivering a shock or the energy may arc between the electrodes. The AED can be used safely if the patient is lying on snow or ice.

Metal is another good conductor of electricity. Be careful with patients on metal flooring, catwalks, stretchers, and other items with metal components. Ensure that no one else is directly in contact with metal that is touching the patient before you administer a shock.

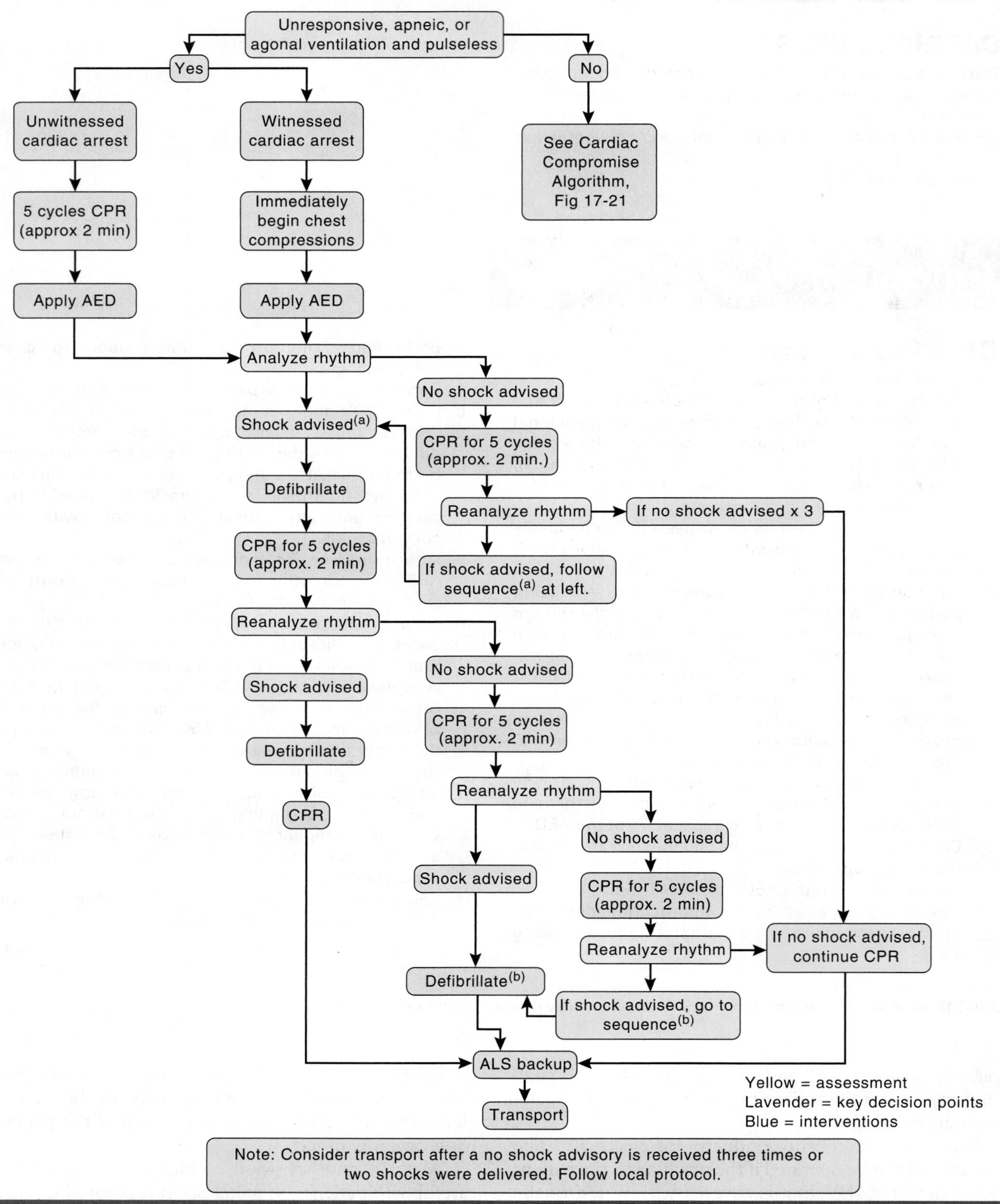

FIGURE 15-17 ✱ Emergency care algorithm: automated external defibrillation.

Objective 15-25
Describe the safety precautions to be taken to protect yourself, other EMS providers, the patient, and bystanders in resuscitation situations.

Objective 15-26
Explain the importance of AED maintenance, EMT training and skills maintenance, and medical direction in the Chain of Survival of cardiac arrest.

If a patient has a transdermal medication patch on his chest (such as nitroglycerin, nicotine, or analgesics), remove it quickly while wearing gloves and wipe the site with a towel or gauze pad before applying the defibrillator pad. Minimize the delay to defibrillation and interruption of chest when doing so. Do not place AED pads over the medication patch. The patch may reduce the effectiveness of the shock by blocking the energy or may cause burns to the skin. (The shock may cause the plastic in the patch to melt and ignite.) Be sure to wipe the nitroglycerin completely from the skin prior to defibrillation.

An extremely hairy chest, another problem that may be encountered, is not necessarily a safety issue but rather an effectiveness issue. If the patient has a very hairy chest, it is possible that the electrodes will stick to the hair and not the skin. This will reduce the amount of energy delivered to the patient and may cause the AED to continuously prompt you to "check the electrodes" for failure of good contact. If you should receive a "check electrodes" message after applying the AED, you can attempt to correct the problem by trying one of the following steps:

- Firmly press down on the pad in an attempt to stick it to the chest wall skin.
- If this does not work, pull the original set of electrodes off. This will remove some of the hair in the area. Apply a second, new set of electrodes with firm pressure applied to the pad.
- If the AED continues to give you a "check electrode" message, consider clipping chest hair with scissors or shaving the area with a disposable razor. Then apply a third, new set of electrode pads.

Keep several extra sets of electrodes and razors in the AED case. Without good contact between the electrodes and the chest, the defibrillation may not be effective or the AED will not allow the energy to be discharged. Be sure to minimize the delay to defibrillation and interruption of chest compressions when doing so.

AED Maintenance

Scheduled maintenance of the AED is crucial to ensuring that the machine functions properly. Follow your local protocols and the manufacturer's directions when maintaining the AED.

You should be aware that AED failure is most commonly attributed to improper maintenance, especially battery failure. Operators of the AED must ensure that batteries are properly maintained and replaced on a set schedule to guarantee proper energy levels. The AED, its batteries, and the system self-check status indicator should be checked at the beginning of each shift. Extra, fully charged batteries should always be available.

To assist in maintenance, a panel of experts has compiled a list of items in addition to batteries that must be checked regularly to ensure proper AED operation. This Operator's Shift Checklist (Figure 15-18∗) should be completed by EMTs (or other AED operators) at the beginning of every shift. Completing the checklist will help ensure that your AED will work when you need it. Doing so will also provide documentation of your maintenance, if necessary.

Training and Skills Maintenance

In addition to ensuring that the AED functions properly when needed, EMTs must also ensure that they can use the device properly when called on to do so. This can be accomplished through continuing education and skills maintenance programs. One recommendation is that an AED operator should refresh or practice his skills with the device every 90 days.

Operators should review incidents of AED use in the system, study any new protocols, and, most importantly, practice working with the system's device. More information regarding updated research on AED procedures can be obtained from several sources, including EMS journals, state EMS offices, and the AHA.

Medical Direction and the AED

Medical direction must play a significant role in the provision of AED services. EMTs use AEDs under the authority of the medical director's license. Medical direction thus has a great stake in ensuring that a system's AED program functions properly. Medical direction's involvement might include the following:

- Making sure that the EMS system has all necessary links in the AHA Chain of Survival
- Overseeing all levels of EMTs
- Reviewing the continual competency skill review program
- Engaging in an audit and/or quality improvement program

AUTOMATED DEFIBRILLATORS: OPERATOR'S SHIFT CHECKLIST

Date: ____________ **Shift:** ______________________ **Location:** ______________________

Mfr/Model No.: ____________________ **Serial No. or Facility ID No.:** ____________________

At the beginning of each shift, inspect the unit. Indicate whether all requirements have been met. Note any corrective actions taken. Sign the form.

	Okay as found	Corrective Action/Remarks
1. Defibrillator Unit		
Clean no spills, clear of objects on top, casing intact		
2. Cables/Connectors		
a. Inspect for cracks, broken wire, or damage b. Connectors engage securely		
3. Supplies		
a. Two sets of pads in sealed packages, within expiration date b. Hand towel c. Scissors d. Razor * e. Alcohol wipes * f. Monitoring electrodes *g. Spare charged battery *h. Adequate ECG paper *i. Manual override module, key or card *j. Cassette tape, memory module, and/or event card plus spares		
4. Power Supply		
a. Battery-powered units (1) Verify fully charged battery in place (2) Spare charged battery available (3) Follow appropriate battery rotation schedule per manufacturer's recommendations b. AC/Battery backup units (1) Plugged into live outlet to maintain battery charge (2) Test on battery power and reconnect to line power		
5. Indicators/*ECG Display		
* a. Remove cassette tape, memory module, and/or event card b. Power on display c. Self-test ok * d. Monitor display functional *e. "Service" message display off *f. Battery charging; low battery light off g. Correct time displayed — set with dispatch center		
6. ECG Recorder		
a. Adequate ECG paper b. Recorder prints		
7. Charge/Display Cycle		
* a. Disconnect AC plug — battery backup units b. Attach to simulator c. Detects, charges and delivers shock for "VF" d. Responds correctly to non-shockable rhythms *e. Manual override functional f. Detach from simulator *g. Replace cassette tape, module, and/or memory card		
8. *Pacemaker		
a. Pacer output cable intact b. Pacer pads present (set of two) c. Inspect per manufacturer's operational guidelines		
☐ **Major problem(s) identified** **(OUT OF SERVICE)**		

**Applicable only if the unit has this supply or capability*

Signature: ______________________

FIGURE 15-18 ✱ Operators Shift Checklist for AEDs. (© Laerdal)

Objective 15-27
Discuss the use of an AED in patients with cardiac pacemakers and automatic implanted cardioverter-defibrillators.

As part of the quality review and improvement program, the system's medical director or a designated representative should review all incidents of AED use. Such reviews can reveal steps that might be taken to speed the entry of cardiac arrest patients into the system, to improve AED training, or to coordinate more effectively AED operation with ACLS backup. These reviews may be accomplished through the following:

- Written reports
- Review of the voice and/or ECG tapes if the system's AED is equipped with that feature
- Review of solid-state memory modules and magnetic tapes if the system's AED is so equipped

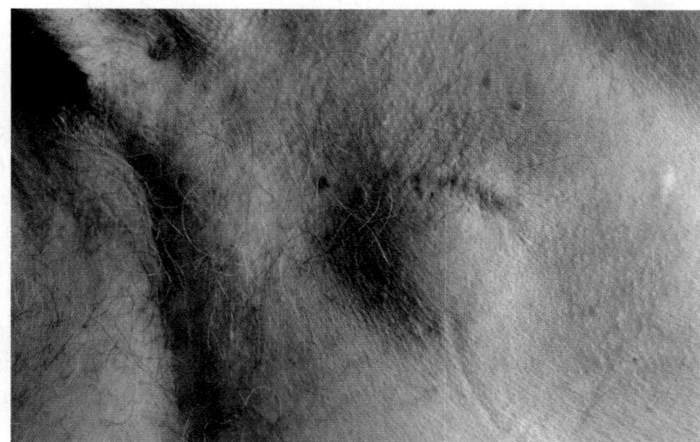

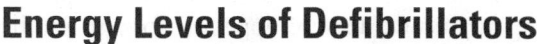

FIGURE 15-19a * An implanted pacemaker in an adult patient. (© Michal Heron)

Energy Levels of Defibrillators

Defibrillators, semiautomated or manual, deliver electrical current to the heart through the chest wall. Electrical current for defibrillators is measured in units called joules. Manual monophasic waveform defibrillators can deliver a range of current levels, usually from 5 or 10 joules to 360 joules. Most AEDs have two preset values of 200 and 360 joules programmed into the machine. Biphasic waveform defibrillators use lower energy settings for defibrillators, typically 150–200 joules for a biphasic truncated exponential waveform or 120 joules with a rectilinear biphasic waveform. It is not so important that EMTs know the difference between a "truncated exponential" and "rectilinear biphasic" waveform machine, rather that they deliver the appropriate amount of energy for their type of AED in a time-efficient and safe manner.

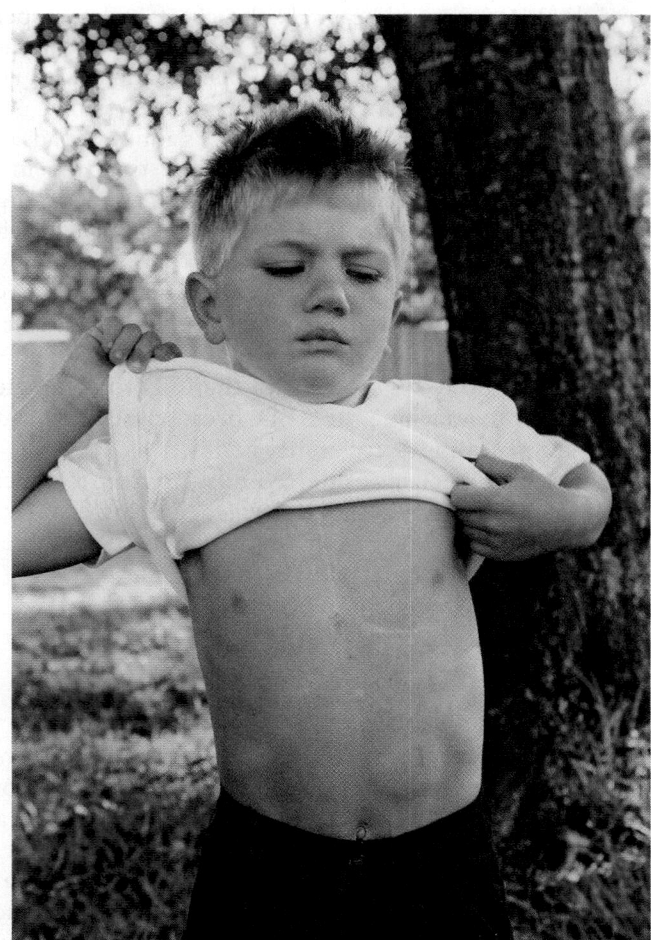

FIGURE 15-19b * Pacemakers may also be found in children. (© Michal Heron)

Cardiac Pacemakers

People whose conduction system cannot sustain a regular and effective rhythm on its own often receive surgically implanted cardiac pacemakers. These devices, powered by long-life batteries, are placed under the skin and have tiny electrodes connecting to the heart. Whenever the patient's heart rate moves outside a certain range, the device takes over the task of setting the heart's pace.

Cardiac pacemakers are usually positioned beneath one of the clavicles. They form a visible lump and can be palpated (Figure 15-19*). If you detect a pacemaker in a cardiac arrest patient, you can still use the AED. However, be sure not to place an adhesive pad directly over the pacemaker.

Objective 15-28
List the advantages and disadvantages of automated chest compression devices, impedance threshold devices, and other circulation-enhancing devices.

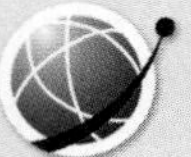

Media Resources
Go to www.bradybooks.com for mykit. Highlights:
- *Video:* Types of Shock
- *Video:* Etiology of Shock
- *Video:* Epi-pen Actions and Use
- *Video:* Bleeding Control/Shock Management

Automatic Implantable Cardioverter Defibrillators

As an EMT, you may encounter automatic implantable cardioverter defibrillators (ICDs) in some patients. These devices are surgically implanted and used in cases of ventricular heart rhythm disturbances that cannot be controlled by medication. The ICD is able to monitor the heart's electrical activity and provide a shock to the heart if it detects a shockable dysrhythmia. Usually the device will deliver four to five shocks. If a patient with an ICD is responsive, he will be able to tell you if he has an ICD and when it is delivering a shock.

If you encounter a responsive cardiac patient with an ICD, allow the device to operate, stabilize the patient, and prepare him for transport. With unresponsive cardiac patients, look for surgical scars on the chest or left upper quadrant of the abdomen. Also look for medical identification tags. Treatment for the unresponsive patient with an ICD is the same as for any other unresponsive cardiac patient. However, when applying the AED's adhesive pads in such patients, do not place them directly over the implanted ICD because the device has an insulated backing that will deflect the shock. Place the electrode pad 1 inch to the side of the ICD, or use an electrode positioning arrangement that avoids the ICD (either the anterolateral or anterior–posterior, arrangement). If the ICD is delivering shocks (indicated by the contraction of the patient's muscles), wait 30 to 60 seconds for the ICD to complete its cycle prior to attaching the AED, because the AED and ICD analysis and shock cycles may conflict.

There have been no reported injuries from contact with ICD patients while the device is delivering a shock. However, a slight tingling sensation may be detectable. Wearing exam gloves may prevent this.

Automated Chest Compression Devices

The efficiency of blood flow in cardiac arrest when external chest compressions are being delivered is a function of how well the chest wall surrounding the heart is being compressed. Even under ideal situations of CPR skill performance, the quality of blood flow from externally applied chest compressions does not parallel normal cardiac output. In addition, CPR efficiency is also hampered by rescuer fatigue, the type of surface the patient is lying on when compressions are being delivered, and the accuracy with which the provider is delivering the compressions (i.e., maintaining good depth, rate, and sequence). When resuscitating a patient, chest compressions require that at least one EMT perform chest compressions. This means that person cannot help ventilate the patient or even help move the patient since that EMT should be doing continuous compressions. Ideally the EMT performing chest compressions would be relieved after every 2 minutes to ensure good chest compressions.

Numerous devices to help deliver external compressions to the patient have been developed in an attempt to improve circulation associated with the compressions. These devices not only allow for increased uniformity in skill provision, but also free up a provider to assist with other patient care tasks. There are many mechanical compression devices still in the research and development stage, waiting to receive federal approval for use in the United States or that have not yet been recommended by the American Heart Association for use in the arrested patient. The efficacy of these devices has not yet been proven.

Mechanical Piston Device

The mechanical piston device is an apparatus that depresses the sternum with a compressed-gas-powered plunger that has been affixed to a backboard. The patient's thorax is positioned supine on the backboard, and the piston device is positioned above the patient with the plunger centered over the portion of the sternum where manual compressions should be applied. The device is then affixed to the backboard.

The device can be configured by the user to deliver a specific rate and depth of compressions. The benefits are that it allows for uniform delivery of compressions, with no diminishment in compression quality from rescuer fatigue, and it frees up an EMS provider to tend to other interventions. Limitations are that some piston devices, especially the first ones on the market, were large, heavy, and cumbersome. Also, since these devices operate on compressed gas, the device becomes useless when the compressed gas runs out. The available evidence can't support routine use of these devices.

Load-Distributing-Band CPR or Vest CPR

This device is composed of a wide band that is applied to the chest circumferentially and, in some models, is attached to the backboard (Figure 15-20∗). The device is either pneumatically or electrically driven to provide an inward constrictive pressure on the thorax, which, in

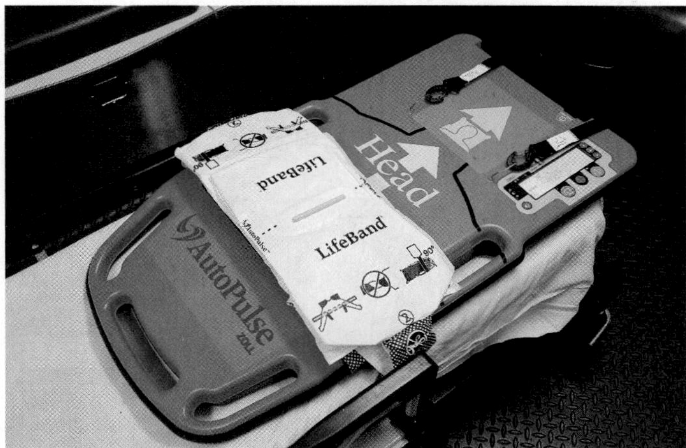

FIGURE 15-20 * The AutoPulse, a load-distributing-band CPR device, compresses the thorax.

turn, compresses the heart. Like the mechanical piston device, the obvious benefit is that it frees up one EMS provider to perform other care interventions. This device is also lighter than the mechanical piston device, is easy to apply, and has been shown to improve coronary and cerebral blood flow over traditional CPR. The available evidence can't support routine use of these devices.

Impedance Threshold Device

An impedance threshold device (ITD) is not a mechanical compression device; however, it has been shown in experimental studies to improve blood flow through the heart during CPR (Figure 15-21*). This device is actually a piece of equipment designed with a valve that limits the amount of air that enters the chest and lungs during the chest recoil phase of active compressions. The device is placed between the cuffed endotracheal tube of an intubated adult patient and the ventilatory adjunct being used to provide artificial ventilations.

Under normal conditions, the recoil of the chest during the relaxation phase of compressions creates a negative intrathoracic pressure. The pressure is then normalized as air rushes into the lungs. With the impedance threshold device, however, air is prohibited from rushing in during the relaxation phase of ventilations, instead allowing the negative intrathoracic pressure to draw more blood toward the heart. This translates into a better cardiac filling for the next active compression. This device may be considered for use by the EMT in a nonintubated adult patient; however, it is absolutely necessary that a tight mask seal is constantly maintained.

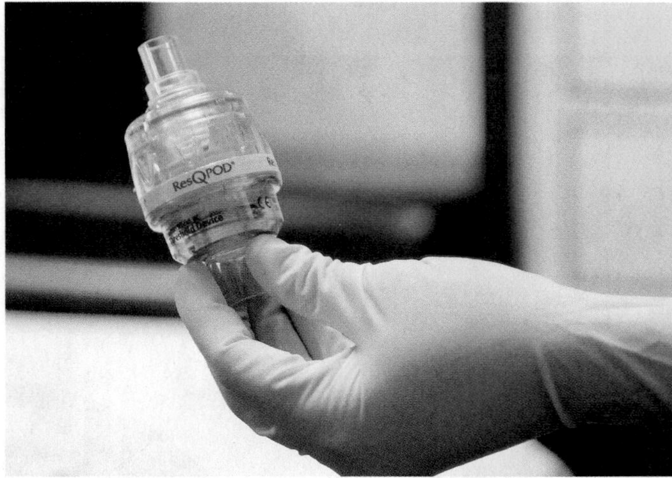

FIGURE 15-21 * The ResQPOD, an impedance threshold device, improves blood flow through the heart during CPR.

Other Circulation-Enhancing Devices

Other circulation-enhancing devices have been developed from the concept of the impedance threshold device. These devices are used to actively compress and also decompress the thorax during resuscitation (Figure 15-22*). The compression phase generates the positive pressure to move the blood out of the heart through the arteries; decompression increases the negative pressure inside the thorax to improve blood return to the heart.

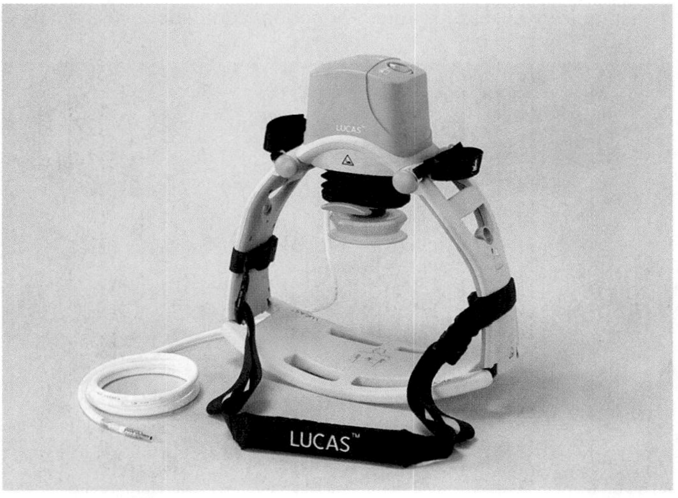

FIGURE 15-22a * The Lucas (Jolife) device actively compresses and decompresses the thorax. (Courtesy of Physio-Control, Inc.)

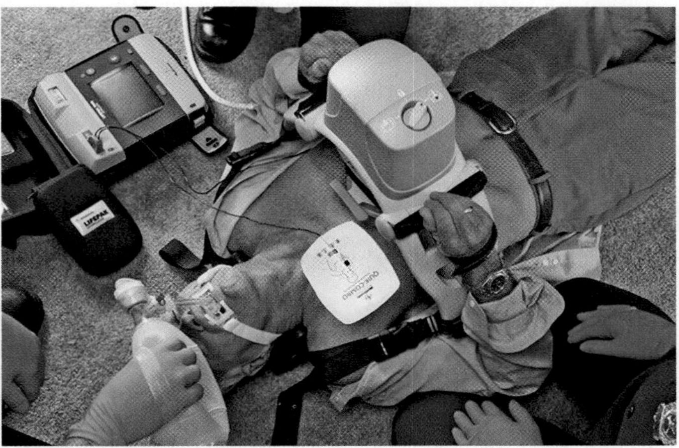

FIGURE 15-22b * The Lucas (Jolife) device applied to a patient. (Courtesy of Physio-Control, Inc.)

EMT skills 15-1 Using a Semiautomated AED

Ideally, at least two EMTs should be present—one to operate the AED, the other to perform CPR.

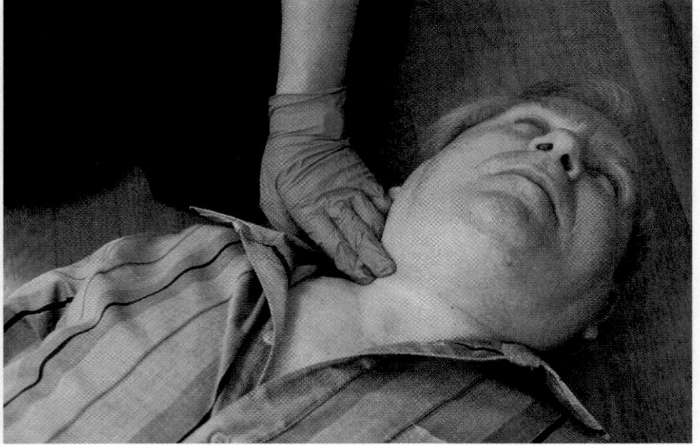

15-1A * In the unresponsive patient suspected of being in cardiac arrest, quickly assess for apnea or agonal ventilations and a pulse.

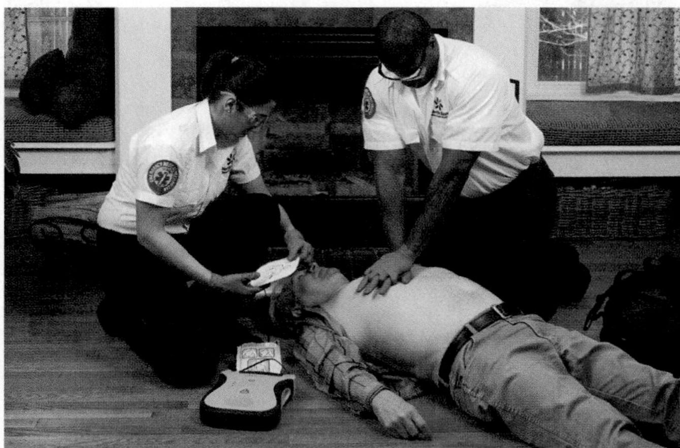

15-1B * One EMT should immediately initiate CPR beginning with chest compressions while the other EMT prepares the AED.

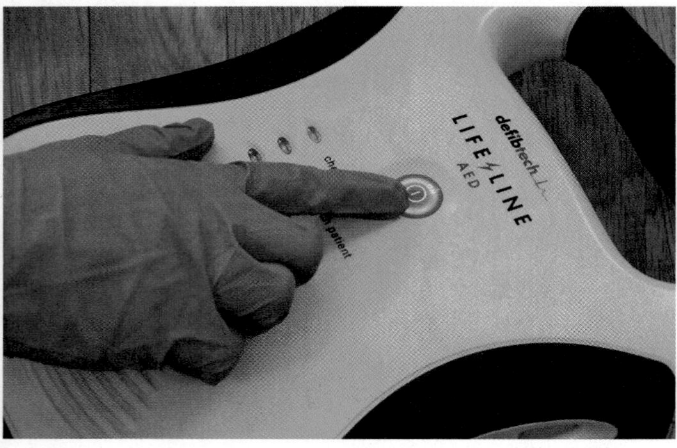

15-1C * Turn on the AED and follow the prompts.

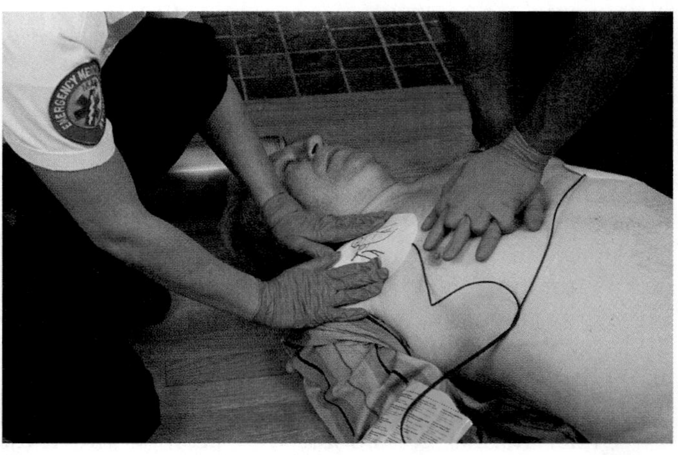

15-1D * Apply the defibrillation pads while chest compressions are being performed. Minimize any interruption in chest compressions.

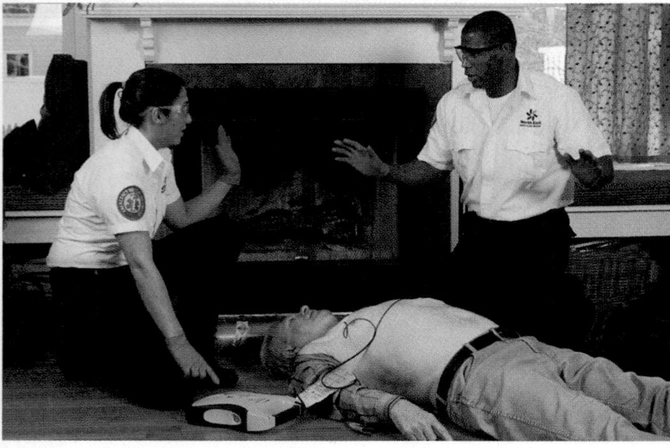

15-1E * Clear the patient for rhythm analysis.

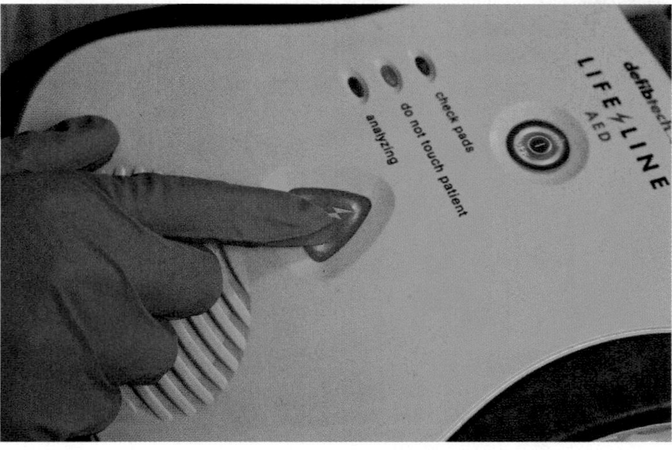

15-1F * Deliver a defibrillation if advised.

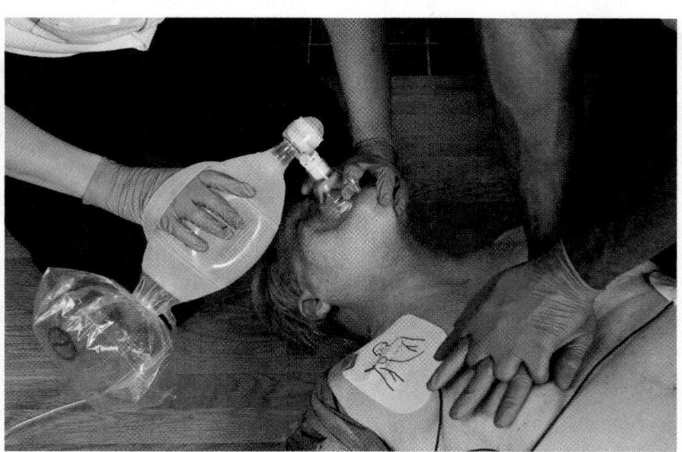

15-1G ✱ Immediately resume CPR beginning with chest compressions following the defibrillation.

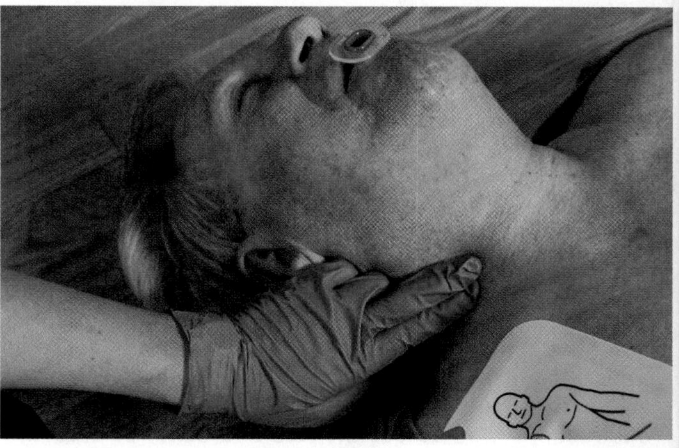

15-1H ✱ After two minutes of CPR, follow the AED prompts to check breathing and pulse in a non-shockable rhythm.

CHAPTER REVIEW

SUMMARY

Shock is a critical condition that is related to a decrease in vascular volume, poor cardiac function, or vessel disturbances. Shock results in an inadequate delivery of oxygen and glucose to cells. This leads to a shift from aerobic to anaerobic cell metabolism. The lack of energy production and the buildup of acid begin to damage cells, tissues, and organs. If not managed effectively, multiple organ systems will fail and lead to death.

Shock is categorized as hypovolemic, distributive, cardiogenic, or obstructive. The names imply the actual etiology of the poor perfusion state. Types of shock include hemorrhagic hypovolemic, nonhemorrhagic hypovolemic, burn, anaphylactic, septic, neurogenic, and cardiogenic. Shock can progress through three stages: compensatory, decompensatory, and irreversible. Irreversible shock will eventually lead to death. The body responds to shock through direct sympathetic nervous system innervation of organs and structures and the release of various hormones. These are all designed to bring the body back to a normal state of perfusion and function. If the shock overwhelms these body responses or the hormones are exhausted, the shock progresses. The management of shock focuses on the airway, ventilation, oxygenation, circulation, and rapid transport.

To increase the survival rate from cardiac arrest, always remember the components of the Chain of Survival. Immediate recognition and activation, early CPR, rapid defibrillation, effective ACLS, and integrated post-cardiac arrest care are all necessary if rates of patient survival from cardiac arrest are going to improve.

When caring for a patient in cardiac arrest, always do your best in each of the interventions you are providing. Remember to "push hard and push fast" with compressions so that the brain and heart can still receive blood flow during the arrest management. Minimize interruptions in chest compressions. Ensure adequate ventilations and provide oxygen during the arrest as well. The automated external defibrillator should be utilized specifically as addressed earlier in the chapter so that those patients in ventricular fibrillation will have the greatest opportunity for survival. Patients in nonventricular fibrillation cardiac arrest (identified by a "no shock" message on the AED) should also receive this high level of care so that they too may have the greatest chance for survival.

Finally, the patient near cardiac arrest, in cardiac arrest, or just coming out of cardiac arrest is probably one of the most challenging and dynamic situations the EMT will ever encounter. It requires a thorough understanding of the body, application of multiple skills simultaneously, and coordination of multiple EMS providers—all done in the shortest time possible so that the patient can be transported to the hospital for definitive care.

CASE STUDY FOLLOW-UP

SCENE SIZE-UP

You have been dispatched for a 26-year-old male patient who has been stabbed in the leg and is bleeding profusely. You are directed into the house by a police officer. You find the patient lying supine on the floor with a large pool of blood around his right thigh.

PRIMARY ASSESSMENT

As you approach the patient, he is not alert and doesn't respond when you call his name. He also appears to be very pale. You instruct a police officer who is also an Emergency Medical Responder to take manual in-line spinal stabilization. The patient moans when you pinch and twist his trapezius muscle. You open the airway using a jaw thrust and inspect inside the oral cavity. The mouth is clear of any obstructions. You assess the rate and depth of breathing by listening for air movement and watching the chest rise. The respirations are rapid and the tidal volume is adequate. You instruct your partner to apply a nonrebreather mask at 15 lpm and to apply the pulse oximeter to attempt to get an SpO_2 reading. The radial pulse is barely palpable and the skin is pale, cool, and clammy. You quickly expose the leg and find a steady flow of blood coming from the wound. You apply direct pressure. You instruct your partner to cut the clothing to expose the remainder of the body.

SECONDARY ASSESSMENT

You recognize the signs the patient is exhibiting to be consistent with hypovolemic shock so you elect to do a rapid secondary assessment. You begin at the head and move systematically down to the toes inspecting and palpating for any other life-threatening injuries. You auscultate the breath sounds and find them to be equal and clear bilaterally. You log roll the patient to place him on a backboard. As you do so, you quickly cut away the clothing to the back and inspect and palpate for any other injuries. You place the patient on the backboard. While your partner finishes applying the immobilization equipment, you obtain a set of vital signs. His blood pressure is 72/58 mmHg, heart rate is 132 bpm, respirations are 26/minute with a good tidal volume, and his skin is pale, cool, and clammy. Once the patient is completely immobilized, you quickly move him to the back of the ambulance and begin rapid transport to the level 1 trauma center.

There was no one at the scene from whom you could have gathered a history. You did not note any medical identification items on his body. The patient still remains only responsive to a painful stimulus; thus, he is not able to provide any history information.

REASSESSMENT

En route to the hospital you reassess the mental status, airway, ventilation, oxygenation, and circulation. You check the pressure dressing on the leg to be sure there is no additional bleeding. You obtain another set of vital signs. You contact the trauma center and provide a radio report of the assessment findings, your emergency care, and the ETA.

Upon arrival to the emergency department, the trauma surgeon meets you to bring the patient into the trauma bay. You provide an oral report and transfer the care of the patient. You then prepare your written report as your partner cleans and prepares the ambulance for another call.

IN REVIEW

1. Define shock.
2. Describe what is needed to maintain adequate cell perfusion.
3. List and describe the three etiologies of shock.
4. List and describe the categories of shock.
5. List and describe each type of shock.
6. List and describe the three stages of shock.
7. Describe the body's neural and hormonal response to shock.
8. Explain the general principles of shock.
9. List the five links in the AHA Chain of Survival.
10. Name and describe the heart rhythms that might benefit from defibrillation.
11. Describe patients for whom use of the AED is appropriate and those for whom it is not.
12. Explain how delivery of CPR is coordinated with use of the AED.
13. Name the procedures an EMT should follow in dealing with an adult patient with no pulse.
14. Explain the basic steps to follow if a resuscitated patient goes back into cardiac arrest during transport.

CRITICAL THINKING

You and your partner, Claire Menzies, have responded to a report of a male in his 50s with breathing difficulty at 115 Clearwater Drive. En route, you receive an update that CPR is being performed at the scene. Dispatch also advises that the ALS team is being contacted and that fire and police vehicles have been sent in support.

Your ambulance and the fire and police vehicles arrive at the scene within moments of each other, 4 minutes after the call came in. There you observe a small crowd gathered around a male patient. A man and a woman are performing CPR. There do not appear to be any hazards associated with this scene, and only one patient is visible. Because the dispatcher advised of CPR in progress, you take the AED when leaving the ambulance. You and your partner have already donned gloves and eye protection while en route.

You find a man, possibly in his mid-50s, lying supine on the ground with effective bystander CPR in progress. The bystanders state that they began CPR immediately upon his collapse and called 911. The patient's skin is slightly cyanotic. Claire begins to set up the semiautomated AED while chest compressions are continued. You decide that this is a priority patient for defibrillation and apply the defibrillation pads to the chest, turn on the AED, and stop CPR. You direct one of two firefighters who have come to the scene to prepare to immediately resume chest compressions, while you instruct the other to prepare for ventilation with a bag-valve mask and high-concentration oxygen.

1. What assessment findings indicate that this patient is indeed in cardiac arrest?
2. Which components of the Chain of Survival have already been met?
3. Why is this patient a candidate for immediate versus delayed defibrillation?
4. What cardiac rhythm is this patient most likely going to show?
5. What is the compression/ventilation ratio going to be for this patient?
6. If the AED indicates that no shock is warranted, what should the next action of the care providers be?

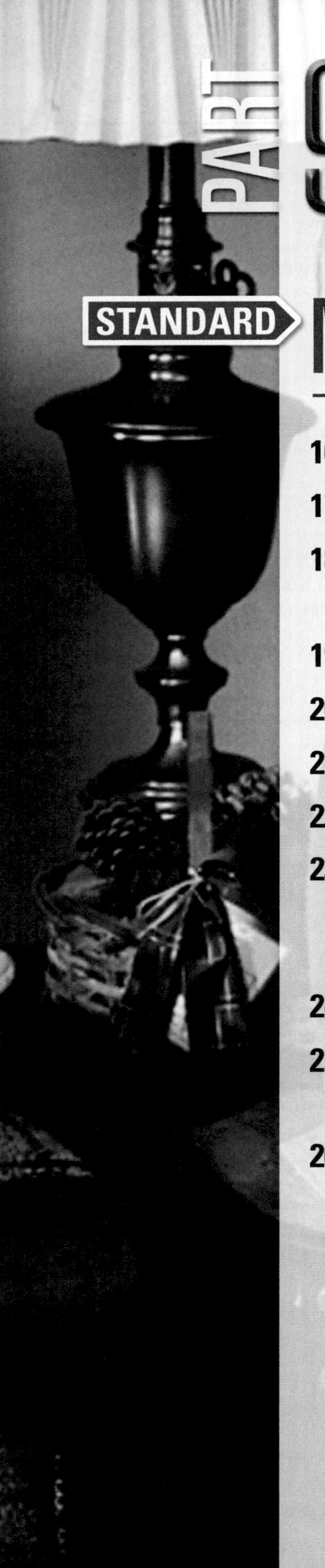

PART 9

STANDARD

Medicine

COMPETENCY

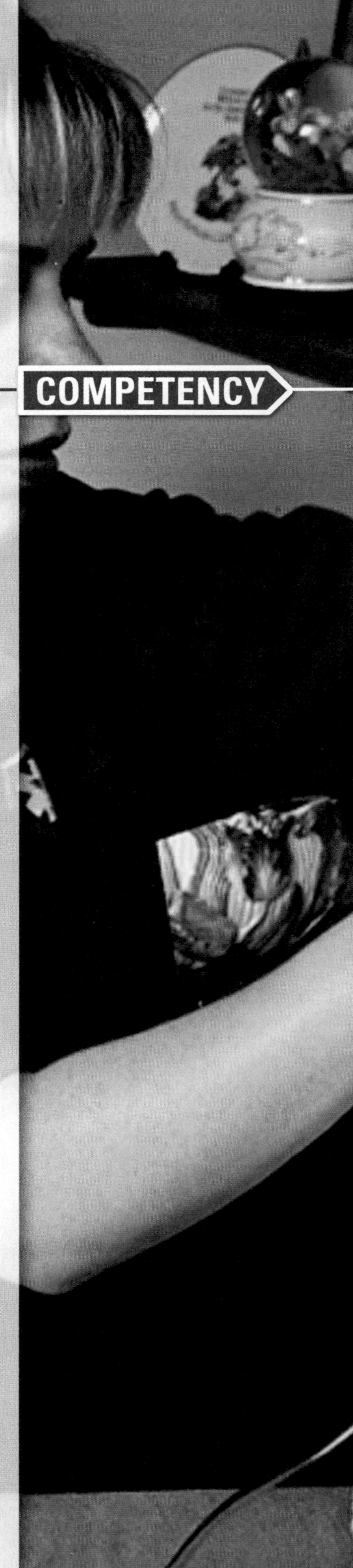

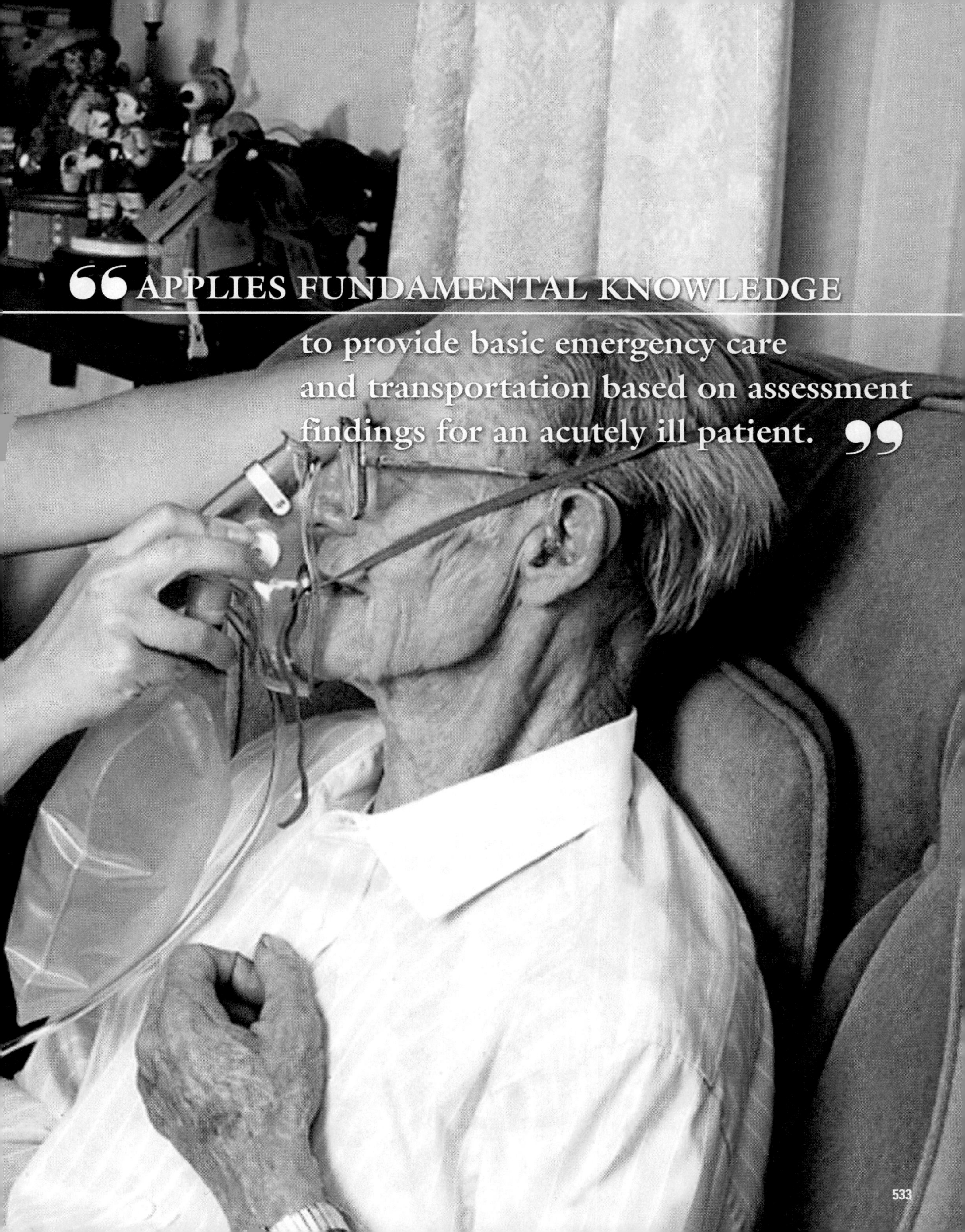

"APPLIES FUNDAMENTAL KNOWLEDGE to provide basic emergency care and transportation based on assessment findings for an acutely ill patient."

CHAPTER 16

Respiratory Emergencies

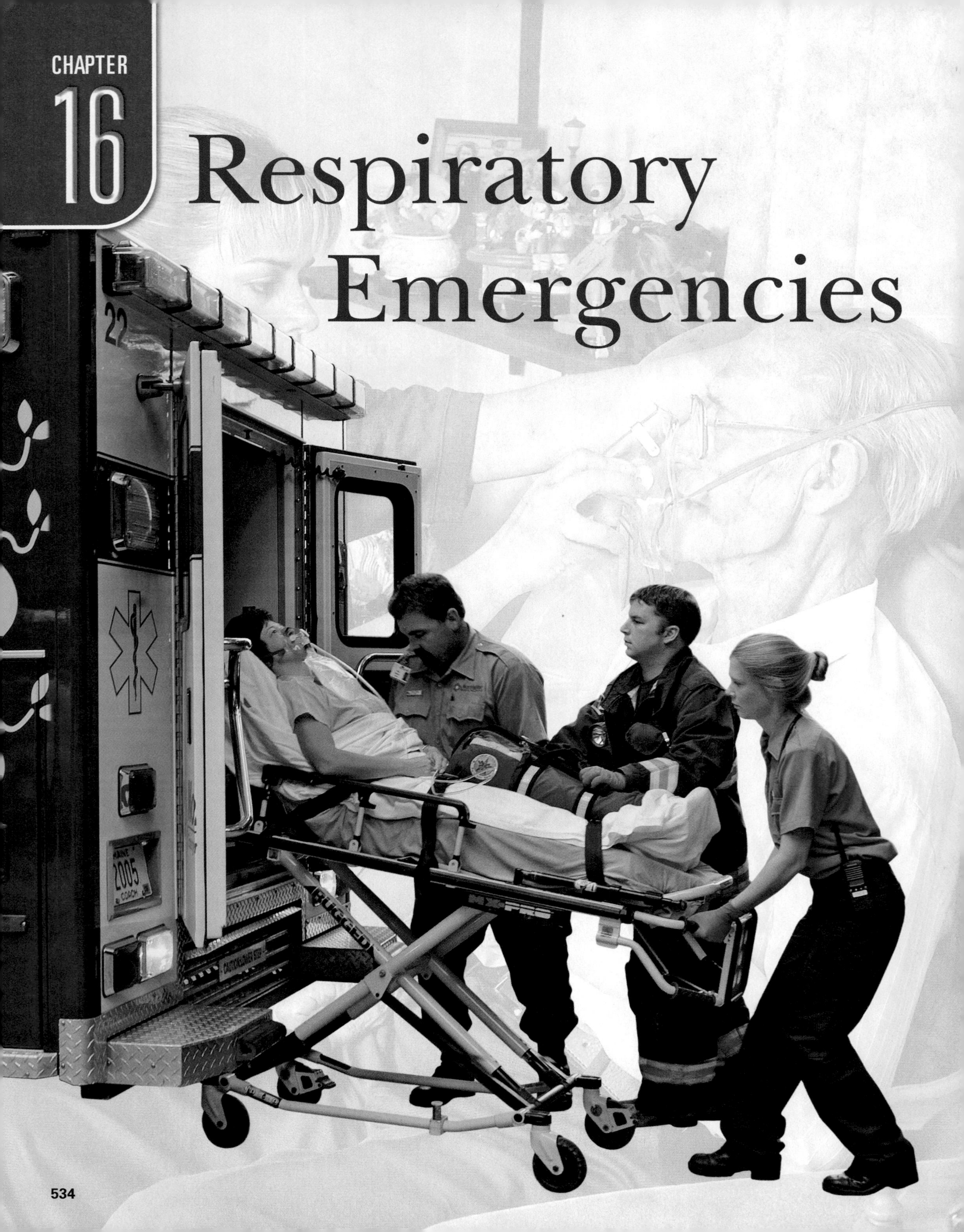

Navigation Guide

The following items provide an overview to the purpose and content of this chapter. The Education Standard and Competency are from the new National EMS Education Standards.

STANDARD **Medicine** (Content Area: Respiratory)

COMPETENCY Applies fundamental knowledge to provide basic emergency care and transportation based on assessment findings for an acutely ill patient.

OBJECTIVES: After reading this chapter, you should be able to:

16-1. Define key terms introduced in this chapter.

16-2. Explain the importance of being able to quickly recognize and treat patients with respiratory emergencies.

16-3. Describe the structure and function of the respiratory system, including:
- **a.** Upper airway
- **b.** Lower airway
- **c.** Gas exchange
- **d.** Inspiratory and expiratory centers in the medulla and pons

16-4. Demonstrate the assessment of breath sounds.

16-5. Describe the characteristics of abnormal breath sounds, including:
- **a.** Wheezing
- **b.** Rhonchi
- **c.** Crackles (rales)

16-6. Explain the relationship between dyspnea and hypoxia.

16-7. Differentiate respiratory distress, respiratory failure, and respiratory arrest.

16-8. Describe the pathophysiology by which each of the following conditions leads to inadequate oxygenation:
- **a.** Obstructive pulmonary diseases: emphysema, chronic bronchitis, and asthma
- **b.** Pneumonia
- **c.** Pulmonary embolism
- **d.** Pulmonary edema
- **e.** Spontaneous pneumothorax
- **f.** Hyperventilation syndrome
- **g.** Epiglottitis
- **h.** Pertussis
- **i.** Cystic fibrosis
- **j.** Poisonous exposures
- **k.** Viral respiratory infections

16-9. As allowed by your scope of practice, demonstrate administering or assisting a patient with self-administration of bronchodilators by metered-dose inhaler and/or small-volume nebulizer.

16-10. Differentiate between short-acting beta$_2$ agonists appropriate for prehospital use and respiratory medications that are not intended for emergency use.

16-11. Describe special considerations in the assessment and management of pediatric and geriatric patients with respiratory emergencies, including:
- **a.** Differences in anatomy and physiology
- **b.** Causes of respiratory emergencies
- **c.** Differences in management

16-12. Employ an assessment-based approach in order to recognize indications for the following interventions in patients with respiratory complaints/emergencies:
- **a.** Establishing an airway
- **b.** Administration of oxygen
- **c.** Positive pressure ventilation
- **d.** Administration/assistance with self-administration of an inhaled beta$_2$ agonist
- **e.** Expedited transport
- **f.** ALS backup

16-13. Given a list of patient medications, recognize medications that are associated with respiratory disease.

16-14. Use reassessment to identify responses to treatment and changes in the conditions of patients presenting with respiratory complaints and emergencies.

continued

Navigation Guide *continued*

KEY TERMS: Page references indicate first major use in this chapter. For complete definitions, see the Glossary at the back of the book.

apnea p. 539
bronchoconstriction p. 539
bronchodilator p. 539
dyspnea p. 539
hypercarbia p. 540
hypoxemia p. 539
hypoxia p. 539
metered-dose inhaler (MDI) p. 554
pulsus paradoxus p. 568
respiratory arrest p. 540
respiratory distress p. 540
respiratory failure p. 540
small-volume nebulizer p. 555
spacer p. 555
tripod position p. 564

MEDIA RESOURCES: Please go to www.bradybooks.com to access mykit for this text. You will find quizzes, critical thinking scenarios, weblinks, animations, and videos related to this chapter—and much more. Look for online information on breath sounds and assessment tips. You will also find animations and video clips on asthma, tuberculosis, ARDS, and COPD.

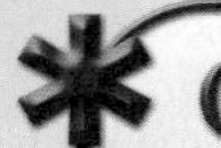

CASE STUDY

The Dispatch

EMS Unit 106—respond to 1449 Porter Avenue, Apartment 322. You have a 31-year-old female patient complaining of respiratory distress. Time out is 1942 hours.

Upon Arrival

You and your partner arrive at the scene and are greeted at the curb by the husband of the patient. As you step out of the ambulance and begin to gather your equipment, you ask, "Did you place the call for EMS, sir?" He states very nervously, "Yes. It's my wife, Anna. She can't breathe. She really doesn't look good." As you and your partner begin walking toward the apartment complex, you ask, "What's your name?" His voice breaks as he tells you, "My name is John Sanders. We've only been married 2 months. Please—you've got to help my wife." You reply, "John, we'll take good care of your wife. But, you'll help us more if you can calm down."

As he leads you up narrow stairs to the third floor of the apartment complex, you scan the scene for safety hazards and note any obstacles that will make it difficult to extricate the patient from the building. Upon walking into the apartment, you note a young woman sitting upright on a kitchen chair, looking very scared, and leaning slightly forward with her arms locked in front of her to hold her up. Before you can even introduce yourself, she begins to speak one word at a time with a gasp for breath in between: "I—can't—breathe."

How Would You Proceed to Assess and Care for This Patient?

During this chapter you will learn about assessment and emergency care for a patient suffering from respiratory distress. Later, we will return to the case and apply the procedures learned.

Introduction

Few things are more frightening to the patient than the inability to breathe easily, and one of the most common symptoms of a respiratory emergency is shortness of breath. A number of other signs and symptoms may accompany difficulty in breathing, which is also known as respiratory distress. Respiratory conditions may present very similarly; this is because many of these findings are from the body's attempt to improve breathing adequacy, not necessarily from the specific respiratory condition. As such, many of your treatment modalities are similar for these conditions. It is important for you to recognize the signs and symptoms of respiratory emergencies, complete a thorough patient interview and physical assessment to determine the cause, and provide immediate intervention.

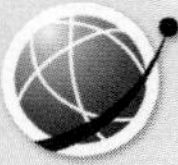

Media Resources
Go to www.bradybooks.com for mykit. Highlights:

- *Animation:* Asthma
- *Video:* Tuberculosis
- *Web Resource:* Asthma Triggers

Objective 16-2
Explain the importance of being able to quickly recognize and treat patients with respiratory emergencies.

Objective 16-3
Describe the structure and function of the respiratory system.

Respiratory Anatomy, Physiology, and Pathophysiology

The respiratory system can be divided into three portions. The first two are the upper and lower airways, with the vocal cords (or glottic opening) being the transition between the two. The primary purpose of the upper and lower airways is the conduction of air into and out of the lungs. The third portion of the respiratory system consists of the lungs and accessory structures, which work in concert with the upper and lower airways to allow the oxygenation of body cells and the elimination of carbon dioxide from the bloodstream.

Normal Breathing

Most patients you encounter as an EMT will be breathing normally. The following findings are consistent with a patient who is breathing adequately:

- An intact (open) airway
- Normal respiratory rate
- Normal rise and fall of the chest
- Normal respiratory rhythm
- Breath sounds that are present bilaterally
- Chest expansion and relaxation that occurs normally
- Minimal-to-absent use of accessory muscles to aid in breathing

The following should also occur in a patient who is breathing adequately, provided that no other condition or injury is involved:

- Normal mental status
- Normal muscle tone
- Normal pulse oximeter reading
- Normal skin condition findings

Abnormal Breathing

Abnormal factors that are present in certain pulmonary (lung) conditions can decrease the efficiency of gas exchange across the alveolar-capillary membrane. They include:

- Increased width of the space between the alveoli and blood vessels
- Lack of perfusion of the pulmonary capillaries from the right ventricle of the heart
- Filling of the alveoli with fluid, blood, or pus

During periods of heightened respiratory effort, the body may employ accessory muscles to help change the size of the thorax (chest cavity) more aggressively in order to move air better. Clinically speaking, many of the findings consistent with respiratory distress come from the use of these accessory muscles during times of disease, stress, or injury.

Other accessory structures that are part of the respiratory system include the inspiratory and expiratory centers in the medulla and pons, located in the brainstem, which exert nervous control of breathing. These respiratory centers receive information about the oxygen and carbon dioxide content of the bloodstream from special sensors in the vascular system. Additionally, stretch receptors in the walls of the lungs provide information to the brain stem to prevent accidental overexpansion injuries, and irritant receptors in the walls of the bronchioles detect the presence of abnormalities such as excessive fluid, toxic fumes or smoke, or significant air temperature changes.

Finally, receptors near the alveoli, called juxtacapillary receptors, detect when the alveolar-capillary beds are becoming abnormally engorged with blood as a result of heart failure. These receptors are believed to play a role in the feeling of shortness of breath the patient may experience, and they may also promote shallow and rapid breathing.

Assessing Breath Sounds

During the physical exam, auscultation of breath sounds may provide additional evidence of breathing difficulty. The general complaint of breathing difficulty can result from a variety of conditions; therefore, being able to describe the type of breath sounds may be helpful to medical direction when you ask for a medication order.

To achieve the most accurate interpretation of breath sounds, it is important to auscultate in the appropriate fashion. Whenever feasible, have the patient sit upright

Objective 16-4
Demonstrate the assessment of breath sounds.

Key Points
It is important to recognize the signs and symptoms of respiratory emergencies, complete a thorough assessment, and provide immediate intervention.

Objective 16-5
Describe the characteristics of abnormal breath sounds.

Key Points
A patient who was initially breathing adequately may deteriorate to a point where breathing is inadequate and insufficient to sustain life.

and, while using the diaphragm end of your stethoscope over bare skin (never auscultate over clothing), instruct the patient to cough one or two times and then take deep rhythmic breaths (inhalation and exhalation) with his mouth open. You may need to instruct the patient a few times to make no airway/vocal sounds while he does this. Place the head of the stethoscope on the patient's thorax, and listen the whole way through the phases of inhalation and exhalation. If necessary, listen to a few of the patient's breaths (each breath including both inhalation and exhalation) at each auscultation location to ensure your interpretation of any abnormal breath sound. Finally, listen to sounds on one location of the body, and then listen to the exact location on the other side (mirror location), before moving on. The photos in EMT Skills 16-1 illustrate common locations for thoracic auscultation. Table 16-1 identifies the significance of these locations.

Three basic types of abnormal breath sounds that you might hear upon auscultation of the thorax may be early indicators of impending respiratory distress:

- *Wheezing* is a high-pitched, musical, whistling sound that is best heard initially on exhalation but may also be heard during inhalation in more severe cases. It is an indication of swelling and constriction of the inner lining of the bronchioles. Wheezing that is diffuse (heard over all the lung fields) is a primary indication for the administration of a beta agonist medication by metered-dose inhaler or by small-volume nebulizer. Wheezing is usually heard in asthma, emphysema, and chronic bronchitis. It may also be heard in pneumonia, congestive heart failure, and other conditions when they cause bronchoconstriction. (These disorders will be discussed later in this chapter.)
- *Rhonchi* are snoring or rattling noises heard upon auscultation. They indicate obstruction of the larger conducting airways of the respiratory tract by thick secretions of mucus. Rhonchi are often heard in chronic bronchitis, emphysema, aspiration, and pneumonia. One characteristic of rhonchi is that the quality of sound changes if the person coughs or sometimes even when the person changes position.
- *Crackles,* also known as *rales,* are bubbly or crackling sounds heard during inhalation. These sounds are associated with fluid that has surrounded or filled the alveoli or very small bronchioles. The crackling sound is commonly associated with the alveoli and terminal bronchioles "popping" open with each inhalation. The bases of the lungs posteriorly will reveal crackles first because of the natural tendency of fluid to be pulled downward by gravity. Crackles may indicate pulmonary edema or pneumonia. This type of breath sound typically does not change with coughing or movement.

Respiratory Distress

The majority of patients you will encounter as an EMT will display an adequate respiratory effort (normal breathing). However, you may encounter a patient with inadequate breathing, or find that a patient who was initially

TABLE 16-1 Auscultation of Breath Sounds: Locations and Significance

Location	Significance
Second intercostal space, midclavicular line (See EMT Skills 16-1A.)	Sounds heard here represent airflow through the larger conducting airways. Airway structures are still supported by cartilage. Abnormal sounds heard best here include stridor and rhonchi.
Third intercostal space, anterior axillary line or Fourth intercostal space, midaxillary line (See EMT Skills 16-1B.)	Sounds heard here represent airflow through smaller conducting airways (bronchioles). You may also be able to hear some airflow into the air sacs (alveoli). The abnormal breath sound heard best in this location is wheezing.
Fifth or sixth intercostal space, posterior midscapular line (See EMT Skills 16-1C.)	While the patient is sitting upright, the sounds heard here represent airflow into the alveoli. This is the best location to hear alveolar airflow. The abnormal sound heard here most commonly is crackles (rales).

Key Terms
hypoxemia decreased oxygen levels in the blood.

Objective 16-6
Explain the relationship between dyspnea and hypoxia.

Key Terms
dyspnea shortness of breath or perceived difficulty in breathing.

apnea absence of breathing; respiratory arrest.

hypoxia the absence of sufficient oxygen in the body cells.

breathing adequately has deteriorated to a point where breathing is inadequate and insufficient to sustain life.

Failing to breathe adequately, even for short periods of time, will result in **hypoxemia** (decreased oxygen in the bloodstream) and cellular death, which will lead to all the other body systems starting to falter as well. For example, with failure of the respiratory system, the neurological system will fail and the patient's mental status will deteriorate. Failure of the respiratory system will also cause the cardiovascular system to fail, causing the patient to display vital sign changes and shock (hypoperfusion). One by one, the body's systems will fail from failure of the respiratory system. If left untreated, a patient with inadequate breathing will die.

Respiratory emergencies may range from "shortness of breath," or **dyspnea**, to complete respiratory arrest, or **apnea**, in which the patient is no longer breathing. These conditions can result from a large number of causes, but most typically they involve the respiratory tract or the lungs. Because quick intervention and appropriate emergency care could be life saving in a respiratory emergency, it is important for you to understand the anatomy and basic physiology of the respiratory tract and lungs and the techniques of airway management and artificial ventilation. For a review of these topics, see Chapter 7, "Anatomy, Physiology, and Medical Terminology," and Chapter 10, "Airway Management, Artificial Ventilation, and Oxygenation."

Shortness of breath, abnormal upper airway sounds, faster- or slower-than-normal breathing rates, poor chest rise and fall—these and other signs and symptoms of respiratory distress may be indications that the cells of the body are not getting an adequate supply of oxygen, a condition known as **hypoxia**.

These and other signs and symptoms may be directly caused by obstructions of airflow occurring in the upper or lower portions of the respiratory tract or from fluid or collapse in the alveoli of the lungs, causing poor gas exchange. If adequate breathing and gas exchange are not present, the lack of oxygen will cause the body cells to begin to die. Some cells become irritable when they are hypoxic, causing the cells to function abnormally. For example, hypoxic cardiac cells become irritable and begin to send out abnormal impulses, leading to cardiac dysrhythmias (abnormal heart rhythms).

Following is a listing of common findings the patient with respiratory distress may display:

- Subjective complaint of shortness of breath
- Restlessness
- Increased (early distress) or decreased (late distress) pulse rate
- Changes to the rate or depth of breathing
- Skin color changes
- Abnormal breathing, lung, or airway sounds
- Difficulty or inability to speak
- Muscle retractions (suprasternal, supraclavicular, subclavicular, intercostal)
- Altered mental status
- Abdominal breathing (excessive use of abdominal muscles)
- Excessive coughing (with or without expectorating material)
- Tripod positioning
- Decrease in pulse oximetry (blood oxygen saturation) reading, especially below 95%

Many complaints of breathing difficulty result from significant narrowing of the bronchioles of the lower airway from inflammation, swelling, or constriction of the muscle layer, a condition known as **bronchoconstriction** or *bronchospasm*. This narrowing causes a drastic increase in resistance to airflow in the bronchioles, making inhalation and particularly exhalation extremely difficult and producing wheezing. The patient may be prescribed a medication in aerosol form that can be inhaled during this episode of breathing difficulty. This medication, known as a **bronchodilator**, is designed to dilate (relax and open) the bronchioles, which results in an increase in the effectiveness of breathing and relief from the signs and symptoms.

Breathing difficulty may also be a symptom of injuries to the head, face, neck, spine, chest, or abdomen. A high index of suspicion and accurate assessment are required so no life-threatening injuries are missed. In addition, cardiac compromise, hyperventilation associated with emotional upset, and various abdominal conditions may produce difficulty in breathing.

Although several factors could lead to a patient complaining of dyspnea, the most common cause of this sensation of shortness of breath is dysfunction in the respiratory system. The sensation of shortness of breath occurs when the metabolic demands of the body are not being met. It is usually caused by one of the following:

1. *Mechanical disruption to the airway, lung, or chest wall* that prevents effective mechanical ventilation. Examples of conditions that may cause a disruption

Objective 16-7
Differentiate respiratory distress, respiratory failure, and respiratory arrest.

Objective 16-8
Describe the pathophysiology by which various conditions lead to inadequate oxygenation.

Key Terms

bronchoconstriction constriction of the smooth muscle of the bronchi and bronchioles.

bronchodilator a drug that relaxes the smooth muscle of the bronchi and bronchioles and reverses bronchoconstriction.

in mechanical ventilation include airway obstruction, flail chest (two or more adjacent ribs fractured in two or more places), chest muscle weakness, neuromuscular diseases, and lung collapse (pneumothorax).

2. *Stimulation of the receptors in the lungs.* Such stimulation will produce a sensation of shortness of breath. Conditions that will stimulate the receptors include asthma, pneumonia, and congestive heart failure.
3. *Inadequate gas exchange at the level of the alveoli and capillaries* causing a decrease in the oxygen content in the blood (hypoxemia) or a rise in the level of carbon dioxide. This may be due to:
   - *a ventilation disturbance:* an inadequate amount of oxygen-rich air entering the alveoli and passing across the alveolar membrane to the capillary;
   - *a perfusion disturbance:* an inadequate amount of blood traveling through the pulmonary capillaries, which decreases the number of red blood cells available to pick up the oxygen and transport it to the cells; or
   - *both a ventilation and a perfusion disturbance in the lungs,* leading to hypoxemia (decreased oxygen levels in the blood) and **hypercarbia** (increased carbon dioxide levels in the blood)

Regardless of the cause, a complaint of breathing difficulty requires your immediate intervention. Time is critical because of the detrimental effects of low oxygen levels on all cells and organs. A patient who is having difficulty breathing but has an adequate tidal volume and respiratory rate is said to be in **respiratory distress**. Because the tidal volume and respiratory rate are still adequate, the patient is compensating and is in need of supplemental oxygen via a nonrebreather mask at 15 lpm.

If either the tidal volume or the respiratory rate becomes or is inadequate, the patient's respiratory status becomes inadequate. The patient is said to be in **respiratory failure**, since the respiratory tidal volume or rate is no longer able to provide an adequate ventilatory effort. This requires you to immediately begin ventilation with a bag-valve-mask device or other ventilation device. Supplemental oxygen must be delivered through the ventilation device. If a patient with inadequate breathing is not treated promptly, it is likely that he will deteriorate to respiratory arrest.

Respiratory arrest is when the breathing effort ceases completely. Respiratory arrest can lead to cardiac arrest in minutes, if not properly managed, because of a lack of oxygen delivery to the brain and heart. Whether breathing difficulty is caused by trauma or a medical condition, your first priority will be to determine if the patient is in respiratory distress and only in need of oxygen therapy, or if he is in respiratory failure or respiratory arrest where he will need immediate ventilation with a bag-valve mask or other ventilation device and supplemental oxygen.

ASSESSMENT Tips

Respiratory distress patients will have an adequate chest rise (tidal volume) and an adequate respiratory rate. Since both the tidal volume and respiratory rate are adequate, the patient has adequate breathing and is only in need of supplemental oxygen. A patient in *respiratory failure* will have inadequate chest rise (tidal volume) or an inadequate respiratory rate or both. If either tidal volume or respiratory rate is inadequate, the respiratory status is inadequate and the patient needs immediate ventilation. Respiratory failure and respiratory arrest are treated the same way, with positive pressure ventilation and supplemental oxygen. ■

Pathophysiology of Conditions That Cause Respiratory Distress

Many conditions may cause a patient to experience respiratory distress. Even though disease processes differ, the assessment and emergency care are basically the same. It is not your responsibility to diagnose the specific condition or disease causing the respiratory distress; however, you are responsible for identifying the signs and symptoms, determining whether the breathing is adequate or inadequate, anticipating deterioration in the patient's status, and providing immediate intervention as necessary to support adequate respiration.

The following sections discuss the pathophysiology of a variety of diseases that may cause respiratory distress:

- Obstructive pulmonary diseases
  - Emphysema
  - Chronic bronchitis
  - Asthma

Key Terms
hypercarbia increased carbon dioxide levels in the blood. Also called *hypercapnia.*
respiratory distress increased respiratory effort resulting from impaired respiratory function.

Key Terms
respiratory failure inadequate respiratory rate and/or tidal volume.
respiratory arrest complete stoppage of breathing.

- Pneumonia
- Pulmonary embolism
- Pulmonary edema
- Spontaneous pneumothorax
- Hyperventilation syndrome
- Epiglottitis
- Pertussis
- Cystic fibrosis
- Poisonous exposures
- Viral respiratory infections

Obstructive Pulmonary Diseases

Responding to a call for a patient complaining of shortness of breath who has an obstructive pulmonary (lung) disease is common in the prehospital environment (Figure 16-1*). An obstructive lung disease causes an obstruction of airflow through the respiratory tract, leading to a reduction in gas exchange. The most severe consequence of reduced airflow is hypoxia.

The three most commonly encountered obstructive pulmonary diseases are emphysema, chronic bronchitis, and asthma. Emphysema and chronic bronchitis are chronic disease conditions that continue to progress. These patients are typically older and exhibit abnormal lung function and signs and symptoms of the disease continuously (chronically). Thus, emphysema and chronic bronchitis are referred to as chronic obstructive pulmonary disease (COPD) (Figure 16-2*). There is a direct causation between cigarette smoking and environmental toxins and the development of emphysema and chronic bronchitis. You may encounter a COPD patient who has a continuous positive airway pressure (CPAP) or a bilevel positive airway pressure (BiPAP) machine on the bedside stand, which the patient uses with a mask applied over the nose to assist in keeping airway passages open and providing adequate oxygenation while the patient is sleeping. Patients who suffer sleep apnea (periods of nonbreathing during sleep) may also use CPAP or BiPAP machines (Figure 16-3*). (For more extensive information on CPAP and BiPAP, review Chapter 10, "Airway Management, Artificial Ventilation, and Oxygenation.")

Asthma patients are typically younger and, unlike emphysema and chronic bronchitis patients, have near normal or normal lung function between asthma attacks. Therefore, asthma is considered an obstructive pulmonary disease, but is not categorized as a chronic obstructive disease. Asthma, which is thought to be passed on genetically, occurs in response to factors within the body (stress, exercise) and factors found in the environment (allergens, chemical fumes).

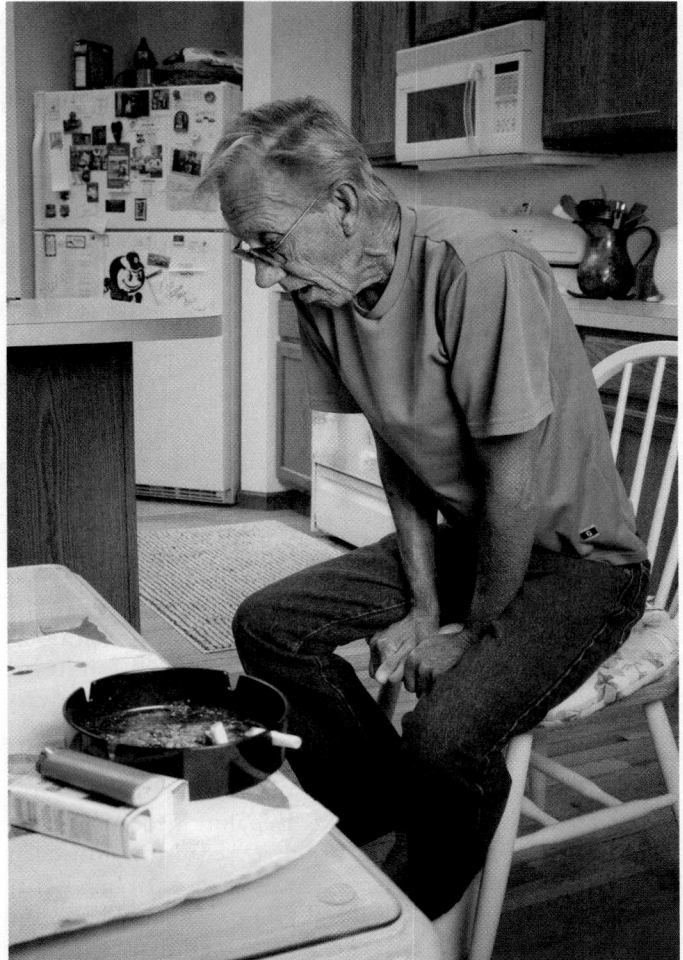

FIGURE 16-1 * Man suffering respiratory distress (indicated by tripod position) from obstructive lung disease.

Emphysema

Emphysema is a permanent disease process that is characterized by destruction of the alveolar walls and distention of the alveolar sacs. It is more common in men than in women. The primary causation factor is cigarette smoking. Persons who are exposed continuously to environmental toxins are also predisposed to developing emphysema.

Key Points
It is not your responsibility to diagnose the specific condition. You are responsible for identifying signs and symptoms, determining if the breathing is adequate or inadequate, anticipating deterioration, and intervening as necessary to support adequate respiration.

Thinking Critically
Since many of the signs and symptoms of emphysema are the same as those for general respiratory distress, how can you determine that the probable etiology for this patient is emphysema, rather than some other cause for his respiratory distress?

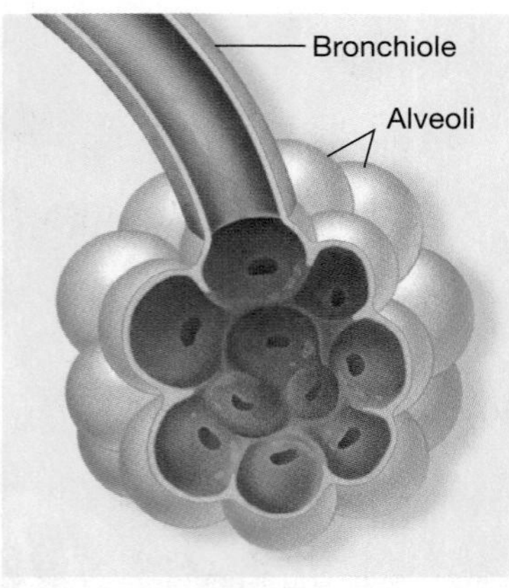

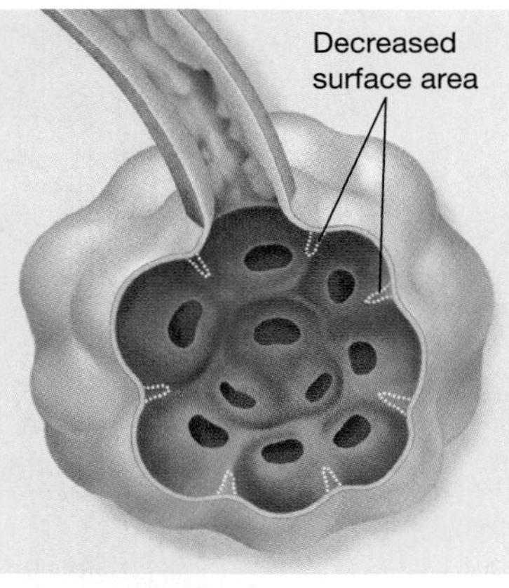

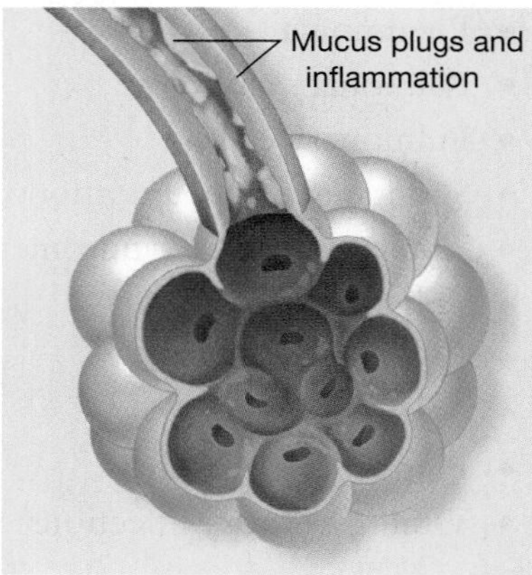

FIGURE 16-2 ✱ Emphysema and chronic bronchitis are chronic obstructive pulmonary diseases.

Pathophysiology In emphysema, the lung tissue loses its elasticity, the alveoli become distended with trapped air, and the walls of the alveoli are destroyed. Loss of the alveolar wall reduces the surface area in contact with pulmonary capillaries. Therefore, a drastic disruption in gas exchange occurs and the patient becomes progressively hypoxic and begins to retain carbon dioxide.

The distal airways also are involved and have a greatly increased airway resistance. Breathing is extremely difficult for the emphysema patient. Exhaling becomes an active rather than a passive process, requiring muscular contraction; therefore, the patient uses most of his energy to breathe. The patient usually complains of extreme shortness of breath upon exertion, which may be simply walking across a room. The loss of lung elasticity and trapping of air cause the chest to increase in diameter, which produces the barrel-chest appearance typical with this disease.

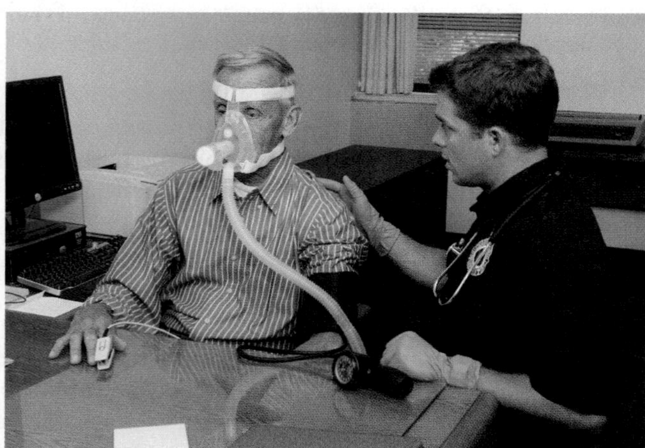

FIGURE 16-3 ✱ CPAP or BiPAP may be used to improve oxygenation.

Assessment Many of the signs and symptoms of emphysema are similar to those listed earlier for respiratory distress and may include the following:

- Thin, barrel-chest appearance
- Coughing, but with little sputum (material that is coughed up)
- Prolonged exhalation
- Diminished breath sounds
- Wheezing and rhonchi (rattles) on auscultation
- Pursed-lip breathing
- Extreme difficulty of breathing on minimal exertion
- Pink complexion (emphysema patients are often called “pink puffers”)
- Tachypnea—breathing rate usually greater than 20 per minute at rest
- Tachycardia (increased heart rate)
- Diaphoresis (sweating; moist skin)
- Tripod position
- May be on home oxygen

Chronic Bronchitis

Chronic bronchitis is a disease process that affects primarily the bronchi and bronchioles. Like emphysema, chronic

Key Points

By definition, chronic bronchitis is characterized by a productive cough that persists for at least three consecutive months a year for at least two consecutive years.

Thinking Critically

What is hypoxic drive? Why do some COPD patients develop it? How should the fact that a COPD patient may be experiencing hypoxic drive affect your decision to administer, or not to administer, oxygen to that patient?

bronchitis is associated with cigarette smoking. By definition, chronic bronchitis is characterized by a productive cough that persists for at least three consecutive months a year for at least two consecutive years.

Pathophysiology Chronic bronchitis involves inflammation, swelling, and thickening of the lining of the bronchi and bronchioles and excessive mucus production. The alveoli remain unaffected by the disease; however, the inflamed and swollen bronchioles and thick mucus restrict airflow to the alveoli so that they do not expand fully, causing respiratory distress and possible hypoxia. Recurrent infections leave scar tissue that further narrows the airway. Like emphysema patients, patients with chronic bronchitis begin to retain carbon dioxide.

A major problem with chronic bronchitis is the swelling and thickening of the lining of the lower airways and an increase in mucus production. The airways become very narrow, causing a high resistance to air movement and chronic difficulty in breathing.

Assessment The following are signs and symptoms of chronic bronchitis:

- Typically overweight
- Chronic cyanotic complexion (chronic bronchitis patients are often called "blue bloaters")
- Difficulty in breathing, but less prominent than with emphysema
- Vigorous productive chronic cough with sputum (material that is coughed up)
- Coarse rhonchi usually heard upon auscultation of the lungs
- Wheezes and, possibly, crackles at the bases of the lungs

This patient frequently suffers from respiratory infections that lead to more acute episodes.

Emergency Medical Care for Emphysema and Chronic Bronchitis Emergency care for the patient with emphysema and chronic bronchitis follows the same guidelines as for any patient suffering from difficulty in breathing. Ensuring an open airway and adequate breathing, position of comfort, and administration of supplemental oxygen are key elements in managing these patients. The patient may also have a prescribed metered-dose inhaler or small-volume nebulizer.

COPD patients may develop a hypoxic drive. Normally, the body's respiratory receptors respond to rising carbon dioxide levels to stimulate breathing. In some COPD patients, constantly high carbon dioxide levels in the blood from poor gas exchange cause the respiratory receptors to respond, instead, to low levels of oxygen. Theoretically, if high concentrations of oxygen are administered to the patient, the receptors pick up the increased oxygen level in the blood and send signals to the respiratory control center to reduce or even stop breathing. This usually occurs when high concentrations of oxygen are administered over a long period of time, but can occur over a short period of time, especially in the chronic bronchitis patient.

In the prehospital setting, this is a rare event and is not a major concern. Oxygen administration should take precedence over a concern about whether the hypoxic drive is going to be lost and cause the patient to stop breathing. (If this should happen, you would initiate positive pressure ventilation with supplemental oxygen, as for any patient with inadequate ventilation.)

If you have categorized the COPD patient as being a high priority, if respiratory distress is evident, and if trauma, shock, cardiac compromise, or other potentially life-threatening conditions exist, high concentrations of oxygen should be delivered by a nonrebreather mask at 15 lpm. If the patient is not in significant distress or is not a priority patient, medical direction may order you to place the patient on a nasal cannula at 2–3 liters per minute. Since many COPD patients are on home oxygen, you may be advised to apply a nasal cannula at the same liter flow or possibly 1 lpm higher than the home oxygen setting. Follow local protocol or medical direction's order for oxygen administration in the COPD patient. *As a general rule, never withhold oxygen from any patient who requires it.* If your protocol allows, in severe cases of respiratory distress consider the use of continuous positive airway pressure (CPAP). (See Chapter 10, "Airway Management, Artificial Ventilation, and Oxygenation.")

Asthma

Asthma is a common respiratory condition that you may be called to the scene to manage. The most common complaint of the asthma patient is severe shortness of breath. Many asthma patients are aware of their condition and have medication to manage the disease and its signs and symptoms. You may be called to the scene for a patient who is suffering an early-onset asthma attack or one in which the patient's medication is not reversing the attack.

Pathophysiology Asthma is characterized by an increased sensitivity of the lower airways to irritants and allergens, causing bronchospasm, which is a diffuse, reversible narrowing of the bronchioles, as well as inflammation to the lining of the bronchioles. The following conditions in the asthma patient contribute to the increasing resistance to airflow and difficulty in breathing (Figure 16-4*):

- Bronchospasm (constriction of the smooth muscle in the bronchioles)
- Edema (swelling) of the inner lining in the airways
- Increased secretion of mucus that causes plugging of the smaller airways

Asthma patients usually suffer acute, irregular, periodic attacks, but between the attacks they usually have either no or very few signs or symptoms. A prolonged life-threatening attack that produces inadequate breathing and severe signs and symptoms is called *status asthmaticus.* Status asthmaticus is a severe asthmatic attack that does not respond to either oxygen or medication. Patients in status asthmaticus require immediate and rapid transport to the hospital. Consider requesting ALS backup.

There are generally two kinds of asthma. Extrinsic asthma, or "allergic" asthma, usually results from a reaction to dust, pollen, smoke, or other irritants in the air. It is typically seasonal, occurs most often in children, and may subside after adolescence. Intrinsic, or "nonallergic," asthma is most common in adults and usually results from infection, emotional stress, or strenuous exercise.

In asthma, the smaller bronchioles have a tendency to collapse when the lungs recoil; therefore, exhalation is much more difficult and prolonged, and air becomes trapped in the alveoli. Because of this, wheezing is heard much earlier upon exhalation. The patient is forced to use energy not only to breathe in but also to eliminate the air from the lungs during exhalation. Thus, exhalation becomes an active process requiring energy that leads to increased breathing workload and eventual exhaustion. Respiratory depression or arrest may shortly follow in severe cases. The loss of wheezing may be an ominous sign of severe bronchoconstriction and deterioration.

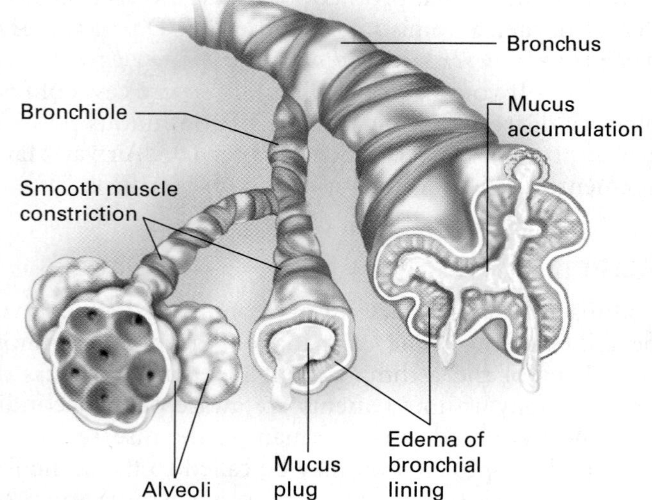

FIGURE 16-4 * Conditions contributing to airflow resistance in asthma.

Assessment The following are signs and symptoms of asthma:

- Dyspnea (shortness of breath); may progressively worsen
- Nonproductive cough
- Wheezing on auscultation (typically expiratory)
- Tachypnea (breathing faster than normal)
- Tachycardia (increased heart rate beyond normal)
- Anxiety and apprehension
- Possible fever
- Typical allergic signs and symptoms: runny nose, sneezing, red or bloodshot eyes, stuffy nose
- Chest tightness
- Inability to sleep
- $SpO_2 < 95\%$ before oxygen administration

The following signs indicate an extremely severe condition with inadequate breathing. Begin positive pressure ventilation with supplemental oxygen:

- Extreme fatigue or exhaustion; the patient is too tired to breathe
- Inability to speak
- Cyanosis to the core of the body
- Heart rate > 150 beats per minute or a slow rate
- Quiet or absent breath sounds on auscultation of the lungs ("silent chest")
- Tachypnea (respiratory rate > 32 breaths per minute)
- Excessive diaphoresis
- Accessory muscle use (neck, chest, abdomen)
- Confusion
- $SpO_2 < 90\%$ with patient on oxygen

Emergency Medical Care During the primary assessment, you would have established and maintained an airway, applied oxygen or begun positive pressure ventilation with supplemental oxygen, and assessed the adequacy of circulation. When providing positive pressure ventilation to a patient suffering a severe asthma attack, the increase in resistance in the bronchioles will make ventilation more difficult to perform. The person operating the bag-valve mask will feel significant resistance when squeezing the bag. Watch for chest rise when providing ventilation to determine the necessary volume and pressure needed to effectively ventilate the patient. You must allow sufficient time for exhalation. Aggressive positive pressure ventilation may increase the amount of air trapped in the alveoli, increasing the pressure inside the chest and causing lung injury. High pressure will also result in reduced cardiac output. Deliver the ventilation with a bag-valve-mask device at a slower rate of 10 times per minute.

During the physical exam, it is necessary to calm the patient to reduce his workload of breathing and oxygen consumption. If the patient has a prescribed metered-dose inhaler or small-volume nebulizer, administration of the beta agonist medication should provide some relief of the breathing difficulty. If your protocol allows, in severe cases of respiratory distress consider the use of continuous positive airway pressure (CPAP). (See Chapter 10, "Airway Management, Artificial Ventilation, and Oxygenation.")

Transport the patient, and continuously reassess the breathing status.

Other Conditions That Cause Respiratory Distress

Pneumonia

Pneumonia is a common cause of death in the United States, especially in the elderly. Patients infected with the human immunodeficiency virus (HIV) and others who are on immunosuppressive drugs, such as transplant patients, are also very prone to pneumonia. Additional risk factors include cigarette smoking, alcoholism, and exposure to cold temperatures.

Pathophysiology Pneumonia is primarily an acute infectious disease, caused by bacterium or a virus that affects the lower respiratory tract and causes lung inflammation and fluid- or pus-filled alveoli (Figure 16-5∗). This leads to poor gas exchange and eventual hypoxia. Pneumonia can also be caused by inhalation of toxic irritants or aspiration of vomitus and other substances.

Assessment The signs and symptoms of pneumonia vary with the cause and the patient's age. The patient generally appears ill and may complain of fever and severe chills. Look for the following signs and symptoms:

- Malaise and decreased appetite
- Fever (may not occur in the elderly)
- Cough—may be productive or nonproductive
- Dyspnea (less frequent in the elderly)
- Tachypnea and tachycardia
- Chest pain—sharp and localized and usually made worse when breathing deeply or coughing
- Decreased chest wall movement and shallow respirations
- Splinting of thorax by patient with his arm
- Crackles, localized wheezing, and rhonchi heard on auscultation
- Altered mental status, especially in the elderly
- Diaphoresis
- Cyanosis
- $SpO_2 < 95\%$

Emergency Medical Care The pneumonia patient is managed no differently from any patient having difficulty in breathing. Ensure adequate oxygenation and breathing. This is an acute infectious disease process that is not usually associated with severe bronchoconstriction, unless it occurs as a complication of asthma or COPD. Therefore, you would not expect the patient to have a metered-dose inhaler or small-volume nebulizer for this condition, nor would you necessarily consider their use unless indications of bronchoconstriction are present. Consult medical direction and follow your local protocol for the use of the metered-dose inhaler or small-volume nebulizer.

Pulmonary Embolism

In pulmonary embolism, an obstruction of blood flow in the pulmonary arteries leads to hypoxia. Patients at risk

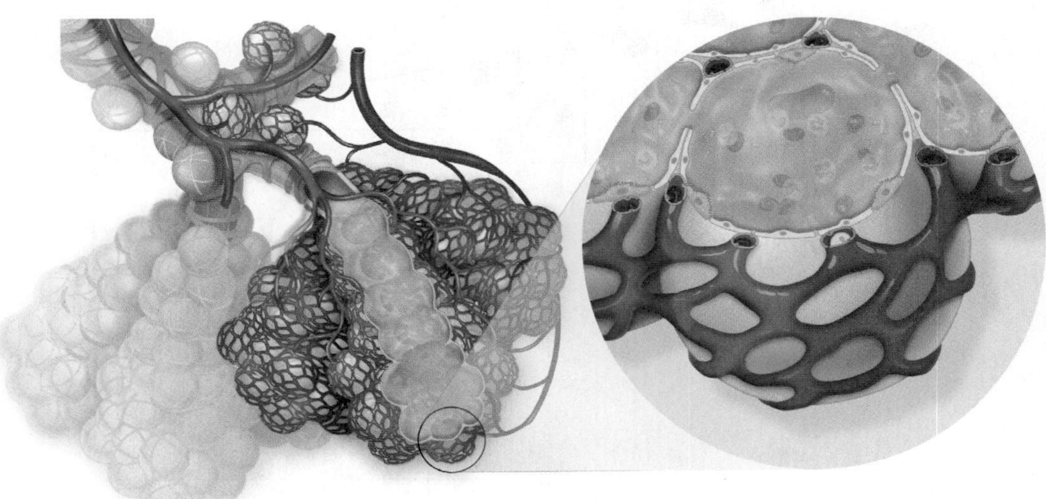

FIGURE 16-5 ∗ Pathophysiology of pneumonia.

for suffering a pulmonary embolism are those who experience long periods of immobility (such as bedridden individuals, those who travel for a long period confined in one position, those with splints to extremities) as well as those with heart disease, recent surgery, long-bone fractures, venous pooling associated with pregnancy, cancer, deep vein thrombosis (development of clots in the veins, most commonly in the legs), estrogen therapy, clotting disorders, history of previous pulmonary embolism, and those who smoke.

Pathophysiology Pulmonary embolism is a sudden blockage of blood flow through a pulmonary artery or one of its branches. The embolism is usually caused by a blood clot, but it may also be caused by an air bubble, a fat particle, a foreign body, or amniotic fluid (Figure 16-6*). The embolism prevents blood from flowing to the lung. As a result, some areas of the lung have oxygen in the alveoli but are not receiving any blood flow. This leads to a decrease in gas exchange and subsequent hypoxia, the severity of which depends on the size of the embolism or the number of alveoli affected.

Assessment Signs and symptoms of pulmonary embolism depend on the size of the obstruction. If a clot obstructs a large artery, gas exchange will be severely impaired and signs and symptoms of respiratory distress will be evident. Suspect pulmonary embolism in any person with a sudden onset of unexplained dyspnea and chest pain (typically sharp and localized to a specific area of the chest) and signs of hypoxia, but who has normal breath sounds and adequate volume. The following are signs and symptoms of pulmonary embolism:

- Sudden onset of unexplained dyspnea
- Signs of difficulty in breathing or respiratory distress; rapid breathing
- Sudden onset of sharp, stabbing chest pain
- Cough (may cough up blood)
- Tachypnea
- Tachycardia
- Syncope (fainting)
- Cool, moist skin
- Restlessness, anxiety, or sense of doom
- Decrease in blood pressure or hypotension (late sign)
- Cyanosis (may be severe) (late sign)
- Distended neck veins (late sign)
- Crackles
- Fever
- $SpO_2 < 95\%$
- Signs of complete circulatory collapse

It is important to note that not all of the signs and symptoms will always be present with pulmonary embolism. The three most common are chest pain, dyspnea, and tachypnea (rapid breathing).

ASSESSMENT Tips

In any patient complaining of shortness of breath, assess for pain, redness, increased warmth, and swelling to the lower leg, especially at the calf. These are signs of a deep vein thrombosis (DVT), a blood clot in a vein of the lower leg that may have broken free, traveled to the lungs, and caused a pulmonary embolism. ■

Emergency Medical Care During the primary assessment, you would have opened the airway and would have initiated positive pressure ventilation with supplemental

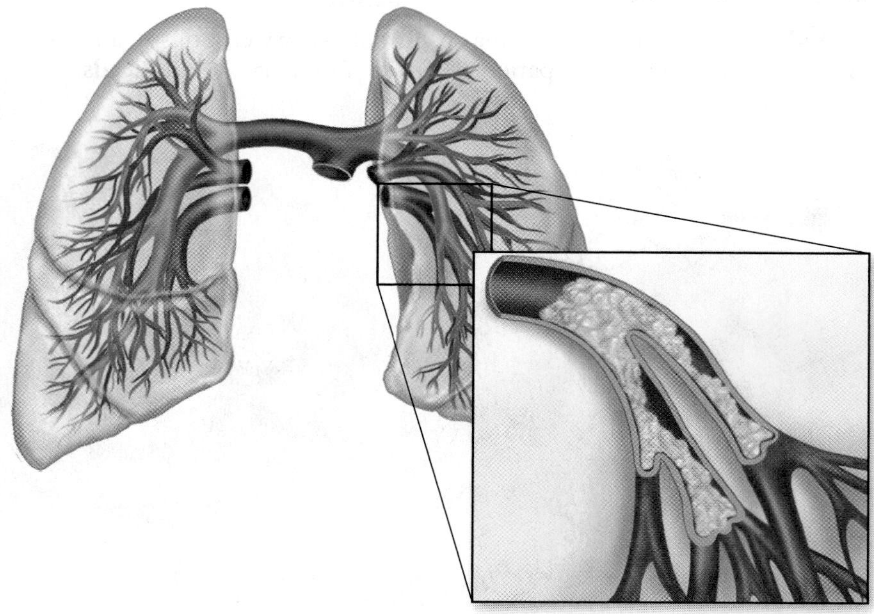

FIGURE 16-6 * A blood clot, air bubble, fat particle, foreign body, or amniotic fluid can cause an embolism, blocking blood flow through a pulmonary artery.

oxygen or applied oxygen by nonrebreather mask. It is important to begin oxygen administration early on and to continuously monitor the patient for signs of respiratory arrest. Immediately transport the patient.

Acute Pulmonary Edema

Pulmonary edema is most frequently seen in patients with cardiac dysfunction leading to congestive heart failure. Other disease processes could also lead to pulmonary edema. The most significant problem associated with pulmonary edema is hypoxia.

Pathophysiology Acute pulmonary edema occurs when an excessive amount of fluid collects in the spaces between the alveoli and the capillaries (Figure 16-7*). This intrusion of fluid disturbs normal gas exchange and leads to hypoxia.

There are two kinds of pulmonary edema: cardiogenic and noncardiogenic. Cardiogenic pulmonary edema is typically related to an inadequate pumping function of the heart that drastically increases the pressure in the pulmonary capillaries, which in turn forces fluid to leak into the space between the alveoli and capillaries and, eventually, into the alveoli themselves.

Noncardiogenic pulmonary edema, also known as acute respiratory distress syndrome (ARDS), results from destruction of the capillary bed that allows fluid to leak out. Common causes of noncardiogenic pulmonary edema are severe pneumonia, aspiration of vomitus, submersion, narcotic overdose, inhalation of smoke or other toxic gases, ascent to a high altitude, and trauma. The causes may differ, but the signs and symptoms are the same.

Assessment The following are signs and symptoms of pulmonary edema:

- Dyspnea, especially on exertion
- Difficulty in breathing when lying flat (orthopnea)
- Frothy sputum
- Tachycardia
- Anxiety, apprehension, combativeness, confusion
- Tripod position with legs dangling
- Fatigue
- Crackles and possibly wheezing on auscultation
- Cyanosis or dusky-color skin
- Pale, moist skin
- Distended neck veins (cardiogenic cause only)
- Swollen lower extremities (cardiogenic cause only)
- Cough
- Symptoms of cardiac compromise (cardiogenic cause only)
- $SpO_2 < 95\%$

ASSESSMENT Tips

Crackles (also called rales) are a sign of pulmonary edema. Be sure to auscultate the posterior lower lobes of the lungs to pick up early indications of crackles and pulmonary edema. If you only auscultate the upper lobes, you may easily miss the condition, since gravity pulls the fluid downward into the lower portions of the lungs. ■

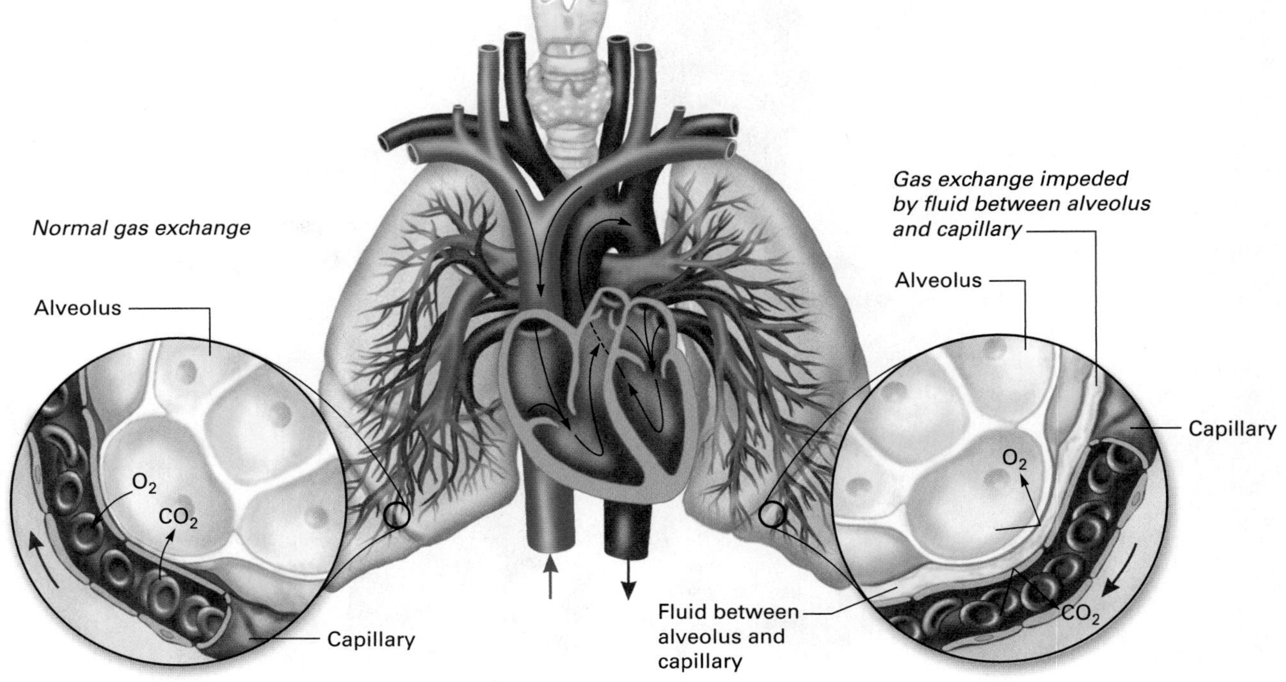

FIGURE 16-7 * Fluid that collects between the alveoli and capillaries, preventing normal exchange of oxygen and carbon dioxide. The fluid may also invade the alveolar sacs.

Emergency Medical Care It is necessary to carefully assess the patient with pulmonary edema. If there is any evidence of inadequate breathing, you need to begin positive pressure ventilation with supplemental oxygen. Even if the patient is still awake and able to talk to you, if the breathing status is inadequate it is vital that you begin ventilation. The positive pressure ventilation will force the oxygen across the alveoli and into the capillaries, which will improve oxygenation and the patient's condition. Explain to the patient what you are doing and why. If your protocol allows, in severe cases of respiratory distress consider the use of continuous positive airway pressure (CPAP). (See Chapter 10, "Airway Management, Artificial Ventilation, and Oxygenation.")

If the breathing is adequate, administer oxygen via nonrebreather mask at 15 lpm and closely monitor the breathing status. Keep the patient in an upright sitting position and transport without delay.

Spontaneous Pneumothorax

A spontaneous pneumothorax is a sudden rupture of a portion of the visceral lining of the lung, not caused by trauma, that causes the lung to partially collapse. Males are five times more likely to suffer a spontaneous pneumothorax than females. Most of these males are tall, thin, lanky, and between the ages of 20 and 40. Many also have a history of cigarette smoking or a connective tissue disorder such as Marfan syndrome or Ehlers-Danlos syndrome. Patients with a history of COPD are more prone to spontaneous pneumothorax as a result of areas of weakened lung tissue called blebs.

Pathophysiology In spontaneous pneumothorax, a portion of the visceral pleura ruptures without any trauma having been applied to the chest. This allows air to enter the pleural cavity, disrupting its normally negative pressure and causing the lung to collapse. The lung collapse causes a disturbance in gas exchange and can lead to hypoxia. It is thought that the reason tall, thin, lanky males are more likely to suffer a spontaneous pneumothorax is that the visceral pleura is stretched within the chest cavity beyond its normal limit. Often the stretched and weakened area ruptures when the patient experiences an increase in intrathoracic pressure from an activity such as coughing, lifting a heavy object, or straining (Figure 16-8*).

Assessment A key finding in spontaneous pneumothorax is a sudden onset of shortness of breath without any evidence of trauma to the chest and with decreased breath sounds upon assessment. The signs and symptoms of a spontaneous pneumothorax are as follows:

- Sudden onset of shortness of breath
- Sudden onset of sharp chest pain or shoulder pain
- Decreased breath sounds to one side of the chest (most often heard first at the apex, or top, of lung)
- Subcutaneous emphysema (may be found)

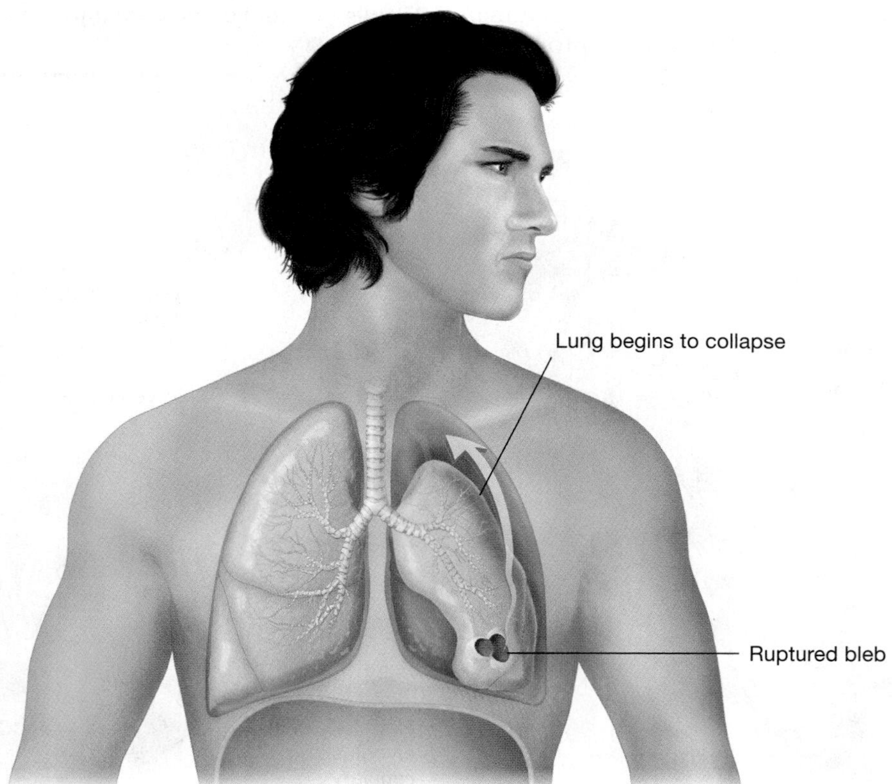

FIGURE 16-8 * A ruptured bleb, or weakened area of lung tissue, causes a spontaneous pneumothorax in which air enters the pleural cavity and travels upward, beginning collapse of the lung from the top.

- Tachypnea
- Diaphoresis
- Pallor
- Cyanosis (may be seen late and in a large pneumothorax)
- $SpO_2 < 95\%$

ASSESSMENT Tips

If a patient presents with a sudden onset of shortness of breath with decreased breath sounds to one side of the chest and no evidence of trauma, you should suspect a possible spontaneous pneumothorax. ■

Emergency Medical Care The patient with a spontaneous pneumothorax requires supplemental oxygen. If the breathing is adequate, apply a nonrebreather mask at 15 lpm. If inadequate breathing is present, it is necessary to provide positive pressure ventilation. Positive pressure ventilation in a patient suffering from a pneumothorax must be performed with great care, since the pneumothorax could easily be converted into a tension pneumothorax (air entering the pleural cavity that cannot escape, eventually causing lung collapse). Use the most minimal tidal volume necessary to ventilate the patient effectively. If cyanosis, hypotension, and significant resistance to ventilation occur, suspect a tension pneumothorax. The pulse oximeter reading will also decline severely with the development of a tension pneumothorax. Contact ALS backup if you suspect a tension pneumothorax.

Hyperventilation Syndrome

Hyperventilation syndrome is frequently encountered in the prehospital setting. It is commonly associated with situations in which the patient is emotionally upset or very excited. Patients suffering "panic attacks" will also suffer from hyperventilation syndrome. Although hyperventilation syndrome is most often associated with an anxious patient, it is important to recognize that hyperventilation syndrome can be caused by a serious medical problem. Therefore, always consider an underlying medical cause of hyperventilation syndrome when assessing and providing emergency medical care.

Pathophysiology The hyperventilation syndrome patient is often anxious and experiences the feeling of not being able to catch his breath. The patient then begins to breathe faster and deeper, causing many of the signs and symptoms of hyperventilation to occur. The true hyperventilation syndrome patient begins to "blow off" excessive amounts of carbon dioxide. A certain level of carbon dioxide is necessary for the body to function normally. When too much carbon dioxide has been eliminated through rapid breathing, the patient begins to experience worsened signs and symptoms of hyperventilation syndrome. The patient becomes more anxious because of the symptoms, and breathes even faster. One result is that the amount of calcium in the body decreases, causing the muscles of the feet and hands to cramp.

Assessment Most often, the patient with true hyperventilation syndrome will be found in an emotionally charged situation that is producing an anxious state in the patient. The following are signs and symptoms of hyperventilation syndrome:

- Fatigue
- Nervousness and anxiety
- Dizziness
- Shortness of breath
- Chest tightness
- Numbness and tingling around the mouth, hands, and feet
- Tachypnea
- Tachycardia
- Spasms of the fingers and feet causing them to cramp (carpopedal spasm)
- May precipitate seizures in a patient with a seizure disorder

Understanding BODY PROCESSES

The light-headedness, dizziness, or fainting experienced by the hyperventilating patient is caused by a drastic reduction of carbon dioxide (the rapid breathing blows off excessive amounts of carbon dioxide). This causes the cerebral arteries to constrict excessively, reducing blood flow to the brain tissue, causing the light-headedness, dizziness, and fainting. ■

Emergency Medical Care The primary management is to get the patient to calm down and slow his breathing. Remove the patient from the source of anxiety or remove the source of anxiety from the scene, if possible. For example, if the scene involves a domestic dispute, removing the other person involved in the dispute may calm the patient. Instruct the patient to consciously slow down his rate of breathing and the amount of air he is breathing. One technique is to have the patient close his mouth and breathe through his nose. You may need to coach the patient to help him slow his rate of breathing.

Do not have the patient breathe into a paper bag or oxygen mask not connected to oxygen to allow him to rebreathe carbon dioxide. These techniques can be fatal if the patient has a true underlying medical condition that is causing the hyperventilation syndrome. Only use a carbon dioxide rebreathing technique if no underlying medical conditions exist and you are specifically instructed by medical direction to do so. Keep in mind that conditions such as pulmonary embolism and myocardial infarction can present very similarly to hyperventilation syndrome. These are two of the conditions in which rebreathing carbon dioxide could be fatal.

In the prehospital setting, it is more common to apply oxygen to the patient. Apply a pulse oximeter to measure the oxygen content of the blood. Never withhold oxygen to a patient.

Epiglottitis

Epiglottitis, an inflammation affecting the upper airway, can be an acute, severe, life-threatening condition if left untreated. Although its incidence is low (estimates are between 10 and 40 cases per million people in the United States), the EMT should always be prepared to handle it because of its potential severity. Conditions that can cause epiglottitis include infectious, chemical, and traumatic agents. In previous years, the most common cause for epiglottitis was *Haemophilus influenzae* type B, and this emergency was almost exclusive to children; however, with the advent of the Hib vaccination, the incidence in children has dropped dramatically. Currently, other organisms such as viruses, fungi, and bacteria are the causes, especially among adults.

Pathophysiology As you recall, the epiglottis is a triangular cartilaginous structure that attaches at its base and closes over the glottic opening (opening to the larynx) during swallowing to prevent food or liquid from getting into the trachea. In certain situations, the epiglottis and base of the tongue can become inflamed. As this progresses, the epiglottis and the structures connected to or immediately surrounding it become inflamed and swollen, leading to a compromised airway and resultant respiratory compromise (Figure 16-9*). If untreated, this partial-to-complete airway obstruction leads to ineffective gas exchange in the lungs, hypoxia, acidosis, and eventually death.

Assessment The following are signs and symptoms of epiglottitis:

- Dyspnea, usually with a more rapid onset
- High fever (although it can occur with only mild fevers)
- Sore throat
- Inability to swallow with drooling
- Anxiety and apprehension
- Tripod position, usually with jaw jutted forward
- Fatigue
- High-pitched inspiratory stridor
- Cyanosis or dusky-color skin
- Trouble speaking
- $SpO_2 < 95\%$

ASSESSMENT Tips

Inspiratory stridor is an indication of an almost completely occluded airway. It is created when the patient breathes in sharply in order to draw air past the airway obstruction. As air passes through the narrowed glottic opening, airflow becomes turbulent and it creates the high-pitched sound. If the inspiratory stridor disappears and your patient's mental status continues to deteriorate, it probably means that total airway occlusion has occurred. ■

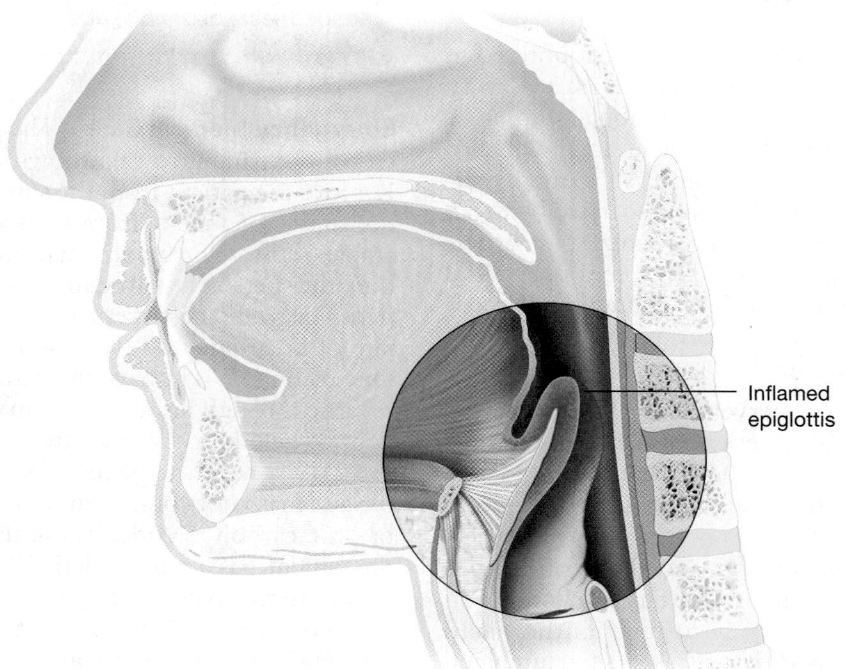

FIGURE 16-9 * Pathophysiology of epiglottitis.

Emergency Medical Care Treatment of epiglottitis is focused on ensuring oxygenation and preventing airway obstruction. If the patient's breathing is still adequate, the first step is administration of high-concentration oxygen at 15 lpm. In addition, and especially for the younger patient, maintaining a calm and quiet environment will help the patient to remain calm, and lessen the burden of respiratory distress. Keep the patient in a position that is comfortable to him, and expedite transport with ALS intercept if possible.

There is absolutely no need to force an inspection of the airway so long as the patient is adequately exchanging air, and it should not be attempted. Any additional irritation to the inflamed epiglottis may result in additional swelling that totally occludes the airway. In fact, attempting airway maneuvers in a patient with epiglottitis is only warranted in those extreme cases of respiratory occlusion from the swollen airway structures.

If the patient continues to deteriorate and requires assisted ventilations with a bag-valve-mask device, squeeze the bag slowly. This will help direct the air past the obstruction and into the lungs rather than into the esophagus to inflate the stomach. If this is not effective in ventilating the patient, it is a situation of complete airway obstruction at the level of the epiglottis, and an ALS provider may need to consider other advanced airway techniques.

Pertussis

Pertussis (also known as "whooping cough") is a respiratory disease that is characterized by uncontrolled coughing. It is a highly contagious disease that affects the respiratory system and is caused by bacteria that reside in the upper airway of an infected person. It is spread by respiratory droplets that are discharged from the nose and mouth during coughing. Pertussis has been found to occur in all age brackets, but it is most reported in children. Generally speaking, the younger the patient, the more severe the clinical condition that develops.

Pathophysiology Pertussis typically starts out seeming very similar to a cold or a mild upper respiratory infection. Because of this, an older patient or the parents of an infant or child may try "waiting it out" before seeking medical care. Thus by the time the patient presents to EMS, the condition may be severe. Within 2 weeks or so of onset, the patient will develop episodes of rapid coughing (15 to 24 episodes in close sequence) as the body attempts to expel thick mucus from the airway, followed by a "crowing" or "whooping" sound made during inhalation as the patient breathes in deeply.

Complications of pertussis include pneumonia, dehydration, seizures, brain injuries, ear infections, and even death. Most deaths occur to younger patients who have not been immunized for this disease, or to those patients who are exposed before finishing the vaccination series. In younger patients, the ongoing and uncontrolled coughing can severely disrupt normal breathing, diminish gas exchange in the alveoli, and promote bacterial pneumonia.

Assessment Signs and symptoms of pertussis are as follows:

- History of upper respiratory infection
- Sneezing, runny nose, low-grade fever
- General malaise (weakness, fatigue, not feeling well)
- Increase in frequency and severity of coughing
- Coughing fits, usually more common at night
- Vomiting
- Inspiratory "whoop" heard at the end of coughing burst
- Possible development of cyanosis during coughing burst
- Diminishing pulse oximetry finding
- Exhaustion from expending energy during coughing burst
- Trouble speaking and breathing (dyspnea) during burst

ASSESSMENT Tips

Pertussis actually has three stages. Stage 1 is characterized by findings consistent with a common cold or upper respiratory infection. In stage 2, coughing continues to worsen to the point that medical care is sought (EMS is summoned), and thus the suspicion for pertussis (whooping cough) is formed. Stage 3 is the recovery stage, and recovery is usually gradual, taking several weeks until a resolution is reached. ■

Emergency Medical Care Treatment of pertussis is similar to the treatment for many other respiratory problems. It is focused on ensuring oxygenation, reversing hypoxemia, and preventing airway obstruction. The patient should remain in a comfortable position, and the EMT should administer high-concentration oxygen at 15 lpm via nonrebreather mask. The EMT should also encourage the patient to expectorate any mucus that is brought up with the coughing. The administration of humidified oxygen may help the mucus become less viscous and be expelled more easily. In addition, the patient will probably be anxious and/or scared, so the EMT should also try to ensure a quiet and calm environment. Expedite transport and consider an ALS intercept.

Finally, remember that this is a very contagious disease, and the EMT should take all precautions necessary to prevent cross-contamination (to include putting a surgical mask on the patient to catch expelled airway droplets), so long as it does not impede the patient's breathing. Following transport of a patient with known or suspected pertussis, consider totally disinfecting the patient compartment of the ambulance.

Cystic Fibrosis

Cystic fibrosis (also known as CF, mucoviscidosis, or mucovoidosis) is a hereditary disease. Although it commonly causes pulmonary dysfunction as a result of changes in the mucus-secreting glands of the lungs, it also affects the sweat glands, the pancreas, the liver, and the intestines.

The pulmonary complications are the most common cause for a patient with this affliction to summon EMS. There is not yet a cure for CF, and many individuals with this disease die at a young age (20s to 30s) as a result of pulmonary failure. In fact, CF is cited as one of the most common life-shortening genetic diseases. Because it is possible to detect CF in a patient at a very young age, it is common for the patient experiencing a crisis to already know of this diagnosis. Fortunately, medical research and treatment is lengthening the life span of some people to as high as 50 years. In terminal stages of the disease, the final medical recourse is lung transplantation when all other interventions have failed.

Pathophysiology Lining most all of the respiratory tree in the body is a layer of tissue that is coated with a mucous lining. This mucous lining is normally watery and helps to warm and humidify inspired air. It also serves to trap any inhaled particles. In cystic fibrosis, however, an abnormal gene alters the functioning of the mucous glands lining the respiratory system and there is an overabundant production of mucus, which is very thick and sticky. As this thick mucus layer develops, there is blockage of the airways as well as an increase in the incidence of lung infections, since bacteria can readily grow in the thick mucus. Repeated lung infections in turn cause scarring of the lung tissue and promote ongoing pulmonary damage. As a result, there is progressive diminishment in the efficiency of respiratory function, which leads to eventual pulmonary failure and death.

Assessment The following are signs and symptoms of cystic fibrosis:

- Commonly a known history of the disease
- Recurrent coughing
- General malaise (weakness, fatigue, not feeling well)
- Expectoration of thick mucus during coughing
- Recurrent episodes or history of pneumonia, bronchitis, and sinusitis
- Gastrointestinal complaints that may include diarrhea and greasy and/or foul-smelling bowel movements
- Abdominal pain from intestinal gas
- Malnutrition or low weight despite a healthy appetite
- Dehydration
- Clubbing of the digits
- Trouble speaking and breathing (dyspnea) with mucus buildup
- Signs of pneumonia

ASSESSMENT Tips

Although the most common complaint patients with CF will have when they present to EMS is difficulty in breathing, many of the other findings are due to dysfunction of other organ systems. The abdominal findings such as dehydration, bowel changes, and poor weight gain are from the damage the disease inflicts on the gastrointestinal tract. Pancreatitis can also cause abdominal pain as does liver damage from the disease. ■

Emergency Medical Care Emergency treatment of a patient suffering from exacerbation of CF is geared toward symptomatic relief of the respiratory distress. If the patient is breathing adequately, he should be provided with high-concentration oxygen at 15 lpm via nonrebreather mask. If the patient is expectorating thick mucus, humidification of the oxygen will help thin the secretions so that expelling them with coughing will become easier. The EMT may also consider administering normal saline through a small-volume nebulizer to aid in this. (Follow local protocol or medical direction.) The patient should remain in a sitting position for comfort and to aid in breathing. Establish ongoing pulse oximetry and, in severe cases, attempt to rendezvous with an ALS unit. If the patient's condition is severe enough that breathing becomes inadequate, the EMT will have to deliver oxygen via positive pressure ventilation.

Poisonous Exposures

Thousands of people die each year from exposures to poisonous substances (Figure 16-10*). *Poisonous inhalation injury* is an umbrella label for any type of inhalation injury that occurs secondary to exposure to toxic substances that can cause airway occlusion and/or pulmonary dysfunction by inhibiting the normal exchange of gases at the cellular level. For example, a patient may

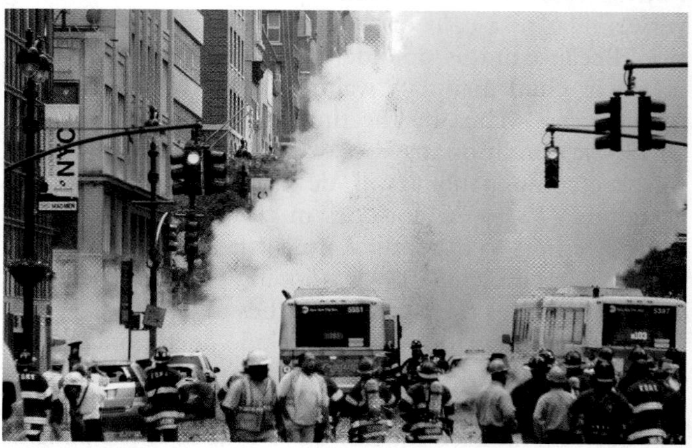

FIGURE 16-10 * Toxic exposure. (© Brendan McDermid/Reuters/Corbis)

be exposed to a volatile chemical through an industrial accident, and this chemical could cause airway edema, alveolar lining damage, or displacement of oxygen. Any of these can result in respiratory failure and death of the patient unless there is immediate and effective treatment.

Pathophysiology The inhalation of any vapors or fumes has the potential for causing some type of compromise to the patient. The majority of toxic inhalation injuries, as will be discussed in Chapter 22, "Toxicologic Emergencies," occur as the result of a fire. Sometimes, though, the toxic exposure may not be evident, since fumes may be present in the environment but undetected by the patient. The first indication of a toxic or poisonous inhalation exposure may be the patient's collapse.

Commonly inhaled poisons that the EMT may be called upon to treat include:

- Carbon monoxide
- Carbon dioxide
- Natural gas
- Chlorine gas
- Liquid chemicals or sprays
- Ammonia
- Sulfur dioxide
- Anesthetic gases
- Solvents
- Industrial gases
- Hydrogen sulfide
- Fumes/smoke from fires
- Paints or Freon
- Glue
- Nitrous oxide
- Amyl or butyl nitrate

These substances can have many effects on the body, as they all lead to cellular hypoxia by some mechanism. They may cause the soft tissue that lines the upper airway to swell to the point that airway occlusion occurs. Some can also cause the displacement of oxygen in the atmosphere and, hence, in the alveoli, also causing hypoxia. The chemicals may be caustic to the point that the alveolar lining is damaged and fluid starts to leak into the alveoli, severely hampering gas exchange. And finally, some inhaled poisons may also exert an action on the body in and of themselves once they cross into the bloodstream. The end result of all these mechanisms, if treatment is delayed, is inadequate cellular respiration, causing cellular death and, in turn, the death of the patient.

Assessment Signs and symptoms of poisonous inhalation injuries are as follows:

- History consistent with an inhalation injury (house fire, industrial accident, and so on)
- The presence of chemicals about the face from the exposure
- Findings of respiratory distress (consistent with either adequate or inadequate breathing)
- Cough, stridor, wheezing, or crackles
- Oral or pharyngeal burns, possible hoarseness
- Dizziness, feelings of malaise
- Headache, confusion, altered mental status
- Seizures
- Cyanosis or other skin color changes
- Nausea, vomiting, abdominal distress/pain
- Copious secretions
- Vital sign changes

ASSESSMENT Tips

Among the most important determinants for patient criticality is the length of exposure to the toxic substance and whether the patient was in an enclosed space. Additionally, exercise great personal caution when entering the scene of a known or potential toxic inhalation unless you are properly trained to do so and protected (i.e., wearing SCBA). ■

Emergency Medical Care Remember that symptoms of respiratory distress are among the most common initial findings consistent with toxic inhalation injuries. The most important primary treatment is to limit the exposure if the patient is still in the toxic environment. Be sure, however, that you can rescue the patient in a manner that is not dangerous to you. If you can't effect a rescue safely, your best action is to remain at a safe distance until properly trained and equipped providers can bring the patient to you.

After ensuring that there is no threat to you, your next goal is to ensure an open airway. If the patient is able to maintain his own airway and there is no associated trauma, place him in a position of comfort. If he is traumatized or unresponsive, place the patient supine and immobilize as needed. Ensure proper oxygenation for the adequately breathing patient by providing oxygen at 15 lpm via nonrebreather mask. If you find the patient is breathing inadequately, provide positive pressure ventilation at a rate of 15 per minute in the adult patient with supplemental oxygen attached. Be sure to properly treat any other injuries or abnormal findings, after ensuring that any compromises to the airway, breathing, and circulatory components are appropriately managed.

Prior to transport, try to ascertain as much information as possible about the inhaled poison for the receiving facility. Because of the criticality of the patient or the potential for rapid deterioration, try to arrange an ALS intercept en route to the receiving facility. Provide early notification to the staff at the receiving facility so they can prepare adequately for your arrival.

Objective 16-9
As allowed by your scope of practice, demonstrate administering or assisting a patient with self-administration of bronchodilators by metered-dose inhaler and/or small-volume nebulizer.

Key Terms
metered-dose inhaler (MDI) device consisting of a plastic container and a canister of medication that is used to form an aerosolized medication that a patient can inhale.

Viral Respiratory Infections

As its name indicates, a viral respiratory infection (VRI) is a condition of the respiratory system caused by a virus. Common VRIs include bronchiolitis, colds, and the flu. In most situations for adults, VRIs are fairly mild, self-limiting, and confined to the upper respiratory system. In children, however, the infection has a greater propensity to spread into the lower airways where more significant infections can occur that will result in patient deterioration.

Pathophysiology Viral respiratory infections are commonly referred to as upper respiratory infections (URIs) by the medical community because the majority of symptoms are found in the nose and throat. In small children, however, VRIs can also cause infections of the lower airway structures such as the trachea, bronchi, bronchioles, or lungs. When an infection involves these lower airway structures, depending on site, the patient may be diagnosed with croup, bronchiolitis, or pneumonia. (See Chapter 38, "Pediatrics," for a discussion of these conditions.)

Known viruses that can cause VRIs include rhinoviruses, parainfluenza and influenza viruses, enteroviruses, respiratory syncytial virus (RSV), and some strains of the adenovirus. These viruses gain entry into the body by way of patient-to-patient contact or, to a lesser extent, through inhalation of respiratory droplets. The major pathophysiology of these viruses is exerted by triggering an inflammatory process with increased mucus production to the upper respiratory structures. There may also be a fever associated with the infection, coughing, runny nose, and findings of mild respiratory distress in the majority of cases. The VRI typically runs its course in about 14 days and, unless extenuating circumstances are present (e.g., a secondary respiratory infection of the lower airways or severe respiratory distress), rarely requires medical attention.

Assessment It is, of course, nearly impossible (nor is it practical) for the EMT to determine if findings of respiratory distress are caused by a VRI or not. There are also no specific treatments for viral infections that the EMT can administer. The mainstay of emergency treatment for respiratory distress secondary to a VRI is supportive.

The following are signs and symptoms of viral respiratory infections:

- Nasal congestion
- Sore or scratchy throat
- Mild respiratory distress, coughing
- Fever (usually around 101°F–102°F)
- Malaise
- Headaches and body aches
- Irritability in infants and poor feeding habits
- Tachypnea
- Exacerbation of asthma if patient is asthmatic

ASSESSMENT Tips

As stated previously, most people do not seek medical attention or summon EMS for a typical VRI because the minimal clinical findings are usually easily treated with over-the-counter cold medications for symptomatic relief. However, if the patient's condition and findings of respiratory distress are severe enough to call EMS, chances are that the infection has spread into the lower airways and is starting to impinge upon normal oxygenation by the lungs. ■

Emergency Medical Care The majority of cases of VRI do not present to EMS because the clinical presentation is confined to nasal and pharyngeal discomfort. In the susceptible patient, however, there may be the presence of concurrent lower tract infections that can cause some degree of respiratory distress. In all but the most severe (and uncommon) of cases, supportive treatment of positioning, oxygen therapy, emotional support, and gentle transport to the hospital is all that is necessary.

If the infection is allowed to persist without medical attention and it develops into a more serious viral infection (especially for the very young or very old), high-concentration oxygen and, occasionally, mechanical ventilation may become warranted. Despite the often minimal presentation, the EMT should always maintain a high index of suspicion for deterioration in a patient who does not respond favorably to supportive measures. As needed, contact ALS for potential medication administration in patients with obvious or potential deterioration.

Metered-Dose Inhalers and Small-Volume Nebulizers

A medication commonly prescribed for the patient with a chronic history of breathing problems is a beta$_2$-specific bronchodilator that comes in a **metered-dose inhaler**

Key Terms
small-volume nebulizer a device that uses compressed air or oxygen to nebulize a liquid medication into a mist that a patient can inhale.

Key Terms
spacer a chamber that is connected to the metered-dose inhaler to collect the medication until it is inhaled.

(MDI) or that can, alternatively, be administered from a **small-volume nebulizer (SVN)**. The medication is dispensed as an aerosol, or mist, that the patient inhales. If the patient has an MDI, the medication is already contained in the device, ready to be dispensed in aerosol form. If the patient, instead, uses an SVN, the liquid medication must be placed into the device where compressed air or oxygen converts it into an aerosol mist. Most people who use prescribed bronchodilator medications will have an MDI, rather than an SVN, because the MDI is more convenient for the patient to use. SVNs are more commonly used in hospital settings, but some patients with chronic conditions will have an SVN for use at home. There are a variety of bronchodilator medications that can be prescribed. These medications can only be administered with the on-line or off-line approval of medical direction.

The most common bronchodilators that can be administered by MDI or SVN are listed in Figure 16-11∗. (Note: All of the medications listed may be used in an MDI. Not all of them are suitable for nebulization in an SVN.) They are considered to be beta$_2$ agonists, which mimic the effects of the sympathetic nervous system. (The exception in the list is ipratropium, which is an anticholinergic bronchodilator rather than a beta$_2$ bronchodilator.) These drugs relax the bronchiole smooth muscle, which dilates the airways. This decreases resistance in the airways and improves the movement of air into the alveoli. Most bronchodilators begin to work almost immediately, and their effects may last up to 8 hours or more. Because of the swift relief they can provide, they are appropriate for prehospital administration by the EMT with the approval of medical direction.

Using a Metered-Dose Inhaler

The MDI, also known as an "inhaler" or "puffer," is a simple device that consists of a metal canister and a plastic container with a mouthpiece and cap. The metal canister that contains the medication fits inside the plastic container. When the canister is depressed, it delivers a precise dose of medication for the patient to inhale. The medication is directly deposited on the bronchioles at the site of bronchoconstriction. See the photos in EMT Skills 16-2, which illustrate administering a medication by MDI.

Some MDIs are connected to a device called a **spacer**. The spacer is a chamber that holds the medication until it is inhaled, thus preventing any loss of medication to the outside and allowing a greater amount of the medication to be delivered to the patient. The spacer device is commonly used by patients who have difficulty using the MDI and is a very effective method of delivering the medication. Spacers are increasingly common as a standard in MDI administration. See the photos in EMT Skills 16-3, which illustrate how to administer an MDI with a spacer.

If the patient is having breathing difficulty that is not related to trauma or a chest injury, and has one of the beta$_2$-agonist bronchodilators in an MDI form prescribed to him by a physician, you should contact medical direction for permission to administer the drug or follow local protocols. Instruct your patient as to what he should do, even if he claims to know how to use the MDI. During the administration, you must coach the patient to breathe in slowly and deeply, to hold his breath as long as he comfortably can, and to breathe out slowly through pursed lips. If the patient is not instructed or coached, the medication may not be effectively administered. If the patient is unable to follow the procedure, even with coaching, you may need to administer the inhaler to the patient. Table 16-2 lists a series of "dos and don'ts" for administering medication from MDIs.

Using a Small-Volume Nebulizer

Some patients who are prescribed beta$_2$ agonists may use a small-volume nebulizer rather than a metered-dose inhaler to dispense the medication. An SVN is a device that has a drug reservoir into which the patient places the beta$_2$ medication in liquid form. The device is then attached to a small electrical compressor that delivers compressed air to the nebulizer by tubing. As an alternative, the supply tubing for the nebulizer can be attached to an oxygen source with the regulator set at 8–10 lpm. As the compressed air or oxygen enters the SVN, it nebulizes the medication (creates a mist) that the patient inhales by way of a mouthpiece attached to the top of the device. (In hospitals and some home settings, the mist may be delivered through a face mask instead of a mouthpiece.)

With an SVN, the patient will continue to inhale the fine mist laden with the medication over a period of time, until the misting stops, rather than in a short measured burst as occurs with the MDI. As with the MDI, the inhaled medication is deposited directly on the bronchiole tissue to promote relaxation. This method of delivery is neither better nor worse than an MDI; it is simply an alternative way of inhaling the medication. Refer to the photos in EMT Skills 16-4 to review the procedure for administration by SVN. The indications for administration, how to coach the patient during medication administration, and

Metered-Dose Inhaler (MDI) / Small-Volume Nebulizer (SVN)

Medication Name

Metered-dose inhalers contain medications with a variety of generic and trade names, including the following. (Note: Not all drugs that are packaged as an MDI are available for nebulization.)

Generic Name	Trade Name
Albuterol	Proventil®, Ventolin®
Metaproterenol	Metaprel®, Alupent®
Isoetharine	Bronkosol®
Bitolterol mesylate	Tornalate®
Salmeterol xinafoate	Serevent®
Ipratropium	Atrovent®
Levalbuterol	Xoponex
Pirbuterol	Maxair

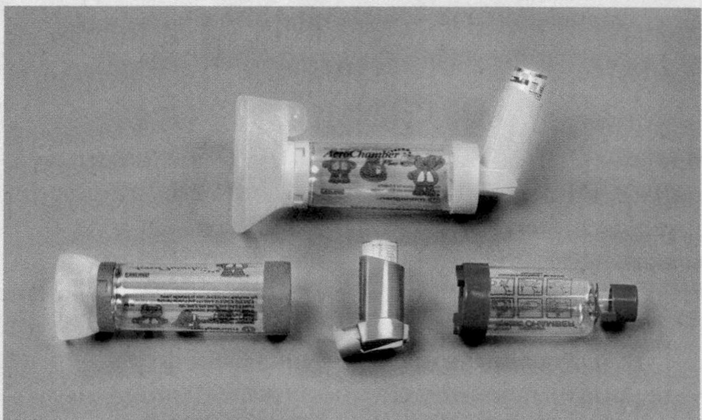

Meter-dosed inhaler.

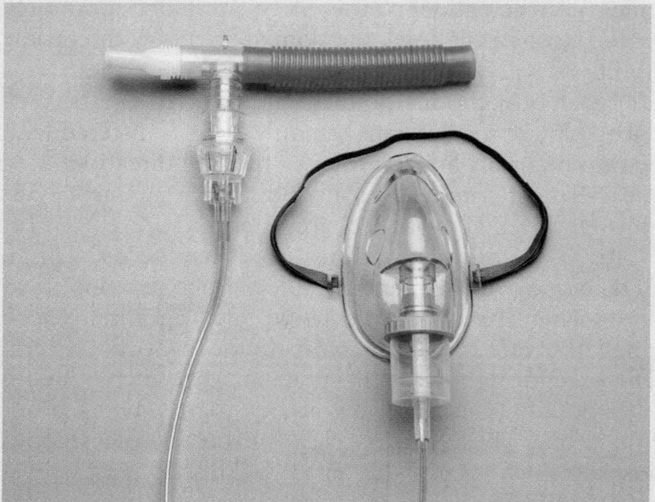

Small-volume nebulizer.
© Carl Leet, YSU

Indications

All of the following criteria must be met before an EMT administers a bronchodilator by metered-dose inhaler (MDI) or small-volume nebulizer (SVN) to a patient:

- The patient exhibits signs and symptoms of breathing difficulty (respiratory distress).
- The patient has a physician-prescribed metered-dose inhaler containing a medication specifically prepared to be delivered by nebulization.
- The EMT has received approval from medical direction, whether on-line or off-line, to administer the medication.

Contraindications

A bronchodilator by MDI or SVN should not be given if any of the following conditions exist:

- The patient is not responsive enough to use the MDI or SVN.
- The MDI or SVN is not prescribed for the patient.
- Medical direction has not granted permission.
- The patient has already taken the maximum allowed dose(s) prior to your arrival.

Medication Forms

Aerosolized medication in an MDI.
Liquid medication packaged to be poured directly into the nebulizer chamber of an SVN (see EMT Skills 16-4C).

Dosage

Each time an MDI is depressed, it delivers a precise dose of medication to the patient. The total number of times the medication can be administered is determined by medical direction. When using an SVN, it usually takes 5–10 minutes for the patient to inhale the medication, depending on the rate and depth of breathing. The medication should be inhaled until the SVN no longer produces a mist.

Administration

To administer a bronchodilator by MDI (EMT Skills 16-2):

1. Ensure right patient, right medication, right dose, right route, and right date. Determine if the patient is alert enough to use the inhaler and if any doses have already been administered prior to your arrival.
2. Obtain an order, either on-line or off-line, from medical direction to assist with the administration of the medication.
3. Ensure that the inhaler is at room temperature or warmer. Shake the canister vigorously for at least 30 seconds.

FIGURE 16-11 ✱ Metered-dose inhaler and small-volume nebulizer.

Metered-Dose Inhaler (MDI) / Small-Volume Nebulizer (SVN)

4. Remove the nonrebreather mask from the patient. Instruct the patient to take the inhaler in his hand and hold it upright. If the patient is unable to hold the device, place your index finger on top of the metal canister and your thumb on the bottom of the plastic container.
5. Have the patient exhale fully.
6. Have the patient place his lips around the mouthpiece (opening) of the inhaler. Another technique is to have the patient open his mouth and place the inhaler 1–1.5 inches from the front of the lips, estimated by two finger widths.
7. Have the patient begin to slowly and deeply inhale over about 5 seconds as he or you depress the canister. Do not depress the canister before the patient begins to inhale. This would allow a majority of the medication to be lost into the air and it will not reach the lower respiratory tract.
8. Remove the inhaler and coach the patient to hold his breath for 10 seconds or as long as comfortable.
9. Have the patient exhale slowly through pursed lips.
10. Replace the oxygen mask on the patient. Reassess the breathing status and baseline vital signs.
11. Reassess the patient and consult with medical direction if additional doses are needed. If an additional dose is recommended, wait at least 2 minutes between each administration or longer based on the medication being administered or medical direction's order.

If using a spacer, follow the same steps with the following exceptions for steps 6 and 7 (EMT Skills 16-3):

6. Remove the spacer cap and attach the inhaler to the spacer.
7. Depress the medication canister to fill the spacer with the medication. As soon as the canister is depressed, have the patient place his lips around the mouthpiece and inhale slowly and deeply. If the inhalation is too fast, the spacer may whistle.

To administer a bronchodilator by SVN (EMT Skills 16-4):

1. Ensure right patient, right medication, right dose, right route, and right date. Determine if the patient is alert enough to use the nebulizer and if any doses have already been administered prior to your arrival.
2. Obtain an order, either on-line or off-line, from medical direction to assist with the administration of the medication.
3. Disassemble the medication chamber from the mouthpiece by unscrewing it. While holding the medication reservoir upright, pour in the medication and reassemble the device.
4. Attach the tubing extending from the bottom of the drug reservoir to the nebulizer compressor and turn it on, or attach the tubing to an oxygen tank with the liter flow set to 8–10 lpm. You should note the mist coming from the mouthpiece almost immediately.
5. Remove the nonrebreather mask from the patient. Instruct the patient to take the nebulizer in his hand and hold it upright. If the patient is unable to hold the device, you may have to do this for the patient, being sure to continuously hold it upright for optimal nebulization of the medication.
6. Have the patient exhale fully.
7. Instruct the patient to place his lips around the mouthpiece of the nebulizer. Another technique is to have the patient open his mouth and place the mouthpiece 1–1.5 inches from the front of the lips, estimated by two finger widths.
8. Have the patient begin to slowly and deeply breathe in the mist.
9. Instruct the patient to occasionally (every 2–3 breaths) hold his breath after inhalation as long as he comfortably can, to assist with medication distribution throughout the respiratory tree.
10. Have the patient exhale normally, and occasionally (every 2–3 breaths) instruct the patient to cough during exhalation to facilitate removal of any mucus or secretions that may be present.
11. You may need to occasionally shake the nebulizer to dislodge any medication that tends to collect on the sides of the drug reservoir. In about 5–10 minutes, the misting of medication should cease and the liquid medication you placed in the nebulizer will be gone. Replace the oxygen mask on the patient.
12. Reassess the patient and consult with medical direction if additional doses are needed. If an additional dose is recommended, wait at least 2 minutes between each administration or longer based on the medication being administered or medical direction's order.

Actions

Beta 2 agonist that relaxes the bronchiole smooth muscle and dilates the lower airways. This reduces the airway resistance and improves airflow into the alveoli.

Side Effects

The side effects associated with the bronchodilator are associated with the drug action itself. The following are common side effects that the patient may complain of or that you may find in your assessment:

- Tachycardia
- Tremors, shakiness
- Nervousness
- Dry mouth
- Nausea, vomiting

continued

FIGURE 16-11 ✱ Metered-dose inhaler and small-volume nebulizer. *continued*

Metered-Dose Inhaler (MDI) / Small-Volume Nebulizer (SVN)

Reassessment

Whenever you administer a bronchodilator to a patient, you must perform a reassessment. The following steps must be included:

- Reassess the vital signs.
- Question the patient about the effect of the medication on the relief of the difficulty in breathing.
- Perform a focused physical exam if changes in the condition or new complaints occur.
- Constantly monitor the airway and breathing status; if the breathing becomes inadequate, begin positive pressure ventilation with supplemental oxygen.
- If the medication has had no or little effect, consult medical direction to consider another dose.
- Document any findings during the reassessment.

FIGURE 16-11 ✱ Metered-dose inhaler and small-volume nebulizer. *continued*

TABLE 16-2 MDI Administration Dos and Don'ts

When administering a metered-dose inhaler, follow these tips:

DO

Instruct the patient to breathe in slowly and deeply.

Be sure the patient is breathing in through his mouth.

Shake the canister for at least 30 seconds before removing the cap.

Depress the canister as the patient begins to inhale.

Coach the patient to hold his breath as long as possible.

Use a spacer device if available and the patient is used to it.

DON'T

Allow the patient to breathe in too quickly.

Allow the patient to breathe in through his nose.

Administer the medication before shaking the canister.

Depress the canister before the patient begins to inhale.

Forget to coach the patient to hold his breath as long as possible.

The patient may experience a variety of side effects from the medication. The most common are an increased heart rate, tremors, and nervousness. More detailed information about bronchodilators and other side effects are listed in Figure 16-11.

how you reassess the patient are identical to those used with a metered-dose inhaler. Following administration, after the misting stops, remove the nebulizer and place the patient back on oxygen if it was removed during drug administration.

Advair: Not for Emergency Use

A drug that is commonly prescribed for patients with uncontrolled asthma is the Advair Diskus (Figure 16-12✱). Unlike the *short*-acting $beta_2$ agonists (for example, albuterol, Xopenex, Bronkosol) that are delivered via an MDI or SVN, Advair is a *long*-acting $beta_2$-specific drug (salmeterol xinafoate) that also contains a steroid (fluticasone propionate) that is used as a maintenance drug. The drug comes in a rotodisk or discus delivery device that requires a different method of administration than the MDI or SVN. Even though Advair is used to treat asthma, *it is not to be used as a rescue inhaler for the pa-*

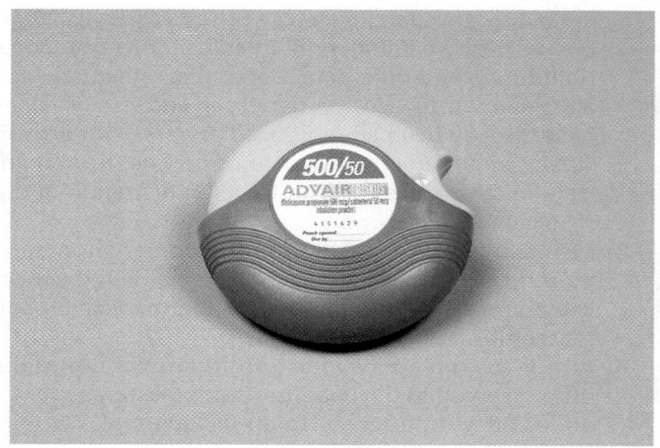

FIGURE 16-12 ✱ The Advair Diskus is commonly prescribed to asthma patients but should *not* be used as a rescue inhaler for the patient experiencing an acute asthma attack.

Objective 16-10
Differentiate between short-acting $beta_2$ agonists appropriate for prehospital use and respiratory medications that are not intended for emergency use.

Key Points
The EMT must remain acutely aware of idiosyncrasies of patients at the extremes of age.

Objective 16-11
Describe special considerations in the assessment and management of pediatric and geriatric patients with respiratory emergencies.

tient experiencing an acute asthma attack. Only a short-acting $beta_2$-agonist drug as listed in Figure 16-11 should be used in the emergency care of the patient experiencing an acute asthma attack.

Age-Related Variations: Pediatrics and Geriatrics

In almost all emergency situations, the EMT must remain acutely aware of idiosyncrasies of patients at both age extremes, the very young and the very old. The incidence and presentation of respiratory disorders in the pediatric patient can be unique because of the differences in anatomy and physiology; similarly, the changes that occur to the anatomy and physiology of the body during aging can alter the incidence and presentation of respiratory distress in the geriatric patient. The goal of the following section is to introduce some of the idiosyncrasies that may be present in patients at the age extremes.

Pediatric Patients

Since infants and children generally have healthy hearts, respiratory failure is the most likely cause of both respiratory arrest and cardiac arrest. This may be prevented if you can recognize the early signs of respiratory distress or respiratory failure and provide the appropriate emergency care.

Respiratory failure for the pediatric patient is defined as inadequate oxygenation of the blood and an inadequate elimination of carbon dioxide from the body. It is usually the result of an inadequate respiratory rate and/or inadequate tidal volume, either of which constitutes inadequate breathing and can lead to respiratory arrest. The root cause is most likely either an upper airway blockage or a lower airway disease. Respiratory conditions in infants and children are discussed in more detail in Chapter 38, "Pediatrics."

Respiratory Distress in the Pediatric Patient: Assessment and Care

Dispatch to an emergency involving an infant or child may provide indications that the patient is suffering from respiratory distress or failure. The time it takes you to arrive at the patient's location should be used to mentally process the points discussed in this section.

Scene Size-Up and Primary Assessment

During scene size-up with the infant or child, as with the adult patient, look for clues to help rule out trauma as a cause of the problem.

Many of the signs and symptoms of breathing difficulty can be spotted as you form your general impression during the primary assessment. Labored or noisy breathing, and a child who is sitting up in a tripod position, lying limply, or unresponsive can be detected "from the doorway," even before you approach the patient. Additional signs and symptoms will be discovered as you contact the infant or child to assess mental status, airway, breathing, and circulation.

Secondary Assessment

Other signs and symptoms may be noted during the secondary assessment of the young patient. (Assessing the infant or child patient will be covered in detail in Chapter 38, "Pediatrics.") Typically, signs and symptoms of respiratory distress will precede respiratory failure in the infant or child. These signs and symptoms will be indications that the body is attempting to compensate for the poor oxygen and carbon dioxide exchange by increasing the work of breathing.

Early Signs of Breathing Difficulty (Respiratory Distress) in the Infant or Child Because *respiratory distress* may quickly proceed to respiratory failure in the infant or child, it is vital that you recognize any of these *early* signs of breathing difficulty:

- Increased use of accessory muscles to breathe
- Sternal and intercostal retractions during inspiration
- Tachypnea (increased breathing rate)
- Tachycardia (increased heart rate)
- Nasal flaring
- Prolonged exhalation
- Frequent coughing—may be present rather than wheezing in some children
- Cyanosis to the extremities
- Anxiety

Thinking Critically
It is important to recognize early signs of respiratory distress. Why is this *especially* critical in an infant or child?

Key Points
Because respiratory distress can rapidly deteriorate into respiratory failure, prompt intervention and transport is critical for the infant or child.

The chest wall is extremely pliable in infants and young children, and the intercostal muscles (muscles between the ribs) are not well developed. Therefore, the child relies heavily on the diaphragm and abdominal muscles to breathe and does not rely very much on the intercostal muscles. Obvious abdominal movement is expected during normal breathing in an infant or young child. In a sense, the intercostal muscles in the infant and young child are viewed more as accessory muscles to breathing. Thus, in the infant and young child, retractions appear to be more prominent *early* in respiratory distress when they begin to use the intercostal muscles to assist in breathing. This is very different from the adult who has a stiffer chest and well-developed intercostal muscles. Retractions in an adult respiratory distress patient are a significant sign of *severe* respiratory distress.

Signs of Inadequate Breathing (Respiratory Failure) in the Infant or Child Signs of *respiratory failure,* which may be similar to those of inadequate breathing, are an indication that the cells are not receiving an adequate oxygen supply. Respiratory compromise, leading to the need to provide positive pressure ventilation, should be recognized in patients who have signs and symptoms of respiratory distress with increased efforts to breathe who continue to deteriorate, or in patients who have inadequate respiratory effort, even with no signs or symptoms of distress.

Respiratory arrest is a condition with no respirations or respiratory effort; however, a pulse is still present.

The signs listed here occur *late* in a respiratory emergency and are an indication that you must immediately intervene and begin positive pressure ventilation with supplemental oxygen:

- Altered mental status—the patient may be listless or completely unresponsive
- Bradycardia (slow heart rate) (Bradycardia would be an initial response in a newborn, a late response in an infant.)
- Hypotension (low blood pressure)
- Extremely fast, slow, or irregular breathing pattern
- Cyanosis to the core of the body and mucous membranes—a late and inconsistent sign
- Loss of muscle tone (limp appearance)
- Diminished or absent breath sounds
- Head bobbing—bobbing of the head with each breath
- Grunting—heard in infants and children during exhalation, indicating diseases that produce lung collapse
- Seesaw or rocky breathing—the chest is drawn inward and the abdomen moves outward, indicating extreme inspiratory efforts
- Decreased response to pain
- Inadequate tidal volume (poor chest rise and fall)

Emergency Medical Care

The emergency medical care for the infant and child is similar to that for the adult. Your goal should be to promptly and efficiently care for the infant or child and minimize the amount of stress. An increased stress level will increase the work of breathing and the body's oxygen demand. Because of the danger that respiratory distress will deteriorate into respiratory failure, *prompt intervention and transport is especially critical for the infant or child.*

For a child who is experiencing difficulty in breathing with adequate breathing (respiratory distress), take the following steps:

1. *Allow the child to assume a position of comfort to reduce the work of breathing and to maintain a more patent airway.* Do not remove the infant or child from his parent (or other caretaker). Allowing the parent to hold the child will reduce the apprehension and stress levels, thereby reducing the breathing workload and oxygen demand.
2. *Apply oxygen by nonrebreather mask to a child who is sitting up in his parent's lap.* If the child does not tolerate the oxygen mask, have the parent hold it near the child's face (Figure 16-13*).
3. *If at any time the infant or child's breathing becomes inadequate (respiratory failure), remove him from the parent, establish an open airway, and begin positive pressure ventilation with supplemental oxygen.* It will be necessary to repeat the physical exam and vital signs.

Just as with adults, a child may also have an MDI or SVN prescribed for respiratory problems associated with the lower airway. These children may present with audible wheezing; diminished breath sounds bilaterally; pale, cool, clammy skin; cyanosis; poor chest rise and fall; and other signs of breathing difficulty. If the child is experiencing breathing difficulty and has a prescribed inhaler or nebulizer, follow the same emergency care procedures for administration of the medication via MDI or SVN as for the adult.

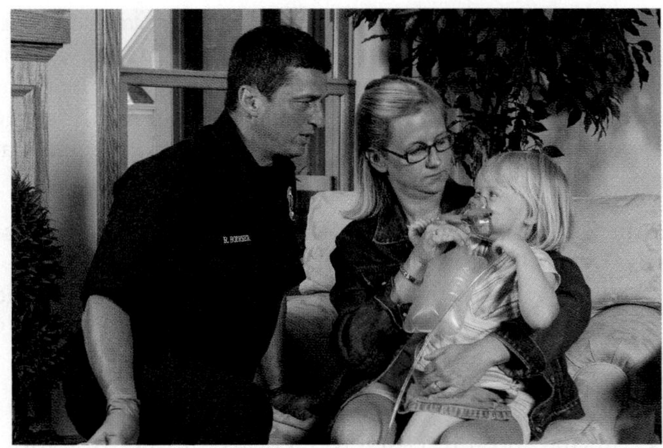

FIGURE 16-13 * If the child does not tolerate the mask, have the parent hold the mask near the child's face.

It is important to bear in mind that the upper airway can be obstructed by foreign bodies or from swelling associated with certain diseases, medical conditions, burns, or toxic inhalations. Stridor and crowing are typical sounds made when the upper airway is partially obstructed by a foreign body or swelling. If a foreign body obstruction is suspected, and the airway is completely blocked, perform foreign body airway obstruction (FBAO) maneuvers to attempt to relieve the obstruction. (Refer to Appendix 1, "Basic Cardiac Life Support," and Chapter 38, "Pediatrics," to review these techniques for the infant and child.) If the airway is partially blocked, place the patient on a nonrebreather mask at 15 lpm and immediately begin transport. Be alert to begin FBAO maneuvers if the partial obstruction becomes complete.

It is important to distinguish blockage caused by a foreign body in the airway from blockage caused by disease. FBAO maneuvers may involve inserting suction devices or the fingers into the airway to remove foreign materials. With some airway diseases, inserting anything into the airway will cause dangerous spasms along the airway, making the condition worse.

Epiglottitis, as described earlier in the chapter, is one condition that can cause obstruction of an infant or child's upper airway when the epiglottis becomes extremely swollen from a localized infection. The epiglottis can swell so much that it completely blocks the opening into the trachea and causes a complete airway obstruction. In this condition, the child usually sits straight up, juts his neck out, and drools because he cannot swallow. He typically has a history of a sore throat, stridor, and fever. This is a life-threatening upper airway emergency—now rare in children, thanks to childhood vaccination. You should apply oxygen by a nonrebreather mask, place the child in a position of comfort, and begin immediate transport. Consider requesting ALS backup. Do not inspect inside the mouth or insert anything inside the airway since it could cause the airway to spasm or completely swell shut. If the patient stops breathing or is breathing inadequately, begin positive pressure ventilation with supplemental oxygen.

Another condition, called *croup (laryngotracheobronchitis)*, commonly seen in children, involves the swelling of the larynx, trachea, and bronchi, causing breathing difficulty. The child typically does not feel well, has a sore or hoarse throat, and has a fever. At night, the condition usually worsens. You might hear a hallmark sign of croup, a cough that sounds like a barking seal. Provide oxygen to the patient, humidified if possible, and begin transport. Usually cool night air will reduce the signs and symptoms somewhat; therefore, the condition may subside slightly after the child is taken outside for transfer to the ambulance. Inadequate breathing can result from croup, so continuously monitor the breathing status.

Gathering a history is especially important when airway blockage is suspected, since it may identify either preexisting diseases that may be causing the airway closure or events that may have led to a foreign body obstruction. (For example, someone witnessed the child choking on food or saw the child put an object into his mouth, or there were small objects around the child that he could have swallowed.) If the blockage was sudden and there was something around that the child could have swallowed and there is no history or other sign of disease, treat the patient for an *upper airway foreign body obstruction*. If the blockage came on gradually, the child has other signs of being ill, or the child has a history of respiratory or other disease, and no one saw the child swallow anything, avoid inserting anything into the airway. Instead, provide oxygen or positive pressure ventilation with supplemental oxygen as necessary.

Reassessment

Transport any infant or child with difficulty breathing or signs of inadequate breathing or airway blockage. Provide reassessment en route. Be prepared to intervene more aggressively if the condition deteriorates.

Geriatric Patients

Respiratory distress can result from any of a number of conditions occurring in the geriatric patient. It can be the primary symptom of a pulmonary problem, or it can be a symptom secondary to failure of a different body system (congestive heart failure, for example, can cause difficulty in breathing). Therefore, difficulty breathing or "shortness of breath" (dyspnea) is one of the more common complaints noted in the elderly. It is important to realize that the elderly already have diminished respiratory function. Therefore, any additional burden can easily overwhelm the respiratory system and lead to inadequate breathing. While shortness of breath can be caused by a number of problems, those listed here represent the most common causes:

Upper Airway Obstruction

- Croup
- Foreign body aspiration
- Epiglottitis
- Tracheostomy dysfunction

Lower Airway Disease

- Asthma
- Bronchiolitis
- Pneumonia
- Foreign body lower airway obstruction
- Pertussis
- Cystic fibrosis

Respiratory Distress in the Geriatric Patient: Assessment and Care

The EMT may have indication that the geriatric patient is suffering from respiratory distress or failure from information received by dispatch. Hints could include the known presence of dyspnea by the caller, but it may also be manifested in complaints such as weakness, inability to ambulate, confusion, chest/abdominal pain, or falls. The time it takes you to arrive at the patient's location should be used to mentally process the points discussed in this section.

Scene Size-Up and Primary Assessment

During scene size-up with the geriatric patient, look for clues to help rule out trauma as a cause of the problem. Many of the signs and symptoms of breathing difficulty can be spotted as you form your general impression during the primary assessment. Labored or noisy breathing, a patient in a tripod position, a patient lying in bed with multiple pillows behind his head, or unresponsiveness can be detected even before you approach the patient. Additional signs and symptoms will be discovered as you contact the patient to assess mental status, airway, breathing, and circulation.

Secondary Assessment

Other signs and symptoms may be noted during the secondary assessment of the geriatric patient. (Assessing the geriatric patient will be covered in detail in Chapter 39, "Geriatrics.") The signs and symptoms of respiratory distress usually briefly precede respiratory failure in geriatric patients. Older patients do not have the compensatory mechanisms a younger adult has, and they typically decompensate much more rapidly. Whenever you see indications of respiratory distress, remember that these indicate the body is attempting to compensate for the poor oxygen and carbon dioxide exchange by increasing the work of breathing, but this compensatory mechanism may be short-lived.

Early Signs of Breathing Difficulty (Respiratory Distress) in the Geriatric Patient Because respiratory distress may quickly proceed to respiratory failure in the geriatric patient, it is vital that you recognize these early signs of breathing difficulty:

- Increased use of accessory muscles to breathe
- Sternal and intercostal retractions during inspiration
- Tachypnea (increased breathing rate)
- Tachycardia (increased heart rate)
- Nasal flaring, breathing with the mouth open
- Prolonged exhalation (with pursed lips)
- Frequent coughing
- Cyanosis
- Anxiety
- Inability to speak in full sentences

The chest wall and points of attachment where the ribs meet the sternum tend to become brittle and more immobile with aging. This means it is more difficult for the geriatric patient to move the rib cage during periods of heightened respiratory effort. The result is more reliance on the diaphragm and abdominal muscles to breathe. The problem is that the geriatric patient's musculature is prone to early fatigue.

Signs of Inadequate Breathing (Respiratory Failure) in the Geriatric Patient Signs of *respiratory failure,* which may be similar to those of inadequate breathing, are an indication that the cells are not receiving an adequate oxygen supply. Respiratory compromise, leading to the need to provide positive pressure ventilation, should be recognized in patients who have signs and symptoms of respiratory distress with increased efforts to breathe who continue to deteriorate, or in a patient who has inadequate respiratory effort, even with no signs or symptoms of distress.

Respiratory arrest is a condition where there are no respirations or respiratory effort; however, a pulse is still present.

The following signs occur *late* in a respiratory emergency and are an indication that you must immediately intervene and begin positive pressure ventilation with supplemental oxygen:

- Altered mental status
- Vital sign changes
- Extremely fast, slow, or irregular breathing pattern
- Cyanosis to the core of the body and mucous membranes

Key Points
Because respiratory distress can deteriorate into respiratory failure, prompt intervention and transport is especially critical for the geriatric patient.

Objective 16-12
Employ an assessment-based approach in order to recognize indications for interventions in patients with respiratory complaints/emergencies.

- Loss of muscle tone
- Diminished or absent breath sounds
- Decreased response to pain
- Inadequate tidal volume (poor chest rise and fall)
- Retractions (suprasternal, supraclavicular, subclavicular, intercostal)

As discussed earlier, the intercostal muscles in the infant and young child are viewed more as accessory muscles to breathing. Thus, in the infant and young child, retractions appear to be more prominent *early* in respiratory distress when they begin to use the intercostal muscles to assist in breathing. This is very different from the geriatric patient who has a stiffer chest and more developed intercostal muscles. Retractions in an adult or geriatric patient with respiratory distress are a significant sign of *severe* respiratory distress.

Emergency Medical Care

The emergency medical care for the geriatric patient is similar to that for the adult. Your first goal should be to reduce any anxiety or stress the patient is experiencing. An increased stress level will increase the work of breathing and the body's oxygen demand. Because of the danger that respiratory distress will deteriorate into respiratory failure, *prompt intervention and transport is especially critical.*

For a geriatric patient who is experiencing difficulty in breathing with adequate breathing (respiratory distress), take the following steps:

1. *Place the patient in a position of comfort to reduce the breathing work and maintain a more patent airway.* Typically this will be a sitting-up position to help the respiratory muscles work more efficiently.
2. *Apply oxygen by nonrebreather mask.*
3. *If at any time the patient's breathing becomes inadequate (respiratory failure), lay him down flat, establish an open airway, and begin positive pressure ventilation with supplemental oxygen.* It will be necessary to repeat the physical exam and vital signs.

Reassessment

Transport any geriatric patient with difficulty breathing or signs of inadequate breathing. Provide reassessment en route. Be prepared to intervene more aggressively if the condition deteriorates.

Assessment and Care: General Guidelines

Assessment-Based Approach: Respiratory Distress

Information provided by the dispatcher may be the first indication that a patient is suffering from a respiratory emergency. The information that the patient is complaining of breathing difficulty should heighten your suspicion of a potential respiratory problem.

Scene Size-Up

Seek clues to determine whether the breathing difficulty is due to trauma or to a medical condition. Be careful not to develop tunnel vision and miss important indications of alternative causes for the breathing difficulty that are not the result of a respiratory problem—for example, a cardiac problem or an open chest wound.

Scan the scene for possible mechanisms of injury. Bystanders who heard gunshots, saw a knife, or heard loud fighting may indicate that the patient's difficulty in breathing may be trauma related. The patient who is found in his house in the middle of the living room may have fallen, struck his chest against the coffee table, and fractured some ribs, causing the lung to collapse. A tall, lanky male patient may have been moving a heavy object or coughing when he experienced a sudden onset of shortness of breath that progressively worsened. Look for oxygen tanks, oxygen tubing, or oxygen concentrators, or medication inhalers or nebulizers at the scene. They usually indicate a chronic respiratory disease. Also scan the scene for alcohol, which is a common contributor to choking and upper airway obstruction and aspiration of vomitus.

Primary Assessment

Form a general impression and assess the mental status, airway, breathing, and circulation.

Key Terms

tripod position a position in which the patient sits upright, leans slightly forward, and supports the body with the arms in front and elbows locked. This is a position commonly found in respiratory distress.

Key Points

An agitated or confused facial expression may indicate inadequate breathing, hypoxia, or hypercarbia.

General Impression Several clues can help you form an impression of a patient who is suffering respiratory distress. These include:

- **The patient's position.** Most frequently, in severe cases of respiratory distress, patients sit upright and lean slightly forward, supporting themselves with their arms, elbows locked in place in front of them between their dangling legs, holding onto the seat. This is referred to as a **tripod position** (Figure 16-14✻).

  The patient in a reclining or supine position could indicate two possible scenarios: (1) the patient is only in mild distress, or (2) the patient is in such severe respiratory distress that he is too exhausted from trying to breathe to hold himself up. This patient requires immediate intervention since respiratory arrest usually follows shortly after development of severe fatigue.

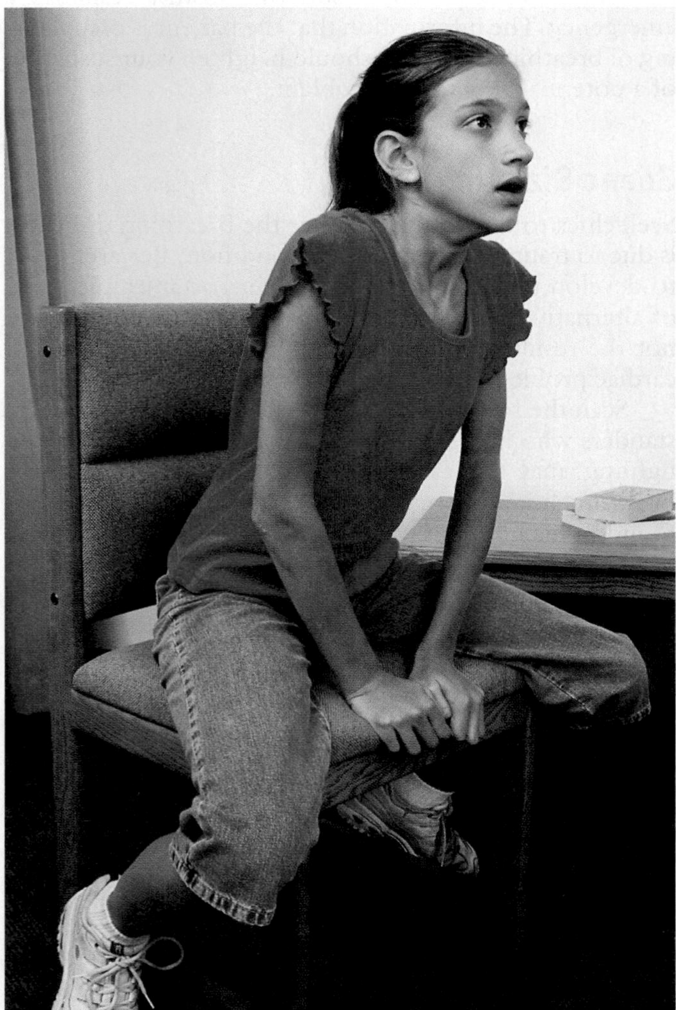

FIGURE 16-14 ✻ A patient in respiratory distress is commonly found in a "tripod" position.

- **The patient's face.** An agitated or confused facial expression may indicate inadequate breathing, hypoxia, or hypercarbia.

Understanding BODY PROCESSES

Hypoxia causes the patient to become agitated and aggressive. Hypercarbia causes confusion, disorientation, and lethargy. ■

- **The patient's speech.** If the speech is normal, assume that the airway is open and clear and the distress is minimal. If the patient is alert and makes eye contact but is unable to speak, consider a severe condition. The patient may speak one or two words and then pause to gasp for a breath. The number of words the patient can speak during one breath usually correlates with the severity of the breathing difficulty.
- **Altered mental status.** A change in the mental status, such as confusion, is a clear indication of inadequate oxygenation of the brain (cerebral hypoxia) and a buildup of carbon dioxide. A sign of imminent respiratory failure is when the patient's eyelids begin to droop and the head bobs with each respiration, as if the patient is beginning to fall asleep while sitting upright. This is a sign that the patient needs positive pressure ventilation immediately.
- **Use of the muscles in the neck and retractions of the muscles between the ribs (intercostal muscles).** Accessory muscle use and retractions are an indication of a significant increased inhalation effort with each breath.
- **Cyanosis.** Cyanosis (bluish gray skin color) is a clear indication of hypoxia but also a sign that may occur late. Look at the area around the nose and mouth when getting the general impression. You will examine many other areas for cyanosis in the physical exam.
- **Diaphoresis.** A patient with respiratory distress commonly is diaphoretic (having sweaty and moist skin

that is inappropriate for the temperature or activity). The patient becomes more diaphoretic the harder he works to breathe.

- **Pallor.** Pale skin color is a sign of hypoxia and severe respiratory distress. Pallor will be seen earlier and more often than cyanosis.

ASSESSMENT Tips

Pale, cool, clammy skin is an *early* sign of hypoxia in the patient. Cyanosis is a clear but *late* sign of hypoxia. ■

- **Nasal flaring.** Flaring of the nostrils with inhalation is another indication that the patient is working hard to breathe in.
- **Pursed lips.** Pursed-lip breathing is when the patient puts his lips together during exhalation as if he is going to whistle. Patients with some chronic respiratory diseases do this subconsciously. This is done to keep the airway pressure in the smaller bronchioles higher during exhalation so they don't collapse but remain open, making the next inhalation a little easier.

Mental Status Restlessness, agitation, confusion, and unresponsiveness are frequently associated with breathing difficulty because the brain is not getting enough oxygen.

Airway Assess the airway for any indication of a complete or partial obstruction from secretions, blood, vomitus, or a foreign body. Listen for snoring, stridor, gurgling, or crowing. Each indicates partial airway obstruction. However, keep in mind that obstructed breathing is not always noisy. Clear the airway with suction, manual maneuvers, and airway adjuncts as needed.

Breathing Carefully assess the breathing. Look at the chest rise and fall, listen and feel for air flowing in and out of the mouth and nose, and quickly auscultate the lungs. Be aware of a chest that is moving up and down upon inspection but produces very little or no air movement from the mouth and nose. Efforts to breathe are being made but are not effective. This patient needs positive pressure ventilation with supplemental oxygen no matter how well the chest is rising and falling. Auscultate the breath sounds on both sides of the chest. Absent or diminished breath sounds are an indication that very little air is moving in and out of the lungs.

Determine an approximate respiratory rate. *If the chest is not rising adequately with each breath or you do not hear or feel an adequate volume of air escaping on exhalation, begin positive pressure ventilation with supplemental oxygen.*

Look for respiratory rates outside the ranges of 8–24 breaths per minute for adults, 15–30 per minute for children, and 25–50 per minute for infants. A respiratory rate that is too slow will not allow enough air to be transported to the alveoli for adequate gas exchange, leading to hypoxia. This patient must be provided positive pressure ventilation.

ASSESSMENT Tips

The average range of normal respiration for an adult patient is 12–20 breaths per minute; however, it is possible for the patient with lower or higher rates to be breathing adequately. Look at the entire patient and assess the tidal volume closely. If the tidal volume (assess chest rise and air movement) is inadequate in high rates, immediately begin ventilation. Elderly patients will have higher resting respiratory rates, typically 20 per minute. ■

On the other hand, a respiratory rate that is too fast does not always compensate for a poor volume of air the patient is breathing. In many cases, the respiratory rate becomes so fast (adult > 40/minute, infant > 60/minute) that it does not allow the patient to take a full enough breath before having to exhale, leading to ineffective volumes of air during inhalation. The respiratory rate will appear faster than normal; however, the chest will not rise adequately or very little air movement will be felt. You must immediately begin positive pressure ventilation. The inadequate chest rise and fall or little movement of air is commonly referred to as shallow breathing. *Shallow breathing is an indication of inadequate breathing.*

In order to have adequate breathing, you must have both an adequate rate and an adequate tidal volume (amount of air moving in and out with one breath). If either the rate or the tidal volume is inadequate, the patient must be provided positive pressure ventilation. If both the rate and the tidal volume are inadequate, you must provide positive pressure ventilation. If the rate and tidal volume are both adequate, you can place the patient on oxygen via a nonrebreather mask at 15 lpm.

You must be aggressive when managing the airway and ventilation status of the patient. Remember that *any* indication of poor or inadequate ventilation must be managed with positive pressure ventilation.

During your assessment, you can summarize the patient's respiratory status as follows:

One inadequate (either rate or tidal volume) = inadequate breathing.

Two inadequates (both rate and tidal volume) = inadequate breathing.

Two adequates (both rate and tidal volume) = adequate breathing.

Remember that a patient who complains of breathing difficulty or presents with signs of hypoxia or hypercarbia may have either adequate or inadequate breathing, as just defined. The patient with inadequate breathing will be

Key Points
Because a patient with difficulty in breathing is considered a priority patient, consider advanced life support backup and expeditious transport.

Objective 16-13
Given a list of patient medications, recognize medications that are associated with respiratory disease.

treated differently from the patient with adequate breathing, as follows:

Inadequate breathing—*Provide positive pressure ventilation* with a bag-valve mask or pocket mask with oxygen connected to the device.

Adequate breathing—*Administer oxygen* via a nonrebreather mask at 15 lpm (Figure 16-15∗).

Circulation Inspect the patient's skin and mucous membranes. Cyanosis, or bluish gray skin, especially to the face, lips, neck, and chest, is an ominous sign of respiratory distress. In people with dark skin, check for cyanosis of mucous membranes under the tongue, at the lining of the mouth, or to the inside of the lower eyelid (conjunctiva). Tachycardia and pale, cool, moist skin are also signs of respiratory distress and hypoxia.

Priority Because a patient with difficulty in breathing is considered a priority patient, consider advanced life support backup and expeditious transport. In the patient with severe respiratory distress, respiratory failure, or respiratory arrest, you will want to transport as soon as possible and continue your secondary assessment en route to the hospital. Signs that you may need to transport expeditiously are evidence of inadequate breathing, an irregular pulse or increased pulse rate (tachycardia) in adults and children, a slow pulse (bradycardia) in newborns with breathing difficulty, and an altered mental status. Also, as stated earlier, cyanosis is an ominous and late sign of respiratory distress, as is a very slow respiratory rate.

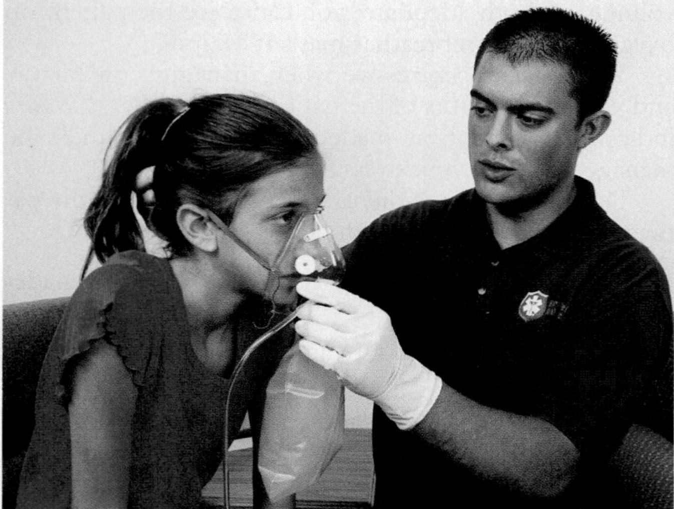

FIGURE 16-15 ∗ Provide oxygen by nonrebreather mask at 15 lpm to the patient who is breathing adequately but with difficulty (respiratory distress).

Secondary Assessment

If the patient is responsive, obtain a history using the OPQRST questions to evaluate the history of the present illness (Table 16-3). If the patient is unresponsive, perform a rapid physical exam and collect as much information as possible from any family or bystanders at the scene.

History The following questions will be particularly helpful in determining your emergency care steps for a patient with respiratory distress:

- *Does the patient have any known allergies to medications or other substances that may be related to the episode of difficulty in breathing?* For instance, some patients may experience a sudden onset of breathing difficulty when they have inhaled substances like dust, dog hair, cat hair, mold, or irritating smoke. An extreme allergic reaction (anaphylaxis), for example, to a bee sting or to something the patient has eaten will cause swelling of the tissues of the upper airway, bronchospasm, and severe respiratory distress.
- *What medications, prescription or nonprescription, is the patient taking?* Gather them to take to the hospital. As discussed earlier, metered-dose inhalers and small-volume nebulizers are devices that that are used to deliver a medication by inhalation. These devices are frequently used by patients with a chronic respiratory disease or recurring breathing problems. Occasionally you might find oral medications used specifically for respiratory problems. Common medications that might be found on the patient or at the scene are found in Table 16-4. It is important to recognize these since they might provide you with a clue that the patient has a history of respiratory problems, and also, medical direction may instruct you to administer one of them. Ask if the patient has already taken any of the medications prior to your arrival, and if so, how many times. Report this information to medical direction or the receiving hospital.

  Note: Medications used by patients with chronic respiratory disease have a variety of side effects. Because many patients self-administer their medication prior to your arrival, this may confuse your assess-

TABLE 16-3 OPQRST for Breathing Difficulty

History	Use the following questions to obtain information about the difficulty in breathing:
Onset	What were you doing when the breathing difficulty started? Did anything seem to trigger the breathing difficulty? Was the onset gradual or sudden? Was the onset accompanied by chest pain or any other symptoms? Was there a sudden onset of pain?
Provocation/palliation	Does lying flat make the breathing difficulty worse? Does sitting up make the breathing difficulty less severe? Is there pain that occurs or increases with breathing?
Quality	Do you have more trouble breathing in or out? Is the pain sharp (knifelike) or dull?
Radiation	If there is pain associated with the breathing difficulty, does it radiate to the back, up the neck, down the arms, or to any other part of the body?
Severity	How bad is this breathing difficulty on a scale of 1 to 10, with 10 being the worst breathing difficulty you have ever experienced?
Time	When did the difficulty in breathing start? How long have you had it? If this is a recurring problem, how long does the breathing difficulty usually last? If the breathing difficulty started other than today, could you recall the exact day and time when this started?

ment slightly since the signs and symptoms now exhibited may result from the medication and not necessarily from the respiratory condition. These side effects are also listed in Table 16-4.

- *Does the patient have a pre-existing respiratory or cardiac disease?*
- *Has the patient ever been hospitalized for a chronic condition that produces recurring episodes of difficulty in breathing?* If so, did he have an endotracheal tube placed down his throat to breathe or require admission to an intensive care unit? This usually indicates that the patient may have a tendency to deteriorate much more rapidly and may require quicker and more aggressive intervention.

Physical Exam The physical exam will give you further information that may indicate the severity of the breathing distress and help you determine whether to simply apply high concentration of oxygen by nonrebreather mask or to proceed with positive pressure ventilation with supplemental oxygen. If the patient is unresponsive, perform a rapid assessment. In the responsive patient, focus the exam on the areas that might provide you with clues as to the severity of the condition.

The posture of the patient is important. As the patient becomes exhausted, you will notice his posture relaxing. This is an indication that he may require artificial ventilation very shortly. Alterations in mental status, combativeness, agitation, and confusion indicate a decreasing level of oxygen getting to the brain and an increasing level of carbon dioxide. A continuous decline would be an indication of the need for aggressive emergency care to include positive pressure ventilation with supplemental oxygen.

TABLE 16-4 Medications Commonly Used for Respiratory Problems

Bronchodilators	Albuterol (Proventil, Ventolin) Bitolterol mesylate (Tornalate) Ipratropium bromide (Atrovent) Isoetharine (Bronkosol) Metaproterenol (Metaprel, Alupent) Salmeterol xinafoate (Serevent) Montelukast (Singulair) Levalbuterol (Xopenex) Pirbuterol (Maxair)	Potential side effects: increased heart rate, nervousness, shakiness, nausea, vomiting, sleeplessness, dry mouth, and allergic skin rash
Mucolytics	Acetylcysteine (Mucomyst)	Potential side effects: nausea, increased wheezing, and altered sense of taste
Steroids	Beclomethasone (Vanceril Inhaler, Beclovent®) Flunisolide (AeroBid) Triamcinolone acetonide (Azmacort)	Potential side effects: dry mouth and increased wheezing

Understanding BODY PROCESSES

Typically, inhalation is an active process requiring energy, whereas exhalation is a passive process requiring no energy. The patient with respiratory distress may have difficulty not only breathing in but also breathing out. He moves to active inhalation and active exhalation, both requiring energy. This may lead to faster muscle fatigue and early respiratory failure. ■

- *Inspect the lips and around the nose and inside the mouth* for cyanosis.
- *Assess the neck* for jugular vein distention, which might indicate an extreme increase in pressure in the chest or venous system. Inspect and palpate for an indrawing of the trachea and tracheal deviation. The trachea pulls inward during inhalation when constricted airflow is present. Tracheal deviation, which is a late sign, is the result of an extreme amount of pressure built up on one side of the chest, collapsing the lung and pushing the mediastinum (the tissues and organs between the lungs, including the heart) and the trachea to the opposite side. This is a sign of a life-threatening emergency.

  Also inspect for retractions, or pulling of the tissue inward, involving the muscles of the neck, at the suprasternal notch, and behind the clavicles. This indicates that the patient is making an extreme effort to breathe and is another situation in which positive pressure ventilation with supplemental oxygen should be considered.

ASSESSMENT Tips

When assessing the neck, look specifically for jugular vein distention during the inhalation phase of respiration. If the jugular veins distend during inhalation, and return to normal during exhalation, this is an indication of a severely increased pressure in the chest or around the heart. It is referred to as *Kussmaul sign.* ■

- *Inspect and palpate the chest* for retraction of the muscles between the ribs, asymmetrical chest wall movement, and also for subcutaneous emphysema, which is air trapped under the subcutaneous layer of the skin. It is felt as a crackling sensation under the fingertips. Unequal chest wall movement may be a sign that air is trapped in one side of the chest cavity and preventing adequate ventilation. Subcutaneous emphysema is a common result of trauma to the neck and chest, indicating a hole in the lung, trachea, bronchus, or esophagus. Inspect for any evidence of trauma.
- *Auscultate the lungs* to determine whether the breath sounds are equal on both sides of the chest. Diminished or absent breath sounds on one side of the chest mean that the lung is not being adequately ventilated because of obstruction, collapse, or surrounding air or fluid. If both lungs have diminished or absent breath sounds, it is an indication that the breathing is inadequate and the patient needs immediate ventilation with supplemental oxygen connected to the ventilation device.

ASSESSMENT Tips

Subcutaneous emphysema can be felt much more easily than it can be seen on inspection. ■

Understanding BODY PROCESSES

Subcutaneous emphysema is an indication that an air leak is present somewhere in an air-containing structure in the neck or chest. Gravity pulls heavier substances downward, forcing the air to travel upward toward the neck and head in the patient who is in a seated position. ■

  Wheezing is a musical whistling sound that is heard in all lung fields upon auscultation of the chest. It is caused by narrowing of the lower airways, primarily the bronchioles, from bronchospasm and edema, or swelling. Wheezing is heard primarily during exhalation. You can expect to hear it most frequently in patients with a history of asthma or emphysema, but it may also be heard when fluid builds up in the lungs. These patients commonly carry medications that can be administered to reverse the bronchospasm and allow for greater air movement. Inspiratory crackles (rales) are indicative of fluid accumulation in the alveoli from a failing heart. This fluid decreases the gas exchange across the alveolar membrane and can lead to respiratory distress or failure. Finally, rhonchi are sounds heard in the larger airways and represent mucus accumulation.

Vital Signs The systolic blood pressure may drop during inhalation. This is related to a drastic increase in pressure inside the chest. When taking the blood pressure by auscultation, watch the needle when obtaining the systolic pressure. If the needle suddenly drops more than 10 mmHg when the patient inhales, it is a significant finding of a severe respiratory condition such as obstructive lung disease. This finding is referred to as **pulsus paradoxus**. You may also note this as a sudden decrease in the amplitude (strength) of the pulse when the patient inhales. As the patient exhales, the pulse strength returns.

The heart rate may be increased (tachycardia) or decreased (bradycardia). Bradycardia in adults, infants, and children is a grave sign of extremely poor oxygenation, impending respiratory failure, and possible cardiac arrest. The

Key Terms

pulsus paradoxus a drop in blood pressure of more than 10 mmHg during inhalation resulting from increased pressure within the chest that suppresses the filling of the ventricles of the heart with blood.

Thinking Critically

In a patient with any indication of respiratory distress, the text states that you should apply a pulse oximeter (if available) early. Why is this important?

skin is usually moist, pale, and cool (lung infections associated with breathing difficulty may produce warm, dry, or moist skin). The breathing rate is typically increased (tachypnea); however, it may decrease as the patient becomes tired and the oxygen levels drop significantly. Cyanosis may be noted in severely hypoxic patients.

Understanding BODY PROCESSES

An increase in the pressure inside the chest will cause a decrease in blood flowing through the veins back to the right side of the heart. This, in turn, will decrease the volume of blood filling the left ventricle, causing a drop in the amount of blood being ejected into the aorta and arteries during the heart's contraction. You will see this as a sudden decrease in systolic blood pressure and pulse amplitude (strength) during inhalation. ■

Early application of a pulse oximeter, if available, is important in a patient with any evidence of respiratory distress, complaint of breathing difficulty, or signs of inadequate breathing. A pulse oximeter reading (SpO_2) of less than 95% in a patient with any breathing difficulty is a concern. This is an indication of hypoxemia (low oxygen levels in the blood). If the pulse oximeter reading is below 90%, this is a significant indication of severe hypoxemia.

Closely evaluate the ventilatory status (respiratory rate and tidal volume). If both are adequate, immediately administer oxygen via a nonrebreather mask at 15 lpm. If either rate or tidal volume is inadequate, begin positive pressure ventilation. You would expect the pulse oximeter reading to increase once the patient is provided oxygen in adequate breathing or following positive pressure ventilation if the patient was breathing inadequately. Therefore, if a pulse oximeter reading can be obtained prior to any administration of oxygen or ventilation, it would provide a baseline reading for you to assess the effectiveness of your treatment.

If the SpO_2 reading continues to remain at 95% or less after the patient has been on a nonrebreather mask for a period of time, it may indicate that the patient is still hypoxic and a disturbance in gas exchange is still present. If this patient were taken off the oxygen, you would expect the pulse oximeter reading to fall below a normal level, indicating severe hypoxemia. Normally, once oxygen has been applied or the patient is being ventilated, the SpO_2 should read 98% or higher. You may still experience a decline once the oxygen is removed. If the SpO_2 reading does not increase to 98% or higher after oxygen administration, be concerned that a hypoxemic state still exists.

At any time you suspect that the patient is not breathing adequately, you must immediately begin to ventilate using a bag-valve mask or other ventilation device with oxygen connected to the device. It is important to note that even though the patient is breathing, he may need to be ventilated. You would integrate your ventilation into the patient's own spontaneous pattern and rate of breathing to produce an effective rate and tidal volume. Do not hesitate to ventilate a spontaneously breathing patient who has an inadequate rate or tidal volume. A poor SpO_2 reading may assist you in making the decision to ventilate. For example, if a patient were breathing at 38 times per minute with a shallow tidal volume and had an SpO_2 reading of 88%, you would immediately make the decision to ventilate the patient with a bag-valve-mask device. You would ventilate at 10–12 times per minute, adding your ventilation to the patient's spontaneous breathing.

Signs and Symptoms A wide variety of signs and symptoms may be associated with breathing difficulty, depending on the location of the obstruction or disease process, the mental status of the patient, and the severity of the respiratory distress. A large number of respiratory conditions, including both medical illness and traumatic injuries, cause signs and symptoms of breathing difficulty. Not all of the signs or symptoms will be present with each patient, nor will you find two cases that are exactly alike. The degree of difficulty in breathing can vary widely from minor to severe.

ASSESSMENT Tips

Respiratory distress may be produced by both medical illnesses and traumatic injuries. Do not assume that a patient in respiratory distress is suffering a medical illness, but expose the patient and inspect for any evidence of traumatic injuries, especially in the patient with a sudden onset of symptoms. ■

It is important to recognize that the degree of shortness of breath or the severity of the complaint of shortness of breath does not correlate with the level of hypoxia. In other words, a patient who states that his severity of dyspnea is a "10" on a scale of 1 to 10, with 10 being the worst, is not necessarily more hypoxic than the patient who complains of "a little shortness of

Thinking Critically

A patient has signs and symptoms of respiratory distress. Should you administer oxygen by nonrebreather mask? Or should you administer positive pressure ventilations with supplemental oxygen? What criteria should you use for making this decision?

Objective 16-14

Use reassessment to identify responses to treatment and changes in the conditions of patients presenting with respiratory complaints and emergencies.

breath" with a severity of "3" on the same scale. It is possible that the patient who perceives the level 3 severity is much more hypoxic than the one who perceives the level 10 severity. A pulse oximeter and a good physical exam would provide the evidence to determine the hypoxia levels of the two patients. Also, remember that hypoxic patients may experience an altered mental status in which they do not complain of the shortness of breath as readily as patients who are not as short of breath.

ASSESSMENT Tips

The severity of shortness of breath does not directly correlate with the level of hypoxia. A severely hypoxic patient may not complain of extreme shortness of breath. Pay close attention to your assessment findings. ■

The key is to recognize the patient who is having *any* difficulty in breathing, perform an accurate assessment, and manage any immediate life threats. The following are common signs of breathing difficulty:

- Shortness of breath (dyspnea)
- Restlessness, agitation, and anxiety
- Increased heart rate (tachycardia) or irregular heart rate in adults and children and a sudden decrease in heart rate (bradycardia) in newborns
- Faster-than-normal breathing rates (tachypnea)
- Slower-than-normal breathing rates (bradypnea)
- Cyanosis to the core of the body, usually seen in the face, neck, and upper chest (This is a late sign of hypoxia. Pale skin is seen earlier than cyanosis as a sign of hypoxia. Flushed, or red, skin may indicate an allergic reaction. With any of these discolorations, the skin is typically moist.)
- Abnormal upper airway sounds: crowing, gurgling, snoring, and stridor
- Audible wheezing upon inhalation and exhalation (In some conditions, wheezing on exhalation will develop before wheezing on inhalation. Auscultation with a stethoscope may reveal wheezing and crackles that cannot be heard by just listening with the ear.)
- Diminished ability or inability to speak
- Retractions from the use of accessory muscles in the upper chest and between the ribs and use of the muscles of the neck in breathing
- Excessive use of the diaphragm to breathe, producing abdominal breathing in which the abdomen is moving significantly during the breathing effort
- Shallow breathing, identified by very little chest rise and fall, and poor movement of air in and out of the mouth
- Coughing, especially if it is a productive cough that produces mucus
- Irregular breathing patterns
- Tripod position
- Barrel chest (Figure 16-16∗) indicating emphysema, a chronic respiratory condition
- Altered mental status—from disorientation to unresponsiveness
- Nasal flaring, when the nostrils widen and flare out upon inhalation
- Tracheal indrawing
- Paradoxical motion, in which an area of the chest moves inward during inhalation and outward during exhalation—a significant sign of chest trauma; can lead to ineffective ventilation
- Indications of chest trauma (e.g., open wounds)
- Pursed-lip breathing, where the lips are puckered during exhalation

Emergency Medical Care

Do not take the time to try to determine the exact cause of the breathing difficulty unless it is in the trauma patient with a possible chest injury that must be managed in addition to the breathing difficulty itself. A trauma patient complaining of difficulty in breathing requires exposure of the chest and back with close inspection for and management of life-threatening injuries. Chest injuries will be discussed in more detail in Chapter 34, "Chest Trauma."

Aside from the management of any chest injuries, you will use the same strategies for managing breathing difficulty and respiratory distress no matter what its cause or underlying disease process.

A patient with breathing difficulty and respiratory distress may deteriorate rapidly. Continuously assess the

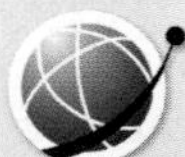

Media Resources

Go to www.bradybooks.com for mykit. Highlights:

- *Animation:* Acute Respiratory Distress Syndrome
- *Animation:* Chronic Obstructive Pulmonary Disease
- *Web Resource:* Breath Sounds and Assessment Tips
- *Web Resource:* Metered-Dose Inhaler

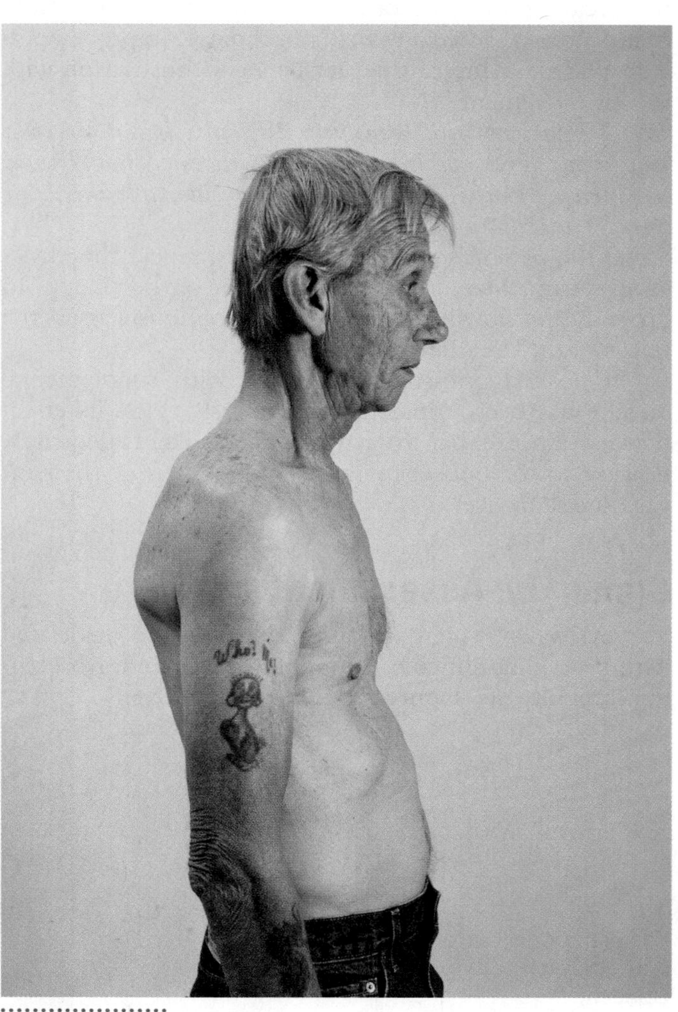

FIGURE 16-16 ✱ Barrel chest in an emphysema patient.

airway for possible obstruction and the ventilation status for inadequacy. Have your ventilation equipment ready and be prepared to control the airway and begin positive pressure ventilation with supplemental oxygen if the patient deteriorates to respiratory failure. Delays in providing adequate ventilation can adversely affect the outcome of the patient in a short period of time. If you are ever in doubt about whether to ventilate, it is better to provide the positive pressure ventilation with supplemental oxygen. Waiting may cost the patient his life.

The following are guidelines for emergency care of the patient with respiratory distress or failure:

Inadequate Breathing (Respiratory Failure)—If signs of inadequate breathing (respiratory failure) are present—poor chest rise and fall, poor volume heard and felt, diminished or absent breath sounds, inadequate rate (too fast or too slow), or severely altered mental status:

1. *Establish an open airway.* Insert an oropharyngeal or nasopharyngeal airway if possible to maintain the airway. If the patient is still responsive, do not insert an airway. Be sure to explain to the patient that you are going to ventilate him to assist and improve his breathing.
2. *Begin positive pressure ventilation with supplemental oxygen.* Check for signs of adequate ventilation (see the next section).
3. *Expeditiously transport* the patient to the hospital.

Adequate Breathing (Respiratory Distress)—If the breathing is adequate (adequate chest rise and fall, good volume of air being breathed in and out, good breath sounds bilaterally, and adequate rate) but the patient complains of difficulty in breathing (respiratory distress):

1. *Continue oxygen administration* at 15 lpm via a nonrebreather mask.
2. *Assess the baseline vital signs.*
3. *Determine if the patient has a prescribed beta$_2$ metered-dose inhaler (MDI).* If so, contact medical direction for permission to administer the medication. Assist the patient with administration of the medication. Be sure to comply with local protocols.
4. *Complete the secondary assessment.*
5. *Place the patient in a position of comfort,* most typically in a Fowler or semi-Fowler (sitting-up) position, and begin transport.
6. *Complete the secondary assessment. If your protocol allows, in cases of severe respiratory distress consider the use of continuous positive airway pressure (CPAP). Current studies show that patients in severe respiratory distress from a variety of conditions may benefit from CPAP. (See Chapter 10, "Airway Management, Artificial Ventilation, and Oxygenation."*

Reassessment

En route to the hospital, perform a reassessment to determine if your emergency care has improved the respiratory distress or respiratory failure or if further intervention is necessary. Better ventilation and oxygenation should improve the patient's mental status. Closely monitor the patient's airway for possible occlusion and the ventilation status for signs of inadequate breathing. If the patient continues to deteriorate, it may be necessary to begin positive pressure ventilation with supplemental oxygen. Monitor the SpO_2 reading. An increase in the SpO_2 indicates improvement in the condition, whereas a decrease may indicate a worsening condition with further hypoxia. Always assess the respiratory rate and tidal volume when there is a decrease in the SpO_2 reading.

Monitor the pulse for changes in the heart rate and regularity. A decreasing heart rate in a patient who has tachycardia may indicate improvement if the mental status is also improving and the respiratory distress is subsiding. If the heart rate is declining along with the mental status, and the respiratory distress is worsening, this is an ominous sign of impending respiratory failure. Increases in the heart rate may be seen with the administration of many of the metered-dose inhalers. These medications mimic the actions of the sympathetic nervous system; therefore, a slight increase in heart rate may be anticipated. This tachycardia would be expected to decrease once the condition improves and the medication begins to wear off.

Understanding BODY PROCESSES

$Beta_2$ metered-dose inhalers also contain trace beta 1 properties. Beta 1 properties increase the heart rate and the force of contraction. An increase in the heart rate following the administration of a $beta_2$ MDI is often a side effect from the trace beta 1 properties. ■

Moist skin (diaphoresis) is a result of the sympathetic nervous system response in the patient with breathing difficulty. An increase in diaphoresis would correlate with a worsening condition.

Reassess and record the blood pressure. Reassess the breath sounds. Improved air movement in the lungs will produce clearer and louder breath sounds on both sides of the chest. Conversely, as the condition deteriorates, the breath sounds become diminished to absent. Note that decreased wheezing may not indicate improvement; it may actually indicate severe bronchoconstriction with less air movement.

The patient with breathing difficulty is considered a priority patient, especially if the condition does not respond to your emergency care. You should consider advanced life support backup.

If the patient's complaint changes, repeat the physical exam and vital signs. Ensure that the oxygen is applied properly and flowing adequately. Continuously assess the status of the breathing.

If positive pressure ventilation with supplemental oxygen has been initiated, continuously assess its effectiveness. Ensure that oxygen is connected and adequately flowing to the pocket mask or the reservoir of the bag-valve-mask device.

Summary: Assessment and Care

To review assessment findings that may be associated with breathing difficulty and emergency care for breathing difficulty, see Figures 16-17∗ and 16-18∗.

Assessment Summary

RESPIRATORY DISTRESS

The following are findings that may be associated with breathing difficulty.

SCENE SIZE-UP

Is breathing difficulty due to a medical or a traumatic cause? Look for evidence of:

- Mechanism of injury—collision, fall, guns, knives, bruising on chest
- Home or portable oxygen tanks or concentrators indicating chronic respiratory problems
- Alcohol or food that may indicate choking

Primary Assessment

General Impression

Position of patient:

- Tripod
- Lying flat

Facial expression:

- Agitated or confused

Speech:

- Patient may gasp for breath between words.

Mental Status

- Alert to unresponsive
- Restlessness
- Agitation
- Disorientation

Airway

- Inspect for incomplete or partial obstruction
- Crowing and stridor (indicate partial obstruction)
- Gurgling (indicates fluid in the airway; suction required)

Breathing

- Signs of inadequate breathing, including poor chest rise and fall, poor volume heard and felt, diminished or absent breath sounds
- Wheezing heard on auscultation

FIGURE 16-17a ∗ Assessment summary: respiratory distress.

Circulation

Tachycardia (more typical in adult with hypoxia)
Bradycardia (more typical in infant or young child with hypoxia)
Cyanosis to mucous membranes, around nose and mouth, nail beds, chest, and neck

Status: Priority Patient

History and Secondary Assessment

History

Signs and symptoms:
Shortness of breath
Restlessness and anxiety
Difficulty in breathing while lying flat
Diaphoresis
Known allergies to medication or other substances
Medications for respiratory conditions
Home oxygen
Prescribed metered-dose inhaler (MDI)
Pre-existing respiratory or cardiac disease
Hospitalized for respiratory condition

Physical Exam

Head, neck, and face:
Cyanosis to face, neck, and mucous membranes
Jugular venous distention (may indicate heart failure or lung injury [tension pneumothorax])
Jugular vein engorgement on inhalation (Kussmaul sign)
Nasal flaring
Pursed-lip breathing
Chest:
Retractions
Accessory muscle use
Wheezing
Productive cough
Barrel chest (indicates emphysema, a chronic respiratory condition)
Abdomen:
Use of abdominal muscles when breathing
Extremities:
Cyanosis to fingers and nail beds
Pale skin
Diaphoresis

Baseline Vital Signs

BP: normal
BP: sudden decrease in the systolic BP by 10 mmHg or greater with inhalation
HR: increased in adults; slow in infants and young children
Pulse: sudden decrease in the pulse amplitude with inhalation
RR: increased; may decrease with greater hypoxia
Skin: cyanosis, paleness, diaphoresis
Pupils: dilated; sluggish to respond to light
SpO_2: 95%

FIGURE 16-17a ✻ Assessment summary: respiratory distress. *continued*

Emergency Care Protocol

RESPIRATORY DISTRESS

1. Establish and maintain an open airway.
2. Suction secretions as necessary.
3. If breathing is inadequate, provide positive pressure ventilation with supplemental oxygen at a minimum rate of 10–12 ventilations/minute for an adult and 12–20 ventilations/minute for an infant or child.
4. If breathing is adequate, apply a nonrebreather mask at 15 lpm.
5. If the patient has signs and symptoms of breathing difficulty and has a prescribed metered-dose inhaler or a nebulization device, administer the beta 2-specific drug as appropriate according to medical direction:
   - Beta 2-specific drugs mimic the sympathetic nervous system and cause bronchodilation.
   - Dose is precisely delivered by the device.
   - Obtain an order from medical direction.
   - Ensure the "five rights" of medication administration.
   - Assemble the equipment (MDI or nebulizer) as discussed previously.
   - Place the device, and instruct the patient how to breathe.
   - Replace nonrebreather mask on patient.
   - Record time and reassess patient.
   - Beta 2 side effects:
     tachycardia
     tremors
     nervousness
     dry mouth
     nausea
6. Consider advanced life support if the condition does not improve.
7. Transport in a position of comfort.
8. Perform a reassessment of the patient's status every 5 minutes.
9. *Complete the secondary assessment.If your protocol allows, in cases of severe respiratory distress consider the use of continuous positive airway pressure (CPAP). Current studies show that patients in severe respiratory distress from a variety of conditions may benefit from CPAP. (See Chapter 10, "Airway Management, Artificial Ventilation, and Oxygenation."*

FIGURE 16-17b ✻ Emergency care protocol: respiratory distress.

Emergency Care Algorithm: Respiratory Distress/Failure/Arrest

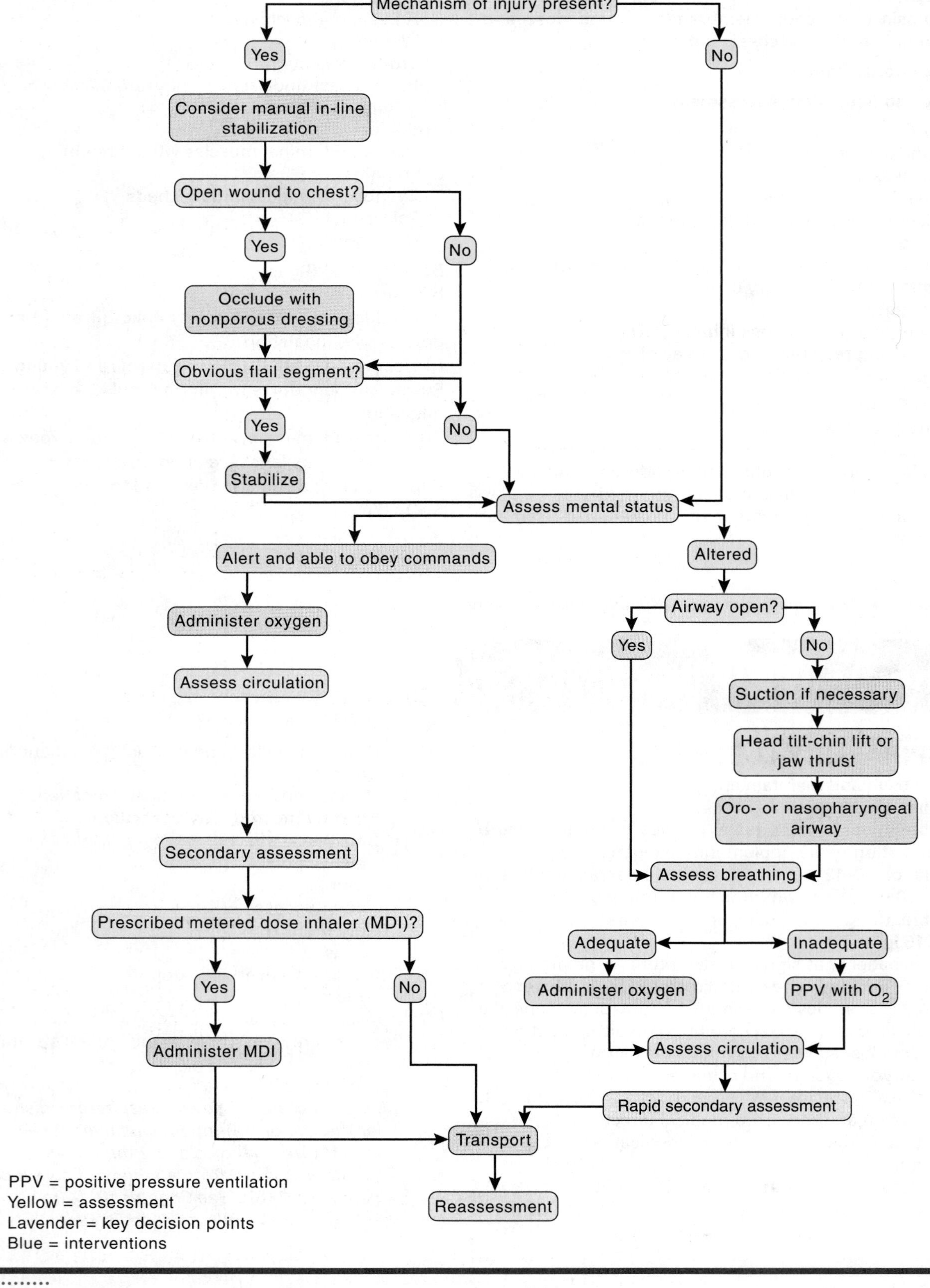

FIGURE 16-18 ✱ Emergency care algorithm: respiratory distress/failure/arrest.

EMT skills 16-1 Auscultating the Chest

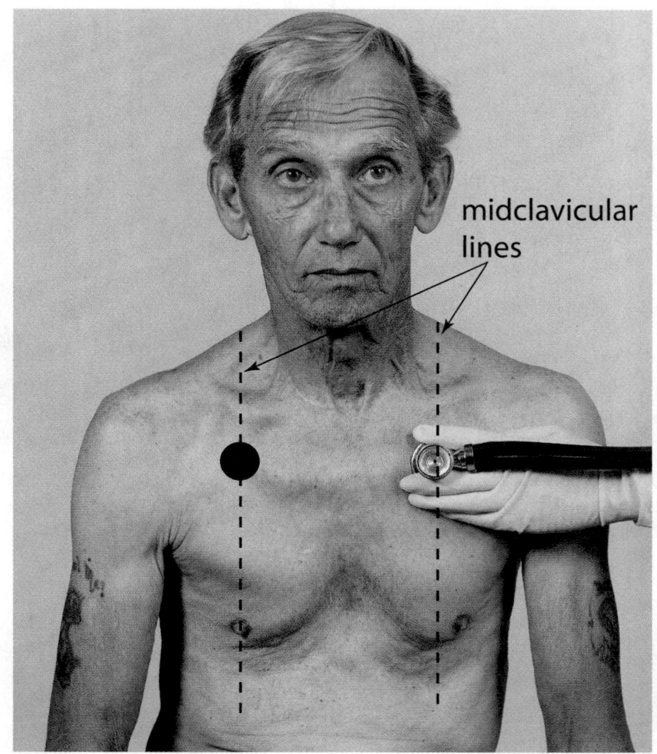

16-1A ✱ Auscultate the anterior chest at the second intercostal space at each midclavicular line.

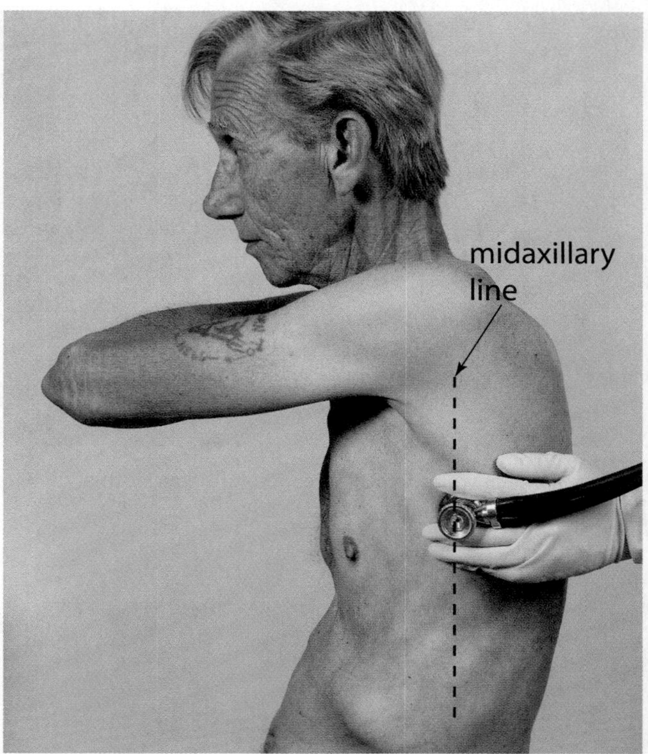

16-1B ✱ Auscultate the lateral chest at the fourth to fifth intercostal space at each midaxillary line.

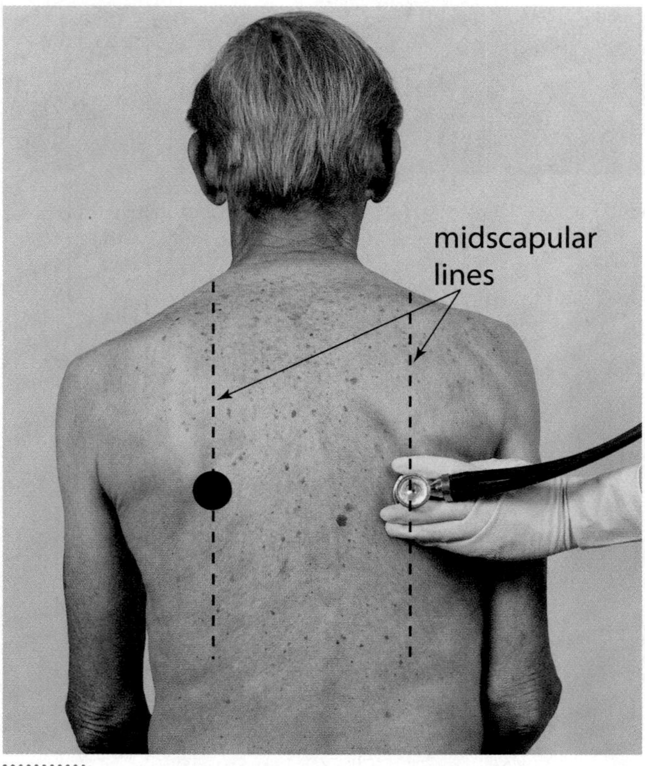

16-1C ✱ Auscultate the posterior chest below the tip of the scapula on each midscapular line.

EMT skills 16-2 Administering Medication by Metered-Dose Inhaler

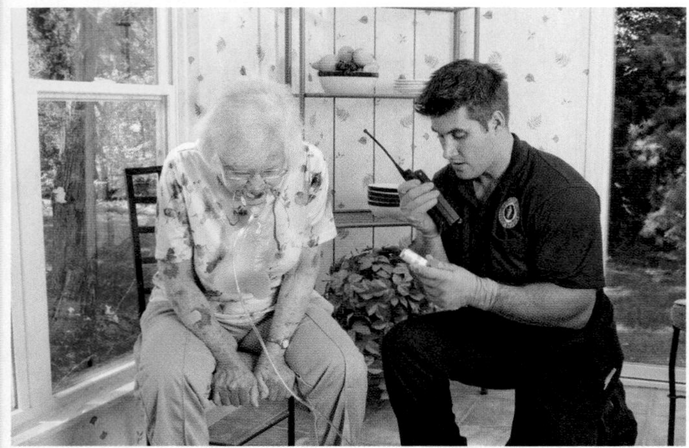

16-2A ✱ Consult with medical direction for an order to administer the medication.

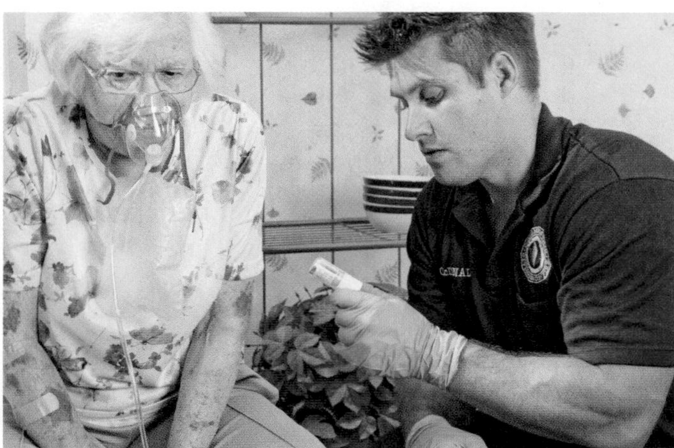

16-2B ✱ Check to make sure the medication is for the patient, that it is the proper one to administer, and that it has not reached its expiration date.

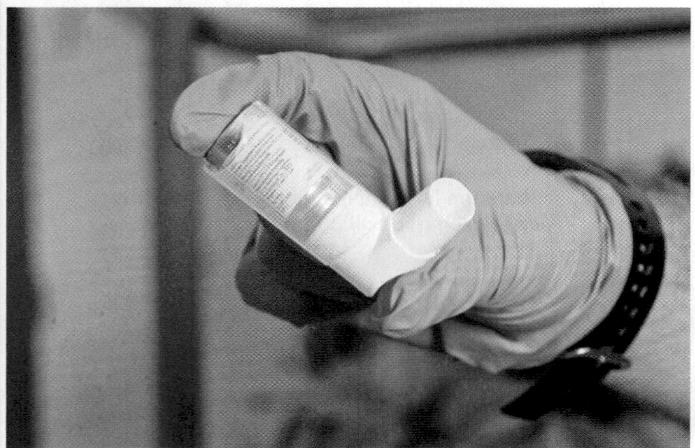

16-2C ✱ Shake the inhaler vigorously for at least 30 seconds.

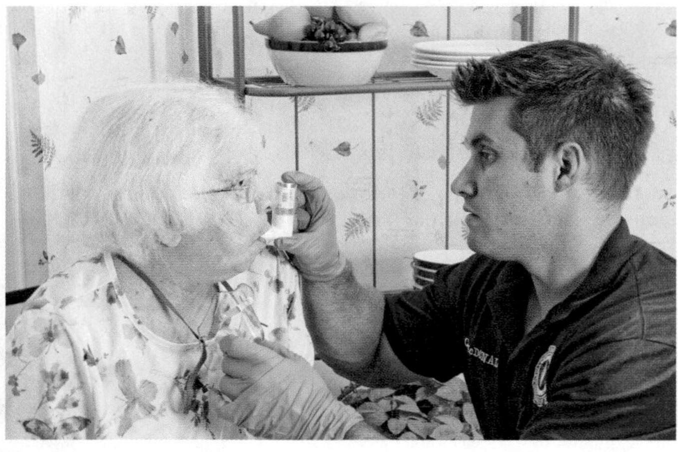

16-2D ✱ Instruct the patient to inhale slowly and deeply for about 5 seconds. As the patient begins to inhale, depress the canister.

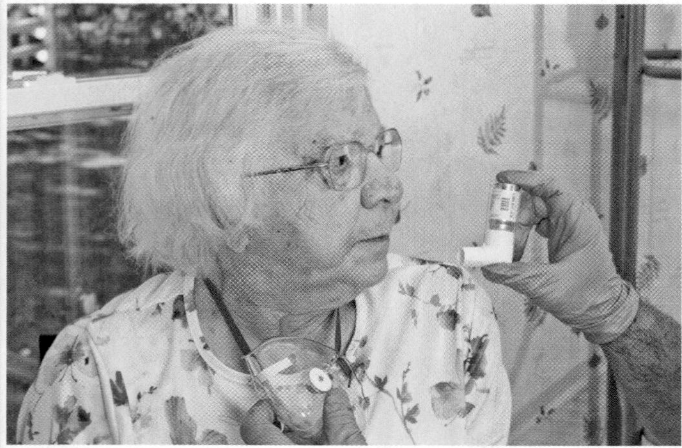

16-2E ✱ Remove the inhaler and instruct the patient to hold the breath for 10 seconds or for as long as is comfortable.

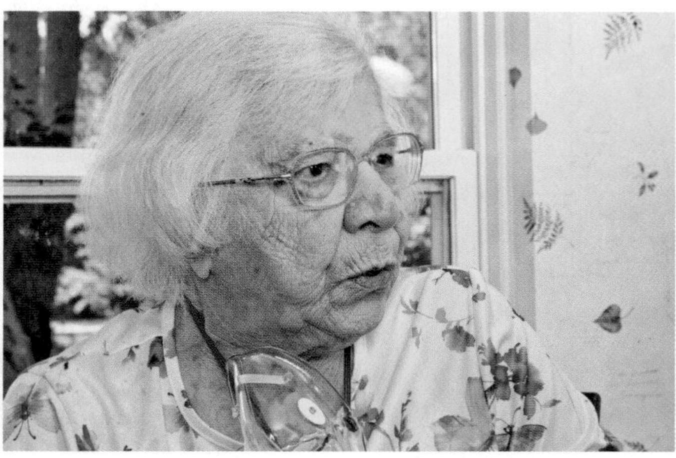

16-2F ✱ Instruct the patient to exhale slowly through pursed lips.

EMT skills 16-2 Administering Medication by Metered-Dose Inhaler *continued*

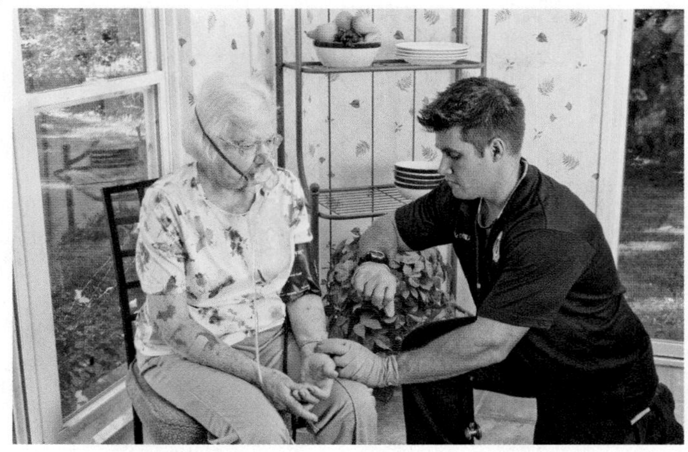

16-2G ✱ Replace the oxygen on the patient. Reassess the breathing status and vital signs.

EMT skills 16-3 Administering a Metered-Dose Inhaler with a Spacer

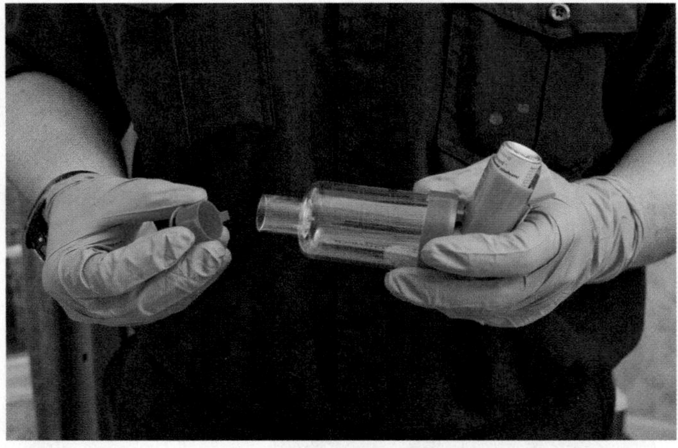

16-3A ✱ Remove the spacer cap. Attach the spacer to the inhaler mouthpiece.

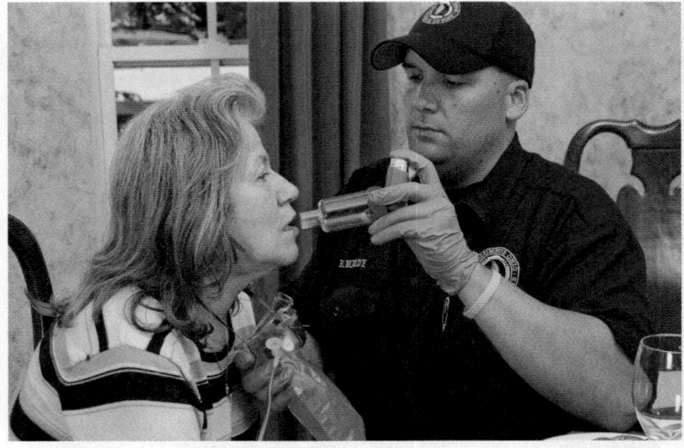

16-3B ✱ Depress the medication canister to fill the spacer with medication.

continued

EMT skills 16-3 Administering a Metered-Dose Inhaler with a Spacer *continued*

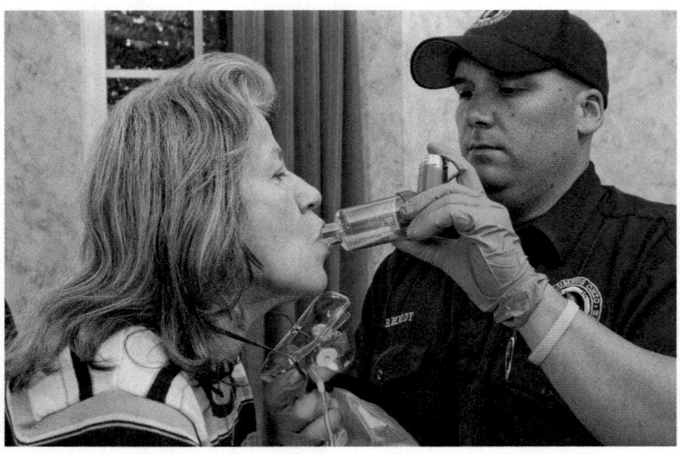

16-3C ✱ Instruct the patient to inhale slowly and deeply. The spacer may whistle if the patient is inhaling too quickly.

EMT skills 16-4 Administering Nebulized Medications

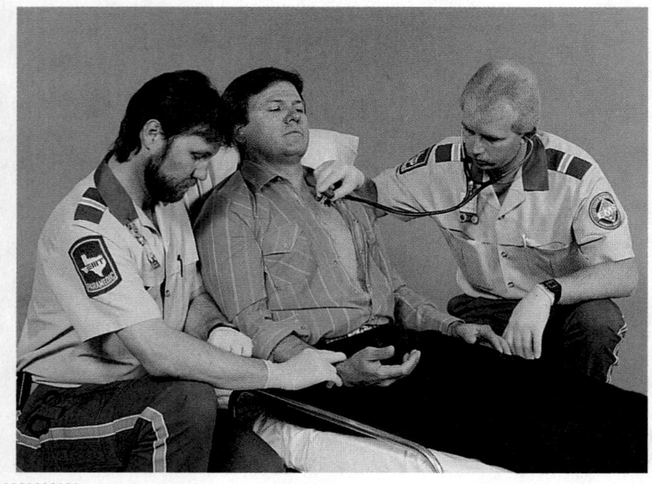

16-4A ✱ Complete the primary assessment and assess the patient's pulse rate and breath sounds.

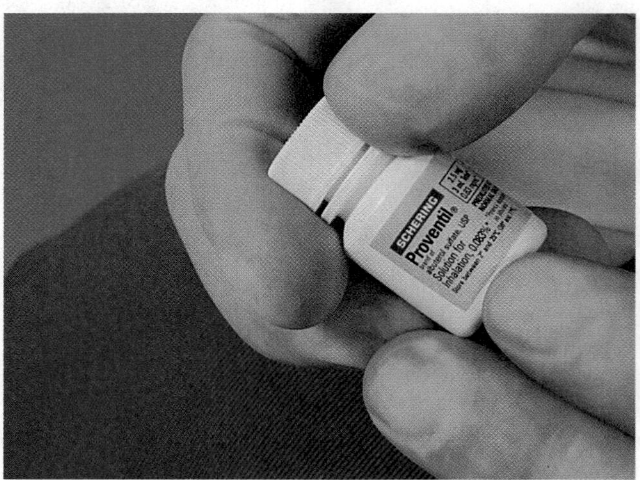

16-4B ✱ Select the correct medication and consult with medical direction for an order to administer the medication.

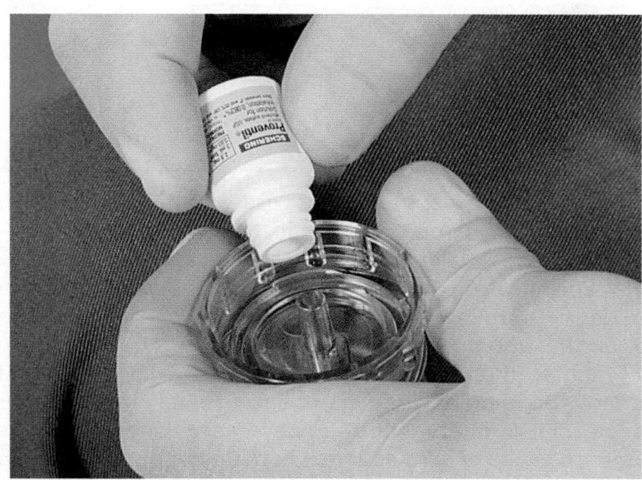

16-4C ✱ Add the medication to the nebulizer chamber.

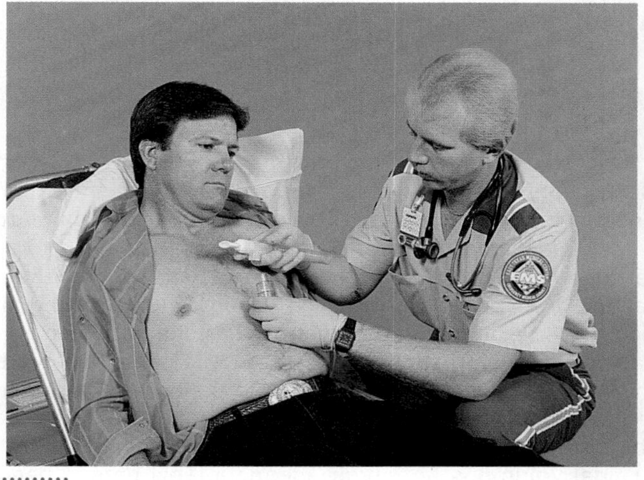

16-4D ✱ Assemble the nebulizer.

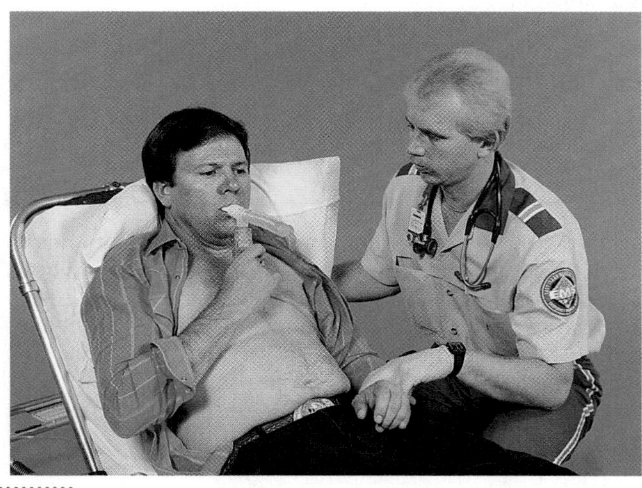

16-4E ✱ Coach the patient to inhale the nebulized medication from the mouthpiece.

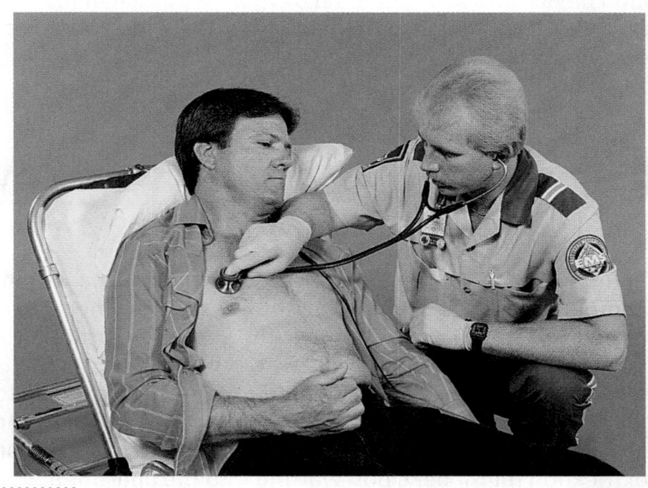

16-4F ✱ Reassess the patient's pulse rate and breath sounds.

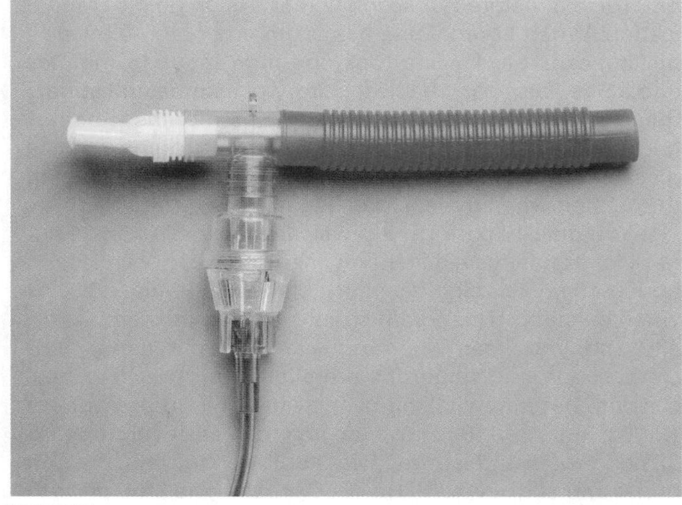

16-4G ✱ Nebulized medications may be administered through a mouthpiece . . .

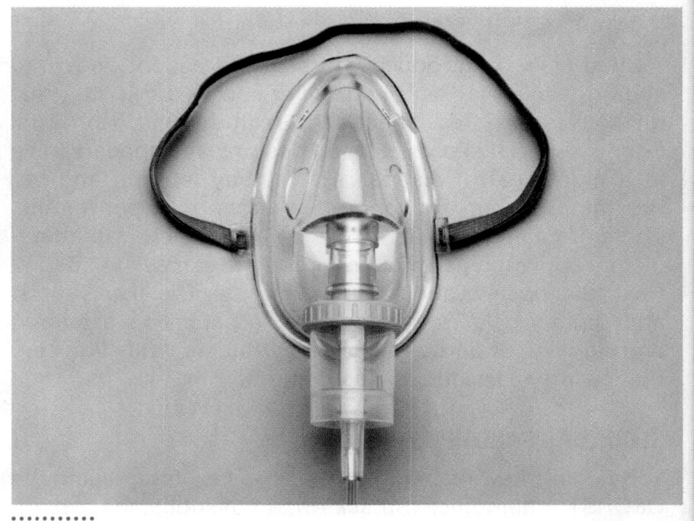

16-4H ✱ . . . or through a face mask. (Photos G and H: © Carl Leet, YSU)

CHAPTER REVIEW

SUMMARY

Respiratory emergencies can range from a patient experiencing respiratory distress to a patient who is in respiratory arrest. It is imperative to effectively assess the patient to determine if the condition is respiratory distress, respiratory failure, or respiratory arrest. The patient with breathing difficulty who is in respiratory distress is still able to compensate for the disturbance and needs supplemental oxygen to improve his oxygenation status. The patient in respiratory failure, as the name implies, has failed to continue to meet the metabolic demands of the body, and the respiratory rate or tidal volume is no longer adequate. This patient needs immediate ventilation with a bag-valve mask or other ventilation device and supplemental oxygen. A patient in respiratory arrest is no longer breathing and also needs immediate positive pressure ventilation.

A patient in respiratory distress who has a history of asthma, emphysema, or chronic bronchitis may have a metered-dose inhaler or home nebulizer unit that delivers a $beta_2$-specific drug. If so, you may assist the patient in using the device to relieve the bronchoconstriction that is impeding airflow into the alveoli.

Infants, children, and geriatric patients may present differently than adults when experiencing a respiratory emergency. Quick intervention is necessary since the most common cause of cardiac arrest in pediatric patients is from an airway or respiratory compromise, and geriatric patients may rapidly deteriorate because of poor compensatory mechanisms.

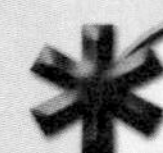

CASE STUDY FOLLOW-UP

SCENE SIZE-UP

You have been dispatched to a 31-year-old female patient complaining of difficulty in breathing. A man nervously greets you at the curb as you gather your equipment. He indicates that the patient is his wife, Anna Sanders, who is having an extremely hard time breathing. You are led up to the third floor of an apartment complex. You do not note any possible hazards, but are looking at how difficult the extrication might be. Upon walking into the apartment you note a young female patient sitting in a tripod position next to the kitchen table.

PRIMARY ASSESSMENT

As you start to introduce yourself, the patient begins to speak, gasping for her breath after each word. With great difficulty she states, "I—can't—breathe." Based on Mrs. Sanders's facial expression and posture, she appears to be in a great deal of distress. Her airway is open and her breathing is rapid and labored at a rate of 34 per minute. There are audible wheezes when she exhales. You immediately apply oxygen via a nonrebreather mask at 15 lpm. Her radial pulse is about 110 per minute. The skin is moist and slightly pale. You recognize the patient as a priority and signal your partner to get the stretcher while you continue with the secondary assessment.

SECONDARY ASSESSMENT

You begin to evaluate the difficulty in breathing using the OPQRST mnemonic. You ask Anna questions she can answer with a nod or a shake of her head to reduce her need to respond by speaking. Some questions you direct to her husband. You ascertain that the breathing difficulty began gradually about 2 hours ago and got progressively worse. She is unable to lie down because this causes her breathing to get much worse, although sitting up is not much better. She has had similar episodes in the past, but none seem to have been this severe. On a scale of 1 to 10, Mrs. Sanders indicates that her difficulty in breathing is about an 8 or 9.

You continue to obtain a history. The primary symptom is severe difficulty in breathing. Mrs. Sanders has an allergy to penicillin. When asked about medications that she takes, Mr. Sanders brings you a prescription of albuterol in a metered-dose inhaler. She is on no other medication. When asked if she has taken any of the albuterol, her husband says, "She took one puff about 15 minutes ago." She has a past medical history of asthma and suffers these attacks maybe once every 4 or 5 months. She has had nothing to eat for about 3 hours but drank a small glass of orange juice about an hour ago. She was cleaning the kitchen when the episode began.

You quickly perform a physical exam. You assess her neck for jugular vein distention. Inspection of her chest and abdomen reveals significant use of the abdominal muscles when exhaling. The breath sounds are diminished bilaterally and you hear wheezing even without using your stethoscope. Her fingertips are slightly cyanotic. You assess the baseline vital signs and find a blood pressure of 134/86; pulse of 118 per minute and regular; respirations at 32 per minute and labored with audible wheezing; the skin moist and slightly pale. Her SpO_2 reading is 88% prior to oxygen administration.

You contact your medical director, Dr. Maxwell, for an order to administer the albuterol by MDI. You check the medication to ensure it is prescribed to Mrs. Sanders, that it is the correct medication, and that it has not expired. You report your physical findings and history to Dr. Maxwell. He gives you an order to administer one dose. If there is no relief of the symptoms, he instructs you to contact him for further orders. Mrs. Sanders is familiar with the MDI and its use, but she is too scared and apprehensive to use it properly. You proceed with the administration by coaching Mrs. Sanders throughout the procedure.

REASSESSMENT

You reassess the vital signs following administration of the albuterol. The blood pressure is 130/84, pulse rate decreases to 90 per minute, and respirations are now 18 per minute and much less labored. Her SpO_2 reading, after oxygen administration, is 96%. The audible wheezes are minimal. The skin is not as moist and both skin and fingernails begin to return to a normal color. You secure Mrs. Sanders in a Fowler position on a stair chair, and you and your partner transport her down to a stretcher your partner has placed on the first floor.

You reassess the difficulty in breathing. Mrs. Sanders is now able to talk in complete sentences and indicates that the shortness of breath is much less severe. She is now only slightly short of breath. You continue oxygen therapy, document your findings and emergency care, and radio the hospital with a report.

Upon arrival at the hospital, you provide the nursing staff with an oral report. You write a prehospital care report form as your partner restocks the ambulance. Before leaving the hospital, you check in on Mrs. Sanders and find her to be relaxed and breathing well. She thanks you for your prompt response and emergency care. You then mark back in service and prepare for the next call.

IN REVIEW

1. List the major signs and symptoms of breathing difficulty.
2. List the signs of adequate breathing.
3. List the signs of inadequate breathing.
4. List the steps of emergency care for a patient who is exhibiting signs and symptoms of breathing difficulty but is breathing adequately (respiratory distress).
5. List the steps of emergency care for a patient who is in respiratory failure.
6. List the signs of adequate positive pressure ventilation and the steps to take if ventilation is inadequate.
7. Explain the steps to administer a medication by metered-dose inhaler and by small-volume nebulizer.
8. List the indications and contraindications for the use of a beta-agonist drug.
9. Describe the early signs of breathing difficulty in the infant or child; list the signs of inadequate breathing and respiratory failure in the infant or child.
10. Explain how to distinguish airway obstruction in the infant or child patient caused by disease, from airway obstruction caused by a foreign body; explain how treatment would differ for the two types of airway obstruction.

CRITICAL THINKING

You arrive on the scene and find a 72-year-old female patient sitting up in her recliner in the living room of her home. She looks very fatigued and appears to be in severe respiratory distress. As you approach her, she appears extremely pale and diaphoretic with circumoral cyanosis. Her head is bobbing with each breath. As you ask her name, she can barely say it. She is gasping with each breath she takes. Her respiratory rate is 36 per minute with a shallow tidal volume. Her radial pulse is weak and rapid. Her skin is pale, very cool, and extremely moist. Her nail beds and fingertips are cyanotic. Her SpO_2 reading is 82%. Her blood pressure is 92/70 mmHg. She has a history of congestive heart failure, two previous heart attacks, and hypertension.

1. What would be the immediate emergency care provided during the primary assessment?
2. What is the respiratory status of the patient?
3. How would you manage the respiratory status of the patient?
4. What would you expect to find upon auscultation of the lungs?
5. What areas of the lungs would be most important to auscultate?
6. What would be the most effective method to increase oxygenation in the patient?

EXPLORE PEARSON **mybradykit**™

Please go to **www.bradybooks.com** to access mykit for this text. You will find quizzes, critical thinking scenarios, weblinks, animations, and videos related to this chapter—and much more. Look for online information on breath sounds and assessment tips as well as animations and video clips on asthma, tuberculosis, ARDS, and COPD.

Register your access code from the front of your book by going to **www.bradybooks.com** and selecting the mykit links.

CHAPTER 17

Cardiovascular Emergencies

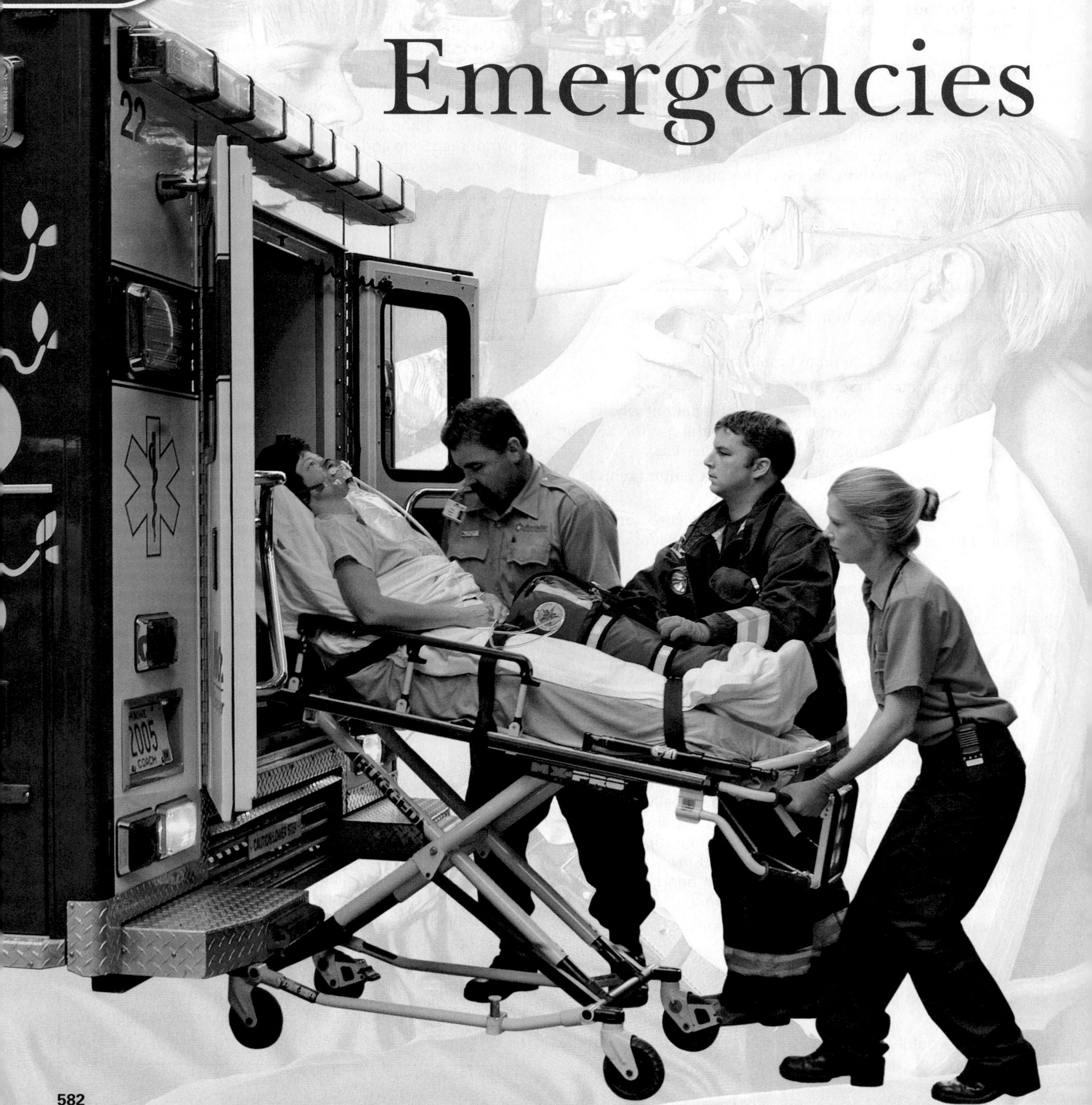

Navigation Guide

The following items provide an overview to the purpose and content of this chapter. The Standard and Competency are from the new National EMS Education Standards.

STANDARD **Medicine** (Content Area: Cardiovascular)

COMPETENCY Applies fundamental knowledge to provide basic emergency care and transportation based on assessment findings for an acutely ill patient.

OBJECTIVES: After reading this chapter, you should be able to:

17-1. Define key terms introduced in this chapter.
17-2. Describe the relationship between chest pain or discomfort, heart disease, and cardiac arrest.
17-3. Describe the structure and function of the circulatory system, including:
- **a.** The cardiac conduction system
- **b.** Conductive tissue and conductivity
- **c.** Contractile tissue and contractility
- **d.** Automaticity
- **e.** Effects of the autonomic nervous system (sympathetic and parasympathetic) on the heart
- **f.** Gross anatomy of the heart
- **g.** Systemic and pulmonary circulation
- **h.** Coronary arteries
- **i.** Plasma and formed elements of the blood

17-4. Explain the relationship between electrical and mechanical events in the heart.
17-5. Describe the processes of depolarization and repolarization, and relate the waves and intervals of a normal electrocardiogram (ECG) to the physiological events they represent.
17-6. Discuss the relationship between hypoxia, damage to the cardiac conduction system, premature ventricular contractions, ventricular tachycardia, and ventricular fibrillation.
17-7. Describe the roles of the heart and blood vessels in maintaining normal blood pressure.
17-8. Explain the importance of early recognition of signs and symptoms and the early treatment of patients with cardiac emergencies.
17-9. Explain the pathophysiology and the appropriate assessment and management of the following conditions that may be classified as cardiac compromise or acute coronary syndrome:
- **a.** Angina pectoris
- **b.** Myocardial infarction
- **c.** Aortic aneurysm or dissection
- **d.** Congestive heart failure
- **e.** Cardiogenic shock
- **f.** Hypertensive emergencies
- **g.** Cardiac arrest

17-10. Explain the typical presentation of myocardial ischemia or infarction in females.
17-11. Explain the indications, contraindications, forms, dosage, administration, actions, side effects, and reassessment for nitroglycerin.
17-12. Explain the special considerations in assessing and managing pediatric and geriatric patients with cardiac emergencies.
17-13. Explain the assessment-based approach to assessment and emergency medical care for cardiac compromise and acute coronary syndrome.
17-14. Discuss the indications and contraindications for fibrinolytic therapy in patients with cardiac emergencies.
17-15. Given a series of scenarios, demonstrate the assessment-based management of a variety of patients with cardiovascular emergencies, including: Explain the indications, contraindications, forms, dosage, administration, actions, side effects, and reassessment for aspirin.

KEY TERMS: Page references indicate first major use in this chapter. For complete definitions, see the Glossary at the back of the book.

acute coronary syndrome (ACS) p. 594
aorta p. 587
arteriole p. 588
artery p. 588
atria p. 585
automaticity p. 585
blood pressure p. 592
capillary p. 588
cardiac compromise p. 593
cardiac conduction system p. 584
circulatory system p. 584
coronary arteries p. 588
heart p. 585
nitroglycerin p. 603
perfusion p. 593
pulmonary artery p. 586
pulmonary vein p. 587
vein p. 588
venae cavae p. 586
ventricles p. 585
venule p. 588

continued

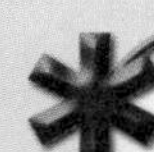

Navigation Guide *continued*

MEDIA RESOURCES: Please go to www.bradybooks.com to access mykit for this text. You will find quizzes, critical thinking scenarios, weblinks, animations, and videos related to this chapter—and much more. Look for online information on heart attacks, congenital heart defects, hypertension, and acute myocardial infarction. You will also find video clips on AEDs, understanding coronary heart disease, and understanding dysrhythmias.

CASE STUDY

The Dispatch

EMS Unit 23—respond to 321 Congress St., Reali's Restaurant. You have a 49-year-old male complaining of chest discomfort. Time out is 1735 hours.

Upon Arrival

You and your partner arrive at 1740 hours and find the patient sitting in a chair at a table clutching his chest. As you approach the patient, you note that he looks very anxious. The scene is secure and he is the only patient. You introduce your partner and yourself. Your patient gives his name as Paul Antak. He states, "I feel like someone is standing on my chest."

How Would You Proceed to Assess and Care for This Patient?

During this chapter, you will learn about assessment and emergency care for a patient suffering from cardiovascular emergencies such as chest discomfort or pain and cardiac arrest. Later, we will return to the case and apply the procedures learned.

Introduction

Some—though certainly not all—patients with chest discomfort or pain are experiencing a heart attack, and some may deteriorate into cardiac arrest at the scene or en route to the hospital. Because of the potential for a severe and often fatal event, the EMT must treat every patient with signs and symptoms of cardiac compromise as a cardiac emergency.

Heart disease is America's number one killer. While the EMT will occasionally be called to a patient who is in cardiac arrest or who goes into cardiac arrest before reaching the hospital, more often the call will be to a responsive patient who has signs and symptoms—particularly chest discomfort or pain—that may be caused by heart disease. Although not every cardiac arrest is preceded by chest discomfort or pain, nor do all patients with chest discomfort or pain proceed to cardiac arrest, for those who do, rapid intervention is vital.

Review of the Circulatory System Anatomy and Physiology

The following is a brief review of the anatomy and physiology of the circulatory system as it pertains more specifically to cardiac emergencies. For a more detailed discussion, review Chapter 7, "Anatomy, Physiology, and Medical Terminology."

The Circulatory System

The **circulatory system**, also known as the *cardiovascular system,* has three major components: the heart, the blood vessels, and the blood. Each of these components may play a significant role in patients experiencing a cardiac-related emergency.

The Conduction System

The heart is more than just a muscle. It contains specialized *conductive* tissue (the **cardiac conduction system**, Figure 17-1*), which generates electrical impulses that are conducted rapidly to other cells of the heart (a prop-

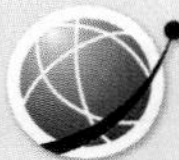

Media Resources

Go to www.bradybooks.com for mykit. Highlights:

- *Web Resource:* Heart Attacks
- *Web Resource:* Hypertension

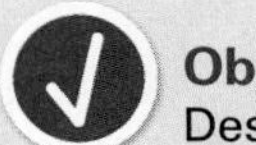

Objective 17-2
Describe the relationship between chest pain or discomfort, heart disease, and cardiac arrest.

Objectives 17-3 and 17-4
Describe circulatory system structure and function and electrical and mechanical events in the heart.

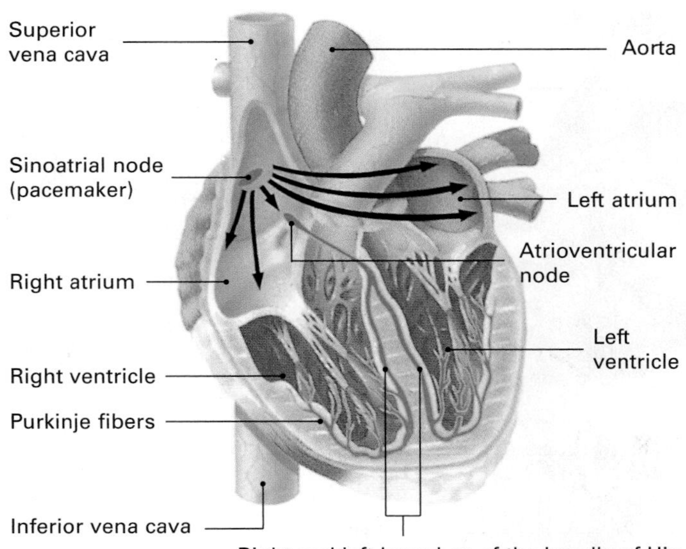

FIGURE 17-1 ✻ The cardiac conduction system.

erty known as *conductivity.* The heart also contains specialized *contractile* tissue that allows the heart muscle to contract when stimulated by the electrical impulses from the conduction system.

Conductive cells are grouped in three areas of the heart—pacemaker sites—where the electrical impulses are created automatically, independent of the autonomic nervous system of the body (a property known as **automaticity**). One pacemaker site is the sinoatrial (SA) node, located in the upper portion of the right atrium. The SA node, known as the primary pacemaker of the heart, generates the impulse that triggers the rest of the heart to contract. A secondary pacemaker site is located at the crux, the point where the walls that separate the upper and lower chambers and the left and right sides of the heart all cross. This pacemaker site, the atrioventricular (AV) node, only creates an impulse if the sinoatrial node fails. The final pacemaker site is widely distributed in the conduction system of the ventricles and is known as the Purkinje fibers or network. These fibers deliver the impulse to the working cells of the heart. If both higher pacemaker sites fail, the Purkinje network can also initiate an impulse to maintain some ventricular contraction.

The heart's electrical impulses travel through the heart from the pacemaker sites via a conduction pathway that is composed of cells that neither initiate an impulse nor contract. Instead, the cells of the conduction pathway rapidly conduct each impulse to the rest of the heart muscle. They do this in a unified fashion so that, rather than the whole heart contracting at once, there is a sequential contraction of the chambers.

In addition to the conductive cells of the heart, there is another group of cells that are often called the "working" cells of the heart, also called contractile cells. Their primary purpose is to contract in response to the electrical impulses provided by the conduction system. These working cells have characteristics of both smooth (involuntary) muscle and skeletal (voluntary) muscle. Like skeletal muscle, they contract strongly when stimulated to help eject blood from the heart. Like smooth muscle, they contract completely, to a very small size, because the heart has to collapse upon itself in order to push blood out of the chambers.

The conduction cells and working cells operate together in unison to fulfill the heart's sole purpose: pumping blood.

The heart's activity is monitored by the body to ensure that it is meeting the body's blood flow requirements. If the heart's activity needs to be modified, assistance is provided by the autonomic nervous system. (Although the heart initiates electrical impulses on its own, the overall heart rate and force of contraction can be influenced by the autonomic nervous system.)

The sympathetic branch of the autonomic nervous system innervates all three pacemaker sites and the working cells of the heart. When the body needs increased blood flow, the sympathetic nervous system is stimulated and causes the heart to beat faster and with greater contractile force, which increases the ejection of blood. The parasympathetic branch of the autonomic nervous system innervates the sinoatrial and atrioventricular nodes. When the parasympathetic nervous system is stimulated, it slows the heart rate and eases the force of contraction. This diminishes cardiac output in situations where strong output is not needed, for example while the body is sleeping or at rest.

The Heart

The **heart** (Figure 17-2✻) consists of four chambers: the **atria** (the two top chambers) and the **ventricles** (the two bottom chambers). As mentioned, the heart has only one purpose: pumping blood within the body. If that single purpose is interrupted, even momentarily, cardiac arrest ensues and the chance of survival is slim.

Key Terms

circulatory system system composed of the heart and blood vessels.

cardiac conduction system contractile and conductive tissue of the heart that generates electrical impulses and causes the heart to beat.

Key Terms

automaticity the ability of cells within the cardiac conduction system to generate a cardiac impulse on their own.

heart the muscular organ that contracts to force blood into circulation through the body.

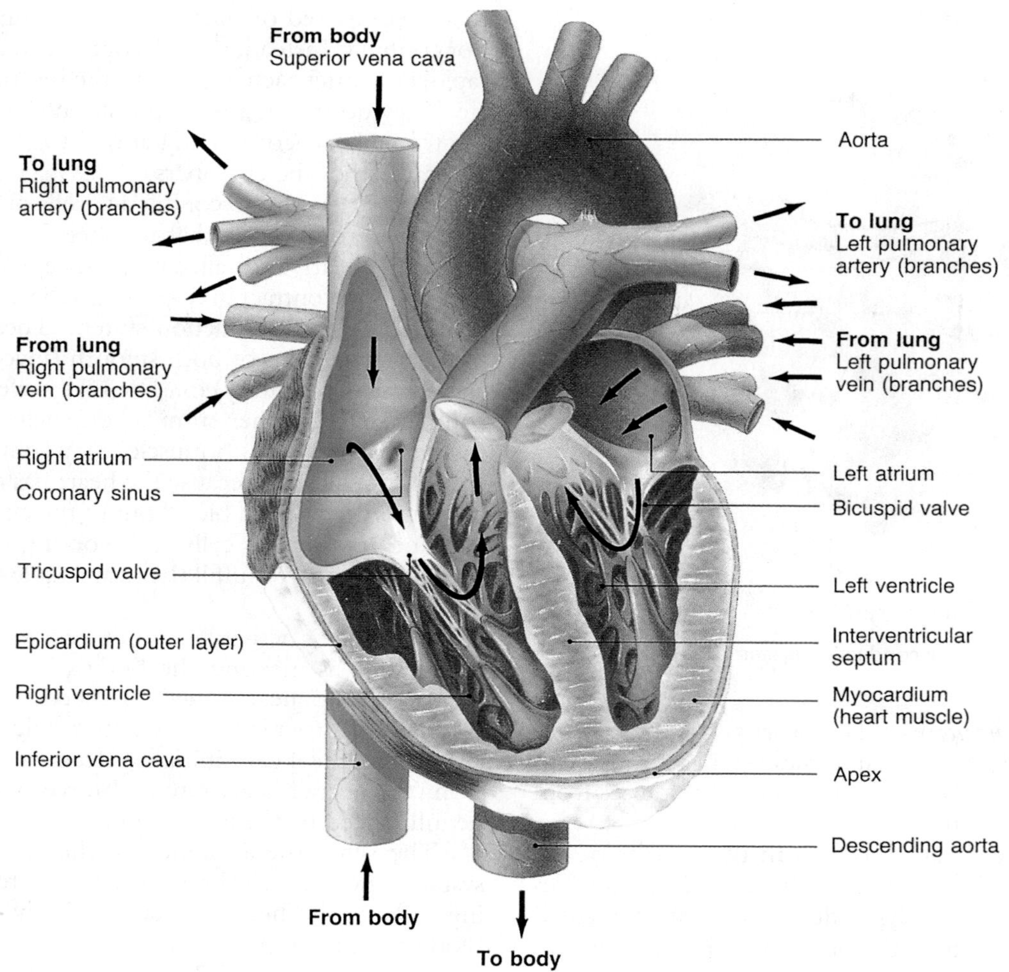

FIGURE 17-2 ✱ The heart.

The right atrium receives deoxygenated blood from the inferior and superior **venae cavae**, the largest veins within the body. Upon contraction, the blood in the right atrium travels through the *tricuspid valve* and into the right ventricle. From the right ventricle, with the next contraction, the deoxygenated blood is ejected through the *pulmonic semilunar valve* and into the **pulmonary arteries**. The pressure in the pulmonary vessels is very low; thus the right ventricle does not have to generate a great deal of force to eject the blood. In some pulmonary (lung) diseases, such as emphysema, however, the pulmonary vessels are compressed or narrowed. This increases the pressure in the pulmonary vessels and makes it much more difficult for the right ventricle to pump the blood out. If this high pressure is sustained over time, the right ventricle begins to weaken and eventually may fail. This is referred to as *right-sided* or *right ventricular heart failure,* also known as *cor pulmonale.*

Understanding BODY PROCESSES

A higher resistance in the pulmonary vessels results in the right ventricle having to contract harder to pump the blood out to the lungs. Over time this causes the right ventricle to weaken and eventually fail, leading to right-sided heart failure. ■

Key Terms

atria the two upper chambers of the heart.

ventricles the two lower chambers of the heart.

venae cavae the two major veins that carry oxygen-depleted blood back to the heart.

Key Terms

pulmonary artery vessel carrying oxygen-depleted blood from the heart's right ventricle to the lungs.

pulmonary vein vessel carrying oxygen-rich blood from the lungs to the left atrium of the heart.

aorta the major artery from the heart.

After the blood is oxygenated in the alveoli of the lungs, it returns to the left atrium via the **pulmonary veins**. The blood in the left atrium is then ejected through the *mitral valve* (also called the *bicuspid valve*) and into the left ventricle upon contraction of the atria. On the next ventricular contraction, the blood is ejected through the *aortic semilunar valve* and into the **aorta**. The blood is then distributed throughout the body to cells and organs (Figure 17-3✻). The pressure in the aorta is very high; therefore, the left ventricle must generate a significant amount of force to eject the blood against this pressure. If the pressure in the aorta is excessively high, as seen in severe hypertensive patients (those with very high blood pressure), or if the blood pressure is simply higher than normal over a long period of time, the left ventricle will begin to weaken and fail. Also, if the left ventricle muscle is damaged due to a blockage of a coronary artery, the ventricle will weaken and will not be able to pump an adequate amount of blood out of the left ventricle. This may lead to *congestive heart failure,* also known as *left-sided* or *left ventricular failure.*

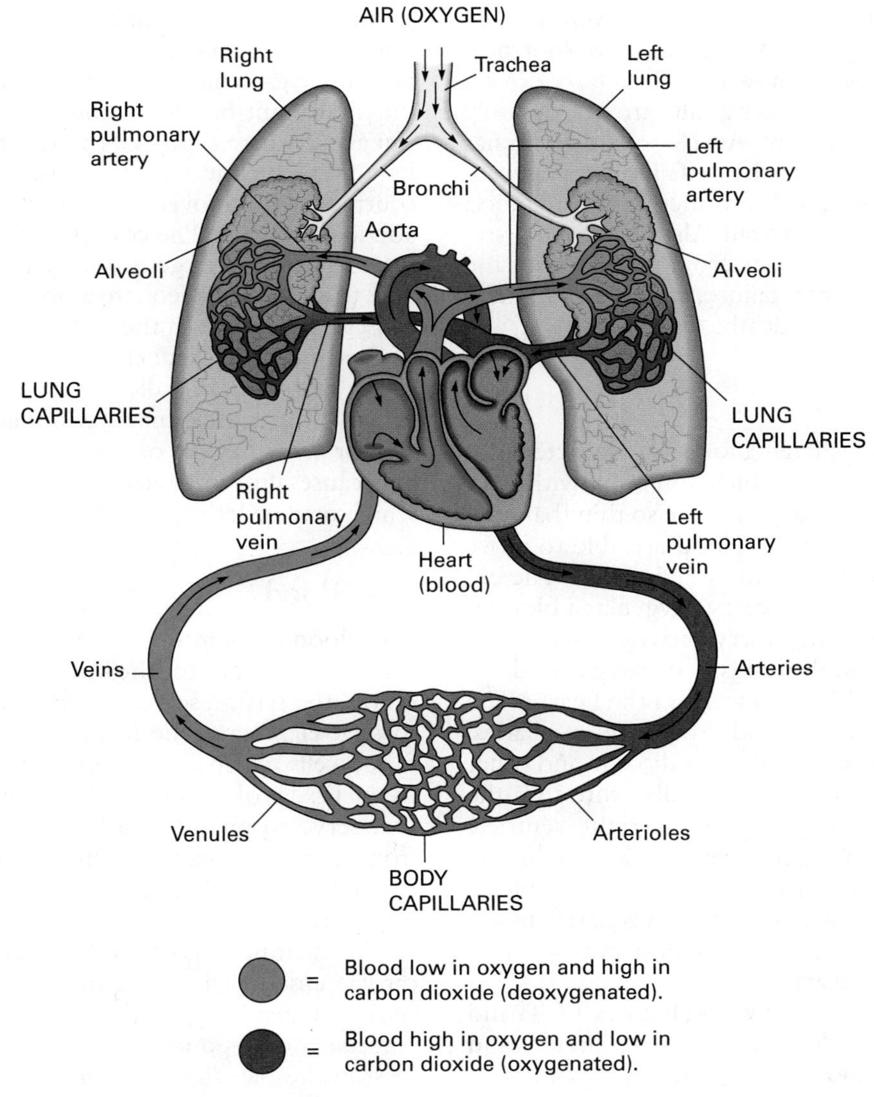

FIGURE 17-3 ✻ Circulation of blood through the cardiovascular system.

Key Terms

artery blood vessel that carries blood away from the heart.

arteriole the smallest branch of an artery.

capillary a tiny blood vessel connecting arterioles to venules.

Key Terms

vein vessel that carries blood toward the heart.

venule smallest vein.

coronary arteries arteries supplying the heart with blood.

Understanding BODY PROCESSES

Left-sided heart failure may result from a constantly high resistance in the arteries causing the ventricle to pump harder or from death to a portion of the left ventricular wall from a coronary artery occlusion. Either circumstance can cause the left ventricle to weaken and eventually fail. ■

When the left ventricle cannot eject the blood effectively, pressure in the left atrium and pulmonary veins begins to build up. This may force fluid out of the capillaries around the alveoli of the lungs, causing a severe gas exchange problem, leading to hypoxia and severe shortness of breath. This condition is known as *pulmonary edema.* It is important to note that older adults are not the only ones to suffer from heart failure. An 18-year-old who has been using cocaine may suffer heart failure from severe vessel constriction that drastically increases the blood pressure and causes the heart to fail. Also, a young person may suffer a heart attack that destroys a portion of the heart muscle, leading to heart failure, cardiac rhythm disturbances, or sudden cardiac death.

The Vessels

The **arteries** carry oxygenated blood to the **arterioles** and then to the **capillaries**, which interface with cells throughout the body. Capillary walls are so thin that oxygen and nutrients carried in the blood are able to move out of the capillaries and into the body's cells. (The exception to the rule that arteries carry oxygenated blood is the pulmonary arteries, which carry deoxygenated blood from the right ventricle to the lungs to be oxygenated. All arteries, however, carry blood away from the heart.) The **veins** carry deoxygenated blood from the capillaries, where the blood has picked up carbon dioxide and other waste products given off by the cells, through the **venules**, to the veins and back to the right ventricle through the inferior and superior vena cava. (Again, the exception to the rule that veins carry deoxygenated blood is the pulmonary veins, which carry oxygenated blood from the lungs back to the left atrium. However, all veins carry blood toward the heart.)

There are many arteries and veins (Figures 17-4a and 17-4b*) as well as smaller arterioles, capillaries, and venules that circulate blood throughout the body.

Coronary Arteries The heart perfuses itself, first, with oxygenated blood before sending the oxygenated blood on to the arteries throughout the body. The **coronary arteries** (Figure 17-5*) are the first two arteries to originate off the aorta and are the same arteries that are associated with many cardiac emergencies. These two arteries branch off from the base of the aorta and are responsible for supplying the heart with a rich supply of oxygenated blood. (The heart gets its blood supply from the coronary arteries, not from the blood that is pumped through its chambers.)

The heart is a muscle that requires a constant supply of oxygenated blood to continue pumping effectively. A good analogy to this concept would be to place a tourniquet around a person's upper arm and ask him to lift a 10-pound weight continuously. How long will he be able to lift the weight before his muscle begins to fatigue without an adequate supply of oxygenated blood? He will not be able to lift the weight for very long at all. Once the tourniquet is removed, the muscle will begin to function adequately again. The concept is the same with the coronary arteries. If a large coronary artery is blocked, it is unable to supply an adequate amount of blood to the heart muscle. Eventually, if the occluded coronary artery is not opened or unblocked, the heart muscle will become hypoxic and begin to die. During the ensuing ischemic process, the muscle may weaken and lead to a *heart attack* or *heart failure,* or the muscle may become irritable and cause abnormal electrical cardiac rhythms, some of which may be lethal.

The Blood

The blood is composed of several components that serve multiple functions for the body. The liquid portion of the blood, the serum, serves as the transport medium for the formed elements. The formed elements include the red blood cells which, among other functions, carry oxygen to the tissues of the body. There are also white blood cells that serve to protect the body and eliminate infections from viruses or bacteria. Platelets are old fragments of destroyed red blood cells whose job is to help in the clotting process to stop bleeding.

These functions of the blood also play a major role in cardiac emergencies. The most significant function in a cardiac emergency is the coagulation process. Blood components respond to injury by forming clots in order to stop the bleeding. The clot that is formed is called a

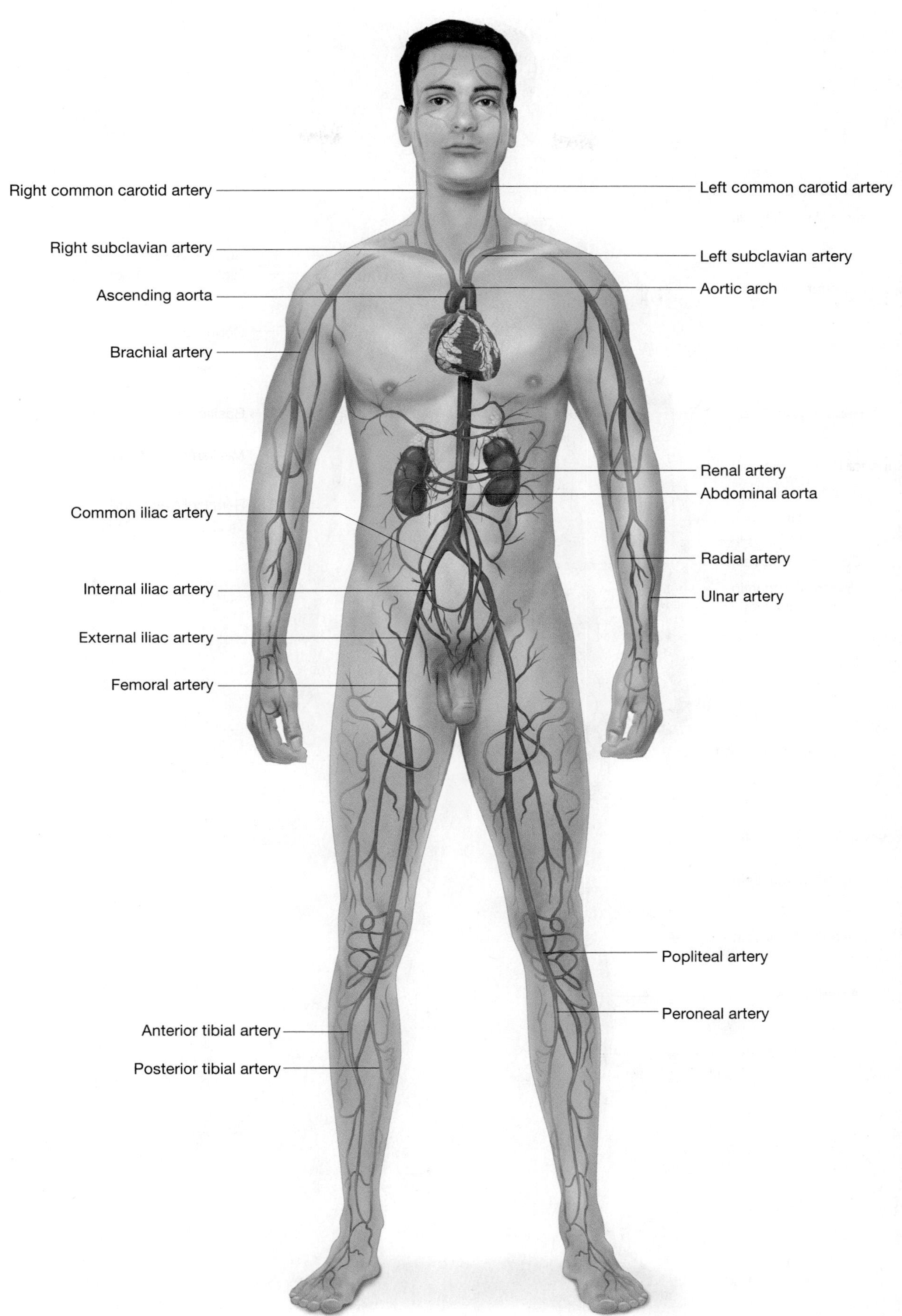
Right common carotid artery
Left common carotid artery
Right subclavian artery
Left subclavian artery
Ascending aorta
Aortic arch
Brachial artery
Renal artery
Abdominal aorta
Common iliac artery
Radial artery
Internal iliac artery
Ulnar artery
External iliac artery
Femoral artery
Popliteal artery
Peroneal artery
Anterior tibial artery
Posterior tibial artery

FIGURE 17-4a ✱ Major arteries.

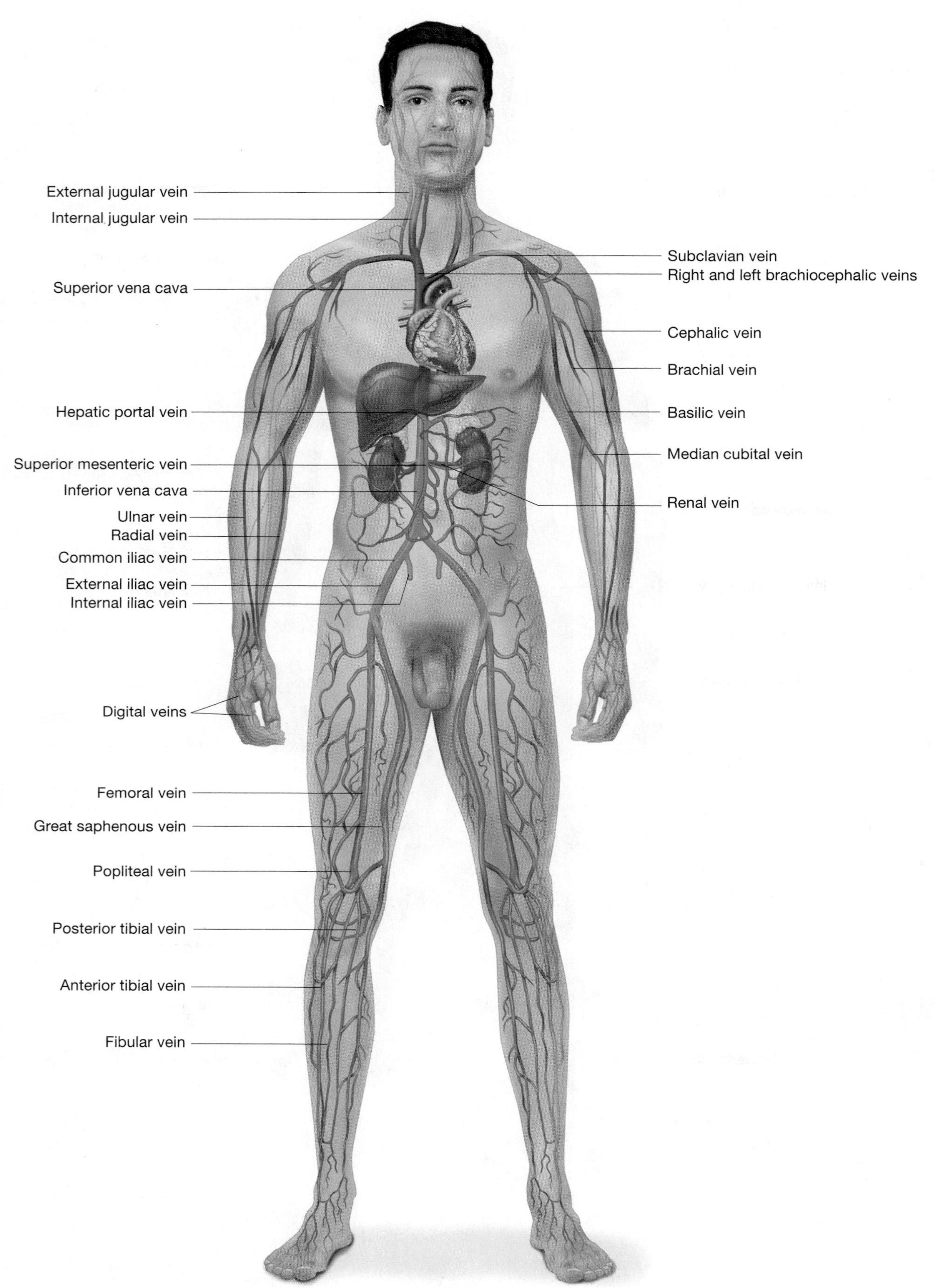
External jugular vein
Internal jugular vein
Superior vena cava
Hepatic portal vein
Superior mesenteric vein
Inferior vena cava
Ulnar vein
Radial vein
Common iliac vein
External iliac vein
Internal iliac vein
Digital veins
Femoral vein
Great saphenous vein
Popliteal vein
Posterior tibial vein
Anterior tibial vein
Fibular vein
Subclavian vein
Right and left brachiocephalic veins
Cephalic vein
Brachial vein
Basilic vein
Median cubital vein
Renal vein

FIGURE 17-4b ✱ Major veins.

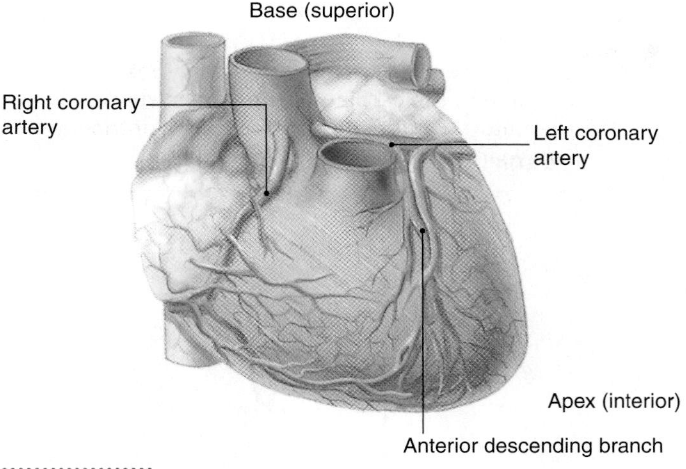

FIGURE 17-5 ✻ The coronary arteries.

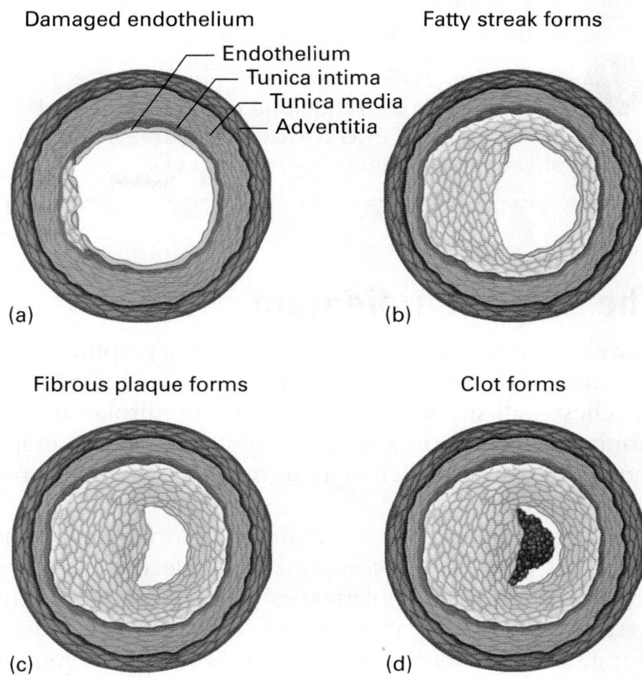

FIGURE 17-6 ✻ The process of artery occlusion (atherosclerosis): **(a)** The endothelium (inner wall) of the artery is damaged as a result of smoking, diabetes, high blood pressure, high blood cholesterol, or other causes. **(b)** Fatty streaks begin to form in the damaged vessel walls. **(c)** Fibrous plaque forms, causing further vessel damage and progressive resistance to blood flow. **(d)** The plaque deposits begin to ulcerate or rupture, and platelets aggregate and adhere to the surface of the ruptured plaque, forming clots that may nearly or totally block the artery.

thrombus. Several components are involved in the clot formation system, the most important of which are *platelets* (disk-shaped elements in the blood that are fragments of cells from the bone marrow), *thrombin* (a protein responsible for activating the formation of a clot), and *fibrin* (strands that are responsible for making the clot stronger).

A thrombus may form within a coronary artery at a site where *plaque* (a fatty deposit) has built up. The thrombus (clot) formation develops in the following way: A plaque deposit inside the coronary artery may weaken over time and rupture. The body views the plaque rupture as an injury and sends out a cascade of substances to form a clot to stop the bleeding at the injury site. Platelets begin to cover the site and thrombin is activated to form a clot. The clot may partially or completely occlude the coronary artery, cutting off or reducing the supply of oxygenated blood to the heart muscle (Figure 17-6✻). The heart muscle becomes deprived of oxygen and may eventually begin to die. This may lead to a heart attack, pump failure, or serious cardiac rhythm disturbances.

Cardiac Contraction

The heart's electrical impulse is first generated in the right atrium at the SA node. It travels through both right and left atria by way of the *Bachmann bundle.* Both atria contract simultaneously as a result of the electrical impulse (a process known as atrial systole), ejecting the blood into the ventricles through the atrioventricular valves that open when the pressure in the atria exceeds the pressure in the ventricles. The impulse then travels to the AV node by way of an *intranodal tract,* located in the area between the atria and the ventricles. There the impulse is inhibited very briefly to allow the blood from the contracted atria to fill the ventricles, and then the impulse travels down the *bundle of His* to the left and right ventricles via the left and right bundle branches.

From the bundle of His and the left and right bundle branches, the electrical impulse travels to the Purkinje fibers, which are embedded in the ventricular muscle, causing the ventricles to contract simultaneously (a process known as ventricular systole). As pressure rapidly increases in the ventricles, it first causes the atrioventricular valves to close. When the pressure exceeds that exerted on the semilunar valves, they open and blood from the right ventricle is propelled toward the lungs while blood from the left ventricle is propelled throughout the body via the aorta.

If the heart rate and force of contraction need to increase or decrease based on the body's demand, the autonomic nervous system facilitates this modification via the sympathetic and parasympathetic nervous systems, as described previously. After the systolic phases of the atria and/or ventricles, there is a diastolic phase in which the heart cells repolarize and await the next impulse, as described in the next section.

When the coronary arteries are occluded, either partially or completely, the conduction system may become irritable from the lack of oxygen. When this occurs, the conduction cells may begin to "fire off" impulses on their own. This may lead to cardiac rhythm abnormalities called *dysrhythmias.* Some of these dysrhythmias may lead to sudden death.

Key Points
The electrocardiogram is a graphic representation of the heart's electrical activity.

Objective 17-5
Describe depolarization and repolarization and explain normal ECG waves and intervals and the physiological events they represent.

Objective 17-6
Discuss the relationship between hypoxia, damage to the cardiac conduction system, premature ventricular contractions, ventricular tachycardia, and ventricular fibrillation.

The Electrocardiogram

The electrocardiogram (ECG or EKG) is a graphic representation of the heart's electrical activity as detected from the chest wall surface. The ECG may be displayed on a monitor screen or on a continuous strip of special graph paper that can record changes in heart activity over a period of time.

Each heartbeat, or mechanical contraction of the heart, has two distinct components of electrical activity: depolarization and repolarization. *Depolarization* is the first, in which electrical charges of the heart muscle change from positive to negative and cause heart muscle contraction. *Repolarization* is the second component, in which the electrical charges of the heart muscle return to a positive charge and cause relaxation of the heart muscle.

The human body acts as a conductor of electrical current. Any two points on the body may be connected with electrodes or electrical "leads" to record the heart's electrical activity. The recording or tracing of this electrical activity produces a graphic representation of depolarization and repolarization in the form of complexes or a series of waves normally occurring at regular intervals. The waves, or deflections, of a normal ECG have three portions (Figure 17-7✱):

- **P wave.** This is the first waveform of the ECG and represents the depolarization (contraction) of the atria.
- **QRS complex.** This is the second waveform and represents the depolarization (contraction) of the ventricles and the main contraction of the heart.
- **T wave.** This is the third waveform and represents the repolarization (relaxation) of the ventricles.

The atria also have a repolarization wave, but it is usually hidden within the QRS complex.

Another portion of the ECG, the PR interval (also referred to as the PRI), is measured in terms of time and used for analysis of the ECG. The PRI is calculated from the beginning of the P wave to the beginning of the QRS complex. It represents the time it takes the heart's electrical impulse to travel from the atria to the ventricles.

In a normally functioning heart, as described earlier, the heart's electrical impulse is generated from the sinoatrial node (review Figure 17-1). The electrical impulse then travels through the heart's conduction system, depolarizing the muscle and producing the contraction that pumps blood into the ventricles and then through the body. This electrical activity is called normal sinus rhythm. It will produce an ECG pattern of regularly spaced peaks that occur between 60 and 100 times each minute, separated by nearly flat lines, as shown in Figure 17-7.

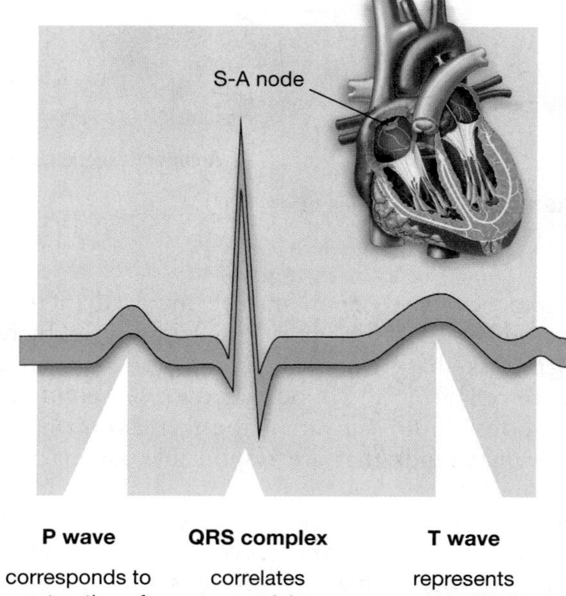
S-A node
P wave
corresponds to contraction of the atria
QRS complex
correlates to ventricles contracting
T wave
represents preparation for next series of complexes

FIGURE 17-7 ✱ An ECG tracing of normal sinus rhythm.

In some cases, the heart muscle becomes hypoxic, is injured, or dies. Also, the electrical conduction system may be damaged or disturbed and may cause the improper functioning of the heart. Sometimes these conditions produce an irritability of the heart that causes the uncoordinated firing of electrical ventricular impulses called premature ventricular complexes (PVCs). When PVCs occur in succession, they may produce ventricular tachycardia (V-Tach), which shows up on an ECG as steep peaks and valleys that are very close together. If left untreated, ventricular tachycardia can degenerate into ventricular fibrillation (VF or V-Fib), which shows up as smaller, uneven, disorganized peaks and valleys.

Blood Pressure

The **blood pressure** is the amount of pressure exerted against the arterial wall during circulation. The *systolic blood pressure* is the measured force exerted during the contraction of the heart, whereas the *diastolic blood pressure* is the pressure inside the artery when there is no contraction, or between contractions of the heart. The

Objective 17-7
Describe the roles of the heart and blood vessels in maintaining normal blood pressure.

Objective 17-8
Explain the importance of early recognition of signs and symptoms and the early treatment of patients with cardiac emergencies.

Objective 17-9
Explain the pathophysiology and the appropriate assessment and management of conditions that may be classified as cardiac compromise or acute coronary syndrome.

vessel's size plays a major role in the blood pressure. A smaller-sized vessel will offer greater resistance, resulting in a higher pressure. Thus, vasoconstriction (constriction of the vessels) will increase vessel resistance and blood pressure. Conversely, the larger the vessel size, the lesser the amount of resistance and the lower the blood pressure. Vasodilation (dilation of the vessels) will cause the resistance to decrease and the blood pressure will fall.

Inadequate Circulation

A properly functioning circulatory system delivers oxygen and nutrients to the body's cells and carries away carbon dioxide and other wastes. These processes take place as blood passes through the capillaries. The delivery of oxygen and nutrients from the blood through the thin capillary walls into the cells, and the removal of carbon dioxide and other wastes, is known as **perfusion**.

Under some conditions, blood does not circulate adequately through all the body's capillaries. The chief result of inadequate circulation is a state of profound depression of cell perfusion, called shock (or hypoperfusion), as described in Chapter 15, "Shock and Resuscitation." The cells become starved for oxygen (hypoxia) and nutrients and become overloaded with carbon dioxide and other waste products.

Hypoperfusion can occur as a result of low blood volume (hypovolemia), insufficient pumping action of the heart (heart failure), or dilated vessels (vasodilation) that may also be leaking. Hypoperfusion from massive vasodilation can also be caused by spinal cord damage that interrupts innervation of the blood vessels. In the absence of stimulation, the smooth muscle in the blood vessels relaxes, which results in massive dilation of the blood vessels, creating a vascular system that is too large overall for the amount of available blood. A more detailed discussion of hypoperfusion and its causes and consequences can be found in Chapter 15, "Shock and Resuscitation."

▶ Cardiac Compromise and Acute Coronary Syndrome (ACS)

The American Heart Association has found that approximately 7 to 8 million people each year will seek treatment in an emergency department in the United States for chest discomfort. Of those patients seeking treatment, approximately 2 million will actually suffer from a cardiac-related condition that involves the coronary arteries. About 1.5 million will suffer an actual heart attack where the coronary artery is occluded and a portion of the heart muscle begins to die. Of those patients, 500,000 will die from the heart attack, 250,000 of whom will die within one hour following the onset of the signs and symptoms. These statistics are definite indications of the significance of cardiac-related emergencies and underscore the importance of the EMT having a good knowledge base regarding cardiac emergencies.

With aggressive management of the patient suffering from a heart attack, including early recognition and expeditious transport to an appropriate facility by emergency medical services, it is possible to reduce the death rate of the heart attack patient, improve the pumping function of the heart, reduce the area of heart muscle that is damaged, and reduce the possibility of the patient suffering from subsequent heart failure.

A key to effective treatment of the patient is early recognition that the patient is suffering from a condition involving the heart and advanced cardiac care delivered within the first few hours after the patient experiences the first symptom of a cardiac problem. Time is a critical element in the survival and improved outcome of many of these patients. Death of a portion of the heart muscle is permanent and irreversible. Thus, it is important for you as an EMT to recognize the signs and symptoms of the many possible cardiac conditions, referred to collectively as **cardiac compromise**, and to provide emergency care and expeditious transport to a medical facility that is prepared to manage a patient with such a condition. Some of these patients may be eligible for drugs (fibrinolytics and antiplatelet agents) or mechanical therapy (angioplasty) that will destroy the clot and restore the blood flow to the heart. The sooner these therapies are delivered, the less the damage that may occur to the heart, and the better the prognosis of the patient's outcome.

Atherosclerosis

To better understand the signs and symptoms of cardiac compromise, it is important to learn some of the basic disease processes related to these conditions. *Arteriosclerosis* is a condition that causes the smallest of arterial structures to become stiff and less elastic. This is often referred to as "hardening of the arteries." A form of arteriosclerosis is *atherosclerosis*. Atherosclerosis is a systemic arterial disease.

Key Terms

blood pressure the force exerted by the blood on the interior walls of the blood vessels.

perfusion delivery of oxygen and other nutrients to the cells resulting from the constant adequate circulation of blood through the capillaries.

Key Terms

cardiac compromise reduced heart function caused by any condition, disease, or injury affecting the heart.

acute coronary syndrome (ACS) signs and symptoms resulting from conditions in which the coronary arteries are narrowed or occluded.

Its name is derived from the Greek word *athere,* meaning "gruel" or "porridge," and *scleros,* which means "hard." It is the underlying pathogenic process in the majority of patients that have coronary artery disease that causes myocardial infarctions as well as the arterial changes that result in stroke. Atherosclerosis alone is the number one killer worldwide, in economically developed countries.

Atherosclerosis is an inflammatory disease that starts with the intimal (innermost) lining of the blood vessels, where endothelial cells become damaged. Common risk factors that are thought to cause this endothelial injury include smoking, diabetes, hypertension, high levels of low-density lipoproteins (LDLs), and low levels of high-density lipoproteins (HDLs).

Once injury occurs, intimal changes and inflammation progress through the following basic pathophysiological events:

- Damage to the intima lining in the vessel allows the movement of blood platelets and other substances in the blood (serum lipoproteins) into the vascular wall. This irritates and inflames the vascular wall.
- As a result of the irritation and inflammation, different types of cells travel to the location, as do smooth muscle cells of the tunica media layer (muscular middle layer of the blood vessel).
- As these cells proliferate, fatty streaks develop in a longitudinal pattern in the lumen (inner opening) of the blood vessels. The blood vessel weakens as the intima and media layers are deprived of nutrients from the expanding plaque.
- In an attempt to "close off" the fatty streaks, smooth muscle cells produce collagen that covers the fatty streak to form a fibrous cap.
- Fibrous caps, however, are not stable and may rupture. The body views the rupture as an injury, which causes the body's clotting mechanism to activate. The development of a thrombus (clot) may occlude the blood vessel.

This progression of vascular disease ties together many of the cardiac, pulmonary, and neurological emergencies seen in the prehospital environment. Although this disease process can affect all arteries in the body, it is not until there is a resulting specific organ dysfunction that the damaging effects to the body become obvious.

When a patient has a buildup of fatty deposits (atherosclerosis) on the inside of the coronary arteries, the condition is called *coronary artery disease (CAD).* The narrowing of the coronary blood vessel increases the resistance to blood flow through the artery and decreases the amount of blood flow to the distal heart muscle. The fatty deposits reduce the coronary arteries' ability to dilate (become larger) and deliver additional blood flow to the heart when needed, such as in an increase in heart rate or more forceful pumping action.

Acute Coronary Syndrome

Acute coronary syndrome (ACS) results from a variety of conditions that can affect the heart in which the coronary arteries are narrowed or occluded by fat deposits (plaque), clots, or spasm. The word *acute* refers to a sudden onset, *coronary* refers to a condition affecting the coronary arteries, and *syndrome* indicates a group of signs and symptoms produced by the condition. Two conditions that are part of any acute coronary syndrome are *unstable angina* and *myocardial infarction* (heart attack). A heart muscle that is not receiving an adequate amount of oxygenated blood because of narrowing of the coronary arteries by plaque or spasms, clot formation inside the coronary artery blocking the blood flow, an increase in the work of the heart that demands more blood flow than can be supplied through the coronary arteries, or any combination of these, results in *cardiac cell hypoxia,* also known as *myocardial ischemia.* The prefix *myo-* refers to muscle and *cardio* refers to the heart. *Ischemia* refers to a deficient supply of oxygenated blood. Myocardial ischemia is a state in which there is inadequate delivery of oxygen to the heart muscle.

The typical response of the heart to ischemia is chest discomfort, commonly referred to as "chest pain" by many health care professionals, although the patient normally refers to the sensation as more of a feeling of discomfort rather than pain. Chest discomfort or pain that is a result of heart muscle ischemia is referred to as ischemic-type chest pain. However, you may ask the patient if he is experiencing "chest pain" and he may answer "no." More often, the patient feels a crushing chest pressure that is described as "dull and aching" and not as "pain." The pain or discomfort may be localized to the area of the sternum and radiate to the jaw, arms, shoulders, or back—which is considered the "typical" chest discomfort in cardiac compromise—or it may be a diffuse chest or back discomfort or ache. Any time you are collecting a history on a patient suffering a suspected cardiac compromise, it is most appropriate to ask if the patient is experiencing "chest discomfort" and not chest pain.

Thinking Critically

Your patient began having chest pain while weeding the garden. She took some of her prescribed nitroglycerin and rested for awhile and reports that the pain has subsided. Do you or do you not suspect that she may be experiencing an acute coronary syndrome emergency? Why or why not?

Key Points

Angina pectoris is a symptom of inadequate oxygen supply to the heart muscle, or myocardium.

Angina Pectoris

Angina pectoris (which means, literally, "pain in the chest") is a symptom commonly associated with coronary artery disease. Many patients suffer from angina-type pain. Classic angina typically occurs upon an increased workload placed on the heart. This may be from an increase in the heart rate or contractile function. *Unstable angina* has a variety of definitions, but usually indicates angina discomfort that is prolonged and worsening, or that occurs without exertion and when the patient is at rest.

Pathophysiology Angina pectoris is a symptom of inadequate oxygen supply to the heart muscle, or myocardium (Figure 17-8✱). As noted earlier, it results from a decrease in oxygen delivered to the myocardium, which is often caused by partial blockage of the coronary arteries, which causes ischemia (reduced delivery of oxygenated blood) that, in turn, results in tissue hypoxia (oxygen deficiency in the tissues). The lack of oxygen causes the discomfort, sometimes described as "crushing," or "squeezing," or as a "tightness" by the patient.

Generally, angina pectoris occurs during periods of stress, either physical or emotional. Once the stress is relieved or removed or the patient rests, the pain will usually go away. The pain is usually felt under the sternum and may radiate to the jaw, down either arm, to the back, or to the epigastrium (upper center region of the abdomen). The pain usually lasts for about 2–15 minutes. Many patients will be able to tell you that they have had angina as part of their past medical history and will have nitroglycerin prescribed for this condition. Prompt relief of the symptoms after rest and administered nitroglycerin is typical of angina.

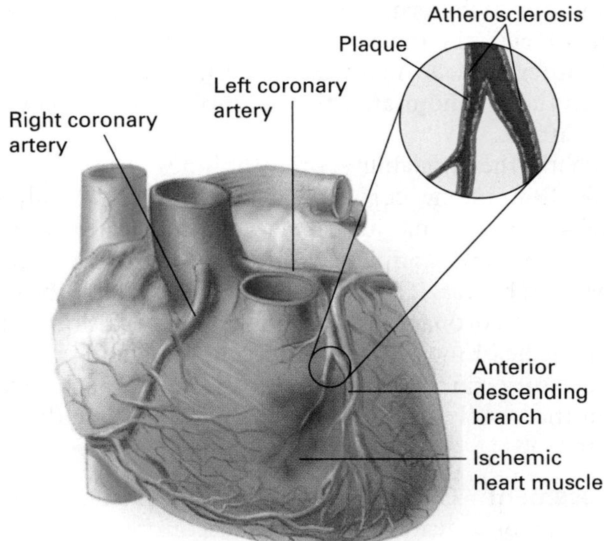

FIGURE 17-8 ✱ Atherosclerotic plaque formation in the coronary arteries results in ischemia distal to the blockage, which causes angina (chest pain).

Assessment The signs and symptoms of angina pectoris (Figure 17-9✱) are similar to those of any cardiac compromise and may include the following:

- Steady discomfort, usually located in the center of the chest but may be more diffuse throughout the front of the chest
- Discomfort that is usually described as pressure, tightness, aching, crushing, or heavy
- Discomfort that may radiate to the shoulders, arms, neck, jaw, back, or epigastric region (upper center abdomen)
- Cool, clammy skin
- Anxiety
- Dyspnea (shortness of breath)
- Diaphoresis (excessive sweating)
- Nausea and/or vomiting
- Complaint of indigestion pain

Women, diabetics, and the elderly may not have the typical presentation of signs and symptoms of angina. The discomfort may appear to be more diffuse or may be described more vaguely. These patients may not have any chest pain or discomfort but may instead complain of shortness of breath, fainting, weakness, or light-headedness.

Classic angina is typically relieved with rest and nitroglycerin. If the classic angina following exertion is not relieved after rest or after three nitroglycerin tablets or sprays over a 10-minute period, you should recognize this as an acute coronary syndrome emergency and provide prompt treatment and transport.

Characteristics of unstable angina may include pain or discomfort that occur at rest, is continuing without relief, or is prolonged. If the patient experiences angina that occurs at rest and lasts for greater than 20 minutes, angina with a recent onset that is getting progressively worse, or angina that wakes the patient at night (nocturnal angina), you should view it as an acute coronary syndrome emergency and provide prompt treatment and transport.

Emergency Medical Care Emergency care for the patient suffering from angina should be provided whether

DISTINGUISHING ANGINA PECTORIS FROM MYOCARDIAL INFARCTION

	Angina Pectoris	Myocardial Infarction
Location of Discomfort	Substernal or across chest	Same
Radiation of Discomfort	Neck, jaw, arms, back, shoulders	Same
Nature of Discomfort	Dull or heavy discomfort with a pressure or squeezing sensation	Same, but maybe more intense
Duration	Usually 2 to 15 minutes, subsides after activity stops	Lasts longer than 10 minutes
Other symptoms	Usually none	Perspiration, pale gray color, nausea, weakness, dizziness, lightheadedness
Precipitating Factors	Extremes in weather, exertion, stress, meals	Often none
Factors Giving Relief	Stopping physical activity, reducing stress, nitroglycerin	Nitroglycerin may give incomplete or no relief

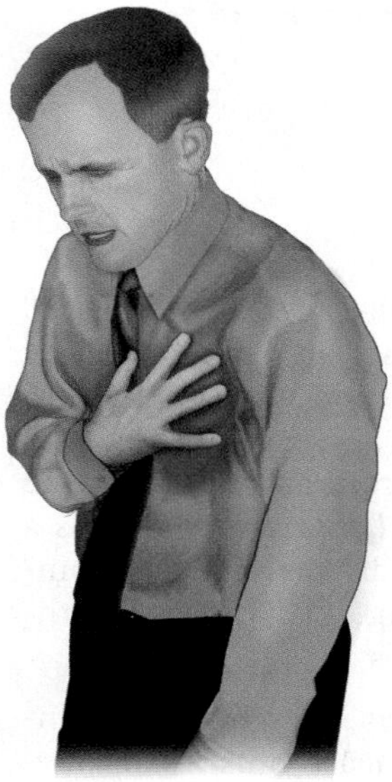

FIGURE 17-9 * Both myocardial infarction and less serious angina can present symptoms of severe chest pain. Treat all cases of chest pain as cardiac emergencies.

signs and symptoms of an acute coronary syndrome emergency exist or not. If so, you should establish an open and patent airway, and immediately provide oxygen via a nonrebreather mask at 15 lpm. If the patient's respirations become inadequate, begin positive pressure ventilation. Apply the pulse oximeter, if available, to monitor the oxygen level. If the patient has prescribed nitroglycerin and his systolic blood pressure is greater than 90 mmHg, place him in a sitting or lying position and administer the nitroglycerin tablets or spray. If the patient is suspected of suffering from a coronary artery occlusion, administer 160–325 mg of aspirin if your local protocol allows it. Consider contacting advanced life support and be prepared to manage a cardiac arrest patient. Continue to perform a reassessment.

Acute Myocardial Infarction

An acute myocardial infarction (AMI) occurs when a portion of the heart muscle dies because of the lack of an adequate supply of oxygenated blood. *Acute* means sudden, *myocardial* refers to heart muscle, and *infarction* refers to death of tissue. An acute myocardial infarction is what the layperson refers to as a heart attack.

Pathophysiology An acute myocardial infarction typically is the result of coronary artery disease that causes severe narrowing or complete blockage of the coronary arteries. A plaque erosion or rupture within the coronary artery may cause the narrowing and blockage to occur. The end result is a portion of heart muscle that does not receive an adequate supply of oxygenated blood. After about 20–30 minutes without adequate perfusion, the heart muscle begins to die. Although rarely, a heart attack could also result from a spasm of the coronary artery. This can be caused by use of a drug such as cocaine.

When the blood flow is blocked, the heart muscle becomes ischemic (hypoxic from inadequate oxygenation). If the blood flow is not restored to that portion of heart muscle, the cells will begin to die. Ischemic heart tissue will become irritable. It may produce abnormal beats in the conduction system that could lead to dysrhythmias. Some dysrhythmias, such as ventricular fibrillation and ventricular tachycardia, may be fatal. Ventricular fibrillation, which is the most common dysrhythmia the patient will suffer initially in cardiac arrest, will usually occur within the first hour after the onset of the symptoms of a heart attack.

With the availability of techniques to re-establish blood flow in the coronary artery by mechanically increasing the internal lumen size and medications called fibrinolytics and antiplatelet agents, commonly referred to as "clot busters," it may be possible to dissolve the clot, reopen the coronary artery, and restore perfusion to the ischemic heart muscle. Prompt recognition and transport is necessary, since the window of time to mechanically open the vessel or to administer the fibrinolytic drugs is limited.

Assessment Chest discomfort is the most significant symptom of a heart attack. The discomfort the patient experiences is similar to that of angina; however, the symptoms last longer. Also, chest discomfort from an acute myocardial infarction will be only partially relieved

Key Points
Diabetics, the elderly, and women are more prone to an atypical presentation of symptoms when suffering a heart attack.

Thinking Critically
In a patient who may be experiencing an aortic dissection, you are cautioned *not* to administer aspirin. Why?

with nitroglycerin or not relieved at all. The boundaries between unstable angina and AMI are not so distinct, and it may be difficult to distinguish between the two conditions.

Signs and symptoms of AMI (review Figure 17-9) include the following:

- Chest discomfort radiating to jaw, arms, shoulders, or back
- Anxiety
- Dyspnea
- Sense of impending doom
- Diaphoresis
- Nausea and/or vomiting
- Light-headedness or dizziness
- Weakness

Remember that diabetics, the elderly, and women are more prone to an atypical (not typical) presentation of symptoms when suffering a heart attack. Many may suffer a "silent MI" where no chest discomfort is experienced. They may complain only of shortness of breath, nausea, light-headedness or weakness.

Emergency Medical Care When the signs and symptoms of an acute myocardial infarction are present, you should proceed rapidly with your assessment and management of the patient. This patient has the potential to go into cardiac arrest; therefore, you should frequently assess the patient and maintain a vigilant watch over the patient's condition. If at all possible, the patient should never be left alone while you are returning equipment to the EMS unit or retrieving and preparing the cot. The automated external defibrillator (AED) must always be available and close to the patient.

Ensure a patent airway and provide positive pressure ventilation with oxygen connected to the device if the breathing is inadequate. If the respiratory rate and tidal volume are both adequate, apply a nonrebreather mask at 15 lpm. Apply a pulse oximeter if available and monitor the oxygen saturation. Place the patient in a position of comfort. If the patient has a prescription for nitroglycerin, administer one tablet every 3–5 minutes up to a total of three tablets. Follow your local protocol. Be sure the systolic blood pressure is above 90 mmHg and remains above 90 mmHg following each nitroglycerin administration. If local protocol allows, administer 160–325 mg of aspirin. Notify the receiving hospital *early* of suspected MIs. Continue to assess the patient en route to the medical facility. Contact ALS for further assistance if available. If the patient becomes pulseless and apneic (no pulse, no respirations), immediately begin cardiac resuscitation and apply the automated external defibrillator. For more detailed information on cardiac resuscitation, see Chapter 15, "Shock and Resuscitation."

Aortic Aneurysm or Dissection

The aorta is the main trunk of the arterial system of the body, carrying blood pumped from the left ventricle of the heart. Branches of the aorta supply blood to the head, neck, and arms before the aorta turns downward through the thorax and abdominal cavity from which arteries branch off to the lower regions of the body.

Two types of life-threatening injuries may occur to the aorta that are often confused with each other: aortic aneurysm and aortic dissection. Both can cause pain that may be confused with the pain of myocardial infarction. Both occur more often in men than in women. However, aortic aneurysm and aortic dissection have distinctly different causes, signs, and symptoms.

Aortic aneurysm occurs when a weakened section of the aortic wall, usually resulting from atherosclerosis, begins to dilate or balloon outward from the pressure exerted by the blood flowing through the vessel. An aneurysm may exist for a long time with no symptoms or signs that the patient is aware of, then suddenly rupture, causing rapid and fatal internal bleeding (Figure 17-10∗). Aortic aneurysms occur most often in the abdominal region. Pain may be felt, especially in the back, when the aneurysm gets large enough, perhaps shortly before rupture occurs. Usually, the aorta cannot be felt on physical examination, but at this final stage it may be felt as a pulsating mass in the abdomen, although this may be difficult or impossible to detect in a heavy-set patient.

Aortic dissection occurs when there is a tear in the inner lining of the aorta and blood enters the opening and causes separation of the layers of the aortic wall (Figure 17-11∗). Aortic dissections occur most often in the area of the thorax. The pain is usually most severe when the dissection first occurs and is most often described as "sharp" pain, or sometimes as a "tearing" or "ripping" pain, often felt in the back, flank, or arm. Syncope may be the only sign in some patients. Depending on the location of the dissection along the aorta, it may cause symptoms similar to stroke or to myocardial infarction and, in fact, may lead to a myocardial infarction

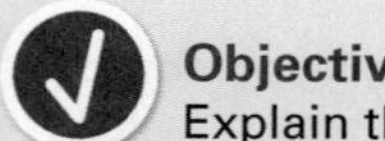

Objective 17-10
Explain the typical presentation of myocardial ischemia or infarction in females.

Key Points
Coronary heart disease is now the single largest cause of death of females in the United States.

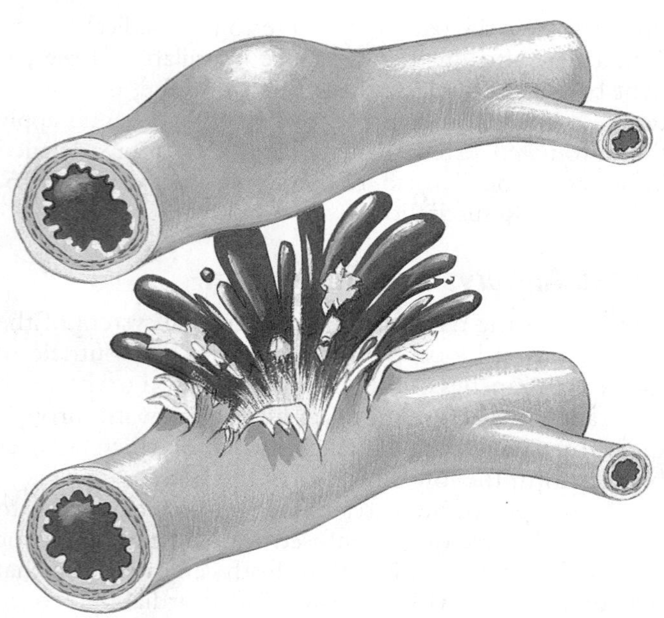

FIGURE 17-10 * Aortic aneurysm leading to aortic rupture.

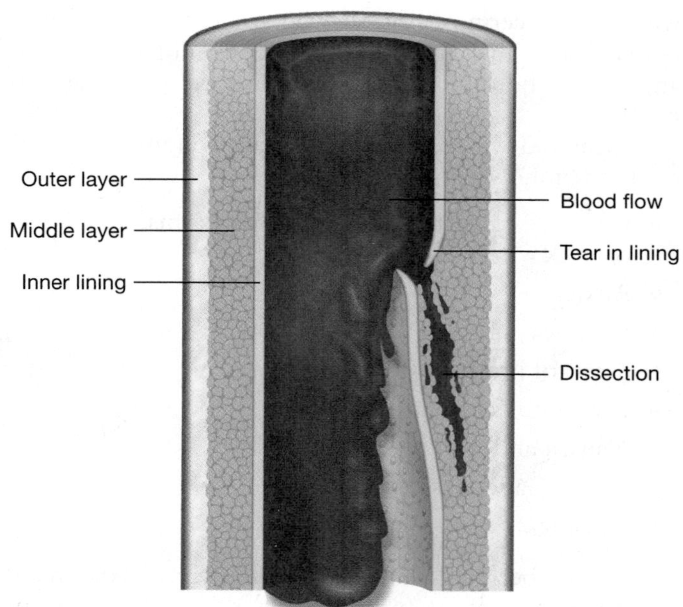

FIGURE 17-11 * Aortic dissection.

or other damage to the heart. A difference of 20 mmHg or greater in the systolic blood pressure reading between the upper arms or a severe decrease or difference in the upper and lower extremity pulse amplitude as compared to central pulses in a patient complaining of back or sharp chest pain should cause you to suspect a possible aortic dissection.

If a pulsating mass is felt and aortic aneurysm is suspected, administer oxygen and transport the patient immediately, as only surgery can prevent or repair rupture of the aneurysm. For a chest or back pain that may result from an aortic dissection or that may be a symptom of myocardial infarction, administer oxygen and assist the patient with prescribed nitroglycerin if the blood pressure is greater than 90 mmHg and no signs of hypovolemia are present. If aortic dissection is suspected, *do not* administer aspirin.

Acute Coronary Syndrome in Females

Of special concern is the presentation of myocardial ischemia or infarction in females. Almost all common descriptions of how an acute coronary syndrome presents clinically have been taken from male cases. This is in part because medical literature at one time described only males with ACS, because they were primarily the ones who suffered cardiac events. However, as females have gained a more prominent presence in the workforce, higher rates of smoking, poor nutrition habits, higher stress levels, and so forth, they are now suffering from heart attacks at rates approaching the rates among males.

Coronary heart disease in females is now the single largest cause of death of females in the United States. In fact, since the incidence of myocardial infarctions in females is greater at older ages than in males, females are almost twice as likely to die from a myocardial infarction or its complications within the first few weeks following the event. The female may present with different signs and symptoms from a male when she is experiencing a cardiac event; however, the event is just as dangerous and can be as deadly. Therefore, the EMT must recognize some of the more subtle signs and symptoms that females suffering from acute coronary syndromes experience.

The following list of symptoms is common for females suffering from a cardiac ischemia or infarction. Although some descriptions are the same as for males, many others are not:

- "Classical" findings (not necessarily *common* findings)
  Dull substernal chest pain or discomfort
  Respiratory distress
  Nausea, vomiting
  Diaphoresis

- "Nonclassical" or "atypical" findings (not necessarily *uncommon* findings)
  Neck ache
  Pressure in the chest
  Pains in the back, breast, or upper abdomen
  Tingling of the fingers
  Unexplained fatigue or weight gain (water weight gain)
  Insomnia

Since the death rate for females who suffer heart attacks is higher than males when the event occurs, the EMT should have a high index of suspicion of ACS when gathering a history from the female patient. Err on the side of the patient and provide emergency care for a potential myocardial infarction or ACS, despite a presentation of "atypical" signs of ischemia or infarction.

Note that diabetics and the elderly are also high-risk groups that may present with atypical findings.

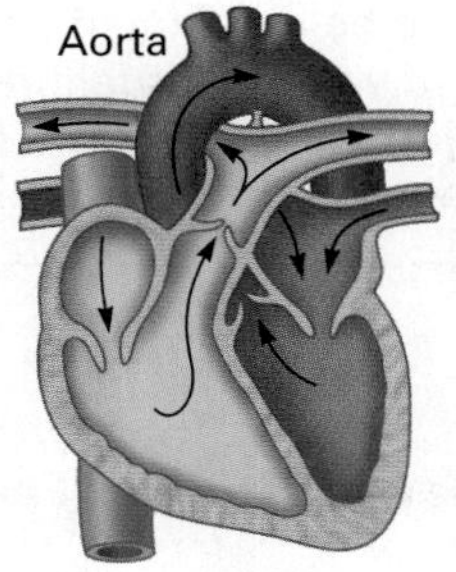

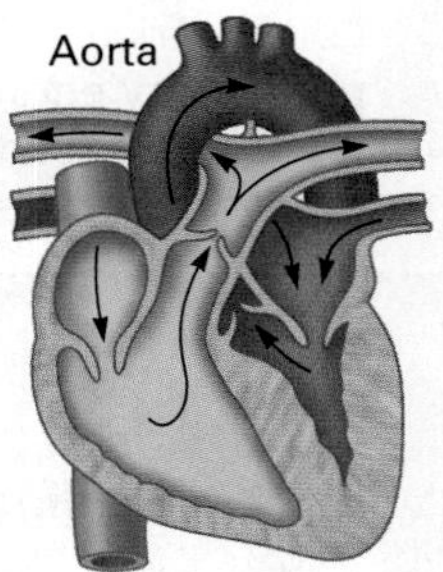

FIGURE 17-12 ∗ Left ventricular hypertrophy (enlargement of the heart muscle) compromises the ability of the left ventricle to pump adequately, causing a decrease in cardiac output and a decrease in blood pressure.

Other Causes of Cardiac Compromise

Heart Failure

When the heart no longer has the ability to adequately eject blood out of the ventricle, it is considered to be failing. The heart failure may be a result of a heart attack that affected a large portion of muscle because, when the heart muscle dies, it no longer contributes to the pumping function of the heart. Heart failure may also be caused by a valve disorder, hypertension, pulmonary embolism, cardiac rhythm disturbances, and certain drugs.

Pathophysiology Heart failure can be categorized as *left ventricular failure* or *right ventricular failure.* The consequences of left or right ventricular failure can be understood by recalling the functions of two sides of the heart: The left side of the heart receives oxygenated blood from the lungs and sends it out to the body's arteries, while the right side of the heart receives deoxygenated blood from the body's veins and sends it to the lungs to pick up oxygen.

Left ventricular failure occurs when the left ventricle cannot pump blood out of the left ventricle effectively (Figure 17-12∗). This reduces blood flow to the arteries and the perfusion of blood to the cells throughout the body. Furthermore, blood waiting to enter the left ventricle from the left atrium and blood waiting to enter the left atrium from the lungs backs up in a sort of "traffic jam." When the left ventricle fails to eject the normal amount of blood with each contraction, the blood pressure begins to build up in the left atrium. The increase in pressure in the left atrium, in turn, causes an increase in pressure in the pulmonary veins, which are responsible for delivering blood from the lungs to the heart. The increase in pressure in the pulmonary veins creates a higher pressure in the capillaries in the lungs. Remember that the capillaries in the lungs are the sites of gas exchange with the alveoli. When the pressure in the capillaries is increased, fluid begins to leak out between the capillary and the alveoli. The fluid collects between the capillary and around the alveoli and distal bronchioles. This causes the space between the capillary and the alveoli to widen, making gas exchange more difficult. The poor gas exchange leads to hypoxia. This condition is referred to as pulmonary edema.

When the right side of the heart fails, the blood backs up into the venous system. The right side of the heart may fail due to failure of the left ventricle. It may also fail due to hypertension (high blood pressure). Chronic obstructive pulmonary disease (COPD) may increase the pressure in the pulmonary vessels in the lungs and cause the right ventricle to work much harder. Over time, this may cause the right ventricle to fail. Signs include peripheral edema, jugular vein distention, and liver enlargement.

Another problem than can occur with left or right heart failure is a condition known as *cardiogenic shock.* This is a clinical state (not a diagnosis) in which the left or right ventricle fails to pump out enough blood to meet the demands of the body. The most common cause for this is myocardial damage that occurs secondary to a heart attack. Other less common reasons include sustained hypertension, valve damage, extremes in heart rate (too fast or too slow), and other cardiac muscle diseases (cardiomyopathies). Cardiogenic shock can be from the pumping inadequacy of either the left or right ventricle.

When the left ventricle fails, the cardiac output drops and there is a diminishment in the perfusion pressure to the rest of the body's organs. Common findings include a drop in systolic blood pressure (to include frank hypotension), diminished or absent peripheral pulse amplitude, altered mental status, changes in the heart rate, poor urinary output, respiratory distress, inspiratory rales, and possible pulmonary edema.

The right ventricle can also fail for any of the same reasons as the left, but has slightly different presentation. Remember that the right ventricle pumps blood to the

Thinking Critically
Left ventricular failure tends to be associated with pulmonary edema, while right ventricular failure tends to be associated with jugular vein distention and peripheral edema. Explain these differences.

Key Points
Patients suffering heart failure will commonly say that they are taking a "water pill," or diuretic.

TABLE 17-1 Findings in Right and Left Heart Failure

	Pure Right Heart Failure	Pure Left Heart Failure
Systolic blood pressure	Low to normal	Normal to high
Breath sounds	Clear sounds	Inspiratory rales
Peripheral edema	JVD and peripheral edema	No JVD or peripheral edema

lungs for reoxygenation. If the right-sided cardiac output starts to drop, then the lungs may be hypoperfused, which can lead to hypoxia and respiratory distress. Also, as the blood starts to accumulate in the ventricle from poor ejection, it will eventually back up into the atrium and subsequently into the vena cava. Findings of this may include jugular venous distension and peripheral edema. One other change in normal physiology is that if the right side is pumping inadequately, then the left side of the heart will receive an insufficient amount of blood. Since the left ventricle can only pump as much blood as it receives, the patient may also display many of the aforementioned findings of poor peripheral perfusion. There is, however, a triad of findings that may help delineate pure left heart failure from pure right heart failure. They are identified in Table 17-1.

Congestive heart failure (CHF) is a medical diagnosis that refers to the condition in which there is a buildup of fluid (congestion) in the body resulting from the pump failure of the heart. In essence, it represents the condition where the left, the right, or both ventricles are failing to meet the body's needs. It may be a chronic condition that presents over a period of time, or it may be more acute, as associated with a large heart attack that affects the left ventricle. Congestive heart failure commonly leads to pulmonary edema and edema (swelling) in other areas of the body. The edema will often be seen in the feet and ankles, the hands, and the presacral area (lower lumbar region) of the supine patient. The fluid may also accumulate in the liver, causing it to enlarge, and also in the abdomen. When fluid collects in the abdomen, the abdomen may become distended and feel like a sponge. Often, these patients will sit upright and dangle their legs, feet, arms, and hands so that the blood can pool in the extremities and lessen the amount the heart has to pump out.

Assessment The signs and symptoms of heart failure depend on the severity of the condition and whether it is an acute-onset or a long-term problem (Figure 17-13∗). The signs and symptoms of heart failure include the following:

- Marked or severe dyspnea (shortness of breath)
- Tachycardia (rapid heart rate greater than 100 bpm)
- Difficulty breathing when supine (orthopnea)
- Suddenly waking at night with dyspnea (paroxysmal nocturnal dyspnea)
- Fatigue on any type of exertion
- Anxiety
- Tachypnea (rapid respiratory rate)
- Diaphoresis (sweating)
- Upright position with legs, feet, arms, and hands dangling
- Cool, clammy, pale skin
- Chest discomfort
- Cyanosis
- Agitation and restlessness due to hypoxia
- Edema (swelling) to the hands, ankles, and feet (Figure 17-14∗)
- Crackles and possibly wheezes on auscultation
- Decreased SpO_2 reading
- Signs and symptoms of pulmonary edema
- Blood pressure may be normal, elevated, or low
- Distended neck veins—jugular venous distention (JVD) (late) (Figure 17-15∗)
- Distended and soft spongy abdomen

Commonly, these patients will tell you that they are taking a "water pill." This is a diuretic that is used to reduce the amount of fluid in the body. They may also be on other drugs to strengthen the force of contraction of the heart and reduce the response of the sympathetic nervous system.

SIGNS AND SYMPTOMS OF
CONGESTIVE HEART FAILURE

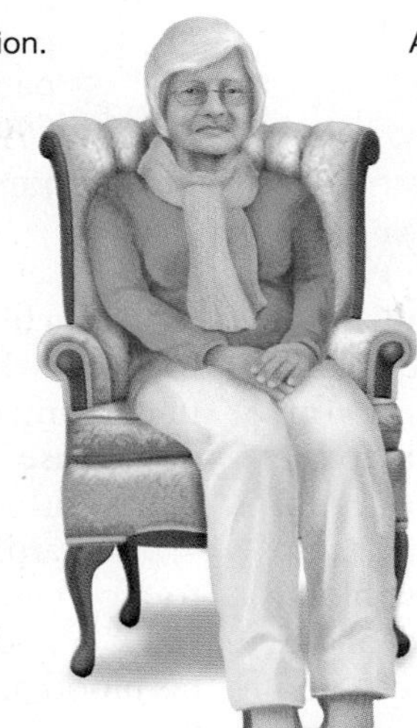
Mild to severe confusion.
Cyanosis.
Tachypnea.
May cough up pink sputnum.
Low, normal, or high blood pressure.
Rapid heart rate.
A desire to sit upright.
Anxiety.
Distended neck veins. (Late)
Crackles.
Shortness of breath (dyspnea).
Pale, cool, clammy skin.
Abdominal distention.
Pedal and lower extremity edema.

FIGURE 17-13 ✱ Signs and symptoms of congestive heart failure.

Emergency Medical Care The treatment for the patient with heart failure is basically the same as for the patient with an acute myocardial infarction. Ensure the patient has a patent airway. Provide positive pressure ventilation with supplemental oxygen connected to the device if the breathing is inadequate.

The heart failure patient with pulmonary edema will benefit significantly from positive pressure ventilation. It will increase the effectiveness of gas exchange by forcing the oxygen to cross over the alveoli and the space between the alveoli and the capillary. You may see drastic improvement in the patient's condition following positive pressure ventilation. If the patient will tolerate positive pressure ventilation and medical direction allows it, attempt to provide ventilation early.

If the patient has an adequate respiratory rate and tidal volume, apply a nonrebreather mask at 15 lpm. If

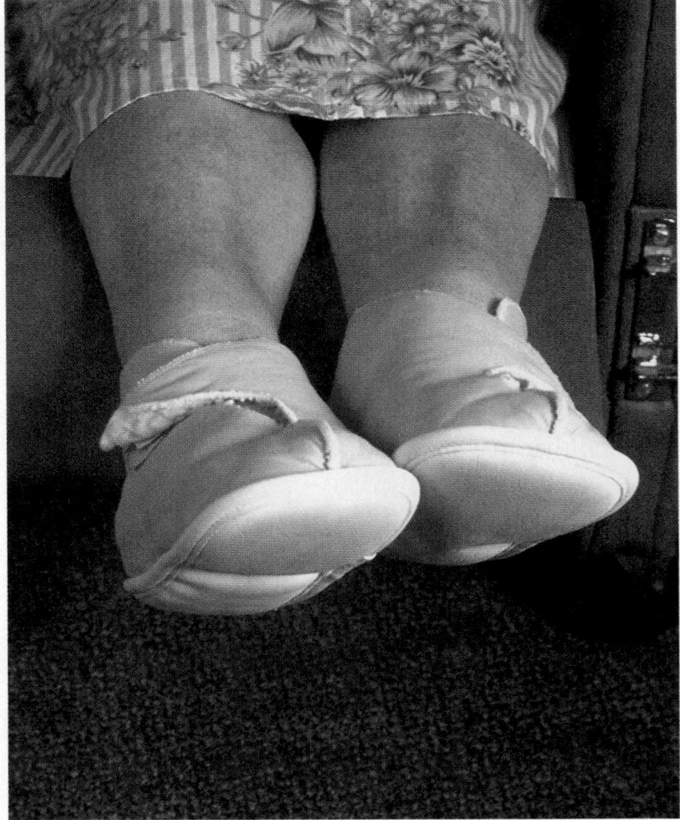

FIGURE 17-14 ✱ Edema to the lower extremities is a classic sign of congestive heart failure.

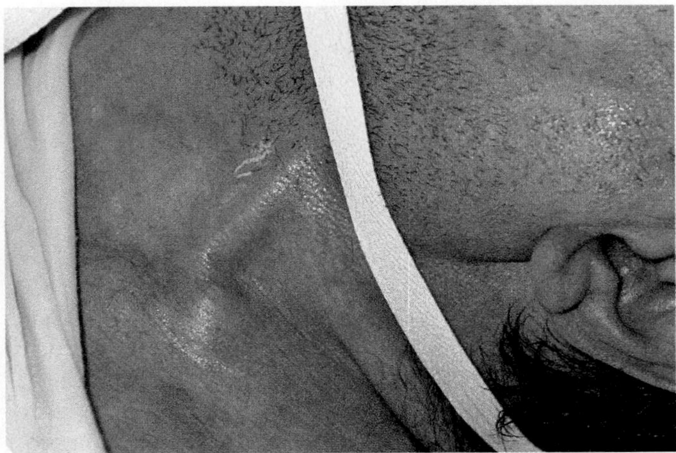

FIGURE 17-15 ✱ Jugular vein distention is a late sign of congestive heart failure. (© David Effron, MD)

Key Points
Some patients have chronically elevated blood pressures. The EMT should only evaluate a patient's current blood pressure in light of what a "normal" blood pressure is for him.

the patient is experiencing chest discomfort and has a prescription for nitroglycerin, administer one tablet every 3–5 minutes to a total of three tablets. Follow your local protocol. Nitroglycerin will also be beneficial to the patient by reducing the pressure in the arteries of the body, making it easier for the left ventricle to pump the blood out. Any venous dilation will cause less blood to return to the heart and reduce the workload of the ventricles. Ensure that the patient has a systolic blood pressure of greater than 90 mmHg prior to administration of nitroglycerin.

Continuously assess the patient and be prepared for respiratory failure and cardiac arrest. Be sure to let the patient assume a position of comfort. Never force the patient to lie flat, since this will commonly worsen the dyspnea.

Hypertensive Emergencies

A hypertensive emergency is defined as a severe, accelerated hypertension episode with a systolic pressure greater than 160 mmHg, and/or a diastolic blood pressure greater than 94 mmHg. Hypertension usually does not produce any clinical findings until there are vascular changes to the heart, brain, lungs, or kidneys. Although hypertension is a common finding in the United States, affecting about 25 percent of the population, episodes of hypertensive emergencies are, fortunately, rare. This is an important point to note. For example, a patient with chronic hypertension may be experiencing a stroke, and you are summoned to care for the stroke, not the elevation in blood pressure. It is just coincidental that the patient's blood pressure is up (which in that situation, is "normal" for him). Conversely, if a rapid increase in blood pressure occurs to a patient who does not have chronic elevations, he may present with signs and symptoms related directly to the hypertensive crisis. It is key to ascertain a thorough patient history in these patients to help make that decision.

Pathophysiology There are two types of hypertensive patients, those with "primary" hypertension and those with "secondary" hypertension. Primary hypertension is most common, and is characterized by a hypertensive state in which no specific cause for the hypertension has been identified (idiopathic), although theories do exist as to the cause. The patient with primary hypertension most likely will be taking medications designed to keep the blood pressure low, and be on a diet that limits certain foods such as sodium. "Secondary" hypertension is said to occur when a patient is hypertensive from some other underlying disease process. For example, patients with renal disease are usually chronically hypertensive, as are patients with certain thyroid disorders.

Regardless of the cause, it is important for the EMT to ascertain from the patient if he has chronic elevations in his blood pressure. If he does, chances are that he has his blood pressure tracked and documented on a card that he carries with him. The EMT should only evaluate his current blood pressure in light of what a "normal" blood pressure is for him. For example, a patient may be experiencing a seizure but coincidently has a diagnosis of high blood pressure that he takes medicine for. A normal blood pressure for him might be 168/90 mmHg. If his actual blood pressure during this emergency is near his average blood pressure, then the EMT should focus treatment on the seizure, and not the blood pressure itself. However, if a patient is found to be experiencing a seizure, but his normal blood pressure is 110/60 mmHg, and you find that his current blood pressure is 168/90 mmHg, then the blood pressure must be considered during the assessment as a possible etiology or sign of a condition causing the seizure such as stroke.

Assessment If the patient has the signs and symptoms listed next, with a blood pressure consistent with his normal blood pressure, treat the underlying cause. If the patient's blood pressure is significantly higher than his normal blood pressure, consider the findings to be related to the hypertension. Signs and symptoms of a hypertensive emergency are:

- Strong, often bounding pulse
- Skin that may be warm, dry, or moist
- Severe headache
- Ringing in the ears
- Nausea and/or vomiting
- Elevated blood pressure
- Respiratory distress
- Chest pain
- Seizures
- Focal neural deficits
- Indications of organ dysfunction (stroke, heart attack, pulmonary edema)
- Possible nosebleed

Key Points
The primary risk factor for cardiac arrest is coronary artery disease. However, cardiac arrest can result from many other conditions, including trauma, overdose, stroke, and seizure.

Key Terms
nitroglycerin medication that dilates the blood vessels, increasing blood flow and decreasing the workload of the heart.

Emergency Medical Care In the prehospital setting, it is difficult to differentiate an emergency produced by hypertension from an emergency that presents with hypertension but has a different cause. It is difficult to make these distinctions without diagnostic tests that are available in the emergency department. Nevertheless, always remember to support lost functions to the airway, breathing, oxygenation, and circulation in any of these patients.

Oxygen administration should be guided by the SpO_2 reading, signs and symptoms of a possible underlying condition, and signs of hypoxia in a patient with adequate breathing. If the patient is breathing inadequately, positive pressure ventilation should be initiated immediately at a rate of 10–12 per minute with supplemental oxygen applied to the ventilation device. The patient should also be placed in a position of comfort, but encourage a semi-Fowler position if there are no airway concerns. Consider contacting ALS for backup or intercept as medications do exist to lower the elevated blood pressure should the patient meet certain criteria. If you suspect the hypertensive patient might be having a stroke, the blood pressure will not be lowered in the prehospital setting; thus, it may not be prudent to delay transport to wait for ALS. Finally, provide emotional support and reassurance while transporting the patient.

Cardiac Arrest

Cardiac arrest is the worst manifestation of cardiac compromise from an acute coronary event. It occurs when the heart, for any of a variety of reasons, is not pumping effectively or at all, and no pulses can be felt. As discussed previously, the primary risk factor for an acute coronary syndrome is coronary artery disease. Although cardiac arrest is commonly caused by an acute coronary syndrome, it can also be caused by a myriad of other conditions. For example, a traumatized patient may be in arrest following severe multisystem trauma or significant blood loss. A person who accidentally or purposely overdoses on his medication may be in arrest as a result of the effects of the medication. Even a stroke or seizure patient may go into cardiac arrest secondary to the initial emergency. The EMT must remain acutely aware of the patient's clinical status whenever he is unstable because any patient has the potential to go into arrest. For more detailed information on cardiac arrest, refer to Chapter 15, "Shock and Resuscitation."

Nitroglycerin

While patients with known cardiac problems may be on a variety of medications, the most common will be **nitroglycerin**. Nitroglycerin is a potent vasodilator (agent that increases the diameter of blood vessels). It works in seconds to relax the muscles of the blood vessel walls. This action dilates arteries, increasing the blood flow through the coronary arteries and oxygen supply to the heart muscle and decreasing the workload of the heart.

Understanding BODY PROCESSES

Nitroglycerin dilates coronary arteries, peripheral arteries, and veins, causing an increase in coronary artery blood flow, a decrease in peripheral vascular resistance, and a decrease in the myocardial workload. ■

Nitroglycerin can be in the form of either a sublingual (under-the-tongue) tablet or a sublingual spray. A paste form of nitroglycerin is also available, but it is not considered appropriate for administration by an EMT, because the onset of action is too long.

If the patient with a history of heart problems is suffering from cardiac-related chest pain and has nitroglycerin that has been prescribed for him by a physician, you may assist the patient in taking this medication after receiving authorization from medical direction. Because nitroglycerin lowers blood pressure, it must not be given to a patient whose systolic blood pressure is less than 90 mmHg or no more than 30 mmHg lower than the baseline systolic blood pressure. Also, have the patient lie or sit down prior to administration. Do not administer the nitroglycerin to a patient with extreme bradycardia (<50 bpm) or tachycardia (>100 bpm). Follow your local protocol when considering the administration of nitroglycerin. If the patient has taken tadalafil (Cialis), vardenafil (Levitra), or sildenafil (Viagra) within the last 24 hours or longer depending on the drug, *do not* administer nitroglycerin because it may cause a potentially fatal drop in systolic blood pressure. Instead, contact medical direction for orders.

If the patient experiences no relief after one dose, another dose may be administered after 3–5 minutes if authorized by medical direction, to a maximum of three

Objective 17-11
Explain the indications, contraindications, forms, dosage, administration, actions, side effects, and reassessment for nitroglycerin.

Objective 17-12
Explain the special considerations in assessing and managing pediatric and geriatric patients with cardiac emergencies.

ASSESSMENT Tips

A systolic blood pressure of 90 mmHg or a systolic pressure that is 30 mmHg less than the patient's baseline systolic pressure is a contraindication to the administration of any additional nitroglycerin. ■

doses. Find out if the patient has already taken one or more doses prior to your arrival to be sure that you are not inadvertently administering more than the maximum.

Nitroglycerin will often produce a stinging or burning sensation under the tongue or may cause the patient to get a headache following administration. You may have heard that if the patient does not feel the stinging or burning, or does not get a headache, then the nitroglycerin is old and ineffective. This is not true. Just because the patient does not feel any of these sensations, it does not mean the nitroglycerin is no good. However, age and light will inactivate nitroglycerin tablets. The patients are commonly instructed to keep a fresh supply sealed in a bottle in a dark area. If the patient has a prescription for nitroglycerin, ask for the "fresh" supply and assist with the administration of the fresh nitroglycerin. Nitroglycerin spray may be good for up to 2 years. Some nitroglycerin may be working but appear to be ineffective because the coronary artery disease is so severe.

See EMT Skills 17-1 for information on how to assist a patient with prescribed nitroglycerin. See Figure 17-16∗ for a detailed summary of the criteria and techniques for the administration of nitroglycerin.

Age-Related Variations: Pediatrics and Geriatrics

Patients who are at the age extremes (the very young and very old) can also experience an acute coronary event, but its presentation and etiology may be somewhat dissimilar than the typical adult patient. Remember that the skills and interventions employed on most adult cardiac arrest patients may not always be appropriate for some of these age-related variations. The goal of the following section is to introduce some of these idiosyncrasies that may be present in patients at the age extremes.

Pediatric Considerations

Pediatric patients do not typically have acute coronary syndromes such as a myocardial infarction or ischemic episode as adult patients do. (However, it is possible.) Typically when a pediatric patient experiences a cardiac disturbance, it is from some congenital heart condition that the family usually knows about. In these situations, it is best to contact medical direction as early as possible and seek advice about the best course of action for the pediatric patient experiencing a cardiac emergency secondary to a congenital heart condition. Whatever additional course of action is recommended, always remember to support any lost function to the airway, breathing, or circulation components of the body. See Chapter 38, "Pediatrics," to learn more about pediatric emergencies related to the cardiovascular system.

Pediatric patients may also experience cardiac arrest, but its frequency is much lower than in adults, and the underlying cause is typically respiratory in nature, rather than cardiovascular as with the adult patient. Infants and children still have a healthy heart at a young age, and it is unlikely to fail. What typically puts a young patient into cardiac arrest is an emergency that leads to airway occlusion or ventilatory insufficiency. As the young patient becomes more and more hypoxic and acidic, the heart will eventually fail and the patient will slip into cardiac arrest. Even with early and appropriate resuscitation, cardiac arrest survival rates for children are much lower than for adults, because the arrest typically occurred after a long period of hypoxemia, acidosis, and ventilatory insufficiency.

These facts underscore the importance for the EMT to remain vigilant about establishing and maintaining an airway in a pediatric patient as well as ensuring adequate ventilation. The best treatment for cardiac arrest in a pediatric patient is to prevent it entirely by ensuring an open airway, adequate breathing, and oxygen supplementation. See Chapter 38, "Pediatrics" to learn more about pediatric respiratory emergencies and cardiac arrest management.

Geriatric Considerations

Geriatric patients will represent the highest number of patients you treat who are experiencing some form of acute coronary syndrome. The emergency may be as minimal as mild respiratory distress and chest discomfort or as severe as full cardiopulmonary arrest. The EMT should

Nitroglycerin

MEDICATION NAME

Nitroglycerin is the generic name. Some of the trade names of nitroglycerin are:

- Nitrostat
- Nitro-Bid
- Nitrolingual Spray

INDICATIONS

All of the following criteria must be met before an EMT administers nitroglycerin to a patient:

- The patient exhibits signs and symptoms of chest pain.
- The patient has physician-prescribed nitroglycerin.
- The EMT has received approval from medical direction, whether on-line or off-line, to administer the medication.

CONTRAINDICATIONS

Nitroglycerin should not be given if any of the following conditions exist:

- The patient's baseline systolic blood pressure is below 90 mmHg systolic or the systolic blood pressure has decreased greater than 30 mmHg from the baseline.
- The heart rate is less than 50 bpm or greater than 100 bpm.
- The patient has a suspected head injury.
- The patient is an infant or a child.
- Three doses have already been taken by the patient.
- The patient has taken tadalafil (Cialis), vardenafil (Levitra), or sildenafil (Viagra) within the past 24 hours.

MEDICATION FORM

Tablet, sublingual spray.

DOSAGE

The dosage for EMT administration of nitroglycerin is either one tablet or one spray under the tongue. The most commonly prescribed dose is either 0.3 mg per tablet (or metered spray), or 0.4 mg per tablet (or metered spray). Regardless of the individual dose unit, the administered dose may be repeated in 3–5 minutes if (1) the patient experiences no relief; (2) the blood pressure remains greater than 90 mmHg systolic or does not fall more than 30 mmHg below the baseline systolic pressure; (3) the heart rate remains above 50 bpm and below 100 bpm; and (4) medical direction gives authorization. The total dose is three tablets or sprays, to include what the patient took prior to your arrival.

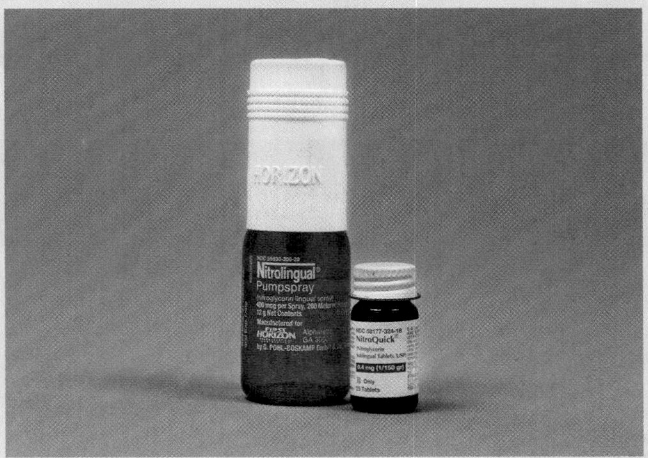

ADMINISTRATION

To administer nitroglycerin (EMT Skills 17-1):

1. Complete the history and physical exam of the cardiac patient and determine that the patient has his own nitroglycerin. Be sure the patient is sitting or lying supine.
2. Assess baseline vital signs to ensure that the systolic blood pressure is greater than 90 mmHg or greater than 30 mmHg below the systolic baseline, and the heart rate is above 50 bpm and less than 100 bpm (follow local protocol).
3. Obtain approval from medical direction, either on-line or off-line, to administer nitroglycerin.
4. Check the patient's medication to ensure that it is nitroglycerin prescribed in the patient's name and to learn the dose and route of administration.
5. Be sure that the patient is alert and responsive.
6. Check the expiration date on the nitroglycerin.
7. Ask the patient when he took his last dose of medication and what its effects were. Also be sure that the patient understands how the medication will be administered.
8. Wear gloves when handling nitroglycerin. As the patient lifts his tongue, place or spray the medication under the tongue. Alternatively, have the patient place the tablet or spray under the tongue himself.
9. Remind the patient to keep his mouth closed and not to swallow until the medication has dissolved.
10. Perform a reassessment of the patient's blood pressure in 2 minutes after the nitroglycerin administration, and before your next dose.
11. Record your actions, including the dosage, the time of administration, and the patient's response.

continued

FIGURE 17-16 ✱ Nitroglycerin.

Objective 17-13
Explain the assessment-based approach to assessment and emergency medical care for cardiac compromise and acute coronary syndrome.

Thinking Critically
During one week you are called to two possible cardiac emergencies. On the first call, the patient is unresponsive with no respiration or pulse. On the second call, the patient is responsive and complaining of chest discomfort. What emergency care do you provide during the primary assessment of each patient?

Nitroglycerin—*continued*

ACTIONS

- Dilates blood vessels
- Decreases workload of the heart
- Decreases cardiac oxygen demand

SIDE EFFECTS

The aim of administering nitroglycerin is to dilate blood vessels in the heart, but blood vessels in other parts of the body are dilated as well. This dilation can cause:

- Headache
- A drop in blood pressure
- Changes in pulse rate as the body compensates for the changes in blood vessel size

REASSESSMENT

Whenever you administer nitroglycerin to a patient, you must perform a reassessment. The following steps must be included:

- Monitor blood pressure frequently during treatment and transport.
- Question the patient about the effect of the medication on the relief of pain.
- Obtain approval from medical direction prior to readministration of the medication.
- Constantly monitor the airway and breathing status; if the breathing becomes inadequate, begin positive pressure ventilation with supplemental oxygen.
- If the medication has had no or little effect, consult medical direction to consider another dose.
- Document any findings during the reassessment.

FIGURE 17-16 ✱ Nitroglycerin. *continued*

remain alert for findings that could indicate acute deterioration in the geriatric population.

There may be some differences in presentation or management of these patients should an acute coronary event occur, or if they go into cardiac arrest, based on the patient's medical history and current medical conditions. Table 17-2 outlines some of these considerations.

Assessment and Care: General Guidelines

Assessment-Based Approach: Cardiac Compromise and Acute Coronary Syndrome

Dispatch information can provide you with the first indications that a patient may be suffering from cardiac compromise. When you are directed to patients complaining of chest pain or chest discomfort and/or difficulty in breathing, suspect the possibility of cardiac problems. Remember that any adult patient with chest pain or chest discomfort should be treated as a cardiac emergency until proven otherwise.

Scene Size-Up

On arrival, perform the scene size-up to ensure that the scene is secure, and then proceed rapidly with the primary assessment.

Primary Assessment

Form a general impression of the patient and his mental status as you approach the scene. Generally, patients experiencing cardiac emergencies fall into two categories: (1) unresponsive patients with no respiration and no pulse (cardiac arrest) and (2) responsive patients who appear to be in minor, moderate, or severe distress.

When you encounter an unresponsive patient with no ventilations, or agonal respirations, and no pulse, immediately begin chest compressions followed by airway management and ventilation (CAB). If the cardiac arrest was not witnessed, immediately initiate CPR beginning with chest compressions for about 2 minutes (which equates to five cycles of 30:2 for a lone rescuer). During the five cycles of CPR, the automated external defibrillator (AED) is applied without interruption to the chest compressions. After the fifth cycle, activate the AED to analyze the rhythm. If the cardiac arrest was witnessed, immediately begin chest compression and apply the AED as soon as it

TABLE 17-2 Special Considerations in Geriatric Cardiac Events

History of diabetes mellitus	A geriatric patient with diabetes has long-term damage to the nerve endings in the body. This causes the typical pain from an MI to be perceived poorly, if at all, by the diabetic patient. Therefore, the diabetic patient experiencing an MI may complain only of respiratory distress or dizziness when standing or even excessive weakness and dyspnea on exertion. It is important for the EMT to identify the patient with diabetes as potentially having an acute coronary event and to treat him appropriately. Contact ALS early, follow your local protocol, and ascertain if additional or alternative therapies are desired by medical direction.
History of trauma	If the geriatric patient is a trauma patient, there must be a high index of suspicion for cardiac involvement as well. Geriatric patients who are traumatized can slip quickly into cardiac arrest and do not respond well to typical interventions. Geriatric patients with head trauma, chest trauma, abdominal trauma, or extremity trauma with severe bleeding are especially susceptible to cardiac arrest.
History of asthma	If a patient with a history of asthma goes into cardiac arrest, the cause may be acute bronchoconstriction that led to hypoxemia, acidosis, and cardiac arrest. Until the bronchoconstriction is reversed, the patient will not regain a pulse or breathing. Early intercept or backup by an ALS unit will allow the administration of medications that may help reverse this condition.
History of COPD	Elderly patients commonly have some form of COPD (emphysema or chronic bronchitis). The arrest may have been caused by an exacerbation of the COPD, which led to hypoxemia, acidosis, and then arrest. ALS backup is needed during the resuscitation of this patient. Remember also that COPD disorders can weaken the lung tissue and cause the development of a pneumothorax and collapse of the lung. (This too may precipitate a cardiac arrest.) Be alert for the presence or the development of a pneumothorax during positive pressure ventilation, which may cause a bleb on the lung tissue to rupture.

is available. Continue with chest compressions until the defibrillation pads are applied. The key to CPR is to limit the interruption of chest compressions; therefore, it may be necessary to work around the compressor until the AED prompts the EMT to "stand clear." Follow the AED protocol. For cardiac arrest patients up to 8 years of age, it is highly desirable that the AED have a dose-attenuating system that will deliver a reduced shock. If a pediatric dose-attenuating system is not available, apply the adult AED and proceed with the AED sequence. (An expanded discussion of AED use is in Chapter 15.)

With responsive patients, first ensure adequate airway, breathing, oxygenation, and circulation. Note the patient's skin color, temperature, and condition. Note also the type, location, and intensity of any pain and presence of other signs or symptoms related to acute coronary syndromes. Apply oxygen if any of these is present:

- Signs of respiratory distress or dyspnea
- Signs of hypoxia
- Signs or symptoms of heart failure
- Signs or symptoms of shock
- An altered mental status
- An SpO_2 reading of <94% (The AHA 2010 guidelines recommend oxygen therapy if the SpO_2 is below 94%; but many EMS protocols call for oxygen therapy below 95%. Follow your local protocol).

Make a decision on whether early transport is needed and contact ALS as appropriate.

Secondary Assessment

Following the primary assessment, you will proceed with the secondary assessment.

History If the patient has an altered mental status and is unable to answer questions appropriately, attempt to obtain history information from the family or bystanders at the scene. If the patient is able to answer questions appropriately, you will obtain a history from the patient and then proceed with the secondary assessment. As previously discussed, the information gained in the history of the medical patient provides the basis for further assessment and emergency care.

You should suspect that any patient complaining of chest discomfort, shortness of breath, fainting, general weakness, or fatigue on exertion may be suffering from a possible cardiac compromise or an acute coronary syndrome. Obtain a history to identify information pertinent to the condition. When conducting a history of the chief complaint and other associated symptoms, such as chest discomfort and shortness of breath, use the OPQRST mnemonic to obtain the information. Chest discomfort is the most common chief complaint and most important signal of patients suffering from cardiac compromise and an acute coronary syndrome.

- **Onset.** *What were you doing when the chest discomfort started? What triggered the discomfort? Was the onset sudden or gradual?*

Thinking Critically
In a patient suffering chest discomfort, what responses to each of the OPQRST questions would be consistent with acute coronary syndrome?

Objective 17-14
Discuss the indications and contraindications for fibrinolytic therapy in patients with cardiac emergencies.

There is a misconception that most acute coronary syndromes occur during physical exertion. According to the American Heart Association, only 10–15 percent occur during exercise or other physical activities. The majority of acute coronary syndromes occur at rest or with normal daily moderate activity. However, very strong emotional events such as death of a spouse, loss of a job, and divorce have commonly been experienced by those suffering a heart attack.

- **Provocation or palliation.** *What makes the chest discomfort worse? What makes the chest discomfort better?*

  Many patients with any type of acute coronary syndrome complain that the discomfort is made worse by exertion. Upon rest, the discomfort is completely relieved or it may have subsided to a lesser intensity. Some patients may complain of the discomfort at rest that worsens with any activity. Some chest discomfort is completely relieved after taking nitroglycerin, but, in worse conditions, the nitroglycerin provides only some relief or no relief of the chest discomfort. You may be called to the scene late at night for a patient who complains of chest discomfort that wakes him from his sleep. This may be a condition called nocturnal (refers to night) angina or it may actually be a heart attack.

- **Quality.** *Describe the chest discomfort. Is it a dull, aching, pressure-type discomfort? Is it pressure, squeezing, crushing, or burning? Is it sharp or stabbing?*

  The chest discomfort is most commonly described as a crushing pressure. It is also often described as dull, aching, squeezing, or burning. Many patients state, "It feels like someone is sitting on my chest." Other patients present with their fist clenched over the center of their chest. This is called the *Levine sign*. It is an indication of severe chest discomfort. The chest discomfort may be described as being a more diffuse dull and aching-type sensation located in the back between the scapulae (shoulder blades). Again, it is important to ask about a "discomfort" and not just "pain." Many patients may deny they are having pain, since the sensation is much more a feeling of pressure and not a true sharp or stabbing pain.

- **Radiation.** *Does the discomfort radiate; that is, does it travel to any other part of the body? Do you feel it anywhere else in the body?*

  Typically, in an acute coronary syndrome, the discomfort may radiate to the arms (most often the left arm), shoulders, jaw, epigastrium (upper middle portion of the abdomen just below the xiphoid process), neck, or back.

- **Severity.** *On a 1-to-10 scale, with 10 being the worst, describe the discomfort.*

  Remember that the 1-to-10 scale is subjective, since many patients have differing perceptions and tolerances for pain. Be sure to ask if the patient has ever experienced this pain previously. If the patient states that he had the same type of pain or discomfort in the past and was diagnosed with a heart attack, it is almost certain that the same presentation of discomfort or pain is due to another heart attack. If the patient presents with his fist tightly clenched over his chest, he is typically suffering from severe discomfort. Be sure to determine the severity both before and after rest and nitroglycerin.

- **Time.** *When did the chest discomfort start? How long have you had the discomfort? Has the discomfort been constant or does it come and go (intermittent)?*

  Because so many patients wait to seek help when experiencing chest discomfort, it may be necessary to determine the actual day and time the discomfort started if it started before the day the call was placed for EMS.

Fibrinolytic Therapy and the EMT's Role One advantage of interviewing the patient in the prehospital setting is the ability to gather information that is important to ongoing management of the patient in the hospital setting. Patient care for a myocardial infarction can be greatly enhanced if the hospital receives certain patient information necessary to make patient care decisions. One important decision the hospital staff needs to make is whether the patient is a candidate for fibrinolytic therapy. Fibrinolytics are a type of drug that, upon administration, dissolve the newly formed clot that is occluding the coronary artery and causing the heart attack. With rapid removal of the clot, distal perfusion can be resumed and the extent of myocardial damage can be minimized or even inhibited. One concern with these medications, however, is that they don't just dissolve clots in the heart; they can dissolve clots no matter where they are located in the vessels of the body. For this reason, recent stroke patients, patients with a history of recent surgery, and similar patients cannot receive fibrinolytic drugs because of the risk that they may cause internal hemorrhage or other life-threatening complications.

As an EMT, you can assist in decision making by attaining answers to important questions that will determine if fibrinolytics are appropriate for this patient. These

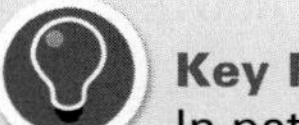

Key Points
In patients with signs and symptoms of cardiac compromise or acute coronary syndrome, an key role for the EMT is to help identify those patients who may benefit from early fibrinolytic therapy.

are questions you will normally ask during the history, including the OPQRST history. The only additional task is documenting them on a specific "fibrinolytic checklist" and presenting it to the emergency department staff as early as possible.

The following list represents the absolute and relative contraindications for fibrinolytic therapy. This information is taken from the most current research available from the American Heart Association:

- Absolute contraindications
  History of prior intracranial hemorrhage
  Known diagnosis of a cerebral vascular lesion
  Diagnosis of a malignant intracranial neoplasm
  Suspected aortic dissection
  Active bleeding (excluding menstrual cycles)
  Bleeding disorders
  Closed head trauma or facial trauma within the past 3 months
  Ischemic stroke within the past 3 months (except acute ischemic stroke within the past 3 hours)
- Relative contraindications
  History of chronic, severe, or poorly controlled hypertension
  Uncontrolled systolic hypertension (>180 mmHg) on presentation
  Uncontrolled diastolic hypertension (>110 mmHg) on presentation
  History of intracranial pathology not covered in absolute contraindications
  Traumatic or prolonged CPR (>10 minutes)
  Major surgery (<3 weeks)
  Internal bleeding within last 2–4 weeks
  Noncompressible vascular punctures
  For streptokinase/anistreplase: prior exposure (>5 days ago) or prior documented allergic reaction to these agents
  Pregnancy
  Active peptic ulcer disease
  Current use of anticoagulants

Although it may appear by this list of contraindications that many patients will be excluded, normally one patient is excluded for a number of different reasons. Even with the criticality and specificity of these contraindications, the use of fibrinolytics has made a significant impact on reducing the morbidity and mortality from acute coronary syndromes. The role of the EMT is to help identify those patients who may benefit from early fibrinolytic therapy.

During your assessment of the patient with cardiac-related chest pain, you may find that a large number of patients, more often males than females, will make excuses as to why the chest discomfort they are experiencing is not a true heart attack. Many people claim the discomfort is nothing more than indigestion, so they take antacids. Many believe they are too healthy to suffer a heart attack. Others feel that if they indicate they are having chest discomfort it will frighten those in the household. Many do not want the embarrassment of having the fire department, First Responders, and EMS crews at their house. Others just feel that it cannot happen to them. This denial extends the period of time before people seek help when experiencing the symptoms of a heart attack. Remember that more than one-half of the patients who suffer a heart attack die outside of the hospital. A majority of those who die do so within the first hour of the onset of the symptoms of the heart attack.

Many times you will find that a family member, friend, or bystander will take the initiative to place the call to EMS, and not at the patient's request. Therefore, many patients will continue to downplay their symptoms. Some patients may be so convincing that not only do they convince themselves, their family, and bystanders, but they also convince the EMS crew. Be firm with the patient and do not let him persuade you that the condition is only a minor or temporary problem. Recognize the signs and symptoms and treat the patient aggressively. This will, potentially, save the patient's life.

Use the following as general guidelines for those patients who have denied the seriousness of their condition and have waited to contact the EMS crew. *These patients must be treated as a cardiac compromise and acute coronary syndrome patient and transported immediately:*

- A patient who has a history of angina (steady chest discomfort that is brought on by activity, exercise, or stress, and usually lasts 2–15 minutes) who is having chest discomfort at rest that lasts longer than 20 minutes
- Recent onset of angina that progressively worsens
- Nocturnal angina (patient who is awakened by the pain at night)
- Angina unrelieved by rest or three nitroglycerin tablets over 10 minutes
- Chest discomfort that lasts greater than 5–10 minutes after rest

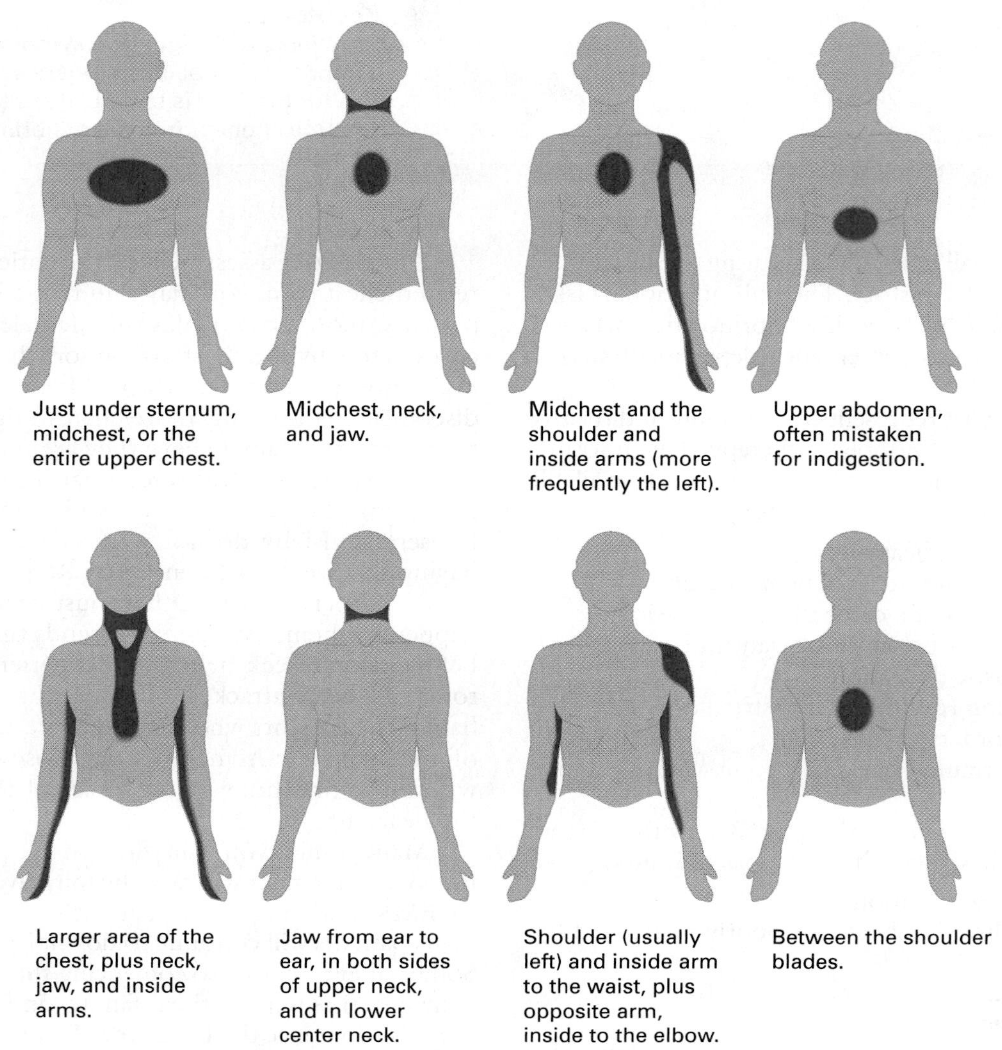
EARLY SIGNS OF ACUTE CORONARY SYNDROME (HEART ATTACK)
Just under sternum, midchest, or the entire upper chest.
Midchest, neck, and jaw.
Midchest and the shoulder and inside arms (more frequently the left).
Upper abdomen, often mistaken for indigestion.
Larger area of the chest, plus neck, jaw, and inside arms.
Jaw from ear to ear, in both sides of upper neck, and in lower center neck.
Shoulder (usually left) and inside arm to the waist, plus opposite arm, inside to the elbow.
Between the shoulder blades.

FIGURE 17-17 ✱ Typical locations and radiation of chest discomfort associated with cardiac emergencies.

Keep in mind that, in some patients, the presentation of an acute coronary syndrome, such as a heart attack, may not follow a typical pattern of signs or symptoms (Figure 17-17✱). These are considered *atypical presentations.* The elderly, diabetics, and women often have atypical presentations when suffering a heart attack. These patients may only feel weak or short of breath or lightheaded, and they will not present with chest discomfort or pain. Some patients, both men and women, suffer a "silent" heart attack, where there are no signs or symptoms that are truly recognizable. Also, the patient may not "look bad" in your general impression. He may appear to be relatively well aside from the chest discomfort or other complaints. The patient may present with one, two, or three of the symptoms. He does not have to have all of the symptoms to be categorized as an acute coronary syndrome or heart attack. One patient may present with only one symptom, whereas the next patient may have five symptoms. As always, err to benefit the patient and treat and transport expeditiously.

Physical Exam and Baseline Vital Signs You will perform a physical exam on the responsive patient suffering from a possible acute coronary syndrome such as chest discomfort or breathing difficulty. During the exam, assess the following:

- **Pupils.** Sluggish or dilated pupils may suggest hypoxia and poor perfusion.
- **Oral cavity.** Cyanotic mucous membranes indicate hypoxia.
- **Neck.** Congestive heart failure or cardiac tamponade (fluid in the sac surrounding the heart) may produce jugular venous distention.
- **Chest.** Auscultate for abnormal breath sounds, especially crackles, which may indicate fluid in the alveoli from left ventricular heart failure.
- **Lower and upper extremities.** Assess for peripheral edema, suggesting heart failure, and peripheral cyanosis, usually indicating vessel disease.

- **Posterior body.** Presacral edema to the lower back is another indicator of heart failure that may be more prominent in the patient who is sedentary and commonly in a supine or lying position.

In addition to performing the focused physical exam, obtain and record the patient's vital signs.

Signs and Symptoms Signs and symptoms associated with cardiac compromise or acute coronary syndrome may vary widely. However, the most common are these:

- Chest discomfort or pain that radiates to any of the following areas: chest, neck, jaw, arm, or back; also epigastric (upper abdomen) pain that may be described as indigestion. (Review Figure 17-17.)
- Sudden onset of sweating (This may be a significant finding by itself.)
- Cool, pale skin
- Difficulty in breathing (dyspnea)

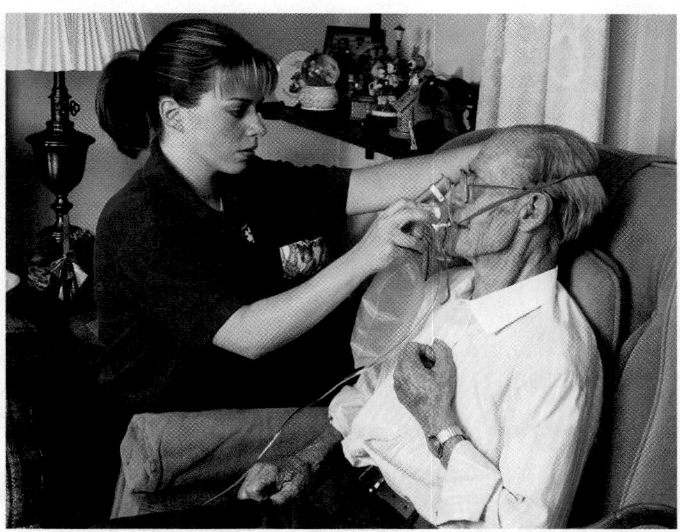

FIGURE 17-18 * Administer oxygen by nonrebreather mask in acute coronary syndrome patients who are hypoxic.

ASSESSMENT Tips

Increased respiratory rate and heart rates in the acute coronary syndrome patient indicate hypoxia or may be only a response to the chest pain or discomfort. ■

- Light-headedness or dizziness
- Anxiety or irritability
- Feelings of impending doom
- Abnormal or irregular pulse rate
- Abnormal blood pressure
- Nausea and/or vomiting

Emergency Medical Care

The American Heart Association Guidelines of 2010 emphasize the need to quickly recognize cardiac arrest and immediately begin chest compressions. Thus, the intervention sequence in the cardiac arrest patient has changed from ABC to CAB: immediate initiation of chest compressions followed by opening the airway and providing ventilation, along with AED application. It is also recognized that many of the interventions can be accomplished simultaneously with enough EMTs or emergency medical personnel on the scene. It is extremely important to reinforce that upon recognition of cardiac arrest the resuscitation must begin immediately with chest compressions. During the resuscitation, the EMT must ensure minimal interruption of chest compressions while providing other interventions or assessments.

1. If the patient appears to be unresponsive, with no breathing or no normal breathing (gasping or agonal breaths), quickly assess the carotid pulse in the adult and child, brachial pulse in the infant (no more than 10 seconds). If no signs of life are present, immediately begin chest compressions. Apply the AED as soon as it is available without interruption to chest compressions until the AED indicates a "stand clear" or analysis of the rhythm. Follow the AED prompts. Also, delay ventilation until after the first set of compressions is delivered.
2. Decrease the patient's anxiety by providing calm reassurance and placing him in a position of comfort (often sitting up; let the patient tell you how he feels most comfortable).
3. Assist the patient who has prescribed nitroglycerin.
4. If local protocol permits and the patient does not have a known aspirin allergy, administer 160–325 mg of uncoated aspirin. Have the patient chew the aspirin. Aspirin reduces the incidence of coronary arteries reoccluding and has antiplatelet effects. (See Figure 17-19* for the criteria and techniques for the administration of aspirin.)
5. Call for ALS backup; initiate early transport.

Reassessment

Although not all patients with chest pain/discomfort or cardiac compromise will deteriorate into cardiac arrest, be ready for this possibility. Closely reassess the breathing and pulse as you perform reassessment during transport. Be prepared to perform CPR and, as appropriate, use automated external defibrillation (as described in Chapter 15, "Shock and Resuscitation") in the event that cardiac arrest does occur.

Summary: Assessment and Care

To review assessment findings that may be associated with cardiac compromise and emergency care for cardiac compromise, see Figures 17-20a*, 17-20b*, and 17-21*.

Aspirin

MEDICATION NAME

Aspirin is the generic name. This is the same aspirin that is purchased over the counter. Trade names of aspirin include:

- ASA
- Bayer
- Ecotrin
- St. Joseph's
- Bufferin

INDICATIONS

All of the following criteria must be met before an EMT administers aspirin to a patient:

- The patient exhibits chest discomfort that is suggestive of a heart attack.
- The EMT has received approval from medical direction, whether on-line or off-line, to administer the medication.

CONTRAINDICATIONS

Aspirin should not be given to a patient who is known to be allergic (hypersensitive) to the drug.

MEDICATION FORM

Tablet.

DOSAGE

The dosage of aspirin is 160–325 mg as soon as possible after the onset of the chest discomfort and symptoms of heart attack. It is recommended that 160–325 mg of a nonenteric aspirin be chewed and swallowed.

ADMINISTRATION

To administer aspirin:

1. Complete the history and physical exam of the cardiac patient and determine that the patient is suffering from an acute coronary syndrome that is suggestive of a heart attack.
2. Obtain approval from medical direction, either on-line or off-line, to administer the aspirin.
3. Be sure that the patient is alert and oriented.
4. Have the patient chew a 160–325 mg nonenteric tablet.
5. Reassess the patient and record the vital signs.

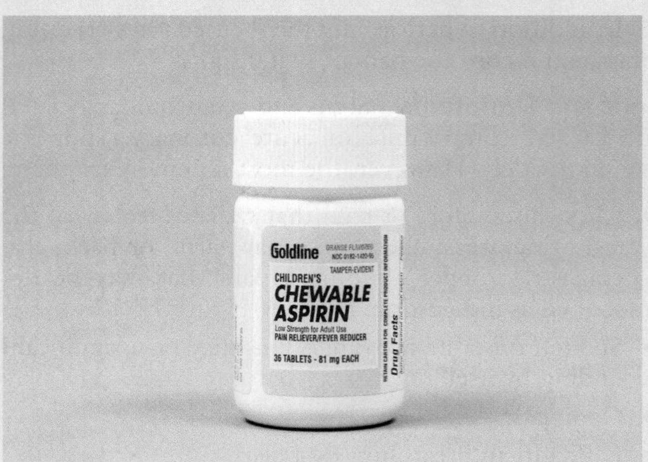

ACTIONS

Aspirin (acetylsalicylic acid [ASA]) is a medication that produces a rapid antiplatelet effect. This effect decreases the ability of platelets to clump together during the clotting cascade and reduces the formation of a clot in the coronary artery at the site of the blockage. The medication also reduces the incidence of coronary reocclusion and recurrent ischemic event following in-hospital therapy with fibrinolytic agents. The aspirin is not used in this situation for its analgesic (pain relief) effects, and should be the nonenteric (not coated) type.

SIDE EFFECTS

When used in this situation, aspirin has very few side effects. The patient may experience stomach irritation or heartburn, nausea, or vomiting. Although typically not used in the prehospital setting, there are aspirin suppositories (300 mg each) that are considered safe and effective for patients with severe nausea, vomiting, or a history of upper gastrointestinal tract disorders.

REASSESSMENT

When you administer aspirin to a patient, you should conduct a reassessment. The aspirin is used in this situation not as a pain reliever but as a drug to prevent platelets from continuing to clump together and occlude the artery. Thus, there may not be an immediate relief in pain such as occurs with nitroglycerin. Be sure to record any changes in the patient's condition and the reassessment findings.

FIGURE 17-19 ✱ Aspirin.

Assessment Summary

CARDIAC COMPROMISE AND ACUTE CORONARY SYNDROMES

The following findings may be associated with cardiac compromise and acute coronary syndromes.

SCENE SIZE-UP

Look for evidence of:
- Home or portable oxygen tanks or concentrators indicating chronic respiratory problems

Primary Assessment

General Impression

Position of patient:
- Tripod (may indicate pulmonary edema)
- Patient may have look of impending doom.
- Patient may be clutching chest.

Mental Status
- Alert to unresponsive
- Restlessness
- Agitation and irritability
- Anxiety

Airway
- Possibly occluded in patient with altered mental status

Breathing
- Signs of inadequacy or difficulty in breathing
- Abnormal sounds may be heard on auscultation (indicating heart failure)

Circulation
- Tachycardia or bradycardia
- Irregular
- Weak peripheral pulses
- Cyanosis to mucous membranes, around nose and mouth, nail beds, chest, neck
- Pale, cool skin

Status: Priority Determination

Secondary Assessment

History

Signs and symptoms:
- Discomfort or pressure sensation in middle of chest that may radiate to neck, to jaw, down arms, or to the back
- Difficulty in breathing
- Light-headedness or dizziness
- Anxiety and irritability
- Nausea and vomiting
- Known allergies to medication or other substances
  - Medications for cardiac conditions:
  - Prescribed nitroglycerin
  - Pre-existing cardiac disease
  - Hospitalized for cardiac condition
  - History of past heart attack

Physical Exam

Head, neck, and face:
- Cyanosis to face, neck, and mucous membranes
- Jugular venous distention (may indicate heart failure or cardiac tamponade)
- Nasal flaring
- Pupils sluggish to respond to light

Chest:
- Inspect for scars indicating previous cardiac surgery
- Retractions
- Breath sounds

Abdomen:
- Use of abdominal muscles when breathing

Extremities:
- Cyanosis to fingers and nail beds
- Pale skin
- Diaphoresis
- Peripheral edema

Other Signs and Symptoms:
- Nausea and vomiting
- Light-headedness or dizziness
- Sense of impending doom

Baseline Vital Signs
- BP: normal, high, or low
- HR: normal, tachycardia, bradycardia, irregular
- RR: increased
- Skin: pale and cool, diaphoresis, maybe cyanosis
- Pupils: dilated, sluggish to respond to light
- SpO_2: readings: may be normal or $< 95\%$

FIGURE 17-20a ✱ Assessment summary: cardiac compromise and acute coronary syndromes.

Objective 17-15
Explain the indications, contraindications, forms, dosage, administration, actions, side effects, and reassessment for aspirin.

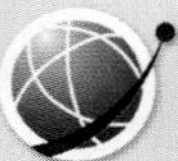

Media Resources
Go to www.bradybooks.com for mykit. Highlights:

- *Video:* Information about AEDs
- *Video:* Understanding Coronary Heart Disease
- *Video:* Understanding Dysrhythmias

Emergency Care Protocol

CARDIAC COMPROMISE AND ACUTE CORONARY SYNDROMES

1. Establish and maintain an open airway.
2. Suction secretions as necessary.
3. If breathing is inadequate, provide positive pressure ventilation with supplemental oxygen at a minimum rate of 10–12 ventilations/minute for an adult and 12–20 ventilations/minute for an infant or child.
4. Apply a pulse oximeter if available and monitor the SpO_2.
5. If the breathing is adequate, administer oxygen to keep the SpO_2 above 94%.
6. Place the patient in position of comfort (sitting or lying).
7. If the patient has signs and symptoms typical of cardiac-type chest discomfort and has prescribed nitroglycerin:
   - Nitroglycerin is a vasodilator and will reduce workload of the heart, dilate coronary arteries, and supply more oxygen to the heart.
     Note: DO NOT ADMINISTER NITROGLYCERIN IF:
       Systolic BP is less than 90 mmHg or greater than 30 mmHg lower than the baseline systolic blood pressure.
       The heart rate is less than 50 bpm or greater than 100 bpm.
       The patient has a suspected head injury.
       The patient has already taken three doses.
       The patient has recently taken tadalafil (Cialis), vardenafil (Levitra), or sildenafil (Viagra) (consult medical direction).
   - Obtain an order from medical direction.
   - Be sure the prescription is the patient's.
   - Wear gloves when touching nitroglycerin.
   - Remove the nonrebreather mask from the patient.
   - Have the patient lift his tongue.
   - Place nitroglycerin tablet or spray under the tongue.
   - Instruct the patient not to swallow.
   - Replace the nonrebreather mask on the patient.
   - Record time and reassess the patient.
   - Side effects:
       Headache
       Decrease in blood pressure
       Changes in heart rate
8. Administer 160–325 mg of aspirin (according to local protocol).
9. Consider advanced life support.
10. Transport in a position of comfort.
11. Perform a reassessment of the patient every 5 minutes.

FIGURE 17-20b ✱ Emergency care protocol: cardiac compromise and acute coronary syndromes.

Emergency Care Algorithm: **Cardiac Compromise**

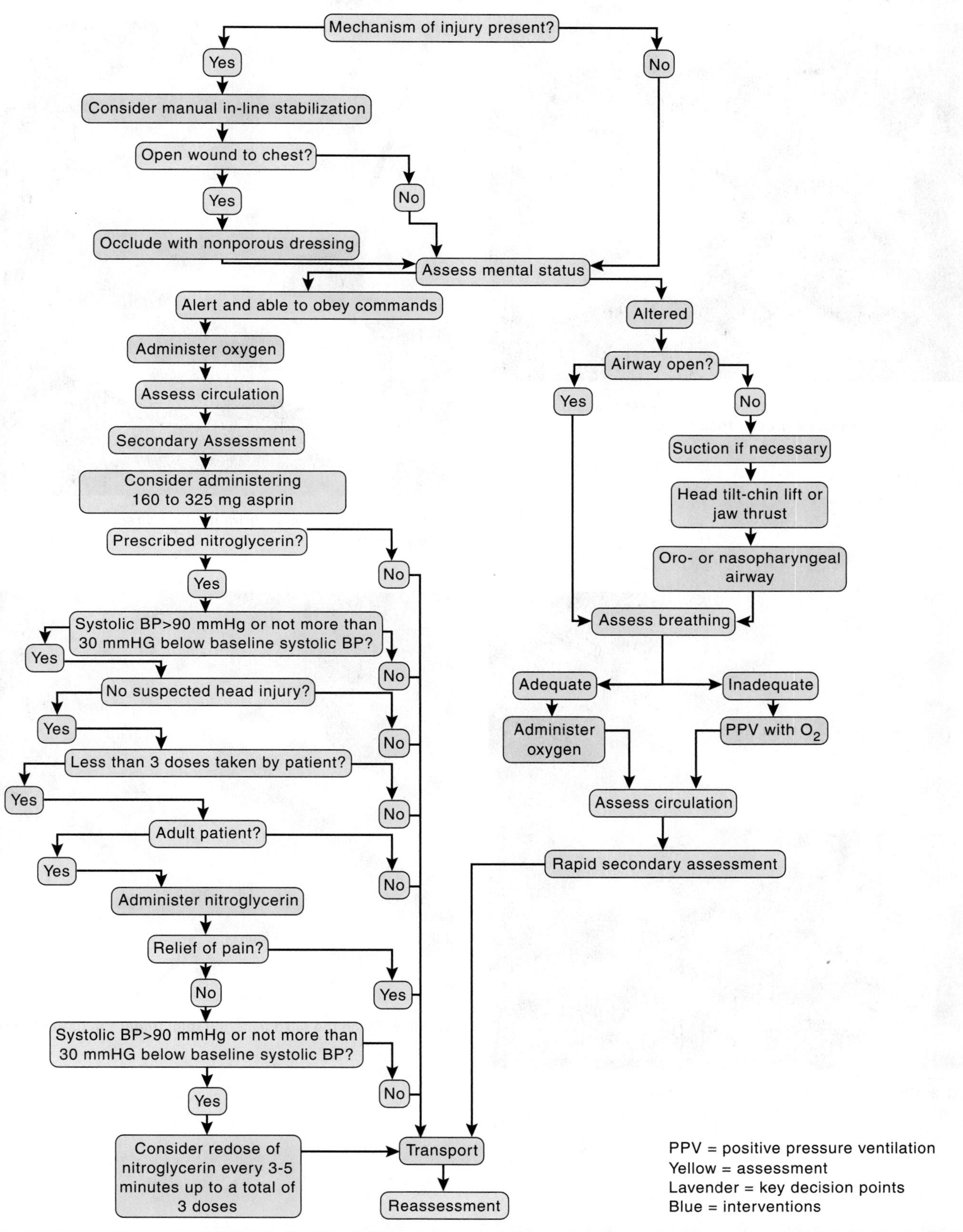

FIGURE 17-21 ✱ Emergency care algorithm: cardiac compromise.

EMT skills 17-1 Assisting a Patient with Prescribed Nitroglycerin

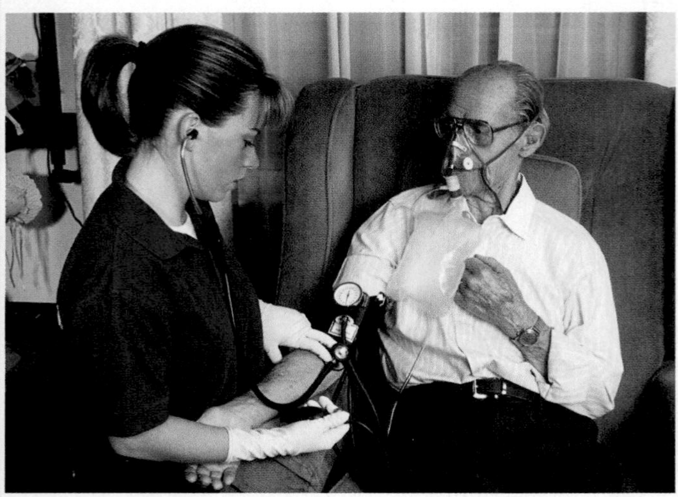

17-1A * Have the patient sit or lie down. Assess blood pressure. Systolic pressure must be greater than 90 mmHg.

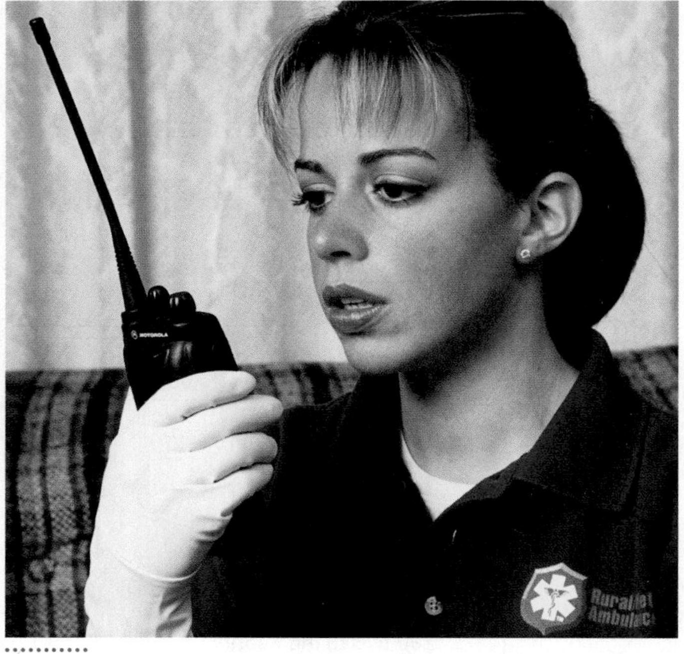

17-1B * Obtain an order from medical direction to administer the nitroglycerin.

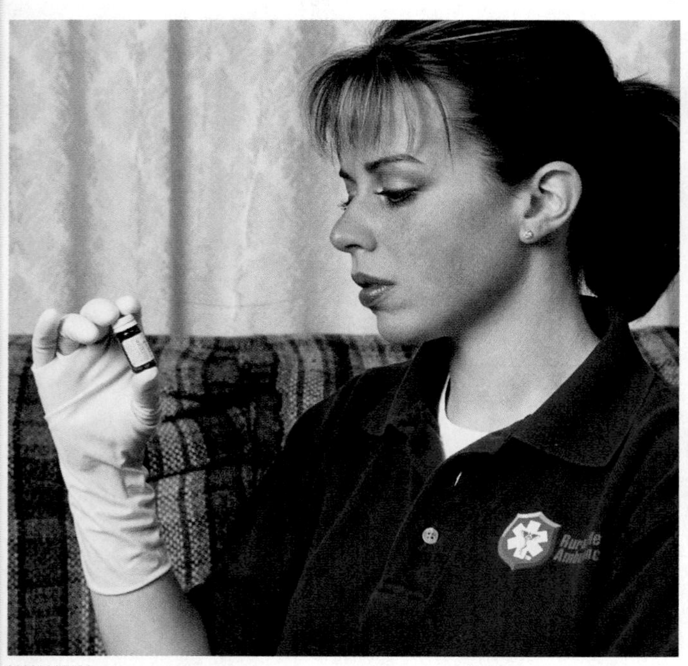

17-1C * Check the medication to ensure that it is prescribed to the patient, it is the proper medication, and it has not expired.

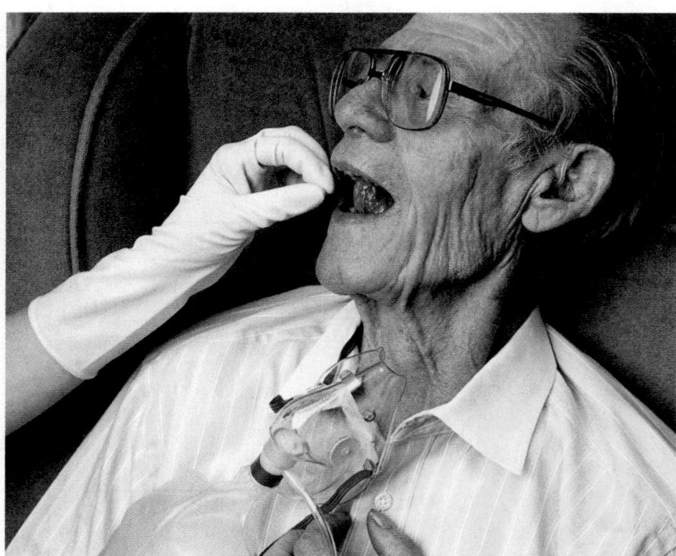

17-1D * Place the nitroglycerin tablet under the patient's tongue.

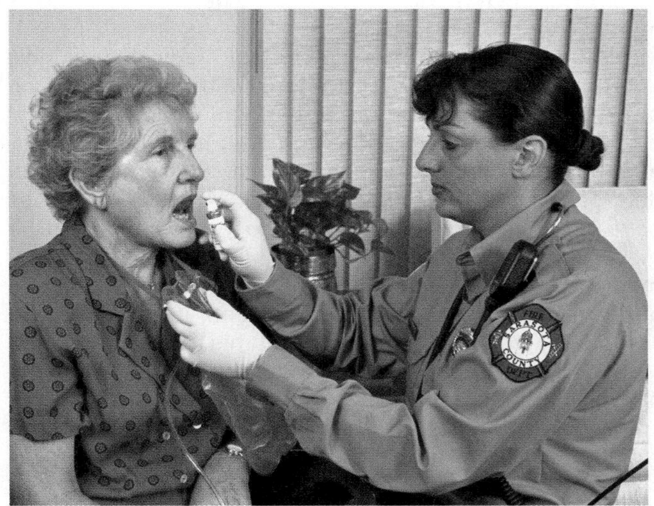

17-1E ✱ To administer nitroglycerin spray, depress the container and deliver one spray under the tongue.

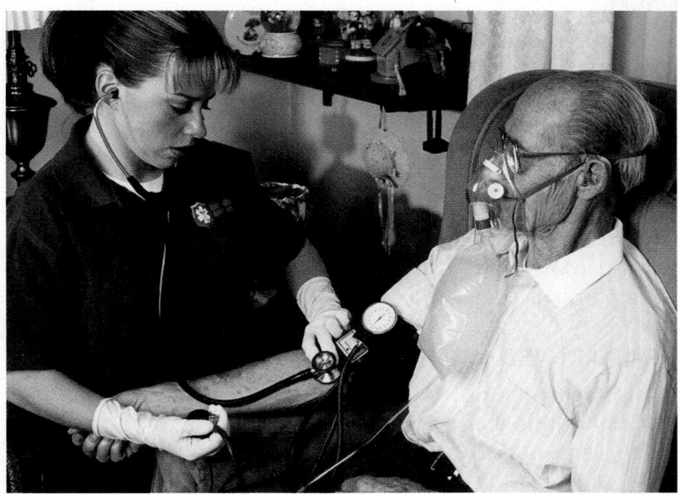

17-1F ✱ Reassess blood pressure within 2 minutes of administering the nitroglycerin.

CHAPTER REVIEW

SUMMARY

Patients suffering from an acute coronary event may be among the most challenging patients encountered by the EMT. They may present anywhere on the continuum from being alert and oriented with only minimal symptoms to being unresponsive and just moments from cardiac arrest. Compounding this picture is that the cardiac patient may go from one extreme to the other very quickly, without much warning for the EMT. Therefore, the EMT must always maintain a high degree of suspicion with cardiac patients that they may deteriorate into cardiac arrest very suddenly.

Treatment for cardiac-related chest pain and other coronary emergencies must be delivered in a timely manner, without error. Patient outcomes are always better if they do not degrade into cardiac arrest. If they should arrest, outcomes are generally poor, carrying with them a low rate of successful resuscitation. To increase the survival rate should your patient be in cardiac arrest on your arrival (or arrest in your presence), always remember the components of the Chain of Survival. Early recognition and access, early BCLS (CPR), early defibrillation, and early ACLS are all necessary if rates of patient survival from cardiac arrest are going to improve.

When caring for a patient in cardiac arrest, always do your best in each of the interventions you provide. Remember to "push hard and push fast" with compressions so that the brain and heart can still receive blood flow during the arrest management. Ensure adequate ventilations and provide oxygen during the arrest as well. The automated external defibrillator should be utilized specifically as addressed earlier in the chapter so that those patients in ventricular fibrillation will have the greatest opportunity for survival. Patients in nonventricular fibrillation cardiac arrest (identified by a "no shock" message on the AED) should also receive this high level of care so that they too may have the greatest chance for survival.

The patient near cardiac arrest, in cardiac arrest, or just coming out of cardiac arrest is probably one of the most challenging and dynamic situations the EMT will ever encounter. It requires a thorough understanding of the body, application of multiple skills simultaneously, and coordination of multiple EMS providers—all done in the shortest time possible so that the patient can be transported to the hospital for definitive care.

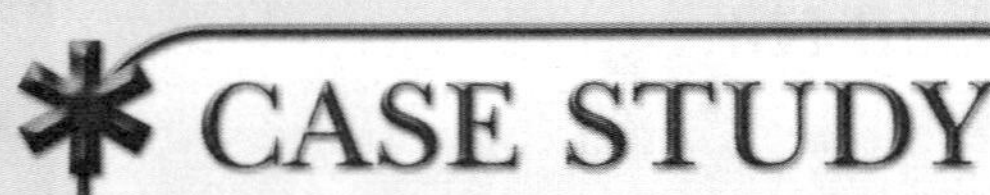

FOLLOW-UP

SCENE SIZE-UP

You have been dispatched to a 49-year-old male patient complaining of chest pain while eating dinner at a local restaurant. You don your gloves and grab the jump kit and oxygen as you leave the vehicle. You approach the patient and notice a moderately crowded dining room with several people around one particular table. There do not appear to be any hazards to your safety. You determine that there is only one patient. Upon arrival at the table you introduce your partner and yourself to the patient, who gives his name as Paul Antak.

PRIMARY ASSESSMENT

After introducing yourself, you note that the patient is clutching his chest and ask, "What seems to be the problem, Mr. Antak?" The patient states, "I feel like someone is standing on my chest." The patient is responsive, alert, and oriented. His airway is open and his breathing is rapid but adequate. Your partner initiates oxygen at 4 lpm by nasal cannula. The patient's pulse is palpable. His skin is pale, cool, and slightly moist. There are no obvious signs of any injuries or other problems. You direct your partner to get the stretcher while you continue with the secondary assessment.

SECONDARY ASSESSMENT

You begin the history using the OPQRST format to assess Mr. Antak's chest discomfort. Mr. Antak describes his discomfort as sudden in onset about 20 minutes ago. Nothing has made it better or worse. At first, he thought it was indigestion, but it did not go away. He describes it as a dull, squeezing pain that radiates to his left arm. He rates this as an 8 on a 1-to-10 scale of pain.

You obtain the rest of the history. His signs and symptoms are chest discomfort with some radiation to the left arm, an extremely irregular pulse, and sweaty and pale skin. He has no known allergies. He does take medication for high blood pressure, and his physician gave him nitroglycerin to take in case of severe chest discomfort. Mr. Antak states that, although he has the nitroglycerin with him, he has not taken any yet. There is no past medical history other than the high blood pressure. He was in the middle of his meal. There were no similar events prior to this incident.

Your physical exam reveals pupils that are equal and responsive to light, but slightly sluggish. The oral mucosa is normal in color. The jugular veins are normal. The breath sounds are equal and clear bilaterally. The abdomen is soft, not tender, and not distended. The pulses are present in all extremities. There is no edema to the feet, ankles, hands, or sacral area. You assess Mr. Antak's baseline vital signs: radial pulse—irregular rate of 98; blood pressure—180/110 mmHg; breathing—28 per minute; skin—cool and moist. The SpO_2 reading is 95% while he is on the supplemental oxygen.

You contact your base hospital for medical direction's approval to assist in administration of nitroglycerin and aspirin. This is granted by Dr. Settler. You ask Mr. Antak for his medication container and note that it contains sublingual nitroglycerin, prescribed for him, with an expiration date of 1 year from today's date. Mr. Antak says he has never taken nitroglycerin before, so you explain that he may get a headache or become light-headed from the medication. You explain that he will need to keep the tablet under his tongue and not swallow until it has dissolved completely. You ask the patient to lift his tongue and when he does, you place one tablet under the tongue. Once the nitroglycerin is dissolved, you then administer 160 mg of chewable aspirin and ask the patient to chew the tablet.

While you are preparing to move Mr. Antak from his chair to the stretcher, he tells you that he is suddenly feeling worse. You verbally reassure him; however, he suddenly loses consciousness and has a seizure that lasts about 5 seconds. You assess him for a verbal response and find none. Your partner simultaneously checks for a pulse and breathing and also finds none. Your patient is now in cardiac arrest. You and your partner then move him carefully to the floor, and your partner immediately initiates chest compressions as you apply the AED. During this brief time of rhythm analysis, you call dispatch on your portable radio to obtain an estimated time of arrival of the backup ALS unit.

The AED indicates a shockable rhythm and begins to charge up for the defibrillation attempt. After ensuring that you, your partner, and all bystanders are clear from the patient, you depress the "shock" button on the AED. You note some muscular contraction to the chest wall with the defibrillation. Immediately after the shock delivery, you resume CPR with chest compressions for five cycles of 30 compressions and 2 ventilations. Following this 2-minute period of CPR, you stop to reassess the breathing and pulse and find a palpable carotid and radial pulse; however, the patient is still unresponsive and is not yet breathing. You continue to ventilate Mr. Antak once every 6 seconds. The ALS providers arrive on scene and ask, "Where are you at with your cardiac arrest management?"

REASSESSMENT

By the time the ALS crew has provided advanced airway management, intravenous access, and some medication administration, you are en route to the hospital. Your partner is driving the ambulance and one of the ALS providers is in the back with you. On the way to the hospital you constantly ensure that the pulse is present, the airway device is inserted properly, and the oxygen is always flowing. The pulse oximetry currently reads 98%, and you notice that the patient is starting to display some random extremity movement. The blood pressure is currently 102/84 mmHg, the heart rate is 102 and still irregular, and you are ventilating the patient at 10 times per minute with a bag-valve-mask device connected to supplemental oxygen. You radio the hospital with an update on Mr. Antak's condition and your estimated time of arrival.

IN REVIEW

1. Define the cardiovascular system.
2. Explain the exchange that takes place between the capillaries and the body's cells.
3. Define perfusion and shock (hypoperfusion).
4. Name the common signs and symptoms of cardiac compromise.
5. Describe the standard emergency medical treatment for patients with signs and symptoms of cardiac compromise.
6. Explain the dosage of aspirin in a cardiac emergency and how it is administered.
7. Explain under what conditions the administration of nitroglycerin is indicated.

CRITICAL THINKING

You arrive on the scene and find a 59-year-old male patient complaining of chest discomfort and shortness of breath. The patient has assumed a tripod position while sitting at the edge of his bed. You notice that he has four pillows on the side of the bed where he sleeps. His complexion appears to be ashen gray and he is extremely diaphoretic. His breathing is very labored, and he speaks two to three words followed by a gasp for a breath. His radial pulse is present and his skin is extremely cool and clammy. His heart rate is 134 bpm, blood pressure is 178/100 mmHg, and respirations are 32 per minute and labored. His SpO_2 reading is 72%. He has a history of three previous myocardial infarctions. He has crackles in the lower and middle lobes of both lungs. His hands and ankles are swollen.

1. What emergency care would you provide during the primary assessment?
2. What condition do you suspect the patient is experiencing?
3. What medication may improve the patient's condition?
4. How would you move the patient from the second-floor bedroom to the ambulance stretcher on the first floor?
5. In what position would you transport the patient?
6. What oxygen device would you apply and at what liter flow?
7. What is causing the crackles in the lungs?

EXPLORE PEARSON **mybradykit**™

Please go to **www.bradybooks.com** to access mykit for this text. You will find quizzes, critical thinking scenarios, weblinks, animations, and videos related to this chapter—and much more. Look for online information on heart attacks, congenital heart defects, hypertension, and acute myocardial infarction. You will also find video clips on AEDs, understanding coronary heart disease, and understanding dysrhythmias.

Register your access code from the front of your book by going to **www.bradybooks.com** and selecting the mykit links.

CHAPTER 18

Altered Mental Status, Stroke, *and* Headache

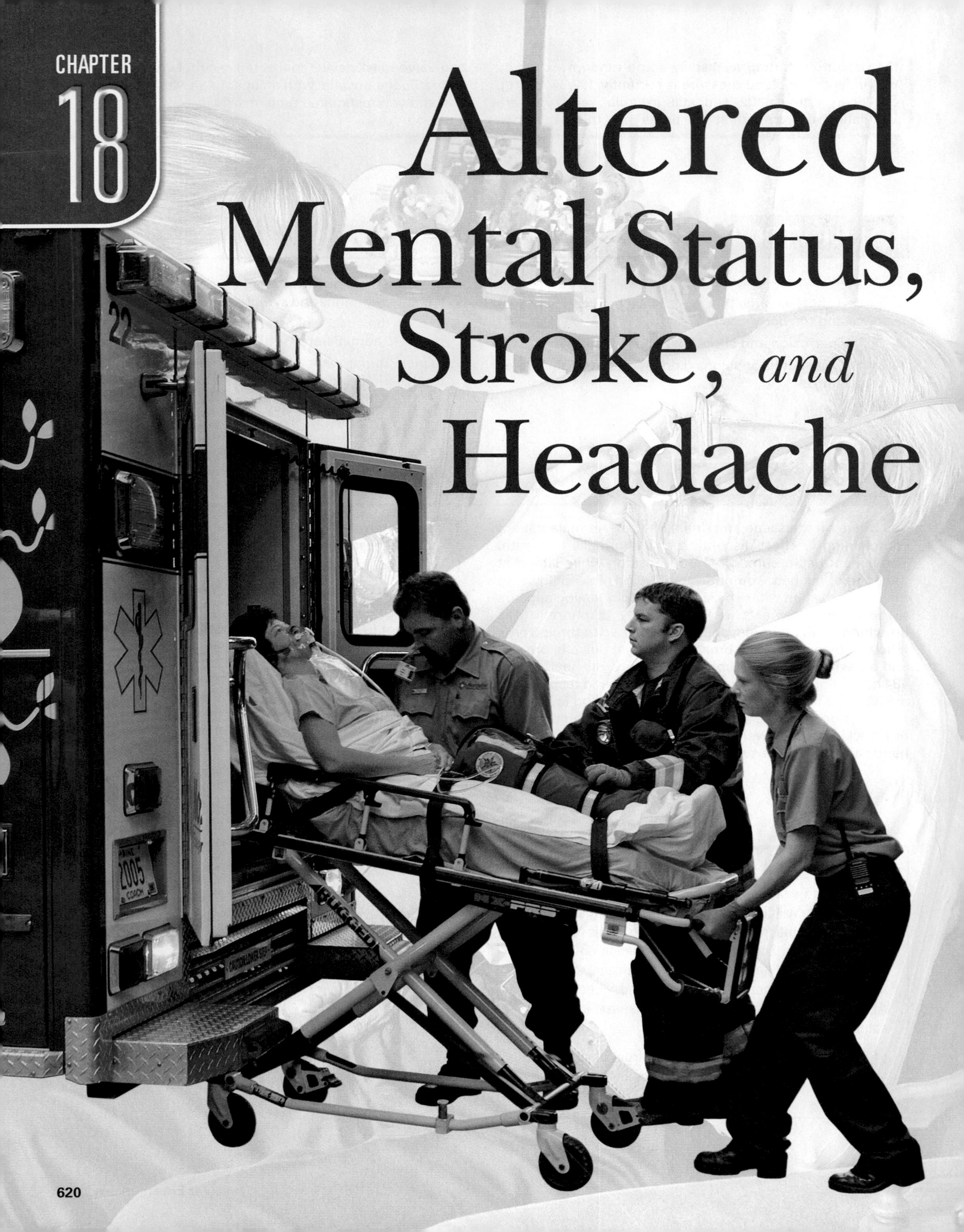

Navigation Guide

The following items provide an overview to the purpose and content of this chapter. The Standard and Competency are from the new National EMS Education Standards.

STANDARD **Medicine** (Content Area: Neurology)

COMPETENCY Applies fundamental knowledge to provide basic emergency care and transportation based on assessment findings for an acutely ill patient.

OBJECTIVES: After reading this chapter, you should be able to:

18-1. Define key terms introduced in this chapter.
18-2. List possible structural, toxic-metabolic, and other causes of altered mental status.
18-3. Describe an assessment-based approach to altered mental status. Obtain information.
18-4. Explain the reason for paying particular attention to airway assessment and management in patients with altered mental status.
18-5. List signs and symptoms of altered mental status commonly associated with:
 a. Trauma
 b. Nontraumatic or medical conditions
18-6. Determine the need for the following interventions in patients with altered mental status:
 a. Manual spinal stabilization
 b. Opening and maintaining the airway
 c. Oxygenation
 d. Ventilation
 e. Positioning
 f. Transport
18-7. Explain the responsibilities of the general public and EMS in the care for a stroke patient that are identified by the American Heart Association as "Detection," "Dispatch," and "Delivery."
18-8. Describe the pathophysiology of stroke and distinguish between ischemic strokes and hemorrhagic strokes.
18-9. Describe the relationship between stroke and transient ischemic attack.
18-10. Describe an assessment-based approach to stroke and transient ischemic attack.
18-11. Discuss the use of the Cincinnati Prehospital Stroke Scale and the Los Angeles Prehospital Stroke Screen.
18-12. Discuss the role of blood glucose determination in the assessment of patients with altered mental status and neurological deficits.
18-13. Describe ways of communicating with patients who have difficulty speaking.
18-14. Recognize indications that a headache may have a potentially life-threatening underlying cause, such as toxic exposure, hypertension, infectious disease, or hemorrhagic stroke.
18-15. Describe the appropriate emergency medical care for a patient suffering from headache.

KEY TERMS: Page references indicate first major use in this chapter. For complete definitions, see the Glossary at the back of the book.

altered mental status p. 622
coma p. 622
embolic stroke p. 627
hemorrhagic stroke p. 627
ischemic stroke p. 627
neurological deficit p. 626
nontraumatic brain injury p. 626
reticular activating system (RAS) p. 622
stroke p. 626
thrombotic stroke p. 627
transient ischemic attack (TIA) p. 630

MEDIA RESOURCES: Please go to www.bradybooks.com to access mykit for this text. You will find quizzes, critical thinking scenarios, weblinks, animations, and videos related to this chapter—and much more. Look for online information on strokes, stroke prevention, and TIAs.

continued

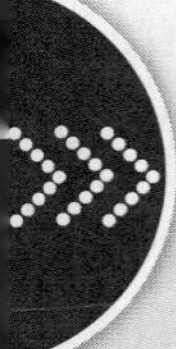

CASE STUDY

The Dispatch

EMS Unit 102—respond to 48 Delason Avenue—you have a 73-year-old female patient who has slurred speech and is unable to move her right arm or leg. Time out is 0840 hours.

Upon Arrival

Upon your arrival you find an elderly woman, who is not alert, lying in bed. Her husband tells you that when she woke up she was "talking funny and slurring her words." Also, he noticed that she was unable to move her right hand, arm, leg, or foot. You also note the smell of urine and feces.

How Would You Proceed to Assess and Care for This Patient?

During this chapter, you will learn about assessment and emergency care for a patient suffering from an altered mental status, stroke, or headache. Later, we will return to the case and apply the procedures learned.

Introduction

It is important for the EMT to recognize that a patient may be having a stroke, provide emergency care, begin rapid transport, and notify the receiving medical facility that the patient is possibly suffering a stroke. Stroke can lead to a compromised airway and inadequate breathing. Early recognition and expeditious transport are vital. You must continuously monitor the airway and breathing and be prepared to intervene.

Headache may be a symptom of an underlying condition or may be a condition in itself. You should consider headache a serious symptom and conduct an assessment looking for an underlying condition as its cause.

Altered Mental Status

In order for a patient to remain in an awake or conscious state, two structures are necessary: an intact reticular activating system and at least one cerebral hemisphere. The **reticular activating system (RAS)** is not an actual structure but a network of nerve cells in the brain stem that constantly transmit environmental and sensory stimuli to and from the cerebrum. If this network is damaged or becomes dysfunctional, the patient will lose consciousness. Similarly, if both cerebral hemispheres are damaged or become dysfunctional, the patient will no longer remain conscious. Thus, in order for the patient to remain in an awake and alert state, the reticular activating system and at least one cerebral hemisphere must be intact.

An **altered mental status** is a significant indication of injury or illness in a patient. The alteration may range from simple disorientation to complete unconsciousness in which the patient is not responsive, even to painful stimuli. An unconscious state where the patient does not respond to painful stimuli is referred to as **coma.** A change in the patient's mental status is an indication that the central nervous system has been affected in some manner. Causes may include trauma, where the brain is injured from a blunt force or penetrating object, or nontraumatic causes such as alterations in the patient's blood sugar level or blood oxygen level.

The cause of an alteration in mental status usually falls into one of two categories: structural or toxic-metabolic. A structural cause of altered mental status results from a space-occupying lesion or depression or from destruction of brain tissue.

Structural Causes of Altered Mental Status

- Brain tumor
- Hemorrhage in the cranium but outside of the brain
- Hemorrhage in the brain tissue
- Direct brain tissue damage from trauma to the brain
- Degenerative disease of the brain
- Brain abscess or infection

Toxic-metabolic causes, as implied by the name, result from circulating toxins or metabolites or from the lack of necessary metabolic substances such as glucose and oxygen.

Toxic-Metabolic Causes of Altered Mental Status

- Severe hypoxia or anoxia (reduced oxygen or no oxygen)
- Abnormal blood glucose conditions (high blood glucose or low blood glucose)

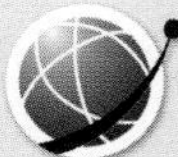

Media Resources
Go to www.bradybooks.com for mykit. Highlights:

- *Web Resource:* Strokes and Stroke Prevention
- *Web Resource:* Brain Tumors

Objective 18-2
List possible causes of altered mental status.

Key Terms

reticular activating system (RAS) nerve cells within the brainstem that control consciousness.

altered mental status a variation from normal function of the mind.

coma an unconscious state in which a person does not respond to any stimulus, including pain.

- Liver failure
- Kidney failure
- Poisoning (e.g., carbon monoxide, cyanide)

There are many other causes of altered mental status that are difficult to fit into one of the categories just listed. These causes may be related to a condition involving drugs, the cardiovascular system, the respiratory system, or infection.

Other Causes of Altered Mental Status

- Shock
- Drugs that depress the central nervous system (e.g., narcotics, alcohol)
- Post seizure (the patient has suffered a seizure and is just beginning to recover)
- Infection
- Cardiac rhythm disturbance
- Stroke

In any patient with an altered mental status, it is vital that you manage any life-threatening injuries or conditions, recognize the mental status change, document it, and continue to monitor the patient for further deterioration.

Assessment-Based Approach: Altered Mental Status

Scene Size-Up

Do a scene size-up to begin to find out why the patient has an altered mental status. Based on the dispatch information and a scan of the scene, determine if the patient has been injured or is suffering from a medical illness. For example, if you arrive on the scene and find an extension ladder next to the house and the patient lying near it, you would immediately expect that the patient has suffered some type of injury from a fall. As you are approaching the patient, inspect the scene for a mechanism of injury that would be significant enough to cause an alteration in mental status. This information may also be gathered from your dispatch information, the patient, relatives, or any bystanders at the scene.

If no mechanism of injury is apparent, you would then suspect that the altered mental status is the result of a medical illness. As you are approaching the patient, look for clues that may indicate the nature of the illness. Alcohol bottles, drug paraphernalia, home oxygen tanks, or chemicals may help explain the cause.

The patient's medications may provide the most valuable information. Have a family member gather the patient's medications while you are performing your assessment. If no family members are present, ask an Emergency Medical Responder or police officer at the scene to look near the kitchen and bathroom sink, kitchen table, and nightstand for both prescription and nonprescription medications. Since insulin, the medication taken to control the blood sugar in diabetes, must be refrigerated, be sure to instruct the individual to look inside the refrigerator. Once the medications have been gathered, they should be kept with the patient. This may provide the emergency department with vital information that would otherwise not be readily available.

If more than one patient at the scene are noted to have an altered mental status, suspect that some type of hazardous gas or poison may be causing the illness. Note any unusual odors. The first priority is to protect yourself so you don't become a patient also. The second priority is to move the patient out of the hazardous environment. If you do not have the proper equipment and training, call for experts to bring the patient out of the danger zone.

Primary Assessment

Stabilize the spine if injury is possible. Pay particular attention to the patient's airway and breathing. Severe alterations in mental status may cause the patient to lose his ability to maintain his own airway. The jaw and tongue become relaxed, fall back, and block the airway. An unresponsive patient commonly has no gag or cough reflex and therefore is unable to keep his airway clear of secretions, blood, and vomitus.

ASSESSMENT Tips

Even though the patient may still have a gag or cough reflex, he may not be able to maintain his own airway if he has an altered mental status. ■

The breathing rate and depth may be inadequate, so be prepared to perform positive pressure ventilation. All patients with altered mental status must initially receive high-concentration oxygen therapy because ensuring an adequate supply of oxygen to the brain is important in

Objective 18-3
Describe an assessment-based approach to altered mental status.

Objective 18-4
Explain the reason for paying particular attention to airway assessment and management in patients with altered mental status.

maintaining or restoring mental function. It is also important to recognize that the poor breathing status or blocked airway may be the cause of the altered mental status as well as the result.

Secondary Assessment

Your partner may take baseline vital signs as you begin gathering information from the patient, relatives, or bystanders regarding the patient's history. It is best to use the patient as the main historian. However, if the patient is disoriented or suffering a severely depressed mental status, he may be unable to provide the necessary answers. During your history, ask the following questions:

- What were the signs and symptoms the patient was complaining of prior to the alteration in the mental status?
- Did the signs and symptoms seem to get progressively worse or better?
- Does the patient have any known allergies?
- What medications, prescription and nonprescription, is the patient taking?
- What is the patient's past medical history? When was the last time he has seen a doctor for his medical condition?
- When did the patient last have something to eat or drink? What did he eat or drink? Did he take any drugs or ingest any alcohol?
- What was the patient doing prior to the onset of the altered mental status?
- Was the onset of signs and symptoms gradual or sudden?
- Did the patient suffer from a seizure, severe headache, or confusion prior to the alteration in the mental status?
- How long has the patient been sick or suffering from these signs and symptoms? When was the patient last well?

If the patient is responsive enough to provide accurate information, collect the history first, followed by the physical examination. Finally, obtain a set of baseline vital signs. If more than one EMT is on the scene, the physical exam can be conducted and baseline vital signs can be obtained by one EMT as the other EMT collects the history. If the patient is unresponsive or is unable to answer history questions appropriately, move directly to the physical examination, collect the baseline vital signs, and then collect the history from any relatives or bystanders at the scene.

The physical exam conducted on a patient with an altered mental status must include examination of the following:

- *Head* for any evidence of possible trauma
- *Pupils* for indications of a head injury (unequal or fixed), drugs (narcotics usually cause pinpoint pupils), hypoxia (sluggish to respond to light)
- *Mouth and oral mucosa* for cyanosis and pallor indicating hypoxia and poor perfusion
- *Chest* for indication of any trauma leading to hypoxia from lung dysfunction
- *Breath sounds* indicating poor gas exchange from injury (pneumothorax) or abnormal breath sounds indicating a possible pulmonary or cardiac condition, for example, crackles (pulmonary edema) or wheezing (asthma attack)
- *Abdomen* for any evidence of intra-abdominal bleeding such as a rigid and tender abdomen (look at the patient's face when palpating the abdomen for grimacing from pain)
- *Lower and upper extremities* for motor and sensory function and pulses
- *Lower extremities* for peripheral edema (may indicate congestive heart failure)
- *Posterior body* for sacral edema (may indicate congestive heart failure)

ASSESSMENT Tips

Narcotics like morphine, heroin, and codeine will typically cause the pupils to constrict and become pinpoint in size. However, the narcotics meperidine (Demerol), propoxyphene (Darvon), pentazocine (Talwin), and some others may not cause the typical constriction of the pupils. ■

The vital signs may also provide clues to the cause of the altered mental status. For example, an extremely rapid heart rate or a very slow heart rate may cause a state of poor perfusion to the brain and lead to an altered mental status. A low blood pressure or an extremely high blood pressure may also provide clues. Altered mental status may result from poor perfusion in a patient with a low blood

Objective 18-5
List signs and symptoms of altered mental status commonly associated with trauma and with nontraumatic or medical conditions.

Objective 18-6
Determine the need for spinal stabilization, airway maintenance, oxygenation, ventilation, positioning, and transport in patients with altered mental status.

pressure, whereas a high blood pressure may be associated with a stroke that is causing the altered mental status. A low pulse oximeter reading may indicate an altered mental status resulting from hypoxia. If a blood glucose monitor (commonly referred to as a glucometer in EMS) is available, check the patient's blood sugar level to determine if a low blood sugar level may be the cause of the altered mental status. (Checking the blood glucose level using a blood glucose monitor will be covered in more detail in Chapter 20, "Acute Diabetic Emergencies.")

Understanding BODY PROCESSES

An extremely fast heart rate, typically greater than 160 beats per minute, may not allow the left ventricle to fill adequately before the next contraction, causing a decrease in blood pressure and brain perfusion. ■

Signs and Symptoms The signs and symptoms associated with an altered mental status will vary depending on the cause, whether from trauma or from a medical cause.

Signs and Symptoms of Altered Mental Status Commonly Associated with Trauma

- Obvious signs of trauma: deformity, contusions, abrasions, punctures or penetrations, burns, tenderness, lacerations, or swelling
- Abnormal respiratory pattern
- Increased or decreased heart rate
- Unequal pupils
- High or low blood pressure
- Discoloration around the eyes (late sign)
- Discoloration behind the ears (late sign)
- Pale, cool, moist skin
- Flexion (decorticate posturing—arms flexed, legs extended) or extension (decerebrate posturing—arms and legs extended)

Signs and Symptoms of Altered Mental Status Commonly Associated with a Nontraumatic or Medical Condition

- Abnormal respiratory pattern
- Dry or moist skin
- Cool or hot skin
- Pinpoint, midsize, dilated, or unequal pupils
- Stiff neck
- Lacerations to the tongue indicating seizure activity
- High systolic blood pressure and low heart rate
- Loss of bowel or bladder control
- Abnormally high or abnormally low blood glucose reading

Emergency Medical Care

If assessment has revealed an injury or set of medical signs and symptoms, perform the appropriate emergency medical care for those specific injuries or medical conditions. In addition, if the patient displays an altered mental status, provide the following care:

1. *Maintain manual spinal stabilization* if trauma is suspected.
2. *Maintain a patent airway.* A patient with an altered mental status may not be able to maintain his own airway. If this is the case, insert a nasopharyngeal or oropharyngeal airway adjunct to help keep the patient's airway open.
3. *Suction any secretions, vomitus, or blood.* Closely monitor the airway by frequently inspecting inside the mouth and suctioning any secretions, blood, or vomitus.
4. *Maintain oxygen therapy.* It is extremely important that the patient continuously receive a concentration of oxygen to maintain his SpO_2 reading above 95% and to eliminate any signs of hypoxia. If there is any question as to how much oxygen to administer, it is better to err to benefit the patient and provide oxygen via a nonrebreather mask at 15 lpm. If the patient continues to breathe adequately, continue oxygen therapy and guide it based on the SpO_2 and signs of hypoxia. A sign of severe hypoxia may be an altered mental status; thus, it may be prudent to maintain oxygen administration via a nonrebreather mask at 15 lpm. If the ventilations are being assisted, make sure the device used to ventilate the patient is properly connected to oxygen.
5. *Be prepared to assist ventilation.* Continuously assess the breathing status. If the breathing rate or depth becomes inadequate, immediately begin positive pressure ventilation with supplemental oxygen connected to the ventilation device.

Key Points
If no mechanism of injury is apparent, suspect that the altered mental status is the result of a medical illness.

Key Terms
neurological deficit any deficiency in the nervous system's functioning.

Key Terms
nontraumatic brain injury a medical injury to the brain, such as stroke, that is not caused by external trauma.

stroke a sudden disruption in blood flow to the brain that results in brain cell damage.

6. *Position the patient.* Patients with an altered mental status should be placed in a lateral recumbent (recovery) position to avoid possible aspiration. If spinal injury is suspected, the patient must be fully immobilized on a long spine board. The spine board and patient may then be rotated as a unit to place the patient on his side if necessary to clear the airway. If the altered mental status patient requires ventilation, do not place him in a lateral recumbent position. It will not be possible to effectively establish and maintain an adequate mask seal and perform bag-valve-mask ventilation with the patient in a lateral position. Place the patient needing ventilation in a supine position and be sure to have suction readily available.
7. *Transport.* Any patient with an altered mental status must be transported to a medical facility for further evaluation. Consider ALS intercept according to local protocols.

Reassessment

Continuously monitor for changes in the patient's mental status, airway, breathing, and circulation. Record the vital signs and communicate your findings to the receiving medical facility. For a patient with an altered mental status, repeat the reassessment every 5 minutes.

Stroke

Neurological Deficit Resulting from Stroke

The ability to be alert and aware of your surroundings, to speak, to feel sensations, and to move are all functions of the brain and nervous system. When the patient loses some or all of these abilities, he is experiencing a **neurological deficit.** A neurological deficit is defined as any deficiency in the functioning of the brain or nervous system. Altered mental status, slurred or absent speech, paralysis, weakness, and numbness are all signs and symptoms of neurological deficit.

A neurological deficit will alert you to the possibility of a condition that is affecting the patient's central nervous system, which is composed of the brain and spinal cord. Thus, you must look for signs and symptoms of both traumatic and medical conditions that may be affecting the brain or the spinal cord. For instance, someone whose spinal cord or brain has been injured by a bullet and someone who has suffered a stroke may both lose the ability to feel sensation or the ability to move the arms or legs. In Chapter 31, "Head Trauma," and Chapter 32, "Spinal Column and Spinal Cord Trauma," you will learn how to assess and care for patients with head and spinal cord injuries caused by trauma (such as from a penetrating wound or a fall). In this chapter, we are primarily concerned with care for the patient with a **nontraumatic brain injury,** or a **stroke,** which is a medical injury to the brain that is not related to trauma.

Acute Stroke

According to the American Heart Association, the third leading cause of death in the adult population is stroke. Approximately 700,000 people each year will suffer a stroke for the first time, or a person with a history of a stroke will suffer another stroke. Of those patients, approximately 158,000 will die as a consequence of the stroke.

Time is a critical factor in the emergency care of stroke. Therefore, emergency medical services play a major role in the management of the stroke patient. One of the most significant factors that make a difference in the care and prognosis of the patient is early recognition of the stroke. Early recognition of a stroke leads to early transport and treatment in the emergency department.

Drugs and mechanical devices are now available that may be used on certain stroke patients to reduce or even reverse the consequences of the stroke by breaking up the clot causing the obstruction. These drugs must be administered within 3 hours from the first sign or symptom of the onset of the stroke. The patient must be delivered to the emergency department at least within 2 hours from the onset of the signs and symptoms of the stroke to allow the emergency department personnel enough time to collect the necessary information to make a decision whether to administer the drugs to destroy the clot causing the stroke. Other therapies to reverse stroke, typically available at specialized centers, can extend the window of opportunity to 6 hours.

ASSESSMENT Tips

The time of onset of a stroke is commonly defined as the last time the patient was seen neurologically intact, meaning without any neurological deficit such as numbness, weakness, paralysis, slurred or stuttering speech, or cognitive problems. ■

Objective 18-7
Explain the responsibilities of the general public and EMS in the care for a stroke patient.

Objective 18-8
Describe the pathophysiology of stroke and distinguish between ischemic strokes and hemorrhagic strokes.

Key Terms

ischemic stroke a stroke caused by obstruction to a vessel in the brain, called a **thrombotic stroke** if caused by a clot or an **embolic stroke** if caused by plaque or other material carried to the brain.

hemorrhagic stroke a stroke caused by rupture of a blood vessel in the brain.

For this reason, the patient or a relative or bystander must recognize signs and symptoms of a stroke and immediately call 911 or call the number to access the emergency medical services. Once emergency medical services arrive at the scene, they must also immediately recognize the signs and symptoms of stroke, assess the patient, provide initial emergency medical care, prepare the patient for rapid transport, and notify the receiving medical facility of transport of a possible stroke patient.

ASSESSMENT Tips

Some stroke patients may exhibit very subtle signs or symptoms at the onset of the stroke, such as simple numbness or tingling in the hand, confusion, stuttering or trouble speaking, dizziness, loss of balance, or difficulty understanding. These are vital to recognize as possible indicators of stroke. ■

The American Heart Association has identified seven "Ds" to describe the best care for the stroke patient. The seven Ds, which address the issue of time as a critical factor in reducing permanent disability and death in the stroke patient, are Detection, Dispatch, Delivery, Door, Data, Decision, and Drug. The first three are the responsibility of the general public and emergency medical services. Detection is the recognition of the signs and symptoms of a stroke either by the patient, a relative at the scene, a bystander, or Emergency Medical Responders. Dispatch is responsible for recognizing the signs and symptoms described by the caller as a possible stroke and prioritizing the call as an emergency. Delivery involves the prompt assessment, emergency care, and transport of the stroke patient. The last four "Ds" deal with the emergency care of the patient in the emergency department, including administration of drugs to break apart the clot causing the stroke.

Pathophysiology of Stroke

Stroke was formerly known as a cerebrovascular accident or CVA. A stroke is similar to a heart attack (myocardial infarction). It is due to an inadequate amount of blood being delivered to a portion of the brain caused by a blood clot obstructing a blood vessel in the brain. Thus, the stroke is often described as a "brain attack," to imply the same general cause and the same level of seriousness as a heart attack. The difference between a stroke and heart attack is the location of the vessel that is occluded by the clot. In a heart attack, a coronary artery is occluded; in a stroke, a cerebral (brain) artery is occluded. Atherosclerosis is usually a contributing factor to clot formation and narrowing of the cerebral arteries.

Types of Stroke

A stroke is caused by interruption of blood flow to the brain. This occurs either by blockage of an artery that is carrying blood to a specific area within the brain or from bleeding within the brain resulting from a ruptured cerebral artery. The blockage is referred to as an **ischemic stroke** and the bleeding is referred to as a **hemorrhagic stroke** (Figures 18-1a and 18-1b*).

Ischemic Strokes

Ischemic strokes occur when the cerebral artery is blocked by a clot or other foreign matter. A clot that develops at the site of occlusion is called a *thrombus*, and the process of clot formation is referred to as *thrombosis*. A stroke resulting from thrombus formation is called a **thrombotic stroke.** A clot or other matter that has traveled from another area of the body is called an *embolus*. When the embolus lodges in a cerebral artery and occludes it, it is known as a *cerebral embolism* and results in an **embolic stroke.**

Thrombosis As the body ages, it is common for plaque deposits to form on the inner wall of arteries and cause them to narrow, reducing the amount of blood they can carry. This process is called atherosclerosis, and the narrowed portions of the arteries are common sites for blood clot formation. Hypertension can also wear away the smooth inner lining of the artery, leaving rough areas. These areas are likely to develop plaque and are also common sites for clot or thrombus formation. When a thrombus forms inside an artery, it can completely block the flow of blood through that artery to the brain. This results in the death of brain tissue, which is a stroke.

Because the narrowing and eventual occlusion of the artery occurs over a longer period of time than an embolic-type occlusion, the onset of signs and symptoms of a thrombotic-type stroke is much slower. This is the most common type of stroke. Severe headache is not a common symptom in a thrombotic stroke.

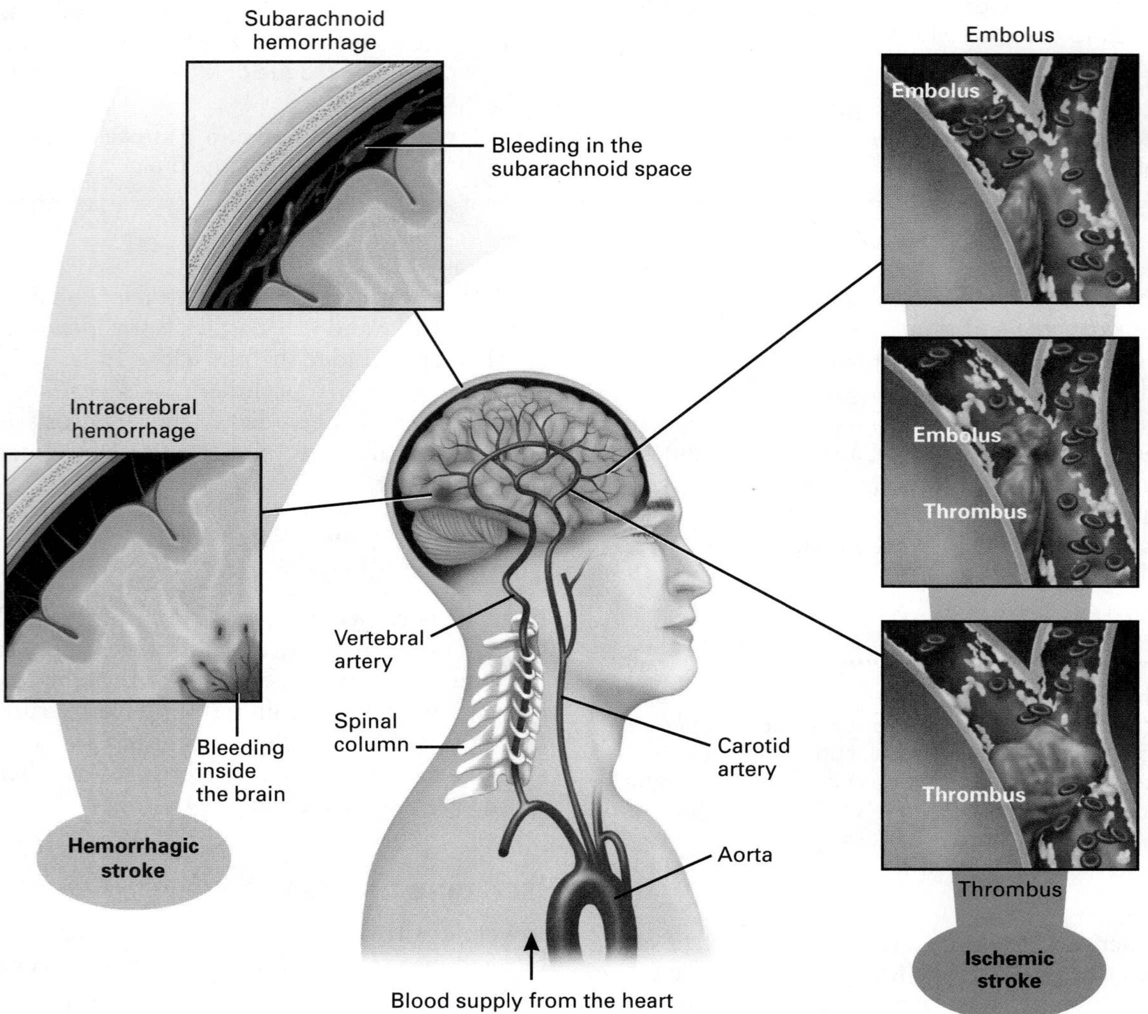

FIGURE 18-1a ✻ **Causes of Stroke** Blood is carried from the heart to the brain via the carotid and vertebral arteries, which form a ring and branches within the brain. A *hemorrhagic stroke* occurs when a cerebral artery ruptures and bleeds into the brain (examples shown: subarachnoid bleeding on the surface of the brain; intracerebral bleeding within the brain). An *ischemic stroke* occurs when a thrombus is formed on the wall of an artery or when an embolus travels from another area until it lodges in and blocks an arterial branch.

Embolism In the stroke patient, an embolus usually originates from the carotid artery in the neck or from the heart. The clot travels until it becomes lodged in a small artery in the brain, blocking blood flow. The brain tissue beyond the point of blockage then begins to die from a lack of oxygen and nutrients. The embolus causing brain tissue death is most often made of clotted blood but may consist of air bubbles, tumor fragments, or fat particles.

Understanding BODY PROCESSES

Atrial fibrillation, an irregularly irregular heart rhythm, is a common risk factor for stroke. The atrial fibrillation itself is not a lethal rhythm and is a common chronic rhythm in the elderly. ■

An embolic-type stroke occurs most often when the patient is awake and active. The onset of signs and symptoms is usually much more sudden than in a thrombotic stroke, and headache, seizure activity, or brief periods of unresponsiveness are more common.

Hemorrhagic Strokes

A hemorrhagic stroke results from the rupture of an artery that causes bleeding within the brain (intracerebral) or in the space around the outer surface of the brain (subarachnoid space). People with hypertension (high blood pressure) are likely candidates for hemorrhagic stroke since ruptures are most likely to occur in arteries that have been damaged by hypertension. The constant high pressure wears away the inner surface of the artery and weakens it, leading to rupture and hemorrhage. An aneurysm, which is a weakened and dilated area within an artery wall, is a common cause of subarachnoid hemorrhages. The weakened area may be a congenital defect that has been present since birth. This is a common cause of strokes in younger, healthy adults.

Key Points
Any patient with sudden onset of headache must be considered serious.

Objective 18-9
Describe the relationship between stroke and transient ischemic attack.

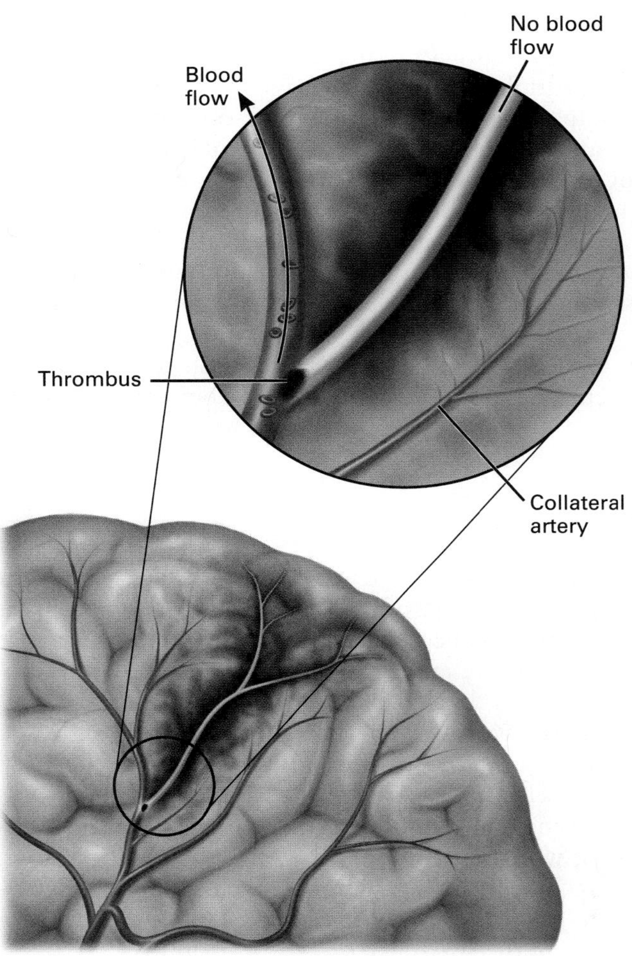

FIGURE 18-1b * Ischemia, Infarction, and Collateral Flow Brain tissues distal to a rupture, thrombus, or embolus receive little or no perfusion and become ischemic (starved of oxygen) and eventually infarcted (dead). When a thrombus grows slowly enough, collateral arteries may form parallel to the blocked artery to perfuse or partially perfuse the oxygen-starved area of the brain.

The onset of signs and symptoms associated with a hemorrhagic stroke is usually very sudden and often occurs during physical activity. Headache is a common and often severe symptom. The patient commonly complains, "This is the worst headache I have ever had." The patient frequently presents with an altered mental status that rapidly deteriorates. Seizures and stiff neck are also common. An atypical picture without mental deterioration is also possible. Hence, any patient with sudden onset of headache must be considered serious.

Understanding BODY PROCESSES

Chronic hypertension (HTN), which is high blood pressure, is a common risk factor for hemorrhagic strokes. ■

It is difficult to distinguish between the two types of stroke—ischemic and hemorrhagic—in the field, because they may present with similar signs and symptoms. However, it is extremely important to collect an accurate history and gather information in the physical exam to pass on to the emergency department, because the information may help the emergency department staff to determine which type of stroke it is. Distinguishing between the types of stroke is critical in the continued care of the patient. The primary difference is that the patient suffering from an ischemic stroke can receive the drug, a fibrinolytic, to break up the clot and restore perfusion to the area of the brain that was not receiving an adequate supply of blood. A hemorrhagic stroke patient cannot receive a fibrinolytic drug because it may increase the amount of bleeding within the brain, worsen the stroke, and possibly lead to the patient's death.

Your role as an EMT is to provide supportive care to the patient by managing any immediate life threats and by collecting the most accurate information possible to report to the emergency department. Your purpose in collecting the information is not to distinguish between the types of stroke but to report it accurately to the emergency department staff. The information you gather at the scene is critical to care of the patient in the emergency department.

Even though you, as an EMT, will not need to determine the type of stroke, it is still important to understand the different types and causes of stroke.

Stroke or Transient Ischemic Attack

Strokes most often affect the elderly who have a history of atherosclerosis (fat deposits in the arteries), heart disease, or hypertension (high blood pressure). According to the American Heart Association Council on Stroke, the most likely candidate for stroke has high blood pressure and a history of brief, intermittent strokelike episodes called transient ischemic attacks (TIAs), which we will discuss in the next section.

The signs and symptoms of stroke are associated with the specific area of the brain that has been affected by a

Key Points
Stroke most commonly involves areas of the brain that control speech, sensation, and muscle function.

Key Terms
transient ischemic attack (TIA) brief, intermittent episode with strokelike symptoms that disappear within 24 hours. TIAs are caused by an oxygen deficit in the brain tissue (ischemia) and are often a precursor to a stroke.

disruption in the blood flow. Most commonly, it involves the areas that control speech, sensation, and muscle function. The onset of the signs and symptoms is usually sudden and may be accompanied by a seizure, headache, or the inability to swallow (dysphagia). The patient may also experience difficulty in breathing (dyspnea).

Paralysis is a common sign in the stroke patient. Another common sign is facial droop, in which there is a loss of facial expression on one side and the facial features droop downward. Typically, the paralysis will affect one extremity (monoplegia) or both extremities on one side of the body (hemiplegia) (Figure 18-2*). Because the nerves on one side of the brain cross over at the level of the medulla (at around the level of the upper lip) and control the movement and sensation on the other side of the body, the damage is usually noticeable on the side opposite the affected area. Therefore, if the stroke occurs on the left side of the brain, the damage is noticeable on the right side of the body; if the stroke occurs on the right side of the brain, the damage is evident on the left side of the body.

It is rare that paralysis from a stroke affects both extremities on both sides of the body. Usually, the face will be paralyzed on one side and the extremities will be weak or paralyzed on the opposite side. The pattern of paralysis is one factor that will help you distinguish stroke from a spinal injury, which, unlike stroke, will frequently cause paralysis to both legs (paraplegia) or to all four extremities (quadriplegia).

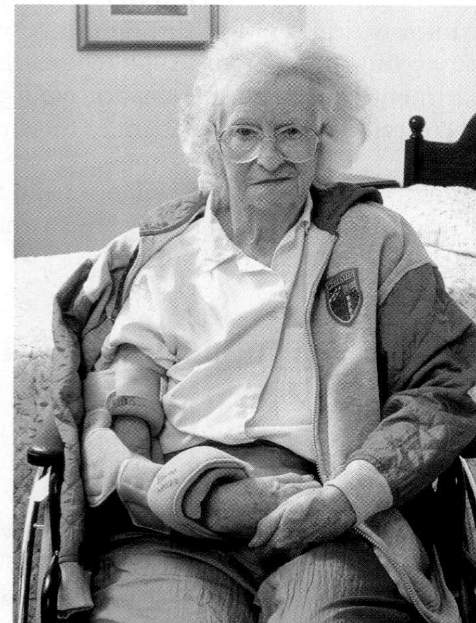

FIGURE 18-2 * The stroke patient will often suffer paralysis affecting the face and extremities on one side of the body.

Some stroke patients experience only weakness in the arms and legs and not paralysis. Carefully monitor the patient because the weakness may progress to complete paralysis.

In stroke patients, alterations in mental status commonly range from alertness to simple confusion or dizziness to complete unresponsiveness. The speech of the patient may be slurred (dysphasia) or completely absent (aphasia). Stroke patients may also speak clearly, uttering nonsensical words (fluent aphasia). The patient may experience double or blurred vision, loss of vision in one eye, or loss of a visual field.

Transient Ischemic Attack

Patients who experience a **transient ischemic attack (TIA)** develop most of the same signs and symptoms as those who are experiencing a stroke. The key difference between a stroke and a TIA is that the signs and symptoms of a TIA disappear typically within 10–15 minutes but almost always within 1 hour of the onset of signs and symptoms. It is unusual for them to last longer than 30 minutes. The TIA always resolves within 24 hours without causing any permanent neurological disability. Ischemia, which refers to an oxygen deficit in the tissues, affects the brain and causes the strokelike signs and symptoms to appear. Reversal of the ischemia leads to disappearance of the strokelike signs and symptoms.

Understanding BODY PROCESSES

A TIA that lasts longer than 10 to 15 minutes is usually a small stroke, not truly a TIA. ■

For example, you arrive on the scene and find a 70-year-old male patient who responds only to verbal stimuli, has right-sided facial droopiness, has slurred speech, and has paralysis to the right arm and leg. You assess the patient and begin your emergency care. By the time you have loaded the patient into the ambulance, 10 minutes have passed. The patient is now alert, able to move his right extremities, and speaking much more clearly, but he still complains of weakness to the right side of his body. When you arrive at the emergency department 13 minutes later, the patient has completely normal motor and

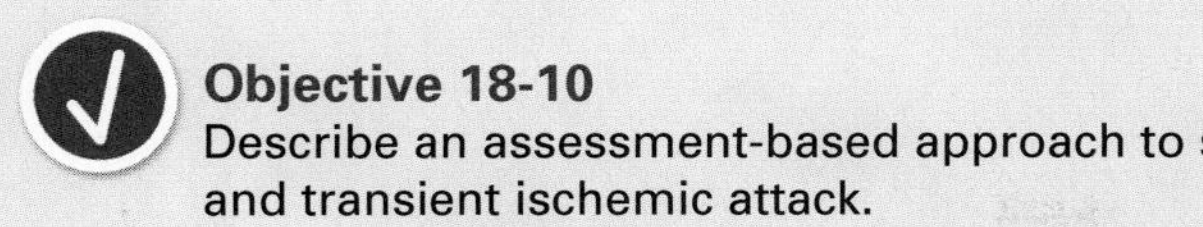

Objective 18-10
Describe an assessment-based approach to stroke and transient ischemic attack.

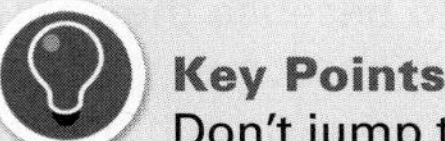

Key Points
Don't jump to conclusions if the patient does not respond to painful stimulus. He may feel it but be unable to move in response to the pain.

sensory function in all extremities and is speaking without any difficulty. The patient has no apparent signs and complains of nothing. In fact, clear documentation by the EMT of the symptoms that prompted the call to EMS may be the only reliable clue to the diagnosis.

This would be typical of a TIA. In contrast, the stroke patient's signs and symptoms would have not disappeared and might have worsened. You should realize that the patient who is experiencing a TIA will be just as frightened as one who is experiencing a stroke. Maintain a reassuring, optimistic, and hopeful attitude in caring for patients with TIA.

TIAs are important to recognize and report. Although this incident is frightening for patients, some may refuse emergency care and transportation to a medical facility because the signs and symptoms disappear. However, almost a third of those who suffer a TIA will eventually have a stroke, and many of those patients will suffer the stroke within a month after the TIA. Therefore, you must encourage the patient to seek further examination and medical care.

The emergency care for the patient suffering a TIA is the same as that discussed later in the chapter for the patient who displays signs and symptoms of a stroke.

Assessment-Based Approach: Stroke and Transient Ischemic Attack

Scene Size-Up

The dispatch information or someone on the scene may alert you to the patient's neurological deficit or altered mental status: sudden weakness of the face, hand, arm, or leg; trouble speaking or stuttering; difficulty seeing in one or both eyes; problem walking or a loss of balance or coordination; confusion; dizziness; or a sudden onset of a severe headache. As you arrive, scan the scene to try to determine whether the neurological deficit is due to trauma or to a medical condition. Look for any signs that would make you suspect that the patient's head or spine has been injured. Scan the scene for alcohol, drugs or drug paraphernalia, and prescription or illegal drugs, which are other possible causes of altered function. Specifically, look for evidence of amphetamines, cocaine, and other stimulants since they are related to nontraumatic brain injury in young adults.

Note where the patient is found and how he is dressed. Many strokes occur at night and the patient awakens with the neurological deficit. You would expect that a patient who is found in bed or wearing nightclothes is more likely to be suffering from a stroke than from a traumatic brain injury. Another clue that the patient has suffered a stroke is a bucket or ice pack next to or near the patient. This could be considered evidence that the patient has experienced nausea, vomiting, or headache, common complaints of many patients with stroke.

Primary Assessment

Immediately inspect the patient's airway and suction any vomitus and secretions. If spinal injury is not suspected, place the patient in a lateral recumbent (recovery or coma) position. If spinal injury is suspected, perform a jaw-thrust maneuver to open the airway and provide manual in-line stabilization with the patient in a supine position. A patient with an altered neurological status may not be able to control his own airway. If the muscles supporting the tongue relax or become paralyzed, the support to both the tongue and epiglottis is lost. The tongue will fall back and occlude the pharynx. The epiglottis will flap forward and partially or completely block the airway at the level of the larynx. The gag reflex may be lost. In the instance of an acute stroke, the muscles of the throat may also be paralyzed. This would prevent the patient from swallowing adequately and could lead to aspiration of secretions.

Insert an oropharyngeal or nasopharyngeal airway if needed. Because the brain controls breathing rate and depth, it is possible to find inadequate breathing or unusual breathing patterns in the stroke patient. If the patient requires ventilation, place the patient in a supine position and begin positive pressure ventilation with supplemental oxygen connected to the device.

In the patient with a neurological deficit, you should not jump to conclusions when assessing the patient's responsiveness. For instance, if you pinch the patient's right hand and he does not respond, you can't assume that he is unable to feel pain or sensation. He may be paralyzed on the right side; that is, he may be able to feel pain but be unable to move in response to the pain. Confirm the finding in another extremity.

Secondary Assessment

Any patient presenting with a sudden weakness of the face, hand, arm, or leg; trouble speaking or stuttering; difficulty seeing in one or both eyes; problem walking or a loss of

Key Points
It is difficult to distinguish between ischemic and hemorrhagic strokes in the field because they may present with similar signs and symptoms. However, it is important to gather information from the history and physical exam to pass on to the emergency department.

balance or coordination; confusion; dizziness; or a sudden onset of a severe headache should be suspected of having suffered a stroke. Some information specific to stroke that can be collected in the physical exam is important to note and report to the emergency department. If the patient is unresponsive, you will perform a physical exam and obtain baseline vital signs before obtaining the history. If the patient is responsive, you will take the history before performing the physical exam and obtaining vitals. Regardless of whether you start with the history or with the physical exam, keep in mind that paralysis or a loss of speech is very frightening to the patient. You must remain calm and confident and continuously reassure the patient.

The physical exam will be a rapid head-to-toe assessment. Any patient with loss of motor or sensory function, speech difficulties, or an altered mental status may be suffering from a head injury. Carefully inspect and palpate the head to determine if there is any evidence of trauma. If evidence of trauma exists, a head injury may be the reason for the neurological deficits being experienced by the patient. However, the patient may have experienced the neurological deficit first, causing him to fall, resulting in an injury to the head. Always have a high index of suspicion and report all your findings, including the scene characteristics.

Inspect the face for a drooped appearance on one side by instructing the patient to look up and smile or show his teeth (see information on the Cincinnati and Los Angeles stroke screens, later). An abnormal finding would be a drooped appearance where one side does not move symmetrically or as well as the other (Figures 18-3a and 18-3b*).

Listen for garbled sounds or slurring when the patient speaks. Have the patient say the following phrase to assess his speech capability: "You can't teach an old dog new tricks." An abnormal finding would be if the patient said the wrong words, slurred words, was not able to say the phrase at all, uttered a completely unrelated phrase, or didn't understand your directions.

Note the patient's ability to obey your commands such as to repeat a phrase or to "Squeeze my fingers" or to "Wiggle your toes." If the patient does not obey all of the commands, it is likely the stroke has affected his thought process and he does not understand what you are asking him to do. If he obeys only certain commands, he may be unable to obey the others because of a neurological deficit such as paralysis to one side of the body.

If you find the patient walking, note his movement and the manner in which he is walking. An abnormality such as unsteadiness can indicate a neurological deficit.

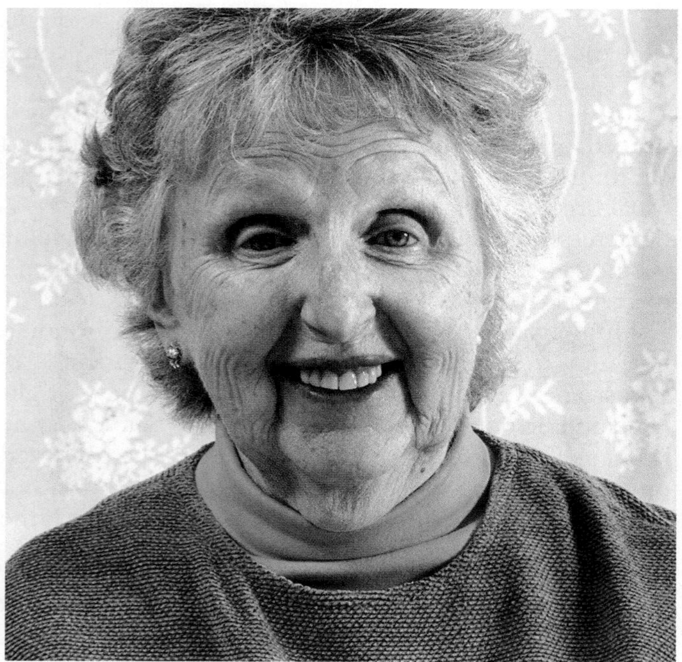

(a)

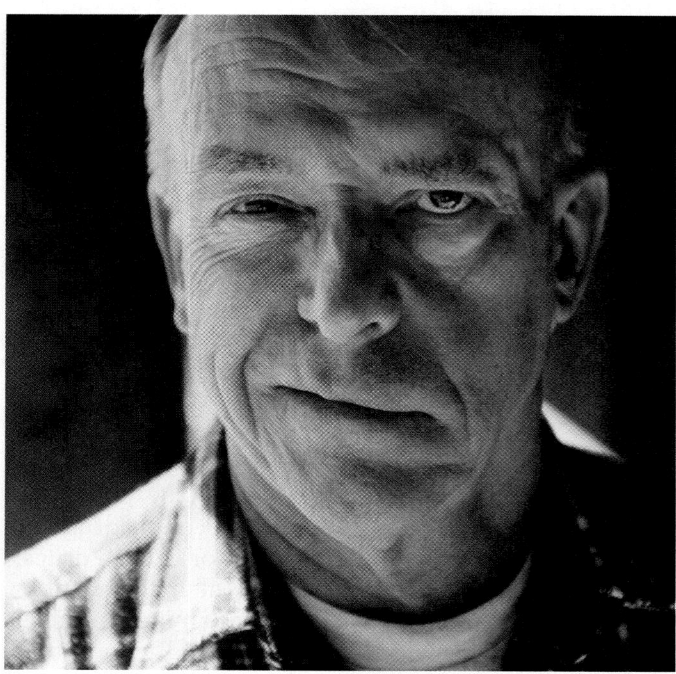

(b)

FIGURE 18-3 * **(a)** The face of a nonstroke patient has normal symmetry. **(b)** The face of a stroke patient often has an abnormal, drooped appearance on one side. (© Michal Heron)

Thinking Critically
In contrast to strokes, TIAs get better by themselves. So why should you and the patient take a TIA seriously?

Objective 18-11
Explain the Cincinnati Prehospital Stroke Scale and Los Angeles Prehospital Stroke Screen.

Key Points
Facial droop, arm drift, slurred words, weak grip—any *one* of these physical exam findings is strongly suggestive of a stroke.

When assessing the extremities, you may find a reduction in the sensory and motor function on one side of the body. The patient may lack the ability to feel your touch or to feel pain and may display weakness or paralysis. Check the grip strength in the upper extremities by having the patient grasp and squeeze your fingers. Have the patient push and pull up against your hands with his feet to assess for equality of strength in the lower extremities. Note any differences in strength between the right and left sides and the upper and lower extremities. Assess for arm drift (Figures 18-4a and 18-4b*) by instructing the patient to extend his arms, palms up, with eyes closed for 10 seconds. Note a downward drift or drop of one extremity.

When performing a neurological examination on a responsive patient who presents with any suspected signs or symptoms of stroke, you should use one of the validated stroke screening evaluation tools, either the Cincinnati Prehospital Stroke Scale or the Los Angeles Prehospital Stroke Screen (LAPSS).

The Cincinnati Prehospital Stroke Scale (Figure 18-5*) tests for (1) facial droop by having the patient show his teeth or make a smile; (2) arm drift by having the patient close his eyes and hold both arms straight out in front of him for 10 seconds; and (3) abnormal speech pattern and muscle paralysis by having the patient say, "You can't teach an old dog new tricks."

The LAPSS takes into consideration other possible causes of altered mental status, such as hypoglycemia, hyperglycemia, or seizures, and also requires a physical test of asymmetry (unequal amount) of strength. The information gathered in the LAPSS (Figure 18-6*) is (1) age greater than 45 years, (2) history of seizures or epilepsy, (3) duration of symptoms, (4) wheelchair or bedridden status of patient, and (5) blood glucose level. Asymmetry of strength is assessed by testing facial smile or grimace, grip, and arm strength.

Both screening tools are highly sensitive and specific. Any one abnormality in the physical tests of either CPSS or LAPSS is highly suggestive of stroke. According to the 2010 American Heart Association guidelines, the presence of a single abnormal finding on the CPSS has a sensitivity of 59 percent and a specificity of 89 percent when scored by prehospital care providers. Similarly, 93 percent of the patients who have suffered an acute stroke will respond *yes* or *unknown* with findings on the LAPSS, and 97 percent of the patients who present with positive findings on the LAPSS will have suffered an acute stroke. It is important to perform one of these evaluations on any patient suspected of having a stroke.

Any one of the following physical exam findings is strongly suggestive of a stroke:

- There is facial droop of one side of the face when the patient is asked to smile or show his teeth.

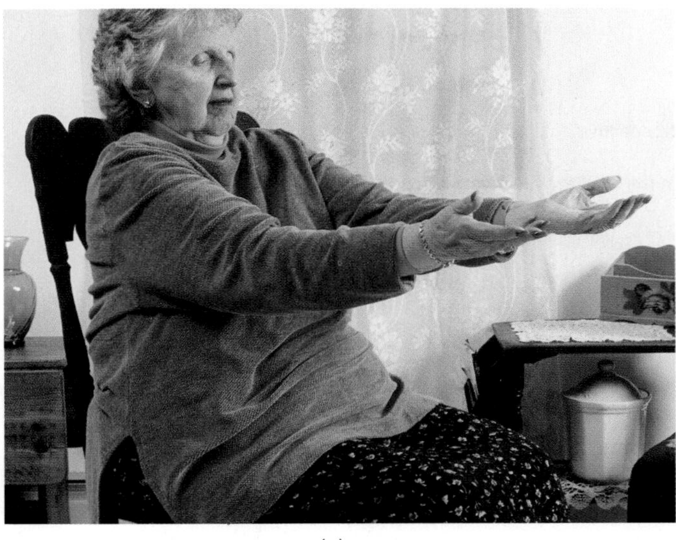

(a)

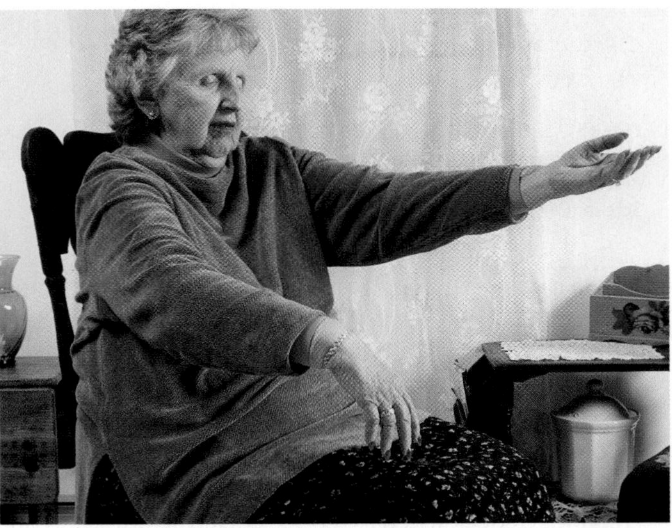

(b)

FIGURE 18-4 * **(a)** A patient who has not suffered a stroke can generally hold arms in an extended position with eyes closed. **(b)** A stroke patient will often display "arm drift" or "pronator drift"; that is, one arm will remain extended, when held outward with eyes closed, but the other arm will drift or drop downward and pronate (turn palm downward).

Cincinnati Prehospital Stroke Scale

Sign of Stroke	Patient Activity	Interpretation
Facial droop	Have patient look up at you, smile, and show his teeth.	*Normal:* Symmetry to both sides. *Abnormal:* One side of the face droops or does not move symmetrically.
Arm drift	Have patient lift arms up and hold them out with eyes closed for 10 seconds.	*Normal:* Symmetrical movement in both arms. *Abnormal:* One arm drifts down or asymmetrical movement of the arms.
Abnormal speech	Have the patient say, "You can't teach an old dog new tricks."	*Normal:* The correct words are used and no slurring of words is noted. *Abnormal:* The words are slurred, the wrong words are used, or the patient is aphasic.

Kothari R. U., Pancioli A., Liu T., Broderick J. Cincinnati Prehospital Stroke Scale: Reproducibility and validity. *Annals of Emergency Medicine.* 1999; 33:373–378.

FIGURE 18-5 ✻ The Cincinnati Prehospital Stroke Scale.

Los Angeles Prehospital Stroke Screen (LAPSS)

Considerations	Yes	Unknown	No
Age **greater than** 45 years			
No history of seizures or epilepsy			
Duration of symptoms is **less** than 24 hours			
Patient is **not** wheelchair bound or bedridden			
Blood glucose level **between 60 and 400 mg/dL**			
Physical exam to determine unilateral asymmetry	**Equal**	**R Weakness**	**L Weakness**
A. Have patient look up, smile, and show teeth		Droop	Droop
B. Compare grip strength of upper extremities		Weak grip	Weak grip
		No grip	No grip
C. Assess arm strength for drift or weakness		Drifts down	Drifts down
		Falls rapidly	Falls rapidly

Kidwell C. S., Saver J. L., Schubert G. B., Eckstein M., Starkman S. Design and retrospective analysis of the Los Angeles Prehospital Stroke Screen (LAPSS). *Prehospital Emergency Care.* 1998;2:267–273.

Kidwell C. S., Starkman S., Eckstein M., Weems K., Saver J. L. Identifying stroke in the field: Prospective validation of the Los Angeles Prehospital Stroke Screen (LAPSS). *Stroke.* 2000; 31:71–76.

FIGURE 18-6 ✻ The Los Angeles Prehospital Stroke Screen (LAPSS).

- One arm does not move or one arm drifts downward when the patient's arms are extended outward for 10 seconds with his eyes closed.
- The patient slurs his words, uses wrong words, or is unable to speak when asked to repeat the phrase "You can't teach an old dog new tricks."
- There is weak or no grip on one side of the body when asked to squeeze your fingers.

When assessing the baseline vital signs, pay attention to the systolic and diastolic blood pressure. Carefully document both readings and repeat every 5 minutes. Hypertension (high blood pressure) may have actually caused the nontraumatic brain injury or may be a sign of increased pressure within the skull. Unequal pupils or abnormal eye movements or gaze are also significant signs of a possible brain injury (either traumatic or nontraumatic).

Objective 18-12
Discuss the role of blood glucose determination in the assessment of patients with altered mental status and neurological deficits.

Objective 18-13
Describe ways of communicating with patients who have difficulty speaking.

Hypoglycemia can sometimes produce signs and symptoms very similar to those of stroke, especially in the elderly. Some hypoglycemic patients may present with confusion and neurological deficits that appear to be due to a stroke. The patient may not have a major alteration in his mental status. If your protocol permits, check the blood glucose level of any patient who presents with an altered mental status or neurological deficits. A patient who has just suffered a seizure may also present with neurological deficits. These deficits, including paralysis, may last up to several hours after the seizure. A good history may provide key information indicating that the paralysis is due to a seizure and not a stroke. However, also keep in mind that strokes may cause seizures.

ASSESSMENT Tips

Some signs and symptoms of stroke are also common to other conditions. The condition that is most commonly misdiagnosed as stroke is hypoglycemia. If possible, assess the blood glucose level in the patient exhibiting signs and symptoms of stroke. ■

During your history, look for medical alert tags, collect the patient's prescription and nonprescription medications, and don't forget to look in the refrigerator for a vial of insulin, used to treat diabetes. Remember that diabetics may be hypoglycemic, and patients who are hypoglycemic may show signs and symptoms similar to those of a stroke patient, especially if the patient is elderly.

Try to gain as much information from the patient as possible. If the speech center of the brain has been affected, the patient may be unable to talk. Yet, don't assume that the patient cannot understand. Determine if the patient can respond to your commands by asking him to blink his eyes or squeeze your finger if he understands. If he is able to understand and make some type of gesture or motion, you can still obtain a history from the patient with the use of questions that can be answered "yes" and "no." For example, you may instruct the patient to blink his eyes twice for yes and once for no. Answers to the following questions will guide you in your emergency care of the patient:

- **When did the symptoms begin?** This is crucial in establishing the time of onset of the stroke. Try to gather from relatives or bystanders when the first sign or symptom appeared. Since the drugs used to dissolve the clot are typically administered within 3 hours of the onset of the stroke, passing this information on to the hospital is critical. The hospital staff can then gauge how much time has expired and the course of treatment. Time is very precious and the transport must occur rapidly to a medical facility that can manage a stroke patient.
- **Is there any recent history of trauma to the head?** Although you may have ruled out trauma while sizing up the scene, it is important to note if the patient has suffered a head injury within the last few weeks.
- **Does the patient have a history of previous stroke?** For instance, the patient may have already lost speech, sensory, or motor function from a previous stroke. In this case the present neurological deficit may be either the result of another stroke or related to some cause other than a stroke or nontraumatic brain injury.
- **Was there any seizure activity noted prior to your arrival?** If so, you should be prepared for the patient to experience a seizure again. (Seizures will be covered in Chapter 19, "Seizures and Syncope.")
- **What was the patient doing at the time of onset of the signs and symptoms?** The activity or lack of activity may point to a traumatic or nontraumatic cause.
- **Does the patient have a history of diabetes?** (Diabetes will be covered in Chapter 20, "Acute Diabetic Emergencies.")
- **Has the patient complained of a headache? A stiff neck?** When collecting the history, it is especially important to note if the patient complained of a headache prior to becoming unresponsive or if the patient is currently complaining of a headache. Ask and document if the patient at any time states, "This is the worst headache I've ever had in my life," or something similar. This is consistent with strokes caused by bleeding in or around the brain.
- **Has the patient complained of dizziness, nausea, vomiting, or weakness?**
- **Has the patient experienced any slurred speech?**

The following questions will provide useful information to the hospital personnel who will be receiving the patient. If the patient's mental status is deteriorating, the hospital staff may be unable to get this information later and will need to rely on the information you are able to obtain.

- Does the patient take any oral anticoagulant drugs?
- Does the patient have a history of hypertension (high blood pressure)?

- Has the patient taken amphetamines, cocaine, or some other stimulant drug?
- Was the onset of signs and symptoms gradual or sudden?
- Did the signs and symptoms get progressively worse or better?
- Did the paralysis or weakness affect one part of the body first and then progress to other areas?
- Does the patient have a history of atrial fibrillation or irregular heartbeat?

Signs and Symptoms The patient can have a wide range of signs and symptoms depending on the extent and location of the stroke. As noted earlier, the three most common findings are facial droop, arm drift, and speech disturbances. Others include (Figure 18-7∗):

- Altered mental status ranging from dizziness or sudden confusion to complete unresponsiveness
- Sudden onset of paralysis (hemiplegia) or weakness (hemiparesis) to the face, arm, hand, or leg, especially to one side of the body
- Numbness or loss of sensation on one side of the body
- Speech disturbances—slurred, garbled, or incomprehensible speech (dysarthria) to complete loss of speech
- Loss of control of the bladder or bowel
- Unequal pupils
- Deterioration or loss of vision in one or both eyes, double vision
- Eyes turned away from the side of the body that is paralyzed
- Nausea and vomiting
- Sudden onset of severe headache
- Seizure activity
- Stiff neck (late symptom)
- Inability to understand what you are saying (sensory or receptive aphasia)
- Inability to form words to talk (expressive or motor aphasia)
- Incoordination of the extremities, usually on one side
- Poor balance, clumsiness, or difficulty in walking (ataxia)
- Hearing loss to one side
- Light or sound sensitivity
- Vertigo
- Dizziness
- Vomiting
- Ignoring one side of the body

In some types of stroke, the signs and symptoms may progress and the patient's condition may continue to deteriorate. This is particularly true of the mental status,

GENERAL SIGNS AND SYMPTOMS OF STROKE

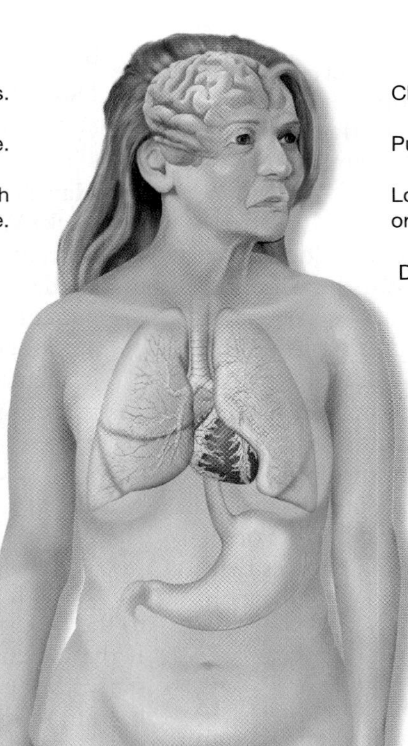
Decreased consciousness.
Severe headache.
Drooping eyelid and mouth on one side of face.
Paralysis or weakness on one or both sides of the body.
Arm drift.
Loss of bowel or bladder control.
Change in personality.
Pupils unequal in size.
Loss of vision, dimness, or double vision.
Difficulty speaking or slurred speech.
Inability to speak.
Nausea or vomiting.
Sudden weakness or paralysis of face, arm, or leg.
Possible seizures.

FIGURE 18-7 ∗ Stroke and transient ischemic attack (TIA) are conditions that may result from nontraumatic brain injury. Loss of speech, sensory, or motor function and altered mental status are among the possible signs and symptoms. Facial asymmetry is a common sign.

ASSESSMENT Tips

Hypotension is a rare finding in the stroke patient. ■

speech disturbance, numbness, weakness, and paralysis. For example, you may find a patient who has weakness to the right arm and leg, has slightly slurred speech, and obeys your commands. By the time you arrive at the hospital the patient is completely paralyzed on the right, is unable to speak, and responds to only painful stimuli.

Emergency Medical Care

If your assessment reveals an injury, provide care for that injury, including spinal stabilization. In addition, if the patient displays an altered mental status or a loss of speech, sensory, or motor function, or if stroke is suspected, provide the following care:

1. **Maintain a patent airway.** Airway compromise in the stroke patient is common. It may be necessary to insert an oropharyngeal or nasopharyngeal airway. Typically, the nasopharyngeal airway is preferred because it is better tolerated by the patient.
2. **Suction secretions and vomitus.** Since vomiting is associated with a brain injury or stroke, be prepared to remove vomitus by suctioning.
3. **Be prepared to assist ventilation.** As the patient deteriorates, breathing may become inadequate. If the rate or quality of breathing is inadequate, begin positive pressure ventilation with supplemental oxygen. It is important to recognize early signs of respiratory failure. Inadequate breathing could drastically increase injury to the brain because of decreased oxygen flow to the brain and a buildup of carbon dioxide.

   If the patient is unresponsive and has unequal pupils or posturing and is breathing inadequately, hyperventilation at a rate of 20 ventilations per minute with supplemental oxygen might be considered. Follow your local protocol or contact medical direction, since hyperventilation of patients with increased pressure inside the skull is considered controversial and may actually worsen the blood flow to the brain.
4. **Maintain oxygen therapy.** According to the AHA 2010 guidelines, if the SpO_2 reading is less than 94%, the patient complains of dyspnea, or signs and symptoms of hypoxia, heart failure, or shock are present, administer oxygen by nasal cannula at 2 to 4 lpm. High-concentration oxygen is no longer considered routine for the stroke patient unless severe signs of hypoxia are present. Many EMS protocols indicate oxygen when the SpO_2 is $<95\%$. Always follow your local protocol.
5. **Position the patient.** If the patient is unable to protect his own airway because of a reduction in his mental status, place him in a left lateral recumbent position (Figure 18-8✱). Place the responsive patient in a supine position. If the patient wants to be placed in a semi-Fowler position, do not elevate the head and chest more than 30 degrees (Figure 18-9✱). If spinal injury is suspected, perform a jaw-thrust maneuver to open the airway and provide manual in-line stabilization with the patient supine. If the patient requires ventilation, place him in a supine position.
6. **Check the blood glucose level** if your protocol permits. If the blood glucose reading is less than 60 mg/dL, suspect a low blood glucose (hypoglycemia) as the possible cause of the signs and symptoms, especially in the elderly patient. (See Chapter 20, "Acute Diabetic Emergencies.")
7. **Protect any paralyzed extremities.** Since the patient cannot move the paralyzed extremity, it is vital to protect the paralyzed extremities from any injury.
8. **Rapid transport.** Transport any patient with suspected stroke to a medical facility capable of immediate computed tomography (CT) imaging and intervention, preferably a stroke center.

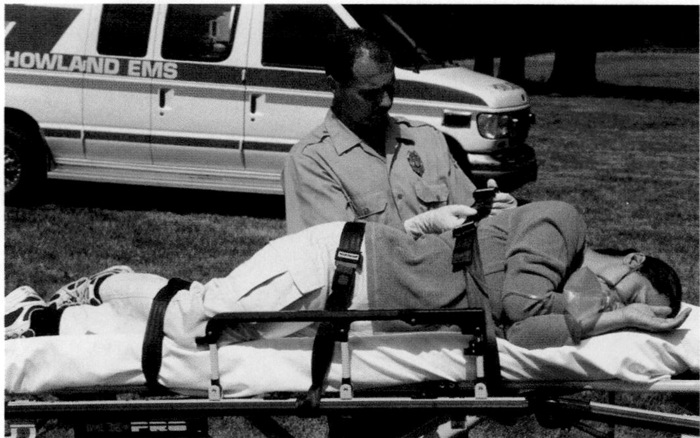

FIGURE 18-8 ✱ Place the unresponsive patient in a left lateral recumbent position if spinal injury is not suspected.

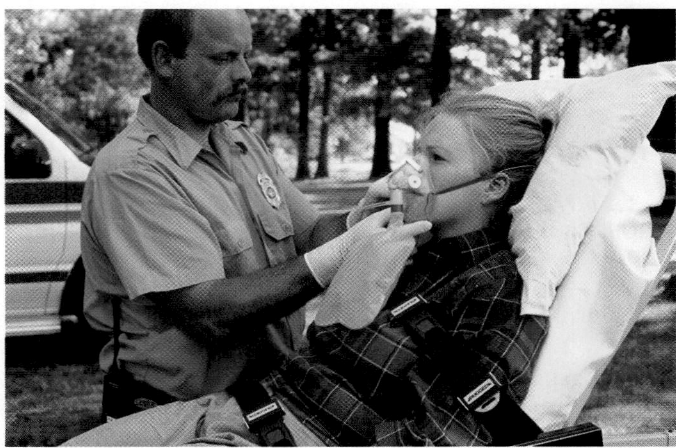

FIGURE 18-9 ✱ Place the responsive patient in a supine position with the head and chest elevated if spinal injury is not suspected.

Assessment Summary

STROKE

The following are findings that may be associated with a stroke emergency.

SCENE SIZE-UP

Is neurological deficit due to trauma or a medical problem?
Look for:
- Mechanism of injury
- Alcohol, drugs, or other substances that are commonly abused
- Position and location of patient
- Bucket or ice pack next to bed

Primary Assessment

General Impression
- Vomitus or secretions in mouth
- Slurred or incomprehensible speech
- Paralysis to one side of body

Mental Status
- Alert to unresponsive
- Able to understand but unable to speak
- Unable to understand or obey commands
- Disoriented

Airway
- Obstruction by tongue
- Obstruction by vomitus or secretions
- (Insert a nasopharyngeal or oropharyngeal airway in the unresponsive patient.)
- Drooling or inability to swallow

Breathing
- Shallow respirations
- Irregular respirations
- Absent respirations

Circulation
- Heart rate may be increased or decreased.

Status: Priority patient

Secondary Assessment

History

Signs and symptoms:
- Altered mental status
- Numbness or loss of sensation to one side of the body
- Weakness or paralysis to the hand, arm, leg, or face on one side of the body
- Speech disturbances (slurred, incomprehensible)
- Loss of bladder and bowel control
- Unequal pupils
- Visual disturbances (loss of vision in one eye, blurred vision, loss of visual field)
- Nausea and vomiting
- Headache (severe in stroke due to hemorrhage)
- Seizure
- Stiff neck
- Facial droop

Ask questions regarding the following:
- Anticoagulant drugs?
- History of hypertension?
- Abuse of amphetamines, cocaine, or other stimulant drug?
- Onset gradual or sudden?
- Signs and symptoms progressively get worse?
- Paralysis affects one side of body first?

Physical Exam
- Head, neck, and face
- Eyelid droop
- Facial droop
- Abnormal eye movements or gaze
- Extremities
- Weak or paralyzed on one side
- Numbness
- Unequal grip strength on one side of body
- Loss of sensation to one side of body
- Arm drift

Baseline Vital Signs
- BP: elevated or normal
- HR: normal or decreased
- RR: normal, decreased, increased, or irregular
- Skin: normal
- Pupils: possibly unequal and dilated
- Blood glucose level: normal

FIGURE 18-10a ✱ Assessment summary: stroke.

During emergency care, explain your procedures—what you are doing to the patient and what the patient should expect next. Even though the patient may appear as if he cannot understand you, he may be aware of everything that is happening and understand everything you are saying.

Reassessment

Perform a reassessment every 5 minutes. Pay special attention to the status of the airway, breathing, circulation, and mental status. This is extremely important since many stroke patients deteriorate rapidly and significantly. Pay par-

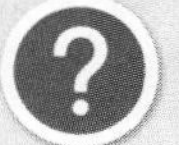

Thinking Critically
Stroke patients sometimes appear to be unaware of what is happening. Nevertheless, you should explain everything you are doing and what to expect. Why?

Emergency Care Protocol

STROKE

1. Establish and maintain an open airway. Insert a nasopharyngeal or oropharyngeal airway if the patient is unresponsive.
2. Suction secretions as necessary.
3. If breathing is inadequate, provide positive pressure ventilation with supplemental oxygen at a minimum rate of 10–12 ventilations/minute for an adult and 12–20 ventilations/minute for an infant or child.
4. According to the AHA 2010 guidelines, if the SpO_2 reading is less than 94%, the patient complains of dyspnea, or signs and symptoms of hypoxia, heart failure, or shock are present, administer oxygen by nasal cannula at 2 to 4 lpm. High-concentration oxygen is no longer considered routine for the stroke patient unless severe signs of hypoxia are present. Many EMS protocols indicate oxygen when the SpO_2 is $<95\%$. Always follow your local protocol.
5. Place the patient in a lateral recumbent position if unresponsive and if no spinal injury is suspected. If responsive and no spinal injury is suspected, elevate the head no greater than 30 degrees.
6. Obtain a blood glucose reading if your protocol permits.
7. Transport.
8. Perform a reassessment every 5 minutes.

FIGURE 18-10b ✱ Emergency care protocol: stroke.

ticular attention to the patient's airway as the mental status changes. Repeat and record vital signs. Communicate any changes in the patient's condition to the receiving facility.

Summary: Assessment and Care

To review assessment findings that may be associated with stroke and emergency care for a patient suspected of having suffered a stroke, see Figures 18-10a✱, 18-10b✱, and 18-11✱.

▸ Headache

A headache may be a condition in itself or a symptom of another condition such as stroke, a brain tumor, or a brain infection. Pain associated with a headache can have a sudden onset, be constant, or continuously recur. The headache may be isolated to one area of the head or may be generalized and felt throughout the head. The pain could be described as mild, moderate, or severe.

Types of Headache

Headaches can be categorized as the following:

- ***Vascular headaches*** occur as a result of dilation or distention of vessels or inflammation within the cranium. Migraine headaches are thought to be caused by spasm of vessels followed by vasodilation and a change in the chemicals that transmit nervous impulses in the brain. Migraines are often described as throbbing and may be generalized or localized to one side of the head. The patient also commonly experiences sensitivity to light (photosensitivity), nausea, vomiting, and sweating. Migraines may be preceded by an aura, such as blind spots, bright shimmering lights, weakness to one side of the body, numbness or tingling to one side of the body, visual or hearing hallucinations, double vision, uncoordination, or syncope. A vascular headache may also be caused by hypertension (high blood pressure) typically reaching 120 mmHg for a headache to occur.
- ***Cluster headaches*** are similar to migraines because they are believed to have a vascular origin. The pain is usually found on only one side of the head or face in the temporal region or around the eye and is excruciating. The patient may also complain of excessive tear production on the side of the pain, nasal congestion or runny nose (rhinorrhea), and nausea. Upon assessment, you might find facial sweating, restlessness or agitation, facial flushing or pallor, scalp or facial tenderness, and drooping eyelids.

Emergency Care Algorithm: **Stroke**

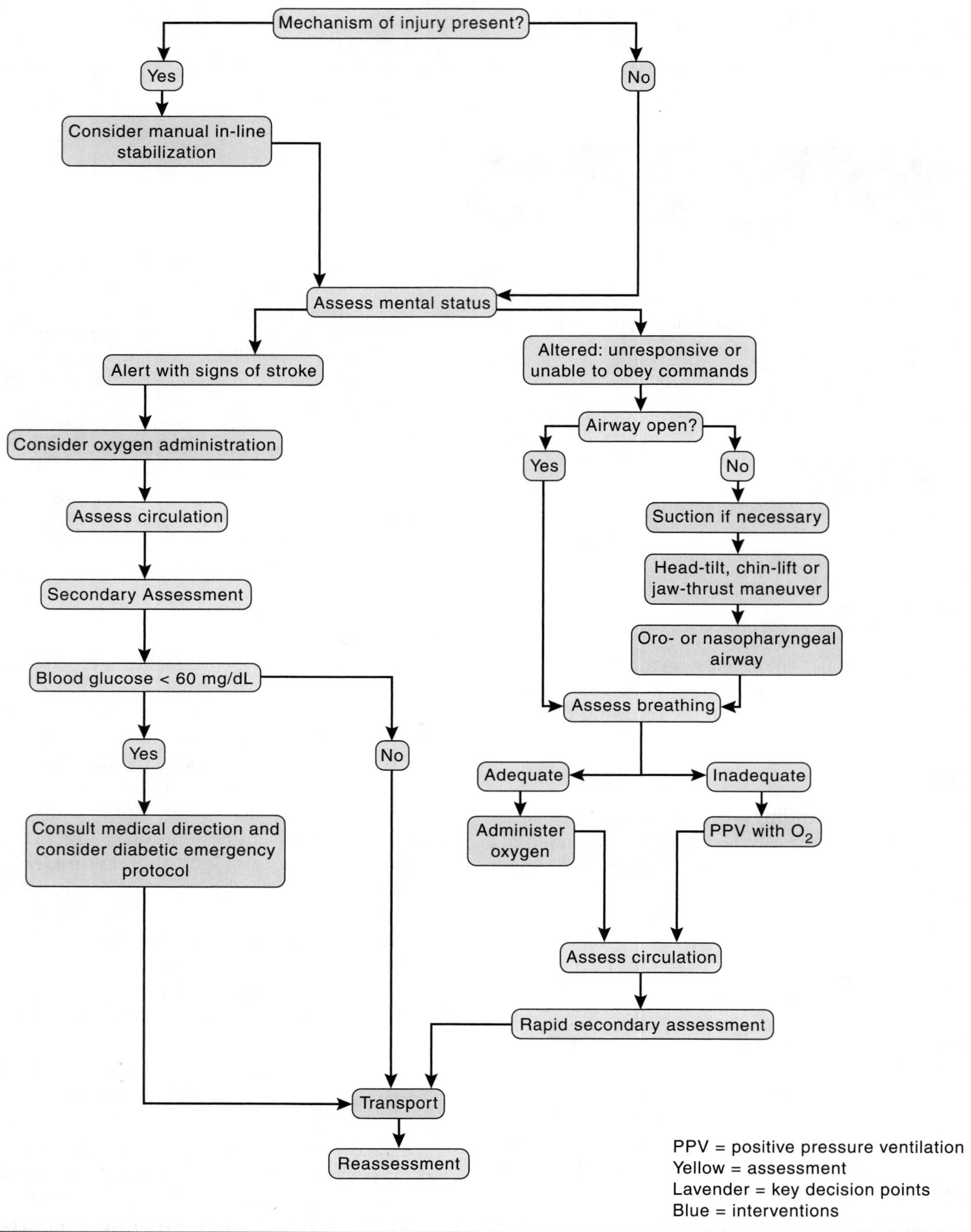

FIGURE 18-11 ∗ Emergency care algorithm: stroke.

Objective 18-14
Recognize indications that a headache may have a potentially life-threatening underlying cause, such as toxic exposure, hypertension, infectious disease, or hemorrhagic stroke.

Objective 18-15
Describe the appropriate emergency medical care for a patient suffering from headache.

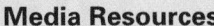

Media Resources
Go to www.bradybooks.com for mykit. Highlights:
- *Web Resource:* Headaches
- *Web Resource:* Transient Ischemic Attacks

- ***Tension headache*** is thought to be caused by contraction of the muscles of the neck and scalp. The pain is usually described as "tight" or "viselike." This is the most common type of recurring headache found in children, adolescents, and adults. The patient may wake in the morning with a headache that worsens throughout the day. The pain occurs to both sides of the head and is described as throbbing, aching, squeezing, or forceful pressure. The pain is usually felt in the frontal, temporal, and occipital regions of the head and often radiates to the neck and shoulders. There is no nausea or vomiting associated with a tension headache; however, the patient may complain that he has no appetite. The onset is usually more gradual than the onset of a migraine.
- ***Organic, traction, or inflammatory headaches*** are a result of tumors, infection, stroke, or inflammatory disorders within the cranium such as meningitis, hemorrhagic stroke, and tumor.

TABLE 18-1 **Serious Causes of Headache**
Tumor
Subarachnoid hemorrhage
Bleeding within the brain
Bleeding around the brain
Meningitis
Hypertension
Hypoglycemia
Carbon monoxide poisoning or other toxic inhalation
Fever
Hypoxemia
Stroke
Depression
Cyanide poisoning

Assessment

During scene size-up, look for clues that a headache may be associated with a toxic exposure. Assess the airway, ventilation, and oxygenation status. Apply oxygen based on the SpO_2 and patient presentation. Oxygen may relieve a cluster headache. Assess pulse and perfusion. Pain will often trigger the sympathetic nervous system and cause tachycardia and pale, cool, clammy skin. Perform a history and secondary assessment looking for any underlying cause of the headache. Assess the blood glucose level if permitted.

With any of the following signs or symptoms, suspect a serious underlying condition (Table 18-1).

- Altered mental status
- Motor or sensory deficit
- Behavior change
- Seizure
- First experience of this type of headache with an abrupt onset
- Worsening of pain with coughing, sneezing, or bending over
- Fever or stiff neck
- Change in the quality of a chronic headache

Emergency Medical Care

1. **Establish and maintain an adequate airway.** This may be necessary if the patient's mental status is deteriorating.
2. **Be prepared to suction.** Vomiting may occur with the headache.
3. **Assess and maintain adequate ventilation.** If the tidal volume or respiratory rate is inadequate, begin positive pressure ventilation with oxygen connected to the ventilation device.
4. **Administer oxygen.** If the ventilation is adequate and the SpO_2 is greater than 95% and no signs of hypoxia or an underlying condition are present, place the patient on a nasal cannula at 2 to 4 lpm. If signs of hypoxia or an underlying condition are present, place the patient on a nonrebreather mask at 15 lpm.
5. **Place the patient in a position of comfort.** The patient may be more comfortable lying flat, on his side, or in a seated position. It may be necessary to keep the lights dim in the back of the ambulance because of the light sensitivity experienced by some patients.
6. **Always be prepared to treat for seizures and transport to a medical facility.**

CHAPTER REVIEW

SUMMARY

Altered mental status may occur as a result of a wide variety of conditions involving both traumatic and medical causes. The causes may be structural or metabolic-toxic. Your primary responsibility is to ensure that you have established and are maintaining an adequate airway, ventilation, oxygenation, and circulation.

Stroke is a common emergency that can lead to devastating and long-term disability for the patient. Some signs and symptoms of stroke are very subtle. Have a high index of suspicion and consider all signs and symptoms when dealing with the possible stroke patient. When providing emergency care, recognition of the stroke, immediate transport, and notification prior to your arrival is crucial. The majority of your actual emergency care will be supportive.

There are two types of stroke: ischemic stroke and hemorrhagic stroke. Ischemic stroke is further categorized as thrombotic or embolic. The most common type of stroke is a thrombotic stroke.

The Cincinnati Prehospital Stroke Scale (CPSS) and the Los Angeles Prehospital Stroke Screen (LAPSS) are two evaluation tools used by EMS to identify possible stroke in a patient. These are both predictive screening tools for stroke. The most common signs and symptoms seen in stroke are sudden onset of weakness, paralysis, or numbness to the arm, hand, leg, or face on one side of the body; confusion or inability of the patient to respond to your questions or commands; trouble speaking; difficulty in vision in one or both eyes; difficulty walking or loss of coordination or balance; or a sudden onset of a severe headache.

Headache may be a condition itself or an indication of a serious underlying condition such as stroke, meningitis, hypertension, poisoning, toxic inhalation, or a number of other conditions. Carefully assess the patient and pay particular attention to any evidence of deterioration in the mental status or vital signs.

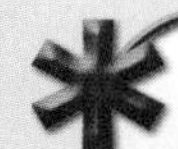

CASE STUDY FOLLOW-UP

SCENE SIZE-UP

You have been dispatched to a 73-year-old female patient who was found by her husband lying in bed. As you arrive on the scene, the husband meets you at the front door, introduces himself as Mr. Stein, and leads you into the house and up to the second floor bedroom. According to her husband, the patient is unable to move the right side of her body. As you scan the scene, you notice nothing out of the ordinary. The house appears to be extremely well kept, yet the smell of urine and feces permeates the air upon entering the bedroom. You notice bottles of prescription medications on the nightstand next to the bed.

PRIMARY ASSESSMENT

The patient is an elderly female who is still in her nightgown. As you approach the patient, you say, "Mrs. Stein?" Mrs. Stein opens her eyes and attempts to answer. Her speech is severely slurred and her face is pulled and drooping on the right side. Her breathing is adequate at a rate of approximately 20 per minute. Her radial pulse is strong and estimated at 70 beats per minute. Her skin is warm and dry.

SECONDARY ASSESSMENT

Mrs. Stein's slurred and garbled speech makes it difficult to understand what she says. She is not alert enough to respond appropriately to your questions, so you decide to begin with the physical exam rather than the history, and you perform a rapid assessment. Her head shows no evidence of trauma. Her pupils are equal and reactive. She has an obvious facial droop to the right side when asked to smile and show her teeth. Her chest is rising and falling symmetrically and the breath sounds are equal bilaterally. Her abdomen is soft and no tenderness or rigidity is noted. Her pelvis is stable with no tenderness on palpation. Mrs. Stein is able to obey your commands, so you check and compare her strength in all four extremities. When asked to squeeze your fingers, she has good grip strength on the left, but grip strength on the right is absent. She cannot lift her right arm when asked to put her arms out in front of her to check for arm drift. When asked to push up against your hands with her feet, the strength is good on the left, but again absent on the right. The posterior of her body shows no abnormalities. You find no medical alert tags.

While you are performing the rapid assessment, your partner is taking baseline vital signs. The blood pressure is 198/110 mmHg. The heart rate is 74 per minute and irregular. The respirations are 22 per minute and of normal depth. The skin is normal in color, warm, and dry. Her SpO_2 is 97%; therefore you elect not to administer oxygen. Her blood glucose level is 98 mg/dL.

Next, you obtain the history, primarily from Mr. Stein. He states that his wife's speech was slurred when she woke up this morning. (Because of this, the time of onset cannot be definitively determined.) Unlike now, however, he was still able to understand her. She complained, "I can't move my right arm or leg," and was disturbed that she had soiled the bed. Mr. Stein immediately went downstairs and called 911. He states, "It seems that she has gotten worse since I found her this way." He does not know of any known allergies his wife has. When asked if she takes any medications, he says, "She does take a water pill, a pill for her heart, and a pill for her blood pressure."

Your partner places the medications from the nightstand into a paper bag to be transported with the patient. According to Mr. Stein, his wife had a heart attack 2 years ago, and she has high blood pressure. He claims that her last oral intake was a cup of coffee last night at about 10:30. He did not notice anything unusual and she did not complain of anything before going to bed or during the night.

You and your partner place Mrs. Stein on her left side on the stretcher. You secure Mrs. Stein to the stretcher, ensuring that the paralyzed extremities are well protected, and transfer her to the ambulance.

REASSESSMENT

Mrs. Stein's mental status does not change while en route to the hospital. Her airway remains open and clear. Her breathing is adequate at a rate of 22 per minute and the radial pulse is strong at a rate of 74 per minute. Her skin remains warm, dry, and a normal color. She continues to attempt to talk, but her speech remains slurred and garbled. The SpO_2 continues to read 97%. You record the vital signs and report Mrs. Stein's condition to the hospital.

Upon arrival at the emergency department, you provide an oral report of Mrs. Stein's condition as you assist in transferring her to the hospital bed. You complete your prehospital care report, restock the ambulance, notify dispatch you are in service, and prepare for another call.

Later that morning, you return to the emergency department to pick up some equipment. While there, you check on Mrs. Stein's status and learn that she has suffered a stroke and is likely to have permanent paralysis to the right side of her body.

IN REVIEW

1. List possible causes of an altered mental status.
2. Explain why the airway and breathing must be closely monitored in a patient with an altered mental status or stroke.
3. List several signs and symptoms of stroke.
4. List the steps in the emergency care of the patient suffering from an altered mental status or stroke.
5. Compare and contrast stroke and TIA with regard to signs and symptoms, how they progress, and emergency medical care.
6. Describe the various types of headache.
7. List signs or symptoms associated with a headache that would indicate a serious underlying cause.

CRITICAL THINKING

You arrive on the scene and find a 68-year-old male patient whose wife states he suddenly began to slur his words. The patient is alert and responding to your questions. You note an obvious slur to his words in addition to a left facial droop. His respirations are 14 per minute with good chest rise. His radial pulse is irregularly irregular at a rate of 108 bpm. His skin is warm and dry. His SpO_2 is 92% on room air. His blood pressure is 242/128 mmHg. His blood glucose reading is 89 mg/dL. He has no known allergies and takes Lipitor. He has no significant medical history and last ate when he had lunch about 2 hours prior to your arrival. The patient was on the phone when the slurring suddenly began. He has obvious facial droop when you ask him to make a smile. His left arm drifts when he attempts to hold both arms out in front of his body. His pupils are equal and reactive. Breath sounds are equal and clear bilaterally. Good pulses are found in all the extremities; however, the left arm and leg exhibit weakness and loss of sensation.

1. What is the oxygenation status of the patient?
2. How would you manage the oxygenation status of the patient?
3. What type of stroke do you suspect the patient suffered?
4. What signs and symptoms would cause you to believe the patient suffered a stroke?
5. How would you manage the patient?
6. What is the significance of the pulse rhythm?

EXPLORE PEARSON **mybradykit**™

Please go to **www.bradybooks.com** to access mykit for this text. You will find quizzes, critical thinking scenarios, weblinks, animations, and videos related to this chapter—and much more. Look for online information on strokes, stroke prevention, and TIAs.

Register your access code from the front of your book by going to **www.bradybooks.com** and selecting the mykit links.

CHAPTER 19

Seizures *and* Syncope

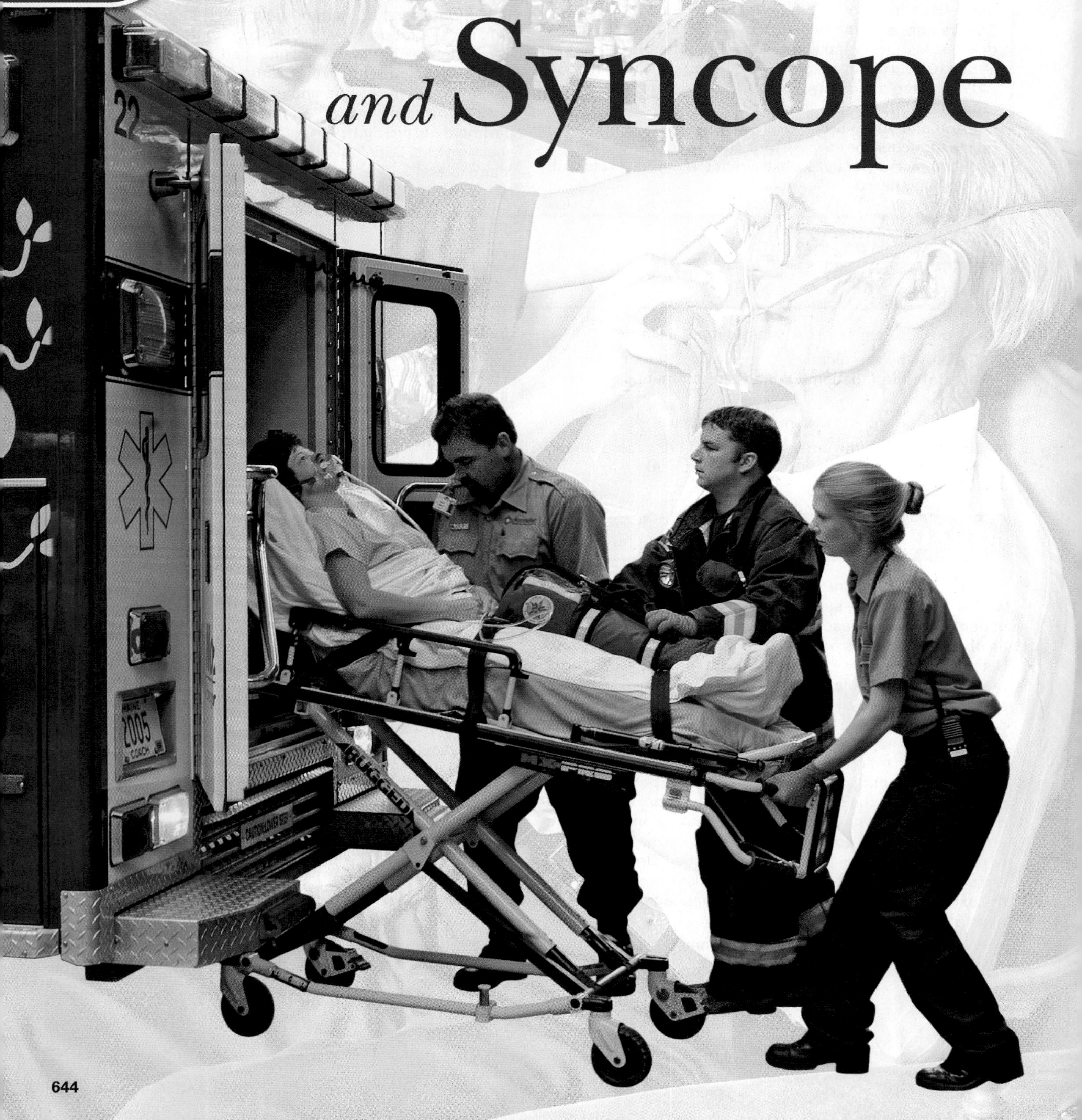

Navigation Guide

The following items provide an overview to the purpose and content of this chapter. The Standard and Competency are from the new National EMS Education Standards.

STANDARD **Medicine** (Content Area: Neurology)

COMPETENCY Applies fundamental knowledge to provide basic emergency care and transportation based on assessment findings for an acutely ill patient.

OBJECTIVES: After reading this chapter, you should be able to:

19-1. Define key terms introduced in this chapter.
19-2. Describe the various ways that seizures can present.
19-3. Discuss the pathophysiology of seizures.
19-4. Explain the concerns associated with prolonged or successive seizures.
19-5. Describe the assessment and emergency medical care of patients with tonic-clonic, simple partial, complex partial, absence, and febrile seizures.
19-6. Anticipate bystander reactions to patients having seizures and take measures to stop unnecessary or inappropriate interventions.
19-7. Describe the assessment and emergency medical care of patients in a postictal state.
19-8. Describe the assessment and emergency medical care of patients who are unresponsive, actively seizing, or in status epilepticus.
19-9. Recognize situations in which the patient who is having or has had a seizure must be a higher priority for transport.
19-10. Discuss the role of blood glucose determination in patients who have had a seizure.
19-11. Discuss relevant questions to ask while gathering a history of the seizure activity.
19-12. Describe common causes of syncope.
19-13. Describe the scene size-up, assessment, and emergency medical care of patients with syncope, including differentiating syncope from seizure.

KEY TERMS: Page references indicate first major use in this chapter. For complete definitions, see the Glossary at the back of the book.

aura p. 648
convulsion p. 646
epilepsy p. 646
generalized tonic-clonic seizure p. 647
postictal state p. 649
seizure p. 646
status epilepticus p. 647
syncope p. 658

MEDIA RESOURCES: Please go to www.bradybooks.com to access mykit for this text. You will find quizzes, critical thinking scenarios, weblinks, animations, and videos related to this chapter—and much more. Look for online information on status epilepticus and syncope. You will also find video clips on seizures and epilepsy.

CASE STUDY

The Dispatch

EMS Unit 106—respond to the Southern Park Mall, main concourse, for a 23-year-old female patient who is seizing. Time out is 1717 hours.

Upon Arrival

You and your partner arrive on the scene within 2 minutes after the alert. A fire department Emergency Medical Responder indicates that the scene is clear of safety hazards and directs you to the location of the patient. As you weave through the shoppers with your equipment and the stretcher, you notice that the mall is unusually crowded because of a holiday craft fair. A large crowd surrounds the patient. You find her supine and actively seizing. A fire department Emergency Medical Responder is cradling her head to protect it. Her sister is at her side holding her hand while providing the fire department with information.

How Would You Proceed to Assess and Care for This Patient?

During this chapter, you will learn special considerations of assessment and emergency care for a patient experiencing a seizure. Later we will return to the case and apply the procedures learned.

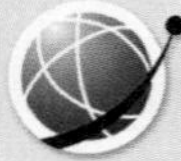

Media Resources
Go to www.bradybooks.com for mykit. Highlights:

- *Web Resource:* Status Epilepticus
- *Web Resource:* Syncope

Key Terms
seizure a sudden and temporary alteration in the mental status caused by massive electrical discharge in a group of nerve cells in the brain.

Objective 19-2
Describe various ways that seizures can present.

Objective 19-3
Discuss the pathophysiology of seizures.

Introduction

A seizure is a sudden onset of random, continuing discharges of electrical activity in the brain, which can lead to unusual manifestations, from staring spells to gross muscle contraction. Most (but not all) seizure activity is accompanied by an altered mental status. Many seizures are self-limiting and last only 2–3 minutes. Most often, the seizure will have stopped by the time EMS arrives on the scene. Frequently, emergency care will consist of assisting the patient during recovery and transporting him to the hospital.

Although seizures occurring in patients who have a history of a seizure disorder can be quite dramatic and frightening to observe, they are often not dangerous in themselves. However, the seizing patient can injure himself by falling or thrashing around. It is important for the EMT to recognize that seizures that are prolonged or are associated with life-threatening conditions or injuries such as head injury or stroke are abnormal and dangerous. Your prompt intervention in the prolonged or abnormal seizure may be life saving.

Seizure

A **seizure** is a sudden and temporary alteration in brain function caused by massive, continuing electrical discharges in a group of nerve cells in the brain. The abnormal electrical discharge typically produces changes in mental activity and behavior ranging from brief trancelike periods of inattention to unresponsiveness and the jerky muscle contractions known as a **convulsion.** A seizure is not a disease in itself but rather a sign of an underlying defect, injury, or disease.

A common cause of seizures is **epilepsy,** a chronic brain disorder characterized by recurrent seizures. There are approximately 125,000 newly reported cases of epilepsy each year. Although epilepsy is often thought of as a childhood disorder, only 30 percent of the new cases occur in children, and these occur most often in early childhood or at the onset of adolescence. Those over the age of 65 are another group with a high new-onset incidence of epilepsy.

If you have never seen a seizing person, you might easily mistake a seizure—or seizure phase—for a stroke, a behavioral disturbance, fainting, or simply daydreaming or lack of attention. What does a seizure "look" like?

The most common type of epileptic seizure, the generalized tonic-clonic seizure, is often called a grand mal seizure. Because these seizures rarely last more than a few minutes, the patient may be in a postictal state by the time you arrive on the scene. The postictal state follows the seizure and is the recovery period for the patient. During this period, the patient may be unresponsive, extremely sleepy, weak, and disoriented or may have strokelike symptoms such as paralysis. Because such a large number of muscles were contracting during the seizure, he will feel extremely tired. He will slowly but progressively regain complete responsiveness and orientation. This phase may last up to 30 minutes.

Epilepsy is only one cause of seizures. Seizures may also result from injuries or medical conditions other than epilepsy and may last much longer than the typical epileptic seizure. Seizure activity that is related to an injury or a medical condition may be an ominous sign of brain injury, even permanent brain damage. It is imperative that you not develop "tunnel vision" and assume that any seizure is caused by epilepsy. Also, patients with epilepsy may develop seizures from other causes, such as head injury. If the patient who suffers a seizure has no known history of a seizure disorder, you should suspect some medical or traumatic cause of the seizure other than epilepsy. During the scene size-up and the remainder of assessment, be alert for any clues to a cause other than epilepsy—for example, an injury that must be managed. Also be aware that a heart attack, stroke, or other medical condition may be confused with a seizure or may produce a seizure.

It is imperative for you to assess and manage the altered mental status associated with the seizure and the postictal state. Prolonged seizures could result in significant airway and breathing compromise. Your task, as an EMT, is not to diagnose the type of seizure, but to assess for and manage any life-threatening conditions and provide reassurance to the patient.

Pathophysiology of Seizures

There are several types of seizures, and each has a variety of signs and symptoms. Some seizures might, at first glance, be mistaken for other conditions. For instance, the patient experiencing an absence seizure can be thought to be simply daydreaming, and the patient who is having a complex partial seizure could be mistaken for someone with a behavioral or psychological disturbance.

Key Terms

convulsion generalized jerky muscle movement.

epilepsy a medical disorder characterized by recurrent seizures.

status epilepticus a seizure lasting longer than 5 minutes or consecutive seizures with no period of responsiveness between them.

Objective 19-4

Explain concerns associated with prolonged or successive seizures.

Objective 19-5

Describe the assessment and emergency medical care of patients with tonic-clonic, simple partial, complex partial, absence, and febrile seizures.

So, while your treatment efforts will be focused on generalized seizure activity and managing any life threats, it is still important for you to recognize the types of seizures.

Seizures are categorized as either primary seizures or secondary seizures. Secondary seizures are also referred to as reactive seizures. *Primary seizures* in adults are usually due to a genetic or unknown cause. Primary seizures are categorized as generalized or partial seizures. *Generalized seizures* involve both hemispheres of the brain and the reticular activating system, which typically results in a loss of consciousness. Generalized seizure activity is usually characterized by rhythmic, tonic-clonic muscle contractions (convulsions). *Partial seizures* are typically related to abnormal activity in just one cerebral hemisphere. Partial seizures are either simple or complex. A patient who is suffering a simple partial seizure will remain conscious, whereas a complex partial seizure will normally produce an altered mental status or unresponsiveness.

Secondary or *reactive seizures* do not result from a genetic cause but occur as the result of an insult to the body, such as fever, infection, hypoxia, hypoglycemia, hyperglycemia, drug intoxication, drug withdrawal, eclampsia in pregnancy, degenerative brain diseases, or imbalances in the electrolytes in the body (Table 19-1). As a rule of thumb, secondary or reactive seizures are generalized in nature and do not produce partial-type seizures. Thus, the patient suffering a seizure from some type of insult to the body will suffer a full convulsive-type seizure. The key with this type of seizure is to identify and treat the underlying cause of the seizure activity. For example, if the seizure activity is due to hypoxia resulting from inadequate breathing, the most important emergency care you can provide that will stop the seizure and prevent it from recurring is to establish an airway and provide effective positive pressure ventilation with supplemental oxygen.

Reactive or secondary generalized seizures that are due to an insult to the body are extremely dangerous and can result in death if not treated promptly. These are totally different from seizures that are primary, in which the patient usually has a diagnosed history of a seizure disorder.

TABLE 19-1 Common Causes of Secondary Seizures

- High fever
- Infection
- Poisoning
- Hypoglycemia (low blood sugar)
- Hyperglycemia (high blood sugar)
- Head injury
- Shock
- Hypoxia
- Stroke
- Drug or alcohol withdrawal
- Dysrhythmias
- Hypertension (high blood pressure)
- Pregnancy complications (eclampsia)
- Blood electrolyte imbalance (sodium, calcium)
- Hyperthermia
- Idiopathic (unknown cause)

Status Epilepticus

A patient who suffers generalized motor seizures that last more than 5 minutes or seizures that occur consecutively without a period of responsiveness between them is considered to be in **status epilepticus.** This is a dire medical emergency that requires aggressive airway management, positive pressure ventilation with supplemental oxygen, and immediate transport to a medical facility. The longer the delay in treatment the greater the chance of the patient suffering permanent brain damage.

Types of Seizures

The type of seizure the patient experiences depends on whether it is primary or reactive and where in the brain the abnormal electrical activity is occurring. The following are the more common types of seizures.

Generalized Tonic-Clonic (Grand Mal) Seizure

A **generalized tonic-clonic seizure** was once referred to as a *grand mal seizure.* This type of seizure usually begins with abnormal electrical activity low in the cerebral cortex that spreads upward, affecting both cerebral hemispheres, and downward, affecting the reticular

Key Terms
generalized tonic-clonic seizure a common type of seizure that produces unresponsiveness and a generalized jerky muscle activity. Also known as a *grand mal seizure.*

Key Terms
aura an unusual sensory sensation that may precede a seizure episode by hours or only a few seconds.

activating system (RAS). The RAS is responsible for wake/sleep activity. If the RAS is disturbed, the patient will lose consciousness. The involvement of both cerebral hemispheres contributes to the loss of consciousness and produces the characteristic jerky, convulsive motor activity.

Understanding BODY PROCESSES

A generalized seizure typically involves both cerebral hemispheres (large lobes) of the brain and the reticular activating system (the wake/sleep system). This is what produces the unresponsiveness during the seizure. ■

The signs and symptoms of a generalized tonic-clonic seizure usually occur in the following six stages (Figure 19-1*):

- **Aura.** The **aura** serves as a warning that a seizure is going to begin and involves some type of sensory perception by the patient. The aura may be a sound, an abnormal twitch, anxiety, dizziness, a smell or odor, an unpleasant feeling in the stomach, visual disturbance, or odd taste. Many patients will tell you that they knew they were going to seize because of the aura. However, generalized seizures do commonly occur without the preceding aura.
- **Loss of consciousness.** The patient loses consciousness sometime after the aura.

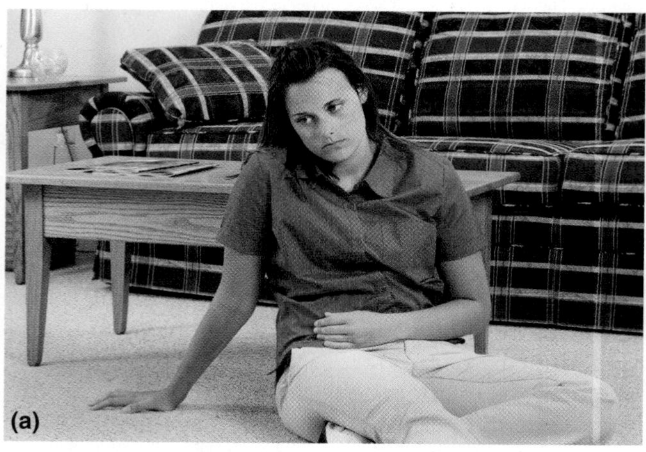

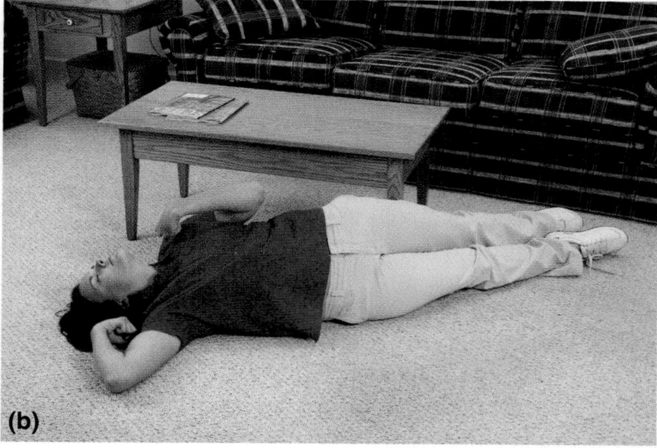

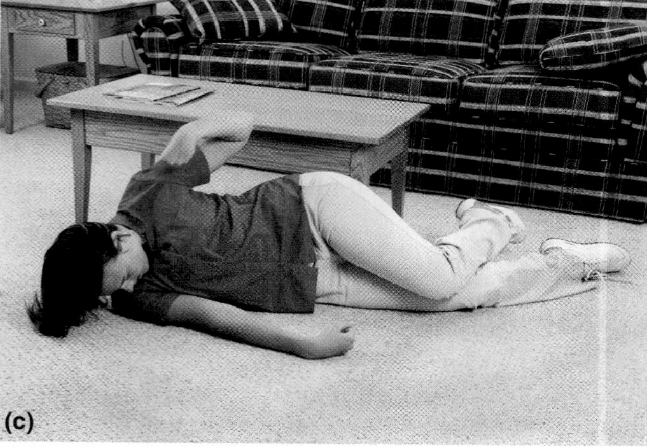

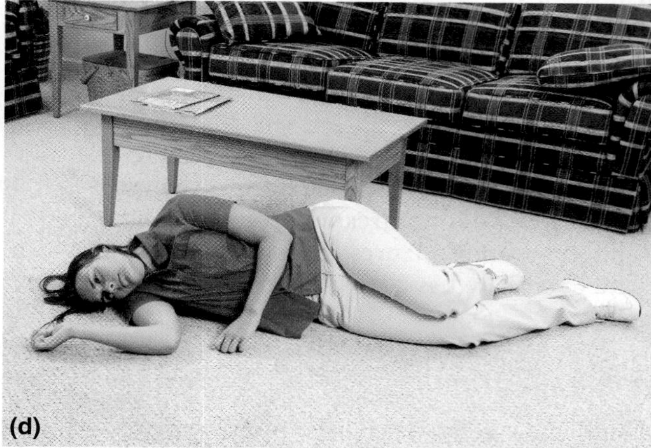

FIGURE 19-1 * A generalized tonic-clonic, or grand mal, seizure is a sign of abnormal release of electrical impulses in the brain: **(a)** aura, **(b)** loss of consciousness followed by tonic phase, **(c)** clonic phase, **(d)** postictal phase.

Key Terms

postictal state the recovery period that follows the clonic phase of a generalized seizure. In a postictal state the patient commonly appears weak, exhausted, and disoriented and progressively improves.

Thinking Critically

Your patient seems drowsy after collapsing suddenly at school. Her friend says, "She was jerking around, having convulsions." "Has this ever happened to you before?" you ask. "No," says the patient, "but I just fainted. It's nothing. I don't want to go to the hospital." What should you do?

- **Tonic phase (muscle rigidity).** The patient's muscles become contracted and tense, and the patient exhibits extreme muscular rigidity with arching of the back.
- **Hypertonic phase.** The patient has extreme muscular rigidity with hyperextension of the back.
- **Clonic phase (convulsion).** Muscle spasms then alternate with relaxation, producing the typical violent and jerky seizure activity of the clonic phase. During the convulsion, a loss of bowel and bladder control may result in involuntary urination and defecation. Also, the tongue, lips, or mouth may be bitten. The breathing may be shallow or absent. This phase usually lasts only 1–3 minutes.
- **Postictal state.** The **postictal state** is the recovery phase. The patient's mental status is altered and may range from complete unresponsiveness to confusion and disorientation. The mental status progressively improves over time. The patient is exhausted and weak. A headache and temporary weakness to one side of the body (hemiparesis) may be present. The postictal phase generally lasts from 10–30 minutes. It could last much longer.

Emergency Medical Care If the patient has a history of epilepsy with recurrent seizures, it is likely that the seizure activity has already stopped and the patient is in a postictal state by the time you arrive on scene. In this case, provide reassurance and conduct a thorough assessment to ensure that the patient did not injure himself and that no abnormal signs or symptoms are present. If this is a typical seizure for the patient, it is likely he will refuse transport. Follow local protocol and contact medical direction if necessary.

If the seizure presents as status epilepticus, provide the emergency medical care outlined in the "Assessment-Based Approach to Seizure Activity" section later in the chapter. Focus on establishing and maintaining an adequate airway, ventilation, oxygenation, and circulation. Remember that status epilepticus is a dire emergency that could result in damage to or death of brain cells, other tissue damage, and organ failure.

Simple Partial Seizure

A *simple partial seizure* is also known as a *focal motor seizure* or *Jacksonian motor seizure*. This type of seizure involves only one cerebral hemisphere. For this reason, it generally produces jerky muscle activity in one area of the body, arm, leg, or face. The patient cannot control the jerky movement. The patient remains awake and aware of the seizure activity because the reticular activating system and both cerebral hemispheres are not involved. The seizure activity may spread from one area of the body to another and sometimes progresses to a generalized tonic-clonic seizure. You should document where the seizure activity began and how it progressed. This information may be extremely helpful in identifying a cause and in the long-term treatment of the patient.

ASSESSMENT Tips

The term "simple" with regard to partial seizures typically refers to a seizure during which the patient retains consciousness. ■

Emergency Medical Care If this is a recurring problem for the patient and not a new-onset condition, emergency care may not be necessary. Contact medical direction or follow your local protocol if the patient refuses care or transport to a medical facility. If the simple partial seizure progresses to a generalized tonic-clonic seizure, follow the emergency care guidelines in the "Assessment-Based Approach to Seizure Activity" section. A patient who suffers a simple partial seizure for the first time must be transported for further medical evaluation.

Complex Partial Seizure

Also known as a *psychomotor* or *temporal lobe seizure*, the *complex partial seizure* usually lasts 1 to 2 minutes. It is termed "partial" because it involves only one cerebral hemisphere. The patient will remain awake; however, he will not be aware of his surroundings. The seizure usually starts with a blank stare, followed by a random activity such as chewing, lip smacking, or rolling the fingers as if moving a marble between them. The patient appears dazed or unaware of his surroundings and mumbles or repeats certain words or phrases. He will not respond to commands. His actions and movements are clumsy and lack direction. He may pick at his clothing, try to remove his clothes, or pick up objects. The patient may run as you approach him or appear afraid of you. Some patients will struggle with you or show abrupt personality changes, such as fits of rage. Although the seizure will last for only

Key Points
Absence seizures, most common in children, are characterized by a blank stare and lack of awareness, then a quick return to full awareness.

Thinking Critically
You are called to assist a patient who has had a seizure in the kitchen at home. Why is it important to conduct a thorough scene size-up?

a few minutes, the postseizure confusion may last much longer. The patient will not remember what happened during the seizure.

Be alert to the possibility of this disorder, even though the patient's behavior may also cause you to suspect intoxication, drug use, mental illness, or disorderly conduct. If the patient does not recover, manage him as a patient with an altered mental status.

ASSESSMENT Tips

The term "complex" with regard to partial seizures typically refers to that which results in an alteration in mental status. ■

Emergency Medical Care Speak calmly and reassuringly. Guide the person gently away from objects that may be hazardous to him or others. Stay with the person until he is completely aware of his surroundings. Because these seizures are recurring in nature, he will most likely refuse transport. Consult medical direction or follow local protocol in this instance.

Absence (Petit Mal) Seizure

Absence or *petit mal seizures,* which are most common in children, are characterized by a blank stare, beginning and ending abruptly, and lasting only a few seconds. There may be rapid blinking, chewing, and lack of attention. The child is unaware of what is occurring during the seizure but then quickly returns to full awareness. No emergency care is necessary for the absence seizure. If this is a first-time observation of the seizure, however, medical evaluation should be recommended.

Febrile Seizure

Febrile seizures, caused by high fever, are most common in children between 6 months and 6 years of age. About 5 percent of children who have a fever will develop febrile seizures. These secondary or reactive generalized seizures are often very short and may not require emergency care; however, always assume that the seizures are serious, because you won't be able to make the diagnosis without a medical evaluation. These seizures will be covered in more detail in Chapter 38, "Pediatrics."

Assessment-Based Approach to Seizure Activity

Scene Size-Up

Because a seizure could be a sign of head injury, look for a mechanism of injury that may suggest blunt or penetrating injury to the head. Also, check the environment for any evidence of poisoning, such as pill bottles and syringes. Look for prescription medications that may indicate a history of epilepsy, diabetes, or heart disease.

ASSESSMENT Tips

Drug or alcohol withdrawal is a common cause of seizures. These are not epileptic seizures and need to be managed immediately. ■

Understanding BODY PROCESSES

A patient with a head injury may not present with seizures until months after the injury. The delayed seizure may be caused by the formation of scar tissue and abnormal electrical connections during the body's attempt to repair brain tissue. ■

The patient may no longer be seizing when you arrive on the scene but may be in a postictal state. Once responsive, the patient may refuse emergency care and transportation. This frequently occurs in public places where the bystanders call EMS. The epileptic patient, however, may be accustomed to the seizure activity and does not necessarily want or need emergency care. If this is the case, you might encourage him to go to the hospital for a checkup if the seizure was abnormal in any way. Always begin with the assumption that the seizure patient needs emergency care.

You can't force a patient to accept transport or treatment, but you do need to document the call and follow the proper patient refusal procedure. A postictal patient (one in the period of recovery from a seizure) may be confused and not in the best state of mind to refuse transport. If this is the situation, contact medical direction for further orders.

Objective 19-6
Anticipate bystander reactions to patients having seizures and take measures to stop inappropriate interventions.

Objectives 19-7 and 19-8
Describe the assessment and emergency medical care of patients in a postictal state and of those who are unresponsive, actively seizing, or in status epilepticus.

ASSESSMENT Tips

The duration of the postictal state will vary from patient to patient and from seizure to seizure in the same patient. The signs of recovery may also vary. ■

If the patient is still seizing when you arrive, you will frequently find bystanders who are attempting to restrain the patient's jerky body movements. The patient's movements should always be guided, rather than restrained, in order to prevent further injury. It may also be necessary to move objects away from the patient (Figure 19-2*). Some people place spoons or other hard objects in the patient's mouth to prevent him from "swallowing his tongue," which is anatomically impossible. Remove these objects immediately because they can easily cause injury to the mouth, tongue, teeth, and jaw or they can break and cause an airway obstruction. It is common for the patient to bite his tongue during the seizure; therefore, you may notice small amounts of blood around his mouth. The smell or sight of urine and feces may also be noted.

Because seizure activity may mimic a heart attack and can result in short periods of apnea (absence of breathing), you may find a bystander performing CPR on the patient on your arrival. Quickly verify a pulse, and immediately stop any unnecessary care. Some cardiac arrests are preceded by seizure activity because of a lack of oxygen and blood to the brain. You should proceed with CPR, application of the automated external defibrillator (AED), and emergency care for cardiac arrest if no pulse is found.

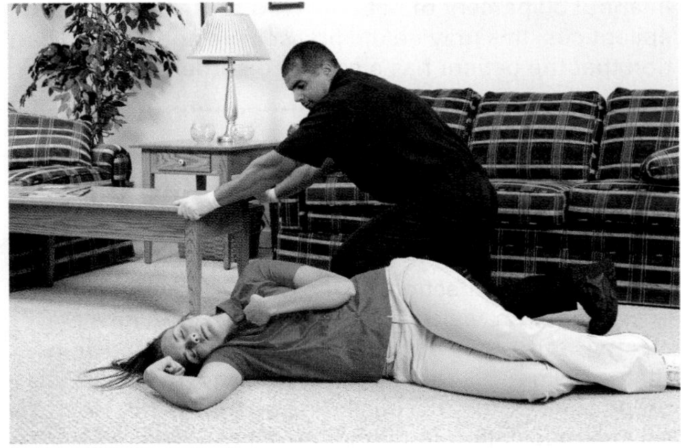

FIGURE 19-2 * Protect the seizing patient from injury by moving furniture and objects away.

Understanding BODY PROCESSES

The convulsive phase of a seizure causes the muscles in the body to contract and relax abnormally. Because the diaphragm is a large muscle, it also contracts and relaxes abnormally. This causes a temporary interruption in the patient's normal ventilatory status. After a convulsive state ceases, the sympathetic nervous system will be activated and cause tachycardia, tachypnea, and possibly hypertension. The hyperventilation may help in restoring the oxygen depletion that occurred during the convulsive phase. ■

Primary Assessment

Form a general impression of the patient as you begin the primary assessment. Whether you find the patient actively seizing or in a postictal state, you should consider both of these an altered mental status that warrants close assessment of the airway, breathing, and circulation. The patient who is not responding to verbal stimuli following the seizure episode, the patient who is actively seizing, or the patient who has suffered more than one consecutive seizure without an intervening period of responsiveness is at the greatest risk for airway, breathing, and circulation compromise. The postictal patient is most often confused, disoriented, weak, and exhausted, but typically has an open airway, is breathing adequately, and has adequate circulation.

Assessing Patients in the Postictal State

- If the patient is talking without distress, it indicates an open airway and adequate breathing. The heart rate is commonly elevated and the skin warm and moist. Continue with the secondary assessment for the medical patient. If the seizure was self-limited and typical for that patient, emergency care may not be required.

Assessing Patients Who Are Unresponsive to Verbal or Painful Stimuli, Actively Seizing, or in Status Epilepticus

- Open the airway with a jaw-thrust or head-tilt, chin-lift maneuver. It may be necessary to insert a nasopharyngeal airway. Large amounts of saliva are produced during the seizure and the tongue is commonly bitten and bleeding. Suction any secretions,

Key Points
High body temperatures are a common cause of seizures in infants and very young children.

Objective 19-9
Recognize seizure patients who are a higher priority for transport.

vomitus, or blood from the airway (Figure 19-3*). Do not place your fingers in the mouth of the seizing patient or any unresponsive patient. He can easily bite down and cause you serious injury. Do not insert an oropharyngeal airway since the patient may regain his gag reflex and vomit.

- During a seizure, the chest wall muscles contract and restrict effective breathing. The patient may appear to have an airway obstruction and may be cyanotic. As long as the seizure does not last longer than 5 minutes or more than one seizure does not occur consecutively, this should not pose a major problem since respiration will quickly return to normal following the abnormal muscle activity. In the following circumstances, you should begin positive pressure ventilation with supplemental oxygen: the patient is severely cyanotic, the seizure has lasted for greater than 5 minutes from the time of onset (not from your arrival), or the breathing does not immediately become adequate following the episode.
- Note the skin temperature and color. High body temperatures are a common cause of seizures in infants and very young children. Hot skin may also indicate a high body temperature resulting from the excessive uncontrolled muscle movement in the adult. Cyanosis is a grave sign of inadequate oxygenation and ventilation. Provide oxygen via a nonrebreather mask at 15 lpm if the breathing is adequate, or, as already noted, positive pressure ventilation with supplemental oxygen if breathing is inadequate.

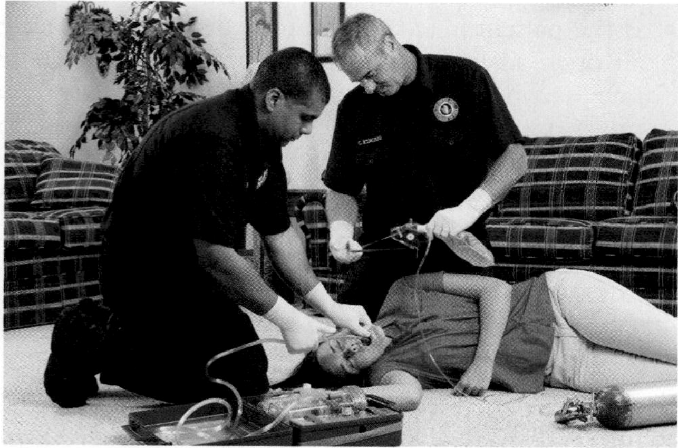

FIGURE 19-3 * Clear the airway of secretions, blood, and vomitus.

- Ensure the presence of a pulse if the patient is unresponsive. Initiate CPR and apply the AED if the patient is pulseless. Check for and manage any serious bleeding that may have resulted from trauma.

The seizure patient should be categorized as a priority for transport if any of the following occurs:

Transport Priority Circumstances

- The patient remains unresponsive following the seizure.
- The airway, breathing, or circulation is inadequate following the seizure activity.
- A second generalized motor seizure occurs without a period of responsiveness between the seizure episodes (status epilepticus).
- A generalized motor seizure lasts longer than 5 minutes (status epilepticus).
- The patient is pregnant, has a history of diabetes, or is injured.
- The seizure has occurred in water, such as a swimming pool or lake.
- There is evidence of head trauma leading to the seizure.
- There is no history of epilepsy or other seizure disorder.
- The seizure is the result of drug or alcohol withdrawal.

ASSESSMENT Tips

In about 30 percent of patients who present with status epilepticus, this may be the first seizure and first indication that the patient has a seizure disorder. ■

Understanding BODY PROCESSES

Causes of status epilepticus may include hypoxia, stroke, tumors, infections to the brain, electrolyte imbalances (sodium, calcium), cocaine use, hypoglycemia, alcohol and other drug withdrawal, and head injury. Status epilepticus in patients with a known seizure disorder often occurs because the patient did not take his seizure medication or did not take it properly. ■

Objective 19-10
Discuss the role of blood glucose determination in seizure patients.

Objective 19-11
Discuss relevant questions to ask while gathering a history of the seizure activity.

Secondary Assessment

In any of the circumstances just listed as transpsort priorities, begin transport immediately following the primary assessment and conduct the secondary assessment en route to the hospital. Perform a rapid assessment if the patient is postictal and still has an altered mental status, or if he does not have a past medical history of epilepsy or seizures. The head must be assessed for possible signs of injury (Figure 19-4∗). The pupils may be unequal if the brain is injured. Look for medical alert tags that might provide information about the patient.

You may find weakness or paralysis on one side of the body or to one area of the body (hand, arm, or leg) following a seizure. This should disappear as the patient slowly becomes more responsive; however, it may last up to 24 hours. If the weakness does not subside or if paralysis is present upon assessment of the motor and sensory function in the extremities, it may be an indication that a stroke or trauma is the actual cause of the seizure activity. The seizure patient usually regains complete recovery of function soon after the postictal episode. Assess the head and extremities for injury that may have occurred as a result of the muscular activity or the fall to the ground. Some muscle contractions are so severe that a bone injury or dislocation may result. Therefore, inspect and palpate for signs of an injured extremity.

ASSESSMENT Tips

Paralysis to one area or one side of the body may occur following a generalized seizure and may last up to 24 hours. This is referred to as Todd paralysis. It may also indicate that a space-occupying problem in the brain is causing the seizure. ■

Assess and record the baseline vital signs. The respirations and heart rate may be elevated. The skin is commonly warm and moist.

Apply a pulse oximeter and determine the SpO_2 reading. If the SpO_2 reading is low, it may be a result of the inadequate breathing the patient suffered during the active seizure period or, alternatively, it may be an indication of hypoxia that possibly caused the seizure. The low SpO_2 reading may also have resulted from aspiration during the seizure or from fluid leaking out of the capillaries in the lungs and into the spaces between the alveoli and the capillaries from increases in the blood pressure during the seizure.

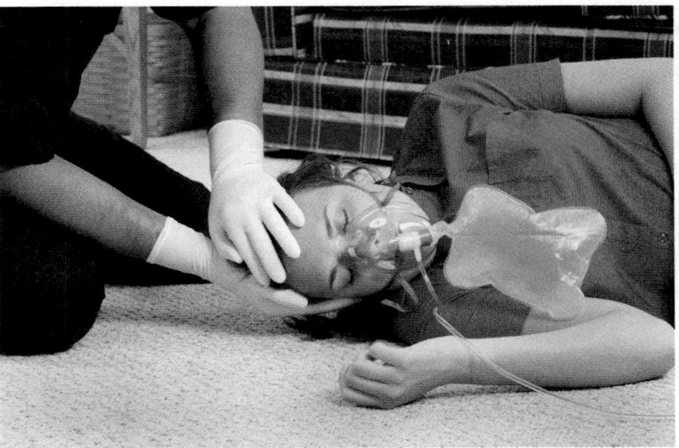

FIGURE 19-4 ∗ Assess the head for any sign of trauma.

Since hypoglycemia may trigger a seizure, if protocol permits assess the blood glucose level by using a glucose meter. If the blood glucose is less than 60 mg/dL, you may suspect the seizure is due to a low blood glucose level. Contact medical direction and request an ALS backup if the patient remains unresponsive or if you are unable to administer oral glucose because of the patient's mental status.

Gather a history from the responsive patient, relatives, and bystanders. If the patient is a priority for transport, you will have to try to gather information from bystanders during the scene size-up or primary assessment or your partner will have to gather it. (Even if the patient is now responsive, he may not recall much, if anything, about how the seizure occurred or progressed.) The following are pertinent questions to ask, and the answers will be important information to pass along to the hospital staff:

- Was the patient awake during the seizure?
- Was the muscle activity a twitching or jerking motion?
- Was the muscle activity isolated to one part of the body or generalized at the time the seizure started? (Most seizures will begin as generalized; some may start focally, then generalize.)
- When did the seizure start?
- How long did the seizure last? (Remember, however, that bystanders tend to overestimate seizure duration.)

- Did the patient experience an aura before the seizure (an unusual sensation that may precede a seizure episode by hours or only a few seconds)?
- Did the patient hit his head or fall?
- Did the patient bite his tongue or mouth?
- Was there a loss of bowel or bladder control?
- Is there any recent history of fever, headache, or stiff neck?
- Is the patient allergic to any medications?
- What medications does the patient take? Are any to control seizures?
- Did the patient take his seizure medication as prescribed?
- Does the patient have a history of epilepsy, previous seizures, diabetes, stroke, or heart disease?
- When was the last time the patient suffered a seizure?
- Was this a typical type of seizure for him to suffer?
- When did the patient last have something to eat or drink?
- What was the patient doing immediately prior to the seizure activity? (Could there have been a fall or injury that caused the seizure, rather than the seizure causing the fall or injury?)

Initially, the postictal patient may not be able to provide you with much of a history. As he progressively improves, the questioning will be easier and the information gathered much more pertinent.

Prescription medications found at the scene or on the patient may provide you with an indication of a medical history of a seizure disorder or epilepsy (Table 19-2). It is important to be familiar with these medications since seizures can be mistaken for other disorders. For instance, some seizures produce behavioral changes that may be interpreted as the patient being drunk or under the influence of drugs.

Signs and Symptoms The most commonly recognized type of seizure activity is the generalized tonic-clonic (grand mal) seizure. The signs and symptoms of each more common type of seizure were described in the previous section. General signs and symptoms that may indicate seizure activity are:

- Convulsions (jerky muscular movement)
- Rigid muscular contraction or muscle spasm
- Bitten tongue
- Excessive saliva
- Urinary or bowel incontinence
- Chewing movement, smacking lips, wringing hands, or some other repetitive activity
- Localized twitching of muscles
- Visual hallucinations (flashing lights, images)
- Olfactory hallucination (smells)

Emergency Medical Care

The EMT must focus on controlling the airway and breathing in the seizing patient. Do not spend unnecessary time trying to determine the exact cause or specific type of seizure. Manage the immediate life threats and transport the patient.

1. **Position the patient.** The postictal patient should be placed in a lateral recumbent (recovery) position to protect the airway and facilitate drainage of secretions. If a spinal injury is suspected, the patient should be properly immobilized in a supine position. However, if the immobilized patient vomits, you should immediately turn the backboard and patient as a unit on the side so that the patient's airway can be cleared more easily. If the patient requires ventilation, position him in a supine position.
2. **Maintain a patent airway.** If the patient is actively seizing or unresponsive, it may be necessary to insert a nasopharyngeal airway. Since the nasopharyngeal airway is flexible, in contrast to the rigid oropharyngeal airway, it is the airway of choice. Do not force anything into the mouth or between the teeth. You may actually do more harm by breaking the teeth. Do not place your fingers in the patient's mouth or place any object between the front teeth.

TABLE 19-2 Medications Commonly Used in the Treatment of Epilepsy

Phenytoin (Dilantin)	Tiagabine (Gabitril)
Phenobarbital	Lamotrigine (Lamictal)
Ethosuximide (Zarontin)	Oxcarbazepine (Trileptal)
Carbamazepine (Tegretol)	Gabapentin (Neurontin)
Valproic acid or divalproex sodium (Depakene or Depakote)	Topiramate (Topamax)
Primidone (Mysoline)	Vigabatrin (Sabril, Keppra)
Clonazepam (Klonopin)	
Clorazepate (Traxene)	
Felbamate (Felbatol)	

If the patient is in status epilepticus—seizing for over 5 minutes or having seizures that occur consecutively without a period of responsiveness between them—open the airway with a head-tilt, chin-lift maneuver and insert a nasopharyngeal airway. Begin positive pressure ventilation with supplemental oxygen. Immediately begin transport and continuously reassess the patient en route to the medical facility.

3. **Suction.** Suction any secretions, blood, or vomitus.
4. **Assist ventilation.** If the seizures last longer than 5 minutes or the breathing status is inadequate during the postictal phase, begin positive pressure ventilation with supplemental oxygen.
5. **Prevent injury to the patient.** Move objects away from the seizing patient so he does not injure himself. Protect the head, arms, and legs. Do not restrain the patient or try to control the movements. Loosen ties, shirt collars, or other tight clothing.
6. **Maintain oxygen therapy.** Continue oxygen therapy via a nonrebreather mask at 15 lpm if the breathing is adequate. Ensure high-concentration oxygen if the patient is being artificially ventilated. Oxygen administration may actually shorten the postictal period.
7. **Transport.** You must contact medical direction or follow local protocol if confronted with a patient who refuses emergency care or transportation. Basically, if this is a normal seizure for the patient, it may not be necessary to seek additional medical treatment, as long as the patient is awake and competent to refuse. However, if anything is abnormal about the seizure, more than one seizure occurred, or the seizure has lasted longer than 5 minutes, the patient must be transported for further evaluation. Follow your local protocol.

Reassessment

Be prepared to manage additional seizures. Monitor the airway, breathing, and circulation. Repeat and record the vital signs. Document and communicate any changes to the receiving medical facility.

Summary: Assessment and Care for Seizures

To review assessment findings and emergency care for seizures, see Figures 19-5* and 19-6*.

Assessment Summary

SEIZURES

The following findings may be associated with seizures.

SCENE SIZE-UP

Is seizure due to trauma or a medical problem? Look for:
- Mechanism of injury
- Alcohol, drugs, or other substances that are commonly abused
- Position and location of patient
- Confined spaces

PRIMARY ASSESSMENT

General Impression
- Is the patient actively seizing?
- Vomitus or secretions in mouth?
- Are all body parts involved in the convulsion?

Mental Status
- Is the patient postictal?
- Alert to unresponsive
- Confused or disoriented

Airway
- Obstruction by tongue
- Obstruction by vomitus or secretions

In an epileptic patient who is unresponsive or actively seizing for greater than 5 minutes, insert a nasopharyngeal airway. If the patient is seizing from a cause other than epilepsy (e.g., severe head injury), immediately insert a nasopharyngeal airway and begin positive pressure ventilation with supplemental oxygen attached to the reservoir.

Breathing
- Shallow respirations
- Absent respirations

Circulation
- Heart rate may be increased.
- Skin may be hot and moist.
- Cyanosis may be present.

Status: Priority Patient If
- Patient has been actively seizing for greater than 5 minutes.
- Patient remains unresponsive between seizures.
- Seizure has a cause other than epilepsy (e.g., hypoxia, head injury).
- Patient is pregnant.
- Patient remains unresponsive following seizure with no improvement.

continued

FIGURE 19-5a * Assessment summary: seizures

Assessment Summary

SECONDARY ASSESSMENT

History

Signs and symptoms of typical epileptic seizure:

- Aura (unusual sensation)
- Unresponsiveness
- Tonic phase (rigid muscles)
- Hypertonic phase (extremely rigid muscles with back arched)
- Tonic-clonic phase (jerky movements)
- Postictal phase (recovery period)
- Other (e.g., hyperventilation, excessive salivation, exhaustion, hemiplegia)

Signs and symptoms of seizure from causes other than epilepsy:

- Unresponsiveness
- Jerky movements (convulsions)
- Excessive salivation
- Hot, wet skin
- Cyanosis

Ask the following questions:

- How long did the seizure last?
- Did the patient have an aura and know he was going to seize?
- Did the patient possibly injure himself?
- Is the patient allergic to any medications?
- Does the patient take seizure medication?
- Did the patient take his seizure medication today?
- When was the last time the patient suffered a seizure?
- Was or is this seizure typical?

Physical Exam

Head, neck, and face:

- Excessive salivation
- Possible cyanosis to mucous membrane and face
- Bitten tongue
- Unequal pupils

Extremities:

- Weak or paralyzed on one side
- General weakness
- Deformities, pain, and swelling from fractures resulting from convulsion
- Unequal grip strength on one side of body

Baseline Vital Signs

- BP: increased or normal
- HR: increased
- RR: increased, irregular, decreased, shallow, or absent
- Skin: warm to hot, moist to wet
- Pupils: possibly unequal and dilated, sluggish to respond
- SpO_2: may be $< 95\%$ as a result of the seizure or as an indication of hypoxia causing the seizure
- BGL: a blood glucose level of < 60 mg/dL may be the cause of the seizure

FIGURE 19-5a ✱ Assessment summary: seizures. *continued*

Emergency Care Protocol

SEIZURES

1. Establish and maintain an open airway. Insert a nasopharyngeal airway if the epileptic patient is unresponsive or has been actively seizing for greater than 5 minutes. Insert a nasopharyngeal airway immediately if the patient is seizing from an etiology other than epilepsy.
2. Suction secretions as necessary.
3. If the patient is actively seizing, or if breathing is inadequate in the postictal phase, provide positive pressure ventilation with supplemental oxygen at a rate of 10–12 ventilations/minute for an adult and 12–20 ventilations/minute for an infant or child. Ventilations may be difficult to deliver because of resistance related to convulsions.
4. If breathing is adequate, administer oxygen by nonrebreather mask at 15 lpm.
5. Place the patient in a lateral recumbent position.
6. Consider advanced life support backup if the patient is actively seizing.
7. Transport.
8. Perform a reassessment every 5 minutes.

FIGURE 19-5b ✱ Emergency care protocol: seizures.

Emergency Care Algorithm: **Seizures**

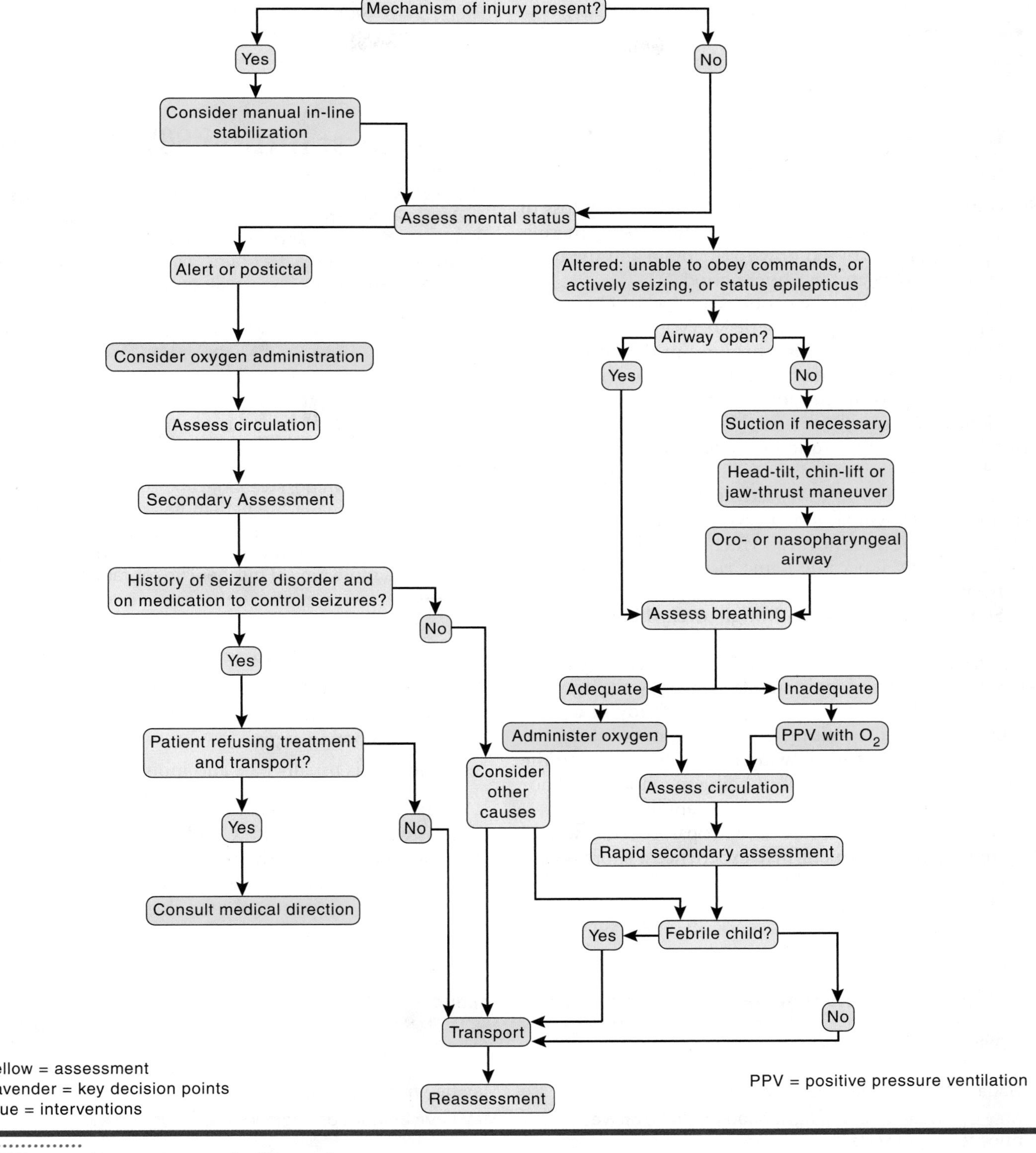

FIGURE 19-6 ✱ Emergency care algorithm: seizures.

Key Terms

syncope a brief period of unresponsiveness caused by a lack of blood flow to the brain; fainting.

Objective 19-12
Describe common causes of syncope.

Objective 19-13
Describe the assessment and care of patients with syncope, including differentiating syncope from seizure.

▶ Syncope

Syncope, or fainting, is a sudden and temporary loss of consciousness. It occurs when, for some reason, there is a temporary lack of blood flow to the brain and the brain is deprived of oxygen for a brief period.

A common cause of syncope is an overwhelming influence of the parasympathetic nervous system that causes blood vessels to dilate throughout the body. With a patient in a standing or seated position, gravity causes the blood to pool in the lower extremities, decreasing blood flow and perfusion to the brain. The hypoperfused brain no longer functions adequately and the patient has a syncopal episode. This type of faint is commonly referred to as a vasovagal faint. A large portion of the parasympathetic nervous system is transmitted through the vagas nerve, which has a dilating effect on the vessels. Hence the name *vaso* (vessel) *vagal* (vagus nerve).

Some patients feel as though everything is going dark, and then they suddenly become unresponsive. Syncope usually occurs when the patient is standing up or when the patient suddenly stands up from a sitting position. The collapse that follows puts the body in a horizontal position, distributing the pull of gravity along the length of the body and allowing blood circulation to the brain to improve. As a result of being in a horizontal position, the patient generally recovers rapidly.

Bystanders may confuse a syncopal episode with a seizure because the patient may experience a short period of jerky muscle movement during the episode (Table 19-3). The difference is that with syncope:

Understanding BODY PROCESSES

Syncope may result when the vessels in the body suddenly dilate. Gravity causes the blood to begin pooling in the extremities and lower areas of the body, decreasing the perfusion to the brain. The decrease in brain perfusion causes the syncopal episode or "faint." The patient recovers quickly when placed supine, which restores circulation to the brain. ■

ASSESSMENT Tips

A typical faint or syncopal episode may be preceded by the patient yawning, sweating, and complaining of dizziness and nausea. If the patient has a sudden syncopal episode (faints) during exertion, it may be an indication that a cardiac rhythm disturbance caused the syncope and not a more typical mechanism for fainting. ■

- The episode usually begins in a standing position.
- The patient remembers feeling faint or light-headed.
- The patient becomes responsive almost immediately after becoming supine.
- The skin is usually pale and moist.

Many patients who faint are afraid that something serious is wrong with them. Conduct primary and secondary assessments. Place the patient in a supine position to allow for improved blood flow to the brain, and provide reassurance. Your protocol may also instruct you to ele-

TABLE 19-3 Differentiation Between Seizures and Syncope

Syncope	Seizure
Usually begins in standing position	May begin in any position
May complain of being light-headed, dizzy, or weak prior to the episode	May have an aura or begin without warning
Sudden loss of consciousness that immediately returns when supine or prone	Sudden loss of consciousness that persists, then has a gradual return to consciousness
May have some muscle twitching	Convulsive muscle activity or repetitive movements during unconsciousness
Skin is usually cool, moist, and pale	Skin may be warm and sweaty

Key Points
Syncope is generally self-correcting, once the patient is horizontal and blood circulation to the brain improves. If the patient does not recover quickly, consider other possible causes for the altered mental status.

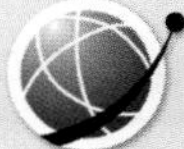

Media Resources
Go to www.bradybooks.com for mykit. Highlights:

- *Video:* Seizures and Epilepsy
- *Video:* Tonic Clonic Seizures

vate the legs 8 to 12 inches. If any complaints, signs, or symptoms are present (in addition to the syncope itself)—based on the SpO_2 reading, complaint, signs, and symptoms—place the patient on oxygen. Keep the patient in a supine position and assess the vital signs.

Because most patients fully recover before you even arrive at the scene, many refuse transport. However, you should encourage them to seek medical attention because of the seriousness of some causes of syncope. See Table 19-4. Consult with medical direction or follow your local protocol in this situation. Document your assessment findings and have the patient and a witness sign a refusal form if the patient is not to be cared for or transported.

Syncope could be a sign of a serious illness or injury. This is particularly true in older patients in whom cardiac and neurological causes are common. If the patient faints, or has an episode of syncope, and is not responding appropriately upon your arrival, consider the condition an altered mental status. Perform primary and secondary assessments and manage the patient's airway, breathing, oxygenation, and circulation as in any altered mental status patient. If the patient has not fallen "flat," or you suspect he may have injured his vertebral column or spinal cord, place him in a supine position for assessment while being careful to maintain manual stabilization of the head and spine.

TABLE 19-4 Some Serious Causes of Syncope

- Myocardial infarction
- Cardiac dysrhythmias
- Stroke or TIA
- Hypovolemia
- Drug use or poisoning
- Pulmonary embolism
- Cardiac tamponade

CHAPTER REVIEW

SUMMARY

A seizure results from abnormal impulses within the brain. The impulses cause certain signs and symptoms to occur based on the type of seizure and what area of the brain is affected. Epilepsy is the most common cause of seizures; however, there are patients in whom there is no known cause for the seizure activity. A convulsion is the jerky muscular movement most often associated with seizure activity. This is only one phase of the seizure and usually lasts for 1–2 minutes. The typical generalized tonic-clonic seizure patient has an aura, a tonic phase, a hypertonic phase, a clonic phase, and then a postictal phase. Most seizures are self-limited and last for only a few minutes. If the seizure lasts longer than 5 minutes or if the patient seizes and then seizes again without a period of consciousness between, he is experiencing status epilepticus. This is a severe condition and a dire emergency that requires immediate and aggressive emergency care and transport.

There are two major categories of seizures: generalized and partial. Generalized seizures typically involve both hemispheres of the brain or the wake/sleep area, causing unconsciousness. Partial seizures usually only involve one cerebral hemisphere, thus the patient maintains some level of consciousness during the seizure. A simple partial seizure does not produce a loss of consciousness, whereas a complex partial seizure is associated with an altered mental status.

Syncope, or fainting, is a condition that may be fairly benign or may be an indication of a serious underlying medical problem. The patient who experiences a simple episode of syncope will recover quickly once he is placed in a supine position and adequate blood flow returns to the brain.

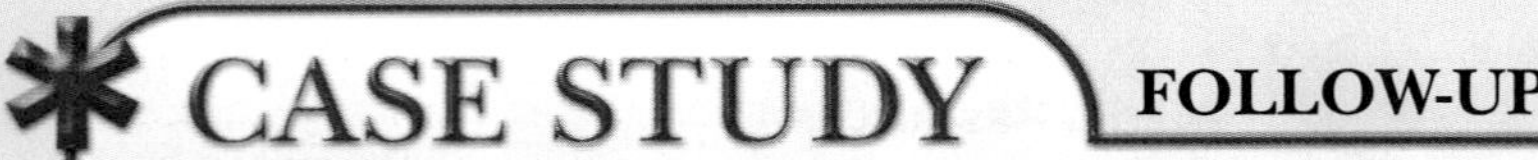

SCENE SIZE-UP

You have been dispatched to the mall for a 23-year-old female patient who is seizing. Your response time is only 2 minutes. The fire department first-response unit is on the scene. Firefighter Wright indicates that there is a large crowd in the mall, but the scene is safe. You and your partner gather the jump kit, suction unit, backboard, head immobilization device, and a set of cervical spinal immobilization collars, and load them onto the stretcher.

As you approach, a large crowd surrounds the patient. She is supine and actively seizing. Firefighter Demarco is cradling her head to protect it from striking the hard floor and maintaining an airway with a jaw thrust. The patient's sister is at her side, holding her hand. You and your partner introduce yourself as EMTs and ask for the patient's name. The sister states, "She is my sister and she is an epileptic. Her name is Carmen Escobar." In an attempt to determine if the patient has injured herself, you ask, "Did she fall to the ground or strike anything as she began to seize?" The sister indicates that Carmen said she felt a seizure coming on, and her sister gently helped Carmen to the ground. There are no immediate indications of a mechanism of injury.

PRIMARY ASSESSMENT

Your general impression of the patient is a young adult female who has a history of epilepsy. The patient is having generalized seizure activity throughout her body. Your partner assesses the airway, breathing, and circulation. The airway has been opened and is being maintained by the firefighter Emergency Medical Responder. Carmen's breathing is irregular and shallow at approximately 18 per minute. The pulse is strong at a rate of approximately 110 per minute. Firefighter Wright places a nonrebreather mask on the patient, providing oxygen at 15 lpm. You ask, "How long has she been seizing?" The sister answers, "About 3 minutes." You ask, "Do you know if this is a typical type seizure for her?" She replies, "Carmen gets this unusual taste in her mouth, then goes unconscious, seizes for a few minutes, and then becomes real tired and weak."

Carmen's seizure activity abruptly stops. You immediately reassess her airway, which appears to be patent. The breathing is deep at a rate of about 20 per minute. The pulse remains strong at approximately 110 per minute. The skin is warm and moist.

Carmen makes incomprehensible sounds. You ask, "Can you tell me your name?" She mumbles, "Carmen."

SECONDARY ASSESSMENT

You begin by gathering a history. Carmen appears to be slowly regaining her orientation, so you first direct the questions to her. When she is unable to answer some questions, you then seek an answer from her sister. In your questioning, you determine that Carmen has recurring seizures as a result of her epilepsy, and that they are controlled with her medication.

She states that this seizure was normal for her condition, and she experienced nothing unusual. She states, "I had this metallic taste in my mouth, so I knew I was about to seize. I told my sister to help me to the floor. After that, I don't remember anything until I woke up and saw you here." You ask, "How do you feel right now?" Carmen responds, "I feel like I just did aerobics for about 3 hours! I'm totally exhausted, and I just feel like sleeping. I also feel so embarrassed."

She has no allergies and is on Tegretol to control the seizures. You ask, "Have you taken your medication as prescribed?" Carmen states, "Yes, I took it this morning. I have about one seizure a month even with the medication." She has no other pertinent past medical history and her last intake of food or drink was about an hour prior to the episode. She was simply walking down the concourse in the mall looking at crafts when she experienced the aura and subsequent seizure.

Carmen's baseline vital signs are as follows: breathing normal at 16 per minute; radial pulse strong at 92 per minute; skin warm, normal color, and slightly moist; pupils equal and reactive; and blood pressure 134/82 mmHg. The pulse oximeter reveals an SpO_2 of 98%. The BGL is 86 mg/dL when checked on the glucose meter.

REASSESSMENT

Carmen is helped up to a nearby bench. She refuses to be transported to the hospital. You contact medical direction and report the history and physical exam findings. Medical direction instructs you to document your history and physical exam findings on an EMS report form, inform the patient that you are requesting that she be transported to the medical facility, and have her and her sister sign the refusal form. The patient complies. You remove the oxygen, and quickly reassess the vital signs. Before you leave, you ask Carmen if she is feeling any abnormal symptoms. She says, "No, this is a typical seizure for me, and I'm used to it. I don't know why they called the ambulance anyway. Thanks for your help, though."

"If you should suffer another seizure, be sure to contact us," you say. As you pack up your equipment, Carmen and her sister walk off into the crowd.

IN REVIEW

1. Explain why the airway is frequently compromised in the actively seizing or postictal patient.
2. List pertinent questions to ask the seizure patient, relatives, or bystanders during the history.
3. Name the five stages of a generalized tonic-clonic seizure and the signs and symptoms associated with each stage.
4. Describe the emergency care steps recommended for treating a generalized seizure.
5. Define status epilepticus and describe how you would care for a patient who is in status epilepticus.
6. List the common conditions or injuries that may cause seizures.
7. Define and describe syncope and explain how you can distinguish it from a seizure.

CRITICAL THINKING

You arrive on the scene of a construction accident and find a 34-year-old male patient who was struck in the head by a falling brick. You note obvious trauma to the head. The patient is having convulsive-type movement. Blood and vomitus are coming from his mouth. The radial pulse is 142 bpm. The skin is moist and warm with cyanosis noted to the nail beds. You don't note any other injury to the body.

1. How would you manage the airway in this patient?
2. Would spinal injury management be a consideration?
3. What type of seizure do you suspect the patient is experiencing?
4. What do you suspect is the cause of the seizure?
5. What emergency care would you provide for the patient?

PEARSON

EXPLORE mybradykit™

Please go to **www.bradybooks.com** to access mykit for this text. You will find quizzes, critical thinking scenarios, weblinks, animations, and videos related to this chapter—and much more. Look for online information on status epilepticus and syncope as well as video clips on seizures and epilepsy.

Register your access code from the front of your book by going to **www.bradybooks.com** and selecting the mykit links.

CHAPTER 20

Acute Diabetic Emergencies

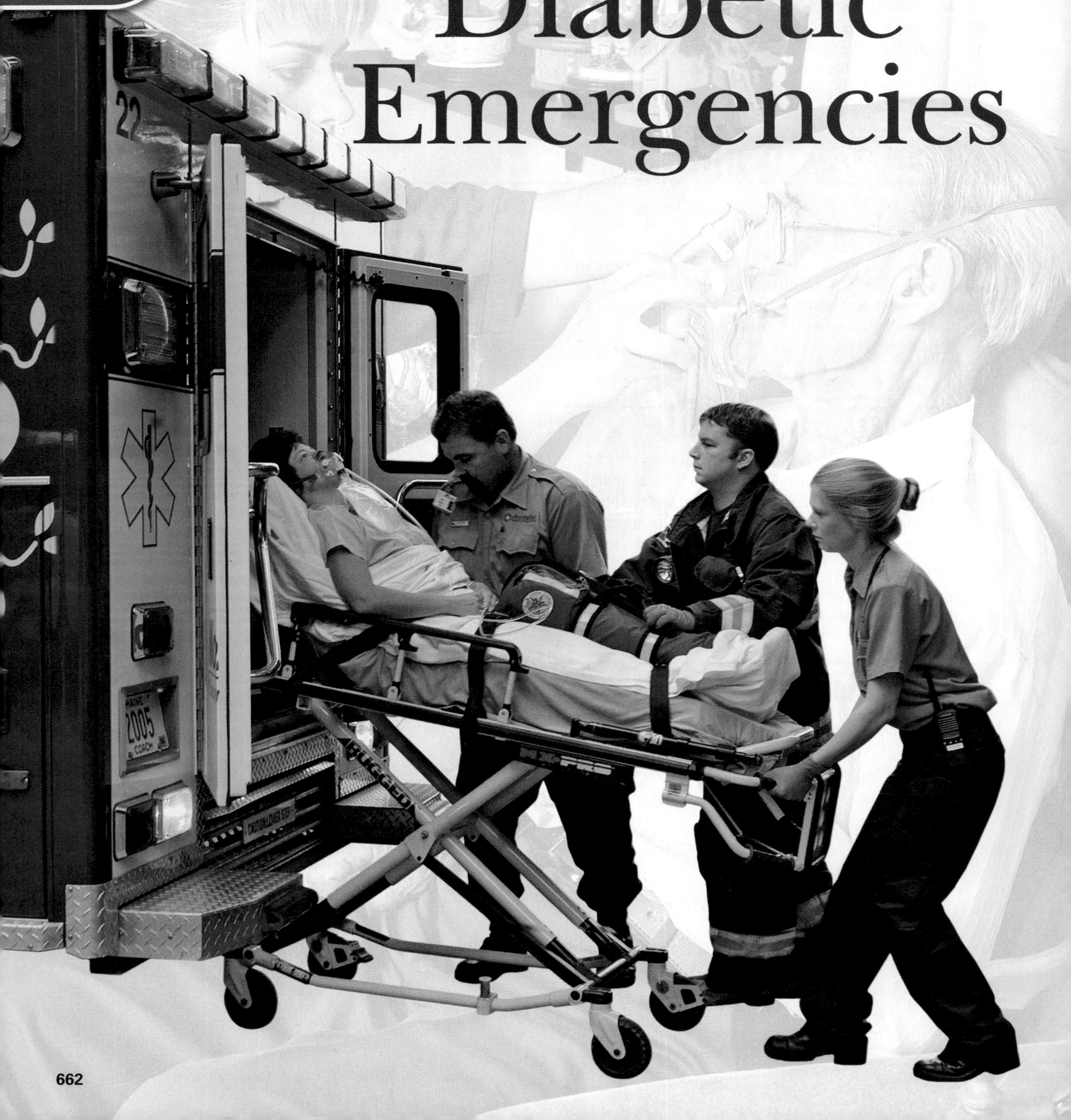

Navigation Guide

The following items provide an overview to the purpose and content of this chapter. The Standard and Competency are from the new National EMS Education Standards.

STANDARD **Medicine** (Content Area: Endocrine Disorders)

COMPETENCY Applies fundamental knowledge to provide basic emergency care and transportation based on assessment findings for an acutely ill patient.

OBJECTIVES: After reading this chapter, you should be able to:

20-1. Define key terms introduced in this chapter.
20-2. Describe the following regarding glucose:
- **a.** The function of glucose in the body
- **b.** Response of brain cells and other body cells to insufficient glucose levels
- **c.** Relationships of glucose and water

20-3. Describe how insulin and glucagon function to control blood glucose levels.
20-4. Describe how glucose levels are regulated in normal metabolism.
20-5. Explain the purposes and process of checking blood glucose levels.
20-6. Discuss the pathophysiology of diabetes mellitus (DM) and contrast type 1 insulin-dependent diabetes mellitus (IDDM) with type 2 non-insulin-dependent diabetes mellitus (NIDDM).
20-7. Discuss the pathophysiology, assessment, and emergency medical care of a hypoglycemic emergency.
20-8. Identify indications and contraindications to the administration of oral glucose.
20-9. Discuss the pathophysiology, assessment, and emergency medical care of diabetic ketoacidosis (DKA).
20-10. Compare and contrast the speed of onset and the signs and symptoms of hypoglycemia and hyperglycemia.
20-11. Describe the primary differences between DKA and hyperglycemic hyperosmolar nonketotic syndrome (HHNS).
20-12. Discuss the pathophysiology, assessment, and emergency medical care of HHNS.
20-13. Discuss the assessment-based approach to a patient with an altered mental status in a diabetic emergency.

KEY TERMS: Page references indicate first major use in this chapter. For complete definitions, see the Glossary at the back of the book.

diabetes mellitus (DM) p. 664
diabetic ketoacidosis (DKA) p. 670
glucagon p. 666
glucose p. 664
hyperglycemia p. 668
hyperglycemic hyperosmolar nonketotic syndrome (HHNS) p. 670
hypoglycemia p. 668
insulin p. 665
oral glucose p. 672
type 1 diabetes p. 670
type 2 diabetes p. 670

MEDIA RESOURCES: Please go to www.bradybooks.com to access mykit for this text. You will find quizzes, critical thinking scenarios, weblinks, animations, and videos related to this chapter—and much more. Look for online information on insulin resistance and hypoglycemia. You will also find video clips on diabetes and how to use a blood glucose meter.

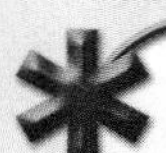

CASE STUDY

The Dispatch
EMS Unit 106—proceed to 514 Chicago Avenue—you have a 66-year-old male patient who appears to be disoriented and belligerent. Be advised, the neighbor placed the call. Time out is 1402 hours.

Upon Arrival
As you and your partner approach the house, a woman walks out the front door. She says, "It's Mr. Bennet. I found him in my garden next door. When I asked what he was doing, he began cursing at me.

continued

He's always such a nice man. I can't believe how he's acting. Now he isn't making much sense when I talk to him." You proceed into the house and find the patient sitting on the edge of the couch mumbling incomprehensible words.

How Would You Proceed to Assess and Care for This Patient?

During this chapter, you will learn about assessment and emergency care for a patient suffering from an acute diabetic emergency. Later, we will return to the case and apply the procedures learned.

Introduction

Diabetes mellitus (DM) is a disease that frequently causes changes in the patient's mental status resulting from alterations in the blood glucose (blood sugar) level. The mental state may range from disorientation to complete unresponsiveness. Significant deterioration of the mental status from acute diabetic emergencies can lead to serious airway and breathing compromise. Brain cell damage and death may occur if the blood glucose reaches a very low level. Acute diabetic emergencies may include hypoglycemia, where the blood glucose level is too low, or diabetic ketoacidosis or hyperglycemic hyperosmolar nonketotic syndrome, where the blood glucose level is excessively high. It is important for the EMT to recognize and provide emergency care for patients who are experiencing an acute diabetic emergency.

More than 10 million Americans have been diagnosed with diabetes mellitus. Unfortunately, approximately 5.4 million other Americans have diabetes but have not yet been diagnosed. Many times, a person's first indication of having the disease is a change in mental status, such as confusion, disorientation, or even loss of consciousness. Prompt recognition and appropriate emergency care of a patient who has an altered mental status because of an acute diabetic emergency is crucial. Long-term complications of diabetes mellitus may include vascular disease leading to stroke, heart attack, and peripheral vascular disease; kidney disease; nerve dysfunction; and retinal nerve disease leading to blindness.

Understanding Diabetes Mellitus

In order to have a basic understanding of diabetic emergencies, it is first necessary to understand normal metabolism—that is, how sugar acts within the body and how some of the hormones from the endocrine system control the movement and maintain the level of glucose in the blood when the body is functioning normally.

Glucose (Sugar)

There are three major food sources for the body's cells. They are carbohydrates, fats, and proteins. Carbohydrates are a primary energy source for the cells. Three major sources of carbohydrates are sucrose (table sugar), lactose (milk and dairy products), and starches (potatoes, bread). These sugars are called complex sugars because of their structure. In the body, the complex sugars are broken down into simple sugars to be absorbed through the digestive tract and into the bloodstream. The simple sugars are **glucose**, galactose, and fructose.

After carbohydrate digestion, approximately 80 percent of the simple sugar is in the form of glucose. Following absorption by the digestive tract, close to 95 percent of the simple sugar entering the body to be used by the cells is in the form of glucose. Therefore, glucose is by far the most important sugar in the body. This is why the sugar levels in the blood are referred to as the blood glucose level.

Glucose is a major source of fuel for the cells. Maintenance of the glucose level in the blood is crucial to normal function of cells. Some cells are able to use fats and proteins as energy sources if little or no glucose is available in the blood; however, the brain cells are not able to use anything but glucose. Thus, cells in the rest of the body can continue to function by using other energy sources, whereas the brain cells (which do not store glucose), when deprived of glucose, will dysfunction, shut down, and eventually begin to die. When cells other than brain cells use other energy sources such as fats, they produce harmful by-products that eventually affect the cell function adversely.

Brain cells are extremely sensitive to a lack of glucose. They are almost immediately affected and will respond quickly to the decrease in available glucose. The brain cells cannot make glucose, they cannot store glucose for more than a few minutes, nor can they collect glucose in a concentration from the blood. As already noted, the consequences of the lack of glucose to brain cells for a short period of time are brain cell dysfunction. The most common sign of brain cell dysfunction is an altered mental status. As the glucose becomes more depleted, the mental status deteriorates further. If the drop in the

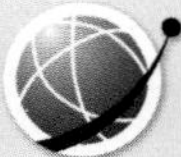

Media Resources

Go to www.bradybooks.com for mykit. Highlights:

- *Web Resource:* Insulin Resistance
- *Web Resource:* Hypoglycemia

Objective 20-2

Describe the function of glucose in the body.

Key Terms

diabetes mellitus (DM) a disease of altered relationships between glucose and insulin.

glucose a form of sugar that is the body's basic source of energy.

insulin a hormone that promotes the movement of glucose from the blood into the cells.

blood glucose level is severe and prolonged, the brain cells will eventually die.

Because glucose is a large molecule, it has a tendency to attract water when it moves, an action known as osmotic pressure. It acts similarly to sodium, in a sense. There is a familiar saying, "Where sodium goes, water goes." This means that when sodium crosses into a cell, water will follow it and cause the cell to swell. If the patient is losing large amounts of sodium from urination or sweating, the sodium will draw out a large amount of water, and the patient will become dehydrated from the water loss.

The glucose molecule will also cause water to follow it. Thus, if a large amount of glucose moves across a membrane, a large amount of water will follow it. This is one reason why glucose administration is dangerous and proven to be detrimental in patients with a head injury or stroke. By giving glucose, the brain allows more glucose to cross into the cells and the glucose brings water with it. This causes brain cells to swell, leading to more edema (swelling) within the skull, which worsens the head injury or stroke.

Understanding BODY PROCESSES

As glucose molecules cross over a membrane, they pull water with them. The fact that glucose will move directly into brain cells without the aid of insulin explains how glucose can worsen edema in the patient with a head injury or stroke. An increase in glucose may also increase the demand for oxygen, because the cells of the body require oxygen to help convert glucose into energy. ■

Frequently, excess glucose spills off into the urine and the patient urinates large amounts of glucose, excreting with it water that was not reabsorbed into the body because the glucose molecule drew it into the urine. The patient may eventually become dehydrated, which is a common complication in a diabetic patient.

Hormones That Control Blood Glucose Levels

The two hormones primarily responsible for controlling levels of blood glucose are *insulin* and *glucagon*, both of which are secreted by the pancreas. Insulin and glucagon have opposite effects on blood glucose level.

Insulin

Insulin is secreted when the blood glucose level is elevated. It has three main functions:

1. It increases the movement of glucose out of the blood and into the cells.
2. It causes the liver to take up the glucose out of the blood and convert it into glycogen, the stored form of glucose.
3. It decreases the blood glucose level by the actions listed in 1 and 2: facilitating the movement of the glucose into the cells and the liver.

Many people believe that insulin carries glucose into the cells. That is not true. What occurs is that insulin attaches to the cell at a specific (receptor) site and causes another channel on the cell membrane to open. A protein then carries the glucose into the cell through this channel. Thus, insulin facilitates the movement of glucose into the cell. If insulin is not available, glucose moves into the cell at a rate approximately 10 times slower. This causes glucose to build up in the bloodstream, causing the blood glucose level to increase. Ironically, as the blood glucose level is drastically increasing because of the lack of the insulin necessary to facilitate moving it into the cells, the cells are beginning to starve because they have no fuel or energy source. The cells begin to look for an alternative energy source, which is normally fats and proteins (Figure 20-1*).

One organ that does not need insulin to help move glucose into the cells is the brain. Glucose will cross the blood-brain barrier readily, whether insulin is present or not. However, while the other cells can use fats and proteins for energy, the brain can only use glucose. As glucose becomes depleted in the blood, the brain begins to suffer severely and begins to dysfunction as it loses its energy source. If left untreated, the brain cells will eventually die. Therefore, a patient with a low blood glucose level is in a serious condition and requires immediate emergency care.

Understanding BODY PROCESSES

Insulin is not required to move glucose across the blood-brain barrier and into the brain cells. In a diabetic with a high blood glucose level and a low or absent insulin level, the brain will continue to get glucose from the blood while the other cells in the body are starving for glucose and beginning to use fat and protein for energy. ■

Objective 20-3
Describe how insulin and glucagon function to control blood glucose levels.

Objective 20-4
Describe how glucose levels are regulated in normal metabolism.

Key Terms
glucagon a hormone that stimulates the liver to convert stored glycogen and other substances into glucose.

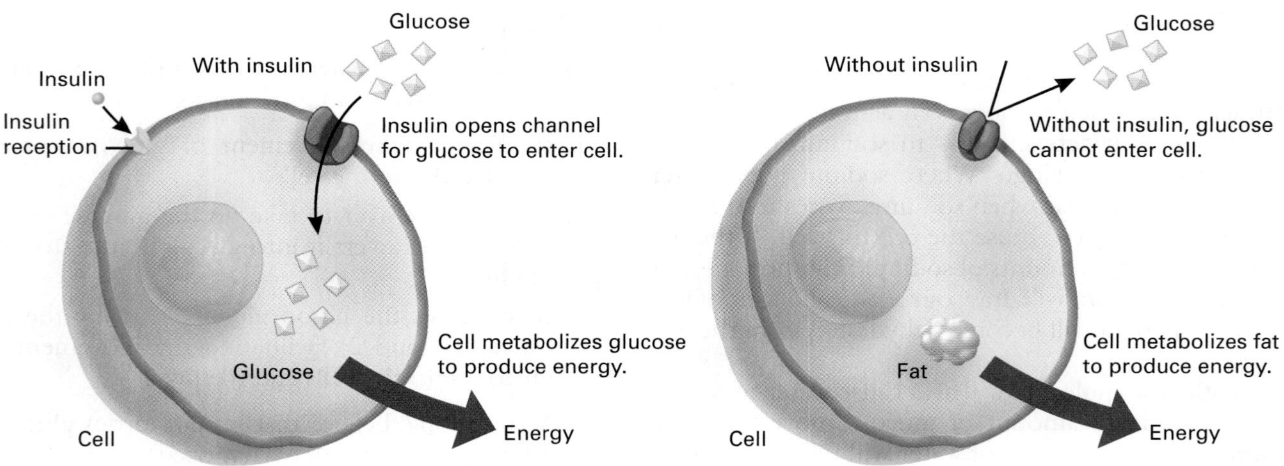

FIGURE 20-1 * Glucose movement into the cell with insulin and the inability of glucose to get into the cell without insulin.

Glucagon

As mentioned earlier, the function of **glucagon** is exactly the opposite of insulin's function. Insulin is secreted when the blood glucose level is high and works to decrease the blood glucose level (by helping to move glucose out of the blood and into the cells). Glucagon, on the other hand, is secreted when the blood glucose level is low and will work to increase the blood glucose level. The major functions of glucagon are:

1. It converts glycogen stored in the liver back into glucose and releases it into the blood.
2. It converts other, noncarbohydrate substances into glucose.
3. It increases and maintains the blood glucose level by the actions listed in 1 and 2: converting glycogen and other substances into glucose.

Glucagon's major role in the body is to raise and maintain the blood glucose level. When the blood glucose level decreases to approximately 70 mg/dL, glucagon is secreted. As just noted, glucagon then begins to convert liver glycogen and other substances into glucose to raise and maintain the blood glucose level until the next meal.

Understanding BODY PROCESSES

Insulin and glucagon have opposite functions. Insulin decreases the blood glucose level by moving glucose out of the blood into the cells as well as into the liver, where it is stored as glycogen. Glucagon raises the blood glucose level by converting the glycogen stored in the liver back into glucose to be released into the blood, as well as converting noncarbohydrates into glucose. ■

Other Hormones

Many other hormones are also released to help maintain the blood glucose level. One of these hormones is epinephrine (adrenaline). Epinephrine is released by the adrenal glands when the blood glucose level decreases to a dangerously low level. Epinephrine stops the secretion of insulin and promotes the release of stored glucose from the liver as well as the conversion of other substances into glucose. Many of the signs you see in a patient with a low blood glucose level are caused by epinephrine. We will discuss the signs and symptoms later in the section on hypoglycemia (low blood glucose).

Normal Metabolism and Glucose Regulation

The blood glucose level of a person who has fasted for 8–12 hours would normally read 80–90 mg/dL. Because patients are not always in a fasting state when you

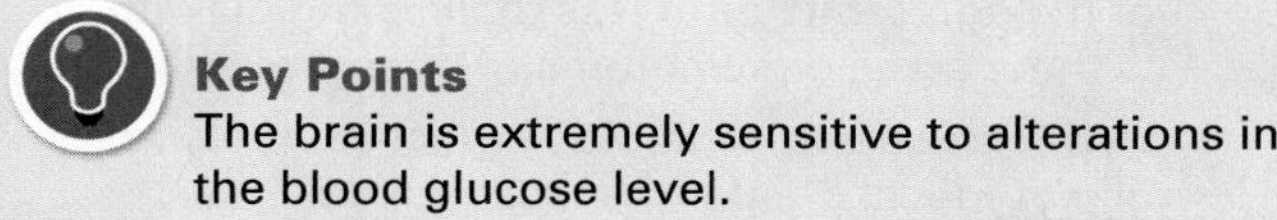

Key Points
The brain is extremely sensitive to alterations in the blood glucose level.

Key Points
The blood glucose level rises when a meal is eaten. A few hours after the meal, the blood glucose level returns to normal.

test their blood glucose level, many sources use much wider ranges of 70–120 mg/dL as a normal blood glucose level.

Because the brain is extremely sensitive to alterations in the blood glucose level, it is necessary for the body to maintain the blood glucose level within this very narrow range. As already explained, this is accomplished primarily by insulin and glucagon (Figure 20-2*). Within 1 hour after a meal, a person's blood glucose level increases to 120–140 mg/dL. When the blood glucose rises, it triggers the pancreas to secrete insulin, which is released from the pancreas and immediately begins to increase the movement of the glucose into the cells. About two-thirds of the glucose is taken up by the liver, which converts it to glycogen to be stored by the liver and muscles for later use. The brain takes up as much glucose as it needs without the aid of insulin. Obviously, these processes of moving glucose out of the bloodstream and into the body cells, the liver, and the brain deplete the blood of glucose—in other words, lower the blood glucose level. Consequently, a few hours after a meal, the blood glucose level drops back to a normal level. As the blood glucose level decreases, the amount of insulin being secreted from the pancreas also decreases.

Eventually, as the cells continue to require and use insulin in the hours after a meal, the blood glucose level drops near the lower end of the normal range. The pancreas recognizes the decreased blood glucose level and secretes glucagon. The glucagon causes the liver to begin converting the glycogen (stored glucose) back into glucose and releasing it into the bloodstream. Other, noncarbohydrate substances will also be converted into glucose. This will raise the blood glucose level and maintain it in that normal range until the next meal.

Glycogen stores in the liver can last for up to 24–48 hours. After that, there is typically no more glycogen left in the liver to be converted into glucose and the blood glucose may drop drastically, while fats and proteins will begin to be used by the body cells at a high rate for energy.

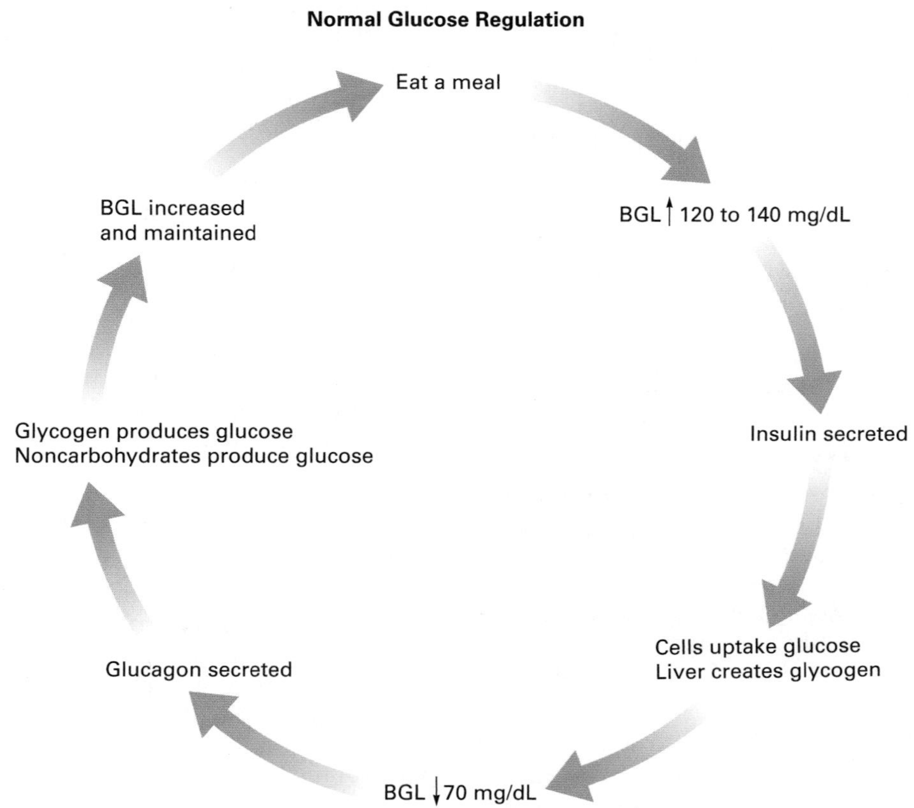

FIGURE 20-2 * Normal glucose regulation.

Thinking Critically

When assessing the blood glucose level, it is important to determine when the patient last had something to eat or drink. Why?

Objective 20-5

Explain the purposes and process of checking blood glucose levels.

Key Terms

hypoglycemia low blood glucose. A blood glucose level of 60 mg/dL with signs or symptoms of hypoglycemia or of less than 50 mg/dL with or without signs or symptoms of hypoglycemia.

hyperglycemia high blood glucose. A blood glucose level greater than 120 mg/dL.

Checking the Blood Glucose Level

Portable blood glucose meters, commonly referred to as glucometers by EMS personnel, are available to both the EMS crew and the diabetic patient. These devices can fairly accurately determine the blood glucose level (BGL): the amount of glucose in the blood. (Glucose is a simple form of sugar; therefore, the terms *glucose* and *sugar* are usually used interchangeably.) The glucose meter analyzes a drop of capillary blood, typically obtained from a finger stick to the patient, and provides a numerical reading that indicates the concentration of glucose in the blood.

Blood glucose is measured in milligrams per deciliter (mg/dL). A normal blood glucose range is 80–120 mg/dL. A reading less than 80 mg/dL may indicate a lower-than-normal level of glucose (sugar) in the blood, whereas a reading greater than 120 mg/dL may indicate a higher-than-normal amount of glucose in the blood.

It is important to determine when the patient last had something to eat or drink. The blood glucose level in a nondiabetic patient following a meal will typically rise to 120–140 mg/dL. Thus, this is not considered abnormal. Likewise, after an 8- to 12-hour fast, a nondiabetic patient's glucose will typically read 80–90 mg/dL. However, in the diabetic patient, the blood glucose may be as high as 120 mg/dL after an 8- to 12-hour fast. Blood glucose readings as high as 200 mg/dL may be normal in a diabetic patient.

Hypoglycemia is typically defined as a BGL of 60 mg/dL or less with signs or symptoms of hypoglycemia or a BGL of less than 50 mg/dL with or without signs or symptoms of hypoglycemia. The primary sign of hypoglycemia is an altered mental status. **Hyperglycemia** can be defined as a persistent BGL greater than 120 mg/dL.

ASSESSMENT Tips

Determine when the patient last had something to eat or drink when you are checking the blood glucose level. In a nondiabetic patient, the blood glucose will normally rise to 120–140 mg/dL following a meal containing carbohydrates. This would not be considered abnormally high. If the blood glucose level was 120–140 mg/dL after an 8- to 12-hour fast, however, it would be considered abnormally high. ■

The blood glucose meter should be used as an adjunct to your assessment and emergency medical care. It is possible to get an inaccurate reading from improper use of the glucose meter, expired test strips, or a poorly calibrated device. Use the blood glucose reading in conjunction with the information collected in the history and the signs found in the physical examination to make a determination on whether to treat the patient as a diabetic emergency.

It is very important to determine whether medical direction and local protocol allow the EMT to test the patient's blood glucose level on the blood glucose meter. If the EMT is permitted to check the patient's BGL with a glucose meter, the EMT must learn the proper use of the particular device carried by his EMS service, since many models are available and in use. As easy as it is to obtain a blood glucose reading with the device, it is just as easy to make a mistake and get an inaccurate reading if the device is improperly used.

Testing the Blood Glucose Level with a Glucose Meter

The blood glucose level should be tested prior to the administration of any oral glucose or sugar-containing solution. In order to test the blood glucose level with a glucose meter, you will need the following supplies and equipment:

- Glucose meter
- Glucose meter test strips
- Lancet
- Lancet device (optional)
- Alcohol swabs

To get an accurate glucose reading, you need to get a good blood sample. To obtain a good blood sample, follow the steps in Table 20-1. Also see EMT Skills 20-1.

Diabetes Mellitus (DM)

Diabetes mellitus (DM) is a condition in which there is disturbance in the metabolism of carbohydrates, fats, and proteins. The primary problem in this condition is either (1) a lack of insulin being secreted by the pancreas or (2) the inability of the cell receptors to recognize the insulin and allow the glucose to enter at a normal rate.

If there is no insulin or a minimal amount of insulin in the blood, the cells will take up glucose at a much slower rate. Or, if there is enough insulin but there is a deficit in the cell receptor sites that prevents them from recognizing

Key Points

When there is a deficiency of insulin, body cells are deprived of glucose but the brain is not, because insulin is not required for glucose to cross over into the brain.

Objective 20-6

Discuss the pathophysiology of diabetes mellitus (DM) and contrast type 1 insulin-dependent diabetes mellitus (IDDM) with type 2 non-insulin-dependent diabetes mellitus (NIDDM).

TABLE 20-1 Steps for Glucose Measurement

1. **Prepare the lancet and lancet device.** A lancet alone could be used to prick the finger; however, it is usually more comfortable for the patient and easier for the EMT to use a lancet device to stick the finger to obtain the blood sample. The lancet device makes it easier to gauge the depth of the stick and provides an extremely quick prick of the finger.
2. **Let the arm hang down at the patient's side if possible.** This will allow for better blood flow to the fingers. If the fingers are cold, attempt to quickly warm the fingers by placing them in your hands for a brief period. This will provide better blood flow to the finger and a better sample.
3. **Remove a new test strip from the vial. Insert the test strip.** The glucose meter will turn on automatically. (This step may vary, depending on the type of glucose meter. Follow the manufacturer's recommendations.)
4. **Match the code number** on the LED screen to the code number on the test strip vial.
5. **When the blood drop symbol flashes on the LED screen,** you are ready to continue with the test.
6. **Grasp the finger near the site to be pricked.** Cleanse it with an alcohol swab and let it dry completely before pricking the site. Squeeze the finger, forcing blood into the tip for 3 seconds.
7. **Keeping the hand downward, if possible, prick the side of the fingertip** and squeeze gently until a drop of blood is formed. Waste the first drop of blood onto a dressing and use the second drop for the test.
8. **Drop the blood onto the specified area on the test strip.** Some test strips may require that the finger be brought to the edge of the test strip, where the blood is absorbed by the strip. Be sure you completely understand the type of test strip you are using and the manufacturer's recommendations on its use. (There is a wide variety of test strips that may require blood placement in different areas on the strip. If the designated test area is not completely covered, it may be necessary to apply a second drop of blood to the site. Typically, this has to be done within 15 seconds of the first drop.)
9. **The blood glucose value will be displayed,** normally within 40–45 seconds. Record the value.
10. **Remove the test strip and place it in a biohazard container.** Turn the glucose meter off.

and attaching insulin, this will also cause a drastic reduction in the amount of glucose that is allowed to enter the cell. Either of these situations will cause an excessive amount of glucose to collect in the blood and raise the blood glucose level. In both situations, because the glucose is not able to enter the cells at a normal rate, the cells begin to starve for energy and must use other sources, such as fat. Even though the blood is filled with glucose molecules, they are not available to the cells for energy production.

One point that you must remember: Although the cells in the body are deprived of glucose, the brain is not, because insulin is not required for glucose to cross over into the brain cells. Therefore, in this situation, the brain has more glucose than it needs while the body cells are starving for glucose.

A patient with diabetes mellitus typically has an abnormally elevated blood glucose level because of a lack of insulin. An elevated blood glucose level is referred to as hyperglycemia. When the blood glucose level increases to about 185 mg/dL, the kidneys cannot reabsorb the high amount of glucose and begin to spill it out into the urine. Once the patient reaches a blood glucose level of 225 mg/dL, a significant amount of glucose will be lost in the urine. Remember the properties of glucose. It is a large molecule and will draw water to it. The excess glucose in the urine will draw water to be urinated out with it, leading to large amounts of body water loss. Over a period of time, this can lead to dehydration.

Because of the higher-than-normal loss of body water, diabetes mellitus patients typically complain of frequent thirst (polydipsia) and frequent urination (polyuria). Also, because the cells are starving for energy, the patient is typically hungry (polyphagia). This is referred to as the three Ps. The three Ps are signs that commonly alert physicians to a possible diagnosis of diabetes mellitus. Unfortunately, the first sign of the patient's diabetes mellitus may be one of the severe hyperglycemic conditions that we will discuss later in the section.

There are four types of diabetes mellitus. The two that you will most often find in the prehospital environment

Key Terms

type 1 diabetes condition in which the pancreas typically does not secrete any insulin; *insulin-dependent diabetes mellitus (IDDM)*.

type 2 diabetes diabetes that can be regulated by diet, exercise, and drugs other than insulin; *non-insulin-dependent diabetes mellitus (NIDDM)*.

Key Terms

diabetic ketoacidosis (DKA) hyperglycemia with low-to-absent insulin level, resulting in dehydration and a buildup of acid.

hyperglycemic hyperosmolar nonketotic syndrome (HHNS) hyperglycemia with some insulin, causing dehydration but no acid buildup.

Understanding BODY PROCESSES

Diabetic patients with high blood glucose levels have a tendency to lose large amounts of body water through excessive urination. If a patient presents with signs of dehydration, check the blood glucose level. ■

are **type 1 diabetes** and **type 2 diabetes**. Type 1 is also referred to as *insulin-dependent diabetes mellitus (IDDM)*, since these patients are required to inject or inhale insulin to regulate their blood glucose levels. The type 1 patient's pancreas usually does not secrete any insulin. These patients are typically younger when the diabetes occurs, most commonly under the age of 40. The peak age for onset of type 1 diabetes mellitus is 10–14 years. The patients are typically lean from weight loss. Their blood glucose levels are extremely high if untreated. These patients will suffer from the three Ps. Type 1 diabetics often have difficulty keeping their blood glucose level within the normal range, with the possibility of having too high or too low a blood glucose level. Therefore, they are prone to suffering from a hyperglycemic condition called **diabetic ketoacidosis (DKA)**. They may also suffer from hypoglycemia (low blood glucose). Type 1 diabetes is less common than type 2 diabetes.

Type 2 diabetes is also referred to as *non-insulin-dependent diabetes mellitus (NIDDM)*, because type 2 patients usually do not have to take insulin. However, they do have to regulate their diet and exercise and take oral drugs to help the pancreas secrete more insulin or to make the insulin that is secreted more effective in facilitating movement of glucose into the cells. Type 2 diabetic patients are usually middle-aged or older. They are typically overweight. Like type 1 diabetics, they suffer from high blood glucose levels if untreated and they may also present with a history of the three Ps. These patients are prone to a hyperglycemic condition called **hyperglycemic hyperosmolar nonketotic syndrome (HHNS)**.

It is estimated that 1–2 percent of the population has a true form of diabetes mellitus. Of these, approximately 25 percent suffer from type 1 (IDDM) and the remaining 75 percent suffer from type 2 (NIDDM). Diabetes mellitus is more common in Caucasians than in non-Caucasians.

The patient with diabetes mellitus is prone to a wide variety of diseases and disorders involving the blood vessels—such as heart attack, stroke, and kidney failure—from blockage of the vessels by fat deposits. The blood glucose level is typically high in the patient with diabetes mellitus. A blood glucose reading that is randomly taken may be greater than 200 mg/dL, compared to 70–120 mg/dL in a patient without diabetes mellitus. A fasting blood glucose level in a patient with diabetes mellitus averages greater than 140 mg/dL, as compared to 80–90 mg/dL in the patient without diabetes mellitus.

▶ Acute Diabetic Emergencies

The emergency conditions that you may be called to manage in the prehospital environment are related to a patient suffering from either a low blood glucose level (hypoglycemia) or a high blood glucose level (hyperglycemia). They are at two ends of a continuum of blood glucose levels (Figure 20-3∗).

Hypoglycemia

Hypoglycemia is the term for a low blood glucose level (*hypo* = low, *glyco* = glucose, *emia* = blood). This condition is more common in type 1 IDDM patients than in type 2 NIDDM patients. Hypoglycemia is the most dangerous acute complication of diabetes mellitus. It is estimated that 9–120 episodes of hypoglycemia will occur per 100 diabetic patients per year. It is one of the most common causes of coma in the diabetic patient.

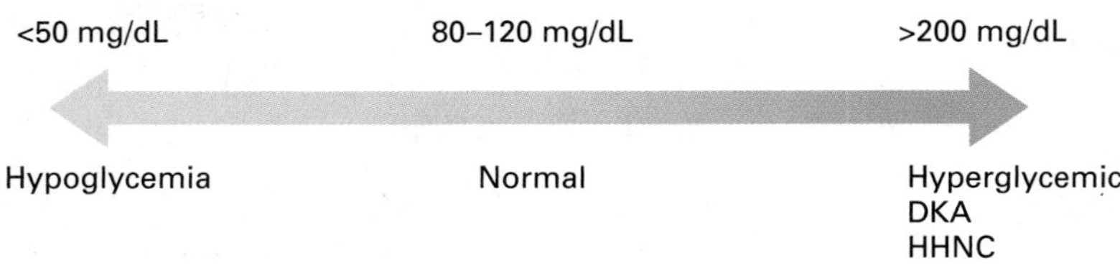

FIGURE 20-3 ∗ Diabetic emergency conditions.

Objective 20-7
Discuss the pathophysiology, assessment, and emergency medical care of a hypoglycemic emergency.

Key Points
The signs and symptoms of hypoglycemia result mainly from the body's release of epinephrine and from brain dysfunction.

Pathophysiology of Hypoglycemia

Hypoglycemia occurs when the amount of glucose in the blood falls below the normal lower limit. As noted earlier, it is typically defined as a blood glucose level less than 60 mg/dL with signs and symptoms of hypoglycemia or less than 50 mg/dL with or without signs and symptoms. The most common sign of hypoglycemia is an altered mental status. This is due to the sensitivity of the brain to a drop in the blood glucose level. As already discussed, the brain cells can use only glucose as an energy source, unlike other cells that can burn fat and protein for energy. As the blood glucose level continues to drop, the mental status of the patient continues to deteriorate. If the blood glucose level is not restored, the brain cells will begin to die.

Hypoglycemia usually occurs in type 1 IDDM where the patient must take insulin to regulate his blood glucose levels. This patient takes his insulin, but with excessive results (blood glucose levels decrease too much), for one of the following reasons:

- The patient takes his insulin and does not eat a meal.
- The patient takes his insulin, eats a meal, but drastically increases his activity beyond normal.
- The patient takes too much insulin—either takes too much at one time or forgets and takes an extra dose.

Type 2 NIDDM patients can also suffer hypoglycemia. The oral medications that they take can cause the blood glucose level to drop too far, resulting in hypoglycemia. Because these oral medications have long-lasting effects, hypoglycemia can be prolonged or can recur if these patients are not monitored.

When there is too much insulin in the blood—either because the patient did not eat after injecting the insulin or he took too much for the amount he ate—the insulin causes the cells in the body to take up most of the glucose from the blood, leaving very little for the brain. Remember that one of insulin's major functions is to help move glucose into the cell. If the patient takes his insulin, eats a meal, and then decides to run 5 miles, which is not a normal activity for the patient, the high activity will cause body cells to use the glucose at a much faster rate, leaving little behind in the blood for the brain. Either of these imbalances—too much insulin or too much exercise—will deplete the blood of glucose and cause the brain cells to begin to fail.

Deterioration of the mental status is a gauge of low blood glucose level and brain cell dysfunction. As the brain cells become more and more deprived of glucose, the mental status will deteriorate further. The patient's brain needs an influx of glucose quickly to reverse the brain cell dysfunction and prevent brain cell death.

Assessment Findings in Hypoglycemia

Hypoglycemia has commonly been referred to as "insulin shock" because of the shocklike signs and symptoms commonly seen with the condition. Many of these are caused by release of epinephrine.

As the blood glucose level drops, epinephrine is secreted at higher levels. The effect of the epinephrine is to shut down secretion of insulin and to stimulate secretion of glucagon, which, in turn, converts stored glycogen and other noncarbohydrate substances into glucose. As a result, many of the signs and symptoms seen in hypoglycemia are associated with the epinephrine circulating in the body. These signs and symptoms appear to be very similar to those in a patient in shock from poor perfusion.

Understanding BODY PROCESSES

When the blood glucose level is decreasing, epinephrine (adrenaline) is released. This produces the tachycardia, diaphoresis, and pale, cool skin typically seen in the hypoglycemic patient. The bizarre behavior, agitation, disorientation, and other mental status changes seen in hypoglycemic patients are due directly to an inadequate amount of glucose being provided to the brain cells. ■

The other signs and symptoms seen in hypoglycemia are from the brain dysfunction. The onset of hypoglycemia signs and symptoms is rapid, from a few minutes to about 20 minutes in most patients who become hypoglycemic. This is due to the rapid decline of brain function and secretion of epinephrine associated with the lack of glucose.

Signs and Symptoms Caused by Epinephrine Release

- Diaphoresis (sweating)
- Tremors
- Weakness
- Hunger
- Tachycardia (increased heart rate)
- Dizziness
- Pale, cool, clammy skin
- Warm sensation

Thinking Critically
What steps are the same and what steps are different for a hypoglycemic patient who is unresponsive and for one who is responsive?

Key Points
The severity of the signs and symptoms as correlated to the blood glucose level varies from patient to patient.

Key Terms
oral glucose a form of sugar often given as a gel, by mouth, to raise the blood glucose level.

Signs and Symptoms Caused by Brain Cell Dysfunction

- Confusion
- Drowsiness
- Disorientation
- Unresponsiveness
- Seizures (may occur in severe cases)
- Strokelike symptoms including hemiparesis

The hypoglycemic patient may present with bizarre or even violent behavior and, for this reason, the patient's condition may be mistaken for a behavioral or psychiatric disorder, drug use, or alcohol intoxication. This is potentially a tragic mistake since hypoglycemia can be fatal if not recognized and treated quickly. There are numerous cases of patients dying as a result of misinterpretation of the signs and symptoms of hypoglycemia. These patients are generally unaware of their actions. Coma (which is unresponsiveness to any noxious stimuli such as pain) may also result from hypoglycemia. Look for a medical identification bracelet, anklet, or necklace during your physical examination.

The severity of the signs and symptoms as correlated to the blood glucose level varies from patient to patient. One patient may be completely unresponsive at a blood glucose level of 45 mg/dL, whereas another at the same blood glucose level may still be responsive but confused. Have a high index of suspicion and do not develop tunnel vision when treating patients. Any patient who presents with an altered mental status, bizarre behavior, violence, or an intoxicated appearance, even if alcohol is smelled on the breath, must be assessed for possible hypoglycemia. This is when the glucose meter provides some valuable information. If the patient appears to be intoxicated and the blood glucose reading comes back as 58 mg/dL, you would treat the patient for hypoglycemia. If the same patient had a blood glucose reading of 124 mg/dL, you would treat him as intoxicated. As a note of interest, alcohol will inhibit the body's ability to convert other noncarbohydrate substances into glucose during hypoglycemia, allowing the blood glucose level to decrease more rapidly. So a diabetic who has been drinking may, as a consequence, also be hypoglycemic.

Hypoglycemia Unawareness

Patients with long-term diabetes mellitus usually recognize their own signs and symptoms that occur when their blood glucose levels are decreasing and they are becoming hypoglycemic. They will ingest a high-sugar food to raise the blood glucose level. Over time, however, the signs and symptoms of hypoglycemia may begin to change. They may not recognize the change, continuing to look for the old signs and symptoms. This may cause them to allow their blood glucose levels to drop significantly without any intervention as the signs and symptoms go unrecognized, and they suddenly experience hypoglycemia.

Emergency Care for Hypoglycemia

The patient suffering from hypoglycemia must be given sugar to increase the blood glucose level as quickly as possible to prevent the brain cells from dying. You would provide the same treatment as outlined earlier in the chapter for a patient with an altered mental status and unknown history. Your management is based on the patient's mental status.

If the patient is unresponsive, is unable to swallow, or is unable to obey your commands:

1. Establish an open airway.
2. Provide oxygen via a nonrebreather mask at 15 lpm if the breathing is adequate.
3. Provide positive pressure ventilation if the breathing is inadequate (either an inadequate rate or an inadequate tidal volume).
4. Contact advanced life support.
5. Assess the blood glucose level.

If the patient has an altered mental status but is responsive, is able to swallow, and is able to obey your commands:

1. Ensure the airway is patent.
2. Assess the blood glucose level if your protocol permits.
3. Administer one tube of oral glucose.

Be sure to continuously reassess the patient's condition for improvement or deterioration. Pay particular attention to the airway and breathing status.

Oral Glucose

Oral glucose is the medication of choice in the emergency medical care of the diabetic patient with an altered mental status. Once it is administered, this heavy sugar

Objective 20-8
Identify indications and contraindications to the administration of oral glucose.

Key Points
Oral glucose may be administered *only* if the patient has *all three* of these: (1) an altered mental status, (2) a history of diabetes controlled by medication or a BGL < 60 mg/dL, and (3) the ability to swallow.

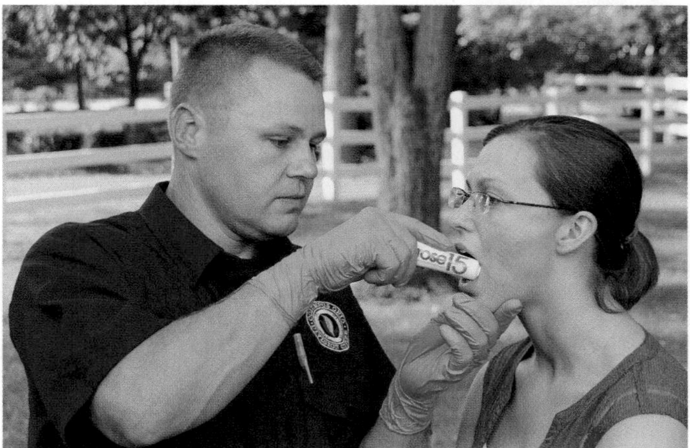

FIGURE 20-4 * One method of administering oral glucose is to squeeze the tube of oral glucose between the patient's cheek and gum.

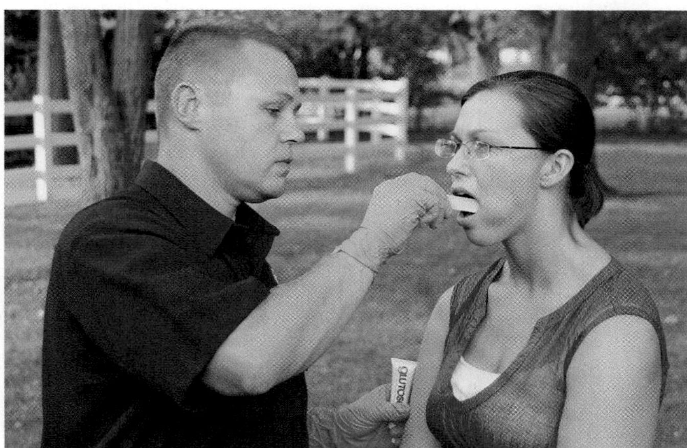

FIGURE 20-5 * One method of administering oral glucose is to squeeze the glucose onto the end of a tongue depressor, which can then be placed between the patient's cheek and gum.

gel raises the amount of glucose circulating in the blood, which increases the amount of glucose available to the brain. Since the brain cells need glucose to function, lowered levels of glucose alter their ability to function properly, causing a decrease in mental status. When the blood glucose level increases, the brain receives an increased amount of glucose and is able to restore brain cell function, bringing about an improvement in mental status.

See Figures 20-4* and 20-5* which illustrate methods of administering or assisting a patient with oral glucose. See Figure 20-6* for a detailed summary of the criteria and techniques for administration of oral glucose.

Oral glucose may be administered only if the patient meets all of the following three criteria: (1) has an altered mental status, (2) has history of diabetes controlled by medication or a blood glucose reading less than 60 mg/dL, and (3) has the ability to swallow. Some patients may meet one or two of these criteria, but not all three. For example, the patient may have an altered mental status and be able to swallow but have no known history of diabetes mellitus or have a blood glucose reading greater than 60 mg/dL. Or the patient may have an altered mental status and a history of diabetes controlled by medication or a blood glucose level less than 60 mg/dL but his level of responsiveness is so depressed that he cannot swallow safely. When using a glucose meter, follow your local protocol. Some protocols require the administration of glucose when the BGL is less than 70 mg/dL.

In cases like the ones just described, in which all three criteria are not met, do not administer oral glucose. Instead, provide emergency medical care for a patient with altered mental status and an unknown history: Maintain an open airway, suction as needed, maintain oxygen therapy, be prepared to assist ventilations, place the patient in a lateral recumbent position, and transport. Contact medical direction for further orders.

Hyperglycemia

Hyperglycemia is the term for a high blood glucose level (*hyper* = high, *glyco* = glucose, *emia* = blood). There are two conditions that may result from extreme hyperglycemia: *diabetic ketoacidosis (DKA)* and *hyperglycemic hyperosmolar nonketotic syndrome (HHNS)*. As noted earlier, DKA is more commonly seen in the type 1 diabetic, whereas HHNS is more common in the type 2 diabetic. In both conditions, the blood glucose level increases drastically. Unlike hypoglycemia, which is a lack of glucose in

Understanding BODY PROCESSES

Hyperglycemic patients have too much glucose in the blood and not enough insulin. The cells in the body are starving, even though the blood glucose level may be extremely high, because there is not enough insulin to move the glucose into the cells. At the same time, however, the brain is getting more than an adequate amount of glucose. ■

Oral Glucose

MEDICATION NAME

Oral glucose is the generic name. Two of the trade names of oral glucose are:

- Glutose
- Insta-Glucose

INDICATIONS

Oral glucose should be administered to a patient who meets all three of the following criteria:

- An altered mental status
- A history of diabetes controlled by medication or a blood glucose level less than 60 mg/dL
- The ability to swallow the medication

CONTRAINDICATIONS

Oral glucose should not be administered to a patient who:

- Is either unresponsive or unable to swallow the medication
- Has a confirmed blood glucose level greater than 60 mg/dL

MEDICATION FORM

Gel, in toothpaste-type tubes.

DOSAGE

Oral glucose is a viscous gel typically packaged in toothpaste-type tubes. The typical dosage is one tube.

ADMINISTRATION

To administer oral glucose:

1. Obtain an order from medical direction. Off-line medical direction would allow the EMT to administer the oral glucose without direct consultation with medical direction. An on-line order may be given by direct consultation with medical direction via phone or radio prior to the administration of the medication.
2. Ensure the signs and symptoms are consistent with hypoglycemia. If protocol permits, obtain a blood glucose reading.
3. Ensure that the patient is responsive and able to swallow the medication and protect his airway. Monitor the patient's airway closely during the administration to avoid accidental blockage by or aspiration of the oral glucose.
4. There are two ways to administer the medication. One way is to hold back the patient's cheek and squeeze small portions of the contents of the tube into the mouth between the cheek and gum (Figure 20-4). The other way is to place small portions of the oral glucose on a tongue depressor, pull back the cheek, and slide the tongue depressor to deposit the medication between the cheek and gum (Figure 20-5). An alternative method is to have the patient squeeze the glucose himself into his mouth. This ensures he is alert enough to swallow it.

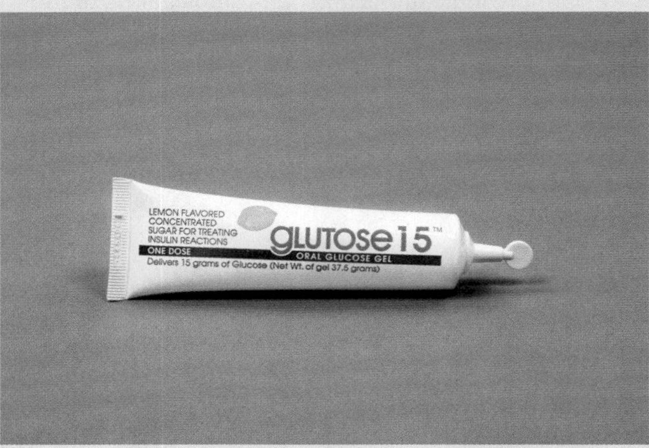

Whichever method you choose, do not squeeze a large amount of glucose into the patient's mouth at one time. This may cause the patient to choke or aspirate the contents. Also, lightly massage the area between the cheek and gum to disperse the gel and increase absorption.

ACTIONS

Increases blood glucose level. Increases glucose available to the brain.

SIDE EFFECTS

There are no side effects of oral glucose when administered properly. However, the thickness of the gel may cause an airway obstruction or the substance may be aspirated in the patient without a gag reflex.

REASSESSMENT

If the patient loses responsiveness or has a seizure, remove the tongue depressor from the mouth and be prepared to suction. Reassess the patient's mental status to determine if the medication has had an effect. Remember, it may take more than 20 minutes before you start seeing any improvement in the patient's mental status following the administration of oral glucose. Reassess the blood glucose level if protocol permits. If the patient's mental status continues to deteriorate, manage the airway and breathing. Make sure that oxygen is flowing to the patient at the highest possible concentration. Constantly monitor the patient's airway and breathing.

FIGURE 20-6 ✱ Oral glucose.

Objective 20-9
Discuss the pathophysiology, assessment, and emergency medical care of diabetic ketoacidosis (DKA).

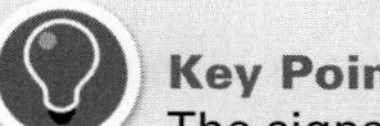

Key Points
The signs and symptoms of DKA are produced primarily by the dehydration and acid buildup.

the blood, in hyperglycemic conditions there is a lack of insulin and an excessive amount of glucose in the blood. In hyperglycemic conditions, the brain has more glucose than it knows what to do with.

Hyperglycemic Condition: Diabetic Ketoacidosis (DKA)

Pathophysiology of DKA

The name itself, *diabetic ketoacidosis,* indicates what is occurring in the condition. The blood glucose level is elevated, typically greater than 350 mg/dL, because of an inadequate amount of insulin. The brain has an excess amount of glucose; therefore, it is not suffering from low blood glucose. However, the other cells in the body are starving for glucose, because there is an inadequate amount of insulin to help move the glucose out of the blood and into the cells at a fast enough rate. The cells begin to burn fat for energy as the glucose collects in the blood.

This causes two problems within the body. First, the excess glucose from the blood begins to spill into the urine, drawing large amounts of water with it. The patient begins to urinate frequently as a consequence of the excessive glucose, simultaneously eliminating large amounts of water attracted to the glucose. This leads to dehydration in the patient. Second, in place of the glucose they can't take in, the cells burn fat for energy, which produces a by-product called ketones. The ketones produce a form of a strong acid. As the cells burn more fat, acid levels in the body begin to increase to dangerous levels (acidosis).

These two problems, dehydration and acidosis, lead to many of the signs and symptoms seen in DKA and may eventually cause the brain to fail. In addition to dehydration and acidosis, an electrolyte imbalance develops, which may lead to cardiac disturbances. Since it takes quite a bit of time for the effects of the acid and dehydration to occur, the signs and symptoms of DKA usually do not occur for up to several days.

You might expect to find one of the following factors:

Factors Causing Hyperglycemia in the Diabetic Ketoacidosis (DKA) Patient

- The patient is suffering from an infection that has upset the insulin and glucose balance.
- The patient takes an inadequate dose of insulin.

Understanding BODY PROCESSES

An altered mental status in the diabetic ketoacidosis patient is not from a lack of glucose to the brain; rather, the altered mental status results from dehydration, fluid shift, and acidosis affecting the brain cells. It takes time for the dehydration, fluid shift, and acidosis to build to critical levels; thus, the onset of signs and symptoms is usually days in hyperglycemia, not minutes as in hypoglycemia. ■

- The patient is taking medications such as thiazide, Dilantin, or steroids.
- The patient has suffered some type of stress such as surgery, trauma, pregnancy, or heart attack.
- The patient had a change in diet in which he has overeaten or increased his carbohydrate or sugar intake.

Assessment Findings in DKA

The signs and symptoms of DKA are produced primarily by the dehydration and acid buildup. The name of the condition explains the signs and symptoms one would expect from the condition. The word *diabetes* means excessive urination. *Ketoacidosis* refers to the production of ketones, which also produces strong acids, from the cells' use of fat as an energy source. Diabetic ketoacidosis is a condition with excessive urination and a buildup of acid from ketone production. Therefore, look for signs of dehydration and acid buildup.

Signs and Symptoms of Diabetic Ketoacidosis (DKA)

- Polyuria (excessive urination)
- Polyphagia (excessive hunger)
- Polydipsia (excessive thirst)
- Nausea and vomiting
- Poor skin turgor
- Tachycardia
- Rapid deep respirations (called Kussmaul respirations)
- Fruity or acetone odor on the breath
- Positive orthostatic tilt test
- Blood glucose level (BGL) > 350 mg/dL

Objective 20-10
Compare and contrast the speed of onset and the signs and symptoms of hypoglycemia and hyperglycemia.

Thinking Critically
Explain why oral glucose should be considered for *both* the hypoglycemic patient *and* the hyperglycemic patient who meets the criteria (altered mental status, history of diabetes, able to swallow).

- Muscle cramps
- Abdominal pain (in 50 percent of patients; more common in children with DKA)
- Warm, dry, flushed skin
- Altered mental status
- Coma (very late)

ASSESSMENT Tips

Poor skin turgor in elderly patients is caused by the normal loss of skin elasticity. Therefore, poor skin turgor does not tell you much about the elderly patient's hydration status. ■

As mentioned previously, DKA progresses slowly over a few days. The signs or symptoms related to dehydration are polyuria, polydipsia, poor skin turgor, tachycardia, and positive orthostatic tilt test. The nausea, vomiting, and muscle cramps are typically due to electrolyte disturbances from the loss of sodium, potassium, and magnesium. The acid in the body will produce Kussmaul respirations, warm and dry skin, and the fruity odor on the breath.

Kussmaul respirations are a pattern of very deep and rapid breathing that is commonly seen in the patient with DKA. It is an attempt by the body to blow off carbon dioxide to reduce the acid load in the body. Carbon dioxide will produce another form of acid called carbonic acid. If the patient can blow off large amounts of carbon dioxide by hyperventilating (deep and rapid breathing), he can then reduce the amount of carbonic acid and thus reduce the total amount of acid in the body. As the ketone acid in the body increases, the patient will breathe deeper and faster in an attempt to keep the acid load under control. The fruity odor, which smells like Juicy Fruit gum or acetone, is from the ketones building up in the body.

ASSESSMENT Tips

Many people are unable to smell acetone; thus, you or your partner may not be able to smell the fruity odor on the DKA patient's breath. ■

Both the dehydration and the acid load endanger the normal function of the body. The altered mental status is produced by the brain becoming dehydrated and from the effects of acid on the brain cells. Remember, the brain in the patient with DKA has more glucose than it can deal with. That is why the progression of the signs and symptoms of DKA occurs over a few days, since it can take a much longer period of time for the dehydration and acid to affect the brain. This is unlike hypoglycemia, which has an onset of only a few minutes to 20 minutes because of the more acute effects of low blood glucose levels on the brain.

Emergency Care For DKA

As an EMT, you may not be expected to distinguish between hypoglycemic and hyperglycemic conditions unless you are able to use a glucose meter. Although the signs and symptoms may differ dramatically between hypoglycemia and hyperglycemia, both conditions may produce an altered mental status (Table 20-2). The patient will typically have a history of diabetes mellitus and will usually be on either an injectable or inhalable form of insulin or an oral hypoglycemic agent to manage the blood glucose.

The patient with diabetic ketoacidosis is typically dehydrated and acidotic. Thus, the treatment is aimed at reducing the blood glucose level and rehydrating the patient. It may be prudent to contact an advanced life support unit to begin rehydration in the field. Follow your local protocol.

In the patient with diabetic ketoacidosis, the prehospital emergency medical care will include the following:

1. Establish and maintain a patent airway.
2. If breathing is adequate, administer oxygen based on the SpO_2 reading and patient signs and symptoms. If the SpO_2 reading is greater than 95% and no signs or symptoms of hypoxia or respiratory distress are present, oxygen may not be necessary. In this case, you may choose to apply a nasal cannula at 2 to 4 lpm. If signs of hypoxia or respiratory distress are present, or the SpO_2 reading is less than 95%, place the patient on a nonrebreather mask at 15 lpm.
3. If the breathing is inadequate (either an inadequate rate or an inadequate tidal volume), provide positive pressure ventilation with oxygen connected to the ventilation device.
4. If your protocol permits, determine the blood glucose level.
5. If you are unsure about the condition, administer oral glucose if the patient is able to swallow.
6. Contact medical direction for further orders.

TABLE 20-2 Signs and Symptoms of Diabetic Emergency Conditions

Sign or Symptom	DKA	HHNS	Hypoglycemia
Onset	Slow, over days	Slow, over days	Sudden, over minutes
Heart rate	Tachycardia	Tachycardia	Tachycardia
Blood pressure	Low	Low	Normal
Respirations	Kussmaul	Normal	Normal or shallow
Breath odor	Sweet and fruity	None	None
Mental status	Coma (very late)	Confusion	Bizarre behavior, agitated, aggressive, altered, unresponsive
Oral mucosa	Dry	Dry	Salivation
Thirst	Intense	Intense	Absent
Vomiting	Common	Common	Uncommon
Abdominal pain	Common	Uncommon	Absent
Insulin level	Low	Low	High
Blood glucose level	High	Very high	Very low
Emergency care and patient needs	**DKA**	**HHNS**	**Hypoglycemia**
Basic care	Oxygen	Oxygen	Oxygen, oral glucose
ALS care	Fluids	Fluids	IV glucose
Patient needs	More insulin	More insulin	Glucose

Oral glucose should be considered in *any* patient who has a history of diabetes who presents with an altered mental status, whether that patient is suffering from hypoglycemia or from hyperglycemia—you may not know which if a glucose meter is not used. If your protocol allows you to measure the blood glucose, do so to determine if the patient is hypoglycemic or hyperglycemic.

You may wonder why it is acceptable to give oral glucose to a patient who may be suffering from a hyperglycemic condition (too much glucose in the blood) when no glucose reading is available. The reason why oral glucose may be given to a patient who has a history of diabetes who is possibly hyperglycemic is that if the patient is not a confirmed hyperglycemic patient and turns out to be hypoglycemic, the patient may suffer possible brain cell damage if glucose is withheld. Remember, when brain cells are deprived of glucose during hypoglycemia they will begin to die. On the other hand, if oral glucose is administered to a hyperglycemic patient, the amount of glucose given is not going to raise the blood glucose drastically and will have little effect on the brain. In other words, the hypoglycemic patient could end up dead if not treated with glucose, while the additional glucose will usually not harm the hyperglycemic patient. Therefore, it is better to err on the side of hypoglycemia and administer glucose to the patient if the condition is unclear or if your orders instruct you to do so.

ASSESSMENT Tips

When possible, glucose administration should be guided by a glucose meter reading. It is well documented that administering glucose to a patient with a stroke, head injury, or other intracranial problem may worsen the neurological outcome. A low blood glucose measurement will help to rule out those conditions and ensure that glucose administration is both needed and safe for the patient. ■

Hyperglycemic Condition: Hyperglycemic Hyperosmolar Nonketotic Syndrome (HHNS)

Pathophysiology of HHNS

The pathophysiology of HHNS is similar to diabetic ketoacidosis. Again, the name of the condition provides an understanding of what is occurring and how the two conditions differ. HHNS is a hyperglycemic condition that causes the blood glucose level to increase drastically. The blood glucose will typically rise to 600–1,200 mg/dL, thus the *hyperglycemic* reference in the name. Because of the high blood glucose level, the kidneys begin to spill off large amounts of glucose in the urine. The glucose draws large amounts of water with it into the urine, which is called a *hyperosmolar* effect. This causes the patient to suffer from significant dehydration.

HHNS is more common in the type 2 NIDDM patient. This is because the type 2 patient's pancreas is able to produce and secrete some insulin, so some glucose is

Objectives 20-11 and 20-12
Describe the primary differences between DKA and hyperglycemic hyperosmolar nonketotic syndrome (HHNS) and discuss the pathophysiology, assessment, and emergency medical care of HHNS.

Key Points
The emergency medical care for HHNS is basically the same as for DKA. If you are unsure which condition is present, treat the patient as if he is hypoglycemic.

still getting into the cells. The glucose entering the cells keeps the amount of fat being burned for energy to a lesser amount than is seen in DKA. If there is not a significant amount of fat being used, then there will be a lesser production of ketones as a by-product of fat breakdown. Therefore, there is not a collection of a large amount of ketones that would cause an acid load in the body, thus the *nonketotic* reference in the name.

The word *syndrome* in the name refers to a set of signs and symptoms. HHNS is a condition in which the patient becomes severely dehydrated from an extremely high blood glucose level. However, since the patient does not produce a massive amount of ketones, the patient will present with the signs of significant dehydration but with no signs of acidosis. The patient's mental status will be altered because of dehydration of the brain tissue and not because of acidosis or a lack of glucose.

An episode of HHNS may be the first indication that a patient has a diabetic condition. It is most commonly found in type 2 NIDDM patients who are elderly. HHNS may also be precipitated by trauma, burns, dialysis, drugs, heart attack, stroke, infection, and head injuries. HHNS carries a fairly high mortality rate. HHNS patients are more likely to have seizures than are hypoglycemic patients.

Assessment Findings in HHNS

The signs and symptoms of HHNS are similar to those of DKA with the exception that those caused by the acidosis in DKA are not present in HHNS (Table 20-2).

Signs and Symptoms of Hyperglycemic Hyperosmolar Nonketotic Syndrome (HHNS)

- Tachycardia
- Fever
- Positive orthostatic tilt test
- Dehydration
- Thirst (polydipsia)
- Dizziness
- Poor skin turgor
- Altered mental status
- Confusion
- Weakness
- Dry oral mucosa
- Dry, warm skin
- Polyuria (if dehydrated, the urine output will be scanty [oliguria])
- Nausea and vomiting

Note that there are no Kussmaul respirations or fruity odor on the breath with HHNS because there is no significant buildup of ketones in the body and therefore no significant acid load.

Emergency Medical Care for HHNS

The emergency medical care for HHNS is basically the same as for DKA. Once again, if you are unsure or if your protocol does not permit you to attempt to distinguish between hypoglycemia, DKA, and HHNS, treat the patient as if he is hypoglycemic. Administering oral glucose to this patient will not drastically elevate his already high blood glucose level. Withholding glucose from a hypoglycemic patient that you mistake as DKA or HHNS may potentially result in brain damage or even the patient's death. Err to benefit the patient and treat as hypoglycemia when unsure of the condition. Other signs and symptoms that may help you distinguish between hypoglycemia, HHNS, and DKA are listed in Table 20-2.

Emergency medical care for HHNS includes these steps:

1. Establish and maintain a patent airway.
2. Provide oxygen via a nonrebreather mask at 15 lpm if the breathing is adequate.
3. If the breathing is inadequate (either an inadequate rate or an inadequate tidal volume), provide positive pressure ventilation with oxygen connected to the ventilation device.
4. If your protocol permits, determine the blood glucose level.
5. If you are unsure about the condition, administer oral glucose if the patient is able to swallow.
6. Contact medical direction for further orders.

Like the DKA patient, the HHNS patient needs to be rehydrated with fluids. It may be necessary to call for advanced life support for this purpose. Follow your local protocols.

Objective 20-13
Discuss the assessment-based approach to a patient with an altered mental status in a diabetic emergency.

Key Points
When gathering a history for a patient with an altered mental status, be sure to ask the "M" question and be prepared to recognize medications that would help to establish a history of diabetes.

Assessment-Based Approach: Altered Mental Status in a Diabetic Emergency

The patient with an altered mental status who you suspect is experiencing an acute diabetic emergency is assessed in the same manner as the altered mental status patient with no known history. However, the patient may have prescription medications to control diabetes mellitus or you may have obtained a blood glucose level that indicates hypoglycemia. If you are unable to assess the blood glucose level with a glucose meter, you have to rely solely on your assessment findings to determine whether the patient is experiencing an acute diabetic emergency and what kind of diabetic emergency he is experiencing. If you are unsure or cannot confirm the condition with a glucose reading, it is better to err on the side of caution and administer oral glucose. If you are unable to confirm the blood glucose level and the actual acute diabetic emergency, an assessment-based approach to the patient is warranted.

Scene Size-Up and Primary Assessment

If clues gathered during the scene size-up and primary assessment lead you to suspect that the patient may be diabetic, look for medical alert tags or other medical identification that confirms a diabetic history (Figure 20-7*). Some patients with insulin-dependent diabetes may be found wearing an insulin pump (Figure 20-8*).

History and Secondary Assessment

While asking the SAMPLE history questions, remember especially to ask the "M" question about medications. It is very important that the EMT recognize the prescribed medications that a diabetic patient might be taking. Presence of such a medication will help to establish the history of diabetes. Be sure to document and report such a medication to hospital personnel. Medications often taken by diabetics include:

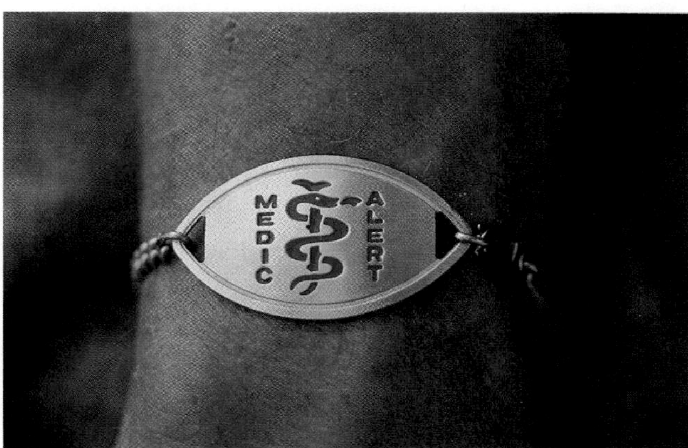

FIGURE 20-7 * A medical identification tag may indicate that the patient is a diabetic.

- Insulin (Humulin, Novolin, Iletin, Semilente)
- Actos
- Diabinese, Glucamide
- Orinase
- Micronase, DiaBeta

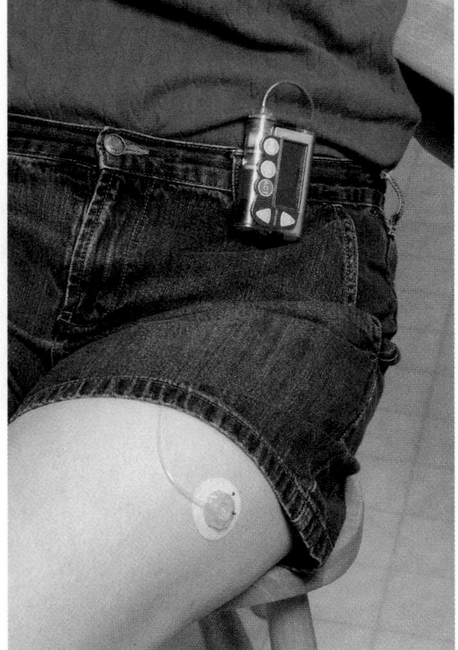

FIGURE 20-8 * Some insulin-dependent diabetics wear an insulin pump.

- Tolinase
- Glucotrol
- Humalog
- Glucophage
- Glynase
- Exenatide (Byetta)
- Lantus
- Exubera (inhaled insulin)

It is particularly important to determine—from the patient, family, or any bystanders—the answers to the following questions, with emphasis on the first four:

- *Did the patient take his medication the day of the episode?*
- *Did the patient eat (or skip any) regular meals on that day?*
- *Did the patient vomit after eating a meal on that day?*
- *Did the patient do any unusual exercise or physical activity on that day?*
- Was the onset of altered mental status gradual or fast?
- How long has the patient had the signs and symptoms?
- Are there any other signs or symptoms associated with the altered mental status?
- Is there any evidence of injury that might be the cause of the altered mental status?
- Was there any period in which the patient regained a normal mental status and then deteriorated again?
- Did the patient suffer a seizure?
- Does the patient appear to have a fever or other signs of infection?

An altered mental status from hypoglycemia will typically have a sudden onset. The signs and symptoms may progress rapidly over 5 to 30 minutes.

Signs and Symptoms

Signs and symptoms commonly associated with a patient who has an altered mental status and has a history of diabetes are (Figure 20-9*):

- Rapid onset of an altered mental status after missing or vomiting a meal, unusual exercise, or physical work
- Intoxicated appearance—from staggering or slurred speech to complete unresponsiveness
- Tachycardia (elevated heart rate)
- Cool, moist skin
- Hunger

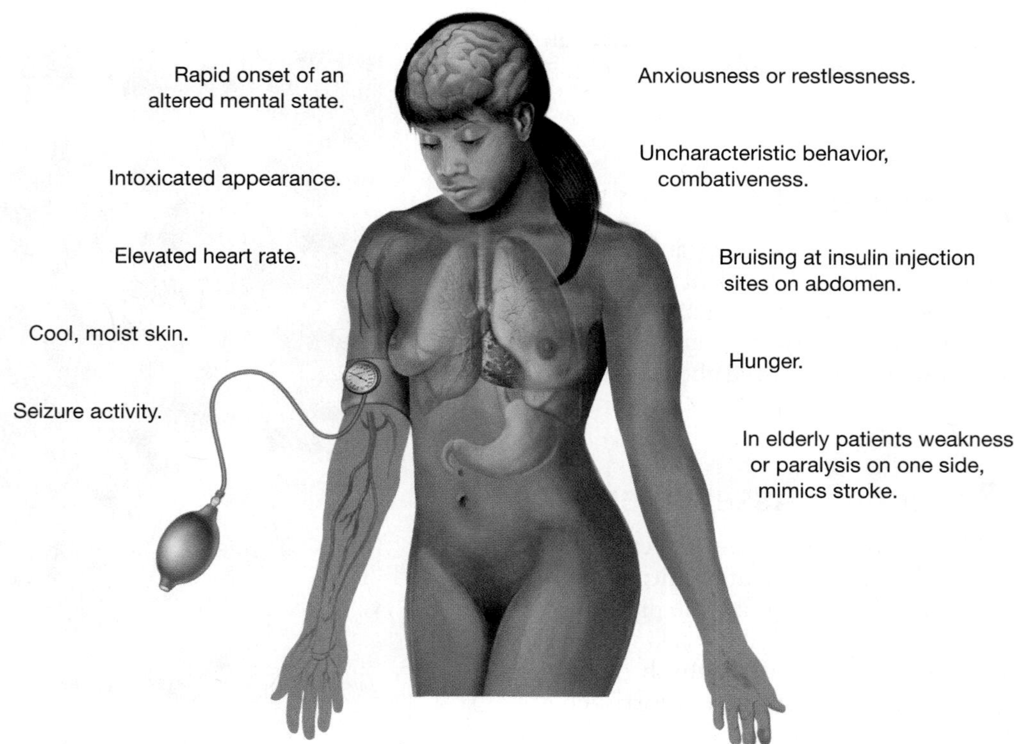
SIGNS AND SYMPTOMS OF HYPOGLYCEMIA
Rapid onset of an altered mental state.
Intoxicated appearance.
Elevated heart rate.
Cool, moist skin.
Seizure activity.
Anxiousness or restlessness.
Uncharacteristic behavior, combativeness.
Bruising at insulin injection sites on abdomen.
Hunger.
In elderly patients weakness or paralysis on one side, mimics stroke.

FIGURE 20-9 * Common signs and symptoms of altered mental status/diabetes.

Key Points
It may take 20 minutes before you start seeing any improvement in the patient's mental status following administration of oral glucose.

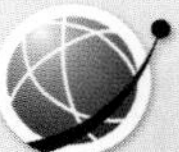

Media Resources
Go to www.bradybooks.com for mykit. Highlights:

- *Video:* Diabetes
- *Animation:* Use of Oral Glucose
- *Video:* Blood Glucose Meter

- Seizure activity
- Uncharacteristic or bizarre behavior, combativeness
- Anxiousness or restlessness
- Bruising at insulin injection sites on the abdomen
- Blood glucose reading of < 60 mg/dL

In addition, elderly patients frequently suffer signs and symptoms that mimic a stroke, such as weakness or paralysis on one side of the body. Keep in mind that some medications (beta blockers) may hide the signs of hypoglycemia.

Emergency Medical Care

Once you have confirmed an altered mental status and suspect a diabetic emergency that is likely a result of hypoglycemia, you will concentrate emergency care on correcting any life-threatening conditions and reversing the low blood glucose level that is likely to be the cause of the altered mental status.

1. **Establish and maintain an open airway.** If the patient's mental status is severely altered, it may be necessary to suction the airway to clear secretions or vomitus and to insert an oropharyngeal or nasopharyngeal airway. Administer oxygen by nonrebreather mask at 15 lpm. If breathing rate or depth is inadequate, assist breathing by positive pressure ventilation with supplemental oxygen. If breathing is adequate, administer oxygen based on the SpO_2 reading and patient signs and symptoms. If the SpO_2 reading is greater than 95% and no signs or symptoms of hypoxia or respiratory distress are present, oxygen may not be necessary. In this case, you may choose to apply a nasal cannula at 2 to 4 lpm. If signs of hypoxia or respiratory distress are present, or the SpO_2 reading is less than 95%, place the patient on a nonrebreather mask at 15 lpm.
2. **Determine if the patient is alert enough to swallow.** Oral glucose, the medication administered to the diabetic patient with a low blood glucose level, is given by mouth. If the patient is unable to swallow, you risk the chance that the patient will aspirate the medication or that the thick, sticky glucose will block the airway. One method to ensure that the patient is alert enough to swallow is to hand him the tube of glucose and instruct him to squeeze the contents into his mouth and swallow. Because the patient might be disoriented, it might take some coaching on your part to get the patient to comply with your command. If he is not alert enough to hold onto the tube or squeeze it in his mouth then you might want to reconsider the administration of glucose.
3. **Administer oral glucose.** Follow protocols established by your local or state medical direction. *If the patient is no longer alert during the administration of oral glucose, stop the administration of the medication. Immediately reassess the patient's airway, breathing, and circulation. Prepare to suction.*
4. **Transport.**

Reassessment

Once the oral glucose has been administered, reassess the patient's mental status to determine if the medication has had an effect. Remember, it may take more than 20 minutes before you start seeing any improvement in the patient's mental status following the administration of oral glucose. If local protocol permits, retest the blood glucose level, using the glucose meter, to determine if the blood glucose level is increasing.

If the blood glucose level is increasing and the mental status is improving, it is likely the patient is suffering from a low blood glucose level. If the blood glucose level is increasing but the patient's mental status is not improving, the patient may be suffering from another condition in addition to the low blood glucose level, such as a stroke. If the blood glucose level remains low, it may indicate that the oral glucose has not yet reached the bloodstream and is not yet effective. If the patient is still able to swallow and alert enough to obey your commands, consult with medical direction for an order to administer an additional tube of oral glucose.

If the patient's mental status continues to deteriorate or does not improve, manage the airway and breathing. Continue to oxygenate the patient. Communicate and record any changes in the patient's condition.

Summary: Assessment and Care

To review assessment findings and emergency care for diabetic emergencies, see Figures 20-10a*, 20-10b*, and 20-11*.

Assessment Summary

ACUTE DIABETIC EMERGENCY: SUSPECTED HYPOGLYCEMIA

The following are findings that may be associated with suspected hypoglycemia that presents with altered mental status.

SCENE SIZE-UP

Is altered mental status the result of a medical or a traumatic cause? Look for evidence of:

- Mechanism of injury
- Home or portable oxygen tanks or concentrators
- Alcohol and drug paraphernalia
- Chemicals at or around the scene
- Enclosed spaces
- Improperly vented heating devices in the winter months
- Medications

PRIMARY ASSESSMENT

General Impression

- Unusual behavior for situation
- Patient may have agitated or confused facial expression

Mental Status

- Alert to unresponsive
- Restlessness
- Agitation
- Disorientation
- Bizarre behavior
- Aggressiveness

Airway

- Secretions and vomitus
- Occlusion from tongue

Breathing

- Signs of inadequate breathing

Circulation

- Tachycardia
- Pale, cool, clammy skin

Status: Priority Patient

SECONDARY ASSESSMENT

Sample History

Signs and symptoms:

- Rapid onset of altered mental status
- Intoxicated appearance
- Tachycardia
- Pale, cool, clammy skin
- Hunger
- Seizures
- Bizarre behavior, restlessness, anxiety

Medications to control diabetes:

- Insulin (Humulin, Novolin, Iletin, Semilente)
- Actos
- Diabinese, Glucamide
- Orinase
- Micronase, DiaBeta
- Glynase
- Tolinase
- Glucotrol
- Humalog
- Glucophage
- Glynase
- Exenatide (Byetta)
- Lantus
- Exubera (inhaled insulin)

Key questions to ask: Did the patient . . .

- Take his medication this day?
- Eat or skip any regular meals?
- Vomit after eating a meal this day?
- Do any unusual exercise or physical activity this day?

Physical Exam

Head, neck, and face

- Dilated pupils

Abdomen

- Sensation of hunger

Extremities

- Pale, cool skin
- Diaphoresis

Other Signs and Symptoms

- Bruising at insulin injection sites
- Weakness or paralysis on one side (especially elderly)
- Blood glucose reading

Baseline Vital Signs

- BP: normal to low
- HR: increased (tachycardia)
- RR: may be increased, normal, or low
- Skin: pale, cool, and diaphoretic
- Pupils: dilated; sluggish to respond

FIGURE 20-10a ✱ Assessment summary: altered mental status—diabetic emergency.

Emergency Care Protocol

ACUTE DIABETIC EMERGENCY

1. Establish and maintain an open airway.
2. Suction secretions as necessary.
3. If breathing is inadequate, provide positive pressure ventilation with supplemental oxygen at a minimum rate of 10–12 ventilations/minute for an adult and 12–20 ventilations/minute for an infant or child.
4. If breathing is adequate, apply a nonrebreather mask at 15 lpm. If the patient becomes alert and oriented and the SpO_2 is greater than 95% and no signs of hypoxia are present, apply a nasal cannula at 2 to 4 lpm.
5. If the patient has an altered mental status with signs and symptoms of hypoglycemia, has a history of medication to control diabetes or has a blood glucose reading less than 60 mg/dL, and is alert enough to swallow, administer oral glucose.
   - Oral glucose (Glutose or Insta-Glucose) is a concentrated sugar solution that is absorbed and raises the blood glucose level.
   - Obtain an order from medical direction.
   - Ensure the patient is alert enough to swallow.
   - Obtain a blood glucose reading if protocol permits prior to the administration of glucose.
   - Squeeze contents of tube between the cheek and gum or place it between the cheek and gum with a tongue depressor or have the patient self-administer the glucose.
   - No side effects should be seen with oral glucose.
6. Consider advanced life support.
7. Transport in a lateral recumbent (coma or recovery) position.
8. Reassess every 5 minutes.
9. Oral glucose may take up to 20 minutes to get a response from the patient.

FIGURE 20-10b ✱ Emergency care protocol: acute diabetic emergency.

Emergency Care Algorithm: Acute Diabetic Emergency

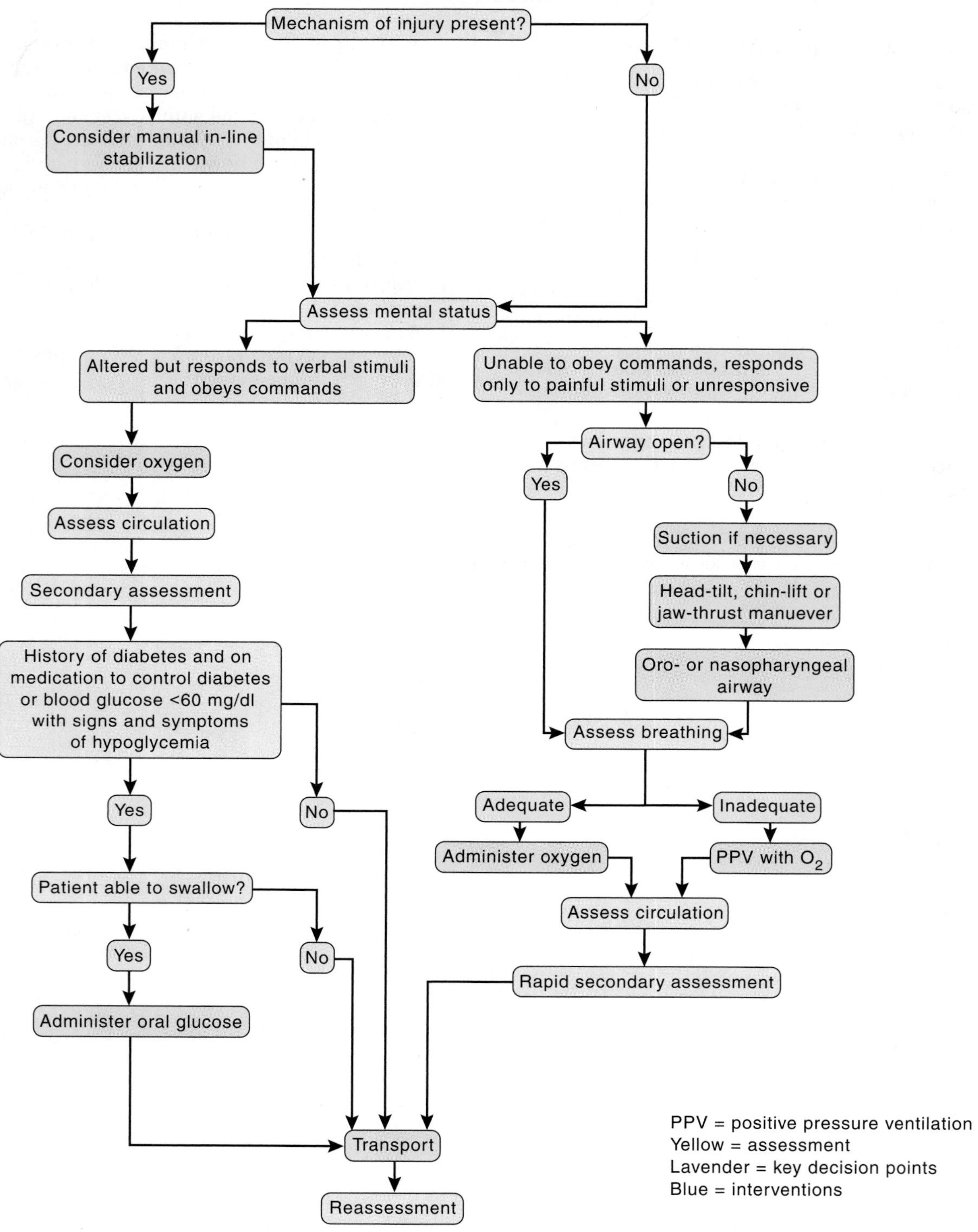

FIGURE 20-11 ✻ Emergency care algorithm: acute diabetic emergency.

Testing the Blood Glucose Level with a Glucose Meter

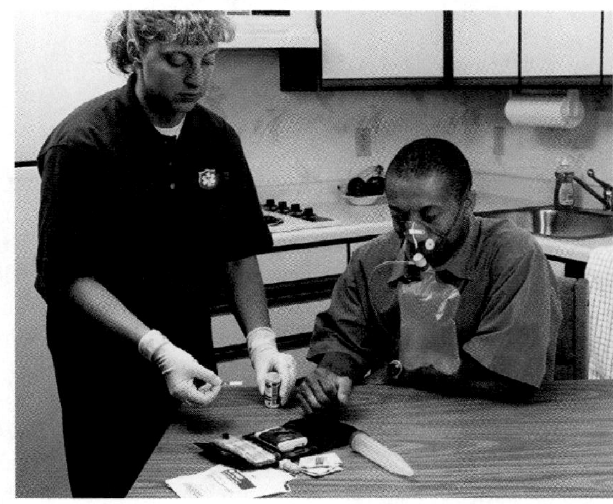

20-1A * Prepare the glucometer.

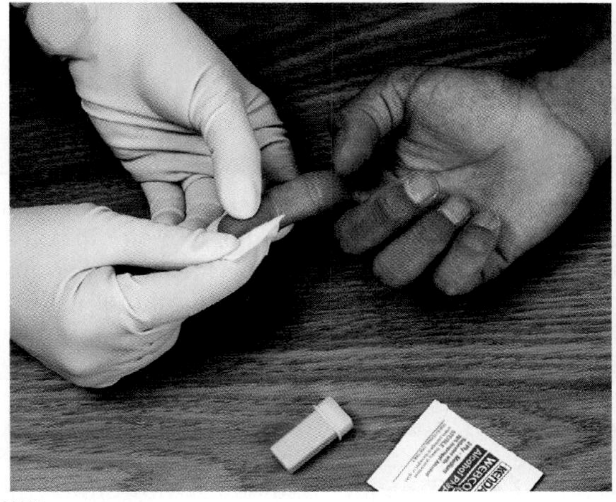

20-1B * Clean the site.

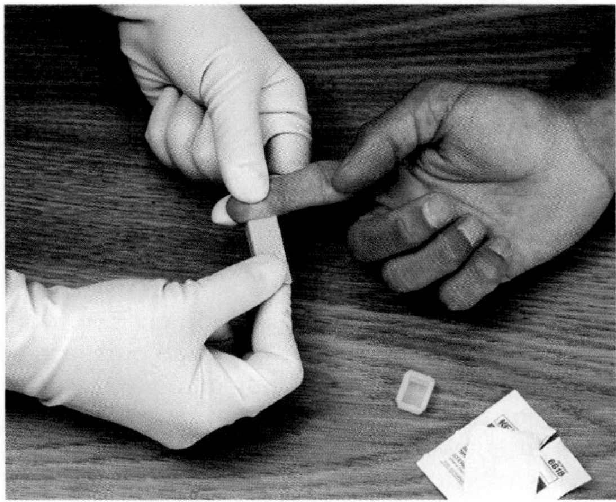

20-1C * Perform the finger stick.

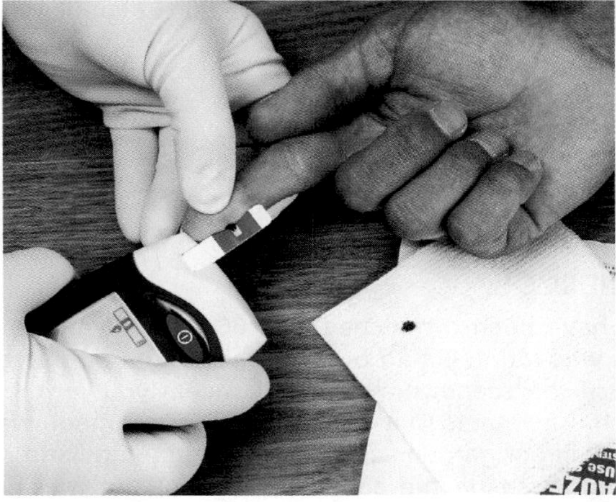

20-1D * Waste the first drop of blood onto a dressing. Drop the second blood drop onto the test strip.

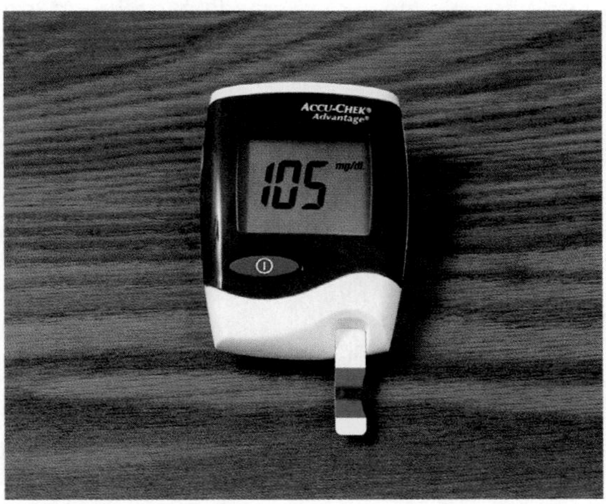

20-1E * Read the blood glucose value displayed on the glucometer.

CHAPTER REVIEW

SUMMARY

An altered mental status resulting from an acute diabetic emergency, especially hypoglycemia, is a significant medical condition that requires prompt assessment and emergency care. The patient with an altered mental status may not be able to protect his own airway. Place the patient in the lateral recumbent position to facilitate drainage of secretions or vomitus from the airway. Carefully assess the ventilatory status of the patient. If the ventilation is inadequate, even if the patient is still breathing, place the patient in a supine position and begin ventilation with supplemental oxygen and with suction available.

Your local protocol may not allow you to distinguish between the diabetic emergency conditions hypoglycemia, DKA, and HHNS, although there are fairly significant differences among them. Primarily, hypoglycemia patients experience a rapid onset of an altered mental status (minutes), whereas the DKA or HHNS patient suffers an altered mental status only after being ill for a day or two or more. The skin may also provide a good clue to the different conditions. The hypoglycemic patient has pale, cool, clammy skin from the release of adrenaline (epinephrine) in the body. The DKA or HHNS patient presents with warm, dry skin. The DKA patient may present with rapid deep respirations (Kussmaul respirations) and a fruity odor on the breath. In hypoglycemia and HHNS, the respirations are typically normal. In hypoglycemia, the respirations may become slow and shallow as the brain cells begin to die from the lack of glucose.

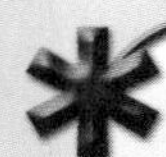

CASE STUDY FOLLOW-UP

SCENE SIZE-UP

You have been dispatched to a 66-year-old male patient who was found acting oddly by his neighbor. As you approach the scene, the neighbor meets you on the front porch. She states that her neighbor, Mr. Bennet, was out earlier in her garden acting extremely strange and now is in his house on the couch talking but not making any sense. You proceed into the house with caution and find the patient in the living room. The scene appears to be in order with no sign of trauma. As you approach the patient to begin the primary assessment, you ask your partner to check the house for medications. Your partner finds digoxin near the kitchen sink and insulin in the refrigerator.

PRIMARY ASSESSMENT

Your general impression is that the patient appears to be pale and perspiring profusely. As you approach you ask him his name. He responds with mumbled words. You assume the airway is open, and his breathing appears to be adequate. The respirations are at approximately 15 per minute. However, because Mr. Bennet's mental status appears to be altered, your partner places a nonrebreather mask on him at a liter flow of 15 lpm. You assess the radial pulse, which is approximately 100 and strong. His skin is moist and cool.

SECONDARY ASSESSMENT

Since Mr. Bennet is not able to respond appropriately to your questions, you perform a rapid secondary assessment. His pupils are equal and respond sluggishly to light. No jugular vein distention is noted in the neck. The breath sounds are equal bilaterally. His abdomen is soft and no tenderness is noted. Mr. Bennet has good pulses in all extremities. He is able to obey your commands. The grip strength is equal but weak in both upper extremities. The strength in the lower extremities is equal but weak. You find no evidence of trauma anywhere on the body. You find no medical alert identification tag.

Mr. Bennet's blood pressure is 102/60 mmHg. His heart rate is 108 per minute. Respirations are 16 per minute and of normal depth. His skin is pale, cool, and moist. His SpO_2 reading is 97% on room air. You record the baseline vitals.

During the secondary assessment, you gather a SAMPLE history. Upon questioning, the neighbor states that she found the patient out in her garden about 15 minutes prior to calling EMS. She says, "Mr. Bennet was acting strange and not himself." The neighbor thinks the patient has a heart and sugar problem. She does not know much more about him. Mr. Bennet is disoriented and does not know his name, where he is, who his neighbor is, or what day it is.

By now you are able to determine that Mr. Bennet has an altered mental status, is able to swallow adequately, has a history of diabetes, and is taking medication for the diabetes (as indicated by his neighbor's mention of "a sugar problem" and the insulin your partner found). His blood glucose level is 48 mg/dL on the glucometer. You administer one tube of oral glucose according to standing orders from medical direction, place the patient so that he is lying on his left side on the ambulance cot, and begin transport.

REASSESSMENT

En route to the hospital you notice that Mr. Bennet is beginning to respond more quickly to commands and questions. He can tell you his name and where he is. His airway is clear and breathing remains adequate. His pulse rate decreases to 86 per minute and his skin becomes less pale, drier, and warmer. You reassess the vital signs and record them. The pulse oximeter reading is 99% and he is showing no signs of hypoxia, so you switch him over to a nasal cannula at 2 lpm.

As you arrive at the hospital, Mr. Bennet is alert and oriented to person, place, and time. He has no complaints and appears in no distress. You give the hospital an oral report of the change in the patient's condition and help transfer him to the hospital bed. You and your partner complete a prehospital care report, restock the ambulance, and prepare for another call.

IN REVIEW

1. Describe the disease process associated with hypoglycemia.
2. Name the common signs and symptoms of a patient with hypoglycemia.
3. Describe the emergency medical care for a patient who is hypoglycemic.
4. Explain why airway management is a major concern in the patient with an altered mental status that results from hypoglycemia.
5. List the indications for oral glucose.
6. List the contraindications for oral glucose.
7. Describe two methods of administering oral glucose.
8. Describe the role of medical direction in emergency care for the diabetic patient.
9. Discuss the disease process associated with diabetic ketoacidosis (DKA).
10. Name the common signs and symptoms of a patient with diabetic ketoacidosis.
11. Describe the emergency medical care for a patient with diabetic ketoacidosis.
12. Discuss the disease process associated with hyperglycemic hyperosmolar nonketotic syndrome (HHNS).
13. Name the common signs and symptoms of a patient with hyperosmolar nonketotic syndrome.
14. Describe the emergency medical care for a patient with hyperosmolar nonketotic syndrome.

CRITICAL THINKING

You arrive on the scene and find a 34-year-old female patient lying supine on the couch. As you enter the scene, you note that the patient is pale and very diaphoretic. She is not alert, and you hear sonorous sounds on inhalation. She responds to painful stimuli with moans. Her respirations are 12 per minute with adequate chest rise. Her radial pulse is 122 bpm. The skin is pale, cool, and clammy. Her BP is 108/62 mmHg. The neighbor who called 911 brings you the patient's medications, which include Zoloft and Novolin. She doesn't know any medical history regarding the patient. She states the patient called her about 20 minutes ago and told her she wasn't feeling well. The neighbor decided to come check on her and found her on the couch and not responding.

1. What emergency care would you provide during the primary assessment?
2. Based on the signs, what condition do you suspect the patient is experiencing?
3. What other assessment procedures would be helpful to you in this patient?
4. What would you expect the blood glucose reading to be in the patient?
5. Why is the onset of the altered mental status significant in this patient?

CHAPTER 21

Anaphylactic Reactions

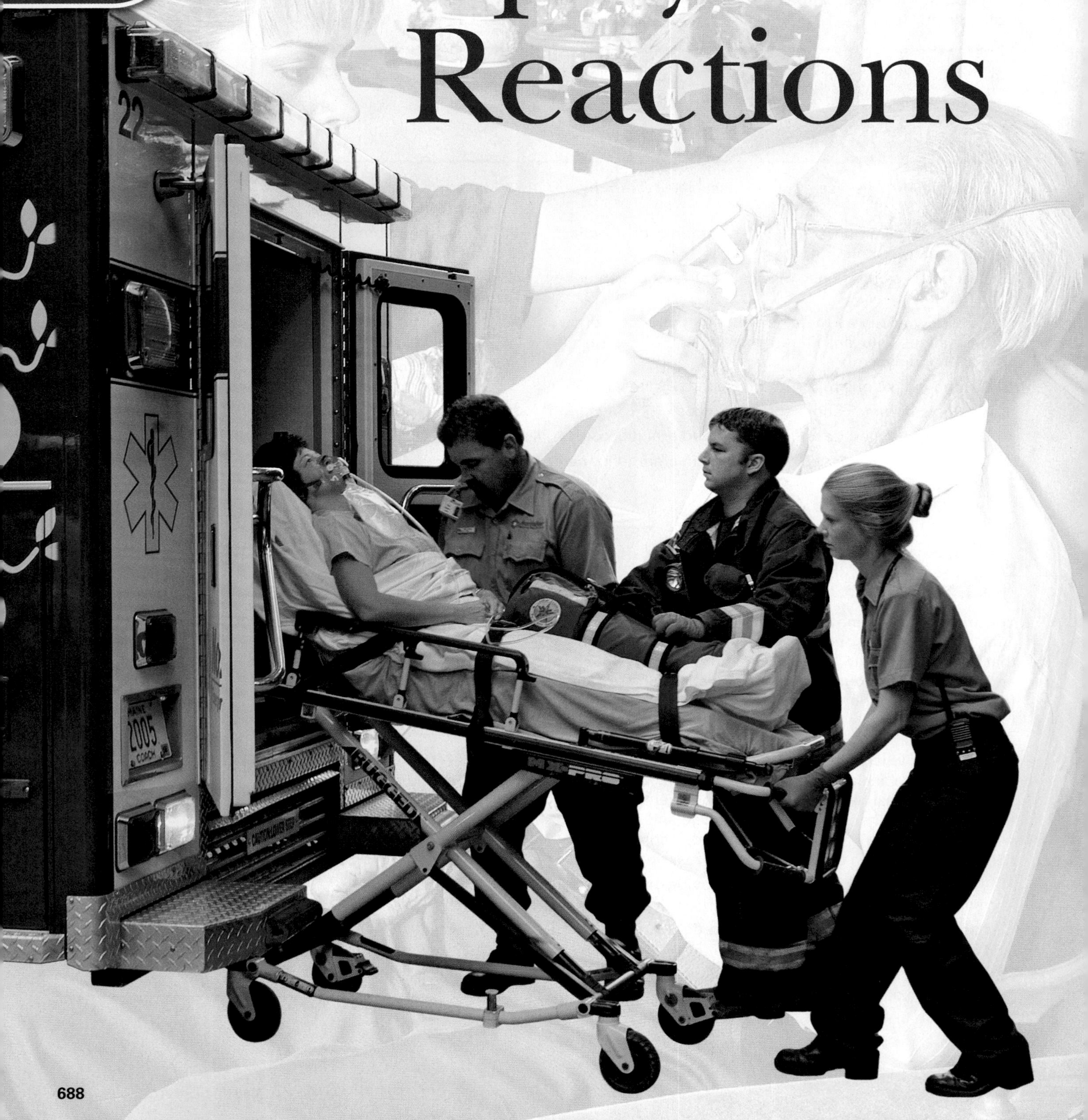

Navigation Guide

The following items provide an overview to the purpose and content of this chapter. The Standard and Competency are from the new National EMS Education Standards.

STANDARD **Medicine** (Content Area: Immunology)

COMPETENCY Applies fundamental knowledge to provide basic emergency care and transportation based on assessment findings for an acutely ill patient.

OBJECTIVES: After reading this chapter, you should be able to:

21-1. Define key terms introduced in this chapter.
21-2. Explain the importance of being able to recognize and treat anaphylactic reactions.
21-3. Describe the pathophysiological process by which exposure to an antigen results in anaphylaxis.
21-4. Explain the life-threatening mechanisms of anaphylaxis, including airway compromise, impaired ventilation and oxygenation, and impaired perfusion.
21-5. Describe the difference between an anaphylactic and an anaphylactoid reaction.
21-6. Discuss the ways that an antigen can be introduced into the body and substances that commonly cause anaphylactic or anaphylactoid reactions.
21-7. Explain an assessment-based approach to anaphylactic reaction including scene size-up, primary and secondary assessments, and reassessment.
21-8. Recognize the signs and symptoms of anaphylactic reaction..
21-9. List the two key categories of signs and symptoms that specifically indicate a severe anaphylactic reaction.
21-10. Develop a treatment plan for the patient with an anaphylactic reaction.
21-11. Describe the role of epinephrine in the treatment of anaphylaxis and the criteria and procedure administration of epinephrine.

KEY TERMS: Page references indicate first major use in this chapter. For complete definitions, see the Glossary at the back of the book.

allergen p. 690
allergic reaction p. 690
anaphylactic reaction p. 690
anaphylactic shock p. 690
anaphylactoid reaction p. 692
anaphylaxis p. 690
antibodies p. 690
antigen p. 690
auto-injector p. 701
endotracheal intubation p. 694
epinephrine p. 701
histamine p. 691
hives p. 694
hypersensitivity p. 691
immune response p. 690
immune system p. 690
malaise p. 694
sensitization p. 691

MEDIA RESOURCES: Please go to www.bradybooks.com to access mykit for this text. You will find quizzes, critical thinking scenarios, weblinks, animations, and videos related to this chapter—and much more. Look for online information on the immune system and allergic reactions. You will also find an animation on anaphylaxis.

CASE STUDY

The Dispatch

EMS Unit 204—proceed to the Veterans' Pavilion at Mill Run Park. You have a 25-year-old male patient complaining of breathing difficulty. Be advised, the Metropark Police are on the scene. Time out is 0714 hours.

Upon Arrival

Upon arrival, you quickly scan the scene to ensure your safety and to look for a mechanism of injury or clues to a possible nature of illness. You exit the ambulance with your emergency kit in hand and proceed to the patient. The scene appears to be safe,

continued

Navigation Guide *continued*

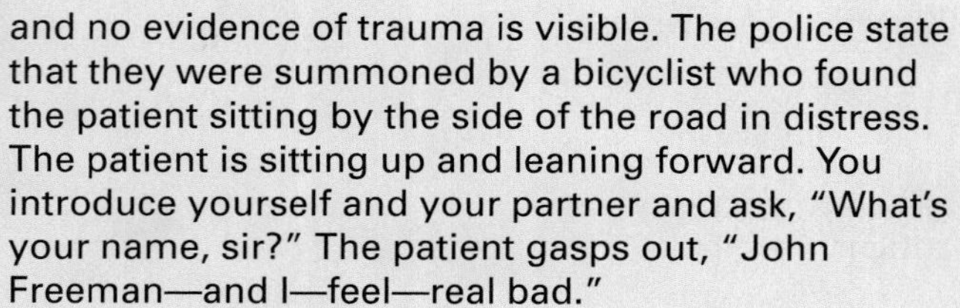

and no evidence of trauma is visible. The police state that they were summoned by a bicyclist who found the patient sitting by the side of the road in distress. The patient is sitting up and leaning forward. You introduce yourself and your partner and ask, "What's your name, sir?" The patient gasps out, "John Freeman—and I—feel—real bad."

How Would You Proceed to Assess and Care for This Patient?

During this chapter, you will learn about assessment and emergency care for patients suffering from allergic reaction. Later, we will return to the case and apply the procedures learned.

Introduction

Allergic reactions can occur at any time and to anyone. A wide variety of substances can produce such reactions. Foods, medications, insect stings—even exercise—are common causes. An allergic reaction may be as mild as a runny nose or mild skin rash. At the other end of the spectrum, however, is the life-threatening allergic reaction that is known as an *anaphylactic reaction.*

An anaphylactic reaction is a severe, exaggerated, systemic, allergic reaction that is associated with severe swelling of the upper and lower airways, constriction of the bronchioles, leakage of fluid from the capillaries, systemic vessel dilation, and an increased production of mucus. An anaphylactic reaction may be so severe that the upper airway closes, the respirations become very labored because of high airway resistance from swollen and constricted bronchioles, and the blood pressure becomes dangerously low because of the dilation of the vessels and leakage of fluid from the capillaries.

Another frightening aspect of anaphylactic reactions is that they typically develop and become life threatening very quickly, within minutes after exposure to the cause of the reaction.

Because anaphylactic reactions are often hard to predict and have the potential to so quickly become life threatening, it is important for the EMT to recognize an anaphylactic reaction in a patient promptly and to manage it swiftly and effectively. Delay in emergency care can easily and rapidly lead to deterioration in the patient's condition and even to death.

Anaphylactic Reaction

The body has a defense mechanism, known as the **immune system**, to fight off invasion by foreign substances. Foreign substances, called **antigens** (including a specific type of antigen called n **allergens**), are recognized by the cells of the immune system and eventually destroyed. In most cases, this immune response takes place with no allergic reaction or with just a mild allergic reaction. Occasionally there is a severe, life-threatening anaphylactic reaction.

Pathophysiology of Anaphylactic Reaction

An antigen can enter the body through the skin, the gastrointestinal tract, or the respiratory tract. When one does, it sets off an **immune response** in which the immune system detects the antigen and produces **antibodies**. Antibodies are proteins that search for the antigen, combine with it, and help to destroy it.

Most antigens that enter the body are easily fought off by the immune system with no allergic response, that is, without producing any noticeable effects. If, however, the type of antigen called an allergen enters the body, the effect is quite different. Although allergens are often quite common and harmless to most individuals, they cause an abnormal response by the immune system known as an **allergic reaction**.

An allergic reaction is a misdirected and excessive response by the immune system to an allergen. The immune system overestimates the danger of the allergen and produces a greater-than-necessary response. The response can be local—that is, a response isolated to one area of the body—or it can be systemic—that is, producing effects throughout the body. The response of the immune system to an allergen is often rapid, leading to the sudden onset of the allergic reaction.

The allergen itself is usually harmless to the patient, and most allergic reactions are mild, producing nothing more than discomfort, such as itching, a runny nose, and watery eyes—results of the body's attempts to eliminate the allergen or antigen. Occasionally, however, a severe, life-threatening immune response occurs. Such a severe, life-threatening allergic reaction is known as an **anaphylactic reaction** and is also known as **anaphylaxis** or **anaphylactic shock**.

In an anaphylactic reaction, the entire body is affected by the release of chemical substances by the immune system. These chemical substances produce life-threatening

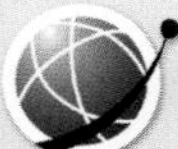

Media Resources

Go to www.bradybooks.com for mykit. Highlights:

- *Web Resource:* Immune System and Allergic Reactions
- *Video:* Allergic Rhinitis

Objectives 21-2 to 21-4

Recognize and explain the pathophysiology and mechanisms of anaphylaxis.

Key Terms

immune system the body's defense mechanism against foreign substances (**antigens**), including those that cause allergic reactions (**allergens**).

reactions in the airway, lungs, blood vessels, and heart. Swelling in the upper airway can cause obstruction and a reduction of air to the lungs. Bronchoconstriction and swelling in the lower airways can cause severe breathing difficulty and possible hypoxia. Blood vessels dilate and capillaries can begin to leak, decreasing the blood pressure and causing shock (hypoperfusion). An increase in mucus production leads to a further restriction of air movement, increased airway resistance, and the potential for plugging of smaller bronchioles.

An anaphylactic reaction is a life-threatening condition that requires prompt recognition and intervention and commonly leads to death without proper treatment.

Understanding BODY PROCESSES

The life-threatening signs and symptoms seen in anaphylactic reactions are produced by bronchoconstriction, increased capillary permeability, and vasodilation. Your emergency care for the patient with an anaphylactic reaction is geared toward reversing those three conditions. ■

Sensitization

An allergic reaction usually does not occur the first time the body is exposed to and produces antibodies against a particular antigen. However, during that first exposure, a condition known as **hypersensitivity** develops, which means that at some subsequent time, when the person is again exposed to that same antigen, an allergic reaction will occur. This process of developing hypersensitivity on first exposure to an antigen is known as **sensitization**. (In some cases, an *anaphylactoid* reaction can occur the first time an antigen is introduced into the body. This type of reaction will be discussed in the next section.)

This is how sensitization works: When an antigen is introduced into the body, the body recognizes it as a foreign or "nonself" substance and forms antibodies to fight off the antigen. The antibodies attach themselves to two types of cells in the body: mast cells and basophils. Mast cells are located in connective tissue and are concentrated around the heart, lungs, and vessels. Basophils are immature mast cells that circulate in the blood. The antibody may stay attached to the mast cells and basophils for minutes, days, weeks, months, or years. As long as the antibody is attached, the patient is said to be "sensitized" to the substance that generated the antibodies.

Once sensitization occurs, the patient is primed for a possible anaphylactic reaction. It may take several exposures to a foreign substance over a long period of time. For example, you may encounter a patient who had eaten crab meat for years without any noticeable reaction, but his consumption of crab on this occasion produced an anaphylactic reaction and a call to EMS. Because of such variations in sensitization, it is difficult to predict who is at risk of developing an anaphylactic reaction. However, once a patient has had an anaphylactic reaction, it should be assumed that he will react in a similar fashion to another exposure to the same antigen.

When the antigen is reintroduced into the body, it attaches to the antibodies that are now located on the mast cells and basophils. The mast and basophil cell membranes break down and release chemical substances, referred to as chemical mediators. These chemical mediators then cause a cascade of events to occur that can lead to specific signs and symptoms and the life-threatening condition of anaphylaxis. The primary chemical mediator released from mast cells and basophils is **histamine**. Histamine causes bronchoconstriction, vasodilation, and an increase in capillary permeability (leakage).

Understanding BODY PROCESSES

The direct attachment of the antigen to the antibody located on the mast cells and basophils causes the cell membrane to break down and release the chemical mediators that produce the anaphylactic reaction. ■

As already noted, the life-threatening responses that are directly produced from the release of the chemical mediators are bronchoconstriction, increase in capillary permeability, and vasodilation (Figure 21-1∗). These produce the signs and symptoms seen in anaphylaxis. If the bronchoconstriction, increase in capillary permeability, and vasodilation can be reversed, the life-threatening condition and the signs and symptoms will be reversed.

Anaphylactoid Reaction

In some reactions the chemical mediators can be released from the mast cells and basophils the first time the antigen is introduced into the body without the patient ever being sensitized. The antigen itself causes the release of the

Key Terms

immune response production of **antibodies** to fight foreign substances. An **allergic reaction** or life-threatening **anaphylactic reaction** (**anaphylactic shock; anaphylaxis**) is an abnormal response.

Objective 21-5

Explain anaphylactic and anaphylactoid reactions.

Key Terms

hypersensitivity altered reactivity to an allergen that causes an allergic reaction, after the **sensitization** that occurs on first exposure.

histamine chemical mediator, released from mast cells, in an anaphylactic reaction.

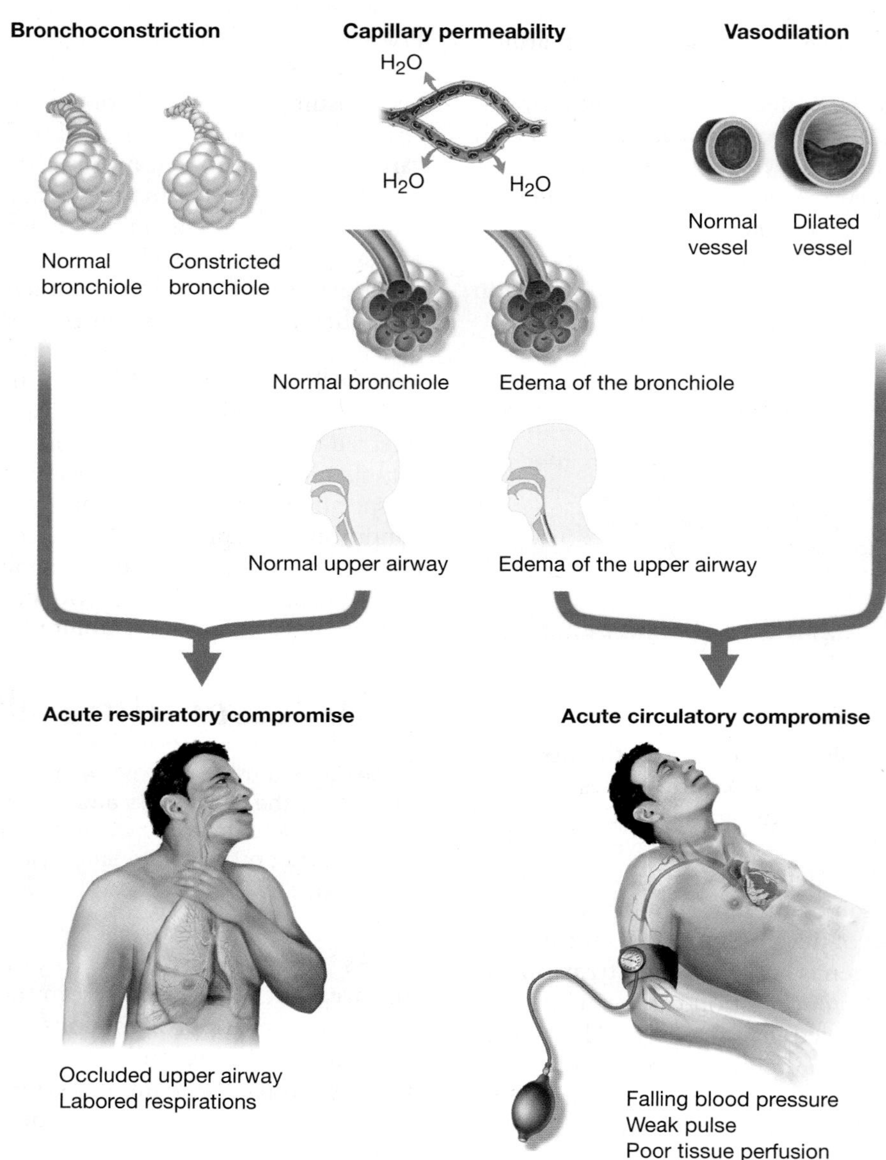

FIGURE 21-1 * Life-threatening responses in anaphylactic reaction: bronchoconstriction, capillary permeability, vasodilation, and an increase in mucus production.

chemical mediators. This reaction, where no sensitization is required, is referred to as an **anaphylactoid reaction**. The body's responses (bronchoconstriction, increased capillary permeability, and vasodilation) and the signs and symptoms are exactly the same as for a true anaphylactic reaction. Thus, the treatment is exactly the same. The primary difference, when you collect the history from the patient, is that he will not have had a previous exposure to the antigen, as the patient suffering from a true anaphylactic reaction would have had. See Table 21-1 for substances that commonly cause anaphylactoid reactions. For purposes of discussion in this chapter, reference to severe

Objective 21-6
List ways an antigen can be introduced into the body and substances that commonly cause anaphylactic or anaphylactoid reactions.

Objective 21-7
Explain an assessment-based approach to anaphylactic reaction.

Key Terms
anaphylactoid reaction reaction similar to an anaphylactic reaction that may occur on first exposure without prior sensitization.

TABLE 21-1 Substances That Commonly Cause Anaphylactoid Reactions

Radiopaque contrast media
Nonsteroidal anti-inflammatory drugs (NSAIDs)
Aspirin
Opiates
Thiamine

allergic reaction and anaphylactic reaction includes anaphylactoid reaction, since the signs and symptoms and treatment are exactly the same.

Causes of Anaphylactic Reaction

An anaphylactic reaction can be triggered by any of a large number of substances. The most common cause is medications that are either taken orally or injected. Some cases of anaphylactic reaction are idiopathic, which means that their causes cannot be identified. This is a difficult situation for the patient, since he does not know what substance may trigger another reaction.

An antigen may enter the body by:

- **Injection.** The substance is introduced directly into the body by bites, stings, needles, or infusions.
- **Ingestion.** The patient swallows the substance.
- **Inhalation.** The patient breathes the substance into his lungs.
- **Contact (absorption).** The antigen is absorbed through the skin.

Injection, especially intramuscular or intravenous injection, is the route most often associated with anaphylactic reactions. Penicillin is the most common cause of anaphylactic reactions. Some of the common causes of anaphylactic reactions are:

- *Venom* from insect bites or stings, especially of wasps, hornets, yellow jackets, and fire ants. Other bites or stings often causing reactions include those of deer flies, gnats, horse flies, mosquitoes, cockroaches, and miller moths. Snake and spider venom may also cause an anaphylactic reaction.
- *Foods,* including peanuts, other nuts, milk, eggs, shellfish, whitefish, food additives, chocolate, cottonseed oil, and berries.

TABLE 21-2 Medications That Commonly Cause Anaphylactic Reactions

Antibiotics	Penicillin
	Tetracycline
	Cephalosporins
	Aminoglycosides
	Sulfonamides
	Amphotericin B
	Nitrofurantoin
Local anesthetics	Procaine
	Lidocaine
	Novocaine
Vitamins	Thiamine
	Folic acid

- *Pollen* from plants, especially ragweed and grasses.
- *Medications* (see Table 21-2), including antibiotics, local anesthetics, aspirin, seizure medications, muscle relaxants, nonsteroidal anti-inflammatory agents, and vitamins. Insulin and tetanus and diphtheria toxoids may also produce an anaphylactic reaction. Remember, however, a side effect of a medication is *not* an allergic reaction to the drug (e.g., nausea after codeine administration).
- *A large number of other substances,* such as glue, can produce an anaphylactic reaction.
- *Exercise* may accentuate the anaphylactic response when certain foods have been ingested close to the time of exercise.
- *Latex,* most often found in examination gloves and other medical devices.

Assessment-Based Approach to Anaphylactic Reaction

Because the signs and symptoms of allergic reaction are similar to those for many other medical problems, you may or may not be able to determine that the cause of the problem is an allergic reaction. However, an anaphylactic reaction should be obvious from its characteristic extreme signs and symptoms.

Thinking Critically
Why is the primary assessment especially important in the case of an allergic reaction?

Key Terms
malaise a general feeling of weakness or discomfort.

Key Terms
endotracheal intubation placement of a tube down the trachea to facilitate airflow to the lungs.

hives raised red blotches associated with allergic and anaphylactic reactions.

Scene Size-Up

During the scene size-up, you must be certain that your own safety is not in jeopardy, especially if the anaphylactic reaction is the result of a bite or sting. You might encounter a patient who disrupted a yellow jacket or wasp nest and was stung several times. The yellow jackets or wasps may still be at the scene and will attack once you exit the ambulance, exposing you to the risk of an anaphylactic reaction from the stings. If you detect the presence of large numbers of wasps or yellow jackets, you may have to wait until they settle or disperse before approaching the patient. It may be necessary to warn bystanders away from the scene to prevent them from becoming patients.

Because so many different substances may cause an anaphylactic reaction, the scene size-up may not provide any obvious clues as to the nature of the illness. A response to a restaurant or a home for a patient complaining of difficulty in breathing and itching after eating may cause you to suspect a possible anaphylactic reaction. Medications found at the scene may provide some clues. A patient at a health club, gym, or park who was exercising following ingestion of food may increase your suspicion that an anaphylactic reaction may be involved.

Primary Assessment

Because an anaphylactic reaction can be life threatening, the primary assessment is an extremely important part of the patient contact. In gathering your general impression of a patient with an anaphylactic reaction, you may note that he complains of "not feeling well" or of **malaise**, a generalized feeling of weakness or discomfort. Such a patient may display a sense of "impending doom." The patient's mental status may be anywhere on the continuum from responsive and alert, to responsive but disoriented, to unresponsive.

Closely assess the airway for signs of obstruction. Stridor or crowing sounds indicate significant swelling to the upper airway. Inserting an airway adjunct may not help relieve the obstruction if the swelling is at the level of the larynx. It may be necessary to provide positive pressure ventilation to force the air past the swollen upper airway. You may also find a swollen tongue that interferes with the airway. Wheezing may be prominent upon assessment of breathing. If a patient is severely disoriented, unresponsive, or breathing inadequately, immediately begin positive pressure ventilation with supplemental oxygen. If the breathing is adequate, place the patient on a nonrebreather mask with an oxygen flow of 15 liters per minute.

Understanding BODY PROCESSES

Wheezing is caused by constriction and inflammation of the lining of the bronchioles, which results in an increase in airway resistance, which makes it more difficult for the patient to move air in and out of the alveoli. ■

Delivery of ventilations may be difficult because of the bronchoconstriction, inflammation, increased mucus production, and drastically increased resistance in the lower airway. You might find it hard to squeeze the bag of the bag-valve-mask device. If a pop-off relief valve is present on the bag-valve-mask device, it may be necessary to deactivate it or to place your thumb over it in order to deliver a sufficient tidal volume of air to ventilate the patient effectively.

Management of the airway may require **endotracheal intubation**, the placement of a tube in the trachea to facilitate breathing. In most jurisdictions, this must be performed by an advanced life support (ALS) team. Consider calling for ALS backup.

The pulse in a patient suffering from an anaphylactic reaction may be weak and rapid. The radial pulse may not be present because of the low blood pressure. Edema, or swelling, may be obvious in the face, neck, lips, tongue, hands, and feet (Figure 21-2a*). The skin may be red and warm, or the patient's skin may be cyanotic from inadequate breathing. You may notice **hives**, raised red blotches, all over the skin (Figures 21-2b and 21-2c*). Hives are usually accompanied by severe itching. Hives

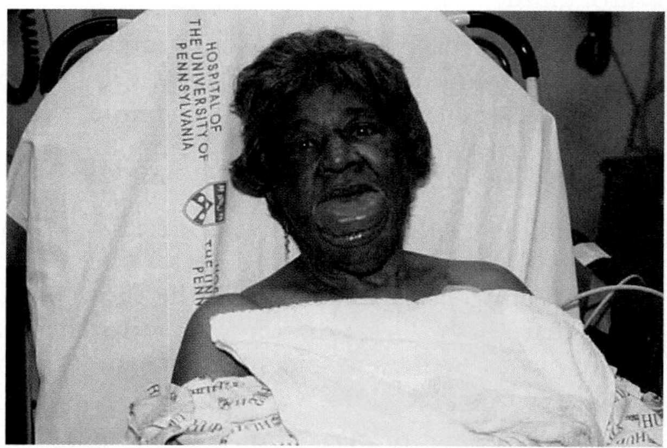

FIGURE 21-2a * Localized angioedema to the tongue from an anaphylactic reaction. (© Edward T. Dickinson, MD)

Key Points
The quicker an allergic reaction develops, the more severe it is likely to be.

Key Points
If the patient exhibits signs of a severe allergic reaction, do not delay transport to complete the secondary assessment.

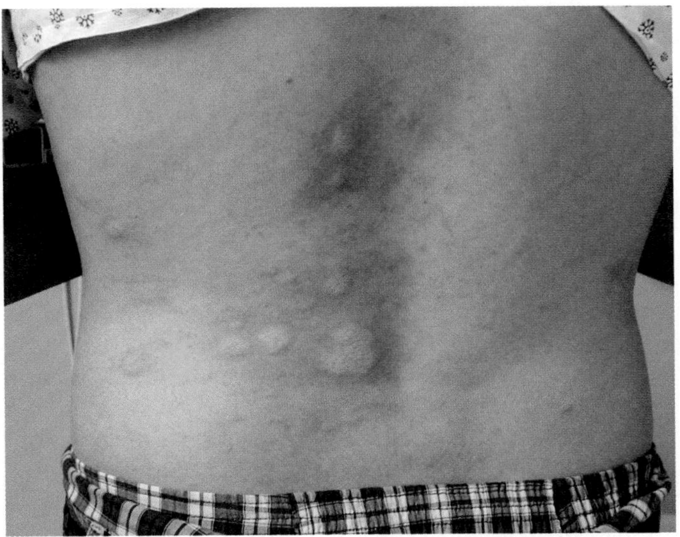

FIGURE 21-2b ✱ Hives (urticaria) from an allergic reaction to a penicillin-derivative drug. (© Charles Stewart, MD, & Associates)

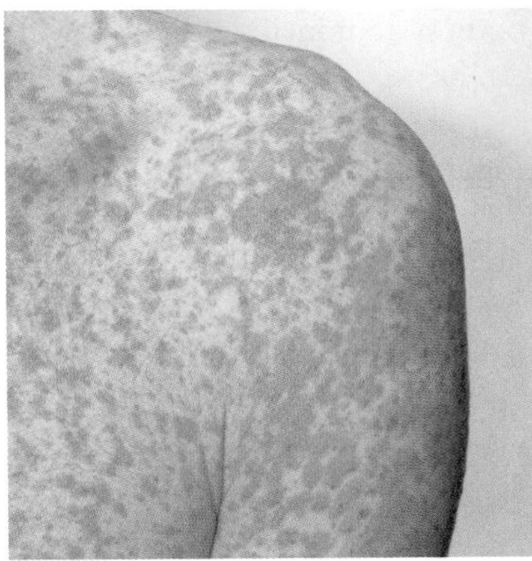

FIGURE 21-2c ✱ Hives to the upper body. (Medical-on-Line/ Alamy)

(urticaria) and itching (pruritus) are the hallmark signs and symptoms of an allergic reaction.

Some of the most immediately noticeable signs of severe allergic responses have the following causes:

- *Rapid and weak pulse* results from fluid loss from the permeable and leaking capillaries and from vasodilation (dilation of the blood vessels), which causes a decrease in the blood pressure and perfusion.
- *Warm, flushed skin* is caused by vasodilation, which allows warm red blood to pool in the vessels in the skin.
- *Hives* result from capillary permeability and leaking in the epidermis (outer layer) of the skin.
- *Edema (swelling) of the skin and other tissues such as the lips and tongue (angioedema or angioneurotic edema)* is caused by capillary permeability and leaking in the dermis (deeper layer) of the skin.

Because of the potential seriousness of an anaphylactic reaction and its effects on the airway, lungs, blood vessels, and heart, the patient is considered a priority and should be prepared for immediate transport. If the patient exhibits signs of anaphylactic reaction—that is, respiratory distress and/or shock (hypoperfusion)—before leaving the scene, determine if the patient has a prescribed epinephrine auto-injector. Inquire of relatives or any bystanders if the patient is unresponsive. If he has a prescribed epinephrine auto-injector, locate it (or them, if he has more than one) immediately.

Secondary Assessment

The secondary assessment should be conducted whether the patient's signs and symptoms indicate a mild, moderate, or severe allergic reaction; however, if the patient exhibits signs of severe reaction, do not delay transport of the patient to complete the secondary assessment. Instead, perform the secondary assessment en route to the hospital.

History Assess the history of the present illness through the OPQRST line of questioning. Information about the onset of the reaction is especially important. What was the patient doing prior to the onset? What seemed to trigger the signs and symptoms? Such questioning may actually identify the antigen causing the reaction. Determine if anything makes the signs or symptoms better or worse. Did the patient take any medications in an attempt to relieve the symptoms?

Time can be a critical factor in dealing with patients with an anaphylactic reaction. Most anaphylactic reactions are apparent within 20 minutes after exposure to the antigen; however, reaction time can vary from seconds to hours. As a general rule, the quicker the patient develops signs and symptoms after exposure, the more severe the reaction will be. Thus, if the reaction occurred within minutes after exposure, you should suspect and be prepared to manage a very severe anaphylactic reaction.

Obtain a SAMPLE history from the patient. If he is unable to speak or is unresponsive, try to obtain as much information as possible from relatives or bystanders while preparing the patient for transport, but without delaying

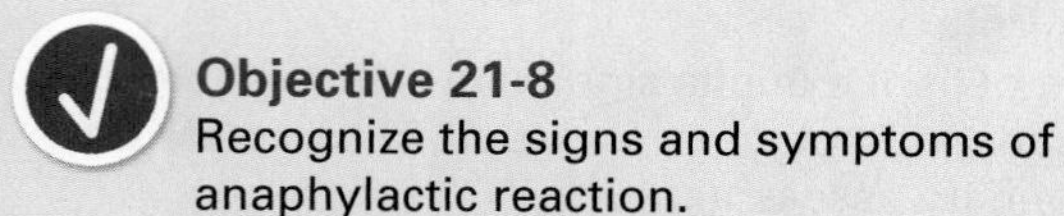

Objective 21-8
Recognize the signs and symptoms of anaphylactic reaction.

Key Points
The signs and symptoms of an anaphylactic reaction usually involve the skin and the respiratory, cardiovascular, gastrointestinal, central nervous, and genitourinary systems.

ASSESSMENT Tips

The faster the onset of the signs and symptoms of an anaphylactic reaction, the more severe and prolonged the reaction will probably be. ■

transport if the patient's signs and symptoms indicate severe reaction. When taking the SAMPLE history, it is important to determine the following:

Signs and Symptoms

- Are the signs and symptoms consistent with an anaphylactic reaction?
- Do the signs and symptoms indicate a mild, moderate, or severe reaction?
- Are the signs and symptoms getting progressively worse or better?

Allergies

- Does the patient have a history of allergies to food, medications, plants, insect stings or bites, or other? Prior anaphylactic reaction? To what?

Medications

- Does the patient have a prescribed epinephrine auto-injector? (This must be determined early in the assessment for a patient with signs and symptoms of a severe reaction.)
- Has the patient taken any medications to relieve the current signs or symptoms, including over-the-counter medications such as Benadryl?
- What other medication is the patient taking? Any new medications prescribed?

Pertinent Past History

- Has the patient ever suffered an anaphylactic reaction in the past?
- How severe was the last reaction?
- Does the patient have any other significant illnesses?

Last Oral Intake

- When was the last time the patient had anything to eat or drink? What did he recently eat or drink?
- How much food or drink did the patient consume?

Events Prior to Illness

- What was the patient doing prior to onset of the anaphylactic reaction?
- What was the patient exposed to that may have caused the anaphylactic reaction?
- What was the route of exposure—injection, ingestion, inhalation, or contact?

Signs and Symptoms The signs and symptoms of an anaphylactic reaction usually involve the skin, respiratory system, cardiovascular system, gastrointestinal system, central nervous system, and genitourinary system. The signs and symptoms vary with the severity of the reaction. An anaphylactic reaction can produce serious compromise of respiratory function or circulatory function (shock, or hypoperfusion) or both. If hypoperfusion or shock is present along with other signs and symptoms of anaphylaxis, it is usually referred to as anaphylactic shock. You would see a decrease in the blood pressure in the patient. Common signs and symptoms of an anaphylactic reaction by body system include the following:

Skin

- Warm, tingling feeling in the face, mouth, chest, feet, and hands (early symptom)
- Intense itching (pruritus), especially of hands and feet (hallmark symptom)
- Hives (urticaria) (hallmark sign)
- Flushed or red skin
- Swelling to the face, lips, neck, hands, feet, and tongue
- Cyanosis (severe cases)

Respiratory System

- Patient complaints of a "lump in the throat"
- Tightness in the chest
- High-pitched cough
- Tachypnea (increased breathing rate)
- Labored breathing
- Noisy breathing (wheezing, stridor, or crowing)
- Impaired ability to talk or hoarseness
- Excessive amounts of coughed-up mucus
- Partially or completely occluded airway
- Difficulty in breathing

Objective 21-9
List the two key categories of signs and symptoms that indicate a severe anaphylactic reaction.

Key Points
Focus the physical exam on the patient's complaints regarding the airway, breathing, and circulation.

Thinking Critically
After a bee sting, your patient has developed respiratory distress and very weak pulses. Is she a candidate for epinephrine? Why or why not?

Cardiovascular System

- Tachycardia (increased heart rate)
- Hypotension (decreased blood pressure)
- Irregular pulse
- Absent radial pulse (severe shock)

Central Nervous System

- Increased anxiety
- Light-headedness
- Unresponsiveness
- Disorientation
- Restlessness
- Seizures
- Headache

Gastrointestinal System

- Nausea/vomiting
- Abdominal cramping
- Diarrhea
- Difficulty in swallowing
- Loss of bowel control

Genitourinary System

- Urgent need to urinate
- Cramping of the uterus

Generalized Signs and Symptoms

- Itchy, watery eyes
- Runny or stuffy nose
- Sense of impending doom
- Complaints of "not feeling well"
- General weakness or discomfort

Physical Exam Focus the physical exam on the patient's complaints involving the airway, breathing, and circulation. If the patient is unresponsive, conduct a rapid secondary assessment. Your major concerns in both the responsive and unresponsive patient are a compromised airway, inadequate breathing, and shock (hypoperfusion). Inspection of the face and neck typically reveals a swollen appearance and hives. The lips may also be swollen and cyanotic.

The two key categories of signs and symptoms that specifically indicate a severe anaphylactic reaction are:

- **Airway and respiratory compromise.** Airway occlusion; respiratory distress or respiratory failure with possible wheezing or stridor
- **Shock (hypoperfusion).** Absent or weak pulses; rapid heartbeat; decreased blood pressure; deteriorating mental status

This patient needs immediate intervention and administration of epinephrine, if possible.

ASSESSMENT Tips

If the face, neck, tongue, and lips are swollen, it is likely that the mucous lining of the larynx of the upper airway is also swollen. Stridorous sounds with respiration would be an indication of this swelling. ■

Understanding BODY PROCESSES

When the lining of the larynx swells, it swells inward, partially occluding the airway and increasing the resistance to airflow. This creates the stridorous sounds. ■

Retractions and poor rise and fall of the chest may be noted upon inspection. Diffuse wheezing may be heard on auscultation of the breath sounds. Diminished breath sounds bilaterally are a sign of inadequate respiration and an indication for immediate positive pressure ventilation. The bronchoconstriction may be so severe that air movement is minimal through the bronchioles and into the lungs; therefore, wheezing or breath sounds may not be heard, especially when severe respiratory distress is evident.

Quickly inspect the extremities for bites, stings, or injection marks. Redness may be noted around the bite or sting, providing a clue to the cause of the anaphylactic reaction. Check pulses and skin temperature, color, and condition for indications of shock (hypoperfusion).

Baseline Vital Signs Assess the baseline vital signs, paying particular attention to the breathing, pulse, and blood pressure. The breathing rate may be beyond the

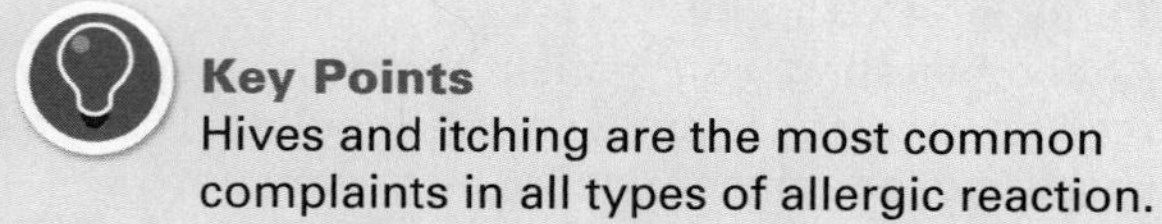
Key Points
Hives and itching are the most common complaints in all types of allergic reaction.

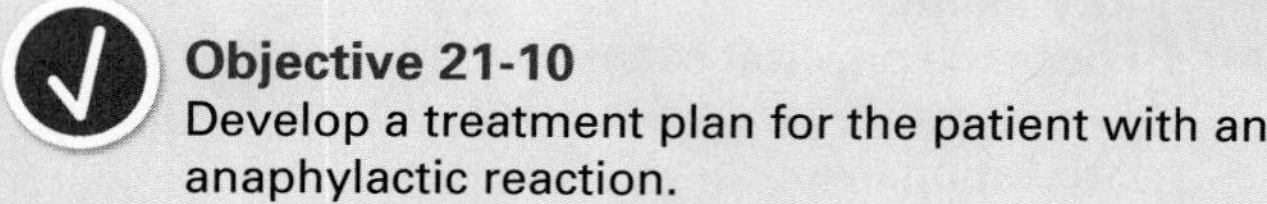
Objective 21-10
Develop a treatment plan for the patient with an anaphylactic reaction.

normal limits. Early in an anaphylactic reaction, you may find that the breathing rate is fast and labored. As the condition progresses and the patient begins to tire, the breathing may become slower than normal and very shallow. Wheezes may be heard without a stethoscope. The breathing may also sound noisy, with a rattling sound on inspiration and exhalation, from the excessive mucus in the larger lower airways. The pulse is rapid and may be weak. In severe cases of anaphylaxis, the radial pulse may be absent or extremely weak. Unlike other types of shock, the skin is usually red, dry, and warm to the touch. Hives and itching are the most common complaints in all types of allergic reaction: mild, moderate, and severe. Hypotension is common in a severe reaction.

Understanding BODY PROCESSES

In a moderate-to-severe allergic reaction, in addition to the bronchoconstriction and edema (swelling) of the bronchiole lining in the lower airways, there is also an increase in mucus production. This mucus may begin to occlude the smaller bronchioles. ■

ASSESSMENT Tips

What appears to be a mild allergic reaction can progress to a severe, life-threatening anaphylactic reaction within minutes. ■

Never underestimate the severity of an anaphylactic reaction. Because death can occur within minutes, immediate intervention is imperative. Do not mistake anaphylaxis for other conditions with similar signs and symptoms such as hyperventilation, anxiety attacks, alcohol intoxication, or hypoglycemia.

Emergency Medical Care

The key to emergency care in cases of allergic reaction is for the EMT to distinguish between mild and moderate-to-severe reactions (Table 21-3). The mild reaction typically does not require aggressive intervention or administration of medication by the EMT. In a patient with a mild reaction, you will maintain an open airway, provide oxygen, and transport the patient as soon as pos-

TABLE 21-3 Differentiating Between a Mild and a Moderate-to-Severe Allergic Reaction

Sign or Symptom	Mild Reaction	Moderate-to-Severe (Anaphylactic) Reaction
Itching	Yes	Yes—usually widespread
Hives	Yes	Yes—usually widespread
Flushed skin	Localized	Widespread
Cyanosis	No	Yes
Edema	Mild to moderate	Severe to face, lips, tongue, neck, and extremities
Heart rate	Normal or slightly increased	Significantly increased
Blood pressure	Normal	Decreased
Peripheral pulses	Present and normal	Very weak or absent
Mental status	Normal	Decreased to unresponsive
Breathing rate	Normal or slightly increased	Significantly increased with poor air movement and severe respiratory distress, or decreased with little air movement, or absent
Wheezing	No or very slight	Present throughout all lung fields
Stridor	No	Yes

Key Points
Patients experiencing a moderate-to-severe allergic reaction require an immediate, aggressive intervention by the EMT.

Key Points
Reassessment is critical. Constantly monitor the patient with a mild reaction for indications that the reaction is worsening and requires further interventions.

sible. Your major concern is that the mild reaction may rapidly progress to a moderate-to-severe, or anaphylactic, reaction. Be prepared to manage the worst-case scenario and continuously reassess the patient's condition.

Patients experiencing a moderate-to-severe reaction require immediate and aggressive intervention by the EMT. Provide the following emergency care:

- **Maintain a patent airway.** The patient may initially present with airway compromise associated with swelling of the tissues lining the larynx. Since airway adjuncts are not effective in managing the obstruction, it may be necessary to force air past the swollen tissues by positive pressure ventilation. If using a bag-valve-mask device, you may find it much harder to compress the bag to deliver the contents. It may be necessary to deactivate the pop-off valve in order to deliver adequate ventilations. Inserting an oral or nasal airway in the unresponsive patient will help to prevent the tongue from occluding the airway.
- **Suction any secretions.** In the severe anaphylactic reaction, heavy secretions may be present. Clear the mouth of secretions by suction when necessary.
- **Maintain oxygen therapy.** It is vital that the patient continuously receive a high concentration of oxygen. If the breathing is adequate, the oxygen should be delivered by a nonrebreather mask at 15 lpm. If the patient is being artificially ventilated, supplemental oxygen must be delivered through the ventilation delivery device.
- **Be prepared to assist ventilation.** Patients with a mild allergic reaction may not exhibit any respiratory distress during the length of your contact. On the other hand, a patient's condition may progress very rapidly over minutes, or more slowly over hours, and eventually produce severe respiratory distress. Have your ventilation equipment ready and prepared to begin positive pressure ventilation, if necessary. Continuously reassess the patient's breathing status for signs of inadequate breathing.
- **Administer epinephrine by a prescribed auto-injector.** In a moderate-to-severe (anaphylactic) reaction, obtain an order from medical direction to administer the patient's prescribed auto-injector. The order may be obtained on-line or off-line. If the patient is suffering from a mild allergic reaction and there are no signs of respiratory compromise (such as respiratory distress, stridor, or wheezing) or shock (weak pulses, decreasing mental status, or low blood pressure), do not administer epinephrine. Consult with medical direction for further orders. If an epinephrine auto-injector is not available, immediately begin transport.
- **Consider calling for advanced life support.** Because of the potential for severe compromise to the airway, breathing, and circulation, it may be necessary to request ALS for advanced airway control and further administration of medication.
- **Initiate early transport.** Do not unnecessarily delay transport of the patient. Continued assessment and emergency care can be done en route to the hospital.

Reassessment

Reassessment is extremely important in the management of mild, moderate, and severe allergic reactions. The patient with a mild reaction should be constantly monitored for indications that the reaction is worsening and that further intervention, such as epinephrine injection or airway control, may be needed. The patient with a moderate-to-severe reaction who has received an epinephrine injection should be reassessed to determine if the injection has been effective in reversing the life-threatening condition.

Regardless of the severity of the reaction, closely reassess the airway, breathing, and circulation status. Signs of deterioration are wheezing or stridor, increased hoarseness or difficulty in speaking, signs of inadequate breathing, decreasing mental status, decreasing blood pressure, increasing heart rate, and weak or absent radial pulses. Reassess and record the baseline vital signs and other reassessment findings.

Reassess the patient 2 minutes after the injection of epinephrine. Look for improvement in the patient's ability to breathe, improvement in his mental status, and an increase in the blood pressure. If the condition has not improved, it may be necessary to consult with medical direction about a second injection if another epinephrine auto-injector is available.

Summary: Assessment and Care

To review assessment findings that may be associated with allergic reaction and emergency care for allergic reaction, see Figures 21-3* and 21-4*.

Assessment Summary

ANAPHYLACTIC REACTION

The following findings may be associated with an anaphylactic reaction.

SCENE SIZE-UP

Ensure your own safety.
Look for evidence of cause of anaphylactic reaction:
- Injection (venom, medications)
- Ingestion (foods, medications)
- Inhalation (pollen, chemical irritants)
- Absorption (chemicals, plants)
- Location of patient may provide clues as to cause (e.g., home, physician's office, outdoors, restaurant).

Primary Assessment

General Impression
- Feeling of impending doom
- Malaise
- Weakness
- Discomfort

Mental Status
- Alert to unresponsive
- Decreasing mental status
- Increased anxiety
- Disorientation
- Restlessness
- Seizure activity

Airway
- Signs of laryngeal edema (stridor, crowing)
- Swollen tongue

Breathing
- Inadequate ventilation
- Wheezing

Circulation
- Weak pulses
- Tachycardia
- Red, warm, dry skin
- Cyanosis

Status: Priority Patient

Secondary Assessment

SAMPLE History

Signs and symptoms:
- Tightness in chest
- High-pitched cough
- Impaired ability to talk or hoarseness
- Urgent need to urinate
- Uterine cramping
- Hives and itching
- Red flushed skin
- Stridor or crowing respirations
- Wheezing on auscultation
- Swelling to face, hands, and feet

Ask questions regarding the following:
- Does the patient have a history of allergy?
- When did the exposure to the allergen occur?
- Can the allergen be identified?
- Has the patient ever suffered an anaphylactic reaction before?
- If so, how severe was the reaction?
- Does the patient have an epinephrine auto-injector?

Physical Exam

Head, neck, and face:
- Edema to face, hands, neck, and lips
- Hives
- Itching
- Warm, tingling feeling
- Cyanosis
- Difficulty in swallowing
- Itchy and watery eyes
- Runny or stuffy nose
- Coughed-up mucus
- Headache

Chest:
- Retractions
- Accessory muscle use
- Wheezing in all lung lobes

Abdomen:
- Nausea/vomiting
- Abdominal cramping
- Diarrhea
- Loss of bowel control

Extremities:
- Warm, tingling feeling in hands and feet
- Itching, especially hands and feet
- Edema (swelling) to hands and feet
- Red, warm, dry skin
- Weak or absent peripheral pulses

Baseline Vital Signs
- BP: hypotension
- HR: tachycardia with weak peripheral pulses
- RR: tachypnea with wheezing and labored breathing
- Skin: red, warm, dry, hives, itching
- Pupils: normal to dilated and responsive to light
- SpO_2: <95%

FIGURE 21-3a ✱ Assessment summary: anaphylactic reaction.

Key Terms
epinephrine a natural hormone that, when used as a medication, constricts blood vessels to improve blood pressure, reduces leakage from blood vessels, and relaxes smooth muscle in the bronchioles.

Objective 21-11
Describe the role of epinephrine in the treatment of anaphylaxis and the criteria and procedure administration of epinephrine.

Key Terms
auto-injector a device with a spring-loaded needle, used for injecting a single dose of medication.

Emergency Care Protocol

ANAPHYLACTIC REACTION

1. Establish and maintain an open airway.
2. Suction secretions.
3. If breathing is inadequate, provide positive pressure ventilation with supplemental oxygen via reservoir at 10–12 ventilations/minute.
4. If breathing is adequate, administer oxygen via nonrebreather mask at 15 lpm.
5. If signs and symptoms of moderate or severe (anaphylactic) reaction, including respiratory distress and/or hypotension, administer epinephrine by the patient's prescribed auto-injector:
   - Epinephrine is an alpha and beta drug that mimics the sympathetic nervous system and constricts blood vessels, tightens the capillaries, dilates bronchioles, and increases heart rate and contractility.
   - Epinephrine adult dose: 0.3 mg (over 66 lb)
   - Epinephrine pediatric dose: 0.15 mg (up to 66 lb)
     a. Obtain order from medical direction.
     b. Check medication.
     c. Remove safety cap.
     d. Press injector firmly against lateral thigh midway between knee and hip.
     e. Hold for 10 seconds.
     f. Dispose of injector in biohazard sharps container.
     g. Record time and reassess patient.
   - Epinephrine side effects:
     Increased heart rate
     Pale skin
     Dizziness
     Headache
     Palpitations
     Excitability and anxiousness
     Chest pain
     Nausea and vomiting
6. Consider calling advanced life support.
7. Expedite transport.
8. Perform a reassessment every 5 minutes.

FIGURE 21-3b ✻ Emergency care protocol: anaphylactic reaction.

Epinephrine Auto-Injector

Epinephrine is the drug of choice for the emergency treatment of a moderate-to-severe allergic reaction to insect stings or bites, foods, drugs, and other antigens. The drug mimics the responses of the sympathetic nervous system. If you recall from Chapter 7, epinephrine has four properties: $alpha_1$, $alpha_2$, $beta_1$, and $beta_2$. $Alpha_1$ causes the vessels to constrict. $Alpha_2$ regulates the amount of vasoconstricton. $Beta_1$ increases the heart rate, force of contraction of the heart, and the speed at which the electrical impulses are carried through the heart. $Beta_2$ causes the bronchiole smooth muscle to dilate.

Recall from earlier in this chapter that three of the major responses to the chemical mediators by the body causing the life-threatening anaphylactic condition are an increase in capillary permeability, vasodilation, and bronchoconstriction. Epinephrine's alpha properties cause vasoconstriction and tighten the capillaries, reversing the vasodilation and increased capillary permeability experienced by the anaphylactic patient. The $beta_2$ properties cause bronchodilation, reversing the bronchoconstriction. The $beta_1$ properties will be responsible for side effects from administration. Also, epinephrine has a direct antihistamine effect, reducing the effects of histamine. You can see why epinephrine is the drug of choice in anaphylaxis.

The body's response to epinephrine is rapid; within seconds, the patient will begin to feel relief. However, the duration of the drug's effectiveness is short, only about 10–20 minutes.

Epinephrine comes packaged in a disposable delivery system for self-administration. Common systems prescribed to patients are the EpiPen auto-injector and the Twinject. Each is an **auto-injector**, which has a spring-activated, concealed needle that is designed to deliver a precise dose of epinephrine when activated. The Twinject contains two doses of epinephrine in one device.

Emergency Care Algorithm: **Anaphylactic Reaction**

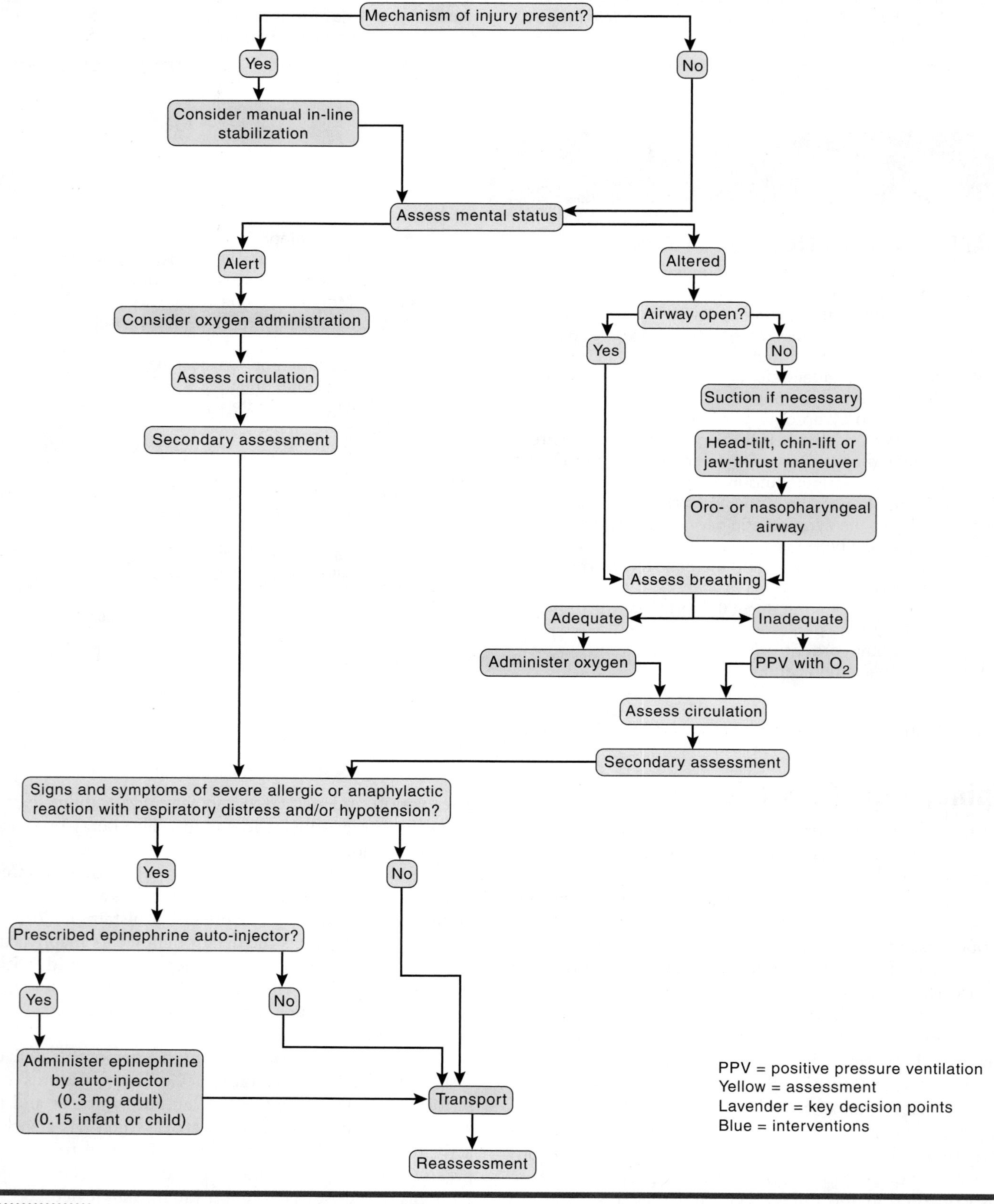

FIGURE 21-4 ∗ Emergency care algorithm: anaphylactic reaction.

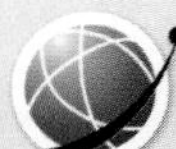

Media Resources

Go to www.bradybooks.com for mykit. Highlights:

- *Web Resource:* EpiPen auto-injector and anaphylaxis
- *Animation:* Anaphylactic Reaction
- *Animation:* Allergic Reactions and Epinephrine

Both epinephrine auto-injectors, the EpiPen and the Twinject, come in two different doses (Figure 21-5*). The 0.3 mg dose of epinephrine is for patients weighing 66 pounds or greater. The injector for infants and children up to 66 pounds delivers 0.15 mg of epinephrine. A child who weighs more than 66 pounds may have an adult epinephrine auto-injector. Because a single dose may not completely reverse the effects of an anaphylactic reaction, the physician may prescribe more than one injector or the Twinject device. If the patient does not have the Twinject device, it is important to determine if the patient has more than one injector so you can take it along and be prepared to deliver a second injection.

The auto-injector is simple to use. It is activated by pressing it against the patient's thigh. The pressure releases a spring-activated plunger, pushing the concealed needle into the thigh muscle and injecting a dose of the drug. If a second dose is needed by the Twinject device, it is necessary to unscrew the gray cap. Hold the blue hub at the needle base and pull the syringe from the barrel. Slide the collar off the plunger. Insert the needle into the thigh and push the plunger all the way down. Remove the needle and dispose of the device in a biohazard puncture-resistant container.

No precise location on the thigh is necessary, but the lateral portion of the thigh midway between the hip and knee is preferred. Do not inject the epinephrine into a vein or into the buttocks. It is preferable to remove clothing from the site of injection. If it is too difficult to remove the clothing or if the situation requires immediate administration, the injection can be given directly through the clothing.

EMT Skills 21-1 provides an illustration of the process of administering the drug using an EpiPen auto-injector. See EMT Skills 21-2 for the process of administering the drug using the Twinject system. See Figure 21-6* for a detailed summary of the criteria and techniques for administration of epinephrine.

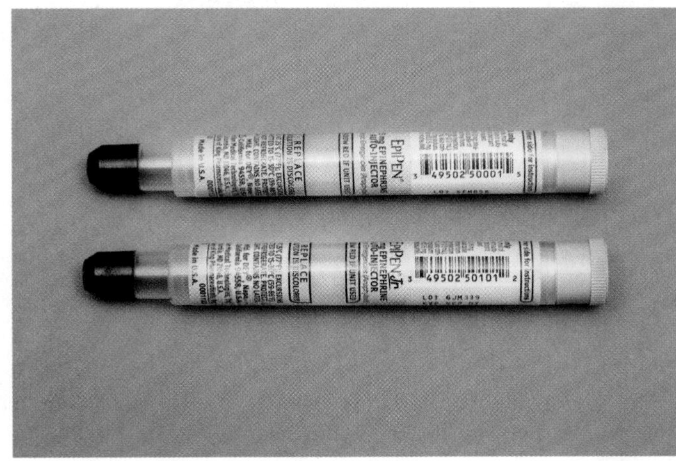

(a)

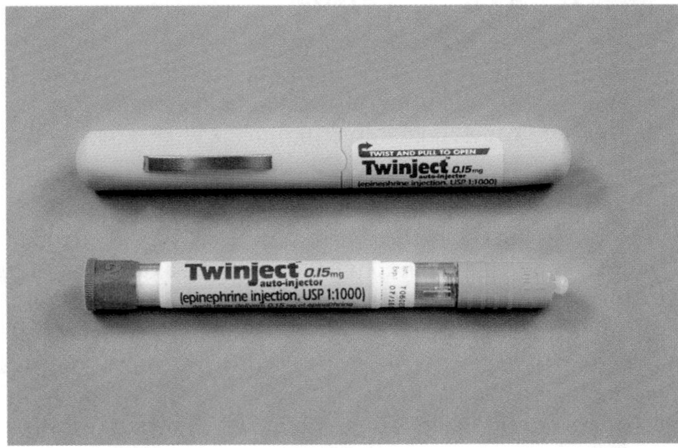

(b)

FIGURE 21-5 * Epinephrine auto-injectors: **(a)** EpiPen auto-injectors for infant/child and adult. **(b)** Twinject auto-injectors for infant/child and adult.

Epinephrine Auto-Injectors

MEDICATION NAME

Epinephrine is the generic name. The trade name is Adrenalin. Trade names of epinephrine auto-injectors are EpiPen, EpiPen Jr., and Twinject (adult and child sizes).

INDICATIONS

All of the following criteria must be met before an EMT administers epinephrine by auto-injector to the patient:

- The patient exhibits signs and symptoms of a moderate-to-severe anaphylactic reaction, including respiratory distress and/or shock (hypoperfusion).
- The medication is prescribed to the patient.
- The EMT has received an order from medical direction for administration, either on-line or off-line.

CONTRAINDICATIONS

There are no contraindications for the administration of epinephrine in a life-threatening anaphylactic reaction.

MEDICATION FORM

Epinephrine is a liquid drug contained within an auto-injector that is designed to automatically inject a precise dose when the safety cap is removed and the auto-injector is pressed firmly against the thigh.

DOSAGE

The adult auto-injector delivers a dose of 0.3 mg (for patient > 66 lb) of epinephrine. The infant-and-child auto-injector delivers 0.15 mg (for child < 66 lb) of epinephrine. A single dose is administered to the patient. It may be necessary in very severe reactions or long transport times to administer a second dose. The EpiPen is capable of delivering only a single dose; however, the Twinject device can deliver a second dose with the same device, if necessary. Consult with medical direction or follow your local protocol for the first dose and before you administer any additional dose beyond the first.

ADMINISTRATION

To administer the epinephrine by auto-injector:

1. Obtain an order from medical direction, either on-line or off-line.
2. Obtain the patient's prescribed auto-injector. Check the medication to be sure that:
   a. The prescription is written for the patient experiencing the anaphylactic reaction. (Medical direction may order administration of epinephrine that is not prescribed to the patient. Some systems carry the EpiPen or Twinject on the EMS unit.)

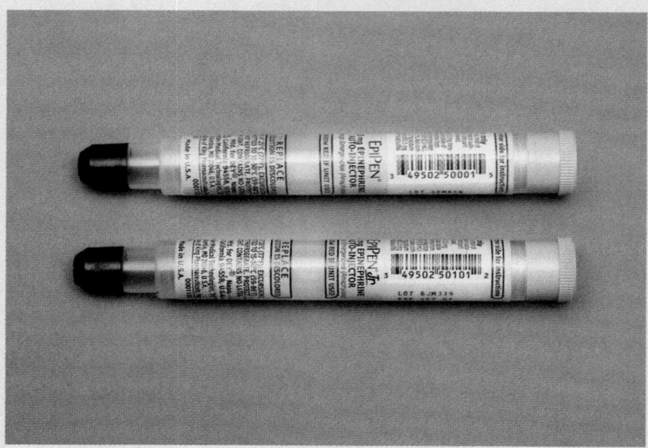

(a)

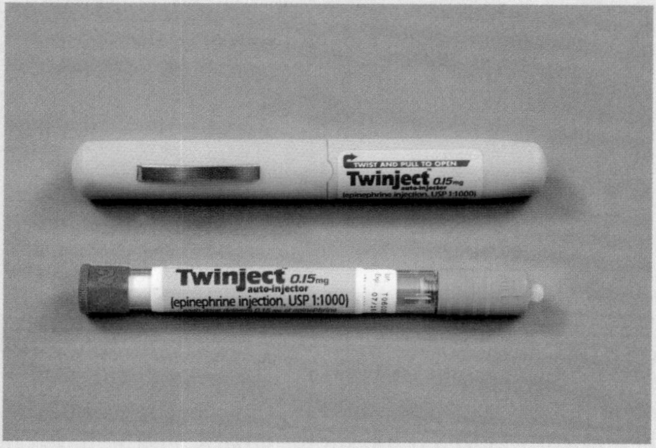

(b)

   b. The medication has not expired, has not become discolored, and does not contain particulates or sediments.
3. Remove the safety cap(s) from the auto-injector.
4. Place the tip of the auto-injector against the lateral aspect of the patient's thigh midway between the hip and knee.
5. Push the injector firmly against the thigh until the spring-loaded needle is deployed and the medication is injected.
6. Hold the auto-injector in place until all of the medication has been injected.
7. Dispose of the single-dose auto-injector in a biohazard container designed for sharp objects. Be careful not to prick yourself since the needle will now be protruding from the end of the injector. Save the Twinject device and transport it with the patient since it contains a second dose. If a second dose is required from the Twinject device, unscrew and remove the gray cap. Be cautious of the exposed needle. Hold the blue

FIGURE 21-6 ✱ Epinephrine auto-injectors. **(a)** EpiPen **(b)** Twinject.

Epinephrine Auto-Injectors—*continued*

hub at the needle base and pull the syringe from the barrel. Slide the yellow or orange collar off the plunger. Insert the needle into the thigh and push the plunger of the syringe completely down. Remove the needle and syringe and dispose of them in a puncture-resistant biohazard container.

8. Record that epinephrine was administered, the dose, and the time of administration.

ACTIONS

Epinephrine mimics the responses of the sympathetic nervous system. The alpha properties quickly constrict blood vessels to improve blood pressure and reduce the leakage from the capillaries. The $beta_2$ properties relax the smooth muscle in the bronchioles to improve breathing and alleviate the wheezing and dyspnea. The $beta_1$, which produces side effects, causes an increase in heart rate and contractility. The drug takes effect within seconds, but the duration of its effectiveness is short, about 10–20 minutes.

SIDE EFFECTS

The patient may complain of side effects following the administration of epinephrine. Possible side effects include the following:

- Increased heart rate
- Pale skin (pallor), especially at the site of injection
- Dizziness
- Chest pain
- Headache
- Nausea and vomiting
- Excitability and anxiousness

REASSESSMENT

Following the administration of epinephrine, it is necessary to reassess the patient. The reassessment should include continued evaluation of the airway, breathing, and circulatory status. Look for the following signs and symptoms that indicate the anaphylactic reaction is worsening:

- Decreasing mental status
- Decreasing blood pressure
- Increased difficulty in breathing and signs of respiratory distress
- Stridor or increased hoarseness

If the condition is worsening, you should consider the following interventions:

- Consult with medical direction about injection of a second dose of epinephrine if a second auto-injector or a Twinject device is available.
- Provide emergency care for shock (hypoperfusion).
- Be prepared to initiate positive pressure ventilation with supplemental oxygen if breathing becomes inadequate.
- Be prepared to initiate CPR and apply the automated external defibrillator (AED) if the patient becomes pulseless.

If the patient's condition improves following the administration of epinephrine, you should continue to reassess. Be aware that the patient may now complain of side effects from the epinephrine. Continue oxygen therapy with a nonrebreather device and treat for shock, if necessary.

Record and document your interventions and reassessment findings. The baseline vital signs should be checked and recorded every 5 minutes.

FIGURE 21-6 ✱ Epinephrine auto-injectors. *continued*

EMT skills 21-1 Administering an EpiPen Epinephrine Auto-Injector

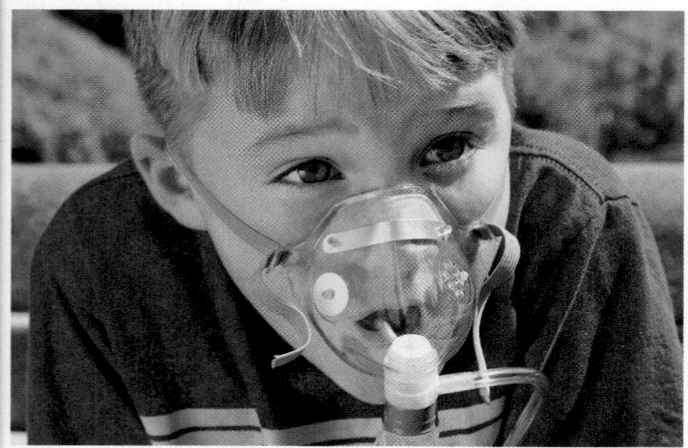

21-1A ✱ Administer oxygen by nonrebreather mask.

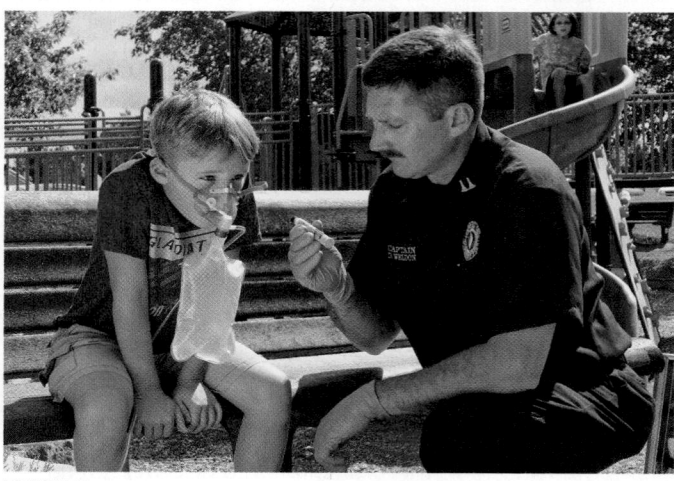

21-1B ✱ Check the EpiPen epinephrine auto-injector to ensure it is prescribed for the patient. Check the expiration date and clarity of the drug.

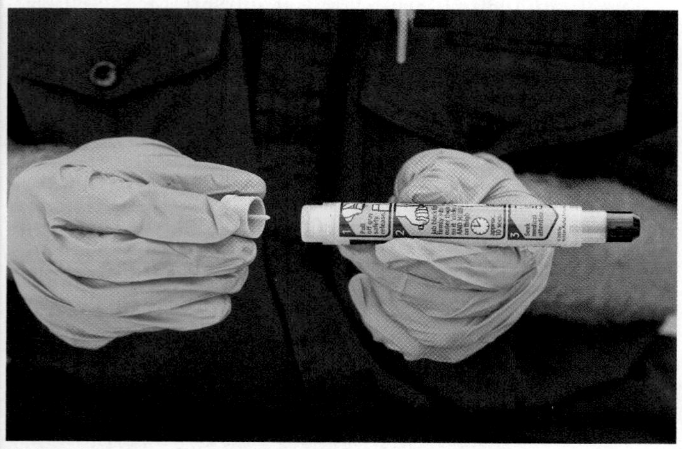

21-1C ✱ Remove the safety cap from the EpiPen auto-injector.

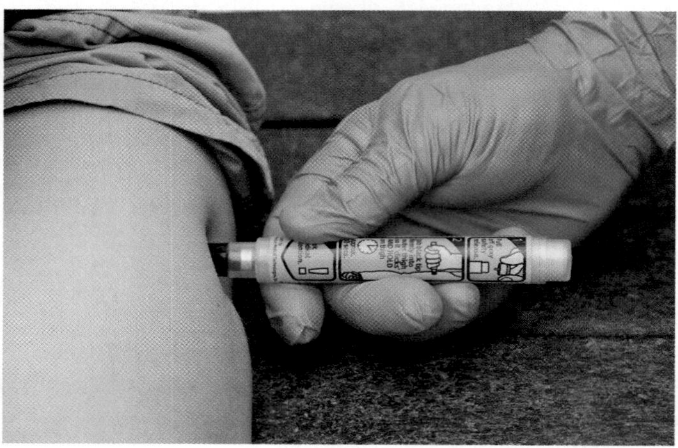

21-1D ✱ Place the tip of the auto-injector on the lateral aspect of the thigh, midway between the hip and knee. Push the injector firmly against the thigh until it activates. Hold it in place until the medication is injected.

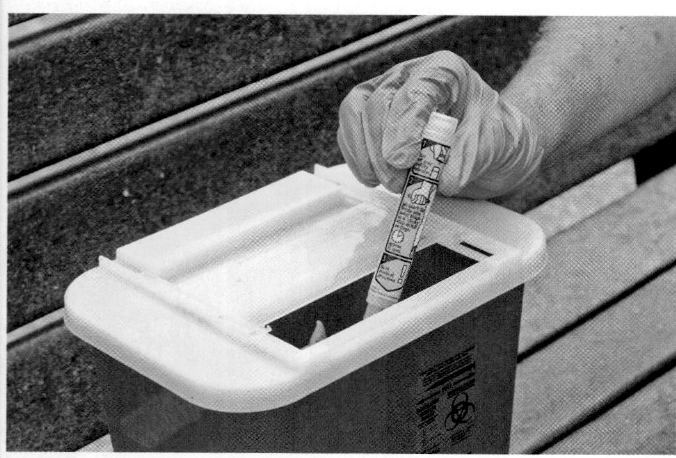

21-1E ✱ Properly dispose of the auto-injector. Then record the time of the epinephrine injection.

Administering a Twinject Epinephrine Auto-Injector

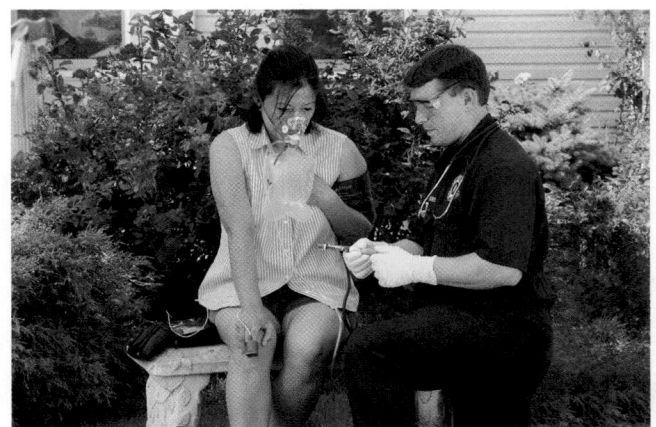

21-2A * Administer oxygen and examine the medication.

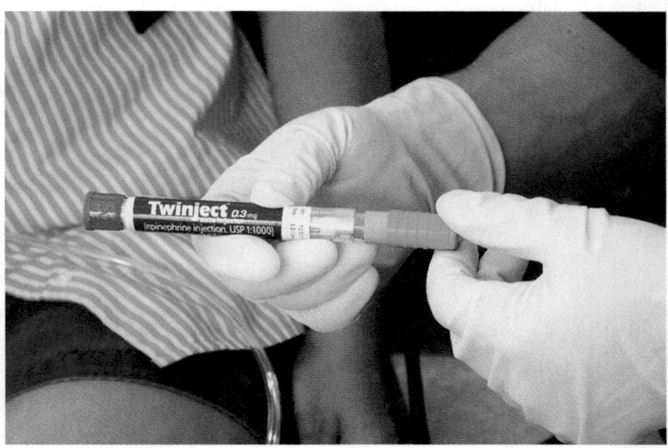

21-2B * To administer the first dose, remove the green cap from the Twinject device.

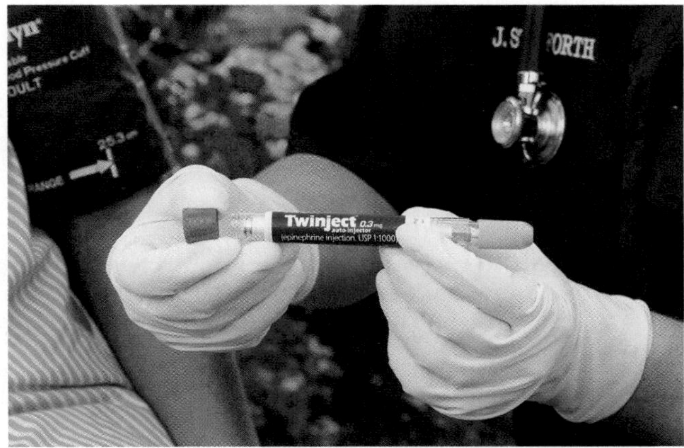

21-2C * Remove the red cap from the back of the Twinject.

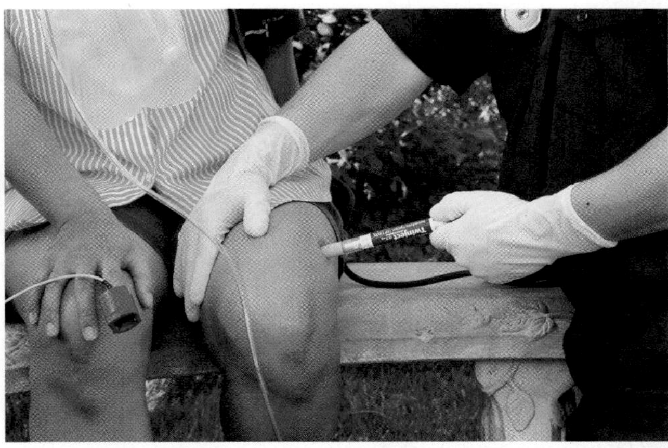

21-2D * Hold the Twinject with the gray cap against the patient's lateral thigh midway between hip and knee to inject the first dose.

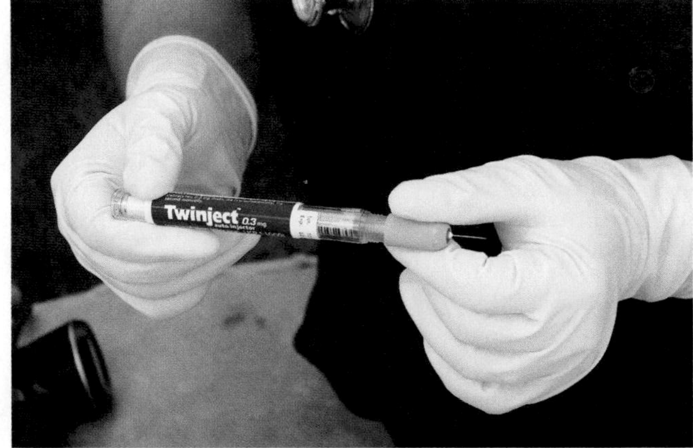

21-2E * To administer a second dose, remove the gray cap.

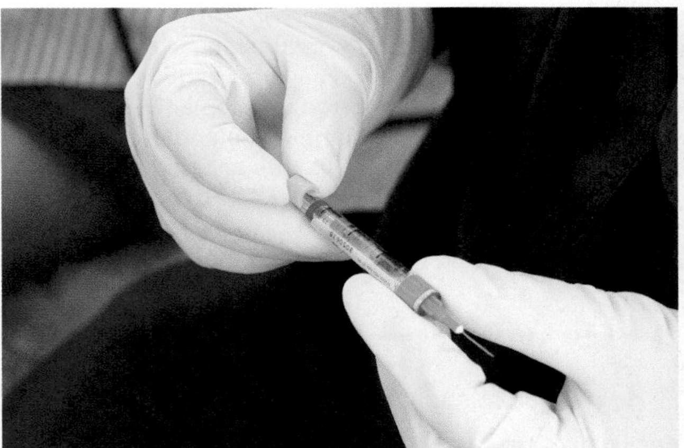

21-2F * Remove the yellow or orange tab from the syringe.

continued

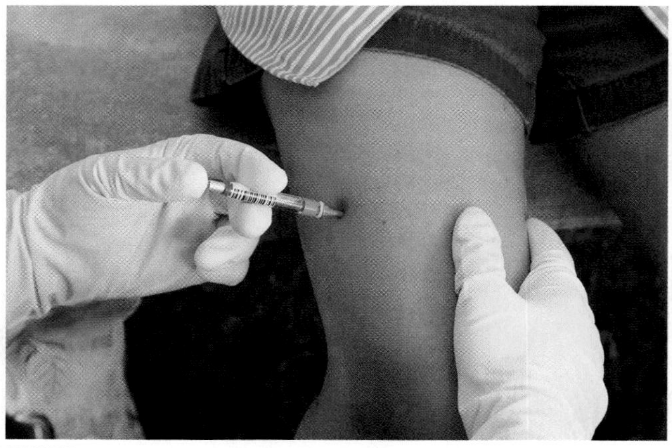

21-2G ✱ Inject the second dose into the lateral thigh on the leg opposite to the one where the first injection was given.

CHAPTER REVIEW

SUMMARY

An anaphylactic reaction is a severe allergic reaction that is an exaggerated immune response to a foreign substance, known as an antigen. For a true anaphylactic response to take place, the patient must first be sensitized by being exposed at least once to the antigen prior to the anaphylactic reaction. Some drugs and other substances do not require sensitization, but will trigger a severe allergic-type reaction on first exposure. This is referred to as an anaphylactoid reaction, and it produces the same signs and symptoms and requires the same treatment as a true anaphylactic reaction.

In order for an anaphylactic reaction to occur, mast cells and basophils must break down and release chemical mediators, of which histamine is the main mediator. The chemical mediators cause the bronchioles to constrict, the vessels to dilate, and the capillaries to leak. These produce most of the signs and symptoms seen in severe allergic and anaphylactic reactions.

Establishing and maintaining an airway, ventilation, oxygenation, and circulation are the key components of emergency care for an anaphylactic reaction. The drug treatment of choice is epinephrine. Epinephrine's alpha properties cause the vessels to constrict and the capillaries to tighten, reversing the vasodilation and increased capillary permeability caused by the chemical mediators. The $beta_2$ properties cause the bronchioles to dilate, reversing the bronchoconstriction.

✱ CASE STUDY FOLLOW-UP

SCENE SIZE-UP

You have been dispatched to a 25-year-old male patient complaining of difficulty in breathing. The patient is located at the Veterans' Pavilion at Mill Run Park. The Metropark Police have been summoned by a bicyclist who found the patient in distress. The scene is safe, and you find the patient sitting on the grass. The police wave frantically for you to hurry. As you approach the patient, you introduce yourselves and ask the patient his name. He is gasping and can barely get out the name "John Freeman." He also offers that he feels "real sick."

PRIMARY ASSESSMENT

Your general impression is that the patient, who is dressed in jogging clothes, appears to be having difficulty in breathing. You also note redness and hives that cover his face and neck. The patient is alert and scratching his arms and legs. John responds to questions in one- or two-word phrases with gasps for breath in between. He states, "I—can't—breathe—and—I itch—all over." You hear stridor as he inhales. Audible wheezes are heard on inhalation and exhalation. His breathing is labored at a rate of 28 per minute. Your partner immediately provides oxygen via a nonrebreather mask at 15 lpm. The radial pulse is barely palpable and is estimated at a rate of approximately 130 per minute. The skin is flushed, dry, and warm to the touch.

SECONDARY ASSESSMENT

You begin your secondary assessment by quickly obtaining a SAMPLE history. You use direct closed-ended questions that require mostly yes and no answers. You determine that John has the following primary symptoms: severe breathing difficulty, itching all over his body, tightness in his throat, and light-headedness. He indicates that he is allergic to yellow-jacket stings. He has a prescribed epinephrine auto-injector in a "fanny pack" around his waist. He suffered a similar reaction about 2 years ago, after which his family physician prescribed the auto-injector. His last reaction was so severe that he had to have an endotracheal tube and spent several days in the hospital. He states that the signs, symptoms, and intensity of this reaction are similar to those of the last one. He last ate at breakfast—a bagel and a cup of coffee.

John states, "I was—jogging on the—trail—when I—felt a sting—in—my left leg. I—ran out of—the woods—to the road. I—felt my—throat—closing and I—began to itch badly." John estimates that it was about 3 minutes from the sting to the onset of signs and symptoms of the reaction.

Your partner is conducting a rapid secondary assessment as you gather the history. He finds what appears to be the injection site. It is extremely swollen and red, and has a large area of hives surrounding it. Your partner indicates the blood pressure is low at 82/50 mmHg and the radial pulse is extremely weak and at a fast rate of 132 beats per minute. The respiratory rate is slightly high at 28 and labored. The skin is warm, dry, and red. Hives are found all over the body. The pulse oximeter reads 88%.

You check the epinephrine auto-injector to be sure it is John's and has not expired. You then contact medical direction at Mercy Hospital for an on-line order to administer the epinephrine. Dr. Westfield gives the order. You recheck the prescription and expiration date and look for any discoloration or sediment. You explain to John that you are going to place the auto-injector against the outer part of his thigh and that he will feel a pinch when the medication is injected. You then administer the epinephrine.

You and your partner place John in a semisitting position on the stretcher, maintaining oxygen therapy, and begin transport.

REASSESSMENT

After about 2 minutes, you reassess the patient and find that the breathing is much less labored and the wheezing has significantly decreased. John says, "Gosh, I feel much better. I can actually breathe now. I feel real nervous though, and my heart is really pounding hard. Is that normal?" You assure him that those are normal side effects from the epinephrine. Your partner indicates that the blood pressure is now higher at 112/68 mmHg and the radial pulse is much stronger and at a slower rate of 109 per minute. The skin looks less red and the hives are beginning to disappear. The SpO_2 reading is 96%. You record your treatment, the time of epinephrine administration, and your reassessment findings.

A few minutes later, you again ask John about the symptoms he is currently experiencing. He says his breathing is much easier now, and he no longer feels dizzy or light-headed. He states, "I'm still pretty itchy though!" You find upon reassessment of the vital signs that the blood pressure is now up to 124/82 mmHg and that the heart rate has decreased to 98 per minute. You contact the hospital and report the patient's condition and give an estimated time of arrival.

Upon arrival at the hospital, you give an oral report to the triage nurse. She says, "Go ahead to Room 9. Dr. Westfield is waiting for you." There, you report to Dr. Westfield the findings of the assessments before and after the epinephrine injection. As you are leaving the room, the doctor joins you for a moment and says, "You know, you've more than likely just saved this guy's life."

With a large grin on your face, you walk back to the ambulance, where your partner indicates that the unit is restocked and set for the next run. You complete your prehospital care report and notify dispatch that you are back in service.

IN REVIEW

1. List and explain the four life-threatening responses of the body to the release of chemical mediators that produce the signs and symptoms seen in an anaphylactic reaction.
2. Explain the meaning of sensitization in relation to an anaphylactic reaction.
3. List the four routes through which an antigen can be introduced into the body.
4. List the major categories of common causes of anaphylactic reaction and give examples of each category.
5. Describe the airway complications that may occur in anaphylaxis and the appropriate management of them.
6. List the common signs and symptoms of anaphylactic reaction in relation to the following body systems/categories: skin, respiratory system, cardiovascular system,

central nervous system, gastrointestinal system, genitourinary system, generalized signs and symptoms.

7. Name the two key categories of signs and symptoms of an anaphylactic reaction.
8. Describe the difference in emergency medical treatment for (a) a mild allergic reaction, and (b) a moderate-to-severe (anaphylactic) reaction.
9. List the indications and contraindications for the epinephrine auto-injector.
10. Describe the method of administration of the epinephrine auto-injector.
11. Describe the actions and possible side effects of the epinephrine auto-injector.

CRITICAL THINKING

You arrive on the scene and find a 38-year-old female patient at home on the steps of her house. She is sitting upright and appears to be alert; however, she is in obvious severe respiratory distress. She gasps after every word, and you hear obvious stridor on inhalation. Her face, lips, and tongue are severely swollen. You note hives on her face and neck. Her respirations are 38 per minute. Her radial pulse is 142 bpm and is very weak. Her skin is warm, dry, and flushed. Her blood pressure is 78/42 mmHg. Her SpO_2 is 76%. Her husband indicates that she suddenly started to experience respiratory difficulty after taking pain medication that was prescribed to her for dental work that she had done a few hours earlier. She has no known allergies and takes no other medications. She has no significant past medical history. Her last oral intake was about 15 minutes prior to your arrival when she took her pain medication. Her husband states that she was sitting in the recliner when the signs and symptoms suddenly appeared. She has hives on her face, neck, and upper chest. You hear wheezing in all lung fields. Her extremities are flushed, warm, and dry. Her pedal pulses are not palpable.

1. What is causing the airway compromise in the patient?
2. What is causing the respiratory distress?
3. How would you manage the airway and ventilation?
4. What would explain the low blood pressure?
5. What emergency care would you provide to the patient?
6. What criteria would you use to determine the need for the administration of epinephrine?
7. What are side effects of epinephrine?
8. What type of reaction is the patient suffering from?

EXPLORE PEARSON **mybradykit**™

Please go to **www.bradybooks.com** to access mykit for this text. You will find quizzes, critical thinking scenarios, weblinks, animations, and videos related to this chapter—and much more. Look for online information on the immune system and allergic reactions as well as an animation on anaphylaxis.

Register your access code from the front of your book by going to **www.bradybooks.com** and selecting the mykit links.

CHAPTER 22

Toxicologic Emergencies

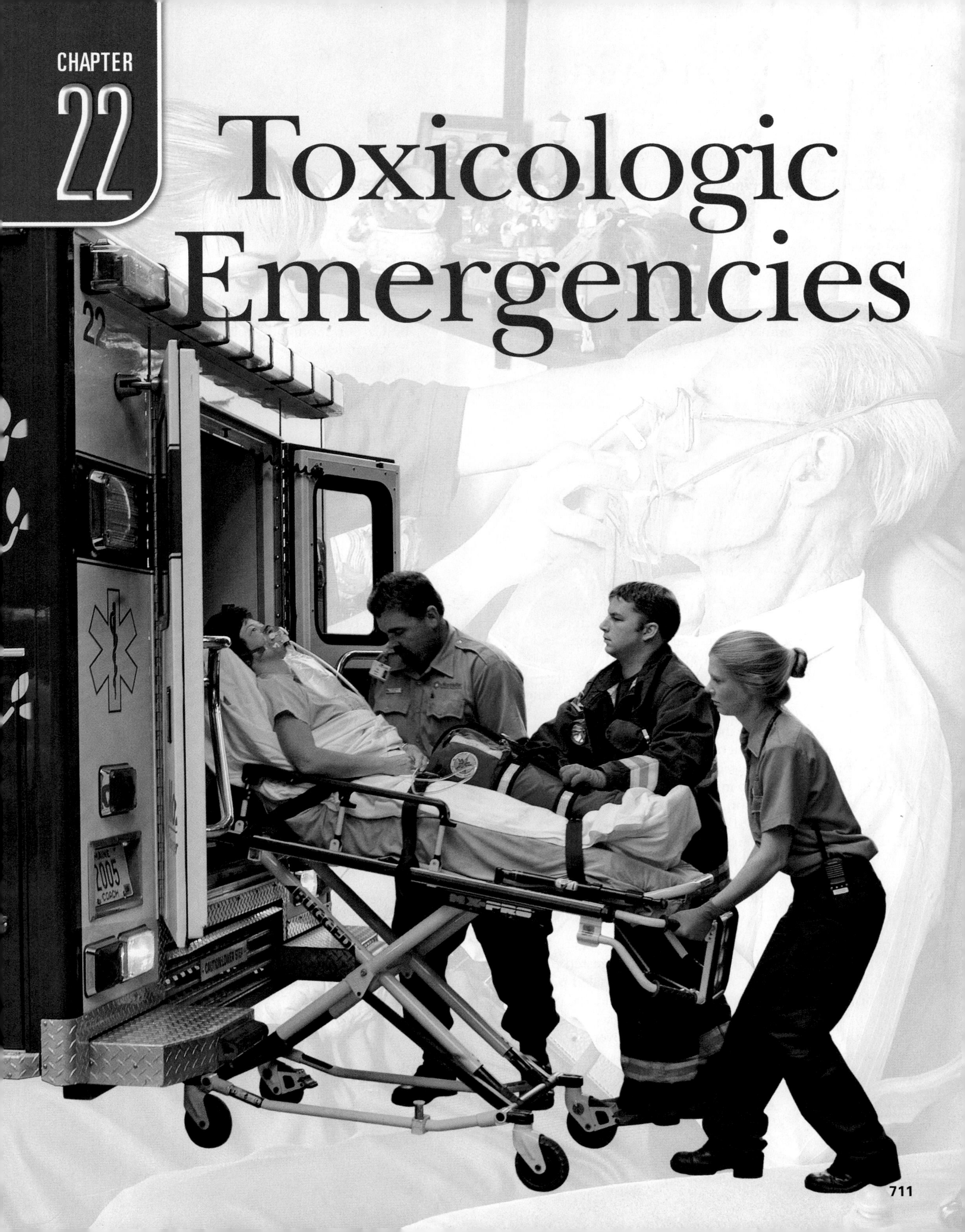

Navigation Guide

The following items provide an overview to the purpose and content of this chapter. The Standard and Competency are from the new National EMS Education Standards.

STANDARD **Medicine** (Content Area: Toxicology)

COMPETENCY Applies fundamental knowledge to provide basic emergency care and transportation based on assessment findings for an acutely ill patient.

OBJECTIVES: After reading this chapter, you should be able to:

22-1. Define key terms introduced in this chapter.
22-2. List the primary concerns of the EMT in managing drug and alcohol emergencies.
22-3. Describe each of the four routes by which a poison can enter the body:
- **a.** Ingestion
- **b.** Inhalation
- **c.** Injection
- **d.** Absorption

22-4. Describe the important steps in managing a poisoning patient, regardless of the specific poison or route of exposure.
22-5. Explain the limited role of specific antidotes in toxicologic emergencies.
22-6. Given a scenario involving a patient who has ingested a poison, describe the steps of assessment-based management.
22-7. Describe the indications, contraindications, mechanism of action, side effects, dosage, and administration of activated charcoal.
22-8. Given a scenario involving a patient who has inhaled a poison, describe the steps of assessment-based management.
22-9. Given a scenario involving a patient who has been exposed to an injected poison, describe the steps of assessment-based management.
22-10. Given a scenario involving a patient who has absorbed a poison, describe the steps of assessment-based management.
22-11. Describe special considerations in assessing and managing patients with each of the following:
- **a.** Food poisoning
- **b.** Carbon monoxide poisoning
- **c.** Cyanide poisoning
- **d.** Exposure to acid or alkali substances
- **e.** Exposure to hydrocarbons
- **f.** Methanol ingestion
- **g.** Isopropanol ingestion
- **h.** Ethylene glycol ingestion
- **i.** Exposure to poisonous plants

22-12. Explain the importance of contacting the poison control center with as complete a patient history as possible, and list specific types of information you should include.
22-13. Given a scenario involving a patient experiencing a drug or alcohol emergency, describe the steps of assessment-based management.
22-14. Describe special considerations in managing violent drug or alcohol abuse patients.
22-15. Describe special considerations in assessing and managing patients experiencing emergencies associated with each of the following:
- **a.** Drug withdrawal
- **b.** Alcoholic syndrome
- **c.** Withdrawal syndrome, including delirium tremens
- **d.** PCP use
- **e.** Cocaine use
- **f.** Amphetamines and methamphetamines
- **g.** Medication overdose
- **h.** Huffing

KEY TERMS: Page references indicate first major use in this chapter. For complete definitions, see the Glossary at the back of the book.

absorbed p. 725
activated charcoal p. 719
antidote p. 713
CNS depressants p. 741
CNS stimulants p. 741
drug abuse p. 736
hallucinogens p. 741
huffers p. 721
ingested p. 715
inhaled p. 721
injected p. 723
narcotics p. 741
overdose p. 736
pharming p. 741
poison p. 713
toxicology p. 713
toxins p. 713
volatile inhalants p. 741
withdrawal p. 736

MEDIA RESOURCES: Please go to www.bradybooks.com to access mykit for this text. You will find quizzes, critical thinking scenarios, weblinks, animations, and videos related to this chapter—and much more. Look for online information on carbon monoxide and poisonous plants. You will also find a video clip on cocaine dependence.

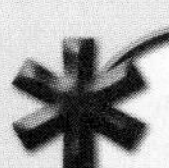

CASE STUDY

The Dispatch
EMS Unit 101—proceed to 1445 Cohasset Drive—you have a 3-year-old patient with abdominal pain. Time out is 1236 hours.

Upon Arrival
A frantic woman holding a child rushes out the door. She seems about 35 years old and identifies herself as Mrs. Horowitz. She tells you that she thinks her daughter, Sophie, ate the leaves of a houseplant and that she is now experiencing bad stomach pains.

How Would You Proceed to Assess and Care for This Patient?
During this chapter, you will learn about assessment and emergency care for patients suffering from various types of poisonings. Later, we will return to the case and apply the procedures learned.

Introduction

Each year in the United States, thousands of people die or become extremely ill from intentional or accidental poisoning. Most calls to poison control centers involve children, especially toddlers who inadvertently swallow poisonous substances while exploring their environment. Poisonings that occur at home usually involve drugs, cleaning substances, and cosmetics. Poisonings may also result from exposure to industrial chemicals, pesticides, and other substances encountered in the workplace or outdoor environment.

Regardless of the cause, when EMS is promptly called and the appropriate assessment, emergency care, and transport are provided, many instances of poisoning can have a successful outcome.

Drugs and alcohol are abused in a number of ways. In general, the emergency management steps for poisoning are applicable to patients in most alcohol and drug emergencies. However, the EMT needs to be aware of special problems associated with drug and alcohol emergencies. For instance, it is possible that drug or alcohol overdose patients will have injured themselves, so you may be treating them for trauma as well. Patients under the influence of, or withdrawing from, alcohol or drugs can be difficult to manage, behaving in an aggressive or even violent manner and posing threats to your safety.

As an EMT, your primary concern in managing drug and alcohol emergencies will be to protect your own safety, maintain an open airway, treat for life-threatening conditions, and offer calm, nonjudgmental assistance.

Poisons and Poisonings

Poisons and Routes of Exposure

A **poison** is any substance—liquid, solid, or gas—that impairs health or causes death by its chemical action when it enters the body or comes into contact with the skin.

There are more than 1 million poisonings every year in the United States. Although some poisonings are intentional and result in a homicide or suicide, most poisonings are accidental and many involve young children. Most often, the substances involved in unintentional or accidental poisonings are household chemicals.

Toxicology is the study of **toxins**, **antidotes**, and the effects of toxins on the body. A toxin is a drug or substance that is poisonous to a human and will cause certain adverse effects that may potentially lead to death. Certain toxins may not be poisonous when used properly, such as prescribed narcotic medications, whereas some toxins are poisonous under all circumstances when in contact with the body, such as sulfuric acid.

Exposure to any harmful substance can be considered a poisoning. However, it is more common for a poisoning to be defined as exposure to a substance other than a drug or medication. The term *overdose* is commonly used

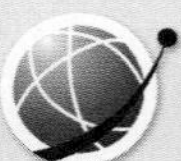

Media Resources
Go to www.bradybooks.com for mykit. Highlights:

- *Web Resource:* Carbon Monoxide
- *Web Resource:* Poisonous Plants

Objectives 22-2 and 22-3
List concerns in managing drug/alcohol emergencies and describe the routes by which a poison can enter the body.

Key Terms
poison any substance that impairs health or causes death by its chemical action.

to describe a poisoning in which the patient has been exposed to an excessive dose of a drug. The drug could be a legally prescribed medication, such as Valium, or it could be an illegal substance such as cocaine. The overdose may be intentional, as in a suicide attempt, or it may be completely accidental. Substance abuse, which can be a form of poisoning, is the inappropriate use of a substance or medication. Substance abuse is addressed later in this chapter.

There are four routes by which a poison can enter the body (EMT Skills 22-1):

- **Ingestion.** A drug or substance can be swallowed with absorption occurring through the gastrointestinal tract (stomach and intestines). This is the most common route of poisoning. A majority of the poison is absorbed from the small intestine and not from the stomach. Thus, it is important to manage the poison before it empties from the stomach into the small intestine. Poisons may remain in the stomach for several hours depending on the circumstances. For example, a larger amount of poison may stay in the stomach longer if it clumps together than if a smaller amount was taken. This will tend to lead to a delayed effect of the poison and signs and symptoms that may not present for several hours.
- **Inhalation.** Breathing a poison, typically a gas, vapor, fume, or aerosol, into the lungs allows for rapid absorption into the body. The poison is transported down the respiratory tract with each inhalation until it reaches the alveoli. Once in the alveoli, the poison can cross the alveolar-capillary membrane and enter the bloodstream, where it is then transported widely throughout the body. This not only produces a more immediate effect than ingestion but also typically causes signs and symptoms to appear earlier with a tendency to be more systemic (throughout the body) in nature. This mechanism produces a variety of signs and symptoms. The inhaled poison can also have direct effects on the pulmonary system by destroying lung tissue. This may lead to pulmonary edema (fluid leaking around and into the alveoli), which inhibits the effective exchange of oxygen and carbon dioxide at the level of the alveoli. Thus, severe respiratory distress in a patient may be an indication of an inhaled poison.
- **Injection.** A poison can be injected under the skin, into the muscle, or directly into a blood vessel. This may result in a local reaction to the poison, which is usually immediate. A local reaction typically causes edema (swelling) at the site of injection, redness, irritation, and sometimes pain. A systemic reaction can occur from injection of a poison, which may be immediate or delayed in its onset, depending on the type of injection and the speed with which it is absorbed and distributed throughout the body. Because of this, a variety of signs and symptoms may occur throughout the body. Injection poisonings may result from drug use, where a person intentionally injects a drug into the body, or from bites and stings. Most insects that can bite or sting are *Hymenoptera*—an order of insects that includes bees, wasps, hornets, yellow jackets, and fire ants. Other injections may result from spiders, snakes, marine animals, ticks, and scorpions. An anaphylactic reaction, the most severe type of allergic reaction, may result from injection of the venom into the body and its interaction with the immune system. (Review Chapter 21, "Anaphylactic Reactions.")
- **Absorption.** A poisonous substance can enter the body when it comes in contact with the skin or mucous membranes. The poisonous substance may be a dry powder or a liquid. Severe absorption poisoning results from pesticides and other lethal substances that come in contact with the skin. Absorption-type poisons may cause local irritation or may result in a systemic effect. As an example, organophosphates are commonly found in certain pesticides. Absorption of an organophosphate through the skin may result in a severe systemic reaction, leading to death.

The signs and symptoms of poisoned patients will depend on the specific poison and the route of entry into the body. One poison may depress the central nervous system, leading to bradycardia, slow, shallow respirations, and hypotension, whereas another poison may stimulate the central nervous system and cause tachycardia, tachypnea, and hypertension. The route of entry may determine how quickly the patient presents with the expected signs and symptoms.

You must always be prepared to handle the patient who suddenly deteriorates from a suspected poisoning. For example, you arrive on the scene and encounter a patient who says he ingested a large quantity of sedatives because he wants to commit suicide. The patient states that he took around 20 sleeping pills. You assess the patient and find that all of his vital signs are normal with no signs of poisoning. You may question whether the patient actually took the pills or if he is seeking attention by saying he did. However, 20 sleeping pills may take up to several

Objectives 22-4 and 22-5
List steps in managing a poisoning patient, regardless of exposure route, and explain the limited role of antidotes.

Key Terms
toxicology the study of toxins, antidotes, and the effects of toxins on the body.

Key Terms
toxins drugs or substances that are poisonous to humans.

antidote a substance that neutralizes the effects of a poison or a toxic substance.

ingested swallowed.

hours to leave the stomach and enter the small intestine for absorption into the body. Not until then will a large amount of the toxic substance be absorbed and the effects begin to be evident. Whatever your suspicions, you must treat the patient as if he truly ingested the poison, contact medical direction for further advice, and constantly monitor the patient's airway and breathing status.

ASSESSMENT Tips

Even if the patient with a suspected poisoning is currently stable, closely monitor the airway, breathing, circulation, and mental status, because acute deteriorations could occur. A sudden decrease in the mental status may indicate rapid patient deterioration. Burns to the lips and inside the mouth suggest that the patient ingested a corrosive poison. Be as thorough as possible while gathering the history from the patient. This information may not be available later if the patient lapses into unresponsiveness. ■

Managing the Poisoning Patient

Regardless of the poison or route, a majority of your emergency care will be supportive. You must establish and/or maintain a patent airway, determine whether the breathing is adequate or inadequate, provide positive pressure ventilation for inadequate breathing or a nonrebreather mask for adequate breathing, assess the circulation, and continue to reassess the patient.

Keeping in mind that these patients can deteriorate quickly, performing a series of reassessments is necessary. Be sure to closely monitor the breathing status and be prepared to ventilate if necessary. Many persons poisoned by ingestion may vomit, which may further complicate the airway. Place the patient in a lateral recumbent position and closely monitor the airway. Remember that the patient could survive the poisoning but die from aspiration of vomitus into the lungs. You can prevent this through positioning, suctioning, and close monitoring of the airway. Basically, you will provide emergency care for the signs and symptoms that the patient presents with.

Antidotes

An antidote is a substance that will neutralize the effects of the poison or toxic substance. Many people think that antidotes are available for a large number of poisons; however, true antidotes are available for only a small number of poisons. The treatment of poisons is generally geared toward limiting or preventing the absorption of the poison, and then managing any other signs and symptoms that may occur. Oftentimes, the treatment is just to support the airway, breathing, and circulation until the poison is eliminated from the body.

An ALS unit may have medications that reverse the effects of certain drugs that may have been injected, ingested, inhaled, or absorbed. For example, an ALS unit carries the drug naloxone (Narcan), which can reverse the effects of a narcotic overdose. Narcan does not remove the drug from the patient's body; instead, it blocks the effects of the narcotic at the cell receptor sites. Narcan usually will wear off much sooner than the typical narcotic, and the patient may relapse until another dose of Narcan can be administered.

Ingested Poisons

An **ingested** poison is one that is swallowed and enters the gastrointestinal system. The poison will usually remain in the stomach for a period of time before entering the small intestine. The length of time the poison remains in the stomach depends on the amount of poison ingested, the amount of food or liquid in the stomach, and the effect of the poison. A majority of the absorption of the poison occurs in the small intestine and not in the stomach. A quicker onset of the poison's effects will occur with a faster emptying of the stomach contents into the small intestine. Thus, it is extremely important to determine the length of time since the patient ingested the poison. This may change the treatment the patient receives.

Poisonous substances commonly ingested are:

- Prescription medications
- Over-the-counter medications (aspirin, acetaminophen, cough syrups)
- Illegal drugs (illicit)
- Household products
- Cleaning agents (soaps, detergents, alkalis)
- Foods
- Insecticides
- Petroleum products
- Plants

Objective 22-6
Given a scenario involving a patient who has ingested a poison, describe the steps of assessment-based management.

Key Points
Most information about an ingested poisoning will be obtained during the secondary assessment.

Many poisonings occur as a result of accidental ingestion. Common causes of accidental ingestion are:

- Taking too much of a medication because of not understanding the directions, particularly in elderly patients
- Combining alcohol with drugs
- Storing poisons in food or drink containers
- Keeping poisonous substances within the reach of children

The ingestion of poisonous plants is a common poisoning emergency, especially in children under the age of 5. Poisonous plants are not necessarily exotic—they include common household and backyard plants, such as morning glory, rhubarb leaves, buttercup, daisy, daffodil, lily of the valley, narcissus, tulip, azalea, English ivy, mistletoe berries, iris, hyacinth, laurel, philodendron, rhododendron, wisteria, and certain parts of the tomato, potato, and petunia plants. A high number of poisonings result from eating wild mushrooms.

Assessment-Based Approach: Ingested Poisons

Scene Size-Up

Clues indicating that there has been an ingested poisoning can often be spotted during scene size-up. You may observe overturned or empty medicine bottles, scattered pills or capsules, recently emptied containers, spilled chemicals, spilled cleaning solvents, an overturned plant or pieces of plant, potting soil or dirt on the floor, the remains of food or drink, or vomitus. Look for a possible suicide note.

Primary Assessment

The primary assessment is a vital step in management of the poisoned patient. The mental status may provide a clue as to the length of time since the patient ingested the substance. Also, it may indicate the effect on the patient. If the patient is experiencing an altered mental status from the poison, it is evident that the poison is already being absorbed into the bloodstream and is having systemic effects on the body. If the patient is still alert and oriented, it may be an indication that the poison has not yet been absorbed in a large quantity or that a large quantity was not ingested by the patient. It is important to constantly monitor for a decreasing mental status to identify patient deterioration.

If the patient has an altered mental status, it is necessary to open and clear the airway. A poisoned patient may deteriorate rapidly. He may be talking while on the scene and deteriorate to complete unresponsiveness en route to the hospital. As noted earlier, the poisoned patient may vomit, which can lead to aspiration. This will complicate the airway and breathing status of the patient. If the patient has an altered mental status, place him in a lateral recumbent position to reduce the possibility of aspiration. The poison itself may have caused burns to the mouth and airway, leading to swelling and a partially occluded airway. Inspect for burns around the mouth and lips and to the oral mucosa inside the mouth. It may be necessary to insert an oropharyngeal or nasopharyngeal airway to effectively ventilate the patient.

Depending on the poison ingested, the patient may have inadequate breathing. Be sure to assess both the respiratory rate and respiratory quality, paying particular attention to how deeply the patient is breathing. Like the airway, the respirations may suddenly become inadequate from the delayed absorption of the poison. Many poisons depress the respiratory drive. Closely monitor the chest rise and fall and the rate of respiration. If either the rate or depth is inadequate, provide positive pressure ventilation with a bag-valve mask or other ventilation device. Also, connect high concentrations of oxygen to the reservoir bag or tube of the ventilation device.

Understanding BODY PROCESSES

A poison that depresses the central nervous system may cause the respiratory, cardiac, and vasomotor centers to dysfunction or fail, leading to ineffective ventilation, bradycardia, and hypotension. ■

Assess the circulatory status of the patient. The heart rate and the skin temperature, color, and condition may provide a clue to the type of poison the patient may have ingested. Also, the circulatory status may indicate the systemic effects of the poison. If the pulse is absent, proceed with the cardiopulmonary resuscitation protocol.

Secondary Assessment

Most information about an ingested poisoning will be obtained during the secondary assessment. If the patient

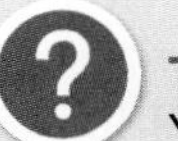

Thinking Critically
Your patient is a teenager whose mother found him swallowing a bottle of her prescription medication. He is alert and answering your questions so you assume he is really OK and may not even need transport to the hospital. Is this a correct assumption on your part?

Key Points
Knowing the length of time since the poison was ingested may change the treatment the patient receives.

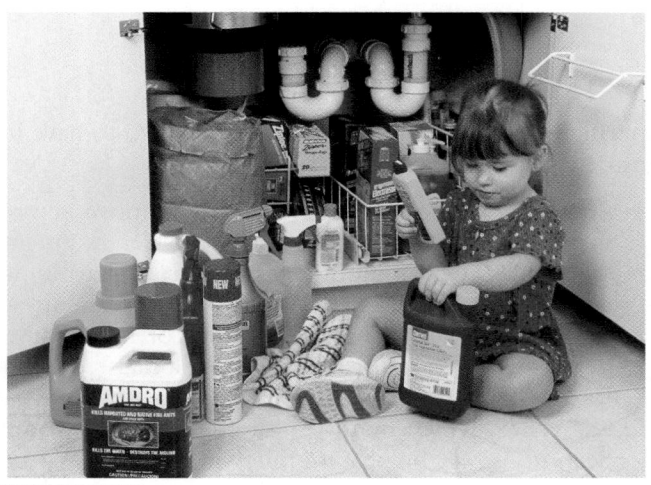

FIGURE 22-1 * Poisoning is the number one cause of accidental death among children.

is a child, other children in the house may have also swallowed the poison, so assess all children carefully. Don't forget that children often ingest more than one poison at a time—especially if they find several bottles of pills or cleaning supplies kept in one place. Watch for the most common poisons ingested by children: plants, cleaning products kept under the kitchen sink (Figure 22-1*), automotive supplies (such as windshield cleaning fluid) kept in the garage, medications (especially liquids), and toiletries (such as cologne, after-shave, and mouthwash).

Understanding BODY PROCESSES

An ingested liquid acid is likely to cause more severe tissue damage to the stomach lining than to the esophagus, because the poison will pass down the esophagus quickly but will then sit in the stomach and continue to burn. ■

Begin the secondary assessment by obtaining information about the patient. Getting a history from a poisoning patient can be difficult, and the history you do get may not be accurate; the patient may be misinformed, may be subject to a drug-induced confusion, or may be deliberately trying to deceive you. Exercise caution with the degree of trust you place in the history gained from a patient who took an intentional overdose. To manage a poisoning patient correctly, however, you need a relevant history. If the patient is unable or unwilling to communicate, you will need to question relatives or bystanders and gather clues from the scene. During the history, ask the following questions:

- *Was any substance ingested?* The answer to this question will help in determining if activated charcoal will be administered. (Remember to ask about over-the-counter medications; these can also be very harmful.)
- *Was any alcohol ingested with the substance?*
- *When did the patient ingest the poison?* (or) *When was the patient exposed to the poison?* This will let you determine the span of time between the exposure and the onset of symptoms. Generally, the faster the onset of symptoms, the more serious the condition.
- *Over what time period was the substance ingested?* (or) *Over what time period was the patient exposed to the poisonous substance?* This is another indicator of the seriousness of the poisoning.
- *How much of the substance was taken?* This is sometimes helpful when determining how quickly the substance may empty into the small intestine and how much antidote is needed at the hospital.
- *Has anyone attempted to treat the poisoning?* Someone may have tried to induce vomiting or give some type of antidote.
- *Does the patient have a psychiatric history that may suggest a possible suicide attempt?*
- *Does the patient have an underlying medical illness, allergy, chronic drug use, or addiction?* Not only will this tell you if the patient may have other conditions complicating the poisoning but it may also give a clue as to what drugs may have been ingested with the poison.
- *How much does the patient weigh?* This is necessary to administer the proper dose of activated charcoal.
- *What medications are available in the house?* This may provide the source of the poisoning if prescription or over-the-counter medications were ingested.

If the patient was able to provide an adequate history, conduct a physical exam of the areas in which the patient has a complaint, sign, or symptom, and of body systems that might be affected in the poisoning. If in doubt, or if the patient is unresponsive or unable to provide an adequate history, perform a complete secondary assessment. Assess the head, neck, chest, abdomen, pelvis, extremities, and posterior body. Inspect and palpate for any abnormalities. This is especially urgent if the patient may have suffered trauma secondary to the poisoning, or vice versa.

Record the vital signs, but realize that vitals have a limited role in establishing the degree of distress caused by a poisoning. You should use other clinical findings indicative of the seriousness of the condition (e.g., diminished mental status, fast or slow heart rate, seizures).

Signs and Symptoms The signs and symptoms of poisoning by ingestion vary, depending on what was ingested. *A seriously poisoned person may have few or no signs or symptoms,* so don't gauge the severity of the emergency on signs and symptoms alone.

The most common signs and symptoms are:

- A history of ingestion
- Swelling of mucosal membranes in the mouth
- Nausea
- Vomiting
- Diarrhea
- Altered mental status
- Abdominal pain, tenderness, distention, and/or cramps
- Burns or stains around the mouth (Figure 22-2*), pain in the mouth or throat, and/or pain during swallowing (corrosive poisons may corrode, burn, or destroy the tissues of the mouth, throat, and stomach)
- Unusual breath or body odors; characteristic chemical odors (such as turpentine) on the breath

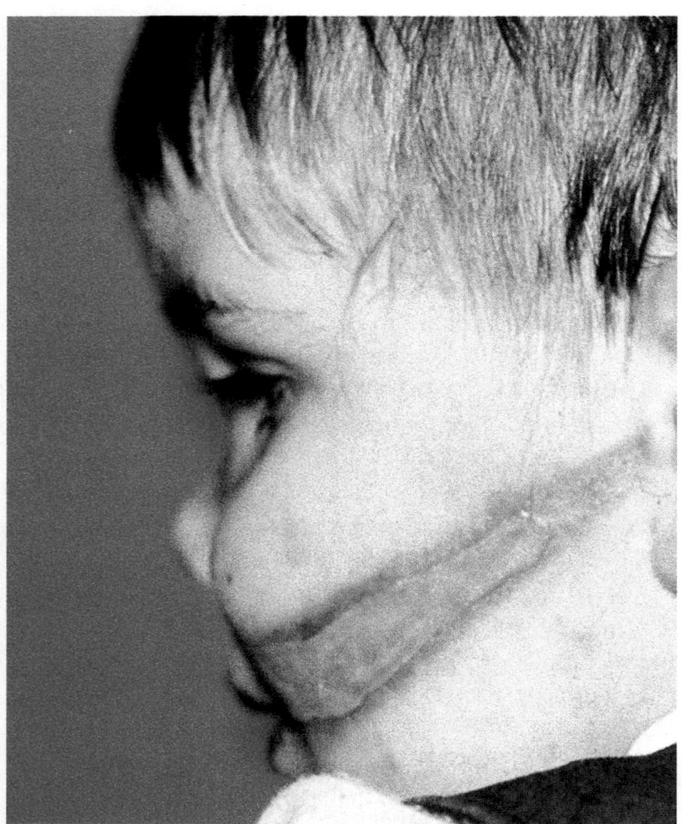

FIGURE 22-2 * Discoloration or burns around the mouth are signs of possible poisoning.

- Respiratory distress
- Altered heart rate (fast or slow)
- Altered blood pressure (high or low)
- Dilated or constricted pupils
- Warm and dry or cool and moist skin
- Altered mental status
- Coma
- Seizures

Emergency Medical Care

Specific treatment for a patient who is known to have ingested a poison is as follows:

1. *Maintain the airway.* Use gloves to remove any remaining pills, tablets, capsules, or other fragments from the patient's mouth, taking care not to injure yourself. If the patient is unresponsive, maintain an open airway with an oropharyngeal or nasopharyngeal airway in conjunction with a manual technique for opening the airway. Be sure not to stimulate the gag reflex, which might cause the patient to vomit. Secretions may be profuse following the ingestion of certain poisons, so be prepared to suction. A poisoning patient's status can change suddenly. Be prepared to protect the patient from aspiration. If possible, place the patient in the lateral recumbent position in case of vomiting.
2. *Provide oxygen or assist ventilations.* Provide positive pressure ventilation with supplemental oxygen if breathing is inadequate. If breathing is adequate, administer oxygen based on the SpO_2 reading and patient signs and symptoms. If the SpO_2 reading is greater than 95% and no signs or symptoms of hypoxia or respiratory distress are present, oxygen may not be necessary. In this case, you may choose to apply a nasal cannula at 2 to 4 lpm. If signs of hypoxia or respiratory distress are present, or the SpO_2 reading is less than 95%, place the patient on a nonrebreather mask at 15 lpm.
3. *Prevent further injury.* If a child has handled or been poisoned by a corrosive, protect yourself while washing the child's hands and fingers and rinsing the child's mouth and lips to remove traces of the corrosive. Be careful when rinsing the mouth that the patient does not swallow the liquid. *Do not flush the mouth of an unresponsive patient as he may aspirate the fluid.*
4. *During transport, consult medical direction* or, if your protocols mandate, contact the regional poison control center. You may be instructed to administer activated charcoal. Follow local protocol. Details on administering activated charcoal are found later in this chapter.
5. *Bring suspected poisons to the receiving facility.* Bring the container and all of its remaining contents, the plant portions or parts that might have been in-

Objective 22-7
Describe the indications, contraindications, mechanism of action, side effects, dosage, and administration of activated charcoal.

Key Terms
activated charcoal a distilled charcoal in powder form that can adsorb many times its weight in contaminants; no longer commonly administered in the emergency care of poisoning patients.

gested, or other specimens to the receiving facility. Remember to bring all possible containers and labels. Prescription bottles with all remaining pills should be transported because they provide a clue to how much was ingested. If a plant was ingested, bring the remaining roots, leaves, stems, flowers, or fruit. If the patient has vomited, bring a sample of the vomitus in a clean, closed container to the receiving facility. Analysis of this material may help the emergency department staff isolate the type of poison involved.

Reassessment

Provide a reassessment with particular attention to the patient's mental status, airway, and breathing. If the patient is unstable, you should repeat the reassessment every 5 minutes. Be sure to contact the receiving hospital so they can prepare for the patient's arrival.

Activated Charcoal

A medication that is rarely used in the emergency medical care of ingested poisonings is **activated charcoal**. Even though the literature has suggested that activated charcoal reduces absorption of the ingested poison, there is no evidence that suggests a better patient outcome. Thus, activated charcoal is rarely administered by emergency medical service personnel in ingested poisons. In some cases of specific medication ingestion that cause a delayed emptying effect, such as opioids, anticholinergic drugs, or medications with a sustained release, medical direction may order the administration of activated charcoal if it is shortly after ingestion. Follow your protocol, medical direction, or the poison control center.

Activated charcoal is a special distilled charcoal that has been treated with superheated steam. It is porous and can adsorb (collect onto its surfaces—or soak up) many times its weight in contaminants. Activated charcoal is produced to have a very small particle size to increase its adsorptive properties. To better illustrate this, consider that a standard 50-gram dose of activated charcoal has roughly the same surface area as ten football fields. The adsorption of the poison by the activated charcoal inhibits the poison from being absorbed into the body. Because of its lack of efficacy, it should be administered within 1 hour of the ingestion and only in specific cases approved by medical direction.

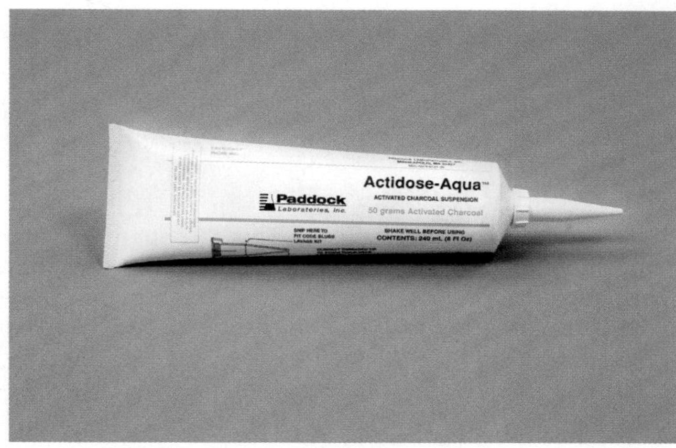

FIGURE 22-3 ✱ Several brands and forms of activated charcoal are available.

Some of the trade names of activated charcoal (Figure 22-3✱) are:

- SuperChar
- InstaChar
- Actidose
- Liqui-Char

Some activated charcoal products contain a laxative agent (cathartic) that helps speed it through the intestinal tract.

Understanding BODY PROCESSES

The use of activated charcoal for the ingested poison is intended to limit the amount of poison absorbed by the intestines due to the charcoal's ability to adsorb the poison while it is still in the stomach or proximal portion of the intestines. However, because of its limited efficacy, it is rarely used and only for specific poisons. ■

See Figure 22-4✱ for a detailed summary of the criteria and techniques for administration of activated charcoal. See EMT Skills 22-2 illustrating how to administer activated charcoal to a patient.

Activated charcoal should be used only for a patient who has ingested poisons by mouth, upon specific orders from medical direction and/or the poison control center. Remember that activated charcoal should not be administered to patients who have an altered mental status because

Activated Charcoal

MEDICATION NAME

Activated charcoal is the generic name. Some of the better known trade names of activated charcoal are:

- SuperChar
- InstaChar
- Actidose
- Actidose-Aqua
- Liqui-Char
- Charcoaid

INDICATIONS

Activated charcoal may be used for a patient who has ingested poison by mouth, upon specific orders from medical direction. It is most effective when administered within 1 hour after the ingestion of the poison and only in very specific cases of poisoning.

CONTRAINDICATIONS

Activated charcoal should not be administered to a patient who:

- Has an altered mental status (is not fully alert) because it may cause aspiration
- Has swallowed acids or alkalis (such as hydrochloric acid, bleach, ammonia, or ethyl alcohol)
- Is unable to swallow
- Overdoses on cyanide

MEDICATION FORM

1. Premixed in water, frequently available in a plastic bottle containing 12.5 grams of activated charcoal
2. Powder—should be avoided in the field

DOSAGE

Unless directed otherwise by medical direction, give both adults and children 1 gram of activated charcoal per kilogram (1g/kg) of body weight. The usual adult dose is 30–100 grams. The usual dose for infants and children is 12.5–25 grams.

ADMINISTRATION

To administer activated charcoal:

1. Consult medical direction or the poison control center, according to local protocol, before administering activated charcoal to any patient. Directions that follow are general. Always follow the orders of medical direction or local protocol.
2. Shake the container of activated charcoal thoroughly; if it is too thick to shake well, remove the cap and stir it until well mixed. The activated charcoal settles to the bottom of the bottle and needs to be evenly distributed.

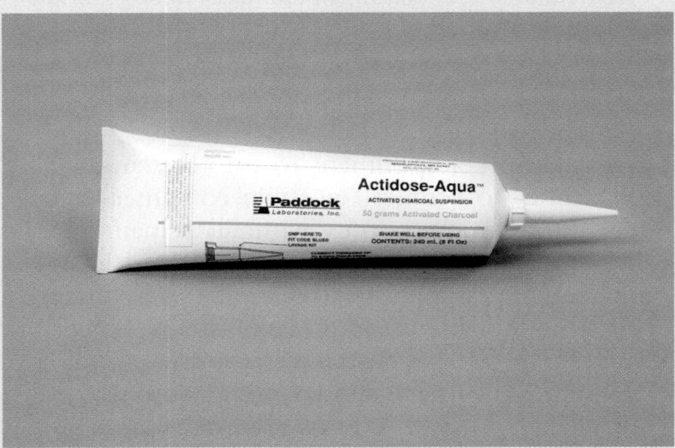

3. Activated charcoal looks like mud. The patient may be more willing to drink it if he can't see it, such as through a straw from a covered opaque container.
4. If the activated charcoal settles, shake or stir it again before letting the patient finish the dose.
5. Record the time and the patient response.
6. If the patient vomits, notify medical direction to authorize one repeat of the dose.

Once you have given a patient activated charcoal, don't let the patient have milk, ice cream, or sherbet. These all decrease the effectiveness of activated charcoal.

ACTIONS

Activated charcoal adsorbs poisons in the stomach, prevents their absorption by the body, and enhances their elimination from the body. The ability of activated charcoal to adsorb poisons is due to the preparation process that makes it extremely porous. Activated charcoal does not bind to (is not effective for) alcohol, kerosene, gasoline, caustics, or metals, such as iron. It is not routinely used for ingested poisoning. Only administer activated charcoal based on medical direction.

SIDE EFFECTS

The most common side effect is blackening of the stools. Some patients, especially those who are already nauseated, may vomit. If the patient vomits, repeat the dose of activated charcoal once. Be alert for further vomiting, and transport as soon as possible. Other side effects are rare.

REASSESSMENT

During administration, ensure that the patient's airway and mental status are adequate so the patient does not aspirate the medication. Check for abdominal pain or distress upon administration. Watch for possible vomiting after administration, and prevent aspiration by placing the patient in a sitting or lateral recumbent position and being prepared to suction.

FIGURE 22-4 ✱ Activated charcoal.

Objective 22-8
Given a scenario involving a patient who has inhaled a poison, describe the steps of assessment-based management.

Key Terms
inhaled breathed in.

Key Terms
huffers people who inhale vapors in order to "get high."

Key Points
Inhaled poisons may destroy lung tissue, so be alert for signs of respiratory distress or failure in this patient.

of possible aspiration, to patients who have swallowed acids or alkalis (such as hydrochloric acid, bleach, ammonia, or isolated ethyl alcohol ingestion), or to patients who are unable to swallow.

In the prehospital environment, use activated charcoal that has been premixed with water. The most common brands contain 12.5 grams of activated charcoal mixed with water in a plastic bottle. Activated charcoal is also available in powder form; however, the powder must be mixed with water before it can be administered to a patient. The use of powdered activated charcoal is discouraged in the field because it is problematic in preparation. Follow local protocol.

Inhaled Poisons

Thousands of people die each year in the United States from inhaling poisonous vapors and fumes, some of which are present without any sign. Most toxic inhalation occurs as a result of fire. It is critical that care be immediate, because the body absorbs inhaled poisons rapidly. The longer the exposure without treatment, the poorer the prognosis.

Common **inhaled** poisons include the following:

- Carbon monoxide
- Carbon dioxide from industrial sites, sewers, and wells
- Chlorine gas (common around swimming pools)
- Fumes from liquid chemicals and sprays
- Ammonia
- Sulfur dioxide (used to make ice)
- Anesthetic gases (ether, nitrous oxide, chloroform)
- Solvents used in dry cleaning, degreasing agents, or fire extinguishers
- Industrial gases
- Incomplete combustion of natural gas
- Hydrogen sulfide (sewer gas)
- Nitrogen dioxide from fermented grain

Some poisons are inhaled intentionally in an attempt to "get high." Patients who inhale paints and propellants are commonly referred to as **huffers**. The toxins are inhaled in a variety of ways in an attempt to produce certain expected effects. These substances can have many effects as they displace the oxygen content in the alveoli, leading to hypoxia. They can exert actions of their own after crossing over the alveoli into the bloodstream, or they can cause structural damage to the alveolar surface itself, which can also impair gas exchange. Look for paint or other material on the lips or around the nose of the patient during the physical exam. This may be the only indication of toxic inhalation in an unresponsive patient. Commonly abused inhaled poisons are:

- Paints
- Freon
- Gas propellants
- Glue
- Nitrous oxide
- Amyl nitrate
- Butyl nitrate

Keep in mind that inhaled poisons typically have a more immediate onset than injected poisons and may produce more systemic effects. Remember also that inhaled poisons may destroy lung tissue, leading to severe respiratory compromise and significant respiratory distress or failure.

Understanding BODY PROCESSES

An inhaled toxin can directly damage the alveoli when inhaled. This will cause fluid to leak into the alveoli and disturb gas exchange, leading to hypoxia. ■

ASSESSMENT Tips

Inhaled poisons often cause a rapid onset of signs and symptoms because of the rapid absorption of the poison into the lungs and into the circulation. Inhaled poisons frequently cause respiratory signs and symptoms early after the exposure to the poison. As the poison is absorbed into the blood, the patient may begin to exhibit systemic signs and symptoms. Young children and the elderly will typically present with signs and symptoms of carbon monoxide poisoning before any other patients who have been exposed. ■

Assessment-Based Approach: Inhaled Poisons

Scene Size-Up

During the scene size-up, ensuring your safety is of prime importance. You should be acutely aware of peculiar odors or visible fumes. At the same time, understand that some gases (e.g., carbon monoxide) can be odorless and colorless. The absence of odor does not guarantee safe air for breathing. You need to ensure scene safety so that bystanders and caregivers will not be injured.

If the information given by those present (or their behavior) or the presence of any hazardous materials placards at the scene indicate that toxic fumes may be present, be sure that you are wearing self-contained breathing apparatus before entering the scene. If you are not properly equipped or trained for hazardous materials rescue, call for assistance from those who are. Have those who are properly trained and equipped bring the patient or patients out of the toxic environment (Figure 22-5∗). Do not enter the scene unless they tell you it is safe. As soon as you are able, determine the number of persons at the scene who may have inhaled the poison. There are likely to be more patients than the one for whom EMS was originally called. Call for additional ambulances as needed. Use your senses, read the scene carefully, and proceed with caution. With inhaled poisons, a mistake regarding your safety may well be a fatal one.

Primary Assessment

Of particular importance in the inhaled poison patient is close assessment and management of the patient's airway and ventilation status. Inhaled poisons may rapidly lead to deterioration in the mental status of the patient, which may in turn compromise the airway. If the patient has an altered mental status, manually open the airway and inspect for any evidence of obstruction. Provide a manual maneuver and insert an oropharyngeal or nasopharyngeal airway, if warranted.

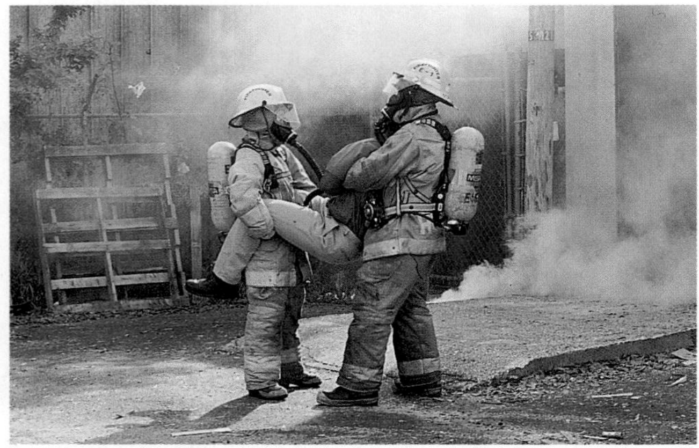

FIGURE 22-5 ∗ Protect yourself. Have trained rescuers remove the patient from the toxic environment.

Closely assess the breathing status, determining the rate and depth of respirations. If the rate is inadequate or the tidal volume (depth) is inadequate as evidenced by shallow breaths and poor chest rise on inhalation, immediately begin positive pressure ventilation with a bag-valve mask or other ventilation device. Maximize oxygenation of the patient during ventilation by connecting oxygen to the ventilation device. If the breathing is adequate in both rate and depth, apply a nonrebreather mask at 15 lpm. It is important to maximize oxygenation in the inhaled poisoning patient who is breathing adequately. Monitor this patient closely since he may deteriorate rapidly and begin to breathe inadequately.

Assess the patient's circulatory status by assessing the pulse and the skin color, temperature, and condition.

Secondary Assessment

During the secondary assessment, get a history from the patient or bystanders and as much information as you can about the substance that has been inhaled. Keep in mind that the patient may be a trauma patient. For example, an explosion could have rendered the patient unresponsive, which caused him to inhale the poisonous fumes from the explosion itself.

Remember to ask the patient or bystanders questions about what was inhaled, when and how long it was inhaled, and what treatments might have been attempted. In addition, you should ask:

- **Does the patient have a history that suggests a possible suicide attempt?** This is more common in apparently intentional carbon monoxide poisonings.
- **Did the exposure occur in an open or a confined space?** A confined space will likely have much higher concentrated amounts of the toxin and may lead to a more severe toxic exposure.
- **How long was the patient exposed?** The severity of the inhaled poisoning is associated with the duration of exposure to the toxin.

Patients who are trapped in a fire are typically exposed to large amounts of toxic substances. Incomplete combustion of products releases toxic fumes, many of which are lethal. Most people who die in a fire do so from inhalation of toxic fumes and not from burns. The second most common cause of death in a fire is from airway injuries secondary to breathing in superheated air. The third most common cause of death in a fire is from trauma.

If the patient is responsive enough to provide you with an adequate history, perform a focused assessment of the areas in which the patient has a complaint, sign, or symptom. If in doubt, or if the patient is unresponsive and unable to provide you with an adequate history, per-

Thinking Critically

An explosion in a factory warehouse has filled the space with toxic fumes. Knowing time is critical, you immediately rush into the facility to rescue patients from the poisonous environment. Have you done the right thing?

Key Terms

injected forced into the body, usually via a syringe, bite, or sting.

Objective 22-9

Given a scenario involving a patient who has been exposed to an injected poison, describe the steps of assessment-based management.

form a complete physical exam. Obtain and record the patient's vital signs.

Signs and Symptoms The following are signs and symptoms of inhaled poisoning:

- A history of inhalation of a toxic substance
- Difficulty breathing or shortness of breath
- Chest pain or tightness; a burning sensation in the chest or throat
- Cough, stridor, wheezing, or crackles
- Hoarseness
- Copious secretions
- Oral or pharyngeal burns
- Dizziness
- Headache, often severe
- Confusion
- Seizures
- Altered mental status, possible unresponsiveness
- Cyanosis
- Respiratory rate faster or slower than normal
- Nausea/vomiting (carbon monoxide poisoning)
- Paint on lips, indicating "huffing"
- Other types of material on face or lips (glue, chemical, and so forth)

Signs of respiratory tract burns include:

- Singed nasal hairs
- Soot in the sputum
- Soot in the throat

Emergency Medical Care

Respiratory symptoms are typically the first to appear with inhalation injuries. Specific treatment to include when treating a patient known to have inhaled poisonous gases/fumes is as follows:

1. *Protect yourself* from exposure to toxic fumes by wearing self-contained breathing apparatus or waiting for a specialized team to make the rescue.
2. *Quickly get the patient out of the toxic environment.*
3. *Place the patient in a supine position or position of comfort.* Loosen all tight-fitting clothing, especially around the neck and over the chest.

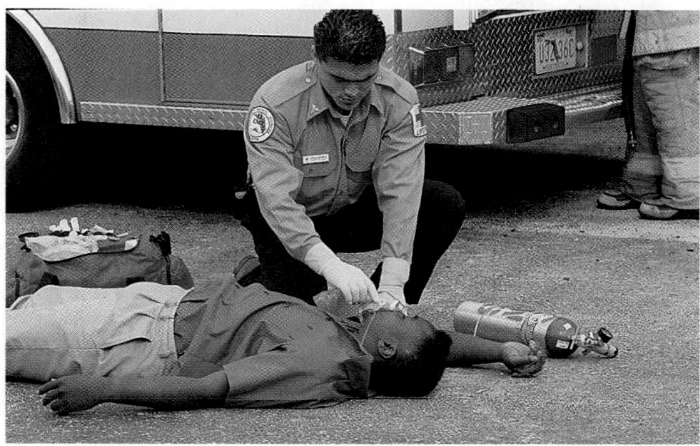

FIGURE 22-6 * Administer oxygen to the inhaled poisoning patient.

4. *Ensure an open airway.*
5. *Start positive pressure ventilation with supplemental oxygen immediately* if the patient is not breathing or has inadequate breathing.
6. *Administer oxygen by nonrebreather mask* at 15 lpm (Figure 22-6*) for all inhaled poisoning patients regardless of the SpO_2 reading.
7. *Bring all containers, bottles, labels, or other clues about the poisoning agent to the receiving facility.*

Reassessment

Provide a reassessment en route to the hospital with particular attention to the patient's airway and breathing. Reassess vital signs and treat any respiratory compromise that may develop.

Injected Poisons

Injected poisons are those that enter the body through a break in the skin—sometimes by the intentional injection of drugs, other times by the bites or stings of animals and insects. Drugs may be injected under the skin, into the muscle, or directly into the bloodstream. Information on specific drug-related emergencies is found later in the chapter. Once the poison is injected into the body, it is usually just a matter of time until it becomes absorbed into the bloodstream and widely distributed throughout the body. Consequently, the findings consistent with an

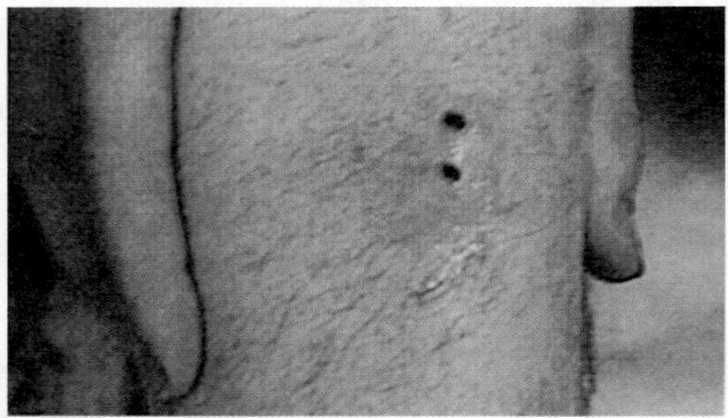

FIGURE 22-7 ✱ Rattlesnake bite.

injected poison could be local (at the site of injection), systemic (throughout the body), or a combination of both. Typically with bites and stings, the first signs and symptoms will be at the site of injection.

The most common sources of injected poisons are bites and stings. Most common are stings from bees, wasps, hornets, yellow jackets, and ants; others include the bites of spiders, ticks, marine animals (such as jellyfish, coral, anemones, and stingrays), and snakes (Figure 22-7✱). Injected poisons generally cause an immediate reaction at the injection site followed by a delayed systemic reaction. Of special note is the threat of anaphylactic shock following the allergic reaction to an insect bite or sting (see Chapter 21, "Anaphylactic Reactions"). More detailed information on bites and stings is found in Chapter 24, "Environmental Emergencies."

Assessment-Based Approach: Injected Poisons

Scene Size-Up

Make note of clues such as discarded syringes or other drug paraphernalia. Consider the possibility of a bite or sting in an outdoor environment (e.g., a sting by a marine life-form at a beach or by an insect at a picnic area). In industrial areas, the patient could also have been accidentally injected by high-pressure equipment with some type of chemical (e.g., paint or an oil-based substance).

Primary Assessment

Carefully assess the patient's airway and breathing. Open the airway, using a manual maneuver, and insert a mechanical airway device, if necessary. If the breathing is inadequate, immediately begin ventilation. Attach oxygen to the ventilation device as quickly as possible. If the breathing is adequate, administer oxygen based on the SpO_2 reading and the patient's signs and symptoms. Assess the mental status and determine if the patient is a high priority for transport. Look for indications of an allergic reaction.

Understanding BODY PROCESSES

Injected poisons are absorbed into the capillaries. Once the poison enters the blood in the capillaries, it is carried throughout the body, where it can affect many organs. ■

Secondary Assessment

During the secondary assessment, get a history from the patient or bystanders and as much information as you can about any substance that may have been injected or about the kind of insect or animal that may have inflicted a bite or sting.

Ask the patient or bystanders the following questions pertaining to injected poisons:

- *Does the patient have a history of drug use?* (Bystanders and the patient may be unwilling to answer this.)
- *Does the patient have a history of allergic reaction to bites or stings?*
- *What was the time lapse between the injection and onset of signs and symptoms?*
- *What type of animal or insect was the patient bitten by?*

If the patient is responsive enough to provide you with an adequate history, perform a secondary assessment. Obtain and record the patient's vital signs.

Signs and Symptoms General signs and symptoms of toxic injection include the following:

- Weakness/lethargy
- Dizziness
- Chills
- Fever
- Nausea/vomiting
- Euphoria
- Sedation
- High or low blood pressure
- Pupillary changes
- Needle tracks
- Pain at the site of injection
- Trouble breathing
- Abnormal skin vitals (color/temperature/condition)
- Possible paralysis
- Swelling and redness at the site of injection

Emergency Medical Care

Treatment for a patient known to have suffered a toxic injection is as follows:

1. *Maintain the patient's airway.* If appropriate, insert an oropharyngeal airway if the patient does not have

Key Points
Injected poisons usually cause an immediate reaction at the injection site with system reactions becoming evident after some elapsed time.

Thinking Critically
Your patient was stung by a bee near a barn. Should you move her away from the barn. Why?

Key Terms
absorbed passed through skin or mucous membranes upon contact.

Objective 22-10
Given a scenario involving a patient who has absorbed a poison, describe the steps of assessment-based management.

a gag reflex. Use a nasopharyngeal airway if the patient has a depressed mental status but will not accept an oropharyngeal airway. Suction vomitus or secretions.

2. *Begin positive pressure ventilations with supplemental oxygen* if the patient's respirations are inadequate. If breathing is adequate, administer oxygen based on the SpO_2 reading and patient signs and symptoms. If the SpO_2 reading is greater than 95% and no signs or symptoms of hypoxia or respiratory distress are present, oxygen may not be necessary. In this case, you may choose to apply a nasal cannula at 2 to 4 lpm. If signs of hypoxia or respiratory distress are present, or the SpO_2 reading is less than 95%, place the patient on a nonrebreather mask at 15 lpm.
3. *Be alert for vomiting.* Position the patient in a lateral recumbent (coma or recovery) position to help prevent aspiration, and be prepared to suction if necessary.
4. *In the case of a bite or sting, protect yourself from injury and protect the patient from repeated injection.* Move the patient away from any insects that are still swarming. Bees can sting only once and then lose their stinger—but wasps, hornets, and yellow jackets can sting repeatedly.
5. *Bring all containers, bottles, labels, or other evidence of poisonous substances to the receiving facility.* If the patient was bitten or stung, try to identify the insect, reptile, or animal that caused the injury (without getting close enough to endanger yourself if it is still alive). If it is dead, bring it to the receiving facility with the patient.

Reassessment

Provide a reassessment with particular attention to the airway and breathing. Monitor the patient for possible development of an anaphylactic reaction. Notify the hospital en route so they can prepare for the patient.

Absorbed Poisons

Absorbed poisons—usually chemicals or substances from poisonous plants that enter through the skin—generally cause burns, lesions, and inflammation. The risk of exposure to a hazardous substance is increasing as more chemicals are used in farming and in everyday objects. A dog's flea collar, for example, could be dangerous to an infant if he put it in his mouth because the chemical in the flea collar could be absorbed by the mucous membranes of the mouth.

Understanding BODY PROCESSES

Absorbed poisons enter the body through the capillaries in the skin or through the mucous membranes in the eyes, nose, or mouth. ■

Skin reactions range from mild irritation to severe chemical burns. Absorbed poisons often cause both local and systemic reactions, which can be severe. Exposure of as little as 2.5 percent of the body surface to 100 percent hydrofluoric acid, for example, can cause death.

Assessment-Based Approach: Absorbed Poisons

Scene Size-Up

Make note of any open containers of chemicals or poisonous plants in the environment. Wear gloves and other protective gear as needed to ensure that the harmful substances do not come into contact with your skin. Call for additional help if more than one patient is injured. Patients should be removed from the dangerous area as soon as possible.

Primary Assessment

Carefully assess the patient's airway and breathing. Some types of absorbed poisons can cause muscle paralysis or weakness and compromise the patient's respiratory status. An altered mental status secondary to the effects of the absorbed poison could cause the jaw and tongue to relax and block the airway. Inspect the patient for any poison that may still be on the person's body or clothes.

Secondary Assessment

Get a history from the patient or bystanders and as much information as you can about any substance that may have been absorbed. Perform a secondary assessment. Obtain and record the patient's vital signs.

Signs and Symptoms The following are signs and symptoms of an absorbed poison:

- A history of exposure to a poisonous substance
- Traces of liquid or powder on the patient's skin
- Burns
- Itching and/or irritation
- Redness
- Swelling

Signs and symptoms of contact with a poisonous plant include the following:

- Fluid-filled, oozing blisters
- Itching and burning
- Swelling
- Possible pain
- A rash (If the rash is scratched, secondary infections can occur.)

Emergency Medical Care

If poison has been absorbed through the skin, the following specific treatment should be included:

1. *Protecting your hands with gloves, move the patient from the source of the poison and remove the patient's contaminated clothing and jewelry.*
2. *Carefully monitor the airway and respiratory status.*
3. *Begin positive pressure ventilations with supplemental oxygen* if the patient's respirations are inadequate. If breathing is adequate, administer oxygen based on the SpO_2 reading and patient signs and symptoms. If the SpO_2 reading is greater than 95% and no signs or symptoms of hypoxia or respiratory distress are present, oxygen may not be necessary. In this case, you may apply a nasal cannula at 2 to 4 lpm. If signs of hypoxia or respiratory distress are present, or the SpO_2 reading is less than 95%, place the patient on a nonrebreather mask at 15 lpm.
4. *Brush any dry chemicals or solid toxins from the patient's skin,* taking extreme care not to abrade the skin or spread the contamination (Figure 22-8∗). Contact medical direction to determine whether to flush the contaminated area.
5. *If the poison is liquid, irrigate all parts of the body with clean water for at least 20 minutes* (a shower or garden hose is ideal). Carefully check "hidden" areas, such as the nail beds, skin creases, areas between the fingers and toes, and hair. If the patient is wearing any jewelry, removing it prior to flushing will ensure that no toxin remains trapped between the jewelry and skin. Continue irrigation en route to the receiving facility if possible. If the poison is a dry powder, brush off the substance and continue the treatment for other absorbed poisons.

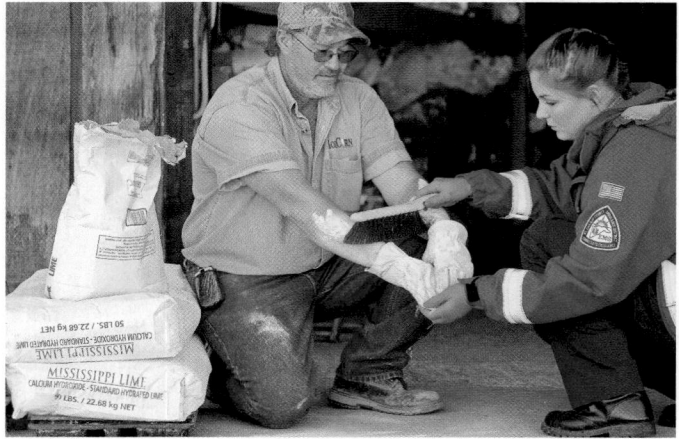

FIGURE 22-8 ∗ Brush dry powder off the patient. Then flush with clean water to remove poison on the surface of the skin.

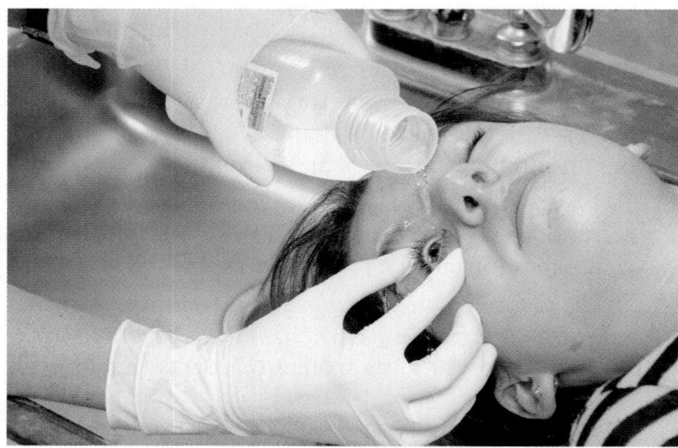

FIGURE 22-9 ∗ Irrigate chemical burns of the eye with clean water for at least 20 minutes.

6. *If the poison entered the eye, irrigate the affected eye with clean water for at least 20 minutes* (Figure 22-9∗); continue irrigation while en route to the receiving facility, if possible. Position the patient so water runs away from the unaffected eye, taking care not to spread the contamination. Further details on treating chemical burns of the eye will be found in Chapter 33, "Eye, Face, and Neck Trauma."

Reassessment

Provide a reassessment en route to the hospital with particular attention to the status of the patient's airway and breathing.

Summary: Assessment and Care

To review assessment findings and care for poisoning emergencies, see Figures 22-10∗ and 22-11∗.

Assessment Summary

POISONING EMERGENCY

The following findings may be associated with a poisoning emergency.

SCENE SIZE-UP

Is the poisoning due to ingestion, inhalation, injection, or absorption (contact)? Look for:

- Mechanism of injury
- Alcohol, drugs, other commonly abused substances
- Empty medicine bottles
- Spilled chemicals, cleaning solvents, other hazardous chemicals
- Pieces of plants
- Position and location of the patient
- Confined spaces
- Peculiar odors
- More than one patient with similar signs and symptoms
- Drug paraphernalia
- Insects, snakes, marine life, other venomous creatures
- Powdered or liquid substance on the skin surface
- Paint or other chemicals on the patient's lips or around the nose

Primary Assessment

General Impression

- Burns to skin from chemical exposure
- Vomitus or secretions in mouth
- Stings or bites to body with areas of swelling

Mental Status

- Alert to unresponsive
- Confused or disoriented

Airway

- Obstruction from swelling from burns to mouth, tongue, upper airway
- Obstruction by vomitus or secretions
- Stridor or hoarseness
- Excessive salivation
- Singed nasal hairs, soot in sputum and throat (carbon monoxide from fire)
- (Insert an oro- or nasopharyngeal airway, if necessary)

Breathing

- Shallow respirations
- Absent respirations
- Wheezing or crackles
- Inadequate or excessive respiratory rates

Circulation

- Heart rate may be increased or decreased
- Skin may be warm, cool, moist, or dry
- Cyanotic, pale, or flushed
- Weak or absent peripheral pulses

Status: Priority Patient

Secondary Assessment

History

Signs and symptoms vary widely, depending on the substance ingested, inhaled, injected, or absorbed.

Ask questions regarding the following:

- What substance was involved?
- When did the exposure occur?
- How long was the duration of exposure?
- How much was ingested, inhaled, or injected?
- Was any antidote or remedy administered?
- Any underlying medical history?
- Any psychiatric history?
- Does anyone else at the scene have similar signs and symptoms?
- Was the patient in a confined space or working with chemicals?
- Has the poison control center been consulted?

Physical Exam

Head, neck, and face:

- Excessive salivation or dry mouth
- Possible cyanosis to mucous membranes and face
- Dilated or constricted pupils
- Swelling
- Flushed, itching, hives
- Burns, discoloration, and swelling to mouth, oral cavity, tongue
- Unusual odors on breath
- Singed nasal hairs
- Soot in mouth and in sputum

Chest:

- Wheezing or crackles
- Respiratory distress

Abdomen:

- Pain and tenderness on palpation
- Distention
- Cramping
- Vomiting
- Diarrhea
- Blood-tinged or bloody vomitus or stool

continued

FIGURE 22-10a ✻ Assessment summary: poisoning emergency.

Assessment Summary

Extremities:
- Weakness
- Numbness
- Cyanosis
- Needle, injection, or bite marks
- Swelling, pain, or irritation at site of injection

Physical Exam

Extremities:
- Burns
- Liquid or powdery substances
- Swelling
- Flushed
- Itching
- Fluid-filled blisters
- Rash

Vital Signs
- BP: increased, normal, or decreased
- HR: increased, normal, or decreased; may be irregular
- RR: increased, irregular, decreased, or absent
- Skin: warm, cool, moist, or dry
- Pupils: dilated, constricted, sluggish to respond

FIGURE 22-10a * Assessment summary: poisoning emergency. *continued*

Emergency Care Protocol

POISONING EMERGENCY

1. Protect yourself from potential exposure by taking necessary Standard (body substance isolation) Precautions and safety precautions.
2. Establish and maintain an open airway.
3. Suction secretions as necessary.
4. If the patient is breathing inadequately, provide positive pressure ventilation with supplemental oxygen at a rate of 10–12 ventilations/minute for an adult and 12–20 ventilations/minute for an infant or child.
5. If breathing is adequate, administer oxygen based on the SpO_2 reading and patient signs and symptoms. If the SpO_2 reading is greater than 95% and no signs or symptoms of hypoxia or respiratory distress are present, apply a nasal cannula at 2–4 lpm. If signs of hypoxia or respiratory distress are present, the SpO_2 reading is less than 95%, or the poisoning was by inhalation, place the patient on a nonrebreather mask at 15 lpm.
6. Place the patient in a lateral recumbent position.
7. Contact the poison control center and/or medical direction to proceed with treatment:

   Ingested Poison

   Establish and maintain an airway, ventilation, and oxygenation.

   Be alert for vomiting and possible airway compromise.

   Inhaled Poison

   Remove the patient from the environment.

   Continue high concentration of oxygen by nonrebreather mask at 15 lpm or via positive pressure ventilation if the patient has inadequate breathing.

   Injected Poison

   Scrape the stinger from the site.

   Watch for signs and symptoms of severe allergic reaction.

   Absorbed (Contact) Poisoning

   Be sure to wear gloves before touching the patient or his clothing.

   Brush off any dry chemicals or solid toxins from the skin.

   Remove contaminated clothing.

   Flush with large amounts of water for at least 20 minutes.
8. Consider advanced life support backup if the patient begins to seize or if status has deteriorated.
9. Transport.
10. Perform reassessment every 5 minutes.

FIGURE 22-10b * Emergency care protocol: poisoning emergency.

Emergency Care Algorithm: **Poisoning Emergency**

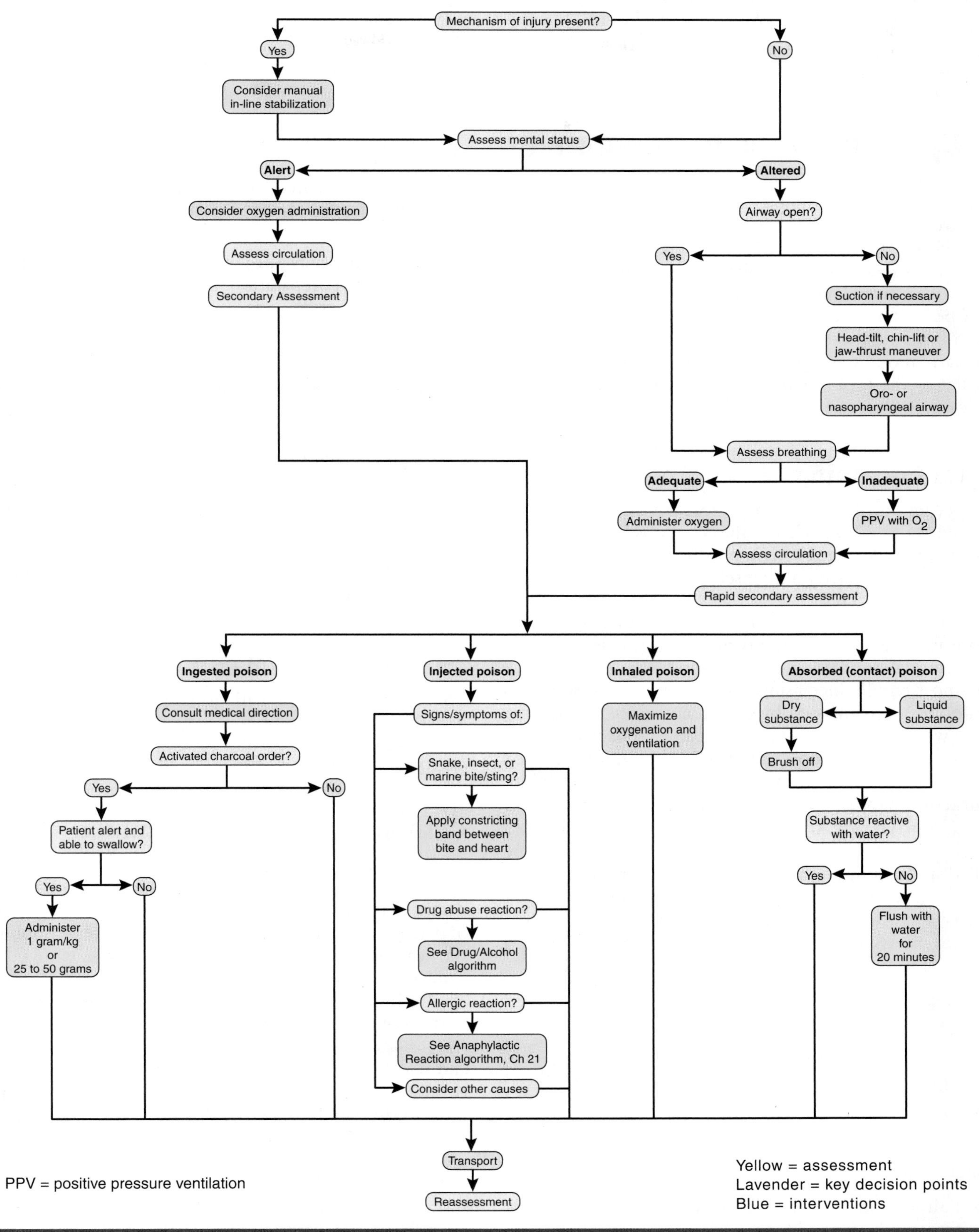

FIGURE 22-11 ✻ Emergency care algorithm: poisoning emergency.

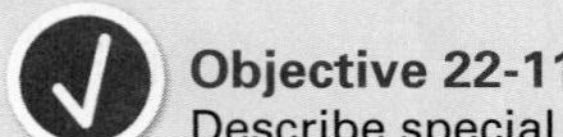

Objective 22-11
Describe special considerations in assessing and managing patients with specific types of poisoning.

Key Points
Children and the elderly are at the greatest risk for severe effects from food poisoning.

Specific Types of Poisoning

The following section provides information regarding the treatment and identification of specific poisonings you will be likely to encounter as well as information on the most valuable resource for poison treatment: poison control centers. This information is provided so that you will be better prepared to recognize and manage common forms of poisoning. You are encouraged, however, to learn about any types of poisonings that may be particular to the area in which you are providing prehospital care.

Food Poisoning

A specific kind of ingested poison is food poisoning—caused by ingestion of food that contains bacteria or the toxins (poisons that bacteria produce). Illness can result from either the bacteria themselves or from the toxins released by the bacteria.

The incidence of food poisoning is increasing dramatically. Each year, millions of Americans develop gastrointestinal disease as a result of food poisoning. One of the most rapidly increasing sources of food poisoning is seafood. Algae ingested by fish create toxins in their tissues, which are then eaten by humans. *Ciguatera,* a commonly reported seafood-related illness in the United States, is caused by eating tainted fish such as dolphin, sturgeon, snapper, grouper, and parrot fish, among others. Unfortunately, the toxins don't make the fish look, smell, or taste any different—and the toxins can't be killed by cooking, freezing, smoking, or drying the fish. In some cases of seafood poisoning, symptoms may spontaneously recur for many years. The food products most commonly associated with poisoning emergencies (which are most prevalent in the summer months) include:

- Eggs
- Chicken
- Ready-to-eat foods (cheese, processed meat)
- Untreated water or unpasteurized milk
- Fish

Some types of foodborne illnesses from these and other foods are:

- **Salmonella.** From contaminated food and water, or from undercooked food
- **Campylobacter.** Common poisoning from contaminated poultry, milk, and water
- **Escherichia coli (E. coli).** Severe gastrointestinal poisoning from numerous contaminated foods, undercooked foods, and untreated (contaminated) water
- **Staphylococcus aureus.** Food poisoning from unhygienic food preparation, associated with foods served cold (such as desserts, custards, and salads)

Signs and Symptoms

Because the signs and symptoms vary greatly, food poisoning can be difficult to detect. The symptoms commonly start hours to days after ingestion and may be severe. The pediatric and geriatric populations are especially at risk for severe signs and symptoms from food poisoning. General signs and symptoms include abdominal cramping, nausea and vomiting, gas, diarrhea, and loud or frequent bowel sounds. More severe findings include increased temperature, blood disorders, muscle cramping or muscle paralysis, and passing blood in the stool.

Emergency Medical Care

To care for a patient with food poisoning, follow the general guidelines for any ingested poison. Do not give the patient anything by mouth, and transport as soon as possible.

Carbon Monoxide Poisoning

Of special concern is carbon monoxide (CO) poisoning by inhalation. Carbon monoxide causes thousands of deaths in the United States each year and sends thousands of persons to the hospital. Carbon monoxide poisoning is the leading cause of death among people who inhale smoke from fires.

Carbon monoxide—formed by the incomplete combustion of gasoline, coal, kerosene, plastic, wood, or natural gas—is completely nonirritating, tasteless, colorless, and odorless. It causes a life-threatening lack of oxygen in two ways: First, it reduces the amount of oxygen carried by the bloodstream because the carbon monoxide molecules replace the oxygen molecules on the red blood cells; and second, it inhibits the ability of body cells to utilize what little oxygen is delivered. The brain, spinal cord, and heart sustain the greatest damage. The danger of carbon monoxide poisoning is increased in an enclosed space.

Key Points
The primary sources of carbon monoxide are home-heating devices and automobile exhaust fumes, but other sources include barbecue grills, charcoal briquettes, kitchen stoves, and faulty water heaters.

Thinking Critically
After being moved outdoors and breathing fresh air, a patient who was exposed to carbon monoxide is feeling much better and refuses transport. How should you respond to this refusal?

The primary sources of carbon monoxide are home-heating devices (including furnaces and wood-burning fireplaces) and automobile exhaust fumes. Other common sources are tobacco smoke, barbecue grills and charcoal briquettes, kitchen stoves, gas lamps, recreational fires, propane-powered industrial equipment, and faulty water heaters, kerosene heaters, and space heaters.

Signs and Symptoms

The initial symptoms of carbon monoxide poisoning are similar to those of the flu, but there is no accompanying fever, general body aches, or swollen and tender lymph nodes. You should consider carbon monoxide poisoning whenever you encounter unexplained flu symptoms (such as headache, nausea, vomiting, and confusion)—especially if the symptoms are shared by other people in the same environment.

The most common signs and symptoms seen early in carbon monoxide poisoning are:

- Headache
- Tachypnea (rapid respiratory rate)
- Nausea and vomiting
- Altered mental status (confusion early, unresponsive late)
- High pulse oximeter reading

Understanding BODY PROCESSES

Carbon monoxide displaces oxygen as it attaches to hemoglobin molecules in the blood. The attached CO turns the color of the hemoglobin extremely red. A pulse oximeter works by reading the color of the hemoglobin. Under normal circumstances, red hemoglobin indicates that oxygen is attached to it. Because CO also turns the hemoglobin red, the pulse oximeter reads the red color and provides an extremely high but false SpO_2 reading. The cells are truly hypoxic even though the SpO_2 reading may be 100%. ■

As the poisoning progresses, the patient may suffer temporary blindness, hearing loss, convulsions, coma, and death. One of the things that makes carbon monoxide poisoning—especially from chronic exposure—so dangerous is that it may easily be mistaken for something else. It takes only a few minutes to die from carbon monoxide poisoning. Death is so certain, in fact, that a great number of suicides are committed with automobile exhaust, which is only 7 percent carbon monoxide.

Emergency Medical Care

If you suspect that someone has carbon monoxide poisoning, evacuate everyone from the enclosed space—even people who apparently have no symptoms. Ideally, patients should be moved at least 150 feet from the suspected sources of the carbon monoxide into open air. All patients with carbon monoxide poisoning must receive medical care; many develop delayed neurological complications after initial recovery. Transport a carbon monoxide patient immediately with a tight-fitting nonrebreather mask at 15 lpm, even if the patient seems to have recovered. Do not rely on the pulse oximeter to guide oxygen therapy. Carbon monoxide monitors (CO-oximeters) are available that can indicate the amount of carbon monoxide in the blood. Just because the patient has awakened or seems more alert does not mean he is better. These findings can be false signs of recovery.

Cyanide

Cyanide is a poison that can be found in a variety of forms. It can enter the body through inhalation, absorption, injection, and ingestion. Cyanide is found in many household products. Rodent poisons, silver polish, and cherry and apricot pits contain cyanide that can be ingested or absorbed. Cyanide salts and long-term sodium nitroprusside therapy are other cyanide-containing sources. Cyanide is also a by-product of incomplete combustion of many plastics, silk, and synthetic carpets. Thus, inhalation of cyanide can occur in fires when these materials are burning. In some areas, firefighters who are treated for smoke inhalation receive cyanide-poisoning antidotes along with basic inhalation treatment as a standard precaution.

Cyanide is an extremely dangerous poison because it interferes with the use of oxygen at the cellular level. Even though initially there is no destruction of lung tissue or disturbance to respiratory mechanics, cyanide poisoning causes severe hypoxia at the level of the cell.

Understanding BODY PROCESSES

Cyanide causes hypoxia at the level of the cell. Oxygen is still being delivered to the cells, but the oxygen cannot be transported and used properly within the cell. ■

Key Points

Cyanide is an extremely dangerous poison that, in large doses, can cause death within minutes.

Key Points

Young children are curious and "get into everything." They are the most frequent victims of ingested poisoning and will often swallow things it is hard for an adult to imagine swallowing, including drain cleaners, floor polish, antifreeze, cosmetics, detergents, and leaves and flowers from poisonous plants.

Signs and Symptoms

Cyanide poisoning in large doses may cause death within a few minutes. The patient may progress quickly from early signs and symptoms to more severe effects. The signs and symptoms of cyanide poisoning are:

Early Signs and Symptoms

- Headache
- Confusion
- Agitation or combative behavior
- Burning sensation in the mouth or throat
- Dyspnea
- Hypertension
- Bradycardia or tachycardia
- Smell of bitter almonds

Late Signs or Symptoms or Those Seen in Large-Dose Cyanide Poisoning

- Seizures
- Coma
- Hypotension
- Pulmonary edema
- Cardiac dysrhythmias
- Acidosis

Emergency Medical Care

Scene safety and personal protection are key elements in management of the patient who suffers from cyanide poisoning. It may be necessary to wear self-contained breathing apparatus to remove the patient from the toxic environment.

Provide the following emergency medical care for a cyanide poisoning:

1. Remove the patient from the toxic environment. Ensure that all rescuers are wearing the necessary personal protective equipment.
2. Remove any contaminated clothing and rapidly decontaminate the patient.
3. Open and maintain a patent airway.
4. Assess the breathing status. If the rate and tidal volume are adequate, apply a nonrebreather mask at 15 lpm if cyanide poisoning is suspected, regardless of the SpO_2 reading. If the respiratory rate or tidal volume is inadequate, immediately provide positive pressure ventilation while maximizing oxygen delivery through the ventilation device.
5. Consider contacting ALS for administration of a cyanide antidote.
6. Rapidly transport the patient.

Acids and Alkalis

Many household products contain strong acids or alkalis. These are commonly referred to as caustic substances. Caustic ingestion poisoning is most common in young children. Strong acids have an extremely low pH. They are commonly found in liquid plumbing drain openers and other bathroom cleaners. Alkalis have an extremely high pH. They are in the form of either a liquid or a solid and are also commonly found around the house in plumbing drain openers.

Acids burn on contact, causing immediate and severe pain. At the burn site, the tissue often dies immediately, producing a protective layer to lessen further burning. If an acid is ingested, a majority of the chemical burn will occur in the stomach and not in the esophagus. The liquid travels down the esophagus quickly, thus allowing very little contact time. Abdominal pain is usually severe and immediate. Bleeding may occur from perforation of the lining of the stomach. Also, the acid may be absorbed by the blood, leading to an acidotic state throughout the body. The patient who has ingested acids may present with burns to and around the mouth. Acids typically burn for only about 1–2 minutes, thereby limiting the damage.

Alkalis also burn on contact; however, it takes longer to recognize the burning sensation. Alkalis have a tendency to burn deeper by continuing to burn through tissue from longer contact times because the burn goes unrecognized for longer periods of time. If ingested, a solid alkali may adhere to the oropharynx or esophagus. This may cause deep burns and possible perforation of the tissue at the site of the burn. Liquid alkalis will most likely injure the stomach tissue, since they pass quickly along the esophagus. The alkali may perforate the stomach and may cause the protective lining to be burned away. Alkalis typically burn for minutes to hours after exposure. Thus, alkalis have a tendency to cause much deeper burns than acids.

Signs and Symptoms

General signs and symptoms associated with caustic poisoning are:

- Burns to the mouth and lips, and around the face
- Dysphagia (difficulty swallowing, drooling)
- Pain to the lips, mouth, and throat
- Abdominal pain
- Hoarseness or dysphasia (difficulty speaking)
- Stridor
- Dyspnea (shortness of breath)
- Evidence of shock from perforation of the stomach or esophagus (pale, cool, clammy skin; tachycardia; decreasing blood pressure; decreased mental status)

Emergency Medical Care

Rapid management and transportation of the patient is necessary when dealing with a caustic poisoning. Take the necessary precautions to protect yourself from coming in contact with the caustic substance. Activated charcoal is not effective in caustic poisoning; therefore, there is no use in administering it in this situation.

Emergency medical care for a caustic substance ingestion is as follows:

1. Ensure that all rescuers are wearing the necessary personal protective equipment.
2. Remove any contaminated clothing and rapidly decontaminate the patient. Flush the contaminated areas with large amounts of water.
3. Open and maintain a patent airway. The burns may have caused edema (swelling) to the upper airway, making it difficult to establish an airway. Insert an oropharyngeal or nasopharyngeal airway if swelling is preventing you from establishing a patent airway. Contact ALS for more advanced airway care, if necessary.
4. Assess the breathing status. If the rate and tidal volume are adequate, apply a nonrebreather mask at 15 lpm. If the respiratory rate or tidal volume is inadequate, immediately provide positive pressure ventilation while maximizing oxygen delivery through the ventilation device.
5. Rapidly transport the patient.

Hydrocarbons

Hydrocarbons are substances that are produced from crude oil, coal, or plant sources. They are commonly found in kerosene, naphtha, turpentine, mineral oil, toluene, and benzene. These substances can be found in common household products such as lighter fluid, glues, paints, lubricants, cleaning and polishing agents, spot removers, cosmetics, pesticides, solvents, and aerosol propellants.

The patients who are most commonly poisoned with hydrocarbons are children under 5 years of age. The toxicity of the hydrocarbon varies widely and is somewhat dependent on the viscosity of the substance. The lower the viscosity, the greater the risk of aspiration and the greater the potential side effects. Hydrocarbon poisoning may occur by ingestion, inhalation, or absorption.

Signs and Symptoms

The signs and symptoms of hydrocarbon poisoning will vary, depending on the type of hydrocarbon and the route of poisoning. If the patient is not exhibiting any signs or symptoms upon your arrival, it is likely the patient will not suffer a serious consequence of exposure to the hydrocarbon. The signs and symptoms may include the following:

- Coughing, choking, crying
- Burns to mouth or contact area
- Stridor
- Dyspnea
- Wheezing
- Tachypnea
- Cyanosis
- Abdominal pain
- Nausea and vomiting
- Belching
- Fever
- Seizures
- Coma
- Altered mental status
- Headache, dizziness, and dulled reflexes (obtunded)
- Slurred speech
- Cardiac dysrhythmias

Emergency Medical Care

Scene safety is of primary importance when treating a patient exposed to a hydrocarbon, especially if the exposure was by inhalation or absorption. Be sure to use the necessary personal protective equipment. Emergency medical care for hydrocarbon poisoning includes the following:

1. Remove the patient from the environment.
2. Remove all contaminated clothing and decontaminate the patient.
3. Open and maintain a patent airway.
4. Assess the breathing status. If the rate and tidal volume are adequate, apply a nonrebreather mask at 15 lpm, regardless of the SpO_2 reading if inhalation of the hydrocarbon is suspected. If the respiratory rate or tidal volume is inadequate, immediately provide

positive pressure ventilation while maximizing oxygen delivery through the ventilation device.

5. Rapidly transport the patient.

Methanol (Wood Alcohol)

Methanol, or wood alcohol, is a poisonous form of alcohol found in a variety of common products such as gasoline antifreeze, windshield washer fluid, paints, paint removers, Sterno and other canned fuels, and shellac. Methanol is a colorless liquid. It is different from ethyl alcohol (also called ethanol or drinking alcohol), which is the form of alcohol that is designed for consumption. Methanol poisoning may occur from ingestion, inhalation, or absorption. Some patients may deliberately ingest methanol alcohol in an attempt to "get drunk" when ethyl alcohol is not readily available. Chronic alcoholics may ingest methanol alcohol to maintain an inebriated state. Children may ingest substances containing methanol alcohol accidentally. Methanol alcohol, when ingested, will cause the liver to produce massive amounts of acid in the body. The onset of signs and symptoms following ingestion will usually occur 40 minutes to 72 hours after ingestion.

Signs and Symptoms

The signs and symptoms are typically related to the central nervous system, gastrointestinal system, and overwhelming acid in the body. Blindness may occur from the ingestion of as little as 4 mL of methanol. The signs and symptoms include the following:

- Altered mental status (confusion, unresponsiveness)
- Seizures
- Nausea and vomiting
- Abdominal pain
- Blurred vision
- Dilated pupils that are sluggish to respond to light
- Visual changes (seeing spots)
- Blindness
- Dyspnea
- Tachypnea

Emergency Medical Care

Emergency medical care for methanol poisoning is primarily supportive. Administration of ethyl alcohol (drinking alcohol) will prevent the methanol from being converted to an acid. An antidote, fomepizole, is now available. Until the patient is at the hospital to receive the aforementioned care, the EMT should provide the following:

1. Open and maintain a patent airway.
2. Assess the breathing status. If the respiratory rate or tidal volume is inadequate, immediately provide positive pressure ventilation while maximizing oxygen delivery through the ventilation device. Adequate ventilation is necessary to help reduce the acidosis in the body. If breathing is adequate, administer oxygen based on the SpO_2 reading and patient signs and symptoms. If the SpO_2 reading is greater than 95% and no signs or symptoms of hypoxia or respiratory distress are present, apply a nasal cannula at 2 to 4 lpm. If signs of hypoxia or respiratory distress are present, or the SpO_2 reading is less than 95%, place the patient on a nonrebreather mask at 15 lpm.
3. Rapidly transport the patient.

Isopropanol (Isopropyl Alcohol)

Rubbing alcohol, the most common form of isopropyl alcohol, is found in many households. Isopropyl alcohol can also be found in many household products such as cosmetics, degreasers, disinfectants, solvents, and other cleaning agents. Poisoning most frequently occurs by ingestion, both accidental and intentional. Alcoholics may ingest isopropyl alcohol as a substitute for ethyl (drinking) alcohol. Isopropyl alcohol is more toxic than ethyl alcohol but less toxic than methanol (wood) alcohol. Following ingestion of isopropyl alcohol, the liver creates acetone. This has a major effect on the central nervous system, gastrointestinal system, and kidneys.

Signs and Symptoms

The signs and symptoms of isopropanol poisoning occur rapidly, usually within 30 minutes following ingestion. Isopropanol acts as a central nervous system depressant, causing respiratory depression. Signs of ingestion include:

- Respiratory depression
- Altered mental status
- Slow respirations, shallow tidal volume
- Abdominal pain
- Bloody vomitus (hematemesis)
- Signs of shock

Emergency Medical Care

Administration of ethyl alcohol does not produce the same beneficial effects with isopropyl alcohol as it does in methanol poisoning. The emergency medical care for isopropanol ingestion includes the following:

1. Open and maintain a patent airway.
2. Assess the breathing status. If the rate and tidal volume are adequate, apply a nonrebreather mask at 15 lpm. If the respiratory rate or tidal volume is inadequate, immediately provide positive pressure ventilation while maximizing oxygen delivery through the ventilation device. Adequate ventilation is necessary to help reduce the acidosis in the body.
3. Rapidly transport the patient.

Ethylene Glycol

Ethylene glycol is commonly found in detergents, radiator antifreeze, windshield deicers, and coolants. Children are commonly susceptible to accidental ingestion of ethylene glycol. The products usually are colorful and have a sweet taste. Therefore, children will ingest the substance containing ethylene glycol with no reason to believe it is harmful. Also, alcoholic patients who are unable to attain ethyl (drinking) alcohol may abuse ethylene glycol. It is fairly common to hear of teenagers who intentionally drink radiator antifreeze to become intoxicated. Very small amounts can be fatal in an adult or a child.

Ethylene glycol has some of the same effects as ethyl alcohol. Thus, the patient may present as if he is intoxicated. However, like methanol and isopropanol alcohols, the by-products of metabolism of ethylene glycol are extremely harmful, primarily affecting the central nervous system, lungs, heart, vessels, and kidneys.

Signs and Symptoms

The signs and symptoms of ethylene glycol poisoning will commonly occur in three stages. The stages are typically associated with the time from ingestion and affect various body systems. The signs and symptoms include the following:

First Stage: Neurological

This stage occurs 30 minutes to 12 hours after ingestion and primarily affects the central nervous system. These signs and symptoms may be mistaken for a person intoxicated on regular ethyl (drinking) alcohol.

- Uncoordinated movements
- Slurred speech
- Altered mental status
- Nausea and vomiting
- Seizures
- Hallucinations

Second Stage: Cardiopulmonary

This stage usually occurs 12–24 hours after ingestion and primarily affects the heart and lungs.

- Tachypnea
- Crackles upon auscultation, indicating pulmonary edema
- Cyanosis
- Dyspnea
- Respiratory distress
- Heart failure

Third Stage: Renal

This stage typically occurs from 24 to 72 hours following ingestion of the ethylene glycol and affects the kidneys.

- Production of very little urine (oliguria) or no urine (anuria)
- Bloody urine (hematuria)
- Pain to the flank areas

Emergency Medical Care

The emergency medical care for ethylene glycol poisoning is primarily supportive. However, administration of ethyl (drinking) alcohol may be considered. Be prepared to manage seizures and respiratory arrest. The emergency medical care includes the following:

1. Open and maintain a patent airway.
2. Assess the breathing status. If the rate and tidal volume are adequate, apply a nonrebreather mask at 15 lpm. If the respiratory rate or tidal volume is inadequate, immediately provide positive pressure ventilation while maximizing oxygen delivery through the ventilation device. Adequate ventilation is necessary to help reduce the acidosis in the body.
3. Rapidly transport the patient.

Poisonous Plants

A fairly common type of absorbed poisoning comes from skin contact with a poisonous plant—usually poison ivy, poison sumac, or poison oak. Poison ivy thrives in sun and in light shade. It usually grows in the form of a trailing vine that sends out numerous kinky brown footlets that are slightly thickened at the tips. It can also grow in the form of a bush and grow to heights of 10 feet or more. You don't need direct contact with the plant to have a reaction from poison ivy; the poisonous element, urushiol, can be carried on animal fur, tools, and clothing. If poison ivy is burned, particles of urushiol are contained in the smoke and can be breathed in or absorbed through the skin. People with an allergy to urushiol—about 75 percent of all Americans—are likely to have severe reactions to contact with poison ivy.

Poison sumac is a tall shrub or slender tree, usually growing along swamps and ponds in wooded areas. Poison oak resembles poison ivy with one important difference: the poison oak leaves have rounded, lobed leaflets instead of leaflets that are jagged. Poison oak is found mostly in the southeastern and western United States.

Other plants that can cause mild to severe dermatitis include stinging nettle, crown of thorns, buttercup, May apple, marsh marigold, candelabra cactus, brown-eyed Susan, Shasta daisy, and chrysanthemum.

Emergency treatment includes scene safety, personal protection measures, and decontamination if any plant substance is still on the person's body. You should first ensure the airway, breathing, and circulatory status. Routine treatment for this type of absorbed poisoning is mainly supportive until arrival at the hospital. You should keep the patient from scratching the site as this may cause a break in the skin, which may allow an infection to set in.

Objective 22-12
Explain information you should provide when contacting the poison control center.

Key Terms
drug abuse self-administration of drugs (or a single drug) in a manner that is not in accord with approved medical or social patterns.

Key Terms
overdose an emergency that involves poisoning by drugs or alcohol.

withdrawal a syndrome that occurs after a period of abstinence from the alcohol or drugs to which a person's body has become accustomed.

▶ Poison Control Centers

Poison control centers have been established across the United States and Canada to assist in the treatment of poison patients. Officials at the center can help you set priorities and formulate an effective treatment plan. Poison center officials can also provide information about any available antidote that may be appropriate for a patient. Any treatment recommended by the poison control center should be discussed with medical direction before it is administered to the patient.

Calls to poison control centers are toll-free, and most are staffed 24 hours a day to assist prehospital personnel as well as the public. Staffed by experienced professionals, each center is also connected to a network of nationwide consultants with access to trained toxicologists who can answer questions about almost any poison. Information on the poison center's computer is updated regularly to provide the latest information on treatment options and antidotes. Centers provide follow-up telephone calls, monitoring the patient's progress and making treatment suggestions until the patient is either hospitalized or no longer has the symptoms.

Be prepared to tell poison center officials the patient's approximate age and weight. Summarize the patient's condition, including level of responsiveness, level of activity, skin color, vomiting, and so on. Give as many specifics about the poison as you can. Again, any directions from a poison control center should be verified by your medical direction. Follow local protocol.

▶ Drug and Alcohol Emergencies

Drug abuse is defined as the self-administration of drugs (or of a single drug) in a manner that is not in accord with approved medical or social patterns. A drug or alcohol **overdose** is an emergency that involves poisoning by drugs or alcohol. A patient's **withdrawal** from alcohol or drugs—a period of abstinence from the drug or alcohol to which the body has become accustomed—can be as serious an emergency as an overdose.

Most drug overdoses you will see in the field involve habitual drug users, but drug overdose can also be the result of miscalculation, of confusion, of using more drugs that interact with each other in a potentially dangerous way, or of intentional use (usually as a suicide attempt) (Figure 22-12∗).

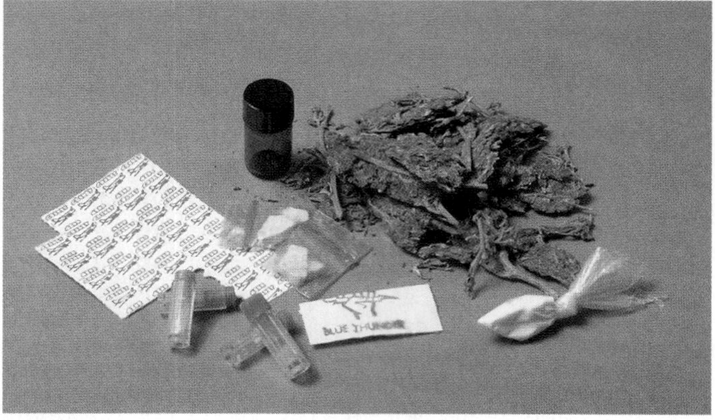

FIGURE 22-12 ∗ A variety of substances may be abused.

Several major medical problems can result from any drug overdose or from sudden withdrawal from a drug. Among the most common findings are altered mental status, respiratory depression, damage to organs such as the kidneys or liver, seizures, cardiac arrest, and hyperthermia or hypothermia. The range of medical problems you may confront in a drug abuse patient is extremely wide and depends upon the type of drug taken. For example, stimulants such as cocaine will increase heart rate and blood pressure, while depressants such as barbiturates will lower them.

Understanding BODY PROCESSES

Drugs with a stimulant effect elevate the heart rate, blood pressure, and respiratory rate and may create a state of excitation. Drugs with a depressant effect may cause a decrease in the heart rate, blood pressure, and respiratory rate and may depress or deepen depression of the mental status. ■

Table 22-1 will give you an idea of the variety of consequences of commonly used drugs. As an EMT, you are not expected to remember everything about each of the drug classes, but the table will help you understand the seriousness and complexity of drug and alcohol emergencies. In drug and alcohol emergencies, the goals are to identify and treat the loss of vital functions caused by the drug—especially impairments to the airway, breathing, oxygenation, and circulation—not the specific effects of the drug itself.

TABLE 22-1 Emergency Consequences of Commonly Abused Drugs

Drug Cluster	Most Common Drug of Abuse	Consequences of Abuse
Stimulants and appetite depressants	Amphetamines Caffeine Cocaine Ephedrine Methylphenidate Nicotine Over-the-counter and prescription drugs Methamphetamine	Moderate dosages cause increased alertness, mood elevation, excitation, euphoria, increased pulse rate and blood pressure, insomnia, and loss of appetite. "Recreational" use of cocaine, even in small doses, can cause severe cardiac toxicity, including angina pectoris, dysrhythmias, and myocardial infarcts. Overdoses can cause agitation, violence, paranoia, increase in body temperature, hallucinations, convulsions, and possible death. Cocaine overdose can cause excitement, euphoria, rapid respiration, elevated blood pressure, cyanosis, paralysis, and loss of reflexes, and can lead to circulatory failure and death. Although the degree of physical addiction is not known, sudden withdrawal can cause apathy, long periods of sleep, irritability, depression, and disorientation.
Cannabis products	Hashish Marijuana THC (tetrahydrocannabinol)	Moderate dosages cause euphoria, relaxed inhibitions, increased appetite, dry mouth, and disoriented behavior. Overdoses can cause fatigue, tremors, paranoia, and possible psychosis. Although the degree of physical addiction is not known, sudden withdrawal can cause insomnia and hyperactivity, and decreased appetite is occasionally reported.
Depressants—narcotics and opiates/opioids	Codeine Heroin Methadone Morphine Fentanyl Oxycodone Hydrocodone Hydromorphone Buprenorphine Opium (90 percent of opiate/opioid-dependent abusers will have a mixed overdose)	Moderate dosages cause euphoria, drowsiness, lethargy, respiratory depression, constricted pupils, constipation, and nausea. Overdoses can cause slow and shallow breathing, clammy skin, watery eyes, runny nose, yawning, restlessness, rapid pulse, elevated blood pressure, diarrhea, loss of appetite, irritability, panic, chills and sweating, cramps, and nausea. Needle tracks are a sign of repeated injections.
Depressants—sedatives and tranquilizers	Alcohol Antihistamines Barbiturates Chloralhydrate Other nonbarbiturate, nonbenzodiazepine sedatives Over-the-counter preparations Diazepam and other benzodiazepines Other major or minor tranquilizers	Moderate dosages can result in slurred speech, drowsiness, impaired thinking, incoordination, disorientation, and drunken behavior without the odor of alcohol. Overdose can result in CNS depression, shallow respiration, cold and clammy skin, sluggish pupils, weak and decreased or rapid pulse, coma, respiratory/circulatory failure, and possible death. Aggressive and suicidal behavior may also occur. Sudden withdrawal results in anxiety, insomnia, tremors, delirium, seizures, and possible death.
Hallucinogens (psychedelic drugs)	DET (N, N-Diethyltryptamine) DMT (N, N-Dimethyltryptamine) LSD (Lysergic acid diethylamide) Mescaline MDA (3, 4 Methylenedioxyamphetamine) PCP (Phencyclidine) STP (DOM-2, 5-Dimethoxy, 4-Methylamphetamine)	Moderate dosages can result in motor disturbances, anxiety, paranoia, delusions of persecution, illusions and hallucinations, and poor perception of time and distance. Overdose can result in longer, more intense "trip" episodes, psychosis or exacerbation of a pre-existing psychiatric problem, and possible death. Flashbacks can occur months or years after the original dose. PCP may also cause paralysis, violence, rage, and status epilepticus.

continued

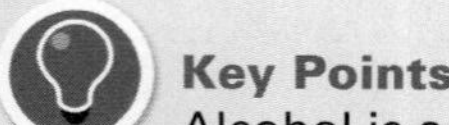

Key Points
Alcohol is a central nervous system depressant that causes an altered mental status and, in large doses, can cause unresponsiveness or death.

Objective 22-13
Given a scenario involving a patient experiencing a drug or alcohol emergency, describe the steps of assessment-based management.

TABLE 22-1 Emergency Consequences of Commonly Abused Drugs *continued*

Drug Cluster	Most Common Drug of Abuse	Consequences of Abuse
Inhalants	Aerosol propellants Gasoline and kerosene Glues and organic cements Lacquer and varnish thinners Lighter fluid Typing correction fluid Medical anesthetics Propane Toluene	Moderate dosages cause excitement, euphoria, feelings of drunkenness, giddiness, loss of inhibitions, aggressiveness, delusions, depression, drowsiness, headache, and nausea. Overdoses can cause a loss of memory, delirium, glazed eyes, slurred speech, drowsiness, hallucinations, confusion, unsteady gait, and erratic heartbeat and pulse. Sudden withdrawal results in insomnia, decreased appetite, depression, irritability, and headache. Death can result from suffocation or from a phenomenon called SSD ("sudden sniffing death"), which is still poorly understood but might follow myocardial infarction.

As you can see in Table 22-1, alcohol is classified as a type of drug. It is a central nervous system depressant that, in moderate doses, causes an altered mental status and, in large doses, can cause unresponsiveness or death. Alcohol is completely absorbed from the stomach and intestinal tract within 2 hours from the time it is ingested and sometimes as quickly as 30 minutes. Once absorbed from the stomach, it is distributed relatively quickly to all body tissues. It is concentrated, however, in the blood and in the brain.

Habitual alcohol abusers, or alcoholics, are prone to a wide variety of illnesses ranging from cirrhosis of the liver to peritonitis. In addition to causing medical problems, alcohol intoxication is a major cause of automobile crashes. Alcohol ingestion, even in smaller doses, is also a major factor in drug overdoses, homicides, burns, drowning, nonaccidental trauma, and general trauma.

Assessment-Based Approach: Drug and Alcohol Emergencies

Scene Size-Up

Conduct a scene size-up. First make sure that the scene is safe, since calls involving drugs or alcohol may involve physical abuse, violent acts, or sudden changes in behavior that may result in violence toward the EMT. In these situations, it may be prudent to call for police backup early so they are on scene with you in case violence erupts. (See "Managing a Violent Drug or Alcohol Abuse Patient," later in this chapter, for specific guidelines on what to do upon encountering a patient who is likely to become aggressive.)

ASSESSMENT Tips

Rapid behavior change may put the EMT at risk. Constantly remain attentive to the dynamics of the scene and the patient. Drug and alcohol emergencies may, at times, erupt in violence that could be directed toward the EMT. ■

Be very careful to note the presence of any potential weapons and not to get stuck with a drug abuser's needle, as most people who share needles also share infectious diseases. Make sure you have taken the appropriate Standard Precautions, since alcoholics and drug abusers may have a higher incidence of bloodborne and airborne diseases. Look for a mechanism of injury that could possibly have caused injury to the patient.

In addition, because drug and alcohol emergencies may mimic other medical conditions, especially stroke and hypoglycemia, you should inspect the area immediately around the patient (and carefully check the patient's pockets) for evidence of drug or alcohol use—empty or partially filled pill bottles or boxes, syringes, empty liquor bottles, prescriptions, hospital discharge orders, or physician's notes that might help you identify what drug the patient has taken. Also check the patient for any medical ID tag that would give information about chronic conditions such as diabetes. Keep any such evidence with the

Thinking Critically
After an evening celebrating with friends at a bar, a woman collapsed in the parking lot on the way to her car. One of her friends found her and called 911. The woman is unresponsive. Should you assume she has simply had too much to drink? How can you begin to narrow in on the possible or probable causes of her condition?

patient since it will be useful for the staff at the poison control center or the emergency department.

Primary Assessment

Begin your primary assessment by forming a general impression. Given the mechanism of injury, take the necessary manual in-line spinal precautions. Quickly scan the patient for any obvious life threats such as gunshot or knife wounds to the chest, major bleeding, or an obstructed airway from vomitus, blood, or other secretions.

The mental status of the drug or alcohol abuse patient can range from extreme excitability to complete unresponsiveness, depending on the substance being abused. If the patient has an altered mental status, open the airway and closely inspect inside the mouth for secretions, vomitus, or other substances that may block the airway or could be aspirated.

Alcohol, narcotics, and other central nervous system (CNS) depressants could easily cause inadequate breathing as a result of slow or absent respiratory rates or decreased inspiratory volume. If the patient is not breathing adequately, as evidenced by either slow breathing (bradypnea), or shallow breathing (hypopnea), provide positive pressure ventilation with supplemental oxygen at a rate of 10–12 per minute. If breathing is adequate, administer oxygen based on the SpO_2 reading and patient signs and symptoms. If the SpO_2 reading is greater than 95% and no signs or symptoms of hypoxia or respiratory distress are present, apply a nasal cannula at 2 to 4 lpm. If signs of hypoxia or respiratory distress are present, or the SpO_2 reading is less than 95%, place the patient on a nonrebreather mask at 15 lpm.

Assess the circulation by palpating for a radial pulse. The heart rate may be decreased or rapid and weak if CNS depressants are abused, whereas the patient may have significantly increased heart rates when CNS stimulants have been taken. The skin in the CNS depressant abuse patient is usually cool, clammy, and pale because of poor perfusion related to hypotension. Assess for major external bleeding that may have occurred as a result of associated trauma.

The odor of alcohol on the patient's breath or clothing may provide a clue to alcohol abuse. However, do not confuse the fruity or acetone odor that is related to a diabetic emergency with the smell of alcohol. In addition, do not automatically decide that an altered mental status or other signs and symptoms are directly related to alcohol ingestion.

ASSESSMENT Tips

The vital signs of a patient who has been abusing drugs may vary widely, based on the type of drug taken. What the EMT may notice, however, is a pattern of signs and symptoms. These patterns may help identify the type of drug, for example, a stimulant or depressant. ■

Other serious medical conditions may be present and not directly related to or caused by the alcohol. Always be suspicious that a condition other than alcohol intoxication may be the cause of altered mental status and other similar signs and symptoms. As an example, the slurred speech that you assume is due to alcohol ingestion may actually be a result of a stroke or head injury.

Understanding BODY PROCESSES

Even though the patient may have taken a drug or ingested alcohol, always consider other possible causes of his condition, such as diabetes, stroke, or even low body core temperature. The EMT should remain suspicious of a wide variety of causes at all times while assessing the patient. ■

It is necessary to prioritize the patient at the end of the primary assessment. *The following six signs and symptoms indicate a high-priority patient* (Figure 22-13*):

- Unresponsiveness
- Inadequate breathing
- Fever
- Abnormal heart rate (slow, fast, weak, or irregular)
- Vomiting with an altered mental status
- Seizures

Secondary Assessment

In the altered mental status or unresponsive patient, conduct a rapid secondary assessment. Examine the patient for any evidence of trauma.

CNS stimulant drugs typically cause dilated pupils, whereas narcotics cause pinpoint pupils. Inspect the mucous membranes inside the mouth for evidence of cyanosis, excessive salivation, or dryness. The membranes may be swollen if volatile chemicals have been inhaled.

DRUG AND ALCOHOL EMERGENCY INDICATORS

If any of the following six danger signs are present, no matter what caused the crisis, the patient's life may be threatened and the patient is a high priority for immediate transport.

1
Unresponsiveness:
The patient cannot be awakened from what appears to be a deep sleep or coma. If awakened for a short period of time, she almost immediately relapses into unresponsiveness.

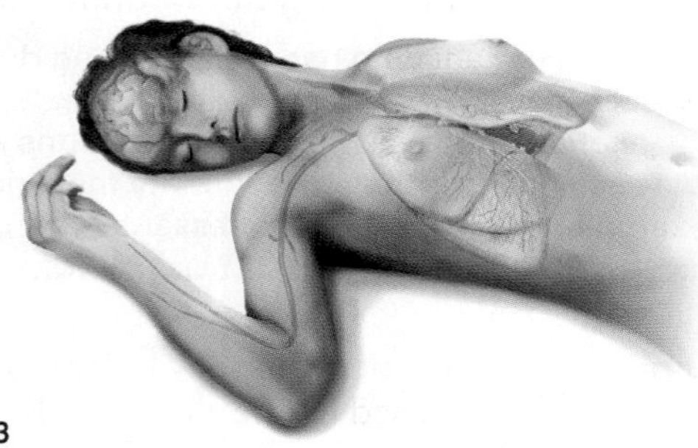

2
Respiratory difficulties:
The pateint's breathing may be very weak, stong and weak cycles, or may stop altogether. Inhalation or expiration may be noisy. If the patient's skin is bluish (cyanotic), she is almost certainly not receiving enough oxygen, but the absence of cyanosis does not necessarily mean that respiratory difficulties are not severe.

3
Fever:
As a guide it may be stated that any temperature above 100° F or 38° C falls into this category.

4
Tachycardia or bradycardia, or an irregular pulse:
Tachycardia, bradycardia or an irregular pulse may be an indication of physiologic instability.

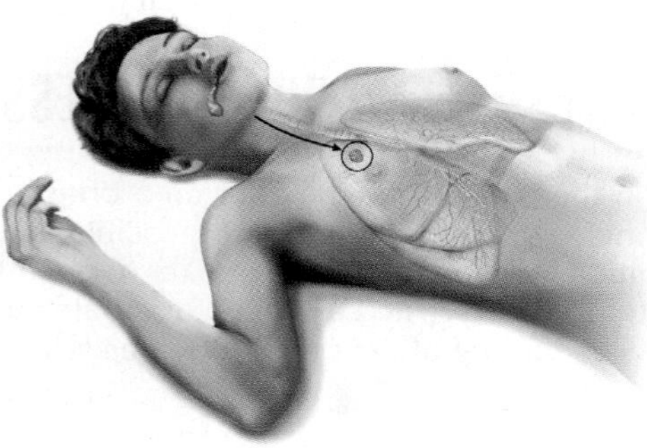

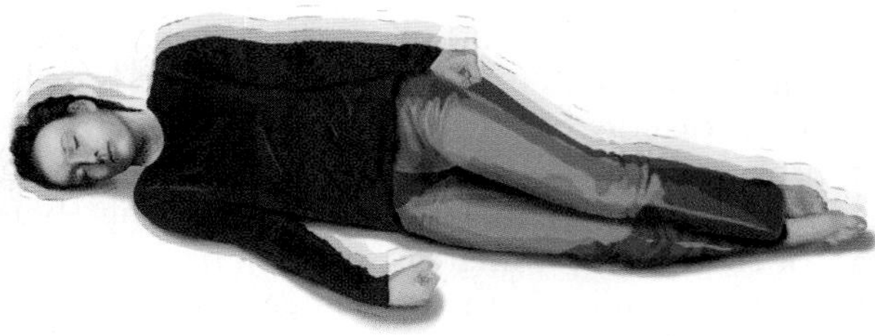

5
Vomiting with altered mental status:
If the patient vomits while not alert or unresponsive, the prime danger consists of the possibility that she may occlude her airway or aspirate vomitus into the lungs.

6
Seizures:
Muscle rigidity, spasm, or twitching of face, trunk muscles, or extremities may indicate an impending convulsion with a series of violent muscle contractions and jerking movements.

FIGURE 22-13 ✱ Drug and alcohol emergency indicators.

As mentioned earlier, "huffers" are patients who inhale paints or propellants in order to "get high" as the poison gets absorbed across the alveolar membrane. These patients are commonly identified by the presence of paint or other material about the mouth and nose. Hallucinogens may cause the face to flush. Jugular venous distention may be found in CNS stimulant or depressant abuse if the patient has suffered heart failure. Auscultate the lungs for abnormal sounds.

Understanding BODY PROCESSES

A huffer may experience a euphoric feeling, or "high," when the paint fumes or gas he inhales displaces the air in his lungs and creates a state of hypoxia. ■

The muscles in the extremities may appear very relaxed and lack any coordination if narcotics were taken. Peripheral pulses may be very weak, rapid, and irregular, if not absent. The skin may appear cool, clammy, and pale in narcotic drug abuse. Look for needle tracks on the extremities (Figure 22-14✱).

Obtain a set of vital signs. The blood pressure may be low with CNS depressants and extremely high with CNS stimulants. The pulse will vary, depending on the drug, and may be elevated, slow, or irregular. The skin may be flushed, pale, or cyanotic. Skin condition may be dry, moist, or normal. The temperature may be cool with CNS depressants and warm with CNS stimulants.

Attempt to gather a history from any relatives, friends, or bystanders at the scene. Look for medical alert tags on the patient.

Key Terms

pharming raiding others' medicine supplies or using faked prescriptions to obtain drugs.

CNS stimulants substances that excite or increase central nervous system functions.

CNS depressants substances that inhibit or decrease central nervous system functions.

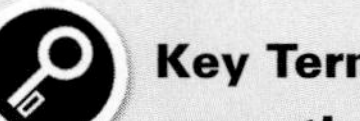

Key Terms

narcotics central nervous system depressants derived from opiates or opioids.

hallucinogens substances that cause hallucinations, or false perceptions.

volatile inhalants substances that are easily vaporized and inhalable.

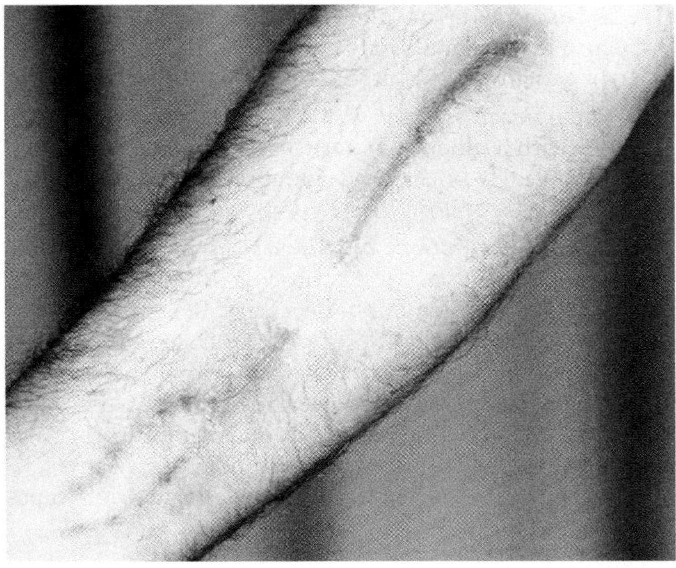

FIGURE 22-14 ✻ Needle track marks on the extremities—a sign of injected drug use.

If the patient is responsive and able to answer your questions and obey your commands, gather a history from the patient before conducting the physical exam and gathering vital signs. During the questioning, attempt to determine what the patient has ingested, injected, inhaled, smoked, or abused in some other manner. Remember, however, that the history may be unreliable because the patient may believe that the EMS provider will get him into trouble with law enforcement. Keep in mind also that patients sometimes abuse more than one substance at a time, using different routes. For example, alcohol is commonly involved with the abuse of other drugs.

The patient may mention **pharming** or a "pharming party." This typically refers to adolescents who raid their parents' or friends' medicine cabinets for prescription medications or who fake symptoms to obtain prescription medications. The teens then attend a pharming party and trade medications and typically take the medications with alcohol to try to obtain a greater high. Painkillers, CNS depressants, anti-anxiety medications, and stimulants are the most popular medications at pharming parties.

Try to establish the past medical history. Determine what prescription medications the patient is taking since these may interact with the substance being abused and worsen the condition or hide certain characteristic signs. Following the history, conduct a physical exam and obtain a set of vital signs.

ASSESSMENT Tips

Painkillers commonly taken at "pharming" parties are OxyContin, Demerol, Darvon, Dilaudid, Percocet, Vicodin, and Tylenol with Codeine. Many of the stimulants taken are those prescribed for attention-deficit disorders, such as Ritalin, Adderall, and Dexedrine. ■

Signs and Symptoms The signs and symptoms can vary widely, depending on the substance or drug that was abused. Many times the patient abuses more than one substance or drug. For example, a patient may take a CNS stimulant, drink large amounts of alcohol, and then take a CNS depressant. This would produce a variety of conflicting signs and symptoms. The following are characteristic signs and symptoms based on the most common types of abused drugs and substances (review Table 22-1):

- **CNS stimulants** excite the central nervous system.
  Signs and symptoms: Excitability, elevated mood, agitation, apprehension, uncooperativeness, tachycardia, tachypnea, dilated pupils, dry mouth, sweating, increased blood pressure, loss of appetite, lack of sleep.
- **CNS depressants** depress the central nervous system.
  Signs and symptoms: Euphoria, drowsiness, sleepiness, decreased breathing rates and volumes, bradycardia, hypotension, dilated pupils that are sluggish to respond to light.
- **Narcotics** are CNS depressants that are derived from opium (opiates) or synthetic opium (opioids).
  Signs and symptoms: Bradycardia, hypotension, inadequate breathing rates and volume, cool, clammy skin, lethargy, constricted pupils, nausea. Respiratory depression or arrest can occur in these patients.
- **Hallucinogens**, sometimes called psychedelic drugs, cause hallucinations.
  Signs and symptoms: Motor disturbances, paranoia, anxiety, visual or auditory hallucinations, tachycardia, dilated pupils, flushed face, poor perception of time and distance.
- **Volatile inhalants** are substances that are inhaled.
  Signs and symptoms: Excitement, euphoria, drunkenness, aggressiveness, depression, headache, drowsiness, nausea, swollen mucous membranes of the nose and mouth, glazed eyes, slurred speech, hallucinations, incoordination, erratic pulse and blood pressure, seizures.

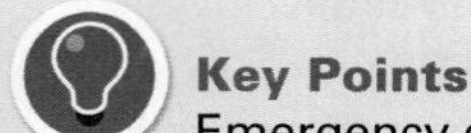

Key Points
Emergency care provided to the drug, substance, or alcohol abuse patient is mostly supportive.

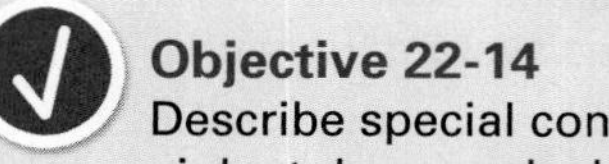

Objective 22-14
Describe special considerations in managing violent drug or alcohol abuse patients.

Emergency Medical Care

The emergency care provided to the drug, substance, or alcohol abuse patient is mostly supportive. Scene safety is a priority at many of these scenes. Close monitoring of the patient is necessary, since a rapid change in his condition may occur from the alcohol, drug, or other substance. Calming the patient may be a primary concern, since people who take stimulants or hallucinogens often become very agitated and excited. In addition to protecting yourself, protect the patient from injuring himself.

The following are steps to manage the drug, substance, or alcohol abuse patient:

1. *Establish and maintain an airway.* If spinal injury is suspected, take manual in-line spinal stabilization. Suction any substance from the mouth. If the patient is unresponsive, consider inserting an oropharyngeal or nasopharyngeal airway.
2. *Administer oxygen.* If the breathing is inadequate, begin positive pressure ventilation with supplemental oxygen attached to the ventilation device at a rate of 10–12 per minute. Closely monitor the breathing status, since many drugs may cause respiratory depression or arrest. This can occur suddenly in some cases. If breathing is adequate, administer oxygen based on the SpO_2 reading and patient signs and symptoms. If the SpO_2 reading is greater than 95% and no signs or symptoms of hypoxia or respiratory distress are present, apply a nasal cannula at 2–4 lpm. If signs of hypoxia or respiratory distress are present, or the SpO_2 reading is less than 95%, place the patient on a nonrebreather mask at 15 lpm.
3. *Position the patient.* The unresponsive patient should be placed in a lateral recumbent position to help protect the airway from aspiration unless a spinal injury is suspected, in which case the patient is positioned supine on a backboard with other spinal precautions taken. If the patient requires ventilation, keep him in a supine position and have suction readily available.
4. *Maintain the body temperature.* Some drugs may cause an increase or decrease in the body temperature. Cover patients with decreased temperatures with a blanket and warm the back of the ambulance. If the patient's temperature is elevated, remove clothing and passively cool the patient, as described in Chapter 24, "Environmental Emergencies." If your EMS service has thermometers available, obtaining an actual temperature may be beneficial to treatment. The use of tympanic thermometers is encouraged, because inserting an oral thermometer into the mouth of a patient with an altered mental status is dangerous.
5. *If your local protocol permits, assess the blood glucose level* with a glucose meter to rule out possible hypoglycemia. If the blood glucose level is less than 60 mg/dL, follow your hypoglycemia protocol.
6. *Restrain the patient only if necessary.* Use restraints according to your local protocols. Request assistance from law enforcement, if necessary. Because the mental status of a drug abuser may result in extreme violence or resistance to your care, you may have to restrain him. Never, however, restrain the patient in a prone position, because this makes monitoring the airway and breathing almost impossible. Many protocols require law enforcement presence prior to patient restraint.

Reassessment

The reassessment is extremely important in drug, substance, or alcohol abuse patients, because their condition can change so rapidly as a result of the influence of the substance. The patient may lose his gag or cough reflex and not be able to maintain his own airway. Closely monitor the airway for vomitus or secretions. The respirations may become inadequate very quickly. The heart rate and blood pressure may fluctuate, either increasing or decreasing excessively. The reassessment should be conducted every 5 minutes to monitor the patient effectively. If the patient is stable, the reassessment may be done at 15-minute intervals, but closely monitor the patient as his condition may rapidly change.

Summary: Assessment and Care

To review assessment findings that may be associated with drug and alcohol emergencies, and emergency care, see Figures 22-15* and 22-16*.

Managing a Violent Drug or Alcohol Abuse Patient

The unusual, always unpredictable, and sometimes violent behavior of the drug or alcohol abuse patient presents special concerns for the safety of the EMS crew, the patient, and bystanders. For more information on how to

Assessment Summary

DRUG OR ALCOHOL EMERGENCY

The following findings may be associated with a drug or alcohol emergency.

SCENE SIZE-UP

Pay particular attention to your own safety.
Look for:
- Mechanism of injury
- Alcohol, drugs, or other commonly abused substances
- Position and location of the patient
- Needles, syringes, or other drug paraphernalia

Primary Assessment

General Impression
- Vomitus or secretions in mouth
- Paint or chemical stains about mouth and nose
- Gunshot or knife wounds to chest
- Excessively excited patient may indicate CNS stimulant drug abuse
- Excessively depressed patient may indicate CNS depressant drug abuse

Mental Status
- Alert to unresponsive
- May appear hyperactive, very nervous or excited, or depressed and lethargic

Airway
- Obstruction by tongue
- Obstruction by vomitus or secretions
- (Insert naso- or oropharyngeal airway if unresponsive)
- Excessive secretions may be present that require suctioning

Breathing
- Respirations shallow, slow, or absent
- Hyperventilation

Circulation
- Heart rate may be increased, decreased, or normal.
- Irregular heart rates may be palpated.
- Skin color may be flushed, pale, or cyanotic.
- Skin temperature may be cool, normal, or warm.
- Skin condition may be wet, dry, or normal.

Status: Priority Patient

Secondary Assessment

General Findings

CNS stimulants:
- Excitability
- Elevated mood
- Agitation
- Apprehension
- Uncooperativeness
- Tachycardia
- Tachypnea
- Dilated pupils
- Dry mouth
- Sweating
- Increased blood pressure
- Loss of appetite
- Lack of sleep
- Dilated pupils

CNS depressants:
- Euphoria
- Drowsiness
- Sleepiness
- Decreased breathing rates and volumes
- Bradycardia
- Hypotension
- Pupils sluggish to respond to light

Narcotics:
- Bradycardia
- Hypotension
- Inadequate breathing
- Cool, clammy skin
- Lethargy
- Constricted pupils
- Nausea

Hallucinogens:
- Motor disturbances
- Paranoia
- Anxiety
- Visual or auditory hallucinations
- Tachycardia
- Dilated pupils
- Flushed face
- Poor perception of time or distance

Volatile inhalants:
- Excitement
- Euphoria
- Drunkenness
- Aggressiveness
- Depression
- Headache
- Drowsiness
- Nausea
- Swollen mucous membranes of nose and mouth
- Glazed eyes
- Slurred speech
- Hallucinations
- Incoordination
- Erratic blood pressure and pulse
- Paint or chemical stains about mouth and nose

continued

FIGURE 22-15a ✻ Assessment summary: drug or alcohol emergency.

Assessment Summary

Drug withdrawal:
- Anxiety and agitation
- Confusion
- Tremors
- Profuse sweating
- Elevated temperature
- Increased heart rate and blood pressure
- Hallucinations
- Nausea
- Seizures
- Abdominal cramps

History

Ask questions regarding the following:
- Did the patient ingest, inhale, inject, or smoke a drug?
- What substance was abused?
- How much was taken?
- How long ago?
- Was the patient given anything in an attempt to reverse the drug?
- Was alcohol ingested?
- If suspected withdrawal, when was the last time the patient had the alcohol or drug?

Physical Exam

Head, neck, and face:
- Dilated, midsize, or constricted pupils
- Pupils sluggish to respond to light
- Dry mouth
- Flushed face
- Swollen mucous membranes of the nose and mouth
- Glazed eyes

Extremities:
- Dry, normal, or clammy skin
- Needle marks

Blood Glucose Level:
- Normal

Vital Signs
- BP: elevated, normal, or decreased
- HR: normal or decreased, possibly irregular
- RR: normal, decreased, increased, or irregular
- Skin: normal, cool and clammy, dry, flushed
- Pupils: possibly dilated, midsize, constricted, and sluggish to respond to light
- SpO_2: Normal to low reading, depending on the respiratory status

FIGURE 22-15a ✱ Assessment summary: drug or alcohol emergency. *continued*

Emergency Care Protocol

DRUG OR ALCOHOL EMERGENCY

1. Establish and maintain an open airway; insert a nasopharyngeal or oropharyngeal airway if the patient is unresponsive and has no gag or cough reflex.
2. Suction secretions as necessary.
3. If breathing is inadequate, provide positive pressure ventilation with supplemental oxygen at a rate of 10–12 ventilations/minute for an adult and 12–20 ventilations/minute for an infant or child.
4. If breathing is adequate, administer oxygen based on the SpO_2 reading and patient signs and symptoms. If the SpO_2 reading is greater than 95% and no signs or symptoms of hypoxia or respiratory distress are present, apply a nasal cannula at 2–4 lpm. If signs of hypoxia or respiratory distress are present, the SpO_2 reading is less than 95%, or the drug abuse route was by inhalation, place the patient on a nonrebreather mask at 15 lpm.
5. Place the patient in a lateral recumbent position if injury is not suspected.
6. Transport.
7. Perform reassessment every 5 minutes with critical patients and at least every 15 minutes with stable patients.
8. For seizures that may occur as a result of withdrawal, refer to the seizure emergency care protocol in Chapter 19.

FIGURE 22-15b ✱ Emergency care protocol: drug or alcohol emergency.

Emergency Care Algorithm: Drug or Alcohol Emergency

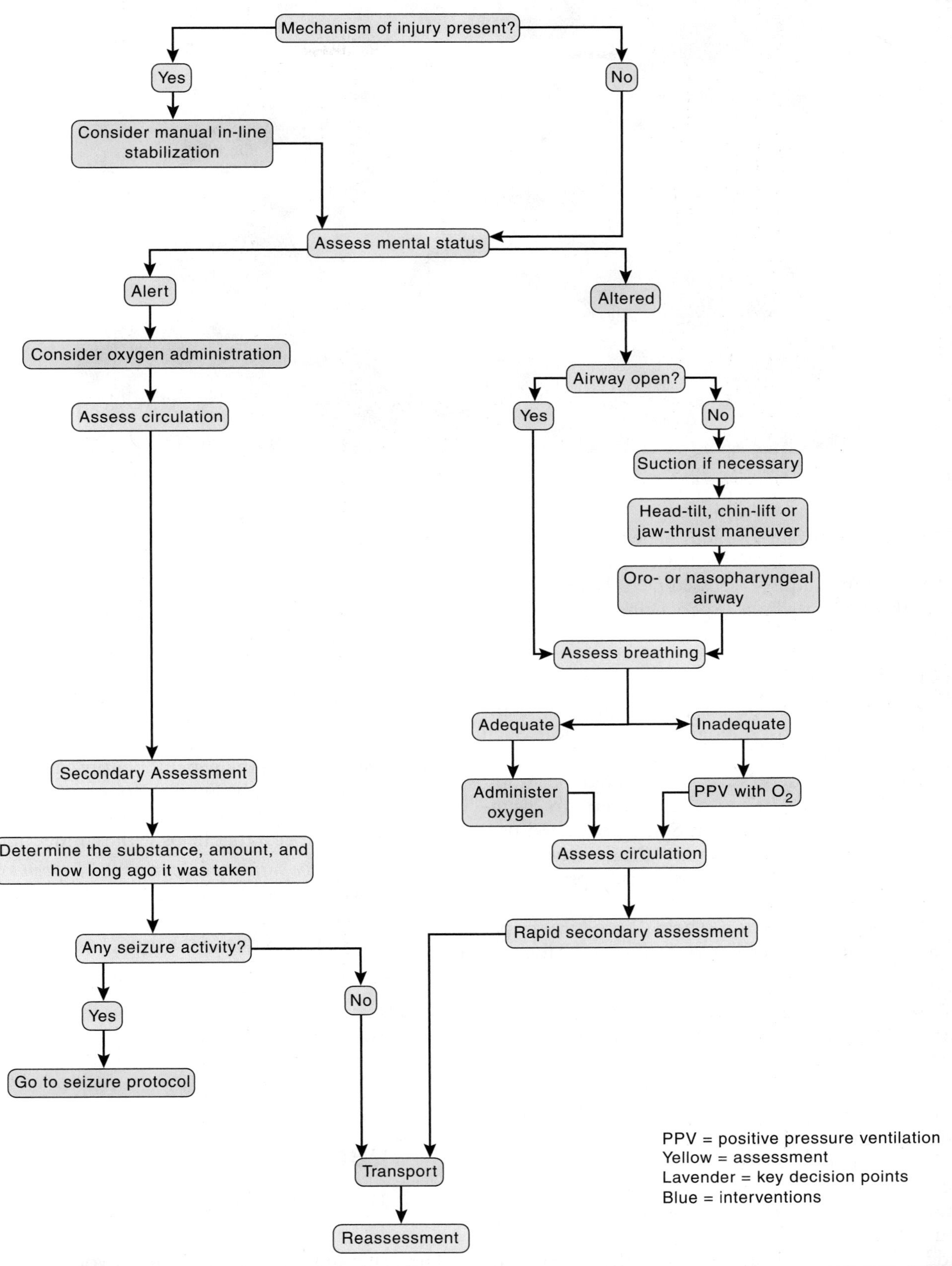

FIGURE 22-16 ✱ Emergency care algorithm: drug or alcohol emergency.

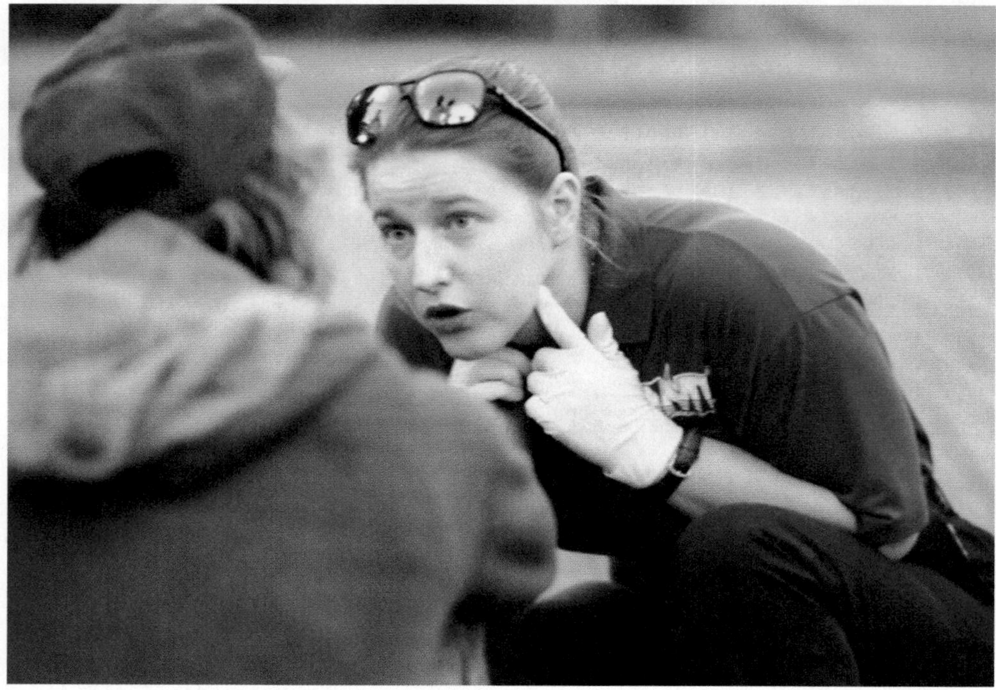

FIGURE 22-17 ✱ Explain who you are and maintain a nonjudgmental attitude. (© Craig Jackson/In the Dark Photography)

interact with and restrain a violent patient (regardless of the reason), see Chapter 26, "Behavioral Emergencies." The talk-down technique, discussed next, is useful when dealing with a patient who is experiencing a "bad trip."

The Talk-Down Technique

Emergencies associated with hallucinogens and marijuana are usually more psychological than physical. Such emergencies may present as intense anxiety or panic states ("bad trips"), depressive or paranoid reactions, mood changes, disorientation, or an inability to distinguish between reality and fantasy. Some prolonged psychotic reactions to hallucinogenic drugs have been reported, particularly with persons already psychologically disturbed.

The talk-down technique can help you reduce the patient's anxiety, panic, depression, or confusion, as follows:

1. *Make the patient feel welcome.* Remain relaxed and sympathetic. Because a patient can become suddenly hostile, have a companion with you. Be calm, but be authoritative and firm.
2. *Identify yourself clearly.* Tell the patient who you are and what you are doing to help. Be careful not to invade the patient's "personal space" until you have established rapport. Try to stay approximately 8–10 feet away until you sense that the patient has some trust in you. Never touch the patient until he gives you permission (Figure 22-17✱) or unless the patient suddenly poses a threat to safety (the patient's or someone else's). Leave yourself a way to safely exit the scene should the patient become violent.
3. *Reassure the patient that his condition is caused by the drug and will not last forever.*
4. *Help the patient verbalize what is happening to him.* Review what is going on. Ask questions. Outline the probable time schedule of events.
5. *Reiterate simple and concrete statements.* Repeat and confirm what the patient says. Orient the patient to time and place. Be absolutely clear in letting the patient know where he is, what is happening, and who is present. Help the patient identify surrounding objects that should be familiar, for example a picture, a person, or maybe even the room or home he is in. This is a process that helps with self-identification.
6. *Forewarn the patient about what will happen as the drug begins to wear off.* There may be confusion one minute, mental clarity the next. Again, help the patient understand that this is due to the drug, not to mental illness.
7. *Once the patient has been calmed, transport.*

Never use the talk-down technique for patients who you know have used the hallucinogen phencyclidine (PCP), because it may further agitate them. (See additional information on PCP patients later in the chapter.)

Specific Substance Abuse Considerations

The drug and alcohol emergencies you encounter may be due to the effect of recently consumed alcohol or drugs, or they may be the result of the cumulative effects

Objective 22-15
Describe special considerations in assessing and managing patients experiencing emergencies associated with alcohol use and withdrawal, drug use and withdrawal, and medication overdose.

Key Points
In problem drinking, alcohol is used to relieve tension or emotional difficulties. In true addiction, abstinence causes physical withdrawal symptoms.

of years of alcohol abuse. While it will not be necessary for you to diagnose the type of alcohol or drug emergency on the scene, it may help to become familiar with various conditions that are caused by consumption of too much alcohol or drugs or by habitual abuse. For instance, the patient who has abused alcohol steadily for years may need treatment not only for acute intoxication but also for medical conditions that have been caused by alcoholism.

What follows are signs and symptoms and special considerations for managing some of the most common types of alcohol and drug emergencies.

Drug Withdrawal

A habitual drug user may develop a *tolerance* to a drug, in which larger doses are required to produce the same desired effects. This quite often leads to a physical or psychological *dependence,* in which the patient experiences a strong need to use the drug repeatedly.

The psychologically dependent person is completely preoccupied with the procurement of the drug. His behavior may be compulsive or neurotic and is geared toward acquiring another dose of the drug. There are, however, no physiological consequences of drug withdrawal for this patient. The physically dependent drug user, on the other hand, undergoes physiological changes within the body that require the drug to be present in his system to prevent withdrawal consequences from occurring. Drugs that commonly produce physical drug dependence are narcotics, sedatives, hypnotics, barbiturates, cocaine, and marijuana.

The following signs and symptoms of drug withdrawal usually begin to occur at about the time when the next drug dose is required, and they usually peak at 48 to 72 hours after the person has stopped taking the drug:

- Anxiety and agitation
- Confusion
- Tremors
- Profuse sweating
- Elevated heart rate and blood pressure
- Hallucinations (visual and auditory)
- Feeling as if there are things on the body that are not there (tactile hallucinations)
- Nausea
- Abdominal cramping

It is important to recognize drug withdrawal as a condition that may cause seizures or a deterioration in the patient's mental status that could result in a blocked airway, inadequate breathing, or poor circulation.

The Alcoholic Syndrome

Alcohol emergencies (Figure 22-18*) are related to the alcoholic syndrome. The alcoholic syndrome usually consists of problem drinking (during which alcohol is used frequently to relieve tensions or other emotional difficulties) and true addiction (in which abstinence from drinking causes physical withdrawal symptoms).

The kind of alcohol used is irrelevant; the heavy beer or wine drinker is as much an alcoholic as the person who drinks too much hard liquor. Alcoholics may abuse alcohol in many forms: Sterno, moonshine, grain alcohol, mouthwash, antifreeze, and rubbing alcohol, to name a few. Frequently, alcoholics are dependent on other drugs as well, especially those in the sedative, barbiturate, and tranquilizer categories. Some alcoholics have underlying psychiatric disorders (especially schizophrenia).

The alcoholic usually begins drinking early in the day, is more prone to drink alone or secretly, and may periodically go on prolonged binges characterized by loss of memory ("blackout periods"). Abstinence from alcohol is likely to produce withdrawal symptoms, such as tremulousness, anxiety, seizures, or delirium tremens (DTs). (See the special segment on delirium tremens later in this chapter.)

As the alcoholic becomes more dependent on alcohol, his performance at work and relationships with friends and family are likely to deteriorate. Absences from work, emotional disturbances, and reckless driving become more frequent.

Be aware that the signs and symptoms of disorders or injuries *unrelated to alcohol*—such as hypoxia, hypoglycemia, hypothermia, recent seizure activity, or head trauma—can easily be confused with the signs and symptoms of intoxication.

Also be aware that alcoholics are prone to injuries and medical conditions brought about by or related to their alcoholism. For example, alcoholics fall down often and are prone to chronic subdural hematomas. Always assess and treat an alcoholic's injuries and medical problems first, before assuming his only problem is "just being drunk."

One of the most serious disorders associated with alcoholism is *Wernicke-Korsakoff syndrome,* a chronic brain syndrome resulting from the toxic effect of alcohol on the central nervous system combined with malnutrition,

ALCOHOL EMERGENCIES

CAUTION: Do not immediately decide that a patient with apparent alcohol on the breath is drunk. The signs may indicate an illness or injury such as epilepsy, diabetes, or head injury.

SIGNS OF INTOXICATION
- Odor of alcohol on the breath
- Swaying and unsteadiness
- Slurred speech
- Nausea and vomiting
- Flushed face
- Drowsiness
- Violent, destructive, or erratic behavior
- Self-injury, usually without realizing it

EFFECTS
- Alcohol is a depressant. It affects judgment, vision, reaction time, and coordination.
- When taken with other depressants, the result can be greater than the combined effects of the two drugs.
- In very large quantities, alcohol can paralyze the respiratory center of the brain and cause death.

MANAGEMENT
- Give the same attention as you would to any patient with an illness or injury.
- Monitor the patient's vital signs constantly. Provide life support when necessary.
- Position the patient to avoid aspiration of vomit.
- Protect the patient from hurting him- or herself.

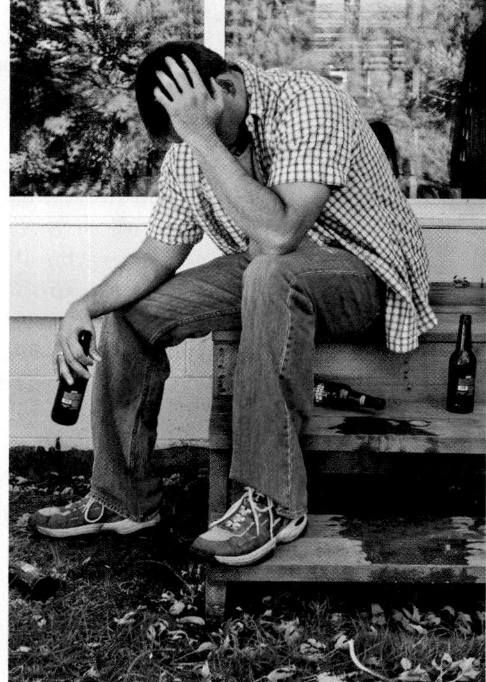

FIGURE 22-18 * Alcohol emergencies.

which is common among alcoholics. Common signs and symptoms of the syndrome include paralysis of the eyes, dementia, hypothermia, the inability to sort fiction from reality, and eventual coma.

Alcoholics often do not eat right, and their health deteriorates. They are more prone to the following illnesses:

- Hypertension
- Altered mental status due to liver malfunction
- Cirrhosis of the liver
- Liver failure (the liver degenerates to fatty material)
- Pancreatitis (including inflammation, abscesses, and necrosis)
- Cardiomyopathy or heart muscle disease
- Peritonitis (inflammation of the abdominal lining)
- Chronic gastric ulcer
- Suppression of the bone marrow's ability to produce red and white blood cells and platelets
- Upper gastrointestinal hemorrhage due to varicose veins in the esophagus, a common cause of death among alcoholics
- Seizures
- Subdural hematoma
- Fractures of the ribs and extremities due to repeated falls
- Hypoglycemia (low blood sugar)
- Pruritus (extreme itching)

The Withdrawal Syndrome

Withdrawal syndrome occurs after a period of abstinence from the drug or alcohol to which a person's body has become accustomed. However, it does not require that the alcoholic or drug abuser stop drinking or taking the drug completely. The withdrawal syndrome can also occur when an alcoholic's alcohol intake falls below the amount usually ingested.

Alcohol withdrawal is dose dependent: The more the alcoholic was drinking, the more severe the syndrome will be. Alcohol withdrawal syndrome (Figure 22-19*), which can mimic a number of psychiatric disorders, is characterized by the following signs and symptoms:

- Insomnia (inability to sleep)
- Muscular weakness
- Fever
- Seizures or tremors
- Disorientation, confusion, and thought process disorders
- Transient visual, tactile, or auditory hallucinations
- Anorexia (a life-threatening loss of appetite)
- Nausea and vomiting
- Hyperthermia (elevated body temperature)
- Sweating
- Rapid heartbeat

ALCOHOL WITHDRAWAL SYNDROME

Delirium tremens constitutes the most extreme form of alcohol withdrawal syndrome. Less severe forms include alcoholic tremulousness, alcoholic hallucinosis, and withdrawal seizures, which generally (but not always) precede delirium tremens.

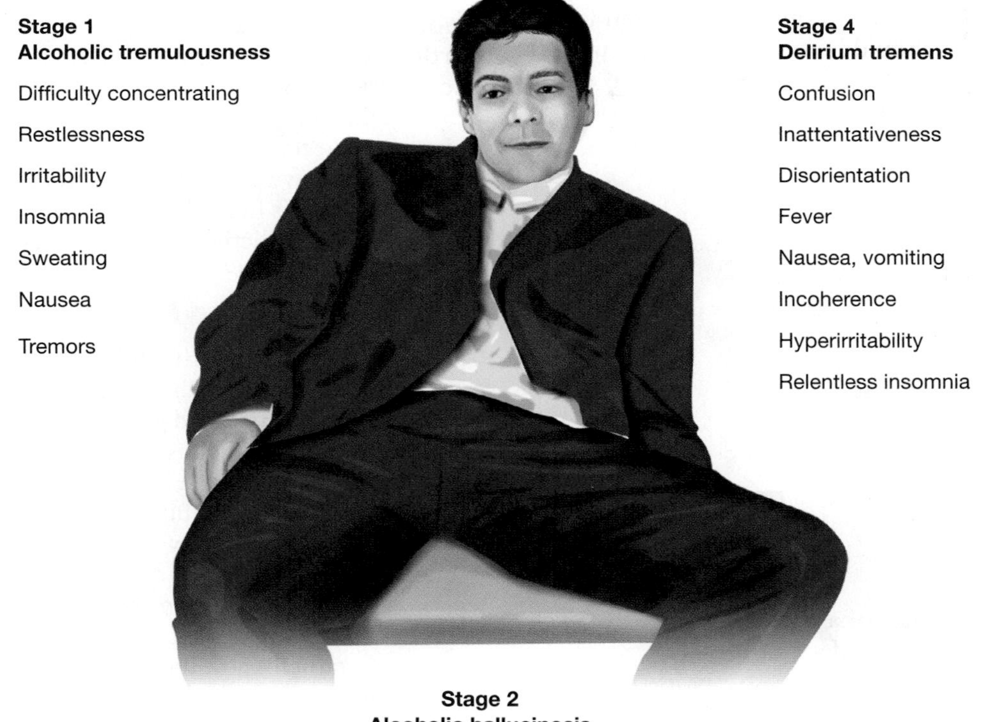

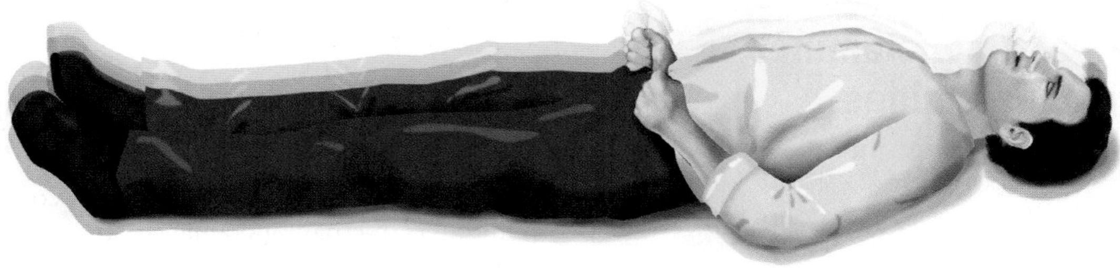

Stage 3
Withdrawal seizures

These are characterized by muscle rigidity and relaxation that usually alternate rhythmically in rapid succession and in groups of 2–6.

FIGURE 22-19 ✱ Alcohol withdrawal.

There are four general stages of alcohol withdrawal:

- *Stage 1,* which occurs within about 8 hours, is characterized by nausea, insomnia, sweating, and tremors.
- *Stage 2,* which occurs within 8 to 72 hours, is characterized by a worsening of stage 1 symptoms plus hallucinations.
- *Stage 3,* which can occur as early as 48 hours following the last alcoholic beverage, is characterized by major seizures.
- *Stage 4* is characterized by delirium tremens (see the next section).

Delirium Tremens

The last stage of alcohol withdrawal, delirium tremens (DTs), is a severe, life-threatening condition with a mortality rate of approximately 5–15 percent. DTs can occur between 1 and 14 days after the patient's last drink, most commonly within 2 to 5 days. A single episode of DTs lasts between 1 and 3 days. Multiple episodes can last as long as a month. DTs should be suspected in any patient with delirium (mental confusion) of unknown cause. Signs and symptoms of DTs are:

- Severe confusion
- Loss of memory
- Tremors
- Restlessness and irritability
- Extremely high fever
- Dilated pupils
- Profuse sweating
- Insomnia
- Elevated blood pressure
- Tachycardia
- Nausea and vomiting
- Diarrhea
- Hallucinations, mostly of a frightening nature (such as delusions of snakes, spiders, or rats)

Seizures are common in alcoholic withdrawal, but not in DTs. However, approximately a third of all those who have seizures in early withdrawal will progress to DTs if left untreated or if treated inadequately. The treatment goals for a patient who is experiencing DTs include psychological as well as physical support (DTs can be a frightening experience).

PCP, Cocaine, Amphetamines, and Methamphetamines

The emergency consequences of commonly abused drugs were discussed in Table 22-1. Because of the unique effects of PCP and cocaine, their use requires special considerations in emergency care.

PCP

One of the most dangerous hallucinogens is phencyclidine (PCP). Known by at least 46 names, it is also called angel dust, killer weed, supergrass, crystal cyclone, hog, elephant tranquilizer, PeaCe Pill, embalming fluid, horse tranquilizer, mintweed, mist, monkey dust, rocket fuel, goon, surfer, KW, or scuffle.

Nothing has so bewildered and amazed researchers as PCP, a drug that is cheap, easy to make, and easy to take, and produces horrible psychological effects (some of which can last for years). PCP is stored in body fat. If a user suddenly loses weight, the drug can be released into the bloodstream and can cause a reaction even if the drug has not been recently taken.

Cocaine

Another drug that deserves special mention is cocaine—partly because of its common use, and partly because of the devastating medical complications of its use.

Cocaine is inhaled through the nose, injected into the veins, and injected into the muscles. An almost-pure form of cocaine known as "crack" is smoked. Another special form of cocaine is heated and inhaled ("free based"). Cocaine is highly addictive, and an overdose can be fatal.

Amphetamines and Methamphetamines

Amphetamines and methamphetamines are abused in a number of forms including tablets, capsules, powders, impregnated in paper, and gelatin. The drug is commonly referred to on the street as "crank" or "go." A crystalline form, referred to as "ice" or "crystal," is smoked, injected, or snorted. Hallucinogenic amphetamines are typically ingested but may be injected or snorted. Street names for hallucinogenic amphetamines include Adam, ecstasy, Eve, essence, harmony, love, tranquility, peace, serenity, and golden eagle.

Amphetamines and methamphetamines stimulate the central nervous system, excite the cardiovascular system, and can produce hallucinations. Hyperthermia, muscle rigidity, or severe excitation may occur, leading to long periods of an awake and excited state. The resulting hypertension, hyperthermia, and increased muscle tone may be life threatening. Methamphetamine use is associated with the sensation of ants or bugs crawling under the skin. The patient often picks at his skin or mutilates himself. Panic attacks and visual and auditory hallucinations may also occur.

Signs and Symptoms of PCP, Cocaine, Amphetamines, or Methamphetamines

Physical signs and symptoms of PCP, cocaine, amphetamines, or methamphetamines are somewhat similar. However, the EMT should remember that emergency management is supportive and not geared toward figuring out exactly what drug was used if the history is unclear. Signs may include:

- Extreme agitation or excitation
- Involuntary horizontal and vertical eye movement
- Unresponsiveness to pain
- Severe muscular rigidity
- Excessive bronchial and oral secretions (leading to choking in some cases)
- Hypertension

- Hyperthermia
- Decreased urinary output
- Seizures
- Respiratory depression or arrest
- Vivid visual or auditory hallucinations
- Sensation of bugs or ants crawling under the skin
- Myocardial infarction (MI), cardiac dysrhythmias, sudden death (these can occur after even small doses and without pre-existing heart disease)
- Aortic dissection (a split of the wall of the aorta)
- Chest pain not related to MI or dissection
- Stroke or intracranial hemorrhage
- Severe headache, unrelated to head injury, that cannot be relieved with analgesics
- Respiratory problems, including hyperventilation, shortness of breath, rapid respiration, Cheyne-Stokes respirations (a repeating pattern of 10–60 seconds of apnea followed by gradually increasing then decreasing depth and frequency of respiration), and respiratory arrest
- Neurological problems, including loss of vision, headache, convulsions, tremors, dizziness, and depressed reflexes
- Psychiatric problems, including anxiety, agitation, euphoria, psychosis, paranoia, hallucinations, suicide, and depression

Before treating any patient suspected of amphetamine, methamphetamine, or cocaine intoxication, take Standard Precautions to prevent the spread of hepatitis B, HIV, and other infectious diseases. These are becoming prominent among amphetamine, methamphetamine, or cocaine users as intravenous use gains popularity.

Emergency Medical Care

You will treat an amphetamine, methamphetamine, cocaine, or PCP overdose as you would any other drug emergency, with the following special considerations.

Your first priority in providing emergency medical care for the patient under the influence of PCP, amphetamine, methamphetamine, or cocaine is to protect yourself and your crew, since the patient may be combative and require restraint. Keep the patient in a quiet, nonstimulating environment.

Check quickly to determine whether there are any injuries that need attention. If there are, administer emergency medical care for those injuries as you would for any trauma patient (ensuring the airway, providing oxygen and ventilations if required, and supporting the circulatory system) before continuing with psychological care. Monitor vital signs regularly and transport the patient as quickly as possible.

Medication Overdose

Another common source of drug overdose is prescription and over-the-counter medications. The overdose may be intentional, where the patient is trying to commit suicide or achieve some type of effect that is not intended for that medication, or it may be accidental. Accidental overdose typically occurs when the patient does not understand the prescription instructions and takes too much of the drug or the patient is forgetful and mistakenly takes the drug more often than is needed. Patients who are on many different medications may suffer synergistic drug interactions when adding a new or an over-the-counter medication. Medications that are commonly involved in overdose are:

- Cardiac medications such as calcium channel blockers, beta blockers, cardioactive steroids, angiotensin-converting enzyme (ACE) inhibitors, and antidysrhythmics
- Psychiatric medications such as benzodiazepines, tricyclic antidepressants (TCAs), selective serotonin reuptake inhibitors (SSRIs), monoamine oxidase inhibitors (MAOIs), and lithium
- Over-the-counter pain relief drugs such as acetaminophen, nonsteroidal anti-inflammatory drugs (NSAIDs), and aspirin
- Antihistamines
- Herbal remedies
- Dietary supplements

Signs and symptoms of medical overdose vary depending on the substance ingested. For example, if beta blockers or calcium channel blockers were involved in the overdose, the heart rate would be bradycardic and the patient would likely be hypotensive; whereas, overdose on acetaminophen will initially not produce any signs or symptoms.

Emergency care for medication overdose focuses on establishing and maintaining an adequate airway, ventilation, and oxygenation. Transport and continuously reassess the patient for changes in his condition. The effects of the medication may continue to increase and cause the patient to deteriorate. This may require you to become more aggressive in your management of the airway, ventilation, and oxygenation.

Huffing

Some poisons are inhaled intentionally in an attempt to "get high." As noted earlier, patients who inhale paints and propellants for this purpose are commonly referred to as "huffers." (See Figure 22-20∗.) The chemical toluene, the agent most commonly used for huffing, is easily found in paints, glues, industrial chemicals, and household chemicals. The toxins are inhaled in a variety of ways in an attempt to produce certain expected effects.

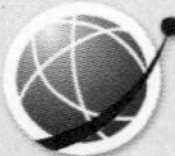

Media Resources

Go to www.bradybooks.com for mykit. Highlights:

- *Web Resource:* American Association of Poison Control Centers
- *Animation:* Cocaine Dependence

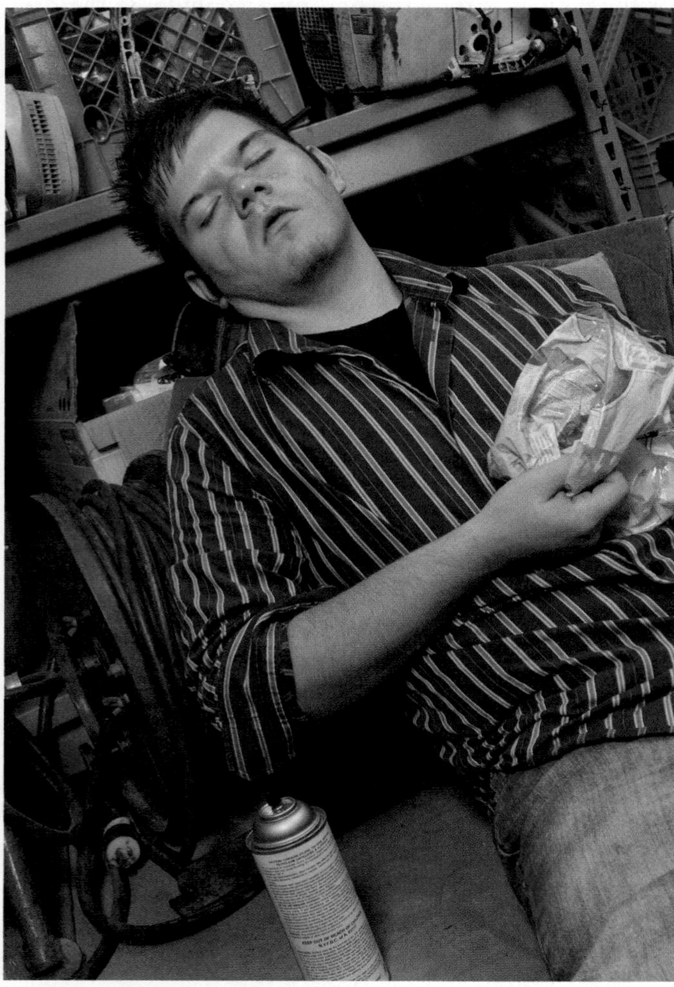

FIGURE 22-20 ✱ A "huffer" inhales poisons deliberately to "get high."

Many of the chemicals used for huffing accumulate in the regions of the brain responsible for feelings of pleasure and reward. After time, they migrate to other regions where they can cause abnormal muscle coordination and alterations in mental status. These substances can also have effects as they displace the oxygen content in the alveoli, leading to hypoxia, or they can cause structural damage to the alveolar surface itself, which can also impair gas exchange. Look for paint or other material on the lips or around the nose of the patient during the physical exam. This may be the only indication of toxic inhalation in an unresponsive patient. Poisons that are commonly used by huffers include:

- Chemicals that contain toluene
- Paints
- Freon
- Gas propellants
- Glue

Keep in mind that inhaled poisons typically have a more immediate onset of effects than injected poisons and may produce more systemic effects. Remember also that inhaled poisons may destroy lung tissue, leading to severe respiratory compromise and significant respiratory distress or failure. Treatment is geared toward removing the patient from the exposure, assessing and treating any loss of vital function caused by the drug (such as airway, breathing, or circulatory deficits), and providing rapid transport to the emergency department.

Routes of Exposure

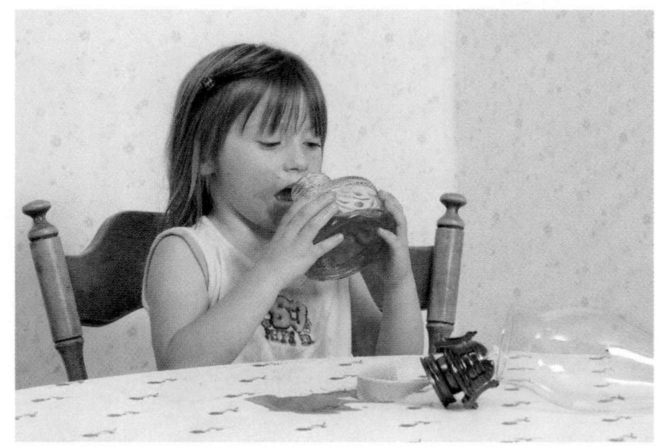

22-1A * Ingestion.

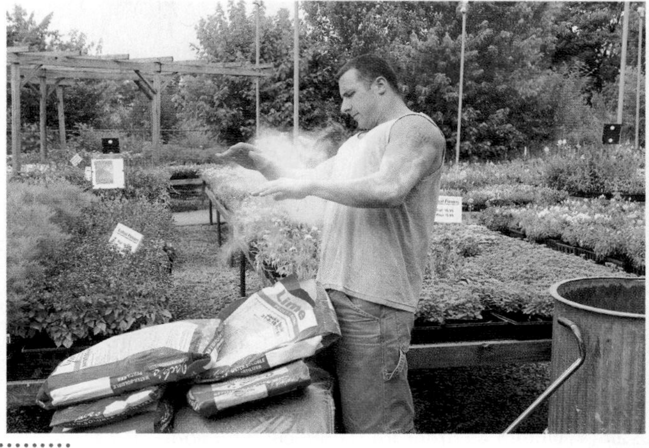

22-1B * Absorption.

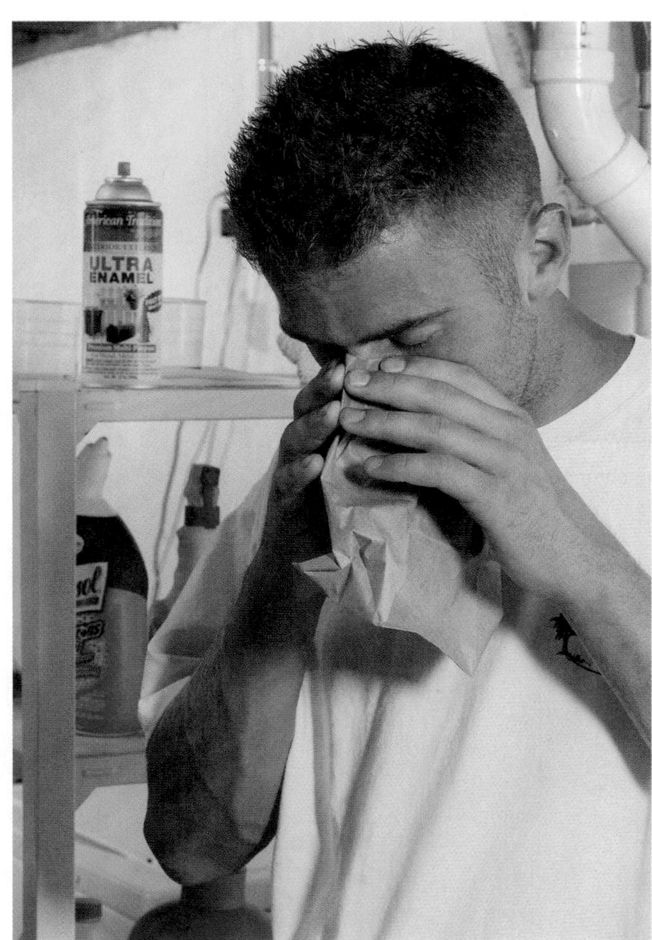

22-1C * Inhalation.

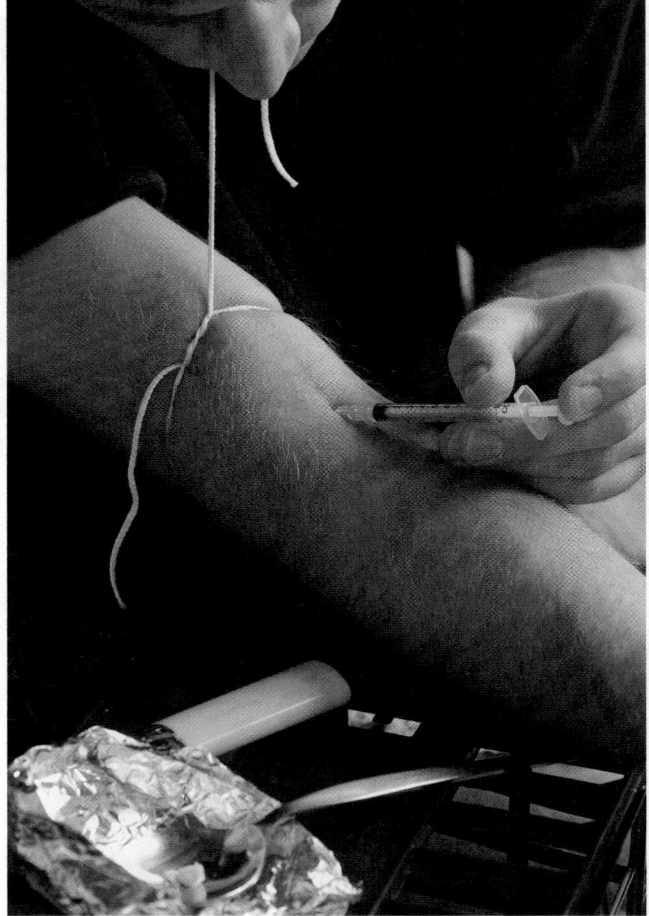

22-1D * Injection.

EMT skills 22-2 Administering Activated Charcoal

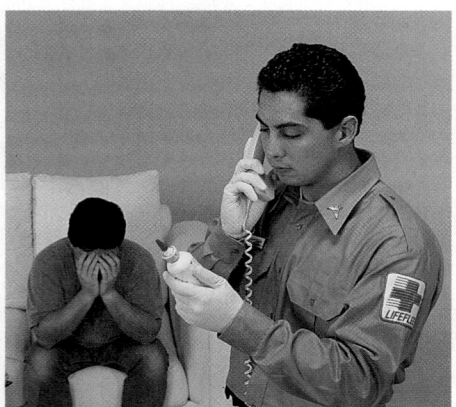

22-2A * Obtain an order from medical direction.

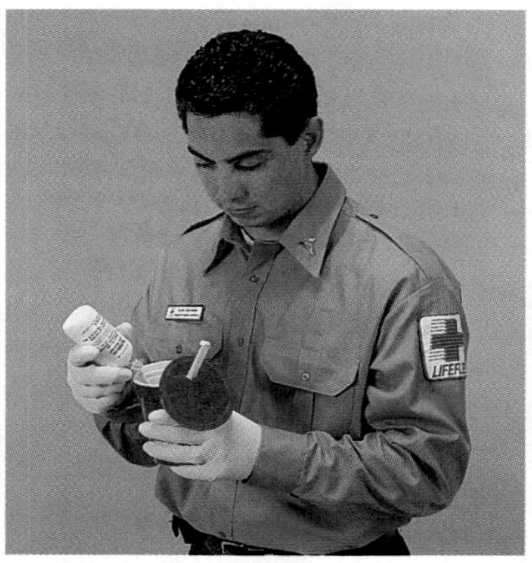

22-2B * Place the activated charcoal in a cup with a lid. A straw may also help to improve the patient's willingness to drink the charcoal.

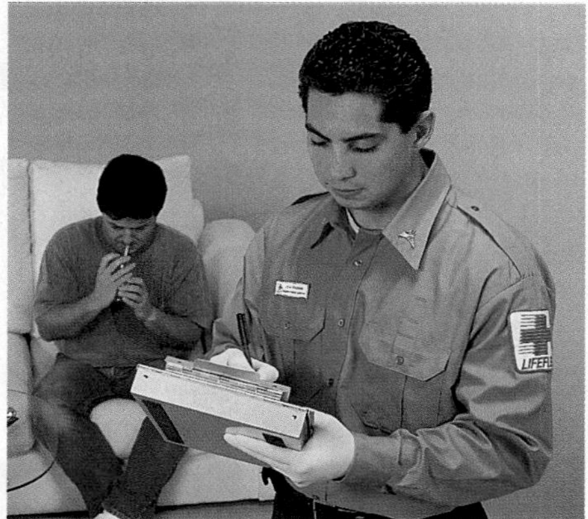

22-2C * Record the dose and time the charcoal was administered.

CHAPTER REVIEW

SUMMARY

Each year in the United States, thousands of people die or become extremely ill from poisonings that occur either accidentally or through some type of intentional act. The greatest number of poisoning emergency patients are children, especially toddlers who swallow some type of poisonous substance as they are exploring their environment. Poisonings often involve prescription or illicit drugs, cleaning substances, and cosmetics. Many other types of poisonings exist. For example, poisonings may result from exposure to industrial chemicals, pesticides, and other substances encountered in the workplace or outdoor environment.

Poisons can gain access to the body by four different routes. Through ingestion, the poison is swallowed and gets absorbed into the bloodstream through the gastrointestinal tract. With inhalation, a poisonous gas or fume becomes absorbed into the bloodstream by way of the alveoli of the lungs. With injections, such as insect stings or injection of illegal drugs, the poison is forcefully inserted through the skin into the tissues. Absorption, typically the slowest route of poisoning, occurs when a poison on the surface of the skin gets absorbed into the tissues.

Regardless of the mechanism, an EMT summoned to a poisoning emergency should approach the situation with a specific process in mind. The first thing to consider is scene safety and ensuring that whatever poison the patient was subjected to will not be a risk to the care providers. After ensuring scene safety, the EMT should complete a primary assessment and ensure that any life threats to the airway, breathing, or circulation are immediately managed. Contact with the poison control center should be made as early as possible, and any treatment recommendations they provide should also be approved by medical direction. The use of activated charcoal for ingested poisonings must meet specific criteria and be approved by medical direction prior to administration. So long as the EMT follows these steps when approaching the patient in a poisoning emergency, many patient outcomes can be successful.

Drugs and alcohol are abused by a variety of people in a number of ways, and the EMT needs to be aware of special problems that are associated with specific drug and alcohol emergencies. For instance, it is possible that drug and alcohol overdose patients will have injured themselves, so you may be treating them for trauma as well as medical consequences. You will also note that patients under the influence of, or withdrawing from, alcohol or drugs can be difficult to manage, oftentimes behaving in an aggressive or even violent manner and posing threats to your safety as well as their own.

While it will not be necessary for you to diagnose the type of alcohol or drug emergency on the scene, it may help for you to become familiar with various conditions or presentation patterns that are caused by consumption of too much alcohol (or drugs) or by habitual abuse. For example, if a patient were to abuse a stimulatory drug, there are usually consistent findings of tachycardia, elevated blood pressure, anxiety, tremors, diaphoresis, and mood elevation. A patient who has abused a depressant drug often presents with a collection of symptoms that includes a decrease in heart rate and blood pressure, cool skin, and a depressed mental status. Patients who are suffering withdrawal symptoms from drug abuse commonly have anxiety and agitation, hallucinations (visual, auditory, or tactile), tremors, sweating, nausea, vomiting, and muscle cramping.

As an EMT, your primary concern in managing drug and alcohol emergencies will be to protect your own safety and, for the patient, to maintain an open airway, treat for life-threatening conditions, and offer calm, nonjudgmental assistance.

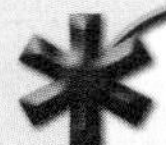

CASE STUDY FOLLOW-UP

SCENE SIZE-UP

You have been dispatched to a 3-year-old patient with abdominal pain. As you approach the patient's residence, you scan the scene, but note no safety hazards. The patient's mother runs out the door, holding the patient, and pulls on your sleeve, saying, "Help! I think my daughter Sophie was eating a plant, and I don't know what to do!" You reassure the mother that you will do all you can to help. As you walk into the living room, you see an overturned plant with dirt and leaves scattered around it. Your partner gathers up some of the leaves, stems, roots, and dirt to keep with the patient and transport to the receiving facility. You have Sophie sit on her mother's lap on the couch.

PRIMARY ASSESSMENT

You assess Sophie while she is on her mother's lap so as not to frighten her. Sophie is hugging her stomach and crying, so your general impression is of a child in pain with an open airway and adequate respirations. She responds appropriately to your simple questions and commands. Using gloves you sweep Sophie's mouth and remove some tiny fragments of the houseplant as well as bits of dirt. You do this to help ensure that Sophie's airway remains open as well as to find evidence of what she has taken into her mouth.

As you examine her oral cavity, you notice that the mucous membranes are beginning to swell and there is some irritation in her throat. Because of the swelling, you will continue to closely monitor her airway patency. Your partner administers oxygen via a nonrebreather mask at 15 lpm. At first Sophie resists the mask, but with encouragement she accepts it.

Sophie's mother gets frightened and starts to cry, blaming herself for the poisoning. "If I would have only watched her better she'd be OK." You reassure Mrs. Horowitz that she did the right thing by calling 911, that breathing the extra oxygen through the mask will help Sophie a lot, and that it's best for her to remain calm so that Sophie will not become frightened and so that you can treat her quickly.

SECONDARY ASSESSMENT

You obtain a history from the mother and determine that she was in the kitchen washing dishes when her daughter toddled off to the living room. About 10 minutes later she heard a crash and her daughter's scream. She ran into the living room and saw the big philodendron overturned and Sophie clutching a handful of leaves. At first she thought Sophie was hurt from the plant tipping over, but when the intensity of Sophie's crying and her complaints of "my tummy hurts" increased over the space of a half hour, she called 911. You ask if she did anything to treat Sophie and she answers that she had Sophie drink some water and spit it out into a basin to rinse her mouth. However, she adds, Sophie did not vomit.

Since the plant that overturned was in a heavy pot, you begin a secondary assessment, checking for any evidence of injury. You don't see any sign of trauma; however, Sophie cringes in pain when you feel for tenderness in her abdomen. You place her on her side on the stretcher, in case of vomiting, while your partner records her vitals. She has a radial pulse rate of 96 bpm. Her respiratory rate is 32 per minute. Her BP is 102/66 mmHg, and her skin is warm and dry. Her pulse oximeter reading is 98%.

You let the mother ride in the ambulance with Sophie, and during transport you contact the poison control center as your protocol indicates for any further orders.

REASSESSMENT

You reassess Sophie's airway, breathing, and circulation and find them adequate. You also check the swelling in the oral cavity and see that the condition of the mucous membranes is not worsening. You reassess her mental status every 5 minutes without noting any change. You reassess her abdominal pain, asking if her tummy hurts more or less or is the same. She nods when you say "same."

You arrive at the emergency department without any further change in Sophie's condition and transfer her to the staff. You and your partner complete a prehospital care report and prepare the ambulance for another call.

IN REVIEW

1. Explain why children are frequent victims of poisoning.
2. List the four ways poisons enter the body.
3. Describe the relationship between poisoning and airway management.
4. Describe the main ways of determining if a poisoning has taken place.
5. Describe the general emergency medical care steps for a poisoning or overdose patient.
6. Give the indications, contraindications, dosage, and administration steps for the administration of activated charcoal.
7. List the general emergency care steps for an ingested poison.
8. List the general emergency care steps for inhaled poisons.
9. List the general emergency care steps for injected poisons.
10. List the general emergency care steps for absorbed poisons (a) to the skin; (b) to the eye.
11. Describe how you can determine whether a patient's condition is alcohol or drug related.
12. Outline the special safety precautions you need to take for a drug or alcohol emergency.
13. List the six indicators that a drug or alcohol patient is a high priority for transport.
14. Explain why the signs and symptoms of alcohol- and drug-related emergencies vary so widely.
15. List the emergency care steps for an alcohol or drug emergency.

CRITICAL THINKING

You are summoned to a residential address for an unknown medical emergency at 1930 hours one cold winter evening. Upon your arrival, you are greeted by the fire and police departments as well as by a middle-aged man who states he is the son of the elderly man inside the home. The son says that he had not been able to reach his father by phone all yesterday or today and was afraid something happened to him. After finding the doors and windows locked, the son has given his permission for the fire and police department to use force in gaining entry into the residence. While you wait outside on the porch, the fire department personnel are first to enter with the police, but they both quickly retreat because of a strong smell of fumes inside the house.

The firefighters then don their self-contained breathing apparatus and re-enter the house. Shortly thereafter, they emerge with an unresponsive elderly male who is wearing pajama bottoms but no shirt. The firefighters report that there was a kerosene heater in the living room and all the burners on the gas stove top and oven were ignited to help heat the downstairs. The son tells you that his father told him a week earlier that his furnace had stopped working and he had to wait until his Social Security check arrived to hire a repairman. You conclude that the patient succumbed to the noxious fumes of the burning gas and kerosene as well as any carbon monoxide that may be present.

The patient responds to painful stimuli with nonpurposeful motion. His pupils are dilated, the airway is patent, breathing is shallow at 38 times per minute, and the peripheral pulses are weak. Blood pressure is 102/88, the pulse oximeter reads 94%, lungs are clear, and the skin is ashen in color. The son is unclear as to what the medical history or medications are for his father, so the fire department is going to re-enter the home in an attempt to find any medication or other clues to his history.

1. Why was it a good idea to allow the fire department to access the home first?
2. What is the underlying mechanism for poisoning in this patient?
3. What is the single greatest intervention you could provide for this patient?
4. Given this type of poisoning, why is the pulse oximeter of little use?
5. What would be the basic tenets of care the patient should receive?

PEARSON

EXPLORE mybradykit™

Please go to **www.bradybooks.com** to access mykit for this text. You will find quizzes, critical thinking scenarios, weblinks, animations, and videos related to this chapter—and much more. Look for online information on carbon monoxide and poisonous plants as well as a video clip on cocaine dependence.

Register your access code from the front of your book by going to **www.bradybooks.com** and selecting the mykit links.

CHAPTER 23

Abdominal, Gynecologic, Genitourinary, *and* Renal Emergencies

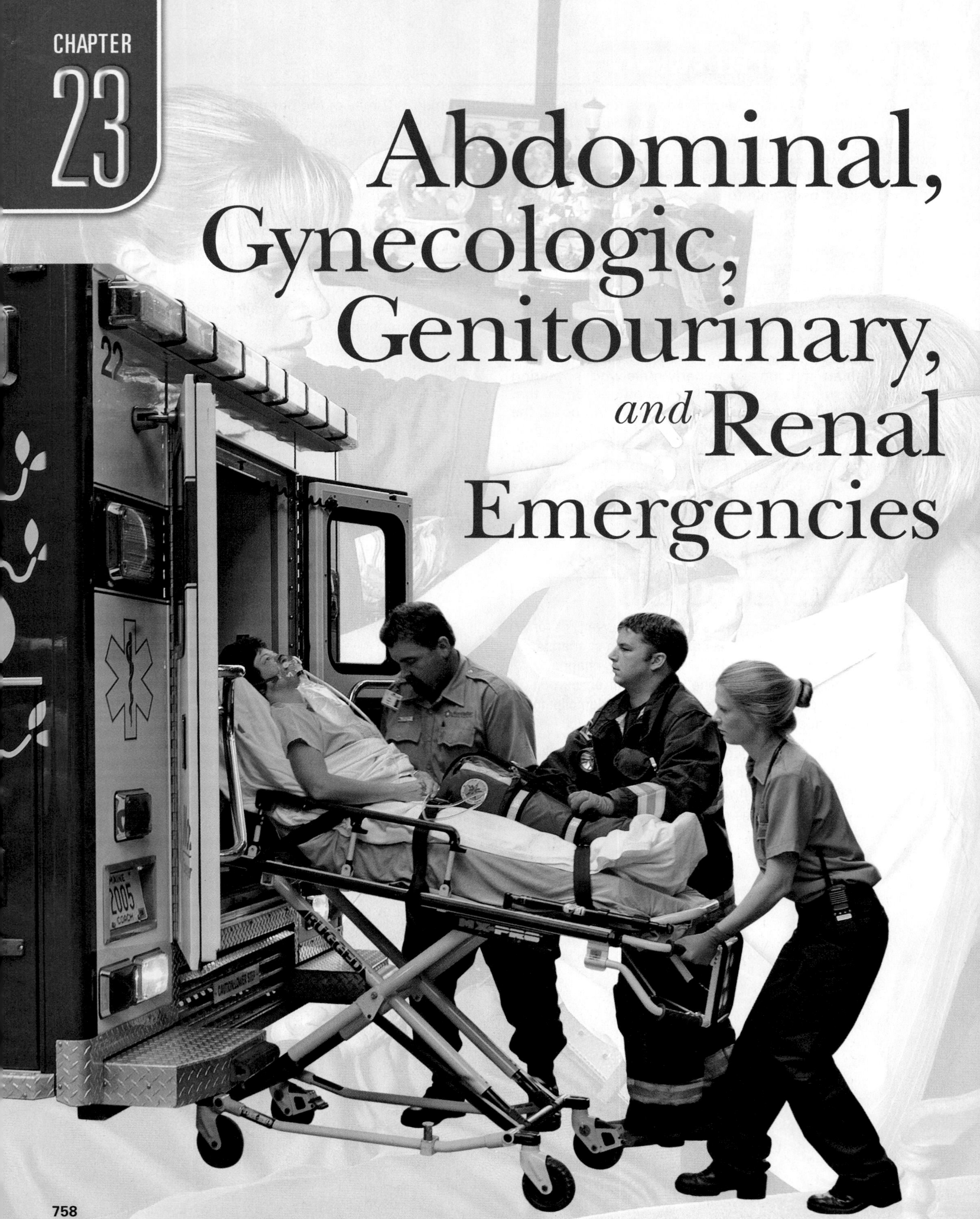

Navigation Guide

The following items provide an overview to the purpose and content of this chapter. The Standard and Competency are from the new National EMS Education Standards.

STANDARD **Medicine** (Content Areas: Abdominal and Gastrointestinal Disorders; Gynecology; Genitourinary/Renal)

COMPETENCY Applies fundamental knowledge to provide basic emergency care and transportation based on assessment findings for an acutely ill patient.

OBJECTIVES: After reading this chapter, you should be able to:

23-1. Define key terms introduced in this chapter.

23-2. Describe the anatomy and physiology of the structures of the abdominal cavity, including:
- **a.** Boundaries of the abdominal cavity
- **b.** Visceral and parietal peritoneum
- **c.** Intraperitoneal and retroperitoneal organs
- **d.** Relationship between the topographic anatomy of the four abdominal quadrants and nine abdominal regions to the location of the organs corresponding to them

23-3. Compare and contrast the general characteristics of hollow and solid organs and vascular structures found in the abdominal cavity.

23-4. List the general mechanisms and types of abdominal pain.

23-5. Describe the pathophysiology and the signs and symptoms associated with common causes of acute abdomen, including:
- **a.** Peritonitis
- **b.** Appendicitis
- **c.** Pancreatitis
- **d.** Cholecystitis
- **e.** Gastrointestinal bleeding
- **f.** Esophageal varices
- **g.** Gastroenteritis
- **h.** Ulcers
- **i.** Intestinal obstruction
- **j.** Hernia
- **k.** Abdominal aortic aneurysm

23-6. Explain the assessment-based approach to acute abdomen, including assessment and appropriate medical care.

23-7. Describe the basic anatomy and physiology of the female reproductive system.

23-8. Describe the pathophysiolgy and the signs and symptoms associated with common gynecologic conditions, including:
- **a.** Sexual assault
- **b.** Nontraumatic vaginal bleeding
- **c.** Menstrual pain
- **d.** Ovarian cyst
- **e.** Endometritis
- **f.** Endometriosis
- **g.** Pelvic inflammatory disease
- **h.** Sexually transmitted diseases

23-9. Explain the assessment-based approach to acute gynecologic emergencies, including assessment and appropriate medical care.

23-10. Describe genitourinary/renal structures and functions.

23-11. Describe the pathophysiology and the signs and symptoms associated with common genitourinary/renal conditions, including:
- **a.** Urinary tract infection
- **b.** Kidney stones
- **c.** Kidney failure

23-12. Describe the purpose of dialysis, how dialysis works, and dialysis emergency management.

23-13. Describe the purposes and types of urinary catheters and urinary catheter management.

23-14. Explain the assessment-based approach to genitourinary/renal emergencies, including assessment and appropriate medical care.

KEY TERMS: Page references indicate first major use in this chapter. For complete definitions, see the Glossary at the back of the book.

abdominal aorta p. 760
abdominal aortic aneurysm (AAA) p. 770
abdominal cavity p. 760
acute abdomen p. 760
appendicitis p. 766
cholecystitis p. 767
dialysate p. 786
dialysis p. 786
dysmenorrhea p. 780
endometriosis p. 780
endometritis p. 780
esophageal varices p. 767
gastroenteritis p. 768
genitourinary system p. 784
guarded position p. 771
gynecology p. 778
hematemesis p. 767
hematochezia p. 767
hematuria p. 785
hernia p. 770
intestinal obstruction p. 769
involuntary guarding p. 773
Markle test p. 765
melena p. 767
menarche p. 779
menses p. 778

continued

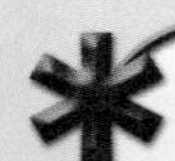

Navigation Guide *continued*

mittelschmerz p. 780
pancreatitis p. 767
parietal pain p. 764
pelvic inflammatory disease (PID) p. 780
peritoneum p. 760
peritonitis p. 765
referred pain p. 764
renal calculi p. 785
rigidity p. 773
somatic pain p. 764
ulcers p. 769
umbilicus p. 761
urology p. 784
visceral pain p. 763
voluntary guarding p. 773

MEDIA RESOURCES: Please go to www.bradybooks.com to access mykit for this text. You will find quizzes, critical thinking scenarios, weblinks, animations, and videos related to this chapter—and much more. Look for online information on genitourinary problems and sexually transmitted diseases. You will also find a video clip on renal failure.

CASE STUDY

The Dispatch
Medic 58—respond to 323 Leslie Place, a single-family dwelling, for a 16-year-old male complaining of "stomach" pain—time out is 0945 hours.

Upon Arrival
Upon arrival at the address you notice a well-kept, single-floor ranch house. There are no apparent safety hazards or signs of trauma. You knock on the door and are greeted by a woman who states, "It's my son, Parker. He's had a fever for the last couple of days. I thought it was the flu or something. But this morning he woke up with a bad pain in his stomach."

How Would You Proceed with This Patient?
This chapter will describe the assessment and emergency medical care for the patient suffering from acute abdominal pain. Later we will return to this case and apply what you have learned.

▶ Introduction

Acute abdominopelvic pain is an emergency you are sure to encounter during your EMS career. It can have any number of causes and may often signal a very serious medical condition. No matter what the cause, in all cases of abdominopelvic pain it is important to assess for life-threatening conditions, make the patient as comfortable as possible, administer oxygen, and get the patient to the hospital quickly.

▶ Acute Abdomen

Acute abdominal pain, sometimes called **acute abdomen**, or *acute abdominal distress,* is a common condition. It may be severe, and it can have any number of causes. Some causes of acute abdominal pain are obvious, but most causes are not that apparent. Medical texts cite approximately 100 different causes of abdominal pain. Acute abdominal pain may arise from the cardiac, pulmonary, gastrointestinal, genital, urinary, reproductive, or other body systems.

Abdominal Structures and Functions

The abdomen, or **abdominal cavity**, is located below the diaphragm and extends to the top of the pelvis. The abdominal cavity is lined with the **peritoneum**. Like the thoracic pleura, the abdominal peritoneum has two layers: the *visceral peritoneum* and the *parietal peritoneum.* The visceral peritoneum is the innermost layer and is in contact with the abdominal organs, whereas the parietal peritoneum is the outer layer. The two layers are separated by a space that contains serous fluid that acts as a lubricant.

The abdominal cavity contains many vital organs (Figure 23-1*). The majority of the abdominal organs—including the stomach, spleen, liver, gallbladder, pancreas, small intestine, and part of the large intestine—are enclosed by the visceral peritoneum. Hence they are termed *intraperitoneal.* However, some organs or portions of organs are located behind the peritoneal space. This area is referred to as the *retroperitoneal space.* The kidneys, ureters, pancreas, and **abdominal aorta** are located in the retroperitoneal space.

Most vital organs of the body, such as the heart, lungs, and brain, are contained within body cavities that are protected by bones. However, just the upper portion of the abdomen is protected by the lower rib cage, while

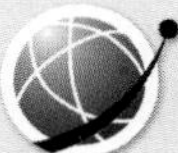

Media Resources
Go to www.bradybooks.com for mykit.
Highlights:

- *Web Resource:* Genitourinary Problems
- *Web Resource:* Dialysis
- *Video:* Renal Failure

Objective 23-2
Describe the anatomy and physiology of the structures of the abdominal cavity.

Objective 23-3
Compare and contrast the general characteristics of hollow and solid organs and vascular structures found in the abdominal cavity.

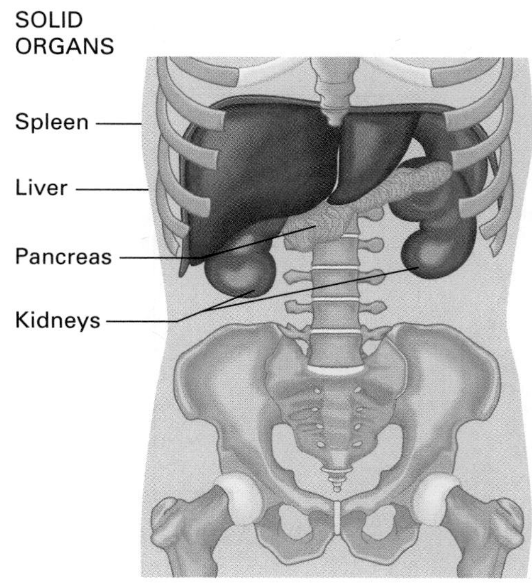

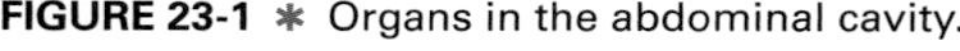

FIGURE 23-1 ✱ Organs in the abdominal cavity.

the remainder of the abdomen is protected only by the muscular layer of the abdominal cavity. When looking at mechanisms of injury, it is easy to see why injuries to the abdomen can be very serious. Trauma to the abdomen is discussed in Chapter 34, "Chest Trauma."

Abdominal Quadrants and Regions

Because you can't use bones as reference points when assessing the abdomen, it is helpful to reference the abdomen by dividing it into quarters, or quadrants, using the navel, or **umbilicus**, as the central reference point (Figure 23-2a✱). In naming the quadrants, right and left are the patient's right and left.

- **Left upper quadrant (LUQ).** Contains most of the stomach, the spleen, the pancreas, and part of the large intestine. The left kidney is behind the abdominal lining.
- **Right upper quadrant (RUQ).** Contains most of the liver, the gallbladder, and part of the large intestine. The right kidney is behind the abdominal lining.
- **Right lower quadrant (RLQ).** Contains the appendix (a worm-shaped structure extending at the beginning of the large intestine), part of the large intestine, and the female reproductive organs.
- **Left lower quadrant (LLQ).** Contains part of the large intestine and the female reproductive organs.

Another way to describe the abdomen is by using a system of nine regions. This is done by drawing four imaginary lines, much akin to a tic-tac-toe board, on the abdomen with the umbilicus in the center of the middle box (Figure 23-2b✱). The regions are (from the patient's right to left, from the top row down):

- Right hypochondriac, epigastric, left hypochondriac
- Right lumbar, umbilical, left lumbar
- Right iliac, hypogastric, left iliac

Types of Abdominal Structures

The abdominal cavity contains three types of structures: hollow organs, solid organs, and vascular structures (Table 23-1). *Hollow organs* contain some type of substance that may leak into the abdominal cavity if the organ is perforated or injured. When a hollow organ is perforated or injured, any substance that leaks into the abdominal cavity may lead to chemical or bacterial peritonitis. Hollow organs typically do not have the same amount of blood supply as solid organs; therefore, they tend not to bleed as much as solid organs.

Solid organs are very vascular (contain a large amount of vessels and blood). Some are covered by a thick fibrous capsule (liver and spleen). When a solid organ is ruptured or injured, it tends to bleed, potentially leading to severe shock.

Key Terms

acute abdomen a sharp, severe abdominal pain with rapid onset. Acute abdomen can have a number of causes.

abdominal cavity the space located below the diaphragm that extends to the top of the pelvis.

peritoneum the lining of the abdominal cavity.

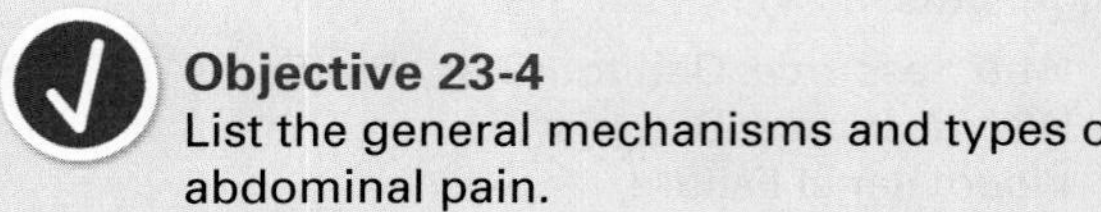

Objective 23-4
List the general mechanisms and types of abdominal pain.

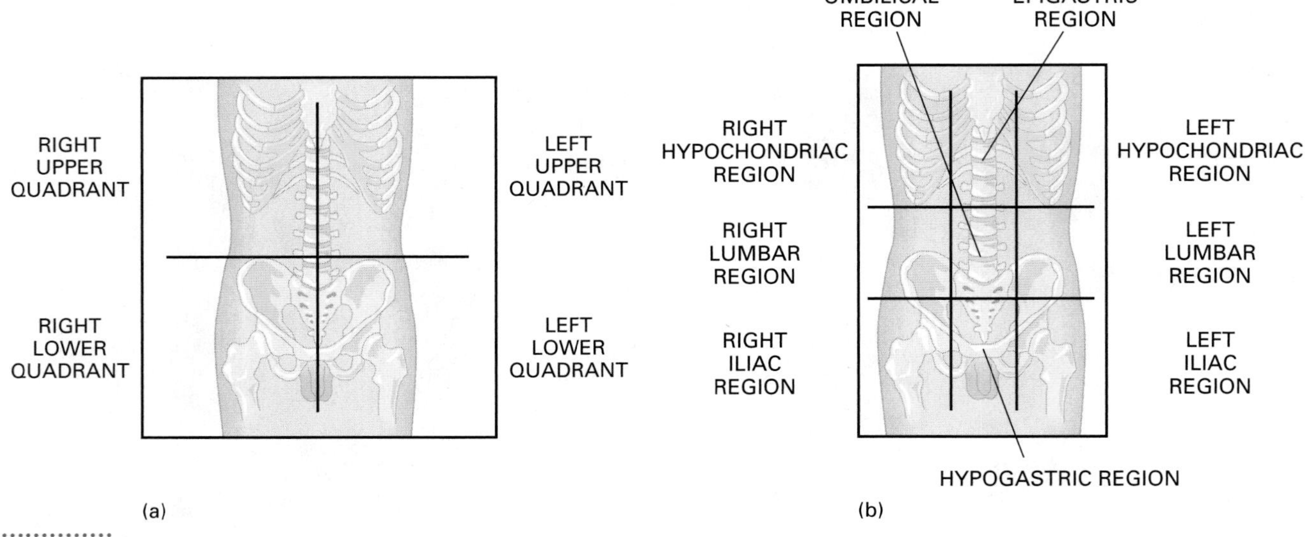

FIGURE 23-2 * **(a)** Abdominal quadrants and **(b)** abdominal regions.

TABLE 23-1 Abdominal Structures

Hollow Organs	Solid Organs	Major Vascular Structures
Appendix	Kidneys	Abdominal aorta
Bladder	Liver	Inferior vena cava
Common bile duct	Ovaries	
Fallopian tubes	Pancreas	
Gallbladder	Spleen	
Intestines		
Stomach		
Uterus		
Ureters		

Vascular structures are the large blood vessels found in the abdominal cavity. Portions of the descending aorta and the inferior vena cava are located in the abdominal cavity. Rupture or injury to either vessel will result in major bleeding, rapid blood loss, and death.

The function of most of the organs contained in the abdomen has to do with digestion of food, absorption of nutrients into the body, and excretion of wastes. Table 23-2 provides a brief list of the organs and their functions. As an EMT, you should not focus on determining which organ or specific illness may be causing a patient's abdominal pain. Your priority is to recognize potential life threats related to acute abdominal pain and provide appropriate emergency medical care.

Abdominal Pain

Pathophysiology of Abdominal Pain

Abdominal pain usually results from one of the following three mechanisms:

- Mechanical forces (stretching)
- Inflammation
- Ischemia (organ and tissue hypoxia)

Abdominal organ emergencies do not typically create a perception of "cutting" or "tearing." The exception is the aorta, which can cause a tearing sensation with certain aortic complications. For the other abdominal viscera, if an organ is torn, the pain will result not from the tearing of the organ itself but from the blood irritating the peritoneum. Certain organs (liver, spleen, and gallbladder) are surrounded by capsules that do contain nerve fibers, and the patient will experience pain if the capsule is stretched by inflammation or swelling.

The rapid distention of an organ will cause a rapid onset of abdominal pain. For example, a patient who is experiencing gas will have a sudden onset of abdominal

Key Terms

abdominal aorta the portion of the descending aorta from the thoracic portion superiorly to the distal point where the aorta divides into the iliac arteries.

umbilicus the navel.

Key Terms

visceral pain poorly localized, intermittent, crampy, dull, or aching pain associated with ischemia or distention of an organ.

TABLE 23-2 Organs of the Abdomen and Their Functions

Stomach	A saclike, stretchable pouch located below the diaphragm that receives food from the esophagus (tubelike structure from the throat). The stomach enables digestion by secreting a specialized fluid to aid in the breakdown and absorption of food.
Duodenum	The first part of the small intestine that connects to the stomach.
Small intestine	A tubelike structure beginning at the distal end of the stomach and ending at the beginning of the large intestine. Its digestive function is to absorb nutrients from intestinal contents.
Large intestine	A tubelike structure beginning at the distal end of the small intestine and ending at the anus. It reabsorbs fluid from intestinal contents, enabling the excretion of solid waste from the body.
Liver	A large, solid organ located in the RUQ just beneath the diaphragm with a slight portion extending to the LUQ. It filters the nutrients from blood as it returns from the intestines, stores glucose (sugar) and certain vitamins, plays a part in blood clotting, filters dead red blood cells, and aids in the production of bile. The liver is proportionally larger in the pediatric patient.
Gallbladder	A pear-shaped sac that lies on the underneath right side of the liver. The gallbladder holds bile, which aids in the digestion of fats.
Spleen	An elongated, oval, solid organ located in the LUQ behind and to the side of the stomach. It aids in the production of blood cells as well as the filtering and storage of blood. The spleen is proportionally larger in the pediatric patient.
Pancreas	A gland composed of many lobes and ducts located in both the RUQ and LUQ, just behind the stomach. It aids in digestion and regulates carbohydrate metabolism.
Kidneys	Paired organs located behind the abdominal wall lining (retroperitoneal), one on each side of the spine. The kidneys excrete urine and regulate water, electrolytes, and acid-base balance.
Urinary bladder	A saclike structure that acts as a reservoir for the urine received from the kidneys.

pain caused by the distention of the intestine. Once the gas is dissipated, the organ is no longer stretched and the pain is eliminated. Therefore, rapid onset of abdominal pain is usually a red flag indicating an acute onset of an abdominal disorder. If the distention of the organ is gradual, as in cirrhosis of the liver where the liver can distend to twice its size, the patient experiences little pain. Thus, pain would not be an early indicator of that condition.

Stretching of the peritoneum will also cause pain. This may be due to distention of an organ that tugs on the peritoneum, adhesions (scar tissue) from surgery or a previous injury, or forceful movement of the small intestine associated with a bowel obstruction. The exception to this is the pregnant patient in her third trimester (last 3 months) of pregnancy. The peritoneum is stretched so far that it is no longer sensitive to stretching. This could be dangerous in a pregnant patient experiencing a condition that would normally cause pain and alert the patient to a problem earlier. The abdominal organs in the pediatric patient are closer together than in an adult.

Pain from stretching a solid organ is usually a steady type of pain. Inflammation of a hollow organ may irritate the lining of the walls of the organ, causing a crampy (colicky) type of pain. Pain associated with ischemia (hypoxia) to an abdominal organ will be steady and severe and will continue to worsen as the organ becomes more hypoxic.

Types of Abdominal Pain

Abdominal pain can be classified as visceral pain, parietal (somatic) pain, or referred pain. The characteristic of pain varies depending on what organ is involved.

Visceral pain occurs when the organ itself is involved. Most organs do not have a large number of highly sensitive nerve fibers; therefore, the pain is usually less severe, is poorly localized (the patient cannot point to the pain with one finger; it is more general in nature), is dull or aching or oppressive, and may be constant or intermittent. Although the pain may not be severe, a serious condition may still exist. This is one of the most important lessons to learn from the differences in the types of pain. Mild and intermittent pain does not mean a mild or insignificant condition. Visceral pain is also associated with nausea and vomiting.

Key Terms
parietal pain localized, intense, sharp, constant pain associated with irritation of the peritoneum. Also called **somatic pain**.

Understanding BODY PROCESSES

Visceral pain is produced by ischemia, inflammation, infection, or mechanical obstruction of an organ. ■

ASSESSMENT Tips

Stimulation of visceral nerve fibers in an organ typically produces pain that is aching, dull, less severe, intermittent, and poorly localized. ■

Parietal pain, also called **somatic pain**, is associated with irritation of the peritoneal lining. Remember, the peritoneum has a larger amount of highly sensitized nerve endings. Thus, one would expect the pain to be more severe and more localized (easier to point to with one finger). Parietal pain is more localized, intense, usually found on one side or the other, sharp, and typically constant. You will typically find the patient lying supine with the knees flexed up toward the chest. This reduces the stretch of the abdominal muscles and puts less pressure on the peritoneum. The patient is usually lying still and breathing shallowly. When the patient breathes deeply, the diaphragm moves lower and pushes on the peritoneum and abdominal organs, causing more pain.

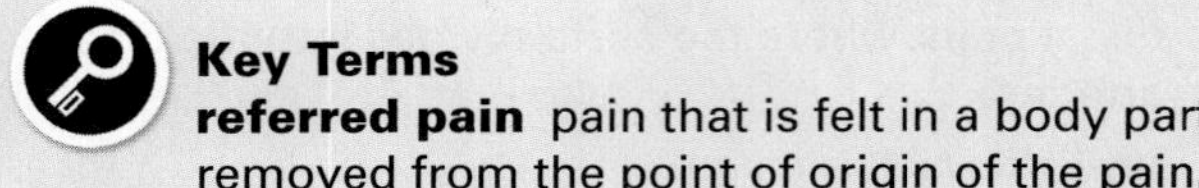

Key Terms
referred pain pain that is felt in a body part removed from the point of origin of the pain.

Understanding BODY PROCESSES

Parietal (somatic) pain is associated with irritation and inflammation of the peritoneal lining of the abdomen. ■

ASSESSMENT Tips

Parietal (somatic) nerve fiber stimulation typically produces sharp, knifelike, intense, constant pain that is highly localized (can be pinpointed). ■

Referred pain is actually visceral pain (pain from the organ itself) that is felt elsewhere in the body. It is usually poorly localized but is felt consistently in the part of the body it is referred to. Referred pain occurs when organs share a nerve pathway with a skin sensory nerve. The brain becomes confused in the interpretation of the impulse and causes the patient to feel pain at a location that may be totally unrelated to the organ involved. As an example, a patient who is experiencing inflammation of the gallbladder (cholecystitis) will typically feel referred pain in his right shoulder and scapular (shoulder blade) area. See Figure 23-3*.

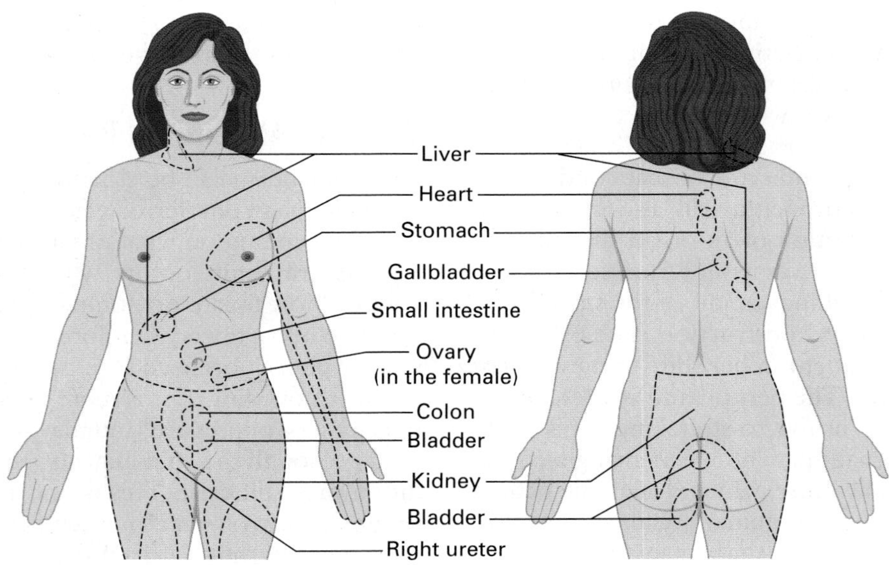

FIGURE 23-3 * Sites of referred pain. The lines point to locations where pain may be felt when there is disease of or injury to the named organ.

Objective 23-5
Describe the pathophysiology and the signs and symptoms associated with common causes of acute abdomen.

Key Terms
peritonitis irritation and inflammation of the peritoneum.

Key Terms
Markle test a test for peritonitis in which the patient stands on his toes, knees straight, then drops to his heels, or in which the heels of a supine patient are struck together or on the bottom. The jarring of the torso will elicit pain when the peritoneal linings are inflamed.

Conditions That May Cause Acute Abdominal Pain

This section is an overview of some of the most common causes of acute abdominal pain or distress. (See Table 23-3.) Definitive care for almost all of these conditions is hospitalization and possibly surgical intervention. These conditions can result in life-threatening complications if left untreated. *You should never spend extended time at the scene trying to determine the exact cause of acute abdominal pain.*

Peritonitis

Irritation and inflammation of the peritoneum is called **peritonitis**. Peritonitis occurs when blood, pus, bacteria, or chemical substances leak into the peritoneal cavity. The onset and type of the abdominal pain a patient experiences is somewhat dependent on the type of substance leaking into the peritoneum. For example, the duodenum contains highly acidic digestive material that usually causes pain that is immediate, severe, sharp, intense, and constant. However, the ileum contains digestive material with a neutral pH (not acidic and not alkalotic). If the ileum is perforated, the material may leak out, but the pain may be delayed for several hours, may be intermittent, or may be not as severe because the material's pH is neutral. Because critical abdominal conditions may present in a variety of ways, it is important to maintain a high index of suspicion when dealing with an acute abdomen.

TABLE 23-3 Some Conditions That May Cause an Acute Abdomen

- Peritonitis
- Appendicitis
- Pancreatitis
- Cholecystitis
- Gastrointestinal bleeding
- Esophageal varices
- Gastroenteritis
- Ulcerative diseases
- Intestinal obstruction
- Hernia
- Abdominal aortic aneurysm

The type or degree of pain often does not indicate the severity of the problem.

Understanding BODY PROCESSES

Abdominal contents that are acidic or alkaline that leak into the abdominal cavity and irritate the peritoneum will produce a sudden onset of severe, sharp, constant abdominal pain. ■

Common Signs and Symptoms of Peritonitis

- Abdominal pain or tenderness
- Nausea, vomiting, or diarrhea
- Fever and chills
- Lack of appetite (anorexia)
- Positive Markle (heel drop or heel jar) test

The Markle "Heel Drop" or "Heel Jar" Test An examination technique called "rebound tenderness" has been used to assess a patient with abdominal pain like that caused by peritonitis and appendicitis. The EMT would push slowly down on a quadrant of the abdomen to slightly compress the tissues beneath and then suddenly release the pressure. When the abdominal contents reassumed their original location, it would make the peritoneal surfaces rub together. If there was inflammation to the peritoneal linings, it would elicit pain in the patient. This technique, however, has fallen into some disfavor because the patient with abdominal pain could be either over-obliging to the test or extremely frightened of someone pushing on his abdomen, and in either case fail to be objective.

As an alternative, the **Markle test** (Figures 23-4a and 23-4b∗) has been shown to be just as reliable but without the number of false positives or negatives seen with the rebound tenderness test. In the Markle technique, the patient is instructed to stand on his feet with his knees straight. Upon request, the patient should raise himself onto his toes and drop suddenly down on his heels, flat-footed, with enough force to produce an audible thump. Since the patient will not know what the EMT is clinically attempting to find out, it is difficult for a skewed response to occur. In fact, many times the patient is very surprised that the heel drop elicits abdominal pain, but the EMT will know that the pain is often felt in the region of the pain's etiology, or cause. This is known as a "heel drop" test.

Sometimes, because of concurrent medical care or the inability of the patient to stand, the test as just described

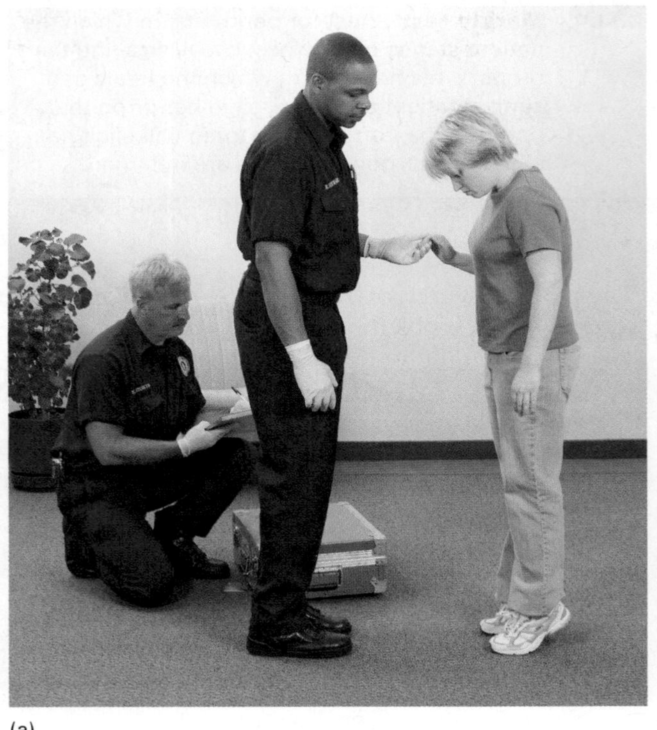
(a)

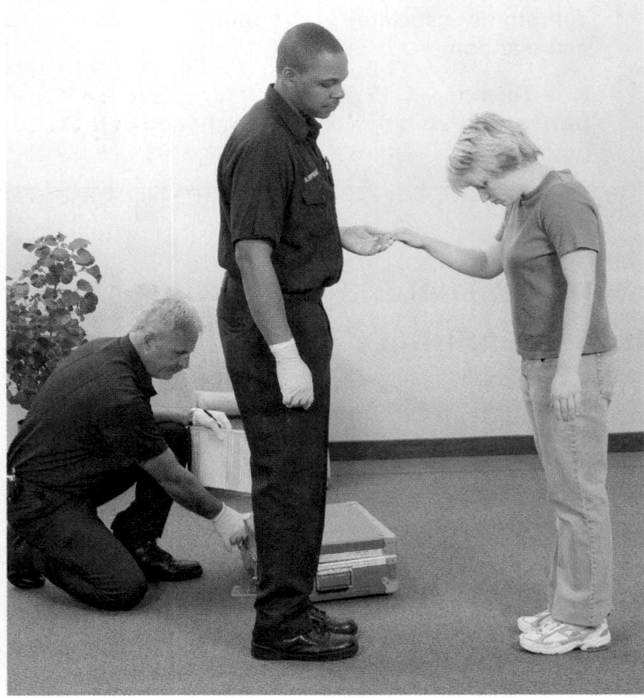
(b)

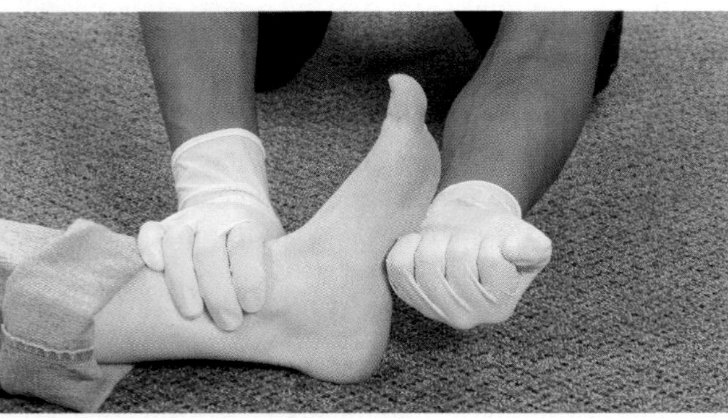
(c)

FIGURE 23-4 ✱ The Markle heel drop test is performed to detect peritoneal irritation. Do not explain the purpose of the test. If the patient can stand **(a)** have her rise onto her toes and then **(b)** drop to her heels forcefully enough to produce an audible thump. **(c)** If the patient is supine, forcefully strike the bottom of the heel. If the peritoneum is irritated, the vibrations transmitted to the abdomen will produce abdominal pain the patient may report or reveal by grimacing.

cannot be performed. In these instances, the EMT can perform a modified Markle test by lifting each of the ankles of the supine patient and knocking the heels together or by making a fist and striking the bottom of the heel (Figure 23-4c✱). This jars the torso, which, in turn, irritates the peritoneal linings and creates the same kind of response as the regular Markle test. This modification is referred to as a "heel jar" test.

When performing either version of the Markle test, be sure to watch the patient's face for a grimace, indicating pain. If the patient moans, ask what hurts. A complaint of abdominal pain is a positive test for rebound tenderness.

Appendicitis

Appendicitis is an inflammation of the appendix that commonly causes an acute abdomen. Appendicitis is usually caused by a blockage in the intestines and results in inflammation and irritation. If left untreated, the inflammation eventually may cause the tissue to die and rupture. This may result in abscess formation (local pus collection), peritonitis, or shock. Appendicitis is common in children because their appendix wall is thinner. This is also true for elderly patients who are prone to perforation. Definitive care for this condition is surgical intervention, ideally before rupture of the appendix contents into the peritoneal cavity.

Common Signs and Symptoms of Appendicitis

- Abdominal pain or cramping—Initially this may be dull, diffuse, and located around the umbilicus. Later this pain is usually localized to the right lower quadrant medial to the iliac crest (pelvic wing), also called the McBurney point.

Key Terms

appendicitis inflammation of the appendix.

pancreatitis inflammation of the pancreas.

cholecystitis inflammation of the gallbladder.

hematemesis vomiting of blood.

hematochezia bright red blood in the stool.

Key Terms

melena dark tarry stools containing decomposing blood normally from the upper gastrointestinal system.

esophageal varices bulging, engorgement, or weakening of the blood vessels in the lining of the lower esophagus.

- Nausea and vomiting
- Low-grade fever and chills
- Lack of appetite (anorexia)
- Abdominal guarding
- Positive Markle (heel drop or heel jar) test

Pancreatitis

Pancreatitis, or inflammation of the pancreas, may cause severe pain in the middle of the upper quadrants (epigastric area) of the abdomen. This abdominal pain sometimes radiates to the back. Pancreatitis may be triggered by a variety of causes including ingestion of alcohol, gallstones, or infection. Complications that may result from pancreatitis include abscesses, sepsis, hemorrhage, tissue death, hypoglycemia or hyperglycemia, and organ failure.

Common Signs and Symptoms of Pancreatitis

- Abdominal pain
- Nausea and vomiting
- Abdominal tenderness and distention
- Mild jaundice (depending on cause)
- Severe abdominal pain with radiation from the umbilicus (navel) to the back and shoulders
- Fever, rapid pulse, and signs of shock (in extreme cases)

Cholecystitis

Cholecystitis, or inflammation of the gallbladder, is commonly associated with the presence of gallstones. This condition is more common in women than men and frequently occurs between the ages of 30 and 50. It rarely occurs in children. In some cases of cholecystitis, the gallstones may actually block the opening of the gallbladder to the small intestine. This blockage causes an increase in pressure inside the gallbladder, which can cause severe pain. Definitive care for this condition is hospitalization and sometimes surgical intervention to remove the gallbladder, stones, or blockage. If left untreated, tissue death, perforation, or pancreatitis may occur.

Common Signs and Symptoms of Cholecystitis

- Sudden onset of abdominal pain located from the middle of the upper quadrants (epigastric area) to RUQ areas (Pain is present more commonly at night and associated with ingestion of fatty foods. Pain may also be referred to the right scapula.)
- Tenderness upon palpation of the RUQ
- Belching or heartburn
- Nausea and vomiting (contents may be greenish)

Gastrointestinal Bleeding

Gastrointestinal bleeding can occur anywhere within the gastrointestinal tract and can be attributed to numerous causes. Gastrointestinal bleeds are usually classified as upper or lower, based on the location of the bleeding. Upper gastrointestinal bleeds are frequently caused by peptic ulcers, gastric erosion, and varices. They are more prevalent in adult males. Lower gastrointestinal bleeds are frequently caused by diverticulosis and occur more in women. Gastrointestinal bleeding most commonly affects people in their 40s to 70s, but children and younger adults may experience it too. Most deaths resulting from gastrointestinal bleeding occur in patients over 60 years of age.

Common Signs and Symptoms of Gastrointestinal Bleeding

- Abdominal pain or tenderness
- **Hematemesis** (vomiting blood, which can be bright red or look like coffee grounds)
- **Hematochezia** (bright red blood in the stool normally signifying a rapid onset)
- **Melena** (dark tarry stools containing decomposing blood normally from the upper gastrointestinal system)
- Altered mental status, weakness, or syncope
- Tachycardia
- Signs of shock

Esophageal Varices

Esophageal varices are a bulging, engorgement, or weakening of the blood vessels in the lining of the lower part of the esophagus. These abnormalities are common to heavy alcohol drinkers or patients with liver disease and are caused by increased pressure in the venous blood supply system of the liver, stomach, and esophagus (Figures 23-5a and 23-5b*). Esophageal varices are

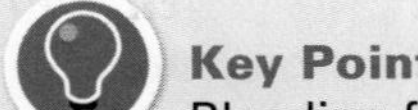

Key Points
Bleeding from esophageal varices can be profuse, leading to shock.

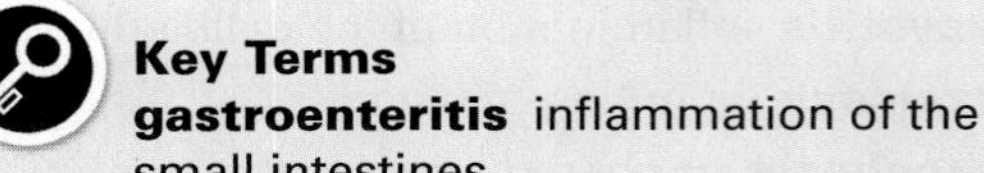

Key Terms
gastroenteritis inflammation of the stomach and small intestines.

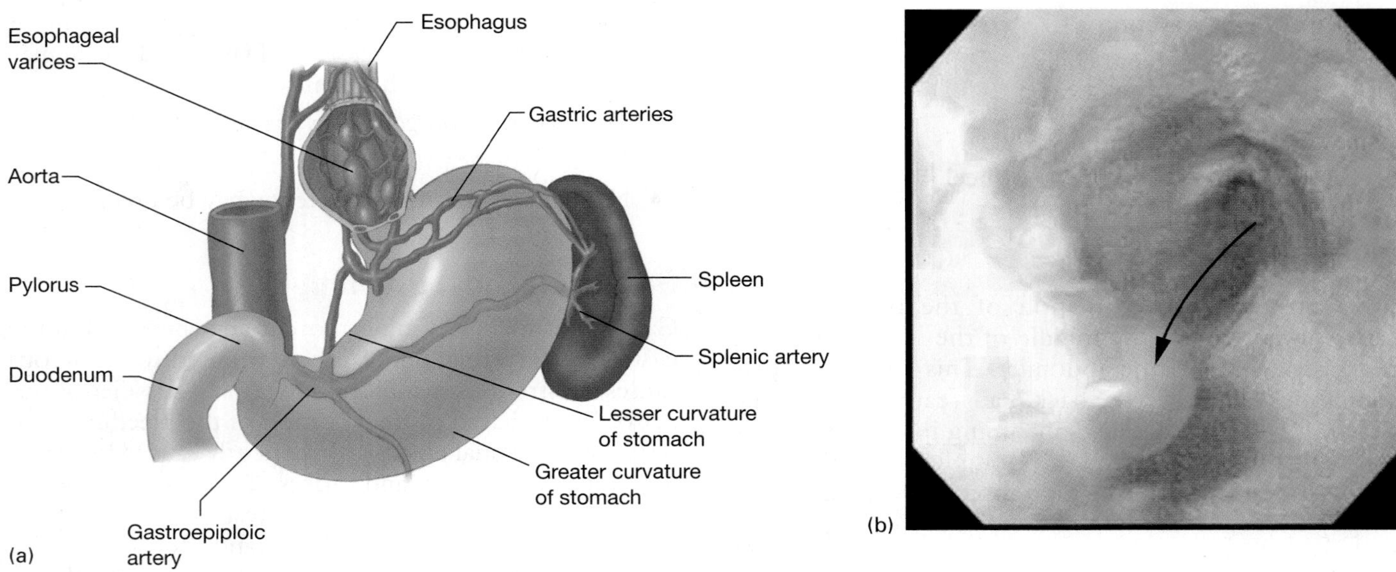

FIGURE 23-5 * **(a)** Esophageal varices are common to heavy alcohol drinkers or patients with liver disease. **(b)** Endoscopic view of an esophageal varix.

usually identified with painless bleeding in the digestive tract. Bleeding can be profuse, leading to shock. Emergency medical care is the same as for any other abdominal pain or distress; however, airway and breathing management may be more challenging.

Common Signs and Symptoms of Esophageal Varices

- Large amounts of bright red hematemesis (vomiting of blood)
- Absence of pain or tenderness in the abdomen
- Rapid pulse
- Breathing difficulty
- Pale, cool, clammy skin
- Other signs and symptoms of shock
- Jaundice (yellowing) of the skin or sclerae of the eyes from liver disease (may be seen in some cases) (Figure 23-6*)

Gastroenteritis

Gastroenteritis, or inflammation of the stomach and small intestines, is commonly associated with the presence of abdominopelvic pain. This condition can be chronic or acute. Chronic gastroenteritis is most commonly a result of an infection. Acute gastroenteritis is normally caused by bacteria and is commonly diagnosed in children. If left untreated, it may result in the breakdown of the mucosal layers in the gastrointestinal tract. This breakdown can lead to dehydration, hemorrhage, ulceration, and perforation. Hematemesis, hematochezia, or melena may be present in severe acute cases. In these severe cases, signs and symptoms of shock will be present.

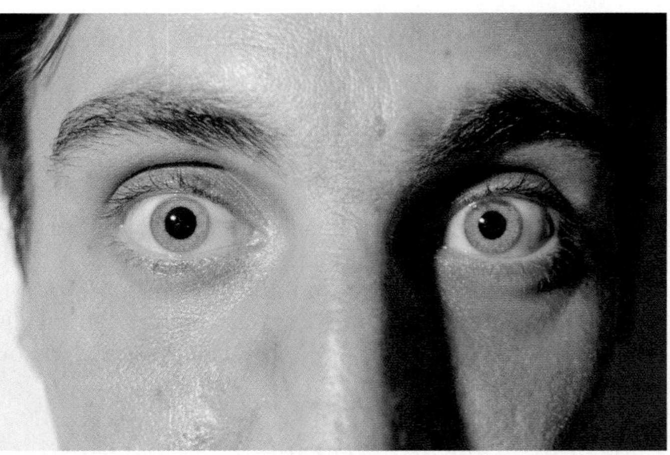

FIGURE 23-6 * Jaundiced sclera of the eyes from liver disease may be seen in some cases of esophageal varices. (© 2008 Vincent Zuber/Custom Medical Stock Photo, All Rights Reserved)

Common Signs and Symptoms of Gastroenteritis

- Abdominal pain or cramping
- Nausea, vomiting, and diarrhea
- Abdominal tenderness
- Fever and dehydration
- In severe cases, signs and symptoms of shock and hemorrhage may be present

Ulcers

Approximately 4 million patients a year are affected by an ulcerative disease. **Ulcers** are open wounds or sores within the digestive tract, usually in the stomach or the beginning of the small intestines (Figures 23-7a and 23-7b*). Ulcers are associated with a breakdown of the lining that normally protects the intestine from the digestive fluids contained inside the digestive tract. This breakdown can cause damage to the stomach or intestine and, in some instances, massive bleeding or perforation. This can result in hematemesis, hematochezia, or melena depending on the location and severity of the bleed. The type of abdominal pain is also affected by the location and severity of the ulcer. Patients with severe ulcerative disease can develop signs and symptoms of shock that are life threatening. Most patients are usually aware of their ulcers and will provide you with this information during the history. In some cases, the patient will take over-the-counter antacids or prescribed medications for this condition.

Common Signs and Symptoms of Ulcers

- Sudden onset of abdominal pain normally in the LUQ and epigastric area, usually described as a burning- or gnawing-type pain before meals or during stressful events
- Nausea and vomiting
- Hematemesis, hematochezia, or melena or coffee-ground emesis in some cases
- Signs or symptoms of shock in cases of massive bleeding
- Peritonitis with a rigid abdomen in cases of perforation

Intestinal Obstruction

An **intestinal obstruction** is a blockage that interrupts the normal flow of the intestinal contents within the intestines. This condition can occur in both the small and the large intestines and can be either partial or complete. Blockages occurring in the small intestines are usually the result of

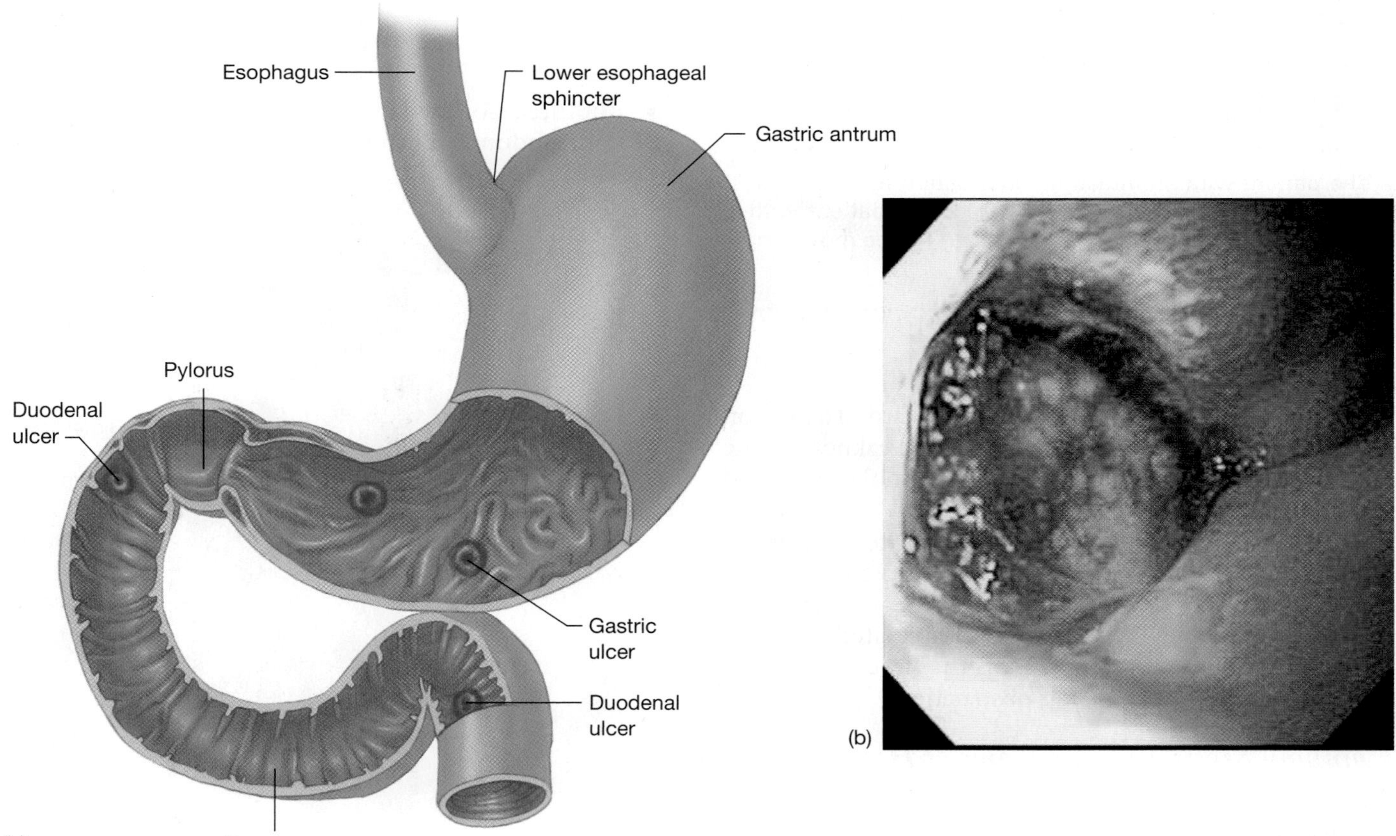

FIGURE 23-7 * **(a)** Ulcers often form in the stomach or the beginning of the small intestines. **(b)** Endoscopic view of an ulcer in the small intestine.

Key Terms

ulcers open wounds or sores within the digestive tract.

intestinal obstruction blockage that interrupts the normal flow of intestinal contents.

Key Terms

hernia protrusion of a portion of the intestine through an opening or weakness in the abdominal wall.

abdominal aortic aneurysm (AAA) a weakened, ballooned, and enlarged area of the wall of the abdominal aorta.

adhesions (a sticking together of the sides of the intestines) or a hernia. Blockages of the large intestines are commonly caused by tumors, fecal impaction, or overloading. If left untreated, intestinal obstructions may lead to sepsis, perforation, intestinal infarction, and peritonitis. Patients over the age of 50 are at increased risk for having an intestinal obstruction. This condition is likely to reoccur in patients who have a history of a previous bowel obstruction.

Common Signs and Symptoms of Intestinal Obstruction

- Abdominal pain, moderate to severe, depending on location of obstruction—typically described as crampy and colicky
- Nausea and vomiting
- Constipation (difficulty in moving bowels)
- Abdominal distention and tenderness
- Abnormally prominent, high-pitched bowel sounds with auscultation in early stages (Bowel sounds may be diminished or absent in some later cases.)

ASSESSMENT Tips

The patient with an intestinal obstruction may want to continue to walk and move, whereas the patient with peritonitis will want to lie very still and not be moved or touched. ■

Hernia

A **hernia** is a protrusion or thrusting forward of a portion of the intestine through an opening or weakness in the abdominal wall. Hernias are most commonly associated with increased pressure in the abdominal cavity during heavy lifting or straining, causing the peritoneum to be pushed into the weakness or opening. Most hernias are not life threatening and can be easily treated. In some cases, however, they may become incarcerated or strangulated, causing the portion of the intestine to be pinched or cut off, producing obstruction.

Common Signs and Symptoms of Hernia

- Sudden onset of abdominal pain (usually after heavy lifting or straining)
- Fever
- Rapid pulse
- Tender mass at point of hernia
- Others similar to intestinal obstruction

Abdominal Aortic Aneurysm

An **abdominal aortic aneurysm (AAA)** is a weakened, ballooned, and enlarged area of the wall of the abdominal aorta. The aneurysm may eventually rupture and is one of the most lethal causes of abdominal pain. Although it can happen at any age, this condition is most common in men over the age of 60. Rupture of the aortic wall generally begins with a small tear of the inner vessel structure, which allows blood to leak between the walls of the aorta (Figure 23-8✱). The process of dissection continues with increasing pressure until, finally, the outer wall is damaged and blood leaks out behind the peritoneum or into the abdominal cavity.

Common Signs and Symptoms of AAA

- Gradual onset of lower lumbar, groin, and abdominal pain
- Rupture associated with sudden onset of severe, constant abdominal pain. May radiate to lower back, flank, or pelvis. May be described as a "tearing" pain.

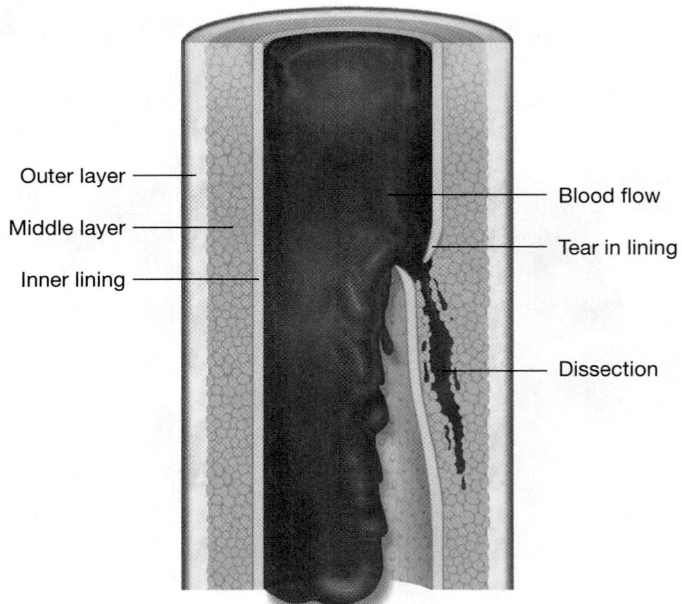

FIGURE 23-8 ✱ Abdominal aortic dissection. The lining of the aorta may weaken, tear, dissect, and eventually rupture.

Objective 23-6
Explain the assessment-based approach to acute abdomen, including assessment and appropriate medical care.

- Testicular pain in the male patient
- Possible nausea and vomiting
- Mottled or spotty abdominal skin
- Pale, cool, clammy, and possibly cyanotic skin in legs from decreased blood and perfusion
- Absent or decreased femoral or pedal pulses
- If the abdomen is soft, a pulsating abdominal mass may be felt. If the aneurysm has burst, the abdomen will be rigid and tender.
- If the aortic aneurysm is starting to rupture, the skin below the waistline may become cyanotic, cold, and mottled. This is from a significant drop in blood flow to the extremities.

If you suspect a patient has an abdominal aortic aneurysm, palpate the abdomen very gently. Pressure or excessive movement may aggravate the aneurysm, causing it to leak or rupture. Assessment for shock is crucial. Transport without delay. If the rupture is in the process of occurring, this is a true emergency.

Vomiting/Diarrhea/Constipation

Vomiting, constipation, and diarrhea are symptoms of many of the conditions previously discussed. In themselves, diarrhea, vomiting, and constipation are rarely medical emergencies but can cause abdominal pain in pediatric and adult patients. The EMT should be concerned when the vomiting or diarrhea has persisted for days (or hours in the case of vomiting) and the patient has become dehydrated. The vomiting mechanism in children is still not fully understood, but the pediatric patient can decompensate very quickly with fluid loss. Infants or children who continue to vomit over a period of one day and adults who continue to vomit for several days may lose significant fluid volume and develop an electrolyte imbalance that is serious enough to cause shock, cardiac dysrhythmias, or other conditions.

Sickle Cell Anemia

Sickle cell anemia is a hereditary blood disorder most often afflicting African Americans and black Africans but also those of Mediterranean, South and Central American, Caribbean, and Middle Eastern origin.

In sickle cell anemia, some red blood cells have abnormal hemoglobin that does not carry adequate oxygen. As a result, the cells take on a crescent (sickle) shape and become fragile, stiff, and rigid. The sickled cells begin to stack up, blocking capillary blood flow. Cells and tissues become ischemic and may die. Patients with this disease often suffer infections from damaged red blood cells blocking the spleen.

Sickle Cell Crisis Almost all patients with the disease suffer painful episodes known as sickle cell crisis. There are four common patterns of acute sickle cell crisis:

- **Bone crisis** typically involves the large long bones in the arm (humerus) and leg (femur and tibia) causing sudden severe pain.
- **Acute chest syndrome** involves a sudden onset of chest pain, possibly with dyspnea and cough, which may be nonproductive, or the patient may cough up blood. A low-grade fever may be present.
- **Abdominal crisis** causes sudden, constant abdominal pain, general or localized. There may or may not also be nausea, vomiting, and diarrhea.
- **Joint crisis** presents with an acute onset of one or more painful, stiff joints.

Other consequences may include stroke, vision disturbances, and detached retina. Almost all sickle cell patients develop kidney damage. Infections occur at higher rates especially in the kidney, lung, bone, and central nervous system. Anemia may cause shortness of breath, lightheadedness and fatigue. Men may have priapism (involuntary and constant erection).

Common Signs and Symptoms of Sickle Cell Crisis

Severe abdominal pain is a frequent complaint leading to EMS response. Other signs and symptoms include:

- Bone pain
- Joint pain
- Fever
- Chest pain
- Shortness of breath
- Fatigue
- Pale skin
- Tachycardia
- Jaundice (yellowed sclera and skin)
- Ulcers on the lower legs
- Excessive thirst
- Priapism
- Frequent urination
- Sudden blindness in one eye

Emergency Care for Sickle Cell Crisis

The emergency care is supportive. Ensure an adequate airway, ventilation, oxygenation, and circulation.

Key Terms
guarded position a position with knees drawn up and hands clenched over the abdomen.

Assessment-Based Approach: Acute Abdomen

As previously stated, it is not important that you try to isolate the exact cause of abdominal pain or distress in the prehospital setting. Rather, you should correctly assess and identify that the patient is suffering abdominal pain and provide suitable emergency medical care based on that symptom.

All patients with abdominal pain should be considered to have a life-threatening condition until proven otherwise. Associated signs of low blood pressure, syncope (fainting), or pale, cool, and clammy skin, coinciding with abdominal pain, are considered very serious and high priority.

Severe abdominal pain is not only very distressing to the patient; it needs to be treated as an emergency. This is especially true if the pain lasts for 6 hours or longer, regardless of its intensity.

Scene Size-Up

Begin by looking out for any potential threats to you, the patient, or other personnel. As you approach the scene, make sure you take Standard Precautions. Use face and eye protection if the patient is vomiting and splash or splatter is anticipated.

Look for any mechanism of injury to rule out trauma as the cause of the abdominal distress. Be alert to any talk or evidence of knives, guns, or other items that could cause penetrating wounds to the abdomen. Also be alert to signs of blunt trauma to the abdomen—for example, any mechanism of injury indicating a fall or auto collision.

Use all your senses to size up the scene. For instance, certain types of bleeding from gastrointestinal causes will have a distinct smell and can be determined as you arrive on the scene. Location of patients may offer clues to their condition. Many EMTs have found that patients who are experiencing abdominal bleeding may faint, and many do so in the bathroom. If you find the patient in the bathroom, you might begin to suspect gastrointestinal bleeding. Look for waste baskets or garbage cans used to catch emesis near the location of the patient. Make sure you note the color and quantity of any vomitus you may see. Look for over-the-counter medications that may have been used to help alleviate abdominal pain before you arrived.

Primary Assessment

As you approach the patient, form a general impression. Stabilize the spine if injury is suspected. A person with an acute abdomen generally appears very ill and will assume a **guarded position** with his knees drawn up and his hands clenched over his abdomen (Figure 23-9*). Start by ensuring that the patient has a patent airway with adequate breathing. Be alert for vomiting and possible aspiration and suction if needed. Apply high-concentration oxygen therapy and assist the patient's ventilations if they are inadequate. Assess circulation by checking the pulse for rate and regularity; checking for obvious or major bleeding; and noting skin color, temperature, and condition.

Look for signs of shock (hypoperfusion): rapid, thready pulse; restlessness; cool, clammy skin; and as a late sign, falling blood pressure. Internal bleeding, peritonitis, and excessive vomiting or diarrhea often lead to considerable fluid loss or shock.

Shock is only one indicator that this is a serious medical emergency. The patient with an acute abdomen should be categorized as a priority for transport if he meets any of the following criteria:

- Poor general appearance
- Unresponsive
- Responsive, not following commands
- Shock (hypoperfusion)
- Severe pain

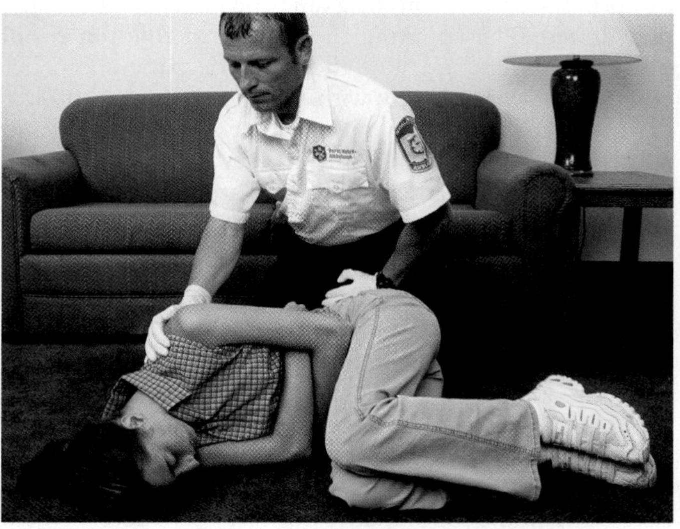

FIGURE 23-9 * Typical "guarded" position for a patient with acute abdominal pain.

Secondary Assessment

In any of the circumstances just discussed, immediately begin transport following the secondary assessment. If the patient is responsive, first conduct the history. If the patient is unresponsive, conduct the history after the physical exam and vitals, gathering information from family or bystanders. If more than one EMT is on the scene, the physical exam can be conducted and baseline vital signs can be obtained by one EMT while the other EMT collects the history.

The following are pertinent questions to ask.

- *Ask the OPQRST questions* (onset, provocation/palliation, quality, radiation, severity, time) to get a full description of the pain, from the pain's onset and what provokes it to its severity and duration or what, if anything, makes it better. When questioning the patient about onset, note if it was sudden and abrupt. If so, it's likely that the patient has a serious medical emergency.
- *Does the patient have any known allergies* to medications, food, or other substances? Is there any medical alert identification tag or information present?
- *Is the patient currently taking any medications,* either over-the-counter or physician prescribed? If so, when was the last time the medications were taken?
- *Does the patient have any pertinent past medical history regarding the abdominal pain or distress?* Has this ever happened to the patient prior to this event and has the patient ever been hospitalized for the same type of abdominal pain? Has the patient had any abdominal surgeries or trauma? Has the patient seen his physician for this pain?
- *When was the last time the patient had anything to eat or drink?* Did the patient ingest large quantities of alcohol or eat very spicy or fatty food? Ask if anyone sharing a meal with the patient is also experiencing abdominal pain.
- *Has the patient's appetite changed?* Is he anorexic? Has there been any weight loss?
- *Has the patient been nauseated?* Ask if he has experienced belching or flatulence. Has he had a fever?
- *Did the patient vomit,* and if so, what was the color and appearance of the vomitus? Ask if vomitus looked like coffee grounds (contains partially digested blood), or if it contained undigested red blood, which indicates a bleeding in the upper gastrointestinal tract. Ask how many times the vomiting has occurred.
- *What was the color of the patient's last stools?* Dark and tarry stools or bright red stools are indicators of gastrointestinal bleeding. Ask how many bowel movements the patient has had. Ask if he has had a change in bowel habits. Ask if he has been constipated or if he has had diarrhea. If he has, ask for its time of onset and frequency.
- *Has the patient had difficulty urinating?* Ask if he has had pain or any changes in the color, frequency, or odor of the urine.
- *Was the patient doing anything prior to the onset that led to the abdominal pain or distress?* Any heavy lifting? Was the patient at rest? Is the patient having any concurrent chest pain?

The physical exam will focus on the abdomen. However, you should still assess the rest of the body for associated signs and symptoms. Remember that some abdominal complaints can be associated with cardiac or pulmonary conditions, especially in the geriatric patient. Other systems can also cause abdominal pain. Perfusion should be assessed in all four extremities.

Perform the physical examination of the abdomen carefully and gently, since the abdomen may be tender. Even the slightest palpation may further aggravate existing pain and make the patient less willing to allow you to examine him. Begin by inspecting the abdomen. Look for any scars indicating previous surgeries. When beginning the exam always ask the patient to point to the area that is the most painful and then palpate each quadrant (Figure 23-10*), beginning with the area of the abdomen that is the least painful and farthest from the site of pain.

- Determine if the patient is restless or quiet and whether pain is increased upon movement.
- Inspect the abdomen to determine if it is distended (enlarged). Ask the patient if this is normal.
- Gently palpate the abdomen using the quadrants as landmarks. Start with the least painful area first and examine the quadrant with specific pain last.
- Assess if the abdomen feels soft or rigid. Normally, the abdomen should be soft and nontender. If the abdomen is rigid, determine if the patient can relax the abdominal muscles upon request. Note any

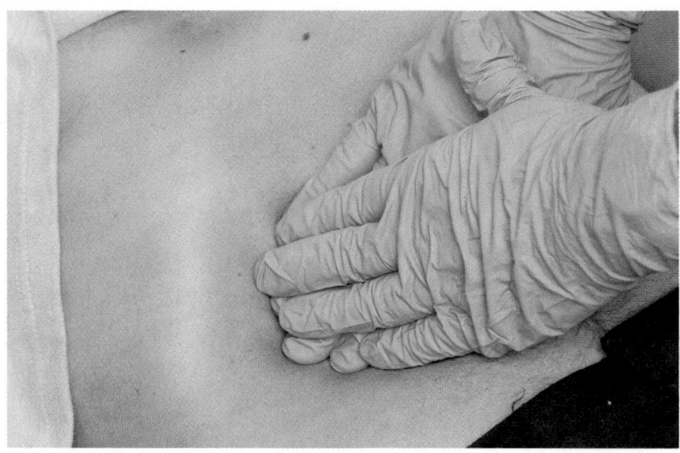

FIGURE 23-10 * Inspect the abdomen, then palpate each quadrant. Note any tenderness, rigidity, or masses.

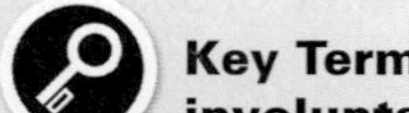

Key Terms
involuntary guarding abdominal wall muscle contraction caused by inflammation of the peritoneum that the patient cannot control. Also called **rigidity.**

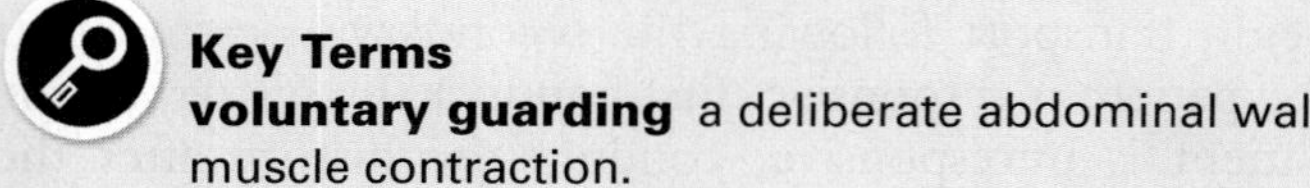

Key Terms
voluntary guarding a deliberate abdominal wall muscle contraction.

involuntary guarding, an abdominal wall muscle contraction that the patient cannot control, resulting from inflammation of the peritoneum. Involuntary guarding is also referred to as **rigidity**. In contrast, **voluntary guarding** is when the patient contracts the abdominal muscles, usually in anticipation of pain or an unpleasant sensation. The problem lies in the difficulty of telling the two apart. Determining if there is true involuntary guarding versus voluntary guarding can be done while you are applying gentle but firm pressure to the abdomen. In either case (voluntary or involuntary guarding) you will notice while you are depressing the abdomen that it is rigid. Ask the patient to take a deep breath. If you feel the abdominal muscles spontaneously relax when the patient breathes in, then the guarding is voluntary. The muscles relax because the brain subconsciously overrides the patient's conscious control and tells the abdominal muscles to relax so it is easier to inhale. If the guarding is involuntary from abdominal irritation, the muscles will remain contracted and rigid even when the patient inhales. Note that geriatric patients may not exhibit rigidity or guarding.

Understanding BODY PROCESSES

Rigidity is an involuntary reflex that causes the abdominal muscles to contract and produce a rigid (boardlike) abdomen. The patient has no control over the muscle contraction. Abdominal guarding is when the patient voluntarily contracts his abdominal muscles. He may relax the muscles after your examination of the abdomen. ■

- Assess if the abdomen is tender or nontender when touched.
- When palpating the abdomen, note any masses that may be present. Are they pulsating?
- Ask the patient if he has any pain in other body areas.
- Document the quadrant in which any pain is located.

Obtain and document the patient's baseline vitals. Expect to find an increased respiratory rate and shallow breathing in patients with acute abdominal pain. Pay attention to blood pressure and heart rate. Decreased blood pressure, increased heart rate, and pale, cool, moist skin are indicators of shock.

Signs and Symptoms The following signs and symptoms may be associated with acute abdominal pain:

- Pain or tenderness—Can be diffuse (widespread) or localized; pain can also be crampy, sharp, aching, or knifelike.
- Anxiety and fear—Very often the patient is anxious and does not want to move for fear of aggravating or creating unbearable pain.
- Position—A patient will draw the feet up to the abdomen (guarded position) while lying on the side in order to relax the abdominal muscles. However, some patients may move about, attempting to find comfort.
- Rapid and shallow breathing—Usually to reduce movement of the diaphragm, which causes more pain
- Rapid pulse—May be from pain or shock
- Blood pressure changes—Sometimes elevated in severe pain but may be low as a late sign of shock
- Nausea, vomiting, and/or diarrhea—Is it excessive?
- Rigid abdomen or guarding—Can this be relaxed upon command?
- Distended abdomen
- Fever or chills
- Belching or flatulence
- Changes in bowel habits or urination—note the frequency, color, odor, and if they have associated pain
- Other signs and symptoms associated with shock
- Signs of internal bleeding—vomiting blood (hematemesis or like coffee grounds), blood in the stool (bright red or dark and tarry; also very distinct smell)

Understanding BODY PROCESSES

Severe abdominal pain activates the sympathetic nervous system. This causes an increase in heart rate, respiratory rate, and blood pressure and may cause the skin to become pale, cool, and clammy. These responses can be mistakenly interpreted as indications of hypovolemia. ■

ASSESSMENT Tips

When assessing blood pressure in the abdominal pain patient, consider the pulse pressure (difference between the systolic and diastolic blood pressure). If it is narrow—along with tachycardia, and pale, cool, clammy skin—it can be a sign of internal bleeding. Inspect inside the mouth of the patient complaining of acute abdominal pain. Pale oral mucosa may indicate the patient has been bleeding over a long period of time. ■

Key Points

In a patient suffering abdominal pain, it is not important to determine the cause of the pain. Instead, keep the airway patent, place the patient in a position of comfort, administer oxygen as appropriate, reassure the patient, treat for shock if appropriate, and transport promptly.

Thinking Critically

Your teenage patient is doubled over with abdominal pain. Her mother produces a bottle of Pepto-Bismol and says, "Here. Give her some of this." Is this good advice?

In infants and children, suspect an acute abdominal emergency if tenderness or guarding upon palpation is present. Do not waste time with extensive exams or palpation prior to initiating transport. Excessive palpation can worsen the pain and aggravate the cause of the abdominal pain or distress.

Emergency Medical Care

Follow these emergency care steps:

1. *Keep the airway patent.* Always be alert for vomiting and the potential for aspiration. It may be necessary to place the patient in the left lateral recumbent position to protect the airway. Be prepared to suction.
2. *Place the patient in the position of comfort.* If the patient is vomiting or has an altered mental status, place him in a lateral recumbent position.
3. *If breathing is adequate, administer oxygen based on the SpO_2 reading and patient signs and symptoms.* If the SpO_2 reading is greater than 95% and no signs or symptoms of hypoxia or respiratory distress are present, oxygen may not be necessary. In this case, you may choose to apply a nasal cannula at 2 to 4 lpm. If signs of hypoxia or respiratory distress are present, or if the SpO_2 reading is less than 95%, place the patient on a nonrebreather mask at 15 lpm.
4. *NEVER GIVE ANYTHING BY MOUTH.*
5. *Calm and reassure the patient.* Provide emotional support.
6. *If signs and symptoms of hypoperfusion are present, treat for shock.* (See Chapter 15, "Shock and Resuscitation.")
7. *Initiate a quick and efficient transport.* Consider ALS intercept based on your protocols.

Reassessment

Perform reassessment during transport. Document and record all vital signs. Communicate all findings to the receiving facility.

Summary: Assessment and Care

To review assessment findings that may be associated with acute abdominal pain and emergency care for acute abdominal pain, see Figures 23-12* and 23-13*.

Assessment Summary

ACUTE ABDOMINAL PAIN

The following findings may be associated with acute abdominal pain.

SCENE SIZE-UP

Pay particular attention to your own safety. Look for:

- Mechanism of injury
- Poisonous substances, especially corrosives
- Position of the patient, typically "guarded," or lying very still with knees drawn up to chest
- Vomitus containing blood or displaying a coffee-ground appearance
- Dark, tarry stool or stool with blood in it
- Location, especially if the patient is found in the bathroom

Primary Assessment

General Impression
- Vomitus or secretions in mouth
- Patient appears ill

Mental Status
- Alert to altered mental status

Airway
- Vomitus may cause obstruction

Breathing
- Shallow and fast respirations

Circulation
- Heart rate is usually increased
- Skin color may be pale, cool, and clammy

Status: Priority Patient

continued

FIGURE 23-12a * Assessment summary: acute abdominal pain.

Assessment Summary

History and Secondary Assessment

History

Signs and symptoms:

- Pain or tenderness to abdomen (crampy, sharp, aching, or knifelike)
- Rigid or distended abdomen
- Anxiety and fear
- Nausea and vomiting
- Dark tarry or bloody stool, possibly diarrhea
- Signs and symptoms of shock

Ask questions regarding the following:

- Onset of pain?
- Any unusual activity at time of onset?
- Was anything taken in an attempt to reduce the pain?
- Any history of abdominal problems?
- Was the patient hospitalized for abdominal problems in the past?
- Any abdominal surgeries or history of trauma?
- Did he eat spicy food or ingest a large amount of alcohol?
- Did he vomit?
- Has his stool changed in color or consistency?
- Have his bowel habits changed? Constipation?
- Any lower back pain?

Physical Exam

Head, neck, and face:

- Pupils sluggish to respond to light

Abdomen:

- Rigid
- Pain on palpation
- Rebound tenderness
- Palpable pulsating mass (abdominal aortic aneurysm)
- Distention
- Discoloration (bruising) around navel or in flank

Extremities:

- Pale, cool, clammy skin
- Reduction in peripheral pulses
- Decrease in strength of femoral and pedal pulses compared to radial or brachial pulses (abdominal aortic aneurysm)

Vital Signs

- BP: decreased
- HR: usually elevated
- RR: usually increased and shallow
- Skin: normal or pale, cool, and clammy
- Pupils: possibly sluggish to respond to light
- SpO_2: may be normal or unreliable if significant blood loss is present

FIGURE 23-12a ✱ Assessment summary: acute abdominal pain. *continued*

Emergency Care Protocol

ACUTE ABDOMINAL PAIN

1. Establish and maintain an open airway. Insert a nasopharyngeal or oropharyngeal airway if the patient is unresponsive and has no gag or cough reflex.
2. Suction secretions as necessary.
3. If breathing is inadequate, provide positive pressure ventilation with supplemental oxygen at a minimum rate of 10–12 ventilations/minute for an adult and 12–20 ventilations/minute for an infant or child.
4. If breathing is adequate, administer oxygen based on the SpO_2 reading and patient signs and symptoms. If the SpO_2 reading is greater than 95% and no signs or symptoms of hypoxia, poor perfusion, or respiratory distress are present, oxygen may not be necessary. In this case, you may choose to apply a nasal cannula at 2–4 lpm. If signs of hypoxia, poor perfusion, or respiratory distress are present, or the SpO_2 reading is less than 95%, place the patient on a nonrebreather mask at 15 lpm.
5. Place the patient in a position of comfort, usually with knees flexed. If the patient is vomiting, place in a left lateral recumbent position only if no spinal injury is suspected.
6. Transport according to the patient's condition.
7. Perform a reassessment every 5 minutes.

FIGURE 23-12b ✱ Emergency care protocol: acute abdominal pain.

Emergency Care Algorithm: **Acute Abdominal Pain**

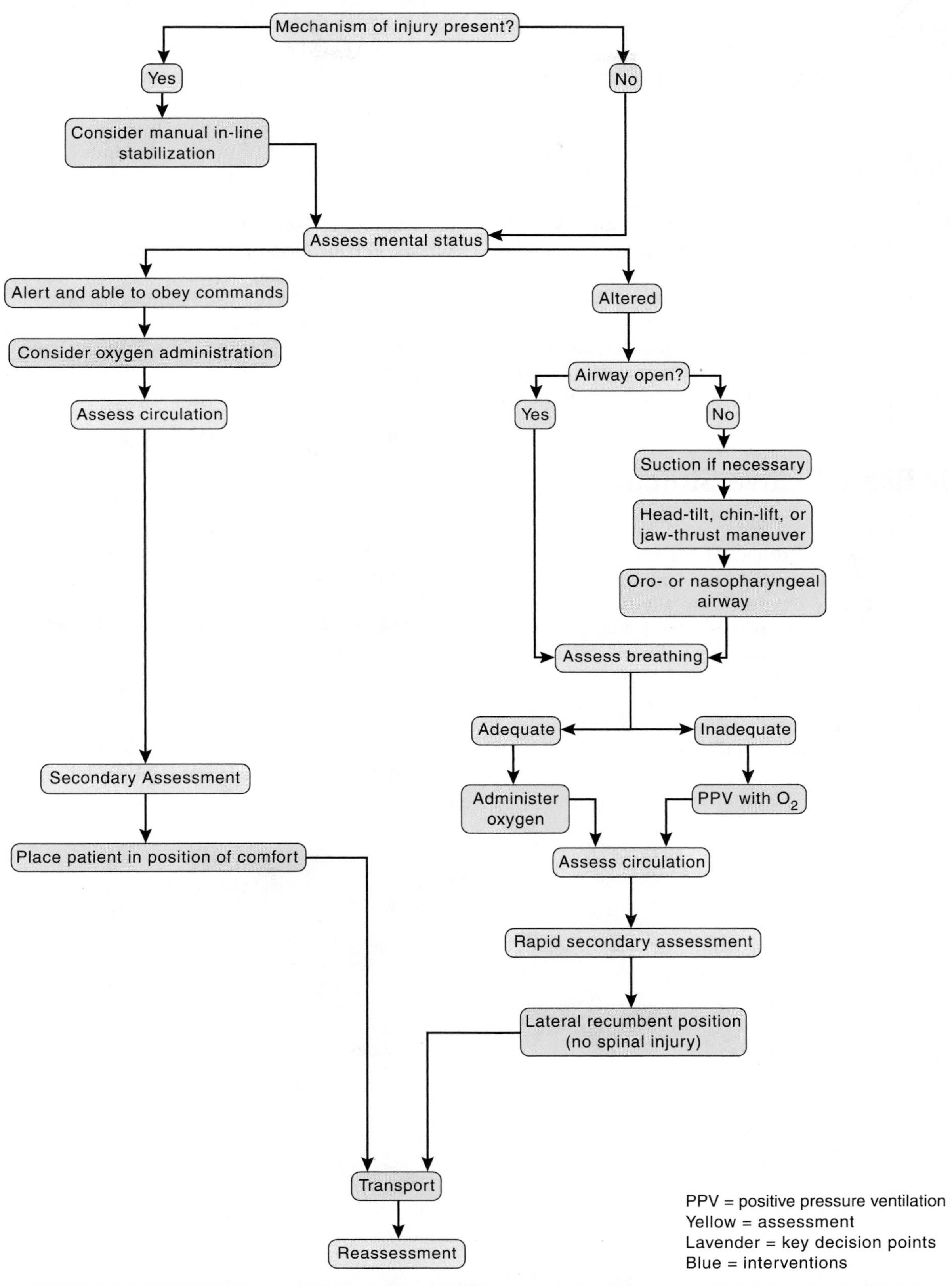

FIGURE 23-13 ✱ Emergency care algorithm: acute abdominal pain.

Key Terms
gynecology branch of medicine that studies health of the female and her reproductive system.

Objective 23-7
Describe the basic anatomy and physiology of the female reproductive system.

Key Terms
menses menstrual period in which the endometrium is sloughed off.

Objective 23-8
Describe the pathophysiolgy and the signs and symptoms associated with common gynecologic conditions.

Gynecologic Emergencies

Gynecology is the branch of medicine that studies health of the female patient and her reproductive system. Female patients who experience gynecologic problems often complain of abdominal pain and vaginal bleeding or abnormal discharge. This pain, bleeding, or discharge may be attributed to various conditions that can be life threatening. Conditions causing abdominal pain in pregnant patients will be discussed in Chapter 37, "Obstetrics and Care of the Newborn."

Female Reproductive Structures and Functions

The female reproductive system (Figure 23-14∗) is composed of the external genitalia and internal organs and structures. The female external genitalia, also called the vulva, consist of vascular tissues called the perineum, mons pubis, labia, and clitoris. The vulva provides accessory functions to the internal organs that are used primarily for reproduction. The internal organs of the female reproductive system are the vagina, uterus, ovaries, and fallopian tubes. The vagina functions as the birth canal during childbirth, receives the penis during sexual intercourse, and serves as a passageway for menstrual flow. The ovaries are the primary sex glands located on each side of the uterus. They excrete hormones and develop and release eggs that are needed for reproduction. The fallopian tubes extend from near each of the ovaries to the uterus. Fertilization of the egg normally occurs here. The uterus is the pear-shaped muscular organ that provides an appropriate site for egg implantation and fetal development during pregnancy. The uterus is lined by the endometrium, which is sloughed off during **menses**, or the menstrual period.

Gynecologic Conditions

This section presents an overview of some of the most common gynecologic conditions that may cause abdominopelvic pain or bleeding. (See Table 23-4.) These conditions can have either medical or traumatic causes. Gynecologic conditions can result in life-threatening complications if left untreated. *Remember that you should never spend extended time at the scene trying to determine the exact cause for acute abdominopelvic pain.*

Sexual Assault

Sexual assault is an act of violence and a crime that is defined differently by each state. Most definitions include sexual intercourse or other sexual activities that are per-

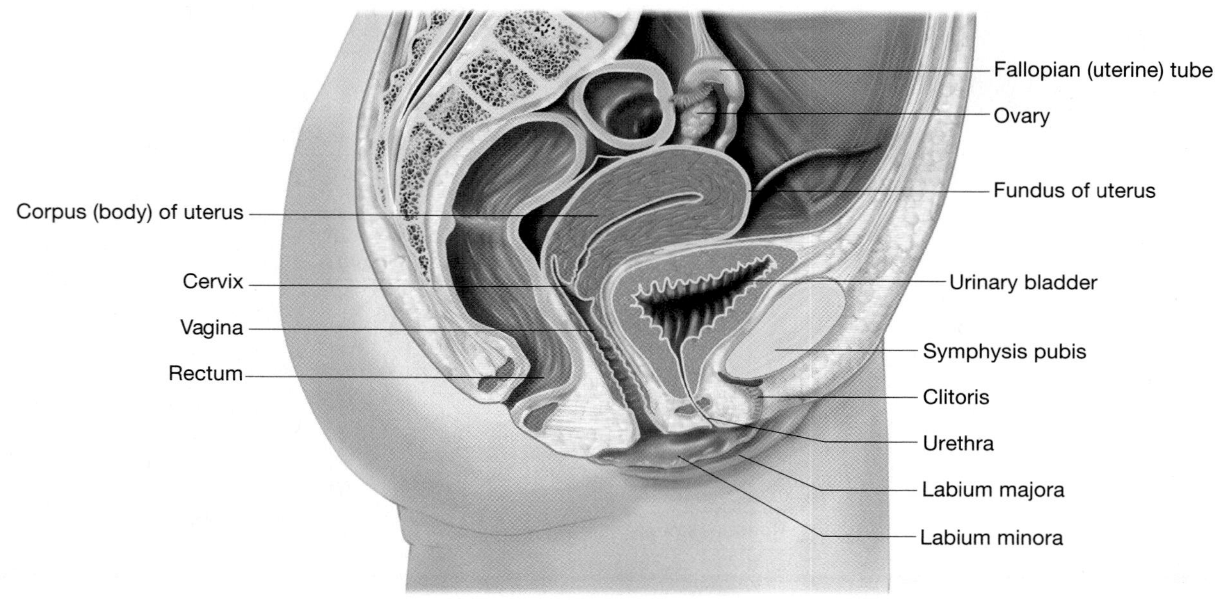

FIGURE 23-14 ∗ Female reproductive anatomy.

Thinking Critically
Sexual assault is a crime in which evidence must be preserved to the extent possible. How should this affect what you say to and how you care for the patient?

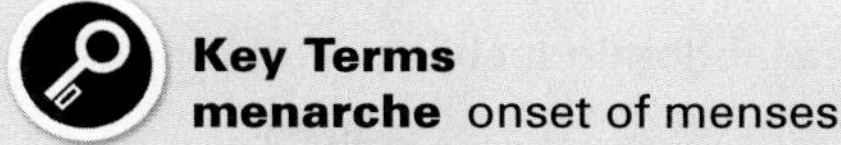

Key Terms
menarche onset of menses.

TABLE 23-4 Gynecologic Conditions That May Cause Abdominal Pain or Bleeding

- Sexual assault
- Vaginal bleeding
- Menstrual pain
- Ovarian cyst
- Endometritis
- Endometriosis
- Pelvic inflammatory disease
- Sexually transmitted diseases

formed without consent. Anyone can be a victim of a sexual assault; however, women are victims more frequently than men. Most victims of sexual assaults know their assailants; however, many will not report the activities to the authorities. As an EMT, you are required to report sexual assault cases to the proper authorities (see Chapter 3, "Medical, Legal, and Ethical Issues"). Make sure you follow your local protocols when dealing with a sexual assault patient.

The effects of rape or sexual assaults are both physical and psychological. Physical effects may include:

- Traumatic injuries from beatings, chokings, and penetrations
- Swelling, bleeding, and pain around the genital or rectal area
- Sexual transmitted diseases
- Possible pregnancy

Psychological effects may include:

- Severe anxiety, depression, or fear
- Inappropriate feelings of guilt
- Flashbacks or nightmares
- Emotional withdrawal, numbness, or irritability

It is important to provide emergency care that addresses both the physical and the emotional needs of the patient. It is also very important that the victims of sexual assaults are evaluated at the hospital and that any evidence related to the crime is preserved to the extent possible. The following guidelines can be applied by the EMT when a sexual assault has occurred:

- Do not allow the patient to change clothes, bathe, comb, or clean any part of her body. If the clothing was changed, collect it, bag it separately, and take it with you.
- Do not cut through any holes or tears in the patient's clothing. Handle the clothing as little as possible.
- Do not touch or change anything at the crime scene unless it impedes emergency medical care.
- Do not clean wounds, if possible. Treat wounds as you would other soft tissue injuries.
- Do not examine the genital area unless there is a life-threatening hemorrhage. Minor bleeding can be absorbed by a pad. Make sure all bloody articles are collected and transported with the patient.

When caring for a patient who has been sexually assaulted, it is important to remain nonjudgmental and objective. Provide a safe environment for the patient. Always maintain patient confidentiality and ask only questions that are pertinent to assessment and emergency medical care. When interviewing the patient, it is not necessary to question her about the specific details of the crime, because your treatment will be based on your assessment findings and your patient's current presentation. Do not touch the patient without her consent or unnecessarily. Respect your patient's wishes and privacy. Obtain vitals and evaluate any other associated injuries that may have occurred. Document all findings objectively and accurately.

Vaginal Bleeding (Nontraumatic)

Vaginal bleeding in female patients may be caused by cancerous lesions, pelvic inflammatory disease, hormonal imbalances, spontaneous abortion (miscarriage), or labor. Vaginal bleeding in female patients occurs naturally with normal menstruation; however, the EMT should not assume any bleeding is occurring from menses. In girls age 10 or older, **menarche**, or the onset of menses, could be the cause of bleeding.

The most common cause of nontraumatic vaginal bleeding other than menses is a spontaneous abortion or miscarriage. Women of childbearing age, of course, are most at risk for a spontaneous abortion. However, menopausal women can also become pregnant and experience spontaneous abortions. More than 20 percent of women who are less than 20 weeks pregnant will have vaginal bleeding. More than 50 percent of these pregnant

Key Terms

dysmenorrhea severe pain or cramps during menstruation.

mittelschmerz abdominopelvic pain during the middle of a menstrual cycle.

Key Terms

endometritis inflammation of the endometrium.

endometriosis the condition in which endometrial tissue grows outside of the uterus.

pelvic inflammatory disease (PID) inflammation of the female reproductive tract.

women with vaginal bleeding will be having or have had a spontaneous abortion. Regardless of the cause, vaginal hemorrhage can be life threatening and should be treated as such.

Common Signs and Symptoms of a Spontaneous Abortion

- Lower abdominal or pelvic pain
- Abdominal tenderness
- Vaginal bleeding
- Rapid pulse
- Signs and symptoms of shock

Menstrual Pain

When the endometrial lining of the uterus is sloughed off during menses, it can be accompanied by strong uterine cramps that cause the severe pain during menstruation called **dysmenorrhea**. Dysmenorrhea is normally caused by hormonal imbalances or other gynecologic conditions. Occasionally, a patient may experience abdominopelvic pain in the middle of her menstrual cycle. This pain is called **mittelschmerz** (German for "middle pain"). It is caused by irritation of the peritoneum by the small amount of bleeding associated with the rupture of ovarian tissue that occurs with release of the mature ovum. Remember that abdominopelvic pain, regardless of the cause, should be treated as an emergency.

Ovarian Cyst

An ovarian cyst is a fluid-filled sac that forms inside or on an ovary. It is formed during ovulation when a follicle containing the egg fails to open as it is supposed to. Ovarian cysts can cause abdominopelvic pain if they rupture, twist, or break open and leak their contents into the abdomen; however, most ovarian cysts are asymptomatic (have no symptoms).

Common Signs and Symptoms of an Ovarian Cyst

- Unilateral abdominopelvic pain that may radiate to the back
- Abdominal tenderness
- Vaginal bleeding that may be irregular or abnormal
- Pain during sexual intercourse or bowel movements

Endometritis

Endometritis is an inflammation of the endometrium. It is most commonly caused by an infection; however, it may also occur from childbirth, abortions, gynecologic procedures, or intrauterine devices. If left untreated, endometritis may lead to peritonitis, abscess formation, septicemia, shock, and infertility.

Common Signs and Symptoms of Endometritis

- Abdominopelvic pain or tenderness
- Fever
- Abdominal distention
- Vaginal bleeding or discharge
- Discomfort during a bowel movement

Endometriosis

Endometriosis is a condition in which endometrial tissue grows outside the uterus. The most common sites for endometrial tissue implantation are the abdomen and pelvis, but the tissue can be implanted anywhere in the body. This endometrial tissue can bleed into the surrounding area and may result in inflammation, scarring, pain, and adhesions. Endometriosis is most commonly diagnosed in women who are 25 to 35 years of age.

Common Signs and Symptoms of Endometriosis

- Abdominopelvic pain or tenderness that may be dull or cramping
- Dysmenorrhea
- Vaginal bleeding
- Pain during sexual intercourse or a bowel movement

Pelvic Inflammatory Disease

Pelvic inflammatory disease (PID) is an infection of the female reproductive tract. Pelvic infections are caused by bacteria, fungi, or viruses. The majority of these infections are caused by the same bacteria that lead to sexually transmitted diseases. Approximately one million women will develop PID each year. Although this condition is spread most often during sex, it can also result from a gynecologic procedure, insertion of an intrauterine device, childbirth, or an abortion.

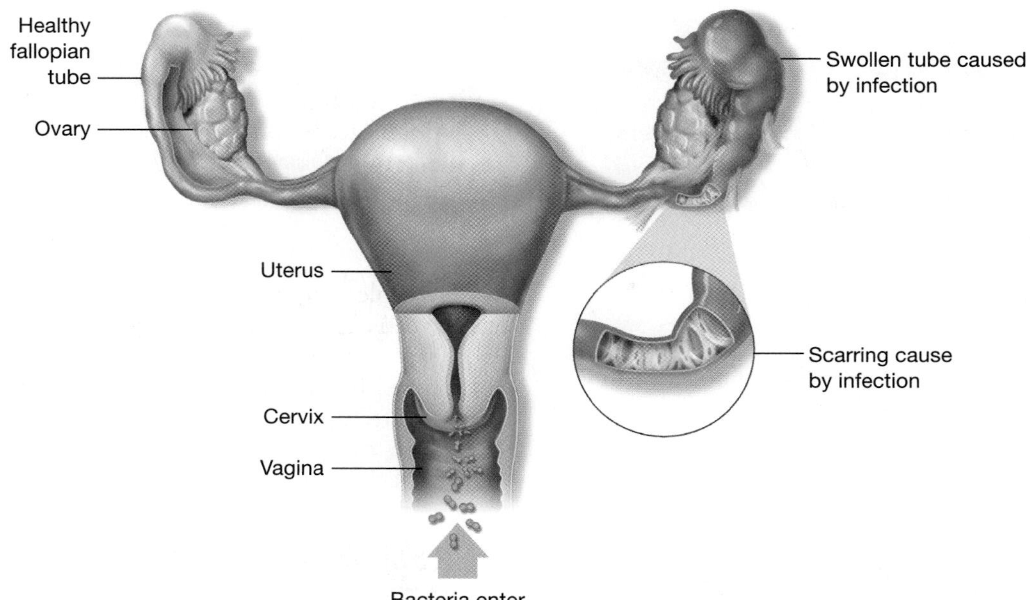

FIGURE 23-15 ✻ How pelvic inflammatory disease (PID) affects the reproductive organs.

Risk factors associated with PID include sexual activity during adolescence, multiple sexual partners, unsafe sexual practices, a recent gynecologic procedure, insertion of an intrauterine device, and a history of sexually transmitted diseases or pelvic inflammatory disease. If left untreated, PID can lead to scarring, infertility, or sepsis (Figure 23-15✻). Although some patients may be asymptomatic, most patients with PID will have abdominopelvic pain.

Common Signs and Symptoms of Pelvic Inflammatory Disease

- Abdominopelvic pain or tenderness
- Vaginal discharge with an abnormal color, consistency, or odor
- Fever and chills
- Anorexia
- Nausea or vomiting
- Irregular vaginal bleeding or cramping
- Pain during sexual intercourse

Sexually Transmitted Diseases

Sexually transmitted diseases (STDs) are infectious diseases that are transmitted through sexual contact. Over 300 million new cases of treatable STDs are diagnosed each year.

Most sexually transmitted diseases are caused by bacteria, viruses, parasites, or fungi. Chlamydia and gonorrhea are the most commonly reported STDs. Some of the most frequent sexually transmitted diseases and their causes are listed in Table 23-5. The treatment for an STD is normally based on the type of organism that causes the infection.

TABLE 23-5 Common Sexually Transmitted Diseases and Their Causes

Sexually Transmitted Disease	Type of Microorganism
Gonorrhea	Bacteria
Syphilis	Bacteria
Chancroid	Bacteria
Chlamydia	Bacteria
HIV	Viral
Herpes	Viral
Genital warts	Viral
Pediculosis	Parasitic
Trichomoniasis	Parasitic

Patients most at risk for developing STDs are those who have multiple sexual partners, do not use condoms, or have had a history of previous STDs or PID. Although some patients with STDs remain asymptomatic, others may complain of abdominopelvic pain and other symptoms. If left untreated, some STDs may lead to sepsis, infertility, abscesses, peritonitis, or other systemic illnesses. It is important to note that the patient and the patient's sexual partners should receive treatment for these conditions.

Common Signs and Symptoms of Sexually Transmitted Diseases

- Abdominopelvic pain or tenderness
- Vaginal discharge with an abnormal color, consistency, or odor

Objective 23-9
Explain the assessment-based approach to acute gynecologic emergencies, including assessment and appropriate medical care.

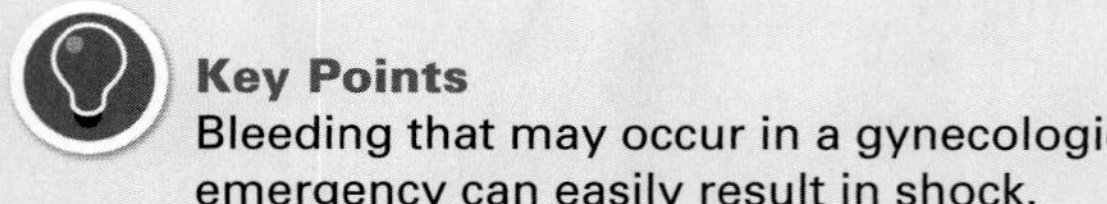

Key Points
Bleeding that may occur in a gynecologic emergency can easily result in shock.

- Fever and chills
- Nausea or vomiting
- Irregular vaginal bleeding or cramping
- Pain during sexual intercourse or urination
- Genital itching, redness, or swelling
- Lesions or ulcers

Assessment-Based Approach: Gynecologic Emergencies

Scene Size-Up

Do a scene size-up and ensure that the scene is safe for you, your partner, and others. Make sure you take all Standard Precautions. Based on the dispatch information and a scan of the scene, determine if the patient has been injured or is suffering from a medical illness. Many gynecologic complaints are called in to dispatch as abdominopelvic pain or vaginal bleeding. If the call appears to be a crime scene, like that encountered from a sexual assault, make sure to call the proper authorities. As you approach the patient, inspect the scene for a mechanism of injury that would be significant enough to cause a possible spinal injury. If no mechanism of injury is apparent, you would then suspect that the gynecologic complaint is a result of medical illness. Remember that patients experiencing a gynecologic emergency may fall or suffer trauma separately from or as a result of their condition.

Primary Assessment

Form a general impression of your patient. If an injury is possible, stabilize the spine. Determine if the patient is alert and oriented or if she has an alteration in her mental status. Because some conditions can result in shock, it is possible for a patient with a gynecologic emergency to be unresponsive. Ensure that your patient has an open and clear airway and use a mechanical airway device if necessary. It may be necessary to suction the airway if vomitus or secretions are present. Determine if the rate, rhythm, and quality of the patient's breathing are adequate.

If breathing is adequate, administer oxygen based on the SpO_2 reading and signs of hypoxia, poor perfusion, or respiratory distress. If breathing is inadequate, provide bag-valve-mask ventilations at 10–12 times a minute with supplemental high-concentration oxygen. Pay particular attention to the patient's perfusion status. Internal and external bleeding that may occur in a gynecologic emergency can easily result in shock. Check the patient's pulse and skin. Look for signs of shock. Identify any major bleeding. If the major bleeding is coming from the vagina, attempt to control the bleeding by placing a pad over the external genitalia to absorb the blood flow. Never pack the patient's vagina.

ASSESSMENT Tips

If the patient has vaginal bleeding, absorb the blood flow with pads and never pack the patient's vagina. ■

Shock is only one indicator that this is a serious medical emergency. The patient with acute abdominal pain or vaginal bleeding as a result of a possible gynecologic emergency should be categorized as a priority for transport if she meets any of the following criteria:

- Poor general appearance
- Unresponsive
- Responsive, not following commands
- Severe pain
- Shock (hypoperfusion)

Secondary Assessment

Make sure you protect the patient's privacy and modesty. It will be necessary to ask questions involving personal issues that some patients may be hesitant or embarrassed to answer. Be patient, compassionate, and professional when communicating with the patient. If the patient is responsive, your partner may take baseline vital signs as you begin gathering information and a history from her. If the patient is unresponsive, perform the physical exam first and then obtain a history and vitals. During your history, ask the following questions:

- What are the signs and symptoms the patient is complaining of?
- Did the signs and symptoms seem to get progressively worse or better?
- How long has the patient been sick or suffering from these signs and symptoms?
- Was the onset of signs and symptoms gradual or sudden?

- What was the patient doing prior to the onset of the complaint?
- Does the patient have any known allergies to medications, food, or other substances?
- When did the patient last have something to eat or drink? What did she eat or drink?
- What medications, prescription and nonprescription, is the patient taking? Is she taking birth control pills or other contraceptives?
- What is the patient's past medical history? When was the last time she has seen a doctor for her medical condition? Has she had any surgeries?
- When was the patient's last menstrual period? Is her cycle regular?
- Does the patient have any vaginal bleeding? If so, how much and for how long? How many pads has she saturated?
- Is there a possibility that she is pregnant? Has she been pregnant before? If so, how many children does she have?
- Does she have any vaginal discharge? If so, what is the color, consistency, and odor like?
- Has the patient had any nausea or vomiting? If so, when and how much?
- Does the patient have any pain associated with urination, defecation, or sexual intercourse?

Signs and Symptoms The signs and symptoms associated with a gynecologic emergency will vary depending on the cause. Abdominopelvic pain and vaginal bleeding are two of the most common signs and symptoms associated with a gynecologic emergency. Others include:

- Vaginal discharge with an abnormal color, consistency, or odor
- Abdominopelvic pain or tenderness
- Nausea and vomiting
- Fever or chills
- Syncope
- Irregular vaginal bleeding or cramping
- Pain during sexual intercourse, urination, or a bowel movement
- Irregular vaginal bleeding or cramping
- Vaginal pain
- Genital itching, redness, or swelling
- Signs of shock

The Physical Exam The physical exam will focus on the gynecologic complaint, which normally involves abdominopelvic pain or vaginal bleeding. However, you should still assess the rest of the body for associated signs and symptoms. You do not need to determine the exact cause of the abdominopelvic pain that may be from a gynecologic condition, but the pain may be from another system. Therefore, all systems should be assessed.

Perform the physical examination of the abdomen carefully and gently, since the abdomen may be tender. You should consider the possiblity that the patient may be pregnant or may have a sexually transmitted disease. Be aware that even the slightest palpation may further aggravate existing pain and make the patient less willing to allow you to examine her.

Begin by inspecting and palpating the abdomen. Ask the patient to point to the area that is the most painful first and then palpate each of the other quadrants before that one. Determine if there is any vaginal bleeding, clots, or tissues. If there is vaginal bleeding, use a pad to absorb the blood and take any tissues with you to the hospital. Document the number of pads that the patient saturates. Obtain and document the patient's baseline vitals. Pay attention to blood pressure and heart rate. Decreased blood pressure, increased heart rate, and pale, cool, moist skin are indicators of shock.

Emergency Medical Care

As previously stated, it is not important that you try to isolate the exact cause of abdominopelvic pain or vaginal bleeding relating to a gynecologic condition in the prehospital setting. Rather, you should correctly assess and identify the pain or bleeding and provide suitable emergency medical care based on the signs and symptoms.

1. *Maintain manual spinal stabilization* if trauma is suspected.
2. *Keep the airway patent.* Always be alert for vomiting and the potential for aspiration. It may be necessary to place the patient in the left lateral recumbent position to protect the airway. Be prepared to suction.
3. *If breathing is adequate, administer oxygen based on the SpO_2 reading and patient signs and symptoms.* If the SpO_2 reading is greater than 95% and no signs or symptoms of hypoxia or respiratory distress are present, oxygen may not be necessary. In this case, you may choose to apply nasal cannula at 2 to 4 lpm. If signs of hypoxia, poor perfusion, or respiratory distress are present, or the SpO_2 reading is less than 95%, place the patient on a nonrebreather mask at 15 lpm.
4. *Control any major vaginal bleeding if present,* if not already started during your primary assessment. Use a pad to absorb the flow and do not pack the vagina.
5. *Place the patient in the position of comfort if no trauma is suspected.* If spinal stabilization is required, fully immobilize the patient on a backboard.
6. *Calm and reassure the patient.* Be supportive and nonjudgmental.
7. *Initiate a quick and efficient transport.* Consider ALS intercept based on your protocols.

Key Terms
urology branch of medicine that studies the urinary system in females and the genitourinary system in males.

Objective 23-10
Describe genitourinary/renal structures and functions.

Key Terms
genitourinary system male organ system that includes both the reproductive and urinary structures.

Reassessment

Continuously monitor the patient for changes in her mental status, airway, breathing, and circulation. For a patient with an altered mental status or signs of shock, repeat the reassessment every 5 minutes. Record the vital signs and communicate your findings to the receiving medical facility.

Genitourinary/ Renal Emergencies

Urology is the branch of medicine that studies the urinary system in females and the genitourinary system in males. The organs of the female reproductive system are separate from those in the female urinary system; however, in males, some of the structures are shared. Because of this, the term **genitourinary system** is referred to in males. Patients with genitourinary or renal conditions frequently experience abdominopelvic pain.

Genitourinary/Renal Structures and Functions

The urinary system is composed of the kidneys, ureters, urinary bladder, and urethra (Figures 23-16*, 23-17a, and 23-17b*). The urinary system produces, stores, and eliminates urine from the body. The kidneys are bean-shaped organs located in the retroperitoneal space. The kidneys filter the blood and excrete waste products in the urine. They also play a role in homeostasis by regulating the body's pH (acid/base levels) and electrolytes, controlling the blood volume, and regulating the blood pressure. The ureters are the tubes that carry urine from the kidneys to the urinary bladder. The urinary bladder houses the urine until it is eliminated from the body via a duct called the urethra. In women, the urethral opening is anterior to the vagina and excretes urine; however, in men the urethra is located at the tip of the penis and eliminates both urine and male reproductive fluid.

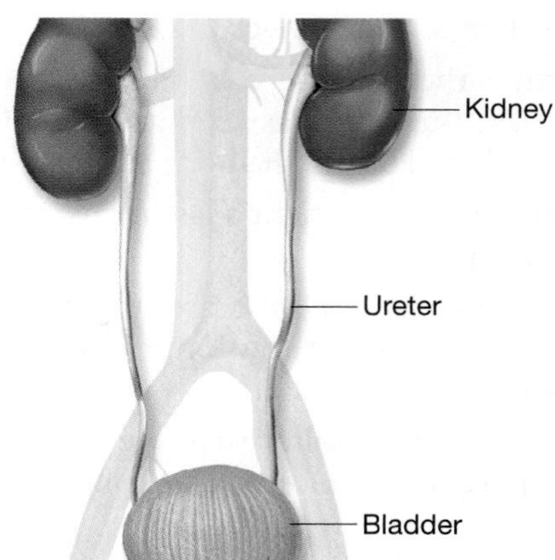

FIGURE 23-16 * The ureters extend from the kidneys to the urinary bladder.

The organs of the male reproductive system include the testes, epididymis, vas deferens, prostate gland, and penis. The testes are the primary male reproductive organs. They produce sperm cells, which are necessary for reproduction and are stored in a small sac called the epididymis. In order for the sperm to leave the body, it

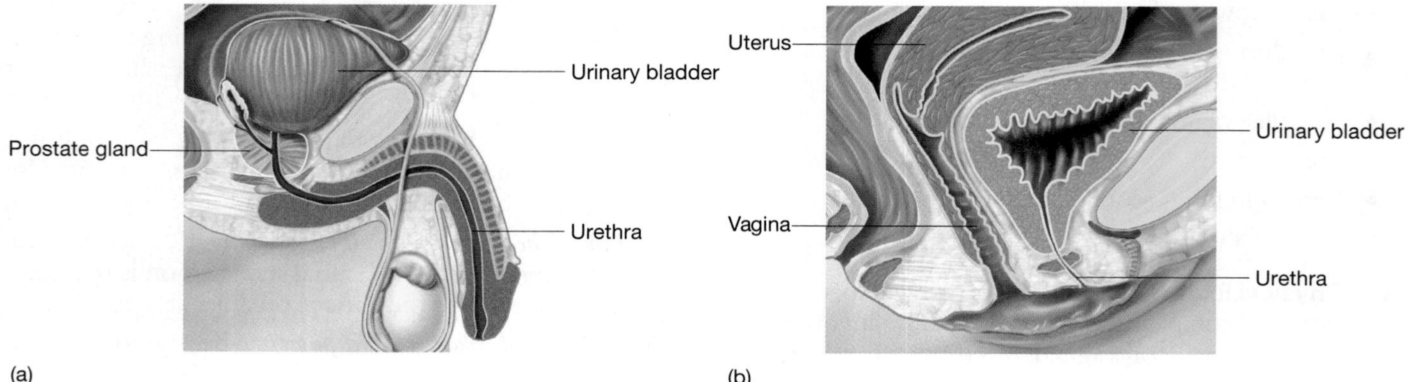

FIGURE 23-17 * **(a)** The male urethra extends from the urinary bladder through the prostate gland and penis. **(b)** The much shorter female urethra extends from the urinary bladder, exiting just in front of the vaginal opening.

Objective 23-11
Describe the pathophysiology and the signs and symptoms associated with common genitourinary/renal conditions.

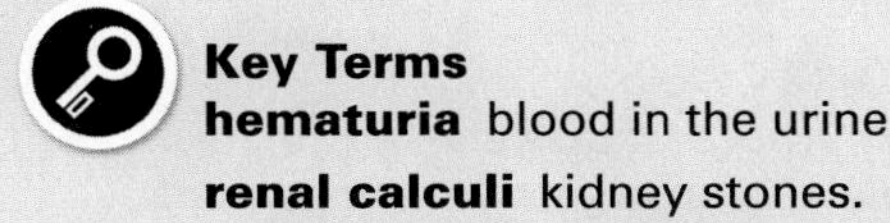

Key Terms
hematuria blood in the urine.
renal calculi kidney stones.

passes through the two ducts called the vas deferens. The sperm then mixes with fluid from the prostate gland before it can be ejaculated from the body. The prostate gland surrounds the male urinary bladder and houses the first part of the male's urethra. The penis is the male organ used for sexual intercourse and urination.

Genitourinary/Renal Conditions

This section presents an overview of some of the most common genitourinary/renal conditions (Table 23-6). It also discusses dialysis and catheter management. Genitourinary or renal conditions can result in life-threatening complications if left untreated. These conditions require the EMT to perform an accurate patient assessment, provide prompt emergency care, and transport the patient.

Urinary Tract Infections

Urinary tract infections (UTIs) can affect the urethra, bladder, ureters, and kidneys. They can also affect the prostate in men. They are most frequently caused by bacteria that enter the urinary system via the urethra. Women, especially those who are pregnant, elderly patients, immobile patients, catheterized patients, and diabetics are prone to urinary tract infections; however, anyone can contract a UTI.

Common Signs and Symptoms of Urinary Tract Infections

- Abdominopelvic pain or tenderness
- Blood in the urine (**hematuria**)
- Urine with cloudiness or a foul or strong odor
- Pain or burning with urination or sexual intercourse
- Frequent or urgent need to urinate
- Genital or flank pain
- Fever or chills
- Nausea or vomiting
- Altered mental status

TABLE 23-6 Common Genitourinary/ Renal Conditions

- Urinary tract infections
- Kidney stones
- Kidney failure

Kidney Stones

Kidney stones, or **renal calculi**, are crystals of substances such as calcium, uric acid, struvite, and crystine that are formed from metabolic abnormalities. They most frequently occur in men between the ages of 20 and 50. Other risk factors associated with renal calculi include family history, hyperparathyroidism, recurrent UTIs, sedentary lifestyle, dehydration, and obesity. Renal calculi are believed to originate in the kidneys and must pass through the rest of the urinary system to be eliminated from the body. Severe pain can occur with renal calculi, especially if the stone is large and is passing through a ureter. If left untreated, renal calculi can lead to loss of kidney function, obstruction of the urinary tract, or kidney damage. The reoccurrence of kidney stones is common and can occur in up to 50 percent of patients who have had them.

Common Signs and Symptoms of Kidney Stones

- Abdominopelvic pain or tenderness
- Flank or back pain that is colicky and severe
- Groin pain
- Abnormal urine color
- Pain with urination
- Frequent or urgent need to urinate
- Fever or chills
- Nausea or vomiting

Kidney Failure

Kidney failure, or renal failure, occurs when the kidneys fail to function adequately. During this condition, the kidneys are not able to filter the wastes and maintain homeostasis as they normally would. Kidney failure is normally classified as either acute or chronic. Acute renal failure (ARF) normally occurs over a period of days and often results from a significant decrease in urine elimination. Some causes of acute renal failure are decreased blood flow to the kidneys, trauma, cardiac failure, surgery, shock, sepsis, and urinary tract obstruction. This condition is sometimes reversible, but many patients will require dialysis.

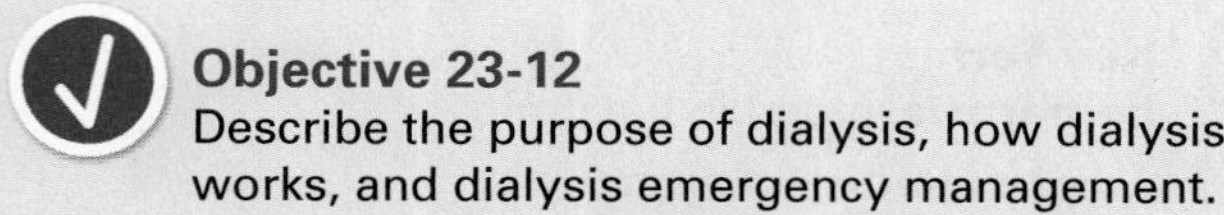

Objective 23-12
Describe the purpose of dialysis, how dialysis works, and dialysis emergency management.

Key Terms
dialysis an artificial process used to remove water and waste substances from the blood.
dialysate a special fluid used for dialysis.

Chronic renal failure (CRF) normally occurs over a period of years, and the symptoms range from mild at first to severe kidney failure. The causes of chronic renal failure are numerous; however, diabetes and hypertension are linked to a majority of the cases. Chronic renal failure results in an accumulation of waste products and fluids that can affect almost every organ system in the body. This condition is permanent and life threatening. Patients with this type of kidney failure ultimately will require dialysis or a kidney transplant for survival.

Some complications that may result from kidney failure are:

- Pulmonary edema
- Cardiac tamponade or pericarditis
- Electrolyte and other metabolic abnormalities
- Cardiac dysrhythmias
- Congestive heart failure
- Hypertension
- Infections
- Hemorrhage
- Liver failure
- Altered mental status
- Seizures
- Uremia

Common Signs and Symptoms of Kidney Failure

- Abdominopelvic or flank pain
- Blood in the urine or stools
- Altered mental status
- Edema of the feet, ankles, and legs
- Decreased urine output or cessation of urination
- Hypertension
- Swelling or easy bruising
- Anorexia
- Tachycardia

Dialysis

Dialysis is an artificial process used to remove water and waste substances from the blood when the kidneys fail to function properly. It generally works through osmosis and filtration of fluid across a semipermeable membrane. In general, the blood containing waste products passes on one side of the membrane while a **dialysate** (special fluid used for dialysis) passes on the other side. When this occurs, the water and waste products travel from the blood across the membrane and into the dialysate thus removing the waste from the patient.

There are two major types of dialysis: hemodialysis and peritoneal dialysis. In hemodialysis, a dialysis machine containing the dialysate is connected to an access site on the patient. The access site may be a shunt, fistula, port, or graft (Figure 23-18*). The patient's blood, which is heparinized, is pumped through the access site and into the machine to have the waste removed. The access site should be treated with care because dialysis cannot occur without it. The EMT should not take the blood pressure of a dialysis patient on the side of the patient's access site. Hemodialysis is commonly performed at an outpatient dialysis facility, but can be performed in other locations.

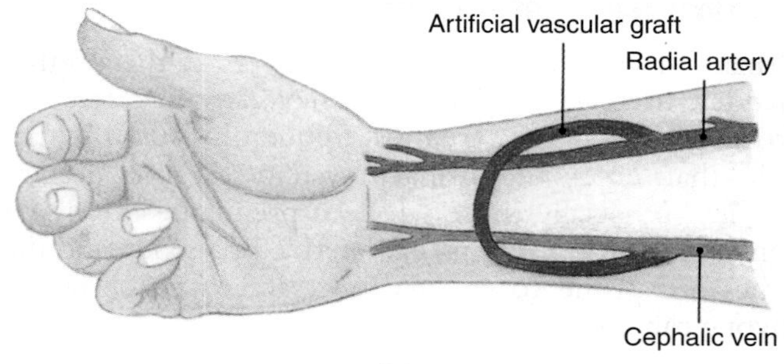

(a)

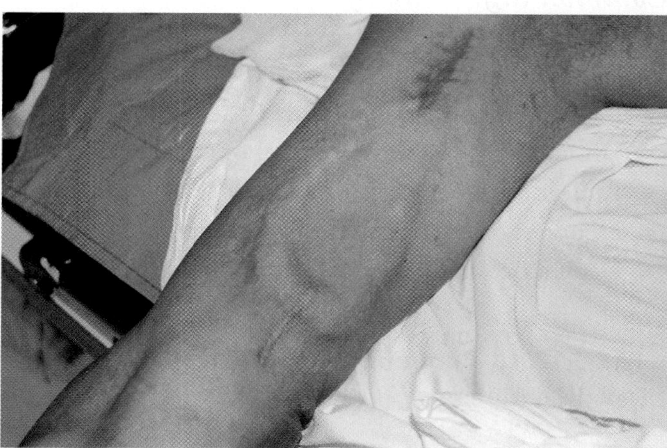

(b)

FIGURE 23-18 * In hemodialysis, a dialysis machine is connected to an access site such as a shunt formed by an artificial graft between an artery and a vein. (Photo: © Edward T. Dickinson, MD)

Key Points
Dialysis can sometimes result in life-threatening complications, but missing a needed dialysis treatment can also be life threatening.

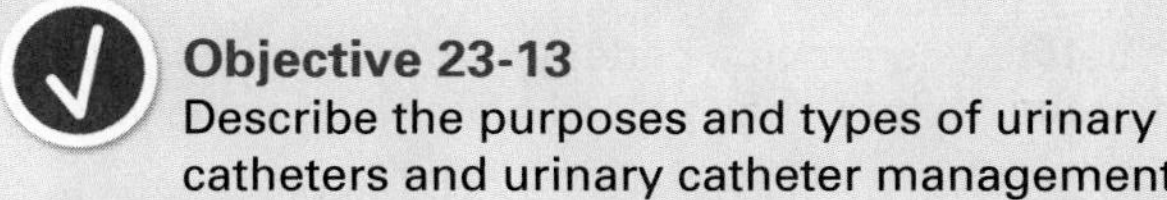

Objective 23-13
Describe the purposes and types of urinary catheters and urinary catheter management.

In peritoneal dialysis, the dialysate is run through a tube into the patient's abdomen (Figures 23-19*). The peritoneal membrane functions as the semipermeable membrane during peritoneal dialysis. The fluid remains in the abdomen for several hours so it can absorb the wastes and then is drained out of the body through a different tube. Peritoneal dialysis is commonly performed at home and is often performed while the patient is sleeping at night. Other peritoneal techniques can be used during the day.

Although dialysis provides a necessary treatment for patients with kidney failure, it has risks that can result in adverse effects and life-threatening complications such as:

- Hypotension
- Muscle cramps
- Peritonitis (especially in peritoneal dialysis)
- Nausea and vomiting
- Hemorrhage (especially from the access site)
- Infection at the access site
- Irregular pulse or cardiac arrest
- Difficulty breathing

In addition to these risks, patients may experience life-threatening problems if they miss their dialysis treatments. The most common problems are weakness and pulmonary edema.

Dialysis Emergency Management Management of a patient with a dialysis emergency involves the following:

1. Maintain the airway, breathing, and circulation.
2. Support ventilation as needed.
3. Provide high-concentration oxygen.
4. Stop any bleeding from the shunt or access site as needed.
5. Position the patient. If the patient has signs of shock, place him in a supine position. If the patient has pulmonary edema, place him upright.
6. Transport.

Urinary Catheters

As an EMT, you may encounter patients who have urinary catheters. There are various types of catheters that serve to collect urine when patients are not capable of eliminating it themselves. Foley or indwelling catheters are the most common. These catheters have a balloon that is inserted into the urinary bladder via the urethra (Figures 23-20a and 23-20b*). The urine drains from

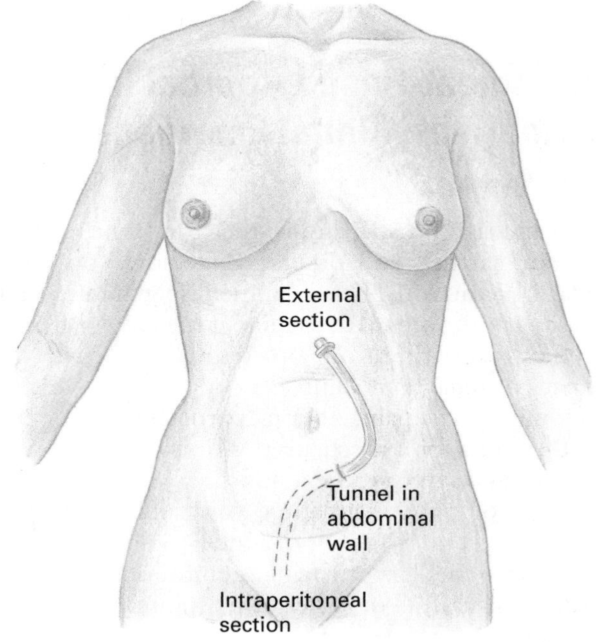

(a)

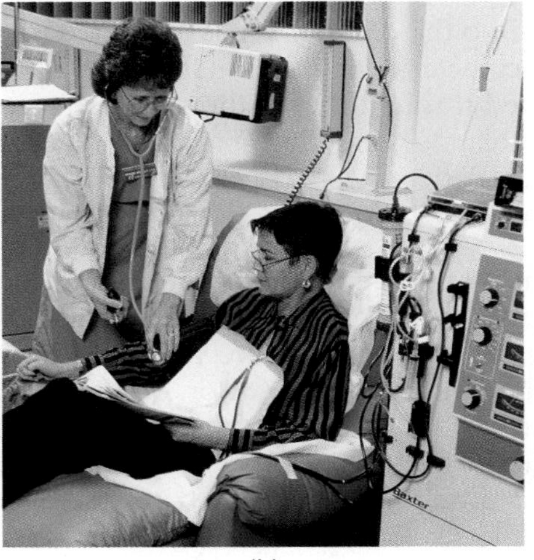

(b)

FIGURE 23-19 * In peritoneal dialysis, dialysate is run through a tube into the patient's abdomen. (Photo: © Michal Heron)

Key Points
Before you move a patient with a urinary catheter, drain the bag, then record how much urine was in the bag and the time you emptied it.

Objective 23-14
Explain the assessment-based approach to genitourinary/renal emergencies, including assessment and appropriate medical care.

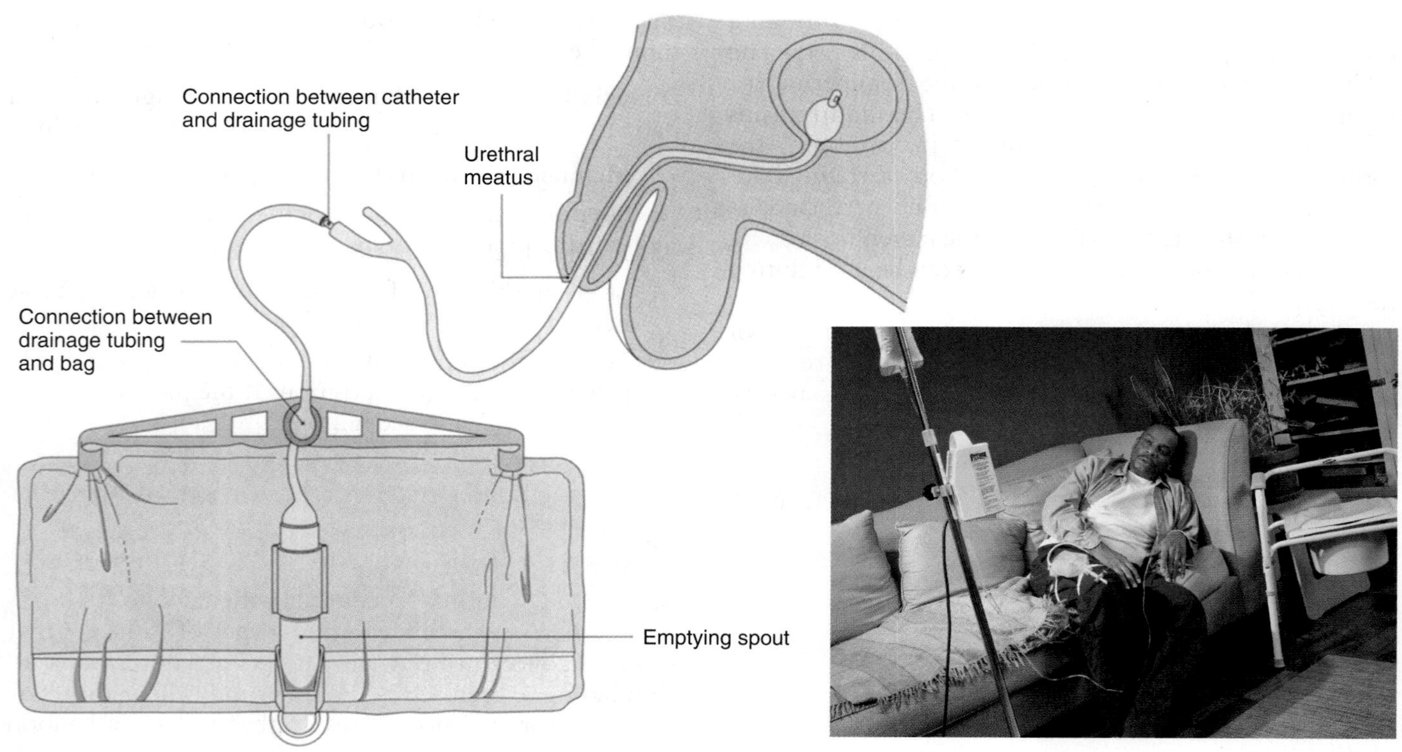

FIGURE 23-20 ✻ Indwelling catheters have a balloon that is inserted into the urinary bladder via the urethra. The urine that drains from the bladder is deposited into an external bag.

the bladder into the catheter and is deposited into a bag. Suprapubic catheters work in a similar way, but instead of being inserted through the urethra they are placed into the urinary bladder directly through the patient's abdominal wall. Patients with catheters are prone to infections and device malfunctions.

Urinary Catheter Management It may be necessary for you to assess and transport patients with catheters. During your assessment, be sure to note any swelling, redness, pain, unusual odor or color, or bleeding around the site. Before you move and transport the patient, you should drain the bag. Record how much urine was in the bag and the time that you emptied it. Make sure that there are no kinks in the device and that it is free from anything it could get caught on before you move the patient. After transferring the patient to either the cot or the bed, make sure that you lower the bag so the urine can freely flow into it.

Assessment-Based Approach: Genitourinary/Renal Emergencies

Scene Size-Up

Do a scene size-up and ensure that the scene is safe for you, your partner, and others. Make sure you take all Standard Precautions. Based on the dispatch information and a scan of the scene, determine if the patient has been injured or is suffering from a medical illness. Many genitourinary or renal complaints may be called into dispatch as abdominopelvic pain. As you approach the patient, inspect the scene for a mechanism of injury that would be significant enough to cause a possible spinal injury. If no mechanism of injury is apparent, you would then suspect that the complaint is a result of a medical illness. Remember that patients experiencing genitourinary or renal emergencies may fall or suffer other trauma as a result of their condition.

Primary Assessment

Form a general impression of your patient. Does he appear to be in major distress? If an injury is possible, stabilize the spine. Determine if the patient is alert and oriented or if he has an alteration in his mental status. Because a genitourinary or renal emergency can have many complications, the patient may be disoriented or unresponsive. Ensure that your patient has an open and clear airway and use a mechanical airway device if necessary. It may be necessary to suction the airway if vomitus or secretions are present. Determine if the rate, rhythm, and quality of the patient's breathing are adequate. If breathing is adequate, apply oxygen based on the SpO_2 reading and signs of respiratory distress, poor perfusion, and hypoxia. If breathing is inadequate, provide bag-valve mask ventilations at 10–12 times a minute with supplemental high concentrations of oxygen. Assess the perfusion status of the patient. Remember that complications from genitourinary or renal emergencies can result in shock. Check the patient's pulse and skin. Look for signs of shock. Identify and control any major bleeding. If the major bleeding is coming from a dialysis shunt, it should also be controlled.

Shock is only one indicator of a serious medical emergency. The patient having a genitourinary or renal emergency should be categorized as a priority for transport if he meets any of the following criteria:

- Poor general appearance
- Unresponsive
- Responsive, not following commands
- Severe pain
- Shock (hypoperfusion)

Secondary Assessment

Protect the patient's privacy and modesty. It will be necessary to ask questions involving personal issues that some patients may be hesitant or embarrassed to answer. Be patient, compassionate, and professional when communicating with them. Your partner may take baseline vital signs as you begin gathering information and a history from the patient if he is responsive. If the patient is unresponsive, perform your physical exam first and then obtain a history and vitals. During your history, ask the following questions:

- What are the signs and symptoms the patient is complaining of?
- Did the signs and symptoms seem to get progressively worse or better?
- How long has the patient been sick or suffering from these signs and symptoms?
- Was the onset of signs and symptoms gradual or sudden?
- What was the patient doing prior to the onset of the complaint?
- Does the patient have any known allergies to medications, food, or other substances?
- When did the patient last have something to eat or drink? What did he eat or drink?
- What medications, prescription and nonprescription, is the patient taking?
- What is the patient's past medical history? When was the last time he has seen a doctor for his medical condition? Has he had any surgeries?
- When was the patient's last menstrual period? Is her cycle regular? Does she have any vaginal bleeding or discharge? Could she be pregnant?
- Is there any genital pain or discharge? If so, what is the color, consistency, and odor like?
- Is there a change in urine? If so, what is the color and odor like?
- Does the patient receive dialysis? If so, when was the last treatment received? When is the next treatment due?
- Does the patient have any abdominopelvic or flank pain?
- Has the patient had any nausea or vomiting? If so, when and how much?
- Does the patient have any pain associated with urination, defecation, or sexual intercourse?

ASSESSMENT Tips

Remember to take the blood pressure of a dialysis patient on the arm without the shunt or access site. ■

Signs and Symptoms The signs and symptoms associated with a genitourinary or renal emergency will vary depending on the cause. They may include the following:

- Urine with an abnormal color, consistency, or odor
- Abdominopelvic pain or tenderness
- Nausea and vomiting
- Fever or chills
- Syncope or altered mental status
- Pain or burning during sexual intercourse, urination, or a bowel movement
- Flank, groin, or back pain
- Frequent or urgent need to urinate or decreased urine output
- Blood in the urine (hematuria)
- Edema of the feet, ankles, and legs
- Hypertension
- Anorexia
- Tachycardia
- Signs of shock

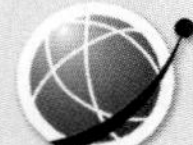

Media Resources
Go to www.bradybooks.com for mykit. Highlights:
- *Web Resource:* STDs
- *Video:* Gonorrhea

The Physical Exam The physical exam will primarily focus on the genitourinary or renal complaint and will normally involve the abdominopelvic area. Genitourinary and renal conditions can affect other body systems; therefore, you must assess related body systems, such as the cardiovascular and respiratory systems, for associated signs and symptoms.

Perform the physical examination of the abdomen carefully and gently. If the patient is a female, you should consider the possibility that she may be pregnant. Begin by inspecting and palpating the abdomen. Remember to ask the patient to point to the area that is the most painful first and then palpate each of the other quadrants before that one. Determine if there is any bleeding, pain, or tenderness. You should also note if the patient has a catheter. If a catheter is present, you should document the amount of urine, color, and odor before emptying it. Remember to keep the catheter free from anything it could get caught on. Obtain and document the patient's vital signs. Remember: Do not obtain a blood pressure in the arm with the fistula or shunt. Pay attention to blood pressure and heart rate. Decreased blood pressure, increased heart rate, and pale, cool, moist skin are indicators of shock.

Emergency Medical Care

As previously stated, it is not important that you try to isolate the exact cause of abdominopelvic pain or a genitourinary or renal condition in the prehospital setting. Rather, you should correctly assess and identify the signs and symptoms and provide the proper emergency medical care as follows:

1. *Maintain manual spinal stabilization* if trauma is suspected.
2. *Keep the airway patent.* Always be alert for vomiting and the potential for aspiration. It may be necessary to place the patient in the left lateral recumbent position to protect the airway if the patient has an altered mental status. Be prepared to suction.
3. *If breathing is adequate, administer oxygen based on the SpO_2 reading and patient signs and symptoms.* If the SpO_2 reading is greater than 95% and no signs or symptoms of hypoxia or respiratory distress are present, oxygen may not be necessary. In this case, you may choose to apply nasal cannula at 2 to 4 lpm. If signs of hypoxia or respiratory distress are present, or the SpO_2 reading is less than 95%, place the patient on a nonrebreather mask at 15 lpm.
4. *Control any major bleeding if present;* recheck the access site for bleeding in a dialysis patient.
5. *Place the patient in the position of comfort if no trauma is suspected.* If spinal stabilization is required, fully immobilize the patient on a backboard. If signs or symptoms of shock are present, then place in a supine position. If pulmonary edema is suspected, place the patient in an upright position.
6. *Calm and reassure the patient.* Be supportive and nonjudgmental.
7. *Initiate a quick and efficient transport.* Consider ALS intercept based on your protocols.

Reassessment

Continuously monitor the patient for changes in mental status, airway, breathing, and circulation. For a patient with an altered mental status or signs of shock, repeat the reassessment every 5 minutes. Record the vital signs and communicate your findings to the receiving medical facility.

CHAPTER REVIEW

SUMMARY

The primary goal in the assessment and management of the patient experiencing acute abdominopelvic pain is to manage any life threats to the airway, breathing, oxygenation, and circulation. Patients with gynecologic, genitourinary, or renal complaints may also complain of pain or bleeding associated with an acute abdomen. It is not the responsibility of the EMT to attempt to determine what the exact condition is or what organ is causing the complaint; however, it is important to recognize the signs and symptoms associated with an acute abdomen, since it can be associated with life-threatening bleeding and hypovolemic shock. Your emergency care for an acute abdominopelvic patient is primarily supportive.

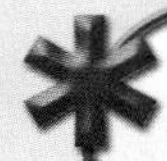

CASE STUDY FOLLOW-UP

SCENE SIZE-UP

You have been dispatched to a 16-year-old male complaining of "stomach" pain. As you approach the home, you scan the scene for any hazards or signs of trauma but find everything in order. You are greeted at the door by the boy's mother. She tells you that her son, Parker, has had a fever for the last couple of days and that he woke up this morning saying his "stomach hurt real bad."

PRIMARY ASSESSMENT

You follow the mother into the boy's bedroom. You note that the patient is lying on his left side, curled up, and holding his stomach. Your general impression is that Parker appears ill. He speaks clearly—confirming a severe pain in his stomach—so you know that he is alert and his airway is open. His breathing is slightly rapid and his skin is flushed. His radial pulse is strong and rapid.

You tell your partner to go ahead and get the stretcher as you administer oxygen at 15 lpm via a nonrebreather mask.

SECONDARY ASSESSMENT

You visually inspect the patient quickly from head to toe as you begin to ask him and his mother some questions. Using the OPQRST mnemonic, you find out the following: The pain began this morning around 5:00; nothing makes the pain better, but lying flat makes it worse; the pain is a dull cramping and is located around the navel, radiating down to the RLQ; Parker says it is "the worst stomach pain" he has ever had; and it has been constant since early this morning.

The history reveals the following: Parker does not have any known allergies; his mother gave him some cold medicine before bed last night; he does not have any significant medical history; he last drank some fluid around 5:30 this morning but vomited shortly thereafter; nothing seems to have led to this condition; his mother states he has not eaten since lunch yesterday; and he has had some nausea with one episode of vomiting. The vomitus was not abnormal and did not contain any blood.

While you are still asking the history questions, you begin the physical exam. You determine that the patient's abdomen is soft but tender to palpation in the RLQ with some guarding. Meanwhile, your partner, who has returned with the stretcher, obtains and documents Parker's baseline vitals. His breathing is adequate but somewhat rapid and shallow with a rate of 28; his radial pulse is strong, regular, and rapid with a rate of 130. His blood pressure is 108/60 mmHg. His skin is warm, dry, and flushed.

You explain to Parker that he needs to go to the hospital. You move him onto the stretcher and allow him to lie in a position that is comfortable for him. His mother elects to drive her own car to the hospital. Once in the ambulance, you prepare for suction in case Parker vomits. Meanwhile, you talk to him about how the football season has been going to help keep his mind off the pain.

REASSESSMENT

While en route to the hospital you continually reassess Parker for any signs of shock, repeat his vital signs, and check to make sure the oxygen is working. Once at the hospital, you give a detailed report regarding Parker's condition to the triage nurse and finish writing your prehospital care report as your partner readies the ambulance for the next call.

Later, while you are at the hospital on another call, you find out that Parker has had successful surgery to remove his inflamed appendix.

IN REVIEW

1. List the organs contained within the abdominal cavity.
2. Using the umbilicus as a reference point, name the quadrants of the abdominal cavity and the organs you would expect to find in each quadrant.
3. List the signs and symptoms of acute abdomen.
4. List the factors that would make you consider a patient who is suffering abdominal pain as a priority for transport.
5. Describe the general guidelines for conducting a physical examination of a patient with acute abdominal pain.
6. Outline the steps for emergency medical care of a patient with acute abdominal pain.
7. List the organs of the female reproductive system.
8. List common gynecologic emergencies that can cause abdominopelvic pain.
9. Describe the guidelines for managing a victim of a sexual assault.
10. List the organs of the renal system.
11. List common genitourinary emergencies.
12. Describe how to manage a patient who has a catheter.
13. Describe hemodialysis and peritoneal dialysis.

CRITICAL THINKING

You arrive on the scene and find a 26-year-old patient who is complaining of vomiting up blood. He tells you that he is an alcoholic and has been drinking for a week or so. He is alert but sluggish in responding to your questions. His respirations are 22 per minute with good tidal volume. His radial pulse is 132 bpm and is very weak. His skin is extremely pale, cool, and clammy. His blood pressure is 86/68 mmHg. He is complaining of abdominal pain to the epigastric region. The pain has been present for about 3–4 weeks; however, it has gotten much worse over the last several days. Today he began to vomit blood. He confirms he has had black, tarry stools. The pain is a "10" on a 1-to-10 pain scale. Nothing relieves the pain. The pain worsens after drinking alcohol. He has not eaten for a few days. The pain is sharp, stabbing, and constant. The pain does not radiate. The patient denies any allergies and takes no medications.

1. What emergency care would you provide during the primary assessment?
2. What assessment findings would lead you to suspect the patient is experiencing an acute abdomen?
3. What are the vital signs indicating?
4. Based on the assessment findings and history information, what might the patient be suffering from?
5. What is the significance of the bowel movement findings?

CHAPTER 24 Environmental Emergencies

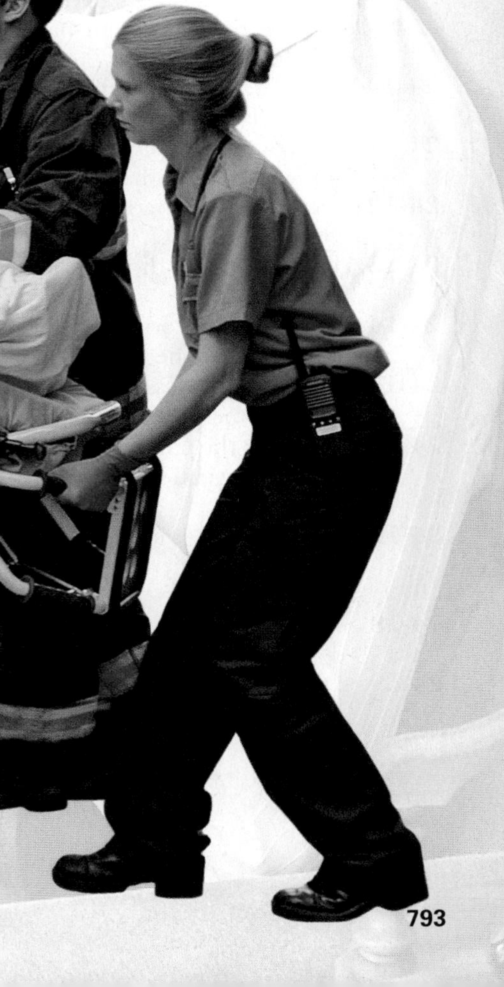

Navigation Guide

The following items provide an overview to the purpose and content of this chapter. The Standard and Competency are from the new National EMS Education Standards.

STANDARD **Trauma** (Content Area: Environmental Emergencies)

COMPETENCY Applies fundamental knowledge to provide basic emergency care and transportation based on assessment findings for an acutely injured patient.

OBJECTIVES: After reading this chapter, you should be able to:

24-1. Define key terms introduced in this chapter.
24-2. Explain the importance of being able to recognize and provide emergency medical care for patients with environmental emergencies.
24-3. Describe the process by which the body maintains normal temperature.
24-4. Explain the mechanisms by which the body loses heat.
24-5. Explain the mechanisms by which the body gains heat.
24-6. Describe the pathophysiology of generalized hypothermia.
24-7. Recognize factors that contribute to a patient's risk for hypothermia, (including immersion hypothermia, urban hypothermia, and myxedema coma or hypothyroidism).
24-8. Describe the pathophysiology of local cold injury, including the stages of local cold injury.
24-9. Discuss the assessment-based approach to cold-related emergencies.
24-10. Describe the emergency medical care for generalized hypothermia.
24-11. Describe the emergency medical care for immersion hypothermia.
24-12. Describe the emergency medical care for local cold injury.
24-13. Describe the pathophysiology of heat-related emergencies.
24-14. Recognize factors that contribute to a patient's risk for hyperthermia.
24-15. Discuss the assessment-based approach to heat-related emergencies.
24-16. Describe the emergency medical care for a heat emergency patient with moist, pale, normal-to-cool skin.
24-17. Describe the emergency medical care for a heat emergency patient with hot skin that is moist or dry.
24-18. Describe the emergency medical care for heat cramps.
24-19. Describe the characteristics of common venomous snakes and factors that affect the severity of a snakebite.
24-20. Recognize the signs, symptoms, and patient history associated with bites or stings of the following:
   a. Black widow spiders
   b. Brown recluse spiders
   c. Scorpions
   d. Fire ants
   e. Ticks
24-21. Discuss the assessment-based approach to bites and stings.
24-22. Describe the signs and symptoms and the emergency medical care for anaphylactic shock resulting from a bite or sting.
24-23. Describe the signs and symptoms and the emergency medical care for a bite or sting.
24-24. Recognize the signs, symptoms, and patient history associated with the bite or sting of a marine animal and the emergency medical care for marine life poisoning.
24-25. Explain the pathophysiology of lightning strike injuries.
24-26. Given a scenario with a patient who has been struck by lightning, predict findings and complications associated with the mechanism of injury.
24-27. Describe the emergency medical care for a patient who has been struck by lightning.
24-28. Describe the signs, symptoms, and patient history associated with acute mountain sicknesses and emergency medical care for acute mountain sickness.
24-29. Describe the signs, symptoms, and patient history associated with high altitude pulmonary edema and emergency medical care for high altitude pulmonary edema.
24-30. Describe the signs, symptoms, and patient history associated with high altitude cerebral edema and emergency medical care for high altitude cerebral edema.

Navigation Guide *continued*

KEY TERMS: Page references indicate first major use in this chapter. For complete definitions, see the Glossary at the back of the book.

active rewarming p. 809
conduction p. 798
convection p. 798
evaporation p. 798
generalized hypothermia p. 799
hyperthermia p. 799
hypothermia p. 797
local cold injury p. 803
myxedema coma p. 803
passive rewarming p. 809
radiation p. 798
respiration p. 799
thermoreceptor p. 796
urban hypothermia p. 802
water chill p. 798
wind chill p. 798

MEDIA RESOURCES: Please go to www.bradybooks.com to access mykit for this text. You will find quizzes, critical thinking scenarios, weblinks, animations, and videos related to this chapter—and much more. Look for online information on hypothermia and hyperthermia.

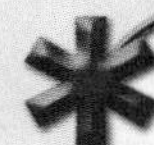

CASE STUDY

The Dispatch
EMS Unit 621—proceed to 2125 Central Avenue. Police are on the scene with a disoriented elderly woman who fell in a snowbank approximately 2 hours ago. Time out is 1314 hours.

Upon Arrival
You arrive at the scene at 1321 hours. A police officer greets you and says he and his partner received a call about a woman found by a neighbor behind a single-family dwelling at 2125 Central Avenue. When they arrived, they found a 62-year-old woman who had apparently been taking out her garbage, wearing a housecoat and slippers, when she slipped and fell. She has been lying in the snowbank for at least 2 hours, according to what she told the police. The officer adds that the woman complained of pain in her left ankle from the fall. As you approach the patient, you note she is responsive and is not shivering.

How Would You Proceed to Assess and Care for This Patient?
In this chapter, you will learn considerations for assessing and managing patients who have suffered from environmental emergencies including exposure to heat and cold as well as bites, stings, and altitude sickness. Later, we will return to the case and apply what you have learned.

Introduction

You will face situations as an EMT that are termed *environmental emergencies.* These are caused when there is a significant disruption in normal physiological activities of the body as a response to a change in some element (or combination of elements) in the patient's natural surroundings. Such emergencies can arise from interaction with the climate, as in exposure to excessive cold or heat. They can also be brought on by contact with creatures living in the environment, as in the bites or stings of snakes or spiders. In addition, going into a high altitude can cause emergencies that would not occur at sea level. These and other causes of environmental emergencies are discussed in this chapter.

Although environmental emergencies happen in large metropolitan areas, they also occur in isolated areas that do not have ready access to an emergency department. Therefore, it is important for the EMT to learn how to assess and provide on-scene or en route emergency medical care for patients affected by environmental emergencies.

Heat and Cold Emergencies

To understand how exposure to heat or cold can create life-threatening situations, you should have a basic understanding of how the body regulates its temperature.

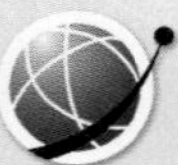

Media Resources

Go to www.bradybooks.com for mykit. Highlights:

- *Web Resource:* Hypothermia
- *Web Resource:* Hyperthermia

Objective 24-2

Explain the importance of being able to recognize and provide emergency medical care for patients with environmental emergencies.

Objective 24-3

Describe the process by which the body maintains normal temperature,

Regulation of Temperature

The human body stubbornly defends its constant core temperature of approximately 98.6°F (37°C). In order to do this, the body must constantly monitor its temperature and balance the amount of heat production and heat loss.

The body temperature is monitored and controlled primarily by the hypothalamus in the brain. The hypothalamus contains a temperature control center called the thermoregulatory center. This center receives input from two different receptors: (1) the central thermoreceptors, which are located on or near the anterior hypothalamus; and (2) the peripheral thermoreceptors, found in the skin and the mucous membranes. A **thermoreceptor** (*thermo* refers to temperature; *receptor* is a sensory nerve ending that receives various types of stimuli) is responsible for sending nerve impulses to the hypothalamus indicating the temperature of the body. The central thermoreceptors measure the core body temperature by monitoring the temperature of the blood, and the peripheral thermoreceptors monitor the body temperature found in the skin and extremities.

When understanding body temperature, the concept of a thermal gradient (transfer of heat or cold) applies. The thermal gradient operates by warmer temperatures moving toward cooler temperatures. In other words, the transfer of heat will always be from hot to cold. As an example, the body skin temperature is normally about 90°F. If the outside temperature is 95°F, heat will be transferred from the outside air to the skin of the body. This causes the body to take on a greater heat load, thereby making the person feel warmer. The heat in this situation is moving down the thermal gradient from the warmer air to the cooler body. If the outside temperature is 65°F, the heat will be transferred from the warmer skin of the body to the cooler outside air. In this instance the thermal gradient is causing the movement of heat down a temperature gradient from the body to the ambient air. If the rate of heat loss starts to exceed the body's heat production, the skin will begin to cool excessively, and the peripheral thermoreceptors will pick up the drop in temperature. In response, the patient begins to feel cool and may try to generate heat by moving about or shivering.

The body must maintain an optimum body temperature so that the cells can continue to function normally. In order to do so, the amount of heat lost by the body must equal the amount of heat gained by the body. If the amount of heat lost exceeds the amount of heat gained, the patient's body core temperature will begin to decrease. Likewise, the amount of heat gained must equal the amount of heat lost. If the amount of heat gained exceeds the ability of the body to lose heat, the body core temperature may begin to increase. The body continuously produces and conserves heat in order to balance heat production and heat loss.

Understanding BODY PROCESSES

The body must maintain an optimum body temperature so that cellular function can continue normally. If at any time the body cannot compensate for the amount of heat that is either gained or lost, resulting cellular and organ damage may lead to an environmental emergency. ■

How is heat produced? The body produces heat mainly through processes of metabolism, including digestion of food. The body also produces heat, increasing it by up to 400 percent, through shivering, which is nothing more than skeletal muscle movement. Skeletal muscle movement is an effective way to produce heat, which is why patients who are losing heat will frequently pace or otherwise move about and jump up and down in place. Keep in mind, though, that shivering will cease when the body core temperature drops to below 90°F (32°C). This is an ominous sign, since cooling occurs very rapidly once shivering has stopped. Hormones such as thyroxin from the thyroid gland and epinephrine from the adrenal gland will increase the metabolic rate of the body and produce heat as a by-product.

How is heat conserved? In a cool or cold environment, the body conserves heat by constricting blood vessels (vasoconstriction) and sending warm blood from the surface of the skin to internal organs. Hair on the skin surface erects (piloerection), thickening the layer of warm air that is trapped immediately next to the skin. (However, piloerection has been shown to have little effect in conserving heat in humans, especially when there is a breeze blowing.) Little or no perspiration is released to the skin surface, preventing cooling by evaporation. The patient may attempt to reduce heat loss by decreasing the surface area of the body through folding his arms across his chest, adding more clothing, or drawing his body up close in a fetal position.

The body also has an elaborate system for cooling itself. There are three organ systems primarily responsible for cooling the body and reducing the body core temper-

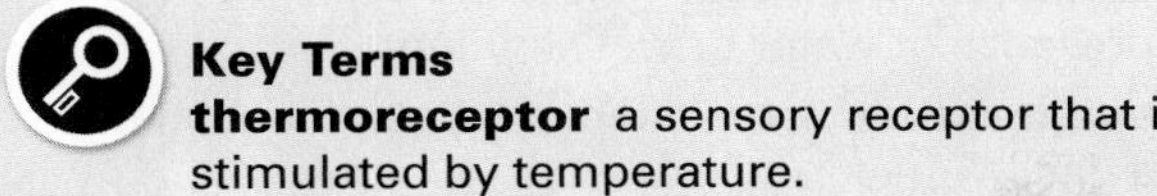

Key Terms
thermoreceptor a sensory receptor that is stimulated by temperature.

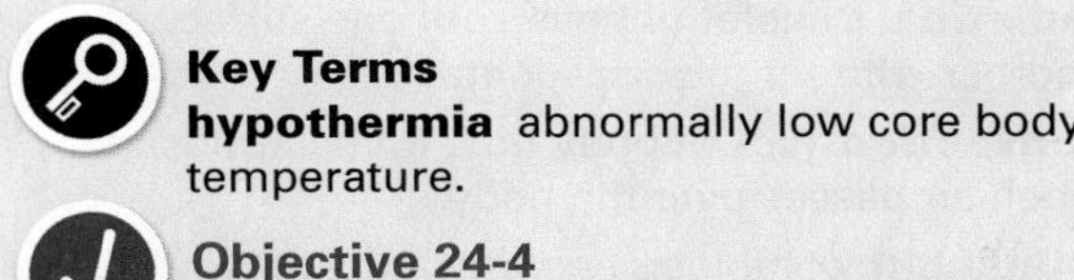

Key Terms
hypothermia abnormally low core body temperature.

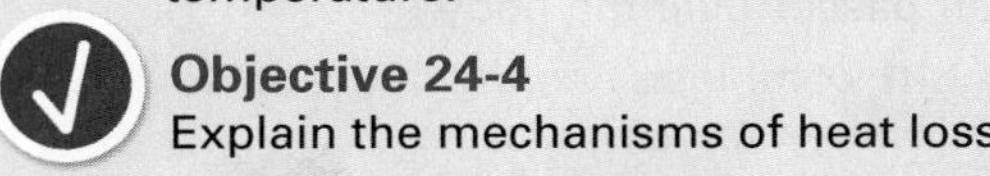

Objective 24-4
Explain the mechanisms of heat loss.

ature: (1) the skin, (2) the cardiovascular system, and (3) the respiratory system. As the core temperature rises, the warmed blood travels to the periphery, and blood vessels near the skin's surface dilate. An increased flow of warmed blood near the skin helps dissipate excess heat through radiation and convection (see the later explanation). However, this cooling system works only if the ambient air is cooler than the skin temperature. If the outside air is as warm as, or warmer than, the temperature of the skin, the body relies on dissipation of the heat through the evaporation of sweat from the skin surface. The cardiovascular system responds to increasing heat loads by elevating the heart rate and increasing the strength of contractions so that more blood can move to the surface of the skin to be cooled. Also, the increase in cardiac output maintains the blood pressure as the peripheral vessels dilate. Finally, the respiratory system contributes to the cooling of the body by eliminating heat through evaporation during exhalation.

Understanding BODY PROCESSES

The body relies on three body systems—skin, cardiovascular, and respiratory—to help maintain a normal temperature when the body becomes too warm. ■

When Heat Lost Exceeds Heat Gained

When the body loses more heat than it gains or produces, the result is **hypothermia**, or low body temperature (<95°F). As mentioned earlier, heat loss occurs through five mechanisms: radiation, convection, conduction, evaporation, and respiration (Figure 24-1*). As an EMT,

MECHANISMS OF HEAT LOSS

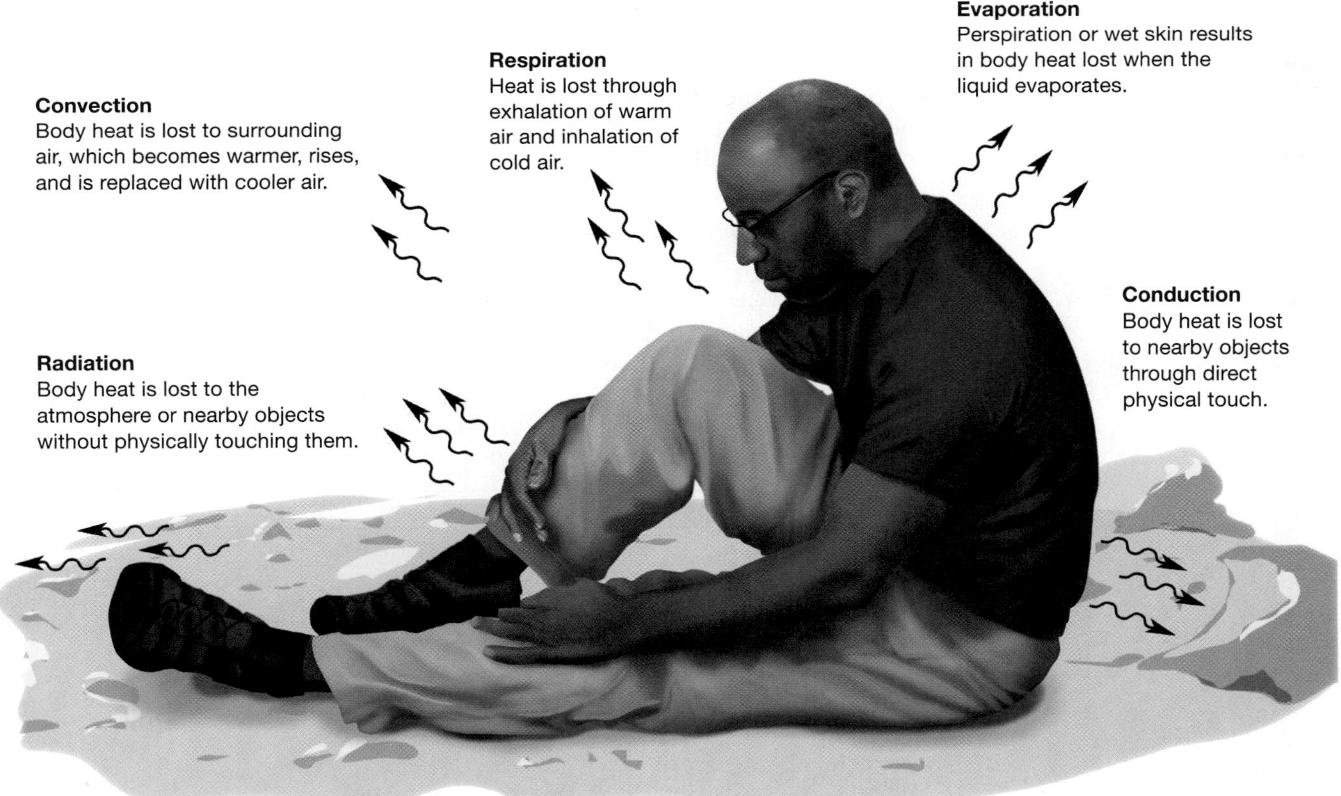

Evaporation
Perspiration or wet skin results in body heat lost when the liquid evaporates.
Respiration
Heat is lost through exhalation of warm air and inhalation of cold air.
Convection
Body heat is lost to surrounding air, which becomes warmer, rises, and is replaced with cooler air.
Conduction
Body heat is lost to nearby objects through direct physical touch.
Radiation
Body heat is lost to the atmosphere or nearby objects without physically touching them.

FIGURE 24-1 * The illustration shows a situation in which a wet, poorly dressed climber has taken shelter in a crevasse or among cold, wet rocks.

Key Terms

radiation transfer of heat from one surface to another without physical contact.

convection loss of body heat to the atmosphere when air passes over the body.

wind chill combined cooling effect of wind speed and environmental temperature.

Key Terms

conduction transfer of heat through direct physical touch with nearby objects.

water chill increase in rate of cooling in the presence of water or wet clothing.

evaporation conversion of a liquid or solid into a gas.

you must be aware of the ways in which heat is lost so that you can be alert to a situation in which a patient may be suffering from hypothermia, and so that you can protect the hypothermic patient from further heat loss.

Radiation The most significant mechanism of heat loss is **radiation**, which involves the transfer of heat from the surface of one object to the surface of another without physical contact. Most heat loss through radiation is from the head, hands, and feet. This is why it is so important to cover a newborn's head after birth.

The amount of heat a person loses through radiation depends also on environmental conditions. In a temperate climate and under normal conditions, a person loses about 55–65 percent of his heat production by radiation. At a temperature of 90°F, however, radiation loss will probably drop to zero. In subzero temperatures, it will drastically increase as body heat is transferred to the atmosphere.

Convection The process of **convection** causes cold air molecules that are in immediate contact with the skin to be warmed. The heated air molecules move away, and cooler ones take their place. Those in turn are warmed, and the process starts all over again. Anything that speeds movement of the air, such as the wind, also speeds the cooling process. That is where the concept of **wind chill** comes into understanding and predicting hypothermia (Figure 24-2*).

A unit of wind chill is the amount of heat that would be lost in an hour from a square meter of exposed skin surface with a normal temperature of 91.4°F. In essence, the wind-chill factor combines the effects of the wind speed and environmental temperature into a number that indicates the danger of exposure. For example, on a windless day, exposed flesh will normally freeze in less than 1 minute at a temperature of –70°F. Because of the wind-chill factor, the same results will occur at a temperature of –20°F if there is a wind speed of between 20 and 25 mph.

Conduction The mechanism of **conduction** causes body heat to be lost through direct contact. Water conducts heat 240 times faster than air, and conduction is the method of heat loss in **water chill**. This means that water and wet clothing will conduct heat away from the body at a much higher rate than air and dry clothing and much more rapidly than the body can produce it. This is an important factor in drowning. Conduction and convection combined produce about 15 percent of heat loss.

Evaporation The process in which a liquid or solid changes to a vapor is called **evaporation.** Evaporation has a cooling effect. When body heat causes the body to per-

WIND-CHILL INDEX

WIND SPEED (MPH)	WHAT THE THERMOMETER READS (degrees °F)											
	50	40	30	20	10	0	–10	–20	–30	–40	–50	–60
	WHAT IT EQUALS IN ITS EFFECT ON EXPOSED FLESH											
CALM	50	40	30	20	10	0	–10	–20	–30	–40	–50	–60
5	48	37	27	16	6	–5	–15	–26	–36	–47	–57	–68
10	40	28	16	4	–9	–21	–33	–46	–58	–70	–83	–95
15	36	22	9	–5	–18	–36	–45	–58	–72	–85	–99	–112
20	32	18	4	–10	–25	–39	–53	–67	–82	–96	–110	–121
25	30	16	0	–15	–29	–44	–59	–74	–88	–104	–118	–133
30	28	13	–2	–18	–33	–48	–63	–79	–94	–109	–125	–140
35	27	11	–4	–20	–35	–49	–67	–82	–98	–113	–129	–145
40	26	10	–6	–21	–37	–53	–69	–85	–100	–116	–132	–148
	Little danger if properly clothed				Danger of freezing exposed flesh			Great danger of freezing exposed flesh				

Source: U.S. Army

FIGURE 24-2 * Wind-chill index.

Key Terms

respiration the exchange of gases between an organism and its environment.

hyperthermia abnormally high core body temperature.

Objective 24-5

Explain the mechanisms of heat gain.

Key Terms

generalized hypothermia an overall reduction in body temperature, affecting the entire body.

Objective 24-6

Describe the pathophysiology of generalized hypothermia.

spire and the perspiration evaporates, the heat that has been absorbed by the sweat is dissipated into the air, and the body surface is cooled. When air temperature equals or exceeds skin temperature, evaporation is the only way the body has of losing heat. Heat loss through evaporation is also affected by the relative humidity of the air. A relative humidity of 75 percent will significantly reduce the effectiveness of evaporation, whereas a relative humidity of 90 percent will cause evaporation to become essentially ineffective. This is evident on humid days when sweat seems to accumulate on the surface of the skin without drying.

The sweating mechanism has its limits. The normal adult can sweat only about 1 liter per hour and can sweat at that rate for only a few hours at a time. In addition, sweating only cools the body effectively if the relative humidity of the air is low. As just mentioned, when the air humidity is high, the water vapor contained in the air inhibits the evaporation of moisture from the skin surface. During intense exercise, about 85 percent of heat loss occurs through sweating. Under normal conditions, however, evaporation combined with heat loss through respiration comprises approximately 20–30 percent of heat loss.

Respiration Breathing, or **respiration**, also produces heat loss. A person breathes in cold air from the atmosphere and breathes out air that has been warmed and humidified inside the lungs and the airway. Some of the body's heat is carried away with the exhalation of this warm, humidified air. Respiration alone comprises about 10–20 percent of heat loss under normal circumstances.

Understanding BODY PROCESSES

Heat loss leading to hypothermia can be from conduction, convection, radiation, evaporation, and/or respiration. ■

When Heat Gained Exceeds Heat Lost

When the amount of heat the body produces or gains exceeds the amount the body loses through the processes just described, the result is **hyperthermia**, or high body temperature. At times, the body may produce more heat than needed even at moderate air temperatures, or may fail to cool the body when needed by not recognizing an increasing core temperature (from certain medical conditions or as a response to certain medications). However, in most cases, hyperthermia occurs in a hot environment. Hyperthermia is most common in situations where the air temperature is high, the humidity is high, and there is little or no breeze.

Understanding BODY PROCESSES

Hyperthermia, or a high body temperature, occurs when the body is unable to cool itself effectively. ■

Exposure to Cold

Exposure to cold can cause two kinds of emergencies. One is generalized hypothermia, also called a generalized cold emergency, which is an overall reduction in body temperature affecting the entire body. The other is local cold injury, or damage to body tissues in a specific (local) part or parts of the body.

Generalized Hypothermia

Generalized hypothermia results from an increase in the body's heat loss, a decrease in the body's heat production, or both. It is the most life-threatening cold injury because it affects the entire body. Mortality (death) from generalized hypothermia can be as high as 87 percent.

Hypothermia can have a sudden onset, as when someone falls through ice, or a gradual onset, as from prolonged exposure to wind, cold air, or cool water.

Pathophysiology of Generalized Hypothermia

In general, thermal control (the ability of the body to regulate its temperature) is lost once the body temperature is lowered to 95°F (35°C). Coma (deep unresponsiveness, severely depressed vital signs) occurs when the body's core temperature reaches approximately 79°F (26°C). Cases have been documented in which patients have survived after reaching a core temperature as low as 64.4°F (17.7°C). Death can occur within 2 hours of the first signs and symptoms of generalized hypothermia (Figure 24-3*). The most important phase of management with hypothermic patients is the first 30 minutes following rescue and during the transport time to the hospital.

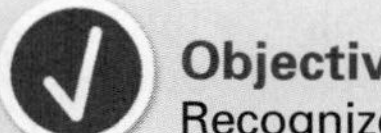

Objective 24-7
Recognize factors that contribute to a patient's risk for hypothermia, (including immersion hypothermia, urban hypothermia, and myxedema coma or hypothyroidism).

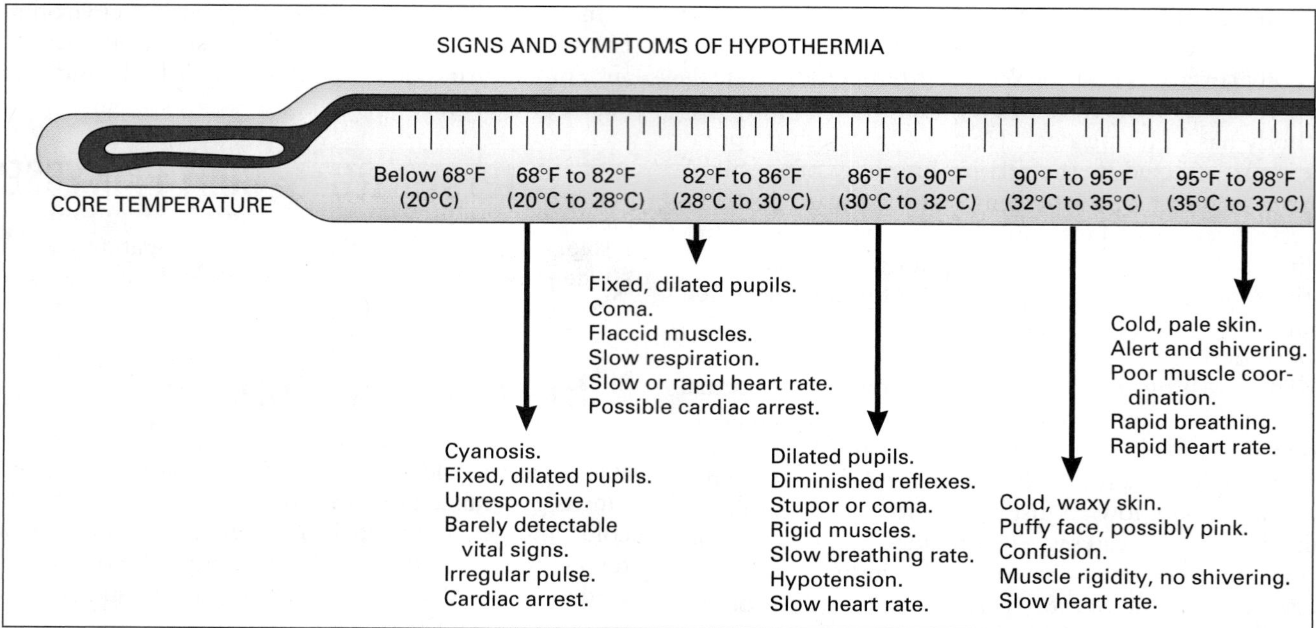

FIGURE 24-3 ✱ Signs and symptoms of a sinking core temperature.

Predisposing Factors

Risk factors for generalized hypothermia include:

- **Ambient temperature, wind chill, and moisture.** Extremely low temperatures are not necessary for hypothermia to occur. It can occur in temperatures as high as 65°F, depending on the wind-chill factor. Wetness, either from perspiration or immersion in water (or rain), always compounds the problem and increases the risk of hypothermia (Figure 24-4✱).
- **Age.** People who are at the extremes of age, such as infants (especially newborns) and toddlers and the elderly, are at increased risk of hypothermia. Infants and young children have a large surface area in relation to their overall size, increasing both the amount and speed of heat loss. The ability to shiver (a heat-producing mechanism) is not well developed in children and does not exist in infants because of their small muscle mass. Both the very young and very old tend to have less body fat, which also contributes to heat loss. The elderly have an impaired recognition of cold, a diminished basal metabolism, and poor constriction of blood vessels in the extremities (a heat-conserving mechanism). This can lead to a condition known as *urban hypothermia* (discussed later), in which an elderly person becomes hypothermic in his own home. Infants and young children are unable to use adaptive behaviors, such as moving to a warm environment or putting on warmer clothing.
- **Medical conditions.** At increased risk for hypothermia are people who have had recent surgery or who have shock, head injury, burns, generalized infection, spinal cord injuries, thyroid gland disorders, and diabetic emergencies such as hypoglycemia. The outcome of a trauma patient with hypothermia is dramatically worsened.
- **Alcohol, drugs, and poisons.** Some drugs, alcohol, and poisons can increase the risk of hypothermia. Substances that impair heat-generating or heat-conserving mechanisms include narcotics, alcohol, antiseizure medications, antihistamines, sedatives, antidepressants, and pain medications such as aspirin, acetaminophen, and nonsteroidal anti-inflammatory drugs.
- **Duration of exposure.** The longer the time a person spends unprotected in a cold environment, the greater the chance that he will become hypothermic.
- **Clothing.** Clothing that is inappropriate for the temperature will allow a person to lose heat at a greater rate than if he had layers of clothing for cold environments. Layers of clothing provide insulation from the cold and protect against excessive heat loss. A hat

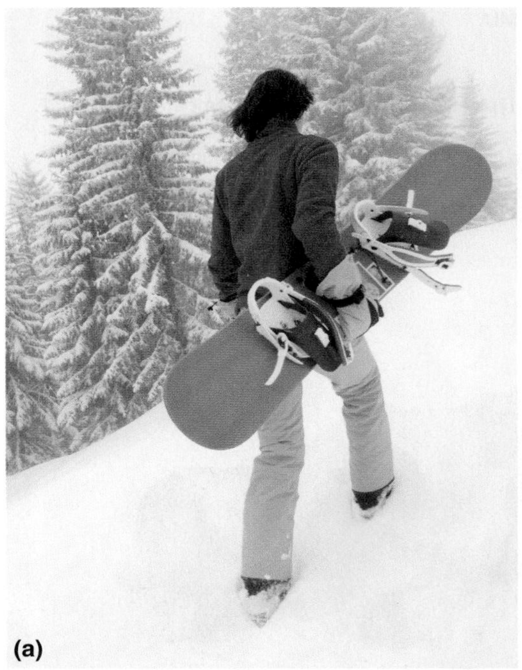
(a)

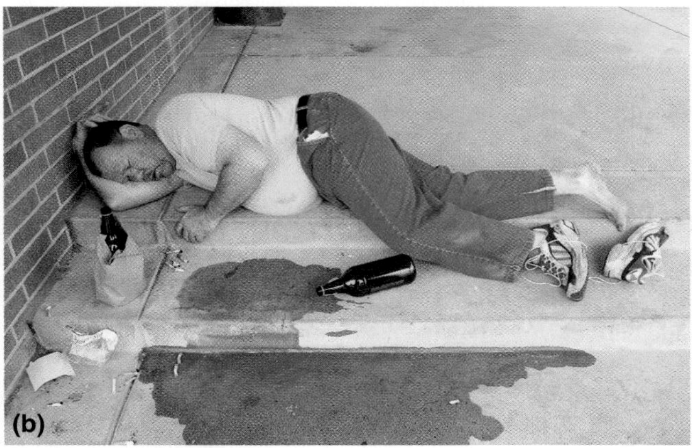
(b)

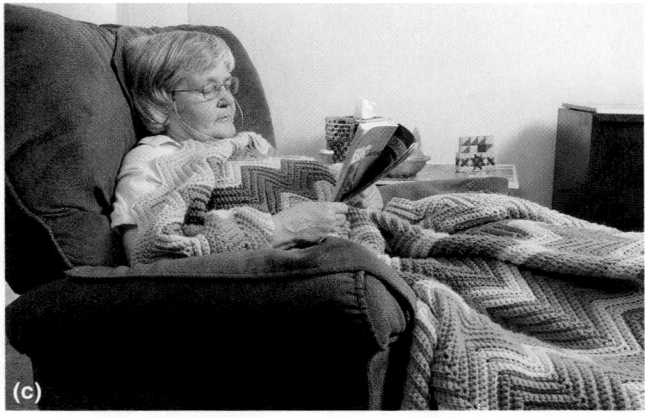
(c)

FIGURE 24-4 ✱ Hypothermia can occur in cold or merely cool environments. All of the persons in these photographs are subject to possible hypothermia: **(a)** a person dressed too lightly for outdoor activity on a very cold day, (Photo a: © Corbis), **(b)** a person sleeping outdoors on a cool surface in cool weather, **(c)** an elderly person living in an inadequately heated home.

reduces heat loss from the head, and appropriate gloves and boots protect against local cold injury. Clothing that doesn't protect against rain and moisture and allows the body to become wet will contribute to the rate of cooling. If in a body of water, it is recommended that a person keep his clothing on to trap a layer of water between the skin and the clothing. This layer of water will be heated by the body and will provide something of a warm insulating water layer.

- **Activity level**. Physical activity requires muscular movement that produces heat as a by-product (thermogenic). Thus, a person who continues to move may generate internal heat that maintains the body's core temperature at a higher level than if he was not moving. In order to continue to move, however, the person must have an adequate amount of fuel in the form of carbohydrates, protein, or fat. In addition, the person must drink an adequate amount of water to remain hydrated. A person in a body of cold water who continues to move may cool faster from convection. As the person continues to tread water, he moves cold water molecules next to his skin, which promotes cooling at a faster rate. If instead he curls into a ball and floats, the water around him will become warmer from his body heat and his curled-up position will lessen the cooling from convection.

Stages of Hypothermia

Hypothermia can occur with little warning and can progress very rapidly. Initial reactions to cold exposure are increases in the basal metabolic rate, muscular shivering, and "goosebumps" (caused by piloerection). All of these are thermogenic in nature. However, in hypothermia, these compensatory mechanisms are not enough to maintain body temperature. As the core temperature drops, the body's thermal-regulating mechanism and perception become confused. A person, even though dangerously cold, may undress, thinking he is too warm. The five stages of hypothermia are illustrated in Figure 24-5✱.

Immersion Hypothermia

Immersion hypothermia occurs as a result of the lowering of the body temperature from immersion in cool or cold water. You should consider the possibility of immersion hypothermia in all cases of accidental immersion. Familiarize yourself with normal spring, summer, fall, and winter river and lake temperatures in your community.

Body temperature can drop to the water temperature in as little as 10 minutes in some circumstances. In fact, body temperature drops 25 to 30 times faster in water than in air of the same temperature (Figure 24-6✱). Extra fat layers tend to insulate people from cooling. Pound

STAGES OF HYPOTHERMIA

Stage 1: Shivering is a response by the body to generate heat. It does not typically occur below a body temperature of 90° F.

Stage 2: Apathy and decreased muscle function. First fine motor function is affected, then gross motor functions.

Stage 3: Decreased level of responsiveness is accompanied by a glassy stare and possible freezing of extremities.

Stage 4: Decreased vital signs, including slow pulse and slow respiration rate.

Stage 5: Death.

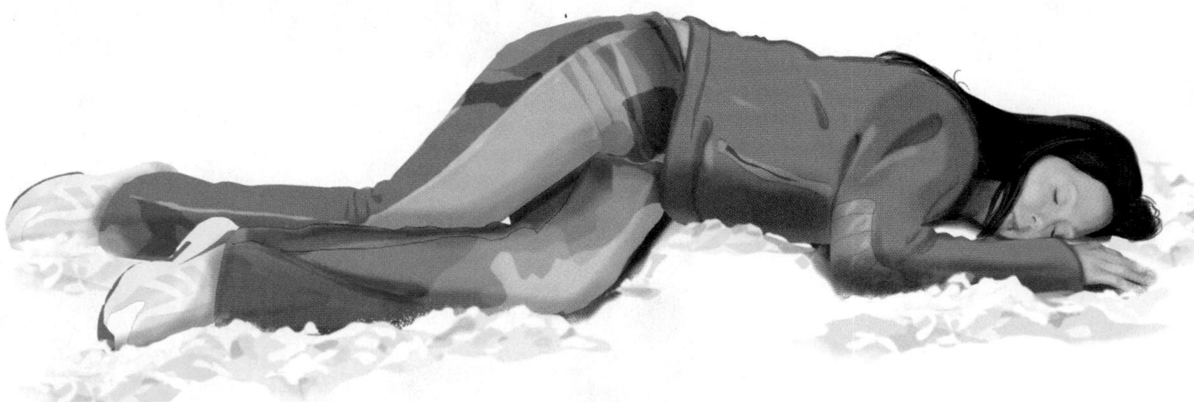

FIGURE 24-5 ✱ Hypothermia is an acute medical emergency requiring immediate attention.

for pound, adult women have greater resistance to heat loss in cold water than men. Similarly, adults can withstand the cold longer than children, and girls have more resistance than boys. Layers of clothing can help to insulate a patient in the water.

Contrary to the popular idea that people die in water only when the water temperature approaches freezing, death can occur within a few minutes when the water is 50°F. The priority with a patient immersed in cool or cold water is getting him out of the water as rapidly as possible and then out of his wet clothes and into a warm environment.

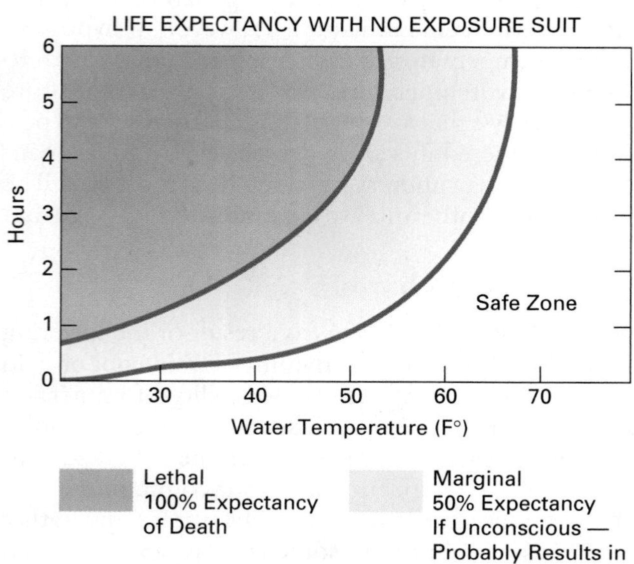

FIGURE 24-6 ✱ Effects of water temperature on survival in cold-water immersion.

Urban Hypothermia

Urban hypothermia, although not clearly defined in medical literature, occurs in those individuals who have a predisposition, disability, illness, or medication usage that renders them more susceptible to hypothermia. Predisposing factors include situations that result in increased heat loss (such as the very young or very old, because of their lower amount of body fat), interference with heat production from medical illnesses or medication use, alterations in mental status, or limited mobility that make the person unable to take protective measures to minimize heat loss.

Urban hypothermia can be further subdivided into two general etiologies: external and internal. The "external" category includes patients who are subject to hypothermia because they do not have the access to a warm environment during the cold months. These are patients who live on the streets or try to take refuge in shelters for the homeless. Because of a lack of access at times during cold temperatures, these patients may be found outdoors in a city without adequate shelter or clothing to keep them warm. This category of patients may suffer from hypothermia not from a medical or traumatic cause, but simply from lack of protection from the cold environment.

Key Terms
urban hypothermia hypothermia precipitated by a too cool indoor or outdoor environment.

Key Points
An elderly person can become hypothermic in an indoor environment that feels comfortable to a much younger EMT.

Key Terms
myxedema coma a life-threatening late complication of hypothyroidism.

local cold injury damage from cold exposure to tissues in a specific part of the body.

Objective 24-8
Describe the pathophysiology of local cold injury.

Urban hypothermia may also occur when the person is indoors. This "internal" category of urban hypothermia includes patients (typically the elderly) who are subject to colder temperatures in the winter months when they attempt to minimize heating bills to save money. Since the elderly commonly have a limited ability to sense cold, coupled with decreased tissue insulation, they may become hypothermic in their own home without realizing hypothermia's insidious onset.

The elderly patient may also be hypothermic even though the outside temperature is warm. Consider the elderly patient who lives in an air-conditioned home in the summer months when it would not be uncommon to have the indoor temperature set at 70°F–72°F. Should this same elderly patient slip while getting out of the shower and fall onto the bathroom floor, resulting in a broken hip, he will be immobile until discovered by someone else. Since most bathrooms have tiled floors, which hold cold temperatures, an elderly patient who is forced to lie on this surface for a prolonged period may become hypothermic. A patient in an air-conditioned environment who has decreased tissue insulation and inability to move from a cold surface is a prime candidate for urban hypothermia, even on a warm day.

ASSESSMENT Tips

Do not overlook the possibility of hypothermia in an elderly (or pediatric) patient who has been subject to the cool ambient temperatures of air-conditioned buildings. ■

Myxedema Coma

As mentioned earlier, certain medical illnesses and diseases may make a person more susceptible to becoming hypothermic. One such disease is hypothyroidism. Hypothyroidism is a clinical syndrome characterized by an absence or severe deficiency of a hormone secreted by the thyroid. The absence of this hormone causes metabolic processes to slow significantly. Symptoms of hypothyroidism can manifest in all organ systems and include a dull facial expression. The voice is often hoarse and the speech may be slow and drawn out. There is commonly facial puffiness and periorbital swelling with droopy eyelids. The hair appears sparse, coarse, and dry, and the skin appears coarse and dry. There is commonly weight gain. The patient's mental status may become altered, and forgetfulness is common. Hypothyroidism may also precipitate sudden psychosis (a condition called myxedema madness). The disease is typically chronic, occurring over months to years.

Myxedema coma is a complication that occurs late in the progression of hypothyroidism and can be fatal. It occurs most commonly in elderly women who present with extreme hypothermia (core temperatures often 75°F–90°F (24°C–32.2°C), seizures, slow reflexes, and respiratory depression. Although myxedema coma occurs rarely (in only 0.1 percent of hypothyroidism patients), it is a true emergency, as death from this complication is likely. Precipitating factors for the condition include exposure to cold temperatures, a recent illness or infection, trauma, and the use of drugs that depress the central nervous system. EMT treatment for this condition is limited to supporting lost functions of airway, breathing, and circulation. It is best if the EMT contacts medical direction regarding the rewarming techniques to be utilized for the severely hypothermic patient with myxedema coma.

Local Cold Injury

Local cold injury, the condition commonly called "frostbite," results from the freezing of body tissue. Local cold injury requires much colder temperatures than are needed to produce generalized hypothermia. Such a local cold injury often accompanies generalized hypothermia; in cases where it does, emergency medical care for hypothermia always takes precedence over care for the local injury.

Pathophysiology of Local Cold Injury

Local cold injury occurs when ice crystals form between the cells of the skin and then expand as they extract fluid from the cells. Circulation is obstructed, causing additional damage to the tissue. Such injuries tend to occur on the hands, feet, ears, nose, and cheeks, which are most commonly exposed to cold.

Predisposing Factors

The following factors can increase the likelihood of a person suffering a local cold injury:

- Any kind of trauma (always check for local cold injury on people injured in cold weather)

- Extremes of age (especially elderly and newborn)
- Tight or tightly laced footwear, which tends to diminish perfusion to the feet
- Use of alcohol during exposure to cold
- Wet clothing
- High altitudes
- Loss of blood
- Arteriosclerosis

Stages of Local Cold Injury

Local cold injuries fall into two basic categories: early or superficial injury and late or deep injury (Figure 24-7*):

- ***Early or superficial cold injury*** usually involves the tips of the ears, the nose, the cheekbones, the tips of the toes or fingers, and the chin. The patient is usually unaware of the injury, which commonly develops after direct contact with a cold object, cold air, or cold water. As exposure time lengthens or temperature drops, the patient will lose feeling and sensation in the affected area, and the skin may begin to turn a waxy gray or yellow color. The skin remains soft but cold to the touch, and normal skin color does not return after palpation. If the affected area is rewarmed, the patient will usually report a tingling sensation as the area thaws and circulation improves.
- ***Late or deep cold injury*** involves both the skin and tissue beneath it. The skin itself is white and waxy in appearance. Palpation of the affected area will reveal a firm to completely solid, frozen feeling. The injury may involve the whole hand or foot. Swelling and blisters filled with clear or straw-colored fluid may be present (Figure 24-8a*). As the area thaws, it may become blotchy or mottled, with colors from white to purple to grayish blue (Figure 24-8b*). Deep cold injury is an extreme emergency and can result in permanent tissue loss.

Assessment-Based Approach: Cold-Related Emergency

Scene Size-Up

Your first step should be to ensure your own safety and that of your partner. Do not put yourself in danger by attempting to make rescues for which you are not properly trained or prepared.

For example, you might be called to a scene at which a skater has fallen through the ice on a pond and is par-

STAGES OF LOCAL COLD INJURY

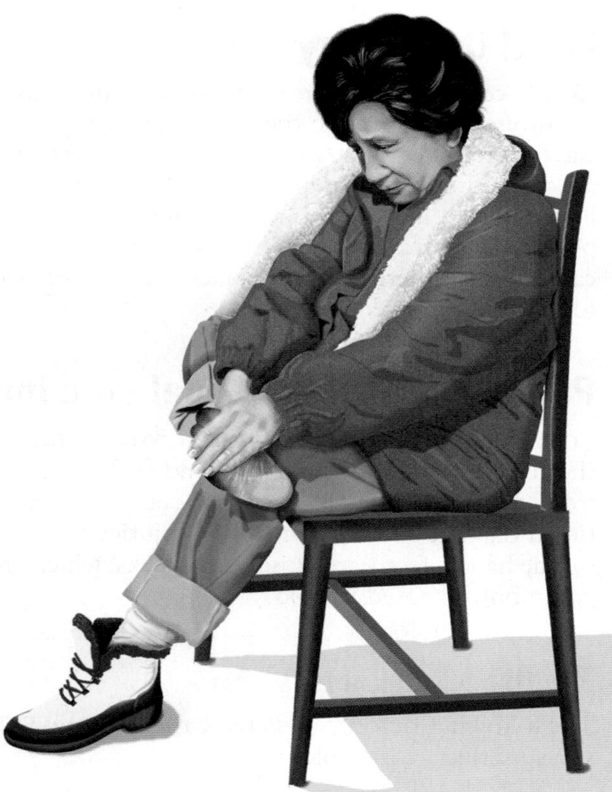

EARLY OR SUPERFICIAL COLD INJURY
usually involves the tips of the ears, the nose, the cheek bones, the tips of the toes or fingers, and the chin. The patient is usually unaware of the injury. As exposure time lengthens or temperature drops, the patient will lose feeling and sensation in the affected area. The skin remains soft but cold to the touch, and normal skin color does not return after palpation. As the area rewarms, the patient may report a tingling sensation.

LATE OR DEEP COLD INJURY
involves both the skin and tissue beneath it. The skin itself is white and waxy with a firm to completely solid, frozen feeling. Swelling and blisters filled with clear or straw-colored fluid may be present. As the area thaws, it may become blotchy or mottled, with colors from white to purple to grayish-blue. Deep cold injury is an extreme emergency and can result in permanent tissue loss.

FIGURE 24-7 * Local cold injuries may progress from early or superficial to late or deep.

Objective 24-9
Discuss the assessment-based approach to cold-related emergencies.

Key Points
Hypothermia can occur after prolonged exposure when the ambient temperature goes no lower than 65°F.

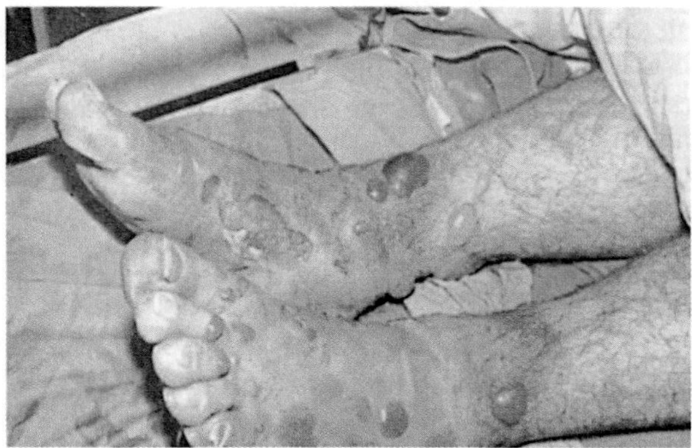

FIGURE 24-8a ✱ In late or deep cold injury, the skin may appear white and waxy and feel firm to solidly frozen. Swelling and blisters may be present.

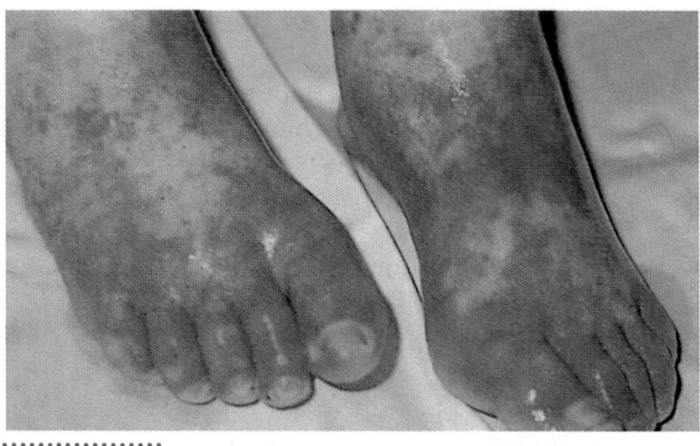

FIGURE 24-8b ✱ As a late or deep cold injury thaws, it may become blotchy or mottled and colored from white to purple to grayish blue.

tially or completely immersed when you arrive. Your first reaction would probably be to go immediately to his aid by walking out onto the ice. You must stop and consider the situation, noting that the ice is obviously unstable, resulting in one person already having broken through. Walking out onto the ice would likely make you a second hypothermia patient at best or a drowning victim at worst. Without adequate ropes and gear such as ladders or boats to reach the patient (and training in how to use them), you should await the arrival of rescuers from the fire department or other agencies.

Cold temperatures and high winds pose hazards for EMT crews. Be prepared for exposure to the cold by putting on layered clothing before leaving the station. You may get called to the scene of an automobile crash where a patient is trapped in the vehicle. The extrication time may be lengthy and you may be exposed to the cold for a prolonged period while treating the patient inside the vehicle.

Cold weather conditions can create or exacerbate unstable environments. Ice may make normally secure surfaces slippery. Snow may pile up on roofs or slopes and suddenly collapse or avalanche. Snow or sleet storms reduce visibility on roads.

Once you have taken appropriate measures to ensure your own safety at the scene, and that of your crew, consider how the characteristics of the scene may have affected the patient. Be alert for signs or evidence of how the patient interacted with the environment before your arrival. Things to look for include the following:

- *Is the patient protected from the cold environment?*
- *Is the ambient (surrounding air) temperature cool or cold?*
- *Does the scene indicate the possibility for urban hypothermia, even though the nature of the call was something different?* As mentioned previously, the EMT may be called for a patient with a suspected broken hip, but upon arrival the patient may also be mildly hypothermic because of the environment.
- *Is the wind blowing?*
- *Does it appear that the patient has been outside for a prolonged period of time?* Is he lying in a driveway, on a porch, or in a garage? Is he in a remote area where a long time might have elapsed before he was discovered? This may be particularly true with snowmobile operators, skiers, hikers, hunters, and people involved in car crashes in remote areas.

Hypothermia can occur after prolonged exposure when the ambient temperature goes no lower than 65°F. You may, for example, encounter a patient who has become intoxicated and fallen asleep on a park bench. The combination of the patient's alcohol consumption and his prolonged exposure, even though the temperature that night never got below 65°F, should alert you to consider the possibility of hypothermia.

- *Is the patient's clothing wet?* This could occur from immersion in a body of water or from rain, snow, sleet, or perspiration.
- *Is the patient properly dressed for the environment?* Finding a patient outside in the snow wearing only a bathrobe should lead you to consider the possibility of hypothermia.

- *What is the temperature inside a residence?* Hypothermia does not occur only outdoors. Many people on low or fixed incomes keep thermostats low to save on heating costs. This practice may again lead to urban hypothermia, especially in the elderly with limited mobility.
- *Is there any evidence that a patient has ingested alcohol or has been using drugs?* These can decrease a person's ability to tolerate or compensate for heat loss.
- *Does the patient have any injury that may interfere with normal thermoregulation such as a spinal injury or a head injury?*

Primary Assessment

Gather a general impression of the patient. Is the patient dressed appropriately for the weather conditions? Is his posture stiff or does he appear to be rigid? The patient may be staggering or appear uncoordinated. His mental status will deteriorate with the level of hypothermia. He may appear drowsy or irrational or may be completely unresponsive in severe cases.

Closely assess the airway, especially in the unresponsive patient. It may be necessary to perform a manual maneuver to establish and maintain an open airway. Early in hypothermia, the breathing rate may be increased and of a normal depth. As the body temperature decreases, however, the respirations will become slow and shallow and eventually absent. As the body core temperature decreases to less than 93°F (34°C), the carbon dioxide production begins to decline as the cell metabolism slows down drastically. At approximately 86°F (30°C), the carbon dioxide production will decrease by about 50 percent for every 8-degree Celsius drop in temperature. Carbon dioxide is the major stimulus to breathe in the normal patient. Thus, a decrease in carbon dioxide production will decrease the drive to breathe, causing the respiratory rate and tidal volume to decrease and eventually become ineffective.

Be prepared to provide positive pressure ventilation with supplemental oxygen if the breathing is inadequate. If the patient is breathing adequately, as evidenced by an acceptable respiratory rate and good alveolar breath sounds, administer oxygen, warmed and humidified if possible, by a nonrebreather mask at 15 lpm. Insertion of a nasal or oral airway was once thought to precipitate cardiac dysrhythmias such as ventricular fibrillation in the hypothermic patient. This belief is now falling into question, as some recent studies are suggesting that aggressive airway management does not increase the risk of precipitating ventricular fibrillation. In either situation, the use of an airway adjunct should be considered if necessary for establishing and maintaining the airway.

Check the carotid and radial pulses carefully. They may be difficult to find in the severely hypothermic patient. Early, the pulse rate may become elevated as the body's cardiovascular system responds to the heat loss, but it will continue to decrease with a falling core body temperature. If the pulse is completely absent, begin chest compressions with artificial ventilation. The skin may appear red early in hypothermia, but as the condition worsens, the skin too will change to pale, then cyanotic, then gray. As the skin continues to cool, it will become firm and cold to the touch.

ASSESSMENT Tips

The pulse, breathing, and blood pressure are difficult to assess in a hypothermic patient. The EMT should exercise due diligence in confirming the presence or absence of vital signs prior to the application of cardiopulmonary resuscitation. ■

The hypothermic patient is a priority for early transport. You should immediately remove the patient from the cold environment, remove any wet clothing, dry the patient thoroughly, and wrap the patient in warm blankets. Since the cold makes the heart very irritable, the patient could easily go into a cardiac dysrhythmia, especially ventricular fibrillation, so handle the patient gently.

Secondary Assessment

The secondary assessment should be conducted in the back of the warmed ambulance. Do not delay moving the patient out of the cold environment to conduct the exam. If the patient is responsive, gather a history. Document complaints of pain or of other symptoms. Determine if the patient is using any medications, especially drugs that might depress the central nervous system or cause blood vessels to dilate. A past medical history is important because the patient with pre-existing diseases or significant medical conditions may deteriorate much faster than the previously healthy individual. Determine the last intake of food and what the patient was doing prior to the incident. Determining how long the patient has been out in the cold is extremely important, because the longer he has been exposed, the more severe the hypothermia is likely to be.

If a mechanism of injury consistent with trauma is suspected or the patient complains of pain to several areas of the body, perform a physical exam. Look for evidence of trauma to the head, neck, or spine, and immobilize the spine. Look for any other evidence of injury to the chest, abdomen, or pelvis if trauma is suspected. Significant burns may lead to hypothermia because the skin's temperature-regulating functions have been destroyed with the destruction of the skin. Feel with your hand the warmth of the abdomen to get an idea of how cold the patient actually is. When assessing the extremities, be alert for signs of local cold injuries. The patient may experience a decrease in sensation in the extremities and may exhibit lack of coordination or difficulty in movement during motor assessment.

Key Points
Factors that predispose people to hypothermia are exposure to cold, age (very young or elderly), pre-existing medical conditions, and use of drugs, alcohol, or poisons.

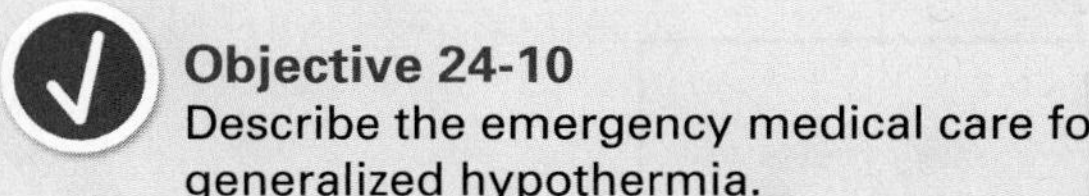

Objective 24-10
Describe the emergency medical care for generalized hypothermia.

The baseline vitals may reveal a blood pressure that decreases with a falling core body temperature. The heart rate will initially be increased but will fall with the temperature decrease. Respirations will be full initially with an increased rate, but will begin to decrease and become shallow as the hypothermia worsens. The skin early on will appear red, then turn pale, then cyanotic, then gray. It will eventually become cold and firm to the touch.

If the patient is unresponsive, perform a physical exam as already described, and attempt to gather information for the history from family or bystanders.

Signs and Symptoms of Generalized Hypothermia It is possible to measure the core body temperature only with a specialized thermometer. This measurement is not always practical in the field, but some EMS systems are using tympanic thermometers rather than the traditional glass thermometers, which must be inserted either orally or rectally. The thermometer used must be of a medical grade that records a broad range of temperatures (rather than traditional home thermometers that only measure a narrow range of temperatures). The tympanic thermometer's accuracy has come under question when it is used in environmental extremes in the prehospital setting. As an alternative, or in conjunction with a thermometer reading, the EMT can rely on presenting signs and symptoms in the assessment of generalized hypothermia.

Remember the factors predisposing people to hypothermia:

- Exposure to a cold environment
- Age (either very young or elderly)
- Pre-existing medical conditions
- Use of drugs (including medications such as beta blockers or antipsychotics), alcohol, or poisons

Be especially cautious for hypothermia when treating a patient who was resuscitated outside. Sometimes rescuers lose track of the time as they work on a patient in a snowbank or on an icy road. Remember that a patient in a motor vehicle is actually inside a microclimate. If the vehicle is involved in a collision, that microclimate can be disrupted, with the heat of the vehicle lost and the patient exposed to environmental conditions similar to those outside the vehicle. For temperature assessment, place the back of your hand on the patient's abdomen beneath the clothing. A patient with generalized hypothermia will have cool abdominal skin.

Signs and symptoms of generalized hypothermia include the following (Figure 24-9*):

- Decreasing mental status correlating with the degree of hypothermia:
  - Amnesia, memory lapses, and incoherence
  - Mood changes
  - Impaired judgment
  - Reduced ability to communicate
  - Dizziness
  - Vague, slow, slurred, or thick speech
  - Drowsiness progressing even to unresponsiveness to verbal or painful stimuli
- Decreasing motor and sensory function correlating with the degree of hypothermia:
  - Joint and/or muscle stiffness; muscle rigidity as hypothermia progresses; stiff or rigid posture
  - Lack of coordination
  - Apparent exhaustion or inability to get up after rest
  - Uncontrollable fits of shivering at first, with little or no shivering as hypothermia progresses
  - Reduced sensation or loss of sensation
- Changing vital signs:
  - Respiratory changes: rapid breathing at first; shallow and slow later; absent near the end
  - Changes in pulse: rapid pulse at first; slow and barely palpable pulse later; irregular or absent pulse near the end
  - Changes in skin color, from red in early stages, changing to pale, then cyanotic, and finally to gray, waxen, and hard; skin that is cold to the touch
  - Slowly responding pupils, typically dilated
  - Low to absent blood pressure

Emergency Medical Care for Generalized Hypothermia

The basic principles of emergency care for generalized hypothermia are:

- Preventing further heat loss
- Rewarming the patient as quickly and safely as possible
- Staying alert for complications

The steps to follow in care are these:

1. *The top priority is to remove the patient from the cold environment and to prevent further heat loss.* Remove any wet clothing, dry the patient, and use

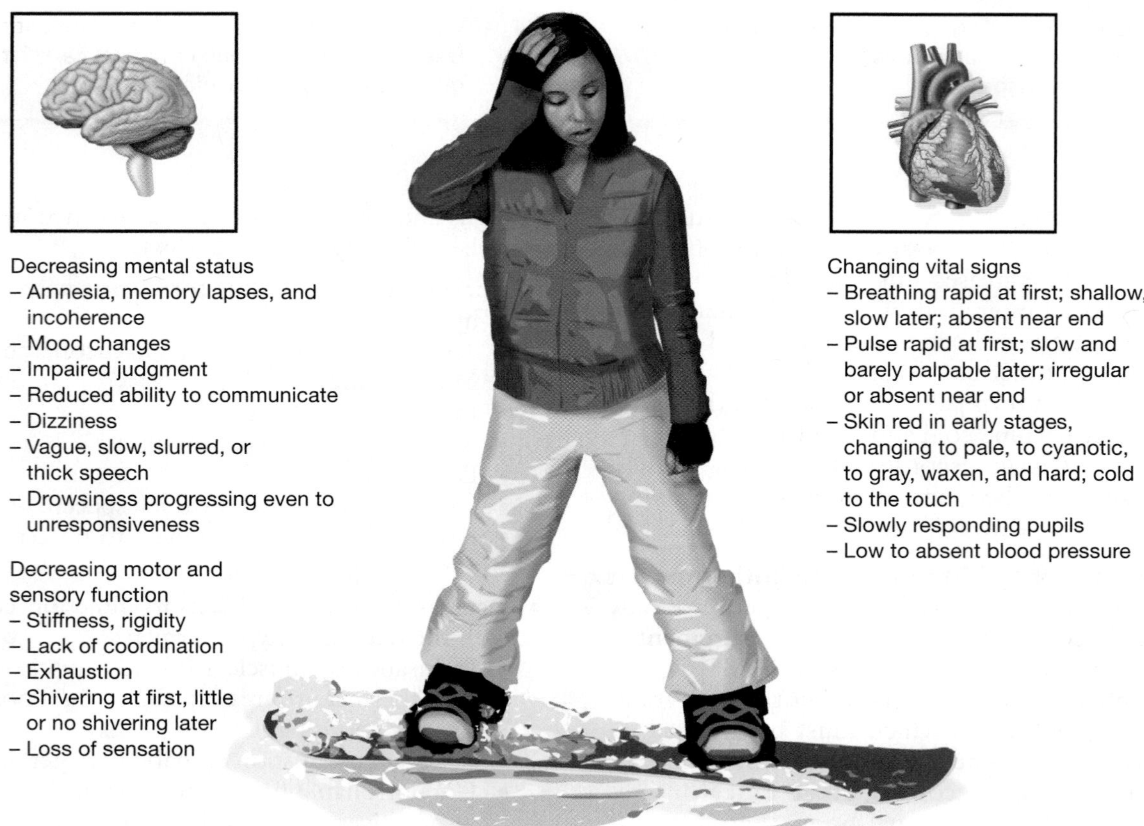
SIGNS AND SYMPTOMS OF HYPOTHERMIA
Decreasing mental status
– Amnesia, memory lapses, and incoherence
– Mood changes
– Impaired judgment
– Reduced ability to communicate
– Dizziness
– Vague, slow, slurred, or thick speech
– Drowsiness progressing even to unresponsiveness
Decreasing motor and sensory function
– Stiffness, rigidity
– Lack of coordination
– Exhaustion
– Shivering at first, little or no shivering later
– Loss of sensation
Changing vital signs
– Breathing rapid at first; shallow, slow later; absent near end
– Pulse rapid at first; slow and barely palpable later; irregular or absent near end
– Skin red in early stages, changing to pale, to cyanotic, to gray, waxen, and hard; cold to the touch
– Slowly responding pupils
– Low to absent blood pressure

FIGURE 24-9 * Signs and symptoms of hypothermia.

blankets to insulate the patient from the cold. Insulate the patient from the ground up; get something underneath the patient as quickly as possible. Remember to insulate the head. Protect the patient from exposure to the wind. You can help prevent further heat loss by using warm, humidified oxygen when possible.

2. *Handle the patient gently.* Rough handling can cause a cardiac dysrhythmia, especially ventricular fibrillation. (Cardiac arrest from ventricular fibrillation is a frequent cause of death in people with severe hypothermia.) Never allow the patient to walk or exert himself in any way. Even minor physical activity can disrupt the rhythm of the heart. Whenever possible, keep the patient in a supine position to increase blood flow to the brain. Elevate the patient's head if the patient has head or chest injuries, shortness of breath, or chest pains, or if the patient needs to be transported over steep terrain.
3. *Administer oxygen* if you have not already done so as part of the primary assessment. If possible, use warm, humidified oxygen. There is increasing evidence that the application of warm humidified oxygen can be extremely beneficial to the hypothermic patient during resuscitation. Do not aggressively ventilate or hyperventilate the patient. A patient with hypothermia has a reduced metabolism and need for oxygen, and unnecessary hyperventilation can cause further cardiac complications. In fact, a spontaneously breathing patient is probably getting adequate ventilation.
4. *If the patient goes into cardiac arrest from ventricular fibrillation or pulseless ventricular tachycardia, immediately initiate CPR beginning with chest compressions and apply the AED.* According to the AHA 2010 guidelines, if ventricular fibrillation or ventricular tachycardia persist after the initial defibrillation, it may be reasonable to continue to defibrillate as the patient is being rewarmed. Follow your local protocol. Continue CPR aggressively, since prolonged survival in cases of hypothermia has been reported. Respiration of only three or four breaths a minute and a pulse of five to ten beats per minute is enough to sustain life in a hypothermic patient.

Thinking Critically

You are participating in the rescue of a patient who fell into a ravine during a winter hike. The patient is clearly hypothermic but insists he can climb out of the ravine on his own two feet with just a bit of help from you. Is this a good idea? Why or why not?

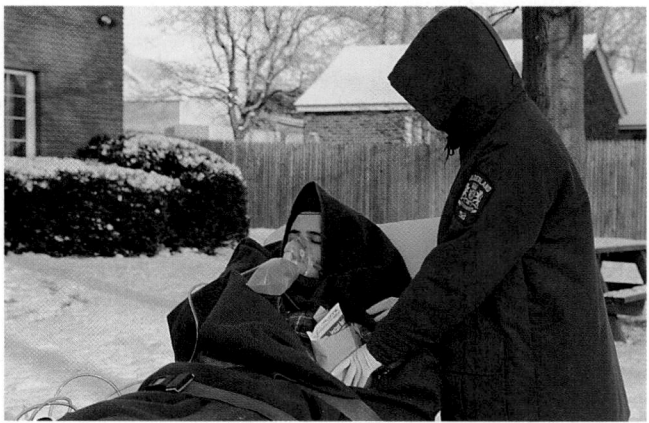

Key Terms

active rewarming technique of aggressively applying external sources of heat to a patient to rewarm his body.

passive rewarming the use of the patient's own heat production and conservation mechanisms to rewarm him.

5. *If the patient is alert and responding appropriately, actively rewarm him.* Note: Some experts advise active rewarming only if you are more than 30 minutes from the receiving facility. Follow medical direction and your local protocol for hypothermia treatment.

 Active rewarming is a technique of aggressively applying heat to warm the patient's body and includes these measures: wrapping the patient in warm blankets; placing heat packs or hot water bottles in the groin, in the armpits, and on the chest (Figure 24-10*); and turning up the heat in the patient compartment of the ambulance.

 Heat should be added to the patient gradually and gently; slower is safer in such cases. *Never immerse a patient in a tub of hot water or in a hot shower.* The body temperature should not be increased more than 1°F per hour. As a general rule, keep the patient's extremities protected from cold, but do not apply heat to them; the object is to rewarm the core body, and rewarming the extremities can be dangerous. Check the patient often to make sure you are not burning his skin with the hot packs or water bottles.

6. *If the patient is unresponsive or is not responding appropriately, do not actively rewarm; use only passive rewarming. Seek medical direction and follow local protocol.* **Passive rewarming** is taking measures to prevent further heat loss and giving the patient's body the optimum chance to rewarm itself. Passive rewarming includes inhibiting further heat loss by wrapping the patient in blankets and then increasing the heat in the patient compartment of the ambulance (Figure 24-11*). All hypothermic patients should receive passive rewarming.

FIGURE 24-10 * One way to actively warm the patient is to place heat packs in the groin, in the armpits, and on the chest. Insulate the packs to prevent burns.

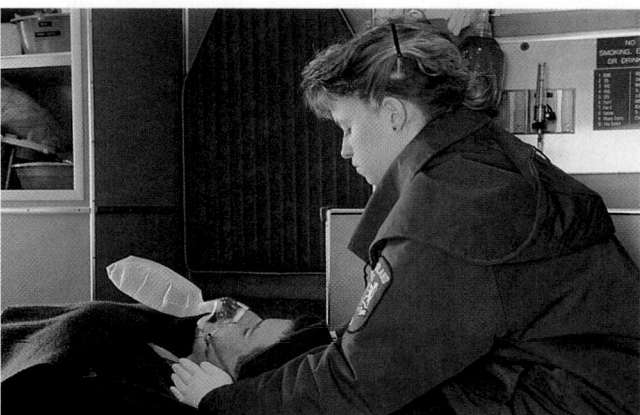

FIGURE 24-11 * Passive rewarming includes wrapping the patient in blankets and turning up the heat in the patient compartment.

7. *Do not allow the patient to consume stimulants,* including tobacco, coffee, or alcohol.
8. *Never rub or massage the patient's arms or legs.* You could force cold venous blood into the heart, resulting in cardiac irritability or cardiac arrest.
9. *Transport as quickly as possible.* The safest rewarming takes place at a medical facility, so transport is the most important factor.

Emergency Medical Care for Immersion Hypothermia

In general, patients with immersion hypothermia should be treated the same as patients with generalized hypothermia with the following steps also taken:

1. *Instruct the patient to make the least effort needed to stay afloat until you reach him.* Turbulence and activity in the water decrease survival time by about 75 percent. If the patient continues to move or struggle, he will cool more quickly because of the increase in the movement of cold water molecules next to the skin and around the body.

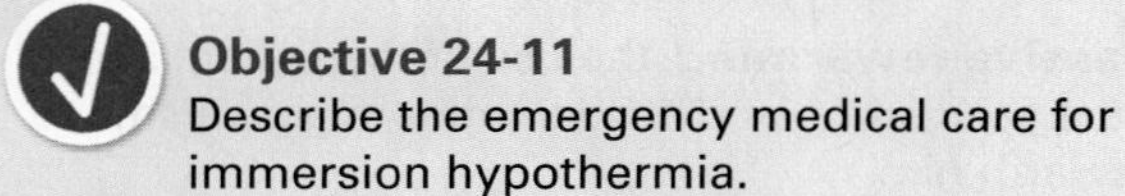
Objective 24-11
Describe the emergency medical care for immersion hypothermia.

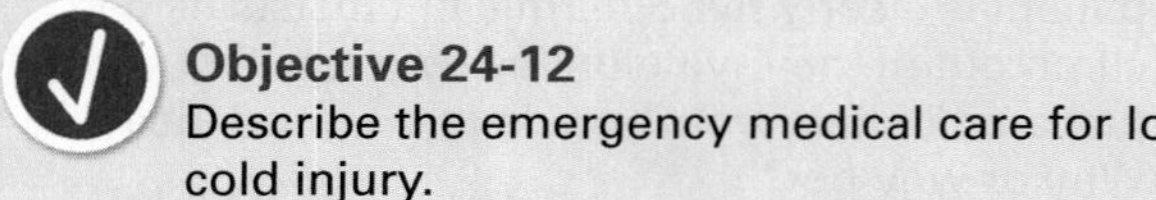
Objective 24-12
Describe the emergency medical care for local cold injury.

2. *Lift the patient from the water in a horizontal or supine position to prevent vascular collapse and provide spinal stabilization if spinal injury is suspected.*
3. *Remove the patient's wet clothing carefully and gently.* Excessive activity can cause the heart to go into ventricular fibrillation. If it is too difficult to remove the clothing, cut it off and layer dry, warm materials around the patient.

Continue treatment as you would for a patient with generalized hypothermia.

Signs and Symptoms of Local Cold Injury Local cold injury can be difficult to assess. While still frozen, even severely affected tissue may appear almost normal with purplish or other abnormal colors appearing only with thawing. The tissue may be completely numb when frozen but will be painful—burning, stinging, and throbbing before it freezes and as it thaws. While you may not be able to assess its severity accurately, you can almost always see a clear demarcation at the site of a local cold injury.

The signs and symptoms of early or superficial local cold injury include the following:

- Blanching of the skin (when you palpate the skin, normal color does not return)
- Loss of feeling and sensation in the injured area
- Continued softness of the skin in the injured area and in the tissue just beneath it
- Tingling sensation during any rewarming

The signs and symptoms of late or deep local cold injury include the following:

- White, waxy skin
- A firm-to-frozen feeling when the skin is palpated
- Swelling
- Blisters
- If partially or wholly thawed, the skin appears flushed with areas of purple and blanching or the skin appears mottled and cyanotic

Emergency Medical Care for Local Cold Injury

The key to emergency care for local cold injury is never to thaw the tissue if there is any possibility of its refreezing. Always seek medical direction and follow local protocol. General guidelines for care include the following:

1. *Remove the patient immediately from the cold environment,* if possible.
2. *Never initiate thawing procedures if there is any danger of refreezing.* Keeping the tissue frozen is less dangerous than submitting it to refreezing.
3. *If breathing is adequate, administer oxygen based on the SpO_2 reading and patient signs and symptoms.* If the SpO_2 reading is greater than 95% and no signs or symptoms of hypoxia or respiratory distress are present, oxygen may not be necessary. In this case, you may choose to apply a nasal cannula at 2 to 4 lpm. If signs of hypoxia or respiratory distress are present or the SpO_2 reading is less than 95%, place the patient on a nonrebreather mask at 15 lpm. (The SpO_2 reading may provide an inaccurate reading or no reading because of the severe peripheral constriction of vessels and lack of adequate perfusion from the cold in the extremities.)
4. *Prevent further injury to the injured part.*

   If the patient has an early or superficial injury:
   - Carefully remove any jewelry or wet or restrictive clothing to prevent causing further injury. If clothing is frozen to the skin, leave it in place.
   - Immobilize the affected extremity to prevent movement and elevate. No part of the injured extremity should be in direct contact with a hard surface.
   - Cover the affected skin with dressings or dry clothing to prevent friction or pressure.
   - Never rub or massage the affected skin.
   - Never re-expose the injured skin to the cold.

   If the patient has late or deep injury:
   - Carefully remove any jewelry or wet or restrictive clothing to prevent causing further injury. If clothing is frozen to the skin, leave it in place.
   - Cover the affected skin with dressings or dry clothing to prevent friction. Avoid pressure.
   - Do not break any blisters or treat them with salve or ointment.
   - Do not rub or massage the affected skin.
   - Never apply direct heat to rewarm the affected part.
   - Do not allow the patient to walk on an injured extremity.

If you are in a wilderness situation or are facing an extremely long or delayed transport, you should initiate active, rapid rewarming of the injured tissue, provided you will be able to keep it thawed. In such circumstances, con-

Thinking Critically

Your patient with a local cold injury is probably a 15-minute ride away from the hospital. Should you massage the frozen area? apply a heating pad? Explain what you should and should not do for this patient.

tact medical direction or follow local protocol. Do not thaw tissue and then allow it to refreeze, because this will completely destroy the tissue. It is also a mistake to thaw frozen tissue gradually; thaw the tissue as rapidly as feasible without causing accidental burning. Slow rewarming has been associated with increased tissue loss.

Rewarming frozen tissue is extremely painful for the patient, and medical direction may want him to take an analgesic, such as aspirin or a nonaspirin product, to help relieve pain during the process. Contacting ALS for this purpose may be warranted because most ALS providers can administer intravenous analgesics to help manage pain.

To rewarm frozen tissue, follow these steps:

1. *Immerse the affected tissue in a warm-water bath* (Figure 24-12✱). The water temperature should be just above body temperature (ideally 104°F). Never use dry heat as it is too difficult to control the temperature.
2. *Monitor the water to make sure it stays at an even temperature.* If possible, use a thermometer. (Water that is too hot can inflict a burn injury.) Keep the water warm by adding warm water. Never heat cooled water with any type of flame or electric unit.
3. *Continuously stir the water to keep heat evenly distributed and constant about the frozen extremity.*
4. *Keep the tissue in warm water until it is soft and color and sensation return to it.* The affected skin should turn a deep red or bluish color, and the skin should be soft and pliable.
5. Following the thawing process, *dress the area with dry sterile dressings.* If the affected area is a hand or foot, place dry sterile dressings between the toes and fingers. Once the skin is thawed, anything that contacts it, including water, must be sterile.
6. *Elevate the affected extremity.*
7. *Protect against refreezing of the warmed part.*
8. *Transport as soon as possible.* Maintain a warm ambient temperature in the patient compartment of the ambulance. ALL patients with frozen tissue require hospitalization.

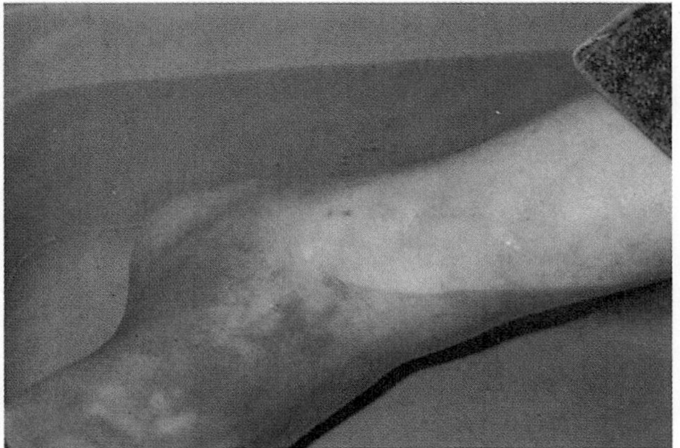

FIGURE 24-12 ✱ Thaw the affected area rapidly in water just above body temperature (100°F–110°F).

Reassessment

During the reassessment of cold emergency patients, it is important to carefully reassess the patient's mental status. A decreasing mental status will indicate deterioration in the patient's condition. Closely monitor the airway and breathing. The breathing rate and depth may continue to decrease to a point of inadequacy where positive pressure ventilation with supplemental oxygen may be required. The pulses may also continue to decrease. Be prepared to begin CPR or to stop the ambulance to defibrillate the patient as warranted. Inspect the skin for changes in color and temperature. The patient may begin to feel sensations and pain if being rewarmed. Repeat and record the baseline vital signs every 5 minutes. Keep the patient warm and try not to re-expose him to the cold.

Summary: Assessment and Care—Cold Emergency

To review assessment findings that may be associated with a cold emergency and emergency care for a cold emergency, see Figures 24-13✱ and 24-14✱.

▶ Exposure to Heat

Just as exposure to cold can produce a variety of medical problems, so too can exposure to heat. Problems created by heat exposure can range from mild discomfort to life-threatening emergencies.

Hyperthermia

Heat-related emergencies are grouped under the name *hyperthermia.* They are brought on by an increase in the body's heat production or by an inability to eliminate the

Assessment Summary

COLD EMERGENCY

The following findings may be associated with a cold emergency.

SCENE SIZE-UP

Pay particular attention to your own safety. Look for:
- Mechanism of injury
- Unstable ice
- Water hazards
- Source of cold exposure
- Ambient temperature
- Wind chill
- Wet clothing
- Alcohol or drugs
- Suspected head or spinal injury
- Exposed areas of skin

Primary Assessment

General Impression
- Is the patient dressed appropriately for the weather?
- Stiff posture
- Staggering or incoordination
- Drowsy or irrational appearance
- Shivering may be apparent if body core temperature is above 90°F or absent if body core temperature is below 90°F.

Mental Status
- Alert to unresponsive based on body core temperature

Airway
- Potentially closed airway if mental status is altered

Breathing
- Initially fast and normal depth, becoming shallow and slow as body temperature decreases

Circulation
- Pulses may be difficult to find and assess.
- Heart rate is usually increased initially.
- Heart rate decreases as body temperature continues to decrease.
- Skin is red early, becoming pale, cyanotic, and mottled as body temperature drops; skin becomes cold to touch.

Status: Priority patient if generalized cold injury (hypothermia) is suspected

Secondary Assessment

Signs and symptoms of generalized cold injury:
- Decreasing mental status
- Decreasing motor and sensory function
- Changes to vital signs

Signs and symptoms of local cold injury—early or superficial:
- Blanching of skin
- Loss of feeling or sensation in injured area
- Underlying tissue remains soft
- Tingling sensation when rewarmed

Signs and symptoms of local cold injury—late or deep:
- White, waxy skin
- Underlying tissue is firm and hard to touch
- Blisters
- Swelling
- Skin purple, blanched, mottled, or cyanotic if thawed

History
- Did the patient ingest alcohol or drugs?
- Does the patient have a circulatory disorder, cardiac disorder, or other medical condition?
- How long has the patient been exposed to the cold?

Physical Exam

Head, neck, and face:
- Pupils may be dilated, sluggish to respond to light
- Slurred speech
- Difficulty forming words and moving mouth
- Red, blanched, cyanotic, or white and waxy if exposed

Abdomen:
- Cold to touch

Extremities:
- Stiff and rigid
- Lack of coordination
- Shivering (body core temperature above 90°F)
- Reduced sensation
- Blanched skin that remains soft to touch (superficial local cold injury)
- Skin white, waxy, cyanotic, swelling, blisters, cold, and firm (deep local cold injury)

Baseline Vital Signs—Generalized Cold Injury
- BP: normal early, continues to decrease, may be absent
- HR: increased early, becoming decreased and barely palpable as body core temperature continues to drop
- RR: initially increased, decreases as body continues to cool
- Skin: red early, becoming pale, cyanotic, gray, waxy, and firm to touch late
- Pupils: dilated; sluggish to respond to light
- SpO_2: in severe cases will not produce a reading because of the severe peripheral vasoconstriction

FIGURE 24-13a ✱ Assessment summary: cold emergency.

Emergency Care Protocol

GENERALIZED COLD EMERGENCY

1. Remove the patient from the cold environment and remove all wet clothing. Prevent further heat loss.
2. Establish and maintain an open airway.
3. Suction secretions as necessary.
4. If breathing is inadequate, provide positive pressure ventilation with supplemental oxygen at a minimum rate of 10–12 ventilations/minute for an adult and 12–20 ventilations/minute for an infant or child.
5. If breathing is adequate, administer oxygen by nonrebreather mask at 15 lpm. If possible, deliver warm humidified oxygen.
6. If no pulse is present, apply the AED. Deliver only one defibrillation and perform CPR. Contact medical direction for further orders.
7. Turn up the heat to maximum in the back of the ambulance. Cover the patient with blankets (passive rewarming).
8. If the patient is alert, actively rewarm by placing hot packs under the armpits, in the groin area, and to the chest. Also perform normal passive rewarming.
9. If the patient is unresponsive or not responding appropriately, perform passive rewarming only.
10. Do not allow the patient to eat or drink stimulants.
11. Do not rub or massage the patient's extremities.
12. Handle the patient gently to prevent stimulation of cardiac dysrhythmias; place in a lateral recumbent position only if spinal injury is not suspected.
13. Transport.
14. Perform a reassessment every 5 minutes.

LOCAL COLD EMERGENCY

1. If you suspect a decreased body core temperature, follow the "Generalized Cold Emergency" protocol before proceeding with the "Local Cold Injury" protocol.
2. Remove the patient from the cold environment and remove all wet clothing; prevent further heat loss.
3. Remove jewelry and wet or restrictive clothing. (Do not remove clothing that is frozen to the skin.)
4. Cover affected skin with dry sterile dressings.
5. For early or superficial injury:
   - Immobilize affected extremity.
   - Do not rub or massage.
   - Do not re-expose to cold.
6. For late or deep injury:
   - Do not rub or massage.
   - Do not break blisters.
   - Do not apply heat or rewarm area.
   - Do not allow patient to walk on affected extremity.
7. If required or instructed to rewarm, follow these guidelines:
   - Immerse affected tissue in warm water bath at 104°F.
   - Monitor water and stir to keep at constant temperature.
   - Keep immersed until color returns and skin and underlying tissue become soft.
   - Dress affected area.
   - Elevate involved extremity. Avoid contact with hard surfaces.
   - Protect against refreezing.
8. Transport.

FIGURE 24-13b ✱ Emergency care protocols: generalized and local cold emergencies.

Emergency Care Algorithm: **Cold Emergency**

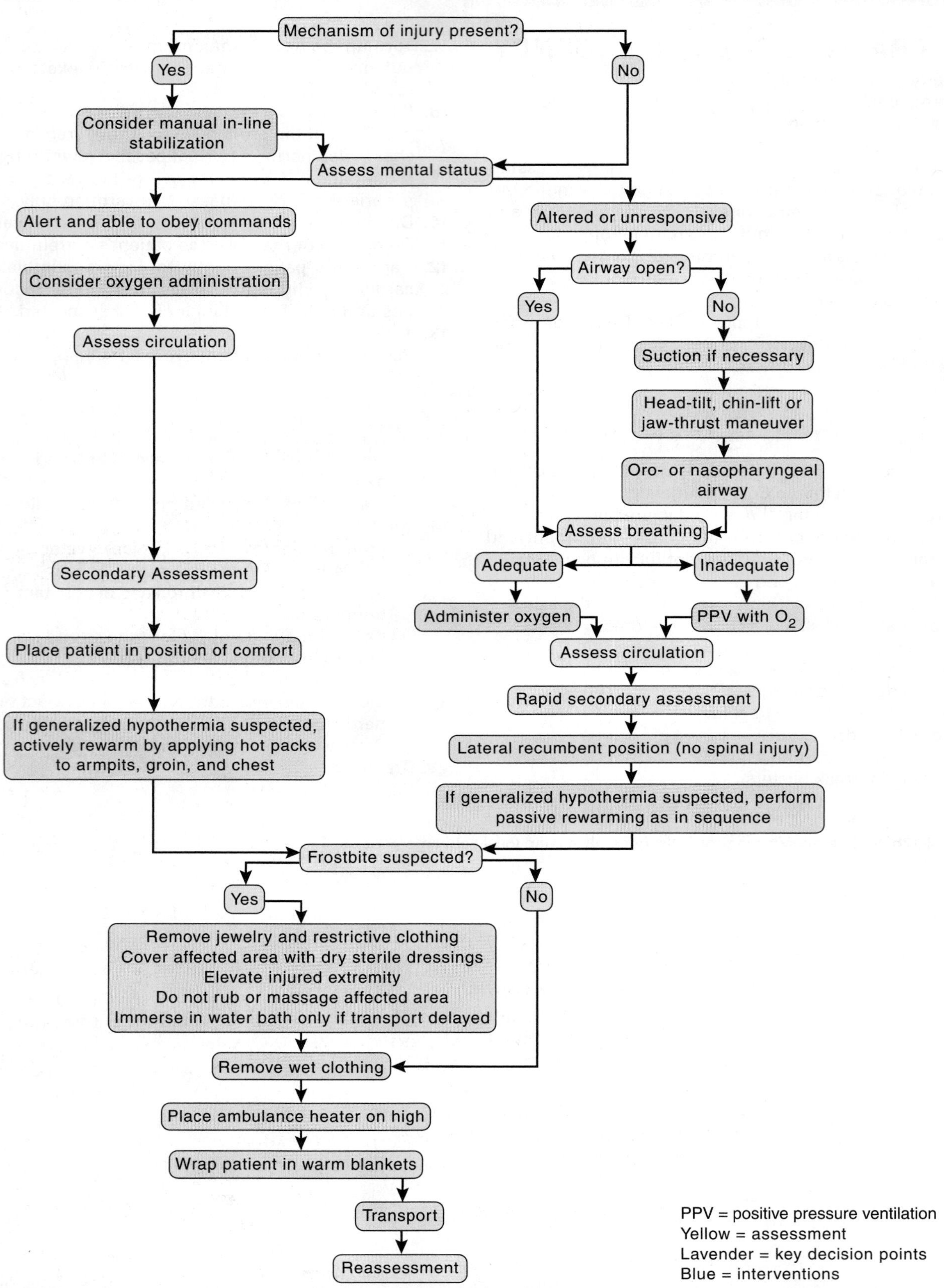

FIGURE 24-14 ✱ Emergency care algorithm: cold emergency.

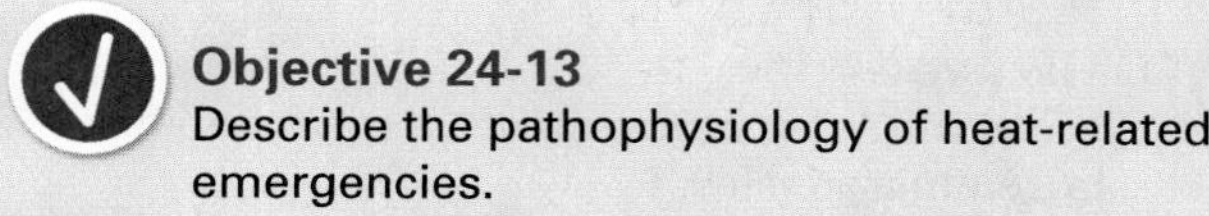

Objective 24-13
Describe the pathophysiology of heat-related emergencies.

Thinking Critically
Your patient has collapsed during a tennis match on a hot day. Her skin is flushed and hot but dry. Could her condition be life threatening? Explain.

heat produced. Most heat injuries occur early in the summer season, before people have acclimated themselves to the season's higher temperatures. Various stages of hyperthermia are commonly called "heat cramps," "heat exhaustion," and "heat stroke."

Pathophysiology of Heat-Related Emergencies

- **Heat Cramps**. The least serious form of heat-related injury is muscle spasms, or cramps, that are thought by some researchers to result from the body losing too much salt during profuse sweating. The cramping is made worse when not enough salt is taken into the body, when calcium levels are low, or when too much water is consumed by the patient. Such cramping is occasionally caused by overexertion of muscles, inadequate stretching or warm-up, and lactic acid buildup in poorly conditioned muscles. This condition is referred to as "heat cramps." Heat cramps characteristically occur to the large flexor muscle groups of the body first, such as the abdominal muscles, gluteus muscles, and hamstrings (large flexor muscles surrounding the femur).

Understanding BODY PROCESSES

Heat cramps are caused by electrolyte imbalance to the muscles, most commonly from overexertion in hot temperatures with excessive diaphoresis (sweating). ■

ASSESSMENT Tips

Heat cramps are the mildest form of the heat emergency and are rapidly identified by muscle spasms and pain to the large flexor muscles of the body. ■

- **Heat Exhaustion**. Extreme physical exertion in a hot, humid environment can affect even an otherwise fit individual. It can produce a disturbance of the body's blood flow, resulting in a mild state of shock. This is brought on by the pooling of blood in the vessels just below the skin resulting from vasodilation as the body works to increase heat loss, but in extreme cases this can also cause excessive blood flow away from the major organs of the body. Prolonged and profuse sweating causes the body to lose large quantities of salt and water. When these are not adequately replaced, blood circulation diminishes, affecting the brain, heart, and lungs. This condition is referred to as "heat exhaustion." *In such cases, a patient's skin will be normal to cool in temperature, either pale or ashen gray in color, and sweaty.* In summary, heat exhaustion is thought to occur when the body has maximized the heat-dissipating mechanisms to a point where other body systems are starting to dysfunction.

Understanding BODY PROCESSES

Heat exhaustion occurs when the body's cooling mechanisms have been expended, and the central nervous system and other systems are starting to show the consequences of this depletion. ■

ASSESSMENT Tips

A patient with heat exhaustion will commonly have slight alterations in mental status, such as dizziness or fatigue, and will present with a normal body temperature and diaphoretic skin. ■

- **Heat Stroke**. If measures are not taken to remove the patient to a cool environment or to stop the physical activity and replace lost fluid, the hypothermic patient's condition can deteriorate into an extreme form of hyperthermia called "heat stroke." This is a life-threatening medical emergency with a mortality ranging from 20–80 percent. It occurs when the body's heat-regulating mechanisms break down and become unable to cool the body sufficiently. The body becomes overheated, body temperature rises, and sweating ceases in about half the patients. Because no cooling takes place, the body stores increasingly more heat, the heat-producing mechanisms speed up, and eventually the brain cells are damaged, causing permanent disability or death. Such patients are commonly unresponsive, and the skin will be hot and red; it may be either moist or dry, since about half the patients in this stage of hyperthermia sweat while about half cease to sweat.

Objective 24-14
Recognize factors that contribute to a patient's risk for hyperthermia.

Objective 24-15
Discuss the assessment-based approach to heat-related emergencies.

The patient with heat stroke does not have to first suffer from heat cramps or heat exhaustion. Heat stroke can occur independently and can be more than an extreme type of heat exhaustion. Classic nonexertional heat stroke (NEHS) occurs typically to elderly patients with sedentary lifestyles, patients who are chronically ill or are on medications inhibiting the temperature-sensing ability of the body, or patients who live in regions of the country that rarely experience heat waves. Exertional heat stroke (EHS) commonly occurs to younger individuals who are engaged in strenuous physical exertion in a very hot environment for prolonged periods. In either instance, heat stroke is a dire medical emergency that carries with it high morbidity and mortality rates if treatment is delayed or inappropriate (up to 80 percent, as previously noted). With effective and timely treatment, morbidity and mortality drops to 10 percent.

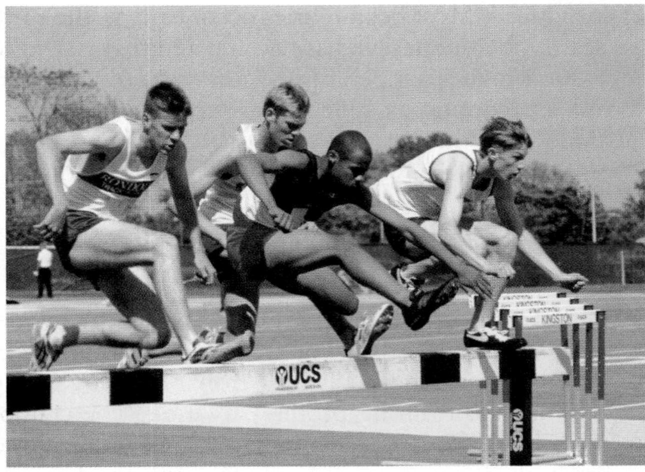

FIGURE 24-15 ✻ Exercise and strenuous activity can cause the loss of more than one liter of sweat per hour. (© Michal Heron)

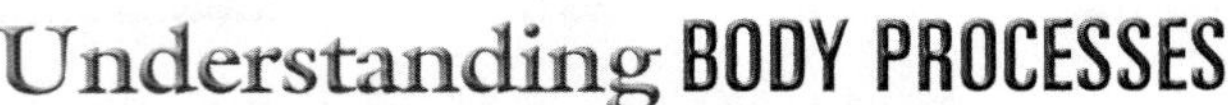

Understanding BODY PROCESSES

Heat stroke occurs when the thermoregulatory mechanism of the body fails to sense and compensate for elevations of the core temperature, and an extremely high core temperature results. ■

ASSESSMENT Tips

Heat stroke should always be considered in a patient with a heat-related emergency coupled with unresponsiveness. ■

Predisposing Factors

Several factors can predispose an individual to heat-related injuries. They include the following:

- **Climate**. Hot temperatures reduce the body's ability to lose heat by radiation; high humidity reduces the body's ability to lose heat by evaporation.
- **Exercise and strenuous activity**. They can cause the loss of more than one liter of sweat per hour and increase heat production (Figure 24-15✻). Exertional heat stroke is the second leading cause of death in high school students, surpassed only by accidental spinal cord injuries.
- **Age**. Individuals at the extremes of age, such as the elderly and infants (especially newborns), have poor ability to regulate body temperature. Elderly patients often take medications that increase the risk of heat injury and may lack the mobility to escape a hot environment. Infants cannot remove their clothing if they get too hot.
- **Pre-existing illnesses**. Including the following:
  - Heart disease
  - Kidney disease
  - Cerebrovascular disease
  - Parkinson disease
  - Thyroid gland disorders
  - Skin diseases, including eczema, scleroderma, and healed burns
  - Dehydration
  - Obesity
  - Infections or other conditions that cause fever
  - Fatigue
  - Diabetes
  - Malnutrition
  - Alcoholism
  - Mental retardation
  - Peripheral vascular disease
- **Certain drugs and medications**. Including alcohol, cocaine, amphetamines, diuretics, barbiturates, hallucinogens, and medications that hamper sweating and increase heat production.

- **Lack of acclimation**. It may take days to weeks to acclimate to a consistently hot environment, especially with a high humidity. Prior to acclimation, the patient is prone to suffering a heat emergency.

Assessment-Based Approach: Heat-Related Emergency

Scene Size-Up

Scan the scene for evidence that the patient is suffering from a heat-related emergency. Probably the most important factors to consider are the ambient temperature and humidity. High temperatures, especially if greater than 90°F, and relative humidity greater than 75 percent, combine to create an environment that renders the body's cooling mechanisms less effective (Figure 24-16*).

Exercise and activity are common precursors to heat-related emergencies. Look for clues to the patient's activities prior to the incident. Where is he found? If you find someone lying in a flower bed in the middle of a humid August afternoon with gardening tools at his side, you could assume that he had been working outside in the hot sun before collapsing.

A person's clothing can also give clues to his activity. If you receive a call to assist a patient in the park in mid-July and find someone dressed in jogging shorts and running shoes, you might assume that he was exercising before the incident. You might find a patient collapsed in a cool, air-conditioned home on a summer day. If he is wearing jogging shorts and running shoes, you might at least suspect that he was outside exercising, felt ill, and returned home to call EMS. Reports of an ill or collapsed patient at an outdoor sporting event held in hot, humid weather should also make you suspect possible heat emergency.

Infants and children left in closed vehicles or in structures that are hot and poorly ventilated are prone to heat emergencies, especially if the infant or child is overdressed and too young to remove his own clothing. Elderly patients, especially those who are not mobile enough to escape their hot environments, are also likely to become victims of a heat emergency.

Look for medications or drugs since these may precipitate a heat-related emergency.

During the scene size-up, recognize your own limits and protect yourself from overexposure to the heat. Dress appropriately and be sure to drink enough water to stay hydrated. If you are on standby at a public event held during the summer or if you have to walk long distances carrying heavy gear on a hot, humid day, you will be exposed to the same environmental extremes as the patients you are expected to treat.

Primary Assessment

While gathering a general impression of the patient, determine if he is dressed inappropriately for the hot environment. The mental status of the patients you encounter

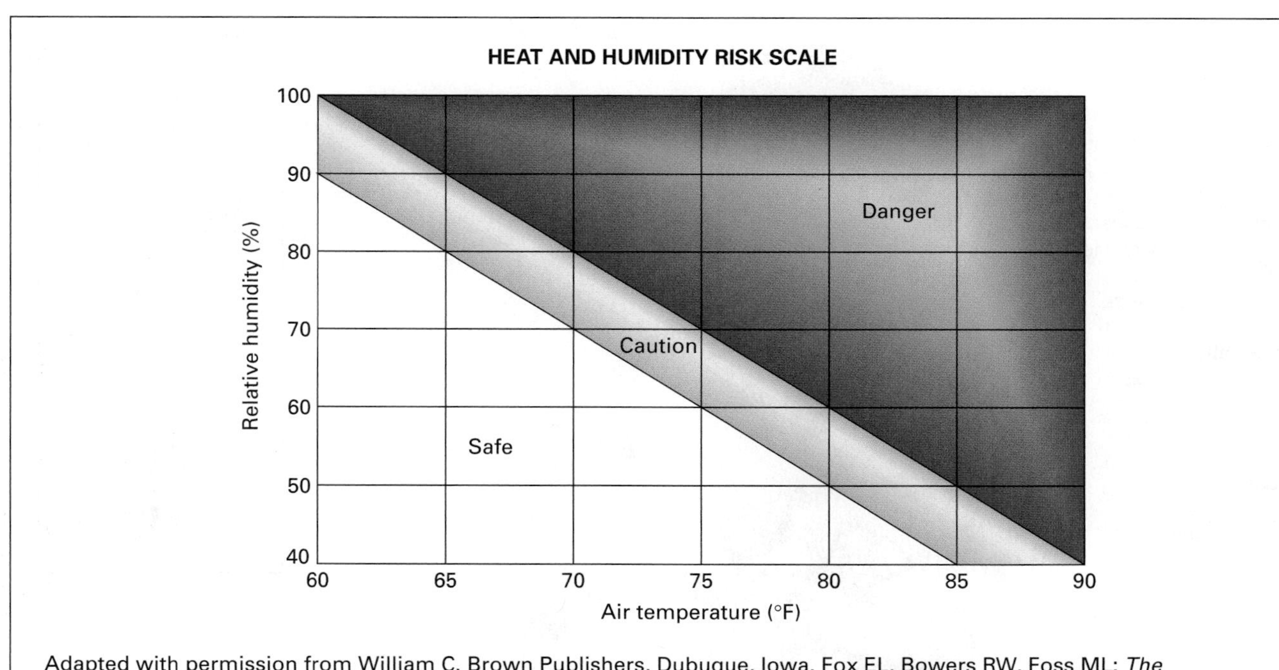

Adapted with permission from William C. Brown Publishers, Dubuque, Iowa. Fox EL, Bowers RW, Foss ML: *The physiological basis of physical education and athletics*, ed. 4. Philadelphia, WB Saunders Co., 1988, p. 503.

FIGURE 24-16 * The risk of illness is increased when heat and humidity produce dangerous conditions. Lower temperatures with high humidity can also cause the body's temperature to rise.

in heat emergencies may range from alert and oriented to completely unresponsive. The patient may complain of dizziness or may have fainted prior to your arrival. The mental status may deteriorate as the condition worsens.

Assess the airway and breathing. Closely monitor the airway and provide oxygen at 15 lpm by nonrebreather mask if the mental status is altered or continues to deteriorate. If the breathing is inadequate, begin positive pressure ventilation with supplemental oxygen.

The patient's radial pulse may be weak and rapid or absent, depending on the level of dehydration. The skin may be moist and pale with a normal-to-cool temperature or hot and dry or moist. *The patient with altered mental status who has hot skin should be considered a priority patient.*

Secondary Assessment

If the patient is found in a hot environment, move him to a cool environment as quickly as possible. If the patient is responsive, gather a history, paying particular attention to the symptoms of which the patient complains. The OPQRST can be modified to gather further information about some of the symptoms. Pay particular attention to medications the patient may be taking, since some can contribute to the heat emergency. Be sure to determine the patient's last oral intake, especially consumption of water or other liquids. Get a description of events that preceded the incident. Conduct a physical exam, targeting areas of complaint that were gathered during the history.

The baseline vital signs may reveal a blood pressure that is normal or low. The heart rate and respirations are typically elevated in heat emergencies. Pulses may be bounding or weak. Skin could be cool, normal, or hot to the touch and either moist or dry. *Hot skin is most alarming, since it indicates the most severe type of heat emergency.*

If the patient is unresponsive, conduct a physical exam, take baseline vital signs, and then gather the history from family or bystanders.

Signs and Symptoms of Generalized Hyperthermia

The general signs and symptoms of heat-related injuries include the following (Figure 24-17*):

- Elevated core temperature
- Muscle cramps
- Weakness or exhaustion
- Dizziness or faintness
- A rapid pulse that is usually strong at first, but becomes weak
- Initial deep, rapid breathing that becomes shallow and weak as damage progresses
- Headache

SIGNS AND SYMPTOMS OF HEAT EMERGENCY

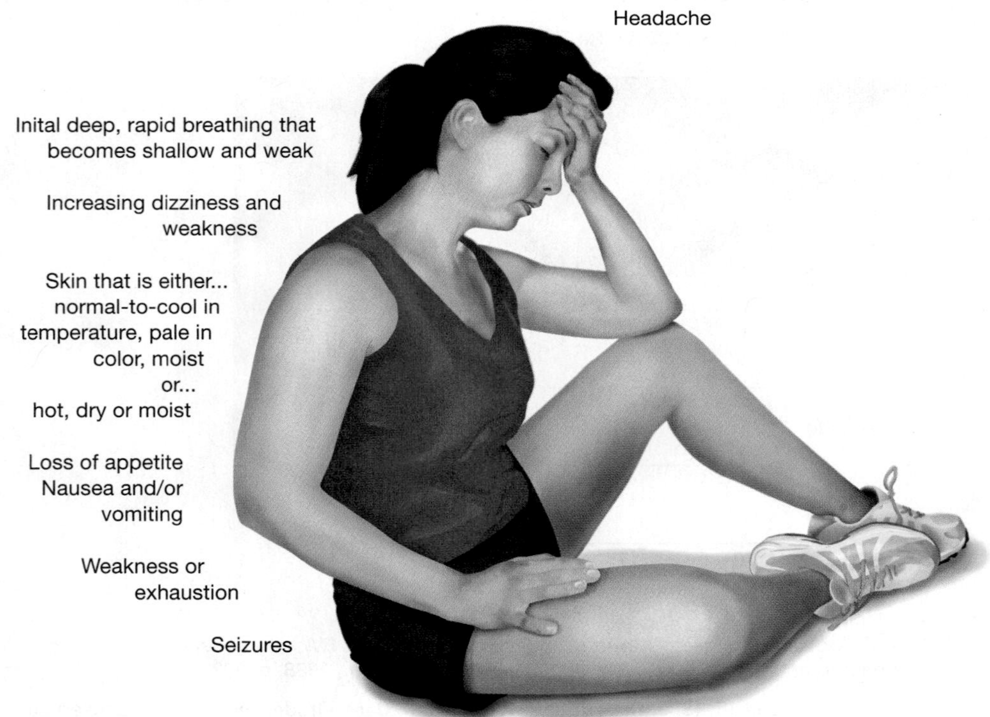

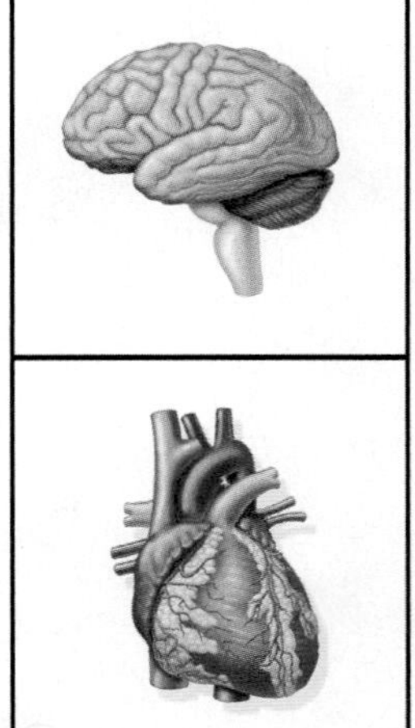

FIGURE 24-17 * Signs and symptoms of a serious heat emergency.

Objective 24-16
Describe the emergency medical care for a heat emergency patient with moist, pale, normal-to-cool skin.

Objective 24-17
Describe the emergency medical care for a heat emergency patient with hot skin that is moist or dry.

- Seizures
- Loss of appetite, nausea, or vomiting
- Altered mental status, possibly unresponsiveness
- Skin that is either moist and pale with a normal-to-cool temperature, or hot and either dry or moist *(Hot skin that is either dry or moist represents a dire medical emergency.)*

Emergency Medical Care for a Heat Emergency Patient with Moist, Pale, Normal-to-Cool Skin

For a patient whose skin is moist and pale, with normal-to-cool skin temperature, provide the following care:

1. *Move the patient to a cool place,* such as the back of an air-conditioned ambulance, away from the source of heat. If no cooler location is immediately available, at least move the patient into the shade.
2. *Administer oxygen.* If breathing is adequate, administer oxygen based on the SpO_2 reading and patient signs and symptoms. If the SpO_2 reading is greater than 95% and no signs or symptoms of hypoxia or respiratory distress are present, oxygen may not be necessary. In this case, you may choose to apply a nasal cannula at 2 to 4 lpm. If signs of hypoxia or respiratory distress are present or the SpO_2 reading is less than 95%, place the patient on a nonrebreather mask at 15 lpm. Provide positive pressure ventilation if needed.
3. *Remove as much of the patient's clothing as you can; loosen what you cannot remove.* The patient should be kept as comfortable as possible.
4. *Cool the patient by applying cold, wet compresses and/or by misting the patient with water and then fanning lightly* (Figure 24-18✱). You want to help cool the patient, but make sure he does not get chilled.
5. *Place the patient in a supine position.* Consider raising the feet and legs 8–12 inches in an attempt to improve blood circulation to the brain and other core organs by reducing pooling in the lower extremities.
6. *If the patient is fully responsive and is not nauseated, have him drink cool water.* Consult with medical direction and follow local protocol.
7. *If the patient is unresponsive or has an altered mental status or is vomiting, do NOT give fluids.*

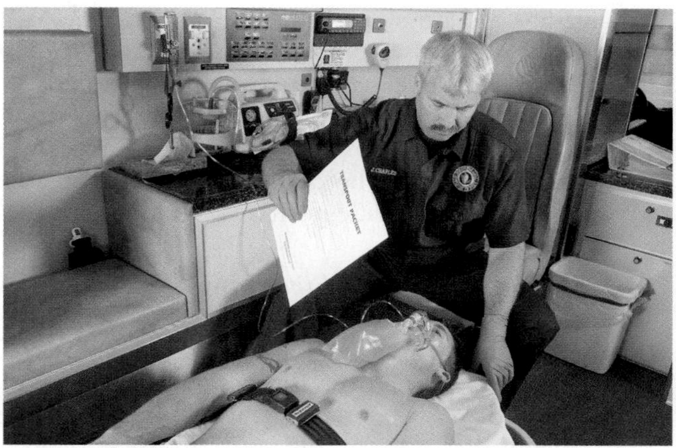

FIGURE 24-18 ✱ If the skin is moist, pale, and normal to cool, place the patient in a cool environment, mist with water or apply cold, wet compresses, and fan to promote cooling.

8. Generally, a hyperthermic patient with moist, pale skin that is normal to cool in temperature needs *transport* when the patient:
   - Is unresponsive or has an altered mental status
   - Is vomiting or is nauseated and will not drink fluids
   - Has a history of medical problems
   - Has a core temperature above 101°F
   - Has a continuously rising temperature
   - Does not respond to therapy (symptoms do not improve)

Emergency Medical Care for a Heat Emergency Patient with Hot Skin That Is Moist or Dry

A patient with hot skin that is either moist or dry represents a dire medical emergency. Cooling the patient takes priority over everything other than airway, breathing, and circulatory management. Provide the following care:

1. *Remove the patient from the source of heat and place him in a cool environment,* such as an air-conditioned room or ambulance. If nothing else, move the patient out of the sun and into the shade.
2. *Remove as much of the patient's clothing as is possible or reasonable.*
3. *Administer oxygen.* If breathing is adequate, administer oxygen based on the SpO_2 reading and patient signs and symptoms. If the SpO_2 reading is greater

Thinking Critically

It's mid-summer and a worker who has been moving heavy boxes in a warehouse with no air conditioning has collapsed. On arrival, you immediately check to see if his skin is cool or hot. Why is this important? How might the findings affect the care you provide?

Objective 24-18

Describe the emergency medical care for heat cramps.

than 95% and no signs or symptoms of hypoxia or respiratory distress are present, oxygen may not be necessary. In this case, you may choose to apply a nasal cannula at 2 to 4 lpm. If signs of hypoxia or respiratory distress are present or the SpO_2 reading is less than 95%, place the patient on a nonrebreather mask at 15 lpm. Provide positive pressure ventilation if needed.

4. *Immediately begin to cool the patient.* Generally, one method alone will not effectively cool the patient, so use a combination of the following (Figure 24-19∗):
   - Pour tepid water over the patient's body. Avoid the use of *cold* water since this may stimulate peripheral thermoreceptors and produce reflexive vasoconstriction and shivering.
   - Place cold packs in the patient's groin, at each side of the neck, in the armpits, and behind each knee to cool the large surface blood vessels.
   - Fan the patient aggressively or direct an electric fan at the patient.
   - Keep the patient's skin wet to promote cooling through evaporation.
5. Because the patient's entire body is involved in the heat emergency, several complications may result from the condition or from the treatment of it. *Be prepared to manage seizures or prevent the aspiration of vomitus.*

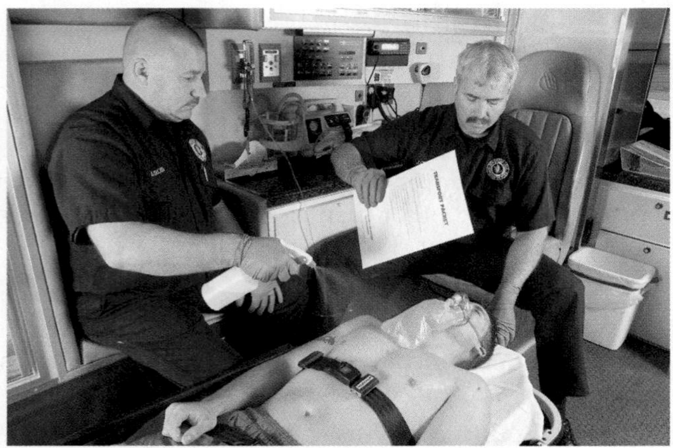

FIGURE 24-19 ∗ If the skin is hot and dry or moist, promote cooling by applying cold packs to the groin, neck, armpits, and backs of knees; fanning the patient; and spraying or pouring tepid water over the patient's body. Then wrap in a wet sheet and continue fanning.

6. Transport immediately, continuing to administer oxygen and cooling methods during transport. *Always transport a hyperthermic patient with hot skin that is moist or dry.* Such a patient always needs hospital care.

Emergency Medical Care for Heat Cramps

As mentioned earlier, one of the symptoms of a heat emergency is muscle cramping. In some patients with the mildest hyperthermia, cramping may be the only symptom. Cramping typically occurs to the muscles of the legs and abdomen.

To treat a patient with heat cramps:

1. *Remove the patient from the source of heat to a cool environment.* If nothing else, move the patient out of the sun and into the shade.
2. *Consult medical direction before giving the patient sips of low-concentration salt water* at the rate of half a glassful every 15 minutes. If possible, use a commercial product, such as Gatorade, with a low glucose content. Salt water is made by diluting one teaspoon of salt in one quart of water. Do not give the patient salt tablets. If in question, either follow local protocol or contact medical direction.
3. *Apply moist towels to the patient's forehead and over the cramping muscles.* Try to gently stretch the involved muscle groups. Some experts advise massaging the involved muscles if it does not cause additional pain. Consult with medical direction and follow local protocol.
4. *Explain to the patient what happened so he can avoid a recurrence of the problem.* Advise the patient to avoid exertion for 12 hours.

Generally, you need to transport a patient with heat cramps only if the patient has other illnesses or injuries, develops other symptoms, or does not respond to your care and deteriorates.

Reassessment

During the reassessment, re-evaluate the mental status, airway, breathing, circulation, baseline vital signs, and treatment. The mental status may continue to deteriorate if the body temperature continues to rise. The mental status may improve once the patient is cooled and treatment is initiated. Closely reassess the airway and breathing. Be prepared to establish an airway and to provide positive pressure ventilation if breathing becomes inadequate, especially in patients with hot skin. Also, be prepared to manage seizures with such patients.

The pulse may continue to weaken, or the rate may increase further. Correlate changes in the pulse rate with the patient's mental status. If the pulse is decreasing and the mental status improving, it is a sign that the treatment is proving effective. If the pulse is rapidly increasing or decreasing and the patient's mental status is declining, it is a grave indication that the patient is deteriorating. Reassess and record the vital signs every 5 minutes. Report your assessment to the receiving hospital.

Summary: Assessment and Care—Heat Emergency

To review assessment findings that may be associated with a heat emergency and appropriate management for heat-related emergencies, see Figures 24-20a*, 24-20b*, and 24-21*.

Assessment Summary

HEAT EMERGENCY

The following findings may be associated with a heat emergency.

SCENE SIZE-UP

Pay particular attention to your own safety. Look for:
- High ambient temperatures, usually greater than 90°F
- Humidity greater than 75 percent
- Evidence of exercise or other activity
- Patient's clothing

Primary Assessment

General Impression
- Is the patient dressed appropriately for the weather?
- Excessive sweating or excessively dry skin
- Dizziness or fainting

Mental Status
- Alert to unresponsive based on body core temperature

Airway
- Potentially closed airway if mental status is altered

Breathing
- Initially fast and normal depth; becoming shallow and slow as body temperature increases

Circulation
- Heart rate is increased.
- Bradycardia may occur very late.
- Skin may be excessively dry or wet, but may be extremely hot (heat stroke).
- Skin may be moist, pale, and normal to cool (heat exhaustion).

Status: Priority patient if hot skin, whether moist or dry, or altered mental status is present

Secondary Assessment

Signs and symptoms:
- Dizziness and weakness
- Headache
- Nausea and/or vomiting
- Seizures
- Muscle cramps
- Hot, dry, or moist skin
- Pale, cool, and moist skin
- Altered mental status

History
- Did the patient ingest alcohol or drugs?
- Does the patient have a circulatory disorder, cardiac disorder, or other medical condition?
- How long has the patient been exposed to the heat?

Physical Exam

Head, neck, and face:
- Pupils may be dilated and sluggish to respond to light
- Slurred speech
- Headache

Extremities:
- Muscle cramps
- Hot skin that is dry or moist (priority patient)
- Cool, pale, and moist skin

Baseline Vital Signs—Heat Emergency
- BP: normal to decreased
- HR: increased; may decrease very late if body core temperature becomes excessively high
- RR: initially increased; may decrease if body core temperature continues to rise excessively
- Skin: may be hot, dry, or moist (priority patient) or cool, moist, and pale
- Pupils: midsize to dilated; sluggish to respond
- SpO_2: 95% or greater core temperature may be normal, lowered, or elevated

FIGURE 24-20a * Assessment summary: heat emergency.

Objective 24-19
Describe the characteristics of common venomous snakes and factors that affect the severity of a snakebite.

Emergency Care Protocol

HEAT EMERGENCY

1. Remove the patient from the hot environment and remove clothing. Prevent further heat gain.
2. Establish and maintain an open airway; insert a nasopharyngeal or oropharyngeal airway if the patient is unresponsive and has no gag or cough reflex.
3. Suction secretions as necessary.
4. If breathing is inadequate, provide positive pressure ventilation with supplemental oxygen at a minimum rate of 10–12 ventilations/minute for an adult and 12–20 ventilations/minute for an infant or child.
5. If breathing is adequate, administer oxygen by nonrebreather mask at 15 lpm.
6. Turn up the air conditioner to maximum in the back of the ambulance.
7. If skin is cool, moist, and pale (heat exhaustion), do the following:
   - Cool patient by applying cold, wet compresses; fan lightly.
   - Place patient in supine position with legs elevated 8–12 inches.
   - If patient is vomiting, place in lateral recumbent position.
   - If patient is responsive and not nauseated, administer water by mouth at a half glass every 15 minutes.
8. If skin is hot and dry or moist (heat stroke), do the following:
   - Pour cool water over patient.
   - Place cold packs in armpits, behind each knee, and at side of the neck.
   - Fan patient aggressively.
   - If patient shivers, slow cooling process.
   - Be prepared to manage seizures.
9. Transport.
10. Perform a reassessment every 5 minutes.

FIGURE 24-20b * Emergency care protocol: heat emergency.

Bites and Stings

Many people who venture into the outdoors fear the possibility of a snakebite. But, in fact, such bites are relatively uncommon and the number of people who die from a snakebite each year is extremely small. Still, the possibility of death or crippling injury from a snakebite does exist and you should be prepared to deal with the situation if you encounter it.

Insect bites and stings are far more common, and luckily most are considered minor. It is only when the patient has an allergic reaction and runs the risk of developing anaphylactic shock that the situation becomes an emergency. Even under those conditions, accurate recognition and prompt treatment can save lives and prevent permanent tissue damage.

Snakebite

About 45,000 people per year are bitten by snakes in the United States; of those, 7,000 receive bites from one of the two types of poisonous snakes: coral snakes and pit vipers (rattlesnakes, copperheads, and water moccasins). More than half the poisonous snakebites involve children, and most occur between April and October during daylight hours.

The bites of nonpoisonous snakes are not considered serious and are generally treated as minor wounds; only bites of poisonous snakes are considered medical emergencies. In only about a third of the cases of bites by poisonous snakes do the snakes inject venom into the victim. When venom is injected, symptoms generally occur immediately. If it is difficult to delineate the poisonous from nonpoisonous snakebite based on the patient's description

Emergency Care Algorithm: **Heat Emergency**

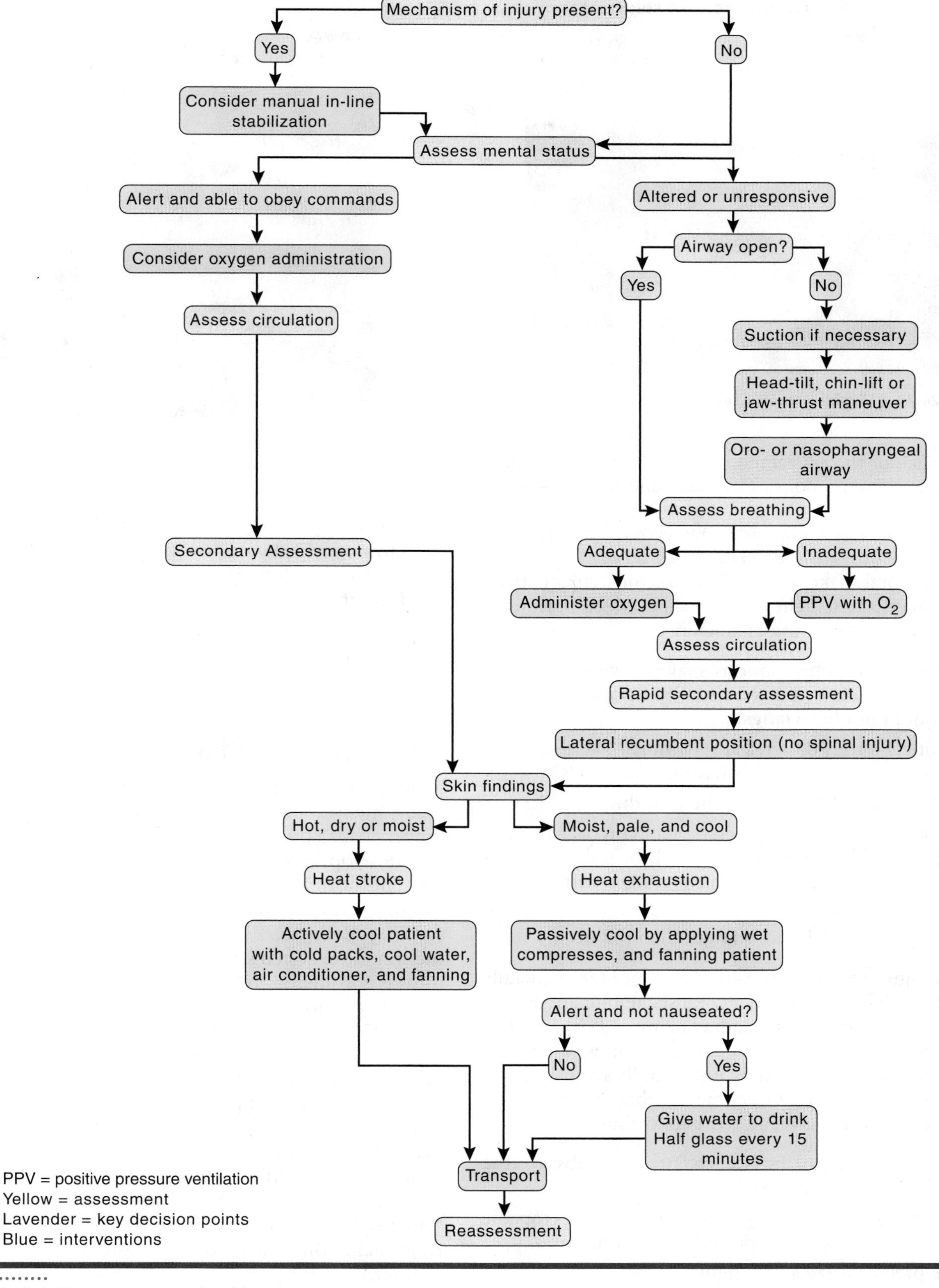

FIGURE 24-21 ✱ Emergency care algorithm: heat emergency.

Objective 24-20
Recognize the signs, symptoms, and patient history associated with bites or stings of black widow spiders, brown recluse spiders, scorpions, fire ants, and ticks.

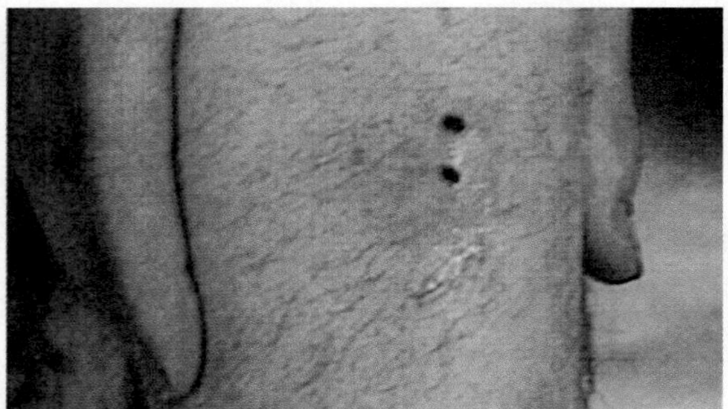

FIGURE 24-22 * Typical rattlesnake bite.

of the snake or the appearance of the bite wound, assume the bite was from a poisonous snake and provide care as appropriate.

A poisonous snakebite is characterized by one or two distinct puncture wounds (Figure 24-22*). The exception is the coral snake, which leaves a semicircular pattern with its teeth as it "chews" the skin. Most poisonous snakes have the following characteristics:

- Large fangs; nonpoisonous snakes have small teeth. The exception is the coral snake, a poisonous snake that does not have fangs.
- Elliptical pupils or vertical slits, much like those of a cat; nonvenomous snakes have round pupils.
- A pit between the eye and the mouth.
- A variety of different-shaped blotches on backgrounds of pink, yellow, olive, tan, gray, or brown skin. The exception is the coral snake, which is ringed with red, yellow, and black.
- A triangular head that is larger than the neck.

The signs and symptoms of a pit viper bite generally occur immediately; those of a coral snake bite are usually delayed by at least 1 hour and as many as 8 hours. The severity of a pit viper bite, depending on how much poison was injected, is gauged by how rapidly symptoms develop (Figure 24-23*). Other factors that determine the severity of a snakebite include the following:

- The location of the bite, since fatty tissue absorbs the venom more slowly than muscle tissue
- Whether pathogens (organisms or substances capable of causing disease) are present in the venom
- The patient's size and weight

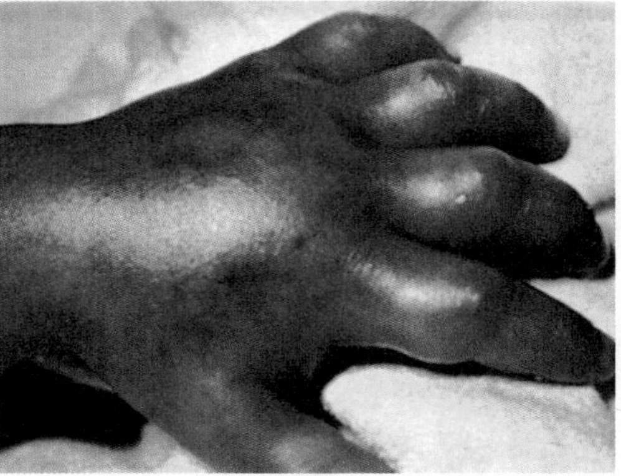

FIGURE 24-23 * Snakebite to the hand.

- The patient's general health and condition
- How much physical activity the patient engaged in immediately following the bite, since physical activity will spread the venom

The emergency medical care for snakebite is the same as general emergency medical care for bites and stings described in the next sections.

Insect Bites and Stings

Most insect bites are treated like any other wound. Generally, medical help is necessary only if the itching lasts longer than 2 days, signs of infection or an allergic reaction develop, or the insect is poisonous.

The normal reaction to an insect sting is a sharp, stinging pain followed immediately by an itchy, painful swelling. Redness, tenderness, and swelling at or around the sting site, even if severe, in the absence of other symptoms is considered to be a local reaction. Local reactions are rarely serious or life threatening and can be treated successfully with cold compresses.

Allergic reactions are another story: Thousands of people are allergic to the stings of bees, wasps, hornets, and yellow jackets. For those people, a sting may precipitate anaphylactic shock. This condition may cause death from within a few minutes to an hour of the sting. For more information on anaphylactic shock, see Chapter 15, "Shock and Resuscitation," Chapter 21, "Anaphylactic Reactions," and the "Assessment-Based Approach: Bites and Stings" section later in this chapter.

Black Widow Spider

The black widow spider is characterized by a shiny black body, thin legs, and a crimson red marking on its abdomen, usually in the shape of an hourglass or two triangles. Of the five species in the United States, only three are black, and not all have the characteristic red marking.

The female black widow spider, larger than the male, is one of the largest spiders in the United States. Males generally do not bite; females bite only when hungry, agitated, or protecting the egg sac. The black widow spider is usually found in dry, secluded, dimly lit areas; it has an extremely strong, funnel-shaped web. They are generally nocturnal, and it is said that they avoid human dwellings. They have been found, however, in outhouses and garages or sheds.

Black widow spider bites are the leading cause of death from spider bites in the United States. Those at highest risk for developing severe reactions to the bites are children under the age of 16, people over the age of 60, people with chronic illness, and anyone with hypertension.

In addition to the general signs and symptoms of bites and stings, black widow spider bites cause the following:

- A pinprick sensation at the bite site, becoming a dull ache within about 30 minutes
- Severe muscle spasms, especially in the shoulders, back, chest, and abdomen
- Rigid, boardlike abdomen
- Dizziness, nausea and vomiting, and respiratory distress in severe cases

When treating patients with black widow spider bite, you should usually provide general wound care and transport.

Brown Recluse Spider

The brown recluse spider is generally brown but can range in color from yellow to dark chocolate brown. The characteristic marking is a brown, violin-shaped marking on the upper back. The bite of the brown recluse spider is a serious medical condition: The bite usually does not heal and may require surgical repair (Figure 24-24*).

Unfortunately, most brown recluse spider bite victims are unaware that they have been bitten, since the bite is often painless at first. Several hours after the bite, it becomes bluish surrounded by a white periphery, then a red halo or "bull's-eye" pattern. Within 7–10 days, the bite becomes a large ulcer.

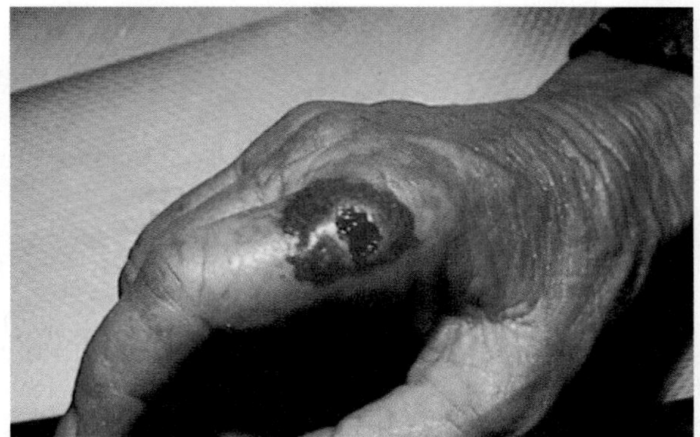

FIGURE 24-24 * Wound from a brown recluse spider bite.

Scorpion

Of the three species of scorpion in the United States that sting and inject poisonous venom, the sting of only one is generally fatal. The severity of the sting depends on the amount of venom injected. Ninety percent of all scorpion stings occur on the hands.

In addition to the general signs and symptoms of bites and stings, scorpion stings cause a sharp pain at the injection site, drooling, poor coordination, incontinence, and seizures.

Fire Ant

Most common in the southeastern United States, the fire ant gets its name not from its red to black color, but from the intense, fiery, burning pain its bite causes. Fire ants bite down into the skin, then sting downwardly as they pivot; the result is a characteristic circular pattern of bites. Fire ant bites produce extremely painful vesicles that are filled with fluid. At first the fluid is clear; later it becomes cloudy. Fire ant bites can also cause a large local reaction, characterized by swelling, pain, and redness that affect the entire extremity.

Tick

Tick bites (Figure 24-25*) are serious because ticks can carry tick fever, Rocky Mountain spotted fever, and other bacterial diseases. Lyme disease, usually transmitted by the

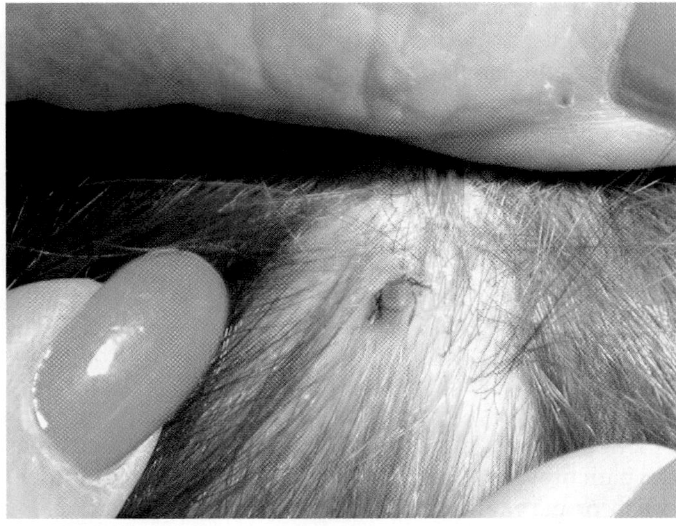

FIGURE 24-25 * A tick embedded in the scalp. (© Charles Stewart, MD, & Associates)

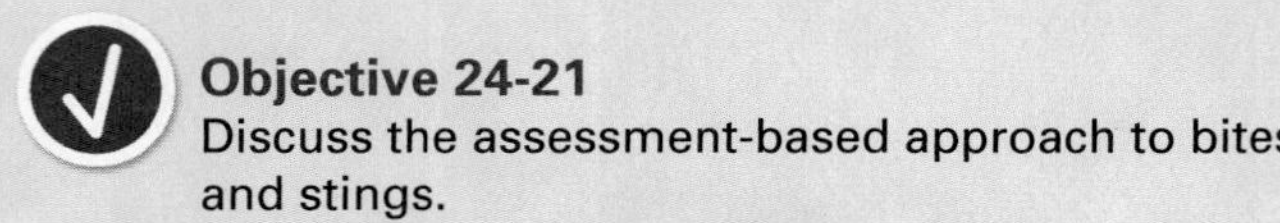

Objective 24-21
Discuss the assessment-based approach to bites and stings.

Objective 24-22
Describe the signs and symptoms and the emergency medical care for anaphylactic shock resulting from a bite or sting.

tiny deer tick but now thought sometimes to be transmitted by the larger dog tick, can cause long-term neurological and other complications if not identified and treated early.

Ticks are visible after they have attached themselves to the skin; they often choose warm, moist areas, such as the scalp, other hairy areas, the armpits, the groin, and skin creases. Many patients are unaware that they have been bitten by a tick.

The only appropriate prehospital treatment for tick bite is prompt removal of the tick, which can help prevent infection. To remove a tick, use tweezers and grasp the tick as close as possible to the point where it is attached to the skin. Pull firmly and steadily until the tick is dislodged. Do not twist or jerk the tick, since that may result in incomplete removal. Never pluck an embedded tick out of the skin, as you may force infected blood into the patient. Avoid squashing an engorged tick during removal, since infected blood may spread contamination. After removal, wash the bite area thoroughly with soap and water and apply an antiseptic.

Assessment-Based Approach: Bites and Stings

Scene Size-Up

Your priority during scene size-up should be to protect yourself and your partner. If your patient has been bitten or stung, you too might fall victim to bites and stings unless you exercise caution.

Rather than going directly to the patient's side, pause and look and listen for swarming bees or hornets. If they are present, you may have to wait until they disperse before approaching.

When you get to the patient's side, scan the ground around him carefully, looking for snakes, ant hills, or openings to underground yellow jacket nests. When you begin to examine the patient, be alert to the possibility that insects have become trapped in his clothing and may bite or sting when you move it.

Once your safety is ensured, look around the scene for evidence of what may have bitten or stung the patient. Is an insect nest visible in a nearby tree, or under the eaves of a house, or in the ground nearby? Are there signs that the patient was engaged in activity such as clearing underbrush or gardening that might have disturbed snakes or insects? Was the patient working in a garage, basement, attic, or shed where spiders and other insects might nest? Are there dead insects on the ground around the patient?

Primary Assessment

During the primary assessment, gather a general impression of the patient and his mental status. If elements of the scene size-up have led you to suspect the possibility of bites or stings, be especially alert when assessing the airway and breathing. Remember that some patients have an allergic reaction to bites and stings that can lead to anaphylactic shock, an emergency that generally has a rapid and life-threatening effect on the airway and breathing.

Secondary Assessment

If you detect the signs and symptoms of anaphylactic shock listed in the next section, continue with assessment and emergency medical care as described in Chapter 21, "Anaphylactic Reactions," and in the sections on anaphylactic shock later in this chapter. If the patient displays the more common signs and symptoms of reaction to bites and stings, continue with the assessment as described in the section on injected poisons in Chapter 22, "Toxicologic Emergencies." Then, provide emergency care as described under "Emergency Medical Care for a Bite or Sting" in this chapter.

Signs and Symptoms of Anaphylactic Shock As noted earlier, anaphylactic shock, a life-threatening medical emergency, may develop following bites or stings. If a patient develops signs and symptoms of this condition, perform the necessary emergency care and transport immediately. Signs and symptoms include the following:

- Hives
- Flushing
- Upper airway obstruction
- Faintness
- Dizziness
- Generalized itching
- Generalized swelling, including eyelids, lips, and tongue
- Difficulty swallowing
- Shortness of breath, wheezing, or stridor
- Labored breathing
- Abdominal or uterine cramps
- Confusion
- Loss of responsiveness
- Convulsions
- Hypotension (low blood pressure)

Objective 24-23
Describe the signs and symptoms and the emergency medical care for a bite or sting.

Objective 24-24
Recognize the signs, symptoms, and patient history associated with the bite or sting of a marine animal and the emergency medical care for marine life poisoning.

Emergency Medical Care for Anaphylactic Shock

Care for anaphylactic shock is as follows:

1. *Maintain a patent airway.* Suction secretions.
2. *Administer oxygen and support breathing.* Provide oxygen at 15 lpm by nonrebreather mask if breathing is adequate. Provide positive pressure ventilation with supplemental oxygen at 10–12 per minute if breathing is (or becomes) inadequate.
3. *Administer epinephrine by a prescribed auto-injector* with permission from medical direction for patients with airway obstruction, wheezing, hypotension, or prior anaphylaxis.
4. *Call for advanced life support.*
5. *Initiate early transport.*

Review the complete description of signs and symptoms and emergency medical care for this condition in Chapter 21, "Anaphylactic Reactions."

Signs and Symptoms of a Bite or Sting General signs and symptoms of bites and stings include the following:

- History of a bite from a spider or snake, or a sting from an insect, scorpion, or marine animal
- Pain that is often immediate and severe or burning; within several hours the area may become numb
- Redness or other discoloration around the bite
- Swelling around the bite, sometimes gradually spreading
- Weakness or faintness
- Dizziness
- Chills
- Fever
- Nausea or vomiting
- Bite marks
- Stinger

Emergency Medical Care for a Bite or Sting

General emergency medical care for bites and stings includes the following steps:

1. *If the stinger is still present, remove it by gently scraping against it* with the edge of a credit card or similar item. Scrape in the direction of the base of the stinger to avoid breaking it off below the skin. Be careful not to squeeze the stinger with tweezers, forceps, or your fingers as doing so can force additional venom from the venom sac into the wound. Make sure you remove the venom sac because it can continue to secrete venom even though the stinger is detached from the insect.
2. *Wash the area around the bite or sting* gently with a mild agent or strong soap solution. If necessary, irrigate the area with a large amount of sterile saline. Make sure contaminated saline flows away from the body. Never scrub the area.
3. *Remove any jewelry or other constricting objects* as soon as possible, ideally before any swelling begins.
4. *Lower the injection site below the level of the heart.*
5. *Apply a cold pack to an insect bite or sting* to relieve pain and swelling. Do not apply cold to snakebites or to injuries inflicted by marine animals.
6. *Some experts advise the use of a constricting band in the treatment of a snakebite, proximal to the bite.* Consult medical direction and follow local protocols.
7. *Observe the patient carefully for the signs and symptoms of an allergic reaction;* in cases of reaction, treat as described in Chapter 21, "Anaphylactic Reactions."
8. *Keep the patient calm, limit his physical activity, and keep him warm. Transport as soon as possible.* If the patient shows any signs of allergic reaction, begin transport immediately.

Reassessment

Most important during the reassessment is to monitor the patient's airway, breathing, and circulation carefully. The signs and symptoms of anaphylactic shock may take minutes to several hours to develop. You should be alert to their appearance and be prepared to provide the emergency medical care for this life-threatening condition as just outlined.

Marine Life Bites and Stings

There are approximately 2,000 poisonous marine animals. While most types live in temperate or tropical waters, some can be found in virtually all waters. Most poisonous marine life is not aggressive; in fact, most cases of such poisoning occur when a person swims into or steps on an animal.

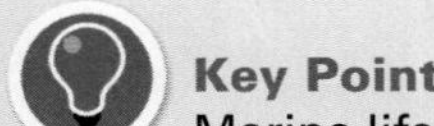

Key Points
Marine life venoms differ from land animal venoms. Marine life venoms can cause more extensive tissue damage, but can be destroyed by heat, requiring application of heat, not ice.

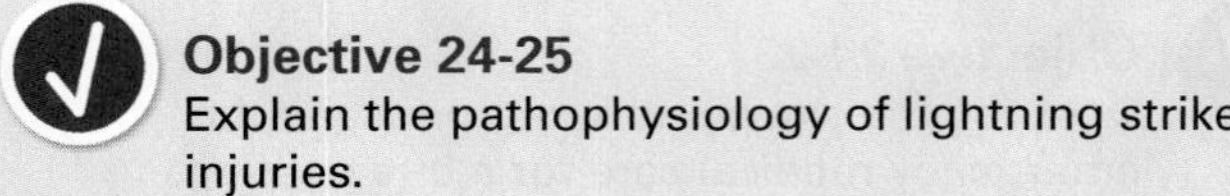

Objective 24-25
Explain the pathophysiology of lightning strike injuries.

There are two important differences between the bites and stings of marine animals and those of land animals. First, the venom of marine life may cause more extensive tissue damage than that of land animals. Second, venoms of aquatic organisms are destroyed by heat; so heat, not ice, should be applied to marine bites and stings.

In cases of marine life bites and stings, try to identify the animal because some very effective antivenins are available.

Emergency Medical Care for Marine Life Poisoning

In general, bites and stings inflicted by marine life should be treated the same as soft tissue injuries. However, follow these specific guidelines as needed:

- Use forceps to remove any material that sticks to the sting site on the surface of the flesh, then irrigate the wound with water.
- Do not attempt to remove spines that are embedded in joints or that are deeply embedded in skin.
- If the patient was stung by a jellyfish, coral, hydra, or anemone, carefully remove dried tentacles and pour vinegar on the affected area to denature the toxin. If meat tenderizer is available, sprinkle the area with it; doing so will help stop the stinging.
- Apply heat or soak the affected area in hot water for at least 30 minutes or throughout transport.

Lightning Strike Injuries

Lightning strikes cause more deaths per year than any other meteorological phenomenon. Approximately 1,000–5,000 people are struck each year in the United States, with 300–500 deaths occurring as a result of the strikes. The highest incidence of a lightning strike is in July, followed by August and June. The highest number of reported lightning strikes occur on Sundays. The second highest incidence occurs on Saturday, followed by Wednesday. These months and days reflect an increase in outdoor activities, including work and recreation. Males are more than eight times more likely to be struck by lightning than females. Children who are playing outside or involved in recreational or sporting activities are frequent victims. A majority of the lightning strikes involve only one person. Approximately 70 percent of lightning deaths involve only one person, whereas 15 percent of lightning deaths involve two people, and 15 percent of the deaths involve three or more victims from the same incident.

Many people believe the highest incidence of lightning strikes is on golf courses. Actually, the majority of lightning strikes, approximately 30 percent, occur in work-related situations, while recreational and open field activities account for 27 percent. Approximately 14 percent of lightning strikes occur to people who are standing under trees. Only 5 percent of all lightning strikes occur when playing golf. Interestingly, talking on the telephone accounts for 2.4 percent of lightning strikes. EMS and other public safety call takers and dispatchers commonly use a headset as part of their communication equipment. The number of call takers and dispatchers struck while connected to the headset is 0.7 percent.

Pathophysiology of a Lightning Strike Injury

Lightning is neither alternating current (AC) nor direct current (DC); however, it acts much more like direct current than alternating current. This has many clinical implications. The current associated with a lightning strike is massive. A lightning bolt's current ranges from 100 million to 2 billion volts with an amperage as high as 200,000. As a point of comparison, standard household current is typically 110–200 volts and 100–200 amps at a breaker box, and 120 volts and 15–20 amps at an outlet. The duration of the lightning strike is 1/100th to 1/1,000th of a second. The speed of a lightning bolt is 1–2 million meters per second. The contact temperature of a lightning bolt is 15,000°F–60,000°F. Even though the contact temperature is so high, the extremely short duration time prevents deep internal and external burns to the body. Contrary to a common misconception, lightning injuries are not typically major burn injuries.

Thunder associated with a lightning bolt is produced by a rapid expansion of the air immediately surrounding the bolt. The rapid explosion and implosion of the superheated and then cooled air, which creates the typical thunder sound, has a major effect on a lightning strike victim. The rapid explosion and implosion of air will propel the person, leading to blunt trauma. Also, the rapid change in air pressure can cause pressure changes in the

Key Points
The heart and nervous tissue are most sensitive to lightning strikes.

Objective 24-26
Given a scenario with a patient who has been struck by lightning, predict findings and complications associated with the mechanism of injury.

body's air-containing cavities, leading to damage and possible rupture. Thus, a lightning strike patient is not only a medical patient but also commonly a trauma patient. Head, neck, chest, abdominal, pelvic, spinal, and extremity trauma must be suspected in lightning strike patients. This is a reason to provide complete immobilization to all suspected lightning strike patients.

There are four major lightning strike mechanisms:

- **Direct strike**. Lightning bolt makes direct contact with the patient.
- **Contact strike**. Lightning strikes an object the patient is in contact with.
- **Splash or side flash strike**. Lightning strikes an object and jumps to a nearby person.
- **Ground current or step voltage strike**. Lightning current energizes the ground.

The direct strike carries the highest rate of injury and death. In a ground current, the farther the patient from the strike, the less the injury and other effects suffered by the patient.

The nervous tissue and the heart are most sensitive to lightning strikes. The lightning will overwhelm and short circuit the body's electrical system. When lightning involves the heart, the heart is depolarized similarly to the depolarization that occurs in a defibrillation. Actually, defibrillation is nothing more than a direct-current shock. If an oscilloscope is present following the defibrillation in a patient, you can note the period of asystole (no rhythm or heart contraction that appears as a flatline on the monitor) following the discharge of energy. The same effect is created by a lightning strike. The heart is depolarized by the massive discharge of energy through the body. Because the energy is so massive, the asystole lasts for a much longer period of time. Since asystole is a condition where there is no cardiac contraction, the result is cardiac arrest. This is called primary cardiac arrest.

The brain is also very sensitive to the lightning strike. The medulla, which houses the respiratory center, is shut down by the lightning strike, and the patient stops breathing. The muscles in the chest, along with all the other muscles in the body, contract severely and for a long period of time. This is similar to defibrillation when the muscular contraction from the shock causes the patient to "jump." Again, the main difference is that the chest muscles during defibrillation only contract for a brief period of time, whereas in a lightning strike, muscle contraction can be prolonged. Another consideration is that the severe muscular contraction may propel the patient, causing blunt trauma.

The heart muscle has properties of automaticity, which means that it can stimulate its own impulse without the help of the brain. What commonly happens in a lightning strike patient is that the heart will begin to beat spontaneously on its own without any intervention; however, the inspiratory centers in the medulla of the brain remain dormant for a much longer time. Despite the patient's heart resuming its beat and regaining a spontaneous pulse, the patient is yet unable to begin to breathe on his own. As the heart beats without any supporting respiration, it begins to circulate severely deoxygenated blood. The heart then becomes hypoxic and acidotic. As the hypoxia and acidosis build up, the heart becomes irritable. The irritability may trigger ventricular fibrillation, leading to a secondary cardiac arrest. This patient will be more difficult to resuscitate, since he will be more severely hypoxic and acidotic.

You, as an EMT, may arrive on the scene and find that the patient—who was in cardiac arrest without pulses, as witnessed by bystanders—has regained a pulse by the time of your arrival with little or no intervention. However, the patient will still not be breathing spontaneously. In this circumstance, aggressive airway management, ventilation, and oxygenation are necessary.

Assessment of the Lightning Strike Patient

The body systems affected by a lightning strike and the related signs and symptoms are:

Nervous System

- Altered mental status—may range from confusion to unresponsiveness
- Retrograde amnesia—cannot remember events before the incident
- Anterograde amnesia—cannot remember events after the incident
- Weakness—most often in the lower extremities
- Pain, tingling, and numbness
- Pale, cool, and clammy skin—may be mottled or cyanotic
- Temporary paralysis
- Dizziness
- Loss of pupillary function

Objective 24-27
Describe the emergency medical care for a patient who has been struck by lightning.

Key Points
Prevention of high-altitude sickness includes ascending gradually. Treatment of high-altitude sickness includes moving the patient to a lower altitude.

- Seizures
- Vertigo

Keep in mind that abnormal nervous system findings may be due to head injury from the blunt trauma and not the lightning strike itself.

Cardiac System

- Asystole or ventricular fibrillation
- Irregular pulse

Respiratory System

- Respiratory distress
- Apnea—absence of breathing

Skin

- Burns—most often are superficial; partial-thickness and full-thickness burns are typically associated with metal on the patient (e.g., chains, coins, hairpins) heating up and causing the burns
- Linear burns—appear as streaks down the body and are associated with sweat on the surface of the body heating up and causing the burns
- Feathering—not a true burn; appears as a nonblanching, reddish brown fern pattern (Figure 24-26*)
- Punctuate burns—appear similar to cigarette burns
- Thermal burns—may occur if the clothing catches on fire

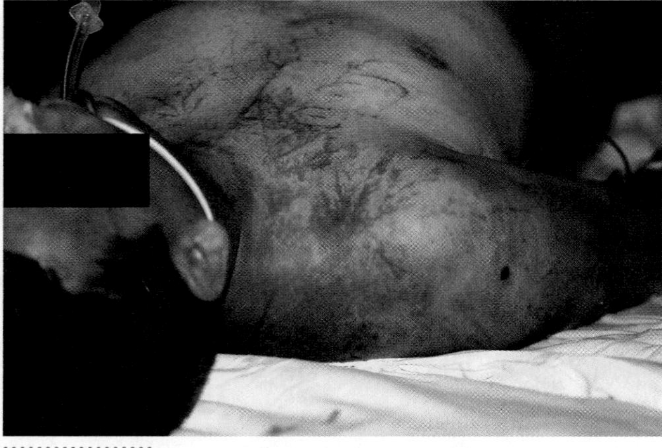

FIGURE 24-26 * A feathering pattern on the skin resulting from a lightning strike. (© David Effron, MD)

Musculoskeletal

- Dislocations
- Fractures

Both dislocations and fractures occur as a result of either the strong muscular contraction or the patient being propelled by the thunder.

Ophthalmic (Eye)

- Unequal pupils
- Drooping eyelid (ptosis)

Otologic (Ear)

- Ruptured tympanic membrane (eardrum)
- Tinnitus (ringing in the ear)
- Deafness

Emergency Care for the Lightning Strike Patient

When managing a lightning strike patient, remember that a lightning strike is not typically a serious burn injury. Rather, you must manage the patient as a medical patient with nervous system and possibly cardiac rhythm dysfunction and as a trauma patient with possible blunt injury. Emergency care includes the following:

- Ensure that the scene is safe; do not become a lightning strike patient yourself.
- If the patient's clothes are on fire, put out the fire.
- Establish in-line manual stabilization.
- Establish an airway if the patient has an altered mental status.
- If the patient is in cardiac arrest, immediately begin CPR and attach the AED. Deliver defibrillation based on the analysis and prompts of the AED after five cycles of 30:2 if the patient's downtime was greater than 4–5 minutes. Provide aggressive ventilation with a high concentration of oxygen.
- If the patient has a pulse but is not breathing or not breathing adequately, begin aggressive positive pressure ventilation at 10–12 per minute. Supply high concentrations of oxygen while ventilating.
- Completely immobilize the patient to a backboard.
- Transport while continuously monitoring the patient's condition.

Objective 24-28
Describe the signs, symptoms, and patient history associated with acute mountain sicknesses and emergency medical care for acute mountain sickness.

Objective 24-29
Describe the signs, symptoms, and patient history associated with high altitude pulmonary edema and emergency medical care for high altitude pulmonary edema.

High-Altitude Sickness

At high altitudes, the pressure of the ambient atmosphere is decreased. As a consequence, the total pressure of oxygen is also decreased, making oxygen less available. An environment with less oxygen may aggravate existing medical conditions, such as angina, congestive heart failure, and respiratory diseases, or it may cause new illnesses to occur. Even healthy individuals can experience illness at a high altitude, especially if the ascent is rapid.

A high altitude is considered to be an altitude above 5,000 feet. At this altitude, the hypoxic environment may be noticeable to the person, but serious illness rarely occurs. An altitude above 8,000 feet is where serious altitude illnesses may present, especially if a rapid ascent is involved. General signs and symptoms of altitude illness are:

- General ill feeling
- Loss of appetite
- Headache
- Disturbance in sleep
- Respiratory distress upon exertion

High-altitude sickness can be prevented by ascending gradually, allowing the body time to acclimate, limiting exertion at high altitude, descending to a lower altitude to sleep, and eating a high-carbohydrate diet. Some people may take acetazolamide (Diamox) or nifedipine (Procardia, Adalat) to try to prevent altitude sickness.

Acute Mountain Sickness

Acute mountain sickness (AMS) typically occurs in people who rapidly ascend to 6,600 feet or greater. Signs and symptoms could develop from 6 to 24 hours after the ascent.

Signs and Symptoms

Signs and symptoms of AMS include:

- Weakness
- Nausea
- Headache
- Shortness of breath
- Light-headedness
- Loss of appetite
- Fatigue
- Difficulty sleeping

Severe signs and symptoms of AMS include:

- Severe weakness
- Decreased urine output
- Vomiting
- Increased shortness of breath
- Altered mental status

These signs and symptoms may worsen if the person ascends higher. Acute mountain illness with often resolve itself within one to two days if the patient does not ascend any higher.

Emergency Medical Care

The primary treatment is to stop the ascent and considering moving the patient down to a lower altitude. Administration of supplemental oxygen may relieve the signs and symptoms. If the case is severe, administer oxygen and move the patient down to a lower elevation.

High-Altitude Pulmonary Edema

High-altitude pulmonary edema (HAPE) is a condition affecting the lungs and gas exchange. Changes in the pressure in the pulmonary vessels cause fluid to be forced out of the capillaries and to collect in and around the alveoli. Children and men are more prone to HAPE. The condition can occur above 8,000 feet; however, it more commonly occurs above 14,500 feet.

Signs and Symptoms

Signs and symptoms of HAPE include:

- Shortness of breath at rest
- Cough
- Fatigue
- Headache
- Loss of appetite
- Tachypnea
- Tachycardia
- Cyanosis
- Crackles or wheezing in at least one lobe of the lung
- Weakness

Objective 24-30
Describe the signs, symptoms, and patient history associated with high altitude cerebral edema and emergency medical care for high altitude cerebral edema.

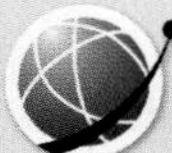

Media Resources
Go to www.bradybooks.com for mykit. Highlights:

- *Web Resource:* Myxedema Coma
- *Web Resource:* Altitude-related Illnesses

Emergency Medical Care

The best emergency care is to move the patient to a lower altitude and administer oxygen. If descent is not possible, administration of oxygen may eliminate the HAPE. This may take 36 to 72 hours to resolve with oxygen therapy alone.

High-Altitude Cerebral Edema

High-altitude cerebral edema (HACE) occurs from the collection of an excessive amount of fluid in the brain tissue. This increases the pressure within the skull and puts pressure on the brain. Most cases occur at altitudes above 12,000 feet; however, cases have been reported at 8,200 feet.

Signs and Symptoms

Signs and symptoms of HACE include:

- Severe headache
- Uncoordination (ataxia)
- Nausea and vomiting
- Altered mental status
- Seizures
- Coma

Emergency Medical Care

The emergency medical care focuses on immediately moving the patient to a lower altitude and administration of supplemental oxygen. In severe cases, it may be necessary to provide positive pressure ventilation with oxygen connected to the ventilation device.

CHAPTER REVIEW

SUMMARY

The environment, loosely defined, is all the surrounding factors that can have an impact on a human. And despite the need for humans to rely on the environment for existence, they also must have certain mechanisms to protect themselves from any abnormalities (or extremes) of the environment. An occasion when environmental influences on a person are so extreme that the body cannot adequately cope is said to be an "environmental emergency." Environmental emergencies as discussed in this chapter include extremes in temperature conditions, which can precipitate either hyperthermia or hypothermia; the adverse effects that result when humans are bitten or stung by insects, snakes, or marine life; lightning strike injuries; and high-altitude sickness.

Although environmental emergencies can affect anyone, they commonly have the most severe effect on patients at either end of the age range (very young or very old), those with significant medical conditions, and individuals taking certain medications.

As an EMT, you must remain acutely aware of environmental influences on every patient you encounter. The first reason is obvious: A person subjected to extreme temperature changes will eventually start to falter, especially if he is not adequately prepared or acclimated to the temperature. Second, a person with either a medical or a traumatic emergency may deteriorate more quickly if the emergency happened in a location where the environmental temperature was abnormally high or low. Third, regarding bites and stings, the person may be unaware for several hours that he was bitten or stung, or he may try to minimize the injury, resulting in a delay of care. Yet another environmental scenario is when the EMT is summoned to care for a patient who was bitten or stung, and the offending agent (e.g., swarming bees) is still within close proximity to the patient. This latter scenario creates a potential environmental concern for the care providers as well as for the patient. When responding to patients who have been struck by lightning, the EMT may be exposed to the possibility of being struck if the storm is still active. High-altitude rescue presents with many complications. Most often, specially trained teams are used to perform high-altitude rescue.

The assessment approach to the patient with an environmental emergency is the same as for any other type of emergency the EMT responds to. The first phase of assessment, the scene size-up, will many times give the EMTs insight as to the type of environmental emergency they may be dealing with. The goal for the EMTs then becomes protecting themselves from the environmental extreme while they are providing care to the patient.

The approach to environmental emergencies, although complex at times, is usually straightforward. First, attempt to remove the environmental influence causing the emergency or remove the patient from the environmental influence. Second, support the body's own compensatory mechanisms. Third, provide specific interventions for any lost function of the airway, breathing, and circulation. And last, determine the best transport destination and continue care en route with ALS backup as warranted.

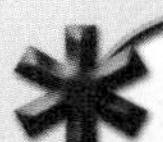

CASE STUDY FOLLOW-UP

SCENE SIZE-UP

Your initial call was for a disoriented elderly woman who fell into a snowbank wearing only a housecoat and slippers approximately 2 hours prior to the call. The woman has also complained of pain in her left ankle.

You pull up at 2125 Central Avenue at 1321 hours. The police radioed in the call, and their presence on the scene assures you that it is secure. It is an overcast afternoon, with gusty winds. The outside temperature is 26°F. Because of information in the dispatch and the weather conditions, you are alert to the probability of generalized hypothermia as well as possible local cold injury and other injuries that might have resulted from a fall. With police on the scene to watch the ambulance, you leave its motor running and the heat turned up in the patient compartment as you get out. One officer stays with the ambulance, while another leads you to the woman.

The scene size-up reveals no obvious hazards; the patient is in the alley behind the house and there are no traffic hazards. Because there is only one patient and the mechanism of injury was a fall, there is no need for additional units.

PRIMARY ASSESSMENT

You approach the woman and say to her, "Hello. My name is Sonia Weill and this is my partner, Jake Gallow. Could you tell us your name and if you're in any pain?" The woman replies, "I'm Harriet Rector. I'm cold. I want to go home. My husband fell once like this, but not for so long. He's dead now. I just want to go inside. I have to feed Fluffy. Nothing hurts. I should have taken out the garbage tomorrow. Is that Thursday? But I hadn't taken it out yesterday. My ankle hurts. On the right. No, the left. Where's my dog?"

In spite of the fact that Mrs. Rector fell into a big, soft snowbank, your partner initiates manual in-line stabilization of her head and neck as a precaution. Your general impression is of an elderly female who is responsive but disoriented. The patient knows her name but is unclear as to the day of the week and exactly where she is. You proceed to assess airway, breathing, and circulation and find no life threats other than the cold environment. You begin oxygen therapy at 15 lpm with a nonrebreather mask and cover the patient with a blanket, making sure to roll her carefully in order to place the blanket under her.

SECONDARY ASSESSMENT

Although the possibility of spine injury is small, you and Jake transfer and immobilize Mrs. Rector to a long spine board and quickly move her into the back of the warm ambulance before undertaking the secondary assessment. You take care to be extremely gentle in moving her.

Once Mrs. Rector is comfortably settled inside the ambulance, you continue questioning her, using the OPQRST format. You determine that her chief complaint is that her left leg hurts from the fall. You attempt to obtain a history, but Mrs. Rector does not respond appropriately to your questions, chiefly asking about her dog. You reassure her that you will get someone to take care of Fluffy.

You perform a physical exam. As you are examining the abdomen, you slide your hand inside Mrs. Rector's housecoat and place the back of your hand on her abdomen. You note that the skin there is cool to the touch, one of the signs of generalized hypothermia. The extremities exam reveals a painful, swollen left ankle. You quickly apply a splint, being sure to check motor function, sensation, and circulation before and after application of the splint.

At the same time, you check for signs of local cold injury. Mrs. Rector was able to keep her hands warm by tucking them under her armpits, but her feet, which were covered only by flimsy slippers, show signs of early superficial cold injury. She has no sensation in her toes. The skin is soft but very cold to the touch, and normal skin color does not return after palpation. You have already removed the slippers and splinted the painful, swollen ankle. Now you splint the other foot as well to prevent movement and protect both feet with dry dressings.

Jake, meanwhile, has finished gathering the vital signs: they are blood pressure 102/60, heart rate 60, respiration rate 12, and skin pale, cold, and firm to the touch.

REASSESSMENT

Once en route to the hospital, you cover Mrs. Rector in an additional warm, dry blanket. You had previously turned up the heat in the patient compartment, producing a suitable environment for passive rewarming.

Your priority is to maintain an airway and breathing and reassess vital signs and mental status. Mrs. Rector continues to speak distractedly about her dog and a number of seemingly unconnected events, indicating that her airway and breathing are adequate but her mental status is still altered. You check to be sure that the nonrebreather mask is securely sealed to her face and that the oxygen flow is adequate. Jake takes another set of vital signs: blood pressure is still 102/60, but the heart rate has increased to 65 and the respiration rate is now 14. The skin is still cool, but it now has a mottled appearance. Mrs. Rector begins to complain that her feet tingle and hurt.

You arrive at Ellis Hospital at 1341 hours. You give your report on the case to the emergency nurse, being sure to include the latest set of vitals taken in the ambulance and to note Mrs. Rector's new complaints about pains in her feet. Then you telephone Mrs. Rector's neighbor who agrees to take care of the dog. Before you leave the hospital, you see the emergency physician and ask about Mrs. Rector's prognosis. She says that they've begun actively rewarming Mrs. Rector, but that it's too early to tell how she will respond.

A few weeks later, you and Jake pass by 2125 Central Avenue on your way back from a call and see Mrs. Rector out walking Fluffy. You return her wave and smile as you go by.

IN REVIEW

1. Name the five processes through which the body loses heat.
2. Explain the difference between hypothermia and hyperthermia.
3. List the signs and symptoms of generalized hypothermia.
4. Explain the steps in treatment of a patient suffering from a local cold injury.
5. Explain the treatment of the patient suffering from a heat emergency.
6. List conditions that would predispose a patient to experience a cold emergency.
7. List conditions that would predispose a patient to experience a heat emergency.
8. Explain the difference between active and passive rewarming.
9. Explain some of the effects of a lightning strike on the nervous, cardiac, respiratory, and musculoskeletal systems, as well as the skin, eyes, and ears.
10. Explain the emergency medical care for the lightning strike patient.
11. List the signs and symptoms associated with bites and stings.
12. Explain the general emergency medical care for a patient suffering from a bite or sting.
13. List the various conditions the patient may suffer when exposed to high altitude.
14. Describe the emergency care for high-altitude conditions.

CRITICAL THINKING

You are called early one summer morning for a patient who has fallen at a gated retirement community near your station. As you proceed to the ambulance, your partner comments on how hot the day is already. You agree, and as soon as you get into your ambulance en route to the scene, you turn on the air conditioning so that the patient compartment is cool. When arriving on scene, you are met at the doorway by a middle-aged female who states she is the patient's daughter. Her father, she explains, did not answer his telephone yesterday afternoon, last night, or this morning, so she became concerned and drove 2 hours to his home to check on him. When she found him, he was lying naked on the bathroom floor.

She escorts you into the home and, as you complete your scene size-up, you note that there are no signs of struggling, the ambient temperature is cool from air conditioning, probably 70°F –72°F, and the entry and egress from the residence will be easy and straightforward. With your gloves on, you and your partner greet the patient, Mr. Ward.

Mr. Ward recounts a history of getting out of the shower yesterday afternoon and stepping onto the tile bathroom floor where he slipped and fell, injuring his hip. This means, by your estimation, that the patient has been lying naked on a cold tile floor in an air-conditioned home for almost 18 hours. You note that the patient is a rather inconsistent historian, and the daughter states to you, "He is just not acting like himself." You assess the area of complaint and find palpable instability, pain, and an overlying contusion to the injured hip.

The patient continues to complain of pain and of being cold, and you note he is becoming less and less compliant to your questioning. The patient's daughter is urging you to hurry up and leave, and the patient wants you to put him in bed and cover him so he can warm up. He now seems not to be concerned with his injured hip at all. At this point, your partner tells you he is going to retrieve the immobilization equipment from the ambulance, and he asks you if, while he is there, he should grab the tympanic thermometer.

1. Does this call initially present as one with an environmental concern?
2. What is the patient's initial emergency that rendered him susceptible to an environmental emergency?
3. What would you expect to find regarding the patient's core temperature with the tympanic thermometer?
4. How might your treatment of this patient change, given a disturbance in his core temperature?
5. Describe the factors that contributed to the potential change in his core temperature.

PEARSON

EXPLORE mybradykit™

Please go to **www.bradybooks.com** to access mykit for this text. You will find quizzes, critical thinking scenarios, weblinks, animations, and videos related to this chapter—and much more. Look for online information on hypothermia and hyperthermia.

Register your access code from the front of your book by going to **www.bradybooks.com** and selecting the mykit links.

CHAPTER 25

Submersion Incidents: Drowning and Diving Emergencies

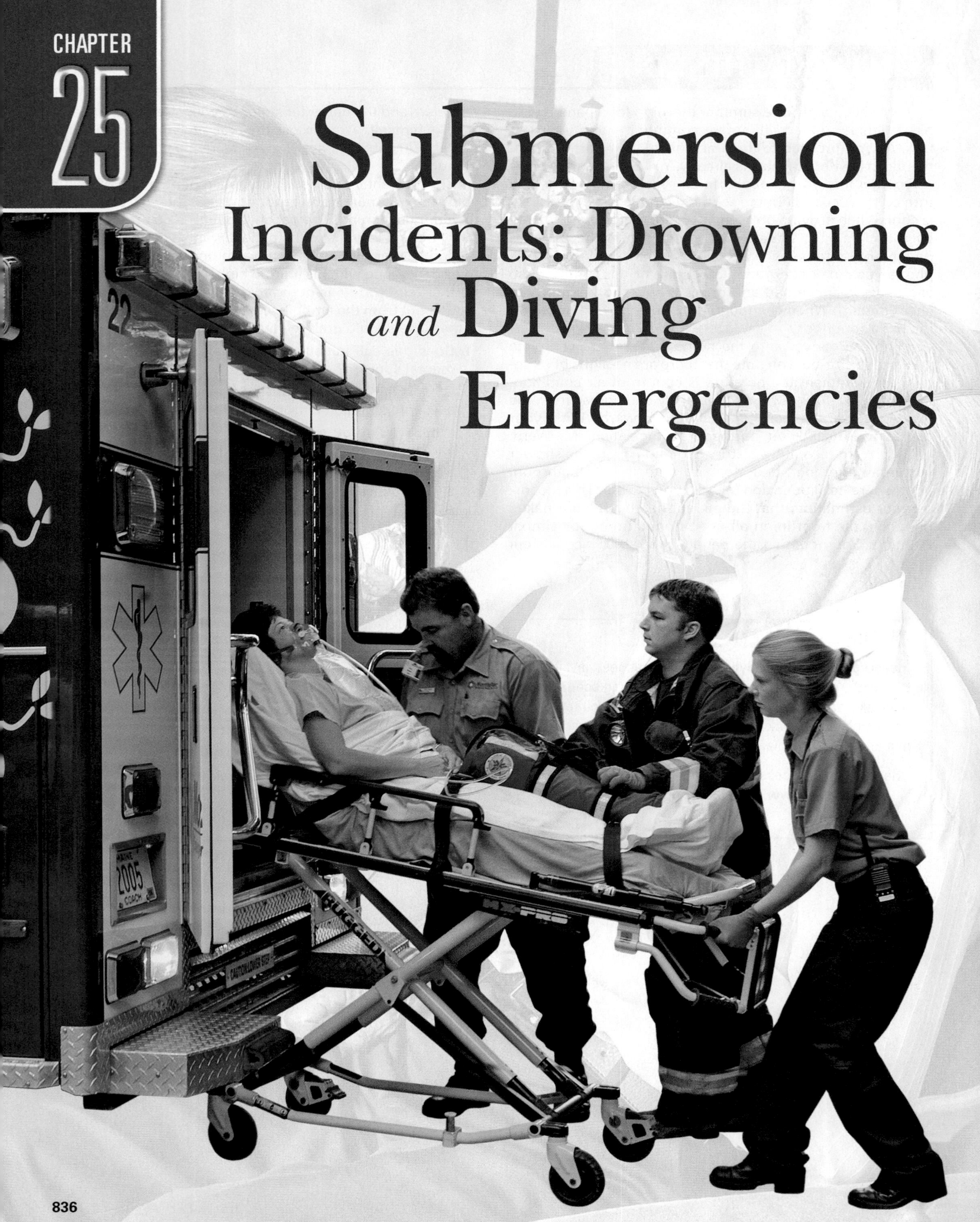

Navigation Guide

The following items provide an overview to the purpose and content of this chapter. The Standard and Competency are from the new National EMS Education Standards.

STANDARD **Trauma** (Content Area: Environmental Emergencies)

COMPETENCY Applies fundamental knowledge to provide basic emergency care and transportation based on assessment findings for an acutely injured patient.

OBJECTIVES: After reading this chapter, you should be able to:

25-1. Define key terms introduced in this chapter.
25-2. Discuss ways to reduce the risk of submersion incidents.
25-3. Describe factors that can lead to submersion incidents in infants, children, adolescents, and adults.
25-4. Explain factors that affect the likelihood of survival from submersion incidents.
25-5. Describe the pathophysiology of drowning.
25-6. Discuss the association between shallow water diving and spinal injuries.
25-7. Explain actions you should take to protect your own safety when responding to a water emergency.
25-8. Explain the necessity of taking spinal precautions to any swimmer or diver who may have suffered trauma.
25-9. Given a scenario in which a patient has suffered a submersion incident, explain how to provide resuscitative care.
25-10. Explain the assessment-based approach to drowning and other water-related injuries, including emergency medical care for the drowning victim.
25-11. Explain the formation and relief of gastric distention in patients involved in submersion incidents.
25-12. Describe laws of physics as they relate to scuba or deepwater diving, including:
- **a.** Boyle law
- **b.** Dalton law
- **c.** Henry law
- **d.** Charles law

25-13. Explain the pathophysiology of decompression sickness.
25-14. Recognize the signs, symptoms, and patient history associated with:
- **a.** Type I decompression sickness
- **b.** Type II decompression sickness
- **c.** Arterial gas embolism

25-15. Explain the pathophysiology of barotrauma injuries.
25-16. Describe the emergency medical care of patients suffering from air embolism, decompression sickness, and barotrauma.

KEY TERMS: Page references indicate first major use in this chapter. For complete defintions, see the Glossary at the back of the book.

drowning p. 838
dysbarism p. 849
gastric distention p. 847
mammalian diving reflex p. 843
surfactant p. 840

MEDIA RESOURCES: Please go to www.bradybooks.com to access mykit for this text. You will find quizzes, critical thinking scenarios, weblinks, animations, and videos related to this chapter—and much more. Look for online information on diving accidents and water-related emergencies.

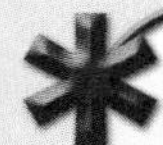

CASE STUDY

The Dispatch

EMS Unit 631—proceed to a submersion incident at 99 Wolf Road in the Delmar Hotel. The manager stated a 25-year-old male is in trouble in the pool. Police are en route at this time. Time out is 2132 hours.

Upon Arrival

Your ambulance arrives at the same time as the police unit. You are met at the hotel entrance by a frantic man who identifies himself as the manager. He leads you back to the pool, saying on the way, "I told them

continued

they couldn't have alcohol in the pool area. But they're so smart. They sneak it in anyway. Then they come running into the office, drunk, yelling for help. One of them thinks he can do a jack-knife into the shallow end. Idiots."

As you reach the pool area, you note a small crowd of young men and women on the deck. Some of them are yelling, "Come on, Robby! Get out, man! Come on!" A couple of paper bags and carry-alls are tipped over near the deck chairs, and empty beer bottles have rolled out from them. The police move the bystanders back and quiet them down.

With the scene secure, you approach the edge of the pool and observe in it a young man floating supine with the support of a hotel employee. The young man appears very scared and tells you he cannot feel his arms or legs.

How Would You Proceed to Assess and Care for This Patient?

During this chapter, you will learn special considerations of assessment and care for patients in water-related emergencies. Later, we will return to the case and apply what you have learned.

Introduction

Water-related incidents make up a category of environmental emergencies posing special challenges for EMTs. Patients in such incidents have often sustained life-threatening injuries. They need emergency medical care as rapidly as possible. But the circumstances in which they have received the injuries may expose medical personnel attempting to assist them to the risk of injury. Caring for patients in such circumstances requires of EMTs not only emergency medical skills but also the ability to recognize and avoid or reduce potential hazards at the scene.

Water-Related Emergencies

While drownings related to swimming are the type of fatality most commonly associated with water emergencies, they are actually responsible for a small number of water-related deaths. The rest are caused mostly by diving and deepwater exploration, boating, and water skiing. Water-related deaths may also result from motor vehicle accidents. In addition to drowning, water-related accidents can cause bleeding, soft tissue injuries, and musculoskeletal injuries.

Drownings do not always occur in large bodies of water. An adult can drown in just a few inches of water, and an infant in even less. Infants often drown in five-gallon buckets; others drown in bathtubs and toilets.

Water emergencies are especially tragic because many of the deaths could be prevented with the wearing of personal flotation devices (PFDs) when in or around water or when boating, with proper adult supervision of swimming pools, and with the provision of locked fences around pools. Prompt and proper application of basic life support techniques by bystanders could also reduce deaths. Commonsense precautions include the following:

- All pools should be fenced.
- Children should be under constant supervision if they are in the area of a lake, pool, pond, or container of water of any significant size.
- Water activities and alcohol do not mix.
- Life preservers or personal flotation devices (life jackets) must always be worn when boating.
- Avoid diving into shallow or unexplored bodies of water.
- Those with seizure disorders must be especially careful when in or around bodies of water.

Definitions

The terms used to describe water-related submersions and deaths vary. The two most common terms that have been used in the past, but commonly misunderstood, are *drowning* and *near-drowning*. According to the *2005 American Heart Association Guidelines for Cardiopulmonary Resuscitation and Emergency Cardiovascular Care*, there has been much confusion regarding the terms used when describing submersion incidents. Because of the confusion and the need for consistent reporting of submersion incidents, drowning is now the only recommended term to be used to describe a submersion event. A **drowning** is an incident in which someone is submerged or immersed in a liquid that results in a primary respiratory impairment. The liquid prevents the patient from breathing air. The patient may live or may die from the event. Regardless of the outcome, it is termed a drowning.

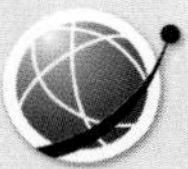

Media Resources
Go to www.bradybooks.com for mykit. Highlights:

- *Web Resource:* Diving Accidents
- *Web Resource:* Water-related Emergencies

Key Terms
drowning submersion causing primary respiratory impairment whether the person survives or dies after the event.

Objectives 25-2 to 25-4
List risks, factors that can lead to submersion, and factors that affect survival.

Incidence of Drowning

There are approximately 4,500 drowning deaths per year in the United States, making drowning the third most common cause of accidental death. Approximately 40 percent of the deaths are in children less than 5 years of age, with the second most common age group being teenagers and the third the elderly. Approximately 85 percent of the drownings are in males. Often, alcohol is involved in the incident.

In children less than 1 year of age, the bathtub is the most common location of drowning. Most often, the child will drown when the parent or primary caregiver leaves the child alone for less than 5 minutes. Keep in mind that drowning that occurs in a bathtub or pail of water may result from child abuse. Look for any other evidence of injury to the child. In children 1 to 5 years of age, the highest incidence of drowning occurs in swimming pools.

Adolescents and young adults most often drown in ponds, lakes, rivers, and oceans. There may be associated trauma, especially cervical spine injuries from diving into shallow water or areas with rock or other obstructions. Alcohol and recreational drugs may also put the adolescent or young adult at greater risk for drowning.

In the adult patient, consider the following conditions that may have led to the submersion:

- Hypoglycemia
- Myocardial infarction (heart attack) from exertion
- Cardiac dysrhythmia
- Syncope
- Seizure
- Depression or a suicide attempt
- Anxiety or a panic disorder
- Arthritis, Parkinson disease, or other neuromuscular disorder that leads to poor body control
- Exhaustion
- Hypothermia
- Alcohol or drug use
- Trauma (especially head or spinal)

Water sports also pose a hazard of submersion and drowning. The use of alcohol and drugs may impair judgment and lead to boating and other water-related accidents. Water skiing, jet skiing, and surfing can cause head or spinal trauma leading to submersion and drowning. Scuba diving accidents from exertion, inexperience, panic, and poor judgment may also cause a drowning. Panic can contribute to a drowning death (Figure 25-1*).

Prognostic Predictors

Quick rescue of the submerged patient from the water and early resuscitation are the most critical factors associated with better outcomes. No single individual characteristic has been found to predict survivability. The following characteristics are part of the Orlowski score that predicts likelihood that a patient would survive neurologically intact. The best chance for survival is in a patient who has two or fewer of the characteristics listed next. If three or more are present, the chance of survival is only 5 percent. The Orlowski predictors of survival are:

- Patient is 3 years of age or older.
- Patient was submerged for greater than 5 minutes.
- Resuscitation did not begin for more than 10 minutes after rescue.
- Patient is comatose on delivery to emergency department.
- Patient's arterial blood is very acidic (pH less than 7.10).

Moderate body core hypothermia associated with submersion is thought to provide a protective mechanism that reduces brain and other organ damage in children. However, most people do not become hypothermic quickly enough after submersion to reduce the severe cerebral injury from hypoxia and ischemia.

Pathophysiology of Drowning

Drowning can be very traumatic for the individual involved. As the person is submerged in water, he attempts to breathe, and either he aspirates water or his larynx spasms and causes him to suffocate. The most significant consequence of a drowning is the lack of ventilation while submerged, which leads to severe and prolonged hypoxia and the accumulation of carbon dioxide in the blood, which may lead to severe acid buildup within the body. The combined hypoxia and acidosis may lead to severe brain injury and cardiac arrest. In any drowning, the factor that has the greatest impact on the patient's prognosis

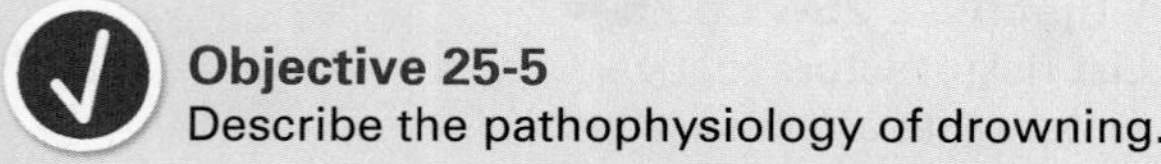

Objective 25-5
Describe the pathophysiology of drowning.

Key Terms
surfactant a substance responsible for maintaining surface tension in the alveoli.

SOMETHING GOES WRONG

Swallowing water
Fatigue
Unable to cope with currents
Injuries
Cold
Entanglement in plants
Loss of concentration

PANIC

INEFFICIENT BREATHING

DECREASED BUOYANCY

EXHAUSTION

DROWNING

CARDIAC ARREST

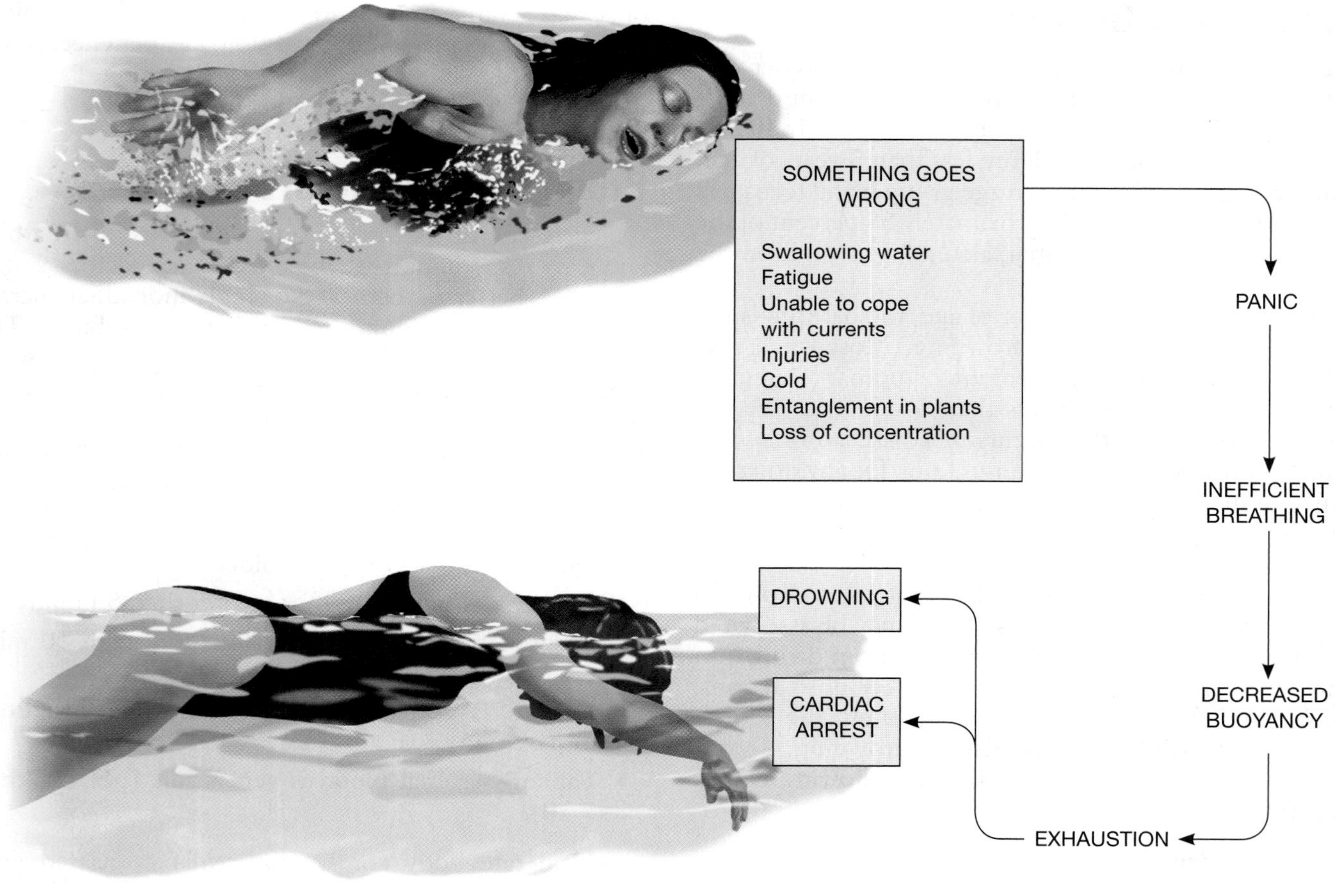

FIGURE 25-1 ✱ Panic can often contribute to the death of the person who loses self-control.

is the duration of the submersion and the consequent severity of the hypoxia. The severe hypoxia associated with the initial drowning event (primary injury) could produce prolonged effects that continue to damage tissue and organs and create an ongoing hypoxia (secondary injury).

Not all patients who are involved in a drowning aspirate water into their lungs. Approximately 10–15 percent of drowning patients are prevented from aspirating water into their lungs during submersion by the spasm and tight closing of the larynx (laryngospasm) that lasts until all inspiratory efforts have ceased. This is referred to as a "dry drowning." Drowning patients who do aspirate water usually aspirate only a small amount that is quickly absorbed by the respiratory tract and into the circulation and does not pose a major problem with airway obstruction.

Thus, the standard practice of performing abdominal thrusts is not necessary during the resuscitation of a drowning patient. In fact, performing abdominal thrusts may lead to regurgitation and aspiration of gastric contents. If water is present in the airway, suction it out. The only time abdominal thrusts should be performed is when a foreign body airway obstruction is suspected in the drowning patient. If the patient vomits during the resuscitation, log roll the patient onto one side and sweep or suction the oropharynx clear of the vomitus.

The issue of salt-water versus fresh-water drowning does not play a major role in resuscitation attempts by emergency medical services. Theoretically, there are differences between salt-water and fresh-water aspiration; however, clinically there is no difference in the resuscitation of the patient. Both types of drowning have a tendency to wash out surfactant.

Surfactant is a substance that maintains surface tension in the alveoli to keep them from collapsing. If surfac-

Key Points

The key to emergency care for drowning is to monitor the breathing status closely and provide positive pressure ventilation to any patient with an inadequate respiratory rate, inadequate tidal volume, or both.

Key Points

If the body core temperature is less than 86°F and the AED indicates a shockable rhythm, attempt just one shock. The patient must be rewarmed to at least 86°F before defibrillation is resumed.

tant is washed out, the alveoli tend to collapse (a condition called atelectasis). The damage to alveolar-capillary structures creates ventilation problems by decreasing functional lung volume and allowing fluid to leak around and into the alveoli, which creates pulmonary edema. The alveolar-capillary damage also interferes with gas exchange, impairing oxygenation of the blood and off-loading of carbon dioxide from the blood. This complication is known as acute respiratory distress syndrome (ARDS).

The key to emergency care is to monitor the breathing status closely and provide positive pressure ventilation to any drowning patient with an inadequate respiratory rate, inadequate tidal volume, or both. Auscultate the lungs for evidence of crackles (rales), which would indicate fluid in and around the alveoli. The patient who is breathing spontaneously but has signs or symptoms of respiratory distress or hypoxia can benefit dramatically from continuous positive airway pressure (CPAP) application. If CPAP is not available, consider early positive pressure ventilation with a bag-valve-mask device.

Maximize the oxygen being delivered to the patient by applying a nonrebreather mask at 15 lpm in the patient who has an adequate respiratory rate and tidal volume. If positive pressure ventilation is being performed, be sure to connect oxygen to the ventilation device and deliver the highest possible concentration.

Understanding BODY PROCESSES

Surfactant is a lipoprotein that lines the inner surface of the alveoli. It maintains a surface-wall tension that keeps the alveoli from completely collapsing. ■

ASSESSMENT Tips

The most important determining factors for patient survival in a drowning are the duration and severity of the hypoxia the patient suffers. ■

Hypothermia is another problem that may be encountered in a drowning patient. Hypothermia may occur as a result of extremely cold water (<41°F or <5°C). This occurs almost immediately and is considered primary hypothermia. Primary hypothermia may actually provide a role in protecting tissues against hypoxia. In other submersion patients, a secondary hypothermia may occur from heat loss through evaporation once the patient is removed from the water and resuscitation is attempted. Secondary hypothermia plays no role in protecting the patient against hypoxia and may cause further detrimental effects on patient outcome.

A patient with a core body temperature of 95°F or less (35°C or less) is considered to be hypothermic. If hypothermia with a body core temperature of less than 86°F is suspected during resuscitation, and the AED indicates a shockable rhythm, a maximum of one shock should be attempted. If the patient remains in a shockable rhythm, continue CPR and rapidly transport. (Follow your local protocols.) The patient must be rewarmed to at least 86°F before defibrillation is resumed.

Hypovolemia (loss of fluid volume within the vascular system) can occur during and after the initial resuscitation period from an increase in capillary permeability (capillaries becoming leaky), producing hypotension (low blood pressure). This may become especially evident when the patient's body begins to rewarm, causing the vessels to dilate. Cardiac dysrhythmias may be present as a result of hypothermia and cardiac hypoxia as well as from an increased amount of acid or a disturbance in the balance of electrolytes (sodium, chloride, potassium) in the blood.

Understanding BODY PROCESSES

If the body core temperature (BCT) is less than 86°F, defibrillation and ALS medications are not effective. The patient must be rewarmed to a BCT above 86°F before proceeding with more than one defibrillation. ■

The important signs, symptoms, or factors to consider in determining the seriousness of a drowning event are the following:

- Persistent cough
- Dyspnea (shortness of breath) or apnea (absence of breathing)
- Altered mental status or loss of consciousness at some point during the submersion
- Vomiting
- Drug or alcohol use
- Pertinent past medical history (e.g., seizures, diabetes mellitus, neuromuscular disorder)
- Hypothermia

Objective 25-6
Discuss the association between shallow water diving and spinal injuries.

Objective 25-7
Explain actions you should take to protect your own safety when responding to a water emergency.

Objective 25-8
Explain the necessity of taking spinal precautions to any swimmer or diver who may have suffered trauma.

- Duration of cardiac or respiratory arrest
- Age of the patient
- Pre-existing disease or conditions

Diving Emergencies

Drowning incidents can be additionally complicated in cases where diving is involved. In most such cases, people sustain injuries as a result of diving into a pool or other relatively shallow body of water. (Other diving emergencies, those resulting from diving in deep water with scuba gear, will be discussed later in this chapter.) Patients who dive into water from a diving board, shore, poolside, boat, or dock often sustain injuries to the head and spine and fractures of the arms, legs, and ribs.

You should always assume that a diver has sustained neck and spine injuries, even if the diver is still responsive. If the patient is still in the water, provide the care as described for a submersion patient under "Emergency Medical Care" later in this chapter. If the patient has left the water, provide care, including resuscitation if necessary, as you would for any other trauma or submersion patient.

Safety Measures in Water-Related Emergencies

In a water-related emergency, you need to reach the patient, but you must do it with utmost concern for your own safety. Certain deepwater accidents require specialized equipment to correct medical complications, but many patients in water-related emergencies can be saved by basic life support measures, such as removing them from the water and suctioning the airway.

Do not let your desire to provide these simple lifesaving measures overwhelm your judgment. You may easily fall victim to the same hazard as the patient. Remember that water can conceal many hazards. Holes, sharp drop-offs, and underwater entanglements such as fallen trees or wire fences may not be visible from shore. In addition, currents in streams, rivers, or storm drains can easily overpower the best swimmer.

Unless a water emergency occurs in open, shallow water that has a stable, uniform bottom, *never go out into the water to attempt a rescue unless you meet all of the following criteria:*

- You are a good swimmer.
- You are specially trained in water rescue techniques.
- You are wearing a personal flotation device.
- You are accompanied by other rescuers.

Failure to follow these guidelines can result in your becoming a patient or a fatality also.

If the patient is responsive and close to shore, use the *reach, throw, row, go* strategy. Make sure you have firm, solid footing and can't slip into the water. Try to reach to the patient by holding out an object for him to grab. You can use an oar, branch, fishing pole, towel, shirt, or other strong object that won't break. Once the patient has grabbed the object, pull him to shore.

If the patient is responsive but too far away to grasp an object you are holding, another way of reaching him is to throw something. The best thing to throw is a rope. Any EMS unit whose territory includes bodies of water should carry 100 feet of polypropylene rope in a throw bag that can be quickly deployed. Make sure you have firm, solid footing and can't slip into the water. Tie a long rope or line to an object that floats and is heavy enough to throw (an inflatable ball, a rescue ring, a thermos jug, a picnic cooler, a capped empty plastic milk jug, or the like). Throw the object underhand to the patient. Once he has grabbed the floating object, pull him to shore (Figure 25-2*).

If the patient is unresponsive or out of reach with a line, you will need to either row to him in a boat if one is immediately accessible (Figure 25-3*) or go to him by wading out or swimming or using a float board.

Never try to go to the swimmer unless you meet the safety criteria listed earlier.

Possible Spine Injury

If the swimmer may have been involved in a diving accident or may have been struck by a boat, water skier, surfboard, or other object, you should suspect possible spine injury. You should also suspect spine injury in any swimmer or diver who has been diving or using a water slide, is suspected of being intoxicated, or has evidence of traumatic injury.

In the case of possible spine injury, the goal is to support the back and stabilize the head and neck as other care is given. It is important to stabilize the patient properly in the water, then to remove him carefully from the water. The American Red Cross suggests that the patient not be removed from the water until a backboard or other rigid support can be applied to the patient for stabilization (see the method outlined under "Emergency Medical Care" later in this chapter).

Thinking Critically

While taking a stroll along the lake shore, you spot a swimmer thrashing and struggling about 50 yards out. Nobody else is around, but you are a good swimmer. Should you attempt a rescue? If not, what should you do instead? What factors should enter into your decision?

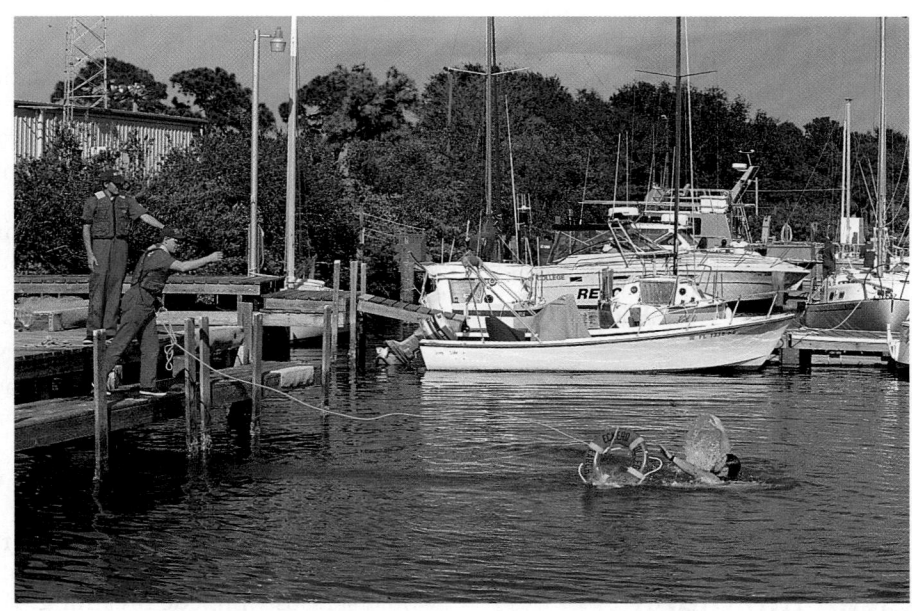

Key Terms

mammalian diving reflex the body's natural response to submersion in cold water in which breathing is inhibited, the heart rate decreases, and blood vessels constrict in order to maintain cerebral and cardiac blood flow.

FIGURE 25-2 ✱ Use an object that floats and is unlikely to break tied to the end of a rope to pull the patient to shore.

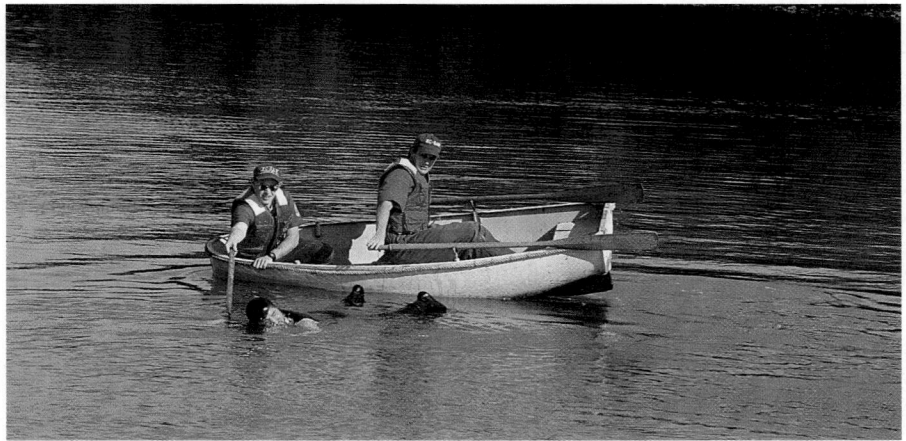

FIGURE 25-3 ✱ Don't become a patient yourself. Use a boat to reach an unresponsive patient.

Resuscitation

There is a significant difference between warm-water and cold-water drowning: When a person dives into cold water (below 70°F or 21°C), the **mammalian diving reflex** may drastically slow down metabolism and make the patient more likely to be resuscitated, even after prolonged submersion. There is controversy regarding the actual benefits of the mammalian diving reflex.

Here is how the mammalian diving reflex works: When the face of a human, or any mammal, is submerged in cold water, the larynx spasms, breathing is inhibited, the heart rate slows, and the blood vessels throughout most of the body constrict. Blood flow to the heart and brain, however, is maintained. In this way, oxygen is sent and used only where it is needed to immediately sustain life. The colder the water, the more oxygen is diverted to the heart and brain. The diving reflex is more pronounced and

Objective 25-9
Given a scenario in which a patient has suffered a submersion incident, explain how to provide resuscitative care.

Objective 25-10
Explain the assessment-based approach to drowning and other water-related injuries, including emergency medical care for the drowning victim.

cooling is more rapid in the young (whose skin surface is greater relative to their body mass). In water at or below 68°F, the body's metabolic requirements are only about half of normal. The brain and heart remain oxygenated for some time and, as a consequence, death can be significantly delayed in the cold-water submersion patient.

Often, patients who have been submerged in cold water—even after 30 minutes or longer in cardiac arrest—can be resuscitated. As a guideline, you should attempt resuscitation on any pulseless, nonbreathing patient who has been submerged in cold water. Remember, hypothermic patients are not pronounced dead until after both rewarming and resuscitation have been performed.

Some experts advise providing resuscitation to every drowning patient, regardless of water temperature, even those who have been in the water for a prolonged period. *Seek medical direction and follow local protocol.*

Assessment-Based Approach: Drowning and Water-Related Emergencies

Scene Size-Up

The scene size-up is especially critical in water-related emergencies. As an EMT, one of your first responsibilities is to ensure your safety and that of your partner; you cannot aid a patient if you yourself become a casualty.

First, study the scene and make sure that it is safe for you to enter. Anytime you are within 10 feet of the water's edge you should consider wearing a PFD. If you choose to go into the water to rescue a patient, be sure you are capable of swimming and do not put yourself in danger. Make sure to take appropriate Standard Precautions, because drowning patients often vomit. Note any relevant mechanism of injury that could contribute to the severity of the situation such as a deep dive in a shallow pool.

Decide if you will need any additional assistance such as a dry team to work on shore and a wet team to immobilize the patient in the water. Be aware that rescues in white water or swift water require specialized techniques and training. If you are not qualified to undertake a rescue, be prepared to contact rescue teams that are.

Survey the scene to determine the number of patients. Usually there will be just one patient, but in some circumstances, such as a car in the water or people struck by a moving boat, there could be more. Call for any extra or expert assistance that may be required.

Primary Assessment

Form a general impression of the patient. Is this a responsive or unresponsive patient? Assess the level of responsiveness and document it, especially noting the reaction to painful stimuli in all four extremities because of the possibility of spinal injury.

Assess the airway, keeping in mind the potential for spinal injury. If the patient is found face down, and a spine injury is suspected, work with a partner or partners, if possible, to carefully turn the patient over while maintaining manual in-line stabilization. Suction water, vomitus, and secretions from the airway. Insert an oral or nasal airway if the airway cannot be managed with manual maneuvers.

Check the breathing to be sure that respirations are present and adequate. Remember that patients with spinal injury often do not breathe if they have a high cervical injury. Assess for any open wounds to the chest that would seriously impede breathing. If the breathing is adequate, administer oxygen via a nonrebreather mask. If breathing is inadequate, provide positive pressure ventilation with supplemental oxygen.

Check the circulation to make sure the patient has a pulse and no life-threatening external bleeding that needs to be controlled. Assess for signs or symptoms of internal bleeding or hypoperfusion (shock). Remember that some patients rescued from the water may have internal injuries, for example from jumping off a bridge into the water.

ASSESSMENT Tips

If the drowning patient is suspected of being hypothermic, assess the pulse for 10 seconds. If no pulse is found, assume it is not present and begin chest compressions and apply the AED. ■

Make a decision on the priority of the patient. Is he a high priority in need of rapid transport to a hospital or is the patient a low priority at this time? Patients with high spinal injuries affecting respirations or who are found in respiratory distress or who are unresponsive are high priority.

Secondary Assessment

Perform a rapid secondary assessment if the patient has an altered mental status or is unresponsive. Also, look for ev-

Key Points
The drowning patient may be categorized as asymptomatic, symptomatic, cardiac arrest, or obviously dead (if there is rigor mortis or dependent lividity).

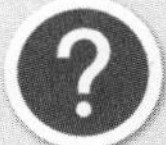

Thinking Critically
Some experts advise providing resuscitation to every drowning patient regardless of water temperature or how long the person has been in the water. Why?

idence of possible injury. If the patient is alert, obtain a history from the patient. If the patient has an altered mental status, attempt to collect a history from relatives, friends, or bystanders at the scene.

Signs and Symptoms For the water-related emergency patient, look for signs and symptoms of any of the following injuries or medical problems:

- Airway obstruction
- Absent or inadequate breathing
- Pulselessness (cardiac arrest)
- Spinal injury or head injury
- Soft tissue injuries
- Musculoskeletal injuries
- External or internal bleeding
- Shock
- Hypothermia
- Alcohol or drug abuse
- Drowning or submersion

Drowning patients may be unresponsive, not breathing, or pulseless, or they may be responsive and possibly gasping or coughing up water.

The drowning patient can be placed into one of the following four categories:

Asymptomatic

- Patient displays no signs or symptoms of the drowning event

Symptomatic

- Altered mental status (may be as slight as confusion)
- Altered vital signs (e.g., tachycardia, bradycardia, tachypnea, bradypnea, hypothermia)
- Respiratory distress or respiratory arrest (respirations may be agonal)
- Dyspnea (no matter how slight, patient is considered symptomatic)
- SpO_2 reading that is $< 95\%$ with or without oxygen support (An SpO_2 reading may be difficult to obtain or may be very low if the patient is hypothermic.)
- Persistent cough
- Wheezing or crackles (rales) upon auscultation of breath sounds
- Decreased body core temperature (hypothermia)
- Cool skin or cyanosis
- Vomiting, diarrhea, or both
- Anxiety

Cardiac Arrest

- No pulses
- Apnea

Approximately half of drowning patients are in asystole (absence of rhythm, which appears as a flat line on the monitor), requiring CPR. Approximately one third are in ventricular tachycardia or fibrillation and in need of CPR and defibrillation.

Obviously Dead

- Rigor mortis
- Dependent lividity (purplish color caused by blood pooling in the lowest areas of the body)

Emergency Medical Care—Drowning Patient

Unless otherwise directed by local protocol or medical direction, do not assume that a patient is dead, even if he is unresponsive and without breathing or pulse and has been submerged for some time. Rather, consider him to be a drowning patient in need of resuscitation. Follow these steps in caring for drowning patients:

1. Remove the patient from the water as quickly and safely as you can. If you suspect that the patient has a spine injury, maintain in-line stabilization and then secure the patient to a backboard before removing him from the water (Figure 25-4*). Follow these steps to remove a patient with a suspected spinal injury from the water:
   - If you find the patient face down, stabilize the patient's head and neck with your arms, then roll the patient over, supporting the back and stabilizing the head and neck.
   - If the patient is not breathing, begin rescue breathing, using a pocket mask if possible.
   - Keeping the head and neck in line with the spinal column, slide a long backboard under the patient; secure the torso and legs to the backboard with straps.

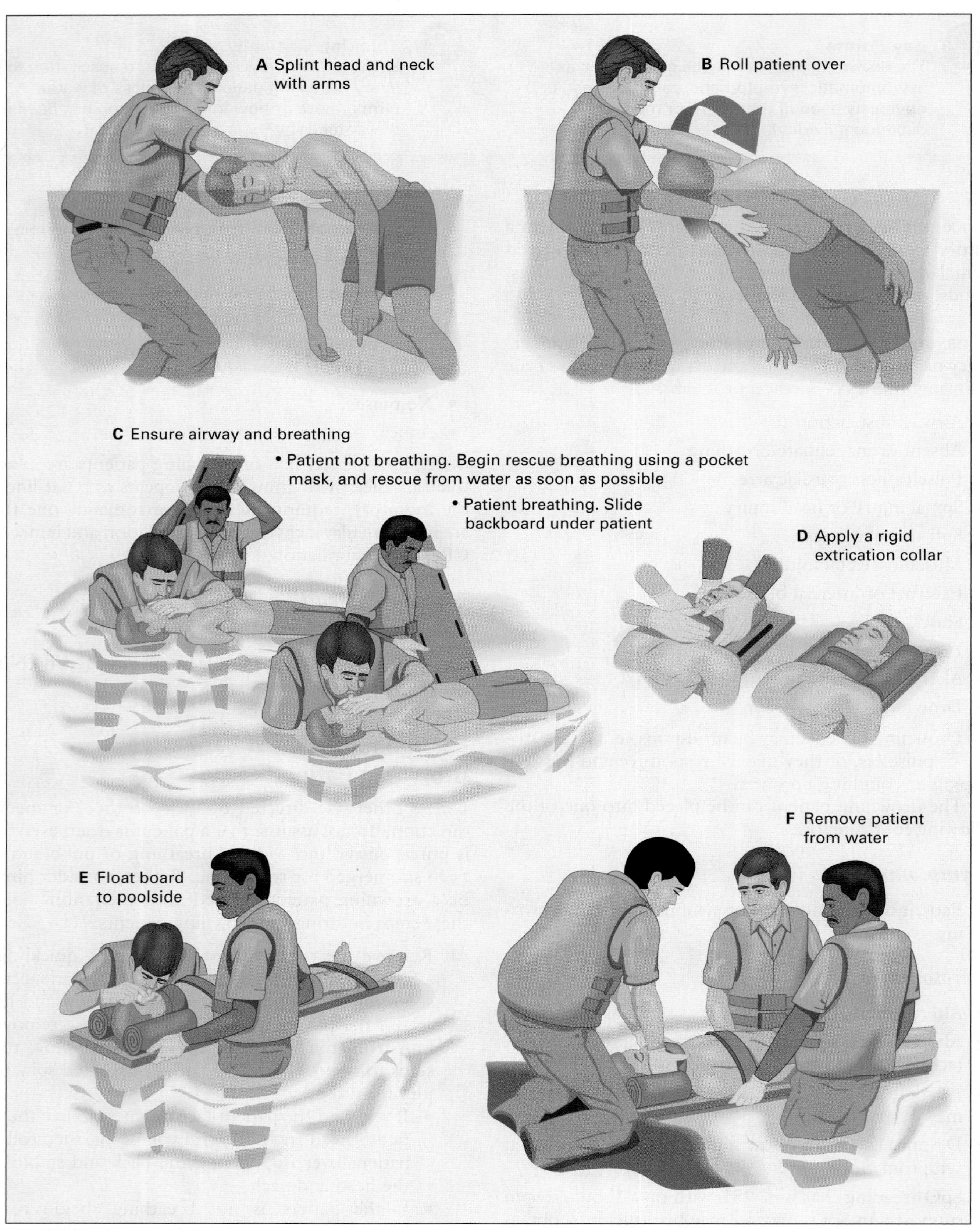
A Splint head and neck with arms
B Roll patient over
C Ensure airway and breathing
• Patient not breathing. Begin rescue breathing using a pocket mask, and rescue from water as soon as possible
• Patient breathing. Slide backboard under patient
D Apply a rigid extrication collar
E Float board to poolside
F Remove patient from water

FIGURE 25-4 ✱ Water rescue, possible spinal injury.

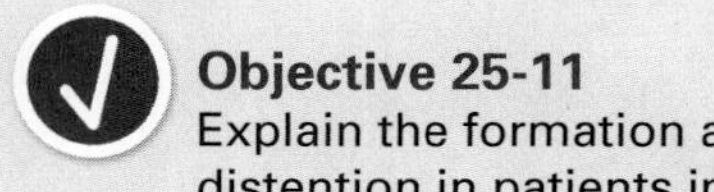

Objective 25-11
Explain the formation and relief of gastric distention in patients involved in submersion incidents.

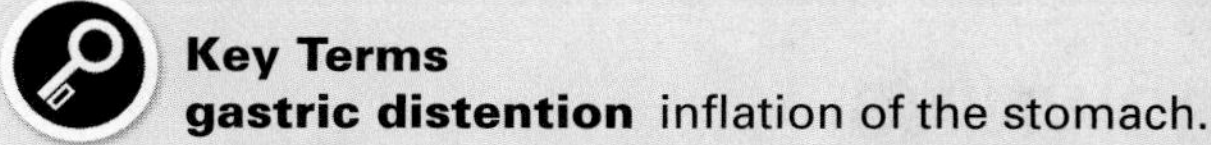

Key Terms
gastric distention inflation of the stomach.

- Apply a cervical spinal immobilization collar and a head immobilization device.
- Float the board to shore or poolside and lift the patient from the water. The chest and head are heavier than the lower extremities, and this results in a tendency for the head of the backboard, and the patient immobilized to it, to slip underwater. Make sure that sufficient support is given to the head end of the backboard.

2. If you do not suspect spine injury, place the patient on his left side so that water, vomitus, and secretions can drain from the upper airway.
3. Be prepared to suction, as these patients often have water in the airways and have a tendency to vomit because of the water that has been swallowed.
4. If the patient is in respiratory arrest or is not breathing adequately, establish an airway and begin positive pressure ventilations with supplemental oxygen as rapidly as you can. *Once you have determined that there are no foreign objects in the airway, provide ventilations with increasing force until you see the patient's chest rise with compression of the bag-valve device.*
5. If the patient is pulseless and apneic and is older than 1 year of age, begin CPR and apply the AED and proceed with the AED protocol. *If hypothermia is suspected* and the AED advises to defibrillate during the resuscitation, deliver only one shock. If this is *not* successful in the suspected hypothermic patient, continue with CPR and immediately begin transport. (Follow local protocols.) In patients less than 1 year of age, perform CPR only and transport immediately.
6. The patient may suffer from severe **gastric distention**, a condition in which the stomach fills with water, enlarging the abdomen to the point that it interferes with the ability to inflate the lungs. Gastric distention can also be caused by air that is forced into the stomach during artificial ventilation when resistance along the airway or too-forceful ventilations cause air to be forced into the esophagus and stomach. When gastric distention reaches the point where it interferes with the ability to ventilate the patient, place the patient on his side. *With suction immediately available,* place your hand over the epigastric area of the abdomen and apply firm pressure to relieve the distention. This will cause regurgitation, which you must immediately manage by positioning the patient on his side (turning the backboard and patient as a unit if the patient is immobilized to a backboard) and suctioning. *Do not apply the Heimlich as a routine maneuver in the submersion or drowning patient. It may lead to vomiting and aspiration. Apply pressure only if the gastric distention interferes with your ability to ventilate the patient effectively.*
7. Manage any other medical or trauma conditions associated with the drowning event, such as soft tissue injuries, seizure, or diabetic emergencies.
8. Transport the patient as quickly as possible, continuing resuscitative measures during transport.

Always transport a drowning patient, even if you think the patient has not suffered any serious effects. A drowning patient can develop complications that lead to death as long as 72 hours after the incident. Approximately 15 percent of all drowning-related deaths result from secondary complications. During transport, you should keep the patient warm and continue to provide high-concentration oxygen.

Reassessment

During reassessment, be alert for signs the patient is deteriorating into respiratory or cardiac arrest, especially if you previously resuscitated this patient. Perform reassessment (repeating the primary assessment, repeating the secondary assessment, repeating vital signs, and checking interventions) every 5 minutes if the patient is unstable, every 15 minutes if the patient is stable.

Summary: Assessment and Care

To review possible assessment findings and emergency care for a drowning emergency, see Figures 25-5* and 25-6*.

Assessment Summary

DROWNING

The following findings may be associated with a drowning emergency.

SCENE SIZE-UP

Pay particular attention to your own safety. Look for:

- Mechanism of injury
- Swift-moving water
- Water hazards
- Cold water
- Cold ambient temperature
- Alcohol or drugs
- Scuba diving equipment
- Is the patient still in the water?
- Do you suspect the patient has a possible spine or head injury?

Primary Assessment

General Impression

- Is the patient moving any extremities?

Mental Status

- Alert to unresponsive

Airway

- Potentially closed airway if mental status is altered
- Vomiting or coughing up water

Breathing

- May be adequate, inadequate, or absent
- Patient may be gasping

Circulation

- Pulses may be present or absent
- Cyanosis may be present
- Cold to touch based on water temperature

Status: Priority Patient (All drowning patients must be transported for further evaluation and management.)

Secondary Assessment

History

Signs and symptoms:

- Altered mental status
- Pulselessness
- Motor or sensory deficits
- Evidence of trauma to head or neck
- Coughing up or vomiting water

History questions:

- Did the patient ingest alcohol or drugs?
- Does the patient have a cardiac disorder or other medical condition?
- How long has the patient been submerged?
- Did the patient dive into the water?

Physical Exam

Head, neck, and face:

- Pupils may be dilated and sluggish to respond to light
- Large amounts of water or vomitus in mouth
- Evidence of trauma to head, neck, or face
- Cyanosis
- Nasal flaring

Chest:

- Persistent cough
- Crackles in lungs on auscultation
- Wheezing
- Decreased breath sounds
- Retractions and accessory muscle use

Abdomen:

- Distended from ingested water
- May be cold to touch if hypothermia is present

Extremities:

- Loss of sensory or motor function in spine-injured patient
- Weak or absent peripheral pulses
- Cyanosis or pallor

Baseline Vital Signs

- BP: normal to decreased; may be absent or extremely difficult to obtain
- HR: normal, increased, decreased, or absent
- RR: normal, increased, decreased, or absent
- Skin: may be pale, cyanotic, cool to cold, depending on water temperature and length of submersion
- Pupils: dilated and sluggish to respond to light
- SpO_2: may be $< 95\%$, indicating hypoxia

FIGURE 25-5a ✱ Assessment summary: drowning.

Thinking Critically

You are an EMT who lives and works inland, far from any deep-water site, so you don't need to know anything about deep-diving emergencies. True or false? Why?

Key Terms

dysbarism a medical condition that results from pressure changes that occur when a person descends in water or ascends in altitude.

Emergency Care Protocol

DROWNING

1. Establish and maintain in-line spinal stabilization if spinal injury is suspected.
2. Begin positive pressure ventilation with a pocket mask in the water, if possible.
3. Float a backboard under the patient and move to shore. Remove the patient on the backboard while maintaining in-line spinal stabilization.
4. Establish and maintain an open airway, insert a nasopharyngeal or oropharyngeal airway if the patient is unresponsive and has no gag or cough reflex.
5. Suction secretions as necessary.
6. If breathing is inadequate, provide positive pressure ventilation with supplemental oxygen at a rate of 10–12 ventilations/minute for an adult and 12–20 ventilations/minute for an infant or child.
7. If breathing is adequate, administer oxygen by nonrebreather mask at 15 lpm. If possible, deliver warm, humidified oxygen if hypothermia is suspected.
8. If no pulse, begin CPR and follow AED protocol. If hypothermia of less than 86°F is suspected, deliver only one shock and continue CPR.
9. If hypothermia is suspected, follow the generalized cold injury protocol.
10. Place the patient in a lateral recumbent position only if spinal injury is not suspected.
11. Always transport a submersion patient.
12. Perform reassessment every 5 minutes.

FIGURE 25-5b ✱ Emergency care protocol: drowning.

Scuba or Deepwater Diving Emergencies

People who take part in scuba or deepwater diving may become victims of drowning incidents such as those described earlier. Scuba diving has evolved into a popular recreational sport for a large number of novice and experienced divers. Also, there is an increasing growth of commercial diving. The growing popularity of recreational and commercial diving has led to an increase in the number of diving incidents and emergencies.

You may not practice as an EMT in or around oceans, but accidents involving diving may occur anywhere. Many people dive in quarries, lakes, rivers, and caves. Air travel has made it easy to dive for an hour, board a plane, and be in a central location away from the ocean within hours. So if you think that—because you do not live or work near the ocean—there is no possibility you will ever have to deal with a diving patient, you are wrong. All EMTs must be prepared to recognize and manage a diving emergency.

The environmental extremes to which deepwater divers are exposed create some special problems. A major complication of deepwater diving emergencies is coma, which may result from asphyxiation, head injury, heart attack, air-tank contamination, intoxication, or aspiration. It can also result from decompression sickness, arterial gas embolism, or barotrauma.

Basic Laws of Physics Related to Scuba or Deepwater Diving Emergencies

Dysbarism is a medical condition that results from the effects on the body of changes in ambient pressure. The pressure changes may occur when a person descends in water or ascends in altitude. Recreational and commercial divers, when descending into depths of water, experience a drastic increase of pressure on the body. The pressure affects only the compressible structures and substances within the body. The body is made up primarily of water, which is noncompressible, but the gas

Emergency Care Algorithm: Drowning Emergency

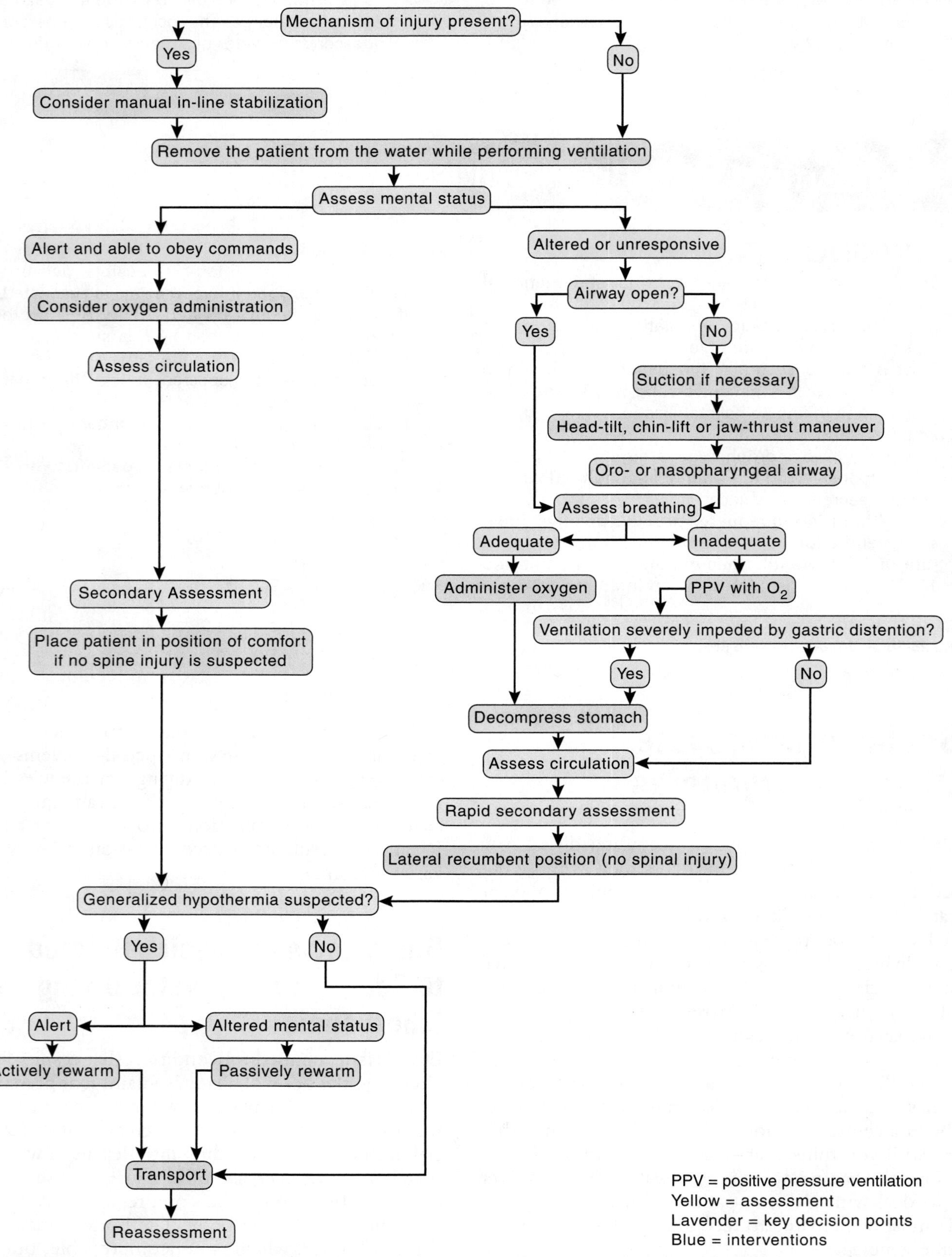

FIGURE 25-6 ✱ Emergency care algorithm: drowning emergency.

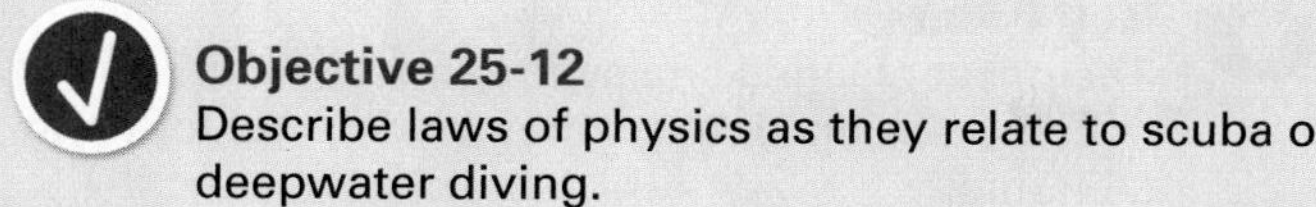

Objective 25-12
Describe laws of physics as they relate to scuba or deepwater diving.

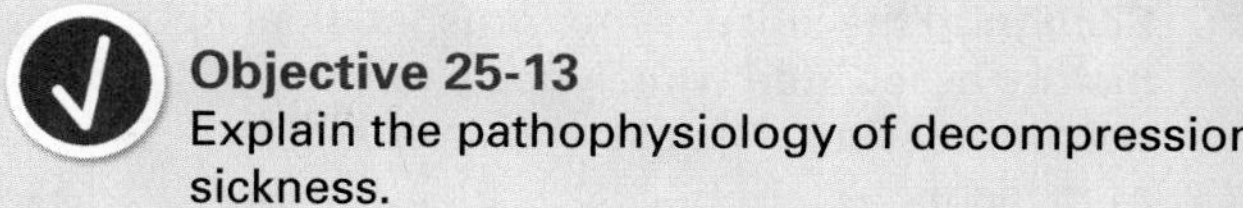

Objective 25-13
Explain the pathophysiology of decompression sickness.

contained within the organs, dissolved in the blood, and found in hollow spaces is compressible and is affected by changes in pressure.

There are four laws of physics that play a major role in the adverse conditions and emergencies experienced by divers. They are:

- **Boyle Law**. At a constant temperature, the volume of a gas is inversely related to the pressure. That is, as the pressure increases, the volume of the gas decreases, and as the pressure decreases, the volume of the gas increases. If the diver breathes in compressed air at a depth where there is a higher pressure on the body and then suddenly ascends, the volume of air in the lungs will rapidly expand because of the decrease in pressure as the diver is ascending. This may lead to barotrauma, or rupture of the alveoli and other lung structures.
- **Dalton Law**. The total pressure of a mixture of gases equals the sum of the partial pressures of the individual gases that make up the mixture. For example, the air we breathe is about 78 percent nitrogen. Since the air pressure at sea level is 760 mmHg, the pressure of nitrogen at sea level (78 percent of the total) is about 593 mmHg. As a diver descends, the total pressure of the air that he is breathing increases, and the pressure of each component gas in the air increases proportionately. As the diver goes deeper under water and the pressure of the inhaled nitrogen increases, the nitrogen begins to dissolve into the blood. (Other gases in the mixture of inhaled air do not have this action.) Nitrogen in the blood will affect the electrical properties of the brain and produce a "nitrogen narcosis" with effects similar to an anesthetic. As a result, every 50 feet of depth is equivalent to one alcoholic drink in its impairment of the diver's judgment.
- **Henry Law**. At a constant temperature, the amount of gas that dissolves in a liquid it is in contact with is proportionate to the pressure of the gas around it. As already noted, when a diver descends and pressure increases, the nitrogen inhaled will tend to dissolve into the body's liquids, mainly the blood plasma. It will then also begin to dissolve into and accumulate in the body fat and tissues. If the diver then ascends too quickly, the dissolved nitrogen is returned to a gaseous state while it is still dissolved, causing bubbles to form in the blood and tissues.
- **Charles Law**. All gases will expand equally upon being heated. Thus, as a diver descends into colder water temperatures, the inhaled and dissolved gases will contract. As the diver ascends, the temperature increases and the gases will expand.

These laws all contribute to the conditions the diver may experience while descending into or ascending from deep water.

Decompression Sickness

Pathophysiology

Decompression sickness (DCS) occurs as the result of the bubbles formed from the expansion of nitrogen in the blood and tissues as described in the Henry law. The bubbles can cause cell damage and lead to organ dysfunction. The bubbles have two primary effects on the body: (1) they act as emboli and cause obstruction in the circulation; and (2) they compress or stretch the blood vessels and nerves. Also, the bubbles may cause coagulation of blood to occur. In response, the vessels and surrounding tissues may release substances as they would in an allergic reaction. These substances may produce signs and symptoms similar to those of an allergic reaction.

Predisposing Factors of Decompression Sickness Factors that increase the risk of a patient developing decompression sickness are:

- Flying or going to a high altitude too soon after a dive (12–24 hours)
- Failure to take the necessary safety stops while ascending from a dive
- Inadequate surface intervals (allows nitrogen to accumulate during a sequence of dives)
- Inadequate decompression or passing the no-decompression limit
- Diving at depths for too long a period of time
- Repeated dives at depth on the same day

Physical characteristics or conditions that predispose an individual to decompression sickness are:

- Poor physical condition
- Obesity (nitrogen dissolves easily in fat)
- Age
- Dehydration

Objective 25-14
Recognize the signs, symptoms, and patient history associated with Types I and II decompression sickness and arterial gas embolism.

Key Points
The onset of signs and symptoms of decompression sickness may be delayed for up to 36 hours.

- Heart or lung diseases or conditions
- Pre-existing musculoskeletal injury
- Fatigue

Other environmental factors that put the diver at risk are:

- Cold water (vasoconstriction decreases the ability of nitrogen to off-load)
- Rough sea conditions (increase workload and effort)
- Heated diving suits (lead to dehydration)
- Heavy work (gas pockets are created in tendons)

Categories of Decompression Sickness

Decompression sickness (DCS) is divided into three categories:

- Type I decompression sickness (mild)
- Type II decompression sickness (serious)
- Arterial gas embolism (AGE)

The pain characteristically associated with decompression sickness has given this disorder its nickname, "the bends." It usually results from a diver ascending too rapidly from a deep, prolonged dive. As noted earlier, gases, typically nitrogen, form bubbles within the blood and tissues, causing obstruction of vessels and compression and stretching of tissue. The onset of DCS may occur up to 72 hours following the dive.

Type I Decompression Sickness Type I DCS is a milder form of decompression sickness. Signs and symptoms include:

- Pain
- Pruritus (itching) and burning sensation of the skin (referred to as "skin bends")
- Skin rash (mottling or marbling of skin)
- Skin has orange-peel appearance (rare)
- Painless pitting edema (uncommon)

Pain (the bends) is the hallmark symptom of DCS. It is seen in approximately 70–85 percent of patients with type I DCS. It is typically a dull, aching, throbbing pain usually in the joints or tendons. It can also be located in other tissue. The shoulder is the joint in which the pain is most commonly experienced. The pain typically begins as mild, or not severe, and then gradually intensifies. Many divers initially think that the pain they experience early on from DCS is due to a pulled muscle or muscle overexertion. A decreased function of the extremities may be seen as a result of muscle splinting. This most often affects the upper extremities.

Type II Decompression Sickness Type II DCS is more serious than type I DCS. The patient experiences more significant signs and symptoms; however, they may be very diverse. The onset of the signs and symptoms is usually immediate, but it could be delayed for up to 36 hours after the incident. The signs and symptoms, which result primarily from effects on the nervous system, the respiratory system, and the circulatory system (hypovolemic shock), are as follows:

Nervous System

- Low back pain that progresses to paresis (weakness), paralysis, numbness or tingling, loss of sphincter control, and girdle pain to the lower abdomen from spinal cord effects—the most common site for type II DCS
- Headache, visual disturbances, dizziness, tunnel vision
- Altered mental status
- Nausea, vomiting, vertigo, tinnitus, partial deafness

Respiratory System

- Substernal burning sensation on inhalation
- Nonproductive cough
- Respiratory distress

The respiratory signs and symptoms are known as the "chokes." The symptoms can begin up to 12 hours following the dive and last for 12–48 hours.

Circulatory System

- Signs of hypovolemic shock, primarily tachycardia and hypotension, resulting from fluid shifting from intravascular (inside the vessels) to extravascular (outside of the vessel)
- Formation of a thrombus from activation of the blood coagulation system

When performing an assessment on the patient, the following may be found in DCS:

- Fatigue
- Signs and symptoms of shock
- Pupillary changes

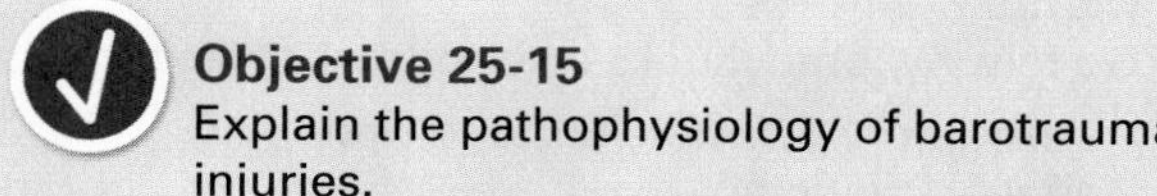

Objective 25-15
Explain the pathophysiology of barotrauma injuries.

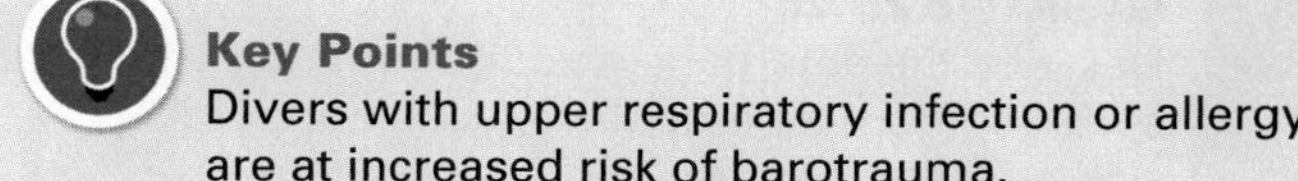

Key Points
Divers with upper respiratory infection or allergy are at increased risk of barotrauma.

- Pallor to the tongue
- Bloody sputum
- Nasal flaring, retraction of the chest, and accessory muscle use
- Tachypnea
- Crackles (rales) upon auscultation
- SpO_2 reading of $< 95\%$ prior to oxygen administration
- Vomiting
- Urinary bladder distention
- Seizure
- Uncoordinated movement (ataxia), weakness, motor and sensory deficits
- Joint pain, decreased range of motion
- Edema
- Cyanosis, pallor, itching, mottling, marbling

Important questions to ask in the history of a suspected DCS patient are:

- Where did the patient dive (river, lake, ocean, cave)?
- What was the lowest depth and for what period of time?
- What were the other depths and for what periods of time?
- What was the rate of ascent from the various depths?
- What has the patient done since the dive? Did the patient fly on an airplane?
- What did the patient do the 72 hours prior to the dive? number of dives? length of dives? time off between dives? surface intervals? water temperature?
- Did the patient do any type of work during the dive?
- What gases did the patient use during the dive?
- Were there any problems experienced by the diver (e.g., entanglement, marine animal bites or stings, equipment problems)?
- What physical condition was the patient in before, during, and after the dive (e.g., fatigue, drug or alcohol use, fever, dizziness, nausea)?
- Was any first aid provided for the patient (e.g., oxygen, position, medications)?

Arterial Gas Embolism

Arterial gas embolism (AGE) is a blocking of blood vessels by an air bubble or clusters of air bubbles. The blockage interferes with perfusion of body tissues with oxygen and nutrients normally supplied by the blood. During a dive, pressure on the diver's body increases and the volume of a gas decreases as he descends. Conversely, that pressure is lessened as the diver ascends. If the diver ascends rapidly while holding his breath, the air in the lungs expands rapidly, rupturing the alveoli and damaging adjacent blood vessels. As a result, air bubbles enter the bloodstream.

The signs and symptoms of air embolism have a rapid onset, often appearing within 15 minutes of a diver's surfacing. They include the following:

- Itchy, blotchy, or mottled skin
- Difficulty in breathing
- Dizziness
- Chest pain
- Severe, deep aching pain in the muscles, joints, and tendons
- Blurred or distorted vision
- Partial deafness, distortion of senses
- Nausea and vomiting
- Numbness or paralysis
- Weakness or numbness on one side of the body
- Staggering gait or lack of coordination
- Frothy blood in the nose and mouth
- Swelling and crepitus in the neck
- Loss or distortion of memory
- Coma
- Cardiac or respiratory arrest
- Behavioral changes (sometimes the only sign)

Barotrauma

Sometimes called "the squeeze," barotrauma occurs during ascent or descent when air pressure in the body's air cavities (such as the sinuses or middle ear) becomes too great. As a result, tissues in the air cavities are injured; for example, the eardrum or sinus may rupture.

Divers with upper respiratory infection or allergy are at increased risk of barotrauma. Signs and symptoms of the condition include the following:

- Mild to severe pain in the affected area
- Clear or bloody discharge from the nose or ears
- Extreme dizziness

Objective 25-16
Describe the emergency medical care of patients suffering from air embolism, decompression sickness, and barotrauma.

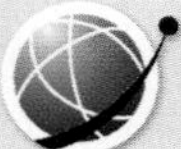

Media Resources
Go to www.bradybooks.com for mykit. Highlights:

- *Animation:* Submersions and Drowning
- *Video:* Drowning

- Nausea
- Disorientation

Patients suffering from barotrauma must be cared for at a medical facility immediately to prevent permanent deafness, residual dizziness, or the inability to dive in the future.

Emergency Medical Care

Follow these steps in caring for a patient who you suspect has an air embolism, decompression sickness, or barotrauma:

1. If any suspected spinal injury exists, establish in-line spinal stabilization. Keep the patient in a supine position if spinal injury is suspected or if the patient is alert. If the patient does not have a suspected spinal injury and has an altered mental status, place the patient in a lateral recumbent position. *Do not place the patient in a Trendelenburg or head-down position.*
2. Open the airway and assess for adequate breathing. If the breathing is adequate, administer oxygen via nonrebreather mask at 15 lpm, even if the SpO_2 reading is greater than 95%. Oxygen is critical in diving emergencies, because it reduces the size of the nitrogen bubbles and improves circulation. Be sure to document the exact time of oxygen delivery. If the tidal volume or respiratory rate is inadequate, begin positive pressure ventilation. Be sure to connect oxygen to the ventilation device to maximize oxygen delivery during positive pressure ventilation.
3. Initiate CPR and apply the AED if indicated.
4. Transport the patient immediately. If it is a diving emergency, try to obtain the patient's diving log and transport it with him to the hospital. Contact medical direction to consider transport to a facility with a recompression chamber. Continue to provide oxygen during transport.

CHAPTER REVIEW

SUMMARY

Drowning is a preventable event that leads to a significant number of accidental deaths, especially in children less than 5 years of age. Often, drowning involves high-risk behavior and alcohol ingestion in teenagers and adults. Water-related sports injuries also contribute to drowning incidences.

The term *drowning* has replaced all of the other terms that have been used in the past to describe a patient who was submerged in water. Drowning is now defined as a person who was submerged or immersed in a liquid substance that impaired his ability to breathe. This definition holds true regardless of whether the patient lives or dies from the incident.

Some drownings may involve the possibility of spinal injury. If spinal injury is suspected, attempt to provide spinal stabilization in the water and during removal of the patient. Emergency care for drowning patients focuses on the airway, ventilation, oxygenation, and circulation. If no pulse is present, begin CPR and apply the AED in patients older than 1 year of age. If hypothermia is suspected and the body core temperature is less than 86°F, deliver only one shock and proceed with CPR. Defibrillation and medications will not be effective until the patient is warmed to at least 86°F.

Scuba diving is a popular sport that can result in decompression sickness, arterial gas embolism, and barotrauma. Even though there may be no scuba diving locations in your response area, it is easy for a patient to have been scuba diving, get on a plane to return home, and suffer his diving emergency in your response area. Be prepared to provide emergency care for the scuba diving patient even though you may not have diving locations in your response area.

CASE STUDY FOLLOW-UP

SCENE SIZE-UP

Your initial call was for a submersion emergency involving a 25-year-old male reported in trouble in the Delmar Hotel pool. Your unit and the police arrive at the same time. You are led to the pool by the hotel manager, who complains that the young man and his friends have been drinking. A crowd of intoxicated bystanders has gathered around the pool and are shouting comments. The police move to clear the crowd. With the only obvious hazard under control, the scene is secure and you approach the pool.

In it is a young man, floating in a supine position supported by a hotel employee. According to the manager, the man had been drinking and suddenly dove into the shallow end of the pool. He floated to the top but said he couldn't move his feet. A hotel employee jumped in and has been supporting him in a supine position in the water, keeping his head, neck, and spine in alignment.

PRIMARY ASSESSMENT

Your general impression is of an adult male in no obvious distress except for his chief complaint, the inability to move his feet, which leads you to suspect a possible spinal injury. There is a lifeguard's float board propped up by the poolhouse. You get it while your partner grabs a cervical spinal immobilization collar. You both slip into the pool, trying not to create unnecessary waves. Your partner takes over manual in-line stabilization from the hotel employee while you assess the airway, breathing, and pulse. The patient keeps up a stream of chatter as you assess, but his speech is somewhat disconnected and slurred. He knows his name, Robby Ash, but not exactly where he is or what day it is.

With Robby's airway and breathing adequate, and no signs of major bleeding or immediate signs of shock, you maneuver the float board into position. You immobilize his torso, then apply the collar and immobilize his head to the board. Then you gently push the board to the side of the pool. There, with the assistance of the employee and two police officers, you remove the board and Robby, as a unit, from the water and set them down on the deck. You and your partner climb out and begin to administer oxygen at 15 lpm by nonrebreather mask. Since the patient is responsive with an adequate airway and breathing, he is not a high priority for rapid transport, so you proceed to the secondary assessment at poolside.

SECONDARY ASSESSMENT

A physical assessment reveals no other injuries aside from a contusion on the top of the head and some point tenderness in the neck. Because of Robby's complaint that he cannot feel his feet, you pay particular attention to the assessment of pulses and motor and sensory function in the extremities. In the upper extremities, radial pulses are present and strong. Robby cannot grip your fingers on command and cannot identify which of his fingers you are touching or pinching. In the lower extremities, pedal pulses are present. Robby cannot move his feet or toes on your command and cannot identify the location of a touch or pinch to any part of either foot.

You take a set of vital signs; they show blood pressure 112/72, a heart rate of 78, and a respiration rate of 15. The SpO_2 reading is 99%. The patient's overall skin color appears normal, but because of his extended time in the pool you cannot accurately assess the temperature of the skin or whether it would be wet or dry if he had not just been removed from the water. His pupils are equal in size and reactive to light.

While your partner, with the assistance of the police officers, proceeds to prepare the patient for transport, you ask the history questions and find out that Robby's only symptom is the lack of feeling in his feet. He has an allergy to penicillin, is taking no medications, and has no pertinent past medical history. His last solid meal was 2 hours ago. He has been drinking beer all night long, which, he agrees, probably led him to attempt the dive into shallow water.

When your partner has finished preparing the patient, you load him into the ambulance and begin transport.

REASSESSMENT

The focus of your care en route to the hospital is to monitor Robby's ABCs and keep him warm. You take another set of vital signs: blood pressure is still 112/72, heart rate is now 76, and respirations 15. His skin is normal color, but still feels cool and damp. The SpO_2 remains at 99%. You check to be sure that the nonrebreather mask is secure, oxygen is flowing adequately, and Robby is well secured to the long spine board.

Because you know Robby has been drinking heavily and probably swallowed a fair amount of pool water, you are prepared for the possibility of vomiting and have suctioning equipment ready. And, in fact, he soon says, "I feel real sick, man." You remove the nonrebreather mask and with your partner's help, turn the board so that Robby is on his left side. You apply suction to clear his mouth and airway as he vomits. When he stops, you return him to the normal position just as you arrive at the hospital.

Upon arrival, you give an oral report to the emergency nurse, being sure to mention the vomiting incident and the latest set of vital signs taken in the ambulance. You fill out the prehospital care report while your partner cleans up and restocks the ambulance. Before you leave the hospital, you see the emergency physician, who tells you that Robby has been taken upstairs for an MRI. He is not optimistic about the possibility that Robby will walk again.

As you pull away from the hospital, you contact dispatch and announce that you are temporarily out of service. You are going back to base so that you can change into dry uniforms.

IN REVIEW

1. List at least five common causes of drowning.
2. Explain the conditions that must apply before an EMT enters the water to attempt a rescue.
3. Describe the four basic methods used in attempting to rescue a patient from the water.
4. Explain why patients who have been submerged in cold water can often be resuscitated after 30 minutes or more.
5. List the injuries and medical problems whose signs and symptoms the EMT should be alert for when assessing the water-related emergency patient.
6. List the steps for removing a drowning patient with a possible spine injury from the water.
7. List the steps of emergency medical care for a drowning patient that should take place after the patient is removed from the water and, if necessary, immobilized to a spine board.

CRITICAL THINKING

It is February and the outside temperature is 34°F. You arrive on the scene of a residence and are directed to the back of the house. You find a 4-year-old male patient lying on the sidewalk next to a swimming pool. The family states that he was outside playing in the snow when he suddenly disappeared. After about 15 minutes of searching, they found the pool cover displaced and found the patient at the bottom of the shallow end of the pool. As you approach the patient, he is extremely pale, cyanotic, and not moving. He is apneic and has no carotid pulse.

1. How would you proceed with the emergency care of the patient?
2. Would you apply the AED and proceed with defibrillation?
3. What are some other special considerations when managing this patient?

CHAPTER 26

Behavioral Emergencies

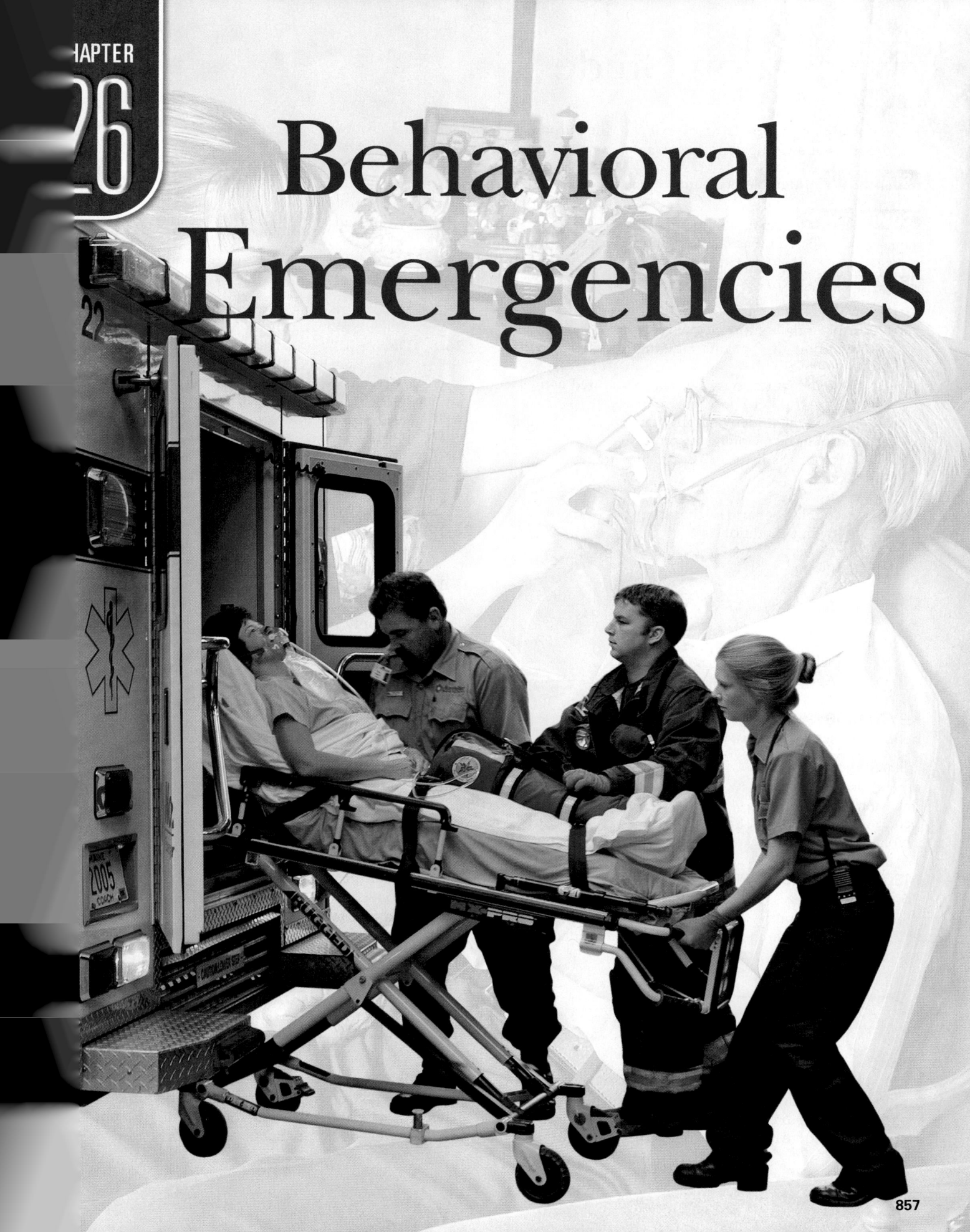

Navigation Guide

The following items provide an overview to the purpose and content of this chapter. The Standard and Competency are from the new National EMS Education Standards.

STANDARD **Medicine** (Content Area: Psychiatric)

COMPETENCY Applies fundamental knowledge to provide emergency care and transportation based on assessment findings for an acutely ill patient.

OBJECTIVES: After reading this chapter, you should be able to:

26-1. Define key terms introduced in this chapter.
26-2. Explain the importance of recognizing and responding to patients suffering from behavioral emergencies.
26-3. Describe indications of danger associated with response to behavioral emergencies.
26-4. Discuss the underlying physical and psychological causes of behavioral emergencies.
26-5. Describe the focus of assessment and history taking for patients who have behavioral emergencies.
26-6. Recognize behavioral characteristics of the following conditions:
- **a.** Anxiety
- **b.** Phobias
- **c.** Depression
- **d.** Bipolar disorder
- **e.** Paranoia
- **f.** Psychosis
- **g.** Schizophrenia
- **h.** Agitated delirium

26-7. Describe risk factors associated with suicide and violence toward others.
26-8. Discuss basic principles related to the assessment and management of patients with behavioral emergencies.
26-9. Recognize indications of attempted suicide during scene size-up and patient assessment.
26-10. Prioritize patient care needs in terms of managing physical and behavioral problems.
26-11. Recognize indications for physical restraint of a patient and follow principles of safe physical restraint of patients.
26-12. Evaluate the need for law enforcement and medical direction involvement in a behavioral emergency situation.
26-13. Document all information pertinent to calls involving behavioral emergencies and patient restraint.

KEY TERMS: Page references indicate first major use in this chapter. For complete definitions, see the Glossary at the back of the book.

agitated delirium p. 863
anxiety p. 860
behavior p. 859
behavioral emergency p. 859
bipolar disorder p. 861
depression p. 861
humane restraints p. 872
paranoia p. 861
phobia p. 861
psychosis p. 861
reasonable force p. 873
schizophrenia p. 862
suicide p. 862

MEDIA RESOURCES: Please go to www.bradybooks.com to access mykit for this text. You will find quizzes, critical thinking scenarios, weblinks, animations, and videos related to this chapter—and much more. Look for online information on panic attacks and also on schizophrenia. You will also find a video clip on how to apply soft restraints.

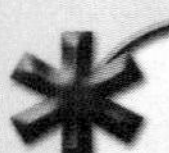

CASE STUDY

The Dispatch

EMS Unit 204—proceed to 3486 East Market Street, King's Motel, Room 22. You have a woman who is cut and bleeding. No other information is available. Time out is 2235 hours.

Upon Arrival

You call back to dispatch and ask to arrange for the motel manager to meet you in the parking lot. You arrive at 2241 hours, position your ambulance, and turn on the scene lights. Because of the report of blood, you take appropriate Standard Precautions. Noting nothing unusual about the scene, you and your partner gather your equipment and exit the ambulance. As you walk toward the motel, a man approaches and says, "Hi. I'm Tom Slavina, the night manager here. Sorry, guys, but I really have no idea what's going on. Your dispatcher called me and asked me to meet you, but I didn't call in a problem and I haven't seen or heard any signs of trouble."

Mr. Slavina leads you to Room 22. The door is closed and the room's drapes are drawn, but there is a light on inside. You pause, but hear no sounds coming from the room. You and your partner stand on opposite sides of the door as you prepare to knock. When you do, your knock swings the door open slightly. You now hear crying from somewhere inside the room, followed by a woman's voice saying faintly, "Please help me. I'm cut and bleeding."

You ask, "Where are you?" and the voice replies, "In the bathroom." You ask, "Is anyone else in the room with you?" The woman sobs for a moment, then gasps out, "No, there's no one here. There's never anyone here. Never. No one cares. No, there's no one."

You cautiously enter the room first, while your partner waits outside. There's no one in the room itself, but you note the closet door is open and a few garments are hanging in it. The bed is rumpled, as if someone had been lying on top of the covers. On the night table by the bed are a lamp, a phone, an opened bottle of rum, and a glass. There are a few dark stains on the carpet between the night table and the bathroom door.

You approach the bathroom and cautiously peer around the corner through the doorway. A woman is sitting on the floor in the middle of the room. Blood from a cut on her left wrist has pooled on the floor and she is holding a large, folding hunting knife in her right hand.

How Would You Proceed to Assess and Care for This Patient?

In this chapter, you will learn special considerations of assessment and emergency care for a patient who has attempted or is threatening suicide as well as for patients suffering other behavioral emergencies. Later, we will return to the case study and apply what you have learned.

Introduction

Emergency care for physical problems is tangible. You can see the wounds you bandage and touch the patient to provide treatments such as splinting bones or restoring breathing. Often, you can see immediately positive results from your efforts.

Care for behavioral emergencies is different. You cannot readily see the comfort that your words or your mere presence provides to someone who is panicked or agitated. It is hard to gauge the immediate results of your care for someone who is depressed. But the care you give patients in behavioral emergencies can just as easily save lives as the care you provide for physical problems.

Behavioral Problems

Behavior is the way a person acts or performs. A person's "behavior" encompasses any or all of that person's activities and responses, especially those responses that can be observed. A **behavioral emergency** is a situation in which a person exhibits "abnormal" behavior—behavior that is unacceptable or intolerable to the patient, the family, or the community. The abnormal behavior that precipitates the emergency may be due to a psychological condition (such as a mental illness), to extremes of emotion, or even to a physical condition (such as a lack of oxygen or low blood sugar).

Patients in the midst of behavioral emergencies may display panic, agitation, and bizarre thinking and actions. Such patients can pose a danger to themselves through suicidal or self-injurious acts, or to others through violent acts or actions whose consequences they may be incapable of understanding.

Behavioral Change

A number of factors may cause a change in a patient's behavior, among them situational stresses, medical illnesses, psychiatric problems, alcohol, or drugs. Some common reasons why behavior may change include the following:

- Low blood sugar in a diabetic, which can cause delirium, confusion, and even hallucinations
- Hypoxia (lack of oxygen)
- Inadequate blood flow to the brain
- Head trauma

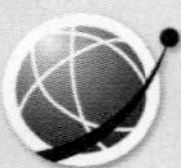

Media Resources
Go to www.bradybooks.com for mykit. Highlights:

- *Video:* Anorexia
- *Video:* Bulimia
- *Video:* How to apply soft restraints

Objectives 26-2 and 26-3
Recognize and respond to behavioral emergencies and associated dangers.

Key Terms
behavioral emergency abnormal **behavior** (actions).
anxiety a state of painful uneasiness.

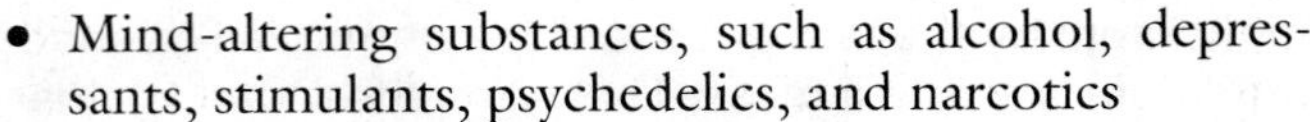

- Mind-altering substances, such as alcohol, depressants, stimulants, psychedelics, and narcotics
- Psychogenic substances, which can cause psychotic thinking, depression, or panic
- Excessive cold or heat
- Infections of the brain or its coverings
- Seizure disorder
- Toxic ingestion or overdose
- Drug or alcohol withdrawal

As obvious as it sounds, you need to be sure you are dealing with a *behavioral,* and not a *physical,* emergency. For example, you may detect what smells like alcohol on a patient's breath. Do not assume the patient is intoxicated; diabetic emergencies can cause alcohol-like odors on the breath, as can Antabuse, a drug used by alcoholics to decrease alcohol dependency.

During the assessment, pay particular attention to the following:

- **General appearance.** Look at the hygiene, clothing, and overall appearance of the patient.
- **Speech.** Listen to the speech pattern for abnormalities, such as slurring. Determine if the responses are appropriate, inappropriate, or incomprehensible.
- **Skin.** The color, temperature, and condition of the skin may provide some indication of the patient's condition.
- **Posture or gait.** Does the patient have a normal posture or is he making unusual movements? When the patient walks, is his gait normal or abnormal?
- **Orientation.** Is the patient oriented to person, place, and time?
- **Memory.** Is the patient able to recall recent and past events?
- **Awareness.** Is the patient aware of his surroundings?
- **Body language.** Is the patient exhibiting any threatening signs, such as a closed fist or angry facial expression?
- **Perception.** Are the patient's thoughts in order? Is there any evidence of hallucinations, delusions, or phobias?
- **Mood.** Is the patient emotionally upset, depressed, elated, anxious, or agitated?
- **Judgment.** Is the patient making rational decisions?

Clues that the problem may be physical rather than psychological include the following:

- The onset of symptoms was relatively sudden; most behavioral problems develop more gradually.
- If the patient has hallucinations, they are visual but not auditory.
- The patient has memory loss or impairment; in most behavioral problems, the memory remains intact and the patient is usually alert, being oriented to person, place, and time.
- The patient's pupils are dilated, constricted, or unequal, or they respond differently to light.
- The patient has excessive salivation.
- The patient is incontinent (has lost bladder or bowel control).
- The patient has unusual odors on his breath.

Behavioral changes and crises often follow (or are a result of) physical trauma or illness. Even if all the clues point to a behavioral problem, assess the patient adequately to rule out a physical cause.

Psychiatric Problems

A number of psychiatric conditions can lead to behavioral emergencies. Among them are anxiety, phobias, depression, bipolar disorder, paranoia, psychosis, and schizophrenia.

Anxiety

Anxiety is a state of painful uneasiness about impending problems. It is characterized by agitation and restlessness and is one of the most common emotions; in fact, anxiety disorders are thought to be the most common form of mental illness. Most clinicians feel that many of the cases are never correctly diagnosed because they so closely mimic other disorders.

One form of anxiety disorder is the panic attack. Patients who are panicked may show intense fear, tension, or restlessness. They often feel overwhelmed and can't concentrate. Their behavior may also cause anxiety among the people around them, so they may be surrounded by a crowd of anxious and excited people when you arrive. These patients often hyperventilate (breathe too deeply), which causes physical symptoms such as

Objectives 26-4 to 26-6
Discuss causes and assessment of behavioral emergencies and recognize behavioral characteristics of psychiatric problems.

Key Terms
phobia an irrational fear of specific things, places, or situations.

Key Terms
depression deep feelings of sadness, worthlessness, and discouragement.

bipolar disorder wide swings between depression and elation; manic-depressive disorder.

paranoia a highly exaggerated or unwarranted mistrust or suspiciousness.

dizziness, tingling around the mouth and fingers, spasms of the hands and feet (carpal-pedal spasms), tremors, irregular heartbeat, palpitations (rapid or intense heartbeat), diarrhea, and sometimes feelings of choking, smothering, or shortness of breath. If severe, anxiety has been known to cause sudden cardiac death.

ASSESSMENT Tips

Panic attack patients usually present with tachycardia, tachypnea, diaphoresis, and pale and cool skin. ■

Phobias

Phobias are closely related to anxiety problems. They are irrational fears of specific things, places, or situations. One of the most disabling is agoraphobia, or "fear of the marketplace," which renders the person terrified of leaving the safety of his own home.

Patients suffering phobias may show evidence of intense fear. Tense and restless, they often wring their hands and pace. They frequently suffer from tremors, tachycardia (rapid heartbeat), irregular heartbeat, dyspnea (difficult breathing), sweating, and diarrhea.

Depression

Depression is one of the most common psychiatric conditions. It is characterized by deep feelings of sadness, worthlessness, and discouragement, feelings that often do not seem connected to the actual circumstances of the patient's life. Depression is a factor in approximately 50 percent of all suicides and may cause other psychological disorders as well.

Depressed patients often present a sad appearance and may have crying spells and listless or apathetic behavior. They feel helpless, hopeless, withdrawn, and pessimistic; they often suffer appetite loss, sleeplessness, fatigue, despondence, and severe restlessness. Believing that no one understands or cares about them or that their problems cannot be solved, they often express the desire to be left alone.

ASSESSMENT Tips

Depression in an elderly patient is considered to be a serious condition in which the patient must be provided care. ■

Bipolar Disorder

Bipolar disorder, also known as manic-depressive disorder, causes a patient to swing to opposite sides of the mood spectrum. During one phase, he has an inflated view of himself; he may feel deliriously happy, elated, and superpowerful. The manic phase alternates with normal moods and a depressive state in which the patient loses interest, feels worthless, worries, and may contemplate suicide. In either the manic or depressive stage, the patient may suffer delusions and hallucinations. Sometimes one phase may last for months; at other times, the patient may swing from one mood to another rather quickly (sometimes within hours).

Paranoia

Paranoia is a highly exaggerated or unwarranted mistrust or suspiciousness. Paranoid patients are often hostile and uncooperative and suffer from the firmly held, but untrue, belief that someone is "out to get them."

Most paranoid patients have elaborate delusions, mostly of persecution. They tend to brood over real or imagined injustices, carry grudges, and recall wrongs done to them years earlier. They seem cold, aloof, antagonistic, hypersensitive, defensive, and argumentative. They cannot accept fault or blame, they avoid intimacy, and they are excitable and unpredictable, displaying outbursts of bizarre or aggressive behavior.

Psychosis

Psychosis is a state of delusion where the patient is out of touch with reality. The patient is truly living within his own world; however, he often mistakes his reality for that which is actually occurring. This may make the patient angry and belligerent or withdrawn. He may be responding to voices only he can hear or reacting to people only he can see. Acute psychosis may result from mind-altering drugs, which is the most common cause, or from intense stress, delusional disorders, or schizophrenia, which is another common cause. The psychosis may last for only a short period of time or may occur as a chronic condition.

Key Terms

psychosis a state of delusion in which a person is out of touch with reality.

schizophrenia a group of mental disorders characterized by distortions of speech and thought, delusions, hallucinations, social withdrawal, and lack of emotional expressiveness.

Key Terms

suicide a willful act designed to end one's own life.

Objective 26-7

Describe risk factors associated with suicide and violence toward others.

Schizophrenia

Schizophrenia is the name given to a group of mental disorders. Patients with this illness suffer debilitating distortions of speech and thought, bizarre delusions, hallucinations, social withdrawal, and lack of emotional expressiveness. Only rarely does schizophrenia manifest as multiple-personality disorder, contrary to common belief.

Violence

Patients in behavioral emergencies brought on by the conditions described earlier or by other circumstances sometimes express their inability to handle the pressures they are feeling through violent acts. Those acts can be directed against themselves or against others.

Suicide

A **suicide** is any willful act designed to end one's own life. Males are four times more likely to die from suicide, but women make three times as many attempts. Fifty-five percent of all suicides are committed with firearms. Among unsuccessful attempts, the most common methods are drug ingestion and wrist slashing.

Suicide is the eighth leading cause of death in the United States among males and the third leading cause of death of young people between the ages of 15 and 24 years. Many people believe that suicide is vastly underreported because of the stigma that still surrounds it.

At least half of all people who succeed at suicide have attempted it previously, and 75 percent give clear warning that they intend to kill themselves. The four most common methods of suicide are (1) self-inflicted gunshot wound, (2) hanging, (3) poisoning by ingestion, and (4) carbon monoxide poisoning.

Many suicide victims make last-minute attempts to communicate their intentions. It is thought that most do not really want to die but use the suicide attempt as a way to get attention, to receive help, or to punish someone. Suicide attempts, however, are too often dismissed as "just trying to get attention." As an EMT, you must understand that the person who attempts suicide, whatever his motive, has a real problem and needs some kind of help or treatment. The patient who attempts suicide unsuccessfully is at high risk of making a successful attempt later if not helped. *Every suicidal act or gesture should be taken seriously, and the patient should be transported for evaluation.*

The following are risk factors and potential signs of impending suicide:

- History of depression and other mental disorders
- Previous suicidal gestures or attempts (80 percent who are successful have made previous attempts)
- Family history of child abuse or maltreatment
- Feelings of hopelessness
- Unwillingness to seek mental health care because of the stigma attached to suicidal thoughts
- Feeling of being isolated from others
- Local epidemic of suicide
- A history of impulsive or aggressive behavior
- Inability to access mental health care
- A recent diagnosis of serious illness, especially an illness that signals a loss of independence
- The recent loss of a loved one, or the loss of a job or money, or a social loss
- Ages between 15 and 24 years and over 40 years
- Alcohol or drug abuse
- Divorced or widowed (five times more likely to commit suicide)
- Person who gives away personal belongings and cherished possessions
- Psychosis with depression
- Homosexuality (higher incidence of depression, HIV infection, alcoholism)
- Major physical stress such as surgery and long periods of sleep deprivation
- Suicide of same-sex partner
- Expression of a clear plan for committing suicide
- Availability of the mechanism to carry out the suicide

ASSESSMENT Tips

Document any statements by the suicide-attempt patient, suicide notes, and any other evidence of suicide attempts at the scene. ■

Key Terms

agitated delirium a mental and physiological state of arousal usually characterized by extreme strength and endurance, tolerance to pain, hostility, and hyperactive behavior; also called *excited delirium.*

Objective 26-8

Discuss basic principles related to the assessment and management of patients with behavioral emergencies.

Key Points

Emotional injury is just as real as physical injury.

Agitated Delirium

Agitated delirium, also known as *excited delirium*, is a mental state and physiological response characterized by:

- Unusual strength and endurance
- Tolerance of pain
- Agitation
- Hostility
- Frenzied and bizarre behavior
- Hot and diaphoretic skin
- Unusual speech

Agitated delirium may be associated with drug use, especially cocaine, methamphetamine, and other central nervous system (CNS) stimulants and psychiatric illnesses.

It may be difficult to differentiate between a patient who is violent and a patient with agitated delirium. In agitated delirium, the patient may suffer a sudden cardiac arrest. Often, the patient fights against the restraints, suddenly appears to relax, and then becomes apneic and pulseless. One potential contributing factor in deaths associated with agitated delirium is allowing the patient to fight against being restrained. Without restraint, the patient is typically violent and a potential danger to you, your partner, bystanders, and himself. Consider early contact with advanced life support for the use of a drug as a chemical restraint to reduce the chance of sudden death.

Violence to Others

Behavioral emergency patients may become assaultive or violent. The angry, violent patient may be ready to fight with anyone who approaches and will probably be difficult to control. Violence can be caused by patient mismanagement (real or perceived), psychosis, alcohol or drug intoxication, fear, panic, or head injury.

Early signs that a person may have lost control and may become violent include:

- Nervous pacing
- Shouting
- Threatening
- Cursing
- Throwing objects
- Clenched teeth and/or fists

Dealing with Behavioral Emergencies

Dealing with patients in behavioral emergencies requires extra sensitivity on the part of the EMT. It is often not the tangible treatment you provide but the intangibles of your interactions with the patient that make the difference between helping the patient through the crisis or deepening it or prolonging it. The way you carry yourself around the patient and how you look at and speak to him are of great importance in these situations.

Basic Principles

Keep the following basic principles in mind whenever you encounter a behavioral emergency:

- **Every person has limitations.** In a behavioral emergency, every person there, including you, is susceptible to emotional injury. Every person has a threshold, and some are able to cope with more than others.
- **Each person has a right to his feelings.** A person who is emotionally or mentally disturbed does not want to feel that way, but at that particular time, those feelings are valid and real.
- **Each person has more ability to cope with crisis than he might think.** For every manifestation of crazed emotion, some strength is probably left within.
- **Everyone feels some emotional disturbance when involved in a disaster or when injured.** You do not know what a particular physical injury might mean to a given individual. A relatively minor hand injury may seem of little consequence, but it could ruin the career or the personal fulfillment of a person who works with his hands as a profession or a hobby.
- **Emotional injury is just as real as physical injury.** Unfortunately, because physical injury is more visible, it is often accepted as being more "real."
- **People who have been through a crisis do not just "get better."** They will probably suffer from their pain and loss for a long time, sometimes for years. Do not expect instantaneous or automatic results; the patient probably will not realize the extent of the event until long after you leave. You're first on the scene,

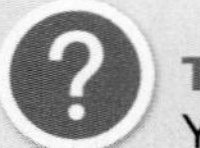

Thinking Critically
Your patient called EMS but on your arrival has locked himself into the bathroom and says he's going to kill himself. His neighbor says, "Oh, he's always doing something dramatic. Just trying to get attention." What do you think of the neighbor's analysis? What steps would you now take?

and your role is to provide a positive beginning to a long, difficult healing process.

- **Cultural differences have special meaning when you are called to intervene in behavioral emergencies.** Come to terms with your own feelings as you approach a situation, and take the time to understand where your patient is coming from.

Techniques for Treating Behavioral Emergency Patients

The situations presented by behaviorally disturbed patients can be difficult. However, there are a number of techniques that can make dealing with those situations easier for you and more helpful to the patient. You can use the following therapeutic interviewing techniques to establish a rapport:

- *Approach the patient slowly and with a purpose.*
- *Engage in active listening.*
- *Be supportive and empathetic.*
- *Limit the interruptions in the interview.*
- *Respect the patient's space.*
- *Limit physical touch until a rapport is established.*
- *Avoid any action the patient may interpret as threatening.*
- *Avoid any questions or statements the patient may construe as threatening.*

Other techniques to use include:

- **Speak in a calm, reassuring voice directly to the patient.** Explain who you are and why you are there.
- **Maintain a comfortable distance between yourself and the patient.** Many patients are threatened by physical contact. Unwanted touching could set off a violent response. After you have established some rapport with the patient, you might then ask if it is okay to touch or to get a little closer, which can be comforting to some patients (Figure 26-1∗).

ASSESSMENT Tips

Touch that may normally be comforting to a patient may trigger an aggressive response in a behavioral emergency patient. ■

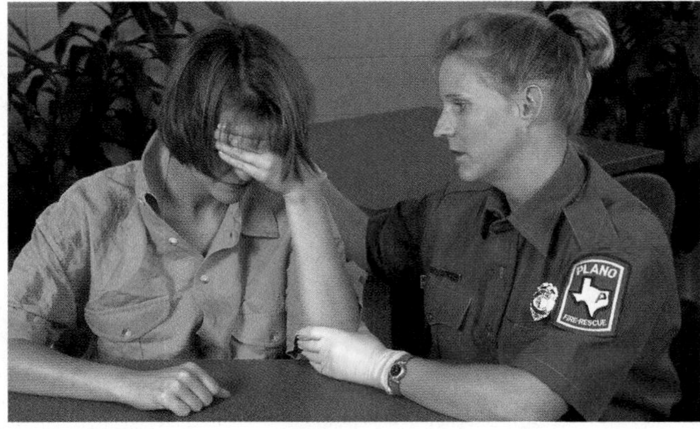

FIGURE 26-1 ∗ Touch may be comforting to some patients, but do not touch the patient suffering a behavioral disturbance without the patient's consent.

- **Seek the patient's cooperation.** Encourage him to explain the problem. Never assume that it is impossible to communicate with a patient until you have tried, even if friends or family members insist it cannot be done. Ask questions. Use gestures to encourage the patient, such as a nod of your head, or use verbal responses, such as "I see" or "Go on," to show you are paying attention.
- **Maintain good eye contact with the patient.** It communicates your control and confidence. The patient's eyes can reflect emotions and tell you whether he is terrified, confused, struggling, or in pain. Furthermore, the eyes can telegraph intentions. If a patient is about to reach for a weapon or make a leap or a dash, his eyes may alert you.
- **Do not make any quick movements.** Act quietly and slowly; let the patient see that you're not going to make any sudden moves (which could precipitate panic or violence on his part).
- **Respond honestly to the patient's questions, but don't foster unrealistic expectations.** Instead of saying, "You have nothing to worry about," say something like, "Even with all the problems you've had, you seem to have lots of people around you who really care about you."
- **Never threaten, challenge, belittle, or argue with the patient.** Many behaviorally disturbed patients will be adept at picking out your weaknesses; they may feel threatened themselves and may try to improve their situation by belittling you. Remain kind and calm and treat the patient with respect. Remem-

Thinking Critically

You might tell a patient: "Oh, come on, don't act like such a baby." Or you might say, "What would you think about coming to the hospital so we could get you some help?" How would each of these communications exemplify (or *not* exemplify) a recommended technique for treating behavioral emergency patients?

Key Points

Always ensure that you have a preplanned and clear route for an exit.

Objective 26-9

Recognize indications of attempted suicide during scene size-up and patient assessment.

ber that the patient is ill, and comments are not directed at you personally.

- **Always tell the truth; never lie to the patient.**
- **Do not "play along" with visual or auditory disturbances.** Reassure the patient that these are temporary and will clear up with treatment.
- **When you can, involve trusted family members or friends.** Some patients are calmed and reassured by the presence of these people, but others may be upset or embarrassed. Let the patient decide.
- **Be prepared to spend time at the scene.** Don't rush to the hospital unless a medical emergency dictates the need for lifesaving care. Avoid panicking the patient.
- **Never leave the patient alone.** All behavioral emergency patients are escape risks, and violence to self or others is a distinct possibility. Once you have responded to the emergency, the patient's safety is one of your primary concerns. Even if the patient pleads to be left alone for just a few minutes, firmly explain that you realize he is capable of handling things, but that you could get into trouble for leaving a patient alone. If the patient needs to go to the bathroom, first check the bathroom for potential weapons (e.g., razors, scissors). Leave the door ajar, but be discreet as you watch. Follow local protocol.
- **Avoid the use of restraint.** Enlist the support of law enforcement or those trained in the use of restraint if you decide restraint is absolutely necessary.
- **Do not force the patient to make decisions.** The patient has probably lost the ability to cope. If necessary, "suggest" things that need to be done (e.g., "How about you lying back so we can take you to the hospital. OK?").
- **Encourage the patient to participate in a motor activity, which helps reduce anxiety.** For example, have the patient gather an extra set of clothing or his medication to take with him.
- **If the patient has attracted a crowd, do what you can to disperse it.** You need to deal with the patient on a one-to-one basis. If the scene is especially hectic, remove the patient from it or remove distressing stimuli from the scene before trying to calm the patient.
- **Always ensure that you have a preplanned and clear route for an exit.** When entering the scene, determine the fastest and safest route of egress from the scene. If there is a family member or bystander blocking that route, politely ask that he move to another location in the room without identifying exactly why you want him to move.

Assessment-Based Approach: Behavioral Emergencies

Behavioral emergencies can be unpredictable, volatile situations. You must make every effort to ensure your safety before you enter such a scene. Remember, if you become a victim, you will not be able to help the patient.

Scene Size-Up

Steps to ensure your safety should begin even before you arrive on the scene. Pay close attention to the dispatch. Does it indicate any violence or potential for violence? Check with dispatch to see whether police are on the way. Begin scene size-up immediately on arrival. Never enter a potentially violent situation without support. Scenes in which EMS providers are most often injured are those that involve drugs or alcohol, behavioral emergency patients, and domestic violence. Injury is most likely to occur in association with sudden behavioral change. Since the behavioral emergency patient is prone to sudden changes in behavior, be extra vigilant when at the scene and during your entire contact with this patient. *If you cannot guarantee your own safety, call the police and wait for them to arrive before you leave your vehicle.*

Also be alert, if you are dispatched to the scene of a suicide or potential suicide, that you do not fall victim to a mechanism that the patient planned to use to end his own life. Running an automobile in a closed garage, blowing out a pilot light and turning on all the burners on a gas stove, and using electrical devices in water are common suicide methods that can pose risks for EMTs.

ASSESSMENT Tips

Scene size-up is extremely important in suicidal patients. If the patient is truly serious about ending his life, he may not hesitate to injure you in order to carry out the plan. ■

Locate the patient visually before you enter the scene (Figure 26-2✱). You can be too easily surprised or even jumped by a patient as you enter the scene if you don't

Key Points
Never let down your guard or turn your back on the behavioral emergency patient.

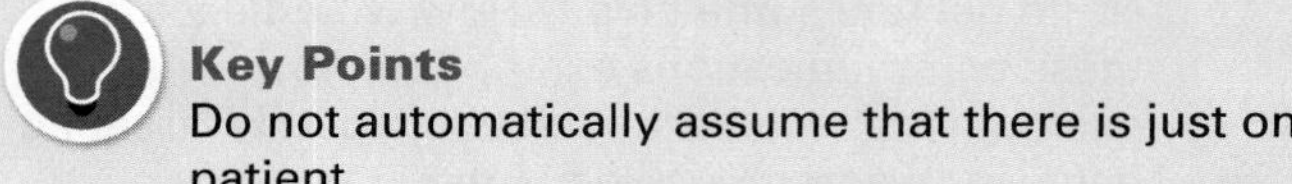

Key Points
Do not automatically assume that there is just one patient.

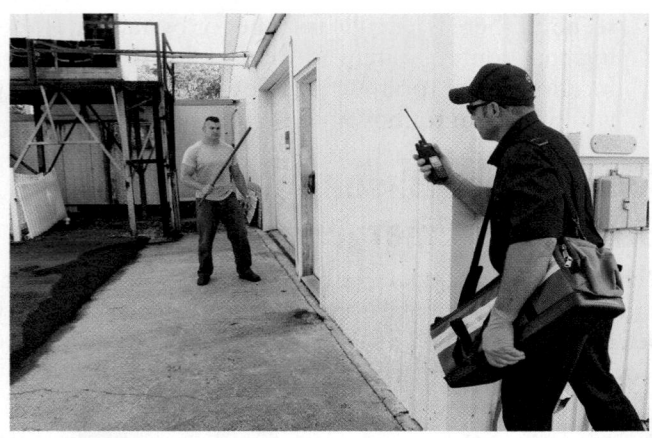

FIGURE 26-2 * Visually locate the patient before approaching. Look for any weapons.

know exactly where he is. You will also be unable to observe his response to your entry if you can't see him. If you can't visually locate the patient, wait for police to enter and secure the scene. Always stay between the patient and an open door so you can exit quickly should the scene deteriorate.

Never let down your guard or turn your back on the patient. Scan quickly for instruments or objects the patient might use to injure himself or others. If you see any dangerous articles, discreetly move them out of the way if possible. If the patient displays a weapon, never ignore or disregard it. Instead, in a calm and nonconfrontational way, tell the patient that you want to help but cannot do so until the weapon is released. Ask the patient to give you the weapon. If he does not, back out of the scene and call or wait for police response. Remember that any weapon can be used against the EMT. Stay outside the danger zone—for a knife, 22 feet; for a gun, much farther.

Early in the assessment, before you physically approach the patient, determine whether you and your partner can handle the situation alone. Even a small person who is sufficiently agitated can be very difficult to handle. If you doubt that you can handle the patient alone, call the police and wait for them to arrive.

If the scene seems secure, scan it for signs of things that may have contributed to the crisis or that the patient might have used in a suicide attempt. Be especially alert for liquor bottles, containers for pills or other medications, or any drug paraphernalia.

What appears to be a behavioral emergency can actually be caused by trauma such as a blow to the head, or by a medical condition such as hypoglycemia. Study the scene for clues that will help you determine the nature of the emergency. Look for a mechanism of injury or a sign of the nature of illness. If a patient has made a suicide attempt, determining either the mechanism of injury (such as a razor blade or handgun) or the nature of illness (such as pills or carbon monoxide poisoning) will be critical.

Do not automatically assume that there is just one patient. Sometimes two or more persons will make a suicide pact. Occasionally a person tries a murder-suicide (attempting to kill someone else and then himself). A method such as carbon monoxide poisoning may have made others ill, too. A person with a violent behavior disturbance may have injured someone else. Always determine the number of patients and call for additional resources as needed.

Primary Assessment

Gather a general impression of the patient. Assess the patient's mental status by asking specific questions that will help you measure the patient's level of responsiveness and orientation. Watch the patient's appearance, level of activity, and speech patterns. Specifically try to determine whether the patient is oriented to time, person, and place.

Pay particular attention to the patient's airway and breathing. Patients who have attempted suicide may have trouble maintaining their airway and respiration. Be prepared to provide oxygen by a nonrebreather mask at 15 lpm or positive pressure ventilation with supplemental oxygen if necessary.

If a patient has attempted suicide, caring for his trauma or medical problem rather than his behavioral problem will be your priority. Proceed with assessment and care based on the mechanism of the suicide attempt. For example, if the patient has taken a large number of pills, or if he attempted to asphyxiate himself in his car, assess and treat him as a poisoning emergency. If he has slit his wrists, treat for bleeding and shock and soft tissue injuries. Make a priority decision regarding further assessment and transport.

Secondary Assessment

Once life threats have been managed, proceed with the secondary assessment. In the patient who is alert and has no significant mechanism of injury, try to obtain a history first. Pay particular attention to medications the patient has taken; they can help you clarify if the situation is a behavioral or medical emergency. Note carefully the events

Key Points
Allow the patient to tell you want happened. Show you are listening by rephrasing or repeating part of what the patient says.

Key Points
When assesing a patient who is potentially violent, observe the patient's posture and body language.

leading to the emergency to help clarify if a suicide attempt is involved.

Inform the patient of what you are doing. Once you have determined what the problem is, explain it to the patient. Without frightening the patient, be honest in explaining what will be done to help. (Uncertainty is likely to make the patient more anxious and fearful.) Ask questions in a calm, reassuring voice. Stay polite, use good manners, show respect, and make no unsupported assumptions.

Allow the patient to tell you what happened. If you can, interview the patient in a quiet room where he has privacy. A patient may be ashamed and hesitant to talk in front of family or friends. Avoid asking questions that can be answered with a simple "yes" or "no." The patient's method of explanation can help you during the assessment.

Show you are listening by rephrasing or repeating part of what the patient says. Look at the patient's eyes, show interest in what the patient is saying, and avoid being judgmental. Give the patient supportive information that is truthful. Acknowledge the patient's feelings. Use phrases such as "I can see that you are very depressed" or "I understand that you must feel frightened." You will have determined the patient's level of responsiveness and orientation during the primary assessment. During the secondary assessment, note any answers to your questions that reveal his general contact with reality, such as an auditory or visual hallucination (the patient is "hearing things" or "seeing things" that are not there). Throughout the assessment attempt to evaluate the following:

- Intellectual function
- Orientation
- Memory
- Concentration
- Judgment
- Thought content (disordered, delusions, hallucinations, worries, fears)
- Language (speech pattern, appropriate words, inappropriate words, incomprehensible)
- Mood (anxiety, depression, elation, agitation, alertness, distractibility)

Determine the patient's chief complaint, then perform a physical exam centered on those areas in which the patient has a complaint. Finally, take a set of baseline vital signs.

If the patient is unresponsive or has an otherwise severely altered mental status or a significant mechanism of injury, you should perform a rapid secondary assessment, head to toe, to seek physical clues or signs as to whether the problem is behavioral, medical, or traumatic. Obtain a set of baseline vital signs. Then try to obtain a history, if not from the patient himself, then from family or bystanders.

Specific tips for assessing suicidal and violent patients and preparing them for transport follow.

Suicidal Patients When performing an assessment on a patient who has attempted or threatened suicide, keep these additional guidelines in mind:

- **Injuries or medical conditions related to the suicide attempt are your primary concern.**
- **Listen carefully.**
- **Accept all the patient's complaints and feelings.** Do not underestimate what the patient may be feeling and do not dismiss what you consider to be minor.
- **Do not trust "rapid recoveries."** Transport the patient even if he seems to be "better."
- **Be specific in your actions.** Do something tangible for the patient such as arranging for a member of the clergy to meet the patient at the hospital.
- **Never show disgust or horror when you care for the patient.** Watch your body language!
- **Do not try to deny that the suicide attempt occurred.** Your denial may be perceived as condemnation of the patient's feelings.
- **Never try to shock a patient out of a suicidal act.** Never try to argue the person out of it, and never challenge the patient to go ahead.

Violent Patients When performing an assessment on a patient who has been violent or seems to offer the potential for violence, keep the following guidelines in mind:

- **Take a history.** Ask bystanders what's been going on. Has the patient been violent or threatened violence? If family members or friends are on the scene, find out if the patient has a history of violence, aggression, or combativeness.
- **Look at the patient's posture.** Anticipate violence if the patient is standing or sitting in a way that threatens anyone (including himself), if the patient's fists are clenched, or if the patient is holding anything that could be used as a weapon.

Key Points
Instruct the patient regarding his behavior. Clearly state the consequences of aggressive behavior before it occurs.

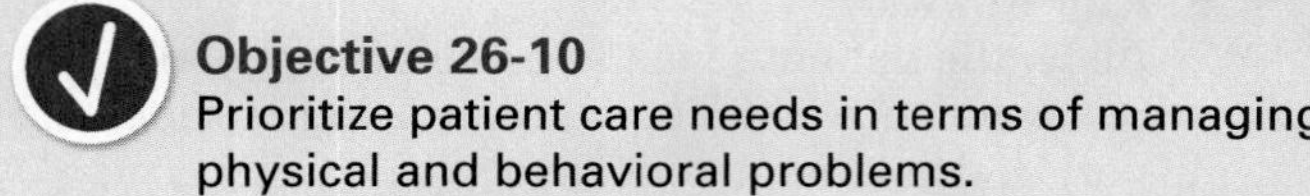

Objective 26-10
Prioritize patient care needs in terms of managing physical and behavioral problems.

- **Listen to the patient.** Anticipate violence if the patient is yelling, cursing, arguing, or verbally threatening to hurt himself or others.
- **Monitor the patient's physical activity.** Signs of potential violence include moving toward the caregiver, carrying a heavy or threatening object, using quick or irregular movements, and having muscle tension.
- **Be firm and clear.** Give the patient instructions regarding his behavior. Clearly state the consequences of an aggressive behavior before such behavior occurs.
- **Be prepared to use restraints, but only if necessary.** See "Restraining a Patient" later in this chapter.

Signs and Symptoms One or more of the following signs and symptoms may indicate a behavioral emergency:

- Fear—of a person or persons, an activity, or a place
- Anxiety—not related to any specific person, place, or situation
- Confusion—may be preoccupied with fears or imaginary attacks
- Behavioral changes—such as radical alterations in lifestyle, values, or relationships
- Anger—inappropriate anger directed at an inappropriate source; usually brief but intense and, often, destructive
- Mania—unrealistically optimistic; prone to take unwarranted risks and display poor judgment
- Depression—crying; inability to function; feelings of worthlessness or hopelessness; threats of suicide
- Withdrawal—loss of interest in people or things previously considered important
- Loss of contact with reality—hallucinations, auditory or visual
- Sleeplessness
- Loss of appetite
- Loss of sex drive
- Constipation
- Crying
- Tension
- Irritability

Emergency Medical Care

Behavioral emergencies come in many forms. A patient may be violent, raving, and threatening others, or depressed and totally withdrawn. One patient may attempt to commit suicide by shooting himself whereas another may take pills. You must be adaptable when providing emergency care for behavioral emergencies. Keep the following guidelines in mind when providing such care:

1. **Your safety is of utmost importance.** Be alert at all times to the possibility that the patient may become violent and do harm to you, others at the scene, or himself. Do not let yourself fall victim to the same mechanism of injury as the patient (e.g., carbon monoxide, electrocution). Never allow a patient to come between you and an exit. Always allow yourself an exit in case the patient becomes violent.
2. **Assess the patient for trauma or a medical condition.** Remember that what seems to be a behavioral emergency may arise from trauma or a medical condition. When patients have attempted suicide, their medical treatment has priority.
3. **Calm the patient, and stay with the patient.** Follow the guidelines discussed earlier for communicating with a patient in a behavioral emergency. Never leave a suicidal patient alone. Never turn your back or drop your guard with a violent or potentially violent patient.
4. **If it's necessary to protect yourself or others, or the patient from harming himself, use restraints.** Never use restraints as a substitute for observation, and never use metal handcuffs if your local protocol does not authorize them and if you are not properly trained in their use. Use restraints only if emergency care would be dangerous or impossible without them. Enlist the aid of trained public safety personnel.
5. **Transport the patient to a facility where he can get the physical and psychological treatment that is needed.** If a patient attempted to commit suicide by drug or medication overdose, be sure to monitor airway, breathing, and circulation carefully and be prepared to assist ventilation. Bring any drugs or medications you find at the scene to the receiving facility with the patient.

Reassessment

Perform a reassessment as warranted by the patient's condition. Monitor the patient's airway, breathing, oxygenation, circulation, and mental status. Repeat vital signs assessment and check any interventions, such as the security of restraints. Continue to calm and reassure the patient.

Summary: Assessment and Care

To review possible assessment findings and emergency care for a behavioral emergency, see Figures 26-3* and 26-4*.

Assessment Summary

BEHAVIORAL EMERGENCY

The following findings may be associated with a behavioral emergency.

SCENE SIZE-UP

Pay particular attention to your own safety. Look for:
- Mechanism of injury
- Weapons
- Hazards in attempted suicide such as a hair dryer in a tub filled with water
- Alcohol or drugs
- Evidence of a medical condition
- Routes of escape

Primary Assessment

General Impression
- Obvious life threats such as open wounds to chest, potentially self-inflicted
- Posture and body language, violent or nonviolent

Mental Status
- Alert
- Confusion or disorientation
- Hyperactivity
- Unresponsiveness

Airway
- Potentially closed airway in attempted suicide from altered mental status or vomitus

Breathing
- Normal
- May be adequate, inadequate, or absent in attempted suicide

Circulation
- Normal
- Pulse may be increased, decreased, or absent in attempted suicide
- Skin normal; may be pale, cyanotic, red, cool, or clammy in attempted suicide

Status: Priority Patient—if attempted suicide with life-threatening injuries or conditions

Secondary Assessment

Physical Exam and History

Signs and symptoms:
- Fear
- Anxiety
- Confusion
- Anger
- Depression
- Withdrawal
- Hallucinations (auditory or visual)
- Irritability
- Excessive crying

History:
- Did the patient ingest alcohol or drugs?
- Does the patient want to commit suicide?
- Is the patient on medications for a behavioral condition?
- Has he taken the medication as prescribed?
- Does the patient have a history of violence, aggression, or combativeness?
- Has the patient had a recent tragic event?

Physical Exam

Head, neck, face:
- Pupils may be dilated, constricted, or midsize.
- Facial expression may indicate anger, depression, or anxiety.

Chest:
- Inspect for evidence of self-inflicted wounds.

Abdomen:
- Inspect for evidence of self-inflicted wounds.

Extremities:
- Inspect for needle marks or self-inflicted wounds.
- Blood glucose level: normal (70–140 mg/dL, depending on last oral intake)

Baseline Vital Signs
- BP: normal or increased, may also be absent or decreased in suicide attempt
- HR: normal or increased, may also be absent or decreased in suicide attempt
- RR: normal or increased, may also be absent or decreased in suicide attempt
- Skin: normal; may be pale, cool, and clammy in patients experiencing fear and anxiousness
- Pupils: normal or may be dilated or constricted in suicide attempt
- SpO_2: 95% or greater in room air

FIGURE 26-3a * Assessment summary: behavioral emergency.

Emergency Care Protocol

BEHAVIORAL EMERGENCY

1. Ensure your own safety and be prepared to retreat if the patient is violent.
2. Assess the patient for possible self-inflicted injury.
3. Establish and maintain in-line spinal stabilization if spinal injury is suspected.
4. Establish and maintain an open airway; insert a nasopharyngeal or oropharyngeal airway if the patient is unresponsive and has no gag or cough reflex.
5. Suction secretions as necessary.
6. If breathing is inadequate, provide positive pressure ventilation with supplemental oxygen at a rate of 10–12 ventilations/minute for an adult and 12–20 ventilations/minute for an infant or child.
7. If breathing is adequate, administer oxygen based on the SpO_2 reading unless an underlying physical condition is suspected that requires higher concentrations of oxygen. If none is suspected and the SpO_2 is $> 95\%$, oxygen is not necessary unless other signs of hypoxia exist. If possible, deliver warm, humidified oxygen.
8. If no pulse is present, begin CPR and follow the AED protocol.
9. If the patient is responding, keep him calm.
10. If the patient becomes violent or threatens to injure himself, you, your partner, or others, restrain the patient.
11. Perform a reassessment every 5 minutes if the patient is unstable or every 15 minutes if stable.

FIGURE 26-3b ✻ Emergency care protocol: behavioral emergency.

Restraining a Patient

The patient who is aggressive and not responding to interventions is a difficult problem for the EMT. *If no one is able to communicate with the patient and you believe that he may present a danger to himself, to you, or to others, you must notify the police. Never leave such a patient alone; unless he is an immediate threat to you, watch him constantly and stay alert for sudden threatening behavior.*

If you need to transport a violent patient against his will, you may need to use restraints. *Even if a violent patient comes with you voluntarily, be prepared to restrain the patient if the situation changes suddenly.*

Restraint should be avoided unless the patient is a danger to himself or others. *Restraints may require police authorization;* seek medical direction and follow local protocol. If you are not authorized by state law to use restraints, wait for someone with the proper authority.

Do not restrain a patient in a prone (face-down) position. Also, never hogtie or hobble-restrain a patient (patient prone, arms tied behind the back, ankles and wrists restrained together). A higher incidence of death has been noted when patients are restrained in a prone position or when hogtied or hobble-restrained. Two significant problems associated with prone restraint of a combative or violent patient are:

- When a patient is placed in a prone position, the weight of the body places upward pressure on the abdomen and forces the abdominal organs to be displaced toward the diaphragm. The added compression prevents a normal downward movement of the diaphragm, leading to the inability of the patient to take in adequate breaths. This results in a decreased tidal volume and inadequate breathing. The inadequate breathing results in hypoxia and acidosis, which may cause further agitation and cardiac arrest.
- With a patient in a prone position, it is impossible to adequately assess the airway and the ventilatory status. You cannot assess for chest rise and adequate tidal volume with the patient in a prone position.

As the prone-restrained patient becomes hypoxic, he will typically begin to struggle more aggressively for a period of time. Remember that hypoxia leads to agitation and aggression, while hypercarbia (buildup of carbon dioxide) leads to confusion and somnolence. As the patient becomes more hypoxic and hypercarbic, he will become more confused and aggressive. This is usually viewed as the patient becoming more violent or combative when, in fact, it is related to the patient's inability to breathe effectively. Subsequently, the patient will become less agitated as he becomes more severely hypoxic and hypercarbic. This is often mistaken by the EMTs as the patient "calming down." Since the patient is in a prone position, it is difficult to see the obvious signs of hypoxia and inadequate breathing. Consequently, a period of time may pass before anyone recognizes that the patient is no longer breathing effectively, is not breathing at all, or is in cardiac arrest.

ASSESSMENT Tips

A patient who begins to "calm down" may be hypoxic from the efforts to fight against the restraints. Carefully and thoroughly assess the patient's airway, ventilation, oxygenation, and circulation. ■

For these reasons, it is necessary to restrain patients in a supine position. If increased upper extremity movement in supine restraint is a problem, take the supine patient's arms over his head and restrain each wrist to the head of the stretcher. This will limit his ability to move. If

Emergency Care Algorithm: **Behavioral Emergency**

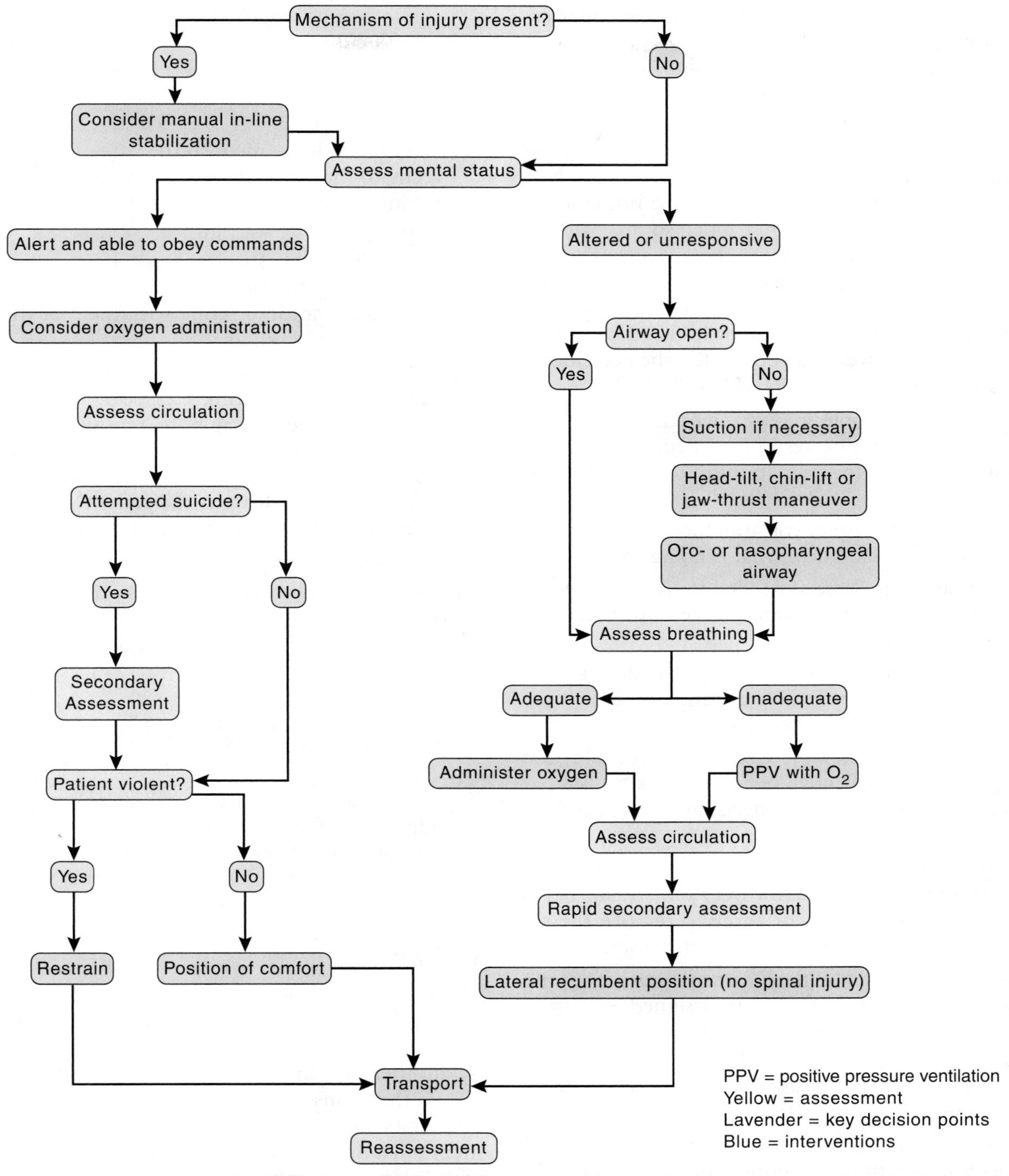

FIGURE 26-4 ✻ Emergency care algorithm: behavioral emergency.

Key Terms

humane restraints padded soft leather or cloth straps used to tie a patient down to keep him from hurting himself or others.

Key Points

Document why you restrained a patient and the technique you used. Always avoid unnecessary force.

vomiting or secretions are a concern, restrain the patient in a lateral position.

Restraints used with a patient should be **humane restraints**. This means that they are padded so they will not injure a patient who struggles against them. Use soft leather restraints, cloth restraints, cravats, or wide roller gauze, but never use metal handcuffs. A violent physical struggle is usually brief, since most people cannot sustain the intensity of such a struggle. However, if you still feel the need for restraints, follow these guidelines (EMT Skills 26-1):

1. Gather enough people to overpower the patient rapidly *before* you attempt restraint. Effective teamwork is more important than the strength of any individual team member.
2. Plan your activities *before* you attempt restraint. Everyone involved should know what is going to happen.
3. Use only as much force as needed for restraint; never inflict pain or use unwarranted force in restraining a patient.
4. Estimate the range of motion of the patient's arms and legs, and stay beyond that range until you are ready to begin imposing restraint.
5. Once you have made the decision to restrain, *act quickly*. A key to effective restraint is taking the patient by surprise; delay or indecision could allow the patient to gain control.
6. One rescuer should talk to the patient throughout the restraining process. However, you should never bargain with the patient or agree to remove the restraints if the patient promises to behave well.
7. Approach the patient with at least four rescuers at the same time; one person should be assigned to each of the patient's limbs. If the patient is taken down in a prone position to gain control, immediately get the patient into a supine position to allow for adequate ventilation and assessment.
8. Secure the patient's limbs with equipment approved by medical direction; as mentioned, restraints should be of soft leather or cloth. If available, use commercial wrist- and ankle-restraining straps.
9. Secure the patient to the stretcher in a supine position with multiple straps—effective placement is around the patient's chest, waist, and thighs. Make sure none of the straps is unduly tight or impairs the patient's breathing. The patient can be restrained to a long spine board or a scoop stretcher, which will allow you to avoid having to undo the restraints on arrival at the emergency department. If the patient is restrained directly to the stretcher, you will have to release the restraints to transfer the patient to the hospital bed.
10. If the patient is spitting on rescuers, cover his face with a disposable surgical mask. If a mask is used, reassess airway and breathing frequently to ensure that the mask is not interfering with them or that the patient has not vomited.
11. Once you have applied restraints, do not remove them—not even during transport. It may be necessary to remove restraints to reposition the patient. This can be done by removing one restraint at a time and controlling the extremity until it is rerestrained to the stretcher. Reassess the patient's circulation frequently to make sure the restraints are not binding.

Make sure you document on the prehospital care report why you felt it necessary to restrain the patient, and thoroughly document the technique you used for the restraint. Again, always avoid unnecessary force.

Legal Considerations

Every time you respond to a call as an emergency care provider, you have a chance of becoming involved with the legal system. That chance becomes greater when you are responding to patients with behavioral problems.

Consent

Consent is permission to treat. Under most state laws, any adult of sound mind has the right to determine whether he will be treated or, more specifically, touched by another person in the course of treatment. In most states, that consent must also be informed. *Informed consent* means that the person who is to receive the treatment must understand what it involves. This means that, with every conscious, mentally competent adult, you must explain the treatment, its nature, and its potential effects before starting it. Under laws in most states, forcing a person to have treatment against his will—that is, without consent—is grounds for a charge of assault and battery.

In most states, anyone age 18 or over is considered an adult, and anyone under the age of 18 who is in the armed services or is married, pregnant, or a parent is also considered an adult (emancipated minor). If the patient

Objective 26-11
Recognize indications for physical restraint of a patient and follow principles of safe physical restraint of patients.

Key Terms
reasonable force the minimum amount of force required to keep a patient from injuring himself or others.

is under the age of 18 and is not an emancipated minor, consent to treat should come from a parent, guardian, or blood relative. Consent should also come from a parent, guardian, or blood relative of a person who is considered to be mentally incompetent.

If you cannot find a responsible adult to consent to the treatment of a minor or of a mentally incompetent patient, or if an adult patient is unresponsive, you can still go ahead and treat. You will act in such cases on the principle of *implied consent.* This is the belief that the person who could grant consent would if he were present or able to do so.

These principles can be difficult to apply in the case of a patient suffering a behavioral emergency. Is he considered mentally competent? Is he able to give, or withhold, informed consent? Consult medical direction and carefully follow local protocols.

Refusal of Care

Emotionally disturbed patients—especially those who are intoxicated or who have taken a drug overdose—commonly refuse treatment. If the disturbed person is alert and oriented, unless considered mentally incompetent, he still must legally provide consent before you can treat him. Under these situations, the patient, not concerned family members, must consent to the care. Depending on state and local law, a patient who is disoriented, in shock, mentally ill, or under the influence of drugs or alcohol may not be considered competent to refuse care.

Your best protection against legal problems when dealing with emotionally disturbed patients is to document carefully and thoroughly all aspects of the encounter. If a patient refuses care, complete a refusal-of-care form (or a similar form used in your jurisdiction), then have it signed and witnessed by a police officer.

If a patient threatens to hurt himself or others *and you can demonstrate reason to believe that the patient's threats are real,* you can transport that patient without his consent. However, you must be able to show that your belief that the patient poses a threat is reasonable. In such cases, make every effort to have law enforcement personnel participate in the transport. They can provide important corroboration for your actions.

Using Reasonable Force

If it proves necessary to restrain a patient or to transport a patient without consent, make sure you use **reasonable force** when doing so. This is defined as the minimum amount of force required to keep the patient from injuring himself or others.

In most areas, police authorization is necessary to use reasonable force in restraining or transporting a patient without consent. Seek medical direction and follow local protocol. In most jurisdictions, an EMT can use reasonable force to defend against an attack by an emotionally disturbed patient without fearing legal consequences. The basic guideline in such circumstances is to avoid any act or use of physical force that may injure the patient during restraint.

The amount of force deemed reasonable depends on the situation. As a general guide, you'll need to consider the following:

- **The size and strength of the patient.** What may seem a reasonable amount of force when used against a 275-pound weight lifter probably wouldn't be considered reasonable when used against a 150-pound person with limited mobility.
- **The type of behavior exhibited by the patient.** You would not be expected to use the same kind of force against a frightened, paranoid person as you would against a belligerent, aggressive person who is loudly and repeatedly threatening to kill you.
- **The mental state of the patient.** It would be considered reasonable to use more force on a patient who is agitated and threatening than on one who is quiet and subdued.
- **The method of restraint.** Soft restraints, commonly called humane restraints, and straps are generally considered reasonable; metal handcuffs are not. Do not use metal handcuffs unless you are specifically trained in their use. If the police apply handcuffs to the patient, ensure that a police officer accompanies the patient in the ambulance or drives directly behind the ambulance in case the handcuffs would need to be removed quickly. If you are not trained in the use of handcuffs, do not take a key to remove them from the patient. A trained individual must be immediately available to remove the handcuffs, if necessary.

Caution: Always be aware that a patient who has become calm following a period of combativeness and aggression may suddenly revert to the earlier behavior. In such cases, you should use reasonable force to restrain the patient even though he has become calm.

Objective 26-12
Evaluate the need for law enforcement and medical direction involvement in a behavioral emergency situation.

Objective 26-13
Document all information pertinent to calls involving behavioral emergencies and patient restraint.

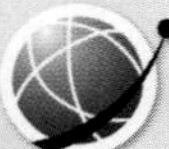

Media Resources
Go to www.bradybooks.com for mykit. Highlights:

- *Web Resource:* EpiPen auto-injector and anaphylaxis
- *Web Resource:* Panic attacks, panic disorders, and agoraphobia
- *Web Resource:* Schizophrenia

Police and Medical Direction

In any case where you might need to use reasonable force or transport without consent, the best way to protect yourself legally is to involve your chain of command. Before you restrain any patient for any reason, seek medical direction. If medical direction advises restraint, you can use that later as justification for your actions, should they be questioned.

Remember that law enforcement personnel should be involved when you need to restrain a patient or transport without consent or if there is any threat of violence. Law enforcement personnel serve a twofold purpose in cases like these: They can help protect you from injury, and they can serve as credible witnesses if a legal case should arise.

False Accusations

The best way to protect yourself against false accusations by a patient is to carefully and completely document everything that happens during the encounter—including detailed aspects of the patient's abnormal behavior. In most jurisdictions, anything documented during the call is considered legally admissible evidence. Anything that is not documented is considered hearsay (not legally admissible).

Another source of protection is to have witnesses, preferably throughout the entire course of treatment, including transport. It is common for emotionally disturbed patients to accuse medical responders of sexual misconduct. To protect against these kinds of charges, consider employing these measures:

- Involve other medical responders who can testify that there was no misconduct.
- Use medical responders that are the same gender as the patient.
- Involve third-party witnesses.
- Carefully document your physical assessment.

Whenever possible, have witnesses sign a written report of the incident.

EMT skills 26-1 Restraining the Combative Patient

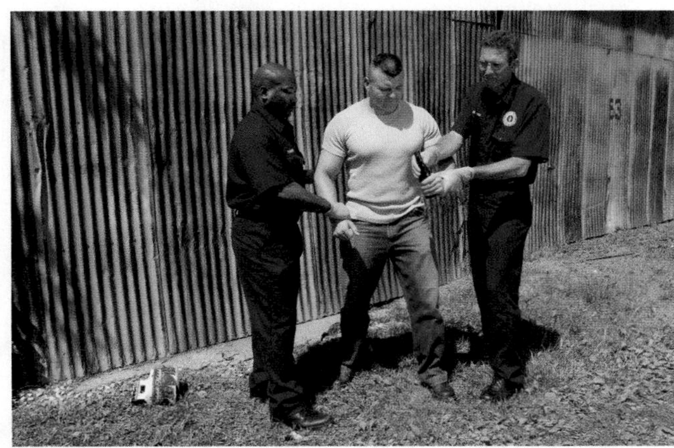

26-1A * If a possibility of danger exists, the patient should be interviewed with another EMT present. Identify yourselves and let the patient know what you expect.

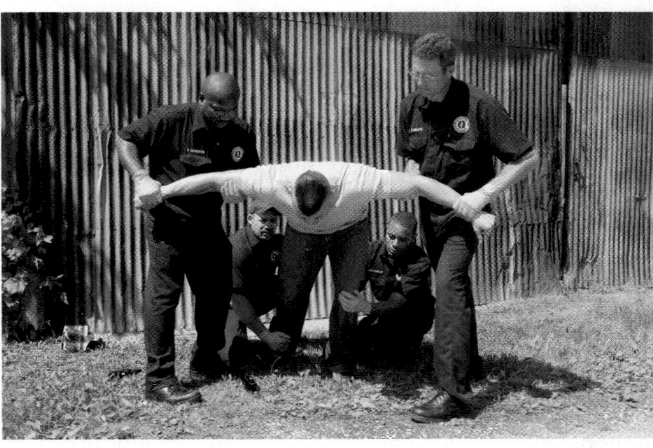

26-1B * Never try to restrain a patient until you have sufficient help and an appropriate plan. If necessary, create a safe zone and wait for police. Follow local protocol.

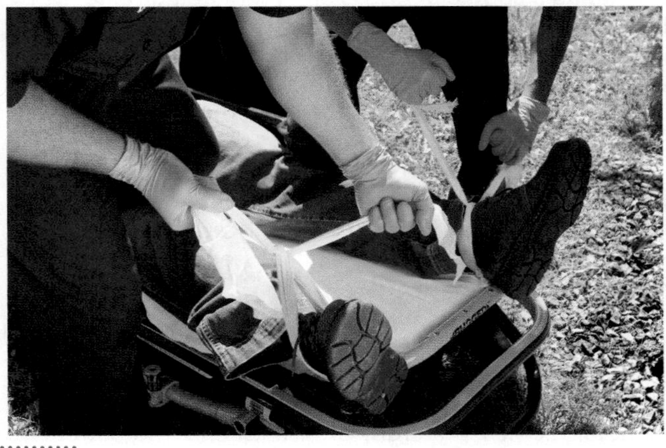

26-1C * Place the patient supine on the ambulance stretcher and apply ankle and wrist restraints. Never restrain the patient in a prone position.

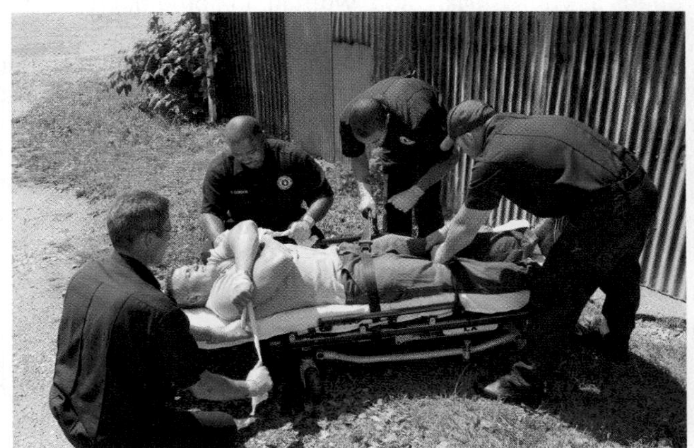

26-1D * One method is to pull arms across the patient's chest and tie on opposite sides of the stretcher frame.

CHAPTER REVIEW

SUMMARY

A behavioral emergency is a situation in which a person exhibits a behavior that is not acceptable or tolerable. Behavioral emergencies may result from a psychiatric disorder or from a medical or traumatic condition. Psychiatric conditions that may cause a behavior change include anxiety, phobias, depression, bipolar disorder, paranoia, psychosis, and schizophrenia. Suicide is a behavioral disorder intended to end the patient's life.

Because behavioral emergencies may involve sudden changes in the patient's behavior, they put the EMT at risk for violence and potential injury. Always remain vigilant on the scene and beware of behavior changes in the patient.

Your primary responsibility in managing a behavioral emergency patient is to provide emergency care for any underlying medical conditions or injuries that may be causing the disorder or that the patient may have inflicted on himself. Know and understand both the patient's limitations and your own limitations.

If the patient is exhibiting aggression and violence, it may be necessary to restrain him. It is best to have law enforcement present prior to the restraint procedure. Follow your local protocol on restraint. Never restrain a patient in a prone position. Never hog-tie or hobble-restrain a patient. Once the patient is restrained, ensure that you have clear access to provide an adequate assessment of his airway, ventilation, oxygenation, and circulatory status, in addition to the ability to perform a secondary assessment. Understand the legal issues involving restraint and patient consent.

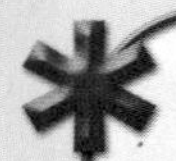

CASE STUDY FOLLOW-UP

SCENE SIZE-UP

You have been dispatched to Room 22 at King's Motel with a report of a woman bleeding. Because blood figures in the report, you take appropriate Standard Precautions. You observe no immediate hazards at the scene and exit the ambulance. The motel manager meets you and leads you to the room, but indicates he has no idea of the problem. The door opens at your knock, and a woman, in some distress, says she's bleeding and asks for help. You enter the room cautiously and find the only occupant, a young woman, sitting on the bathroom floor bleeding from a wound on her left wrist. In her right hand she is holding a large hunting knife.

You say, "Miss, we're emergency medical technicians and we're here to help you. But first, could you please reach up and put the knife on top of the sink and slide back from it a little." The woman is sobbing heavily and doesn't move or give any sign that she's heard you. You say again, "Please, miss, we want to help you, but before we can you have to put the knife down. Just reach up and put it on the sink. Then move back, just a bit." This time, she hears you. She slowly raises her arm and places the knife on the edge of the sink. Then she half turns away and buries her face in her hands. You then move into the bathroom, pick up the knife, and hand it to your partner, who secures it.

PRIMARY ASSESSMENT

You introduce yourself and your partner to the patient and ask her name. She replies, "Maria Foster." You tell her once again that you have come to help her. Your general impression is of a female in her early 20s who appears to be emotionally upset and is crying. She has an open wound to her left wrist. You ask, "Maria? May I call you Maria? Maria, may I please take a look at your wrist?" Maria nods yes, giving consent, and holds her wrist out toward you.

Bleeding from the wound has now stopped. The patient is alert and oriented. Her airway is open and her breathing is adequate. Her right radial pulse is present and her skin is slightly pale, cool, and moist. You explain, "Maria, you have lost some blood. I'd like to give you some oxygen. I think it would make you feel better and help you out a bit. Is that OK?" She nods her head again.

The injury to her wrist is not severe and blood loss has not been extensive. Maria's condition does not warrant a priority transport, so you proceed with the secondary assessment.

SECONDARY ASSESSMENT

You indicate to the motel manager that the situation is under control and ask him to wait outside the room. Then you ask Maria what happened.

She says, "No one cares. I got so tired of it. I just wanted it all over. All of it. I thought I'd come here where nobody knows me and slit my wrists and that would be it. Over. I had a couple of drinks and I was going to do it, I really was. I thought I could go through with it. I did one wrist and then I saw the blood and I chickened out. I called 911. Now I'm sorry I did. No, I'm not. Oh, I don't know. I'm so confused. I don't know . . ." She trails off into sobs.

You have listened carefully to Maria's story. You try to show your concern and acknowledge her feelings by saying, "I'm sorry that you're feeling so bad, Maria. I can understand how confused you feel. If it's OK, I'd like to ask you a few more questions and then see if I can help you with that wrist."

Maria nods her consent, so you go ahead with obtaining a history. You find that Maria has no other physical complaints. She has no known allergies, is on no medications, and has no significant past medical history. She last ate at about 4:00 yesterday afternoon and had about two glasses of rum over the 2 or 3 hours she was sitting in the room before cutting her wrist.

You ask if she inflicted any other wound to her body. She denies doing so. You inspect and palpate the area around the wrist wound. You note that a radial pulse is present. The skin below the wound is slightly pale and cool and dry to the touch. Maria is able to wiggle her fingers of her left hand and she can identify which of her fingers you are touching. You apply a dressing to the wound and bandage it. Your partner, meanwhile, obtains a set of baseline vital signs; they show a blood pressure of 148/84 mmHg, a heart rate of 94 per minute, and a respiration rate of 14 per minute.

You explain to Maria that you and your partner are going to put her on the stretcher and take her to Clarendon Hospital. You ask if there is anyone you can call to meet her at the hospital. Maria says nothing for a minute, then replies softly, "My mother." She gives you her mother's number and your partner calls it. Maria's mother agrees to come to the hospital. You move Maria into the ambulance and begin transport.

REASSESSMENT

En route, you quickly repeat the primary assessment, reassess the wound to the wrist to ensure that it is not bleeding, and get another set of vital signs. You continue to talk to Maria and listen carefully to what she says to you. Upon arrival at the hospital, you transfer care of the patient to the emergency department staff. After completing the prehospital care report and preparing the ambulance to return to service, you go back to see how Maria is doing. Her mother is with her, and they both thank you for your help and showing that you care. Just then you receive a call for another run, so you wish Maria luck as you head back to the ambulance.

IN REVIEW

1. List some of the clues that a behavioral problem may be due to physical rather than psychological causes.
2. Explain some of the causes that can lead to violence in the behavioral emergency patient.
3. Explain basic steps to follow during the assessment of a potentially suicidal patient.
4. Explain basic steps to follow during assessment of a violent patient.
5. List some of the basic signs and symptoms of a behavioral emergency.
6. Explain the basic steps of emergency medical care in a behavioral emergency.
7. Explain the proper way to restrain a violent patient.
8. List factors that would be considered in determining if the force used with a patient was reasonable.
9. Explain the circumstances in which you can transport a patient without his consent.
10. Explain basic steps to protect yourself against false accusations by a patient.

CRITICAL THINKING

You arrive on the scene and find a 26-year-old male patient with multiple self-inflicted stab wounds to his abdomen. The patient refuses your care and will not let you come within 10 feet of him without becoming very aggressive and violent. He is alert and pacing while holding his abdomen. You are unable to conduct any type of assessment on the patient.

1. What scene safety issues are involved?
2. How would you proceed in providing care for this patient?
3. What is your primary responsibility in managing the patient?
4. Would you consider restraining this patient?
5. What criteria would you use to make the decision to restrain the patient?
6. How would you proceed in restraining the patient?
7. What are some hazards involving patient restraint?
8. What legal issues are of concern in this patient?

PEARSON

EXPLORE mybradykit™

Please go to **www.bradybooks.com** to access mykit for this text. You will find quizzes, critical thinking scenarios, weblinks, animations, and videos related to this chapter—and much more. Look for online information on panic attacks and schizophrenia as well as a video clip on how to apply soft restraints.

Register your access code from the front of your book by going to **www.bradybooks.com** and selecting the mykit links.

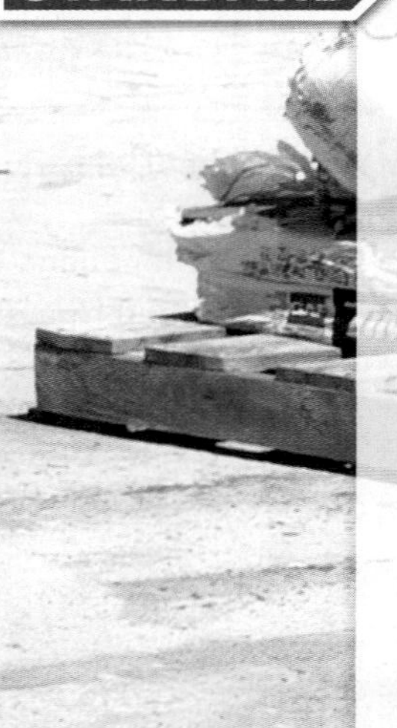
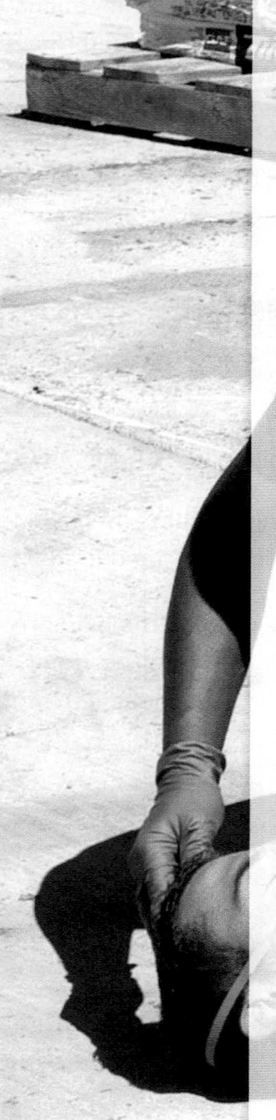

PART 10

STANDARD

Trauma

COMPETENCY

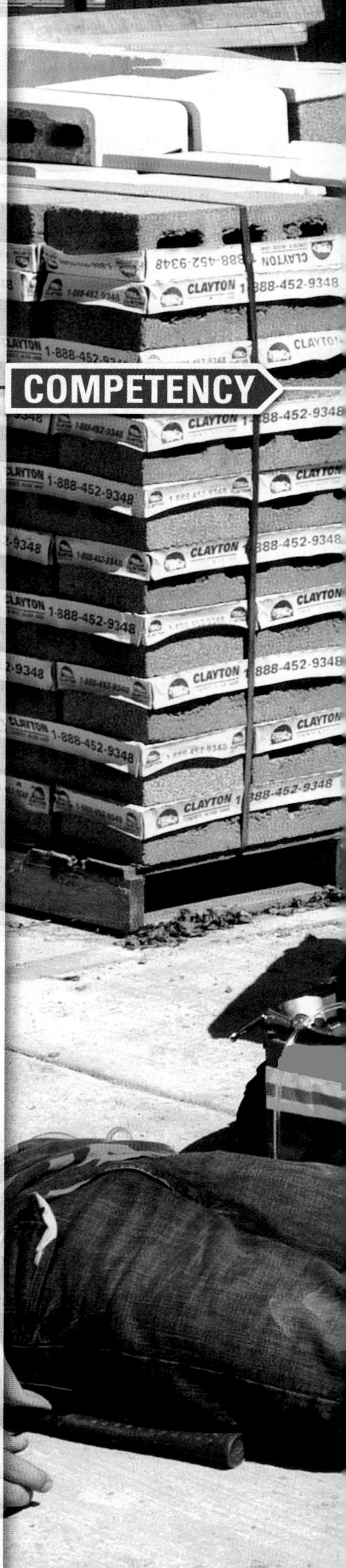

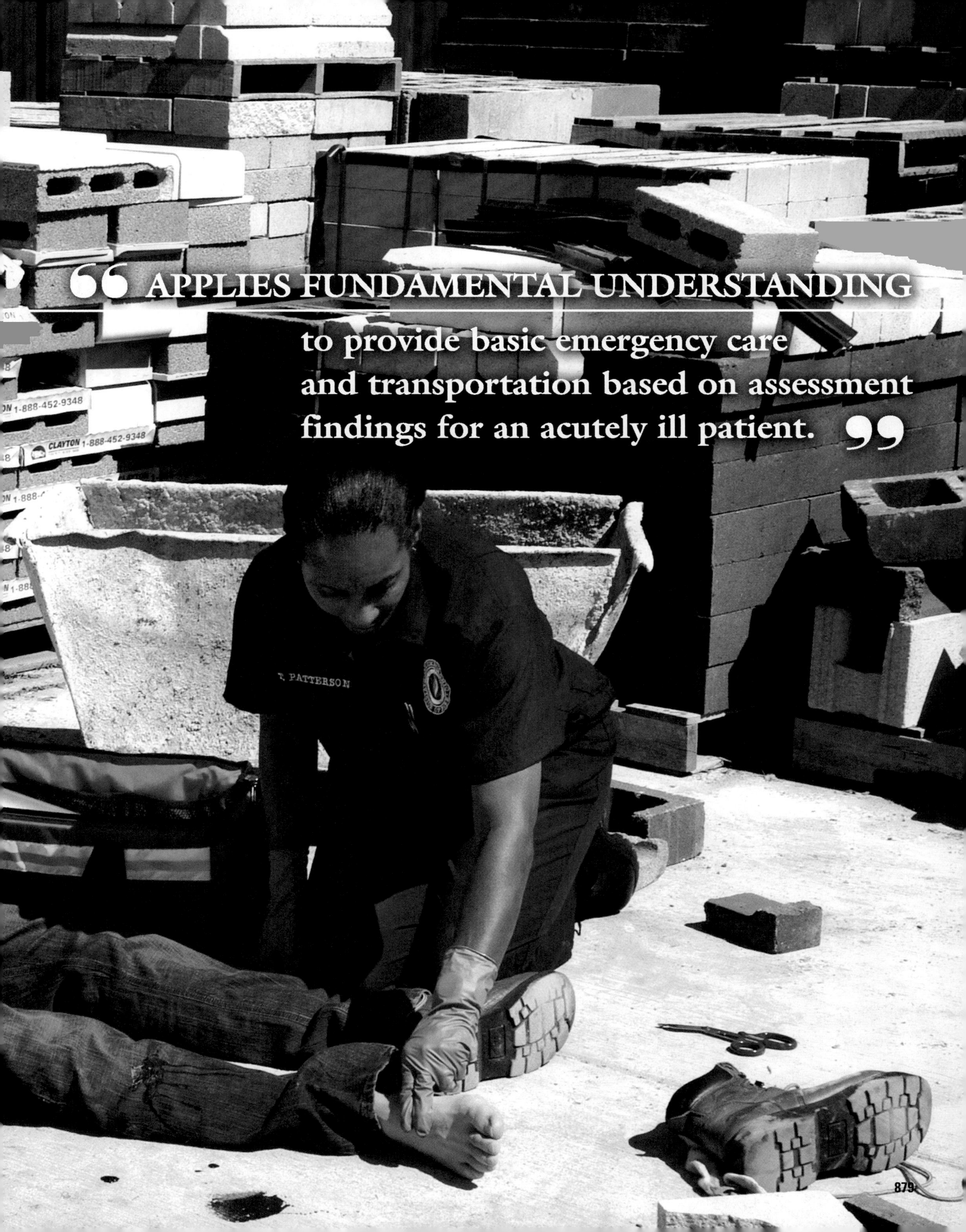

"APPLIES FUNDAMENTAL UNDERSTANDING to provide basic emergency care and transportation based on assessment findings for an acutely ill patient."

CHAPTER 27

Trauma Overview: *The* Trauma Patient *and the* Trauma System

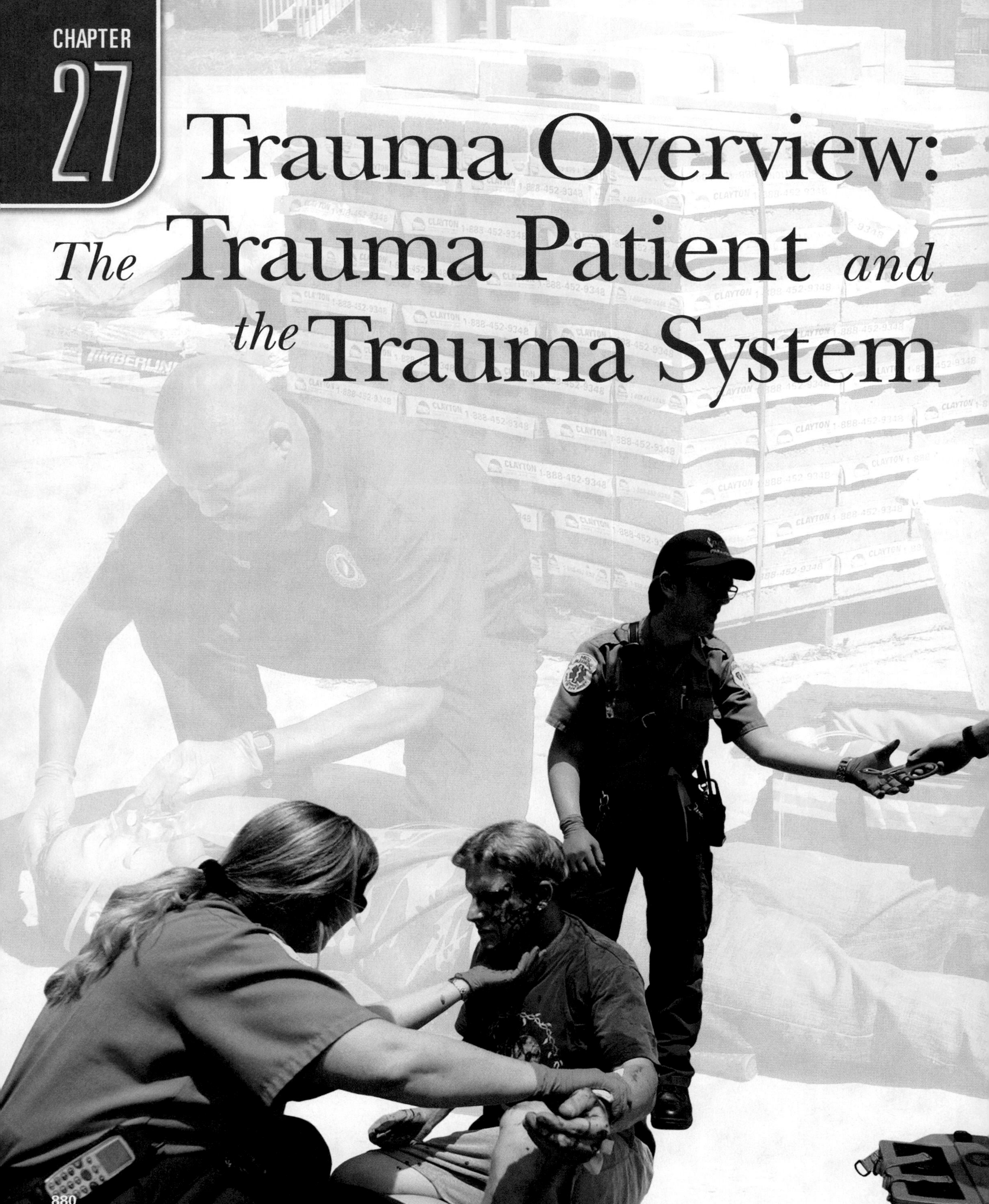

Navigation Guide

The following items provide an overview to the purpose and content of this chapter. The Standard and Competency are from the new National EMS Education Standards.

STANDARD **Trauma** (Content Area: Trauma Overview)

COMPETENCY Applies fundamental knowledge to provide basic emergency care and transportation based on assessment findings for an acutely injured patient.

OBJECTIVES: After reading this chapter, you should be able to:

27-1. Define key terms introduced in this chapter.
27-2. Explain why an understanding of kinetics is helpful to understanding injury and trauma.
27-3. Describe the relationship of mass and velocity to kinetic energy, including the relative contribution of each to the amount of kinetic energy.
27-4. Explain the effects of acceleration and deceleration on kinetic energy and the potential for injury.
27-5. Describe the impacts that take place in a typical motor vehicle collision.
27-6. List situations in motor vehicle collisions in which you should have a high index of suspicion for critical injuries.
27-7. Explain the typical patterns of injury associated with each of the following types of motor vehicle impacts:
- **a.** Frontal
- **b.** Rear
- **c.** Lateral
- **d.** Rotational and rollover
- **e.** Vehicle–adult pedestrian
- **f.** Vehicle–child pedestrian

27-8. Discuss the effects of the use of restraint systems in motor vehicle collisions.
27-9. Explain the typical patterns of injury associated with motorcycle collisions.
27-10. Describe factors that affect the pattern and severity of injury produced in falls.
27-11. Compare and contrast injury patterns produced by low-, medium-, and high-velocity penetrating mechanisms of injury.
27-12. Describe the mechanisms by which blast injuries produce injury.
27-13. Describe the principles of care for multisystem trauma patients.
27-14. Explain the term "golden period" and identify indications for an on-scene time of 10 minutes or less when caring for trauma patients.
27-15. Differentiate the characteristics of Levels I, II, III, and IV trauma centers.
27-16. Identify patients who meet trauma triage criteria for transportation to a trauma center.
27-17. Discuss the "golden principles" and special considerations in trauma care.

KEY TERMS: Page references indicate first major use in this chapter. For complete definitions, see the Glossary at the back of the book.

cavitation p. 896
dissipation of energy p. 896
drag p. 896
fragmentation p. 896
kinetic energy p. 882
kinetics p. 882
kinetics of trauma p. 882
mechanism of injury (MOI) p. 882
profile p. 896
trajectory p. 896

MEDIA RESOURCES: Please go to www.bradybooks.com to access mykit for this text. You will find quizzes, critical thinking scenarios, weblinks, animations, and videos related to this chapter—and much more. Look for online information on gun violence and trauma scenarios. You will also find animations on types of injuries and the mechanisms of injuries in motor vehicle collisions.

continued

CASE STUDY

The Dispatch

EMS Unit 632—proceed to 49 Elm Street—police are on the scene of a minor motor vehicle collision with a driver complaining of pain in his knees. Time out is 1307 hours.

Upon Arrival

The police officer greets you and explains that he was taking a report of a minor rear-end collision when the driver of the car that was struck from behind began to complain of knee pain. As you approach the vehicle you notice that the driver is responsive and there are no cracks in the windshield of his car. Apparently the patient was waiting to make a left turn and another vehicle struck him from behind.

How Would You Assess and Care for This Patient?

During this chapter, you will learn special considerations in sizing up the mechanism of injury. Later, we will return to the case and apply what you have learned.

Introduction

Since the early 1970s, trauma (injury) has been recognized as the leading cause of death for those between the ages of 1 and 40 and is the fourth leading cause of death for all age groups, after cardiovascular disease, stroke, and cancer. Trauma makes up a significant percentage of the calls to which prehospital personnel respond.

With any trauma patient, determining the possible extent of injury is critical to making good priority decisions regarding on-scene assessment and care versus rapid transport with assessment and care continuing en route. To make these judgments, the EMT must not only recognize obvious injuries but also maintain a high index of suspicion for hidden injuries. An understanding of mechanisms of injury is the chief component of this crucial assessment skill.

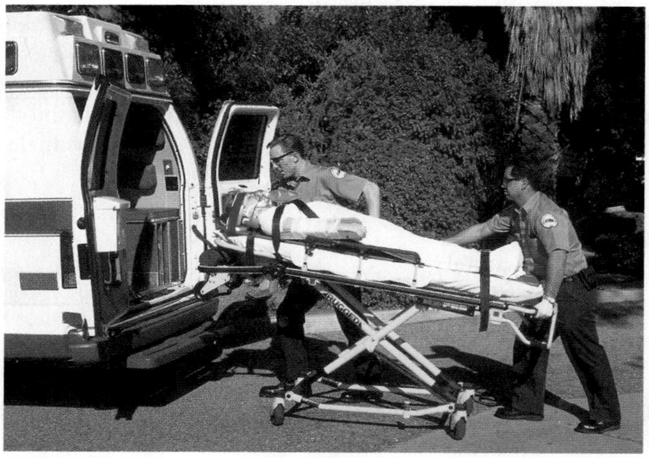

FIGURE 27-1 ✱ Is the patient a priority for transport? Analysis of the mechanism of injury may be a crucial element in the decision.

The Kinetics of Trauma

Mechanism of injury (MOI) refers to how a person was injured. The mechanism may be a motor vehicle collision, a fall, a gunshot, or other. The science of analyzing mechanisms of injury, sometimes called the **kinetics of trauma,** helps you to predict the kind and extent of injuries as a basis for your priority decisions regarding continuing assessment, care, and transport (Figure 27-1✱).

Trauma is nearly always the result of two or more bodies colliding with each other. (Except for blast injuries caused by pressure waves, it is difficult to think of an injury that does not involve a collision of bodies—a passenger's head with a windshield, a knife with someone's chest, and so on.) **Kinetics,** is the branch of mechanics dealing with the movements of bodies. So understanding kinetics is helpful in understanding mechanisms of injury and trauma.

How severely a person is injured depends on the force with which he collides with something—or something collides with him. This force depends partly on the energy contained in the moving body or bodies. The energy contained in a moving body is called **kinetic energy.**

Mass and Velocity

The amount of kinetic energy a moving body contains depends on two factors: the body's mass (weight) and the body's velocity (speed). Kinetic energy in a moving body is calculated this way: the mass (weight in pounds), times

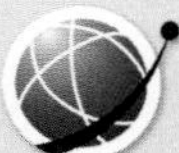

Media Resources

Go to www.bradybooks.com for mykit. Highlights:

- *Web Resource:* Safety Information for Pediatrics
- *Web Resource:* Trauma Scenarios
- *Animation:* Mechanism of Injury in Vehicle Collisions
- *Animation:* Types of Injuries in Vehicle Collisions

Objective 27-2

Explain why an understanding of kinetics is helpful to understanding injury and trauma.

Objectives 27-3 and 27-4

Describe the relationship of mass and velocity and of acceleration and deceleration to kinetic energy and the potential for injury.

the velocity (speed in feet per second) squared, divided by two. The formula can be written like this:

$$\text{kinetic energy} = \frac{\text{mass} \times \text{velocity}^2}{2}$$

This formula illustrates that as the mass of a moving object is doubled, its kinetic energy is also doubled. You would be injured twice as badly if you were hit by a 2-pound rock as if you were hit by a 1-pound rock thrown at the same speed.

However, velocity is a much more significant factor than mass. Suppose you were hit by a rock thrown at a velocity of 1 foot per second, then hit by the same rock thrown again at 2 feet per second. The rock thrown at 2 feet per second would be not twice as harmful as at 1 foot per second, but four times as harmful—because the factor of velocity is squared.

Understanding the factor of velocity is important in evaluating mechanism of injury in vehicle collisions. During your scene size-up, as you try to get an idea of how seriously vehicle passengers may have been injured, it is important to estimate the speed the vehicle or vehicles were going at the time of collision, knowing that a high-velocity collision will almost certainly have caused greater injury.

Understanding velocity also helps in understanding gunshot wounds and knife wounds. The great damage bullets do results not from their mass (a bullet doesn't weigh very much) but from their velocity. A bullet wound is potentially more traumatic than a knife wound (depending on which organs and structures are struck). Even if the bullet is smaller and lighter than the knife blade, a bullet exploding from the barrel of a gun impacts the body at a relatively higher velocity than a knife blade propelled by a human hand.

Acceleration and Deceleration

The *law of inertia,* which is one of the *laws of motion* described by Sir Isaac Newton, states: *A body at rest will remain at rest, and a body in motion will remain in motion, unless acted upon by an outside force.* A person hit by a car and a person thrown several yards by an explosion are examples of bodies at rest that were put into motion by an outside force. Conversely, the person who has fallen onto a concrete pavement and the car that hits a guard rail are examples of bodies in motion that were stopped by an outside force.

The rate at which a body in motion increases its speed is known as *acceleration.* The rate at which a body in motion decreases its speed is known as *deceleration.* While mass and velocity are major factors in determining the force of impact, acceleration and deceleration also play key roles.

A faster change of speed (acceleration or deceleration) results in more force exerted. For example, two cars of the same weight moving at the same rate of speed have the same kinetic energy. If one car is braked to a gradual stop and the other is stopped suddenly by striking a telephone pole, however, the one with the faster rate of deceleration—the one that struck the pole—exerts more force.

As another example, two people of the same size and weight riding in different cars at the same rate of speed have the same amount of kinetic energy. Suppose that one starts moving faster gradually by normal pressure on the gas pedal, and the other starts moving faster suddenly by being struck from behind by an out-of-control tractor trailer. The one with the faster rate of acceleration—the one struck from behind—will have his body jerked out from under his head and neck with sufficient force to cause a severe whiplash injury, while the one that accelerates gradually is not injured at all.

Energy Changes Form and Direction

Energy travels in a straight line unless it meets and is deflected by some kind of interference. If kinetic energy, transmitted to a human body, continues to travel in a straight line without interruption, injury may not occur. However, energy traveling through the human body is frequently interrupted. The interruption may be due to a curve in the bone, an organ that is caught between two hard surfaces, or tissue that is pulled against a fixed point. Energy is then forced to change form because it can no longer travel in a straight line. The result is either blunt or penetrating injury, which is discussed later in the chapter.

Impacts

In the typical vehicular collision, there are actually three impacts, each of which is an opportunity for energy to be absorbed by the vehicle and the patient. First, the vehicle is suddenly stopped and gets bent out of shape (Figure 27-2a∗). This is called the *vehicle collision.* Next,

Objective 27-5

Describe the impacts that take place in a typical motor vehicle collision.

Key Terms

mechanism of injury (MOI) the factors and forces that cause traumatic injury.

Key Terms

kinetics of trauma the science of analyzing mechanism of injury.

kinetics the branch of mechanics dealing with the motions of material bodies.

kinetic energy the energy contained by an object in motion.

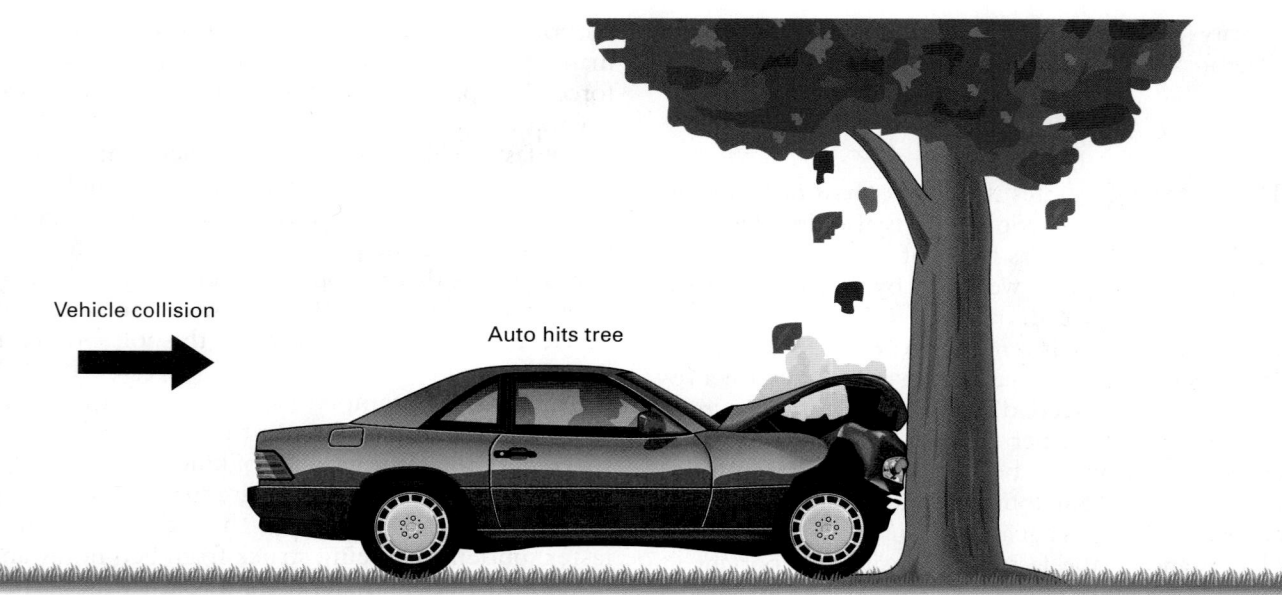

FIGURE 27-2a ✱ Vehicle collision. The vehicle strikes an object.

the patient comes to a quick stop on some part or parts of the inside of the vehicle, such as the steering wheel, causing injury to the chest (Figure 27-2b✱). This is called the *body collision*. Finally, there is the *organ collision* in which the patient's internal organs, which are all suspended in their places by tissue, come to a quick stop, sometimes striking an inside surface of the body (e.g., the inner chest wall or the inner skull) (Figure 27-2c✱).

Occasionally, there may be more impacts, such as a motorcycle rider who hits a car and is thrown. The cyclist hits the handlebars of the motorcycle, then the hood of the car, and finally the ground. With the impact of the cyclist against the handlebars, car, and ground, the internal organs also strike the inner body. So there are six potential

Body collision

Body hits steering wheel causing broken ribs

FIGURE 27-2b ✱ Body collision. The occupant continues forward and strikes the inside of the automobile.

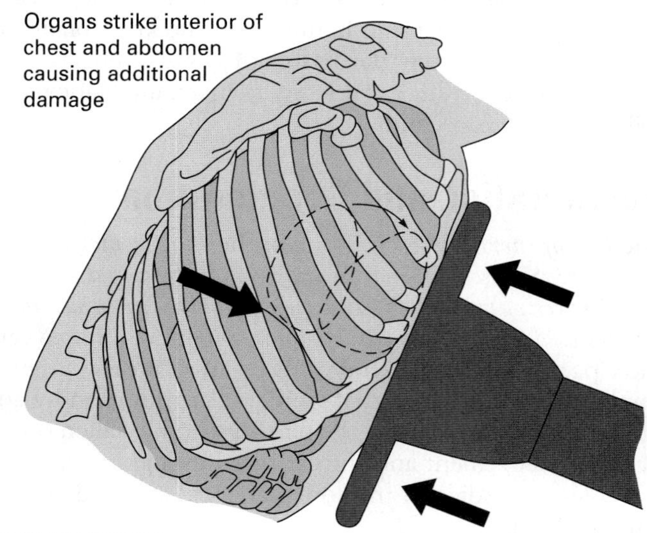

FIGURE 27-2c ✱ Organ collision. The organs continue to move forward and strike the inside of the skull, chest, or abdomen.

Key Points

With a thorough understanding of mechanisms of injury, you can look at a damaged vehicle and determine what types of injuries the patient is likely to have experienced.

Objective 27-6

List situations in motor vehicle collisions in which you should have a high index of suspicion for critical injuries.

impacts—three body collisions and three organ collisions—each of which produces energy and potential injury.

By comparing the number of impacts, it is easy to understand why a person in or on a moving vehicle who gets thrown has a much greater chance for injury than one who is restrained or remains within the vehicle.

Your understanding of the kinetics of trauma also makes it clear why the faster a vehicle is traveling, the greater the kinetic energy—and the higher the rate of acceleration or deceleration, the greater the force. The greater these factors and the greater the number of impacts, the greater the potential for injury.

Mechanisms of Injury

With a thorough understanding of mechanisms of injury, you will be able to arrive on the scene of a vehicle collision and determine, simply from looking at the damaged vehicle, what types of traumatic injuries the patient is likely to have experienced. Or, you will be able to arrive at the scene of a fall and, judging by the patient's position, quickly estimate the types of injuries you will be called upon to treat. (As you read about the injuries that may be caused by various mechanisms of injury in the remainder of this chapter, keep in mind that later chapters will deal with these kinds of injuries in more detail.)

Common mechanisms of injury include vehicular collisions, falls, penetrating gunshots or stabbings, and explosions. The fall is actually the most common mechanism of injury, accounting for more than half of all trauma incidents. However, the fall is not the most lethal mechanism of injury. Over one-third of all deaths from trauma result from vehicle collisions.

Vehicle Collisions

As discussed earlier, velocity is a key factor in mechanism of injury. The greater the speed at collision, the greater the chance of life-threatening injury. If a vehicle collided at high speed, your index of suspicion should include the possibility of the most severe injuries. Immediate assessment, aggressive treatment, and rapid transport are essential to saving occupants involved in these kinds of accidents.

You should also have a high index of suspicion in the following situations:

- **Death of another occupant of the vehicle.** A force severe enough to kill one passenger will almost certainly cause severe injuries, if not death, to all other passengers in the same compartment. Even if another passenger does not appear to be badly injured, maintain a high level of suspicion that this passenger has potentially fatal injuries, which may be internal or otherwise hard to detect.
- **An unresponsive patient or a patient with an altered mental status.** One of the earliest signs of brain injury is altered mental status or unresponsiveness. Consider the patient's mental status prior to your arrival when determining a baseline mental status, especially in the patient with a suspected head injury. A brief period of unresponsiveness or disorientation that is followed by a return of alertness may be a sign of brain injury. If this has been reported to you about a patient whom you then examine and find to be alert, you should still consider him as a patient with an altered mental status. Alternatively, if bystanders report that the patient was alert and talking coherently after the crash, and your baseline mental status assessment indicates that he is not alert after your arrival at the scene but responds to verbal stimuli, this would be an extremely important assessment finding, especially when considering a possible head injury.
- **Intrusion of greater than 12 inches for the occupant site or greater than 18 inches anywhere to the vehicle.** Intrusion of the vehicle is a deformity occurring to the interior compartment. The occupant site is anywhere in the vehicle where the patient was riding.
- **Ejection from the motor vehicle.** A patient who has been partially or completely ejected from a motor vehicle is at a much greater risk of injury than one who has remained inside the vehicle. The ejected patient is exposed to a greater transfer of energy, which increases his risk of multiple or severe injuries. The patient's chance of death increases by 25 times when ejected. There is also a much higher incidence of cervical spine fracture in ejected patients.

A brief period of unresponsiveness or disorientation followed by a return of alertness may be a sign of brain injury. If this has been reported to you about a patient whom you then examine and find to be alert, you should still consider him as a patient with an altered mental status. Or if the bystanders report that the patient was alert and talking coherently after the crash, and your baseline mental status assessment indicates that he is not alert after your arrival at the scene but responds to verbal stimuli, this would be an

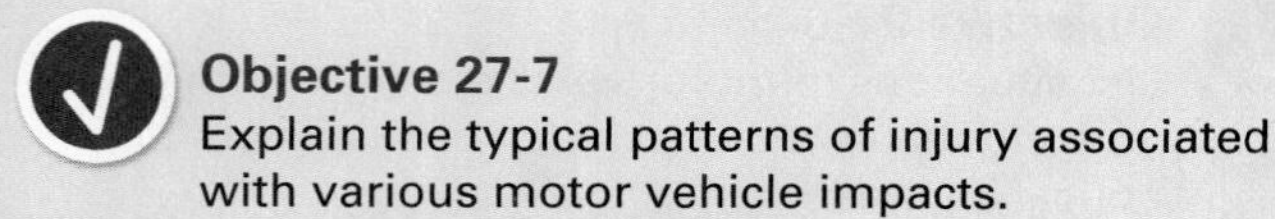

Objective 27-7
Explain the typical patterns of injury associated with various motor vehicle impacts.

Key Points
If unrestrained occupants travel in an up-and-over direction, they may be ejected, or partially ejected, from the vehicle.

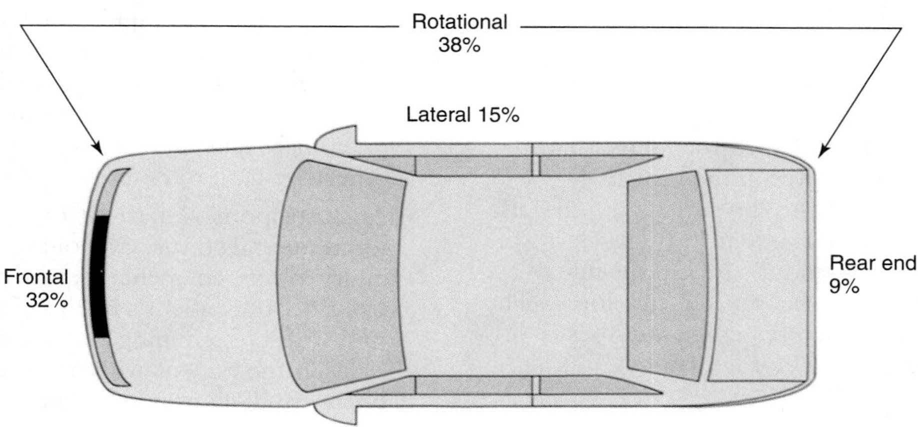

FIGURE 27-3 ✱ Types of impacts in motor vehicle trauma and their incidence of frequency in urban areas (by percentage).

extremely important assessment finding, especially when considering a possible head injury.

Motor vehicle collisions can be classified as frontal, rear-end, lateral, and rotational and rollovers (Figure 27-3✱). Each type has a predictable pattern of injury.

Frontal Impact

In the frontal impact (Figure 27-4✱), the driver will continue to move forward at the same speed the vehicle is traveling (Figure 27-5✱). Then he will proceed to go either up and over the steering wheel, causing injuries to the head, neck, chest, and abdomen and possible ejection through the windshield (Figure 27-6a✱), or he will go down and under the steering wheel, causing injuries to the knees, femurs, hips, acetabulum, and spine (Figure 27-6b✱).

If the unrestrained occupants of a vehicle involved in a collision travel in an up-and-over direction, they may be ejected from the vehicle. Partial ejection is also possible, for example the head protruding through the windshield. Severe soft tissue injuries, including avulsions and crushing injuries, often result. The chance of sustaining a spinal injury or a fatal injury is increased dramatically when the occupant is ejected.

Look for injuries to the abdomen, chest, face, head, and neck (Figure 27-7✱) when there is a frontal impact with the patient following an up-and-over pathway or with either full or partial ejection.

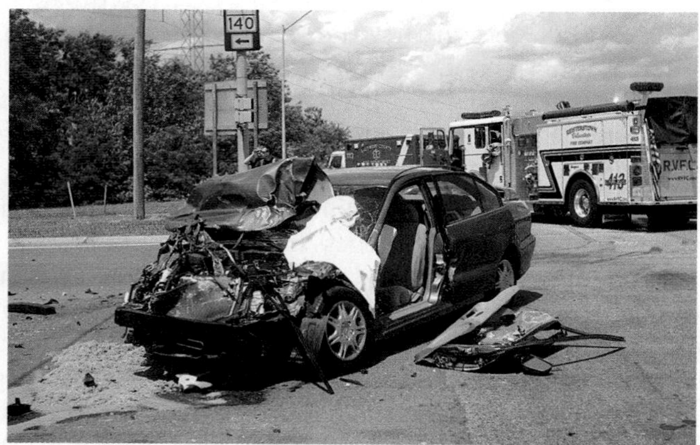

FIGURE 27-4 ✱ Frontal impact. (© Mark C. Ide)

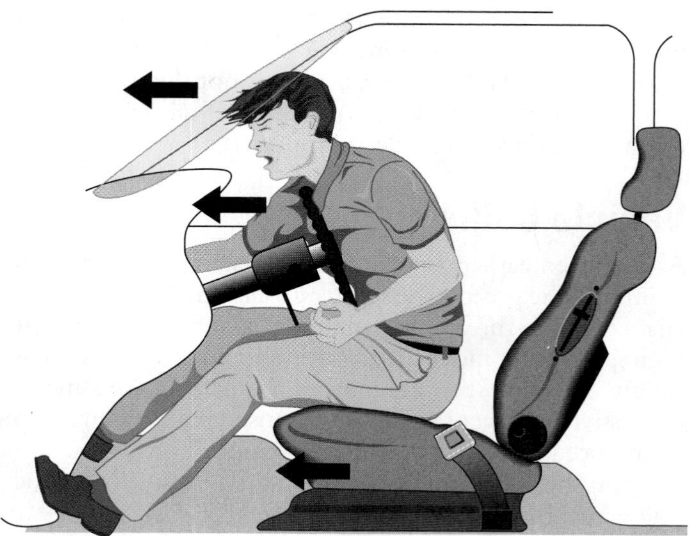

FIGURE 27-5 ✱ In a frontal collision, the occupant continues to move forward at the same speed the vehicle was moving.

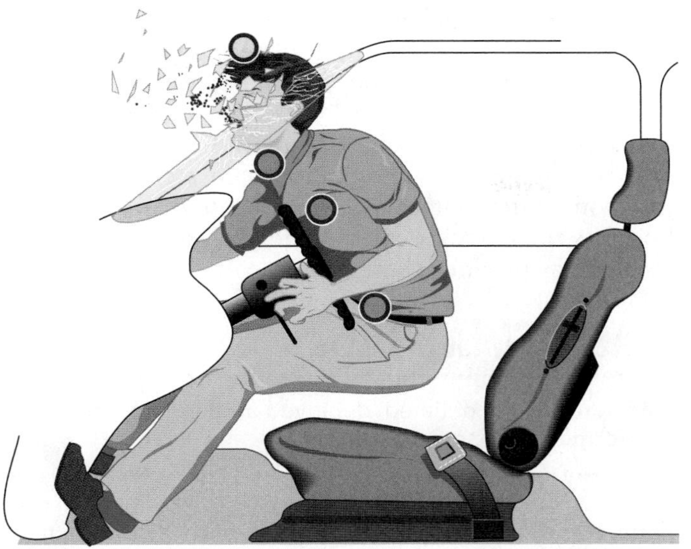

FIGURE 27-6a ✻ The up-and-over pathway causes impact to the head, neck, chest, and abdomen.

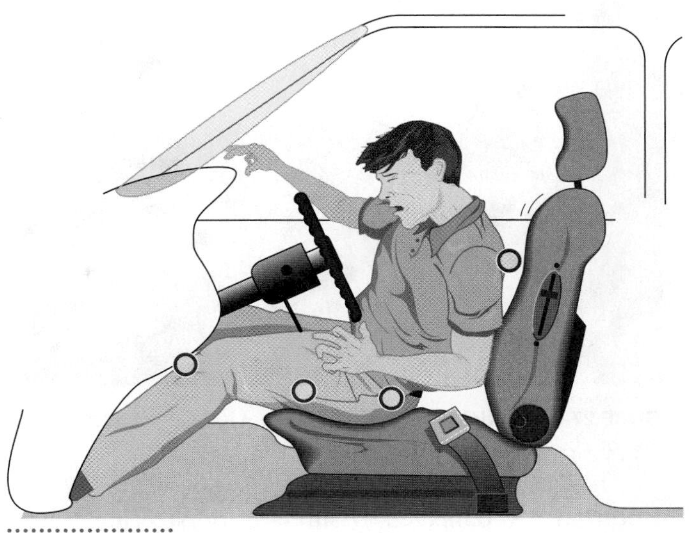

FIGURE 27-6b ✻ The down-and-under pathway causes impact to the knees, femurs, hips, acetabulum, and spine.

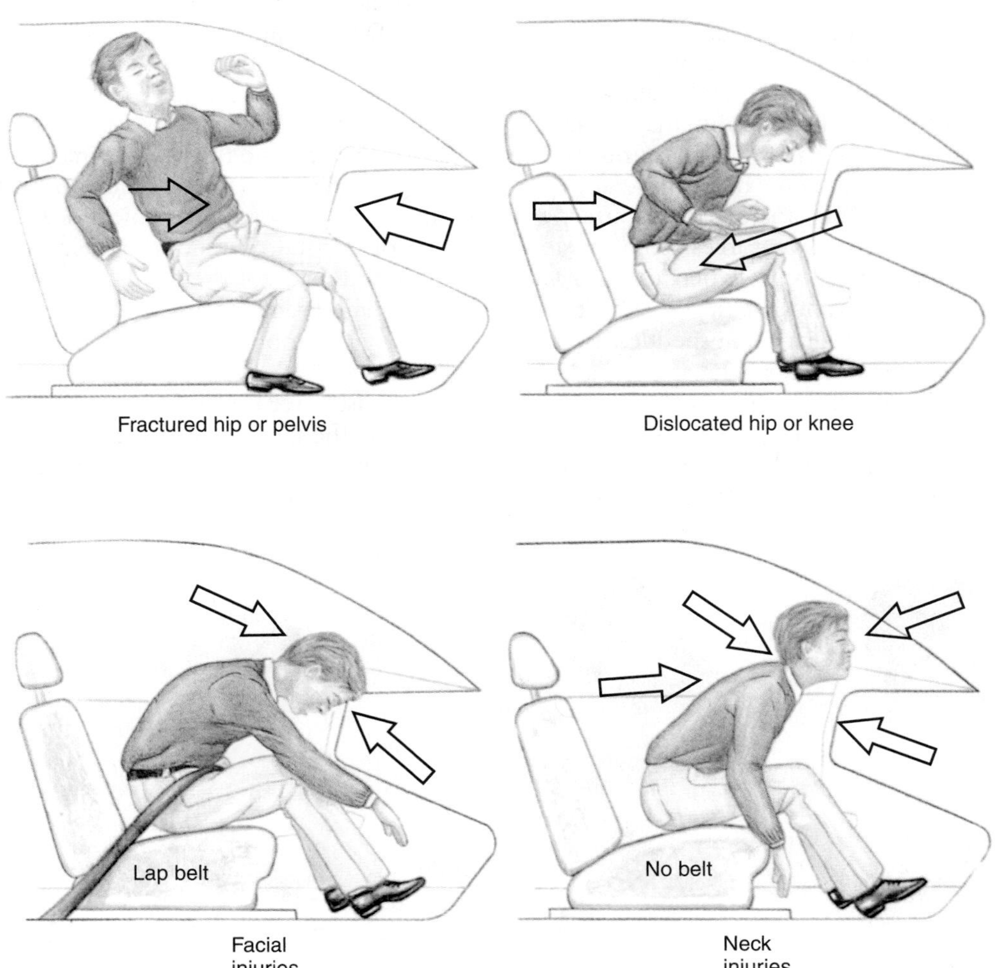

FIGURE 27-7 ✻ Examples of mechanisms of injury associated with frontal impact.

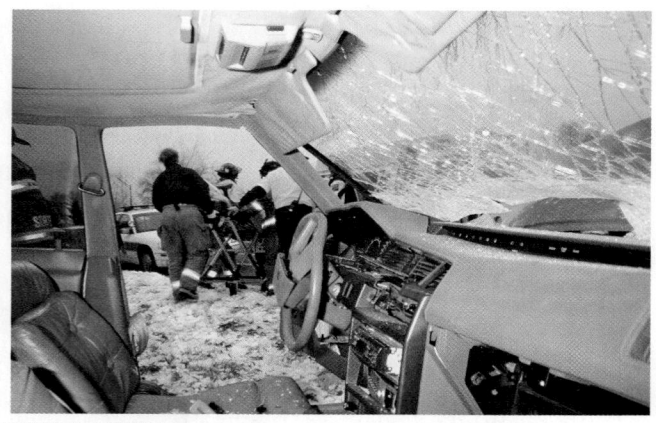

FIGURE 27-8 ✱ A deformed steering wheel indicates possible chest or abdominal injury. (© Jeff Forster)

Abdomen A damaged dashboard or steering wheel (Figure 27-8✱) should cause you to suspect abdominal injury. As the abdomen strikes the dashboard or steering wheel, the liver, spleen, and hollow organs of the abdomen are compressed between the front and back abdominal walls and spine. The hollow organs are more easily displaced, leaving the solid liver and spleen to bear the brunt of the compression.

Chest As the chest hits the dashboard or steering wheel, bones and soft tissues are both affected (review Figure 27-8). The ribs and sternum may break, and the cartilage connecting the ribs to the sternum may separate. A torn intercostal artery can bleed 50 mL per minute into the chest cavity with no blood seen externally.

The heart and lungs are the major organs affected. The heart suffers the effect of two forces: compression and shear. Compression force occurs when the heart is caught between the sternum and the spine, which can bruise the heart muscle. The heart is suspended by the aorta, which is attached posteriorly at the arch by a ligament. Shear force tends to pull the aorta at the ligament, which may tear or transect the aorta.

The lungs can also be affected. Air, trapped in the lungs by sudden closure of the epiglottis, is compressed between the ribs and spine. This kind of compression injury is called a "paper bag injury" because it is like blowing up a paper bag, then popping it between your hands. Air compressed inside the limited areas of a lung can bruise or rupture the lung (Figure 27-9✱).

Patients in a frontal collision who are unrestrained may come into contact with the steering wheel or dashboard as the air bag deploys. The explosive force of the air bag may produce chest injury.

ASSESSMENT Tips

Be sure to lift a deflated, deployed air bag to assess for deformity of the steering wheel. ■

Face, Head, and Neck These parts of the body are next to impact the dashboard, windshield, or window. As you approach the vehicle, always check for the typical "spider web" windshield cracking (Figure 27-10✱) or other impact marks to the windshield, which are usually caused by a head striking the glass. Depending on the impact point and amount of glass, the face may have extensive soft tissue damage. Head injuries usually result when an occupant is ejected from the vehicle, and skull fracture may occur. Depending on the force involved, penetrating bone shards or a depressed skull fracture may result, lacerating the brain tissue.

Even in the absence of bone injury, the force of the impact may damage the brain. First, the floor of the skull is very rough, with many sharp projections. When the brain moves across these projections, it can become lacerated or bruised. Second, the brain may rebound against the opposite side of the skull from the original point of impact. The brain can be bruised on the side of the impact or on the opposite side as the brain hits the wall of the skull.

Because force travels in a straight line, energy not dissipated by the face or head will continue down the neck, with the potential for causing cervical spine injury. If the occupant is thrown forward at such an angle that the neck

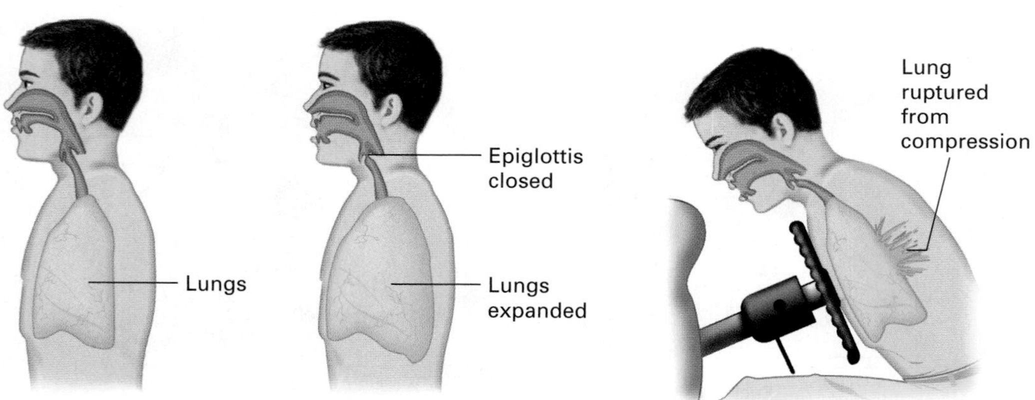

FIGURE 27-9 ✱ The "paper bag" syndrome results from compression of the chest against the steering column.

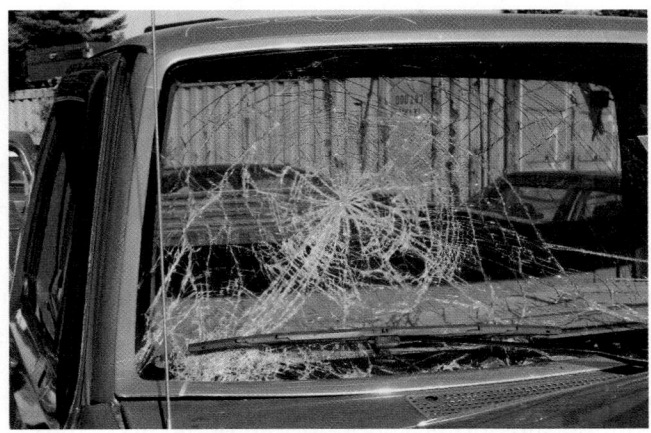

FIGURE 27-10 * Impact marks or cracking to the windshield indicates a possible head injury.

is caught by the steering wheel or the dashboard, the trachea is in direct danger of being injured.

Deployment of the air bag may also cause injury to the face, head, and neck.

ASSESSMENT Tips

"Spider web" or other impact marks to the windshield would heighten your suspicion of a potential head injury. Be aware that the impact mark on the windshield can also be made by an air bag that was deployed during the crash. ■

Rear-End Impact

In a rear-end impact (Figure 27-11*), the patient's head and neck are immediately whipped back. The body is propelled forward by the seat, while the head and neck, following the law of inertia, tend to remain at rest. Additionally, because the weight of the body exceeds that of the head, the body keeps moving while the head slows (Figure 27-12a*).

If there is a headrest that has been properly positioned and seat belts are worn, injury is minimized. However, if the vehicle does not have headrests or they are improperly positioned, the neck is hyperextended and the anterior spinal ligaments are often stretched or torn. This is often referred to as a "whiplash" injury. An improperly positioned headrest that is pushed all the way down to restrain just the neck and not the head can actually contribute to the severity of the injury by creating a fulcrum against which to bend the neck backward.

The injuries to be expected include the initial neck injury followed by either the frontal up-and-over or down-and-under injuries once the vehicle comes to a complete stop and the occupant jolts forward (Figure 27-12b*).

Lateral Impact

When a vehicle is struck laterally, or directly on the side, it can be crushed inward, impinging upon the occupants

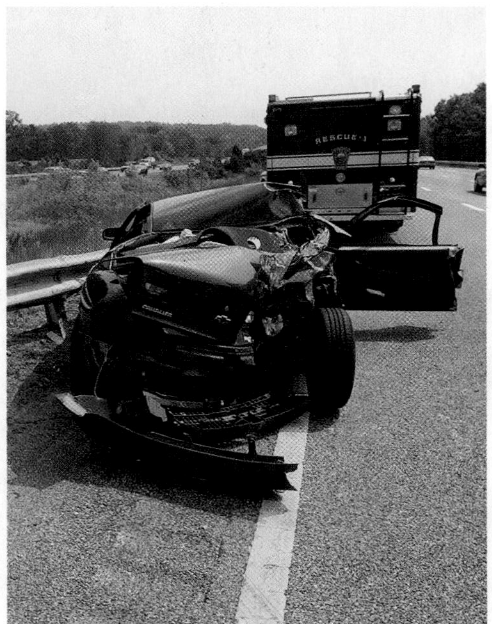

FIGURE 27-11 * Rear impact. (© Mark C. Ide)

(Figure 27-13*). Injuries may occur to the head, neck, chest, abdomen, and pelvis. You need to ask yourself who took the brunt of that collision and very carefully examine the side of the patient's body that bore the brunt of the lateral impact (Figure 27-14*).

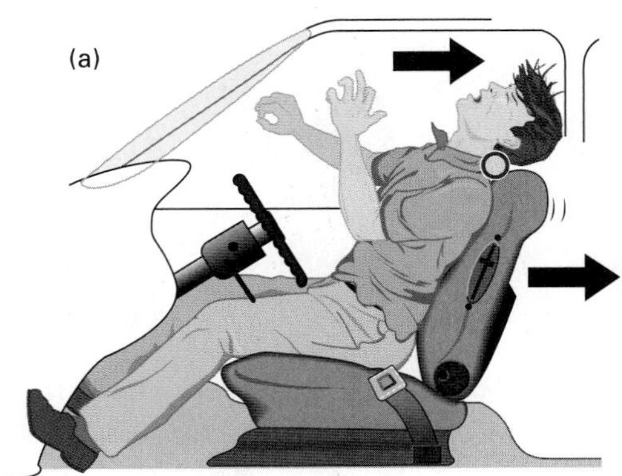

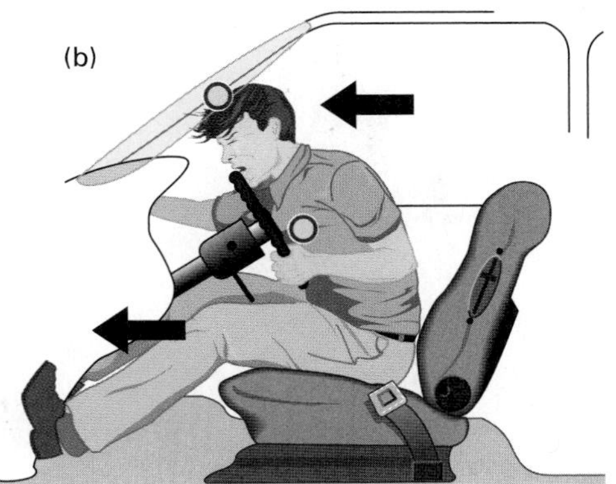

FIGURE 27-12 * **(a)** In a rear impact with an unrestrained occupant, initial movement is backward, causing potential neck injury. **(b)** The occupant then moves forward, causing impact to the head and chest.

Key Points
When the body is pushed laterally from under the head, the head moves in the opposite direction, damaging structures of the lateral neck.

Thinking Critically
Injuries from rotational crashes are the hardest to predict. Why?

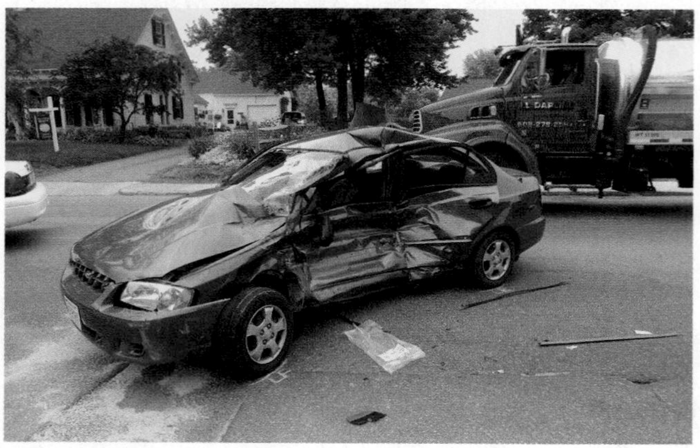

FIGURE 27-13 ✱ Lateral impact. (© Mark C. Ide)

Head and Neck As the energy of the impact is absorbed, the body is pushed laterally, out from under the head. This causes the head to move in the opposite direction. The structures in the lateral areas of the neck are not as strong as in the anterior/posterior portion of the neck, thus resulting in more frequent muscle tears and ligament injuries. The vertebrae are not designed for extreme lateral movement, and vertebral fractures are common. If there is more than one person in the passenger compartment, head injuries are frequently caused when heads collide.

Chest and Abdomen Injuries occur when the door strikes the side of the chest and abdomen. If the impact is on the shoulder, the energy traveling in a straight line may dissipate at the curve in the clavicle, resulting in a fracture. If the arm is caught between the door and chest, or if the door hits the chest, fractured ribs and flail segments are possible. If the fractures occur low in the rib cage, the liver or spleen may be affected.

Pelvis The impact of the vehicle door to the chest wall also causes a lateral impact to the pelvis. Fractures of the pelvis and upper femur usually complete this pattern.

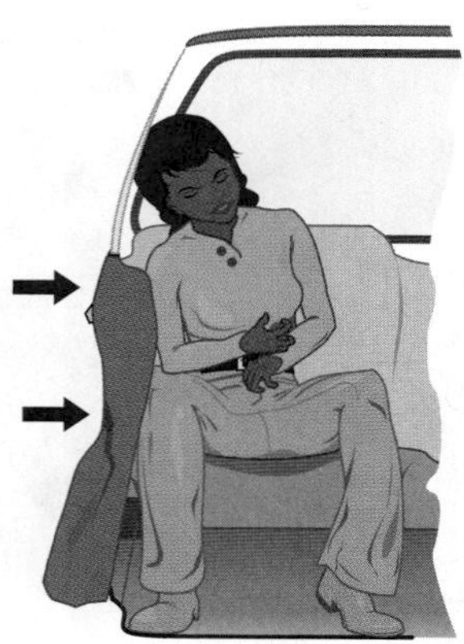

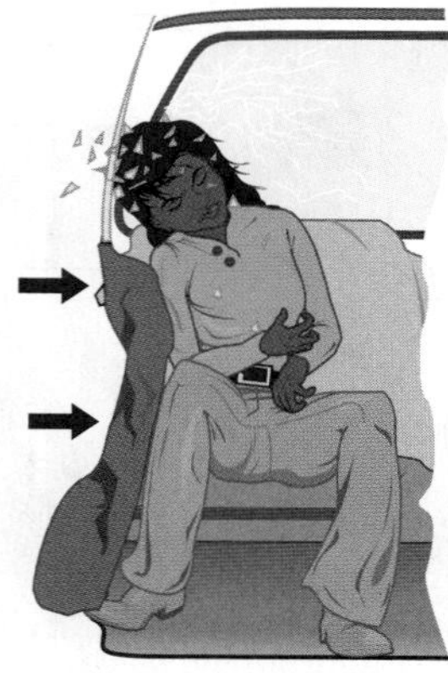

FIGURE 27-14 ✱ Lateral impact causes impact to the head, shoulder, lateral chest, lateral abdomen, lateral pelvis, and femur.

Rotational or Rollover Crash

Injuries from rotational crashes (Figure 27-15✱) are not as easy to predict as those from other crashes. The vehicle spins around the point of impact, causing the occupants who are not restrained to strike the mirror, posts, and doors, resulting in many injuries. Both head-on and lateral injury patterns occur.

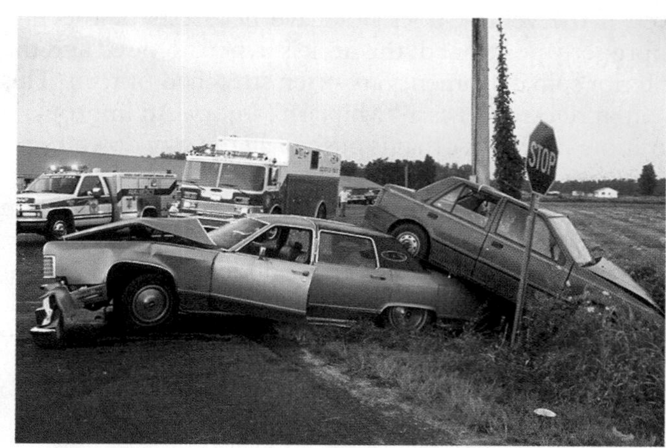

FIGURE 27-15 ✱ Rotational impact. (© Robert J. Bennett)

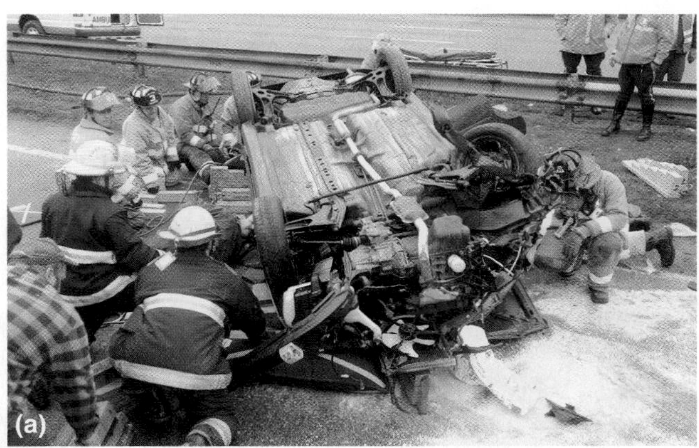

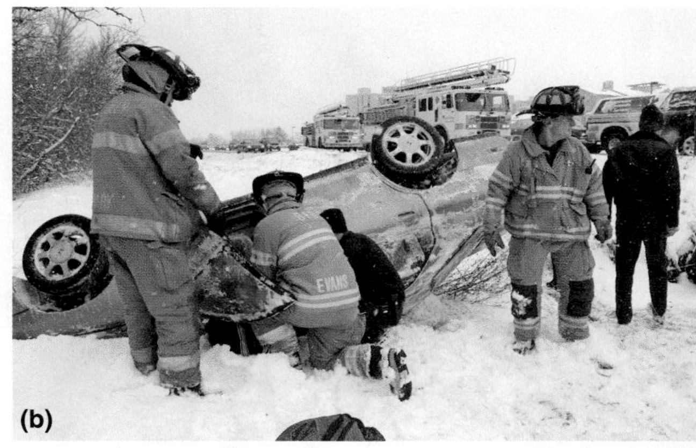

FIGURE 27-16 ✱ Rollover impacts. (Photo a: © Mark C. Ide; photo b: © Jeff Forster)

During a rollover, the vehicle hits the ground multiple times and in various places (Figure 27-16✱). The occupant changes direction every time the vehicle does (Figure 27-17✱). Vehicles with a high center of gravity, such as sports utility vehicles and vans, are more prone to rollovers. Every protruding object in the vehicle, including the rearview mirror, the headrest, and the door handles, becomes a potentially lethal object.

While a specific pattern of injury is impossible to predict in a rollover, there are a few common characteristics. First, multiple systems injury is common. Second, ejection is common if the occupant was not restrained. Finally, crushing injuries to ejected occupants are common. Following the laws of motion, if you go straight through the windshield into the ditch, so does your vehicle, right into the ditch on top of you. Sometimes patients are thrown into other lanes of traffic too fast for oncoming vehicles to avoid.

Vehicle–Pedestrian Collision

When a vehicle hits a pedestrian, the extent of injury depends on how fast the vehicle was going, what part of the pedestrian's body was hit, how far the pedestrian was thrown, the surface the pedestrian landed on, and the body part that first struck the ground. There are likely to be different patterns of injury in children than in adults. This is because adults are larger and have a different weight distribution. Also, children and adults react to an impending collision differently.

A child who is about to be hit by a vehicle—whether the child is walking or riding a bicycle (Figure 27-18✱)—generally turns toward the oncoming vehicle, so injuries from the impact are generally to the front of the body. A common pattern in a child struck by an auto is the combination of injuries to the femur, chest, abdomen, and head. Because a child is small and has a low center of gravity, a child struck by a vehicle is usually thrown in front of the vehicle, and is often subsequently run over by the same vehicle that hit him. A child struck by the bumper may be thrown onto the hood and then, when the vehicle stops, may be thrown off the car.

An adult, on the other hand, usually turns away from an oncoming vehicle, so the most common impact is to the side of the body. The bumper generally strikes the lower leg, typically causing fractures of the tibia and

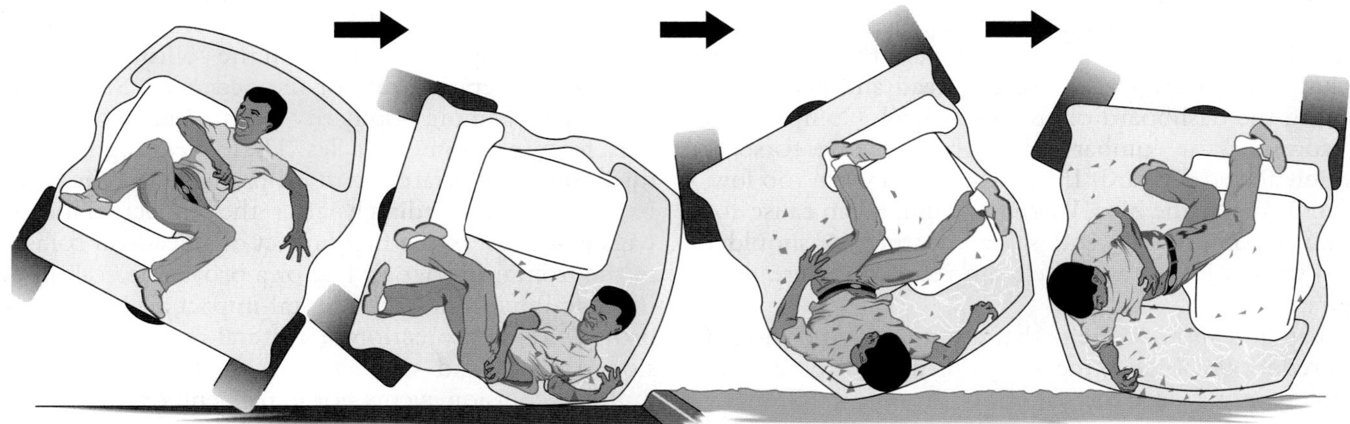

FIGURE 27-17 ✱ In a rollover of an unrestrained occupant, impact to the body is difficult to predict and commonly results in multiple system injury.

Objective 27-8
Discuss the effects of the use of restraint systems in motor vehicle collisions.

Key Points
Air bags are most effective when used with seat belts. In fact, the air bag may not be effective without a seat belt.

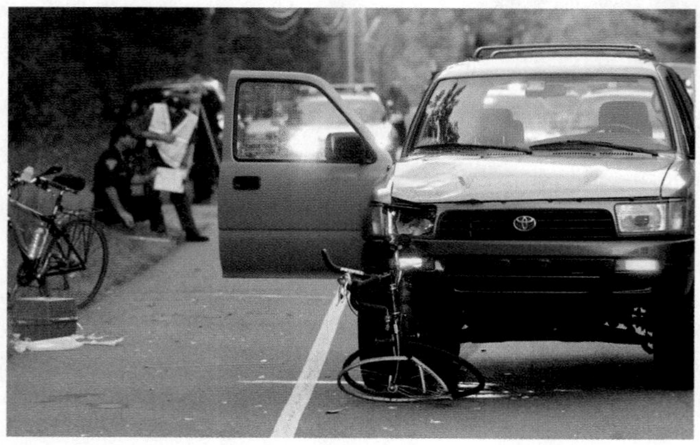

FIGURE 27-18 * A child about to be hit by a vehicle generally turns toward the vehicle. (© Mark C. Ide)

fibula. As the legs are propelled forward from the force of the vehicle, the adult generally falls backward and lands on the hood, resulting in injuries to the back, chest, shoulders, arms, and abdomen. If the adult continues across the hood and collides with the windshield, serious head and neck injuries are possible. Finally, the force of the moving vehicle throws the adult off the hood and to the ground.

Restraints: A Cause of Hidden Injuries

Hidden injuries may occur from the use of restraints in motor vehicles, including air bags and seat belts (Figure 27-19*). Lap belts, when worn properly, distribute force across the iliac crests of the pelvis. The lap belt prevents the occupant from being ejected but, without a shoulder strap, it does not prevent the chest from striking the steering wheel or the head and neck from striking the dashboard or steering wheel. Compression fractures of the lumbar spine occur as the torso is forcibly flexed forward. If the seat belt is worn too low, it can dislocate the hips. Worn too high, it can cause abdominal compression and spinal fracture. A shoulder strap worn without a lap belt can result in severe neck injury.

Lap and shoulder belts that are properly positioned may reduce the force of the impact on any one point and, consequently, reduce the severity of the injuries. Properly applied lap belts and shoulder straps do not, however, prevent the head and neck from moving laterally or forward and back.

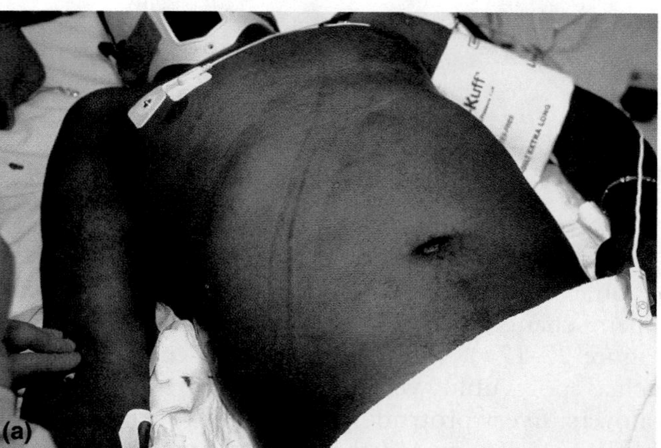

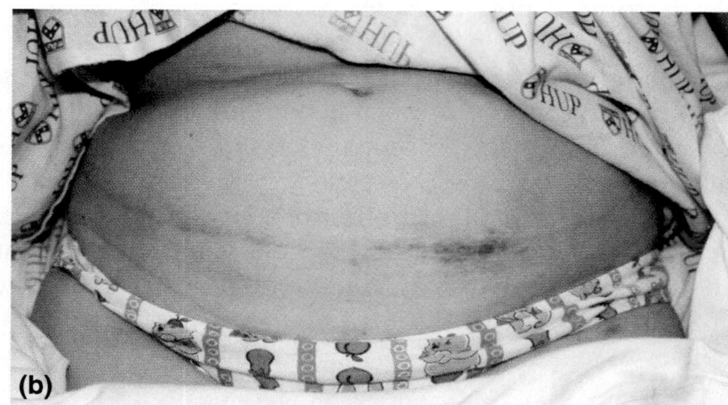

FIGURE 27-19 * Seat belt injuries to **(a)** the upper chest, **(b)** the abdomen. (Both photos: © Edward T. Dickinson, MD)

Frontal air bags are triggered to inflate from the steering wheel or glove compartment when a collision occurs. They cushion the forward motion of the occupant, absorbing the energy from the collision and slowing the deceleration rate of the occupant. Side-impact air bags are gaining popularity and are becoming a standard feature in some vehicles. These are designed to reduce injury associated with a broadside collision. The bag deflates immediately after the impact. Thus, air bags work best in the first impact of a head-on collision in the frontal-impact air bag or a broadside collision in the side-impact air bag. Frontal-impact air bags do not provide much protection in a lateral or broadside collision. Frontal and side air bags do not work well in multiple collision events nor in rear-end or rollover collisions. Air bags are most effective when used with seat belts. In fact, the air bag may not be effective without a seat belt.

Thinking Critically

Air bag manufacturers recommend that, in any collision in which the airbag deployed, rescuers should lift the bag and look beneath it. Why?

Objective 27-9

Explain the typical patterns of injury associated with motorcycle collisions.

Because the air bag deflates immediately after the impact, the driver may still hit the steering wheel. In any collision involving an air bag, the manufacturers of air bags recommend that rescuers lift the deployed air bag and check for deformation of the steering wheel. Any visible deformity of the steering wheel indicates potentially serious internal injury.

An air bag, especially when used without lap and shoulder restraints, may be the cause of injury. If the air bag is deployed in close proximity to the head, neck, or chest, usually 10 inches or less, significant injury may result from the deployment. Head, spine, eye, facial, and arm injuries are associated with air bag deployment. The individuals most prone to injury resulting from air bags are older adults, short adults (less than 5′ 2″), and infants and children less than 12 years of age. As noted in the next section, any child who is less than 12 years of age should ride in the rear seat of the vehicle; an infant in a safety seat must be placed in the rear seat of any vehicle that has a front passenger air bag. There have been a number of deaths associated with air bag deployment; however, the benefits of the air bags far outweigh the risks.

Considerations for Infants and Children The properly secured car seat restrains a child at three points (overhead or T-shield seats) or at five points. During a collision, any part of the body that is not restrained continues forward at the same speed the vehicle was traveling prior to the impact. As the child's head snaps forward, the neck is stretched against the resistance of the shoulder restraints. The result can be a spinal cord injury without injury to the vertebrae, which are pliable in children.

Even if the seat is facing backward, the same kind of injury can happen if the car seat is rotated into a reclining position. To prevent head snapping, the proper position for the car seat is to face backward and reclined to a 45-degree angle. To completely avoid injury from air bag deployment, children should always be restrained in the back seat of the vehicle and not in the front passenger seat.

Motorcycle Collisions

Motorcycle collisions account for a significant number of motor vehicle collisions on and off our nation's highways (Figure 27-20*). The incidence of morbidity (illness or injury) and mortality (death) is greatly affected by whether the rider is wearing a helmet. There are three main types of impact in motorcycle collisions: head-on, angular, and ejection. Ejection is most often associated with the head-on impact.

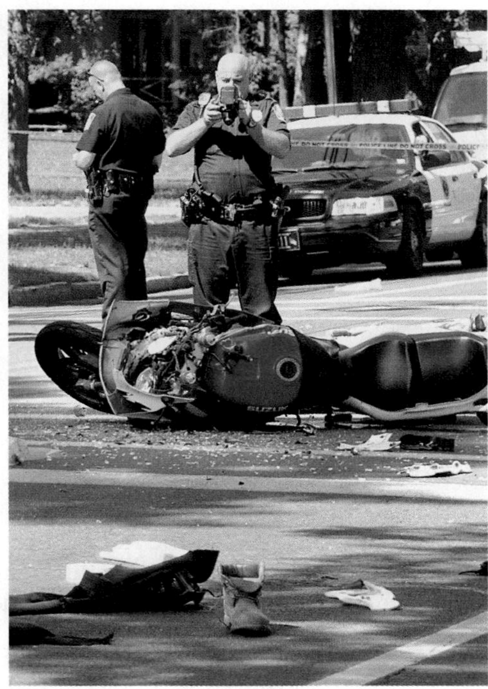

FIGURE 27-20 * Motorcycle collisions can result in multisystem trauma from multiple impacts to the rider. (© CW McKean/ Syracuse Newspapers/The Image Works)

Head-On Impact When this kind of impact occurs, the motorcycle tends to tip forward because of the location of its center of gravity. This causes the rider to travel into the handlebars at the same speed the bike was traveling. Depending on what part of the rider's anatomy strikes the handlebars, a variety of injuries may occur.

Angular Impact In angular motorcycle impacts, the rider strikes an object, usually a protruding object, at an angle. The object impacts whatever body part it comes into contact with, usually breaking or collapsing in on the rider. Examples include the edges of signs, outside mirrors on motor vehicles, or fence posts. The result can be severe avulsion injuries or even traumatic amputations.

Ejection After any motorcycle collision, ejection occurs if the rider clears the handlebars. Ejection continues until a body part impacts with the object of the collision, the ground, or both. Boots, leather clothing, and a helmet help to protect against soft tissue damage, commonly

Key Points
Abrasions can range from superficial to full-thickness and can be complicated by dirt or other particles embedded in the tissue.

Objective 27-10
Describe factors that affect the pattern and severity of injury produced in falls.

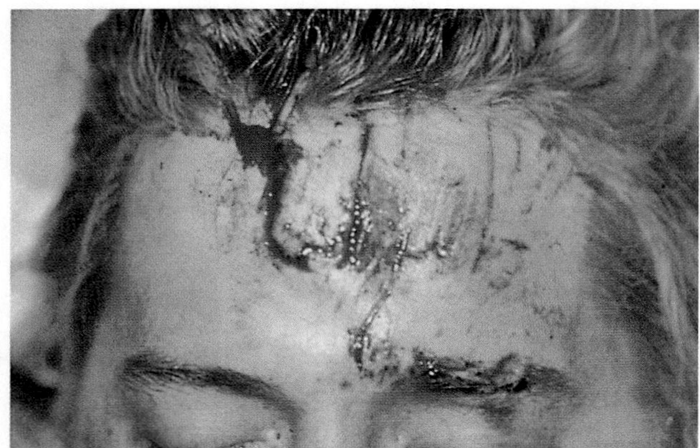

FIGURE 27-21 * Soft tissue injury to the forehead.

called "road rash," and against head and facial injuries (Figures 27-21* and 27-22*). If the rider is not wearing a helmet, the incidence of severe head injury and death increases 300 percent, the same as that for auto ejections.

"Laying the Bike Down" This is an evasive action on the part of the rider, designed to prevent ejection and separation of the driver from the bike in an impending collision. The bike is turned sideways and "laid down" with the driver's inside leg dragging on the pavement or ground. The driver tends to lose speed faster than the bike, thus moving the bike out from under the driver.

Abrasions can range from superficial abrasions, involving only the epidermis, to full-thickness abrasions, which extend through the subcutaneous tissue and, in severe cases, to the covering over the bone. Abrasions can be complicated by particles embedded in the tissue such as dirt, grass, or asphalt.

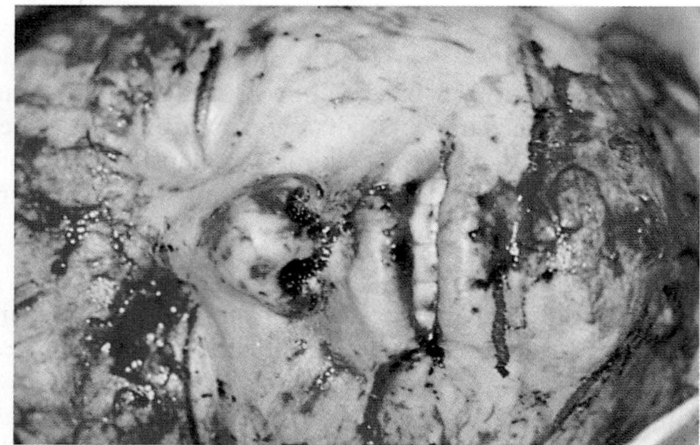

FIGURE 27-22 * Soft tissue injury to the face.

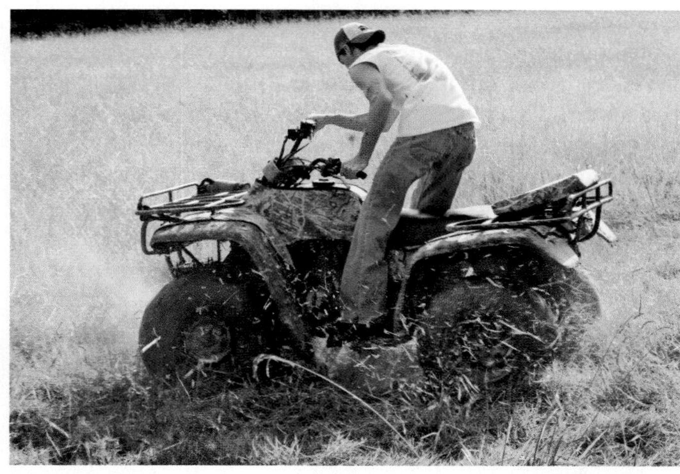

FIGURE 27-23 * All-terrain vehicles (ATVs) can cause multiple injuries from the combination of speed and instability. (© Ken Kerr)

Burns are most often sustained when the inside leg does not clear the bike. The leg becomes caught between the exhaust pipe and the ground. The longer the contact with the hot pipe, the worse the burn.

All-Terrain Vehicles ATVs are very problematic since they are easily tipped over (Figure 27-23*). The three-wheel versions have been pulled off the market. Even the four-wheel ATVs are quite unstable and can easily cause collisions similar to motorcycle collisions.

Falls

Falls are the most common mechanism of injury. The severity of trauma depends on the distance, surface, and body part that impacted first. Associated factors are objects that interrupt the fall prior to landing.

In general, the greater the distance of the fall the more severe the injury, because increased height increases the velocity at impact. Some experts believe that the surface is more of a determining factor of injury than the height. A fall of 20 feet, which is equivalent to two stories of a building, onto an unyielding surface is considered severe for an adult, and a fall of more than 10 feet, or 2 to 3 times the height of the child, can cause severe injuries in a child. Internal organ damage is frequent, and you should have a high index of suspicion regardless of how the patient looks at first.

The pattern of trauma injuries also depends on the body part that impacts first. As we pointed out earlier,

Thinking Critically
Even though the victim of a fall has landed on his feet, he may have sustained spinal and even internal organ injuries. Why?

Objective 27-11
Compare and contrast injury patterns from low-, medium-, and high-velocity penetrating mechanisms of injury.

energy travels in a straight line until it is forced to curve. At that point, energy changes form to dissipate, and injury occurs.

Feet-First Falls

A feet-first landing causes energy to travel up the skeletal system. Fractures of the heels and fractures or dislocations of the ankles are common (Figure 27-24*). If the knees are flexed at the time of impact, the majority of energy will be dissipated at the knees and will preserve the rest of the skeletal system. If the person lands flat-footed with knees locked, however, energy will be transmitted up through the femurs to the hips and pelvis, possibly causing fractures.

If energy remains, the spine will absorb the force at every curve of the lumbar, midthoracic, and cervical spine. The patient who fell three times his height or more will probably have a spinal injury resulting from the transmission of energy up through the legs and hips and into the spine.

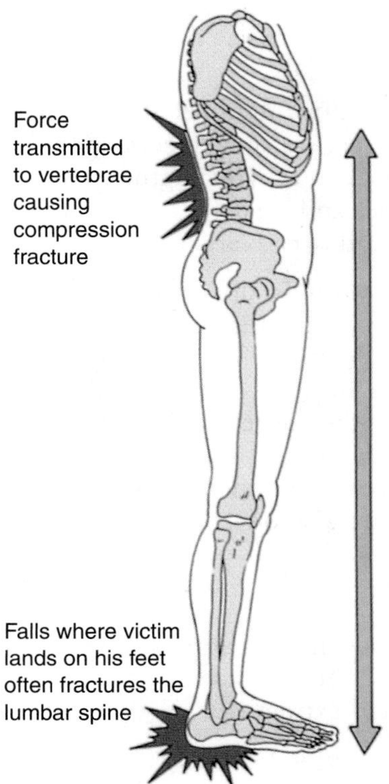

Force transmitted to vertebrae causing compression fracture
Falls where victim lands on his feet often fractures the lumbar spine

FIGURE 27-24 * In falls the energy of impact is transmitted up the skeletal system.

In falls of more than 20 feet, the internal organs are likely to be injured from deceleration forces: the liver, spleen, kidney, aorta, and heart may be affected.

Extending the arms to break the fall as the body is thrown forward is natural. The first point of energy dissipation is at the wrist. A fracture of the wrist bones known as a Colles, or "silver fork," fracture is common. The elbow and shoulder are the next points of potential injury. If the body is thrown backward, the most common injuries are to the head, back, and pelvis.

Head-First Falls

In head-first falls, the pattern of injury begins with the arms and extends up to the shoulders. The head may be forcibly hyperextended, hyperflexed, or compressed, all of which can cause extensive damage to the cervical spine. As the body continues its downward motion, the torso and legs are thrown either forward or backward. Chest, lower spine, and pelvic injuries are also common.

Penetrating Injuries

Penetrating injuries are caused by any object that can penetrate the surface of the body—such as bullets, darts, nails, and knives. The amount of damage that results depends on the amount of kinetic energy transferred to the tissue and the area of the body it penetrates. Of these two factors, the amount of kinetic energy transferred to the tissue is the greatest indicator of potential damage. For example, if the object is a knife, the low kinetic energy limits the damage to just the immediate site of impact and the underlying structures. The higher kinetic energy of a bullet results in tissue damage extending relatively far from the site of impact. If the kinetic energy produced by the bullet is totally absorbed by the body tissues, the bullet will not exit. If kinetic energy remains with the bullet, however, an exit wound will occur.

Penetrating injuries are classified as low, medium, and high velocity (Figure 27-25*).

Low-Velocity Injuries

A knife or other object impaled in the body exerts damage to the immediate area of impact and its underlying structures. As the person tries to defend against an attack, wounds may occur. These are generally slash marks on the hands and arms that occur when the person puts up one or both hands or arms to ward off the attacker or in an attempt to grab the knife.

Key Terms

trajectory the path of a projectile during its travel; a trajectory may be flat or curved.

dissipation of energy how energy is transferred to the human body by the forces acting on it.

drag the factors that slow a projectile.

Key Terms

profile the size and shape of a bullet's point of impact.

cavitation a cavity formed by a pressure wave resulting from the kinetic energy of a bullet traveling through body tissue; also called *pathway expansion.*

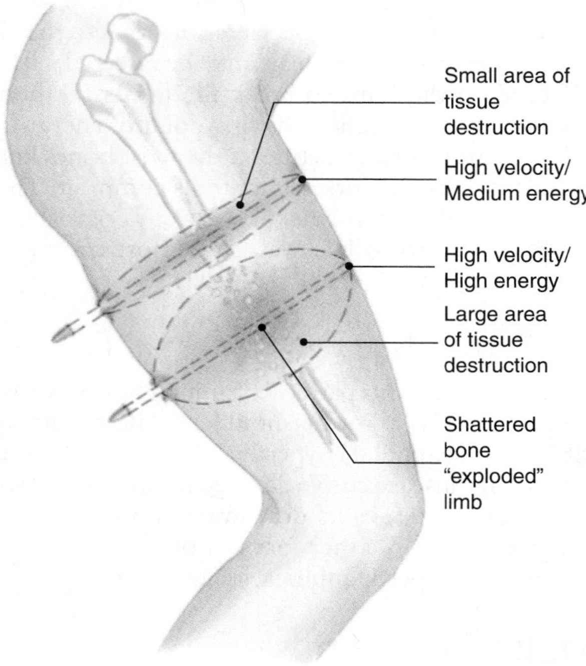

FIGURE 27-25 ✱ The severity of injury caused by penetrating trauma is related to the velocity of the penetrating object.

The length of the object used in the stabbing also provides valuable clues. For example, a person stabbed from behind in the left upper chest with a short (3-inch) paring knife may suffer a pneumothorax (air in the chest cavity). If stabbed with an 8-inch knife, the injuries may include lacerated pulmonary veins, lacerated aorta, and even laceration to the heart itself. If you know the type of knife and its length, you should report it to the hospital staff.

Medium- and High-Velocity Injuries

Medium- and high-velocity projectiles are generally pellets or bullets. Most shotguns or handguns fire at medium velocity. High-velocity weapons include high-power, high-speed rifles such as an M-16 or a 30-30 Winchester.

The damage caused by medium- and high-velocity projectiles depends on two factors: trajectory and dissipation of energy. **Trajectory** is the path or motion of a projectile during its travel. Normally, a bullet, once fired, follows a curved trajectory or path. However, the faster the bullet, the flatter the curve of the trajectory and the straighter the path of the bullet.

Dissipation of energy is the way energy is transferred to the human body from the force acting upon it. In the case of medium- and high-velocity projectile injuries, dissipation of energy is affected by drag, profile, cavitation, and fragmentation.

1. **Drag.** The factors that slow a bullet down, such as wind resistance, constitute drag.
2. **Profile.** The impact point of the bullet is its profile. The greater the size of the impact point, the more energy is transferred.
3. **Cavitation.** Sometimes called pathway expansion, cavitation is the cavity in the body tissues formed by a pressure wave resulting from the kinetic energy of the bullet. Cavitation greatly extends the tissue damage beyond the initial bullet pathway. That is, the hole created in the tissues is larger than the diameter of the bullet. (Cavitation occurs with medium- and high-velocity projectiles but not generally with low-velocity projectiles.) Blown-out tissue caused by cavitation and carried along with the bullet explains why the exit wound is always larger than the entry wound. Always assess for an exit wound. However, EMS personnel should not make judgments about the exact pathway of the bullet or specific organ injury based on entrance and exit wounds.
4. **Fragmentation.** A bullet that breaks up into small pieces or releases small pieces upon impact increases the body damage. The fragments increase the frontal impact area and create greater tissue damage with injuries spread over a larger area of the body.

Shotgun wounds differ significantly from rifle or handgun wounds, because shotguns have multiple pellets that spray in a pattern. The multiple pellets increase the impact surface area, thus increasing the amount of energy transferred to the tissues. Close-range shotgun wounds can cause devastating tissue damage, while long-range wounds may cause no more than relatively minor tissue damage (Figure 27-26✱).

Gunshot Wounds

Of fatal wounds that occur from firearms, 90 percent involve the head, thorax, and abdomen. Wounds also occur to the neck and extremities.

Head The interior of the skull is a fixed space with little-to-no room for expansion. When the energy from a projectile enters the skull and starts to dissipate, brain tissue is severely compressed.

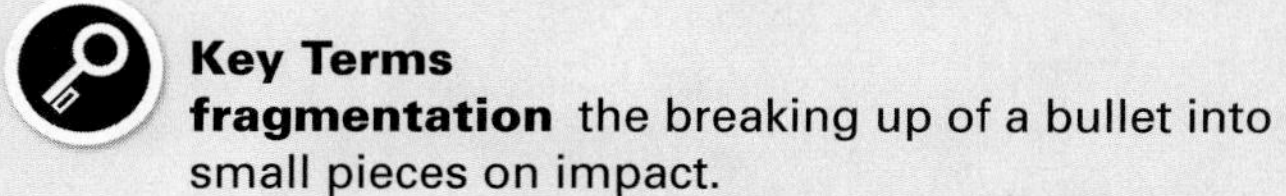

Key Terms
fragmentation the breaking up of a bullet into small pieces on impact.

Objective 27-12
Describe the mechanisms by which blast injuries produce injury.

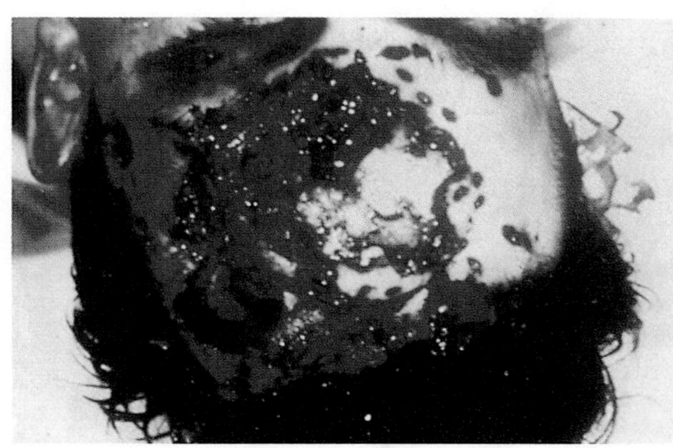

FIGURE 27-26 * A wound resulting from close-range shotgun blast. Note the tattooing of the skin from the gunpowder.

Gunshot wounds to the face generally result in major soft tissue injuries that immediately threaten the airway. It is very difficult to get a good seal when ventilating the patient who is lacking facial contours. Bleeding is extensive, and the airway is difficult to manage.

Chest Lung tissue is relatively tolerant of the cavitation caused by projectiles. The numerous air-filled alveoli form a spongy mass that is easily movable. Pneumothorax is a common result of injury to the chest and/or lung, with air or a combination of air and blood escaping into the chest cavity. Associated rib fractures may also occur.

The heart is not as tolerant of projectiles as are the lungs, but the outer covering of the pulmonary vessels, aorta, and heart is tough and elastic. These tissues may be able to seal themselves off from low-velocity projectile wounds, but medium- and high-velocity projectiles are likely to cause significant wounds to the heart and the great vessels that enter and exit the heart.

The lower boundary between the chest cavity and the abdomen is formed by the diaphragm. If a projectile strikes the lower part of the chest or upper abdomen during exhalation, the projectile is more likely to enter below the relaxed diaphragm and cause an abdominal wound. If the projectile strikes the same area during inhalation, the projectile is more likely to enter above the contracted diaphragm and cause a wound to the chest cavity. Suspect both thoracic and abdominal injury if the entrance wound is between the nipple line and the waist.

Abdomen The abdomen is often secondarily injured when the chest is injured. The abdominal cavity is large and contains structures that are fluid filled (such as the bladder), air filled (such as the stomach), solid (such as the spleen), and bony (such as the pelvic bones). The air-filled and fluid-filled structures are more tolerant of cavitation than are the solid organs. The majority of abdominal wounds are not rapidly fatal, even though a high percentage involving medium-velocity injuries require surgical repair.

Extremities The extremities contain bone, muscle, blood vessels, and nerves. Bone injury from a projectile results in bony fragments becoming secondary missiles, lacerating surrounding vessels, muscles, and nerves. Muscle expands, resulting in capillary tears and swelling. Vessels can be severed, ripped, buckled, and obstructed. As a result, circulation and motor and sensory function to the extremity may be severely or totally compromised.

Blast Injuries

Blast injuries can occur as a result of explosions from, for example, natural gas, gasoline, fireworks, improvised (man-made) explosive devices, and grain elevators (Figure 27-27*). Regardless of the cause, every explosion has three phases: primary, secondary, and tertiary (Figure 27-28*). Each causes specific patterns of injury.

- *Primary phase injuries* are due to the pressure wave of the blast. These injuries primarily affect the gas-containing organs, such as the lungs, stomach, intestines, inner ears, and sinuses. Severe damage and

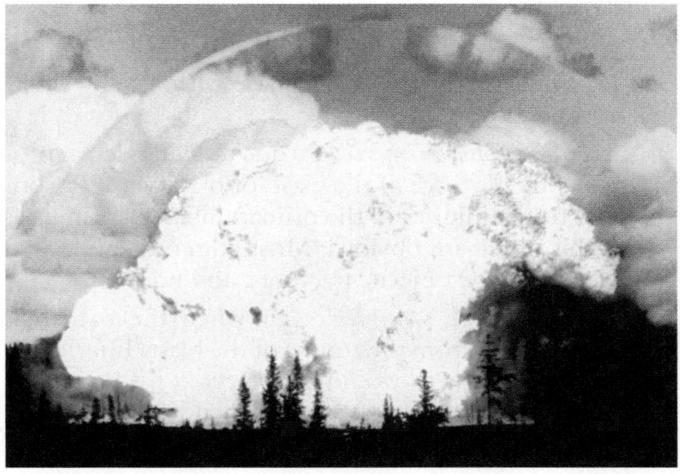

FIGURE 27-27 * An explosion releases tremendous amounts of heat energy, generating a pressure wave, blast wind, and projection of debris.

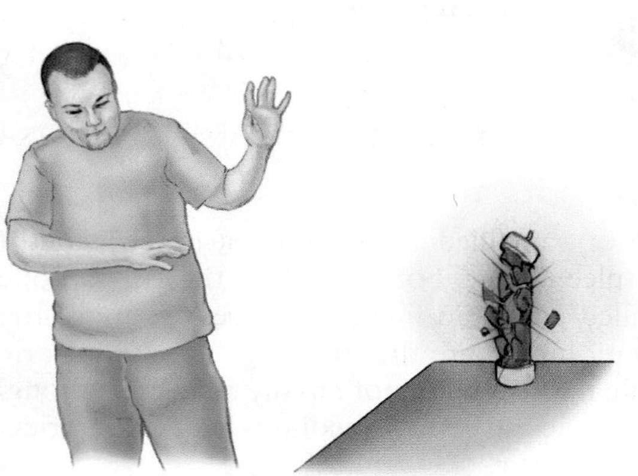

(a) Explosion
Instantaneous combustion of the explosive agent creates superheated gases. The resulting pressure blows the bomb casing apart.

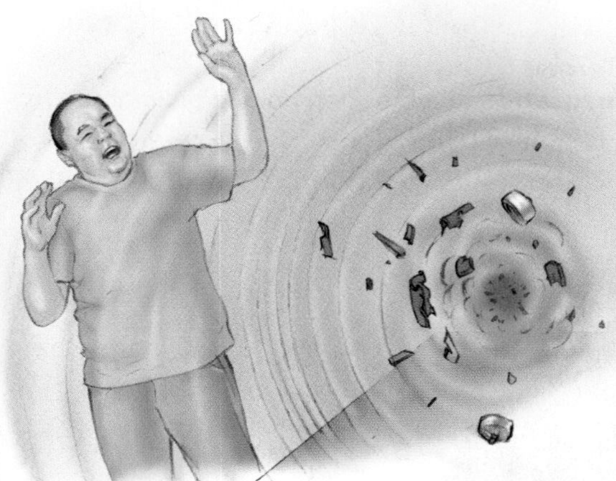

(b) Pressure Wave/Primary Injury
Air molecules slam into one another, creating a pressure wave moving outward from the blast center, causing pressure injuries.

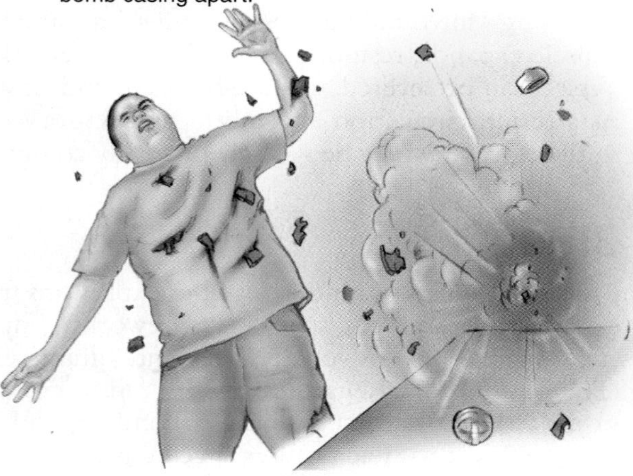

(c) Blast Wave/Secondary Injury
Instantaneous combustion of the explosive agent creates superheated gases. The resulting pressure blows the bomb casing apart. Pieces of the bomb become projectiles that cause injuries by impacting the victim.

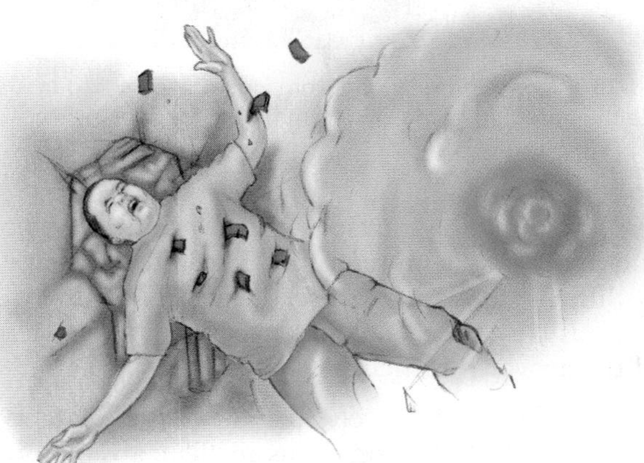

(d) Victim Displacement/Tertiary Injury
The blast wind may propel the victim to the ground or against objects, causing further injuries.

FIGURE 27-28 ✱ Blast injuries can cause injury with the initial blast, when the patient is struck by debris, or by the patient being thrown from the site of the blast.

death may occur from this phase without any external sign of injury.

- ***Secondary phase injuries*** are due to flying debris propelled by the force of the blast, or blast wind. In contrast to the injuries in the primary phase, the injuries of this phase are obvious. Most common are lacerations, impaled objects, fractures, and burns.
- ***Tertiary phase injuries*** occur when the patient is thrown away from the source of the blast. Injuries are much the same as would be expected from ejection from a vehicle. The pattern is dependent on the distance thrown and the point of impact.

Injuries sustained during the secondary and tertiary phases are the most obvious and are more easily accessed and treated. Injuries of the primary phase are most often ignored or unsuspected and, therefore, go untreated. Unfortunately, injuries of the primary phase are just as severe as, if not more severe than, those obtained during the other phases. In general, the index of suspicion on all blast injury patients must remain high, regardless of the initial presentation.

The Multisystem Trauma Patient

Approximately 90 percent of trauma patients have a simple or single injury that involves only one body system, such as a fractured tibia or a soft tissue laceration with no

Objective 27-13
Describe the principles of care for multisystem trauma patients.

Objective 27-14
Explain "golden period" and identify indications for an on-scene time of 10 minutes or less.

Key Points
Severely injured patients have the best chance for survival if intervention takes place as quickly as possible from the time of injury.

major bleeding. A multisystem trauma patient has multiple injuries or involvement of more than one body system. The body systems may include the central nervous, pulmonary, cardiovascular, gastrointestinal, urinary, reproductive, musculoskeletal, and integumentary systems. Multiple organ injuries are considered to be multisystem trauma, even though they may be part of the same body system, such as the small intestine or the liver. For example, a patient with a chest injury involving the lung (the pulmonary system and the lung as the organ) may also have a head injury (the central nervous system and the brain as the organ), or a patient with an abdominal injury (the gastrointestinal system and the small intestine as the organ) may also have a pelvic fracture (the musculoskeletal system).

Multisystem trauma carries a high incidence of morbidity and mortality. It requires the EMT to respond quickly, provide a rapid assessment to identify immediately life-threatening injuries, manage any life threats, rapidly prepare the patient for transport, and expeditiously transport the patient to an appropriate facility that can provide trauma care (Figure 27-29∗). It is important to follow your local, regional, or state destination protocols when making a transport decision for a trauma patient.

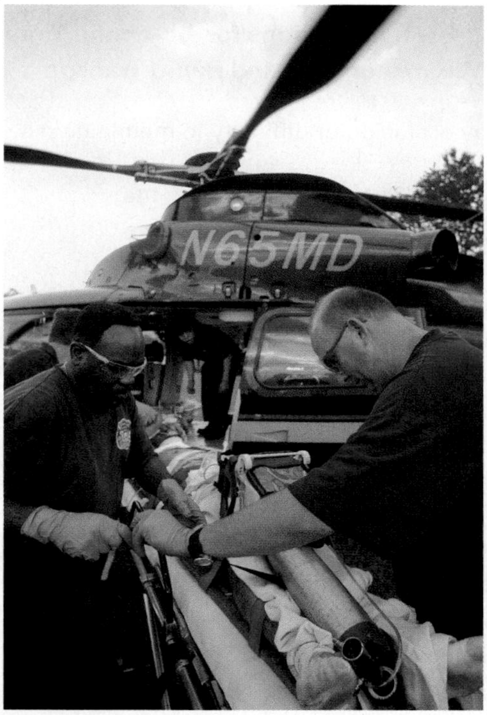

FIGURE 27-29 ∗ The multisystem trauma or other severely injured patient must be transported expeditiously to a trauma center. (© Mark C. Ide)

The Golden Period

The "golden period" has been established as a parameter for emergency care because severely injured patients have the best chance for survival if intervention takes place as quickly as possible from the time of injury. This was once referred to as the "golden hour." However, some injured patients require definitive care in less than an hour to survive; whereas, some patients can survive if care is provided beyond one hour. As an example, a patient with a lacerated spleen will need care in less than an hour to have the best chance of survival because of the extreme blood loss associated with a splenic injury. A patient who is bleeding very slowly from a small torn vessel can still go into shock from the blood loss over time and die; however, he may be able to survive for several hours without definitive care. Thus, the golden period is variable depending on the patient injury. Regardless, the EMT must assess, treat, and transport the injured patient as quickly as possible.

Some EMS systems refer to the "platinum 10 minutes." This means that in cases of severe trauma 10 minutes is the maximum time the EMS team should devote to on-scene activities—with patient assessment, emergency care for life threats, and preparation for transport all being accomplished within 10 minutes of arriving on the scene. The patient should be loaded into the ambulance and transport begun within 10 minutes after arriving on the scene of a severely injured or multisystem trauma patient. However, you must not go to the scene, load the patient, and transport without performing an assessment and providing emergency care. You must assess for life-threatening injuries, provide emergency care for the life threats, and prepare the patient for transport within those 10 minutes.

If a patient is not severely injured (or is without any life-threatening medical problems), more time can and should be devoted to completing normal on-scene assessment and emergency care before transport is undertaken.

The key is determining whether the patient is or is not (possibly) severely injured. It is to the patient's potential benefit to err on the side of overestimating, rather than underestimating, the extent or severity of injuries. The harm that can be done by delaying transport when it

Key Points
The harm that can be done by delaying transport, when needed, outweighs the good that can be done by completing on-scene assessment and care.

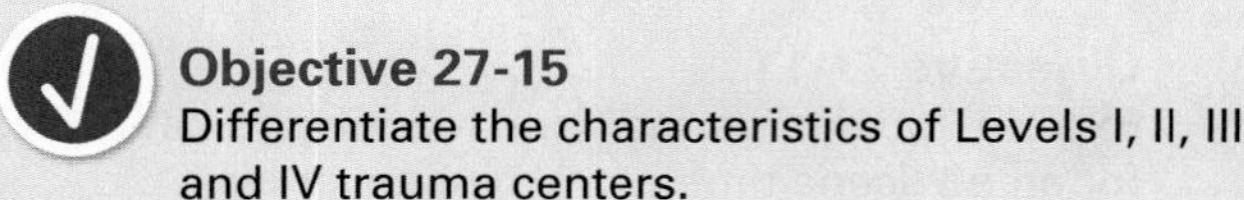

Objective 27-15
Differentiate the characteristics of Levels I, II, III, and IV trauma centers.

TABLE 27-1 Indications for On-Scene Time of 10 Minutes or Less and Rapid Transport

- Airway occlusion or difficulty in maintaining a patent airway
- Respiratory rate < 10 or > 29/minute
- Inadequate tidal volume
- Hypoxia ($SpO_2 < 95\%$)
- Respiratory distress, failure, or arrest
- Suspected skull fracture
- Flail chest
- Suspected pneumothorax, hemothorax, or tension pneumothorax
- Pelvic fracture
- Two or more proximal long-bone fractures
- Crushed or mangled extremity
- Uncontrolled external hemorrhage
- Suspected internal hemorrhage
- Signs and symptoms of shock
- Significant external blood loss with controlled hemorrhage
- Glasgow Coma Scale score 14 or less
- Altered mental status
- Seizure activity
- Sensory or motor deficit
- Any penetrating trauma to the head, neck, anterior or posterior chest or abdomen, and above the elbow or knee
- Amputation of an extremity proximal to the finger
- Trauma in a patient with significant medical history (myocardial infarction, chronic obstructive pulmonary disease, congestive heart failure), $>$ 55 years of age, hypothermia, burns, or pregnancy
- Multisystem trauma
- Open or depressed skull fracture
- Suspected brain injury
- Paralysis

is needed outweighs the good that can be done by completing on-scene assessment and care at a more deliberate pace. That is why EMTs are taught to maintain a "high index of suspicion"—a presumption that a patient has severe injuries if there is any indication at all that this is possible, which is often based on findings at the scene as to the mechanism of injury and the amount of force that may have been delivered.

As you have learned in this chapter, a patient involved in trauma may have hidden, internal injuries. These may be far more serious than any of the external injuries that you can observe. In some cases, there can be internal injuries with no external injuries that you can detect.

In instances of trauma, you must evaluate and rely on the patient's assessment findings and indicators of critical injuries or instability as well as the mechanism of injury in your priority decision. (See Table 27-1.)

The Trauma System

The trauma system was designed to provide immediate surgical intervention for patients with internal trauma. Although this accounts for a small percentage of patients, approximately 10 percent, this care dramatically reduces the morbidity and mortality of these patients.

The trauma system requires significant resources and is expensive to maintain and operate. Hospitals with certain recognized capabilities are considered to be part of the trauma system and are recognized as trauma centers (Figure 27-30*). A common designation of trauma centers according to the American College of Surgeons Committee on Trauma is:

- **Level I—Regional Trauma Center.** Can manage all types of trauma 24 hours a day, 7 days a week.
- **Level II—Area Trauma Center.** Can manage most trauma with surgical capabilities 24 hours a day, 7 days a week. They are capable of stabilizing more specialized trauma patients and then transferring them to a level I center.
- **Level III—Community Trauma Center.** Has some surgical capability and specially trained emergency department personnel to manage trauma. This type of center focuses on stabilizing the seriously injured trauma patient and then transferring to a higher-level center.
- **Level IV—Trauma Facility.** Is typically a small community hospital in a remote area capable of stabilizing seriously injured trauma patients and then transferring them to a higher-level trauma center.

In addition to the aforementioned trauma centers, some facilities carry a specialty center designation. These centers have personnel capable of managing special types

Objective 27-16
Identify patients who meet trauma triage criteria for transportation to a trauma center.

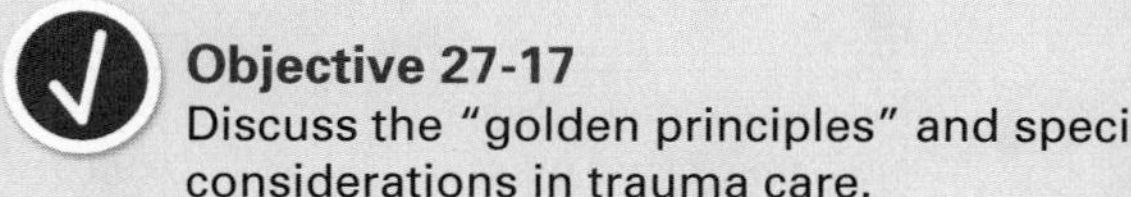

Objective 27-17
Discuss the "golden principles" and special considerations in trauma care.

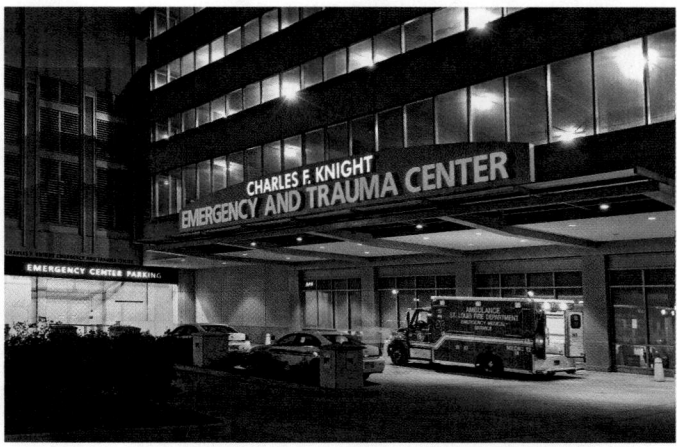

FIGURE 27-30 ✱ A St. Louis Fire Department ambulance pulls up at the Charles F. Knight Emergency and Trauma Center. (© Ray Kemp/911 Imaging)

of trauma, such as spinal cord injuries or burns. Specialty centers may include neurocenters, burn centers, spinal cord injury centers, pediatric trauma centers, and limb reimplantation centers.

EMS interfaces with and is an integral component of the trauma system. It is crucial that EMS personnel triage patients accurately for transport to an appropriate trauma center. See Figure 27-31✱ for field triage criteria regarding transport of trauma patients to an appropriate trauma facility, as developed by the Centers for Disease Control.

Golden Principles of Prehospital Trauma Care

The golden principles of prehospital trauma care apply to all patients who have experienced some type of injury but especially those with multisystem trauma or critical injuries. The principles are:

- Ensure at all times the safety of the EMS personnel, patients, and bystanders.
- Quickly determine the need for additional resources at the scene.
- Determine the mechanism of injury and kinematics involved in producing real or potential injuries.
- Provide a primary assessment to identify and manage immediate life threats.
- Establish and maintain spinal stabilization for patients suspected of having a vertebral or spinal cord injury.
- Establish and maintain a patent airway.
- Establish and maintain adequate oxygenation in the patient with an adequate rate and adequate tidal volume by keeping the SpO_2 reading greater than 95%.
- Provide positive pressure ventilation with a high concentration of oxygen connected to the ventilation device in the patient with an inadequate respiratory rate or inadequate tidal volume.
- Control external hemorrhage with direct pressure followed by a tourniquet if direct pressure is ineffective.
- Treat for shock by maintaining a normal body temperature and splinting fractures when appropriate.
- Consider application of the pneumatic antishock garment (PASG) for decompensated shock (systolic blood pressure less than 90 mmHg) associated with suspected pelvic fracture, intra-abdominal bleeding, or retroperitoneal bleeding or in patients with profound hypotension with a systolic blood pressure less than 60 mmHg.
- Maintain manual spinal stabilization until the patient is completely immobilized on a backboard.
- Transport critically injured or multisystem trauma patients within 10 minutes to the appropriate trauma facility according to the trauma triage criteria. Always follow your local, regional, or state destination protocols.
- Obtain a history from the patient, relatives, or bystanders.
- Perform a secondary assessment to identify all other life-threatening and non-life-threatening injuries and manage each according to priority.

Special Considerations in Trauma Care

The following are special considerations in the trauma patient. Many of these considerations also apply to the medical patient:

- **Your personal safety is of utmost importance when arriving on scene and throughout the entire time you are with the patient.** You must always remain alert for potential scene hazards. These might

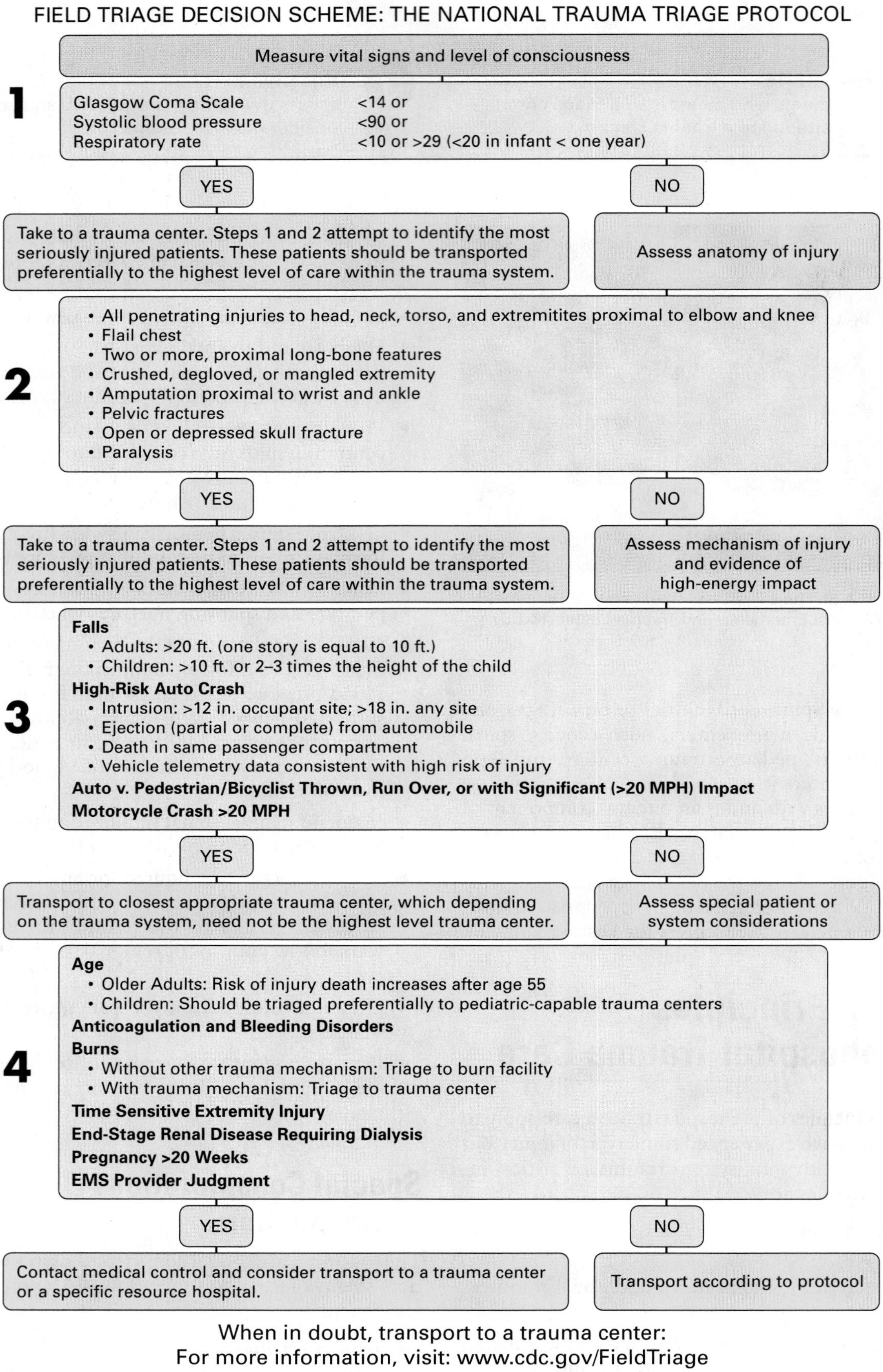

FIELD TRIAGE DECISION SCHEME: THE NATIONAL TRAUMA TRIAGE PROTOCOL

Measure vital signs and level of consciousness

1

Glasgow Coma Scale	<14 or
Systolic blood pressure	<90 or
Respiratory rate	<10 or >29 (<20 in infant < one year)

YES — Take to a trauma center. Steps 1 and 2 attempt to identify the most seriously injured patients. These patients should be transported preferentially to the highest level of care within the trauma system.

NO — Assess anatomy of injury

2

- All penetrating injuries to head, neck, torso, and extremitites proximal to elbow and knee
- Flail chest
- Two or more, proximal long-bone features
- Crushed, degloved, or mangled extremity
- Amputation proximal to wrist and ankle
- Pelvic fractures
- Open or depressed skull fracture
- Paralysis

YES — Take to a trauma center. Steps 1 and 2 attempt to identify the most seriously injured patients. These patients should be transported preferentially to the highest level of care within the trauma system.

NO — Assess mechanism of injury and evidence of high-energy impact

3

Falls

- Adults: >20 ft. (one story is equal to 10 ft.)
- Children: >10 ft. or 2–3 times the height of the child

High-Risk Auto Crash

- Intrusion: >12 in. occupant site; >18 in. any site
- Ejection (partial or complete) from automobile
- Death in same passenger compartment
- Vehicle telemetry data consistent with high risk of injury

Auto v. Pedestrian/Bicyclist Thrown, Run Over, or with Significant (>20 MPH) Impact

Motorcycle Crash >20 MPH

YES — Transport to closest appropriate trauma center, which depending on the trauma system, need not be the highest level trauma center.

NO — Assess special patient or system considerations

4

Age

- Older Adults: Risk of injury death increases after age 55
- Children: Should be triaged preferentially to pediatric-capable trauma centers

Anticoagulation and Bleeding Disorders

Burns

- Without other trauma mechanism: Triage to burn facility
- With trauma mechanism: Triage to trauma center

Time Sensitive Extremity Injury

End-Stage Renal Disease Requiring Dialysis

Pregnancy >20 Weeks

EMS Provider Judgment

YES — Contact medical control and consider transport to a trauma center or a specific resource hospital.

NO — Transport according to protocol

When in doubt, transport to a trauma center:
For more information, visit: www.cdc.gov/FieldTriage

FIGURE 27-31 ✻ Field Triage Decision Scheme: The National Trauma Triage Protocol.

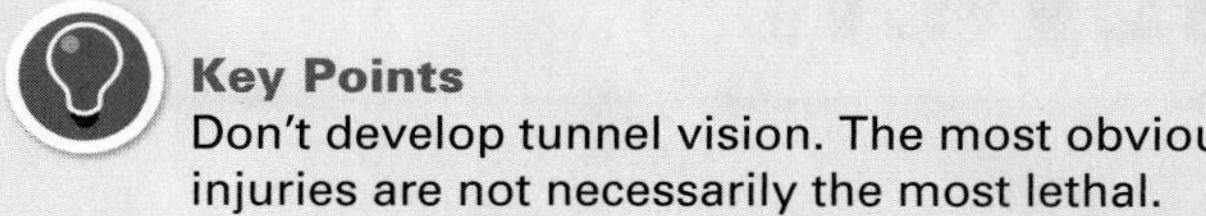

Key Points
Don't develop tunnel vision. The most obvious injuries are not necessarily the most lethal.

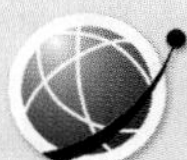

Media Resources
Go to www.bradybooks.com for mykit. Highlights:
- *Web Resource:* Gun Violence
- *Animation:* Entrance and Exit Wounds

involve traffic on the roadway, hazardous materials, hostile environment, unsecured crime scene, and sudden changes of patient behavior. An injured EMT is no longer able to provide care and requires additional resources at the scene.

- **Airway management and adequate ventilation and oxygenation are key elements in managing the trauma patient.** Shock from blood loss results in an inadequate delivery of oxygen to the cells. This causes the cells to convert from aerobic to anaerobic metabolism resulting in little energy production, acid accumulation, and eventual cellular dysfunction and death. Thus, ensuring the patient has an adequate airway, ventilation, and oxygenation contributes to managing and reversing the shock state.
- **Stop significant bleeding.** If a patient is losing a significant amount of blood, the delivery of oxygen and glucose to the cells is impaired. Hemoglobin in the red blood cell is the primary mechanism for oxygen transport. With any type of bleeding, red blood cells and hemoglobin are being removed from the vessels and decreasing the oxygen-carrying capability of the blood. The result is shock. To prevent or reverse shock, you must stop the bleeding as quickly as possible by direct pressure. If this is not effective, a tourniquet is then applied.
- **Assessment of the trauma patient is conducted in a sequence that promotes a systematic approach to the patient.** There are times when you must deviate from the sequence to provide emergency care for a life threat. As an example, airway always is assessed before circulation in the sequence. However, if you identify a major bleed (arterial or venous) during the general impression, you must first control the bleeding prior to moving on in the assessment. Adhering rigidly to a sequence when presented with obvious life threats may contribute to the deterioration of the patient.
- **Rapid transport of the severely injured patient is essential to his survival.** The definitive care for many seriously injured trauma patients is surgery. On-scene time should be limited to 10 minutes if at all possible. Rapid extrication should be used to remove the patient from a vehicle. Use the triage transport criteria to determine the need for rapid transport and the most appropriate medical facility. Consider intercepting with an advanced life support unit or transport by air medical if ground transport is excessive. Notify the receiving facility of the patient's condition and estimated time of arrival.
- **A backboard can serve to secure suspected fractures in an unstable patient who requires rapid transport.** En route, if time or the patient's condition permits, further stabilization of fractures can be accomplished through splinting. Taking the time at the scene to splint suspected fractures will delay transport and may contribute to the deterioration of the patient.
- **Do not develop tunnel vision and become focused on dramatic injuries or dramatic patients.** An open humerus fracture with a bone protruding from the skin at a 90-degree angle will attract your attention. However, if the patient is alert and screaming in pain, you must assume that he has an adequate amount of energy, good perfusion, and an adequate amount of oxygen and glucose delivered to the cells. On the other hand, the patient sitting next to him who barely nods his head in response to your question of "Are you okay?" likely is lacking energy from inadequate perfusion. It may be prudent to assess the quiet patient first. The most obvious injuries are not necessarily the most lethal. Often, the lethal injuries are occult and can be easily missed without a systemic and thorough assessment.

CHAPTER REVIEW

SUMMARY

Mechanism of injury generally refers to how a person was injured. Knowing the mechanism of injury may increase your suspicion that the person might have suffered certain injuries. However, your patient assessment is the most valuable method to determine what injuries the patient has sustained. Mass and velocity determine the amount of kinetic energy applied to the body in various types of mechanism of injury. The change in the kinetic energy is responsible for producing injury.

A force applied to the body will usually result in blunt or penetrating trauma. Blunt trauma is from a force applied to the body in which there is no penetration of the body by an object (for example, a blow to the chest with a baseball bat). Penetrating trauma will produce a break in the continuity of the skin by the object (for example, a knife or a bullet). Vehicle collisions frequently cause blunt trauma and create some typical injury patterns based on the type of impact: frontal, rear-end, lateral, rotational, or rollover. Even though vehicle safety restraints and air bags have saved a large number of lives, they also can produce injuries, such as bruising, fractures, and face and eye trauma. Motorcycle, all-terrain vehicle, and other recreational vehicle crashes produce various typical injury patterns in patients.

The severity of a penetrating trauma injury commonly depends on the mass and the velocity of the object as it strikes the body. The greater the mass and the higher the velocity, the greater the kinetic energy that is produced and the more severe the resulting injury. Velocity has a greater effect than mass. High-velocity weapons are particularly prone to producing massive bodily injury. Blast injuries, resulting from an explosion, are associated with three phases of injury: primary phase injuries (pressure injuries), secondary phase injuries (debris impacts), and tertiary phase injuries (from the person being thrown by the force of the blast).

Trauma systems have been developed to allow for rapid intervention in the injured patient. There are different designations of trauma facilities with various levels of care. Trauma triage criteria have been developed to assist the EMT in recognizing the need for rapid transport of an injured patient and determining the most appropriate facility to transport to.

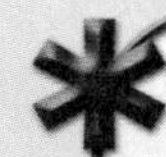

CASE STUDY FOLLOW-UP

SCENE SIZE-UP

Your initial call was for a minor collision with one patient complaining of knee pain. The police officer greeted you and explained that he was taking a report from the driver of a car that was struck from behind when he began to complain of the pain. He estimates the collision occurred at around 30 mph. He tells you that the other driver has been driven to the hospital by a friend.

The scene size-up reveals no obvious hazards; both vehicles have been moved off the road into a parking lot. You see only slight denting to the rear of your patient's vehicle. There is only one patient, and since his car wasn't damaged enough to interfere with the operation of the doors, gaining access to the patient is easy and will not require a rescue unit. You put on your disposable gloves and approach the vehicle.

PRIMARY ASSESSMENT

You introduce yourself to the patient and ask him his name, and he says, "Call me Mike." You explain that, as a safety measure, your partner will get into the back seat and reach from behind to hold Mike's head still. There are no dents or damage to the steering wheel and no cracks in the windshield.

Your general impression is of a 40-year-old male in no obvious severe distress. Mike's chief complaint is pain in the knees, and he tells you privately that he did not have his seat belt on and went down and under the dashboard during the impact. He is alert and oriented. The airway, breathing, and circulation status are all fine. Because the mechanism of injury is not significant—and your general impression is that Mike is not badly injured—you determine that he is a low priority for immediate transport and that you will conduct the secondary assessment at the scene.

You maintain a high index of suspicion, however, and will be ready to change your priority decision if you find out that the mechanism of injury was more severe than seems true at this point, if any potential life threats are identified, or if there is any deterioration in Mike's condition.

SECONDARY ASSESSMENT

You proceed with a rapid secondary assessment and find no signs of injury. The knees, which Mike says continue to hurt, show no evidence of bruising, swelling, or deformity. A quick check of all four extremities reveals no loss of pulses or sensory or motor function. You obtain a set of baseline vitals, which are all within normal ranges. Rapid extrication technique is not warranted in this case, so you work with your partner and a police Emergency Medical Responder to apply a cervical spine immobilization collar and a KED immobilization vest, then transfer and immobilize Mike to a long spine board.

Once he is secured, you reassess Mike's pulses and motor and sensory function in all four extremities. In the ambulance, you proceed to ask Mike history questions and find out he now also has an ache in his lumbar spine, is allergic to sulfa drugs, takes medication for allergies to environmental substances, has a history of asthma that has not been bothering him recently, and last ate and drank at breakfast 2 hours ago. Mike states he was just waiting for the oncoming traffic to clear so he could make a left turn when suddenly the other car struck him from behind.

REASSESSMENT

Because Mike is stable, you conduct a reassessment every 15 minutes on the way to the hospital. You repeat the primary assessment and vital signs. You check to be sure that he is securely immobilized with no loss of function to the extremities. To help him feel a little more comfortable, you apply a cold pack to his knees. You arrive at the hospital, transfer Mike to the care of the emergency department staff, and prepare your ambulance for the next call.

IN REVIEW

1. Based on the formulas for kinetic energy and force, explain how the following are likely to affect the severity of an injury: (a) mass and velocity; (b) acceleration and deceleration.
2. Name and describe, in sequence, the three impacts that take place in a vehicular collision.
3. Name and describe four types of motorcycle collision.
4. Describe the path of energy and possible patterns of injury for each of the following kinds of falls: (a) feet first; (b) landing on outstretched hands; (c) head first.
5. Define cavitation and tell which of the following kinds of weapons would be likely to produce it: knife, handgun, M-16 rifle.
6. Explain the cause of each of the following phases of blast injury: primary, secondary, and tertiary.
7. Name mechanisms of injury that should cause the EMT to have a high index of suspicion of significant injury.
8. List the various types of trauma centers.
9. List anatomical criteria for rapid transport of a trauma patient.
10. List mechanism of injury criteria for rapid transport of a trauma patient.
11. List physiological criteria for rapid transport of a trauma patient.

CRITICAL THINKING

You arrive on the scene and find a 62-year-old male patient who, while driving on the freeway, struck a cement barrier head-on. The police estimate he was traveling at 65 mph upon impact. The windshield has an impact mark on the driver's side, the air bag deployed, and the headrest is completely down. The patient was wearing his lap and shoulder restraints. The patient is unresponsive.

1. Based on the mechanism of injury, what injuries do you suspect the patient possibly has suffered?
2. What type of impact was involved in the collision?
3. What two different pathway patterns of injury may be involved in this collision?

EXPLORE PEARSON **mybradykit**™

Please go to **www.bradybooks.com** to access mykit for this text. You will find quizzes, critical thinking scenarios, weblinks, animations, and videos related to this chapter—and much more. Look for online information on gun violence and trauma scenarios. You will also find animations on types of injuries and mechanisms of injuries in motor vehicle collisions.

Register your access code from the front of your book by going to **www.bradybooks.com** and selecting the mykit links.

CHAPTER 28 Bleeding and Soft Tissue Trauma

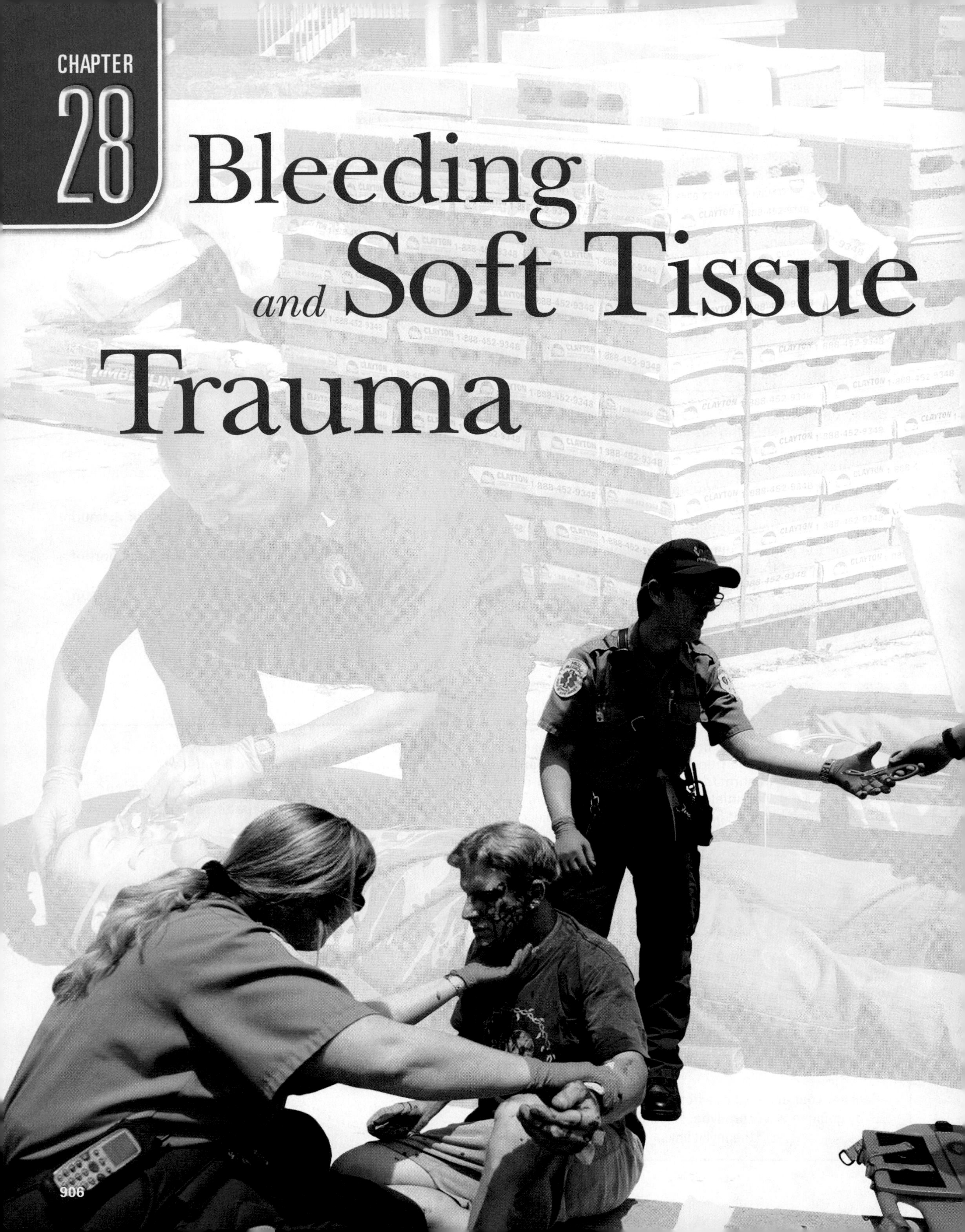

Navigation Guide

The following items provide an overview to the purpose and content of this chapter. The Standard and Competency are from the new National EMS Education Standards.

STANDARD **Trauma** (Content Areas: Bleeding; Soft Tissue Trauma)

COMPETENCY Applies fundamental knowledge to provide basic emergency care and transportation based on assessment findings for an acutely injured patient.

OBJECTIVES: After reading this chapter, you should be able to:

28-1. Define key terms introduced in this chapter.

28-2. Explain the importance of recognizing and providing emergency medical care to patients with soft tissue injuries to control bleeding, prevent or treat shock, and to prevent contamination of wounds.

28-3. Recognize the severity and type of external bleeding.

28-4. Describe methods of controlling external bleeding.

28-5. Describe the assessment-based approach to external bleeding, including emergency medical care.

28-6. Explain why bleeding from the nose, ears, or mouth is of special concern and describe the appropriate care for bleeding from the nose, ears, or mouth.

28-7. Recognize indications of the severity of internal bleeding and describe the assessment-based approach to internal bleeding, including medical care to maintain perfusion and treat for shock.

28-8. Explain factors that may increase bleeding.

28-9. Define hemorrhagic shock and describe the assessment-based approach to hemorrhagic shock, including emergency medical care.

28-10. List types of closed soft tissue injuries and describe the assessment-based approach to closed soft tissue injuries, including emergency medical care.

28-11. List types of open soft tissue injuries and describe the assessment-based approach to open soft tissue injuries, including emergency medical care.

28-12. Explain special considerations and appropriate care for chest injuries, abdominal injuries, impaled objects, amputations, and large neck injuries.

28-13. Describe various types of dressings and bandages, including the purpose and methods of applying pressure dressings, and discuss general principles of dressing and bandaging.

KEY TERMS: Page references indicate first major use in this chapter. For complete definitions, see the Glossary at the back of the book.

abrasion p. 926
air embolism p. 933
amputation p. 927
avulsion p. 927
bandage p. 934
closed injury p. 924
contusion p. 924
crush injury p. 924
dressing p. 934
ecchymosis p. 924
epistaxis p. 914
evisceration p. 932
hematoma p. 924
impaled object p. 932
laceration p. 927
occlusive dressing p. 931
open injury p. 925
penetration/puncture p. 928
sterile p. 934

MEDIA RESOURCES: Please go to www.bradybooks.com to access mykit for this text. You will find quizzes, critical thinking scenarios, weblinks, animations, and videos related to this chapter—and much more. Look for online information on tourniquets and compartment syndrome. You will also find video clips on decubitus ulcers and shock.

continued

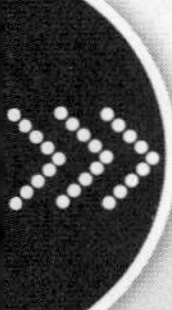

CASE STUDY

The Dispatch

EMS Unit 101—respond to Riverside High School at 1434 River Street for a reported stabbing—time out 1645 hours.

You ask the dispatcher if the police have been alerted. He doesn't know but will check. You and your partner decide that if the police are not on the scene, you will stage at the minimart down the street until the scene is secure.

The dispatcher comes back and advises you that the police are at the scene and have one person in custody. He says your patient is a male with a stab wound to the left upper abdomen with profuse bleeding.

Upon Arrival

You and your partner have put on your gloves and eye protection. As you pull into the high school parking lot, you notice a crowd of teenagers and adults gathered around a young male lying on the ground. You notify dispatch that you are "on arrival." Time is 1651.

A police officer approaches your unit. Your partner asks if the scene is secure. The officer states it is, and tells you they have one teenager in custody. You note that there is only one patient.

As you exit the vehicle and approach the patient, you see the young male, who appears to be a teenager, lying supine on the ground with a large penetrating wound to the left upper quadrant of the abdomen. The wound is bleeding profusely. There is no impaled object. No weapon is visible near the patient.

How Would You Proceed with This Patient?

During this chapter, you will learn about bleeding and shock. Later, we will return to the case study and put in context some of the information you learned.

Introduction

Bleeding can be a significant, life-threatening emergency. As an EMT you must be able to recognize obvious or external bleeding problems, as well as not-so-obvious internal bleeding problems. If either type of bleeding is left untreated, it has the potential to lead to rapid patient deterioration, shock, and death.

Control of severe external bleeding is performed during the primary assessment. Only airway and breathing have a higher priority; however, if major bleeding is recognized during the general impression it should be immediately managed. Internal bleeding and shock are treated immediately following the primary assessment. An important element of the emergency care of bleeding associated with signs and symptoms of shock is to transport the patient to a medical facility as rapidly as possible.

Injuries to the soft tissues—the skin, muscles, and nerves—are often dramatic but rarely life threatening. However, they are serious if they involve large vessels or organs or if they lead to airway or breathing compromise, uncontrolled bleeding, or shock.

In general, emergency medical care emphasizes controlling bleeding, preventing further injury, and reducing the risk of infection. Unless an injury is life threatening, care is usually accomplished after the primary assessment and prior to lifting and moving. Failure to recognize and provide care for soft tissue injuries may lead to severe, uncontrolled bleeding, possible additional injury including hemorrhagic shock, or further contamination of the wound and increased risk of infection.

External Bleeding

Standard Precautions must be taken routinely to avoid exposure of skin and mucous membranes to blood and other body fluids. Wear personal protective equipment, including gloves and eyewear, and wash your hands before and after each run. Standard Precautions are your best defense against transmission of infectious disease. (For more details, see Chapter 2, "Workforce Safety and Wellness of the EMT.") This is true for all EMS calls, but especially in the presence of trauma with external bleeding (Figure 28-1*).

Severity

The severity of blood loss is dependent on several variables:

- Amount of blood loss
- Rate of blood loss

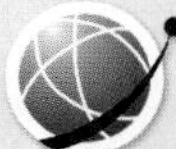

Media Resources
Go to www.bradybooks.com for mykit. Highlights:

- *Web Resource:* External and Internal Bleeding
- *Web Resource:* Contusions and Ecchymoses
- *Web Resource:* Compartment syndrome

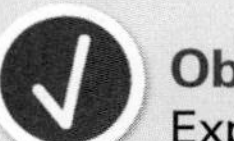

Objective 28-2
Explain the importance of recognizing and providing emergency medical care to patients with soft tissue injuries to control bleeding, prevent or treat shock, and to prevent contamination of wounds.

Objective 28-3
Recognize the severity and type of external bleeding.

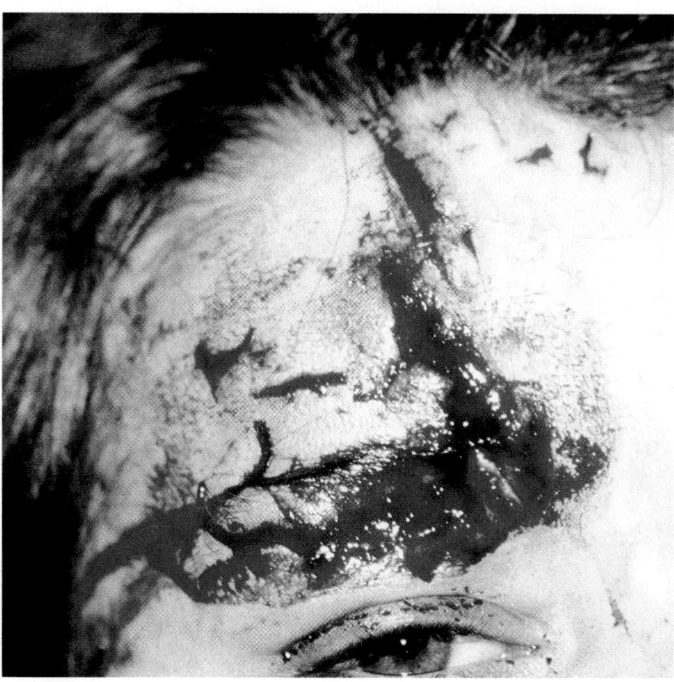

FIGURE 28-1 ✱ External bleeding from a soft tissue injury to the head.

- Other injuries or existing conditions
- Patient's existing medical problems
- Patient's age

The severity of bleeding relative to the amount of blood loss is dependent on the patient. A 500-mL blood loss may not be as severe in a large patient as it would be in a child or smaller adult. An adult patient has 70 mL/kg of blood volume. An average-sized adult is considered to be 154 lb, which is 70 kg. Thus, an average-sized adult has 4,900 mL or 4.9 liters of blood volume (70 mL × 70 kg = 4,900 mL). A loss of 15 percent of blood volume or more is considered significant and can lead to shock. In the 154-lb patient, a loss of 735 mL of blood can lead to a shock state. Infants and young children typically have 80 mL/kg of blood volume. A 22-lb infant (10 kg) would have a total blood volume of 800 mL (10 kg × 80 mL = 800 mL). A 15 percent blood loss would be 120 mL (800 mL × 15% = 120 mL). A 200-mL blood loss in an average-sized adult would represent only a 4 percent blood loss, whereas a 200-mL blood loss in a 10-kg infant would represent a 25 percent blood loss.

ASSESSMENT Tips

The best way to estimate the amount of blood loss is not to look on the ground or at the clothing of the patient but rather to perform an assessment and determine the severity of the signs and symptoms. ■

To conclude that a loss of 500 mL of blood is not significant in an adult would be wrong, since the severity of that volume of blood loss is relative to the patient's weight. The estimate of blood loss must be made based on the patient's signs and symptoms (Table 28-1) and not on what appears to be on the floor, soaked into the patient's clothing, in the toilet, or elsewhere on the scene.

The natural response of the blood vessels to bleeding is vessel constriction and clotting. However, a serious injury can prevent that defense mechanism from working, resulting in uncontrolled bleeding. A vessel that has been cut across, or perpendicular to the vessel, will have a tendency to retract and clot off. A cut along the length of the vessel will cause the vessel to open wider when it contracts. This will cause the vessel to bleed more severely. Remember: *Uncontrolled bleeding or significant blood loss can lead to hemorrhagic shock and quite possibly to death.*

Understanding BODY PROCESSES

The middle layer of a blood vessel is made up of smooth muscle (tunica media) that gives it the ability to constrict when injured. A transverse (across) cut of a vessel will cause the vessel to retract, thickening the smooth muscle layer at the cut end of the vessel and reducing the diameter of the vessel, which reduces blood flow and allows clotting to occur more easily. ■

Types of Bleeding

There are three types of bleeding: arterial, venous, and capillary. Each type can be life threatening. Each has its own characteristics (Figure 28-2✱):

- **Arterial bleeding.** Bright red, spurting blood from a wound usually indicates a severed or damaged artery. The blood is bright red because it is rich in oxygen. Spurting generally coincides with the pulse or contraction of the heart. Arterial bleeding can be

TABLE 28-1 Classes of Hemorrhage

	Class I	Class II	Class III	Class IV
Amount of blood loss	< 15%	15–30%	30–40%	> 40%
Heart rate	↑	↑↑	↑↑↑	↑↑↑↑ or ↓
Vasoconstriction	↑	↑↑	↑↑↑	↑↑↑↑ or ↓↓
Ventilatory rate	Normal	↑	↑↑	↑↑↑
Systolic blood pressure	Normal	Normal	↓	↓↓↓
Pulse pressure	Normal	Narrow	Narrow	Very narrow or wide
Skin	Normal or slightly pale and cool	Pale, cool, and clammy	Severely pale and cool	Severely pale, cold, and mottled

Note: In this table, up arrows indicate an increase, down arrows indicate a decrease, and multiple arrows indicate a greater degree of increase or decrease. For example, two arrows indicate a greater change than one arrow, and so on.

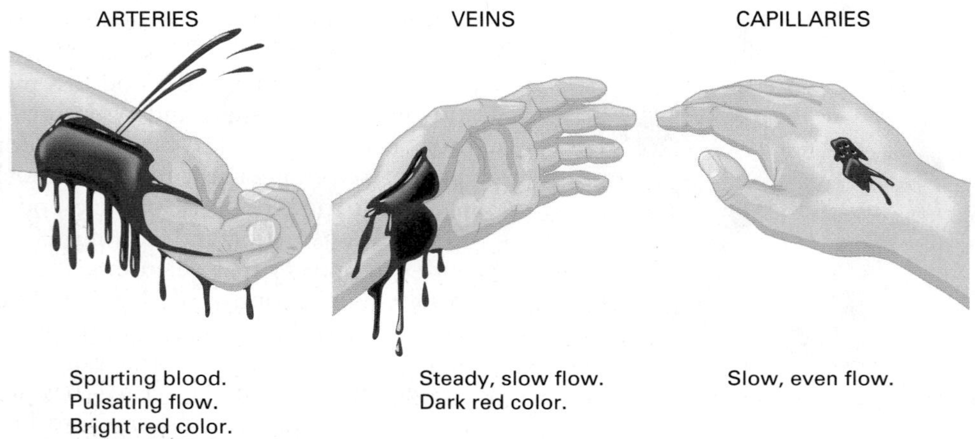

FIGURE 28-2 ✱ Types of bleeding.

more difficult to control than any other type of bleeding because of the higher pressure in the arteries, although the muscular walls may assist in hemostasis. As the patient's blood pressure decreases, the spurting may also decrease and present as a steady flow of blood instead.

- **Venous bleeding.** Dark red blood that flows steadily from a wound usually indicates a severed or damaged vein. When blood is dark red, it is depleted of oxygen. A steady flow usually indicates venous bleeding, because veins are under less pressure than arteries. Venous bleeding may be profuse, but it is usually easier to control than arterial bleeding because of its lower pressure.
- **Capillary bleeding.** Slowly oozing blood that is a dark or intermediate color of red usually indicates damaged capillaries (Figure 28-3✱). In most cases, capillary bleeding is easily controlled. This type of bleeding often clots spontaneously. However, if a large body surface is involved, bleeding may be profuse and the threat of infection great.

Methods of Controlling External Bleeding

Direct Pressure

The first method for controlling bleeding is direct pressure (EMT Skills 28-1A to 28-1C). This is usually accomplished by placing a sterile gauze pad or dressing over the injury site and applying fingertip pressure directly to the point of bleeding. Large, gaping wounds may require packing with sterile gauze and the application of direct hand pressure, if fingertip pressure fails (EMT Skills 28-1D). If, during the primary assessment, you find a major bleed, apply pressure to the site with your gloved hand until dressings can be applied.

If severe bleeding persists while direct pressure is being applied over dressings, remove the dressings and apply direct pressure to the point of bleeding, typically directly to the vessel that is bleeding. If diffuse bleeding is discovered, apply additional pressure. A pressure dressing can be applied to the wound to control hemorrhage. (See the section on pressure dressings later in the chapter.)

Objective 28-4
Describe methods of controlling external bleeding.

Key Points
The first method for controlling bleeding is direct pressure. If bleeding is not controlled with direct pressure, the next step is to apply a tourniquet.

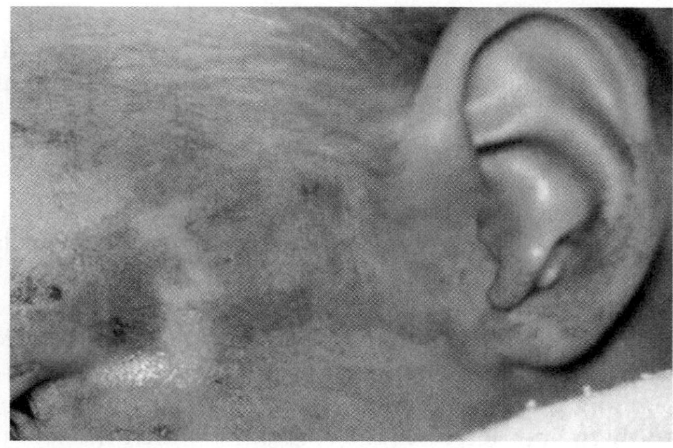

FIGURE 28-3 ∗ Capillary bleeding. (© David Effron, MD, FACEP)

If major bleeding is occurring around an impaled object, apply direct pressure on either side of the object to control the bleeding. Never apply pressure to the object and never remove the object.

Tourniquets

If bleeding is not controlled with direct pressure, the next step is to apply a tourniquet. Many commercial tourniquets are now available (Figures 28-4a and 28-4b∗).

To apply a tourniquet, follow these directions (EMT Skills 28-2A to 28-2D):

1. Use a bandage or commercial device that is 4 inches wide. If using a bandage rather than a commercial device, it should be four to six layers thick.
2. Wrap the tourniquet around the extremity at a point just proximal to the bleeding but as distal on the extremity and as close to the injury as possible. Do not cover the wound with the tourniquet.
3. Tighten the tourniquet until the hemorrhage ceases.
4. Secure the tightening rod or device.
5. Write the time of tourniquet application on tape and secure it to the tourniquet (for example, TK 13:32). Never cover the tourniquet or site of bleeding. Continuously reassess the wound for recurrent bleeding.
6. Notify the receiving medical facility that a tourniquet has been applied.
7. Document the use of the tourniquet and the time it was applied in the prehospital care report.

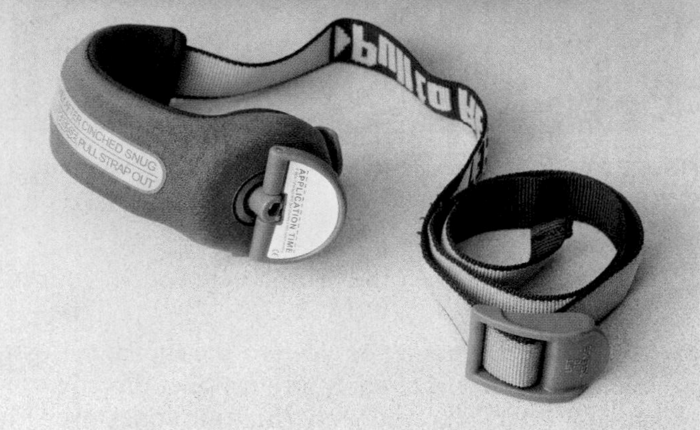

(a)

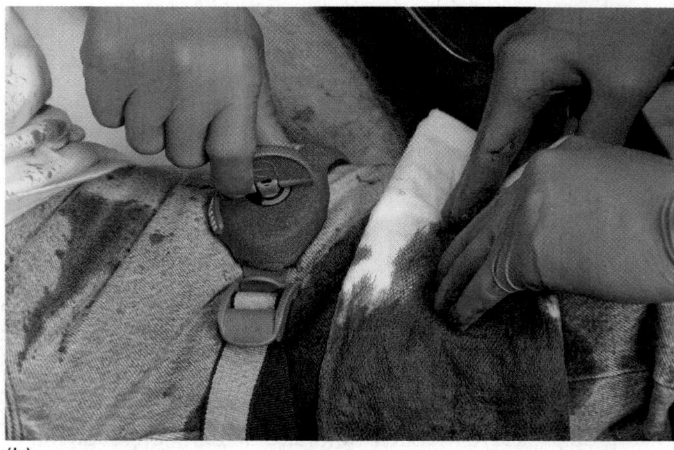

(b)

FIGURE 28-4 ∗ **(a)** Many commercial tourniquets are available. **(b)** If direct pressure has not been effective, a tourniquet may be applied to control bleeding.

In some cases, an inflated blood pressure cuff may be used as a tourniquet until bleeding stops (Figure 28-5∗). Typically, the cuff will be inflated to 20 mmHg beyond the patient's systolic blood pressure. If this technique is used, the cuff needs to be monitored to maintain pressure.

When using any type of tourniquet, consider the following guidelines:

- Always use a wide bandage 4 inches or greater; never use wire, a belt, or any other material that may cut the skin or underlying soft tissue.
- Once it is applied, secure the tourniquet tightly. Do not loosen or remove it unless you are directed to do so by medical direction or local protocol. Prolonged transport, typically greater than 2 hours, may be an

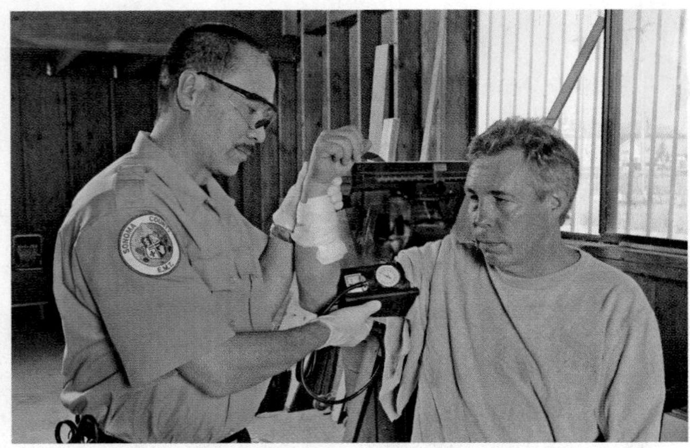

FIGURE 28-5 ✱ In some cases, an inflated blood pressure cuff may be used as a tourniquet.

indication to loosen the tourniquet. Follow your local protocol.

- Apply the tourniquet as close to the injury as possible. However, never apply a tourniquet directly over any joint, and do not apply the tourniquet over the wound itself.
- Always make sure the tourniquet is in open view.
- Document the time of application on a piece of tape and affix it to the tourniquet.
- The tightness needed for a tourniquet to control hemorrhage in a leg is typically greater than that needed to control hemorrhage in an arm.

Understanding BODY PROCESSES

If a tourniquet applied to an extremity does not completely stop arterial blood flow, the arterial blood will continue to flow into the extremity but the venous blood will not be able to flow out. This will build up arterial and venous pressure in the wound and actually increase the amount of bleeding. Be sure the tourniquet completely stops the arterial blood flow once it is applied. ■

Elevation

There is no evidence showing that elevation is an effective method to control or slow bleeding. However, there is also no evidence that shows it is harmful to the patient. Thus, elevation would not be harmful after direct pressure is applied to the wound on the extremity. Elevation can only be considered if it is done in conjunction with direct pressure. Never use elevation alone and never elevate an extremity with a suspected fracture that has not been splinted.

Splints

Bleeding can be life threatening in an open wound to an extremity with a suspected fracture. If left unsplinted, movement of broken bone ends or bone fragments can continue to damage surrounding tissues and blood vessels. Also, movement of the extremity may cause the clots that have formed to be broken, which will allow the vessels to continue to bleed. Splinting the extremity may assist with control of bleeding associated with a possible fracture because the splint will decrease movement at the site of the bleeding wound.

The source of bleeding in some fractures is the bone itself and not the surrounding vessels. This is especially true of the pelvis and femur. When the femur is fractured, it allows the surrounding muscle and tissue to lose tension and increase the diameter of the thigh. Basically, the cylindrical size of the thigh is increased. This allows more bleeding to occur within the thigh. The application of a traction splint serves not only as a splint but also as a method of bleeding control. The traction splint that is applied to a suspected fractured femur attaches to the ankle and at the level of the hip. Traction is applied to the ankle, which pulls the femur back in line. In turn, the traction increases the tension of the muscle and tissue surrounding the femur. This decreases the cylindrical size of the thigh and decreases the space into which the femur and surrounding vessels can bleed. The smaller-sized thigh may tamponade the bleeding with the increased pressure around the femur.

Apply splints on scene to extremity fractures only if the patient is stable and there are no life threats. If the patient is unstable, has any life threats, or exhibits signs of hemorrhagic shock, place the patient on the backboard and align the extremity fractures. Begin rapid transport. If time and the patient's condition permit, splint individual fractures en route to the medical facility.

See Chapter 30, "Musculoskeletal Trauma," for more information on splints and splinting.

Understanding BODY PROCESSES

Up to 1,500 mL of blood can be lost around each femur and 500–750 mL around the tibia and fibula. ■

Topical Hemostatic Agents

New types of dressings continuously being developed and tested are designed with substances on the dressing that promote clotting. The hemostatic dressing has fibrinogen and thrombin on the surface of the dressing to promote clotting and stop bleeding when applied to wounds. The chitosan dressing contains a substance called chitin, which is found in shrimp shells, lobsters, crabs, insects, worms, fungus, and mushrooms. The chitosan on the dressing promotes clotting when it is applied to the wound. These dressings have shown dramatic results when applied to wounds with major arterial and venous bleeding.

There are also hemostatic agents that are poured directly into the wound at the site of bleeding to cause clotting to occur (Figure 28-6✱). These agents are used with

Objective 28-5
Describe the assessment-based approach to external bleeding, including emergency medical care.

Thinking Critically
As you approach a patient who has been ejected from a vehicle, you see that she is bleeding from an open fracture to the femur. "First thing we have to do is control that bleeding," says your partner. What other "first things" need to be done?

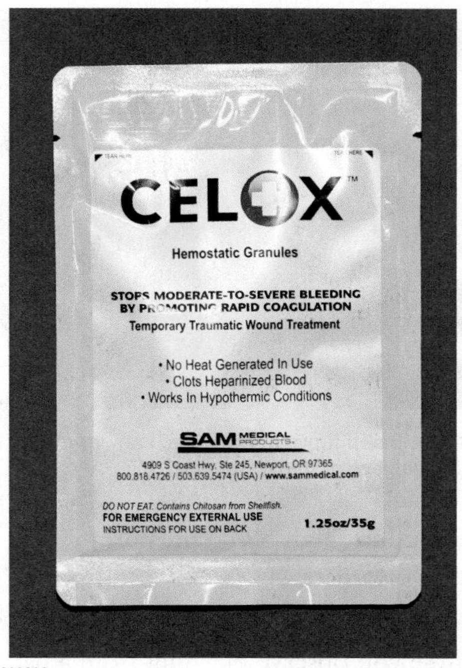

FIGURE 28-6 ✱ Topical hemostatic agents such as Celox can be used with pressure dressings to control bleeding.

pressure dressings to control arterial and venous bleeding. Celox and QuickClot are types of hemostatic agents that come in either a granular form that is poured into the wound at the site of bleeding or as granules contained in a sponge that is applied directly to the wound. TraumaDex is made from plants and contains microscopic beads that are porous and are believed to dehydrate the blood and promote clotting.

The use of hemostatic agents is usually reserved for prolonged transport times. Be sure to follow your local protocol.

Assessment-Based Approach: External Bleeding

Scene Size-Up, Primary Assessment, and Rapid Secondary Assessment

Based on dispatch information, begin preparing for the call while still en route to the scene by putting on gloves and eye protection. If you are responding to a known scene of violence or to an accident, make certain that the appropriate support agencies have been notified (police have secured the scene, for example, or special extrication teams have been notified).

Upon arrival, make sure the scene is safe before you enter, and take notice of any potential mechanism of injury. Also note the number of patients at the scene. If more than one patient has profuse bleeding, more resources may be required to effectively treat them.

As you approach the patient, begin to gather a general impression. Note the posture of the patient and whether he is alert or appears to have an altered mental status. An altered mental status is a sign of poor perfusion and shock. Note any significant bleeding. Significant bleeding is characterized as arterial or venous bleeding or bleeding that flows freely and steadily and is not controlled. If you note significant bleeding as you approach the patient, the first immediate action should be to control the bleeding with direct pressure. As that is being done, you or your partner should continue with the primary assessment.

Ensure that the patient has a patent airway. Assess the breathing rate and tidal volume to determine if breathing is adequate. If the breathing is adequate, immediately apply oxygen via a nonrebreather mask at 15 lpm. This is an early and necessary emergency care procedure for shock and for blood loss. If the breathing is inadequate, begin positive pressure ventilation with supplemental oxygen attached to the ventilation device. Assess the central and peripheral pulses, skin, and capillary refill.

External bleeding has a tendency to be very dramatic. Control the bleeding, but continue with the primary assessment. Do not skip the assessment of the airway, breathing, and circulation because you are distracted by a dramatic, bloody patient. Control the bleeding and proceed with the assessment.

After the primary assessment, perform the rapid secondary assessment in any patient who has suffered significant bleeding, who has an altered mental status, who presents with multiple injuries, or who has suffered a significant mechanism of injury. The rapid secondary assessment will reveal any other potential life threats and will provide further information about the stages of shock. Since bleeding is a serious condition, the rapid secondary assessment should not, if possible, take more than 90 seconds to perform.

Be sure to obtain a set of baseline vital signs for two reasons: (1) The vital signs will indicate the seriousness of the blood loss. (2) The baseline vital signs can be compared to a series of later vital signs measurements to determine if the patient's condition is deteriorating, remaining

Objective 28-6
Explain why bleeding from the nose, ears, or mouth is of special concern and describe the appropriate care for bleeding from the nose, ears, or mouth.

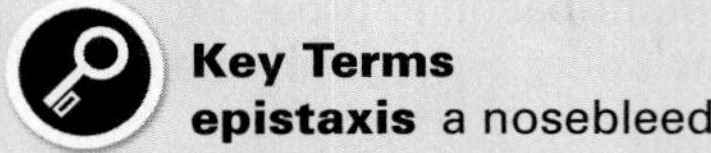

Key Terms
epistaxis a nosebleed.

the same, or improving. Keep in mind that vital signs may be deceiving and may not indicate the seriousness of the condition. Also assess signs of perfusion or hypoperfusion.

Emergency Medical Care

Severe external bleeding should be controlled during the primary assessment, following these steps:

1. *Take the necessary Standard Precautions.*
2. *Apply direct pressure* to the site of the bleeding. Apply a pressure dressing if possible.
3. If direct pressure fails to control the bleeding, *apply a tourniquet*. Be sure to note the time when the tourniquet is applied.
4. *Provide care for shock by administering oxygen via a nonrebreather mask at 15 lpm for adequate breathing or via positive pressure ventilation with supplemental oxygen if breathing is inadequate. Keep the patient warm, and transport immediately.*
5. *Immobilize injured extremities.*

Reassessment

During the reassessment, ensure that the bleeding is still under control. Be alert for wounds that may suddenly begin to bleed again. Repeat the primary assessment, and obtain a set of vital signs every 5 minutes if the patient appears to be unstable. The patient would be considered unstable if any abnormal vital signs are noted, such as persistent tachycardia. Serial vital sign assessments are important to monitor the level of shock and blood loss. Provide additional emergency care and assessment as necessary.

Bleeding from the Nose, Ears, or Mouth

The EMT may encounter patients who are bleeding from the nose, ears, or mouth (Figure 28-7*). These special areas may be cause for concern, because they can indicate a serious condition. Possible causes of bleeding from the nose, ears, or mouth include the following:

- Skull injury
- Facial trauma
- Digital trauma (nose picking)
- Sinusitis and other upper respiratory tract infections

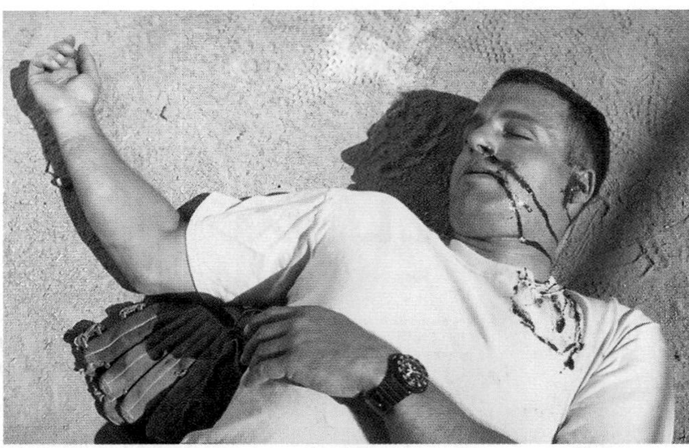

FIGURE 28-7 * Bleeding from the nose, ears, or mouth could be a sign of serious illness or injury.

- Hypertension (high blood pressure)
- Clotting disorders
- Esophageal disease

Any time you observe bleeding from a patient's ears or nose, suspect a possible skull fracture. If the patient has experienced a head injury, you should not attempt to stop the flow of blood, which could create pressure inside the skull, causing even more damage. Instead, place a loose dressing around the area to collect the drainage and limit exposure to sources of infection.

Epistaxis, or nosebleed, is bleeding from the nose, which may result from injury, disease, or the environment. Usually this type of bleeding is more of an annoyance than a threat to life. However, in cases of extreme blood loss, hemorrhagic shock can develop.

To provide emergency medical care for nosebleed, place the patient in a sitting position and have him lean forward. Apply direct pressure by pinching the fleshy portion of the nostrils together (EMT Skills 28-3A and 28-3B). Keep the patient as calm and as still as possible. Apply ice or a cold pack over the bridge of the nose, if possible.

ASSESSMENT Tips

The initial complaint of some patients with epistaxis may be throwing up blood, because the blood will irritate the gastric mucous lining when swallowed and cause the patient to vomit. In this case, recognize that the bleeding is not from the stomach but from the nasopharynx. ■

Key Points
Because internal bleeding is seldom obvious, it can result in severe blood loss with rapid progression to shock and death in just minutes.

Objective 28-7
Recognize indications of the severity of internal bleeding and describe the assessment-based approach to internal bleeding, including medical care to maintain perfusion and treat for shock.

Internal Bleeding

Internal bleeding may result from a variety of causes, including blunt trauma, abnormal clotting, rupture of a blood vessel or vascular structure, and certain fractures (especially pelvic fractures). Because it is not visible and seldom obvious, internal bleeding can result in severe blood loss with rapid progression of hemorrhagic shock and death—all in a matter of minutes.

Severity

The severity of internal bleeding depends on the patient's overall condition, age, other medical conditions, and source of the internal bleeding. The two most common sources of internal bleeding are injured or damaged internal organs and fractured extremities, especially fractures of the femur or pelvis. Always suspect internal bleeding if there are penetrating wounds to the skull, chest, abdomen, or pelvis.

A hematoma is a contained collection of blood. A hematoma the size of the patient's fist equates to approximately 10 percent of the blood volume. A significant amount of internal bleeding can be associated with fractures. A fracture of the tibia, fibula, or humerus can cause a loss of 500–750 mL of blood in the average-sized adult patient. A loss of 1,500 mL of blood can occur around a femur fracture. Body cavities can hold much larger amounts of blood. Approximately 3,000 mL of blood can be lost in the thorax.

The severity of internal bleeding should be estimated based on signs and symptoms. *Always suspect internal bleeding in cases of unexplained signs and symptoms of hemorrhagic shock.*

Assessment-Based Approach: Internal Bleeding

Scene Size-Up and Primary Assessment

During your scene size-up, look for and evaluate potential mechanisms of injury. Your suspicion of internal bleeding may be based on the mechanism of injury you identify. Ask yourself questions such as *Did the patient fall? Is there a weapon or other item that might have caused trauma?* If, for example, the emergency involves a fall, motorcycle or automobile collision, pedestrian impact, or blast, suspect blunt trauma and internal bleeding. Remember that penetrating injuries can result in both external and internal bleeding.

After ensuring that the scene is safe, approach the patient. During your general impression, look for any obvious external bleeding that is considered to be major. If you find a major bleed, immediately control it with direct pressure. As you continue with the primary assessment, assess the patient's mental status. A decreasing mental status is an early sign of both hypoxia and shock. As the patient continues to lose blood, the mental status will continue to deteriorate.

Assess the airway and ensure that it is patent. If it is not, open the airway with either a jaw-thrust or head-tilt, chin-lift maneuver, depending on whether a spinal injury is suspected. Assess the respiratory rate and tidal volume. If both the respiratory rate and tidal volume are adequate, immediately apply a nonrebreather mask and administer oxygen at 15 lpm. If either the respiratory rate or the tidal volume is inadequate, immediately begin positive pressure ventilation with oxygen connected to the ventilation device. The respiratory rate may provide some early clues in your assessment of blood loss. As the patient loses blood, the poor perfusion state, cell hypoxia, and the sympathetic nervous system will cause an increase in the rate and depth of respiration. In the patient with tachypnea, carefully inspect, palpate, and auscultate the chest during the rapid secondary assessment since the rapid breathing may also indicate a chest injury.

After assessing the airway and breathing, assess the pulses, skin, and capillary refill. The quality of the pulse is usually the first thing to indicate a blood loss, even before an increase in the pulse rate. The pulse will become weak and thready. As the bleeding continues, tachycardia will then develop. Depending on how much blood the patient lost before you arrived on the scene, you may find both a weak and thready pulse and tachycardia. If no radial pulse is found, this is an indication of severe hemorrhagic shock. It indicates that the vessels in the extremities have become severely constricted in an attempt to shunt blood to the core of the body, and the volume of blood is significantly decreased.

The skin will become pale, cool, and clammy in a hypoperfusion state. This is also seen as a result of the sympathetic nervous system causing the peripheral vessels to constrict (vasoconstriction) and shunt the blood to the core of the body. As the warm, red blood gets shunted to the core of the body, the skin becomes cooler and paler. The sympathetic nervous system will cause the skin also to become clammy or diaphoretic (sweaty). The capillary

Thinking Critically
You can determine if the patient is in shock based just on information from your quick primary assessment regarding mental status, respiration, pulse, skin, and capillary refill. What signs and symptoms relative to each of these (that could be observed during the primary assessment) would indicate shock?

Key Points
A narrow pulse pressure is an indication of significant blood loss.

refill will be delayed. Be aware of environmental and disease conditions that may affect the capillary refill status. In infants, children, and adult males, capillary refill is typically less than 2 seconds. Adult females have a normal capillary refill of less than 3 seconds. Geriatric patients have a normal capillary refill of less than 4 seconds.

Understanding BODY PROCESSES

When blood loss occurs, almost immediately the nervous system sends signals from the brain to increase the heart rate, strengthen its contraction, and constrict vessels. The brain also stimulates the adrenal glands to secrete epinephrine and norepinephrine, which occurs within a few minutes. The epinephrine and norepinephrine will produce a sustained effect on the heart and vessels. The alpha properties in the epinephrine and norepinephrine will cause the vessels to constrict, creating the pale appearance and coolness of the skin. Alpha will also stimulate the sweat glands, causing the clammy, or diaphoretic, presentation. The effects of alpha stimulation are to constrict the vessels and increase the systemic vascular resistance in an attempt to raise the blood pressure. ■

The information collected in the primary assessment is important in determining if the patient's condition is improving, deteriorating, or remaining the same. Based on this quick assessment, the information gained regarding the mental status; respiratory rate and depth; pulse rate and quality; skin color, temperature, and condition; and capillary refill is enough to make a judgment that the patient is in shock. You would then proceed to a rapid secondary assessment to identify any other life threats and to attempt to determine where the patient is bleeding.

Secondary Assessment

If the potential mechanism of injury and your general impression of the patient suggest internal bleeding, proceed to a rapid secondary assessment following the primary assessment. If there is evidence of contusions, abrasions, deformity, impact marks, swelling, or other trauma, treat the patient for internal bleeding. This is a priority patient; prepare for immediate transport following the rapid secondary assessment and initial emergency care.

Signs and Symptoms Internal bleeding is not visible and may not be easily detectable. In some patients, by the time obvious signs and symptoms are present, the patient may have lost a significant amount of blood. Be on guard for subtle signs and symptoms and changes in the patient's condition. Signs and symptoms of internal bleeding include the following:

- Pain, tenderness, swelling, or discoloration of suspected site of injury
- Bleeding from the mouth, rectum, vagina, or other orifice
- Vomiting bright red blood or blood the color of dark coffee grounds
- Dark, tarry stools, or stools with bright red blood
- Tender, rigid, or distended abdomen

ASSESSMENT Tips

There can be internal bleeding with *no* obvious distention; 1 to 2 liters may distend the abdomen only 1 inch.

Signs and symptoms of internal bleeding that also indicate hemorrhagic shock are as follows:

- Anxiety, restlessness, combativeness, or altered mental status
- Weakness, faintness, or dizziness
- Thirst
- Shallow, rapid breathing
- Rapid, thready pulse (typically > 90/minute in an adult)
- Pale, cool, clammy skin
- Delayed capillary refill
- Narrow pulse pressure (difference between systolic and diastolic pressure)
- Dropping blood pressure

Understanding BODY PROCESSES

As the systolic blood pressure drops from the decrease in blood volume, the systemic vasoconstriction causes the diastolic blood pressure to be maintained or to increase, creating a narrow pulse pressure. A narrow pulse pressure is an indication that a significant amount of blood has been lost. ■

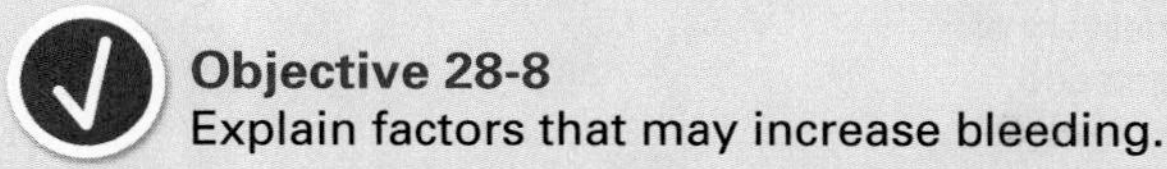

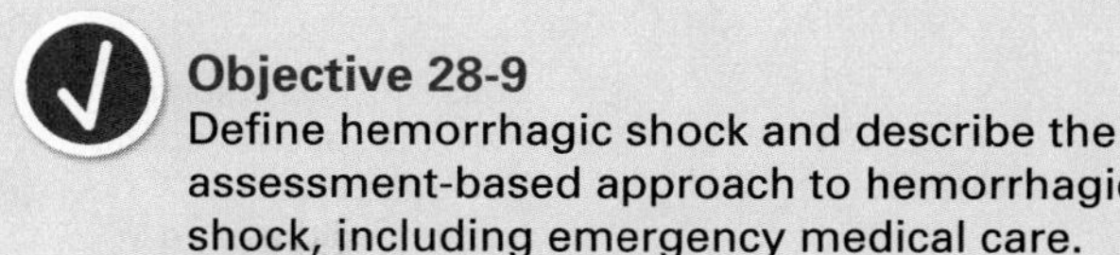

- Dilated pupils that are sluggish in responding to light
- Nausea and vomiting

Emergency Medical Care

The goal of all emergency medical care for internal bleeding is to recognize its presence quickly, maintain the body's perfusion, treat for shock, and provide rapid transport to an appropriate medical facility.

1. *Take Standard Precautions* by wearing appropriate personal protective equipment.
2. *Maintain an open airway and adequate breathing.* Provide positive pressure ventilation if respiratory rate or tidal volume is inadequate.
3. *Administer oxygen by a nonrebreather mask at 15 lpm* if you have not already done so.
4. *Control external bleeding with direct pressure. If direct pressure is unsuccessful in controlling the bleeding, apply a tourniquet.* Splint any extremity that you suspect is fractured. Initial splinting can be achieved by the long backboard when expeditious transport is critical. Once en route, if time and the patient's condition permit, fractures can be more specifically managed.
5. *Provide immediate transport* to critical or unstable patients and those with signs and symptoms of hemorrhagic shock.
6. *Provide care for shock,* as detailed later in this chapter.

Reassessment

Continually re-evaluate the critical patient, performing a reassessment every 5 minutes during transport, or more frequently if needed.

Factors That May Increase Bleeding

The following factors may interfere with the clotting process and lead to an increase in the rate of bleeding or the amount of blood lost:

- **Movement.** Movement can disrupt the clotting process and allow bleeding to continue.
- **Low body temperature.** A low body temperature may make the clotting process slower and less effective. That is one reason why it is necessary to keep the bleeding and shock patient warm.
- **Medications.** Coumadin (warfarin) and other anticoagulant drugs, aspirin, ibuprofen, and other nonsteroidal anti-inflammatory drugs (NSAIDs) will interfere with the clotting process.
- **Intravenous fluids.** Intravenous fluids may increase the blood pressure, causing clots to break free, or the water or other properties of the fluid may interfere with the clotting process.
- **Removal of dressings and bandages.** If the bleeding has been controlled, do not remove the dressing to examine the wound. This may disrupt the clotting and cause the bleeding to begin again.

Hemorrhagic Shock

Shock is most often the direct result of inadequate perfusion of tissue from the loss of blood volume. (As you will recall from Chapter 15, "Shock and Resuscitation," shock from fluid loss is called *hypovolemic shock.* When the fluid loss results from bleeding, or hemorrhage, it is known as *hemorrhagic hypovolemic shock,* or simply *hemorrhagic shock.*) When the cells of the body do not receive the oxygen, glucose, and other nutrients they need, they begin to fail and die. If this condition persists, cell failure, organ failure, and death will follow (Figure 28-8*). It is imperative that hemorrhagic shock is recognized and treated promptly. Immediate transport is necessary.

Certain major organs of the body require an adequate blood flow to function properly. When bleeding continues unchecked, there is a reduction in circulating blood volume. In response, blood may be shunted or redirected from less important organs to more important organs. Since these important organs are located in the head and trunk, peripheral perfusion (to the extremities) and perfusion of the skin, for example, are drastically reduced.

Hemorrhagic shock should be suspected in any patient who has suffered or may have suffered trauma (Figure 28-9*).

Assessment-Based Approach: Hemorrhagic Shock

As in any case with potential for exposure to blood or body fluids, wear the appropriate personal protective

CYCLE OF HEMORRHAGIC SHOCK

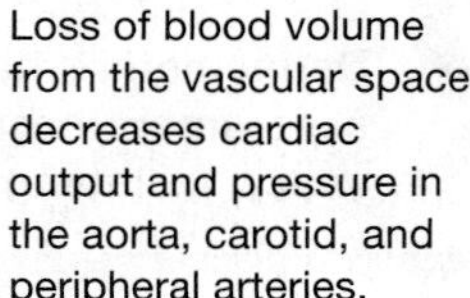

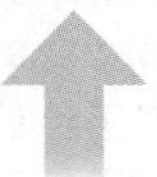
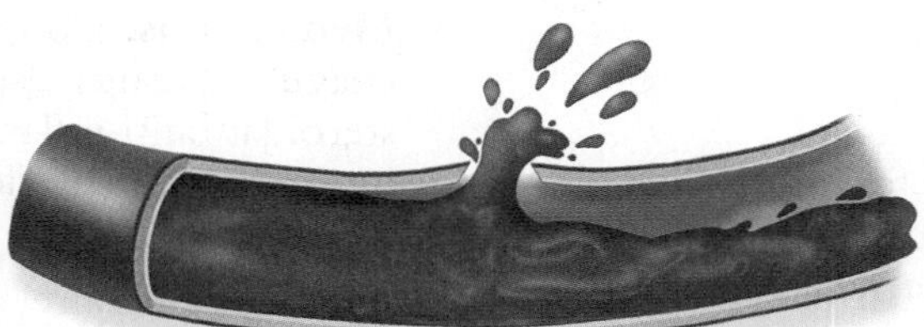

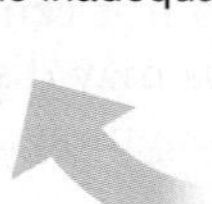

TRAUMA
Loss of blood volume from the vascular space decreases cardiac output and pressure in the aorta, carotid, and peripheral arteries.
Decrease in the delivery of oxygen and glucose to cells and the removal of carbon dioxide.
Baroreceptors trigger hormone release and sympathetic nervous system stimulation to increase cardiac output, blood pressure, and perfusion.
Heart rate and contractility increase, vessels constrict, respiratory rate increases, and urine output decreases in an attempt to compensate and increase cardiac output, blood pressure, and perfusion.
Patient exhibits tachycardia, weak peripheral pulses, decreased mental status, tachypnea, and pale, cool and clammy skin.
Continued volume loss overwhelms compensatory mechanisms and blood pressure falls, tachycardia and tachypnea further increase, peripheral pulses are extremely weak or absent, mental status deteriorates.
Brain becomes ischemic and medulla fails, causing a severe drop in perfusion and blood pressure.
Patient becomes unresponsive, heart rate severely increases and then drops dramatically, blood pressure decreases significantly and may not be obtainable, respirations decrease and become inadequate.
Further decrease in blood volume, perfusion, and blood pressure leads to brain tissue death, multiple organ failure, and eventual patient death.

FIGURE 28-8 ✱ Continuous cycle of shock.

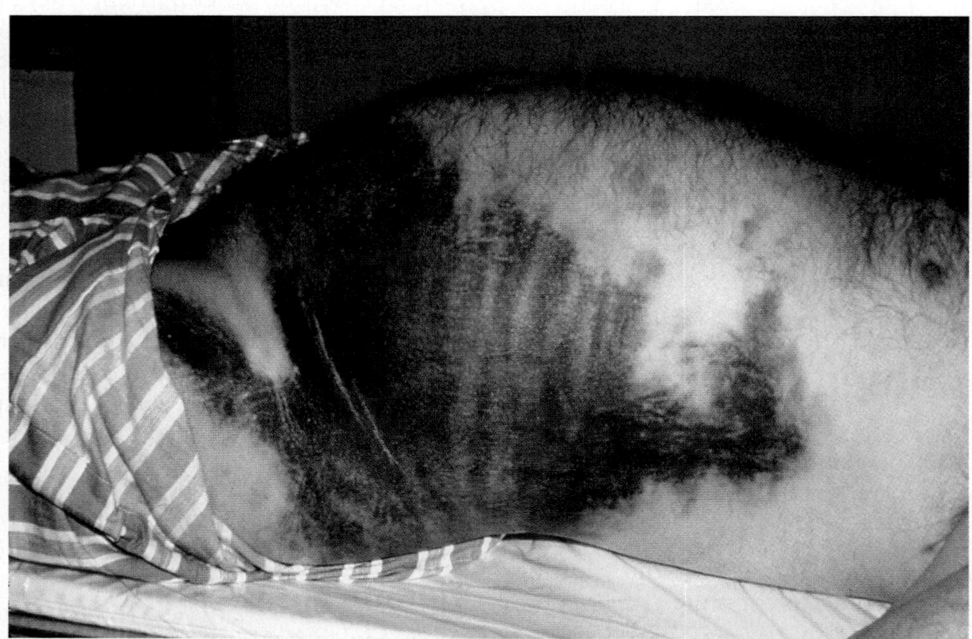

FIGURE 28-9 ✱ Abdominal bruising is a sign of blunt trauma and probable internal bleeding.

equipment. If possible, put it on while en route to the scene to decrease the amount of time it takes to get to the patient.

Scene Size-Up and Primary Assessment

During scene size-up, take note of any potential mechanism of injury that may have caused external or internal bleeding. Penetrating injuries may prompt you to seek law enforcement resources and to re-evaluate scene safety. When it is safe to approach the patient, assess the mental status, airway, breathing, and circulation, noting any abnormalities or signs of shock. Provide high-concentration oxygen if breathing is adequate; provide positive pressure ventilation with supplemental oxygen if breathing is inadequate.

Secondary Assessment

If multiple injuries, internal bleeding, or hemorrhagic shock is suspected, or the patient has an altered mental status, perform a rapid secondary assessment. Assess for signs and symptoms of hemorrhagic shock throughout the assessment. Restlessness, anxiety, thirst, and an altered mental status may be the first signs of shock. If the patient exhibits these signs, assess for internal or external bleeding in the chest, in the abdomen, in the pelvis, around the femur, or to the upper extremities.

Monitor for peripheral perfusion and skin color, temperature, and condition. Peripheral blood flow will be decreased as internal bleeding progresses. This may cause weak, thready, or absent pulses in the distal extremities, and also cause the skin to become pale, cool, and clammy.

Signs and Symptoms A blood loss of greater than 15 percent will affect the patient's vital signs. Establish a baseline as soon as possible. The signs and symptoms of shock are as follows:

- Mental status:
  - Restlessness
  - Anxiety
  - Altered mental status

Understanding BODY PROCESSES

A decrease in blood perfusion to the brain will decrease the delivery of oxygen and elimination of carbon dioxide, causing the patient to present with restlessness, anxiety, and an altered mental status. ■

- Peripheral perfusion and perfusion of the skin:
  - Pale, cool, clammy skin
  - Weak, thready, or absent peripheral pulses
  - Delayed capillary refill
- Vital signs:
  - Increased pulse rate (early sign), with weak and thready pulse (early sign)
  - Increased breathing rate (early sign) that may be deep or shallow, labored, and irregular
  - Narrow pulse pressure
  - Decreased blood pressure (late sign)
- Other signs and symptoms:
  - Dilated pupils (sluggish reaction)
  - Marked thirst

Understanding BODY PROCESSES

When fluid surrounding the cells in the hypothalamus of the brain moves into the blood vessels to try to increase the blood volume, the concentration of the particles (electrolytes) in the fluid changes, causing the patient to experience thirst. ■

  - Nausea and vomiting
  - Pallor with cyanosis to the lips

Note: Infants and children can compensate, or maintain their blood pressure, until their blood volume is depleted by almost one-third. Then their condition will suddenly and radically deteriorate. If a child's blood pressure is dropping, it is an ominous sign.

Emergency Medical Care

The treatment of hemorrhagic shock needs to occur early in the primary assessment and continue until transfer of care to the receiving medical facility is complete. The main priority in the care of this patient is to maintain perfusion to the vital organs and interrupt any progression or worsening of shock.

Emergency medical care of hemorrhagic shock is as follows (EMT Skills 28-4A to 28-4C):

1. *Maintain Standard Precautions* by wearing the appropriate personal protective equipment, including gloves and eye protection.
2. *Maintain an open airway. If breathing is adequate, administer oxygen via a nonrebreather mask at 15 lpm.* If breathing is inadequate, begin positive pressure ventilation with supplemental oxygen connected to the ventilation device.
3. *Control any external bleeding* using the techniques described earlier in this chapter.
4. *Apply and inflate the pneumatic antishock garment (PASG) if signs and symptoms of hemorrhagic shock are present; if the lower abdomen is tender with a suspected pelvic injury (lower abdominal tenderness, pelvic instability) with a systolic blood pressure of* < 90 *mmHg; if there is profound hypotension (systolic blood pressure* < *50 to 60 mmHg); if there is suspected intraperitoneal hemorrhage with hypotension or suspected retroperitoneal hemorrhage with hypotension; and if there is no evidence of chest injury, pregnancy,*

Key Points
Treatment for hemorrhagic shock must begin early in the primary assessment and continue until transfer to the receiving facility is complete. The priority is to maintain perfusion to vital organs and interrupt any progression of shock.

Thinking Critically
Your 3-year-old patient has fallen several feet from a window onto a cement patio. She looks unfazed, her blood pressure is normal, and bleeding from some cuts seems minor. You begin treating her for shock. Why?

evisceration, or cardiac arrest. Always apply and inflate the pneumatic antishock garment (PASG) only in accordance with local protocols and if approved by medical direction. See Figure 28-10∗ and the more detailed section on the PASG that follows.

5. *Place the patient in a supine position.*
6. *Splint suspected bone or joint injuries.* In the hemorrhagic shock patient, transport is critical. Thus, the fractures will be initially stabilized by the long backboard. En route, if time and the patient's condition permit, the fractures can be individually splinted.
7. *Use a blanket to cover any patient suspected of suffering hemorrhagic shock* to prevent loss of body heat. Since the patient may have a decreased blood flow to nonvital organs, the body's heat regulation may be impaired. Warm the patient compartment to 85 degrees during transport to prevent body heat loss. Remove any wet or blood-soaked clothes.
8. *Transport the patient immediately.*

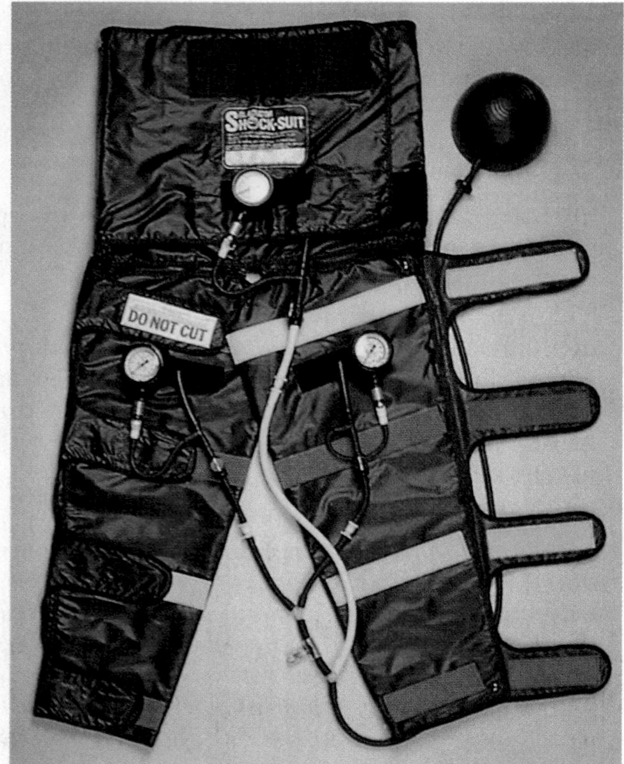

FIGURE 28-10 ∗ A pneumatic antishock garment (PASG).

Note: Because of the ability of infants and children to compensate for shock by maintaining blood pressure, followed by a sudden deterioration into severe and possibly irreversible shock, it is crucial in infants and children not to wait for significant signs of shock to appear but to treat the infant or child based on any suspicion of trauma and subtle signs and symptoms of shock. A child's total blood volume is far less than that of an adult. Even a small loss of blood that would not be considered life threatening for an adult should be considered critical in an infant or child. Immediate transport is crucial.

Remainder of the Assessment

Continue to assess the patient for changes in mental status and vital signs throughout the rapid trauma assessment and reassessment. These may be conducted en route if early transport is initiated because of suspected shock.

Pneumatic Antishock Garment (PASG)

The PASG is a controversial device that is primarily used to control blood loss. Follow your local protocol regarding use of the PASG.

Indications

- Suspected pelvic fracture with hypotension (systolic blood pressure < 90 mmHg)
- Profound hypotension (systolic blood pressure < 50–60 mmHg)
- Suspected intraperitoneal hemorrhage with hypotension (internal abdominal trauma and bleeding)
- Suspected retroperitoneal hemorrhage with hypotension

Contraindications

- Penetrating thoracic trauma
- Splinting of lower extremity fractures
- Eviscerated abdominal organs
- Impaled object in abdomen
- Pregnancy
- Cardiopulmonary arrest

For application and inflation of the PASG, see EMT Skills 28-5A to 28-5G. Once inflated, the PASG should not be deflated in the prehospital setting unless ordered by medical direction. If you suspect the patient has suffered a ruptured diaphragm or if he complains of respiratory distress after inflation, contact medical direction to consider deflation.

Summary: Assessment and Care

To review possible assessment findings and emergency care for bleeding and hemorrhagic shock, see Figures 28-11* and 28-12*.

Hemophilia

There are many different types of blood disorders. One you are likely to encounter is a clotting disorder called hemophilia. This disorder is a congenital disease (one the patient was born with) that prevents activation of the normal clotting mechanisms found in the blood. This means that even the smallest wound or cut in a patient with hemophilia can cause uncontrolled bleeding.

Bleeding in this patient is always considered to be significant. Provide emergency care for bleeding as for any patient. However, for the patient to obtain the special medication necessary to assist clot formation, transport to a medical facility immediately.

Assessment Summary

BLEEDING AND HEMORRHAGIC SHOCK

The following findings may be associated with bleeding and shock.

SCENE SIZE-UP

Pay particular attention to your own safety. Look for:
- Mechanism of injury
- Splatters or pools of blood at the scene
- Blood-soaked clothing
- Penetrating trauma
- Blunt trauma

Primary Assessment

General Impression
- Obvious massive external hemorrhage
- Extremely pale color
- Appears weak and ill

Mental Status
- Alert to unresponsive, based on amount of blood loss and shock
- As blood loss continues, mental status decreases

Airway
- May be closed if mental status is altered
- May be bleeding in airway from trauma

Breathing
- Initially fast and normal to deeper volume
- May become shallow and fast or slow as blood loss and shock progress
- May be absent or inadequate if bleeding in chest or associated with chest injury
- May be fast and shallow if abdominal injury is present

Circulation
- Pulses possibly difficult to find because of extreme blood loss
- Increased heart rate that becomes extremely elevated, then suddenly decreases with continued blood loss
- Pulses becoming extremely weak or absent as blood loss and shock continue
- Skin becoming increasingly pale, cool, and clammy as blood loss and shock progress

Status: Priority Patient

Secondary Assessment

Physical Exam

Head, neck, and face:
- External bleeding
- Blood from ear, nose, or mouth
- Pupils dilated and sluggish to respond to light
- Cyanosis
- Pale oral mucosa

Chest:
- Penetrating or blunt trauma to chest
- Decreased breath sounds if bleeding into chest cavity

Abdomen:
- Rigid, distended abdomen
- Discoloration around umbilicus or in the flank area (late)
- Penetrating or blunt trauma
- Pain on palpation

Pelvis:
- Unstable on palpation
- Pain

continued

FIGURE 28-11a * Assessment summary: bleeding and hemorrhagic shock.

Assessment Summary

Extremities:
- Obvious external bleeding
- Deformity or discoloration around femur(s)
- Poor or absent peripheral pulses
- Pale, cool, clammy skin
- Cyanosis

Baseline Vital Signs

BP: decreasing or absent

HR: increased

RR: increased

Skin: pale, cool, clammy, cyanosis

Pupils: dilated and sluggish to respond

SpO_2: decreased or may get an erroneous or low perfusion reading

History

Signs and symptoms of blood loss and hemorrhagic shock:
- Anxiousness
- Decreasing mental status
- Pale, cool, clammy skin
- Decreasing blood pressure
- Narrow pulse pressure
- Tachycardia
- Tachypnea
- Poor or absent peripheral pulses
- Dilated and sluggish pupils
- Capillary refill greater than 2 seconds in infants, children, and adult males; greater than 3 seconds in adult females; greater than 4 seconds in elderly adults

FIGURE 28-11a ✻ Assessment summary: bleeding and hemorrhagic shock. *continued*

Emergency Care Protocol

BLEEDING AND HEMORRHAGIC SHOCK

1. Control any major life-threatening bleeding.
2. Establish manual in-line stabilization if spinal injury is suspected.
3. Establish and maintain an open airway; insert a nasopharyngeal or oropharyngeal airway if the patient is unresponsive and has no gag or cough reflex.
4. Suction secretions as necessary.
5. If breathing is inadequate, provide positive pressure ventilation with supplemental oxygen at a minimum rate of 10–12 ventilations/minute for an adult and 12–20 ventilations/minute for an infant or child.
6. If breathing is adequate, administer oxygen by nonrebreather mask at 15 lpm.
7. Control bleeding with direct pressure (use fingertip pressure).
8. Splint suspected fractures.
9. Apply a tourniquet if bleeding is not controlled with direct pressure. Note the time the tourniquet was applied and mark it on the tourniquet.
10. Apply sterile dressings and bandages.
11. Maintain body temperature.
12. Consider application of the PASG.
13. Place the patient supine.
14. If spinal injury is suspected, immobilize the patient to a backboard.
15. Transport.
16. Perform reassessment every 5 minutes.

FIGURE 28-11b ✻ Emergency care protocol: bleeding and hemorrhagic shock.

▶ Soft Tissue Trauma

The Skin

Review the description and function of the skin provided in Chapter 7, "Anatomy, Physiology, and Medical Terminology." You may recall that the skin is one of the most durable and largest organs of the body. It is composed of three layers—the *epidermis,* the *dermis,* and a *subcutaneous layer.* It protects the body from the environment, bacteria, and other organisms, and it helps to regulate the body's temperature. The skin also senses heat, cold, touch, pressure, and pain, and it aids in the elimination of water and various salts.

The term *wound* usually refers to an injury to the skin and underlying tissues (EMT Skills 28-6A to 28-6D). Wounds to the skin are categorized as *closed, open, single,* or *multiple.* These types of injuries are discussed in detail on the following pages.

Emergency Care Algorithm: **Bleeding and Shock**

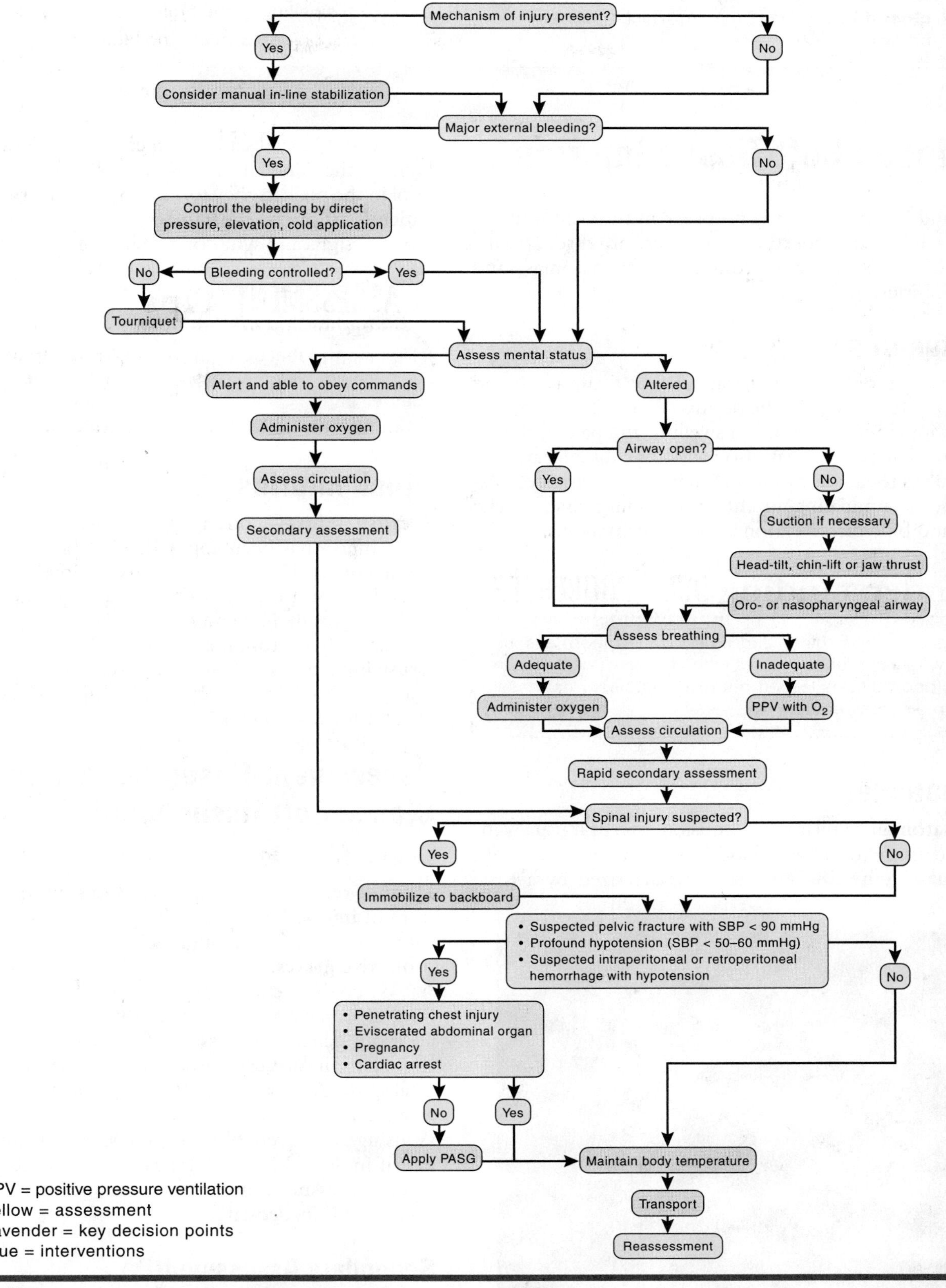

Mechanism of injury present?
Yes
No
Consider manual in-line stabilization
Major external bleeding?
Yes
No
Control the bleeding by direct pressure, elevation, cold application
Bleeding controlled?
No
Yes
Tourniquet
Assess mental status
Alert and able to obey commands
Altered
Administer oxygen
Assess circulation
Secondary assessment
Airway open?
Yes
No
Suction if necessary
Head-tilt, chin-lift or jaw thrust
Oro- or nasopharyngeal airway
Assess breathing
Adequate
Inadequate
Administer oxygen
PPV with O_2
Assess circulation
Rapid secondary assessment
Spinal injury suspected?
Yes
No
Immobilize to backboard
• Suspected pelvic fracture with SBP < 90 mmHg
• Profound hypotension (SBP < 50–60 mmHg)
• Suspected intraperitoneal or retroperitoneal hemorrhage with hypotension
Yes
No
• Penetrating chest injury
• Eviscerated abdominal organ
• Pregnancy
• Cardiac arrest
No
Yes
Apply PASG
Maintain body temperature
Transport
Reassessment
PPV = positive pressure ventilation
Yellow = assessment
Lavender = key decision points
Blue = interventions

FIGURE 28-12 ✻ Emergency care algorithm: bleeding and shock.

Objective 28-10
List types of closed soft tissue injuries and describe the assessment-based approach to closed soft tissue injuries, including emergency medical care.

Key Terms
closed injury any injury in which there is no break in the skin.

Key Terms
contusion a closed injury to the tissue and blood vessels within the dermis characterized by discoloration, swelling, and pain; a bruise; bruising or swelling of the brain.

ecchymosis black and blue discoloration.

▶ Closed Soft Tissue Injuries

A wound in which there is no break in the continuity of the skin is called a **closed injury.** There are three specific types of closed injuries: contusions, hematomas, and crush injuries.

Contusions

A **contusion,** or bruise, is an injury to the tissue and blood vessels contained within the dermis (Figure 28-13*). This type of injury causes localized swelling and pain at the injury site. The patient may also have some discoloration at the injury site caused by blood leaking from damaged vessels and accumulating in the surrounding tissues. The black and blue discoloration is called **ecchymosis.**

Understanding BODY PROCESSES

The ecchymosis (black and blue discoloration) associated with a contusion occurs when the red blood cells in the blood that has leaked out of the capillary or vessel become deoxygenated. ■

Hematomas

A **hematoma** is similar to a contusion, except it usually involves damage to a larger blood vessel and a larger amount of tissue (Figure 28-14*). It is characterized by a large lump with bluish discoloration caused by blood collecting beneath the skin. This blood may also separate tissues and pool in the pockets they form. A hematoma the size of the patient's fist can be equal to 10 percent blood loss, causing minimal signs and symptoms of hemorrhagic shock.

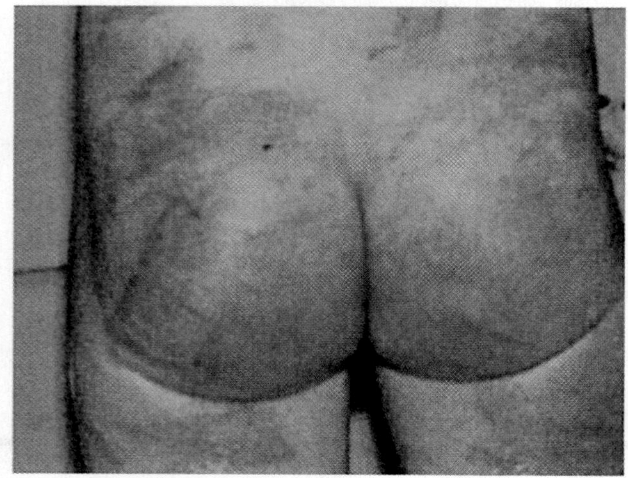

FIGURE 28-13 * Contusions.

ASSESSMENT Tips

Hematomas that occur in the elderly with fragile soft tissue could bleed excessively and become extremely large. ■

Crush Injuries

A **crush injury** is one in which force great enough to cause injury has been applied to the body. Severe blunt trauma or crushing force can cause serious damage to the underlying soft tissues with associated internal bleeding, and may result in hemorrhagic shock. Internal organs may actually rupture if a severe crush injury is sustained. Crush injuries can fall into either category, open or closed injuries. See "Open Soft Tissue Injuries" later in this chapter for more details.

Assessment-Based Approach: Closed Soft Tissue Injuries

Scene Size-Up and Primary Assessment

During your scene size-up, include a scan for the mechanism of injury. Be sure you have taken all Standard Precautions before you approach the patient, including protective gloves.

When the scene is safe, approach the patient and conduct a primary assessment. If the mechanism of injury and your general impression of the patient suggest a possible spinal injury, establish in-line stabilization of the cervical spine. After assessing the mental status and ensuring an adequate airway and breathing, check for and treat obvious signs of severe bleeding and shock. Administer oxygen if indicated in the adequately breathing patient, or positive pressure ventilation with supplemental oxygen if breathing is inadequate.

Secondary Assessment

Perform a secondary assessment, checking for evidence of trauma. Assess baseline vital signs and obtain a history.

Key Terms

hematoma a closed injury characterized by a mass of blood beneath the epidermis.

crush injury an open or closed injury in which high-pressure forces cause serious damage to underlying soft tissues with internal bleeding, resulting in possible hemorrhagic shock.

Key Terms

open injury injury in which the skin is broken.

Objective 28-11

List types of open soft tissue injuries and describe the assessment-based approach to open soft tissue injuries, including emergency medical care.

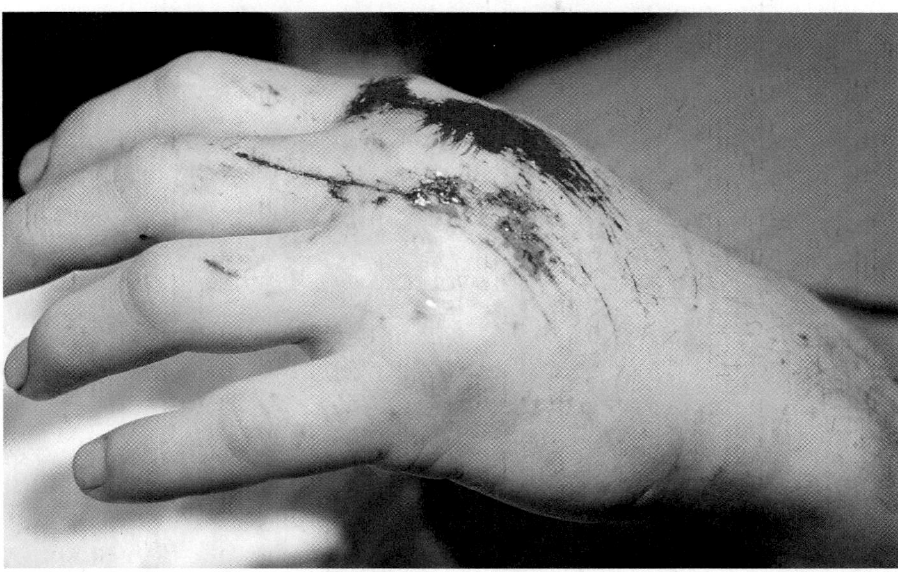

FIGURE 28-14 ✱ Hematoma underlying an abrasion.

Signs and Symptoms Signs and symptoms of closed soft tissue injury include:

- Swelling, pain, and discoloration at the injury site
- Signs and symptoms of internal bleeding and hemorrhagic shock if the underlying organs are injured

Emergency Medical Care

In general, small contusions do not require treatment. They usually heal by themselves. Larger contusions, hematomas, and crush injuries, however, can be an indication of serious underlying internal injuries and blood loss and can lead to compromised blood flow and nerve injury.

Steps to provide emergency medical care for closed soft tissue injuries are as follows:

1. **Take standard precautions.** Since blood or body fluids may be present, wear protective gloves, eyewear, and other appropriate personal protective equipment. Wash your hands thoroughly after the call, even if gloves were worn.
2. **Ensure an open airway and adequate breathing.** Provide oxygen by nonrebreather mask at 15 lpm or positive pressure ventilation with supplemental oxygen as needed.
3. **Treat for shock, if necessary.** If you suspect significant blood loss, provide emergency care based on the mechanism of injury and the patient's signs and symptoms.
4. **Splint suspected fractures.** Prevent a closed injury associated with possible bone fracture from becoming an open injury, reduce the amount of bleeding, and relieve the patient's pain by immobilizing the injured extremity. The injured extremity should also be elevated, if possible.

Reassessment

For the reassessment, repeat the primary assessment, reassess and monitor vital signs, and recheck all interventions.

Open Soft Tissue Injuries

When the continuity of the skin is broken, the wound is called an **open injury.** In open injuries the patient is at risk for external bleeding and contamination with dirt and bacteria, which may lead to infection. The open injury may be the first indicator of a deeper, more serious injury, such as a fracture or ruptured or lacerated organ.

There are six general types of open injuries: abrasions, lacerations, avulsions, amputations, penetrations/punctures, and crush injuries (Figure 28-15✱).

Key Points
Small contusions usually heal without treatment. Larger contusions, hematomas, and crush injuries can indicate serious internal injuries.

Key Terms
abrasion an open injury to the epidermis caused by a scraping away, rubbing, or shearing away of tissue.

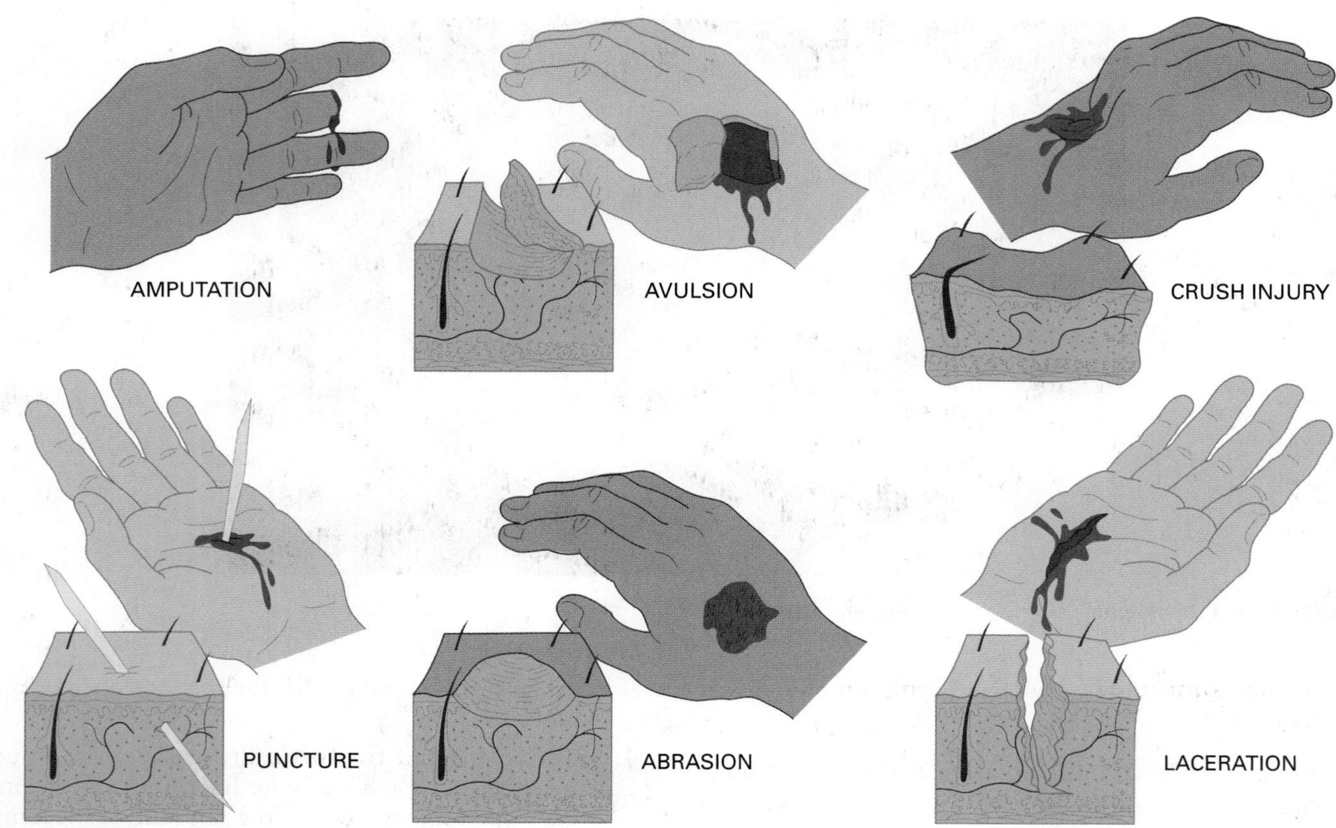

FIGURE 28-15 * Classification of open injuries.

Abrasions

An **abrasion** generally is caused by scraping, rubbing, or shearing away of the epidermis, the outermost layer of the skin (Figure 28-16*). Even though an abrasion is considered a superficial injury, it often is extremely painful because of the presence of exposed nerve endings. In most cases, blood will ooze from the wound (capillary bleeding), which can be controlled easily with direct pressure.

While small abrasions may not be life threatening, abrasions to large areas of the body surface may be cause for concern. For example, as a result of a motorcycle accident, a patient may slide across the pavement, causing head-to-toe abrasions ("road rash"). Bleeding in such a case may not be a serious threat; however, contamination, infection, and the potential for underlying injuries will be significant.

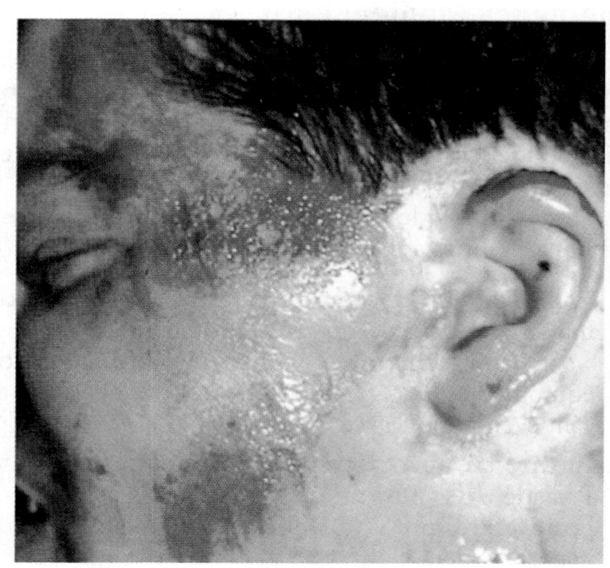

FIGURE 28-16 * Abrasions.

Key Terms

laceration an open injury whose edges may be linear (smooth and regular) or stellate (jagged and irregular); a wound that penetrates the brain.

Key Terms

avulsion an open injury characterized by a loose flap of skin and soft tissue that has been torn loose or pulled off.

amputation an open injury caused by the ripping or tearing away of a limb, body part, or organ.

Lacerations

A break in the skin of varying depth, a **laceration** may be *linear* (regular) or *stellate* (irregular) (Figures 28-17*, 28-18a, and 28-18b*). Lacerations may bleed more than other types of open soft tissue injuries, especially when an artery is involved. Linear lacerations are usually caused by a knife, razor, or broken glass. They usually heal better than stellate injuries because the wound has smooth edges. Stellate lacerations are commonly caused by a blunt object. The edges of the wound will be jagged and healing may be prolonged.

Avulsions

An **avulsion** is a loose flap of skin and underlying soft tissue that has been torn loose (partial avulsion) or pulled completely off (total or complete avulsion) (Figures 28-19a and 28-19b*). Bleeding may be severe because of blood vessel injury, although some blood vessels may tamponade (compress) themselves by retracting into the soft tissue. Healing will be prolonged and scarring may be extensive.

Avulsions are most commonly a result of accidents with industrial or home machinery and motor vehicles. They commonly involve the fingers, toes, hands, feet, forearms, legs, ears, and nose. A small amount of blood loss does not negate the possibility of a serious injury. The severity of an avulsion is directly related to the effectiveness of circulation and perfusion distal to the injury.

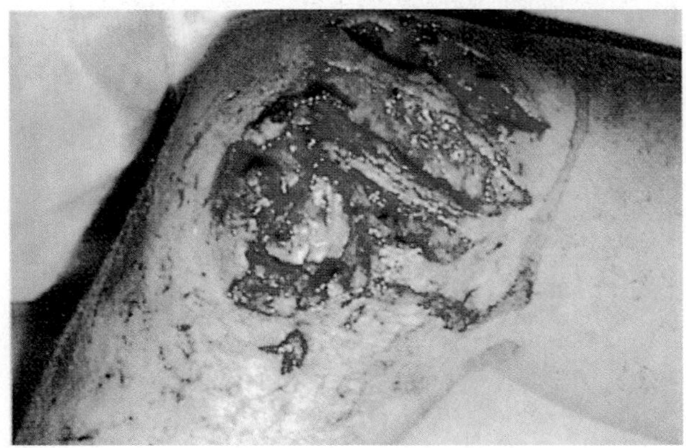

FIGURE 28-17 * Lacerations and deep abrasions.

Amputations

An **amputation** involves a disruption in the continuity of an extremity or other body part (Figures 28-20a to 28-20c*). Amputations are the result of ripping or

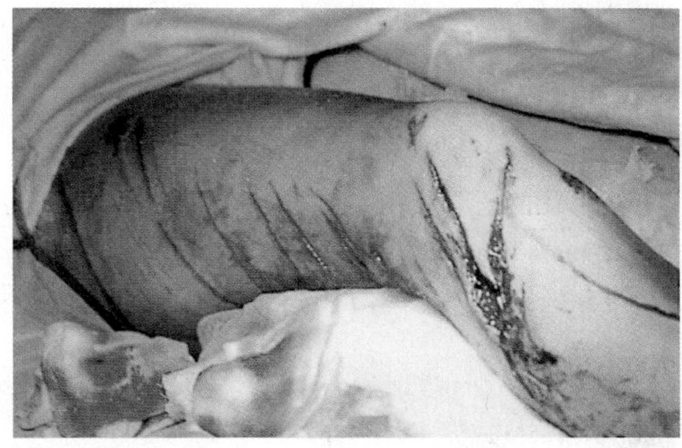

FIGURE 28-18a * Lacerations to the leg.

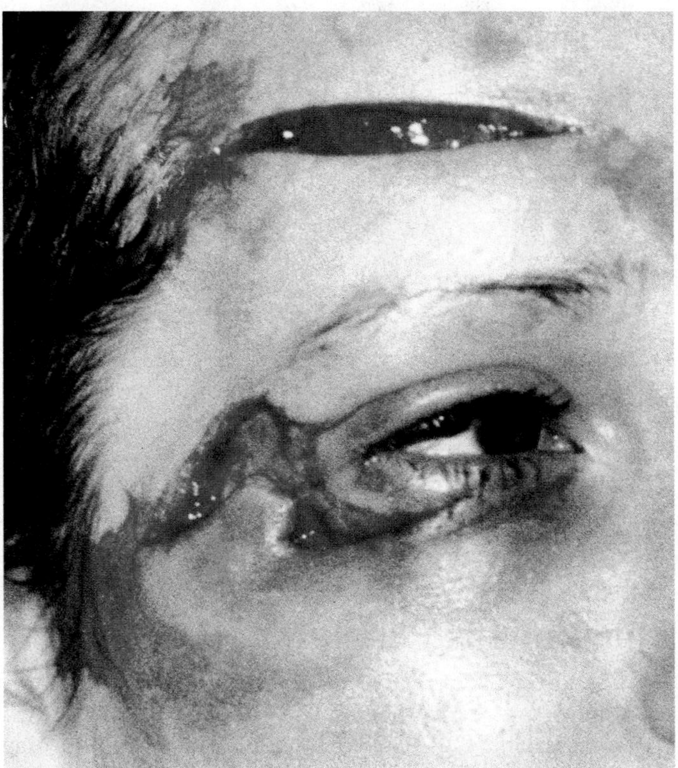

FIGURE 28-18b * Lacerations to the face.

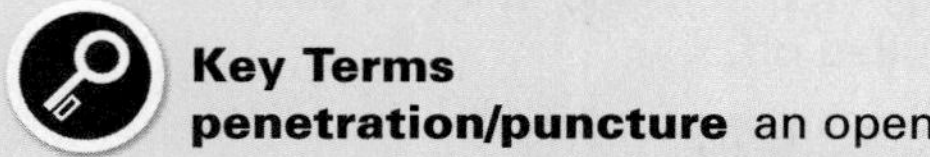

Key Terms
penetration/puncture an open injury caused by a pointed object being pushed into the tissues.

Key Points
A penetration/puncture entry wound may appear small and bleed very little, but the wound may be deep and damaging and cause significant internal bleeding.

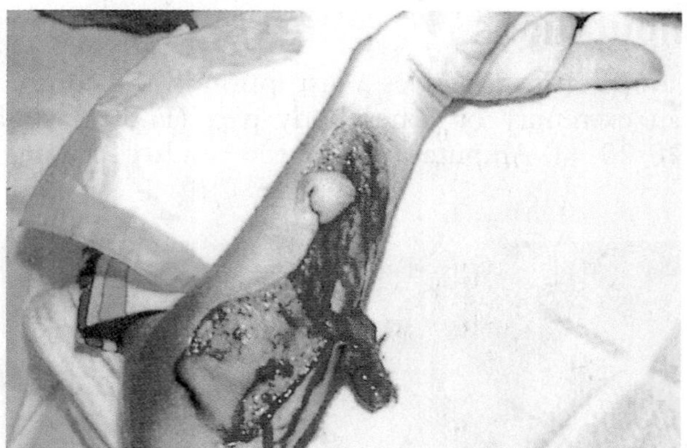

FIGURE 28-19a * Forearm avulsion.

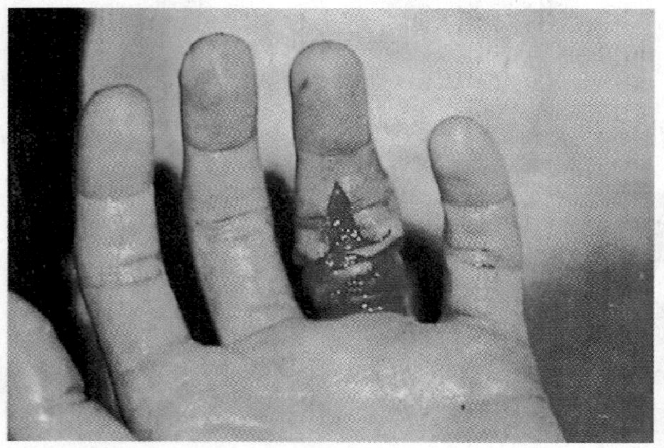

FIGURE 28-19b * Ring avulsion.

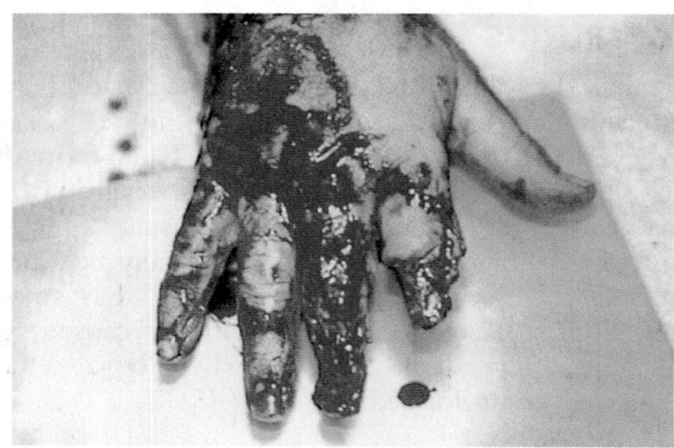

FIGURE 28-20a * Finger amputation.

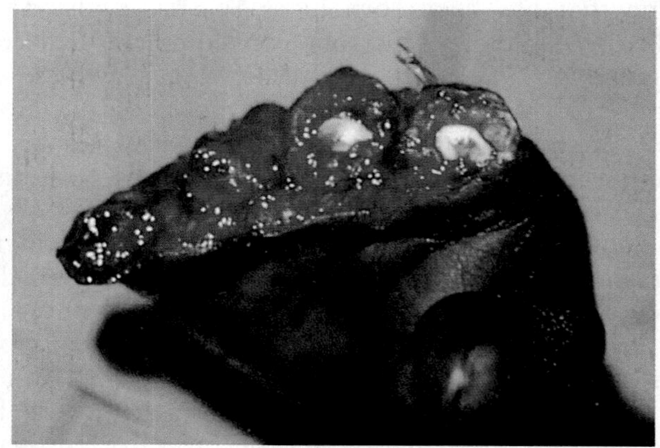

FIGURE 28-20b * Finger amputations.

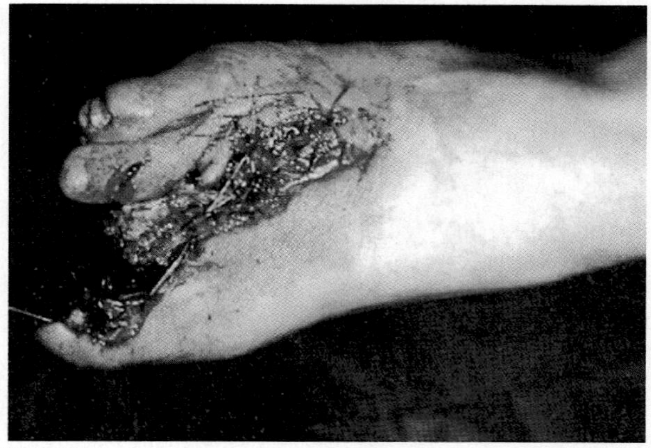

FIGURE 28-20c * Toe amputation.

tearing forces often associated with industrial, agricultural, power tool, or motor vehicle accidents. Bleeding from amputations may be massive. However, in most cases, because of the elasticity of the blood vessels, very little bleeding occurs. An incomplete amputation typically bleeds more than a complete amputation. Always consider shock in cases of amputation.

Penetrations/Punctures

A **penetration/puncture** injury generally is the result of a sharp, pointed object being pushed or driven into the soft tissues (Figure 28-21*). The entry wound may appear very small and cause little bleeding. However, such injuries may be deep and damaging and may cause

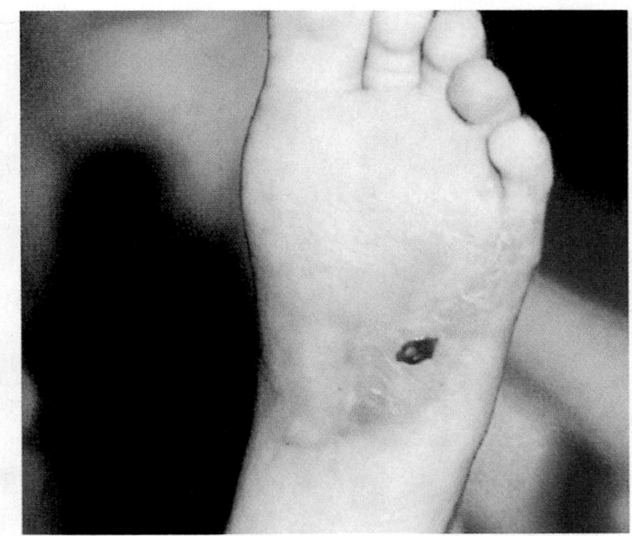

FIGURE 28-21 ✱ Penetration/puncture wound to the foot.

severe internal bleeding. The overall severity of the injury depends on the location, the size of the penetrating object, the depth of penetration, the forces involved, and the structures in the path of the injury. It can be difficult to determine the extent of injury based on the external wound. Therefore, treat these injuries with great caution.

Gunshots may cause both an entrance and an exit wound (EMT Skills 28-7A to 28-7F). In general, the entrance wound is smaller than the exit wound and, if the patient was shot at close range, the entrance wound will be surrounded by powder burns. The exit wound is usually larger and will bleed more profusely. Remember to assess for the possibility of multiple gunshot wounds, especially in areas covered with hair.

Stab wounds may be easily detected or may be small and hidden by clothing or body parts, such as an extremity. Expose the patient and carefully inspect all areas of the body so that a potentially life-threatening injury is not missed. Always assess the patient for underlying internal injuries and hemorrhagic shock.

ASSESSMENT Tips

Fractures to the extremities are often referred to as distracting injuries because the pain and possible deformity might distract the patient and keep him from complaining of wounds and injuries to other areas of the body. This is why it is necessary to completely expose the trauma patient and inspect for wounds. ■

Crush Injuries

Usually the result of blunt trauma or crushing forces, crush injuries may not appear to be serious (Figure 28-22✱). The only external sign may be an injury site that is painful, swollen, and deformed. External bleeding may be minimal or absent. Always suspect that there may be internal injury and severe internal bleeding in the presence of crush injuries.

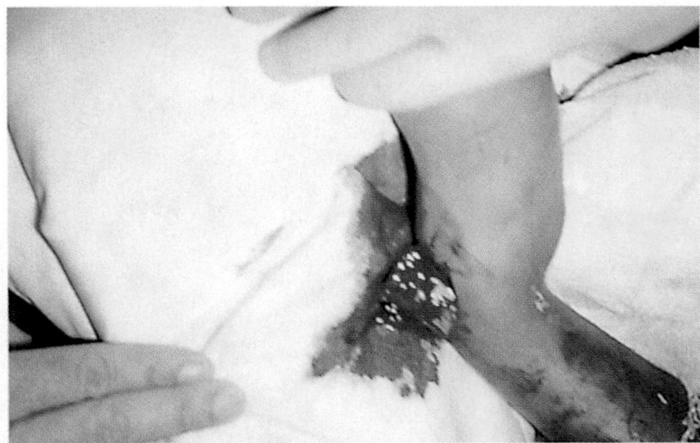

FIGURE 28-22 ✱ Crush injury, open wound.

Patients with crush injuries may appear to be unaffected at first. However, they can deteriorate rapidly into shock. This typically occurs when the object causing the crush injury is lifted from the patient. The object will initially tamponade, or restrict, any bleeding while it is against the body. Then, when released, the blood vessels or internal organs will begin to bleed freely and profusely.

Other Soft Tissue Injuries

Bites

Dog bites are a common type of animal bite. The soft tissue injuries caused by dog bites are usually to the hands, arms, and legs, although some occur on the head and face (Figure 28-23a✱). Complications include infection, *cellulitis* (inflammation of skin cells), and *septicemia* (blood infection). *Rabies* and *tetanus* (lockjaw) are also a concern, although rare. Human bites (Figure 28-23b✱) may cause *hepatitis* (inflammation of the liver).

Generally, bite wounds are a combination of penetration/puncture injuries and crush injuries, which may also involve internal organs and bones. Severity of a bite injury is related to the force of the animal's jaws. The most dangerous bite occurs from injuries over vascular areas. Human bites are probably the most difficult to manage in the long term because of the high rate of infection. (The human mouth carries a greater amount of bacteria.) The most frequent human bite locations are the ears, nose, and fingers.

Emergency care for bites is essentially the same as for other soft tissue injuries. However minor the wound may appear, the bite should be evaluated at a medical facility. Always ensure scene safety first. If possible, arrange for someone to contain or isolate the animal, so that it will not interfere while you provide care to the patient.

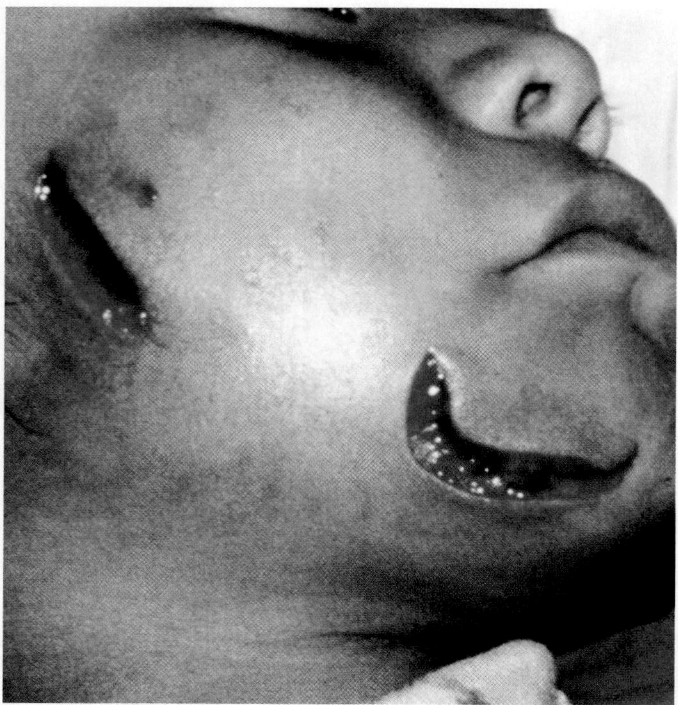

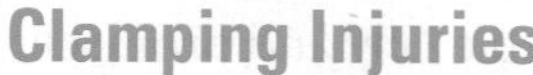

FIGURE 28-23a ✱ Dog bite to a child's face.

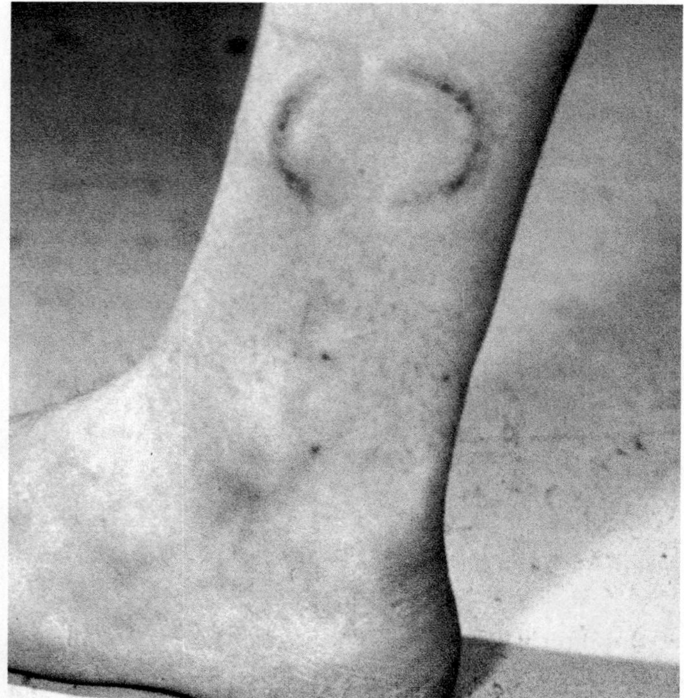

FIGURE 28-23b ✱ Human bite to the lower leg.

Clamping Injuries

A *clamping injury* is a body part that is caught or strangled by some piece of machinery (Figure 28-24✱). Most clamping injuries involve a finger or hand caught in an opening (the mouth of a bottle, for example). Time is a factor because the longer a part remains clamped, the more damage there may be. Also, edema makes removal more difficult over time.

In general, if a body part is trapped in a clamping object and the patient is stable, apply a lubricant (K-Y Jelly, for example) and slowly attempt to wiggle the part loose. If possible, elevate the body part above the level of the patient's head to decrease circulation pressure as you attempt to remove the part.

If a clamping injury causes severe bleeding or shock and if the patient cannot be rapidly disentangled, immediately transport the patient. Lifesaving measures may then be initiated and the clamping object removed later by emergency department personnel. If the clamping object is too large to transport, specialized personnel may be required to cut away parts of the machine or other clamping object and disentangle the patient.

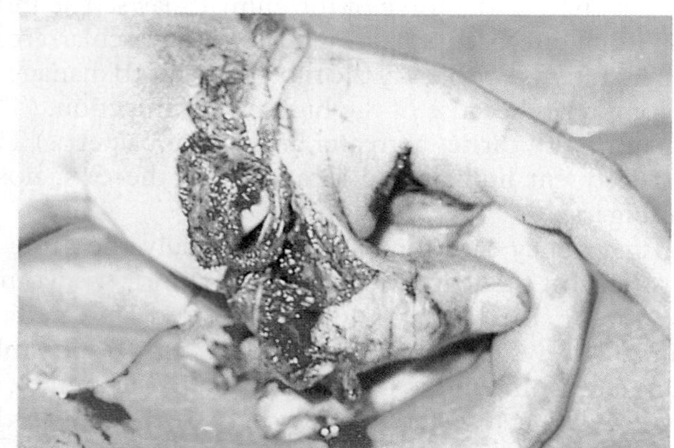

FIGURE 28-24 ✱ Clamping injury.

Assessment-Based Approach: Open Soft Tissue Injuries

If you are responding to a known scene of violence or to an accident, check with dispatch to make certain that the appropriate resources have been marshaled (police have secured the scene, for example, or special extrication teams have been notified). Since there is an increased likelihood of exposure to blood or body fluids when you treat a patient with open injuries, be sure to wear the appropriate personal protective equipment, including gloves and eye protection. In cases of potential splattering, a protective mask should be worn.

Scene Size-Up and Primary Assessment

Make sure the scene is safe before you enter, and take notice of potential mechanisms of injury. Be prepared to stabilize the cervical spine if the mechanism of injury or signs and symptoms suggest it may be necessary.

Get a general impression of the patient and the patient's mental status as you approach. When you reach the patient, ensure an open airway. If severe injuries or hemorrhagic shock are suspected or apparent and breath-

Key Points
Unless bleeding is severe, care for open soft tissue injuries is performed after the primary assessment.

Objective 28-12
Explain special considerations and care for chest and abdominal injuries, impaled objects, amputations, and large neck injuries.

Key Terms
occlusive dressing a dressing that can form an airtight seal over a wound.

ing is adequate, provide oxygen by nonrebreather mask at 15 lpm. If breathing is inadequate, initiate positive pressure ventilation with supplemental oxygen connected to the ventilation device. Bring any severe bleeding under control with direct pressure.

Secondary Assessment

Conduct a secondary assessment. Assess baseline vital signs, and obtain a history. For patients without a significant mechanism of injury, without an altered mental status, and without multiple injuries, perform a modified secondary assessment, using components of the complete secondary assessment for the specific injury site.

Signs and Symptoms The signs and symptoms of open soft tissue injuries include the following:

- A break in the skin and external bleeding
- Localized swelling, pain, and discoloration at the injury site
- Possible signs and symptoms of internal bleeding and hemorrhagic shock

Emergency Medical Care

Unless bleeding is severe, emergency care for open soft tissue injuries is performed after the primary assessment.

1. **Take standard precautions.**
2. **Ensure an open airway and adequate breathing.** Provide oxygen by nonrebreather mask at 15 lpm or positive pressure ventilation with supplemental oxygen as needed.
3. **Expose the wound.** In order to completely assess the wound, expose the entire injury site. Cut away clothing and, if necessary, clear the area of blood and debris with sterile gauze, dressings, or the cleanest material available. Thoroughly assess and evaluate the patient for additional wounds or injuries.
4. **Control the bleeding with direct pressure.** Use a tourniquet if bleeding is not controlled with direct pressure.
5. **Prevent further contamination.** Keep the wound as clean as possible. If there are loose particles of foreign material around the wound, wipe them away with a sterile gauze or similar clean material. Always wipe away from the wound, never toward it. Never pick out embedded particles or debris.
6. **Dress and bandage the wound.** If not already done, apply a dry sterile dressing. Secure it with a bandage. Check distal pulses both before and after applying the bandage to be sure it is not too tight.
7. **Keep the patient calm and quiet.** Remember that an early sign of shock is restlessness and anxiety. The more excited a patient becomes, the higher the heart rate and blood pressure, which may lead to increased bleeding.
8. **Treat for hemorrhagic shock.** If signs and symptoms are present, provide the appropriate care.
9. **Transport.**

Reassessment

Perform a reassessment by repeating the primary assessment, monitoring vital signs, and rechecking interventions.

Special Considerations

All of the emergency care steps just described apply to the specific injuries discussed in detail in the next sections: chest injuries, abdominal injuries, impaled objects, amputations, and large open neck injuries. *In all of these cases, ensure an open airway. Administer oxygen or, if breathing is inadequate, provide positive pressure ventilation with supplemental oxygen attached to the ventilation device.*

Chest Injuries A chest injury may prevent adequate respiration by causing the lung to collapse. In cases of penetrating chest wounds:

1. **Use an occlusive dressing to prevent air from entering the chest cavity through the wound** (a condition known as an *open pneumothorax*). An **occlusive dressing** (one that can form an airtight seal), such as Vaseline gauze, household plastic wrap, or the plastic bag from a dressing or oxygen mask, should be secured with tape on three sides (Figure 28-25*). A commercial device, such as an Asherman chest seal, can also be

ASSESSMENT Tips

A tension pneumothorax will present with signs and symptoms of severe respiratory distress and cardiovascular compromise as evidenced by hypotension, narrow pulse pressure, increasing heart rate, and pale, cool, and clammy skin. ■

Thinking Critically

What is the difference between how you should tape an occlusive dressing to an open chest wound and how you should tape an occlusive dressing to an open abdominal wound? Why are these dressings taped differently?

Key Terms

evisceration a protrusion of organs from a wound.

impaled object an object embedded in the body.

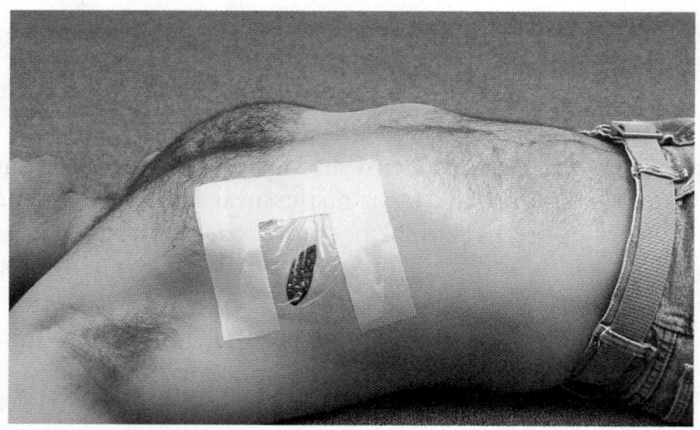

FIGURE 28-25 * Open chest injury with occlusive dressing taped on three sides. (© Shout Picture Library)

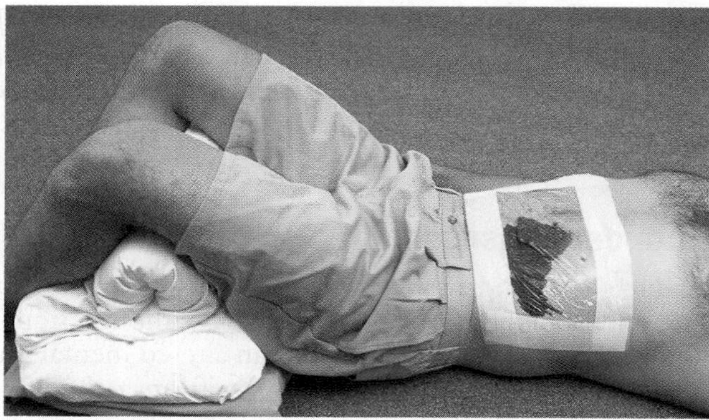

FIGURE 28-26 * Cover the abdominal organs with a moist sterile dressing and an occlusive covering.

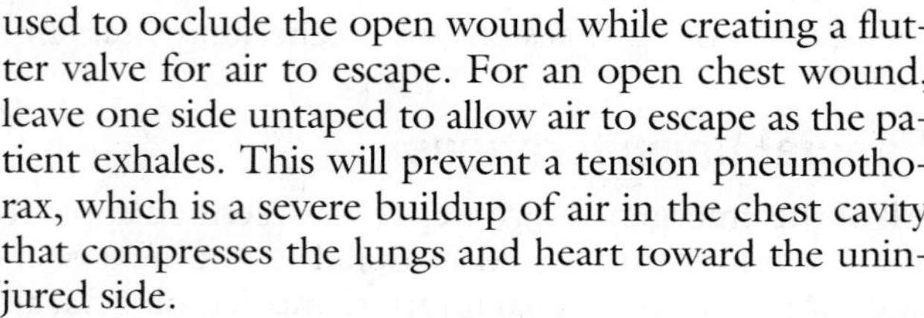

used to occlude the open wound while creating a flutter valve for air to escape. For an open chest wound, leave one side untaped to allow air to escape as the patient exhales. This will prevent a tension pneumothorax, which is a severe buildup of air in the chest cavity that compresses the lungs and heart toward the uninjured side.

2. **If there is no suspected spinal injury, the patient may assume a position of comfort or any position that allows for easiest chest expansion.** (However, with any significant mechanism of injury to the chest, including gunshots, spinal injury should be assumed. Spinal stabilization must be established and maintained until complete spinal immobilization is done.)

Abdominal Injuries Abdominal wounds sometimes result in an **evisceration** (internal abdominal organs protrude through the wound). Follow these guidelines when dealing with such an injury:

1. **Do not touch the abdominal organs or try to replace the exposed organs.** You may cause further damage and increase contamination of the organs and abdominal cavity.
2. **Cover the exposed organs.** Use a sterile dressing moistened with sterile water or saline. The dressing should be large enough to cover all of the protruding organs. Sterile gauze is preferred. Avoid all absorbent materials, such as toilet tissue or paper towels, which may cling to the organs. Then loosely cover the moistened dressing with an occlusive dressing taped on all four sides (Figure 28-26*). Maintain temperature with layers of a more bulky dressing, such as a particle-free bath blanket or towel. Do not apply the PASG if it is used in your system.
3. **Flex the patient's hips and knees, if they are uninjured and if spinal injury is not suspected.** This will help to decrease the tension of the abdominal muscles. Placing pillows or other materials under the patient's knees also may be helpful. (However, suspect spinal injury with a significant mechanism of injury to the abdomen.)

Impaled Objects An **impaled object** (an object still embedded in a wound) should never be removed in the field, unless it is through the cheek or the neck where it is obstructing airflow through the trachea (Figure 28-27*).

Emergency medical care for a patient with an impaled object includes the following (EMT Skills 28-8A to 28-8C):

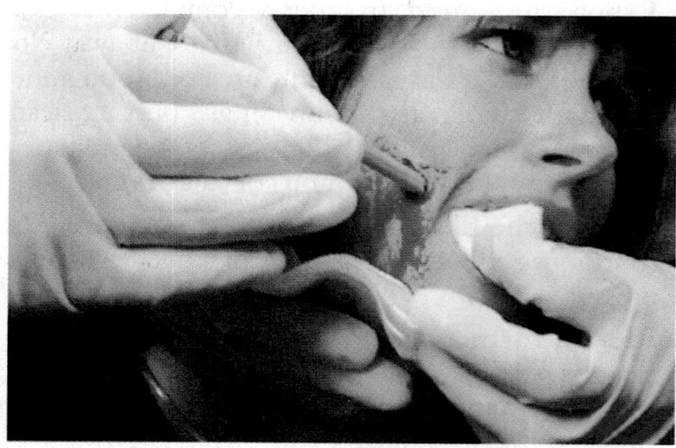

FIGURE 28-27 * An impaled object in the cheek may be removed. Dress outside of wound and inside between cheek and teeth.

1. **Manually secure the object.** Prevent any motion, which can cause further damage and bleeding.
2. **Expose the wound area.** Remove clothing from around the wound, but be careful to cause no further motion of the object.
3. **Control bleeding.** Apply direct pressure to the wound edges. Avoid putting undue pressure on the impaled object.
4. **Use a bulky dressing to help stabilize the object.** Surround the entire impaled object with dressings. Pack them around the object, and tape it securely in place to avoid motion during transport. A dressing formed into a ring or doughnut shape may be used to stabilize the object. If it is in the abdomen, do not use the PASG if it is used in your system.

Amputations In amputation injuries, you must care for the amputated part, as well as for the patient and the injury site. Your handling of the amputated part can have significant impact on the success of surgical reattachment.

First, provide emergency medical care to the patient. Enlist others to look for any missing body parts. Once a body part is located, follow these guidelines (Figure 28-28*):

1. **Remove any gross contamination by flushing the part with sterile water or saline.** Never immerse the part in water or sterile saline, since this may damage it.
2. **Wrap the part in a dry sterile gauze dressing.** (Check with local medical direction, which may dictate the use of moist dressings instead.)
3. **Wrap or bag the amputated part in plastic.** Place it in a plastic bag or plastic wrap in accordance with local protocol. Label the bag with the patient's name, date, and time the part was wrapped and bagged.
4. **Keep the amputated part cool.** Place the wrapped and bagged part in a cooler or other suitable container with an ice pack or ice on the bottom to keep the part cool. Do not place the part directly on the ice pack or ice to avoid any possibility of freezing the part. The container should also be marked with the patient's name, date, and body part.
5. **Transport the part with the patient, if at all possible.** In some cases, however, this may not be possible, especially when the part has not been located. In this instance, arrange for immediate transport of the body part, once it is found, to the same facility to which the patient has been transported.

Note: If an amputation is incomplete and the body part is still partially attached, do not complete the amputation. Care for the wound as previously described, but also make sure that the partially amputated part is not twisted or constricted. Immobilize the injured area to prevent further injury.

Large Open Neck Injuries In addition to severe bleeding from a wound involving the major blood vessels of the neck, there is the danger of air being sucked into a neck vein and carried to the heart, which can be lethal. Bleeding control and prevention of an **air embolism** (air bubble) are the major goals (Figure 28-29*). Assess any neck wound for major blood vessel involvement. Arterial bleeding will be profuse with bright red blood spurting from the wound and is a grave sign. Venous bleeding will be dark red and flowing steadily from the wound.

In general, follow these guidelines for care of a large open neck wound:

1. *Place a gloved hand over the wound to control bleeding.*
2. *Apply an occlusive dressing,* which should extend beyond all wound edges to avoid air or part of the

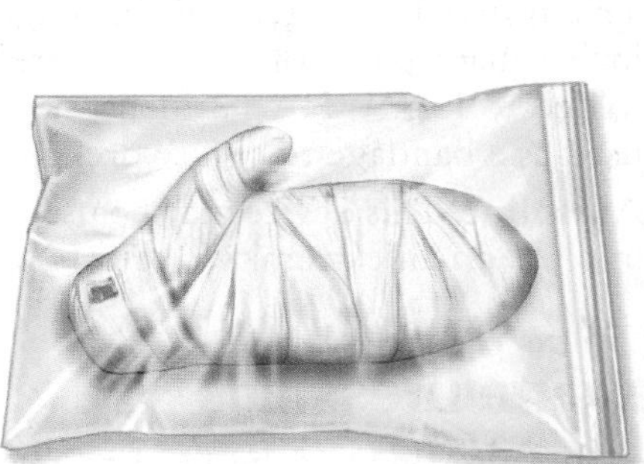

(1) Wrap completely in sterile dressings Place in plastic bag and seal shut.

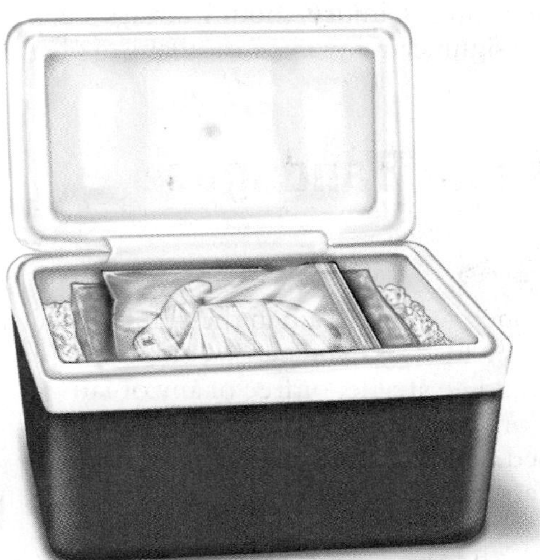

(2) Place sealed bag in a cooler or other suitable container to keep it cool.

FIGURE 28-28 * Emergency care for amputated part. Follow local protocol.

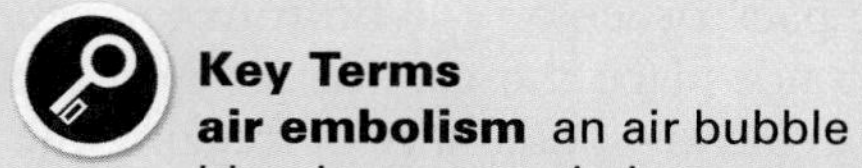

Key Terms
air embolism an air bubble that enters the bloodstream and obstructs a blood vessel.

Objective 28-13
Describe various types of dressings and bandages, including the purpose and methods of applying pressure dressings, and discuss general principles of dressing and bandaging.

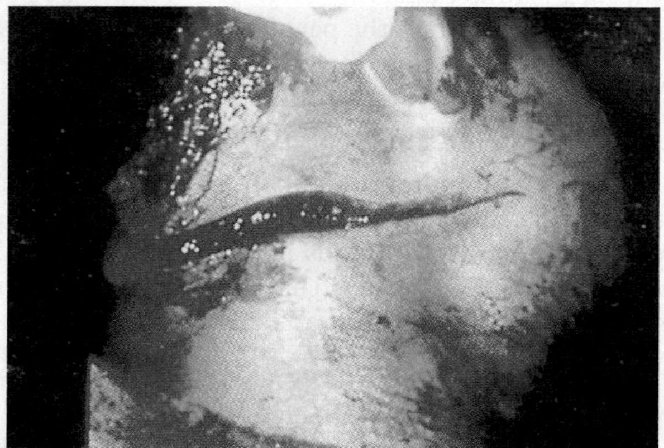

FIGURE 28-29 * Open wound to the neck.

dressing being sucked into the wound. Tape the dressing on all four sides.

3. *Cover the occlusive dressing with a regular dressing.*
4. *Apply only enough pressure to control the bleeding.* Compress the carotid artery only if it is severed and it is necessary to control bleeding.
5. *Once bleeding is controlled, apply a pressure dressing,* taking care not to restrict airflow or compress the major blood vessels in the neck. Such a dressing should not be applied circumferentially around the neck. (Direct pressure is preferred.)
6. *If there is a suspected spinal injury, provide appropriate immobilization.* Spinal injury should always be suspected with any significant injury or mechanism of injury to the neck.

Dressings and Bandages

Dressings

A **dressing** covers an open wound to aid in the control of bleeding and to prevent further damage or contamination. The dressing should be **sterile,** or free of any organisms (bacteria, virus, or spore) that may cause infection. Commercially wrapped and packaged dressings are available in various types and sizes.

The following are common types of dressings (Figures 28-30a to 28-30d*):

- **Gauze pad.** Available in various sizes (2″ × 2″, 4″ × 4″, 5″ × 9″, and so on), a gauze pad is made of layered gauze.
- **Self-adhering dressing.** This type of dressing adheres to itself when overlapped. It is available in various sizes and may also be used as a roller bandage.
- **Universal or multitrauma dressing.** This is a bulky dressing, usually 10″ × 36″, and is used on large areas such as abdominal wounds. (Also called abdominal or ABD pads.)
- **Occlusive dressing.** This dressing creates an airtight seal for open abdominal, chest, and large neck injuries. A petroleum-type occlusive dressing is impregnated with petroleum to prevent adhering to the open wound. An improvised occlusive dressing may be made from sterile plastic wrap, plastic bags, or a similar material.

  Note: Plastic is preferred over aluminum foil as an occlusive dressing, because foil has been found to cause further damage to exposed internal organs, and it is not as pliable as plastic.

Bandages

Once a dressing is applied, a **bandage** is used to secure a dressing in place (EMT Skills 28-9A to 28-9G). In most cases it is not necessary for a bandage to be sterile, but it should be clean and free of debris. Bandages that may be used as dressings are also available in various types and sizes. The following are common types of bandages:

- **Self-adhering bandage.** This type of bandage adheres to itself when overlapped. It may be used as a dressing or as a roller bandage (EMT Skills 28-10A to 28-10C).
- **Gauze rolls.** Available in various sizes, this bandage is rolled meshed gauze.
- **Triangular bandage.** This bandage is usually a 40-inch square piece of cloth (Figure 28-31*). When folded to form a 2- or 3-inch-wide cravat, it may be used as a bandage to secure dressings.
- **Air splint.** This device may be used to hold dressings in place on an extremity (Figure 28-32*).

Pressure Dressings

A pressure dressing can be used to maintain control of bleeding. Apply a pressure dressing in the following way:

1. *Cover the wound with several sterile gauze dressings or a sterile bulky dressing.*

Key Terms

dressing a sterile covering for an open wound.

sterile free from living microorganisms that may cause infection.

Key Terms

bandage any material used to secure a dressing in place.

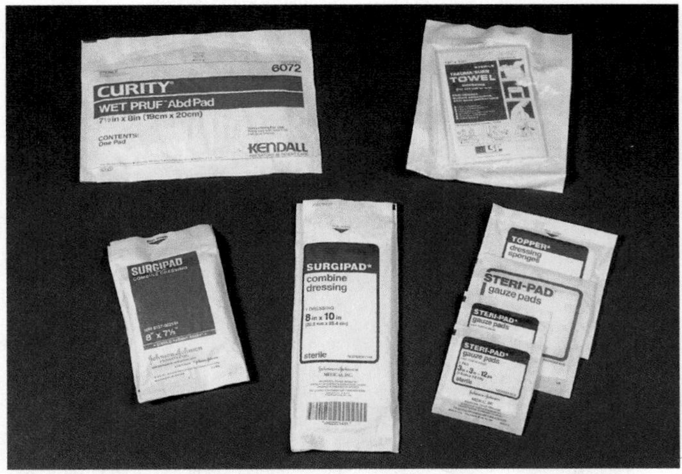

FIGURE 28-30a ✱ Sterile gauze pads.

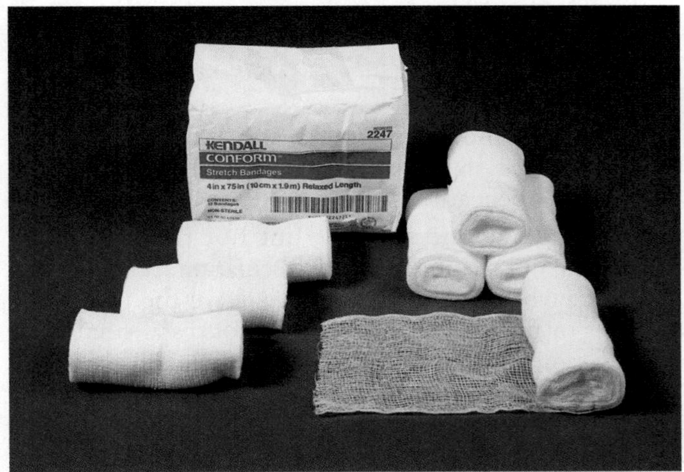

FIGURE 28-30b ✱ Nonelastic, self-adhering dressing and roller bandages.

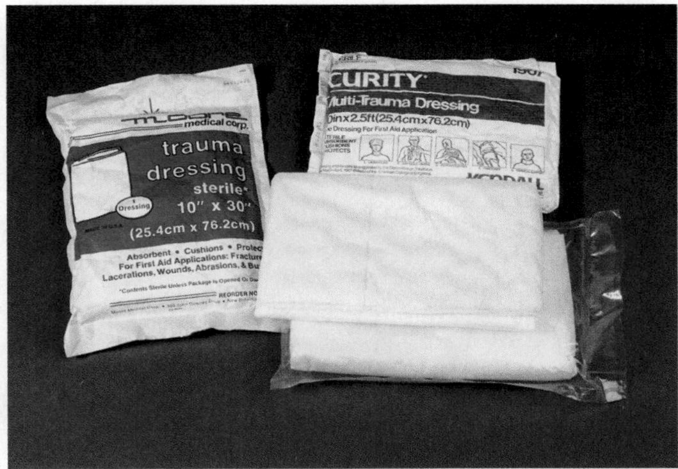

FIGURE 28-30c ✱ Multitrauma dressings.

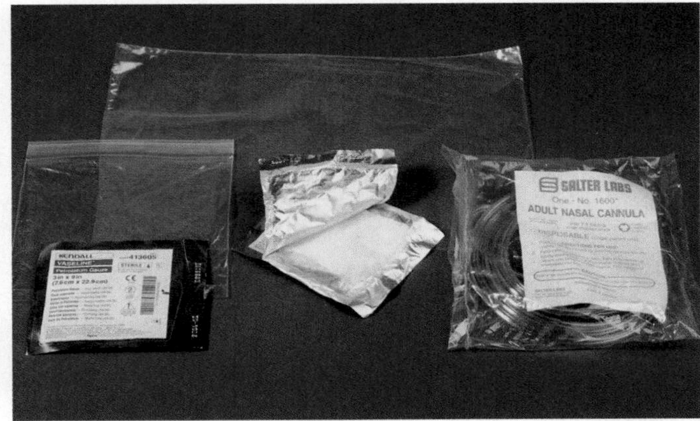

FIGURE 28-30d ✱ Materials that can be used as occlusive dressings.

2. *Apply direct pressure* over the wound until the bleeding is controlled.
3. *Bandage firmly* to create enough pressure to maintain control of the bleeding. Check distal pulses to be sure the bandage is not too tight. An air splint or blood pressure cuff can also be used to hold a pressure dressing in place. If you use a blood pressure cuff, be sure that distal pulses are still present after inflation.
4. *If blood soaks through the original dressing and bandage, indicating continued severe bleeding, remove them and apply direct fingertip pressure.* Once the bleeding is controlled, apply dressings and bandage over the wound again.

General Principles of Dressing and Bandaging

There are no hard-and-fast rules for dressing and bandaging wounds. Often, adaptability and creativity are far more important ingredients. In dressing and bandaging, use the materials you have on hand and the methods you

Key Points

Keep dressings as free of dirt and debris as possible.

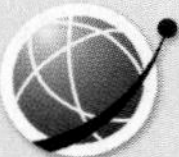

Media Resources

Go to www.bradybooks.com for mykit. Highlights:

- *Web Resource:* Tourniquets
- *Video:* Shock

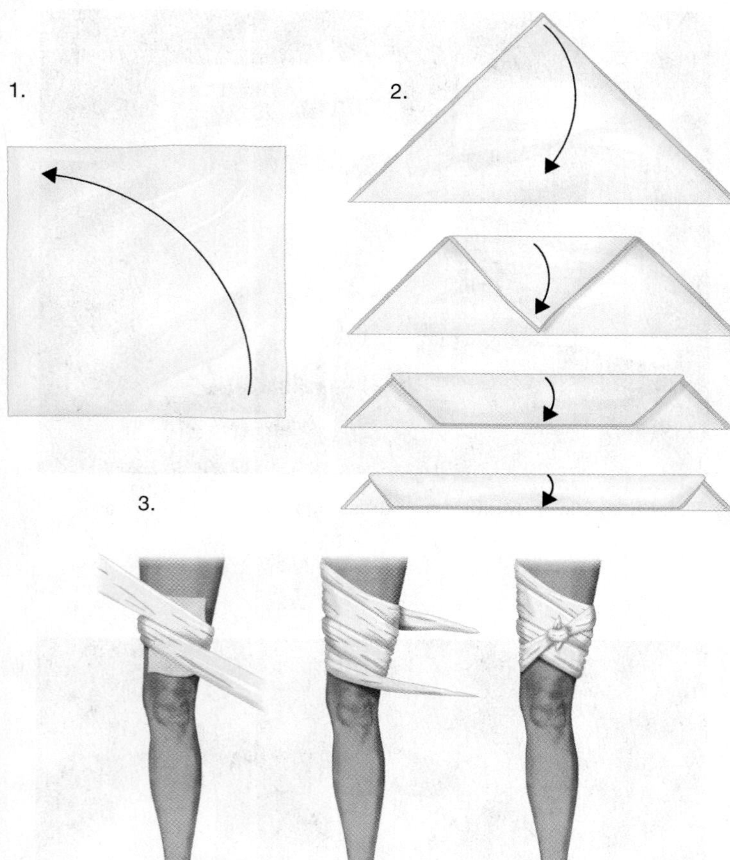

FIGURE 28-31 ✱ Triangular bandage as cravat.

can best adapt, as long as the following conditions are generally met:

- **Dressing materials should be as clean as possible.** Sterile materials are always preferable. When you open dressing packages or handle any materials that you will use as dressings, do so carefully to keep those materials as free of dirt and debris as possible.
- **Do not bandage a dressing in place until bleeding has stopped.**
- **A dressing should adequately cover the entire wound.** All edges of a dressing should be covered by the bandage. Tape bandages in place or secure with a square knot. Make sure there are no loose ends of cloth, gauze, or tape that could get caught when the patient is transported.

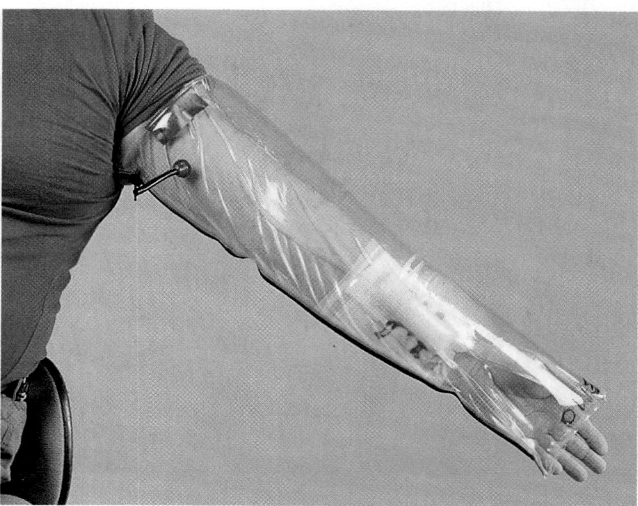

FIGURE 28-32 ✱ An inflatable air splint.

- **If possible, remove all jewelry from the injured body part.** Jewelry may interfere with circulation if swelling occurs.
- **Do not bandage a wound too loosely.** Bandages should not slip or shift and should not allow the dressing beneath to slip or shift.
- **Bandage wounds snugly, but not too tightly.** Be careful not to interfere with circulation. If the injured part involves the hands or feet, leave the tips of the toes or fingers exposed to allow for distal circulation assessments. For circumferential bandages, check distal pulses and motor and sensory function before and after bandage application.
- **If you are bandaging a small wound on an extremity, cover a larger area with the bandage.** This will help avoid creating a pressure point, and it will distribute pressure more uniformly.
- **Always place the body part to be bandaged in the position in which it is to remain.** Avoid bandaging across a joint, and do not try bending a joint after the bandage has been applied.
- **Apply a tourniquet if bleeding is not controlled with direct pressure.** Once in place, a tourniquet must not be removed in the field.

Summary: Assessment and Care

To review possible assessment findings and emergency care for soft tissue injuries, see Figures 28-33✱ and 28-34✱.

Assessment Summary

SOFT TISSUE TRAUMA

The following findings may be associated with soft tissue injury.

SCENE SIZE-UP

Pay particular attention to your own safety. Look for:
- Mechanism of injury
- Splatters or pools of blood at the scene
- Blood-soaked clothing
- Penetrating trauma
- Blunt trauma

Primary Assessment

General Impression
- Obvious massive external hemorrhage
- Extremely pale color
- Open or closed injuries to body

Mental Status
- Alert to unresponsive, based on amount of blood loss and shock
- As blood loss continues, mental status decreases

Airway
- May be closed if mental status is altered
- May be bleeding in airway from trauma

Breathing
- Initially fast and normal to deeper tidal volume
- *May become shallow and fast or slow as blood loss and shock progress*
- May be absent or inadequate if bleeding in chest or associated with chest injury
- May be fast and shallow if abdominal injury is present

Circulation
- Pulses possibly difficult to find if extreme blood loss
- Increased heart rate that becomes extremely elevated, then suddenly decreases with continued blood loss
- Pulses becoming extremely weak or absent as blood loss and shock continue
- Skin becoming increasingly pale, cool, and clammy as blood loss and shock progress

Status: Priority patient if uncontrolled bleeding or shock is suspected

Secondary Assessment

Physical Exam

Head, neck, and face:
- Look for large laceration to neck that may cause air emboli

Chest:
- Open wound to chest

Abdomen:
- Rigid, distended abdomen
- Discoloration around umbilicus or in flank area (late)
- Penetrating or blunt trauma
- Pain on palpation
- Abdominal evisceration

Extremities:
- Obvious external bleeding
- Swelling, pain, and discoloration at injury site
- Flaps or complete avulsions
- Amputations

Baseline Vital Signs

BP: normal; may decrease or become absent in shock
HR: normal or increased in shock
RR: normal or increased in shock
Skin: normal or pale, cool, clammy, cyanotic in shock
Pupils: normal or dilated and sluggish to respond in shock

SAMPLE History

Signs and symptoms of closed soft tissue injury:
- Swelling
- Pain
- Discoloration
- Shock if associated with internal injury

Signs and symptoms of open soft tissue injury:
- Abrasions
- Lacerations
- Punctures
- Avulsions
- Amputations
- Obvious external bleeding
- Shock if associated with significant bleeding

FIGURE 28-33a ✱ Assessment summary: soft tissue trauma.

Emergency Care Protocol

SOFT TISSUE TRAUMA

1. Establish manual in-line stabilization if spinal injury is suspected.
2. Control any major life-threatening bleeding.
3. Establish and maintain an open airway. Insert a nasopharyngeal or oropharyngeal airway if the patient is unresponsive and has no gag or cough reflex.
4. Suction secretions as necessary.
5. If breathing is inadequate, provide positive pressure ventilation with supplemental oxygen at a rate of 10–12 ventilations/minute for an adult and 12–20 ventilations/minute for an infant or child.
6. If breathing is adequate, administer oxygen based on the SpO_2 reading and patient signs and symptoms. If the SpO_2 reading is greater than 95% and no signs or symptoms of hypoxia, respiratory distress, or shock are present, oxygen may not be necessary. In this case, you may choose to apply nasal cannula at 2–4 lpm. If signs of hypoxia, respiratory distress, or shock are present, or the SpO_2 reading is less than 95%, place the patient on a nonrebreather mask at 15 lpm.
7. If there is an open chest injury, apply a nonporous dressing taped on three sides.
8. Control bleeding with direct pressure (use fingertip pressure).
9. Apply a tourniquet if bleeding is not controlled with direct pressure.
10. Apply sterile dressings and bandages.
11. Splint suspected fractures.
12. Maintain body temperature.
13. Consider PASG if indicated.
14. Place the patient supine.
15. If spinal injury is suspected, immobilize the patient to a backboard.
16. Manage specific soft tissue injuries as follows:
    Abdominal evisceration:
    Apply a moist sterile dressing over the wound and cover with a nonporous dressing taped on four sides. Position the patient supine and flex knees.
    Large laceration to neck:
    Apply direct pressure to stop bleeding. Apply a nonporous dressing taped on all four sides.
    Open chest wound:
    Apply a nonporous dressing taped on three sides.
    Impaled object:
    Apply dressings to the wound and stabilize in place. Remove the object only if impaled in the cheek or obstructing ventilation in the neck.
    Avulsion:
    Do not complete avulsion. Rinse the wound to clean off debris if necessary. Apply dressing and bandages to keep the avulsed tissue in place. Splint the extremity to limit movement.
    Amputation (partial):
    Do not complete a partial amputation. Realign the extremity to as normal a position as possible. Apply sterile dressings.
    Splint to immobilize and limit movement. Be prepared to control bleeding.
    Amputation (complete):
    Clean debris.
    Apply direct pressure to the stump to control bleeding. Apply sterile dressings and bandages. Wrap the amputated part in a dry, sterile gauze dressing. Then wrap or bag the amputated part in plastic and place on a cold pack or ice. Do not freeze. Transport with the patient, if possible.
17. Transport.
18. Perform reassessment every 5 minutes if unstable and every 15 minutes if stable.

FIGURE 28-33b ✻ Emergency care protocol: soft tissue trauma.

Emergency Care Algorithm: Open Soft Tissue Trauma

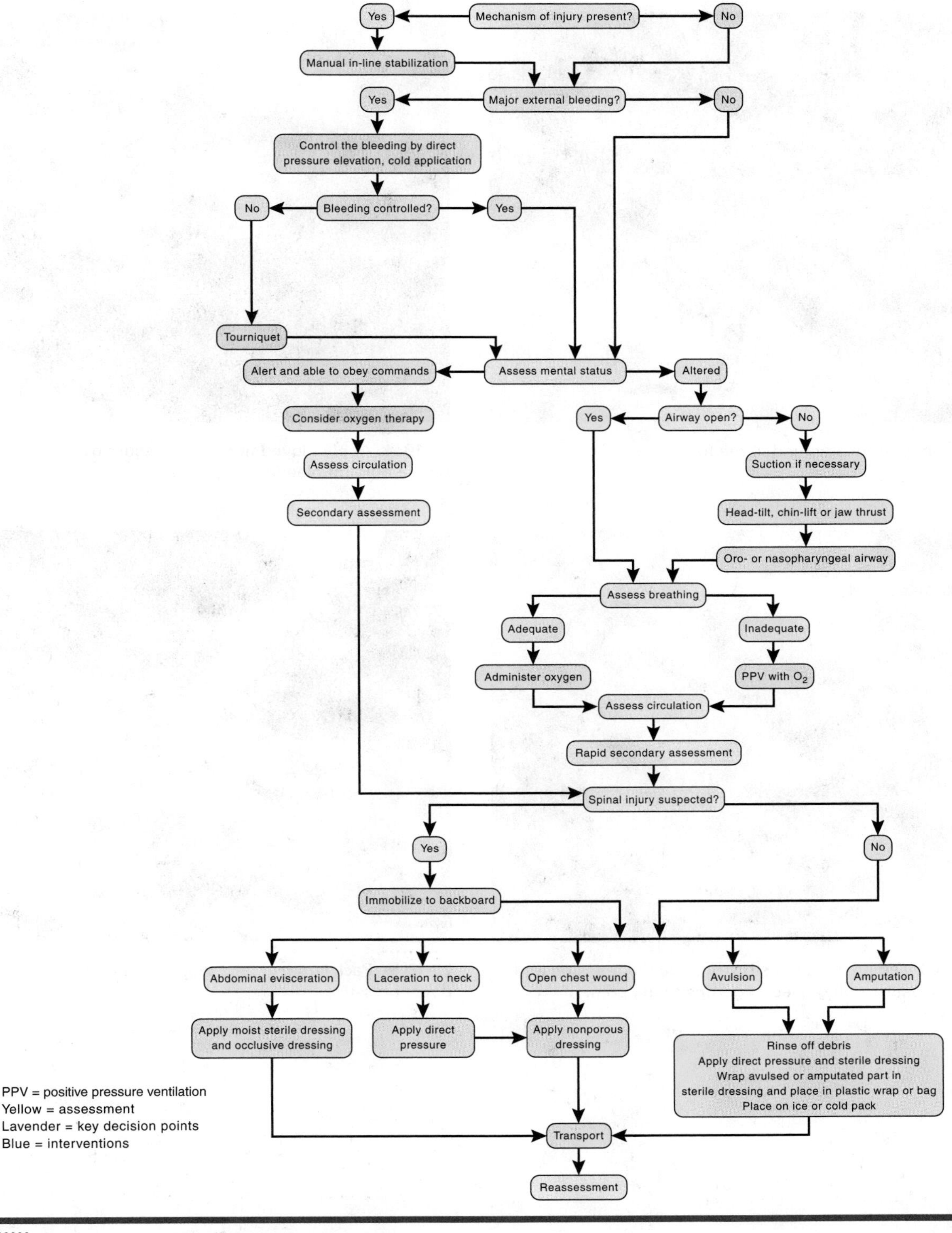

FIGURE 28-34 ✱ Emergency care algorithm: open soft tissue trauma.

EMT skills 28-1 Bleeding Control by Direct Pressure

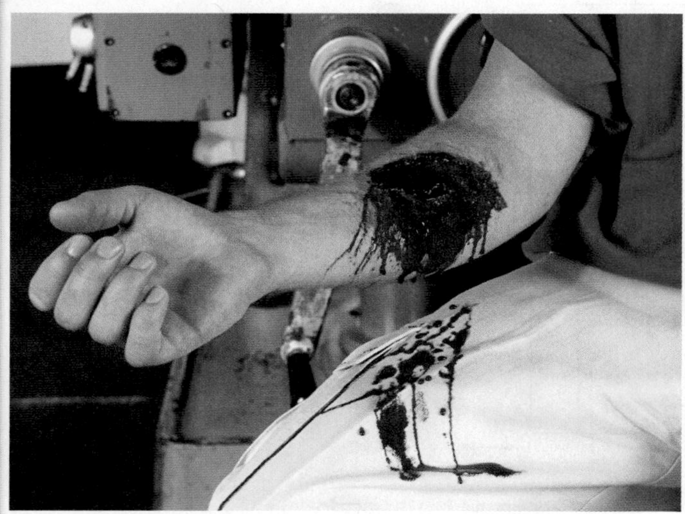

28-1A * Bleeding from a wound to the forearm.

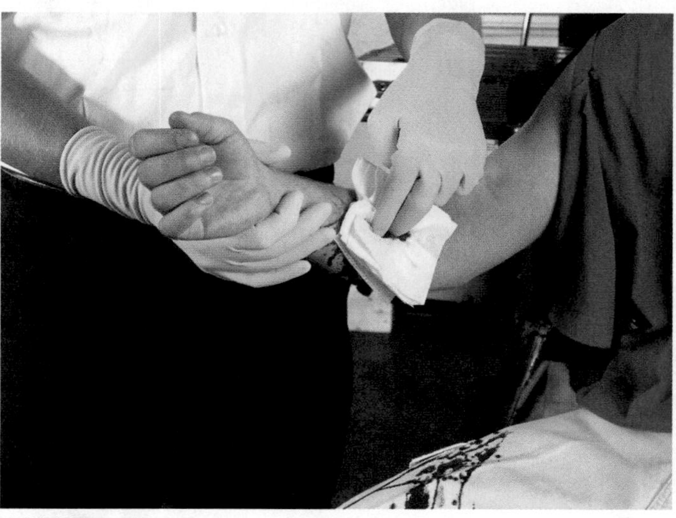

28-1B * Apply gloved fingertip pressure over a dressing directly on the point of bleeding.

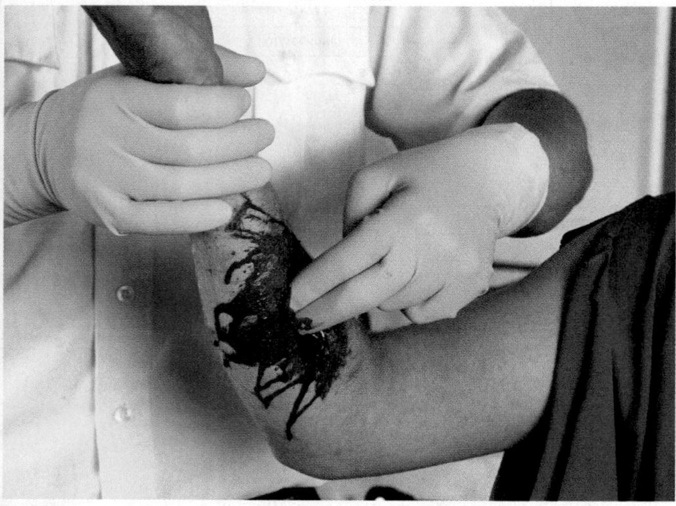

28-1C * If the bleeding does not stop, remove the dressing and apply direct pressure with gloved fingertips to the point of bleeding.

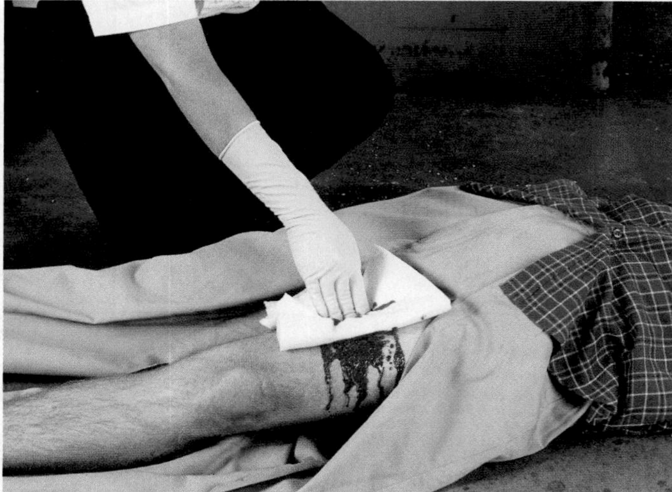

28-1D * Pack large, gaping wounds with sterile gauze and apply direct pressure.

EMT skills 28-2 Application of a Tourniquet

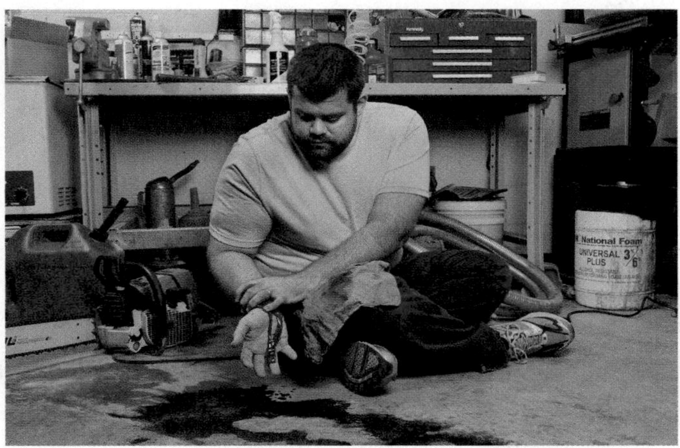

28-2A * First attempt to control bleeding by direct pressure.

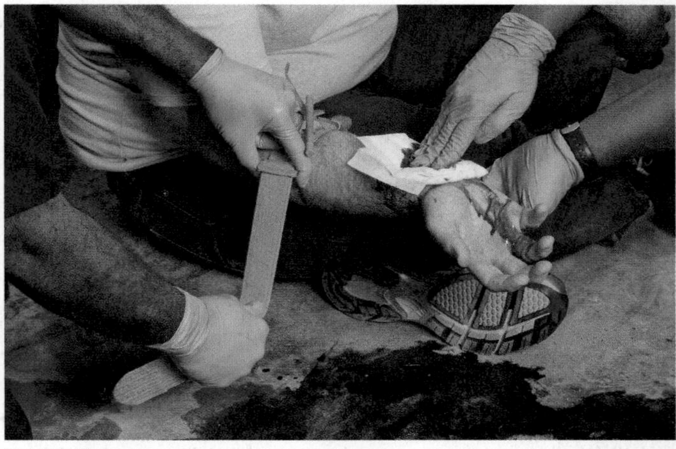

28-2B * If direct pressure is ineffective, apply direct pressure over a thick dressing while preparing the tourniquet.

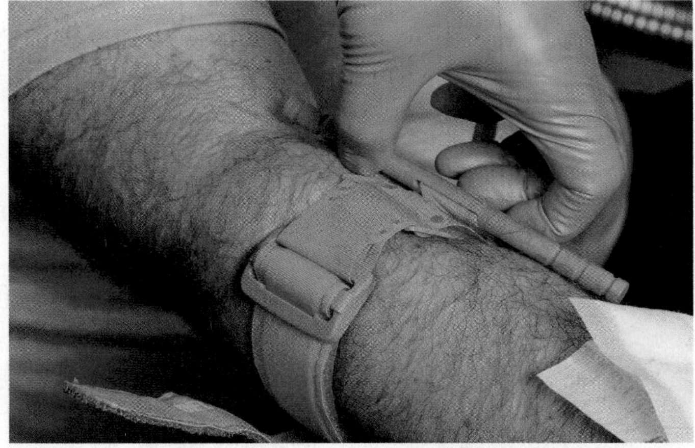

28-2C * Apply the tourniquet proximal to the wound but not over a joint.

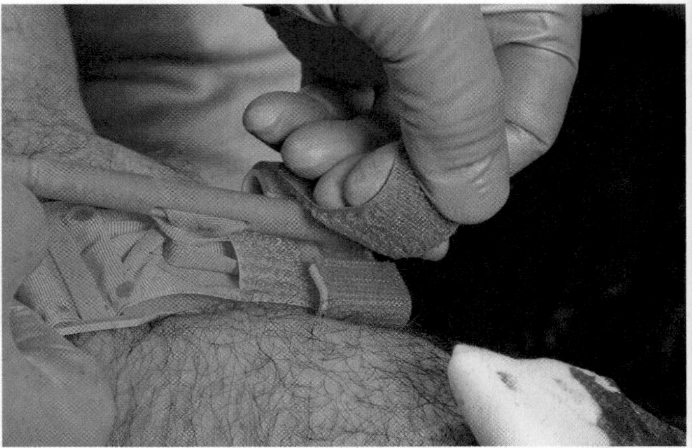

28-2D * Pack large, gaping wounds with sterile gauze and apply direct pressure. Twist the rod to tighten the tourniquet to the extent necessary to control bleeding and secure the tightening rod. Write the time of tourniquet application on tape and apply it to the tourniquet, leaving the tourniquet exposed to view, and notify the receiving facility that a tourniquet has been applied. Continuously reassess the wound for recurrent bleeding. Do not loosen or remove the tourniquet unless directed to do so by medical direction or local protocol.

EMT skills 28-3 Controlling a Nosebleed

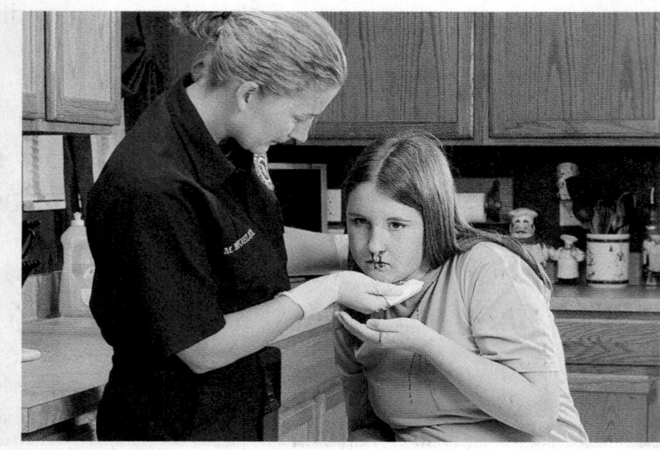

28-3A ✱ Have the patient sit and lean forward.

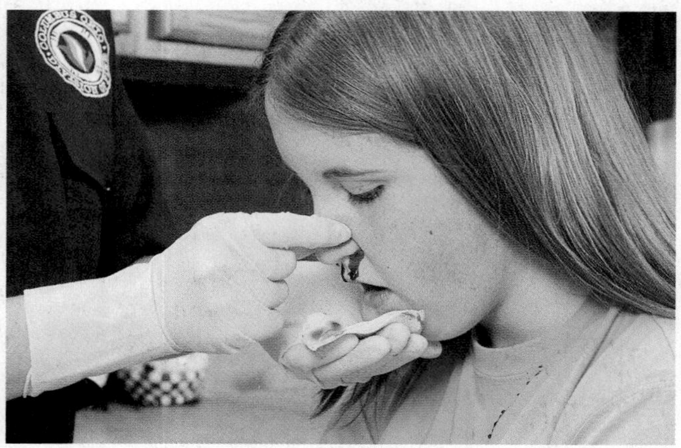

28-3B ✱ Pinch the fleshy part of the nostrils together.

EMT skills 28-4 Emergency Care for Shock

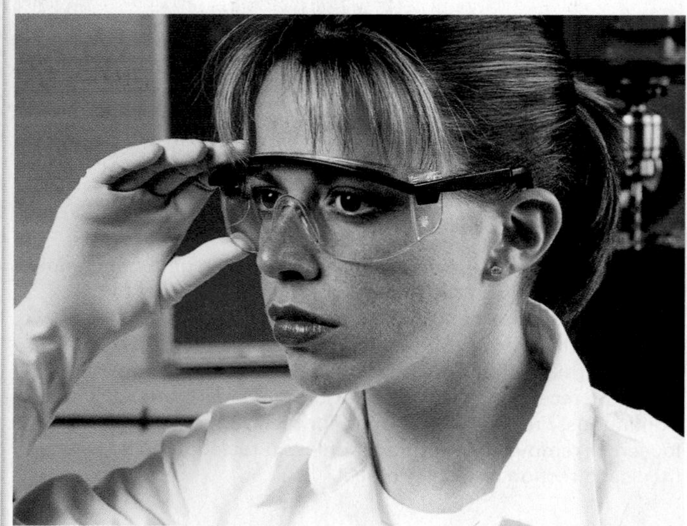

28-4A ✱ Take all necessary Standard Precautions.

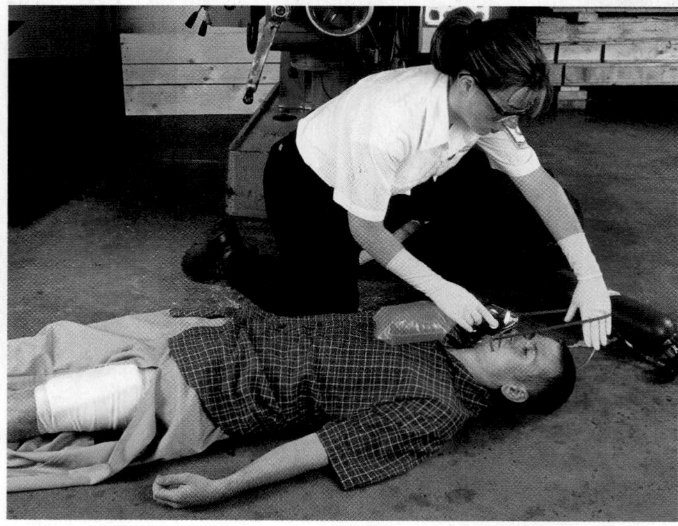

28-4B ✱ Administer oxygen by nonrebreather mask or positive pressure ventilation as needed.

EMT skills 28-4 Emergency Care for Shock *continued*

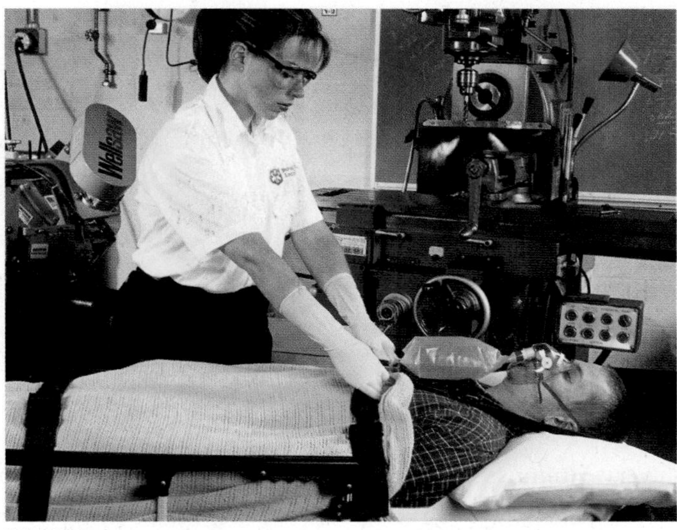

28-4C ✱ Cover the patient to prevent loss of body heat.

EMT skills 28-5 Applying the PASG

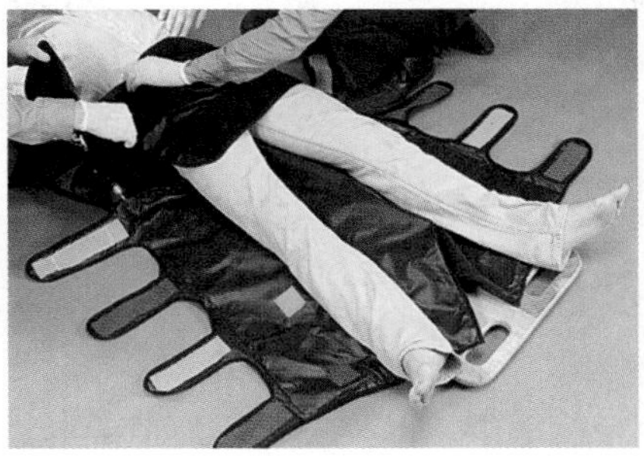

28-5A ✱ Log roll the patient onto the garment so the upper edge is below the patient's bottom rib.

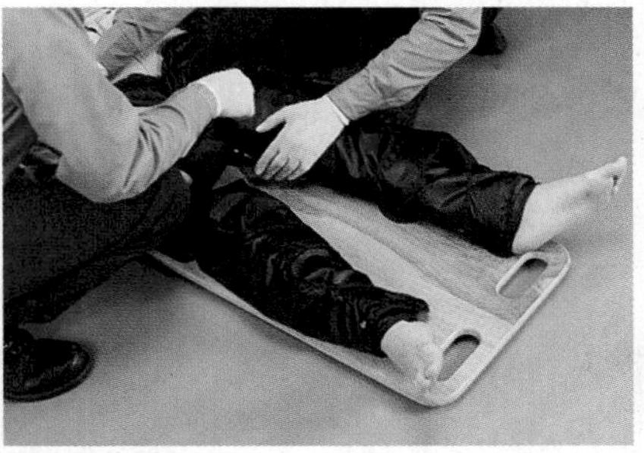

28-5B ✱ Enclose the legs one at a time, securing the Velcro straps.

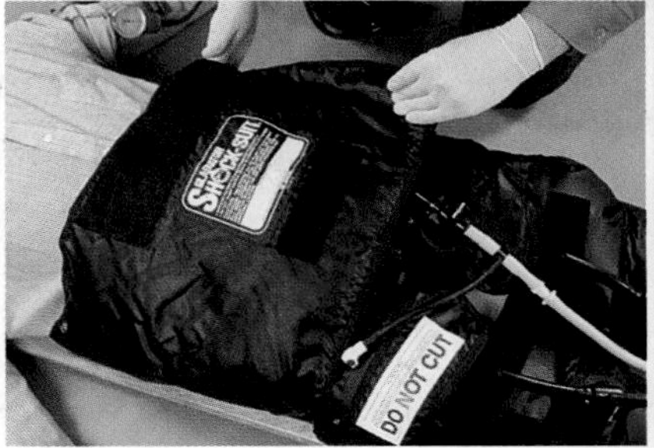

28-5C ✱ Enclose the abdomen and pelvis, securing the Velcro straps.

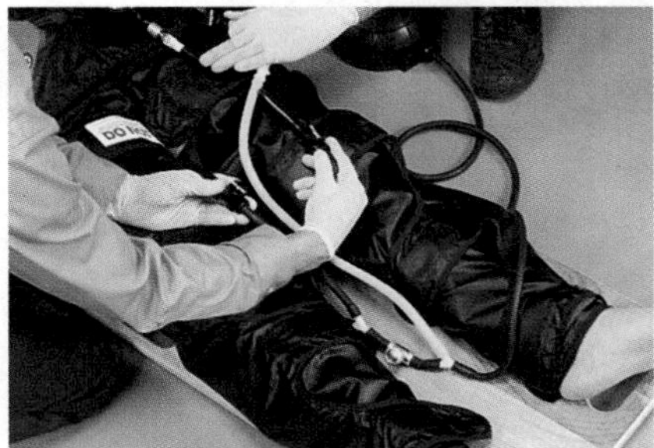

28-5D ✱ Check the tubes. Open the stopcocks to the legs; close the abdominal compartment stopcock.

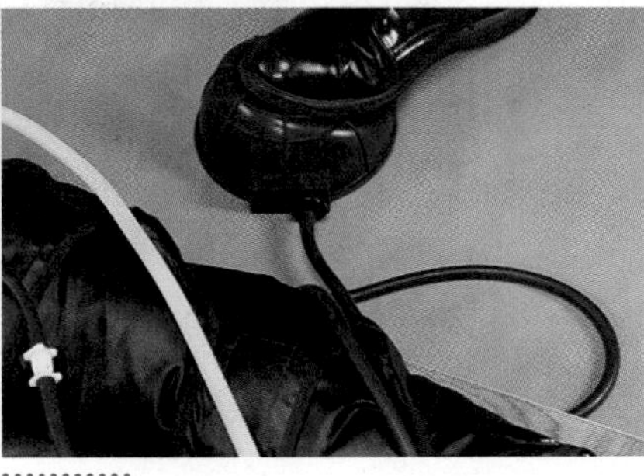

28-5E ✱ Inflate the lower compartments until the Velcro crackles. Close the stopcocks.

continued

EMT skills 28-5 Applying the PASG *continued*

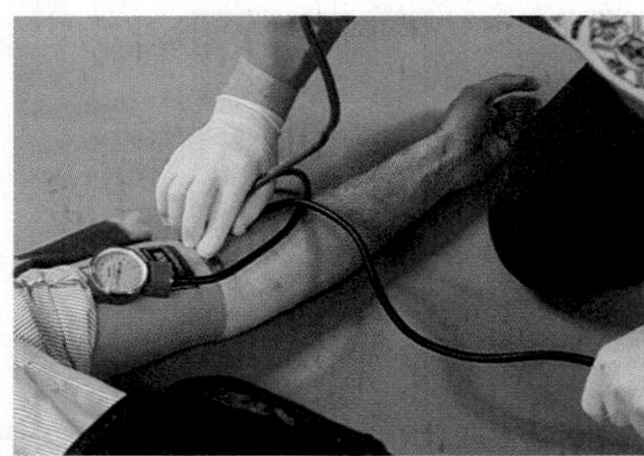

28-5F ✱ If the systolic blood pressure is below 90, open the stopcock, inflate the abdominal compartment, and close the stopcock.

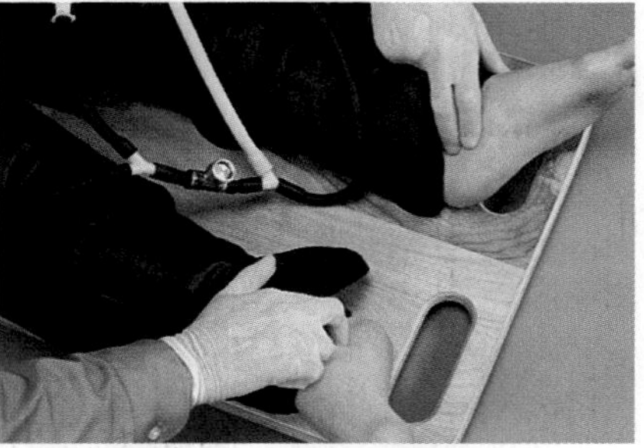

28-5G ✱ Check both extremities for a distal pulse.

Monitor and record vital signs every 5 minutes. If the garment loses pressure, add air as needed. Some protocols call for the inflation of all three compartments of the garment simultaneously. Always follow local protocols. Some systems require medical direction for application of a PASG.

Note: In these photos, the patient's clothing remains on for demonstration purposes. In actual use, clothing should be removed.

EMT skills 28-6 Soft Tissue Injuries

Soft tissue injuries can occur in a variety of ways, as shown in these photos.

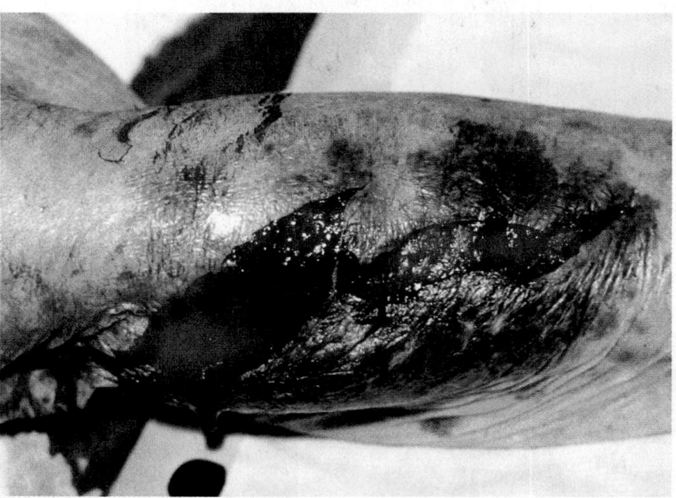

28-6A ✱ During a street altercation, one participant struck the other with a tire iron—blunt trauma resulting in an open soft tissue injury to the arm.

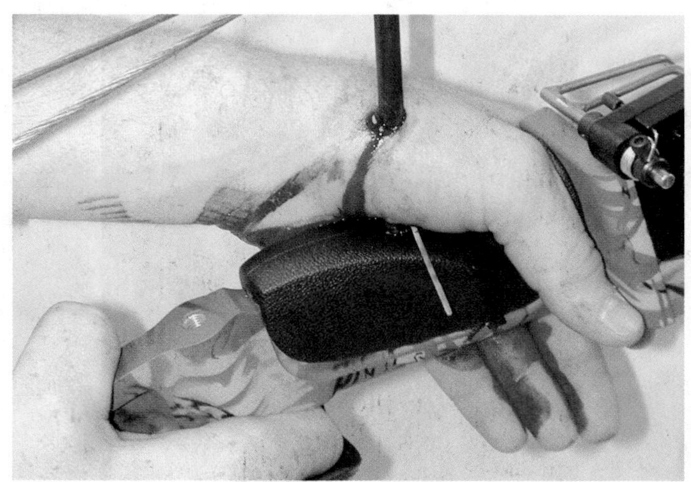

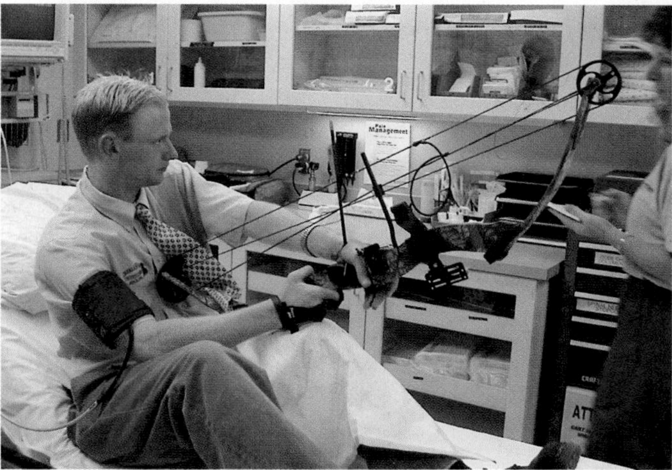

28-6B * **(1)** and **(2)** This patient, a salesman in a sporting goods store, was demonstrating a bow with a carbon fiber arrow. During the demonstration, the apparatus broke, releasing the arrow, which penetrated the patient's hand. (Both photos: © Charles Stewart, MD, and Associates)

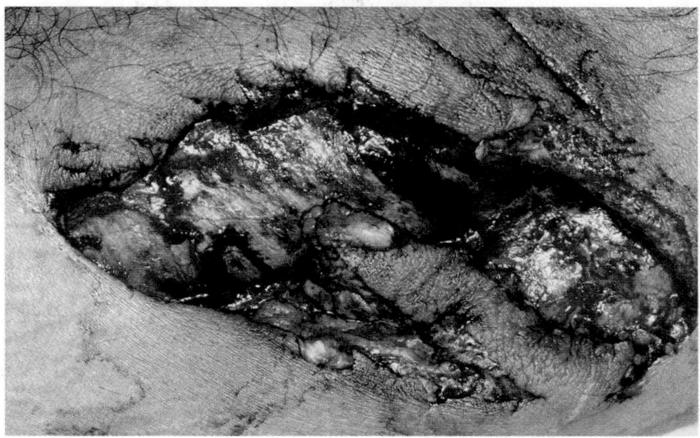

28-6C * Lawnmower accidents are all too common. This one caused a severe laceration to the patient's lower leg. (© Maria A. H. Lyle)

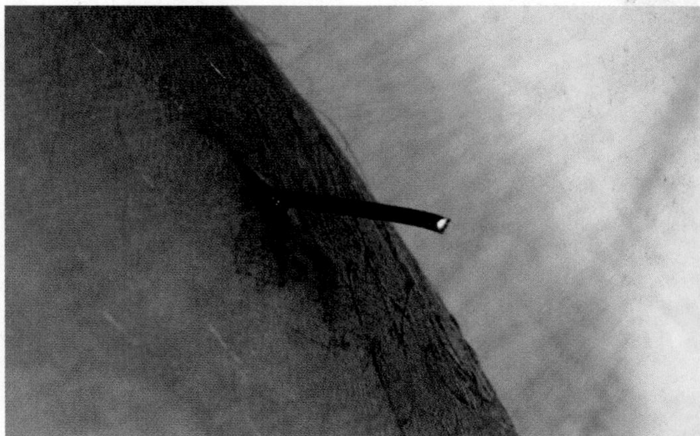

28-6D * A young teenager had a CD player in his room. When it fell from a shelf, a wire became impaled in the patient's leg. (© Maria A. H. Lyle)

Gunshot Wounds

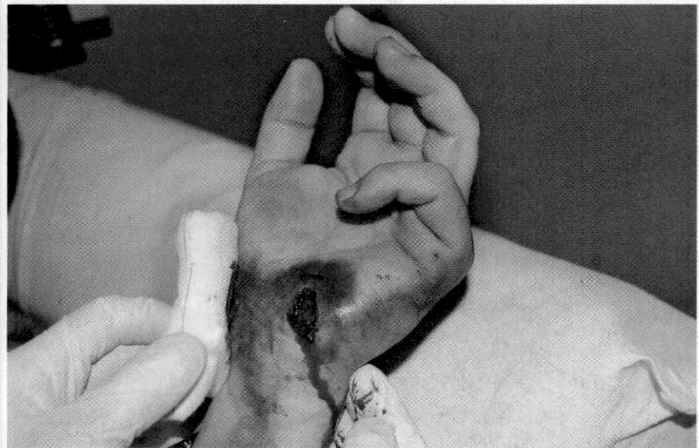

28-7A * Powder burns from gunshot. (© Edward T. Dickinson, MD)

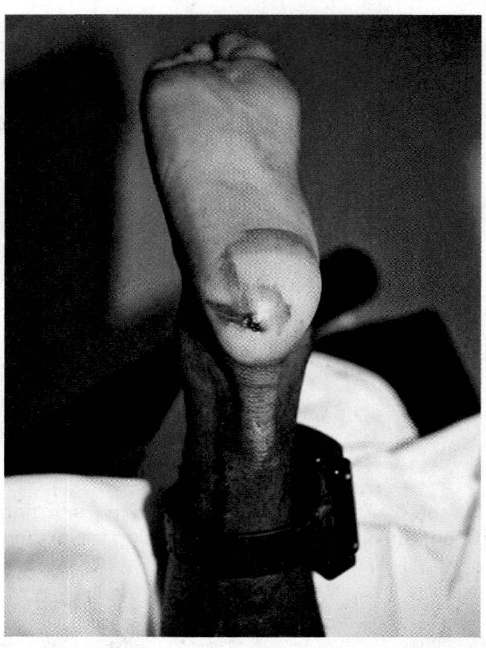

28-7B * Gunshot wound to the foot. (© Edward T. Dickinson, MD)

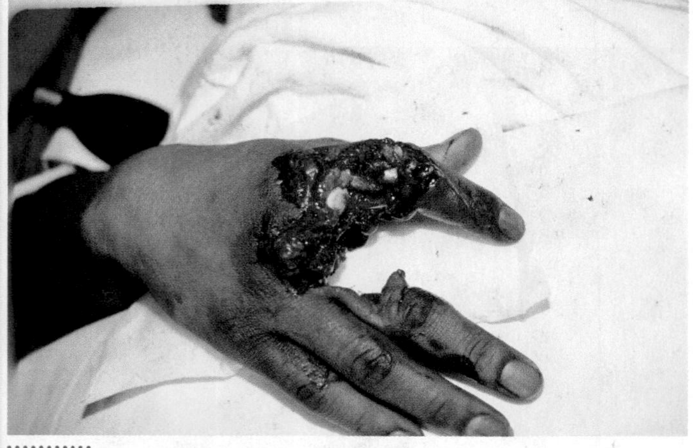

28-7C * Gunshot wound to fingers. (© Edward T. Dickinson, MD)

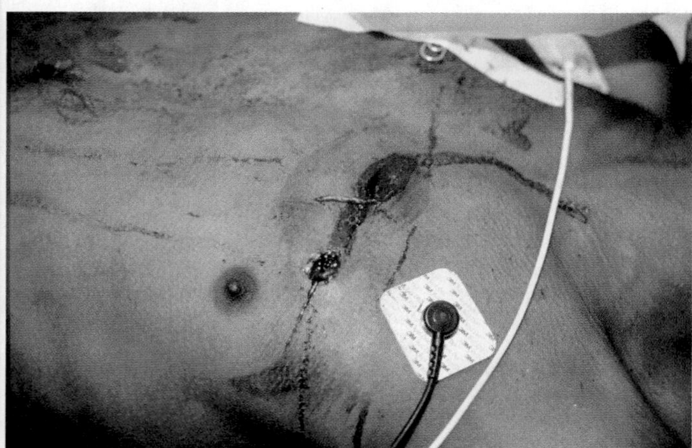

28-7D.1 * Gunshot entrance wound to the chest. (© Edward T. Dickinson, MD)

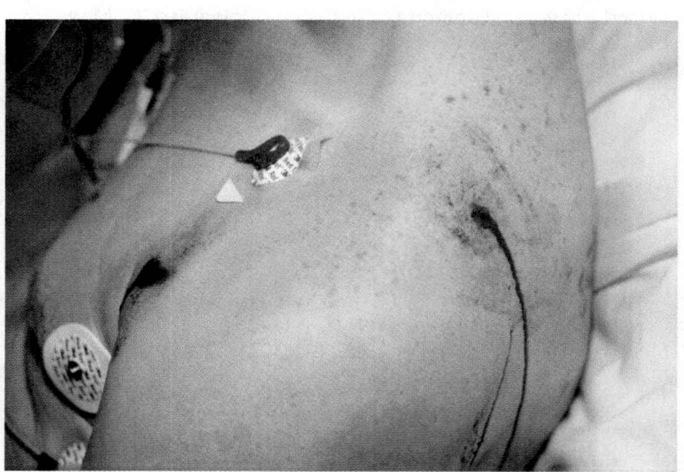

28-7D.2 * Gunshot exit wound from the shoulder. (© Edward T. Dickinson, MD)

EMT skills 28-7 Gunshot Wounds *continued*

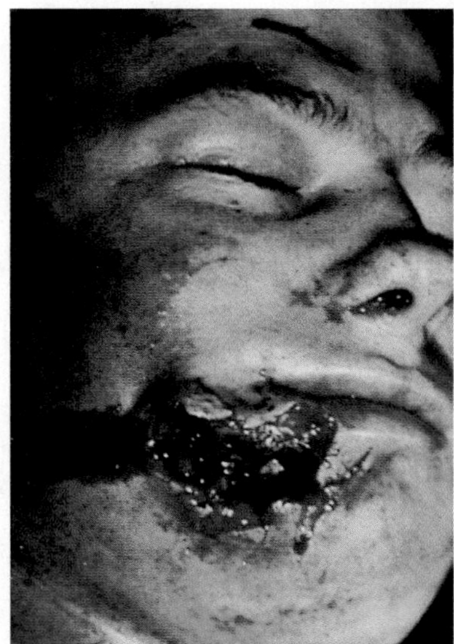

28-7E ✻ Gunshot wound to the chin.

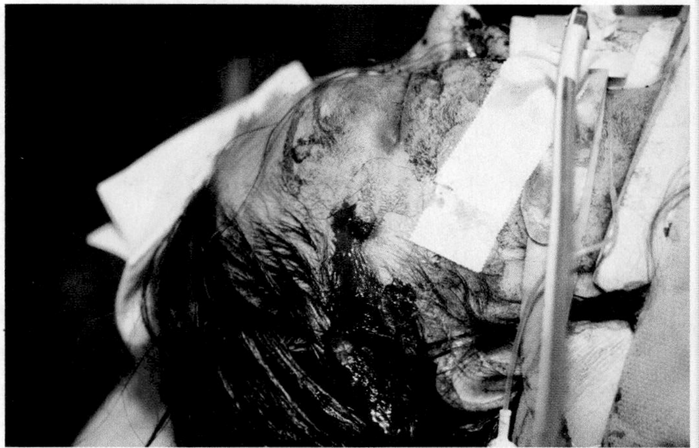

28-7F ✻ Gunshot wound to the side of the head. (© Edward T. Dickinson, MD)

EMT skills 28-8 Stabilizing an Impaled Object

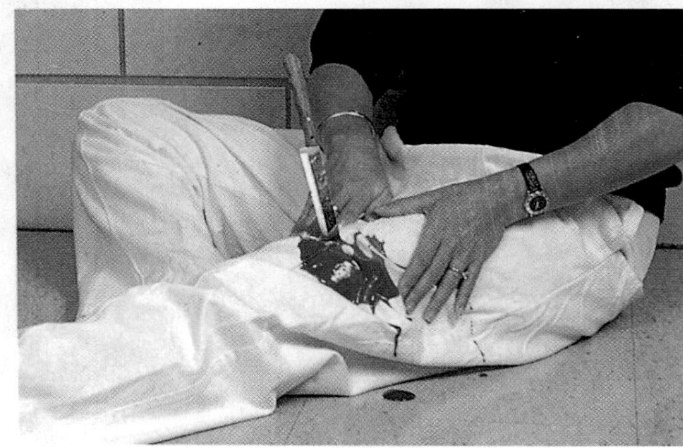

28-8A ✻ An impaled kitchen knife.

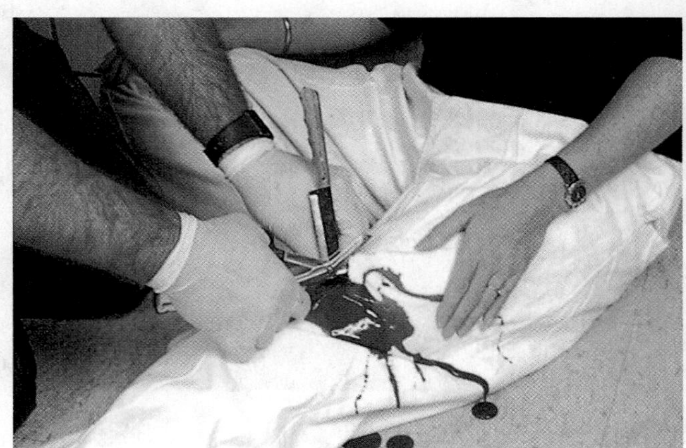

28-8B ✻ Cut away clothing.

continued

EMT skills 28-8 Stabilizing an Impaled Object *continued*

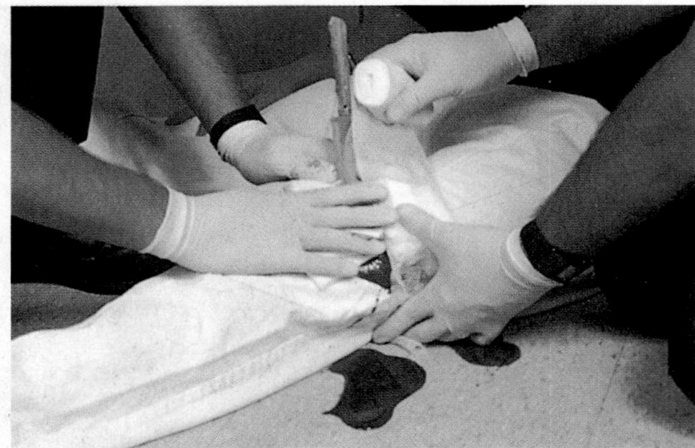

28-8C ✱ Stabilize and bandage the object in place.

EMT skills 28-9 Bandaging

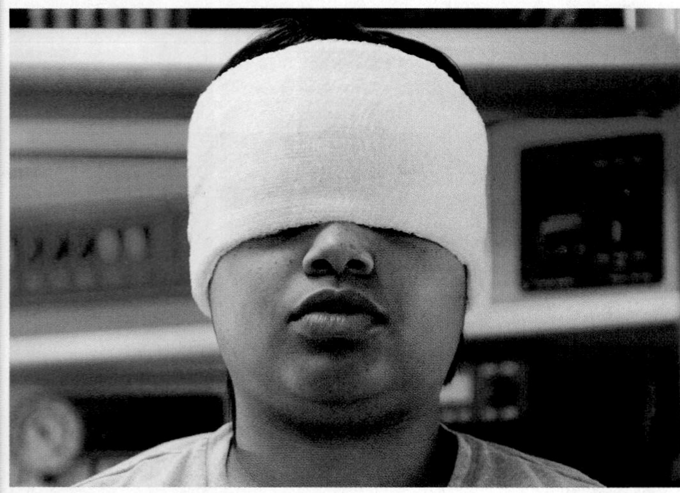

28-9A ✱ Head and/or eye bandage.

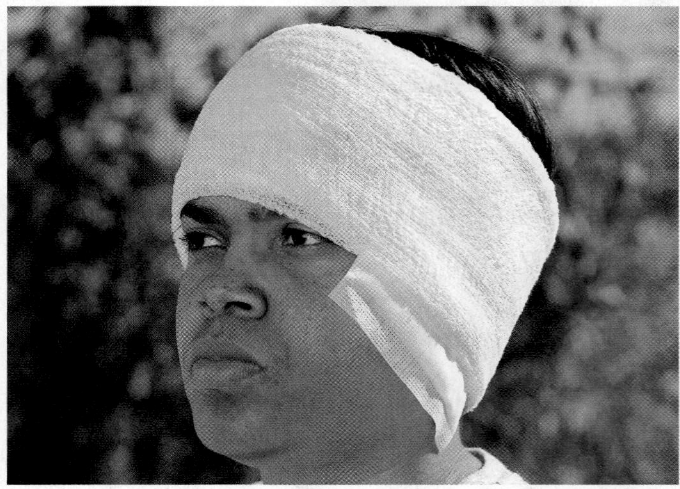

28-9B ✱ Head and/or ear bandage.

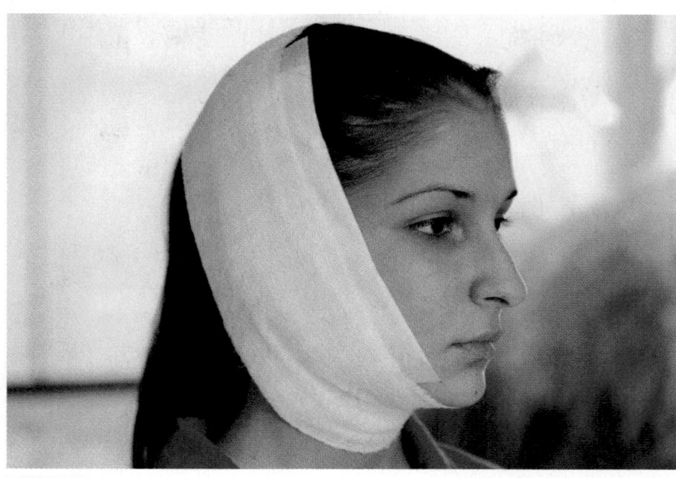

28-9C ✻ Cheek bandage (be sure the mouth will open).

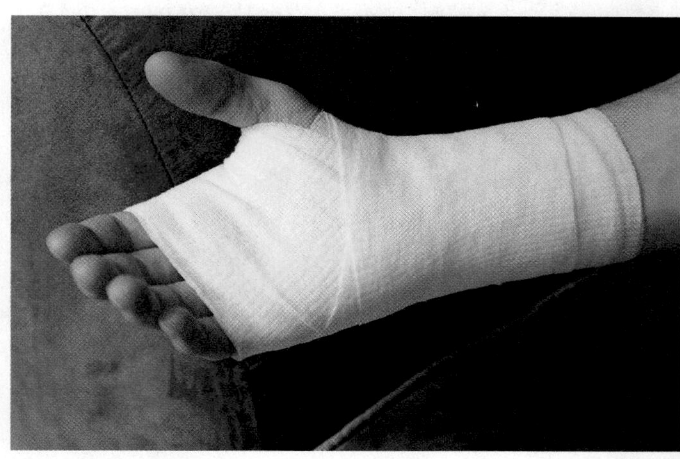

28-9D ✻ Hand bandage.

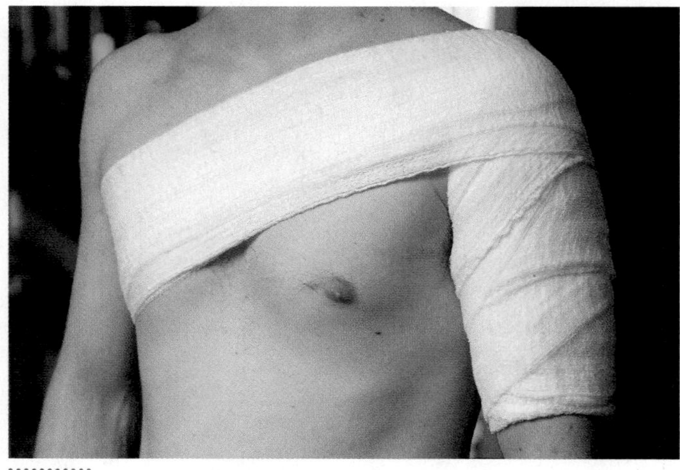

28-9E ✻ Shoulder bandage.

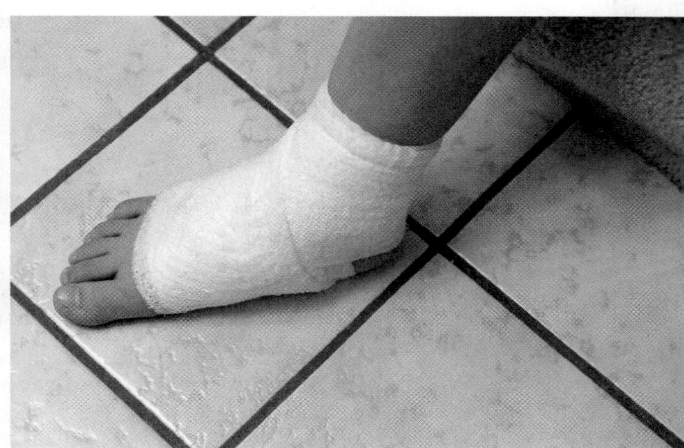

28-9F ✻ Foot and/or ankle bandage.

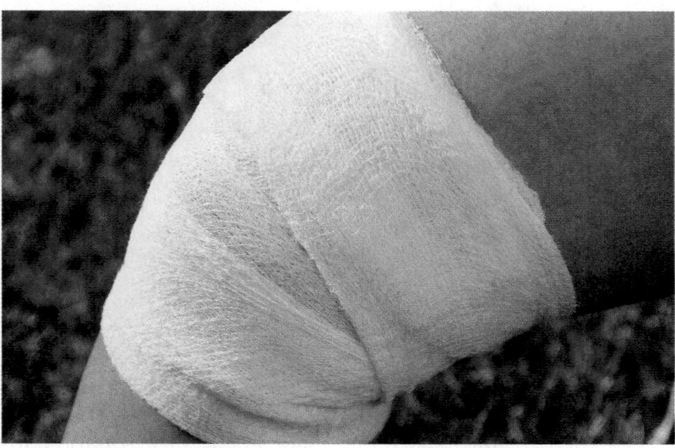

28-9G ✻ Knee bandage.

EMT skills 28-10 The Self-Adhering Roller Bandage

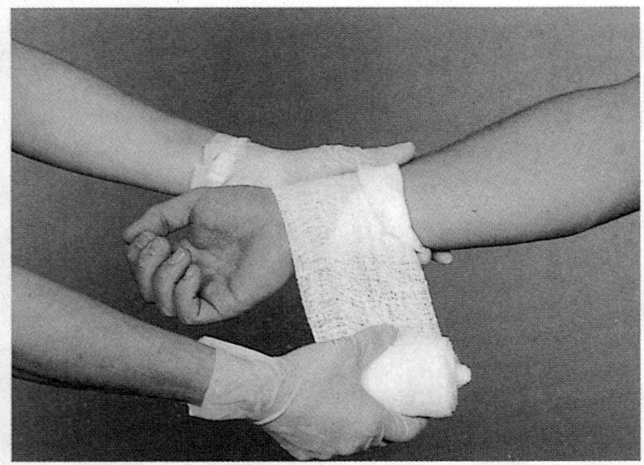

28-10A ✱ Secure the self-adhering roller bandage with several overlying wraps.

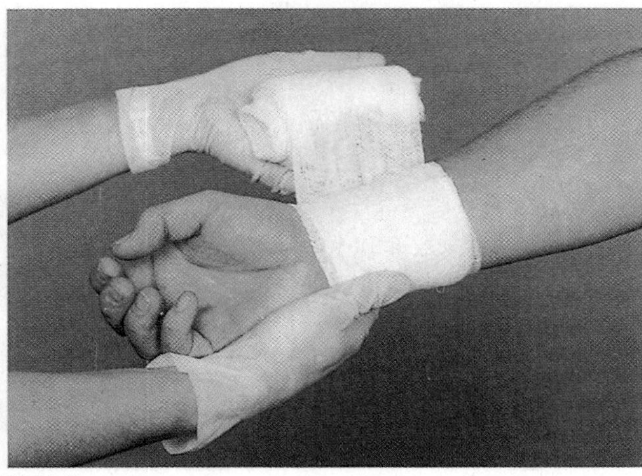

28-10B ✱ Overlap the bandage, keeping it snug.

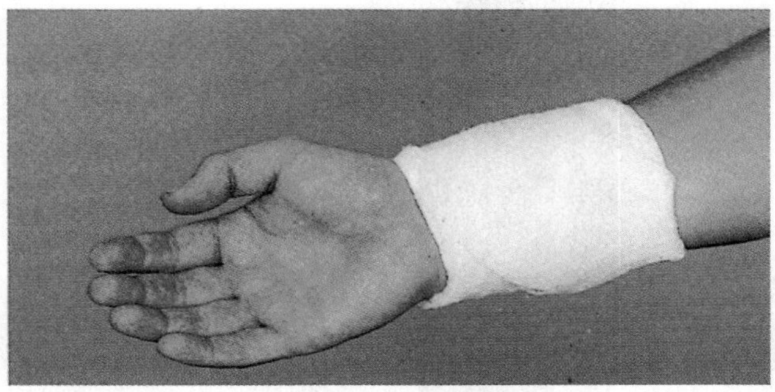

28-10C ✱ When the bandage covers an area larger than the wound, secure with tape or tie it in place.

CHAPTER REVIEW

SUMMARY

Perfusion is the delivery of oxygen, glucose, and other nutrients to the cells and the elimination of carbon dioxide and other waste products. Perfusion occurs from adequate circulation of blood through the vessels and capillaries. If the perfusion becomes insufficient, it is called hypoperfusion or shock. Hypovolemic shock is most often a result of blood loss. If not treated promptly and effectively, shock can rapidly lead to death.

Bleeding may be external or internal. External bleeding is easy to identify, since it can be seen during the patient assessment, whereas internal bleeding cannot be seen and must be suspected based on the patient's signs and symptoms. Bleeding could be arterial, venous, or capillary. Arterial bleeding is the most difficult to control, followed by venous bleeding. Methods to control external bleeding include direct pressure, elevation, pressure points, splinting, pressure splints, and cold application. A tourniquet is used only as a last resort on a severe uncontrolled bleeding wound.

Bleeding may lead to shock. The patient will present with a variety of signs and symptoms. Emergency care includes establishing and maintaining an airway, breathing, oxygenation, and circulation; controlling any bleeding; splinting any suspected fractures; keeping the patient warm; and providing rapid transport.

Soft tissue injuries are often dramatic, but rarely are they life threatening unless they involve organs or major vessels. Soft tissue injuries are classified as open or closed. A complication of an open soft tissue injury is the introduction of bacteria and other contaminants into the wound, increasing the risk of infection. The primary step in emergency care of the soft tissue injury is to stop any major bleeding. Other types of injuries involving the soft tissues that are life threatening are open chest wounds, abdominal evisceration, and large and deep lacerations to the neck.

Dressings are sterile and cover the wound directly, whereas a bandage may or may not be sterile and is typically used to hold the dressing in place. An occlusive dressing is used to prevent air from entering the wound. Bandages should be applied in a manner that securely holds the dressing in place but does not compromise the circulation or the wound.

CASE STUDY FOLLOW-UP

SCENE SIZE-UP

You and your partner have responded to a reported stabbing at Riverside High School. You arrive on the scene to find it has been secured. You approach the patient, an unresponsive male lying supine on the ground with a large penetrating wound to the left upper quadrant of the abdomen. The wound is bleeding profusely. There is no impaled object and no weapon visible.

PRIMARY ASSESSMENT

Your general impression of the teenage patient is that he is critical and will require rapid transport to the hospital. You immediately tell your partner to get the stretcher. You begin to assess the patient's mental status and note that he is unresponsive to verbal stimuli but will grimace to painful stimuli. His airway is patent with rapid and shallow breathing at a rate of 34 per minute. You instruct one of the Emergency Medical Responders to begin bag-valve-mask ventilations with supplemental oxygen at 12/minute.

You cannot feel a radial pulse but you can feel a carotid pulse, which is weak and rapid with a rate of 120 bpm. Dark red blood is flowing profusely from the abdominal wound. You decide to quickly pack the wound with sterile dressings and tape the dressings in place.

Your partner and an Emergency Medical Responder return with the stretcher and a pair of firefighter Emergency Medical Responders who have just arrived on the scene. Since there are no other signs of external trauma, you decide not to use spinal precautions.

SECONDARY ASSESSMENT

Once the patient is on the stretcher and in the ambulance, you conduct a rapid secondary assessment that does not reveal signs or symptoms not already known, other than that the abdomen is rigid to palpation. The patient remains unresponsive.

Your partner obtains a set of vital signs. You notify the hospital via radio of your patient's condition and expected arrival in 7 minutes.

Your partner informs you that blood pressure is 72/56 mmHg, pulse is 134 bpm, breathing is being assisted at a rate of 12/minute, and skin is pale, cool, and clammy. Although the external bleeding was profuse, you know that, because the wound site is the abdomen, the patient is most likely bleeding internally as well as suffering from hypoperfusion shock. You begin a rapid secondary assessment to find any additional wounds.

REASSESSMENT

Transport time is short. There is time for only one reassessment, which reveals no changes in the patient's condition. You arrive at the hospital and quickly unload the patient. You give a quick report to the waiting trauma team as you transfer care to them. You then begin the task of documenting the call on your prehospital care report. Your partner and the firefighters begin to clean and decontaminate the ambulance and equipment used during the call.

On the evening news, you learn that the patient died while in surgery. The next day you get a chance to talk to the emergency physician who explains that the patient had a lacerated splenic artery and an abdomen filled with blood. You ask if you could have done anything different, or better, or faster. The doctor tells you there was nothing anyone could have done for this patient in the prehospital setting that you did not do, and she commends you for your work in attempting to control bleeding, assisting ventilations, and—especially—transporting the patient without delay. The only satisfaction to be gained from this sad case is the knowledge that you gave the young patient the best possible chance.

IN REVIEW

1. Describe arterial, venous, and capillary bleeding.
2. Describe the primary method to control external bleeding.
3. Explain (a) when and (b) how to use a tourniquet to control bleeding.
4. Name the two most common sources of internal bleeding.
5. List the signs and symptoms of internal bleeding, including late signs.
6. Describe emergency medical care of internal bleeding.
7. List the signs and symptoms of hemorrhagic shock.
8. Describe emergency medical care of hemorrhagic shock.
9. Describe each of the three types of closed soft tissue injuries.
10. Identify the general signs and symptoms of closed soft tissue injuries.
11. Outline the general emergency medical care for closed soft tissue injuries.
12. Describe each of the six types of open soft tissue injuries.
13. Identify the general signs and symptoms of open soft tissue injuries.
14. Outline the general emergency medical care for open soft tissue injuries.
15. Describe the special considerations that must be taken when providing emergency medical care to patients with the following injuries: penetrating chest wounds, abdominal evisceration, impaled object, amputated part, and large open injury to the neck.
16. Describe the purpose of a dressing and name several available types.
17. Describe the purpose of a bandage and name several available types.
18. Describe the purpose of a pressure dressing and outline the steps for applying a pressure dressing.

CRITICAL THINKING

You arrive on the scene of a domestic incident. The police direct you into the kitchen of the home where you find a 52-year-old male patient with a knife impaled in his anterior chest on the right side approximately 2 inches inferior to the clavicle on the midclavicular line. He also has a large, gaping laceration to the left side of his neck with a large, steady flow of blood. He is moaning. His respirations are 46 per minute and severely shallow. His radial pulse is absent. The skin is extremely pale, cool, and clammy. His carotid pulse is 132 bpm.

1. What immediate emergency care would you provide for the patient?
2. How would you manage the wound to the neck?
3. What complications may be associated with the neck wound?
4. How would you manage the knife impaled in the chest?

PEARSON

EXPLORE mybradykit™

Please go to **www.bradybooks.com** to access mykit for this text. You will find quizzes, critical thinking scenarios, weblinks, animations, and videos related to this chapter—and much more. Look for online information on tourniquets and compartment syndrome as well as video clips on decubitus ulcers and shock.

Register your access code from the front of your book by going to **www.bradybooks.com** and selecting the mykit links.

CHAPTER 29

Burns

Navigation Guide

The following items provide an overview to the purpose and content of this chapter. The Standard and Competency are from the new National EMS Education Standards.

STANDARD **Trauma** (Content Area: Soft Tissue Trauma)

COMPETENCY Applies fundamental knowledge to provide basic emergency care and transportation based on assessment findings for an acutely injured patient.

OBJECTIVES: After reading this chapter, you should be able to:

29-1. Define key terms introduced in this chapter.
29-2. Explain the concept that burns are not just "skin deep."
29-3. Describe the effects of burns on the following body systems:
  a. Circulatory
  b. Respiratory
  c. Renal
  d. Nervous and musculoskeletal
  e. Gastrointestinal
29-4. Explain the classification of burns by depth and by body surface area involved, for both adult and pediatric patients.
29-5. Discuss considerations of burn depth, location, body surface area involved, the patient's age, and any preexisting medical conditions in determining the severity of burn injuries.
29-6. Discuss each of the following types of burns:
  a. Thermal
  b. Inhalation
  c. Chemical
  d. Electrical
  e. Radiation
29-7. Discuss each of the following mechanisms of burn injuries:
  a. Flame
  b. Contact
  c. Scald
  d. Steam
  e. Gas
  f. Electrical
  g. Flash
29-8. Describe the assessment-based approach to burns.
29-9. Describe special considerations in the scene size-up when responding to calls involving burned patients.
29-10. Explain the concept of stopping the burning process.
29-11. Identify indications of inhalation injury.
29-12. Discuss special considerations for dressing burns, including burns to specific anatomical areas.
29-13. Describe special considerations in responding to, assessing, and managing chemical and electrical burns.

KEY TERMS: Page references indicate first major use in this chapter. For complete definitions, see the Glossary at the back of the book.

burn sheet p. 965
circumferential burn p. 959
eschar p. 958
full-thickness burn p. 958
partial-thickness burn p. 958
rule of nines p. 961
rule of ones p. 962
superficial burn p. 957

MEDIA RESOURCES: Please go to www.bradybooks.com to access mykit for this text. You will find quizzes, critical thinking scenarios, weblinks, animations, and videos related to this chapter—and much more. Under Media Resources, look for online information on burns in children, burn centers, and injuries from fireworks.

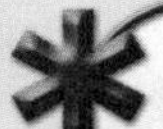

CASE STUDY

The Dispatch

EMS Unit 101—respond with the fire department to 38 Blackstrap Road for a reported structural fire. Time out is 0235 hours.

As you are getting into the ambulance you hear the fire department dispatcher alert the response companies that there is a man trapped on the second floor of the building. Reports are that the house is fully involved and a second alarm response has been requested. You look at your partner and you both know this could be a "bad" call if the patient has severe burn injuries.

Navigation Guide *continued*

Since you know that a fire like this may mean multiple patients, you request two more ambulances to respond to the fire scene for support. You and your partner don your protective clothing, just in case.

Upon Arrival

As you arrive on the scene, you notice that a firefighter is carrying a patient down a ladder from the second floor. Your partner gets the back of the ambulance ready by preparing the stretcher, turning on the heat, and arranging the burn supplies. You meet the firefighter at the bottom of the ladder. He tells you he found the patient, a male, on the second floor near a bedroom window, unresponsive.

How Would You Proceed to Assess and Care for This Patient?

During this chapter, you will learn about assessment and emergency care for a patient suffering from burn injuries. Later, we will return to the case and apply the procedures learned.

Introduction

Each year over 2 million people suffer burn injuries. Burn injuries are complicated because, contrary to what most people think, they are not just "skin deep." In addition to damaging the structure of the skin and compromising its functions, burn injuries impact most of the body's other systems in some way. For instance, burn injuries can impair the body's fluid and chemical balance and body temperature regulation, as well as its musculoskeletal, circulatory, and respiratory functions. Burn injuries may also affect a person's emotional well-being because of possible disfigurement and the need to cope with long healing processes.

In order to properly assess and provide emergency care for burn patients, EMTs need to have a fundamental understanding of the kinds of burns, how burn injuries are classified, and how they affect adult, child, and infant patients.

The Skin: Structure and Function Review

To understand how to classify burns, it is necessary first to understand the structure and function of the skin. (Review the information on the skin in Chapter 7, "Anatomy, Physiology, and Medical Terminology," and Chapter 28, "Bleeding and Soft Tissue Trauma," as well as reading the information in this chapter.)

The skin has a structure of three layers: The outermost layer is the *epidermis,* which provides a watertight and resilient barrier from the external environment; the second layer is the *dermis,* which contains small capillary beds as well as the sensory structures of the skin; and the innermost layer is the *hypodermis* (also called the *subcutaneous layer),* composed of fatty connective tissue and containing larger blood vessels. The layers range in thickness from one cell to several layers of cells. The skin serves multiple functions. For instance, it:

- Provides a physical barrier against the external environment
- Provides a barrier against infection
- Provides protection from bacteria or other harmful agents
- Insulates and protects underlying structures and body organs from injury
- Aids in the regulation of body temperature
- Provides for sensation transmission (hot, cold, pain, and touch)
- Aids in elimination of some of the body's wastes
- Contains fluids necessary to functioning of other organs and systems

All of these functions can be impaired or destroyed by a burn injury.

Airway, Breathing, and Circulation

Most burn patients who die in the prehospital setting will die from an occluded airway, toxic inhalation, or other trauma, and not from the soft tissue trauma of the burn itself. The EMT should first establish and maintain a patent airway, adequate ventilation, and adequate oxygenation, and ensure that any life-threatening bleeding has been controlled. Only then will the EMT turn attention to further assessment and care of the burn.

Objective 29-2
Explain the concept that burns are not just "skin deep."

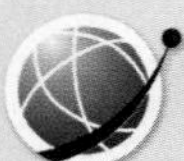

Media Resources
Go to www.bradybooks.com for mykit. Highlights:

- *Web Resource:* Burns in Children
- *Web Resource:* Burn Centers

Objective 29-3
Describe the effects of burns on the circulatory, respiratory, renal, nervous, musculoskeletal, and gastrointestinal systems.

▶ Effects of Burns on Body Systems

Burn injuries can not only impair or destroy the structure and functions of the skin, they can also damage other body systems. This section discusses some of the potential complications from burns to body organ systems other than the skin. The organ systems discussed are all essential for patient survival and successful recovery. Burn injuries that impair any of these functions can have a dramatic effect on the patient's outcome.

By providing the proper emergency medical care of the airway, preventing further contamination, and providing protection from further injury, you can decrease burn patient mortality considerably.

Circulatory System

Burn injuries can cause extreme fluid loss and increased stress on the heart. Burns increase capillary permeability, or the ability of fluid to leak from the vessels, which decreases the fluid volume inside the vessels. As fluid leaks from the damaged tissue cells to areas between the cells, it creates edema (swelling), which can further compromise tissue perfusion to local capillary beds as well as perfusion to distal tissues.

A condition that can occur with moderate to major burns that cover sufficient body surface area (BSA) is called *burn shock*. Burn shock, which develops only after the first few hours, results from extensive vascular bed damage that allows both fluid and protein molecules in the plasma to leak into surrounding tissues. The loss of plasma proteins causes the normal fluid balance of the rest of the vascular system to become disturbed and, as a result, blood plasma starts to seep from all capillary beds (even those not involved in the burn itself). The end result is a large fluid shift out of the vessels and into the spaces surrounding the cells to a point where the total vascular volume is insufficient to meet the body's needs. This also explains the extensive swelling seen in the burn patient. In the first 24 hours after a burn injury, as a result of the fluid loss from the vessels into the tissues, the edema may cause the body to swell to double its normal size.

The fluid loss just described can lead to shock (hypoperfusion). Major burns will require large amounts of fluid replacement during the patient's hospitalization. For example, an average adult patient with a full- or partial-thickness burn area of 50 percent BSA may need as much as 15 liters of fluid in the first 24 hours after a burn injury. However, fluid losses are usually not significant in the early hours of a burn. An EMT who finds a newly burned patient in a state of hypoperfusion should first consider direct blood loss from an associated external or internal hemorrhage.

Respiratory System

Burns may affect the respiratory system in a variety of ways. Swelling of the face or throat may cause airway closure. Inhalation of superheated air may cause the lining of the larynx to swell (laryngeal edema) and may cause fluid to accumulate in the lungs. Smoke and toxic gas inhalation may cause respiratory arrest or compromise or poisoning from noxious fumes. If the patient is in an enclosed space, he would have a higher probability of having an inhalation injury. If the chest is circumferentially burned, eschar (tough, leathery burned skin) may restrict chest expansion.

Renal System (Kidneys)

The decrease in blood flow from fluid loss caused by a burn (see the prior section on the circulatory system) will, of course, cause decreased blood flow to the kidneys and a consequent decrease in urinary output. Also, the burn injury will cause many wastes to form in the blood because of cell destruction, such as myoglobin from muscle destruction. This is particularly true with electrical burns. Since the kidneys are responsible for filtering the contaminated blood, a blockage in the kidneys may also result. In the end this may cause all or parts of the kidneys to stop functioning.

Nervous and Musculoskeletal Systems

Burn injuries can destroy nerve endings in the burn area and cause loss of function to extremities or other body parts. An extremity burn may cause loss of function, long-term muscle wasting, and joint dysfunction because of scarring. Patients who face loss of function, extreme pain, and scarring will also be prone to fear and anxiety. These patients may need both medical and psychological help to aid the healing process.

Thinking Critically
Your patient, just rescued from a burning building, has severe burns over a large body surface area, soot around his nose and mouth, an altered mental status, and copious bleeding from a head wound. In priority sequence, what steps should you take as you assess and care for this patient?

Key Terms
superficial burn burn that involves only the epidermis.

Objective 29-4
Explain the classification of burns by depth and by body surface area involved, for both adult and pediatric patients.

Gastrointestinal System

Although it is a low priority for the EMT, the gastrointestinal system plays an important role in the long-term care and survival of severely burned patients. As blood flow is decreased, blood is rerouted from this system to the rest of the body. Nausea or vomiting are common in burns of greater than 10 percent BSA and can further upset normal chemical balances, and long-term stress may cause ulcers. In order to promote healing and survival of burn patients, the gastrointestinal system must be kept functioning properly to insure adequate nutritional support for healing.

Assessment and Care of Burns

Classifying Burns by Depth

Burns are classified according to depth of the injury. Burn injuries involving the skin are classified as superficial (first-degree), partial-thickness (second-degree), or full-thickness (third-degree) burns (Figure 29-1*). In most cases you can quickly classify the burn as you form your general impression and establish a more detailed evaluation during the secondary assessment. A fourth-degree burn also exists and is commonly associated with electrical injuries.

Superficial Burns

Formerly referred to as a first-degree burn, a **superficial burn** involves only the epidermis. Usually a superficial burn is caused by a flash (a sudden occurrence of heat or flame lasting only a few seconds), hot liquid, or the sun. The skin will appear pink to red and will be dry. In some cases there may be slight swelling, but there will be no blisters. The skin will be soft and tender to the touch.

Although superficial in nature (affecting only the epidermis), these types of injuries may be very painful because the pain receptors in the underlying dermis of the skin are still intact. Superficial burns, generally, will take several days to heal but will not require much emergency medical care if only a small area is injured. The injury may

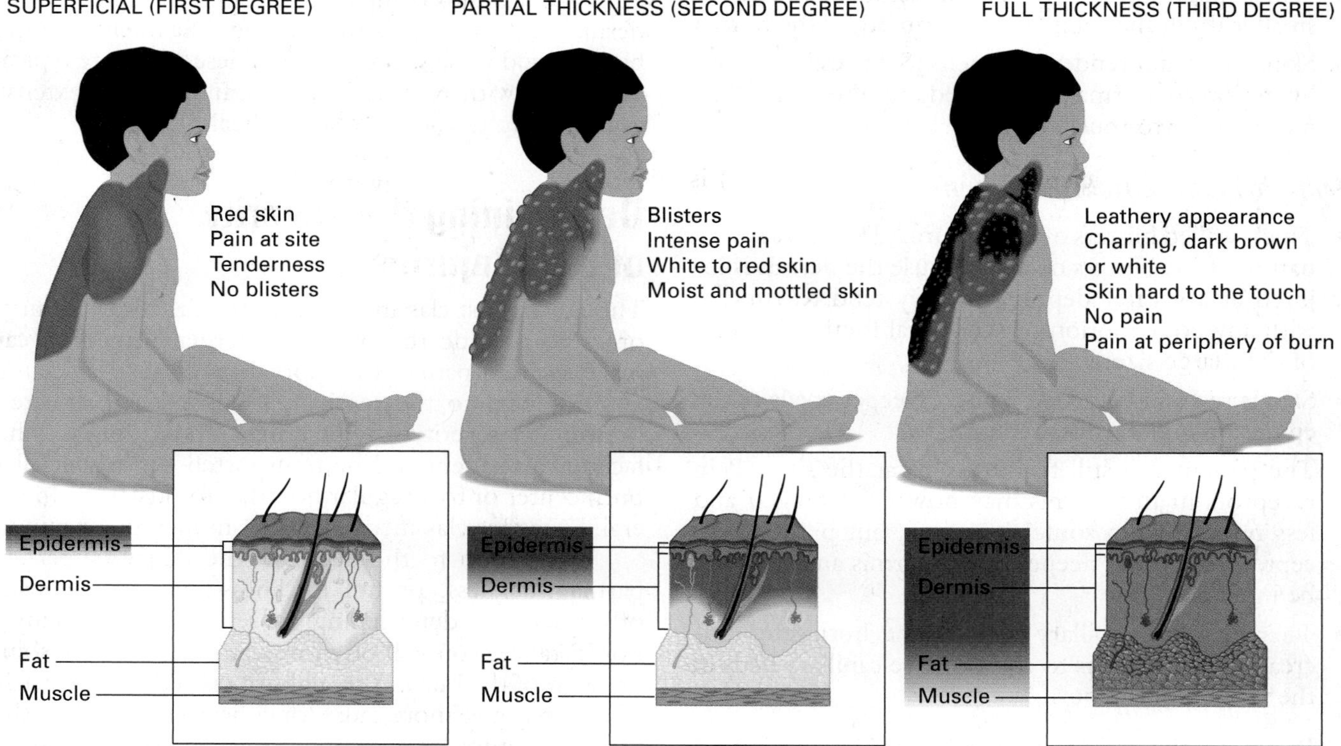

FIGURE 29-1 * Classification of burns by depth.

Key Terms

partial-thickness burn burn that involves the epidermis and portions of the dermis.

full-thickness burn burn that involves all the layers of the skin and can extend beyond the subcutaneous layer into the muscle, bone, or organs.

Key Terms

eschar the hard, tough, leathery dead soft tissue formed as a result of a full-thickness burn.

Objective 29-5

Discuss considerations in determining the severity of burn injuries.

cause the epidermis to peel but not cause any scarring. Examples of superficial burns include sunburn or a minor scald injury.

Partial-Thickness Burns

Formerly known as a second-degree burn, a **partial-thickness burn** involves not only the epidermis but also portions of the dermis. Partial-thickness burns occur from contact with fire (flame or flash), hot liquids or objects, chemical substances, or the sun. In addition, damage to the small blood vessels causes plasma and tissue fluid to collect between the layers of skin and form blisters. Since pain receptors are still intact, the patient will complain of pain from the burn.

Partial-thickness burns are further classified as *superficial partial-thickness* and *deep partial-thickness* burns. The signs and symptoms are as follows:

Superficial Partial-Thickness Burns

- Thin-walled blisters result from superficial dermal layer damage.
- Skin is pink and moist. (The moisture is caused by small leaks in the capillary beds caused by the burn.)
- Skin is soft and tender to touch. (Skin resiliency and hydration are normally preserved, but the skin will be more tender to touch.)

Deep Partial-Thickness Burns

- Thick-walled blisters often rupture. (The more severe nature of the blisters occurs because the dermis is injured at a greater depth, and they tend to rupture with any body motion or accidental friction because of their large size.)
- Skin is red and blanched white. (Deeper levels of the epidermis and dermis are injured.)
- The patient can still feel pressure at the site. (Pain receptors in the dermis may now be damaged and less responsive in some situations, but pressure receptors are found deeper in the dermis and may still be intact.)
- There is poor capillary refill to the burn site. (Increased edema starts to compromise capillary beds in the vicinity of the burn.)

Partial-thickness burns cause intense pain resulting from damage to nerve endings. Examples of partial-thickness burns include thermal flame burns or severe scaldings (EMT Skills 29-1).

Full-Thickness Burns

Formerly known as a third-degree burn, a **full-thickness burn** involves all the layers of the skin. This type of burn results from contact with extreme heat sources such as hot liquids or solids, flame, chemicals, or electricity. The skin will become dry, hard, tough, and leathery and may appear white and waxy to dark brown or black and charred. The tough and leathery dead soft tissue formed in the full-thickness burn injury is called an **eschar.**

Most full-thickness burns are not very painful because nerve endings have been destroyed. However, in most such injuries there will be surrounding areas of partial-thickness and/or superficial burns that may cause intense pain. Full-thickness burns are often evident in patients who have been trapped in a confined space with flames or who have been exposed to a high heat source or chemical contact (EMT Skills 29-2).

Some full-thickness burns may also be categorized as fourth-degree burns. A fourth-degree burn is a very deep burn that extends completely through the epidermis and dermis and deep into the tendons, ligaments, muscle, bone, blood vessels, and nerves. These burns are typically associated with electrical injuries and require extensive skin grafting to allow the site to heal.

Determining the Severity of Burn Injuries

The EMT must classify the severity of the burn injury in order to provide the optimal emergency medical care, make the best patient transport decision, and give an accurate report to the receiving facility. The estimate of burn injury severity may be crucial in deciding to which facility the patient will be transported—to a specialized burn center or to a regular hospital, for instance. In general, burns are classified as critical, moderate, or minor.

In addition to the depth of the injury (superficial, partial thickness, or full thickness), you will consider other factors in determining the severity of a burn injury. For instance, you will often want to consider the source or agent of the burn. A small burn caused by an electrical source may give more cause for concern than a small thermal (heat) burn because of the electrical burn's potential for internal injury. Likewise, a chemical burn will vary in

Thinking Critically

Burns to the eyes, ears, hands, feet, genital/groin area, hips, and shoulders and circumferential burns are especially critical. What are the critical aspects of each of these?

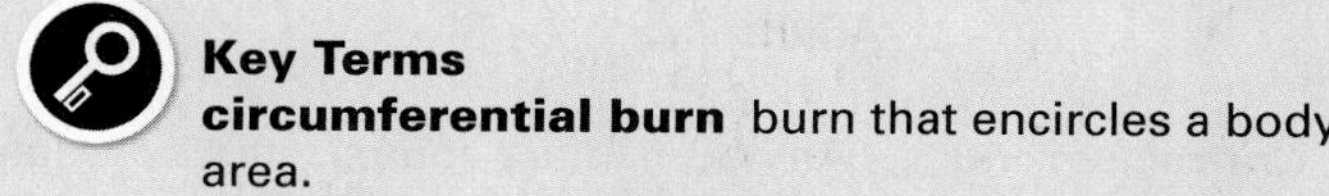

Key Terms

circumferential burn burn that encircles a body area.

severity depending on the type and strength of the chemical. Inhalation injuries or burns involving the airway are always considered critical.

The most important factors to consider in determining burn severity are (Figure 29-2✱ and Table 29-1):

- Depth of burn
- Location of the burn
- Patient's age
- Pre-existing medical conditions
- Percentage of body surface area involved

Burn Injury Location

Just as the depth of the burn injury and its body surface area are important, so too is the location of the burn. Injuries to certain body areas are more critical than those to other areas. Burns of the face (Figure 29-3✱) are considered critical because of the potential for respiratory compromise and long-term cosmetic concerns, as are injuries to the eyes or ears. Hands and feet are also given special consideration because of the potential for loss of function. Burn injuries to the genital or groin region are of concern because of the potential for loss of genitourinary function and increased chances for infection. Finally, burns that occur to regions of the body where there is major joint function (for example, hips and shoulders) may be considered critical because of loss of joint function should the injury not receive appropriate burn care early in the course of recovery.

Circumferential burns, which encircle a body area such as an arm, a leg, or the chest—and especially ones

CRITICAL BURNS

- Full thickness burns involving hands, feet, face, eyes, ears, or genitalia.
- Burns associated with respiratory injury.
- Full-thickness burns covering more than 10% of body surface.
- Partial-thickness burns covering more than 25% of body surface in adults.
- Partial-thickness burns > 20% in children less than 10 years and adults more than 50 years.
- Chemical burns or high-voltage electrical burns.
- Burns complicated by fractures or major trauma.
- Moderate burns in young children or elderly patients.
- Circumferential burns to any body part, such as arm, leg, or chest.

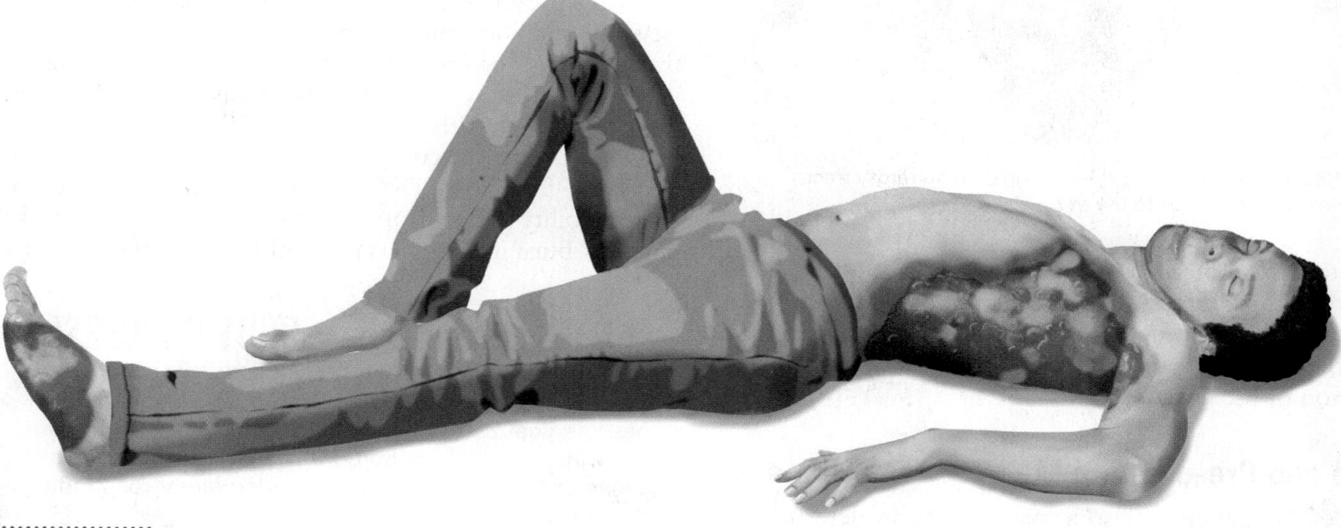

FIGURE 29-2 ✱ Critical burns.

TABLE 29-1 Determining Burn Severity Classification

	Adults	Children Under Age 5
Critical (severe) burns	• Any burn injury complicated by respiratory tract injuries or other accompanying major traumatic injury • Full- or partial-thickness burns involving the face, eyes, ears, hands, feet, genitalia, respiratory tract, or major joints • Any full-thickness burn injury covering 10% or more BSA • Any partial-thickness burn injury covering 25% or more BSA in adults younger than 50 years or 20% or more in adults older than 50 • Burn injuries complicated by a suspected fracture to an extremity • Any burn that encircles a body part (e.g., arm, leg, or chest) • Any burn classified as moderate in an adult younger than 55 is considered critical in an adult older than 55	As for adults plus . . . • Any full- or partial-thickness burn greater than 20% BSA • Any burn, including a superficial burn, involving hands, feet, face, eyes, ears, or genitalia • Any burn classified as moderate for an adult
Moderate burns	• Full-thickness burns with 2–10% BSA excluding the face, hands, feet, genitalia, or respiratory tract • Partial-thickness burns with 15–25% BSA involvement • Partial-thickness burns of 20% or more in adults younger than 50 years or 10% or more in adults older than 50	• Any partial-thickness burn of 10–20% BSA
Minor burns	• Full-thickness burns involving less than 2% BSA • Partial-thickness burns less than 15% BSA • Superficial burns less than 50% BSA	• Any partial-thickness burn less than 10% BSA

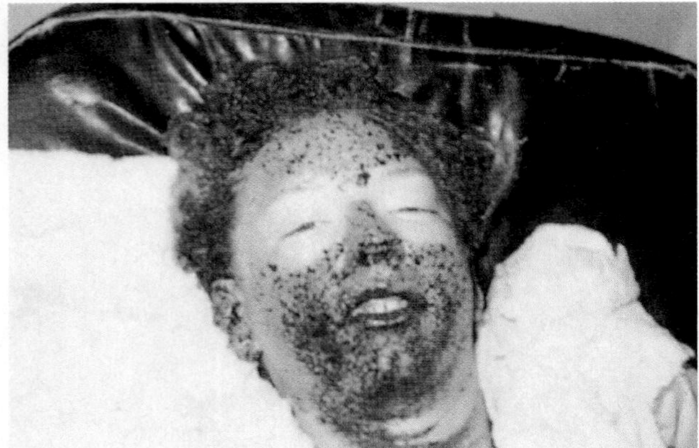

FIGURE 29-3 ✻ Burns to the face suggest respiratory tract involvement or injuries to the eyes.

that encircle joint areas—are critical because of the circulatory compromise and nerve damage that result from constriction or from swelling tissues. Burns that encircle the chest may impede respiratory function by limiting expansion of the chest.

Age and Pre-existing Medical Conditions

Age of the patient is also a major factor in determining the severity of the burn injury. Children under age 5 and adults over age 55 have less tolerance for burn injuries. Children, in addition to BSA percentage differences, face other challenges of growth process impairment. Because of their relatively larger skin surface in relation to body mass, they have the potential for greater fluid loss in burn injuries than adults. Older adults have prolonged healing processes and may have underlying medical conditions that affect their response to burn injuries.

Any pre-existing illness or injury may increase the severity of a burn injury. A patient with an existing respiratory illness or condition may be adversely affected if there is further respiratory compromise from a burn injury. A patient with an existing cardiovascular problem may have increased complications from a burn injury and resulting fluid loss. Diabetes will compromise the patient's ability to heal from the burns. What may seem like a minor burn in an otherwise healthy adult may be more

Understanding BODY PROCESSES

Pre-existing cardiovascular, pulmonary, endocrine, or neurological disease may turn a minor or moderate burn into a critical condition in an elderly patient because of the body's inability to adequately respond to the stress of the burn. ■

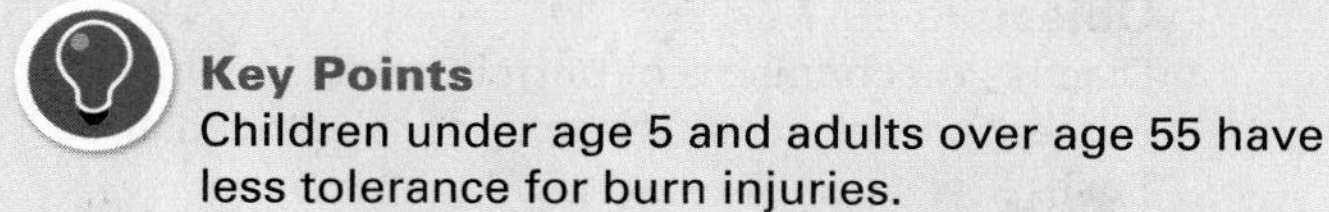

Key Points
Children under age 5 and adults over age 55 have less tolerance for burn injuries.

Key Terms
rule of nines standardized format to identify the amount of skin or body surface area (BSA) that has been burned.

severe in those patients with pre-existing medical conditions. If the patient has experienced other injuries along with a burn injury, the life threat or potential for shock (hypoperfusion) may be increased as well.

Special Considerations for Infants and Children As mentioned earlier, infants and children have a larger body surface in relation to mass than adults. For this reason, burn injuries can have increased effects on infants and children. Fluid and heat loss are also greater in infants and children than in adults. There is a higher risk for shock (hypoperfusion), airway difficulties, and hypothermia with burn injuries to infants. Further differences in burn injury severity classification for children less than 5 years old are outlined in Table 29-1.

In addition to assessment and emergency medical care considerations, you must consider the possibility of child abuse when a child has a burn injury. (See information about assessing for and reporting child abuse in Chapter 38, "Pediatrics.")

Body Surface Area Percentage

The **rule of nines** is a standardized way to quickly determine the amount of skin surface, or the body surface area (BSA) percentage, of a burn (Figure 29-4∗). The rule of nines is only applied to partial-thickness or full-thickness burns. The rule of nines is not applied to superficial burns. In an adult, the head and neck together, each upper extremity, the chest, the abdomen, the upper back, the lower back, the anterior of each lower extremity, and the posterior of each lower extremity each represents a BSA of 9 percent. The genital region represents a 1 percent BSA. This rule will guide you in determining the burn severity, categorizing the patient for triage, and alerting the receiving facility as to the severity of the patient.

In infants and children there are different BSA percentages assigned to body regions because of their different proportional dimensions. The infant's or young child's head is much larger in relationship to the rest of the body than in adults. Therefore, for infants 1 year of age or less, the head and neck are counted as 18 percent (greater than an adult), the chest and abdomen as 18 percent (same as an adult), the entire back as 18 percent (same as an adult), each upper extremity as 9 percent (same as an adult), and each lower extremity as 14 percent (less than an adult). The rule of nines is altered to allow the head to account for more of the total BSA. The larger percentage of BSA for the head was shifted from

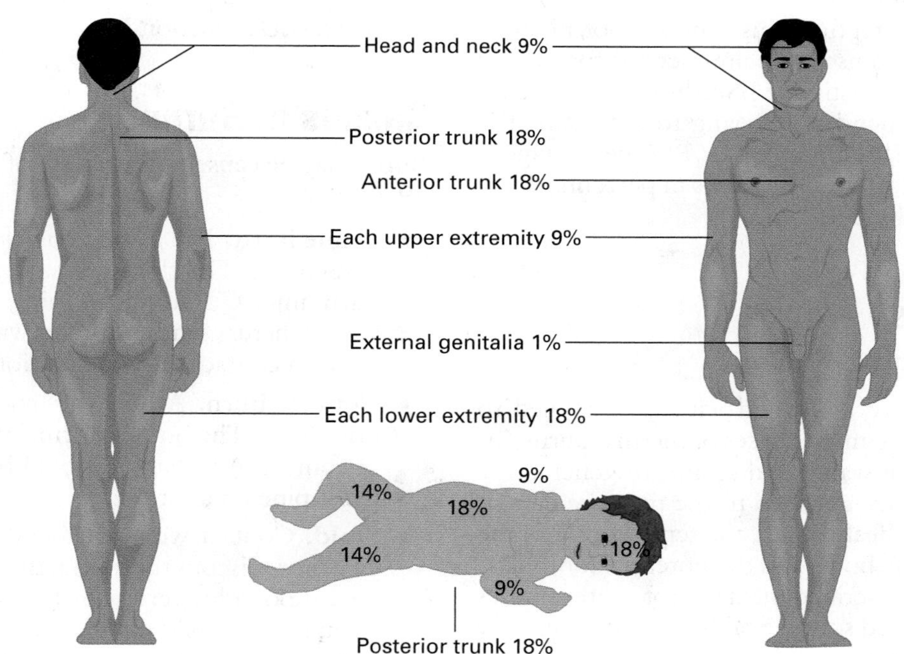

FIGURE 29-4 ∗ The "rule of nines" is a method for estimating how much body surface is burned in the adult or infant patient.

Objective 29-6
Discuss types of burns, including thermal, inhalation, chemical, electrical, and radiation burns.

Key Terms
rule of ones the concept that the area of a patient's palm is equal to about 1 percent of his body surface area (BSA); a way to quickly identify the amount of skin or BSA that has been burned.

Objective 29-7
Discuss mechanisms of burn injuries, including flame, contact, scald, steam, gas, electrical, and flash.

the legs because of the disproportionate size of the head in infants and young children (and their proportionally smaller legs). For children over the age of 1 year, for each year beyond 1, add 0.5 percent to each leg and subtract 1 percent for the head. This formula will be used until the adult rule of nines values are reached. For example, for a 3-year-old child you would add 1 percent (0.5% × 2 years beyond 1) to each leg and subtract 2 percent from the head. Thus, the legs in the 3-year-old would equal a total of 15 percent and the head would equal 16 percent.

ASSESSMENT Tips

The head of the infant or child accounts for more of the total BSA than it does in the adult. This is because the head is proportionally larger in younger patients. ■

An alternative way to determine the BSA estimate is to compare it to the patient's palm (of the hand) surface area, which equals approximately 1 percent of BSA. This is known as the **rule of ones,** also called the *rule of palms.* For example, if the burn area is equal to "seven palm surface areas," then the burn would be estimated at 7 percent BSA. You can use this method to estimate a burn area on a patient of any age.

You may find it helpful to use the rule of nines in larger burn injuries and use the palm method for smaller burns. You can begin to estimate BSA during the primary assessment. Do not spend time trying to determine the exact percentage of BSA injured. The BSA percentage is an estimate only, and slight differences in percentage will not affect prehospital medical care.

Types of Burns

There are five major types of burns:

- ***Thermal burns*** are associated with heat applied to the body. There are many causes of thermal burns, including flame, hot water, and steam. In general, the severity of the burn is related to the time the patient is exposed to the heat source, the temperature of the heat applied to the body, and the potential for inhalation injury (as described next). Hot water causes thermal burns called scalds. Scalds in children may be a form of child abuse.
- ***Inhalation burns*** are associated with high-temperature air or steam that is inhaled and causes damage to the mucosa of the upper airway. This will result in edema that may restrict airflow and lead to an airway obstruction. Another complication is the inhalation of toxic gases such as carbon monoxide and cyanide gas. If the patient is in an enclosed area, he is more likely to suffer an upper airway burn and toxic inhalation.
- ***Chemical burns*** are produced by acids, alkalis, and other heat-generating chemicals. The type of chemical, its concentration, and the duration of exposure to the chemical will determine the severity of the burn. Chemical burns are discussed in more detail later in the chapter.
- ***Electrical burns*** result from resistance to electrical current flow in the body. The burns are primarily internal. The electricity may interfere with the conduction system of the heart and result in cardiac arrest. Electrical burns are covered in more detail later in the chapter. Lightning is both a medical and traumatic event with typically little burn injury. Lightning injuries are covered in Chapter 24, "Environmental Emergencies."
- ***Radiation burns*** occur from the absorption of radiation into the body. Radiation burns are covered in Chapter 43, "Hazardous Materials," and Chapter 45, "EMS Response to Terrorism Involving Weapons of Mass Destruction."

Causes of Burns

Burns may be caused by a variety of mechanisms (Figure 29-5∗):

- **Flame burn.** The patient comes into contact with an open flame. The clothing may ignite, causing further burn injury. Natural clothing fibers typically will burn, whereas synthetic fibers will usually melt, which causes a contact burn in addition to the flame burn.
- **Contact burn.** A burn occurs from contact with a hot object. The burn is normally localized to the area of contact. An example would be touching a hot exhaust pipe on a car.
- **Scald.** Contact with hot liquid causes a scald burn. The more viscous the liquid, the more severe the burn because of a longer contact time. Intentional scalds, often seen in child abuse, typically involve the entire extremity from being immersed and held in the hot

Objectives 29-8 and 29-9
Describe the assessment-based approach to burns and special considerations in the scene size-up when responding to calls involving burns.

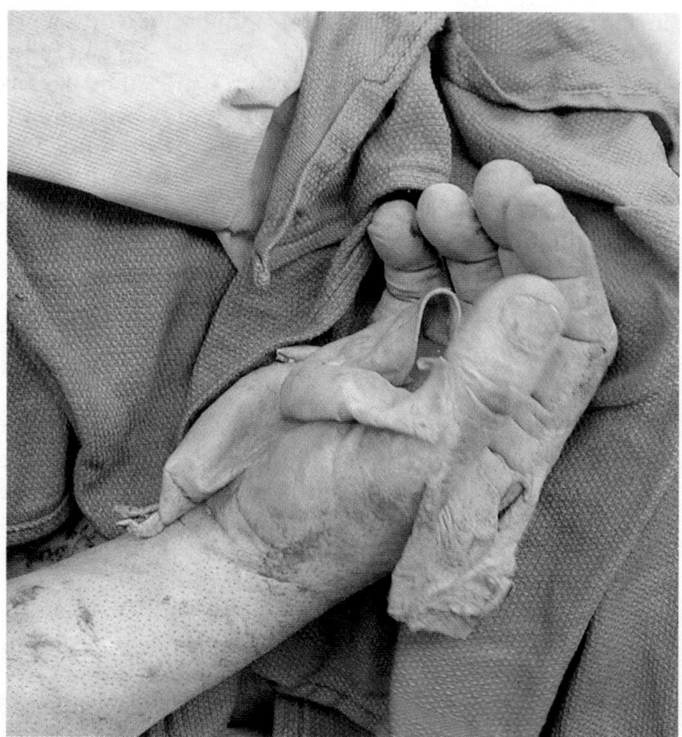

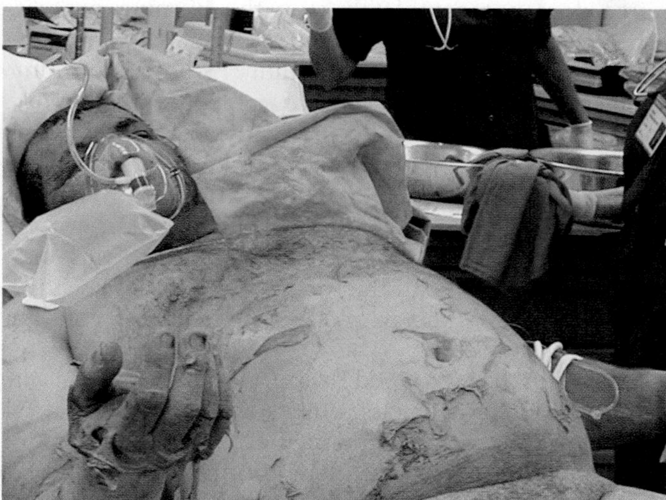

FIGURE 29-5 ✱ Burns can occur by a variety of mechanisms. This patient was doing commercial painting using a spray gun with oil paint in an enclosed area. A spark ignited the paint vapors, causing an explosion. In addition to the obvious burns to the skin, because of the ignition of vapors in an enclosed space, inhalation injuries are also likely to have occurred. (© Charles Stewart, MD, and Associates)

water. Accidental scalds will show patches of burns separated by unburned areas caused by splashing.

- **Steam burn.** Hot steam causes severe burns, often more severe than flame burns, because of the high heat capacity of steam. Typically, these types of burns are found in industrial accidents or in those who inappropriately open a car radiator while it is hot. Steam can cause thermal burns to the distal airways in the lungs.
- **Gas burn.** Hot gases may cause upper airway burns; however, it is not likely that the hot gas will cause distal airway burns. Distal airway injury may occur, however, from the by-products of combustion rather than from the hot gas.
- **Electrical burn.** Because bones, muscles, and other tissues offer resistance to the electrical energy passing through them, the by-product is heat, which results in internal burns. With an electrical burn, the clothing may ignite, resulting in a flame burn.
- **Flash burn.** This is a type of flame burn but is the result of a flammable gas or liquid that ignites quickly. Areas of the body covered by clothing normally are not burned. Inhalation injury may occur if the flash occurs in a closed space. There is a lesser incidence of inhalation injuries when the event occurs outside. A typical flash burn would occur from throwing gasoline on smoldering charcoal to reignite it.

Assessment-Based Approach: Burns

Scene Size-Up

Your first priority is to determine whether the scene is safe to enter. Do not enter scenes for which you are not trained. If the patient is in an unsafe environment, such as a fire-engulfed building, and you do not have the proper equipment or training to enter, you must wait until properly equipped and trained personnel can safely remove the

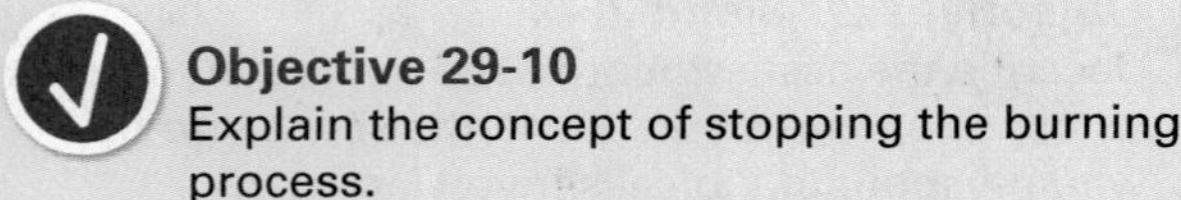

Objective 29-10
Explain the concept of stopping the burning process.

Key Points
During the secondary assessment, check for any injury that may have occurred in addition to the burn.

patient. Once the scene is safe to enter, you must take appropriate Standard Precautions and then begin assessing the mechanism of injury and number of patients.

Primary Assessment

Remember that removing the patient from the burn source does not completely stop the burning process. Burn injuries need to be "cooled down" within approximately the first 10 minutes of injury. Stop the burning process initially by using water or saline. As you work to stop the burning, attempt to remove any smoldering clothing and jewelry, which will still be producing heat and may constrict swollen extremities. If any clothing still adheres to the patient, cut around the area. Do not attempt to remove the adhered portion, since this may cause further damage to the soft tissues. Do not keep the burn immersed, as this may cause hypothermia; cool for 60–120 seconds only.

Once you have stopped the burning process, you can continue your primary assessment and evaluate the patient's airway, breathing, and mental status. Look for any indications that the airway may be injured or compromised, such as sooty deposits in the mouth or nose, singed facial or nose hairs, signs of smoke inhalation, or any facial burns. A burn victim's first reaction when frightened or startled—such as when trapped in a confined space or startled by an explosion—is to inhale deeply. Air in these situations may be superheated and will have an adverse effect on the airway and respiratory function, so you need to consider the likelihood of airway compromise and breathing difficulties. Provide oxygen by nonrebreather mask at 15 lpm or, if breathing is inadequate, provide positive pressure ventilation with supplemental oxygen.

To complete the primary assessment, assess the patient's circulation and determine whether the patient is a priority for transport. Make a rapid estimate of the severity of the burn, taking into account BSA percentage and any information you have gained about the burn source or agent and any information about the age and medical condition of the patient that you have gained from bystanders or the patient himself. Remember not to spend too long estimating the exact BSA percentage of the burn; you can gather more information later in your assessment.

Most burns do not bleed and are not a cause of early shock. If signs and symptoms of shock are present, look for other sources of blood loss or possible spinal injury. As in all traumatic emergencies, a burn injury patient is a priority for transport if he is unresponsive with no gag reflex or is responsive but not following commands, if he has airway compromise or difficulty breathing, if he shows signs of shock or uncontrolled bleeding, or if he presents with severe pain. A patient with a "critical" burn, as discussed earlier, should also be treated as a priority patient even though he may not present as unstable initially.

Remember that critical burns themselves are not immediately life threatening. Immediate causes of death are airway swelling and inhalation injury.

Secondary Assessment

After treating all life-threatening injuries, conduct the secondary assessment, beginning by reassessing the mechanism of injury and chief complaint. Perform a physical exam. Check for evidence of any injury that may have occurred in addition to the burn, and get a more accurate estimate of BSA percentage than the one you determined during the primary assessment. As you examine the patient, continue to remove his clothing and jewelry, but do not attempt to remove debris or any adhered clothing. Record the patient's baseline vital signs.

ASSESSMENT Tips

The determination of an accurate BSA burned can be delayed until the physical exam is completed. Prior to this, the EMT should focus on establishing and maintaining the airway, breathing, oxygenation, and circulation. ■

Obtain a history from the patient or from family and any bystanders. However, if the patient's burn is considered critical or if he is a priority for transport for other reasons, you may not have time to obtain the answers to your questions at the scene. If possible, ask the following questions:

- How did the burn happen?
- What caused the burn?
- Was the patient exposed to an explosion or other significant mechanism of injury?
- Did the patient lose consciousness at any time?
- Was the patient confined in an enclosed space or found to inhale copious amounts of smoke?

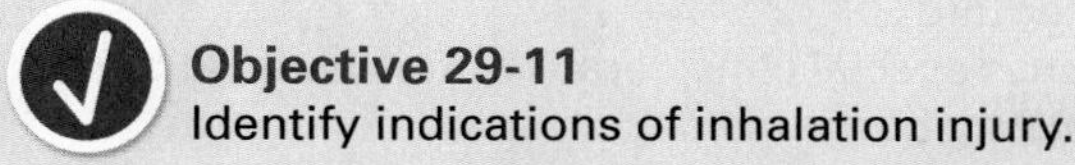

Objective 29-11
Identify indications of inhalation injury.

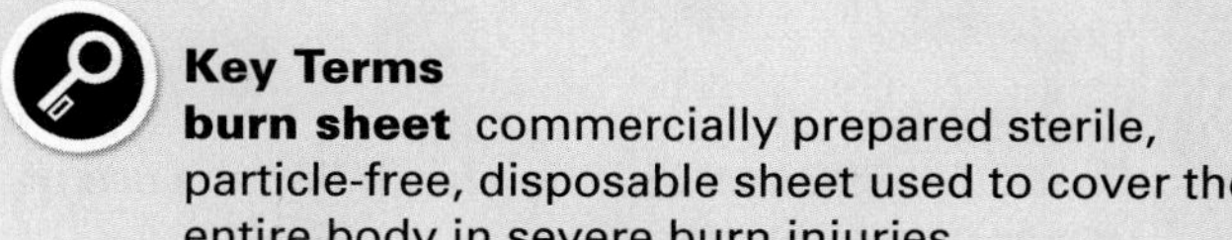

Key Terms
burn sheet commercially prepared sterile, particle-free, disposable sheet used to cover the entire body in severe burn injuries.

- How long ago was the patient burned?
- What care was given by bystanders?
- If the burn involved chemicals, what chemical?
- If the burn was a scald, how did it happen? (If a scald or burn injury involves an infant, child, or elderly patient, consider the possibility of abuse.)
- Does the patient have any history of significant heart disease, pulmonary problems, diabetes, or any other condition that might increase the burn severity or complicate treatment?

Signs and Symptoms In addition to estimating BSA and noting location of the burn injuries, watch for the following signs and symptoms of burn depth and possible inhalation injuries:

Superficial Burns

- Pink or red, dry skin
- Slight swelling
- Pain and tenderness to touch

Partial-Thickness Burns

- White to cherry red skin
- Moist and mottled skin
- Blistering and intense pain

Full-Thickness Burns

- Dry, hard, tough, and leathery skin that may appear white and waxy to dark brown or black and charred (eschar)
- Inability to feel pain because of damaged nerve endings
- Pain on peripheral edges of burns

Inhalation Injuries

- Singed nasal hairs
- Facial burns
- Burned specks of carbon in the sputum
- A sooty or smoky smell on the breath
- Respiratory distress accompanied by restriction of chest wall movement, restlessness, chest tightness, stridor, wheezing, difficulty in swallowing, hoarseness, coughing, and cyanosis
- The presence of actual burns of the oral mucosa

Emergency Medical Care

There are many ways to care for burn injuries. Check with your local medical director to determine the most appropriate emergency medical care for burn injuries in your region. The following steps in emergency medical care for burn injuries represent a general protocol in providing care. Particular attention is paid to preventing further contamination and injury.

1. *Remove the patient from the source of the burn and stop the burning process.* As mentioned earlier, you should not attempt to enter an unsafe environment and extricate the patient unless you have the proper training and equipment. Once the patient has been removed from the source of the burn, you can stop the burn process by using water or saline (Figure 29-6a*), but do not keep it immersed. If the burn source is a semisolid or liquid (e.g., tar, grease, or oil), cool the burn with water or saline to stop the burning process but do not attempt to remove the substance since this could cause further tissue damage. Dry chemicals should be brushed away before flushing with copious amounts of water. Remove any smoldering clothing and any jewelry. If any clothing remains adhered to the patient, cut around the area (Figure 29-6b*). Do not attempt to remove the adhered portion.
2. *Establish and maintain an airway and breathing.* Pay particular attention to evidence of inhalation injury to the patient's upper airway. Maintain an open airway and administer oxygen by nonrebreather mask at 15 lpm, especially if inhalation of toxic gases is suspected. If breathing is inadequate, provide positive pressure ventilation with supplemental oxygen at a rate of 10–12 breaths per minute in an adult and 12–20 per minute in an infant or child.
3. *Classify the severity of the burn and transport immediately if critical.* Take into account the factors mentioned earlier: BSA percentage, source or agent of the burn, location of the burn, age of the patient, and preexisting medical conditions. (Review Table 29-1.)
4. *Cover the burned area with a dry sterile dressing* (Figure 29-6c*) or a sterile, particle-free disposable **burn sheet** or an approved commercial burn dressing. A clean white sheet is acceptable if no burn sheet is available. Continual use of a wet or moist dressing may cause hypothermia because of the loss of heat regulation in the burned area. However, some EMS

Key Points
Check with medical direction regarding the use of wet or moist dressings.

Objective 29-12
Discuss special considerations for dressing burns, including burns to specific anatomical areas.

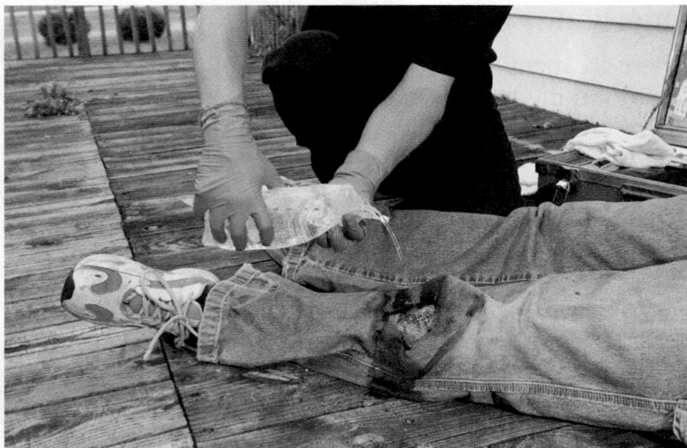

FIGURE 29-6a * Stop the burning process.

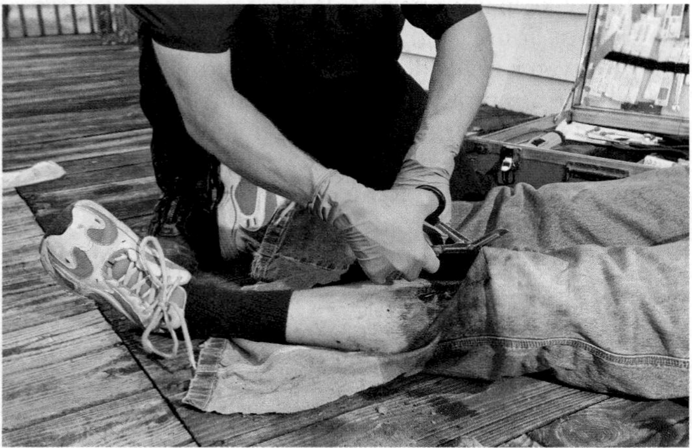

FIGURE 29-6b * Remove the smoldering clothing.

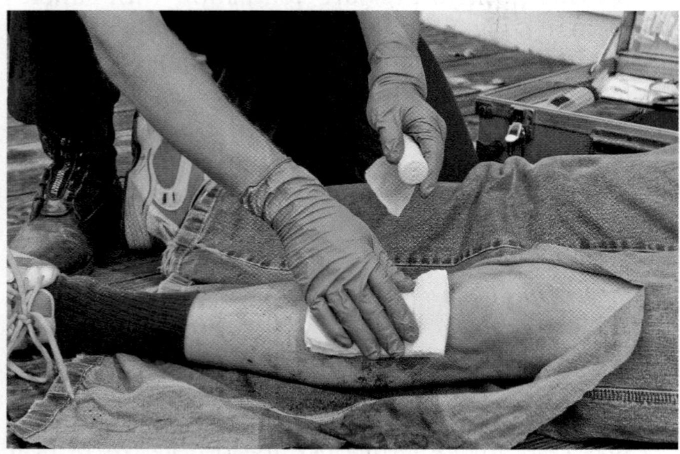

FIGURE 29-6c * Cover with dry, sterile dressings.

TABLE 29-2 Burn Unit Referral Criteria

- Inhalation injury
- Partial-thickness burn of greater than 10% BSA
- Full-thickness burn
- Burns involving hands, feet, face, genitalia, perineum, or major joints
- Electrical burns
- Lightning strike injury
- Chemical burns
- Burns in patients with pre-existing medical conditions or other trauma where the burn is the major injury

Source: American College of Surgeons Committee on Trauma.

systems may use a moist dressing on a 10 percent BSA or less partial-thickness burn. Check with local medical direction regarding the use of wet or moist dressings.

5. *Keep the patient warm and treat other injuries as needed.* Remember, the burn injury will impair or destroy the skin's heat regulation function and may be accompanied by other injuries.
6. *Transport the patient to the appropriate facility,* depending on the severity of the burn and local protocol for burn injuries. See Table 29-2 for burn unit referral criteria.

Special Considerations for Dressing Burns

In dressing a burn, follow these guidelines:

- Avoid using any material that shreds or leaves particles since this may further contaminate the burn.
- Never apply any type of ointments, lotions, or antiseptics to burn injuries. This may cause heat retention and hospital personnel would most likely have to vigorously cleanse the area of any debris material.
- Never break or drain blisters. This may cause further contamination and potential for fluid loss.

Special areas of concern when applying burn dressings are the hands, the toes, and the eyes. In those areas, follow these guidelines:

Key Points
Always consider ALS response when dealing with airway complications in burn injuries.

Objective 29-13
Describe special considerations in responding to, assessing, and managing chemical and electrical burns.

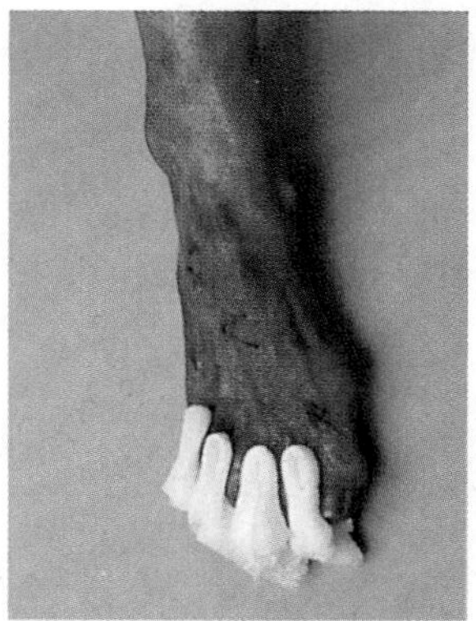

FIGURE 29-7a * Separate burned toes with dry, sterile gauze.

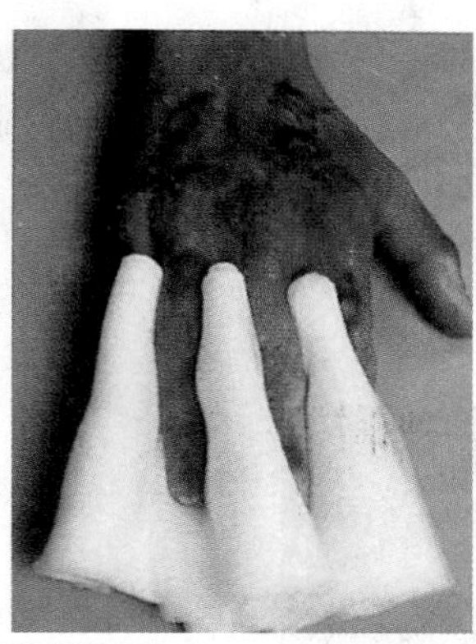

FIGURE 29-7b * Separate burned fingers with dry, sterile gauze.

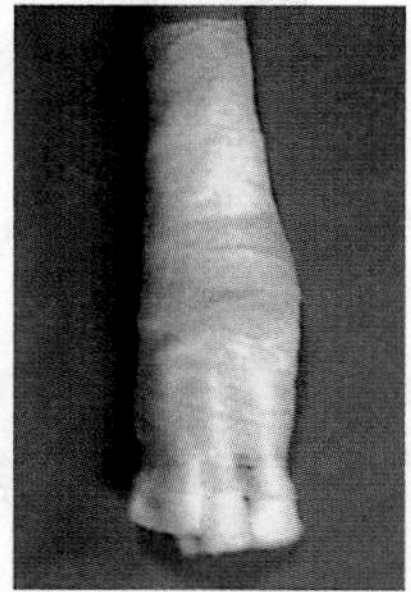

FIGURE 29-7c * Cover the burned fingers or toes completely with dry, sterile dressings.

For Burns of the Hands and Toes

- Remove all rings and jewelry, which may constrict with swelling after the burn injury. Separate all digits with dry, sterile dressing material to prevent adhering of burned areas (Figures 29-7a to 29-7c*).

For Burns of the Eyes

- Do not attempt to open eyelids if they are burned. Determine if the burn is thermal or chemical. If thermal, apply a dry, sterile dressing to BOTH eyes to prevent simultaneous movement of both eyes (Figure 29-8*). Chemical burns should be flushed with water while en route to the hospital. Flush the eye from the medial to the lateral side to avoid washing the chemical into the opposite eye. See more about chemical burns in the following section.

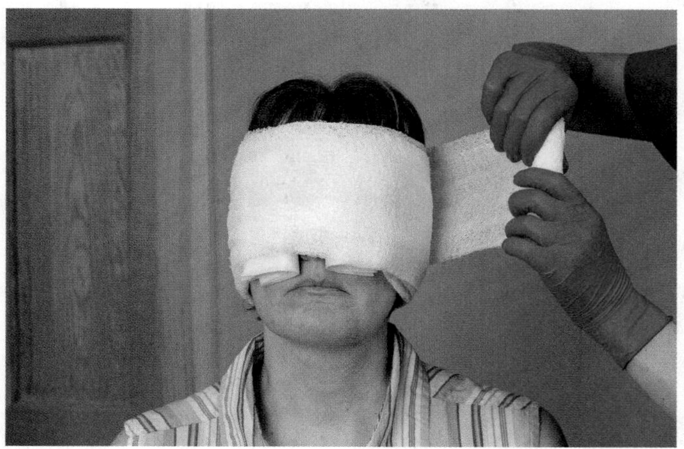

FIGURE 29-8 * Apply sterile gauze pads to both eyes.

Reassessment

Perform the reassessment. Monitor vital signs and check interventions every 5 minutes for unstable patients and every 15 minutes for stable patients. Continually evaluate the airway, especially if there are any burns to the face.

Note: Swelling or closure of the airway may be rapid, and emergency medical care will need to be quickly accomplished. Always consider advanced life support (ALS) response when dealing with airway complications in burn injuries.

Chemical Burns

Chemical burns require immediate care, since the longer the chemical is in contact with the skin the greater the potential for injury (Figure 29-9*). In many cases, emergency medical care may be started by people at the scene. Industrial sites may have special response teams or Emergency Medical Responders and equipment available to provide initial emergency medical care. However, you should follow these rules when dealing with chemical burn injuries:

- *Protect yourself first.* As with other burn emergencies, never enter an unsafe scene. Chemical burns may involve a hazardous material incident that you may not be prepared to handle or that may cause you to become exposed. Wear gloves and eye protection at a minimum. In cases of a large exposure you may have

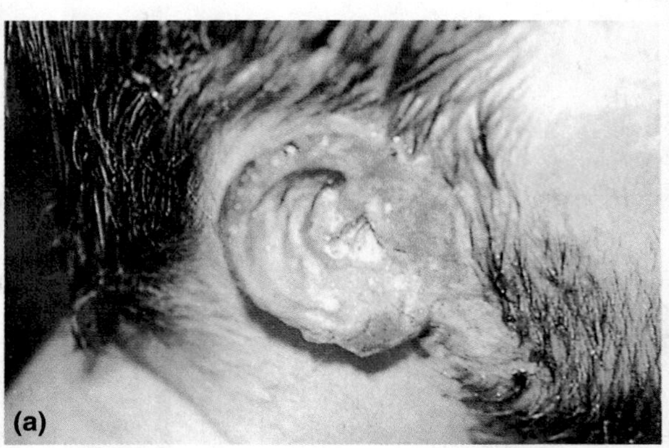

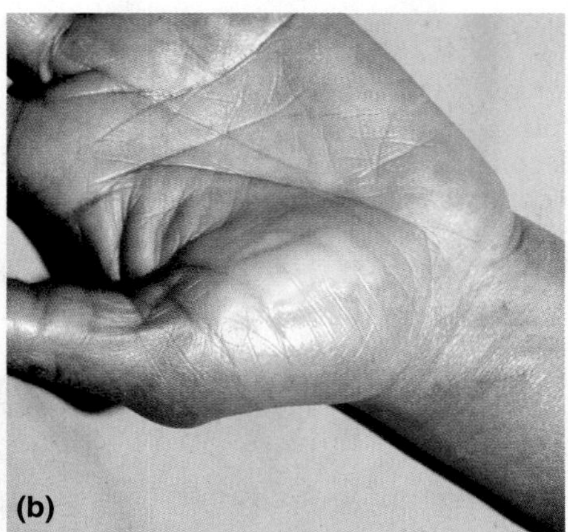

FIGURE 29-9 ✱ **(a)** Chemical burn to the face and ear. **(b)** Chemical burn to the hand. (Both photos: © David Effron, MD, FACEP)

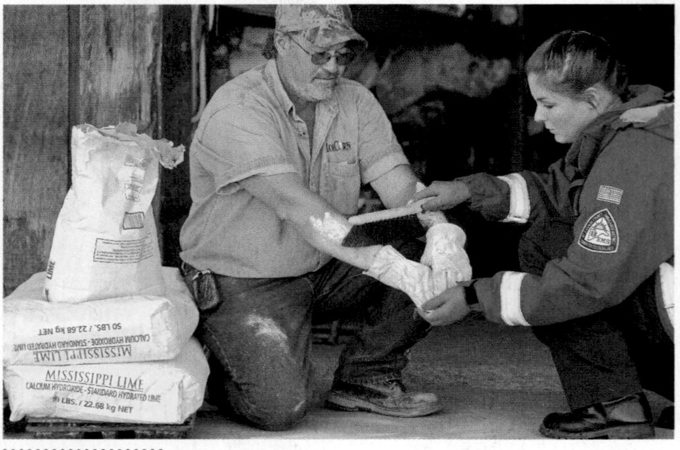

FIGURE 29-10 ✱ Lime powder should be brushed off the skin before flushing with water.

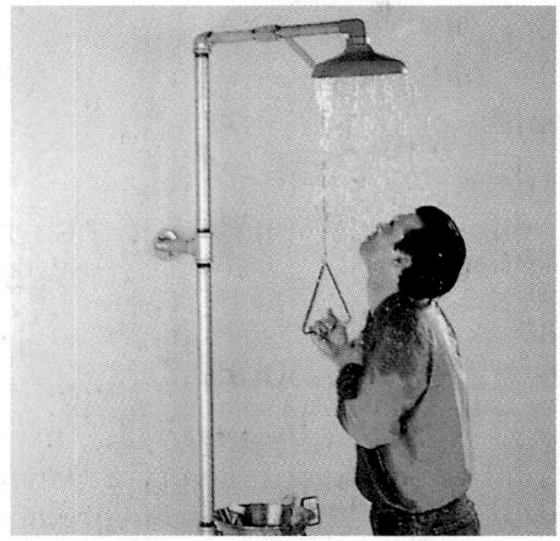

FIGURE 29-11 ✱ Flushing a chemical burn patient under an emergency wash/shower system at the worksite. (© Lab Safety Supply)

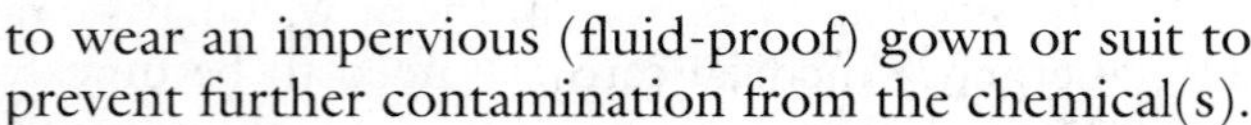

to wear an impervious (fluid-proof) gown or suit to prevent further contamination from the chemical(s).

- *Dry chemicals (e.g., dry lime) should be brushed off before flushing with water* (Figure 29-10✱).
- *Most chemical burns can be flushed with copious amounts of water* (Figures 29-11✱ and 29-12✱). Always ensure that the chemical is one that may be diluted with water. (Consult a hazardous materials

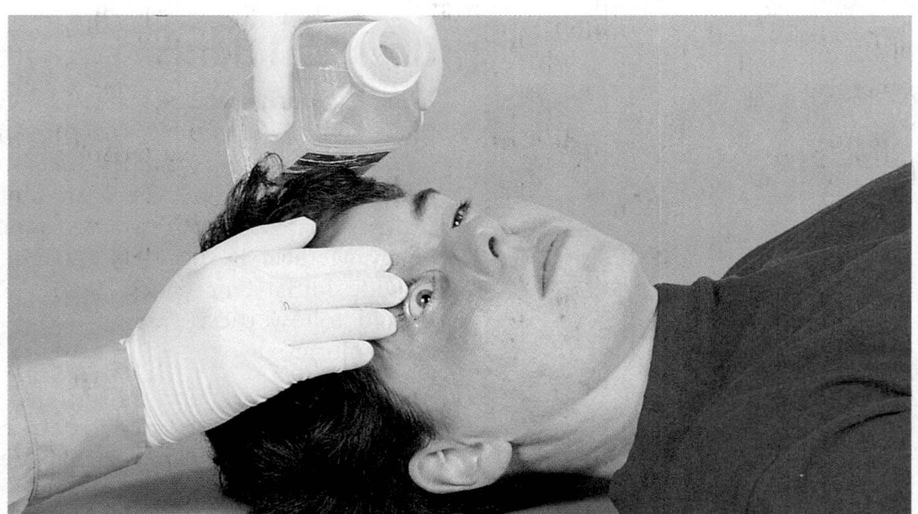

FIGURE 29-12 ✱ Flushing a chemical burn to the eye.

Key Points
Always assume the electrical source is still charged unless you have reliable information that the power source has been completely shut down.

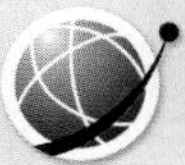

Media Resources
Go to www.bradybooks.com for mykit. Highlights:
- *Web Resource:* Injuries from Fireworks

guidebook.) Some chemicals may produce combustion when they come into contact with water. Minimize further wound contamination by making sure fluid runs away from the injury and not toward any uninjured areas. Remove all clothing and jewelry as in other burn injuries. Continue to flush while en route to the hospital.

Electrical Burns

Electrical burns, including those caused by electrical currents and lightning, can cause severe damage not only to soft tissues but to the body as a whole.

Electrical energy will always seek to flow to the ground. As the energy enters the body, it will seek the path of least resistance to exit the body. All tissues between the entrance and exit of the current will potentially be injured due to the extreme heat created by the resistance of body structures to the electricity (Figure 29-13* and EMT Skills 29-3). Since the body, especially the heart, produces its own electrical energy from chemical reactions, electrical injuries can disturb or destroy these functions, causing irregular heartbeat or even cardiac arrest.

Scene safety is crucial in electrical burn injuries because of the extremely hazardous nature of the electrical source. Always assume the electrical source is still charged unless you have received reliable information that the power source has been completely shut down.

When caring for electrical burn injuries:

- *Never attempt to remove a patient from an electrical source unless trained and equipped to do so.*
- *Never touch a patient still in contact with the electrical source.*
- *Administer oxygen* by nonrebreather mask at 15 lpm or positive pressure ventilation with supplemental oxygen, if necessary, at a rate of 10–12 per minute in an adult and 12–20 per minute in an infant or child.
- *Monitor the patient for cardiac arrest.* Be prepared to administer CPR and apply an automated external defibrillator (AED) if the patient deteriorates to cardiac arrest.

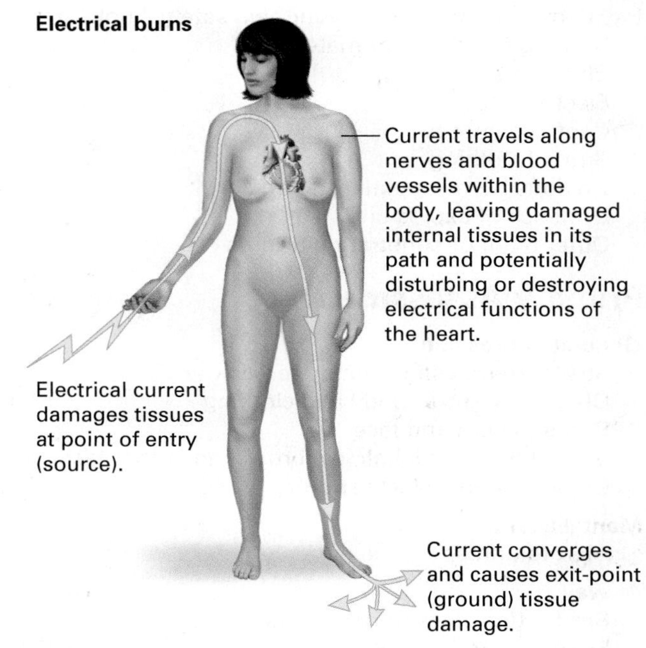

Electrical burns
Current travels along nerves and blood vessels within the body, leaving damaged internal tissues in its path and potentially disturbing or destroying electrical functions of the heart.
Electrical current damages tissues at point of entry (source).
Current converges and causes exit-point (ground) tissue damage.

FIGURE 29-13 * Look for two separate burns when electricity is the cause of injury.

- *Assess the patient for muscle tenderness* with or without twitching and any seizure activity.
- *Always assess for an entrance and exit burn injury.* All tissue in between is suspect for injury even if not readily visible. Emergency medical care for entrance and exit injuries is the same as for other thermal burns.
- *Transport the patient as soon as possible.* Most electrical burn injuries have a slow onset, and underlying tissue or organ damage may not be readily apparent. These patients should be assumed to have critical injuries, even if burns appear insignificant.

Summary: Assessment and Care

To review possible assessment findings and emergency care for burn emergencies, see Figures 29-14* and 29-15*.

Assessment Summary

BURN EMERGENCY

The following findings may be associated with a burn emergency.

SCENE SIZE-UP

Pay particular attention to your own safety. Look for:

- Burning structures or material
- Chemicals
- Electrical sources
- Confined spaces
- Burned clothing
- Obvious burns to patient's body
- Evidence of explosion
- Other blunt or penetrating trauma

Primary Assessment

General Impression

- Stridor or crowing from upper airway
- Obvious burns to body and clothing
- Burns to neck and face
- Singed hair, nasal hair, eyebrows, and other facial hair
- Carbonaceous (black) sputum

Mental Status

- Alert to unresponsive

Airway

- Stridor (indicates upper airway burn)
- Edema to oral mucosa and tongue
- Burns around neck and face
- Black inside mouth

Breathing

- Normal to increased if airway or respiratory tract is not involved
- Increased or decreased, labored, and shallow if airway or respiratory tract burns

Circulation

- Increased; may be decreased if severely hypoxic
- Skin normal in unburned areas; may be cool, clammy, and pale

Status: Priority patient if large body surface area burns, airway or respiratory tract is involved, critical burns are apparent, or burns involve hands, feet, face, genitalia, or major joint locations

Secondary Assessment

Physical Exam

Head, neck, and face:

- Burns
- Singed hair, eyebrows, facial and nasal hair
- Dark black (carbonaceous) sputum
- Swelling of tongue and oral mucosa
- Hoarseness
- Coughing (may cough up black sputum)
- Cyanosis
- Stridor
- Burns to the oral mucosa

Chest:

- Burns
- Wheezing
- Circumferential burns around thorax may impede ventilation
- Blunt or penetrating trauma if explosion or fall involved

Abdomen:

- Burns
- Blunt or penetrating trauma if explosion or fall involved

Extremities:

- Burns (the appearance of the burn is largely determined by the burning mechanism, for example, thermal versus chemical)
- Circumferential burns may reduce distal circulation
- Swelling, pain, and discoloration if explosion or fall involved

Baseline Vital Signs

- BP: normal, may decrease with severe burns after a few hours (if BP decreased at the scene, look for evidence of other trauma)
- HR: normal or increased
- RR: normal; increased and labored if respiratory tract burn involved
- Skin: normal in unburned areas (if pale, cool, clammy immediately after burn may indicate shock from other trauma)
- Pupils: normal
- SpO_2: may be less than 95% if inhalation injury or toxic inhalation has occurred

History

Signs and symptoms of superficial burns:

- Skin that is pink or red, and dry
- Slight swelling
- Pain

Signs and symptoms of partial-thickness burns:

- Skin that is white to cherry red
- Moist and mottled
- Blisters
- Intense pain

Signs and symptoms of full-thickness burns:

- Skin that is dry, hard, tough, and leathery
- White and waxy, dark brown, or charred
- No pain in burned area
- Usually pain around the site of full-thickness burn

Signs and symptoms of inhalation injury:

- Facial burns
- Singed nasal and facial hair and eyebrows
- Black sputum
- Respiratory distress with labored breathing
- Coughing, hoarseness, cyanosis, stridor

FIGURE 29-14a ✱ Assessment summary: burn emergency.

Emergency Care Protocol

BURN EMERGENCY

1. Remove the patient from the source of burn and stop the burning process.
2. Establish manual in-line stabilization if spinal injury is suspected.
3. Establish and maintain an open airway; insert a nasopharyngeal or oropharyngeal airway if the patient is unresponsive and has no gag or cough reflex.
4. Suction secretions as necessary.
5. If breathing is inadequate, provide positive pressure ventilation with supplemental oxygen at a minimum rate of 10–12 ventilations/minute for an adult and 12–20 ventilations/minute for an infant or child.
6. If breathing is adequate, administer oxygen by nonrebreather mask at 15 lpm if inhalation of a toxic gas or upper airway burn is suspected. If the burn is isolated to an area of the body and does not involve the face or a possible inhalation injury or toxic exposure, base your oxygen administration on the SpO_2 reading and signs of hypoxia.
7. Estimate body surface area burn (percent BSA) using the rule of nines.
8. Determine depth of burn: superficial, partial thickness, or full thickness.
9. Apply sterile dressings and bandages or a burn sheet.
10. If the burn is less than 10 percent BSA, dress wet per protocol. Dress all other burns dry.
11. Maintain body temperature.
12. Manage other associated injuries as appropriate.
13. If spinal injury is suspected, immobilize the patient to a backboard.
14. Manage specific burns as follows:
    Dry chemical burn:
    Remove affected clothing, brush off dry chemical, then irrigate with large amounts of water.
    Liquid chemical burn:
    Remove affected clothing; irrigate with large amounts of water if the chemical is one that does not react to water.
    Burns to the hands and feet:
    Remove all rings and jewelry; dress between digits.
    Chemical burns to the eyes:
    Flush with large amounts of water and continue to flush en route.
    Thermal burns to the eyes:
    Do not attempt to open eyelids; apply dry, sterile dressing to both eyes.
    Electrical burns:
    Carefully monitor pulse and respiration; inspect for entrance and exit wounds; assess for muscle tenderness; apply AED if patient is in cardiac arrest.
15. Transport.
16. Perform a reassessment every 5 minutes if unstable and every 15 minutes if stable.

FIGURE 29-14b ✱ Emergency care protocol: burn emergency.

Emergency Care Algorithm: **Burn Emergency**

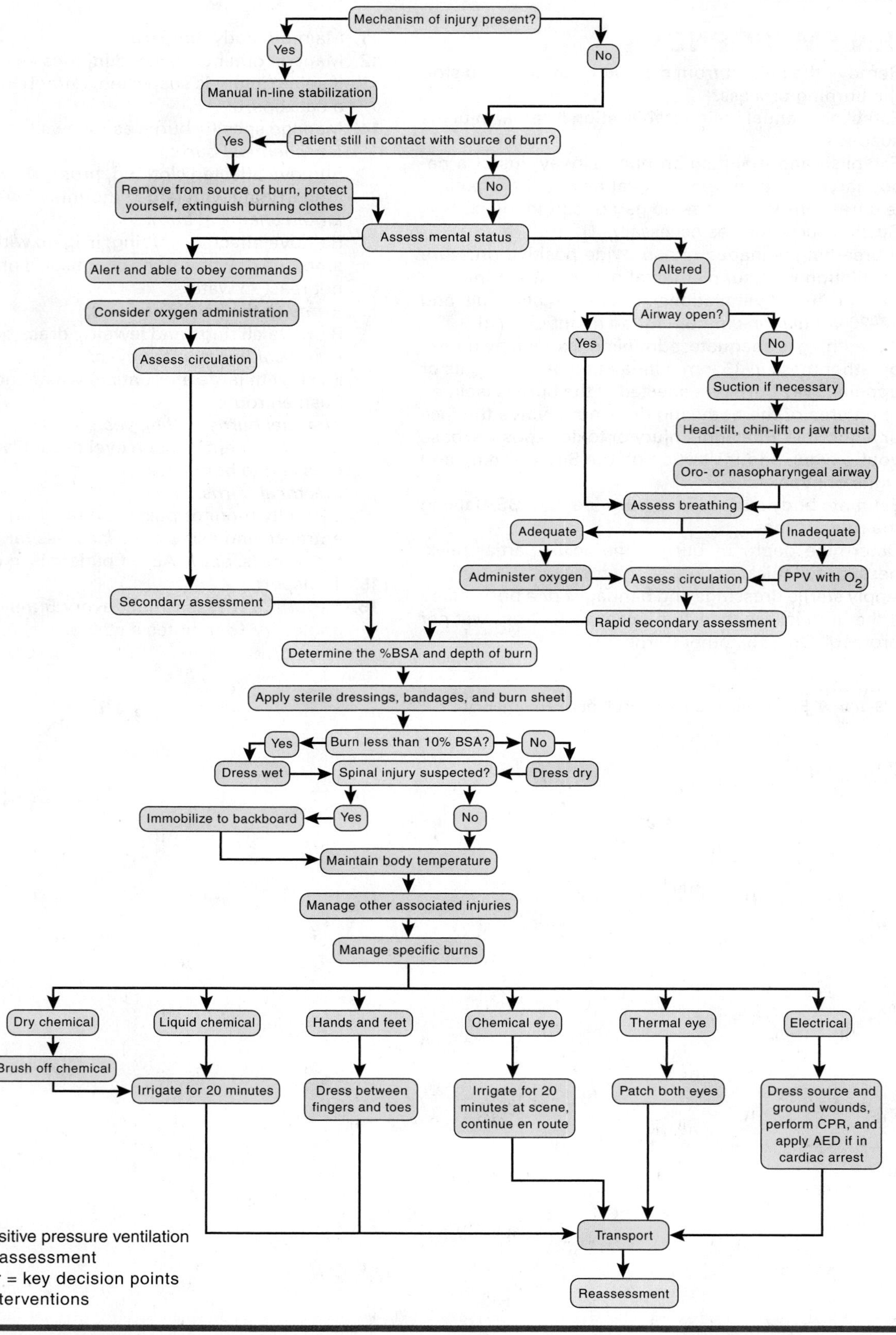

FIGURE 29-15 ✱ Emergency care algorithm: burn emergency.

EMT skills 29-1 Partial-Thickness Burns

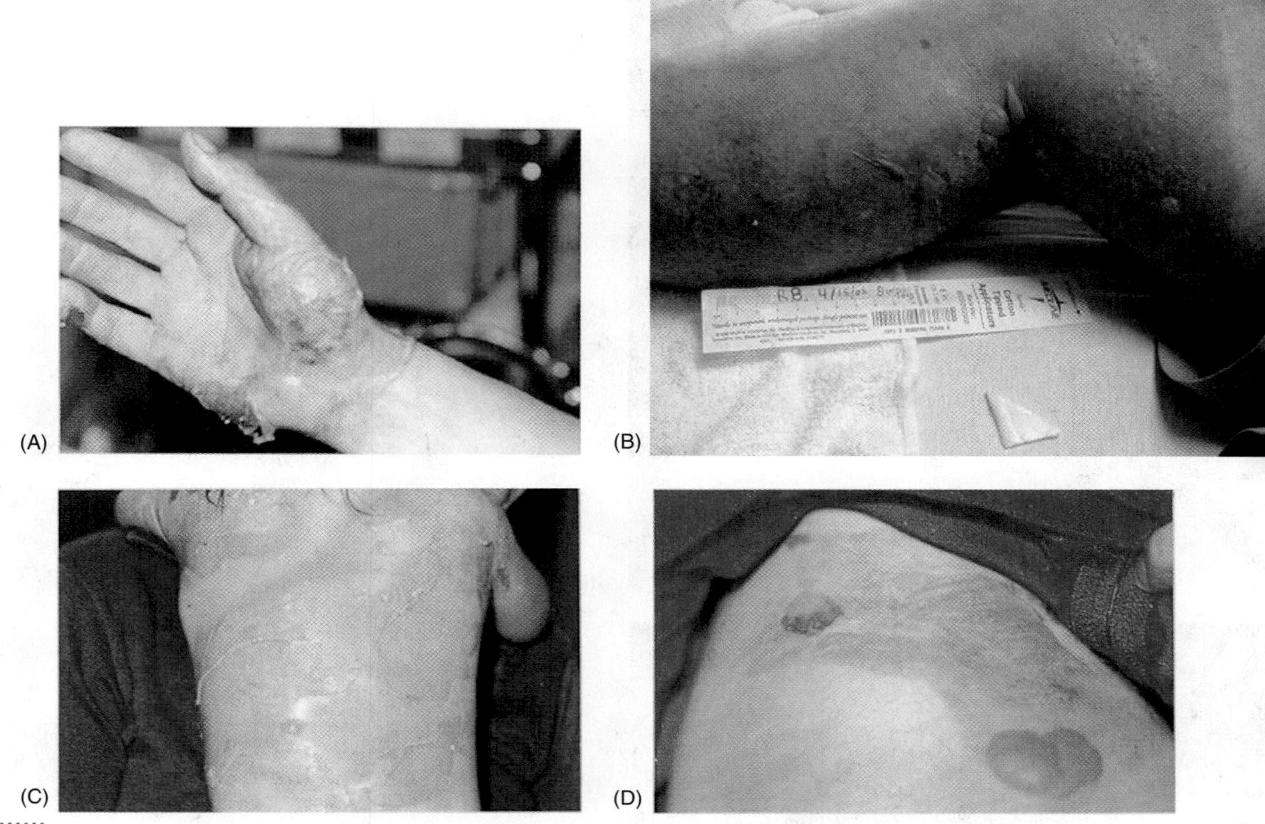

29-1 * (Photo B: © Maria A. H. Lyle/Sarasota Memorial Hospital)

Full-Thickness Burns

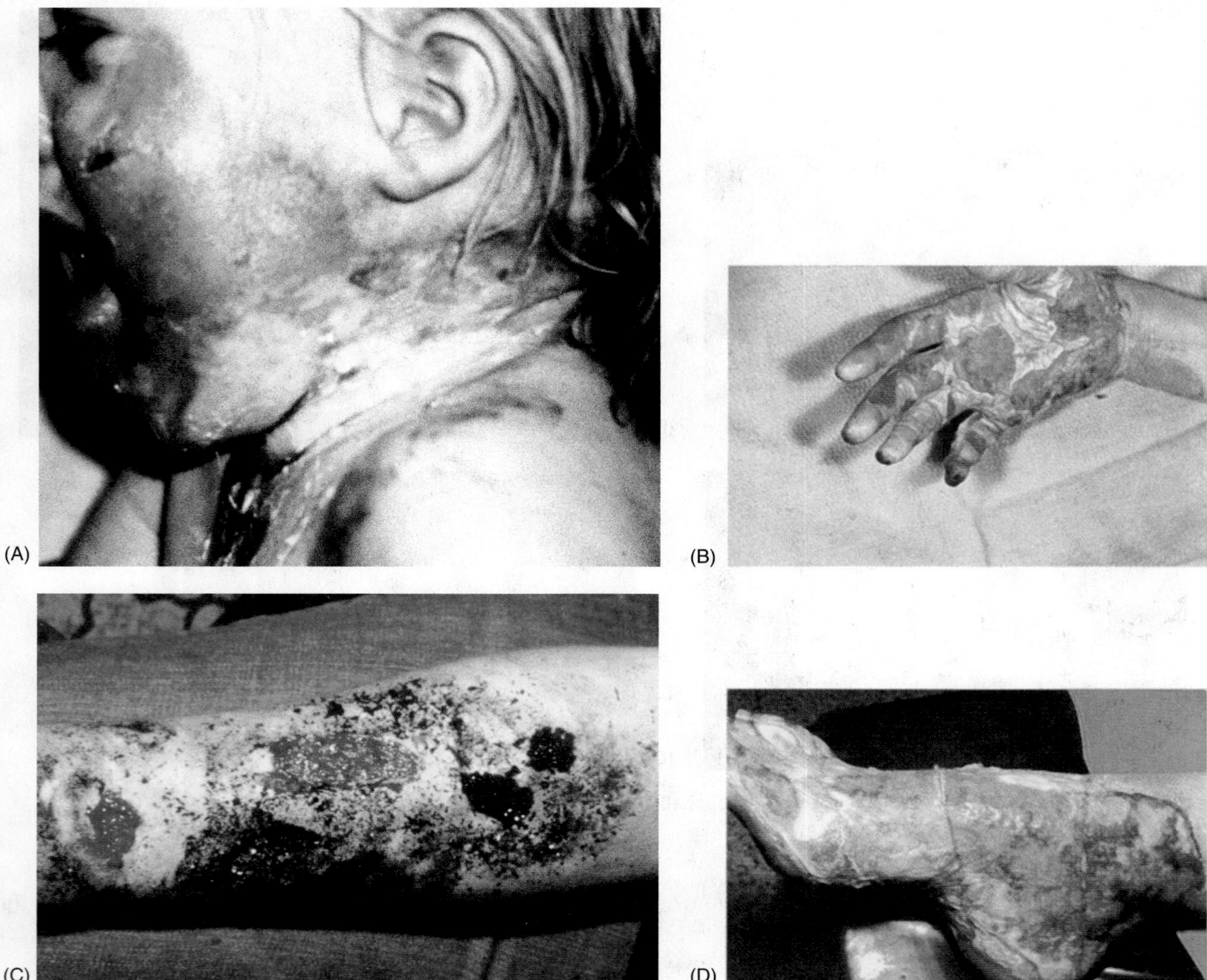

29-2 *

EMT skills 29-3 Electrical Burns and Lightning Injuries

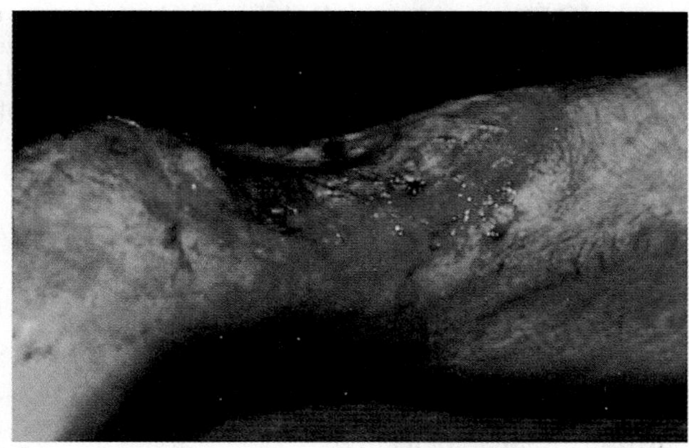

29-3A ✱ Full-thickness electrical burn.

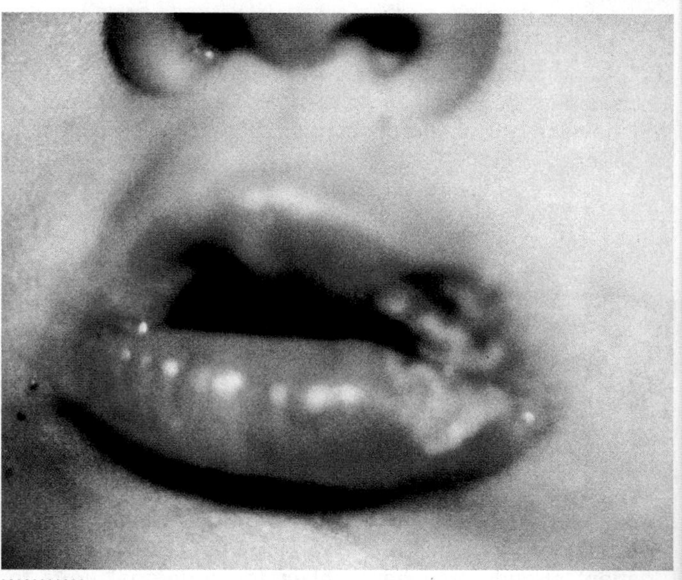

29-3B ✱ Electrical burn caused by chewing on an electrical cord.

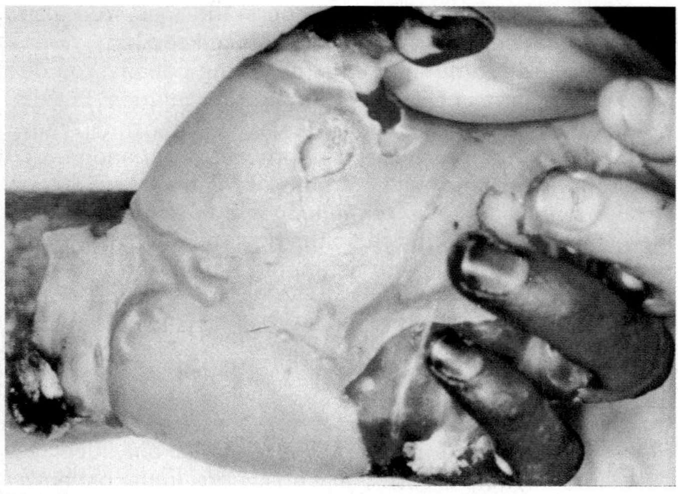

29-3C ✱ Burn associated with lightning injury.

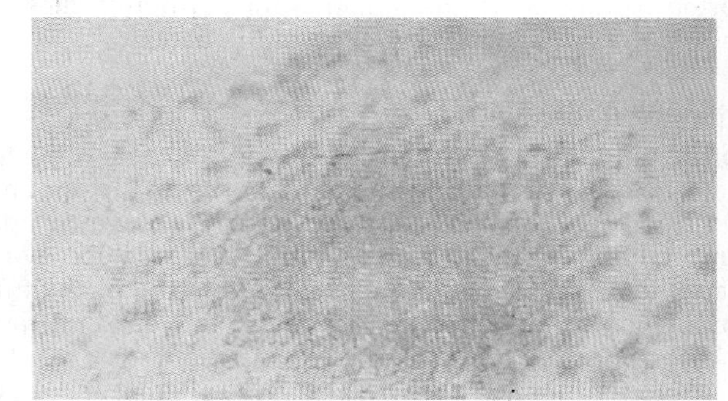

29-3D ✱ Abnormal skin pattern associated with lightning injury.

CHAPTER REVIEW

SUMMARY

Although burns are not the most common mechanisms of trauma that EMTs see in the prehospital setting, they usually present with a dramatic clinical impression. While the obvious manifestations of burns are frequently impressive, the EMT must remember that these patients may have associated injury to the airway, breathing, or circulatory system that is of greater risk to life and limb, initially, than the burn is. Only after ensuring that all life threats found during the primary assessment are properly managed should the EMT focus attention on the burn injury itself. Initial management at the scene (and during transport) is the prime determinant of survival for any type of burn.

Inhalation burns are of significant concern, because if the patient is not properly assessed, is not provided with adequate airway or ventilatory management, or is not oxygenated as needed, the inhalation injury will easily contribute to patient morbidity and mortality. The EMT must be aware of the unique metabolic and cardiovascular problems that accompany burn injuries. Although some of these concerns cannot be initially managed by the EMT, these factors will have important implications, especially in respect to transport.

Providing care for the critically injured burn patient will include the use of many of the EMT's assessment and management skills, and the quality of prehospital care rendered during the first hours after a burn injury will have a major impact on long-term outcome. By being vigilant in the evaluation and management of these patients, particularly with regard to airway management and ventilatory support, the EMT can provide the patient with the greatest chance of a meaningful recovery and return to a functional life.

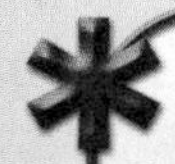

CASE STUDY FOLLOW-UP

SCENE SIZE-UP

You and your partner have been dispatched to a reported structural fire. You have arrived on the scene of a fully involved structure fire with one patient trapped on the second floor. You have donned your gloves, mask, and eye protection. Since this is a "working" fire with one known patient already, you have called for additional units for assistance.

As you arrive, you spot a firefighter carrying the reported patient down the ladder. Your partner readies the back of the ambulance as you go to the patient.

PRIMARY ASSESSMENT

You begin your assessment by noting that the patient, a male, has severe charring and other burns on the right half of his body and that he is unresponsive. His airway is open but breathing is shallow and rapid. His face is somewhat blackened. You immediately place him in the back of the ambulance on the stretcher. His pulse is weak and rapid and you consider him a high-priority patient.

Your partner has inserted an airway adjunct and set up the bag-valve unit for positive pressure ventilation with supplemental oxygen. He begins ventilations while you stop the burning process. You pour sterile saline over the patient's burned areas and at the same time begin to assess the severity of the burn. There are full-thickness burns over the patient's right chest and abdomen both front and back, right arm, and leg. There is singed nasal hair and blackened areas around the face. You quickly estimate this to be about a full-thickness burn over a 50 percent BSA and classify the patient as critical in terms of burn severity.

You begin to remove clothing and jewelry, continuing to stop the burning process, then immediately begin transport to the local trauma center.

SECONDARY ASSESSMENT

The patient remains unresponsive as you begin to further assess and treat him. You have cooled the burn down and now cover the patient with a sterile burn sheet and place sterile dressings between his fingers and toes. You also cover the patient with several blankets to keep him warm. Your partner is continuing to ventilate the patient. You do a physical exam, checking for any further injuries, but do not find any. You assess the patient's vital signs, and they are BP 98/68 mmHg, pulse 124 bpm and rapid and weak, respirations assisted at 12 breaths per minute. The SpO_2 is 87%. Upon auscultation of the lungs you discover wheezing in all lung fields. You radio the hospital to advise them of the patient's status and estimated time of arrival. You are unable to obtain a history because the patient is unresponsive and his critical condition did not allow you time to question bystanders at the scene.

REASSESSMENT

Since transport time is short, you conduct only one reassessment. There is essentially no change in the patient's status and the positive pressure ventilations seem to be helping. At the hospital, you give a quick report to the hospital staff as you take the patient to the trauma room. The emergency physician immediately prepares to intubate the patient as other personnel start fluid replacement.

You next begin the task of completing the prehospital care report as your partner readies the vehicle. The dispatcher advises you that you will be required back at the fire scene as quickly as possible.

IN REVIEW

1. Define and list the characteristics of superficial, partial-thickness, and full-thickness burns.
2. Define the rule of nines and describe how it is used on both adult and infant or child burn injury patients.
3. Using the rule of nines, name the percentage of body surface area (BSA) burned if (a) a 4-year-old child has superficial burn injuries to the front and back of both legs as well as the chest, abdomen, and back; (b) an adult has partial-thickness burn injuries to the front of one lower extremity and to the front and back of the other lower extremity.
4. Determine the burn severity classification for patients "a" and "b" in question 3.
5. Describe the basic emergency care steps for burn injuries.
6. List the three things an EMT should not do when applying dressings to a burn injury patient.
7. List the emergency medical care guidelines for chemical burns.
8. List the emergency medical care guidelines for electrical burns.

CRITICAL THINKING

You are called to a local university where a female student was working on an experiment under the protective hood in her chemistry lab. When she was removing a beaker of solution from under the hood, the beaker bumped the edge of the sash and splashed her face and chest with an alkali chemical, ammonium hydroxide. Although the student was wearing safety glasses, the solution splashed behind her glasses and soaked into her lab jacket and clothing underneath.

The laboratory assistant immediately got her to the safety shower and began the flushing process before calling 911. By the time you arrive, the patient is sitting down on a chair with a wet towel wrapped around her bare chest, and she is holding her hand over her closed eyes in an attempt to shield them from the bright light in the laboratory. Upon assessment and questioning, she complains only of a severe burning to her eyes. She has no observable burns to her face or oral cavity, and the chemical that splashed onto her chest did not seem to penetrate to her skin.

1. Would these burns be considered mild, moderate, or severe?
2. What is your rationalization for your answer to question 1?
3. How are the eye injuries best managed while en route to the hospital?
4. What is the process recommended for flushing chemical eye injuries?
5. If there was a community hospital within 2 minutes of the university, and a regional burn/trauma center within 15 minutes of the university, which facility should the EMT elect to transport to?

EXPLORE PEARSON **mybradykit**™

Please go to **www.bradybooks.com** to access mykit for this text. You will find quizzes, critical thinking scenarios, weblinks, animations, and videos related to this chapter—and much more. Look for online information on burns in children, burn centers, and injuries from fireworks.

Register your access code from the front of your book by going to **www.bradybooks.com** and selecting the mykit links.

CHAPTER 30

Musculoskeletal Trauma

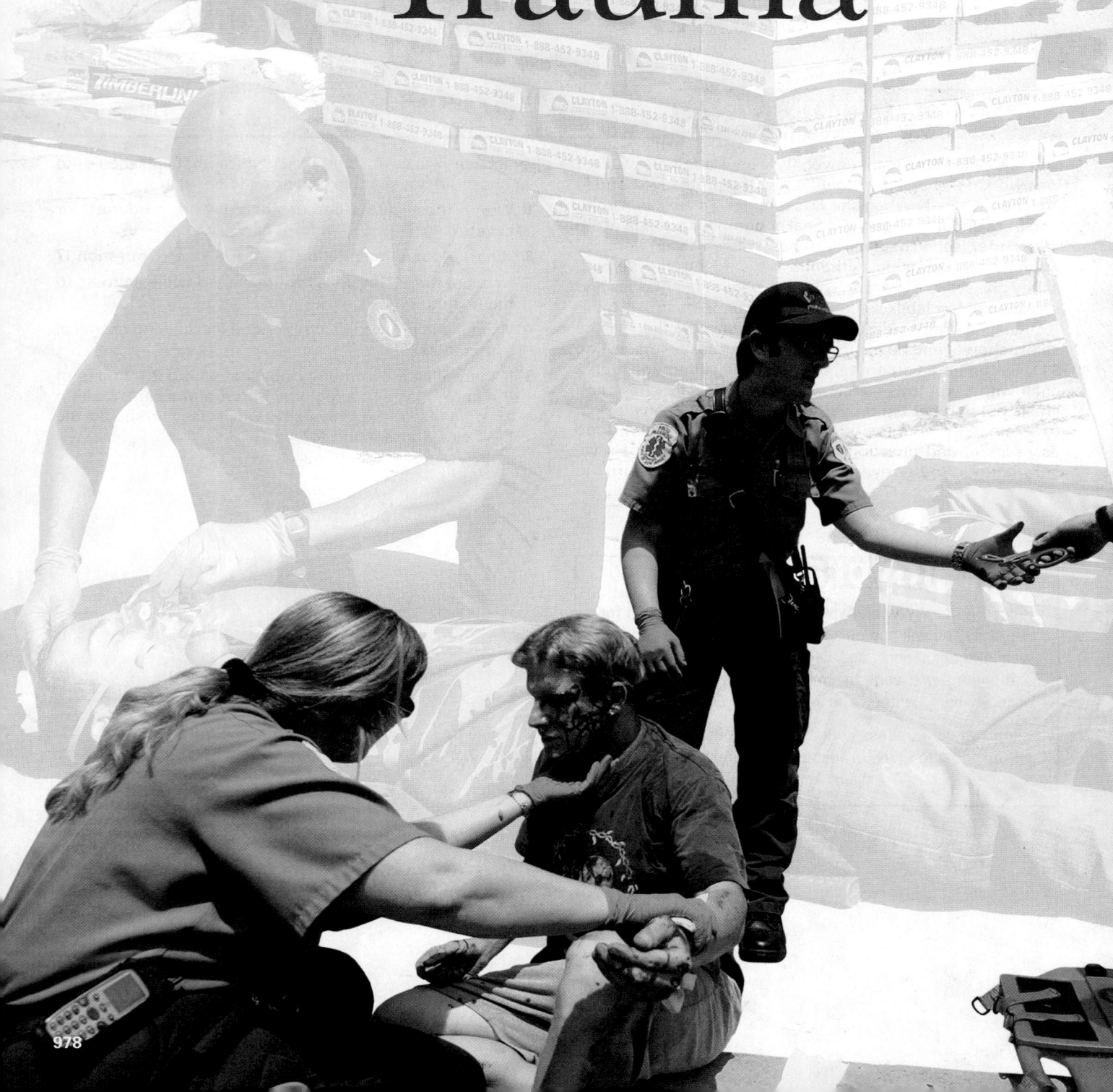

Navigation Guide

The following items provide an overview to the purpose and content of this chapter. The Standard and Competency are from the new National EMS Education Standards.

STANDARD **Trauma** (Content Area: Orthopedic Trauma)

COMPETENCY Applies fundamental knowledge to provide basic emergency care and transportation based on assessment findings for an acutely injured patient.

OBJECTIVES: After reading this chapter, you should be able to:

30-1. Define key terms introduced in this chapter.
30-2. Describe the structures and functions of the musculoskeletal system, including:
- **a.** Bones
- **b.** Skeletal muscle
- **c.** Tendons
- **d.** Ligaments
- **e.** Cartilage
- **f.** Joints

30-3. Describe each of the following types of injuries and their associated signs and symptoms:
- **a.** Fractures
- **b.** Strains
- **c.** Sprains
- **d.** Dislocations

30-4. Give examples of direct, indirect, and twisting forces that can produce musculoskeletal injuries.
30-5. Explain why fractures of the femur and pelvis are considered to be critical fractures.
30-6. Describe the assessment-based approach to bone and joint injuries.
30-7. Establish the priority for assessing and treating musculoskeletal injuries with respect to a patient's overall condition.
30-8. Discuss the significance of assessing a musculoskeletal injury for each of the following findings:
- **a.** Pain
- **b.** Pallor
- **c.** Paralysis
- **d.** Paresthesia
- **e.** Pressure
- **f.** Pulses

30-9. Explain the rationale for splinting musculoskeletal injuries.
30-10. Compare and contrast the characteristics and uses of various types of splints, including:
- **a.** Rigid splints
- **b.** Pressure (air or pneumatic) splints
- **c.** Traction splints
- **d.** Formable splints
- **e.** Vacuum splints
- **f.** Sling and swathe
- **g.** Spine board
- **h.** Improvised splints

30-11. Discuss hazards of improper splinting.
30-12. Discuss special considerations in splinting long bone injuries, splinting joint injuries, and traction splinting.
30-13. Discuss special considerations in splinting pelvic fractures.
30-14. Describe the basic pathophysiology of compartment syndrome.

KEY TERMS: Page references indicate first major use in this chapter. For complete definitions, see the Glossary at the back of the book.

compartment syndrome p. 999
crepitus p. 989
direct force p. 986
indirect force p. 986
osteoporosis p. 985
paresthesia p. 997
pathologic fracture p. 984
splint p. 991
twisting force p. 986

MEDIA RESOURCES: Please go to www.bradybooks.com to access mykit for this text. You will find quizzes, critical thinking scenarios, weblinks, animations, and videos related to this chapter—and much more. Look for online information on fractures. You will also find video clips on joint injuries, long bone injuries, and splints.

continued

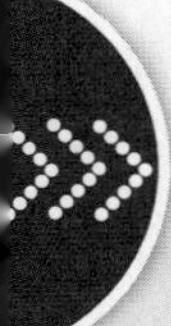

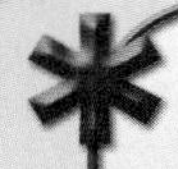

CASE STUDY

The Dispatch
Medic One—respond to the Peninsula High football field—you have a 17-year-old male patient complaining of leg pain. Time out is 1634 hours.

Upon Arrival
You are met by the football coach. He tells you his quarterback was tackled very hard. The patient cries out in pain, "My leg, my leg!"

How Should You Proceed to Care for This Patient?
During this chapter, you will learn how to assess and treat a painful, swollen, or deformed extremity. Later we will return to the case and apply the knowledge and skills learned.

Introduction

Injuries to muscles, joints, and bones are some of the most common emergencies you will encounter in the field. They can range from simple and non-life-threatening injuries (such as a broken finger or sprained ankle) to critical and life-threatening injuries (such as a fracture of the femur or spine). Regardless of whether the injury is mild or severe, your ability to provide emergency care efficiently and quickly may prevent further painful and damaging injury and may even keep the patient from suffering permanent disability or death.

Musculoskeletal System Review

The two main parts of the musculoskeletal system, as is obvious from its name, are the muscles and the skeleton. The functions of the musculoskeletal system are:

- To give the body shape
- To protect the internal organs
- To provide for movement
- To store salts and other materials needed for metabolism
- To produce red blood cells necessary for oxygen transport

The musculoskeletal system was presented in Chapter 7, "Anatomy, Physiology, and Medical Terminology," which you may wish to review. Some major points about the musculoskeletal system are summarized in the following sections.

The Muscles

There are three kinds of muscles: voluntary (skeletal), involuntary (smooth), and cardiac. Involuntary muscles are found in the walls of organs and help move food through the digestive system. Cardiac muscle is found only in the walls of the heart.

The kind of muscle that is pertinent to the topic of this chapter, musculoskeletal injuries, is voluntary muscle. Voluntary muscles are those that are under control of a person's will. They make possible all deliberate acts, such as walking, chewing, swallowing, smiling, frowning, talking, or moving the eyeballs. Often referred to as skeletal muscles, most voluntary muscles are generally attached at one or both ends to the skeleton.

The voluntary muscles form the major muscle mass of the body. Movements of the body are the result of work performed by the muscles. What enables muscle tissue to work is its ability to contract—to become shorter and thicker—when stimulated by a nerve impulse. In addition to enabling us to move, muscles help give our bodies their distinctive shapes.

Muscles can be injured in many ways. Overexerting a muscle may break fibers, and muscles subjected to trauma can be bruised, crushed, cut, torn, or otherwise injured, even if the skin is not broken. Muscles injured in any way tend to become swollen, tender, painful, or weak.

Tendons and Ligaments

Tendons and ligaments (Figure 30-1*) are, in a sense, the glue that holds the body together. Composed of specialized connective tissue, *tendons* connect muscle to bone while *ligaments* connect bone to bone. Tendons and ligaments, as well as muscles, can be bruised, crushed, cut, or torn, and are included in the category of musculoskeletal injuries.

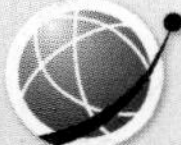

Media Resources
Go to www.bradybooks.com for mykit. Highlights:

- *Web Resource:* Fractures and Sprains
- *Web Resource:* Osteoporosis and Fractures

Objective 30-2
Describe the structures and functions of the musculoskeletal system, including bones, skeletal muscle, tendons, ligaments, cartilage, and joints.

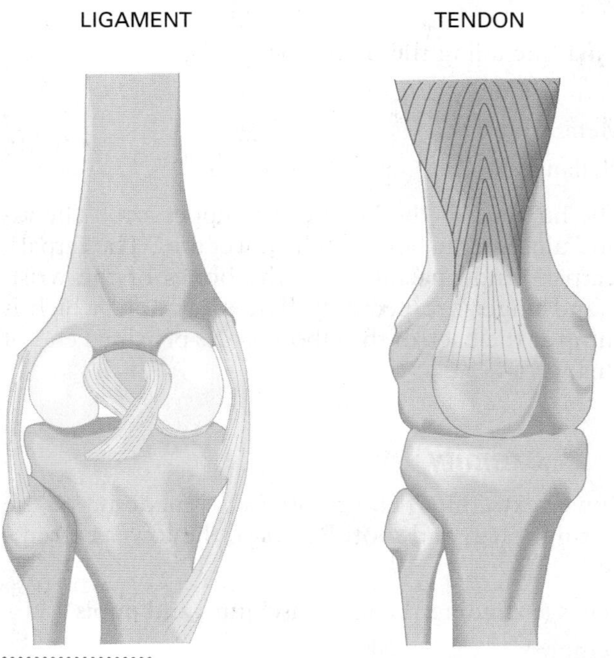

FIGURE 30-1 ✻ Ligaments connect bone to bone. Tendons attach muscle to bone.

Cartilage

Cartilage is an extension of the bone end and is composed of connective tissue. It is a strong, smooth, flexible, compressible, and slippery substance found at the point of articulation of two bones (Figure 30-2✻). Cartilage allows the bones to ride over each other during movement with relatively little friction. Cartilage also acts somewhat as a shock absorber between the bone surfaces. Cartilage can be injured, leading to joint pain.

The Skeletal System

The skeletal system (Figure 30-3✻) supports the body, allowing it to stand erect. Without its bones, the body would collapse. As the body's structural framework, the skeleton must be strong to provide support and protection, jointed to permit motion, and flexible to withstand stress. A major element in motion is the body's *joints,* or places where bones meet. Joints allow for several different types of motion:

- **Flexion.** Bending motion that moves the extremity toward the body
- **Extension.** Bending motion that moves the extremity away from the body

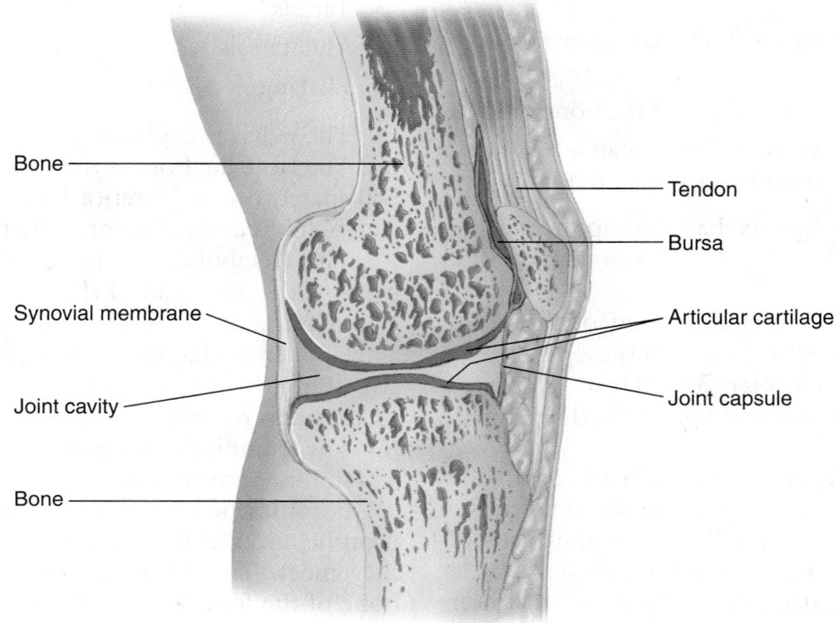

FIGURE 30-2 ✻ Structure of a joint.

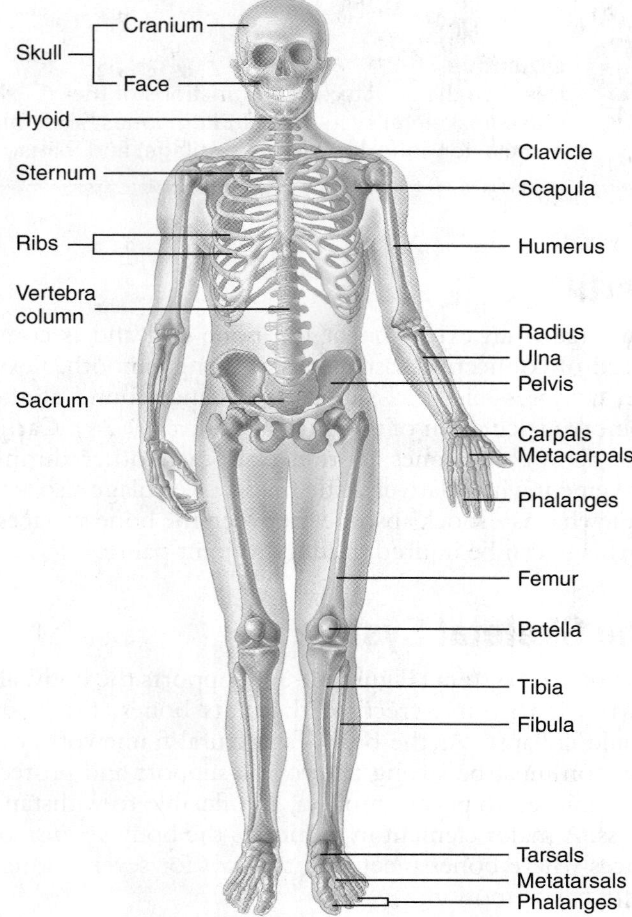

FIGURE 30-3 ✻ The skeletal system.

- **Adduction.** Movement of a body part toward the midline of the body
- **Abduction.** Movement of a body part away from the midline of the body
- **Rotation.** Turning along the axis of the bone or joint
- **Circumduction.** Movement through an arc of a circle or in a circular motion from a central point

The skeletal system has six basic components: the skull, spinal column, thorax, pelvis, lower extremities, and upper extremities.

The axial skeletal system is composed of the head, thorax, and vertebral column. Injury to these structures is covered in detail in Chapter 31, "Head Trauma," Chapter 32, "Spinal Column and Spinal Cord Trauma," and Chapter 34, "Chest Trauma."

The appendicular skeletal system is made up of the bones in the extremities, to include the shoulder girdle and the pelvis. Injuries to these bones are the focus of this chapter. The appendicular skeleton can be divided into bones of the upper extremity and bones of the lower extremity.

Upper Extremity

The upper extremity (Figure 30-4✻) consists of the shoulder girdle, arm, forearm, and hand. Bones of the upper extremity are:

- Clavicle (collarbone)
- Scapula (shoulder blade)
- Humerus
- Radius
- Ulna (including the olecranon)
- Carpal bones
- Metacarpals
- Phalanges

The humerus is the bone of the upper arm. The radius and ulna are the bones of the lower arm. The carpals, metacarpals, and phalanges are the bones of the wrist, hand, and fingers, respectively. The olecranon, which is the bump at the back of the elbow, is the proximal end of the ulna.

Lower Extremity

The lower extremity (Figure 30-5✻) is made up of the pelvis, thigh, leg, and foot. Bones of the lower extremity are:

- Pelvis (including the ilium, ischium, and pubis)
- Femur
- Patella (kneecap)
- Tibia
- Fibula
- Calcaneus (heel bone)
- Tarsals
- Metatarsals
- Phalanges

The pelvis is made up of the ilium, ischium, and pubis. The large flat bone is the ilium. The iliac crest is what is palpated on the anterior-lateral body at the belt line. The ischium and pubis form the floor of the pelvis.

The acetabulum is a hollow depression in the lateral pelvis where the head of the femur (the thighbone) fits, creating a joint. All of the bones create the pelvic girdle. The greater trochanter is a process of the proximal femur. It is the bony projection that is felt on the lateral upper thigh, often referred to as the hip.

The femur is the bone of the upper leg, while the tibia and fibula are the bones of the lower leg. The patella covers the joint where the femur and tibia meet. Condyles are protuberances at the sides of the tibia and femur where they meet. The calcaneus, or heel bone, is the largest bone of the foot. The tarsals, metatarsals, and phalanges are the bones of the ankle, foot, and toes, respectively.

Objective 30-3
Describe fractures, strains, sprains, and dislocations and their associated signs and symptoms.

Key Points
An open fracture has an associated open wound that is vulnerable to contamination and infection.

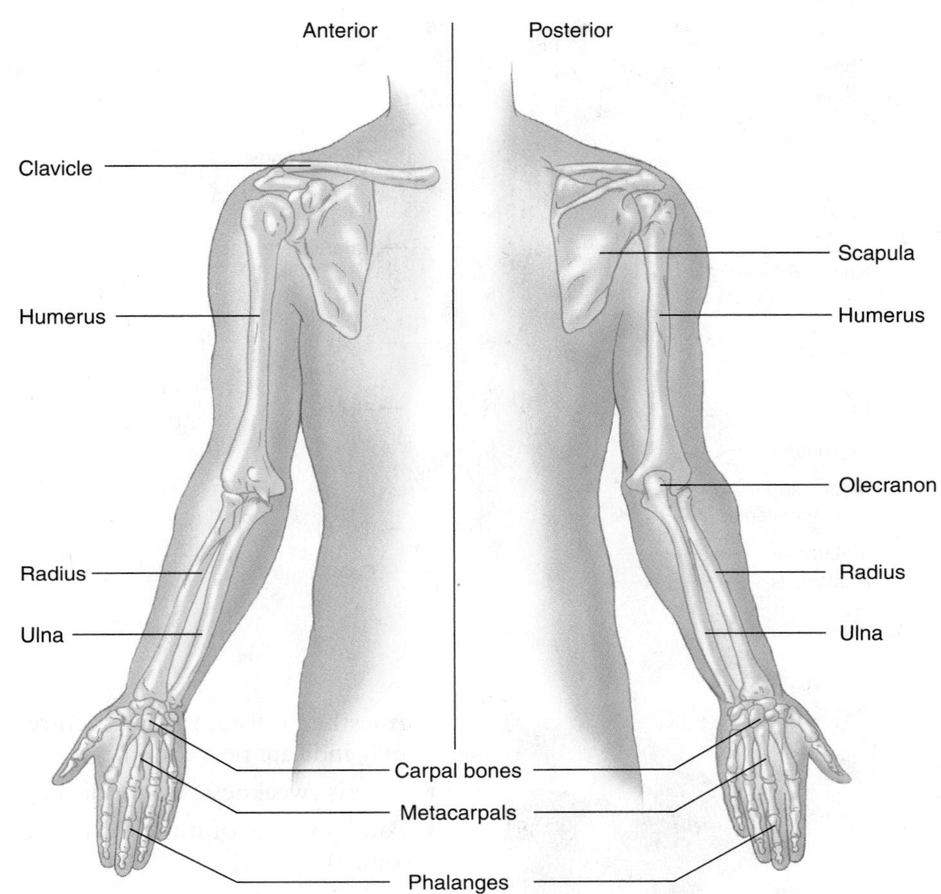

FIGURE 30-4 ✱ Bones of the upper extremity.

▶ Injuries to Bones and Joints

Types of Injuries

Several kinds of musculoskeletal injuries are possible. The first to come to mind is a *fracture* or, simply, a broken bone (Figure 30-6✱). Although many of the signs and symptoms are similar, the injury may not involve a fracture but may be a strain, sprain, or dislocation.

Fracture

A fracture is a break in the continuity of a bone. Fractures occur as a result of a variety of mechanisms of injury, including direct force, indirect force, and twisting force. These forces are discussed later in the section.

A fracture is generally categorized as open or closed. An open fracture is a fracture with an associated open wound. The open wound may have been caused by the bone end punching through the muscle, soft tissue, and skin, or it may have been caused by the force that caused the fracture, such as a bullet. If there is no break in the skin, the fracture is considered to be closed. An open fracture is additionally complicated by the introduction of bacteria and other contaminants that may lead to infection.

If the bones become displaced, there may be damage to surrounding nerves, blood vessels, muscles, ligaments, and tendons.

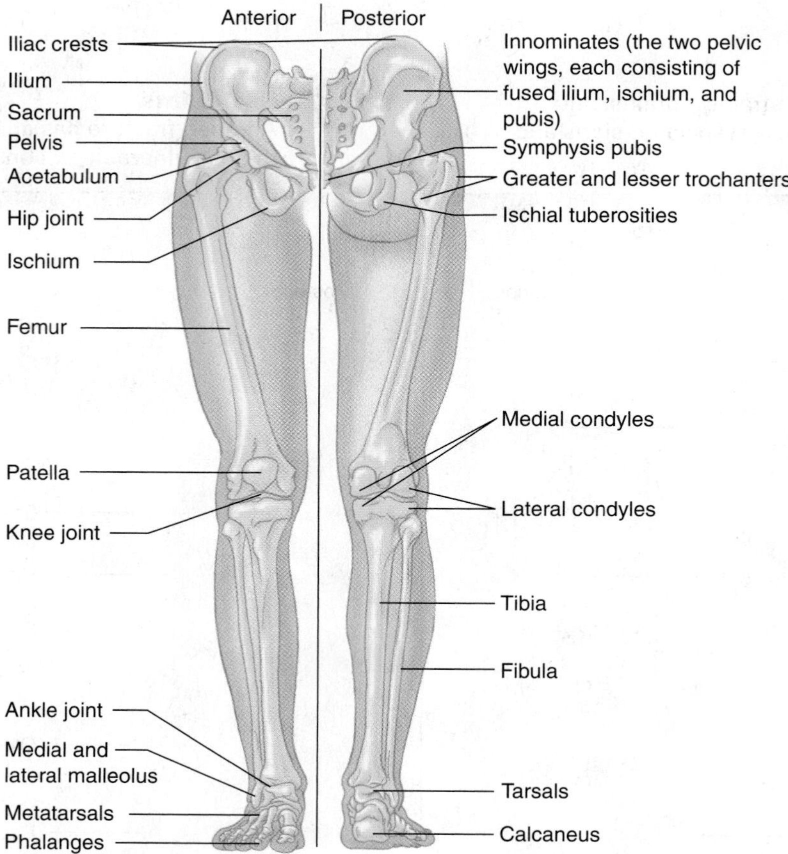

FIGURE 30-5 ✱ Bones of the lower extremity.

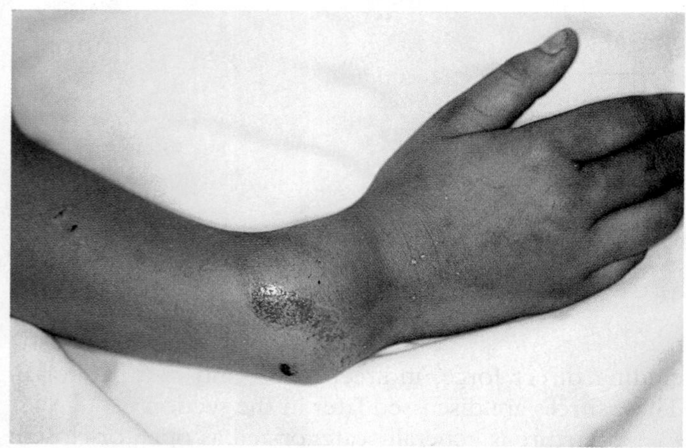

FIGURE 30-6 ✱ Fracture of the wrist. (© Charles Stewart, MD, and Associates)

Signs and symptoms of a fracture may include:

- Pain
- Tenderness
- Deformity
- Discoloration
- Paresthesia distal to the fracture site (tingling or abnormal sensation; may indicate nerve injury)
- Anesthesia distal to the fracture site (loss of feeling; may indicate nerve injury)
- Paresis (weakness; may indicate nerve injury)
- Paralysis (loss of muscle control; may indicate nerve injury)
- Inability to move the extremity (may indicate muscle or tendon damage)
- Decreased pulse amplitude, increased capillary refill time, paresthesia, or pale, cool skin distal to the fracture site (may indicate vessel injury)

There are several types of fractures (Figure 30-7✱). You can distinguish the type of fracture only through an X-ray. A hairline fracture is a small crack in the bone that doesn't create instability. The patient may present only with pain and tenderness. A **pathologic fracture** results from a disease that causes degeneration and dramatically weakens the bone and makes it prone to fracture. These fractures often occur without a significant force being applied. A patient may be walking normally across the room and suffer a pathologic fracture. Patients with a past medical history of cancer often suffer pathologic fractures.

Complications that may result from a fracture include hemorrhage from the bone itself; instability of the extremity leading to an increased incidence of tissue, nerve, or vessel damage; surrounding tissue damage; infection

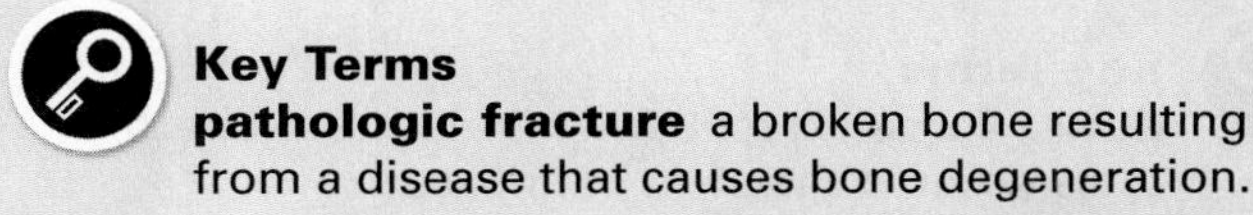

Key Terms
pathologic fracture a broken bone resulting from a disease that causes bone degeneration.

Key Terms
osteoporosis a degenerative bone disorder associated with an accelerated loss of minerals, primarily calcium, from the bone.

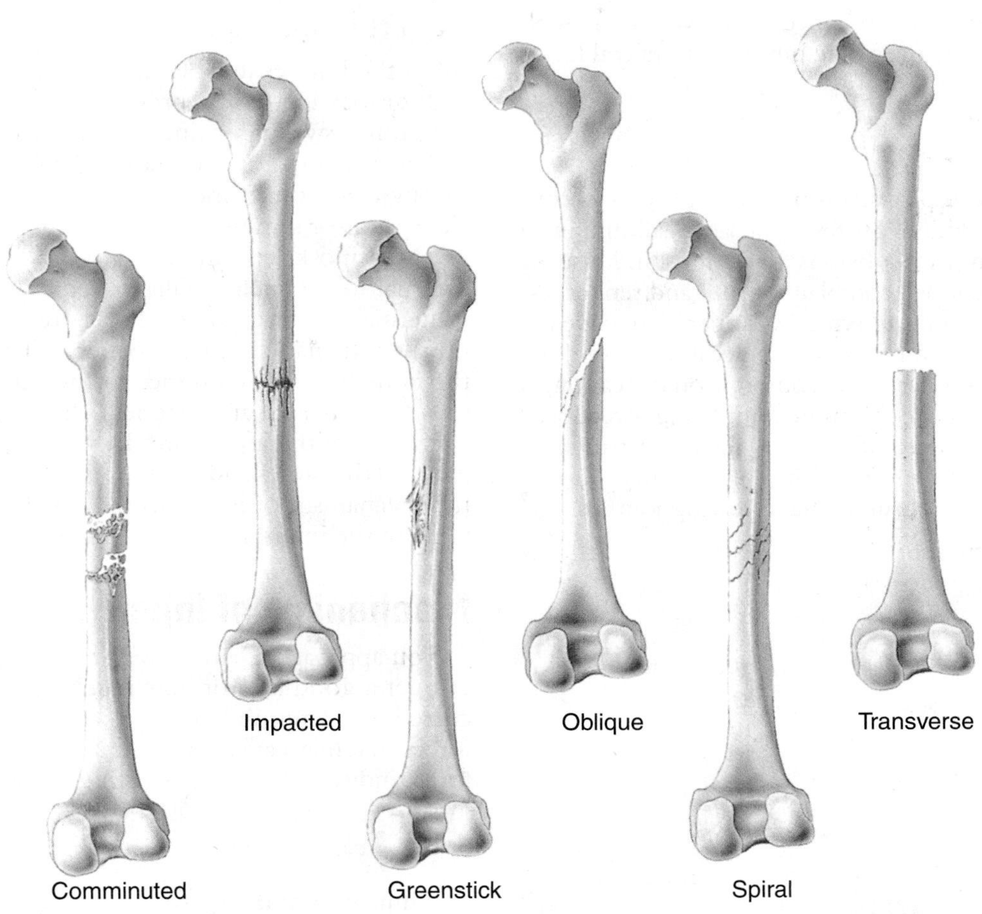

FIGURE 30-7 ✻ Types of fractures.

associated with an open fracture; and interruption of distal blood supply.

Geriatric patients are especially prone to fractures because of changes in their bone structure. After 40 years of age, bones start to become less flexible, more brittle, and more easily fractured. **Osteoporosis** is a degenerative bone disorder associated with an accelerated loss of minerals, primarily calcium, from the bone. This condition dramatically weakens the bones and makes them susceptible to fracture. Osteoporosis typically affects women more than men and occurs most often after menopause.

Strain

A strain is an injury to a muscle or a muscle and tendon, possibly caused by overextension, or overstretching. Overstretching tears muscle fibers and causes pain that typically increases with the muscle use. A strain may also occur as a result of extreme muscle stress or fatigue associated with overuse. Because there is no bleeding, the injury does not present with edema or discoloration. Typically, the patient complains of pain on palpation, usually localized to a specific site, and pain or weakness with use of the muscle.

Sprain

A sprain is an injury to a joint capsule, with damage to or tearing of the connective tissue, and usually involves ligaments. The shoulder, knee, and ankle are the joints most vulnerable to sprains. The patient typically experiences immediate pain and tenderness at the joint upon injury.

Thinking Critically
A child who fell from a tree has swelling, pain, and discoloration of her upper arm. A man braced himself with one arm when he fell to the sidewalk but has no swelling, discoloration, or pain. Can you tell if either patient has a fracture, sprain, or dislocation? Why or why not?

Objective 30-4
Give examples of direct, indirect, and twisting forces that can produce musculoskeletal injuries.

Key Terms
direct force direct blow. Injuries from direct force occur at the point of impact.

The joint then becomes inflamed and swollen. Discoloration usually occurs over time but not for several hours after the injury.

Dislocation

A dislocation is the displacement of a bone from its normal position in a joint (Figure 30-8*). The joint is found in an abnormal position with obvious deformity and usually swelling. The patient will complain of pain and tenderness at the site of dislocation and typically is unable to move the extremity. A dislocation is dangerous because it can damage blood vessels and nerves by compression or tearing. A dislocation usually occurs from the joint being forced well beyond its normal range of motion; thus, the patient is likely to also have ligament or joint capsule injury.

Dislocations may occur at the following joints:

- Acromioclavicular
- Sternoclavicular
- Shoulder
- Elbow
- Wrist
- Hand
- Metacarpal-phalangeal
- Hip
- Knee
- Ankle
- Foot
- Metatarsal-phalangeal

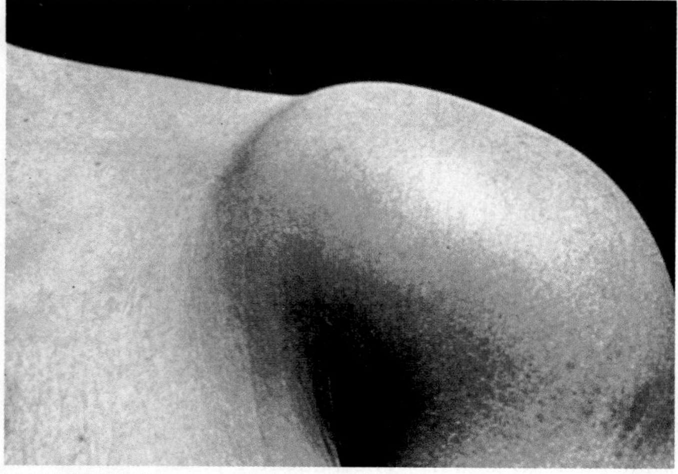

FIGURE 30-8 * Dislocation of the shoulder joint.

General Injury Considerations

All of the injuries just discussed—fracture, strain, sprain, and dislocation—may present with similar signs and symptoms: swelling, pain, or deformity. Sometimes there will be discoloration. Sometimes broken bones will break through the skin. Some fractures do not produce any obvious signs or symptoms.

Musculoskeletal injuries are usually associated with external forces such as falls or vehicle collisions, though some may occur through disease (e.g., bone degeneration), particularly in elderly patients. The force applied to the body may cause injuries to the surrounding soft tissues (e.g., nerves and arteries), and even to body areas distant from the injury site. In assessing and treating injuries to the bones and joints, it is important to determine the mechanism of injury as well as the signs and symptoms of the injury itself.

Mechanism of Injury

As you approach a patient with an injured extremity, you can get a good idea of how much damage may have occurred by determining the mechanism of injury. The forces that may cause bone and joint injury include direct force, indirect force, and twisting force.

Direct Force

The injury from **direct force**, or a direct blow, occurs at the point of impact. For example, a man in an automobile accident who is not wearing a seat belt is thrust forward, the knees hitting the dashboard. As a result, the patella may be fractured.

Indirect Force

With **indirect force**, the force impacts on one end of a limb, causing injury some distance away from the point of impact. For instance, a woman is thrown from a horse and lands on two outstretched hands. One arm sustains a fractured wrist, while the clavicle (collarbone) at the end of the other arm is fractured.

Twisting Force

In **twisting force**, one part of the extremity remains stationary while the rest twists. Take the case of the child running across a field who steps into a hole. The child's foot is rammed snugly into the hole and stays stationary

Key Terms

indirect force a force that causes injury some distance away from the point of impact.

twisting force a force that twists a bone while one end is held stationary.

Objective 30-5
Explain why fractures of the femur and pelvis are considered to be critical fractures.

Objective 30-6
Describe the assessment-based approach to bone and joint injuries.

while her leg twists, fracturing the tibia and/or fibula. Bone and joint injuries from twisting force occur commonly in football or skiing accidents.

Critical Fractures: The Femur and the Pelvis

Most fractures are not considered critical injuries and can be managed with standard splinting procedures. However, two specific fractures are associated with a high incidence of serious bleeding and the potential for the patient to develop shock. A fracture to the femur or pelvis is considered a critical injury and must be managed not only to immobilize the bones but also to reduce the associated bleeding. The bones of both the femur and the pelvis contain a large blood supply (Figure 30-9✻). When fractured, the bones have a tendency to bleed heavily. Also, the bones are in close proximity to other large vessels that may be lacerated by the bone ends, leading to serious bleeding.

Understanding BODY PROCESSES

Severe bleeding associated with a fractured pelvis or femur often occurs from the bone itself and not from a lacerated vessel outside of the bone. ■

When the femur fractures, the bone bleeds heavily. A patient can easily lose approximately 1,500 mL or 1.5 liters of blood around each femur. Furthermore because the tension on the muscles in the thigh is lost, the diameter of the thigh is allowed to increase. This permits a larger volume of blood to be housed within the thigh, and it also allows the bone to bleed more freely. A principle in splinting a fractured femur is not only to immobilize the bone ends but also to reduce the amount of bleeding. A traction splint, which is discussed in detail later in the chapter, is applied to accomplish two goals: (1) The bone ends will be realigned, which will help prevent further injury and reduce pain, and (2) the size (diameter) of the thigh will be decreased, which will allow less blood to accumulate and will also indirectly put pressure on the bleeding bone ends.

Understanding BODY PROCESSES

A traction splint is thought to reduce the compartment size that the femur can bleed into, thereby decreasing the amount of blood loss associated with the fracture. ■

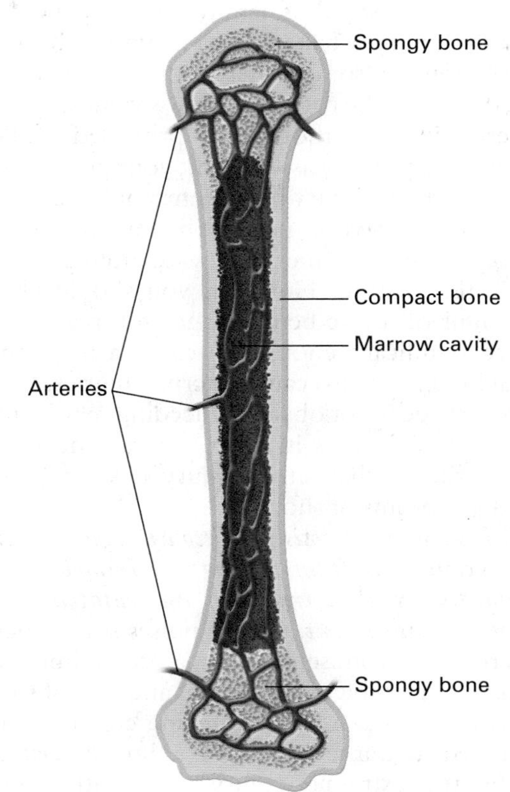

FIGURE 30-9 ✻ The bones are highly vascular and can bleed profusely if injured, as illustrated with the long bone shown. The bones of both the femur and the pelvis contain a large blood supply with a tendency to bleed heavily when fractured.

The pelvis, like the femur, has a rich blood supply. If it is fractured, a large amount of bleeding will occur from the fractured pelvic bone. Two liters of blood can be lost within the pelvic cavity. Application of the pneumatic antishock garment, which will be discussed in more detail later in the chapter, will not only stabilize the fracture but also decrease the size of the compartment into which the pelvis can bleed, which may tamponade the bleeding pelvis.

Assessment-Based Approach: Bone or Joint Injuries

Scene Size-Up and Primary Assessment

As you approach the patient with a possible bone or joint injury, take appropriate Standard Precautions and consider the mechanism of injury. During your scene size-up,

Objective 30-7
Establish the priority for assessing and treating musculoskeletal injuries with respect to a patient's overall condition.

Key Points
A fracture is considered a "distracting injury" because it may draw attention away from other, more serious problems.

ask questions of bystanders, family, and the patient. Is the cause of the injury a fall, ejection from a vehicle, high-speed collision, or some other traumatic force? Try to imagine the forces the patient's body was subjected to and the direction in which those forces propelled the body.

During the primary assessment, your general impression of the patient's injury helps determine the priority of care and whether your patient has a life-threatening emergency. Joint and bone injuries are often dramatic but rarely life threatening. However, you should check for obvious signs of severe hemorrhage and treat for shock. Any force significant enough to cause a major musculoskeletal injury can also cause internal injuries. When severe hemorrhage is not obvious, bleeding may be internal to the injury site. This is often the case during blunt trauma. If the mechanism of injury is severe, look for signs and symptoms of shock.

Pulselessness or cyanosis distal to an injured extremity is a serious condition. If this is apparent, immobilize the injury immediately, then transport immediately following your secondary assessment. Absent pulses sometimes indicate arterial compromise, which may cause impaired tissue perfusion, possible tissue death, and loss of the limb.

If the patient has a life-threatening condition that requires immediate transport but is not directly related to or caused by the extremity injury (e.g., intra-abdominal trauma), you will initiate transport and, if time and the patient's condition permit, immobilize the extremity injury en route. If the patient is immobilized to a spine board, this will provide temporary stability to the injured extremity.

Secondary Assessment

If the patient is unresponsive or there are multiple injuries or the mechanism of injury is significant, conduct a rapid secondary assessment. If the patient is responsive and oriented, multiple injuries are not suspected, and the mechanism of injury is not significant, conduct a modified secondary assessment, inspecting and gently palpating the injured bone or joint. Assess the joints above and below any bone injury or the bones above and below any joint injury. As you examine the patient, be gentle and reassuring because musculoskeletal injuries can be frightening for the patient. Check for deformity, contusions, tenderness, swelling, discoloration, and open wounds at the injury site. Assess the skin temperature, color, and condition; assess the pulse amplitude; and check the capillary refill time distal to the site of injury. Keep in mind that a fracture must be *suspected* in the field by these signs; a fracture can only be definitively diagnosed by X-rays at the hospital (Figure 30-10*) unless obvious bone ends are protruding from the skin.

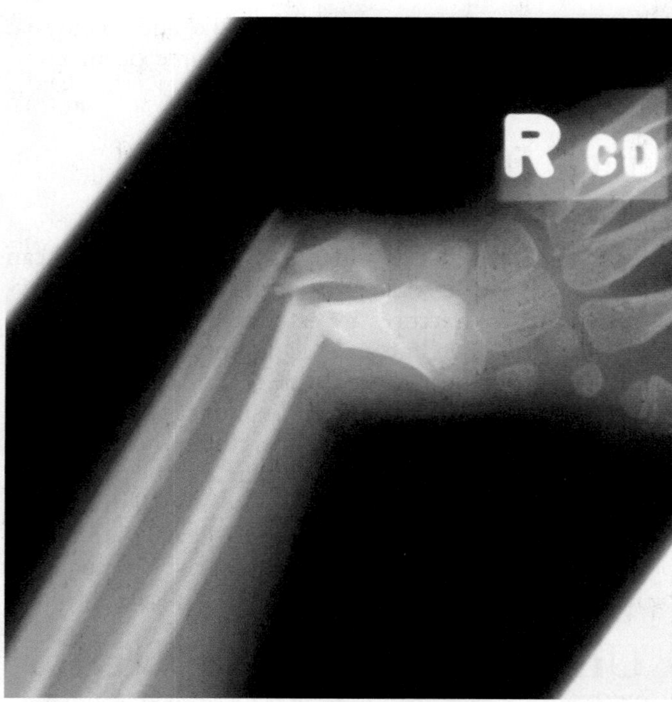

FIGURE 30-10 * A fracture can only be definitively diagnosed by X-ray. In the field, a suspected fracture is identified by the presence of deformity, pain, tenderness, swelling, discoloration, and angulation.

ASSESSMENT Tips

The severe pain associated with a fracture to an extremity may distract the patient from complaining of other more significant pain, such as abdominal pain or spinal pain. For this reason, fractures are referred to as distracting injuries. ■

Assess the baseline vitals and obtain a history from the patient. Don't forget to ask such basic questions as:

When did the injury occur?

What happened?

Where does it hurt?

What did you feel at the time of injury?

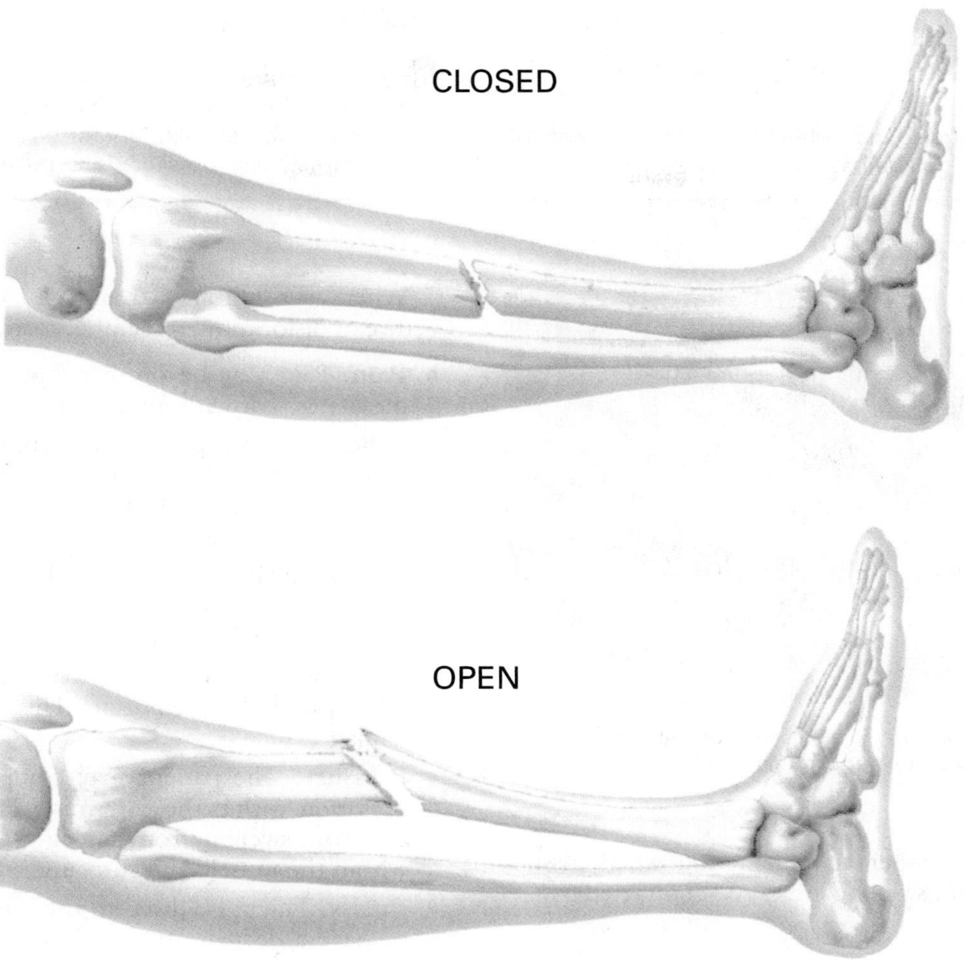

FIGURE 30-11 * Closed and open injuries.

Most patients with significant musculoskeletal injury will complain of pain localized to the area of injury. The patient may also report feeling or hearing something snap.

Signs and Symptoms Bone and joint injuries can be one of two types, closed or open (Figure 30-11*):

- **Closed.** In which the overlying skin is intact (Figure 30-12*)
- **Open.** In which an open wound is associated with the fracture; bone may or may not protrude through the wound (Figure 30-13*)

The signs and symptoms of bone and joint injury may include (Figure 30-14*):

- Deformity or angulation (When compared to the normal extremity, there is a difference in the size or shape or the injured extremity is in an unnatural position.)
- Pain and tenderness
- Grating, or **crepitus**, the sound or feeling of broken fragments of bone grinding against each other
- Swelling

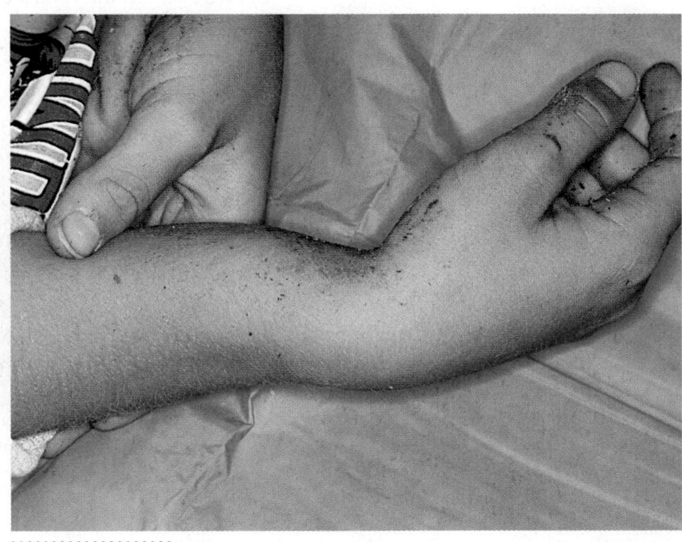

FIGURE 30-12 * A closed fracture has no associated open wound. (Shown here, a Colles fracture to the wrist, also called a silver fork deformity because the deformed wrist looks like an inverted fork.) (© Charles Stewart, MD, and Associates)

Key Terms
crepitus the sound or feel of broken fragments of bone grinding against each other.

Objective 30-8
Discuss the significance of assessing a musculoskeletal injury for pain, pallor, paralysis, paresthesia, pressure, and pulses.

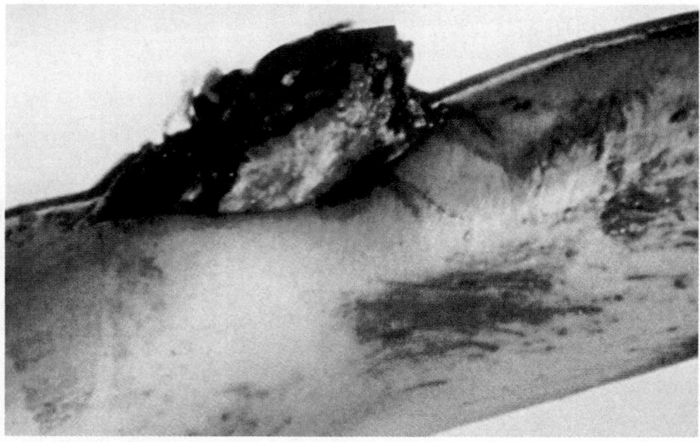

FIGURE 30-13 * An open fracture presents with an open wound, often with a bone end protruding through the skin.

- Disfigurement (either an indentation where tissues have separated or swelling indicating contracted tissue)
- Severe weakness and loss of function
- Bruising (discoloration)
- Exposed bone ends
- Joint locked into position

When assessing an extremity for the possibility of a fracture or dislocation, remember to evaluate the six "Ps":

- **Pain.** Pain may be on palpation (tenderness), with movement, or without movement.
- **Pallor.** The skin distal to the injury site may be pale and capillary refill delayed if an artery is compressed or torn. If a vein is blocked by the fracture, the distal extremity may appear warm, red (flushed), and swollen.
- **Paralysis.** The patient is unable to move the extremity. This may be from nerve, muscle, tendon, or ligament damage.
- **Paresthesia.** The patient may complain of numbness or a tingling sensation. This may indicate nerve damage.
- **Pressure.** The patient may complain of a pressure sensation within the extremity. This may be associated with swelling from damaged tissue or blood loss within the muscle and surrounding structures.
- **Pulses.** The pulse distal to the injury may be absent or have a decrease in amplitude. This may indicate damage to an arterial vessel.

It is often not possible to diagnose the nature of the injury in the prehospital setting. Do not waste time try-

SIGNS AND SYMPTOMS OF BONE OR JOINT INJURIES

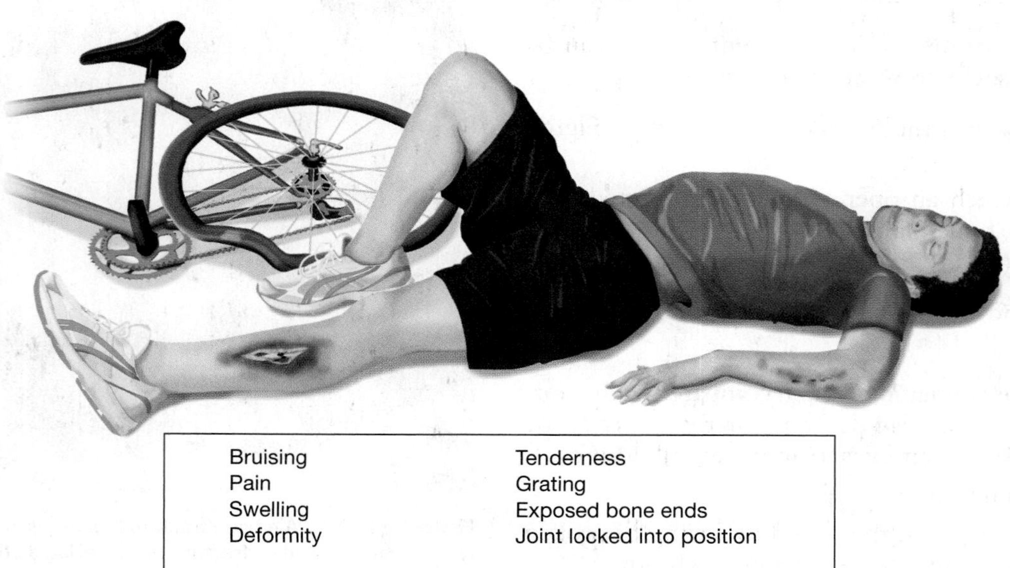

Bruising	Tenderness
Pain	Grating
Swelling	Exposed bone ends
Deformity	Joint locked into position

FIGURE 30-14 * Signs and symptoms of bone or joint injuries.

Key Points
Always check a patient's distal pulses, motor function, and sensation both before and after splint and document your findings.

Key Terms
splint any device used to immobilize a body part.

Objective 30-9
Explain the rationale for splinting musculoskeletal injuries.

ing to figure out which kind of injury it is. Any painful, swollen, or deformed extremity should be given the emergency care that is outlined next.

ASSESSMENT Tips

Suspect a dislocation when deformity and pain are found at a joint. ■

Emergency Medical Care

In some cases, the bone injury is the chief complaint. If the patient has a life-threatening condition caused by or directly related to the extremity injury, such as a femur or pelvic fracture with hypotension or an open fracture with severe bleeding, you will immobilize the injured extremity during your primary or secondary assessment if the appropriate resources are available and it does not cause a delay in transport of the patient, and transport immediately. If the patient has a life-threatening condition not directly related to the extremity injury (e.g., intra-abdominal trauma), you will initiate transport immediately and immobilize the extremity en route if time and critical patient care permit.

Perform the following steps to immobilize a suspected fracture:

1. *Use proper Standard Precautions,* such as disposable gloves, before you approach the patient.
2. *Administer oxygen, if needed.*
3. *Maintain in-line spinal stabilization* if spinal injury is suspected.
4. *Splint bone and joint injuries.* Check the patient's distal pulses, motor function, and sensation both before and after splinting. Document your findings in the prehospital care report. Specifics on splinting are detailed in the next section.
5. *Apply cold packs to the painful, swollen, or deformed extremity* to reduce pain and swelling.
6. *Elevate the extremity* (if spinal injury is not suspected) and keep it elevated throughout transport.
7. Transport.

Reassessment

Perform the reassessment, including a recheck of the patient's vital signs and interventions. Is the injured extremity properly immobilized? Make sure that the patient's distal pulses, motor function, and sensation have improved or have not deteriorated as a result of immobilization.

Summary: Assessment and Care

To review possible assessment findings and emergency care for musculoskeletal injuries, see Figures 30-15∗ and 30-16∗.

Basics of Splinting

Any device used to immobilize a body part is a **splint**. A splint can be soft or rigid. It can be commercially manufactured or it can be improvised from virtually any object that can provide stability.

There are two basic reasons for splinting a bone or joint injury. First, splinting prevents movement of any bone fragments, bone ends, or dislocated joints, reducing the chance for further injury. Second, splints usually reduce pain and minimize the following common complications from bone and joint injuries:

- Damage to muscles, nerves, or blood vessels caused by movement of bone fragments or bone ends
- Conversion of a closed fracture to an open fracture (by breaking through the skin)
- Restriction of blood flow as a result of bone ends or dislocations compressing blood vessels
- Excessive bleeding from tissue damage caused by movement of bone ends
- Increased pain associated with movement of bone ends or dislocated bones
- Paralysis of the extremities resulting from a damaged spine

General Rules of Splinting

Regardless of where you apply the splint, follow these general rules (EMT Skills 30-1):

- *Both before and after you apply the splint, assess the pulse, motor function, and sensation distal to the injury.* (Keep the mnemonic PMS for pulse, motor function, and sensation in mind as you manage a suspected fracture.) You should evaluate these signs every 15 minutes after applying the splint to make sure the splint is not impairing circulation to the extremity.

Assessment Summary

MUSCULOSKELETAL INJURY

The following findings may be associated with a musculoskeletal injury.

SCENE SIZE-UP

Pay particular attention to your own safety. Look for:

- Mechanism of injury
- Ejection from a vehicle
- High-speed collision
- Sports injury
- Fall
- Crushing force
- Gunshot wounds
- Evidence of other trauma

Primary Assessment

General Impression

- Major bleeding associated with suspected fracture
- Open fracture sites
- Obvious deformity to extremities

Mental Status

- Alert to unresponsive based on other injuries

Airway

- Clear and open unless associated with facial fractures or other injuries

Breathing

- Normal; increased if extreme pain or associated with shock or other injury

Circulation

- Pulse is normal; may be increased in response to pain or shock
- Skin is normal; may be cool, clammy, pale, and cyanotic in extremity if bone injury disrupts distal blood flow

Status: Priority patient if distal pulses are not present or if bone injury is associated with other life-threatening injuries such as severe blood loss, shock, or internal injuries

Secondary Assessment

Physical Exam

Pelvis:

- Pain
- Instability on compression
- Deformity

Extremities:

- Pain
- Deformity
- Tenderness on palpation
- Crepitus
- Loss of function distal to injury
- Open wounds
- Discoloration
- Exposed bone ends
- Abnormal inward or outward rotation of foot and leg (hip dislocation or femur fracture)

Baseline Vital Signs

- BP: normal, or may be decreased if there is other trauma and shock
- HR: normal, or may be increased in response to pain or other injuries, bleeding, or shock
- RR: normal, or may be increased in response to pain, other injuries, bleeding, or shock
- Skin: normal, or may be pale, cool, clammy, and cyanotic if the bone injury is interfering with distal circulation or associated with bleeding and shock
- Pupils: normal or may be dilated and sluggish if associated with bleeding and shock

History

Signs and symptoms of an open fracture:

- Pain, deformity, swelling to long bone
- Open wound associated with suspected fracture site
- Exposed bone ends

Signs and symptoms of a closed fracture:

- Pain, deformity, swelling to long bone

Signs and symptoms of a dislocation:

- Pain, deformity, swelling to a joint
- Abnormal rotation of foot and leg (hip dislocation)

FIGURE 30-15a ✱ Assessment summary: musculoskeletal injury.

- Immobilize the joints both above and below a long bone injury. (If the forearm is fractured, immobilize the wrist and the elbow.) Immobilize the bones above and below a joint injury. (If the elbow is injured, immobilize the humerus of the upper arm and the radius and ulna of the forearm.)
- Remove or cut away all clothing around the injury site with a pair of bandage scissors so you won't accidentally move the fractured bone ends and complicate the injury. Remove all jewelry around the injury site, especially distally, because it may become entrapped by swelling. Bag the jewelry and either give it to a family member or see that it is transported with the patient. Carefully document the disposition of the patient's jewelry.
- Cover all wounds, including open fractures, with sterile dressings before applying a splint, then gently bandage. Avoid excessive pressure on the wound.

Emergency Care Protocol

MUSCULOSKELETAL INJURY

1. Establish manual in-line stabilization if spinal injury is suspected.
2. Establish an open airway, and insert a nasopharyngeal or oropharyngeal airway if the patient is unresponsive and has no gag or cough reflex.
3. Suction secretions as necessary.
4. If breathing is inadequate, provide positive pressure ventilation with supplemental oxygen at a rate of 10–12 ventilations/minute for an adult and 12–20 ventilations/minute for an infant or child.
5. If breathing is adequate, administer oxygen based on the SpO_2 reading and patient signs and symptoms. If the SpO_2 reading is greater than 95% and no signs or symptoms of hypoxia or respiratory distress are present, oxygen may not be necessary. In this case, you may choose to apply nasal cannula at 2 to 4 lpm. If signs of hypoxia or respiratory distress are present, or the SpO_2 reading is less than 95%, place the patient on a nonrebreather mask at 15 lpm.
6. Control any major bleeding.
7. If a priority patient, splint suspected fractures and dislocations en route to the medical facility.
8. If a spinal injury is suspected, immobilize the patient to a backboard.
9. Follow the general rules of splinting:
   a. Assess pulses and motor and sensory function distal to injury before and after splinting.
   b. Immobilize joints above and below in a long bone injury, and bones above and below in a joint injury.
   c. Dress and bandage all open wounds before splinting.
   d. If a suspected fracture is grossly deformed or no distal circulation is present, apply gentle traction and attempt to realign. If excruciating pain or resistance is met, stop and splint in the position found.
   e. Splint suspected dislocations in position found unless distal pulses are absent. If no distal pulses, apply gentle traction and realign unless extreme pain or resistance is met. Splint in position found.
   f. Cold can be applied to the deformity to reduce swelling and pain.
   g. Elevate the extremity slightly to reduce swelling. Remove all jewelry and constrictive clothing on the affected extremity.
   h. Reassess pulses and motor and sensory function.
10. Suspected fractures or dislocations requiring special equipment or procedures:
    Hip Dislocation or Fracture:
    Pad between legs and bind legs together or apply long board splints; place the patient on a backboard.
    Pelvis:
    Apply PASG and inflate all three sections to splinting pressure, or pad between legs and bind legs together; place the patient on a backboard. A pelvic binder or an improvised pelvis wrap can be applied.
    Femur:
    Apply a traction splint; place on a backboard.
    Shoulder:
    Sling and swathe if in a relatively normal position. Vacuum splint, wire ladder splints, or board splints if severely deformed.
    Clavicle:
    Sling and swathe.
11. Transport.
12. Perform reassessment every 5 minutes if unstable and every 15 minutes if stable.

FIGURE 30-15b ✱ Emergency care protocol: musculoskeletal injury.

- If there is a severe deformity or the distal extremity is cyanotic (bluish) or lacks pulses, align the injured limb with gentle manual traction (pulling) before splinting. As a general rule, make one attempt to align the extremity. *If pain, resistance, or crepitus increase, stop.* Generally, you should not try to align a wrist, elbow, knee, hip, or shoulder—major nerves and arteries close to these joints increase the chance of causing further damage. *Follow local protocol.*
- Never intentionally replace protruding bones or push them back below the skin. (Occasionally, during realignment, these will be drawn into the wound.)
- Pad each splint to prevent pressure and discomfort to the patient.
- Apply the splint before trying to move the patient. Do not release manual traction until after the splint has been applied.
- When in doubt, splint the injury.
- If the patient shows signs of shock, align the patient in the normal anatomical position. Treat for shock and transport immediately without taking the time to apply a splint. If the femur or pelvis is suspected to be fractured, splinting should be considered as a bleeding control measure. Splint the femur or pelvis at the scene only if enough resources are present so that a delay in transport does not occur.

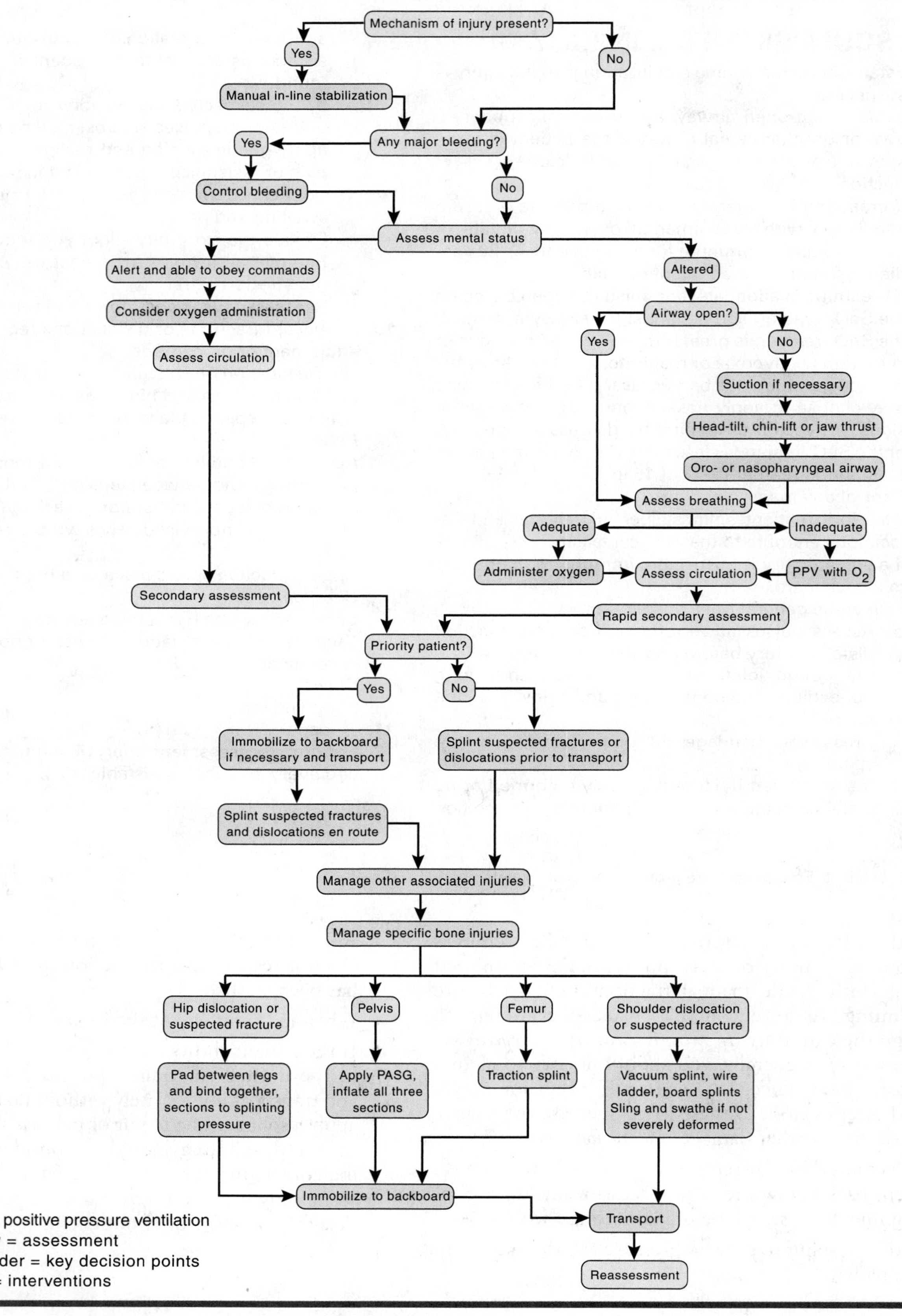

FIGURE 30-16 ✱ Emergency care algorithm: musculoskeletal injury.

Key Points
Some splints are more suitable to certain types of injuries; others are interchangeable. Follow your local protocols about which splints to use in given situations.

Objective 30-10
Compare and contrast the characteristics and uses of various types of splints.

Splinting Equipment

Some splints are more suitable to certain types of injuries than others, but many are interchangeable (Figure 30-17*). Follow your local protocol in such cases. The general types of splints are rigid splints, pressure splints, traction splints, formable splints, vacuum splints, sling and swathe, spine board, and improvised splints.

Rigid Splints

Rigid splints are commercially manufactured splints made of wood, plastic, cardboard, or compressed wood fibers. Some are designed in specific shapes for arms and legs and are equipped with Velcro closures; others are pliable enough to be molded to fit any appendage. Some come with washable pads, but others must be padded before being applied.

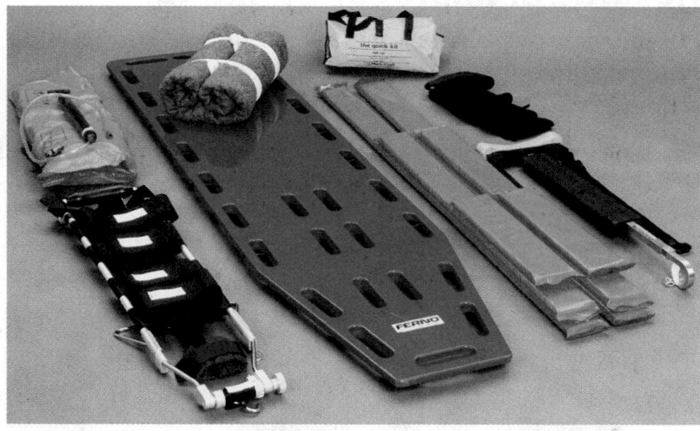

FIGURE 30-17 * Examples of splints.

Pressure (Air or Pneumatic) Splints

The main type of pressure splints are air or pneumatic splints. Air splints are soft and pliable before being inflated but rigid once they are applied and filled with air. Air splints cannot be sized, may impair circulation, may interfere with the ability to assess pulses, and may lose or gain pressure with temperature and altitude changes. Seek medical direction and follow local protocol regarding their use.

Traction Splints

Traction splints (Figure 30-18*) provide a counterpull, alleviating pain, reducing blood loss, and minimizing further injury. Traction splints are not intended to reduce (correct) the fracture, but simply to immobilize the bone ends, reduce the diameter or container size of the thigh, and prevent further injury. Several types of traction splints are available, and procedures vary according to the manufacturer. Specifics about traction splinting are detailed later in this chapter.

Formable Splints

Formable splints are a type of rigid splint that is malleable enough to form to a deformed or angulated extremity. The splint is shaped to the deformed extremity instead of making the extremity fit the splint. Once shaped to the injured extremity, it is fixed in place with cravats or Velcro straps. Formable splints are typically made of wire, thin aluminum, or another metal that can bend.

Vacuum Splints

Vacuum splints (EMT Skills 30-2) are soft, pliable splints that are easily formed to deformed extremities. The air is

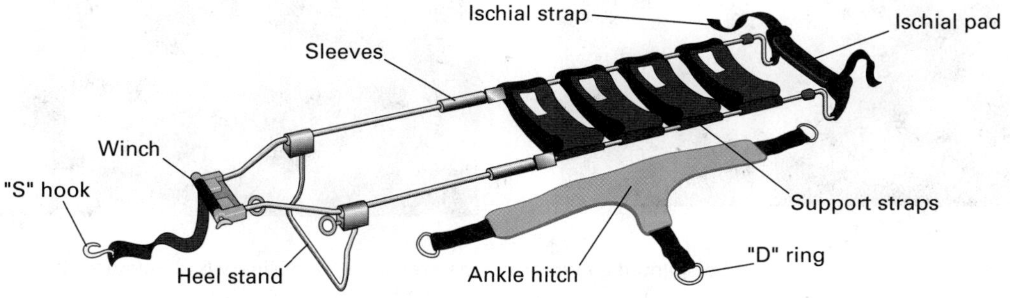

FIGURE 30-18 * A bipolar traction splint.

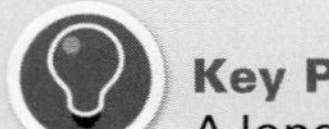

Key Points
A long spine board is a full body splint and provides some stabilization when individual fractures cannot be splinted.

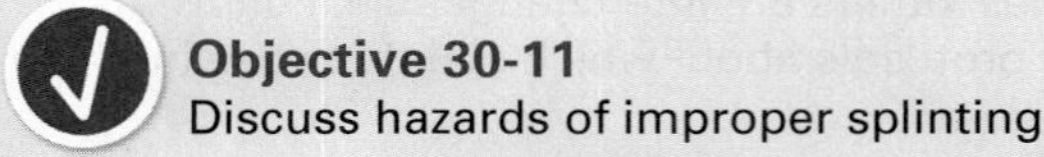

Objective 30-11
Discuss hazards of improper splinting.

then sucked out of the splint, causing it to become rigid in its position of placement. Vacuum splints are considered to be a type of formable splint.

Sling and Swathe

A sling and swathe is often used to provide stability to a painful and tender shoulder, elbow, or upper humerus injury. A sling is a triangular bandage. The sling supports the patient's arm, while a swathe of cloth holds the patient's arm against the side of the chest. This minimizes the pain and further injury associated with arm and shoulder movement. (See instructions for applying a sling and swathe under "Splinting Specific Injuries" later in this chapter.)

Spine Board

A long spine board is a full body splint. In the case of a critical injury when extremity fractures cannot be splinted at the scene, placing the patient on a long spine board will provide some stabilization through the limitation of movement. This is not an ideal method of splinting; however, uncomplicated fractures are not a priority in critically injured or unstable patients. Rapid transport will take precedence over splinting extremity injuries. A short spine board or vest-type immobilization device may also be used as a splint. A vest-type immobilization device is sometimes used to splint a suspected pelvic injury when turned upside down.

Improvised Splints

You may be forced to improvise at the scene. Improvised splints can be made from a cardboard box, cane, ironing board, rolled-up magazine, umbrella, broom handle, catcher's shin guard, or any similar object. An effective improvised splint must be:

- Light in weight, but firm and rigid
- As wide as the thickest part of the fractured limb
- Long enough to extend past the joints and prevent movement on either side of the fracture
- Padded well so the inner surfaces are not in contact with the skin

An ordinary bed pillow or blanket roll (Figures 30-19a and 30-19b*) can be an effective improvised splint when wrapped around the area and secured with several cravats.

Hazards of Improper Splinting

For all their obvious benefits to the patient with a bone or joint injury, splints can also cause complications if they are applied in the wrong manner. Improper splinting can:

- Compress the nerves, tissues, and blood vessels under the splint, aggravating the existing injury and causing new injury

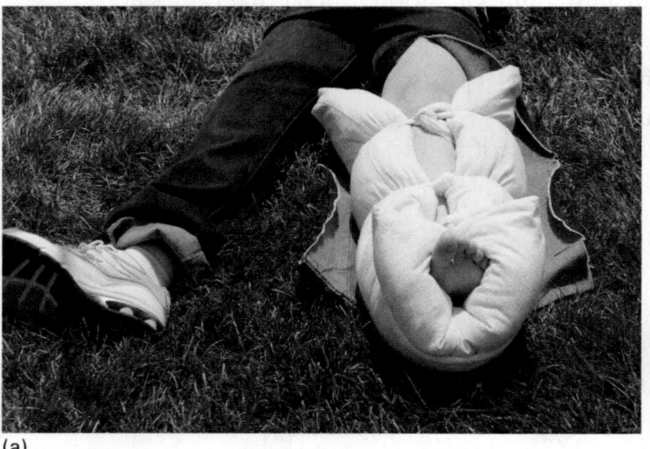

(a)

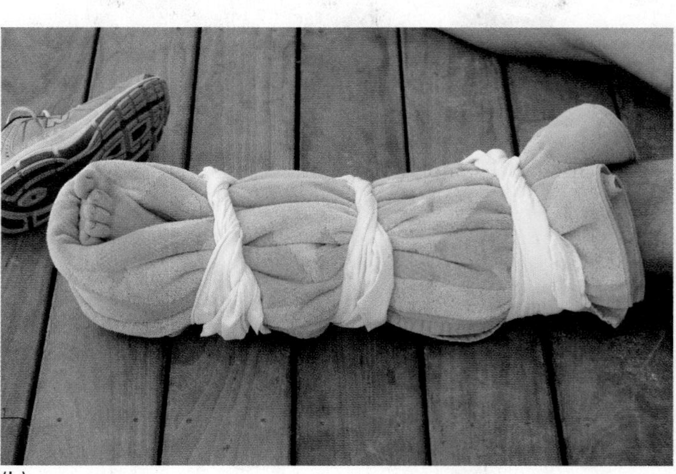

(b)

FIGURE 30-19 * An injured foot or ankle may be splinted by wrapping the area in **(a)** an ordinary bed pillow, or **(b)** a heavy towel or blanket.

Objective 30-12
Discuss special considerations in splinting long bone injuries, splinting joint injuries, and traction splinting.

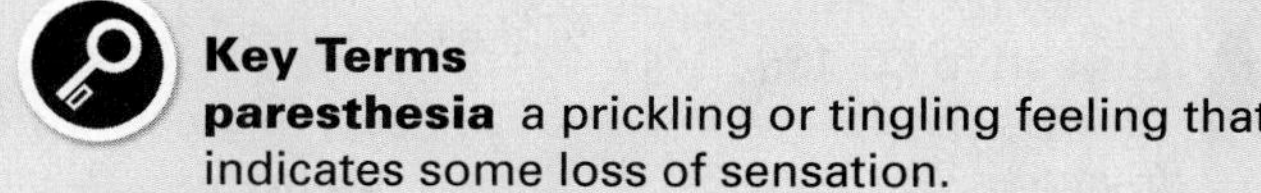

Key Terms
paresthesia a prickling or tingling feeling that indicates some loss of sensation.

- Delay the transport of a patient who has a life-threatening injury
- Reduce distal circulation, compromising the viability of the extremity
- Aggravate the bone or joint injury by allowing movement of the bone fragments or bone ends or by forcing bone ends beneath the skin surface
- Cause or aggravate damage to the tissues, nerves, blood vessels, or muscles from excessive bone or joint movement
- Cause damage to the skin from improper padding

Splinting Long Bone Injuries

Special considerations must be taken into account when splinting long bones or joints. Remember that some long bone injuries may lead to serious internal bleeding. As you assess for evidence of trauma, look for the following signs and symptoms of long bone injury:

- Exposed bone ends
- Joints locked in position
- **Paresthesia**, a pricking or tingling feeling that indicates some loss of sensation
- Paralysis
- Pallor of the injury site
- Loss of distal pulse

Assess the pulse and motor and sensory function below the injury site. Assess the radial pulse for an upper extremity, the dorsal pedal or posterior tibial pulse for a lower extremity. Sensation is intact if the patient can tell you, without looking, which finger or toe you are touching and can feel painful stimuli. If the injury involves an upper extremity, motor function is intact if the patient can make a fist, undo the fist, spread the fingers, and make a hitchhiking sign with the thumb. If the injury involves a lower extremity, motor function is intact if the patient can tighten the kneecap (patella) and move the foot up and down as if pumping an automobile accelerator.

If the limb is severely deformed, is cyanotic, or lacks distal pulses, align it with gentle traction. Provide steady, gentle pressure along with traction. If pain or crepitus increases, stop.

For specific guidelines on splinting a long bone injury, see EMT Skills 30-3. In EMT Skills 30-3E, you will see that the hand (or foot) must be immobilized in the position of function. The position of function for a hand is with the fingers curled as if holding a ball. You can put a roll of bandage in the patient's hand to support this position. The position of function for the foot is at a 90-degree angle to the leg with the foot bent at the normal angle to the leg, not pushed downward or upward toward the shin.

ASSESSMENT Tips

If the foot or ankle is injured, having the patient push down and pull back with the great (big) toe will give you the same results as if the entire foot were tested. ■

Splinting Joint Injuries

A common joint injury is the displacement of a bone end from the joint, or dislocation. In a dislocation, the ligaments holding the bones in proper position are often stretched and sometimes are torn loose. Dislocations cause serious pain because the joint surfaces are rich in nerves.

The principal signs and symptoms of any type of joint injury are pain, swelling, deformity, and possible rigidity and loss of function. As with long bone injuries, assess the pulse and motor and sensory function below the injury site. Look for paresthesia or paralysis. If the distal extremity is cyanotic (bluish) or lacks pulses, align the joint with gentle traction. If pain or crepitus increases, stop. Do not spend time trying to differentiate a joint injury from a bone injury since it may be difficult to distinguish between the two; for both you will need to splint and transport.

For specific guidelines on splinting a joint injury, see EMT Skills 30-4.

Traction Splinting

Fractures of the femur can be successfully immobilized with a traction splint. A fractured femur is complicated because of the amount of bleeding that can occur from the fractured bone. A fractured femur is also complicated because the large muscle mass of the thigh contracts and pulls the fractured femur ends so that they override, or pass each other. This allows the thigh to increase in

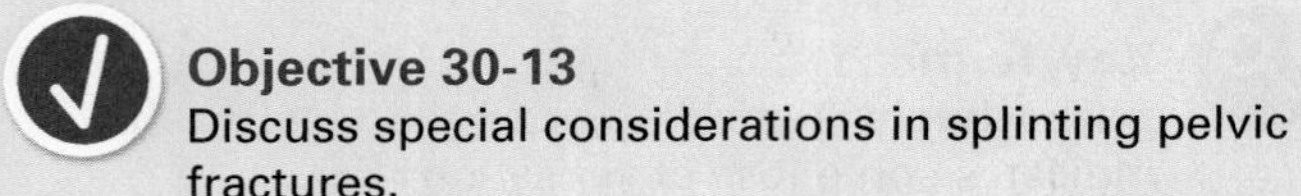

Objective 30-13
Discuss special considerations in splinting pelvic fractures.

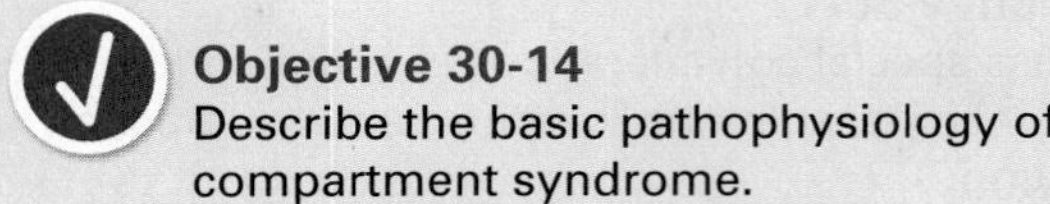

Objective 30-14
Describe the basic pathophysiology of compartment syndrome.

diameter, which permits more blood loss to occur within the thigh, causing great pain in addition to a lot of internal soft tissue injury.

Traction splinting reduces the diameter of the thigh, decreases the space in which bleeding can occur, and realigns the fractured femur. This helps to tamponade the bleeding, relieve pain, and reduce the incidence of internal injuries that would occur if the patient were transported without immobilization. *Remember that you don't have to be certain the femur has actually been fractured. If the thigh is painful, swollen, or deformed, you should treat as if the femur is fractured.*

In general, you should not use a traction splint if:

- The injury is within 1–2 inches of the knee or ankle.
- The knee itself has been injured.
- The hip has been injured.
- The pelvis has been injured.
- There is partial amputation or avulsion with bone separation, and the distal limb is connected only by marginal tissue. (In such a case, using a traction splint would risk separation.)

See EMT Skills 30-5 for instructions on applying a bipolar traction splint. See EMT Skills 30-6 for instructions on applying a unipolar traction splint.

Splinting Specific Injuries

Special techniques may be applied to the splinting of suspected bone and joint injuries to specific sites. Splinting techniques are illustrated in EMT Skills 30-7 for the shoulder and EMT Skills 30-8 for the upper arm, elbow, forearm, wrist, hand, fingers, pelvis, hip, thigh, knee, lower leg, ankle, and foot.

Pelvic Fracture

Pelvic fractures may be associated with significant pain and bleeding. The pneumatic antishock garment (PASG) is a device that can be used to splint the pelvis and decrease the compartment size to reduce bleeding (Figure 30-20a*). Another method to stabilize the fracture and tamponade the bleeding is to use a commercial pelvic splint (Figure 30-20b*). If a PASG or commercial pelvic splint is not available, an improvised pelvic wrap may be applied. To apply an improvised pelvic wrap:

1. Fold a sheet lengthwise to approximately an 8-inch width.
2. Slide it under the small of the back and then down under the pelvis until it is centered and the ends of the sheet are of equal length on both sides of the patient.

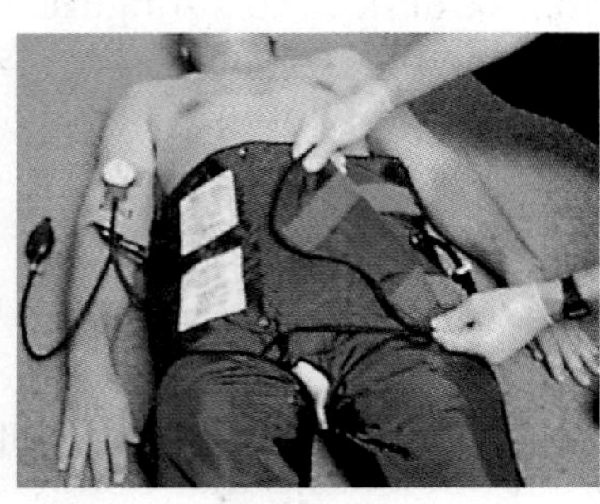

(a)

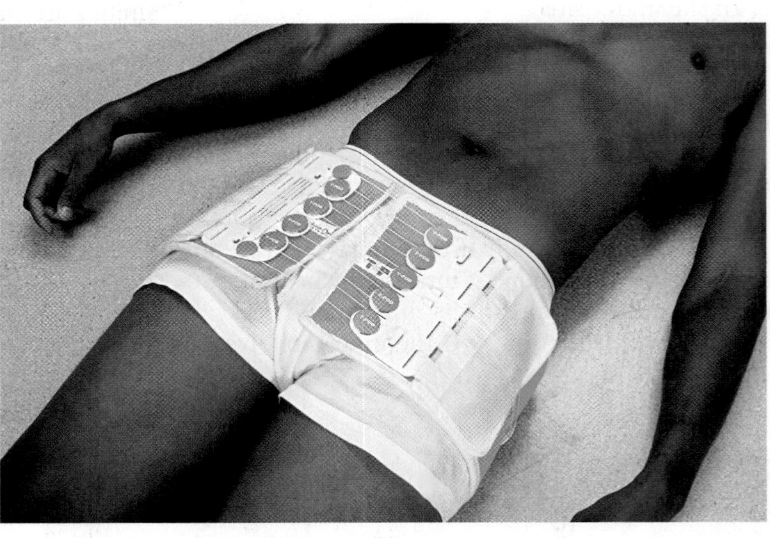

(b)

FIGURE 30-20 * A pelvic fracture can be effectively splinted with **(a)** a PASG, or **(b)** a commercial pelvic splint. A pelvic splint may also be improvised from a sheet.

Key Terms
compartment syndrome tissue pressure in a confined space causing decreased blood flow, leading to hypoxia and possible muscle, nerve, and vessel impairment.

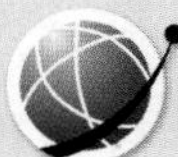

Media Resources
Go to www.bradybooks.com for mykit. Highlights:

- *Video:* Joint Injuries
- *Video:* Long Bone Injuries and Splints
- *Video:* Application of a Sager Splint

3. Cross the tail ends over the patient and twist the ends until the sheet is tightly secured around the pelvis.
4. Tuck the sheet ends under the patient or tie the ends into a square knot.
5. Place the patient on a backboard or rigid device.

An example of a commercial device used to splint the pelvis in the same manner as the pelvic wrap is the London pelvic splint.

Compartment Syndrome

Compartment syndrome may occur when an extremity is fractured or injured. It may also occur in the buttocks and abdomen of the body. When an injury occurs, swelling and bleeding in the space between the tissues is usually present. If the pressure in the space around the capillaries exceeds the pressure needed to perfuse the tissues, the blood flow is cut off and the cells become hypoxic, leading to **compartment syndrome**. The hypoxic cells release chemicals that cause the capillaries to leak, leading to further swelling. If the pressure continues, the cells eventually die, resulting in the loss of muscle, nerves, and vessels in the affected area.

Compartment syndrome usually develops over time as edema around an injured area increases, so it may not be seen at the initial stages of injury. It is commonly associated with fractures, arterial and venous bleeding from penetrating or blunt trauma, crush injuries, and high-energy trauma. Signs and symptoms of compartment syndrome include the following:

- Severe pain or burning sensation
- Decreased strength in the extremity
- Paralysis of the extremity
- Pain with movement
- Extremity feeling hard to palpation
- Distal pulses, motor, and sensory function possibly normal

Emergency care focuses on treating any life-threatening injuries first. Immobilize and splint the affected extremity. Elevate the extremity and apply a cold pack or ice. It is extremely important to transport the patient, since he may lose the limb if compartment syndrome is not treated quickly and effectively.

EMT skills 30-1 General Splinting Rules

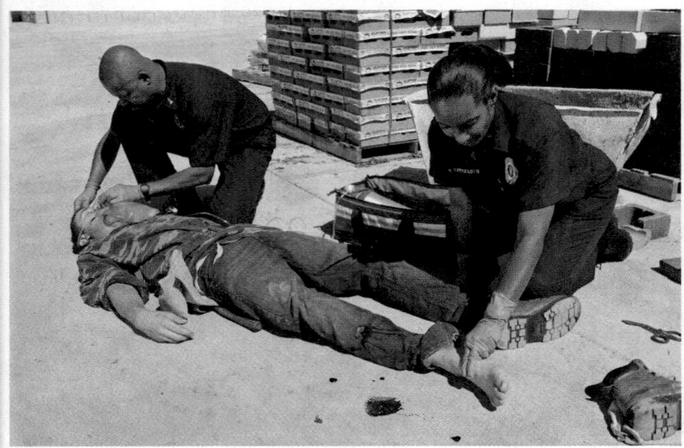

30-1A ✱ Assess the distal pulse and motor and sensory function.

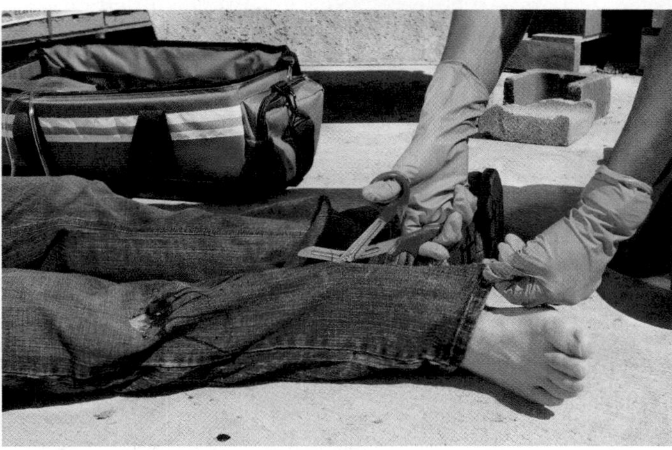

30-1B ✱ Cut away clothing to expose the injury site.

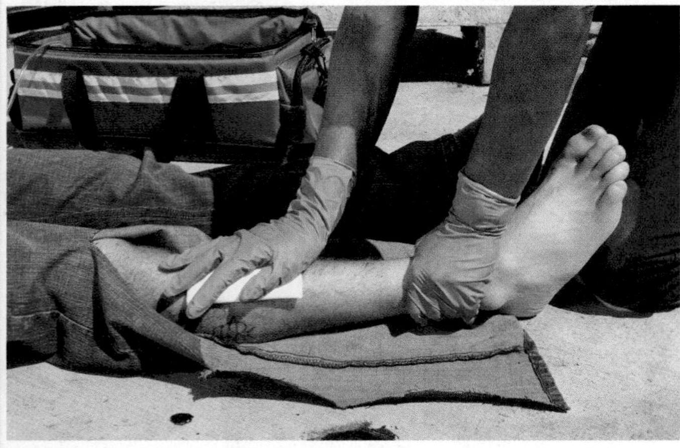

30-1C ✱ Place a sterile dressing over the open wound.

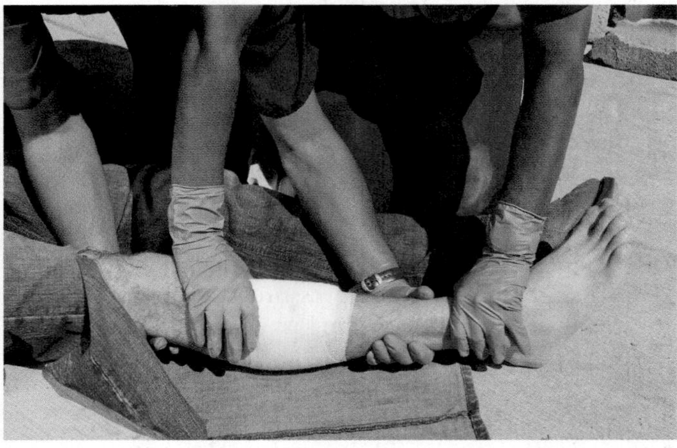

30-1D ✱ Align the extremity with gentle traction if there is severe deformity, absence of distal pulses, or cyanosis.

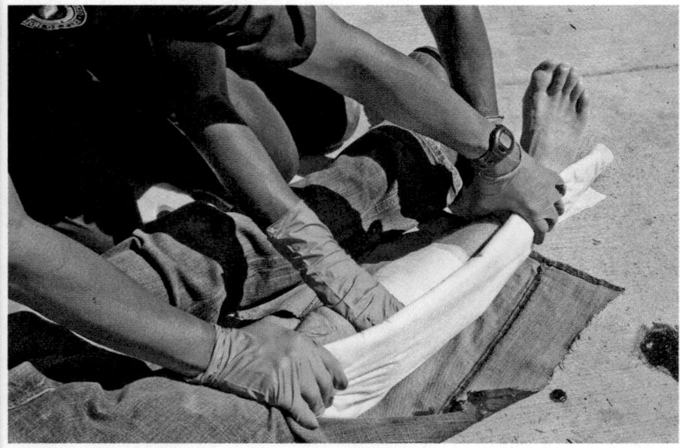

30-1E ✱ Pad the splint to prevent discomfort and unnecessary pressure. The correct size splint will immobilize the joint above and below the site of a bone injury.

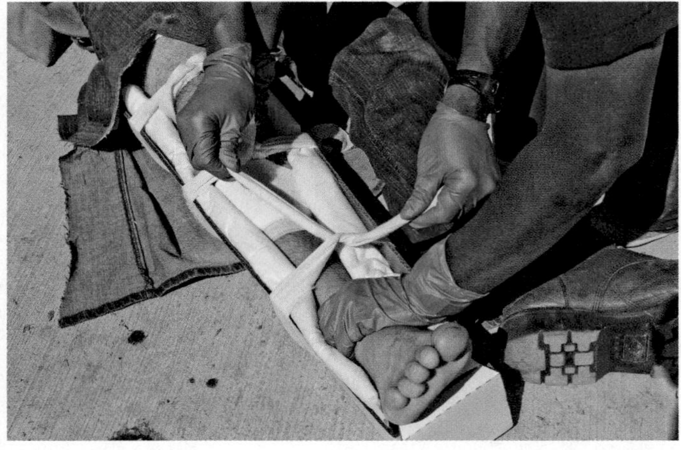

30-1F ✱ Maintain manual traction. Do not release until the splint has been applied. Assess distal pulse and motor and sensory function after the splint has been applied.

EMT skills 30-1 General Splinting Rules *continued*

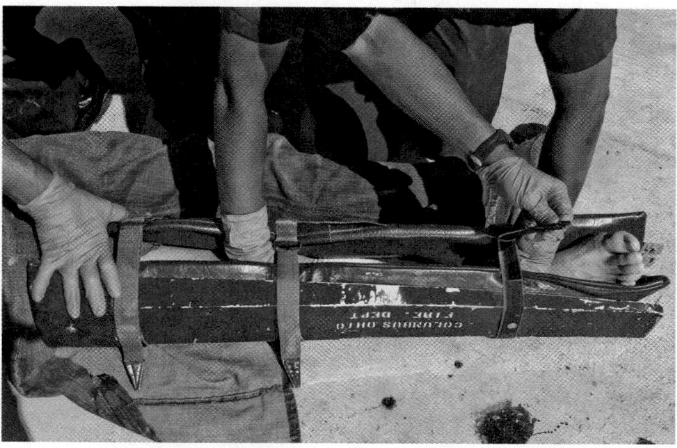

30-1G ✱ If your service uses commercially prepared prepadded splints, skip the padding step, but maintain manual traction in any case.

EMT skills 30-2 Applying a Vacuum Splint

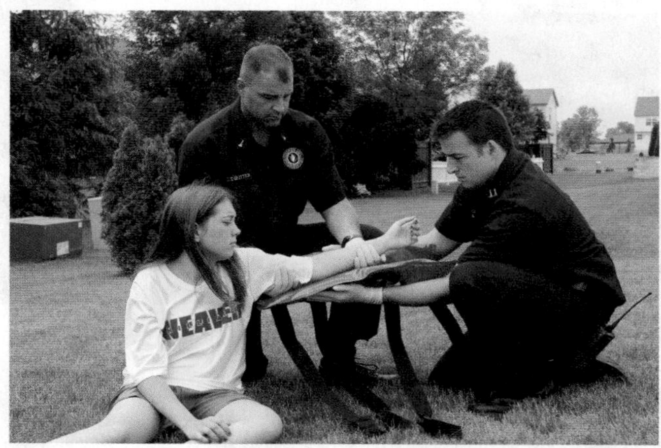

30-2A ✱ Manually stabilize the suspected fracture and assess pulse and motor and sensory function.

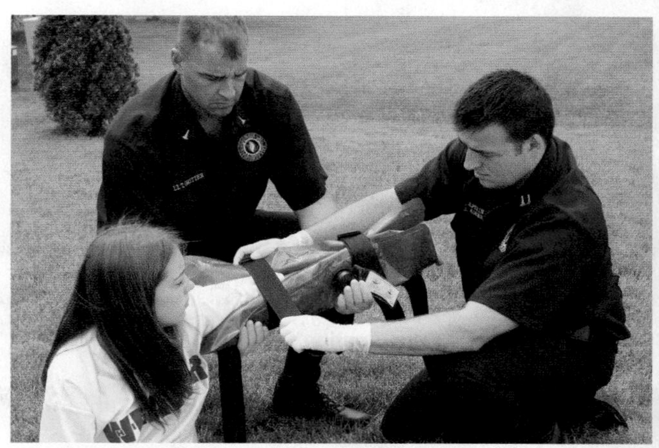

30-2B ✱ Apply the splint and secure it to the extremity.

continued

EMT skills 30-2 Applying a Vacuum Splint *continued*

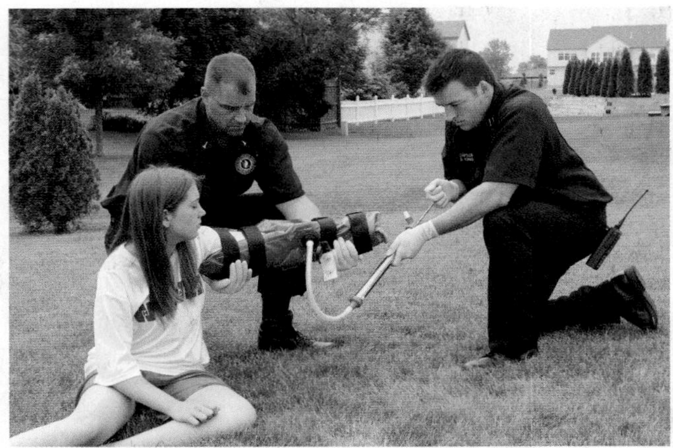

30-2C ✱ Suction the air out of the splint until it is rigid. Reassess pulse and motor and sensory function.

EMT skills 30-3 Splinting a Long Bone

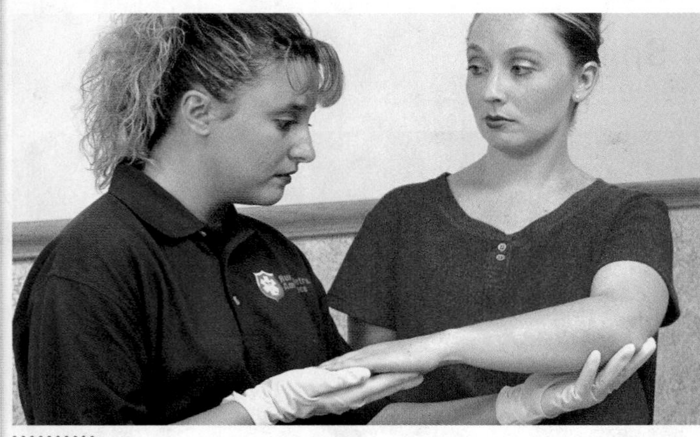

30-3A ✱ Apply manual stabilization to the injured extremity.

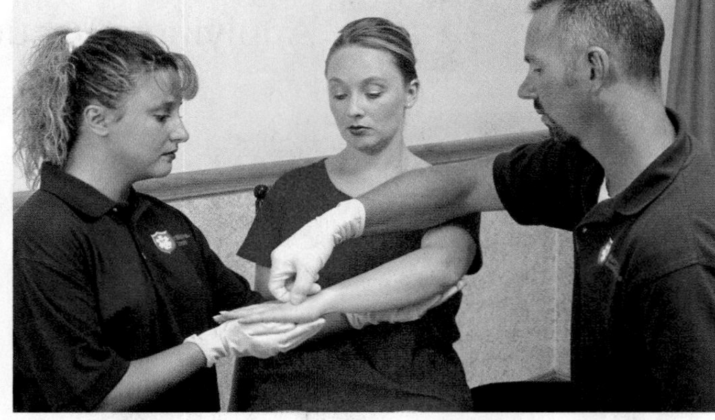

30-3B ✱ Assess the distal pulse and motor and sensory function.

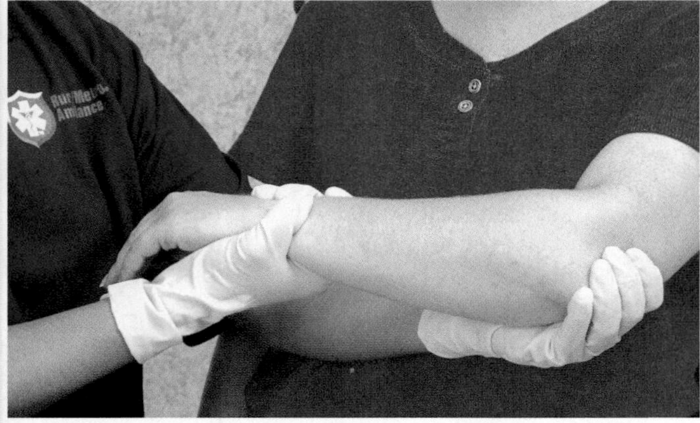

30-3C ✱ If the deformity is severe, distal pulses are absent, or the distal extremity is cyanotic, align with gentle manual traction.

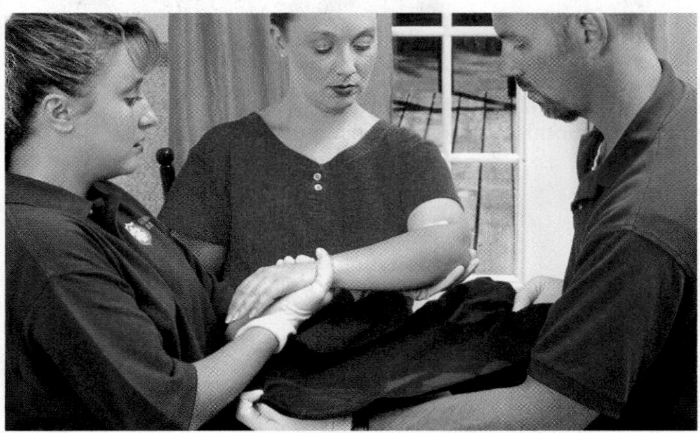

30-3D ✱ Measure the splint for proper length.

EMT skills 30-3 Splinting a Long Bone *continued*

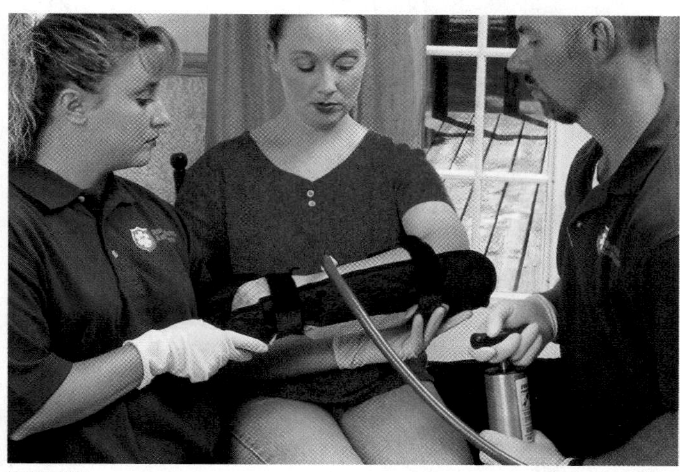

30-3E * Secure the entire injured extremity. The hand (or foot) must be immobilized in the position of function.

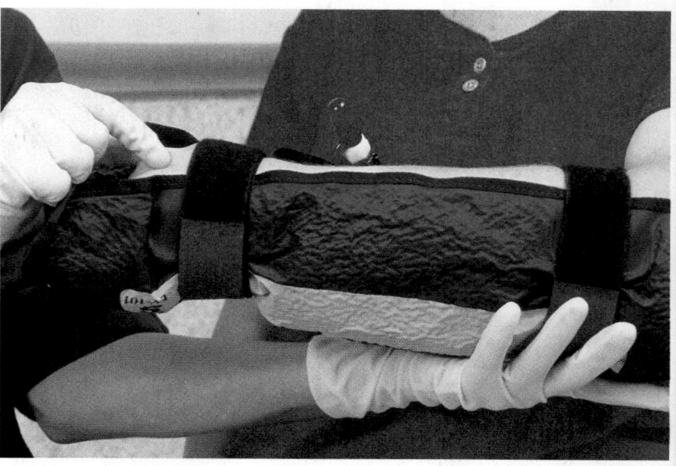

30-3F * Reassess the pulse and motor and sensory function.

EMT skills 30-4 Splinting a Joint

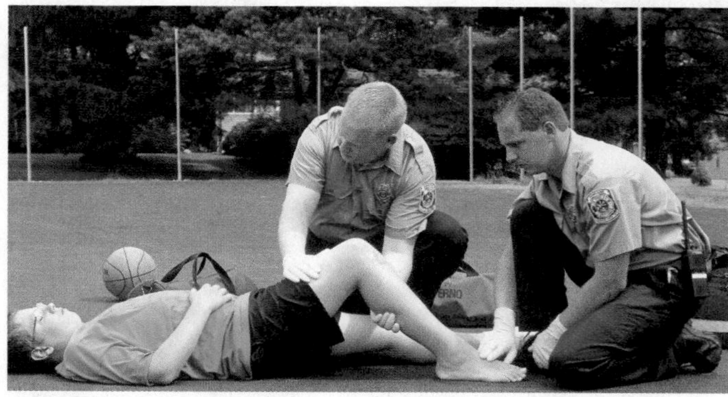

30-4A * Manually stabilize the joint in the position found. Then assess distal pulse and motor and sensory function.

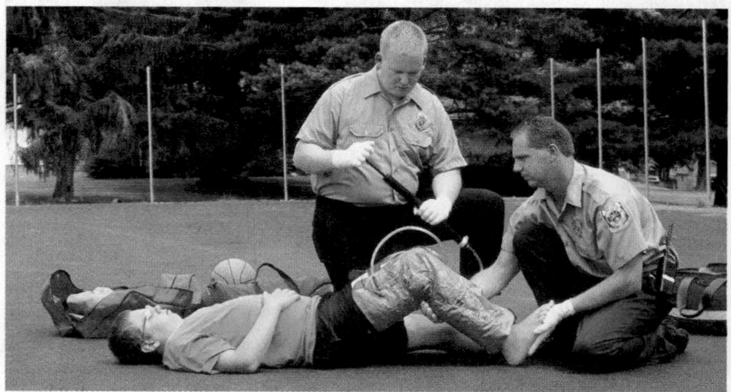

30-4B * Apply the splint to immobilize the bone above and below the joint.

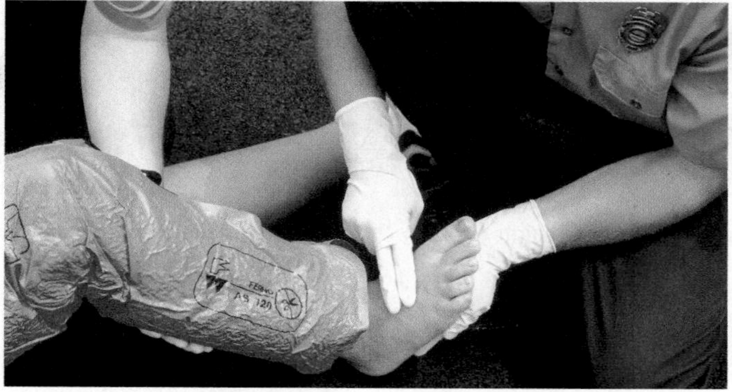

30-4C * Reassess sensory function, pulses, and motor function after the splint is applied.

EMT skills 30-5 Applying a Bipolar Traction Splint

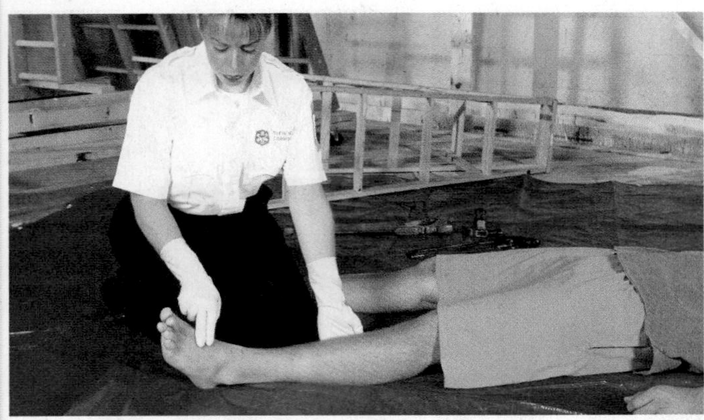

30-5A ✱ Assess distal pulses and motor and sensory function.

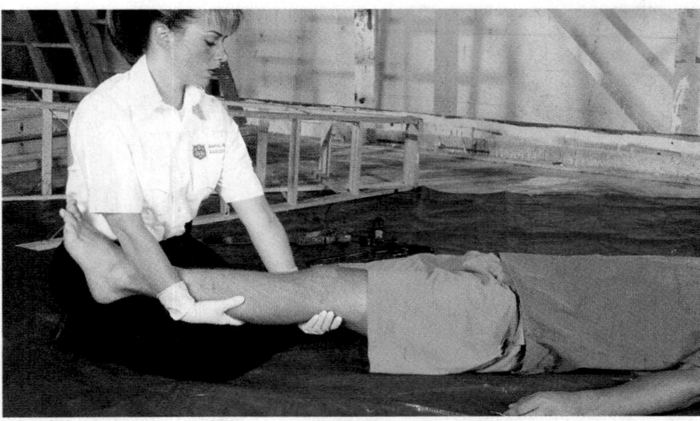

30-5B ✱ Stabilize the injured leg by applying manual traction.

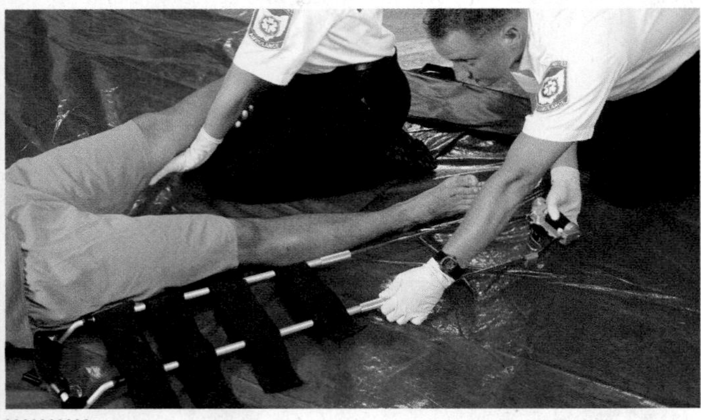

30-5C ✱ Adjust the splint for proper length, using the uninjured leg as a guide.

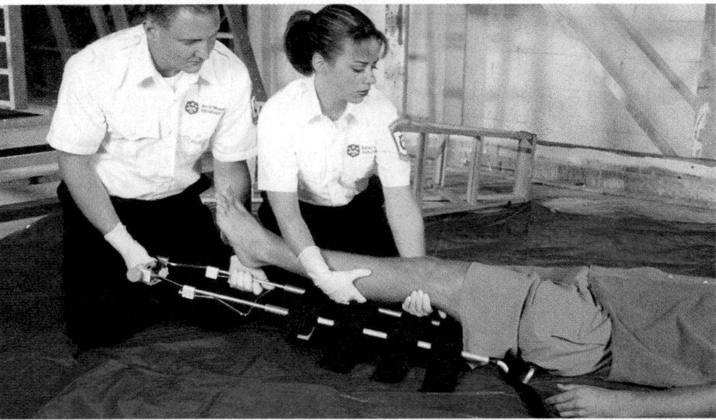

30-5D ✱ Position the splint under the injured leg until the ischial pad rests against the bony prominence of the buttocks. Once the splint is in position, raise the heel stand.

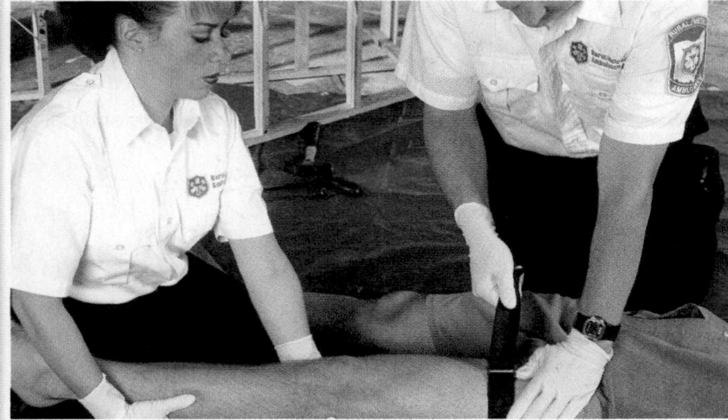

30-5E ✱ Attach the ischial strap over the groin and thigh.

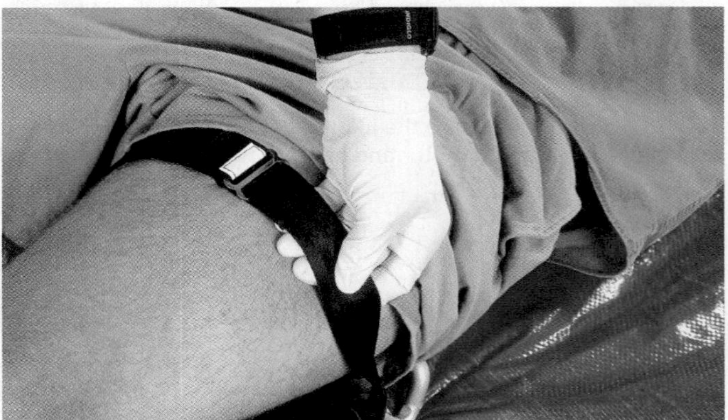

30-5F ✱ Make sure the ischial strap is snug but not tight enough to reduce distal circulation.

Applying a Bipolar Traction Splint *continued*

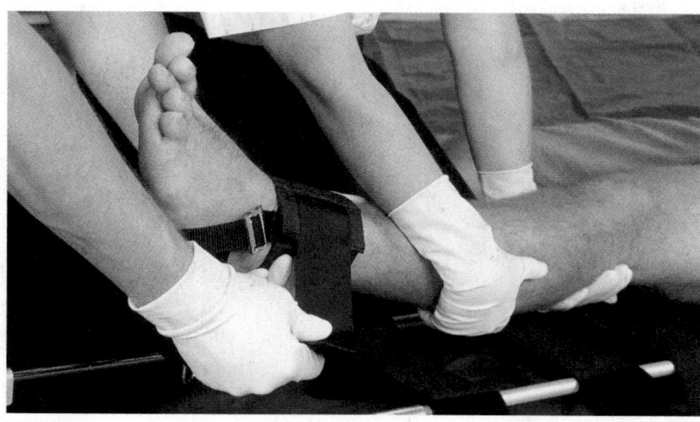

30-5G ✱ With the patient's foot in an upright position, secure the ankle hitch.

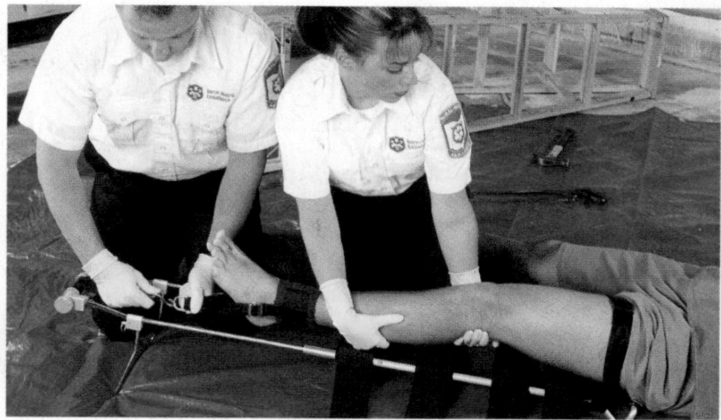

30-5H ✱ Attach the "S" hook to the "D" ring and apply mechanical traction. Full traction is achieved when the mechanical traction is equal to the manual traction and the pain and muscle spasms are reduced. In an unresponsive patient, adjust the traction until the injured leg is the same length as the uninjured leg.

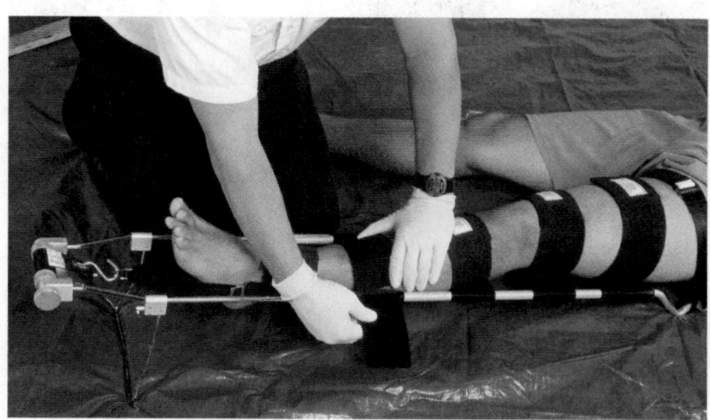

30-5I ✱ Fasten the leg support straps.

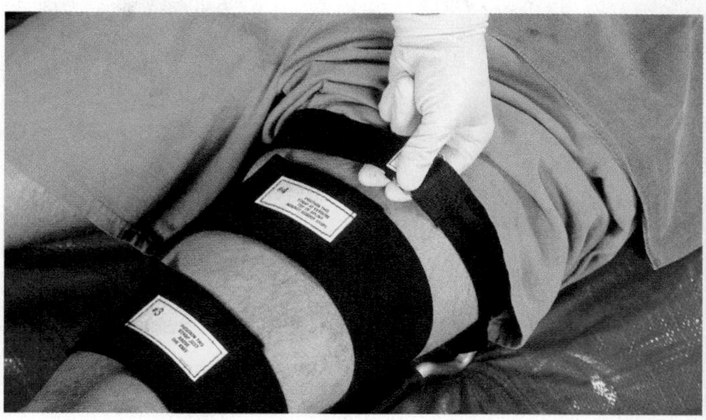

30-5J ✱ Re-evaluate the ischial strap and ankle hitch to ensure that both are securely fastened.

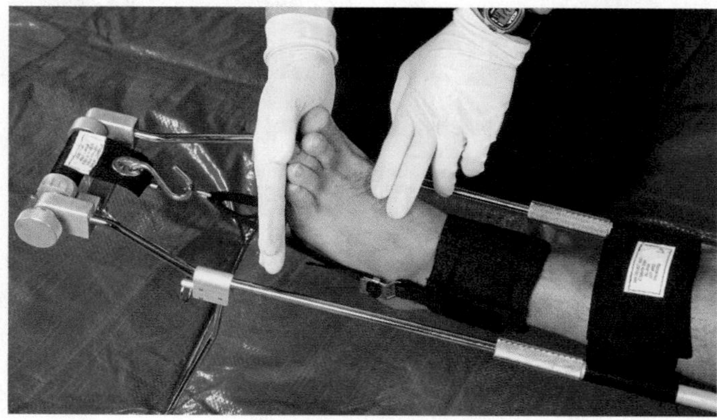

30-5K ✱ Reassess distal pulses and motor and sensory function.

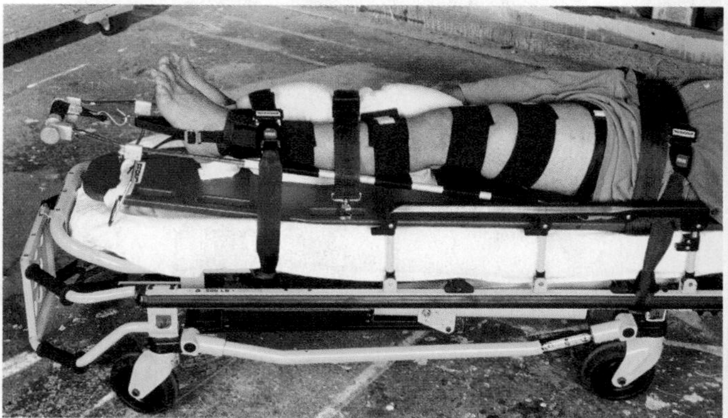

30-5L ✱ Place the patient on a long board and secure with straps. Pad between the splint and uninjured leg. Secure the splint to the backboard.

EMT skills 30-6 Applying a Unipolar Traction Splint

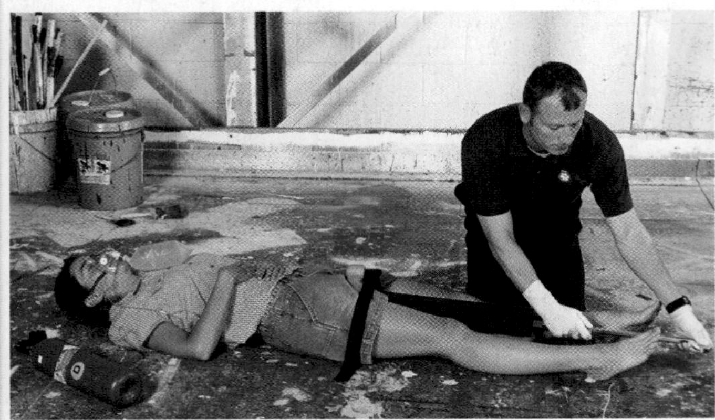

30-6A ✱ Assess distal perfusion and motor and sensory function. Place the splint along the medial aspect of the injured leg. Adjust it so that it extends about 4 inches beyond the heel.

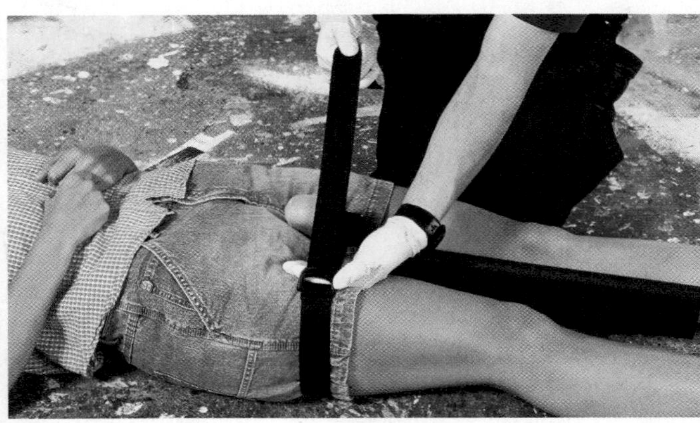

30-6B ✱ Secure the strap to the thigh.

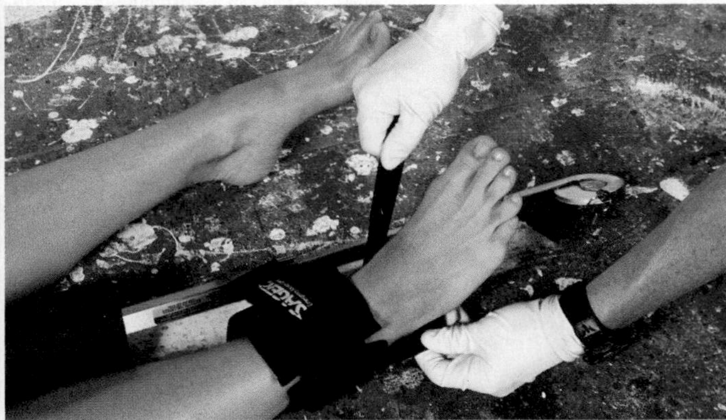

30-6C ✱ Apply the ankle hitch and attach it to the splint.

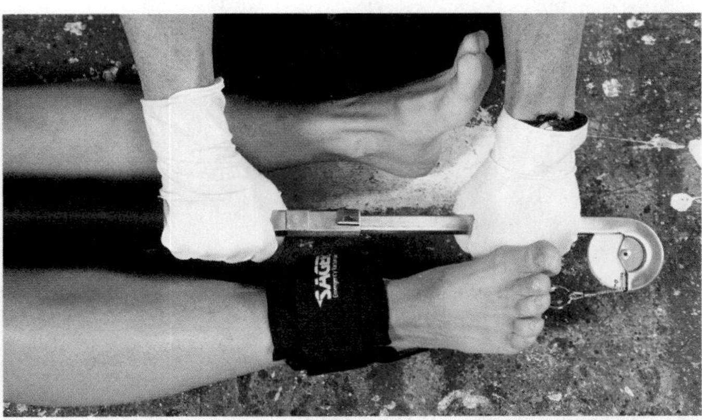

30-6D ✱ Apply traction by extending the splint. Adjust the splint to 10 percent of the patient's body weight.

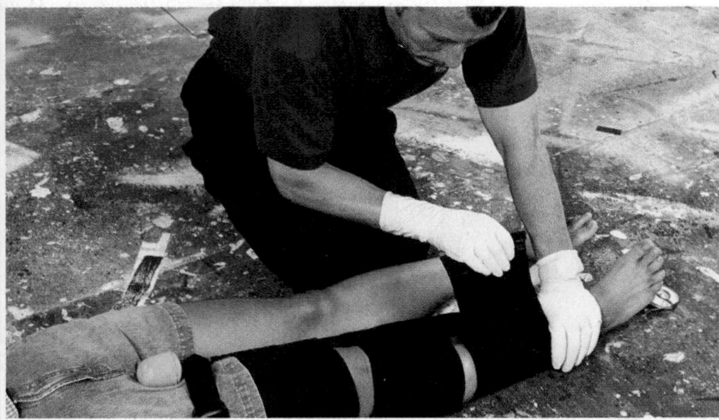

30-6E ✱ Apply the straps to secure the leg to the splint. Reassess distal pulses and motor and sensory function.

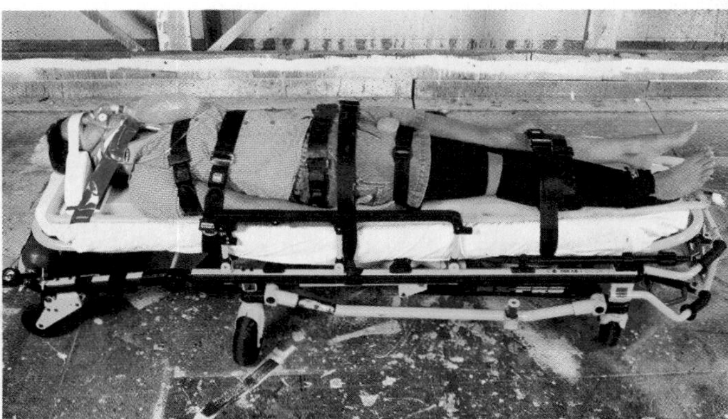

30-6F ✱ Place the patient onto a long backboard. Strap the ankles together and secure to the board.

EMT skills 30-7 Applying a Sling and Swathe

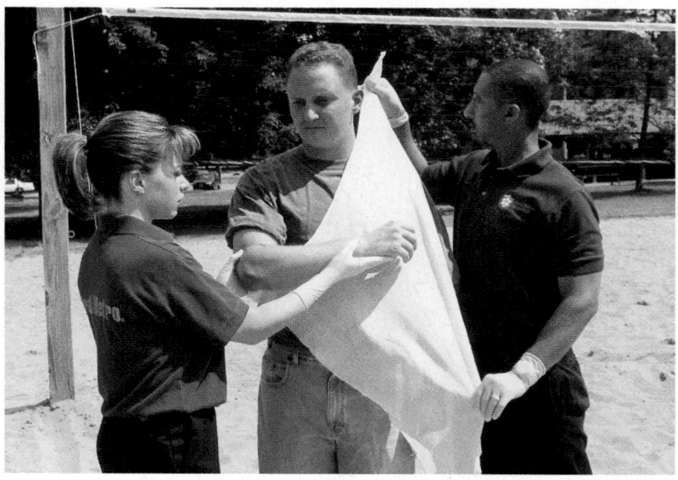

30-7A * First, place one end of the base of an open triangular bandage across the shoulder of the uninjured side, with the apex behind the elbow of the injured arm. Bend the arm at the elbow with the hand elevated 4–5 inches.

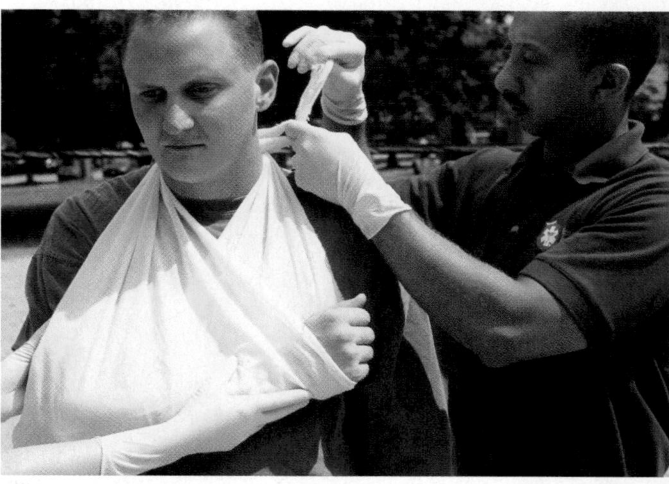

30-7B * Bring the lower end of the bandage over the shoulder of the injured side. Tie it in a knot at the back of the neck.

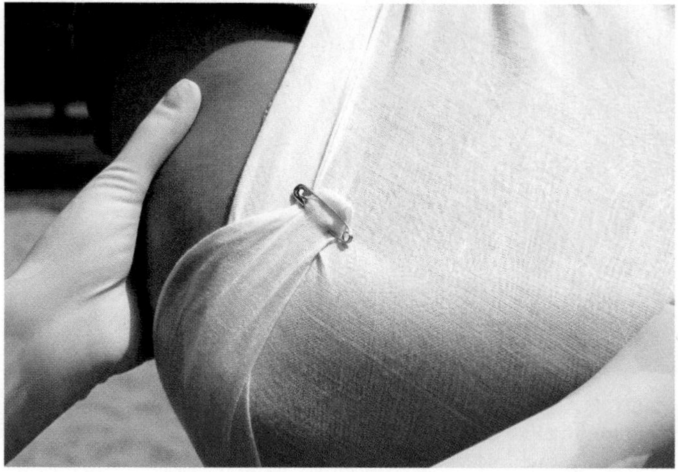

30-7C * Pin the apex to form a pocket at the elbow.

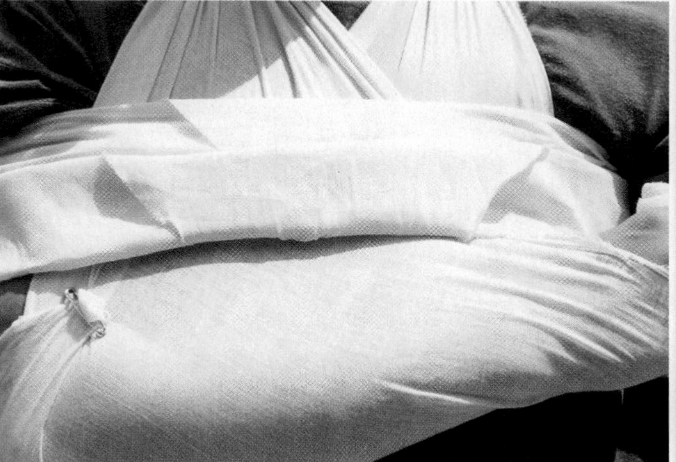

30-7D * Immobilize the injured arm to the body with a swathe.

EMT skills 30-8 Splinting Specific Injuries

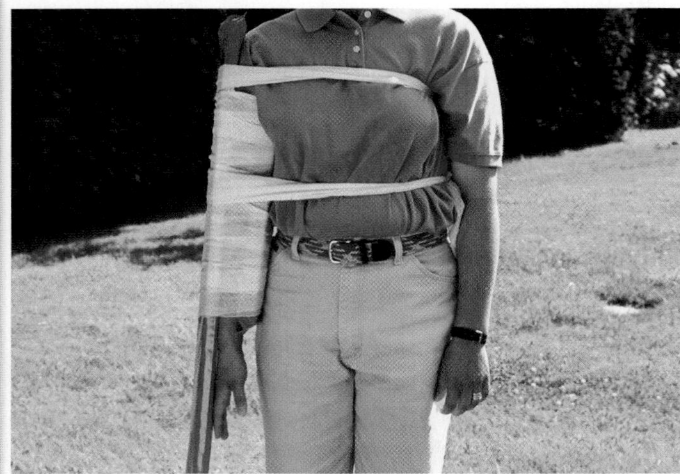

30-8A * Fixed splint for humerus injury.

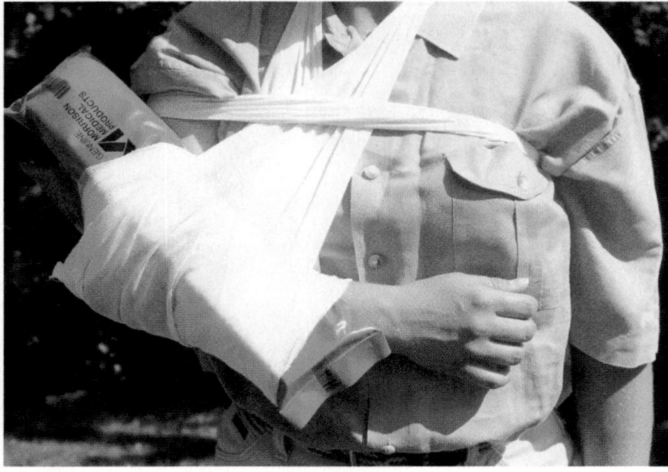

30-8B * Fixation of rigid splint with a sling and swathe.

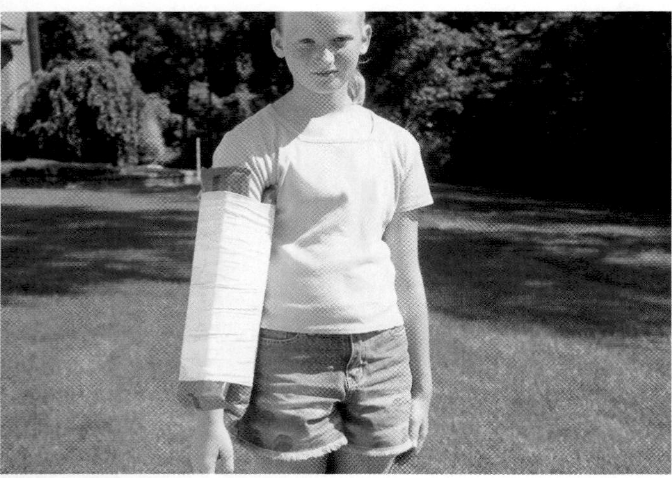

30-8C * Application of a fixed splint for a humerus injury to a child.

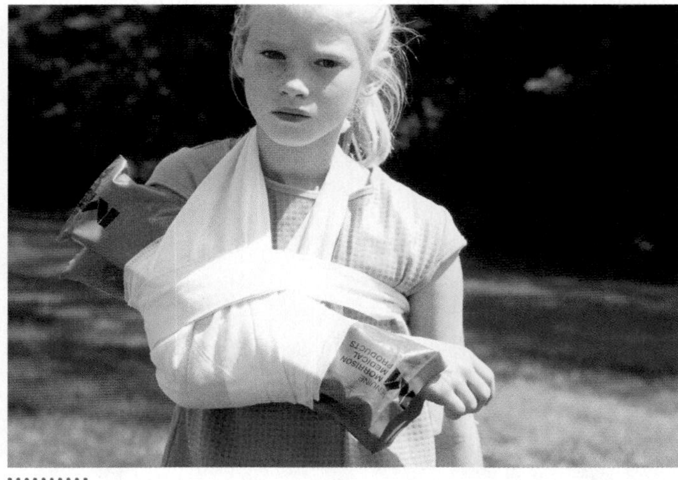

30-8D * Application of a rigid splint with sling and swathe to a child for an elbow injury.

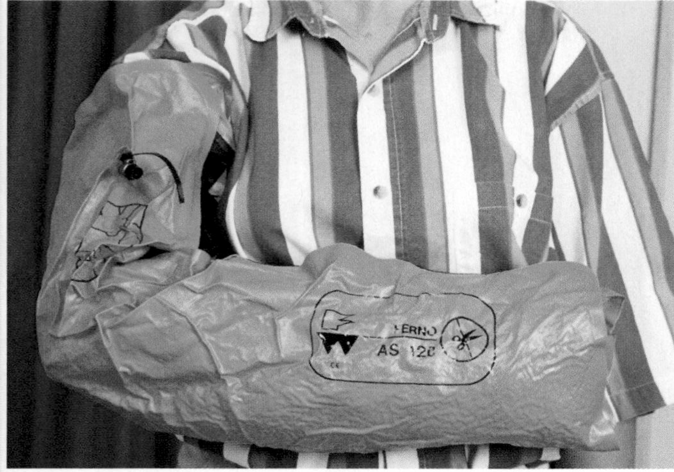

30-8E * Immobilization of an elbow injury with a vacuum splint in a bent position.

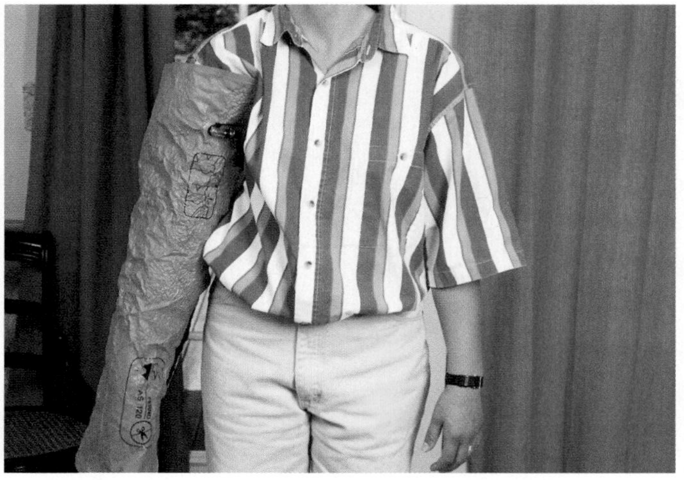

30-8F * Immobilization of an elbow injury with a vacuum splint in a straight position.

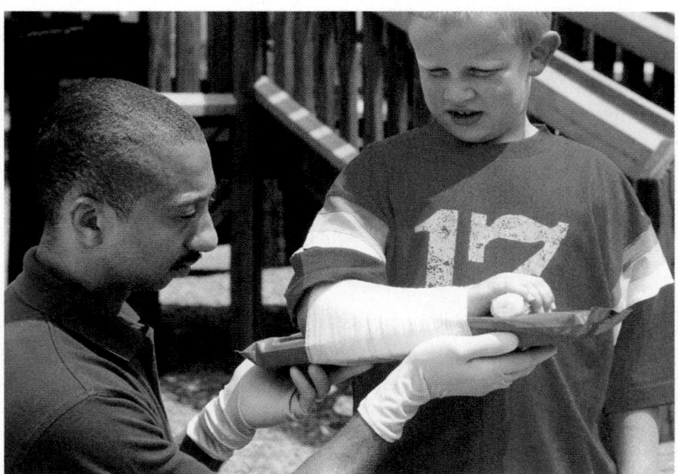

30-8G ✱ Immobilization of a bone injury to the forearm, wrist, or hand.

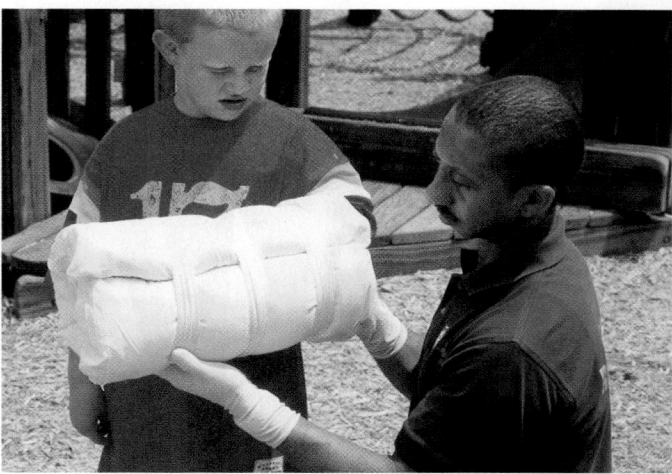

30-8H ✱ Immobilization with a blanket roll splint of a bone injury to the forearm, wrist, or hand.

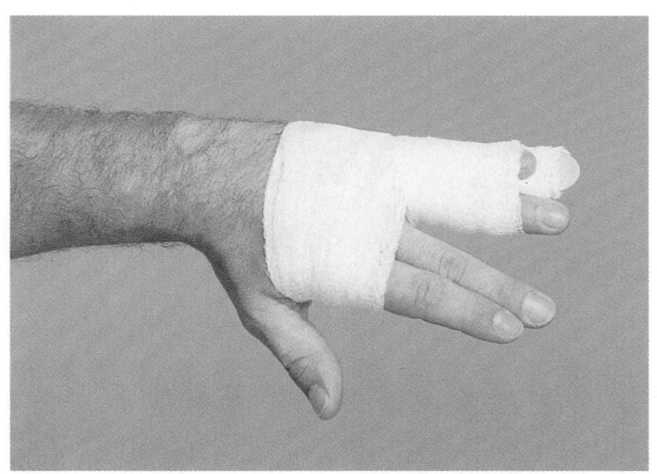

30-8I ✱ Bone injury to the finger splinted with a tongue depressor.

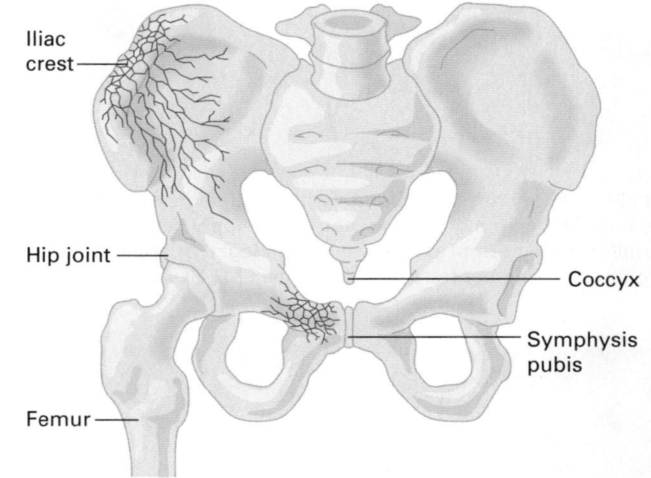

30-8J ✱ Common sites of injury to the pelvis.

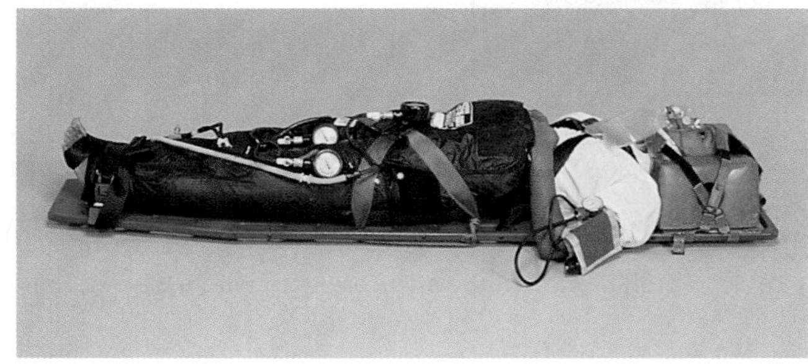

30-8K ✱ Use of the PASG is recommended to splint a suspected pelvic injury.

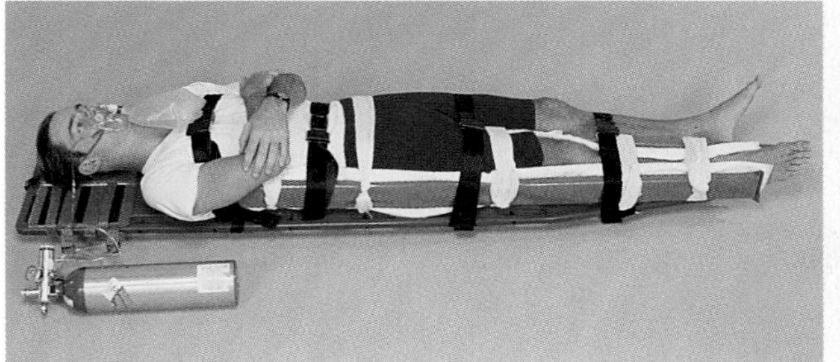

30-8L ✱ Rigid splint for hip injury.

continued

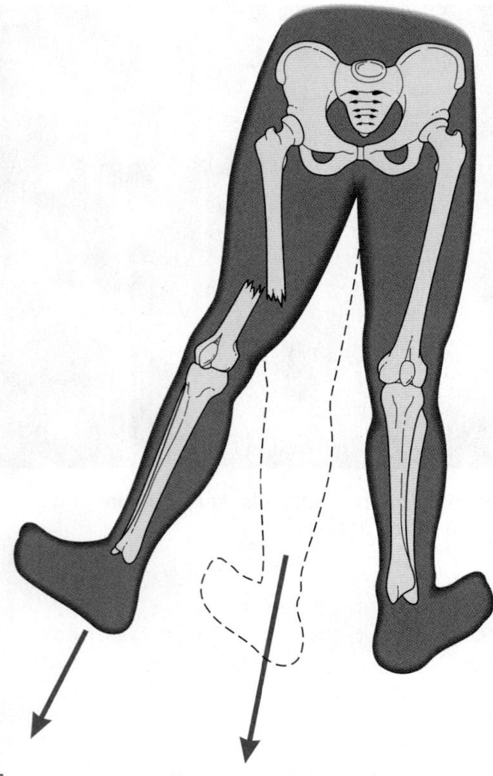

30-8M ✱ Injury to shaft of femur with angulation, shortening, and rotation of the limb below the injury site. Apply gentle traction parallel to the normal axis of the injured leg. (For application of bipolar and unipolar traction splints, see EMT Skills 30-5 and 30-6.)

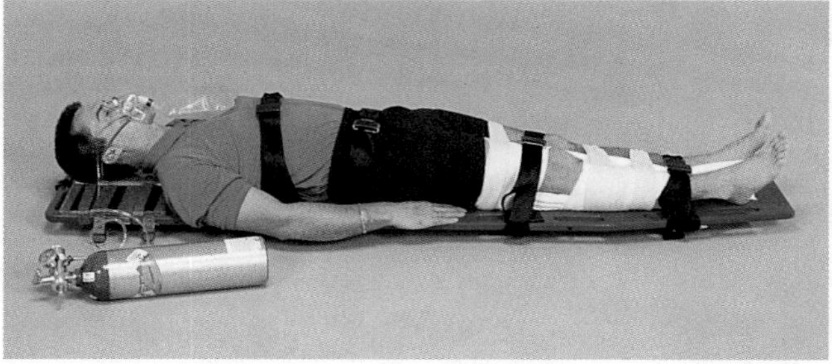

30-8N ✱ Immobilized knee injury in straight position.

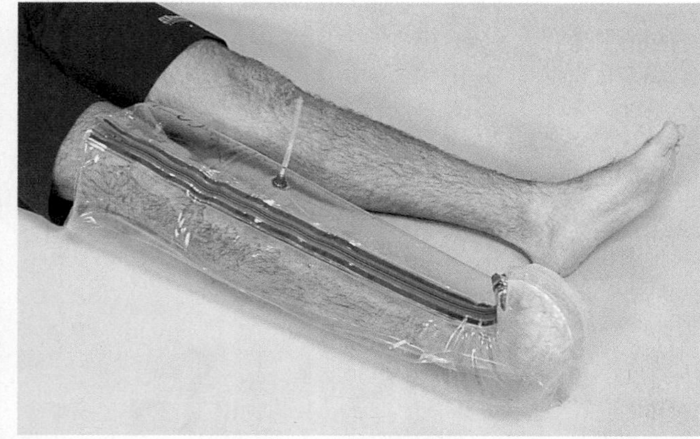

30-8O ✱ Immobilization of a lower leg injury with an air splint.

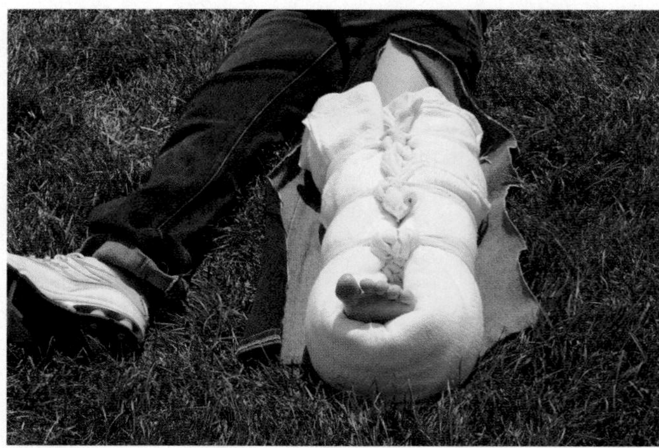

30-8P ✱ Immobilization of the ankle and foot with a blanket roll.

CHAPTER REVIEW

SUMMARY

A fracture is a break in the continuity of the bone. Some fractures present with obvious signs and symptoms, whereas others may have a more subtle presentation. Fractures can be open or closed. Other associated injuries are dislocations, sprains, and strains. The two main purposes of splinting are to prevent movement and reduce pain. When splinting a joint, be sure to immobilize the bone above and below the joint. When splinting a long bone, you must immobilize the joint above and below the injured bone. Always assess motor and sensory function and distal pulses both prior to and after splinting an extremity.

There are a variety of splints, including rigid, pressure (air or pneumatic), traction, vacuum, improvised, and sling and swathe. Select the proper splint for the injury. Improperly applied splints may aggravate or cause further injury.

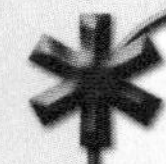

CASE STUDY FOLLOW-UP

SCENE SIZE-UP

You and your partner have just arrived at the high school football field. You have been dispatched to a 17-year-old male patient complaining of leg pain. The scene appears safe as you put on your disposable gloves and remove the stretcher from the ambulance. Your partner grabs the trauma kit. As you wheel the stretcher onto the field you are met by the football coach who tells you his quarterback, Tom Cvitanovic, was tackled. "He can't move his right leg. He got tackled pretty hard." The coach's remarks lead you to believe the mechanism of injury may mean a fracture caused by direct force. You approach Tom and introduce yourself. Your partner asks, "What happened, and where is the pain?"

PRIMARY ASSESSMENT

Tom complains of severe right leg pain and says his right arm hurts, too. Because he is talking clearly, you assume his airway is open. His breathing is adequate; his radial pulse is strong and 103 per minute. You do not believe he has a life-threatening condition. Tom then lets out a groan, and says, "Oh, man, can't you do anything for the pain?!!" He seems frightened so you reassure him that he'll get care quickly. Your partner is at Tom's head maintaining manual in-line spinal stabilization. He is alert and oriented, is exhibiting no signs of respiratory distress or hypoxia, has no complaints of shortness of breath, and has an SpO_2 reading of 99% on room air; therefore, you decide not to place him on oxygen.

SECONDARY ASSESSMENT

While your partner continues spinal stabilization, you perform a secondary assessment and assess for signs of injury. Tom denies any neck pain. However, because of the mechanism of injury, you apply a cervical spine immobilization collar as your partner continues to maintain manual stabilization.

You find that Tom's right arm is tender and swollen. Approximately 6 inches below Tom's right knee you see bone ends protruding through a fracture site. Pulse, motor, and sensory function are good below both injury sites.

You apply a cold pack to Tom's right arm and then take his baseline vitals. His blood pressure is 142/70 mmHg, respirations are 20 per minute, pulse is 120 per minute, and skin is warm and slightly sweaty. Skin color is normal. You obtain a history and learn that Tom denies any further pain or injury. He says he is allergic to aspirin and doesn't take any medication. He tells you that 3 years ago he broke the same leg and was hospitalized for almost a week. He had his last meal at noon. Then he describes how he was tackled by two, maybe three, other football players.

Following your local protocols, you decide to apply a vacuum splint to Tom's right arm. You cover the protruding bone ends below the knee with a trauma pad and note that there is very little bleeding. Following local protocols, and with your partner's assistance, you apply padded board splints to Tom's right leg. You recheck the pulse and motor and sensory function of Tom's injured arm and leg. There is no change. Once Tom is fully immobilized to a backboard, you load him into the ambulance for transport.

REASSESSMENT

You perform a reassessment and find that Tom remains alert and oriented. His airway, breathing, and circulation remain adequate. You reassess vital signs and then recheck your medical interventions. The vacuum splint is rigid, and the padded board splints are secure. You reassess pulses, motor function, and sensation to Tom's right arm and leg. You radio your report to the emergency department, continue your reassessment, and reassure Tom that you are only 5 minutes away from the hospital.

A few weeks later, when you are reading the sports page, you spot a picture of Tom on the team bench with crutches propped up beside him. The season is nearly over, but Tom is only a junior and is expected to quarterback the team again next year.

IN REVIEW

1. List three functions of the musculoskeletal system.
2. Explain the difference between an open and a closed bone injury.
3. List the indications that would lead you to suspect a bone or joint injury.
4. Explain the reasons for splinting a bone or joint injury.
5. List the emergency medical care steps for treating a bone or joint injury.
6. Outline the general rules for splinting a bone or joint injury.
7. Describe the complications that can arise from improper splinting of a bone or joint.
8. List contraindications for (reasons for not using) a traction splint on a suspected femur fracture.

CRITICAL THINKING

You arrive on the scene and find a 24-year-old female patient who was riding her bike when she was struck by a car. She was thrown from her bike to the ground. She is alert and moaning loudly. Her airway is open and her respirations are 26 per minute with good chest rise. Her radial pulse is weak and her skin is pale, cool, and clammy. Her heart rate is 128 per minute. During the rapid trauma assessment, you note that her pelvis is unstable and she complains of severe pain when it is palpated. You also note a deformed right lower leg. Her blood pressure is 96/72 mmHg.

1. What initial emergency care would you provide to the patient?
2. What specific injuries do you suspect?
3. How would you manage the possible fractures?
4. What complications would occur with the suspected fractures?

PEARSON

EXPLORE mybradykit™

Please go to **www.bradybooks.com** to access mykit for this text. You will find quizzes, critical thinking scenarios, weblinks, animations, and videos related to this chapter—and much more. Look for online information on fractures as well as video clips on joint injuries, long bone injuries, and splints.

Register your access code from the front of your book by going to **www.bradybooks.com** and selecting the mykit links.

CHAPTER 31

Head Trauma

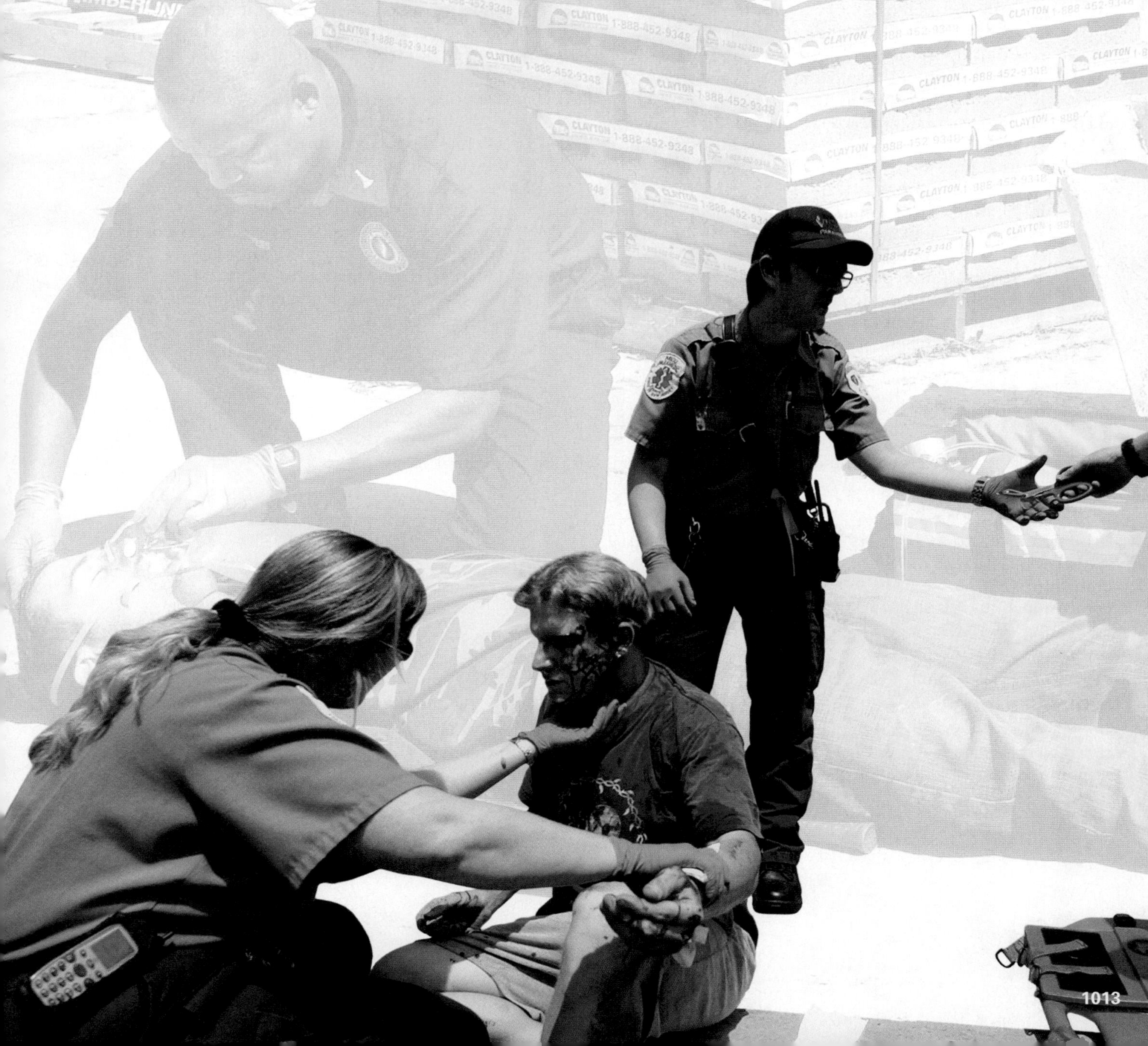

Navigation Guide

STANDARD **Trauma** (Content Area: Head, Facial, Neck, and Spine Trauma)

COMPETENCY Applies fundamental knowledge to provide basic emergency care and transportation based on assessment findings for an acutely injured patient.

OBJECTIVES: After reading this chapter, you should be able to:

31-1. Define key terms introduced in the chapter.
31-2. Explain the importance of recognizing and providing emergency medical care to patients with injuries to the head.
31-3. Identify the anatomy of the skull.
31-4. Identify the meningeal layers and the spaces into which intracranial bleeding can occur in relationship to the meninges, skull, and brain.
31-5. Associate each of the major anatomical portions of the brain with its functions.
31-6. Explain the pathophysiology and key signs and symptoms of injuries to the scalp, skull, and brain, including:
- **a.** Scalp lacerations
- **b.** Skull fractures
- **c.** Cerebral concussion and diffuse axonal injury
- **d.** Cerebral contusion
- **e.** Coup/contrecoup injury
- **f.** Cerebral and intracranial hematomas
- **g.** Cerebral laceration

31-7. Identify and, where possible, manage factors that can worsen traumatic brain injuries, including:
- **a.** Hypoxia
- **b.** Hypercarbia
- **c.** Hypoglycemia
- **d.** Hyperglycemia
- **e.** Hyperthermia
- **f.** Hypotension

31-8. Describe the goals of emergency treatment of patients with traumatic brain injuries.
31-9. Describe the pathophysiology and key signs of increased intracranial pressure and brain herniation.
31-10. Describe the neurological assessment of patients with suspected traumatic brain injury.
31-11. Discuss the focus of history taking and assessment for patients with injuries to the head.
31-12. Assess and provide emergency treatment to patients with injuries to the head.
31-13. Explain the importance of reassessment of the patient with an injury to the head.
31-14. Document information relevant to the assessment and management of patients with injuries to the head.

KEY TERMS: Page references indicate first major use in this chapter. For complete definitions, see the Glossary at the back of the book.

anterograde amnesia p. 1029
Battle sign p. 1027
brainstem p. 1016
cerebellum p. 1016
cerebrospinal fluid (CSF) p. 1015
cerebrum p. 1016
concussion p. 1019
consensual reflex p. 1027
contusion p. 1019
Cushing reflex p. 1029
diplopia p. 1029
epidural hematoma p. 1021
extension posturing p. 1024
flexion posturing p. 1024
herniation p. 1022
laceration p. 1021
meninges p. 1016
raccoon sign p. 1027
retrograde amnesia p. 1029
subdural hematoma p. 1020

MEDIA RESOURCES: Please go to www.bradybooks.com to access mykit for this text. You will find quizzes, critical thinking scenarios, weblinks, animations, and videos related to this chapter—and much more. Look for online information on traumatic brain injuries. You will also find a video clip on applying a cervical collar.

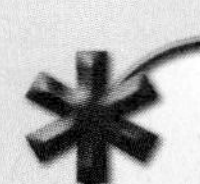

CASE STUDY

The Dispatch
EMS Unit 504—proceed to 2516 Elmwood Street—unresponsive 18-year-old male. Time out is 1230 hours.

Upon Arrival
Family members are waiting outside as your unit approaches the house. An anxious woman begins to speak as soon as you open your door: "My son, we can't wake him up. We found him on his bed and we can't wake him up! He just came home 20 minutes ago. He laughed and said he'd bumped his head playing basketball. But he seemed fine. I went to get him for lunch and we couldn't wake him up. He's in his room. Please hurry!"

How Would You Proceed to Assess and Care for This Patient?
In this chapter, you will learn about assessment and care for a patient suffering from head injury. Later, we will return to the case study and apply the procedures learned.

Introduction

Injuries to the head pose some of the most serious situations you will face as an EMT. The patient is often confused or unresponsive, making assessment of his condition difficult. Drug and alcohol use will also cloud the assessment and make head injury diagnosis difficult. Head injuries to a patient can occur days or weeks before the onset of any signs or symptoms. In addition, many injuries to the head are life threatening. Such injuries are, in fact, a leading cause of death among this nation's young people. Many patients who survive head injuries suffer permanent disability. The cost of failing to recognize or properly treat such injuries can be very high.

Head injuries must be looked at with concern because the skull encases the structures of the central nervous system. The central nervous system, made up of the brain and the spinal cord, coordinates the functions of other body systems. Injury to it can have severe consequences.

Anatomy of the Skull and Brain

The skull is the portion of the skeletal system that contains and protects the brain and the portion of the spinal cord that exits from the brain. At this point, you may want to review the information about the skeletal and nervous systems that was presented in Chapter 7, "Anatomy, Physiology, and Medical Terminology."

The Skull

The brain, which occupies 80–90 percent of the space inside the skull, is surrounded by plates of large, flat bones that are fused together to form a helmetlike covering called the *cranial skull.* The remainder of the skull is made up of facial bones. Composed of 14 irregularly shaped bones, it is made up of the cheek, nose, and jaw bones (Figure 31-1*). The *basilar skull,* or floor of the skull, is made up of many separate pieces of bone and is the weakest part of the skull. Some of its bones are thin and perforated extensively by the spinal cord, nerves, and blood vessels. The basilar skull has many bony ridges that can cause injury to the brain. Also, the skull tightly encloses the brain, severely limiting the swelling and bleeding that can occur around the brain.

The Brain

Within the skull, the brain is cushioned in a dense, serous substance called **cerebrospinal fluid (CSF).** Produced by the brain, this fluid protects the brain and spinal cord against impact. The cerebrospinal fluid is clear and colorless, circulates throughout the skull and spinal column, and is reabsorbed by the circulatory system. The fluid not only cushions and protects but also performs a function similar to lymph fluid in combating infection and cleansing the brain and spinal cord. When both the skull and the membrane surrounding the brain are broken, cerebrospinal fluid leaks out, often through the nose, ears, or both—a classic sign of basilar skull fracture.

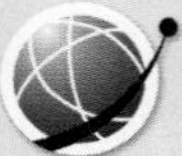

Media Resources

Go to www.bradybooks.com for mykit. Highlights:

- *Web Resource:* Traumatic Brain Injury
- *Web Resource:* Types of Brain Injuries

Objective 31-2

Recognize and treat patients with head injuries.

Objectives 31-3 and 31-4

Identify the anatomy of the skull and meninges.

Key Terms

cerebrospinal fluid (CSF) a clear fluid that surrounds the brain and the spinal cord.

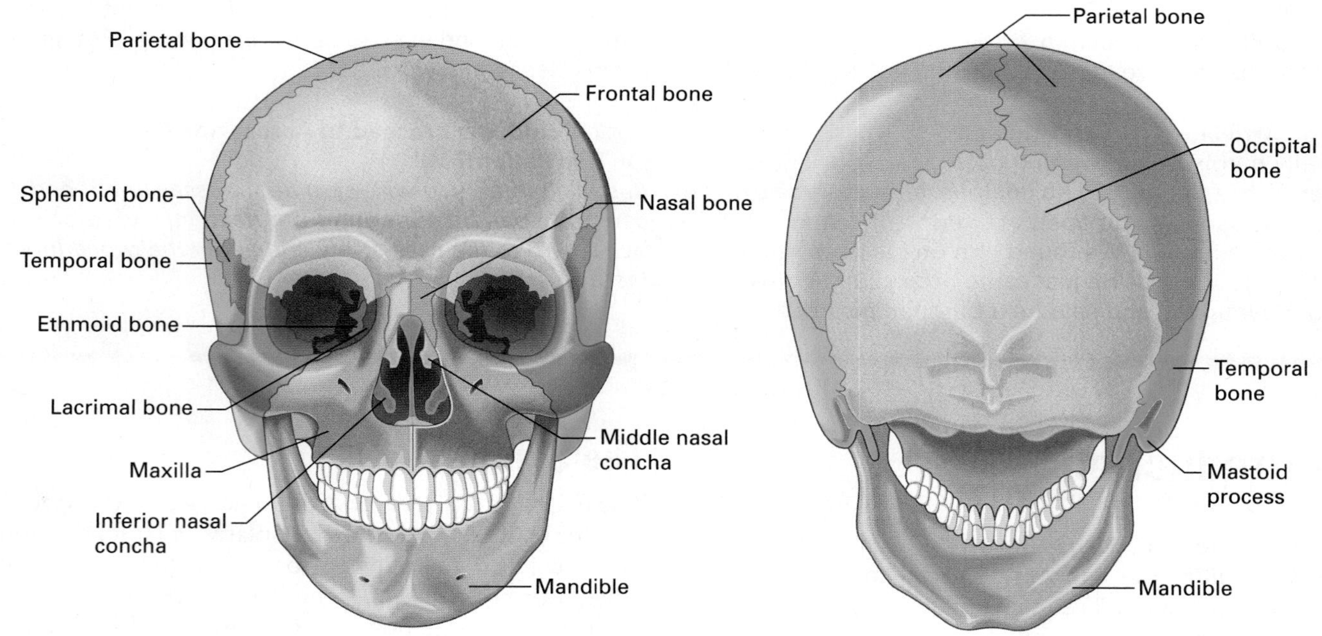

FIGURE 31-1 ∗ The skull.

The Meninges

Inside the skull, the surface of the brain is protected from injury by three **meninges,** or layers of tissue, that enclose the brain (Figure 31-2∗). The outermost is the *dura mater* ("hard mother"), composed of a double layer of tough, fibrous tissue. The next layer is the *arachnoid*. Beneath that, in contact with the brain, is the *pia mater* ("soft mother"). All three layers enclose not only the brain, but the brainstem and the spinal cord as well. The arachnoid membrane and the pia mater are separated by a lattice of fibrous, spongy tissue filled with cerebrospinal fluid called the *subarachnoid space*.

Bleeding that occurs between the dura mater and the skull is called *epidural* and usually involves the brain's outermost arteries. Recognized and treated early, such bleeding may have no permanent consequences. *Subdural* bleeding, on the other hand, occurs beneath the dura and is usually venous. Bleeding that occurs between the arachnoid membrane and the surface of the brain is called *subarachnoid hemorrhage*. It can be fatal in minutes.

Parts of the Brain

The brain is divided into three anatomical components:

- The **cerebrum**—The largest part of the brain, the cerebrum, comprises three-fourths of the brain's volume. It is divided into two hemispheres (right and left). Each hemisphere is made up of four distinct lobes: a frontal lobe (anterior), a parietal lobe (middle), an occipital lobe (posterior), and a temporal lobe (side). The cerebrum is responsible for most conscious and sensory functions, the emotions, and the personality. The cerebrum is not attached to the inside of the skull.
- The **cerebellum**—Sometimes called the "little brain," the cerebellum controls equilibrium and coordinates muscle activity. Tucked underneath the cerebrum, it controls muscle movement and coordination, predicts when to stop movement, and coordinates the reflexes that maintain posture and equilibrium.
- The **brainstem**—The brain's funnel-shaped inferior part, the brainstem, is the most primitive and best

Objective 31-5
Associate each of the major anatomical portions of the brain with its functions.

Key Terms
meninges layers of tissue protecting the brain. They include the dura mater, the arachnoid, and the pia mater.

Key Terms
cerebrum part of the brain controlling conscious and sensory functions, emotions, and personality.

cerebellum part of the brain controlling equilibrium and muscle coordination.

brainstem part of the brain that controls most automatic functions of the body.

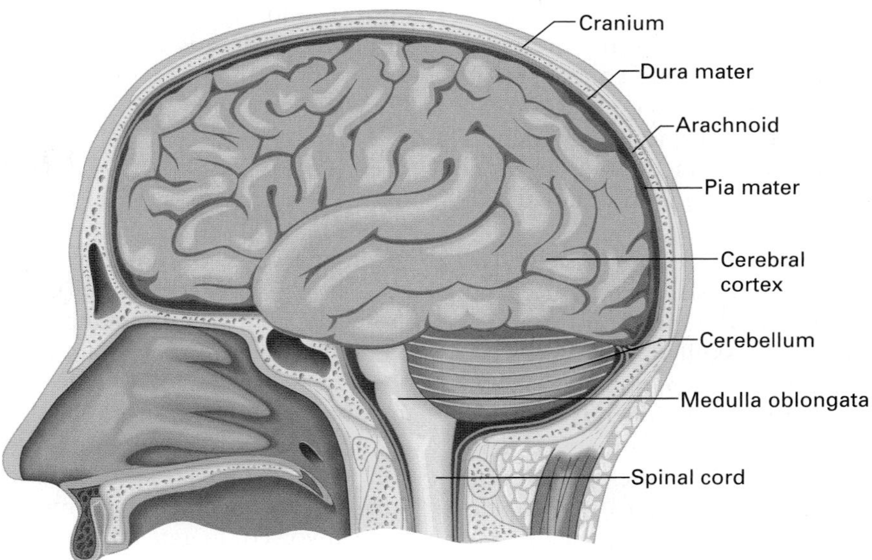

FIGURE 31-2 ✱ The meninges and brain.

protected part of the brain. Tethered to the skull by numerous nerves and vessels, it controls most automatic functions of the body, including cardiac, respiratory, vasomotor (blood pressure), and other functions vital to life. The brainstem is made up of the pons, the midbrain, and the medulla, or medulla oblongata, which physically connects the brain to the spinal cord. All of the messages between the brain and the spinal cord pass through the medulla.

▶ Head Injury

Head injuries can involve the scalp, the skull, the brain itself, or combinations of these.

Scalp Injuries

The scalp may be injured in the same way as any other soft tissue; it may be contused, lacerated, abraded, or avulsed. Because of the rich supply of blood vessels to the scalp, injuries of the scalp tend to bleed very heavily. In addition, the underlying fascia may be torn while the skin stays intact. Bleeding then occurs under the skin and may be confusing at first as you try to assess the patient. (The presence of blood under intact skin can mimic skull deformity.)

Understanding BODY PROCESSES

The vessels in the scalp are not able to constrict as effectively as other blood vessels in the body; thus, they bleed more heavily when injured, which can lead to shock if uncontrolled. The skull is covered by a layer of fascia (fibrous membrane) and then by the scalp. The fascia adheres to the skull loosely, more easily creating a scalp avulsion. ■

ASSESSMENT Tips

When palpating the skull, you may identify a depressed skull fracture that doesn't really exist—or fail to detect a depressed skull fracture that actually does exist. The reasons: The fascia, which lies under the scalp but above the skull, can rupture and become depressed and feel, on palpation, like a depressed skull fracture. Conversely, blood may fill the area between a depressed skull fracture and the scalp, making the skull feel normal and not depressed during palpation. ■

Skull Injuries

Because of the skull's spherical shape and thickness, it is generally deformed only if the trauma is extreme. A

Key Points
Head injury can cause bleeding, swelling, and increased pressure within the skull, resulting in reduced perfusion of the brain.

Objective 31-6
Explain the pathophysiology and key signs and symptoms of injuries to the scalp, skull, and brain.

linear skull fracture, which is the most common type, resembles a line. There is no gross deformity in a linear fracture and it can only be diagnosed through a radiograph. A *depressed skull fracture* occurs when the bone ends are pushed inward toward the brain. Typically, the depression can be palpated in the area of fracture. A depressed skull fracture may pose harm if the bone ends damage the brain tissue.

Skull fractures can be open or closed. A *closed skull fracture* is an injury in which the skull is fractured but there is no open wound to the overlying scalp. An *open skull fracture* is a fracture of the skull with an associated open wound to the scalp. The open wound allows for the possibility that bacteria and other contaminants will enter the skull and infect the brain. If the dura mater is damaged, cerebrospinal fluid may leak from the open wound.

A *basilar skull fracture* is a fracture to the floor or bottom of the cranium. This fracture often begins as a linear temporal fracture that extends downward and continues into the base of the skull. Basilar skull fractures often cause leakage of cerebrospinal fluid from the ears, nose, or mouth. Ecchymosis (bruise-type discoloration) around the eyes and behind the ears often occurs with a basilar skull fracture; however, it often takes several hours for the bruising to become apparent.

A skull deformity itself does not cause disability or death; rather, it is any underlying damage to the brain that leads to serious consequences. In short, the skull deformity presents no danger if it is not accompanied by brain injury, hematoma, cerebrospinal fluid leakage, or subsequent infection.

Understanding BODY PROCESSES

The thinnest portion of the skull is the temporal region, which is therefore very prone to fracture. Often, linear temporal fractures extend to the bottom of the skull, creating a basilar skull fracture. ■

Brain Injuries

As already explained, the brain is enclosed within the skull—a rigid, unyielding case. Injury can cause swelling of brain tissue or bleeding within the skull. Both conditions can cause increased pressure inside the skull and decreased perfusion of the brain, resulting in an inadequate delivery of oxygen and glucose to and removal of carbon dioxide and other waste products from the brain tissues. A brain injury caused by trauma is often referred to as a traumatic brain injury (TBI).

Pathophysiology of Traumatic Brain Injury

Brain injury may be direct (from penetrating trauma), indirect (from a blow to the skull), or secondary (for example, from a lack of oxygen, buildup of carbon dioxide, or change in blood pressure). The injury may be closed or open.

In cases of *closed head injury* (Figure 31-3*), the scalp may be lacerated but the skull remains intact and there will be no opening to the brain. *Brain damage within the intact skull can, nonetheless, be extensive.* The amount of injury depends mainly on the mechanism of injury and the force involved. In general, brain tissue is susceptible to the same kinds of injury as any soft tissue, especially contusion and laceration. (As noted earlier, under "Skull Injuries," there can also be a closed fracture of the skull in which the scalp overlying the fractured skull remains intact. If either the scalp or the skull remains intact, there will be no open path to the brain for entry of bacteria or other contaminants, but various types of brain injury can occur.)

An *open head injury* (Figure 31-4*) involves a break in the skull as well as a break in the scalp, such as that

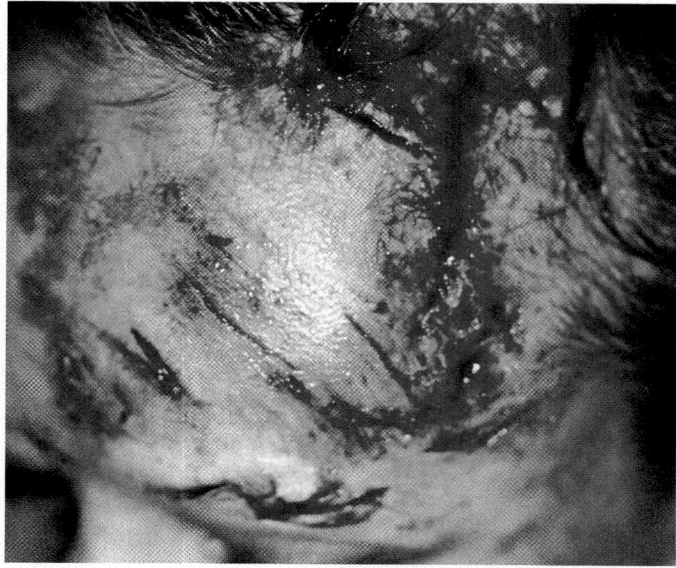

FIGURE 31-3 * Closed head injury.

Key Terms
concussion mild injury that causes temporary loss of brain function.

Key Terms
contusion injury that causes bruising or swelling of the brain.

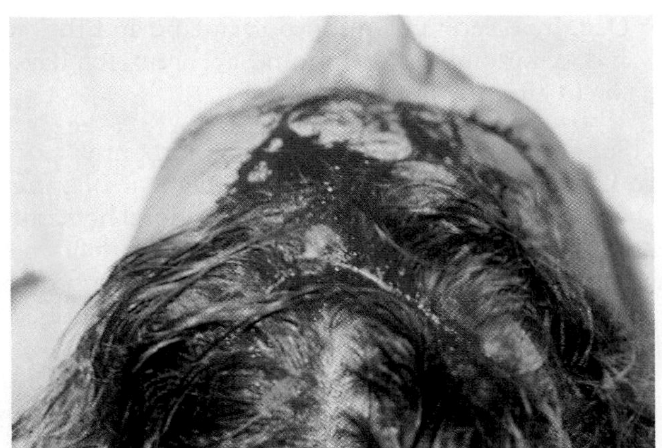

FIGURE 31-4 * Open head injury.

caused by impact with a windshield or by an impaled object. It involves direct local damage to the involved tissue, but it can also result in brain damage from infection, laceration of the brain tissue, or punctures of the brain by objects that invade the cranium after penetrating the skull.

Injury to the brain that results from shearing, tearing, and stretching of nerve fibers is called a *diffuse axonal injury (DAI)*. This type of injury interferes with the communication and transmission of nerve impulses throughout the brain. DAI is most common in auto crashes and pedestrians struck by autos. The severe acceleration and deceleration causes the shearing, tearing, and stretching injury. DAI is categorized as mild, moderate, or severe. A concussion is a mild diffuse axonal injury. A severe diffuse axonal injury involves the brainstem.

Specific types of brain injuries include *concussion,* a temporary loss of the brain's ability to function; *contusion,* bruising or swelling of the brain; *hematoma,* pooling of blood within the brain; and *laceration,* or tearing of the brain tissue.

Concussion

A **concussion** normally causes some disturbance in brain function ranging from momentary confusion to complete loss of responsiveness, and it usually causes headache. If there is a loss of consciousness, it is usually brief (lasting only a few minutes) and does not recur.

A concussion is a mild diffuse axonal injury which, as just noted, involves stretching, tearing, and shearing of brain tissue. As a general rule, a concussion presents with an altered mental status that progressively improves. If the mental status does not improve, if it improves and then worsens, or if it deteriorates from when you arrived on the scene, suspect a type of head injury other than concussion. Concussion patients may lose consciousness immediately following the impact to the head but not minutes or hours after. A loss of consciousness that occurs several minutes or hours after the impact results from some type of injury other than concussion.

Depending on where the force is absorbed by the brain, the signs of simple concussion might include the following:

- Momentary confusion
- Confusion that lasts for several minutes
- Inability to recall the incident and, sometimes, the period just before it (retrograde amnesia) and after it (anterograde amnesia)
- Repeated questioning about what happened
- Mild to moderate irritability or resistance to treatment
- Combativeness
- Inability to answer questions or obey commands appropriately
- Nausea and vomiting
- Restlessness

Remember that the key distinguishing characteristic of concussion is that its effects appear immediately or soon after impact, and then they gradually disappear. An injury that causes symptoms that develop several minutes after an incident or symptoms that do not subside over time is not a concussion, but a more serious injury.

Contusion

A **contusion,** or bruising and swelling of the brain tissue, can accompany concussion. A contusion causes bleeding into the surrounding tissues and may or may not cause increased intracranial pressure, even in cases of open head injury. Contusion is usually caused by coup/contrecoup or acceleration/deceleration injury.

In *coup/contrecoup injury,* there can be damage at the point of a blow to the head and/or damage on the side opposite the blow as the brain is propelled against the opposite side of the skull. In *acceleration/deceleration injury,* typical of a car crash, the head comes to a sudden stop but the brain continues to move back and forth inside the

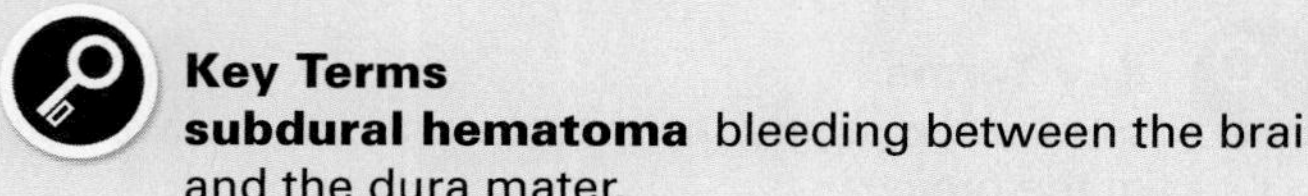

Key Terms
subdural hematoma bleeding between the brain and the dura mater.

Thinking Critically
A teenager trying to start his father's motorcycle runs it into a tree. The parents call EMS two hours after the collision. "He was fine right after," says the father, "but about 10 minutes ago he kind of passed out. It's probably just a concussion." Is the father's diagnosis correct? Why or why not?

skull, resulting in bruising (possibly very severe) to the brain.

Signs and symptoms of contusion include the initial signs and symptoms of concussion plus one or more of the following:

- Decreasing mental status or unresponsiveness
- Paralysis
- Unequal pupils
- Vomiting
- Alteration of vital signs
- Profound personality changes

Contusion can lead to swelling of the brain tissue, which can result in permanent disability or death. You may improve the patient's chances for recovery by aggressive airway management, ensuring adequate ventilation and oxygenation to prevent hypoxia, and reversing and preventing hypotension.

Subdural Hematoma

Subdural hematoma is a collection of blood between the dura mater and the arachnoid layer of the brain (Figure 31-5a∗). It typically is due to low-pressure venous bleeding from small bridging veins that are torn during the impact to the head. Bleeding occurs above the brain. Subdural hematomas are commonly associated with cerebral contusion. Cerebral injury may be caused by pressure that is applied to the brain tissue from the formation of the hematoma and increased intracranial pressure.

There are two types of subdural hematoma:

- **Acute.** Signs and symptoms begin almost immediately after the injury
- **Occult.** Bleeding continues over time and the signs and symptoms don't become apparent for days to weeks after the injury

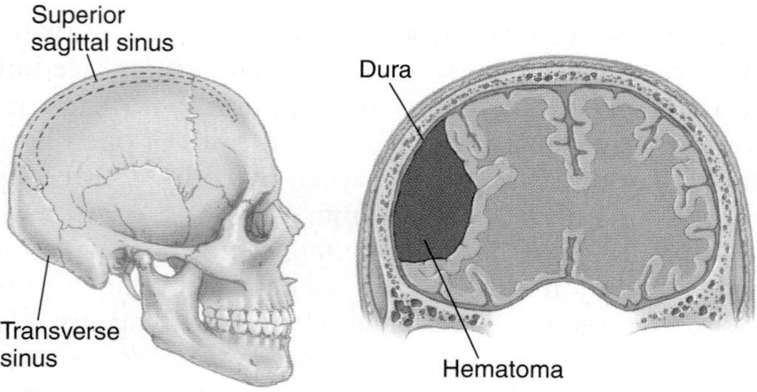

FIGURE 31-5a ∗ Subdural hematoma.

Subdural hematoma is the most common type of severe head injury. Approximately 33 percent of patients with severe head injury suffer from a subdural hematoma. Subdural hematoma is more common in patients older than 60 years. The older the patient gets, the more fragile the bridging veins become, making injury more likely when an impact occurs to the head.

Anytime a patient has suffered an impact to the head, you should suspect a subdural hematoma. Patients with a subdural hematoma typically will lose consciousness, but they may not. However, the level of consciousness will progressively deteriorate. An occult (hidden, or not obvious) subdural hematoma may be difficult to identify, since many patients do not remember any impact or injury to the head. These patients, who tend to be older, frequently complain of headache, personality changes, weakness, paralysis, or other signs of increasing intracranial pressure.

Any patient with an abnormally long blood-clotting time, which prolongs the period of bleeding, is particularly susceptible to subdural hematoma. For example, hemophiliacs are prone to a subdural hematoma, even with minimal impact to the head, as a result of their clotting disorder. Alcoholics have prolonged clotting times and are also more subject to falling and striking their heads. Patients who are taking anticoagulant drugs such as Coumadin are also prone to subdural hematoma with minimal trauma to the head.

Signs and symptoms of subdural hematoma include the following:

- Weakness or paralysis to one side of the body
- Deterioration in level of responsiveness
- Vomiting
- Dilation of one pupil
- Abnormal respirations or apnea
- Possible increasing systolic blood pressure
- Decreasing pulse rate
- Headache
- Seizures
- Confusion
- Personality change (chronic subdural hematoma)

Key Terms

epidural hematoma bleeding between the dura mater and the skull.

laceration a wound that penetrates the brain.

Objective 31-7
Identify and, where possible, manage factors that can worsen traumatic brain injuries.

Objective 31-8
Describe the goals of emergency treatment of patients with traumatic brain injuries.

Epidural Hematoma

Epidural hematoma accounts for only about 2 percent of all head injuries that require hospitalization. However, it is an extreme emergency. It most commonly occurs from low-velocity impact to the head or from deceleration injury. It is almost always associated with a skull fracture, especially in the temporal region because of the location of the meningeal arteries.

In an epidural hematoma, arterial or venous bleeding pools between the skull and the dura (protective covering of the brain) (Figure 31-5b*). Bleeding is usually rapid, profuse, and severe. The bleeding expands rapidly in a small space, causing a dramatic rise in intracranial pressure. Approximately 66 percent of the bleeding is arterial.

Signs and symptoms of epidural hematoma include the following:

- Loss of responsiveness followed by return of responsiveness (lucid interval) and then rapidly deteriorating responsiveness (a presentation that occurs in only 20 percent of cases)
- Decreasing mental status (a more common presentation than the classic lucid interval)
- Severe headache
- Fixed and dilated pupil
- Seizures
- Increasing systolic blood pressure and decreasing heart rate
- Vomiting
- Apnea or abnormal breathing pattern
- Systolic hypertension and bradycardia (Cushing reflex)
- Posturing (withdrawal or flexion)

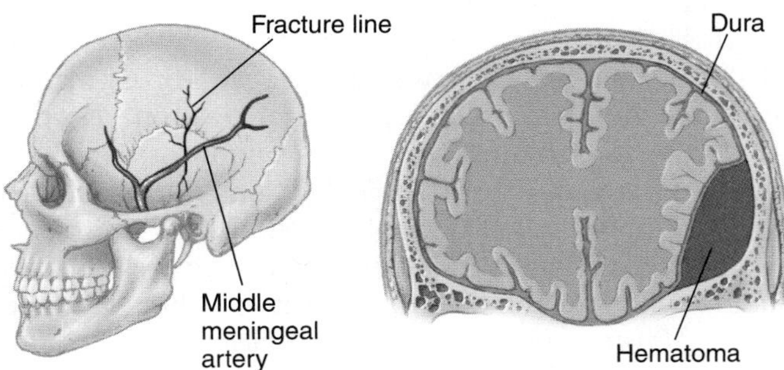

FIGURE 31-5b * Epidural hematoma.

Late signs can include fixed and dilated pupils, absent reflexes, and decreasing vital signs. Immediate surgical repair is needed in cases of epidural hematoma. If it is treated early, the prognosis is generally good, since underlying brain damage is usually minimal.

Laceration

Like a contusion, a **laceration** of brain tissue can occur in either an open or a closed head injury. Often it occurs when an object penetrates the skull and lacerates the brain. It is a permanent injury, almost always results in bleeding, and can cause massive disruption of the nervous system.

Remember that with isolated head trauma, a patient's blood pressure may go up and the pulse rate down (a late finding). If your patient has a subdural or epidural hematoma or laceration, but his blood pressure is dropping, you must consider that he is bleeding somewhere else in the body. If this is the case, treat the underlying shock resulting from blood loss, attempt to maintain the systolic blood pressure above 90 mmHg, and maintain oxygenation at an SpO_2 reading of 95% or greater. When providing emergency care to the patient with a traumatic brain injury, it is imperative to understand that the brain injury may be worsened by any one of the following:

- Hypoxia
- Hypercarbia (high level of carbon dioxide)
- Hypoglycemia (blood glucose level < 60 mg/dL)
- Hyperglycemia
- Hyperthermia
- Hypotension (systolic blood pressure < 90 mmHg)

Emergency care of a traumatic brain injury patient, regardless of the cause or type, should focus on establishing and maintaining:

- A patent airway
- Adequate ventilation
- Adequate oxygenation (SpO_2 of 95% or greater)
- A systolic blood pressure greater than 90 mmHg
- A normal body core temperature
- A normal blood glucose level

Seizure activity in the traumatic brain injury patient could lead to worsening of the injury, increased hypoxia

Key Terms
herniation compression and pushing of the brain through the foramen magnum.

Objective 31-9
Describe the pathophysiology and key signs of increased intracranial pressure and brain herniation.

Key Points
Be alert for signs of head injury and cervical spine injury at the outset of assessment.

and hypercarbia levels, increased hypoglycemia, and an increase in the core body temperature. Seizures must be stopped as quickly as possible. If the patient seizes, consider contacting an ALS unit.

Brain Herniation

The brain is enclosed in a rigid container: the skull. In addition to the brain, cerebrospinal fluid and blood occupy the limited space. There is very little room for any other mass to collect. If a hematoma or cerebral swelling develops within the cranium, the added mass will cause some other substance or structure to be pushed out. Initially, blood and cerebrospinal fluid are squeezed out of the brain. If the swelling or hematoma continues to develop, pressure inside the skull (called the intracranial pressure, or ICP) rises. With a rise in ICP, the brain is eventually compressed and pushed out of its normal position, downward toward and through the foramen magnum, which is the large opening in the base of the skull. This process is referred to as **herniation**.

Compression of the brain will cause it to dysfunction. Pushing the brain downward and out of the foramen magnum compresses the brainstem, destroying vital functions including the heartbeat, respirations, and blood pressure. Thus, herniation is an extremely serious and potentially deadly condition.

Signs and symptoms specific to brain herniation are:

- Dilated or sluggish pupil on one side
- Weakness or paralysis
- Severe alteration in consciousness
- Abnormal posturing (decorticate, also called flexion; decerebrate, also called extension)—also known as nonpurposeful movement
- Abnormal ventilation pattern
- Cushing reflex (increased systolic blood pressure and decreased heart rate)

If signs of herniation are evident, controlled hyperventilation of the patient may be considered. Hyperventilation has been shown to reduce the blood flow in the brain; thus, it is controversial and may not be included in your protocol. Hyperventilation should not be performed if the patient is hypotensive. Hyperventilation will be discussed in greater detail later in the chapter.

Assessment-Based Approach: Head Injury

You have studied many of the elements of assessment that apply to head injury—for example, the AVPU method of assessing mental status—in earlier chapters. We review and develop these assessment elements on the following pages with particular emphasis on how they apply to a patient who has, or may be suspected to have, a head injury (Figure 31-6*).

Scene Size-Up

Because head injuries can be so serious, always be alert for signs of them during the scene size-up. Unresponsiveness or altered mental status, especially in trauma patients, should always suggest the possibility of head injury. Never assume that mental status changes in a trauma patient are due to drug or alcohol intoxication. Other signs of head injury can be more obvious. These might include bleeding from the scalp or face or an apparent mechanism of injury, such as a fractured windshield at the scene of an automobile crash, a deformed helmet at a bicycling crash, or evidence of a fall (Figures 31-7a and 31-7b*).

Nontraumatic injuries to the brain can be caused by clots or hemorrhaging. Such injuries can cause altered mental status and present signs and symptoms similar to those in trauma cases. (See Chapter 18, "Altered Mental Status, Stroke, and Headache.")

Primary Assessment

When performing the primary assessment, be alert for cervical spine injury. Forces applied to the head may have been strong enough to injure the cervical spine as well. Manual in-line stabilization of the spine should be your first step (Figure 31-8*).

If the patient is unresponsive or has an altered mental status, establish an airway using a jaw-thrust maneuver while holding in-line spinal stabilization. Keep in mind that head injuries often involve injury to or blockage of the airway (Figure 31-9*). Maintain the patient's airway and provide oxygen by nonrebreather mask at 15 lpm if breathing is adequate, or positive pressure ventilation with supplemental oxygen if breathing is inadequate. *Maintaining an adequate airway and providing oxygen are vital, because head injuries can become worse if there is an inadequate supply of oxygen to the brain.*

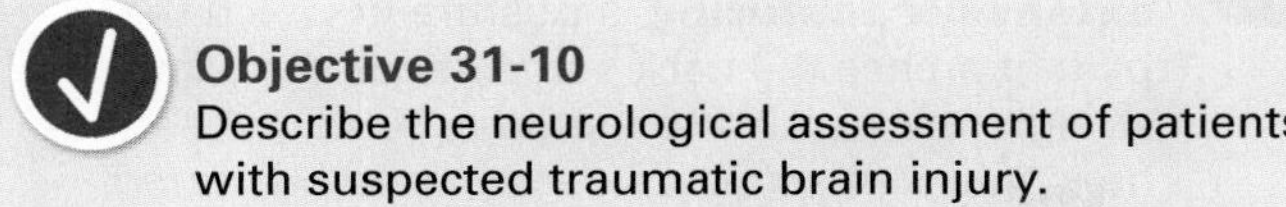

Objective 31-10
Describe the neurological assessment of patients with suspected traumatic brain injury.

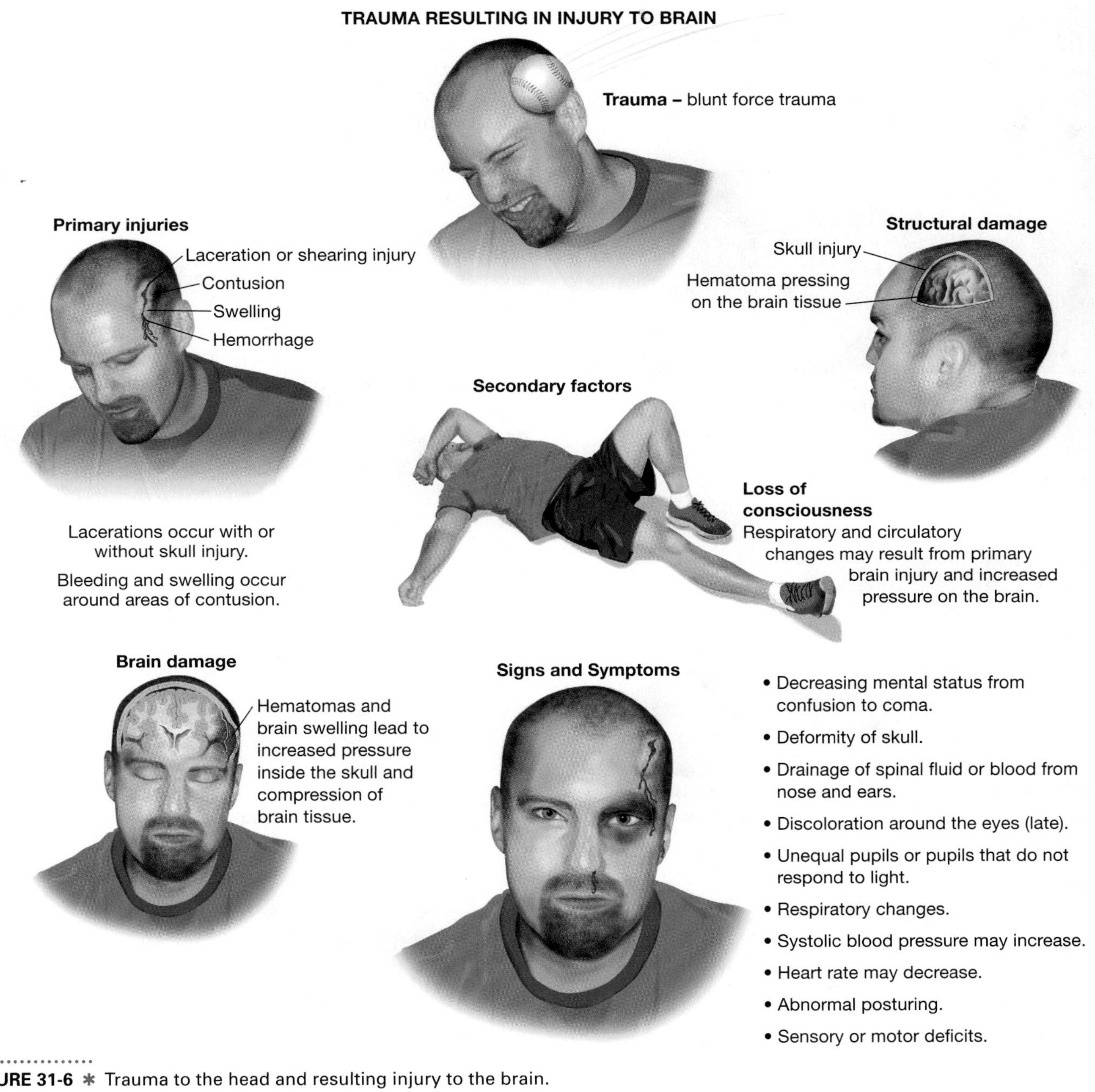

TRAUMA RESULTING IN INJURY TO BRAIN

Trauma – blunt force trauma

Primary injuries

Laceration or shearing injury
Contusion
Swelling
Hemorrhage

Lacerations occur with or without skull injury.

Bleeding and swelling occur around areas of contusion.

Structural damage

Skull injury
Hematoma pressing on the brain tissue

Secondary factors

Loss of consciousness
Respiratory and circulatory changes may result from primary brain injury and increased pressure on the brain.

Brain damage

Hematomas and brain swelling lead to increased pressure inside the skull and compression of brain tissue.

Signs and Symptoms

- Decreasing mental status from confusion to coma.
- Deformity of skull.
- Drainage of spinal fluid or blood from nose and ears.
- Discoloration around the eyes (late).
- Unequal pupils or pupils that do not respond to light.
- Respiratory changes.
- Systolic blood pressure may increase.
- Heart rate may decrease.
- Abnormal posturing.
- Sensory or motor deficits.

FIGURE 31-6 ✻ Trauma to the head and resulting injury to the brain.

Mental Status A decreasing mental status is the most important sign in cases of suspected head injury. The mental status is initially assessed using the AVPU mnemonic. Keep in mind that the patient's mental status may change. For example, the patient may be alert but deteriorate slowly, or he may respond to verbal stimuli and deteriorate to responding to painful stimuli only.

A patient who responds to pain may do so in two ways. The patient may try to move away from or remove the pain. This is a *purposeful* response. Or the patient may

Key Terms
flexion posturing a posture in which the patient arches the back and flexes the arms inward toward the chest. A sign of serious head injury. Also called *decorticate posturing.*

Key Terms
extension posturing a posture in which the patient arches the back and extends the arms straight out parallel to the body. A sign of serious head injury. Also called *decerebrate posturing.*

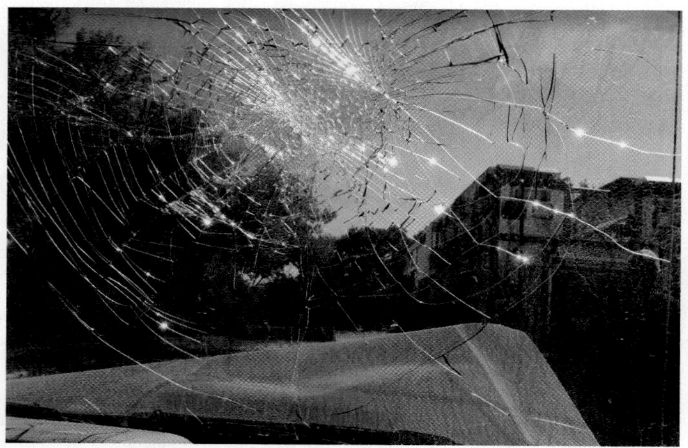

FIGURE 31-7a * A fractured windshield indicates a probable head injury.

respond by inappropriately moving parts of his body, reacting to the pain but not trying to stop it. This is a *nonpurposeful* response.

A nonpurposeful response to pain indicates a deeper state of unresponsiveness. Patients who respond nonpurposefully will usually do one of two things. They will posture by flexing their arms across their chest and extending their legs (**flexion posturing** or decorticate posturing), which indicates an upper-level brainstem injury, or they will extend both arms down at their sides, extend their legs, and sometimes arch their backs (**extension posturing** or decerebrate posturing). Decerebrate posturing represents the lowest level of nonpurposeful pain response, indicating a lower-level brainstem injury.

The lowest level on the AVPU scale is "unresponsive." A patient at this level exhibits no response at all to verbal or painful stimuli. This is an ominous sign in head injury.

Record your observations of mental status accurately, noting the types of stimuli administered and the patient's

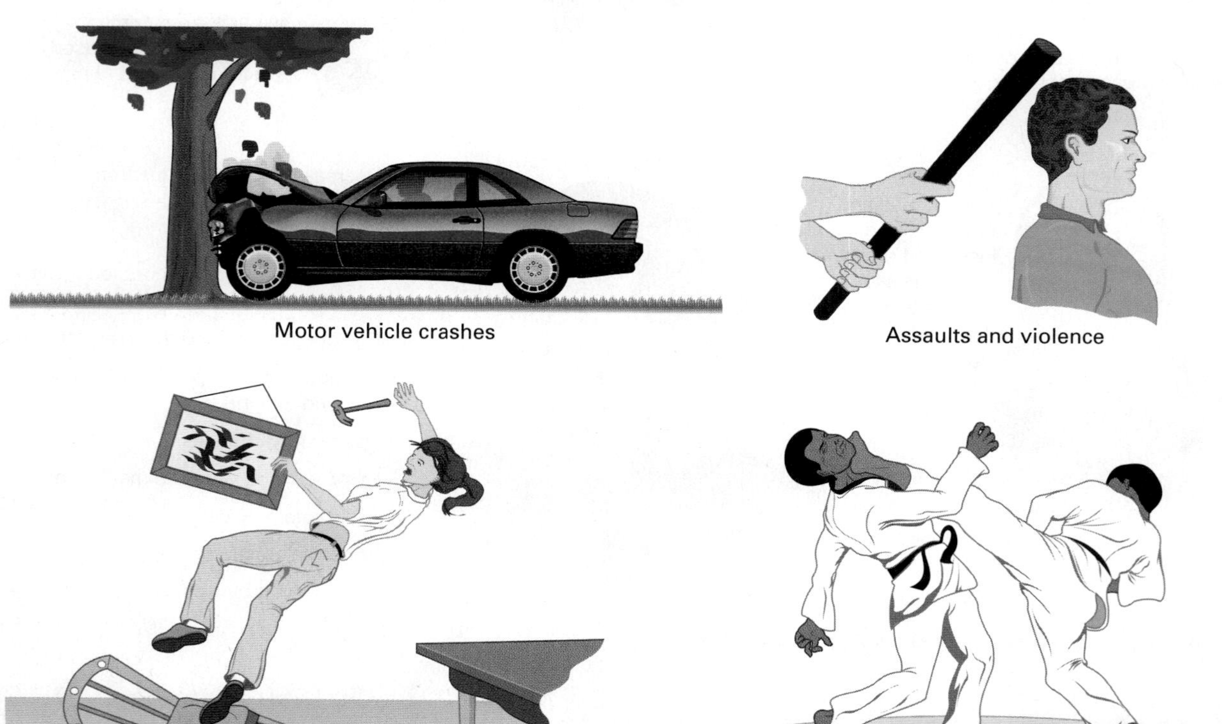

FIGURE 31-7b * Mechanisms of head injury.

Key Points
In the prehospital setting, the numerical values on the Glasgow Coma Scale are not as important as the types of response to specific stimuli.

Key Points
During assessment, remember that a patient with a head injury may not experience or respond to pain that would normally be experienced.

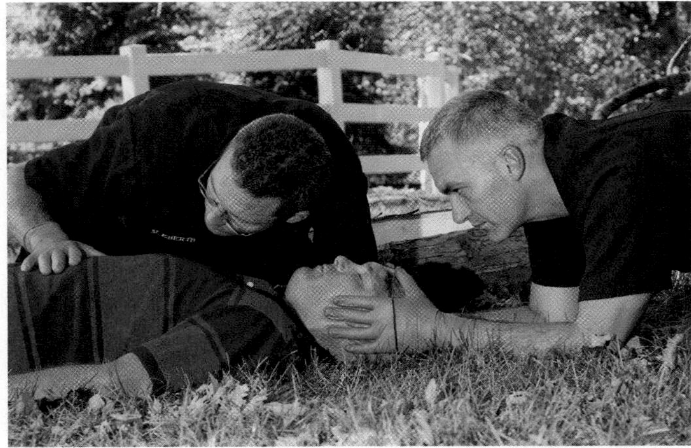

FIGURE 31-8 * Establish and maintain spinal stabilization. Then open the airway and assess breathing.

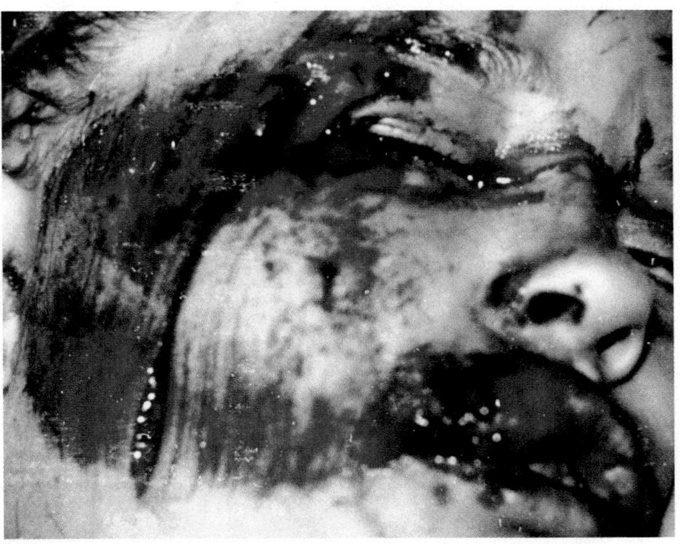

FIGURE 31-9 * Head injuries, especially injuries to the face, often cause airway blockage.

responses. You must determine a baseline for level of responsiveness and check repeatedly for signs of deterioration. For example, a patient who first responds to the loud calling of his name, but later only responds to a shoulder pinch with decorticate posturing, has a deteriorating level of responsiveness. Such deterioration of level of responsiveness in cases of head injury can be a sign of a serious problem.

A useful and more discriminating tool for determining a patient's level of responsiveness is the Glasgow Coma Scale (Tables 31-1 and 31-2). The scale is a measure of the patient's eye opening, verbal response, and motor response to different stimuli. In the prehospital setting, the numerical values on the scale are not as important as the types of response to specific stimuli.

TABLE 31-1 Glasgow Coma Scale

Eye Opening	
Spontaneous	4
To verbal command	3
To pain	2
No response	1
Verbal Response	
Oriented and converses	5
Disoriented and converses	4
Inappropriate words	3
Incomprehensible sounds	2
No response	1
Motor Response	
Obeys verbal commands	6
Localizes pain	5
Withdraws from pain (flexion)	4
Abnormal flexion in response to pain (decorticate rigidity)	3
Extension in response to pain (decerebrate rigidity)	2
No response	1

Secondary Assessment

When dealing with trauma patients who have head injuries, or suspected head injuries, you will perform a physical exam. A patient with a head injury may not complain of pain or other symptoms of trauma. Therefore, it is extremely important to perform a complete physical exam in the patient with a head injury in an attempt to identify signs of trauma and injury to other areas of the body. When performing the assessment, keep in mind that the patient may not respond even if the area is injured. As an example, the head-injured patient with an abdominal injury may not experience or respond to the pain when you palpate the abdomen. This may allow you to miss potentially serious injuries.

Thinking Critically
A bystander says that your patient passed out after running his bike into a lamppost but adds, "He was only out for a minute. I don't think he needs to go to the hospital." Is the bystander right? Why or why not?

TABLE 31-2 Pediatric Glasgow Coma Scale

		> 1 Year	< 1 Year	
Eye opening	4	Spontaneous	Spontaneous	
	3	To verbal command	To shout	
	2	To pain	To pain	
	1	No response	No response	
		> 1 Year	**< 1 Year**	
Best motor response	6	Obeys		
	5	Localizes pain	Localizes pain	
	4	Flexion-withdrawal	Flexion-withdrawal	
	3	Flexion-abnormal (decorticate rigidity)	Flexion-abnormal (decorticate rigidity)	
	2	Extension (decerebrate rigidity)	Extension (decerebrate rigidity)	
	1	No response	No response	
		> 5 Years	**2–5 Years**	**0–23 Months**
Best verbal response	5	Oriented and converses	Appropriate words and phrases	Smiles, coos, cries appropriately
	4	Disoriented and converses	Inappropriate words	Cries to pain
	3	Inappropriate words	Cries and/or screams	Inappropriate crying and/or Screaming
	2	Incomprehensible sounds	Grunts	Grunts
	1	No response	No response	No response

Following the physical exam, you will check vital signs and obtain a history. Be aware, however, that patients with a head injury may become disoriented or unresponsive. If a patient is alert and oriented, you or your partner might wish to gather the history while the other performs the physical exam.

Remember that any patient who loses consciousness, even briefly, must be evaluated at the hospital. *A patient whose mental status worsens at any stage of the assessment or treatment process needs immediate transport and continuous monitoring during transport.*

Physical Exam Perform a physical exam, paying particular attention to the following parts of the exam in cases of suspected head injury:

- **The Head.** Use extreme care in checking the patient's head (Figure 31-10✱). Palpate for deformities, depressions, lacerations, or impaled objects around the head and face (Figure 31-11✱). Be careful not to jab or apply pressure to skull depressions or deformities.

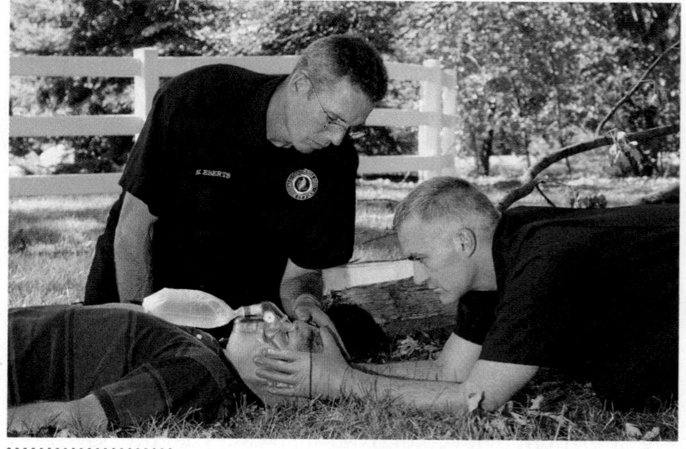

FIGURE 31-10 ✱ Inspect and carefully palpate the patient's head.

Key Terms
consensual reflex same or similar reaction of the unstimulated pupil when the other pupil is stimulated, as when a light is shined into one pupil and both pupils contract.

Key Terms
raccoon sign discoloration of tissue around the eyes suggestive of basilar skull injury.

Battle sign discoloration of the mastoid suggesting basilar skull fracture.

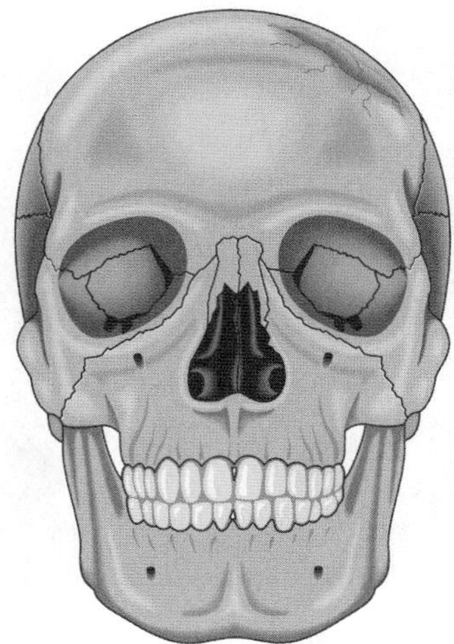

Soft area or depression.

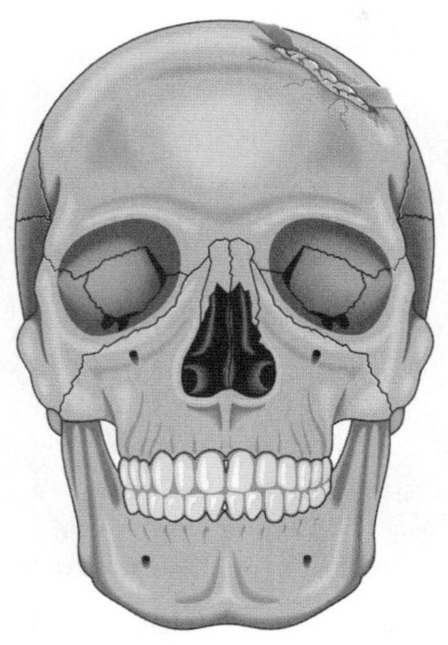

Open wound with bleeding and/or exposed brain tissue.

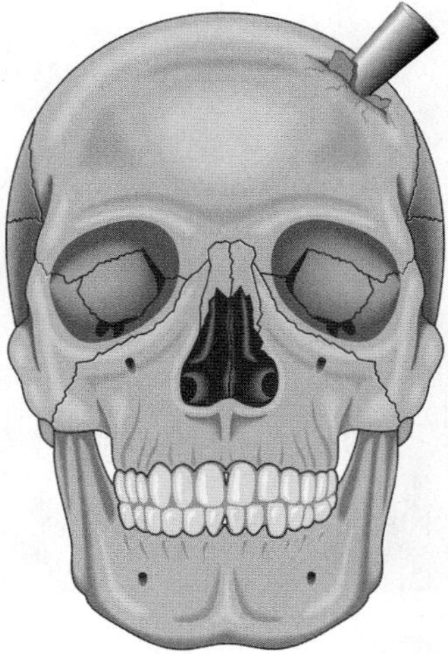

Impaled object in skull.

FIGURE 31-11 * Examine the head for deformities, depressions, lacerations, or impaled objects.

- **The Eyes.**
  1. Check the patient's pupils with a bright light (Figure 31-12*). Are they equal in size? Do they react equally? Both pupils should react the same when a light is shined in only one of the pupils. This reflex in the unstimulated eye is known as a **consensual reflex.** If one or both pupils are fixed and dilated, this may signal an increase in pressure in the brain.
  2. Check eye movements. Do the eyes track (follow movement normally)? Is one eye positioned downward and outward?
  3. Is there any discoloration? A purplish discoloration (bruising) of the soft tissues around one or both eyes—**raccoon sign**—may be an indication of intracranial injury. It is a delayed sign of skull fracture that usually does not appear for up to 4–6 hours after the injury.

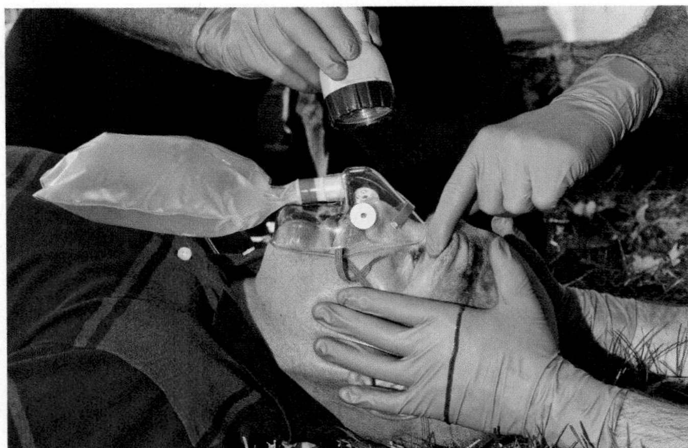

FIGURE 31-12 * Assess pupils for size, equality, and reactivity.

Understanding BODY PROCESSES

A fixed and dilated pupil in a patient with a brain injury is usually the result of compression of the third cranial nerve in the lower area of the brain and indicates severe compression of brain tissue. ■

ASSESSMENT Tips

In a brain injury, the affected pupil is usually on the same side as the injury. ■

- **The Ears and Nose.**
  1. Check both ears for leakage of blood or clear fluid; skull fracture or intracranial bleeding can cause both (Figure 31-13*).
  2. **Battle sign,** a purplish discoloration (bruising) of the mastoid area behind the ear, is another delayed and very late sign of a basilar skull fracture.

Key Points
Any discharge from the nose or ears must be taken seriously.

Key Points
If definite signs of brain herniation exist, begin positive pressure ventilation and consider controlled hyperventilation at 20/min with supplemental oxygen. (Warning: Prolonged hyperventilation at a rate above 20 may reduce cerebral blood flow and worsen the head injury.)

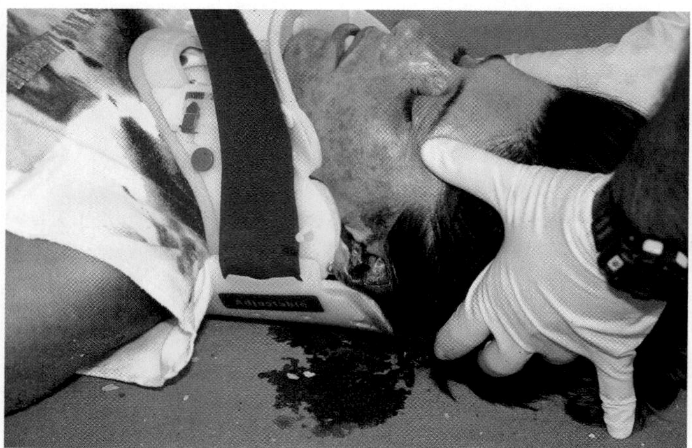

FIGURE 31-13 ✱ This patient was riding on a BMX track, doing flips on a bicycle without a helmet or other protective gear. She fell backward and hit her head, causing a cranial injury. Note the blood leaking from her ear. (© Maria A. H. Lyle)

3. Check the nose for leakage of blood or clear fluid, which can indicate skull fracture or intracranial injury.

ASSESSMENT Tips

To distinguish a clear fluid leaking from the ears or nose from tears or nasal secretions, check the fluid for glucose. Cerebrospinal fluid contains glucose; tears and nasal secretions do not. The glucose reading in cerebrospinal fluid will be about half of the blood glucose reading. Note, however, that ANY discharge from the ears or nose must be taken seriously. ■

- **Motor/Sensory Assessment.** To examine motor and sensory function, if the patient is alert, check his ability to move his fingers and toes. Have him squeeze your fingers with both hands simultaneously to test for equal grip strength. Ask the patient to tell which finger or toe you are touching without watching what you are doing. Pinch each extremity and ask if he can identify the pain. Ask if the patient feels any weakness on one side of the body compared to the other (Figure 31-14✱).

If the patient is only responsive to verbal or painful stimuli, motor and sensory function cannot be as accurately assessed, but watch for a response such as a grimace or withdrawal from a painful stimulus.

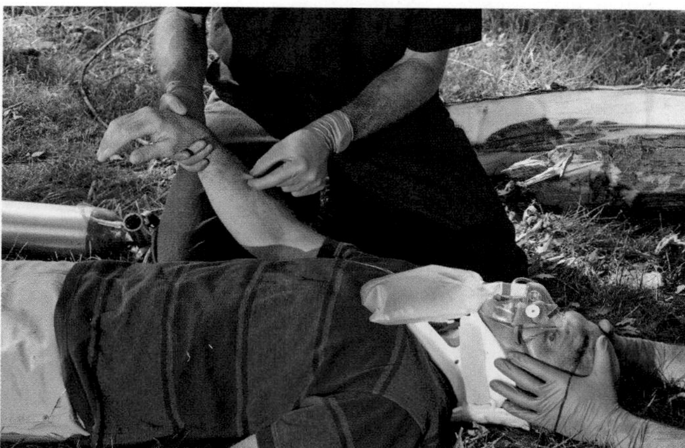

FIGURE 31-14 ✱ Assess motor and sensory function.

Vital Signs Check and record vital signs every 5 minutes, staying alert to any changes. In cases of possible head injury, be alert to the following:

- **Blood Pressure.** If the systolic blood pressure is high or rising, suspect pressure inside the skull; if it is low or dropping, suspect blood loss that has led to shock. Low blood pressure very early in a patient with a head injury almost always is due to bleeding elsewhere in the body (there is not enough space in the brain to permit enough bleeding to reduce blood pressure). It should be a signal to check the rest of the body for bleeding. However, a low blood pressure may also be an ominous sign that the head injury is so severe that the brain can no longer maintain an adequate blood pressure because of brainstem failure. Hypotension needs prompt attention, as it worsens the brain injury.
- **Pulse.** If the pulse is fast or increasing, suspect hemorrhage elsewhere in the body or early onset of hypoxia. If it is slow or decreasing, suspect pressure inside the skull or severe hypoxia.
- **Respiration.** Assess the rate, depth, and pattern of respiration. The patient may display several different respiratory patterns if the brain is compressed from increased intracranial pressure resulting from swelling and/or bleeding inside the skull. The respirations may be extremely fast and shallow, completely irregular, or absent (apnea).

If definite signs of brain herniation exist (unequal pupils, posturing, fixed pupil, Cushing reflex, hemiplegia or hemiparesis, decrease in the Glasgow Coma Scale of

Key Terms
Cushing reflex syndrome of increased systolic pressure, decreased heart rate, and changed respiratory pattern indicating severe head injury.

Objective 31-11
Discuss the focus of history taking and assessment for patients with injuries to the head.

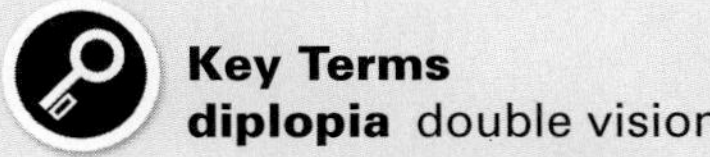

Key Terms
diplopia double vision.

retrograde amnesia inability to remember circumstances prior to an incident.

anterograde amnesia inability to remember circumstances after an incident.

two points or more), and if you have not already done so, begin positive pressure ventilation and consider controlled hyperventilation at a rate of 20 ventilations per minute with supplemental oxygen. (Hyperventilation at a rate > 20 for a prolonged period may reduce cerebral blood flow and worsen the head injury.) A sign of severe head injury, increasing intracranial pressure, and possible herniation is the **Cushing reflex,** in which the systolic blood pressure increases and the heart rate decreases. The respiratory pattern may also change.

Understanding BODY PROCESSES

In the Cushing reflex, the systolic blood pressure increases from an attempt to force blood flow into the brain to maintain perfusion of brain cells that are being compressed from the injury. ■

ASSESSMENT Tips

There is very little room for bleeding into the brain. So in the patient with trauma to the head, if the blood pressure is decreasing, the pulse pressure is narrow, the heart rate is elevated, and the respiratory rate is increased (signs of hemorrhage), suspect shock, but look for evidence of bleeding in an area of the body other than the brain. ■

If positive pressure ventilation is needed but significant signs and symptoms of severe brain injury and herniation are not present, ventilate at a rate of 10–12/minute.

History The history can provide vital information about the mechanism of injury. A patient with a head injury may experience a deteriorating mental status. If he is unable to answer questions appropriately, try to obtain information from others at the scene. The following questions are particularly relevant in cases of head injury:

- When did the incident occur?
- What is the patient's chief complaint? Did he feel pain, tingling, numbness, or paralysis? Where? How have symptoms changed since the accident?
- How did the accident occur?
- *Did he lose consciousness at any time? This information is critically important in assessing a brain injury.* How long was the period of unresponsiveness? When did it occur in relation to the injury? Did the patient suddenly lose consciousness and then gradually reawaken, or did he pass out immediately, suddenly wake up, then gradually lose consciousness again?
- Was the patient moved after the incident?
- Is there any history of a previous injury to the head? If so, when did it occur? Was the patient knocked unconscious? Sometimes an injury to the head days or weeks after an incident in which a patient was knocked unconscious can reinjure the brain.

Signs and Symptoms Signs and symptoms of head injury include the following:

- Altered mental status—disorientation to unresponsiveness that doesn't improve or that continues to deteriorate
- Decreasing mental status
- Irregular breathing pattern (severe)
- Increasing blood pressure and decreasing pulse (Cushing reflex, a late finding) (severe)
- Obvious signs of injury—contusions, lacerations, or hematomas to the scalp or deformity to the skull
- Visible damage to the skull (visible through laceration in the scalp)
- Pain, tenderness, or swelling at the site of injury
- Blood or cerebrospinal fluid from ears or nose
- Discoloration (bruising) around the eyes in the absence of trauma to the eyes (raccoon sign—very late)
- Discoloration (bruising) behind the ears, the mastoid process (Battle sign—very late)
- Absent motor or sensory function (severe or poor response)
- Nausea and/or vomiting; vomiting may be forceful or repeated
- Unequal pupil size with altered mental status (severe) (Figure 31-15*)
- **Diplopia**—double vision
- Possible seizures
- Nonpurposeful response to painful stimuli (severe) (Figure 31-16*)
- **Retrograde amnesia**—the patient is unable to remember circumstances leading up to the incident
- **Anterograde amnesia**—the patient is unable to remember circumstances after the incident

Objective 31-12
Assess and provide emergency treatment to patients with injuries to the head.

Thinking Critically
Your head injury patient has one dilated pupil, displays extension posturing, has an increased blood pressure reading, a decreased heart rate, and a decreased mental status. You begin positive pressure ventilation with supplemental oxygen. Should you hyperventilate him?

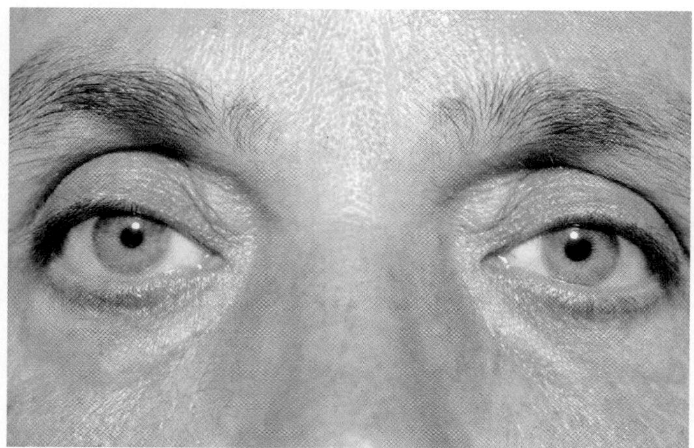

FIGURE 31-15 ✱ Unequal pupils. (© Medscan/Corbis)

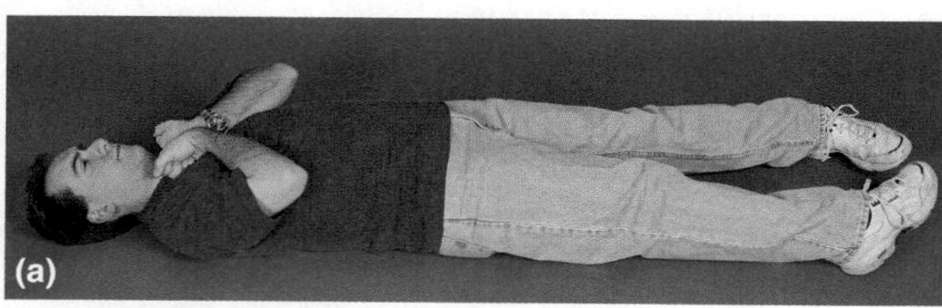

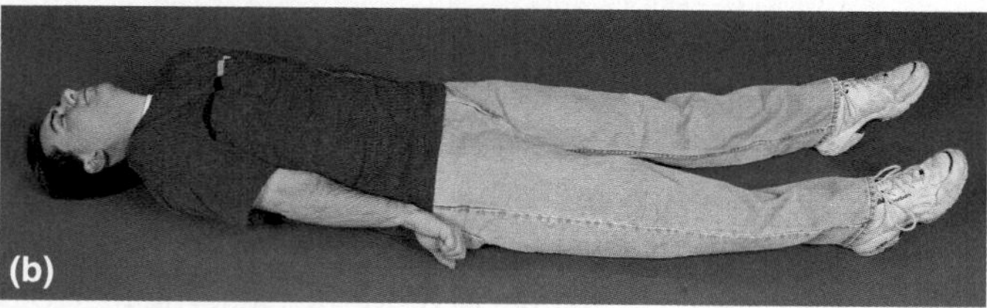

FIGURE 31-16 ✱ Nonpurposeful responses to painful stimuli include **(a)** flexion (decorticate) posturing and **(b)** extension (decerebrate) posturing.

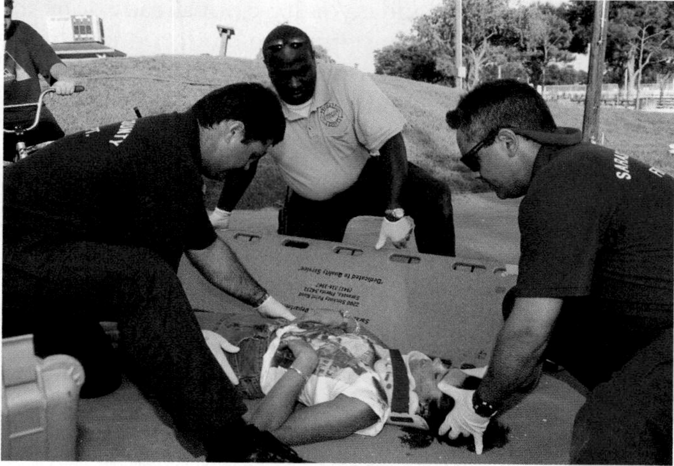

FIGURE 31-17 ✱ The patient who incurred a head injury while doing flips on a bicycle is prepared for transport by helicopter to a trauma center. Note that manual spinal stabilization is being maintained while the patient is transferred to a backboard. (© Maria A. H. Lyle)

Emergency Medical Care

To treat a patient with a head injury:

1. *Take Standard Precautions.*
2. *Establish manual in-line spinal stabilization.*
   - Maintain neutral positioning of the head and neck manually, even after a cervical collar is applied, until the patient is completely immobilized to a backboard (Figure 31-17✱).
3. *Maintain a patent airway, adequate breathing, and oxygenation.* Oxygen deficiency in the brain is the most frequent cause of death following head injury.
   - Use a jaw-thrust maneuver to open the airway.
   - Remove any foreign bodies from the mouth, and suction blood and mucus.
   - Protect against aspiration by having suction available at all times and by being prepared to roll the secured patient to clear the airway.
   - Administer oxygen by nonrebreather mask at 15 lpm if breathing is adequate, or positive pressure ventilation with supplemental oxygen at 10–12/minute if breathing is inadequate. Maintain the SpO_2 reading at 95% or greater.
   - Consider controlled hyperventilation at a rate of 20 breaths per minute if signs of *severe* head injury and brain herniation are present—such as unequal pupils, increased systolic blood pressure, irregular or absent breathing (or Cushing reflex: increased systolic blood pressure with decreased heart rate and changed breathing pattern), absent motor or sensory function on one side of the body, weakness on one side of the body, seizures, abnormal posturing (nonpurposeful movement), or a decrease in the Glasgow Coma Scale of two points or more.
4. *Monitor the airway, breathing, pulse, and mental status for deterioration.* Any patient who deteriorates must be transported immediately.

Objective 31-13
Explain the importance of reassessment of the patient with an injury to the head.

Objective 31-14
Document information relevant to the assessment and management of patients with injuries to the head.

5. *Control bleeding.* Face and scalp wounds may bleed heavily, but such bleeding is usually controlled easily.
   - Do not apply pressure to an open or depressed skull injury; doing so can drive pieces of fragmented bone into the brain tissue.
   - Dress and bandage open head wounds as indicated in the treatment of soft tissue injuries.
   - Do not attempt to stop the flow of blood or cerebrospinal fluid flowing from the ears or nose. Instead, cover loosely with a completely sterile gauze dressing to absorb, but not stop, the flow.
   - For other wounds, use gentle, continuous direct pressure with sterile gauze only as needed to control bleeding.
   - Never try to remove a penetrating object. Instead, immobilize it in place and dress the wound.
6. *Be prepared to provide emergency care for seizures.*
7. *Transport immediately.*

Reassessment

Provide a reassessment during transport, paying close attention to the airway and mental status of the patient. Repeat the reassessment every 5 minutes.

Summary: Assessment and Care

To review possible assessment findings and emergency care for injuries to the head, see Figures 31-18* and 31-19*.

Assessment Summary

HEAD INJURY

The following are findings that may be associated with a head injury.

SCENE SIZE-UP

Pay particular attention to your own safety. Look for:
- Mechanism of injury
- Ejection from a vehicle
- High-speed collision
- Sports injury
- Fall
- Crushing force
- Gunshot wounds

Evidence of other trauma
- Impact mark on windshield
- Deformed helmet
- Obvious scalp and skull injuries

Primary Assessment

General Impression
- Altered mental status
- Open fracture sites to skull
- Obvious deformity to skull

Mental Status
- Alert to unresponsive based on type and degree of head injury
- Unresponsiveness or decreasing mental status associated with trauma to the head (a hallmark sign of head injury)
- Decorticate or decerebrate (nonpurposeful) posturing to painful stimuli
- Garbled or slurred speech

Airway
- Assume airway is closed if patient has an altered mental status
- May be occluded by bleeding associated with facial fractures
- Be prepared to manage vomiting

Breathing
- May be absent, inadequate, or normal
- Abnormal breathing patterns may occur

Circulation
- Pulse may be normal or decreased
- Skin is normal

Status: Priority patient if patient never regains consciousness or has a decreasing mental status

continued

FIGURE 31-18a * Assessment summary: head injury.

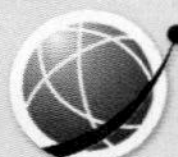

Media Resources
Go to www.bradybooks.com for mykit. Highlights:

- *Web Resource:* Documentary on Traumatic Brain Injuries
- *Video:* Applying a Cervical Collar

Assessment Summary

Secondary Assessment

Physical Exam

Head:
- Open or closed wounds to the head or face
- Leakage of blood or cerebrospinal fluid from ears, nose, or mouth
- Discoloration around eyes (raccoon sign) or behind ears (Battle sign) (late signs)
- Unequal pupils or fixed and dilated pupil

Extremities:
- No response to pain or light touch
- Inability to move extremities

Blood glucose level:
- Normal

Baseline Vital Signs
- BP: normal, may have a significantly increased systolic BP (Cushing reflex)
- HR: normal or bradycardia (Cushing reflex); tachycardia may be associated with shock associated with bleeding from other injuries
- RR: normal, irregular, decreased, or absent (Cushing reflex)
- Skin: normal or may be pale, cool, and clammy if other injuries are present with bleeding and shock
- Pupils: may be equal or unequal, reactive or unreactive; may be fixed and dilated
- SpO_2: normal—may be < 95% if respirations are abnormal or decreased

History

Signs and symptoms of an open or closed skull fracture:
- Pain, deformity, swelling
- Open wound associated with suspected fracture site
- Exposed bone ends
- Facial trauma
  - Penetrating injuries or impaled objects in the head
  - Cushing reflex (triad): increased systolic blood pressure, decreased heart rate, abnormal respiratory pattern
  - Nausea and vomiting
  - Abnormal motor/sensory response
  - Patient loses responsiveness after impact to the head
  - Loss of responsiveness, followed by a lucid interval, then a gradual loss of responsiveness

FIGURE 31-18a ✱ Assessment summary: head injury. *continued*

Emergency Care Protocol

HEAD INJURY

1. Establish manual in-line stabilization.
2. Establish and maintain an open airway. Insert an oropharyngeal airway if patient is unresponsive and has no gag or cough reflex. (A nasopharyngeal airway is not recommended, especially if there is cerebrospinal fluid leakage from the nose or injury to the face.)
3. Suction secretions as necessary.
4. If breathing is inadequate, provide positive pressure ventilation with supplemental oxygen at a rate of 10–12 ventilations/minute for an adult and 20 ventilations/minute for an infant or child. Consider controlled hyperventilation at 20 ventilations/minute if signs of brain herniation are present and the patient is not hypotensive.
5. If breathing is adequate, administer oxygen by nonrebreather mask at 15 lpm. Maintain an SpO_2 of 95% or greater.
6. Control any major bleeding. Be careful not to apply excessive pressure to open or depressed skull fractures.
7. Immobilize patient to backboard.
8. Transport.
9. Perform a reassessment every 5 minutes if unstable and every 15 minutes if stable. Be prepared for vomiting and seizures.

FIGURE 31-18b ✱ Emergency care protocol: head injury.

Emergency Care Algorithm: **Head Injury**

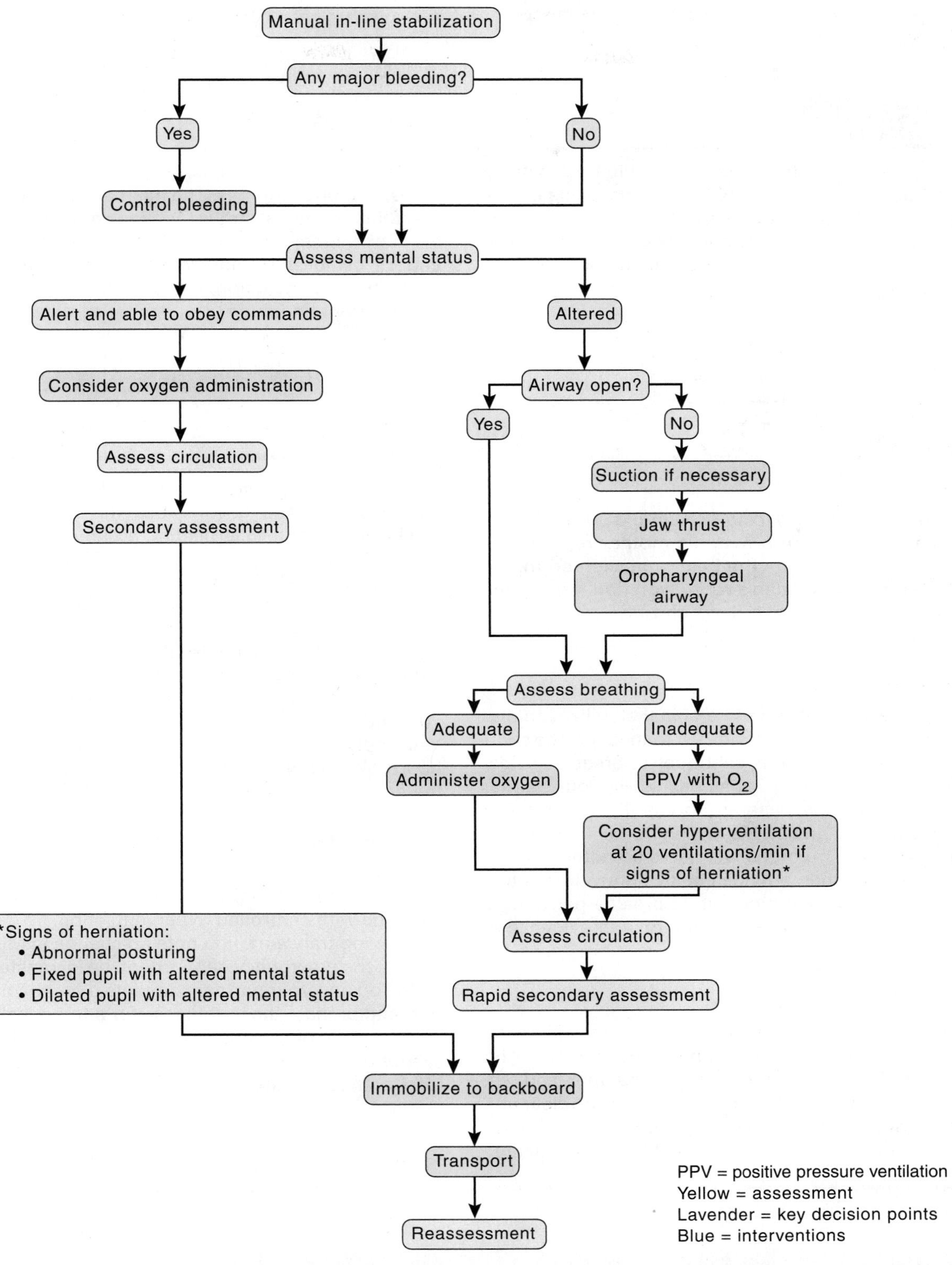

FIGURE 31-19 ✻ Emergency care algorithm: head injury.

CHAPTER REVIEW

SUMMARY

A head injury is a devastating injury that could lead to death or permanent disability. The rigid skull encapsulates the brain and provides significant protection. The same protective rigid skull does not provide any flexibility, and this can lead to severe increases in pressure within the skull, leading to compression and death of brain cells.

Head injuries are classified as scalp injuries, skull injuries, and brain injuries. The hallmark sign of a brain injury is an altered mental status that does not improve or that deteriorates. Emergency care focuses on protecting the spine and on establishing and maintaining an airway, effective ventilation, oxygenation, and circulation to prevent or limit secondary brain injury.

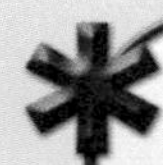

CASE STUDY FOLLOW-UP

SCENE SIZE-UP

You have been dispatched to an 18-year-old unresponsive male, Mike Ryan. As you arrive, his mother reports that he experienced a bump on the head that seemed minor. As you enter the young man's room, you find him supine on his bed. His breathing is deep and fast with snoring respirations.

PRIMARY ASSESSMENT

You immediately establish in-line spinal stabilization and open Mike's airway using a jaw-thrust maneuver. The snoring sounds disappear, but he continues to breathe rapidly and deeply. While holding his airway open, your partner pinches his shoulder muscle and holds it. His arms flex across his chest, he arches his back, and his legs stiffen. Your partner inserts an oral airway. It is accepted without any gag reflex. You then provide positive pressure ventilation with supplemental oxygen at 20 breaths per minute because you suspect severe head injury with evidence of flexion posturing.

SECONDARY ASSESSMENT

Your partner performs a physical exam and takes vital signs. Mike's left pupil is dilated and nonreactive to light. Vital signs are BP 190/72 mmHg, pulse is 62 bpm, and respirations are assisted at 20 per minute. Lungs are clear and there are no signs of injury to the rest of his body. SpO_2 is 99% after positive pressure ventilation has been initiated.

You obtain a history from the family. It reveals that Mike was knocked unconscious for about 3 minutes 2 weeks ago after a rollerblading accident. He said he was fine and never sought medical care. This morning he was playing basketball and, according to his brother Sean, was hit in the head with an elbow. After that, the two brothers walked home. Sean states he noticed that Mike was walking oddly and complained of being tired. Once home, Mike went up to his room to lie down.

When the exam and history findings are recorded, you and your partner prepare the patient for transport. You apply a cervical collar and move him onto a backboard. When immobilization is complete, Mike is taken to the ambulance.

REASSESSMENT

En route to the hospital, you monitor Mike's airway, breathing, circulation, and level of responsiveness. You continue with controlled hyperventilation.

During transport, you note no change in Mike's condition. At the emergency department, he is transferred to the staff. You and your partner complete a prehospital care report and prepare the ambulance for another call.

A couple of months later, as you are passing the high school on the way to another call, you are happy to spot Mike and Sean walking toward the school. Mike seems to be fine.

IN REVIEW

1. Name the two parts of the central nervous system.
2. Define the meninges and name the three layers of the meninges.
3. Name the three anatomical components of the brain.
4. Describe an open and a closed head injury.
5. Name other types of injury that may be present and related to a head injury.
6. Name some of the major types of brain injury.
7. Explain why determining a baseline level of responsiveness is important in cases of head injury.
8. Explain why a history is important in cases of head injury.
9. List the signs and symptoms of head injury.
10. Outline the steps of emergency medical treatment in cases of head injury.
11. List signs of brain herniation.

CRITICAL THINKING

You arrive on the scene and find a 33-year-old male patient who startled an intruder when arriving home. The intruder stabbed the patient in the head with a screwdriver. The screwdriver is impaled in the skull. The police are on the scene. The patient responds to painful stimulus by flexing his arms, arching his back, and contracting his legs. He has blood in his mouth, and you hear gurgling sounds. His respirations are irregular at a rate of approximately 22 per minute with minimal chest rise and fall. Your partner indicates the radial pulse is strong and the HR is 42 bpm.

1. What immediate emergency care would you provide for the patient?
2. What do the vital signs indicate?
3. Would you hyperventilate the patient or not? Based on what criteria would you make the decision?
4. How would you manage the impaled screwdriver?

CHAPTER 32

Spinal Column and Spinal Cord Trauma

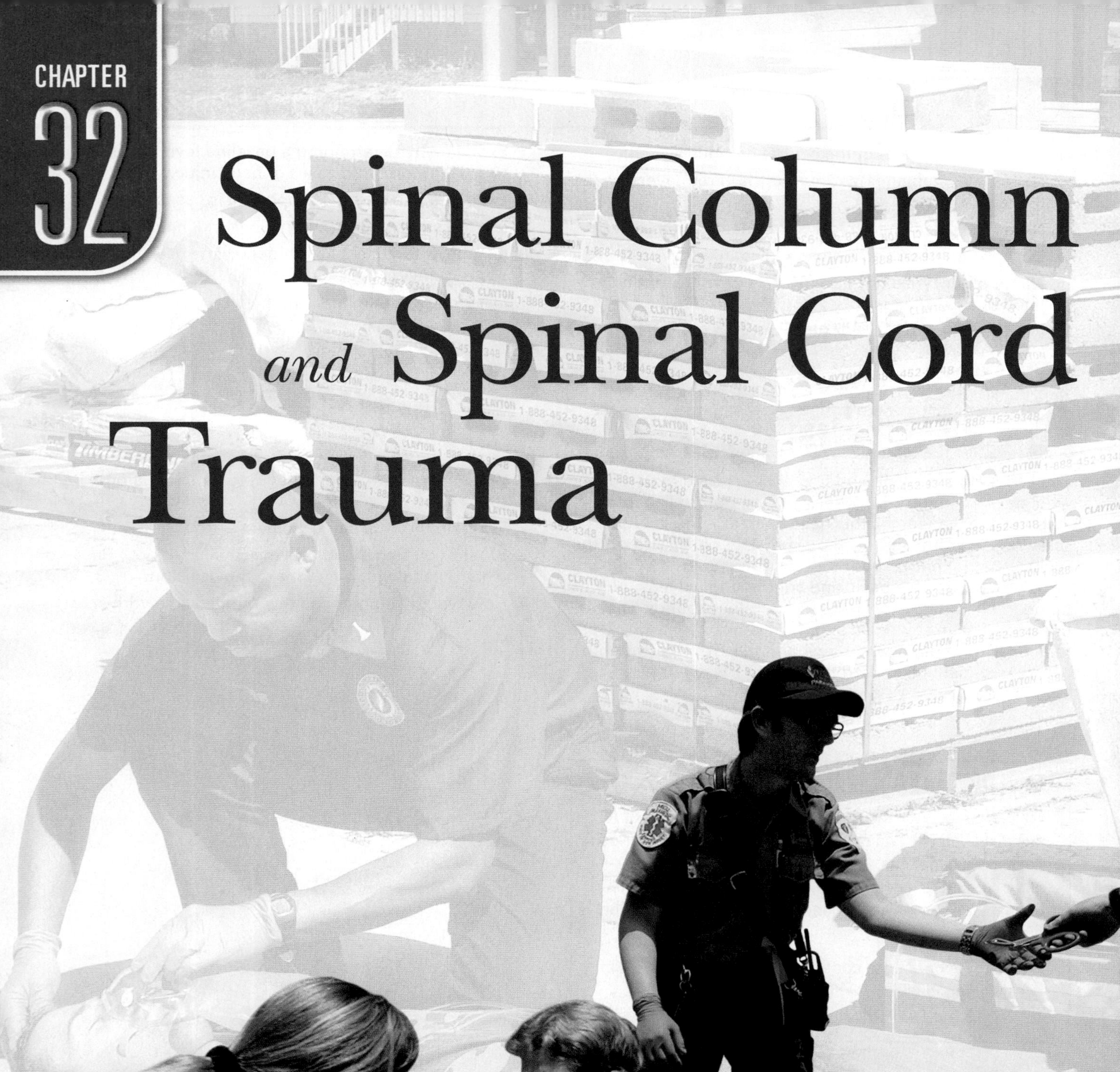

Navigation Guide

The following items provide an overview to the purpose and content of this chapter. The Standard and Competency are from the new National EMS Education Standards.

STANDARD **Trauma** (Content Area: Head, Facial, Neck, and Spine Trauma)

COMPETENCY Applies fundamental knowledge to provide basic emergency care and transportation based on assessment findings for an acutely injured patient.

OBJECTIVES: After reading this chapter, you should be able to:

32-1. Define key terms introduced in this chapter.
32-2. Describe the structure and function of the spinal column, spinal cord, and tracts within the spinal column.
32-3. Recognize common mechanisms of spinal injury and describe the incidence of neurological deficits in patients with spinal column trauma.
32-4. Give examples of forces that would produce each of the following mechanisms of spinal injury:
- **a.** Compression
- **b.** Flexion
- **c.** Extension
- **d.** Rotation
- **e.** Lateral bending
- **f.** Distraction
- **g.** Penetration

32-5. Differentiate spinal column injury and spinal cord injury.
32-6. Describe the concept of complete spinal cord injury and differentiate between the concepts of spinal shock and neurogenic hypotension.
32-7. Describe the concept of incomplete spinal cord injury and syndromes that may result from incomplete spinal cord injury.
32-8. Use scene size-up, patient assessment, and patient history to develop an index of suspicion for spinal injuries.
32-9. Given a series of scenarios, demonstrate the assessment-based management of patients suspected of having an injury to the spine.
32-10. Demonstrate the assessment of pulse, motor function, and sensory function in the extremities of a patient who is suspected of having an injury to the spine.
32-11. Recognize signs and symptoms of injury to the spinal column and spinal cord.
32-12. Explain how complications of spinal injury may result in inadequate breathing, paralysis, and inadequate circulation.
32-13. Describe appropriate emergency medical care for the patient with suspected spinal injury.
32-14. Describe correct immobilization techniques for the following:
- **a.** Supine or prone patient
- **b.** Standing patient
- **c.** Seated patient

32-15. Describe the indications for rapid extrication and the correct procedures for rapid extrication.
32-16. Explain special handling and immobilization considerations when spinal injury is suspected for the following:
- **a.** Helmet removal
- **b.** Football injuries, including removal of face mask and immobilization
- **c.** Infants and children, including extrication from a car seat

KEY TERMS: Page references indicate first major use in this chapter. For complete definitions, see the Glossary at the back of the book.

anterior cord syndrome p. 1045
Brown-Séquard syndrome p. 1045
central cord syndrome p. 1044
cervical spine p. 1039
coccyx p. 1040
complete spinal cord injury p. 1043
disk p. 1039
incomplete spinal cord injury p. 1044
lumbar spine p. 1040
neurogenic hypotension p. 1043
priapism p. 1043
sacral spine p. 1040
spinal column p. 1039
spinal cord p. 1040
spinal shock p. 1043
thoracic spine p. 1040
vertebrae p. 1039

continued

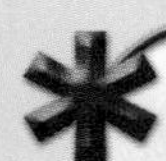

Navigation Guide *continued*

MEDIA RESOURCES: Please go to http://www.bradybooks.com/ to access mybradykit for this text. You will find quizzes, critical thinking scenarios, weblinks, animations, and videos related to this chapter—and much more. Look for online information on spinal cord injuries. You will also find an animation on cervical injuries and application of a cervical collar.

CASE STUDY

The Dispatch
EMS Unit 106—respond to Rita's Dance and Gym, 1403 Lisbon Road. You have a 12-year-old female patient who has fallen. Time out is 1552 hours.

Upon Arrival
Upon your arrival, an assistant at the gym tells you that a young girl fell during a gymnastics meet. She directs you into an open gymnasium. Across the floor, you see a crowd of people around a young girl lying on a mat. A woman is holding the girl still. The woman says, "She missed a maneuver off the top bar. She fell and hit the bottom bar with the middle of her back, then landed head first on the floor." The young girl is crying.

How Would You Proceed to Assess and Care for This Patient?
During this chapter, you will learn special considerations of assessment and emergency care for a patient suffering from a possible spine injury. Later we will return to the case and apply the procedures learned.

Introduction

Spine injuries are among the most formidable and traumatic you will manage as an EMT. Yet you may face the probability of such injuries on almost a daily basis. Automobile crashes, shallow-water diving accidents, motorcycle crashes, and falls are common causes of spine injury. Likewise, accidents during skiing, sledding, football, and gymnastics can result in spine injury. It is your job as an EMT to recognize injuries that could damage the spinal column or spinal cord and provide appropriate emergency care. You must be aware that improper movement and handling of patients in such situations can lead to permanent disability or even death.

Anatomy and Physiology of Spine Injury

To appreciate the potential severity of spine injuries, you should begin by understanding the relationship between the nervous system and the parts of the skeletal system most closely related to it, the skull and the spinal column, also referred to as the vertebral column. Before continuing, you may want to review the information about the skeletal and nervous systems that was presented in Chapter 7, "Anatomy, Physiology, and Medical Terminology," Chapter 30, "Musculoskeletal Trauma," and Chapter 31, "Head Trauma."

The Nervous System

Injuries to the spine have the potential for severity because within the spinal column is the spinal cord. This structure carries nerve impulses from most of the body to the brain and back to the body. A single spinal cord injury can affect several organs and body functions.

Parts of the Nervous System

The nervous system has two major functions: communication and control. It enables the individual to be aware of and react to his environment. It also coordinates the responses of the body to changes in the environment and keeps body systems working together.

The nervous system consists of nerve centers and nerves that branch off from the centers and lead to tissues and organs. Most nerve centers are in the brain and spinal cord.

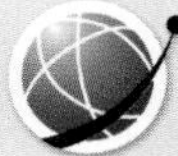

Media Resources

Go to www.bradybooks.com for mykit. Highlights:

- *Web Resource:* Spinal Cord Injury and Research
- *Web Resource:* Central Cord Syndrome

Objective 32-2

Describe the spinal column, cord, and tracts.

Key Terms

spinal column the 33 vertebrae that enclose and protect the spinal cord.

vertebrae bony segments of the spinal column.

disk fluid-filled cartilage pad between vertebrae.

The structural divisions of the nervous system (Figure 32-1∗) are:

- The *central nervous system (CNS)*, which consists of the brain and the spinal cord.
- The *peripheral nervous system*, which consists of nerves located outside of the brain and spinal cord.

The functional divisions of the nervous system are:

- The *voluntary nervous system*, which influences the activity of voluntary (skeletal) muscles and movements throughout the body.
- The *autonomic nervous system*, which is automatic and influences the activities of involuntary muscles and glands; the autonomic system is partly independent of the rest of the nervous system. The sympathetic nervous system and parasympathetic nervous system are included in the autonomic nervous system.

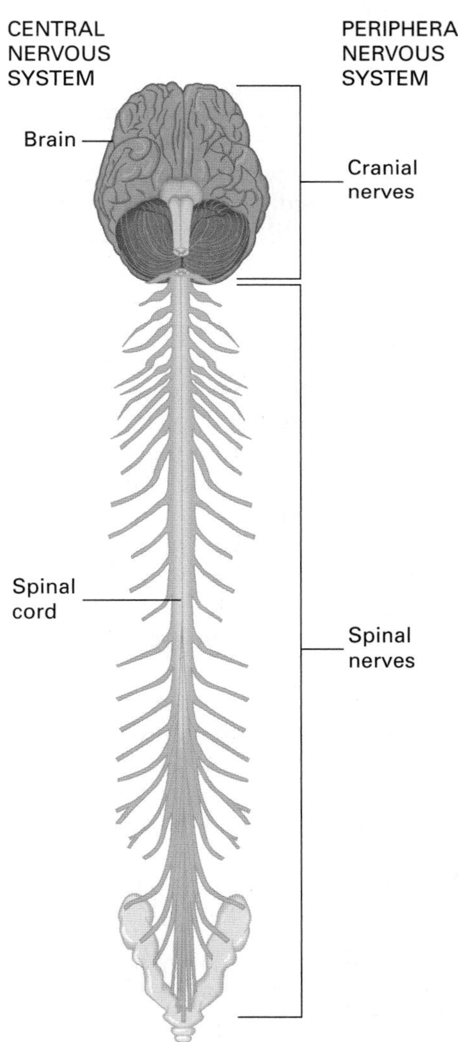

FIGURE 32-1 ∗ Components of the central and peripheral nervous systems.

The Skeletal System

The *skeletal system* gives the body its framework, supports and protects vital organs, and permits motion. The bony framework of the body is held together by *ligaments*, tough, fibrous connective tissue. The skeleton is flexible enough to absorb and protect against impacts and stress. The parts of the skeletal system that protect the most important parts of the nervous system are the skull and the spinal column.

The Skull

Resting at the top of the spinal column, the skull contains the brain. The skull has two parts: the cranium (or brain case) and the face.

The Spinal Column

The **spinal column**, or *vertebral column,* is the principal support system of the body. Ribs originate from it to form the thoracic cavity, and the rest of the skeleton is directly or indirectly attached to the spine.

Amazingly mobile, the spinal column is made up of 33 irregularly shaped bones called **vertebrae**. The *body* of a vertebra is the bulky portion that faces anteriorly in the spinal column. The posterior aspect of a vertebra is the *spinous process.* The spinous processes can be felt as the bony projections along the spinal column. Lying one on top of the other to form a strong, flexible column, the vertebrae are bound firmly together by strong ligaments. Between each two vertebrae is a fluid-filled pad of tough elastic cartilage called a **disk** that acts as a shock absorber. The spinal column, which surrounds and protects the spinal cord, is divided into five parts (Figure 32-2∗):

- The **cervical spine**—The first seven vertebrae that form the neck. The cervical vertebrae are the most mobile and delicate; injury to the cervical spine is the most common cause of spinal cord injury.

Key Terms
cervical spine the first seven vertebrae; the neck.

thoracic spine the 12 vertebrae that comprise the upper back.

lumbar spine the five vertebrae that form the lower back.

Key Terms
sacral spine the five fused vertebrae at the posterior pelvis.

coccyx the four fused vertebrae that form the lower end of the spine; the tailbone.

spinal cord nervous tissue that extends from the brain to level L2 within the spinal column.

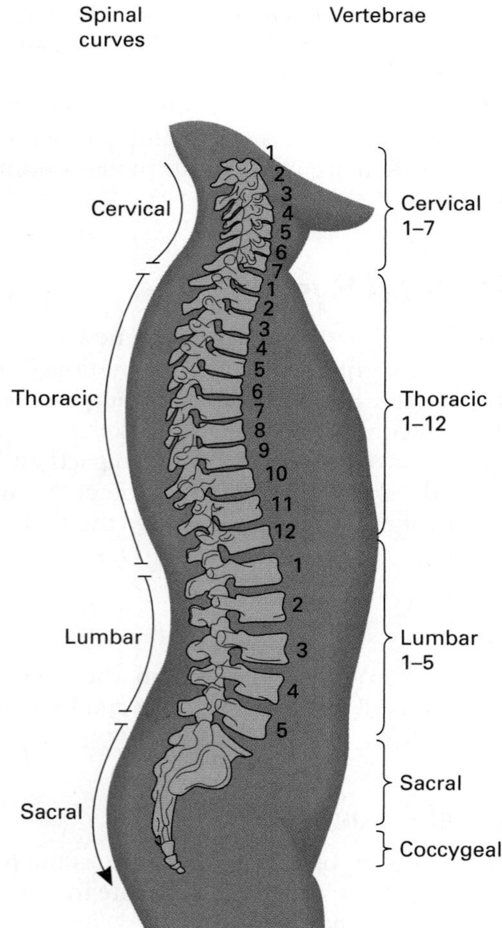

FIGURE 32-2 ✱ The spinal (vertebral) column.

- The **thoracic spine**—The 12 vertebrae directly below the cervical vertebrae that comprise the upper back.
- The **lumbar spine**—The next five vertebrae that form the lower back.
- The **sacral spine** (sacrum)—The next five vertebrae that are fused together and form the rigid posterior portion of the pelvis.
- The **coccyx** (tailbone)—The four fused vertebrae that form the lower end of the spine.

The **spinal cord**, composed of nervous tissue, exits the brain through an opening at the base of the skull. The cord is surrounded by a sheath of protective membranes (meninges) and a cushioning layer of cerebrospinal fluid. The cord narrows as it goes, filling 95 percent of the spinal column "canal" in the cervical vertebrae (neck) but only 60 percent in the lumbar area (lower back). All nerves to the trunk and extremities originate from the spinal cord. The spinal cord carries messages from the brain to the various parts of the body through nerve bundles.

There are three main types of tracts within the spinal cord that are tested in the assessment to determine if spinal cord injuries exist. The *motor tracts* carry impulses down the spinal cord and out to muscles. As their name implies, motor tracts are tested by having the patient move. The motor tracts on the right side of the spinal cord carry the impulses that allow the patient to move on the right side of the body; the motor tracts on the left side allow movement on the left side of the body.

The *pain tracts* carry impulses from pain receptors up the spinal cord to the brain. The pain tracts are tested by applying pain to the patient. Upon entering the spinal cord, a pain tract crosses over and carries the impulse up the opposite side of the cord. Thus, pain applied to the right side of the body is actually carried up the left side of the spinal cord. To test the right pain tract in the spinal cord, you must apply pain to the left side of the body; to test the left pain tract, apply pain to the right side of the body.

The last set of tracts carry light touch impulses from sensory receptors up the spinal cord to the brain. The *light touch tracts* are tested by applying light touch to the patient. The light touch sensation is carried up the same side of the spinal cord as the side where the touch is applied. If you apply light touch to the right side of the body, the light touch is carried up the right side of the spinal cord; light touch applied to the left side of the body is carried up the left side of the cord.

Since light touch and pain are carried by different tracts, it is possible for the patient to be unable to feel light touch but able to feel the pain of a pinch. This finding may be present if the spinal cord is partially but not completely injured.

Studying the spinal cord tracts to understand where they are located and what impulses are carried by them

Understanding BODY PROCESSES

Motor and light touch tracts carry the impulse on the same side of the spinal cord as the extremity that is being tested, whereas pain is carried up the opposite side of the spinal cord from the extremity the pain is applied to. This may create what appear to be conflicting assessment findings in the incomplete spinal cord injury. ■

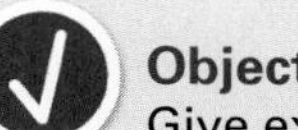

Objective 32-3
Recognize common mechanisms of spinal injury and describe the incidence of neurological deficits in patients with spinal column injury.

Objective 32-4
Give examples of forces that would produce compression, flexion, extension, rotation, lateral bending, distraction, and penetration of the spine.

Objective 32-5
Differentiate spinal column injury and spinal cord injury.

will help you better understand assessment findings associated with incomplete spinal cord injuries, which will be discussed later in the chapter. Also, knowing that various tracts within the spinal cord carry different impulses will reinforce and help you better understand the steps in the neurological assessment.

ASSESSMENT Tips

You cannot assume that just because a patient cannot feel light touch he will also not be able to feel pain, since light touch and pain sensations are carried by different spinal tracts. ■

Common Mechanisms of Spine Injury

The most common cause of spinal injuries is automobile crashes. These make up close to half (48 percent) of all spinal injuries. The next most common cause is falls (21 percent). Gunshot wounds and recreational activities such as diving and football are the next most frequent causes of spinal injuries. Any patient with a gunshot wound to the neck; the anterior, lateral, or posterior chest; the abdomen; or the pelvis must be suspected of having a possible spinal injury.

It is important to note that only 14–15 percent of patients who have spinal column fractures or dislocations will have a spinal cord injury that results in neurological deficits (motor or sensory dysfunction). This means that 85–86 percent of the patients who actually have a spinal fracture or dislocation will not present with a neurological deficit. When you arrive on the scene and find the patient walking about, it does not mean the patient did not suffer a spinal injury. The patient could have suffered a spinal column injury with no spinal cord involvement. Improper management of this patient, however, can convert a spinal column injury into a spinal cord injury. The result, which may be permanent paralysis, is catastrophic. Conversely, it is important to note that a patient can have a spinal cord injury without any spinal (vertebral) column damage. This specific condition is referred to as spinal cord injury without radiologic abnormality or SCIWORA. Do not become complacent in the management of any patient with a significant mechanism of injury for spinal trauma or one who displays any signs or symptoms of spinal column or cord injury.

Elderly patients may suffer fractures much more easily with less force applied to the spine. C1 and C2 dislocations may be more common in elderly patients who suffer from rheumatoid arthritis, and may be more common in Down syndrome patients because of abnormal development of the odontoid (second cervical vertebra).

The spine is quite strong and flexible, but it is particularly susceptible to injury from the following mechanisms (Figure 32-3∗):

- **Compression.** When the weight of the body is driven against the head. This is common in falls, diving accidents, motor vehicle crashes, or other accidents where a person impacts an object head first.
- **Flexion.** When there is severe forward movement of the head in which the chin meets the chest, or when the torso is excessively curled forward.
- **Extension.** When there is severe backward movement of the head in which the neck is stretched, or when the torso is severely arched backward.
- **Rotation.** When there is lateral movement of the head or spine beyond its normal rotation.
- **Lateral Bending.** When the body or neck is bent severely from the side.
- **Distraction.** When the vertebrae and spinal cord are stretched and pulled apart. This is common in hangings.
- **Penetration.** When there is injury from gunshots, stabbings, or other types of penetrating trauma that involve the cranium or spinal column.

You must suspect spine injury in any case that may involve one or more of these mechanisms. Suspect spine injury even if the patient appears to be able to move normally. Injured vertebrae that are still aligned, but unstable, can become unstable at any moment and damage or sever the spinal cord.

Spinal Column Injury Versus Spinal Cord Injury

A *spinal column injury* is an injury to one or more vertebrae, that is, the portion of the spine composed of bone. Whether it is a fracture or a dislocation, a spinal column injury is a bone injury. One thing we know about fractures and dislocations is that they hurt! If a patient has an injury to the spinal (vertebral) column, which is the bony portion of the spine, it will produce a complaint of pain or tenderness somewhere along the spine. Remember, pain is what the patient complains of, and tenderness is

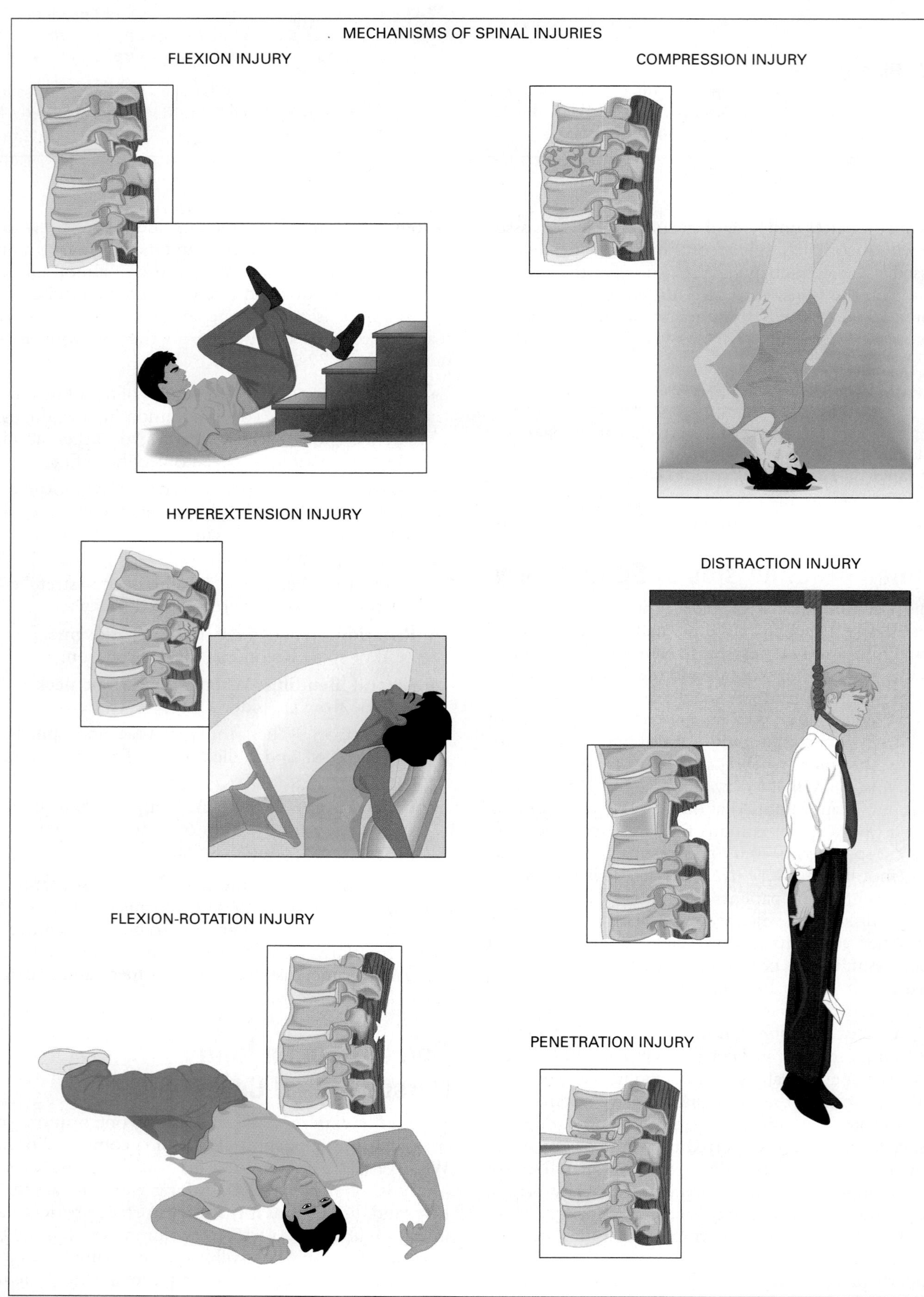

FIGURE 32-3 ✱ Mechanisms of spine injury.

Objective 32-6

Describe complete spinal cord injury, spinal shock, and neurogenic hypotension.

Key Terms

complete spinal cord injury spinal cord injury causing complete loss of motor, sensory, and autonomic function below the level of injury.

Key Terms

spinal shock paralysis, loss of sensation, and possible vasodilation caused by spinal cord injury.

priapism a persistent erection of the penis.

neurogenic hypotension vasodilation and relative hypovolemia caused by spinal cord injury.

pain elicited on palpation. You must gently palpate the length of the spine, feeling for any gross abnormalities, while also checking for tenderness. If at any point the patient complains of pain or tenderness along the length of the spinal column, it is an indication of potential injury. The patient must receive complete spinal immobilization, which is described later in the chapter.

A *spinal cord injury* involves damage to the nervous tissue that is enclosed inside the hollow center of the bony spinal column: the spinal cord. As discussed previously, the spinal cord contains motor tracts that transmit impulses from the brain that cause muscle movement, and sensory tracts that transmit impulses of light touch, pain, and pressure to the brain. If the spinal cord is injured, a disruption in one or more of the motor or sensory tracts is likely. Thus, the patient with a spinal cord injury would experience a loss of motor or sensory function or both.

Although a patient complaining of pain to the spinal column likely has a vertebral (spinal column) fracture or injury, pain does not indicate a spinal cord injury. Conversely, a loss of motor or sensory function indicates a spinal cord injury; however, it does not imply a vertebral fracture or injury. This is because a spinal column injury can occur without a spinal cord injury, and a spinal cord injury can occur without a spinal column injury. So a patient may experience a loss of motor or sensory function but have no pain. Or the patient may complain of pain but have no loss of motor or sensory function. In either case—pain/tenderness along the spinal column or loss of motor/sensory function—the patient would be considered to have a spinal injury and must be completely immobilized.

Complete Spinal Cord Injury

A **complete spinal cord injury** results when an area of the spinal cord has been completely transected (cut crossways) either physically or physiologically. The injury, having severed the motor and sensory tracts, prevents any motor impulses from passing down from brain to body or sensory impulses from passing up from body to brain through the injured area of the cord. Therefore, there is a total loss of motor and sensory function below the level of injury. The patient presents with the inability to move or feel sensations of pain, light touch, and crude pressure below the level of injury. The patient will also likely present with a loss of bowel and bladder control because autonomic function is blocked.

When a patient presents with complete loss of motor and sensory function distal to the cord injury, however, it may not always indicate complete spinal cord injury. The patient may, instead, be experiencing spinal shock.

Spinal Shock

Spinal shock is a temporary concussion-like insult to the spinal cord that causes effect below the level of the injury. Such an injury usually occurs high in the cervical region. Below the level of injury there is a loss of muscle tone (flaccid muscles), the patient is unable to feel sensations of light touch or pinch (anesthetic effect), and the patient is unable to move the extremities or any voluntary muscles (paralysis). The patient will typically lose control of the bladder and bowel. A male patient may have an involuntary erection of the penis called **priapism**. The vessels below the site of injury may dilate, leading to a decreased blood pressure (neurogenic hypotension, explained in the next section). Temperature regulation is also disrupted by the loss of vessel tone.

Spinal shock usually resolves within 24 hours after the incident but may last for several days. This patient should be managed as one with a spine injury, even if the dysfunction begins to resolve while you are managing the patient.

ASSESSMENT Tips

A patient in spinal shock may present with complete paralysis that may resolve within 24 hours to several days after the injury. ■

Neurogenic Hypotension from Spinal Shock **Neurogenic hypotension** from spinal shock, also called *spinal-vascular shock* or *neurogenic shock*, results from an injury to the spinal cord that interrupts nerve impulses to the arteries. When the arteries lose nervous impulses from the brain and spinal cord, they relax and dilate (enlarge). This vasodilation causes a relative hypovolemia within the circulatory system. That is, there is more space than there is blood to fill the arteries. Because of this, the patient becomes hypotensive (has lowered blood pressure).

With spinal shock, sympathetic nerve impulses to the adrenal glands are lost, which prevents the release of epinephrine and norepinephrine. This causes vessel dilation (red skin) and a lack of sweat gland stimulation (causing

Objective 32-7
Describe incomplete spinal cord injury and syndromes that may result from incomplete spinal cord injury.

Key Terms

incomplete spinal cord injury injury to some but not all spinal cord tracts so that some functions are lost and others are intact.

central cord syndrome loss of function in upper extremities from central cord injury.

the skin to remain dry). With the blood pooling in the periphery and the lack of circulating hormones (epinephrine and norepinephrine), the patient's physical signs are different from those of classic hypovolemic shock (shock from fluid loss). Instead of pale, moist skin as would develop with hypovolemia, the spinal shock patient's skin will be warm and dry and may appear slightly pink or red. In spinal shock, where sympathetic impulses are impaired, the patient's pulse is typically 60–80 beats per minute. This differs from the rapid rates that usually result from sympathetic nervous system stimulation in hypovolemia.

Treatment for spinal shock is much the same as for any other shock. Cervical spinal stabilization must be applied and the patient must be kept warm and completely immobilized.

Incomplete Spinal Cord Injury

Incomplete spinal cord injury occurs when the spinal cord is injured—but not completely through all of the three major tracts (motor, light touch, and pain tracts). That means that some of the tracts are spared and retain function. Because some tracts are injured and some are not, the patient may present with conflicting or confusing signs of spinal cord injury. Some of the spinal cord is not injured; therefore, some function is retained. The patient may be able to move some areas of the body and not move other areas of the body, or the patient may retain the sensation of pain to some areas of the body but not to others. Unlike a complete spinal cord injury, which causes complete loss of motor and sensory function below the level of injury, the incomplete spinal cord injury produces only loss of some function in some areas of the body.

The three most common types of incomplete spinal cord injury result in distinctive patterns of signs and symptoms (syndromes). They are central cord syndrome, anterior cord syndrome, and Brown-Séquard syndrome.

Central Cord Syndrome If the central portion of the spinal cord is injured (Figure 32-4a*), the patient may present with weakness or paralysis and loss of pain sensation to the upper extremities while the lower extremities have good function. This is opposite to what is expected in a patient with a complete spinal cord injury, which is loss of function below the site of injury. The reason for the loss of function in the upper extremities and not the lower is that the medial (inner) aspects of the motor and pain tracts control the upper extremities, whereas the lateral (outer) portions of the tracts control the lower extremities. In **central cord syndrome,** the medial or middle portion of the spinal cord is injured, causing a dysfunction in the inner tracts that control upper extremity motor and sensory function. Central cord syndrome is more commonly seen in elderly patients.

ASSESSMENT Tips

In central cord syndrome, the patient presents with a loss of motor function or weakness and loss of pain sensation to the upper extremities while motor and sensory function remain normal in the lower extremities. ■

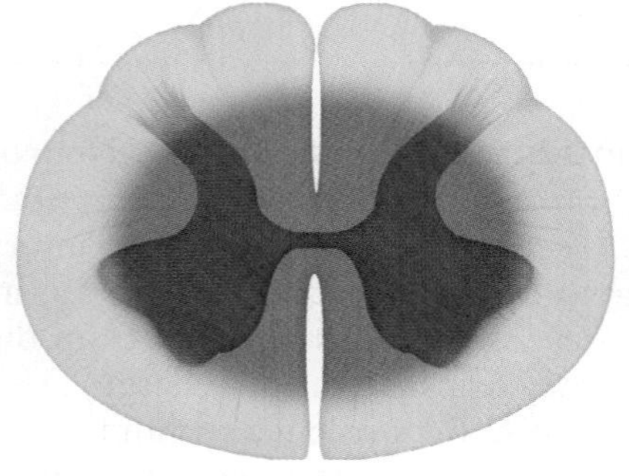

(a) Central cord syndrome

(b) Anterior cord syndrome

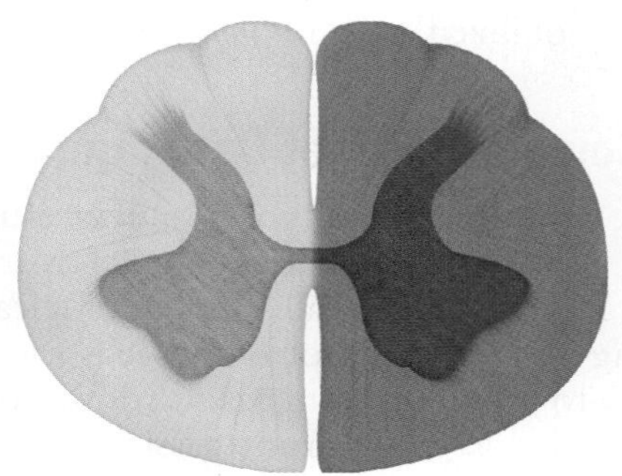

(c) Brown-Séquard syndrome

FIGURE 32-4 * Cross sections of the spinal cord showing the H-shaped gray matter surrounded by white matter. Illustrated here are the three most common types of incomplete spinal cord injury. (The areas of injury are highlighted in red.) Each results in a distinctive syndrome, or pattern of sensory and motor deficits. **(a)** Central cord syndrome results from injury to the central cord. **(b)** Anterior cord syndrome results from injury to the anterior cord. **(c)** Brown-Séquard syndrome results from injury to the right or left half of the cord.

Key Terms

anterior cord syndrome loss of most function below site of anterior cord injury.

Brown-Séquard syndrome loss of different functions on opposite sides of the body from injury to one side of the spinal cord.

Objectives 32-8 and 32-9

Use assessment information to develop an index of suspicion and the assessment-based approach to management of patients with suspected spine injury.

Anterior Cord Syndrome **Anterior cord syndrome** results from injury of the sensory and motor tracts located in the anterior portion of the cord (Figure 32-4b∗). The posterior portion of the cord, where the tracts for light touch are located, is not injured. The patient will present with the loss of sensation to pain and loss of motor function below the site of cord injury; however, the patient will retain the ability to feel light touch.

ASSESSMENT Tips

In anterior cord syndrome, the patient loses the ability to feel pain and crude touch below the site of injury and also likely experiences the loss of motor function below the injury site. However, the patient retains the ability to feel light touch both above and below the site of injury. ■

Brown-Séquard Syndrome An injury to a hemisection—the right or left half—of the spinal cord (Figure 32-4c∗) disrupts the spinal tracts on only one side of the cord. The patient experiences motor and sensory losses below the injury site, but the distinctive feature of **Brown-Séquard syndrome** is that the effects differ on the two sides of the body. The patient loses motor function and light touch sensation on one side but loses pain sensation on the opposite side. As an example, on the right the patient may be unable to move and unable to feel light touch but is able to feel pain. On the left he is able to move and feel light touch but does not feel pain. As you will recall from earlier in the chapter, the pain tracts cross over upon entering the spinal cord and carry the impulse up the opposite side of the cord, but the motor and light touch tracts carry the impulse up the same side as where they entered the cord. This explains the different assessment findings on opposite sides of the body.

ASSESSMENT Tips

In Brown-Séquard syndrome, the patient loses motor function and light touch sensation on one side of the body while retaining pain sensation on that same side. On the opposite side of the body, the patient retains motor function and light touch sensation while losing pain sensation. ■

A complete spinal cord injury will result in the classic findings: total paralysis and loss of sensation below the level of injury. Any time you get abnormal motor function or sensation results from your assessment, findings that conflict with the classic findings, suspect incomplete cord injury. In either case, however, your emergency care must remain the same. *The patient who has suffered any spinal cord injury—whether complete or incomplete—requires complete immobilization!*

Emergency Care for Suspected Spine Injury

Assessment-Based Approach: Spine Injury

Scene Size-Up

Because suspicion of, and emergency care for, spine injury are most often based on mechanism of injury, the scene size-up is an extremely important phase of patient assessment.

Likely Mechanisms of Spinal Injury Be especially alert to the possibility of spine injury when called to any of the following scenes, since all of them are likely to produce the mechanisms that may result in spinal injury:

- Motorcycle crashes
- Motor vehicle crashes
- Pedestrian–vehicle collisions
- Falls
- Blunt trauma
- Penetrating trauma to the head, neck, or torso
- Sporting injuries
- Hangings
- Diving or other water-related accidents
- Gunshot wounds to the head, neck, chest, abdomen, back, or pelvis
- Unresponsive trauma patient
- Electrical injuries

Gunshot wounds to the head, neck, chest, abdomen, back, or pelvis should always cause suspicion of injury to the vertebrae or spinal cord. Even if entrance and exit wounds are closely aligned and appear to indicate a clean, straight-through wound, the bullet could have ricocheted and caused an injury to the vertebrae or spinal cord. Also,

Key Points
Gunshot wounds to the head, neck, chest, abdomen, back, or pelvis should always cause suspicion of spine injury.

Thinking Critically
At the scene a passenger from a collision vehicle is sitting on a roadside bench. As you begin manual stabilization of her head and spine, a bystander says, "That's not necessary. She was walking around, so her spine isn't hurt." Should you discontinue stabilization? Why or why not?

exploding fragments from other bones could have injured the spine. With any gunshot wound to the body, immediately establish manual in-line spinal stabilization and take the necessary spinal precautions during your emergency care.

Also suspect spine injury with any serious blunt injury to the head, neck, chest, abdomen, back, or pelvis—and even to the legs or arms. The energy of the impact can travel up the extremity to the spinal column.

Clues to Mechanism of Injury Upon arrival, scan the scene closely for evidence of a mechanism of injury that could cause damage to the vertebrae or spinal cord. Look up, down, and around the patient for signs that an injury has occurred. If an unresponsive patient is lying on the ground near a tree, assume that the patient fell out of the tree until proven otherwise.

Even though there may be no overt signs of trauma to the patient, a spine injury may nevertheless exist. In such a situation, opening the airway using a head-tilt, chin-lift maneuver (which requires extension of the head and neck) or failing to provide proper manual in-line spinal stabilization may produce catastrophic permanent injury or even be lethal to the patient. These dire results can be avoided if you perform a thorough assessment of the scene for mechanism of injury and maintain a high index of suspicion of spine injury.

You must deduce the mechanism of injury from the evidence at the scene and determine if such a mechanism could have injured the spine. For example, on arrival at the scene of an automobile collision, you may note damage to the front of the car. As you quickly scan the car, you note an impact mark on the front windshield on the driver's side, apparently made by the driver's head (Figure 32-5*). You also note that the patient is not wearing his lap or shoulder restraint.

This evidence should create a high index of suspicion that the patient was propelled forward in the crash and struck his head on the windshield. This would likely have caused the head and neck to bend (flex) forward during the forward movement and bend backward (hyperextend) during the rearward movement. Both motions are significant mechanisms of injury that might not be suspected if the damage to the vehicle was not observed.

You may arrive at a collision scene and find the patient walking around or sitting in the back of a police car. This does not rule out the possibility of spine injury, especially an incomplete spinal cord injury or a vertebral injury.

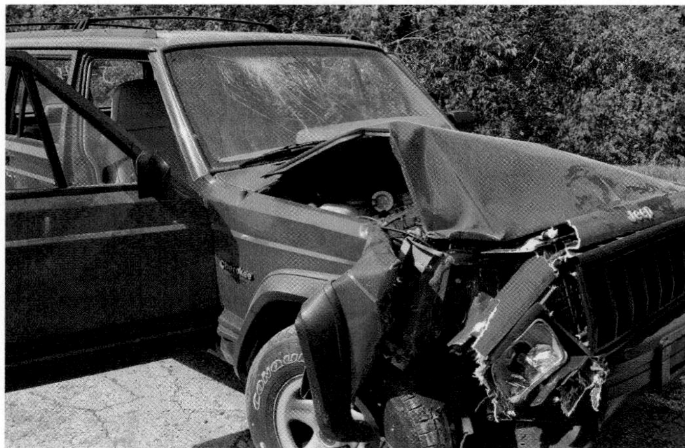

FIGURE 32-5 * Front-end damage and a driver's side windshield fracture indicate that the driver was probably thrown head first into the windshield.

Many times, a patient with a stable spine injury does not exhibit signs and symptoms consistent with injury to the spine. Improper movement by either the patient or the EMT can easily cause the stable injury to become unstable, resulting in permanent neurological damage or even death. You must maintain proper in-line spinal stabilization, even if the patient has moved prior to your arrival.

Suspicion of injury to the spine based on the mechanism of injury sets the standard for subsequent emergency care for the patient. All assessment and care must be conducted with extreme caution to avoid excessive movement and manipulation of the body. In-line spinal stabilization must be maintained throughout the entire patient contact.

Primary Assessment

When performing the primary assessment, the general impression may not lead you to suspect a spine injury, since the signs and symptoms may not be apparent. *Regardless of the lack of obvious trauma or patient complaints, you must adopt a high index of suspicion and initiate immediate manual in-line spinal stabilization if the scene size-up has suggested a mechanism of injury that could cause spine injury. Manual stabilization must not be released until the patient is securely strapped to a backboard with his head and neck immobilized or until a spinal injury has been ruled out through your assessment if your protocol permits.*

An important factor to consider in the patient with a possible spine injury is the mental status. If the mental

Key Points
When the mechanism of injury suggests possible spinal injury, responses from a patient with an altered mental status are unreliable. In this situation, assume spinal cord injury and completely immobilize the patient.

Key Points
A patient who is unresponsive, is unable to obey commands, has an abnormal respiratory pattern, or has signs of spine injury such as numbness or paralysis must be considered a high priority for prompt transportation.

status is altered, it may be an indication of a head injury, alcohol intoxication, drug influence, shock, hypoxia, or other causes. An altered mental status does not allow the patient to respond adequately to questions or physical assessment or to provide complaints of pain, numbness, tingling, weakness, paralysis, or other signs of neurological dysfunction. In the case of an altered mental status, the patient is considered unreliable and you should always assume a spinal cord injury and completely immobilize that patient.

If the patient has other injuries, especially extremity fractures, the pain associated with these injuries may distract from any pain or tenderness the patient is experiencing to the spinal column. Thus, the patient does not complain of pain to the spinal column, allowing the EMT who is not prudent to miss the possible spinal injury. Be careful not to be drawn away from spinal assessment by other injuries, known as "distracting injuries." Any patient with injuries above the clavicles (head, face, neck) should be assumed to have cervical spine injury.

Furthermore, if a patient has trouble communicating with you because of a language barrier, deafness, or other reasons, he may not be able to complain of symptoms or respond appropriately to your assessment.

Whenever spine injury is suspected, you must open the airway using the jaw-thrust maneuver instead of the head-tilt, chin-lift maneuver. Do not turn the patient's head to the side to facilitate drainage of fluids from the airway. Instead, suction any secretions, blood, or vomitus from the patient's mouth.

Spinal cord damage from a cervical spine injury can block nerve impulses traveling from the brain to the diaphragm and intercostal muscles, which are necessary for adequate respiration. Inadequate or absent breathing may result. There may be very little or no movement of the chest and only slight movement of the abdominal muscles, or you may note excessive abdominal muscle movement. Be prepared to provide positive pressure ventilation with supplemental oxygen.

Understanding BODY PROCESSES

An injury to the cervical spine in the area of the third (C3) to fifth (C5) cervical vertebrae may injure the phrenic nerve that controls the function of the diaphragm. Since the diaphragm provides more than 60 percent of the effort to breathe, the patient will develop respiratory failure and will require ventilation. An injury to the spinal cord at this level will also eliminate impulses to the intercostal muscles, because the nerves that control these muscles exit at the seventh cervical (C7) to first thoracic (T1) vertebrae. ■

The patient's pulse and skin color, temperature, and condition may appear normal in spite of injury to the vertebrae. However, an injury to the spinal cord can interrupt the transmission of impulses from the brain to the heart and the blood vessels that control blood pressure. You may find the radial pulse weak or absent because of a reduced blood pressure. The skin may be warm and dry below the site of spinal cord injury and cool, pale, and moist above the site of injury. This is relatively rare.

Understanding BODY PROCESSES

The warm and flushed skin is due to massive vasodilation below the site of injury and the loss of sympathetic tone provided to those vessels, allowing the blood to pool in the vessels in the skin and extremities. ■

ASSESSMENT Tips

The skin may initially appear flushed and warm in the patient with a spine injury; however, as the pooled blood begins to deoxygenate and cool, the skin will become mottled and cool. ■

The mental status of a patient with a spine injury may range from completely alert and oriented to unresponsive.

Based on the mechanism of injury, categorize the patient as either high or low priority for emergency care or transport. If the patient is unresponsive, is responsive but unable to obey your commands, or displays an abnormal respiratory pattern or obvious signs of spine injury such as numbness or paralysis, you must consider the patient a high priority for emergency care and prompt transportation.

Secondary Assessment

Conduct the secondary assessment. Continue manual in-line spinal stabilization and reassess the patient's mental status. Conduct a physical exam, then assess vital signs and gather a history.

Objective 32-10
Demonstrate the assessment of pulse, motor function, and sensory function in the extremities of a patient who is suspected of having an injury to the spine.

Key Points
A wooden Q-tip can be used to check both pain and light touch. Break the stick in half. Use the jagged end to test for pain and the cotton tip to assess for light touch.

Physical Exam Instruct the patient to be still and not attempt to move. Do not attempt to unbutton or unzip clothing to expose the patient. Instead, reduce unnecessary movement by cutting clothing away. Conduct a physical exam. Inspect and palpate the head, neck, chest, abdomen, pelvis, extremities, and posterior body for evidence of trauma.

When spine injury is suspected, pay particular attention to the following during the exam:

- **Injuries Associated with Spine Injury.** Watch for evidence of trauma to the head, posterior cervical region, anterior neck, chest, abdomen, back, and pelvis. Injuries to these areas also frequently cause spine injury.
- **Cervical Spine Immobilization Collar.** Following your assessment of the neck, apply the cervical spine immobilization collar (CSIC). The cervical collar is only an adjunct to full spinal immobilization; it does not provide complete immobilization by itself. Do not release manual in-line spinal stabilization until the patient is fully immobilized on a backboard. This will be done after the secondary assessment.
- **Assessing Pulses and Motor and Sensory Function.** In the responsive patient, assess the pulses and motor and sensory function (EMT Skills 32-1) of each extremity. While assessment of pulses and motor and sensory function is being performed, maintain manual spinal stabilization.

To assess the pulses, do the following:

Pulse Assessment

- Check for the presence and strength of the radial pulses for the upper extremities, the pedal pulses for the lower extremities.

To assess for motor function, ask the patient to do the following:

Motor Function Assessment: Upper Extremities

- "Flex your arms (bend the arms at the elbows) across your chest" (tests motor function at C6).
- "Extend your arms (straighten the arms to the side of the body)" (tests motor function at C7).
- "Spread your fingers out on both hands and don't let me squeeze them together" (tests motor function at T1).
- "Hold out both arms and don't let me push your hand down" (done while you support the hand under the wrist) (tests motor function at C7).

Motor Function Assessment: Lower Extremities

- "Push down against my hands with your feet" (place your hands under the feet) (tests motor function at S1 and S2).
- "Pull up against my hands with your feet" (place your hands on the tops of the feet) (tests motor function at the level of L5).

A wooden Q-tip can be used for checking both pain and light touch. Break the stick in half. Use the jagged broken end to test for pain and the soft cotton tip to assess for light touch. If you don't have a Q-tip, you can pinch the skin for pain and lightly touch the skin for light touch.

Test for Pain Perception

- Have the patient close his eyes. With the sharp end of the wooden Q-tip stick, poke one of the hands. When the patient grimaces, moans, or responds in some other way, ask "Where does it hurt?" Repeat the test on the other hand and then on each foot.

Test for Light Touch Perception

- Have the patient again close his eyes. Lightly touch the patient's fingers on one hand, then the other. As you perform this test for light touch to the fingers, ask:
  - Can you feel me touching your finger?"
  - "Can you tell me what hand and which finger I'm touching?"

  You would repeat the test on one of the toes on each foot. As you test for light touch on the toes, ask:

  - "Can you feel me touching your toe?"
  - "Can you tell me which foot and what toe I'm touching?"

If the patient is unresponsive, pinch the foot and hand to determine a sensory response. Compare the sensory function and strength in the upper and lower extremities. It is more common for spine injuries to cause paralysis to all four extremities (*quadriplegia*) or to the lower half of the body only (*paraplegia*). Loss of function confined to the right or left side of the body (*hemiplegia*) is more typical of a brain injury or stroke. Conflicting or

Key Points

If the brain or spinal cord is damaged, baseline vital signs may be affected by neurogenic hypotension with a low blood pressure and normal or bradycardic heart thythm.

Key Points

Because of the seriousness of a spine injury, try to reduce time at the scene by taking the history while the physical exam is being conducted.

partial loss of motor or sensory function may be an indication of an incomplete spinal cord injury.

Understanding BODY PROCESSES

Pain applied to an extremity may travel through a nerve tract, enter the spinal cord, and be immediately turned around and sent back out through a motor tract, causing the patient to move even though the impulse never reached the brain. Thus, the motor response to this *does not* tell you about the integrity of the brain and the nerve tracts, which is what it is intended to do. ■

- **Posterior Exam.** Carefully log roll the patient with in-line spinal stabilization to assess the posterior body. Palpate the area of the spine very gently. Evidence of deformity, tenderness, contusions, lacerations, punctures, or swelling to the spine or around the spine should heighten your suspicion that a spinal column injury exists. Muscle spasms along the spinal column are a protective reflex and a common indication that a spine injury has occurred.

Baseline Vital Signs Obtain and record a set of baseline vital signs. If the brain or spinal cord is damaged, baseline vital signs may reflect neurogenic hypotension. The blood pressure will be low and the heart rate normal or bradycardic. The hypotension associated with spinal shock is not usually severe but mild, with a systolic blood pressure usually no lower than 80 mmHg. As noted earlier in the chapter, in spinal shock the skin is warm and dry and the patient will present with motor and/or sensory deficit. Closely reassess the patient for deterioration and report these findings to the emergency department. If the hypotension is severe and the patient has tachycardia, suspect bleeding as the cause of shock and treat accordingly. Hypovolemia and spinal cord injury can both be present in the same patient; therefore, be cautious in your assessment, since spinal cord injury may prevent the typical signs of hypovolemic shock from occurring.

Understanding BODY PROCESSES

The hypotension in spinal shock is due to massive vasodilation and pooling of blood in peripheral vessels. No blood or fluid is lost from the vessels; however, the increase in the vessel size reduces the vessel resistance, the blood pressure, and perfusion. This produces a distributive type of shock. ■

ASSESSMENT Tips

Neurogenic hypotension resulting from vasodilation in a spinal injury rarely produces a systolic blood pressure of less than 80 mmHg. ■

History Obtain a history from the responsive patient. Because of the seriousness of a spine injury, try to take this history as the physical exam is being conducted. Questions that might be asked in cases of suspected spine injury include the following:

- Does your neck or back hurt?
- Where does it hurt?
- Can you move your hands and feet?
- Do you have any pain or muscle spasms along your back or to the back of your neck?
- Do you have any numbness or tingling sensations in either of your arms or legs?
- Was the onset of pain associated with a fall or other injury?
- Did you move or did someone move you before our arrival?
- Were you up walking around before our arrival?

Assess for allergies, medications, past medical history, and the last intake of food or drink. Remember to ask about events prior to the onset of signs or symptoms, because they may provide evidence of or clarify the mechanism of injury.

If the patient is unresponsive, obtain the history from the bystanders at the scene. Try to determine the patient's mental status before your arrival, if the patient was moving any extremities, or if the patient was moved prior to your arrival.

Signs and Symptoms Most often, you will take spinal precautions based solely on the mechanism of injury rather than on specific signs and symptoms of spine injury. It is imperative for you to recognize that a patient's lack of pain in the spinal column or his ability to walk, to move his extremities, and to feel sensations does not rule out the possibility of spinal column (vertebral) or incomplete spinal cord injury.

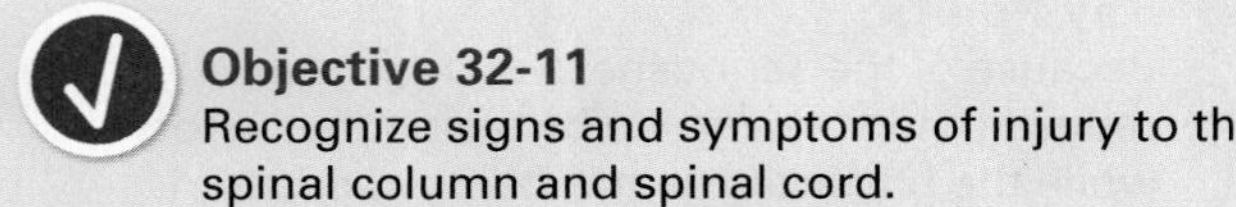

Objective 32-11
Recognize signs and symptoms of injury to the spinal column and spinal cord.

The following are signs and symptoms of spine injury (Figure 32-6∗):

- Tenderness in the area of injury, specifically along the spinal column.
- Pain associated with movement from spine injury that may be localized. Ask the patient to pinpoint the location (by telling you where it is, not by trying to point to it). *Do not ask the patient to move to try to elicit a pain response. Do not move the patient to test for pain.*
- Pain independent of movement or palpation along the spinal column or in the lower legs. Such pain is generally intermittent instead of constant and may occur anywhere along the spinal column from the base of the head to the extreme lower back. If the lower spinal column is injured, the patient may complain of pain to the legs.
- Obvious deformity of the spine upon palpation. This is a rare assessment finding.
- Soft tissue injuries. Those from trauma to the head and neck are associated with cervical spine injury. Soft tissue injuries to the shoulders, posterior thorax (back), or abdomen are associated with thoracic or lumbar spine injury. Lower extremity trauma is associated with lumbar and sacral spine injury.
- Numbness, weakness, tingling, or loss of sensation or motor function in any of the arms or legs.
- Loss of sensation or paralysis below the suspected level of injury or in the upper or lower extremities. Paralysis of the extremities is a reliable sign of spine injury.
- Loss of bowel or bladder control (incontinence).
- Priapism, a persistent erection of the penis resulting from injury to the spinal nerves to the genitals. It

SIGNS AND SYMPTOMS OF POSSIBLE SPINAL INJURY

• PAIN	Unprovoked pain in area of injury, along spine, in lower legs.
• TENDERNESS	Gentle touch of area may increase pain.
• DEFORMITY (rare)	There may be abnormal bend or bony prominence.
• SOFT TISSUE INJURY	Injury to the head, neck, or face may indicate cervical-spine injury. Injury to shoulders, back, and abdomen may indicate thoracic- or lumbar-spine injury . Injury to extremities may indicate lumbar- or sacral-spine injury.
• PARALYSIS	Inability to move or inability to feel sensation in some part of body may indicate spinal fracture with cord injury.
• PAINFUL MOVEMENT	Movement may increase pain. Never try to move the injured area.
• ALSO:	Loss of bowel or bladder control, priapism, impaired breathing.

FIGURE 32-6 ∗ Signs and symptoms of possible spine injury.

Objective 32-12
Explain how complications of spinal injury may result in inadequate breathing, paralysis, and inadequate circulation.

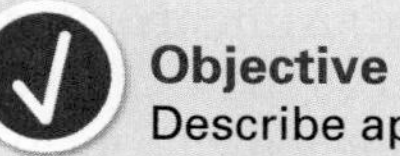

Objective 32-13
Describe appropriate emergency medical care for the patient with suspected spinal injury.

occurs soon after injury and is a classic sign of cervical spine injury.

- Impaired breathing, especially breathing that involves little or no chest movement and only slight abdominal movement. This is an indication that the patient is breathing with the diaphragm alone. Diaphragmatic breathing is indicative of cervical spine injury. If injury to the nerve that controls the diaphragm occurs, you may see either no breathing effort or an attempt to breathe using only the abdominal muscles.

Complications of Spine Injury Spine injury may produce catastrophic permanent damage. Three major complications of spine injury are these:

- **Inadequate Breathing Effort.** Paralysis of the respiratory muscles may occur with injury to the cervical spine. Rapid deterioration of the patient's condition and death may result without quick intervention by the EMT. The diaphragm may continue to function even if the chest wall muscles are paralyzed. The patient will display shallow, inadequate breathing with little movement of the chest or abdomen. Continuous positive pressure ventilation is necessary.
- **Paralysis.** Paralysis may occur below the site of spinal cord damage. If the damage is to the spinal cord below the cervical region, paralysis is isolated to the lower half of the body (paraplegia). Damage to the cervical spinal cord can produce complete paralysis of the entire body (quadriplegia or tetraplegia). Paralysis and complete loss of sensation to only one side of the body (hemiplegia) is more common in head injuries and stroke; however, an incomplete spinal cord injury may cause loss of motor and sensory function in different areas of the body.
- **Inadequate Circulation.** Blood pressure and perfusion may be poor in the patient with spine injury as a result of spinal shock. If the spinal cord nerve fibers traveling from the medulla in the brain to the blood vessels are damaged, the blood pressure control center (vasomotor center) can no longer maintain the muscle tone in the blood vessels. Below the point of spinal cord injury, the blood vessels dilate (increase in size) and lower their resistance. Subsequently, blood begins to pool in the dilated vessels, the blood pressure drops, and the perfusion of other tissues of the body is reduced. Because of the blood vessel dilation, the skin is usually warm and dry, even though the tissue perfusion is poor. The heart rate typically remains normal or decreases slightly. In this case, be sure to look for other reasons for the low blood pressure.

ASSESSMENT Tips

Pain or tenderness along the vertebral column is a significant sign of possible spinal column (vertebral) fracture. ■

Emergency Medical Care

In cases of suspected spine injury, it is not the role of the EMT to diagnose the condition or the site of the injury. The EMT must instead ensure that life-threatening conditions are cared for, that the possibility of further injury is reduced by careful handling of the patient, and that the patient is properly immobilized to a backboard and expeditiously transported to a medical facility.

When in doubt, immobilize the patient.

It is safer to err on the side of caution and completely immobilize a patient if spine injury is suspected. Immobilization devices can always be removed at the emergency department once the physician or radiographic studies determine that no spine injury exists. Paralysis resulting from failure to immobilize a patient because he did not display signs and symptoms of spine injury cannot be so easily undone.

The general guidelines for emergency care of a patient with a suspected spine injury are these:

1. **Take necessary Standard Precautions.**
2. **Establish manual in-line spinal stabilization immediately upon making contact with the patient** (EMT Skills 32-2). Ensure that the head is in a neutral, in-line position. That means bringing the head into a position in which the nose is in line with the navel (belly button) and the head is neither flexed forward nor extended backward. This manual stabilization must be maintained until the patient is completely secured and immobilized to the backboard.

   If the patient complains of severe pain to the neck or cervical spine, or the head does not easily move, stabilize and maintain the head in the position found.

   If an Emergency Medical Responder is holding manual in-line spinal stabilization upon your arrival, instruct him not to let go. If he can continue with the stabilization, evaluate the position of the patient's head and make any necessary readjustments. If the Emergency Medical Responder needs to be relieved, you should take over the in-line stabilization in a controlled manner. Replace the Emergency Medical Responder's hands on the patient's head with yours one at a time so that stabilization is never lost or uncontrolled.

3. **When performing the primary assessment, open and maintain the airway with the jaw-thrust maneuver.** Insert an oropharyngeal or nasopharyngeal airway, if necessary. Suction secretions without turning the patient's head. Provide positive pressure ventilation or oxygen via a nonrebreather device while manual in-line stabilization is maintained.
4. **Assess the pulse, motor function, and sensation (both pain and light touch) in all extremities.** Record these and document any differences or changes in the neurological status during your contact with the patient.
5. **Assess the cervical region and the neck before applying the cervical spine immobilization collar.** Gently palpate the cervical region for any deformities or tenderness.
6. **Apply a cervical spine immobilization collar.** Be sure that you are familiar with the type of cervical collar you are using. Refer to the manufacturer's instructions on proper sizing since each device is different. An improperly sized collar can cause more harm to the patient, compromise the airway, and further aggravate a potential spine injury. Information about sizing and applying the cervical spine immobilization collar is given on the following pages.

   If the cervical spine immobilization collar does not fit properly, use a rolled towel or blanket instead. Loosely wrap the towel or blanket around the patient's neck to take the place of the cervical collar, taping the towel or blanket to the backboard. Maintain manual in-line stabilization.
7. **Immobilize the patient to a long backboard.** Steps for immobilization in a variety of different circumstances are illustrated and explained on the following pages.
8. **Once the patient is immobilized, reassess, record, and document the pulses and motor and sensory function in all extremities.**
9. **Transport to the hospital.**

Reassessment

Perform a reassessment every 5 minutes en route to the hospital. Ensure that the airway is clear and that breathing is adequate. Reassess and record the vital signs. Look for any changes in the pulse, skin condition, or blood pressure.

Because a spine injury is rarely an isolated injury, look for signs of shock (hypoperfusion): The skin becomes pale, cool, and moist; the blood pressure falls; the heart rate increases; and the patient's mental status decreases. Remember that a decreasing level of responsiveness is an early sign of head injury, while a rising systolic blood pressure and decreasing heart rate are late signs of head injury.

If the patient has any further complaints, repeat those necessary parts of the physical exam. Be aware of complaints of tingling, numbness, loss of sensation, or paralysis anywhere in the body. Re-evaluate any airway adjuncts, positive pressure ventilation devices, mask seal, oxygen therapy, splints, and immobilization devices. Record your findings in the prehospital care report and communicate them to the emergency department.

Summary: Assessment and Care

To review possible assessment findings and emergency care for injuries to the spine, see Figures 32-7* and 32-8*.

Guidelines for Immobilization

As an EMT, you will encounter patients with spine injury or suspected spine injury in a variety of different circumstances. Some may be lying unresponsive on the ground. Others might be responsive, but seated in wrecked automobiles. Still others might be walking about. No matter what the circumstances, your task when you encounter a patient with suspected spine injury is to immobilize that patient safely and swiftly and transport him to a receiving facility. Mastering a variety of tools and techniques will help you carry out this task successfully.

Tools

The basic tools you will use in immobilizing patients are cervical spine immobilization collars, long backboards, and both rigid and vest-type short backboards.

Cervical Spine Immobilization Collars

A cervical spine immobilization collar should be used any time you suspect injury to the spine based on the mechanism of injury, the patient's history, or the signs and symptoms. There are several types of cervical collars (EMT Skills 32-3). *Never use a soft collar; it permits too much movement.*

The collar by itself does not immobilize the patient. The purpose of the collar is not to prevent the head from moving, but rather to prevent the head from moving in relation to the spine and to reduce the compression of the cervical

Assessment Summary

SPINE INJURY

The following findings may be associated with a spine injury.

SCENE SIZE-UP

Pay particular attention to your own safety. Look for:
- Mechanism of injury
- Automobile crash
- Motorcycle crash
- Pedestrian–vehicle collision
- Fall
- Blunt trauma
- Penetrating trauma to the head, neck, and torso
- Hanging
- Diving accident or submersion incident
- Gunshot wound to head, neck, chest, abdomen, or pelvis
- Electrical injury

Primary Assessment

General Impression
- Assume spinal injury based on mechanism of injury
- Patient may be paralyzed and not moving

Mental Status
- Alert to unresponsive, based on type and degree of injury

Airway
- Assume airway is compromised if patient has an altered mental status

Breathing
- May be absent, inadequate, or normal
- Little or no movement of chest with slight or excessive abdominal muscle use, depending on level of spinal cord injury

Circulation
- Pulse and skin color vary, depending on injury
- Pulse may be normal or decreased
- Skin may be normal, or may be pale, cool, and clammy above site of injury and flushed, warm, and dry below site of injury

Status: Priority patient if evidence of a spinal injury or altered mental status exists

Secondary Assessment

Physical Exam

Head and neck:
- Open or closed wounds to the head, neck, or face

Chest:
- Blunt or penetrating trauma to chest

Abdomen:
- Blunt or penetrating trauma to abdomen

Pelvis:
- Blunt or penetrating trauma to pelvic area

Extremities:
- No response to pain or light touch
- Inability to move extremities
- Numbness or tingling sensation in extremities

Posterior body:
- Deformity to spinal column
- Evidence of trauma
- Swelling around spinal column
- Tenderness on palpation of spinal column
- Muscle spasms along spinal column
- Blunt or penetrating trauma to back

Baseline Vital Signs

BP: normal, or may be low

HR: normal, or bradycardia

RR: normal, irregular, decreased, or absent

Skin: normal, or may be pale, cool, and clammy above site of injury and flushed, warm, and dry below site of injury

SpO_2: 95% or greater unless poor perfusion status or breathing status is affected by cord injury

Pupils: equal and reactive, may be sluggish to respond to light

Note: If the blood pressure is low, heart rate is elevated, and skin is pale, cool, and clammy, suspect hypovolemic shock. Look for other trauma and treat for shock.

History
- Tenderness in area of injury
- Pain
- Deformity to the spine
- Soft tissue injuries to posterior body, neck, or cervical region
- Numbness, tingling, weakness, or paralysis in arms and/or legs
- Loss of bowel and bladder control
- Priapism (persistent erection of penis)
- Inadequate breathing or abnormal breathing patterns

FIGURE 32-7a ✻ Assessment summary: spine injury.

Key Points
A collar that is too small will not restrain the head adequately. A collar that is too large may cause extension of the neck and aggravate a spine injury.

Emergency Care Protocol

SPINE INJURY

1. Establish manual in-line stabilization. Do not release it until the patient is immobilized onto the backboard.
2. Establish and maintain an open airway. Insert a nasopharyngeal or oropharyngeal airway if the patient is unresponsive and has no gag or cough reflex.
3. Suction secretions as necessary.
4. If breathing is inadequate, provide positive pressure ventilation with supplemental oxygen at a rate of 10–12 ventilations/minute for an adult and 12–20 ventilations/minute for an infant or child.
5. If breathing is adequate, administer oxygen if the SpO_2 is less than 95% or any signs of respiratory distress or hypoxia are present.
6. Control any major bleeding.
7. Apply a cervical spine immobilization collar.
8. Place the patient on the backboard, pad any voids, and apply a minimum of three straps, at chest, hips, and above knees. Once the torso is secured, secure the head in a head immobilization device.
   - Standing patient: Immobilize using standing immobilization technique.
   - Seated patient with critical injuries: Perform rapid extrication and immobilize to a backboard.
   - Seated patient with no critical injuries: Apply a vest-type immobilization device. Extricate and immobilize to a backboard.
   - Supine or prone patient: Log roll the patient onto a backboard and immobilize.
9. If blood pressure and heart rate are low and skin is flushed below the level of injury, suspect spinal shock with neurogenic hypotension. Treat for shock.
10. If blood pressure is low, heart rate is elevated, and skin is pale, cool, and clammy, suspect hypovolemic shock. Look for other injuries and treat for shock.
11. Transport.
12. Perform a reassessment every 5 minutes if unstable and every 15 minutes if stable. Be prepared for vomiting and seizures.

FIGURE 32-7b * Emergency care protocol: spine injury

spine during movement and transport of the patient. Even if you believe that the injury is only to the cervical (neck) area, the cervical collar is not enough. The entire spine must be stabilized and then immobilized. After a collar is applied, in-line manual stabilization must be maintained until the patient is fully secured to a backboard.

Sizing of the collar to the patient is based on the design of the device (EMT Skills 32-4). Be sure to use a collar of the proper size for the patient.

Using a collar that is too small will not restrain the patient's head adequately. Using a collar that is too large may cause extension of the patient's neck and aggravate the spine injury.

Cervical spine immobilization collars should be applied by two rescuers: One stabilizes the neck manually in the neutral position while the other applies the collar. Placement of the cervical collar should never obstruct the patient's airway. See EMT Skills 32-5, EMT Skills 32-6, EMT Skills 32-7, and EMT Skills 32-8 for detailed descriptions of how to apply a cervical spine immobilization collar.

Full Body Spinal Immobilization Devices

Several different types of long board immobilization devices exist to provide stabilization and immobilization of the head, neck, torso, pelvis, and extremities (EMT Skills 32-9A and 32-9B). Generally, long backboards are used to immobilize patients who are found in a lying or standing position. They may also be used in conjunction with short backboards. For proper immobilization of a patient, padding, straps, and cravats are also used with the long board.

Short Spinal Immobilization Devices

The most common short spine device is the commercially made vest-type device with supplied straps for the head, chest, and legs (EMT Skills 32-9C). A device now less commonly used than in the past is the rigid short spine board. This device requires the addition of backboard straps, padding, tape, or cravats to secure the patient. Both vest-type and rigid devices provide stabilization and immobilization to the head, neck, and torso. They

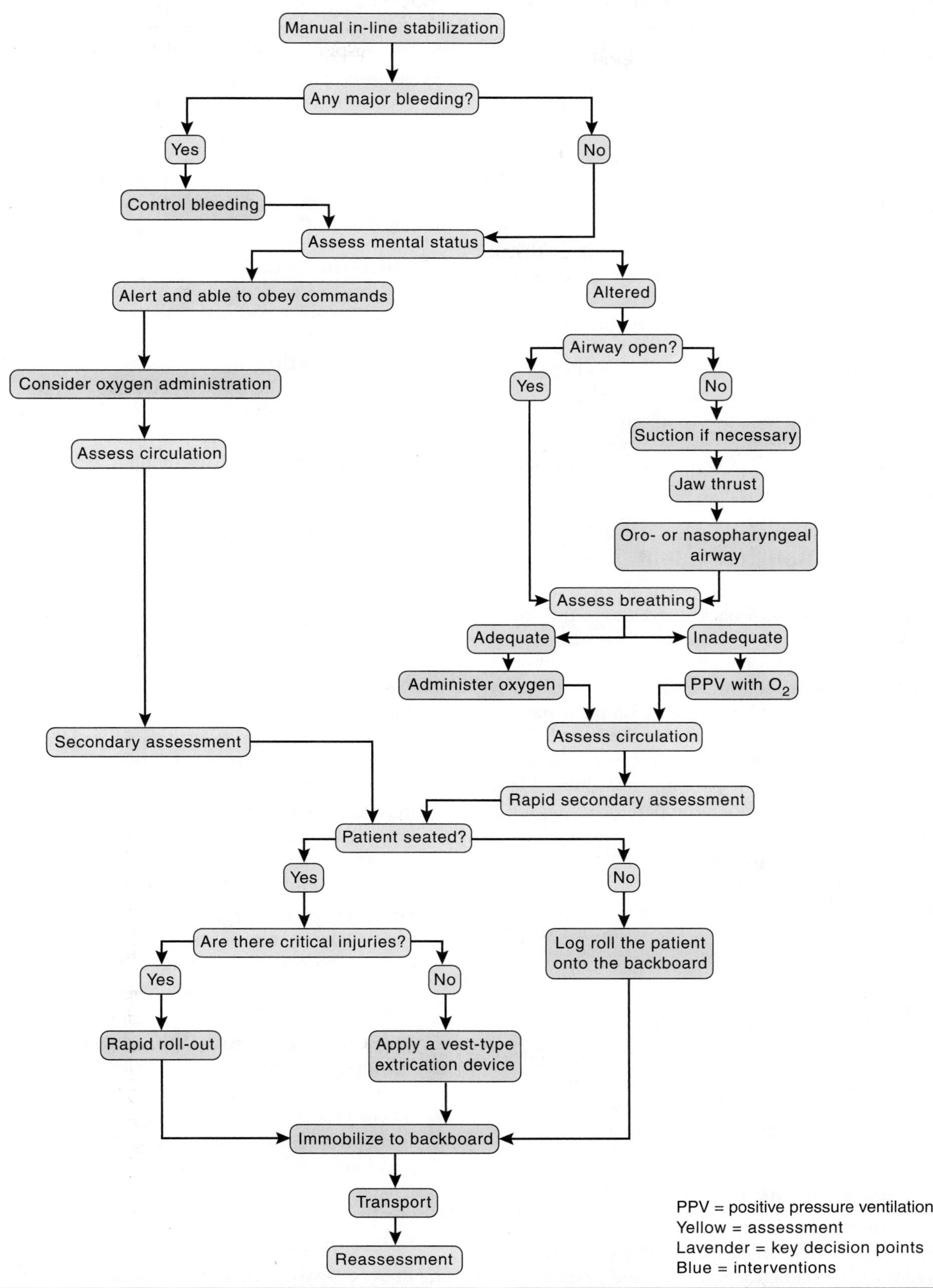
Manual in-line stabilization
Any major bleeding?
Yes
No
Control bleeding
Assess mental status
Alert and able to obey commands
Altered
Airway open?
Yes
No
Suction if necessary
Jaw thrust
Oro- or nasopharyngeal airway
Consider oxygen administration
Assess circulation
Assess breathing
Adequate
Inadequate
Administer oxygen
PPV with O2
Assess circulation
Secondary assessment
Rapid secondary assessment
Patient seated?
Yes
No
Are there critical injuries?
Yes
No
Log roll the patient onto the backboard
Rapid roll-out
Apply a vest-type extrication device
Immobilize to backboard
Transport
Reassessment
PPV = positive pressure ventilation
Yellow = assessment
Lavender = key decision points
Blue = interventions

FIGURE 32-8 ✱ Emergency care algorithm: spine injury.

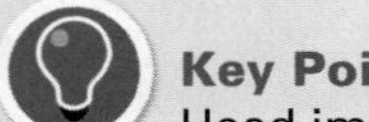

Key Points
Head immobilizers and straps or cravats are used to keep the patient's head and body from rolling, slipping, or sliding up, down, or laterally on the backboard.

Objective 32-14
Describe correct immobilization techniques for a supine or prone patient, a standing patient, and a seated patient.

require a significant amount of time to apply and are most commonly used to immobilize noncritical sitting patients with suspected spine injuries, not critical patients who require rapid transport.

It is very important to be completely familiar with the proper use of these devices to avoid further injury to the patient. For vest-type devices, follow all of the manufacturer's instructions regarding application and use of the device.

Both vest-type and rigid short boards should be used only to immobilize the patient while moving him from a sitting position, then immediately to a long board. Short devices cannot adequately immobilize a patient because they can't immobilize the surrounding joints of the head, torso, and legs.

Other Immobilization Equipment

Whenever a patient is placed onto a backboard, he must be secured to the board with backboard straps and some type of head immobilizer. Techniques for using this equipment to immobilize a patient to a long backboard are discussed in the next section.

Straps or cravats should be placed to keep the patient from sliding up and down or laterally on the board. Place straps across the chest and under the armpits in a manner that does not interfere with the patient's breathing. Place straps across the pelvis and above the patient's knees.

Deceleration straps are another important adjunct to immobilization. These straps are fastened across the patient's shoulders. They help prevent the patient's torso from sliding up the backboard and compressing the cervical spine when the ambulance slows or stops during transport.

Immobilization Techniques

You will encounter patients with suspected spine injuries in a variety of circumstances. The guidelines that follow tell you how to use the tools we have just described to immobilize patients in the most common situations.

Immobilizing a Supine or Prone Patient

When you encounter a supine or prone patient with a suspected spine injury, first ensure that all life-threatening situations have been managed, establish and maintain in-line manual spinal stabilization, and apply a cervical spine immobilization collar. Then you must immobilize the patient to a long backboard. A brief description of the four-rescuer log roll and immobilization procedures are provided in EMT Skills 32-10 and EMT Skills 32-11.

1. **Move the patient onto the spine board by log rolling the patient.** This move is ideally performed by at least four rescuers. One rescuer at the patient's head directs the movement and maintains in-line stabilization of the patient. One to three other rescuers actually move the patient onto the backboard. As the patient is rolled onto his side, his posterior body should be carefully assessed if this has not been done during the primary assessment.
2. **Position the long spine board under the patient by sliding the board under the patient during the log roll.** Then place the patient on the board at the command of the rescuer who is maintaining in-line stabilization. Use a slide, proper lift, log roll, or scoop stretcher to position the patient on the backboard so that movement is as limited as possible. (The method used will depend on the situation, the scene, and available resources.)
3. **Place padding in the spaces between the patient and the board.** In an adult, pad under the head and torso, taking care to avoid extra movement. In an infant or child up to approximately age 8 years, pad under the shoulders (because the child's relatively larger head will otherwise cause the neck to flex forward) and anywhere along the length of the body as necessary to maintain a neutral position.
4. **Immobilize the patient's torso to the board with straps.** The strap across the chest should be tight enough to prevent shifting of the torso but not so tight that it inhibits movement of the chest muscles and impairs breathing.
5. **Immobilize the patient's head to the board with a commercial head/cervical immobilization device or through the use of blanket rolls and tape.** Never place padding behind the neck itself. If the patient vomits, your strapping technique should be good enough to enable you to roll the patient onto his left side several times without any change in body position on the board.
6. **Secure the patient's legs to the board with straps.**
7. **Proceed with care as described earlier under "Emergency Medical Care."**

If only two or three rescuers are available, the log roll can be done using the techniques shown in EMT Skills 32-12 and EMT Skills 32-13.

Immobilizing a Standing Patient

It is not uncommon to find patients with suspected spine injuries standing or walking around at the scene of an accident. Never permit such patients to sit down or to walk to the cot and lie down on a backboard. In such cases, you should instead use a standing long board technique to assist the patient from a standing to a supine position while keeping his spine aligned. This technique is outlined here and also illustrated in EMT Skills 32-14.

1. **One EMT should immediately take normal manual in-line spinal stabilization measures while another EMT applies a cervical collar.**
2. **Position the long board behind the patient.** Examine the back carefully.
3. **Two EMTs should stand on either side of the patient to support him.** Each should place one arm under the patient's armpit and grasp the highest reachable handhold on the long board. The EMTs' other hands should be holding the patient's elbows to steady and support him. The third EMT maintains in-line manual stabilization.
4. **The EMTs at the sides of the patient should each place a leg behind the board.** They should then slowly tip the board backward and begin lowering it to the ground while the third EMT maintains stabilization. Be sure to inform the patient what you are going to do before you tip the board backward.
5. **Once the board is lying level on the ground, one EMT maintains manual stabilization while the others perform the necessary assessment and care.** The patient is then immobilized on the backboard following the guidelines for prone and supine patients given earlier.
6. **Proceed with care as described earlier under "Emergency Medical Care."**

This technique can also be adapted for use by two EMTs, as illustrated in EMT Skills 32-15.

Immobilizing a Seated Patient

If the patient with a suspected spine injury is found in a seated position, a short spinal immobilization device will be used. This will minimize movement and aggravation of potential spine injury while the patient is being transferred to a long board for complete immobilization.

The following are general steps to follow. The steps involved in using a vest-type device are illustrated in EMT Skills 32-16.

1. **Use manual in-line spinal stabilization and apply a cervical collar.** Assess pulses and motor and sensory function in all four extremities.
2. **Position the short spinal device behind the patient.** Examine the back carefully. Be careful that the EMT who is holding in-line spinal stabilization does not move excessively or move the patient as the device is positioned. You should slide the board behind the patient and as far into the seat as you can. The top of the board should be level with the top of the patient's head, and the bottom of the board should not extend past the coccyx. The body flaps should fit snugly under the patient's armpits.
3. **Secure the device to the patient's torso.** Make sure the straps are tight enough to prevent movement of the device laterally or vertically. If the device has straps that circle the legs, apply and tighten these after the chest straps are applied.
4. **Pad behind the patient's head to ensure neutral alignment of the head and neck with the remainder of the spine.** Excessive padding will cause the head and neck to flex forward, whereas lack of padding will allow the head and neck to be extended.
5. **Secure the patient's head to the device.** Maintain manual in-line spinal stabilization even though the head is secured to the device. Securing the head is the last step in the application of the device.
6. **Position a long backboard under or next to the patient's buttocks and rotate him until his back is in line with the backboard.** Lower the patient onto the backboard while maintaining manual in-line spinal stabilization. If it is not possible to get a long backboard next to the patient, lift the patient under his arms and legs and lower him onto the long board.
7. **Follow the guidelines for immobilizing a patient to a long backboard.** Release manual in-line spinal stabilization only when the patient is completely secured to the backboard. Assess pulses and motor and sensory function and record your findings on the prehospital care report.
8. **Proceed with care as described earlier under "Emergency Medical Care."**

There are several special considerations to be aware of when using a short spinal device:

- Do any assessment of the back, scapula, arms, or clavicles before you apply the board.
- Angle the board to fit between the arms of the rescuer who is stabilizing the patient's head without jarring the rescuer's arms.
- As already mentioned, push the spine board as far down into the seat as possible. If you don't, the board may shift and the patient's cervical spine may compress. The top of the board must be level with the top

Objective 32-15
Describe the indications for rapid extrication and the correct procedures for rapid extrication.

Objective 32-16
Explain special spinal handling and immobilization considerations, when spinal injury is suspected, for helmet removal, for football injuries, and in infants and children.

of the patient's head; the base of the board must not extend past the coccyx.

- Never place a chin cup or chin strap on the patient. They will prevent the patient from opening his mouth if he needs to vomit.
- When applying the first strap to the torso, take care not to apply the strap too tightly, which could cause abdominal injury or impair breathing.
- Always tighten the torso and leg straps before securing the patient's head to the device. This prevents accidental movement of the patient's cervical spine.
- Never allow buckles to be placed midsternum where they would interfere with proper hand placement if CPR becomes necessary.
- Never pad between the cervical collar and the board; doing so creates a pivot point that may cause hyperextension of the cervical spine when the head is secured.
- Assess pulses and motor and sensory function before and after applying the device.

Rapid Extrication

There are times when you will have to move a patient with a suspected spine injury before immobilizing him to a long backboard or even to a short spinal device. The three situations in which such movement is permissible are as follows:

- The scene is not safe (because of the threat of fire or explosion, chemical spills, or gunfire, for example).
- The patient's condition is so unstable that you need to move and transport him immediately.
- The patient blocks your access to a second, more seriously injured patient.

In these circumstances—when the time saved by immediate extrication will make the difference between life and death—a *rapid extrication* is performed. Rapid extrication eliminates the delay inherent in the use of spinal immobilization devices. Time is critical in the situations just described; therefore, the benefit of rapid transport outweighs the risk of movement during extrication.

Rapid extrication requires constant cervical spine stabilization and good communication among the EMTs moving the patient. The patient's entanglement with seat belts, wreckage, or other objects can complicate rapid extrication procedures, so all rescuers need to be aware of the patient's position as well as any potential problems as the extrication is proceeding.

In rapid extrication, the patient is brought into alignment with manual in-line spinal stabilization and a cervical spine immobilization collar is applied. A long backboard is positioned next to him. The patient is quickly transferred to the long backboard while manual in-line spinal stabilization is maintained. The rapid extrication procedure is described in more detail in EMT Skills 32-17A to 32-17D.

The rapid extrication technique requires EMTs to improvise at the scene based on the type of car, location of the roof support posts, console between the seats, and size of the patient. If time, resources, and patient condition permit, removal of the roof will allow for much better access to the patient and for easier removal using the rapid extrication technique, as illustrated in EMT Skills 32-17E and 32-17F.

Special Considerations

Handling and immobilization of patients with suspected spine injuries can be complicated by a variety of factors. Two of the more common situations you will encounter involve suspected spine injury in people wearing helmets and suspected spine injury in infants and children.

Helmets

Activities such as bicycle riding, motorcycle riding, and playing football can easily lead to accidents that can produce spine injury. People taking part in such activities often wear helmets, and you may arrive at an accident scene to encounter a patient still wearing a helmet. Thorough assessment of a patient is difficult under any circumstances; the presence of a helmet makes the task still more difficult. But removal of a helmet should not be an automatic step. Such removal could risk aggravating the spine injury, if one exists. You should first assess the patient wearing the helmet in the following areas:

- Assess the patient's airway and breathing.
- Assess the fit of the helmet and the likelihood of movement of the patient's head within the helmet.
- Determine your ability to gain access to the patient's airway if intervention should be necessary to assist his breathing.

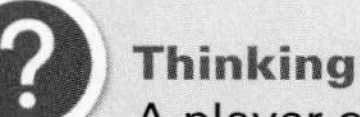

Thinking Critically
A player on the local high school football team has collapsed on the field after a rough tackle. He is responsive but unable to obey your commands. You pull out your extractor tool to cut the clips of his face mask, but your partner says, "Let's get him loaded. We can get the mask off en route." Is your partner right? Why or why not?

Key Points
For an injured football player, decisions about removing or not removing shoulder pads and helmet should take into account airway alignment as well as access for assessment and treatment.

You should *leave the helmet in place* if your assessment reveals the following:

- The helmet fits well, and there is little or no movement of the patient's head inside the helmet.
- There are no impending airway or breathing problems.
- Removal of the helmet would cause further injury to the patient.
- You can properly immobilize the spine with the helmet in place.
- The helmet doesn't interfere with your ability to assess and reassess airway and breathing.

You should *remove the helmet* if your assessment reveals the following:

- The helmet interferes with your ability to assess or reassess airway and breathing.
- The helmet interferes with your ability to adequately manage the airway or breathing.
- The helmet does not fit well and allows excessive movement of the head inside the helmet.
- The helmet interferes with proper spinal immobilization.
- The patient is in cardiac arrest.

Helmet Removal

There are two basic types of helmets: sports helmets (such as those worn for football) and motorcycle helmets. Typically, sports helmets have an opening in the front and allow much easier access to the airway. Face masks on football helmets can be removed either by cutting the plastic clips that hold the mask to the helmet or by unsnapping the face mask retainers. Motorcycle helmets, on the other hand, generally cover the full face and have a shield that prevents access to the airway.

The techniques for the removal of motorcycle and sports helmets are illustrated in EMT Skills 32-18 and EMT Skills 32-19. The general steps for removal of a helmet are these:

1. Take the patient's eyeglasses off before you attempt to remove the helmet.
2. One rescuer should stabilize the helmet by placing hands on each side of the helmet with fingers on the mandible (lower jaw) to prevent movement.
3. A second rescuer should loosen the chin strap.
4. The second rescuer should place one hand anteriorly on the mandible at the angle of the jaw and the other hand at the back of the head.
5. The rescuer holding the helmet should pull the sides of the helmet apart (to provide clearance for the ears), gently slip the helmet halfway off the patient's head, then stop.
6. The rescuer who is maintaining stabilization of the neck should reposition, sliding his hand under the patient's head to keep the head from falling back after the helmet is completely removed.
7. The first rescuer should remove the helmet completely.
8. The patient should then be immobilized as described earlier.

Football Injuries

When dealing with football injuries, the EMT has to take into consideration the equipment football players wear. In most cases, an injured player is wearing not only a helmet but also shoulder pads. Usually the shoulder pads and the helmet elevate the player's head, neck, and shoulders off the ground, almost in a neutral position. Because of this, you should leave the helmet on the player unless it is absolutely necessary to remove it. Removing the helmet while leaving the shoulder pads on will cause the head to drop and hyperextend the neck. Removal of the shoulder pads is difficult because the player is usually on his back and the attempt may cause unnecessary movement, risking aggravation of his injury.

According to the Inter-Association Task Force for Appropriate Care of Spine-Injured Athletes, the face mask of the helmet should be removed at the earliest possible point, but before transportation. The face mask should be removed any time a spinal injury is suspected, regardless of the mental status and airway or respiratory status of the patient. As already noted, the helmet should only be removed in specific situations.

Removal of the Face Mask If you are expected to respond to or stand by at football events, it is important that you have the proper tools to remove the face mask of the helmet in the quickest way with the least amount of movement (EMT Skills 32-20). Several different types of tools, such as the FM extractor, Trainer's Angel, knives, pruning shears, and PVC pipe cutters, can be used to remove the face mask. Even though the plastic clips holding the face

Key Points
In a collision involving a child in a car seat, you must extricate the child from the car seat. You cannot immobilize a child in a car seat for transport.

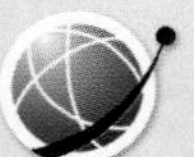

Media Resources
Go to www.bradybooks.com for mykit. Highlights:

- *Animation:* Cervical Injuries and Application of a Cervical Collar
- *Video:* How to Use a KED
- *Video:* When to Use a Long Board

mask are typically screwed in place, a screwdriver is *not* recommended to take off the face mask. Unscrewing the clips causes excessive movement of the head, especially if the screws have been in place for some time and are rusted. DuraShears, EMT shears, and a seat belt cutter are also not recommended because these tools take too much time to cut the plastic clips. A simple pruning tool used for gardening often is the best device to use.

The face mask of the helmet is usually secured by four plastic loop-clips or loop-straps that are screwed into the helmet. By cutting these plastic straps or clips, the face mask can be completely removed. This allows the EMT complete access to the airway for assessment and intervention. A common practice has been to cut the side clips or straps and lift or "peel" the face mask upward. By this method, the face mask is said to be "retracted" or "swung away." This is no longer recommended, since it causes excessive movement of the head and neck during the process. It is now recommended that all four clips or straps be cut and the face mask completely lifted off the helmet.

Immobilization of the Player One EMT or trainer will maintain in-line spinal stabilization by grasping the helmet and holding the head and neck in a neutral in-line position. The helmet, chin straps, and pads should be left in place. A second EMT will remove the face mask. Once the face mask has been removed, the patient assessed, and emergency care provided, the patient must be completely immobilized to a backboard.

Every attempt must be made to apply a cervical spine immobilization collar. However, it may be impossible to apply a cervical collar with the football equipment in place. Do not remove the helmet or shoulder pads to apply a cervical collar. Instead, if the collar cannot be applied with the helmet and pads in place, pad with towels, blanket rolls, or other such material to reduce movement.

A six-person lift is recommended to move the patient onto the backboard. Once on the backboard, straps must be applied to secure the chest, pelvis, and lower extremities above the knees. Acceleration/deceleration straps should be used to reduce movement during braking and acceleration of the ambulance. The helmet should be taped to the backboard to prevent movement. Keep the chin strap in place the entire time, even after the patient is completely immobilized. Any gaps between the patient and the backboard should be filled in with towels, pillowcases, or other items.

There are only two circumstances in which the helmet should be removed: (1) if it does not adequately secure the head because it is too large for the patient, or (2) if you cannot gain access to the airway. If the helmet is removed, padding must be added behind the head to ensure that the head and shoulder pads are kept in a neutral in-line position. Except in the noted circumstances, it is not recommended to remove the helmet.

Infants and Children

When treating infants or children, use a rigid board appropriate for the child's size, following the guidelines outlined earlier for general immobilization. However, the following special considerations should apply when immobilizing infants or children:

- Pad from the shoulders to the heels of an infant or a child, if necessary, to maintain neutral in-line immobilization. The larger head of the infant or young child usually up until 8 years of age causes the head and neck to flex when supine. Use padding behind the shoulders and upper back to eliminate flexion and maintain neutral alignment of the head, neck, and spine.
- Make sure the cervical collar fits properly before applying it to an infant or child. If you don't have a collar that fits, immobilize the neck with a rolled towel, tape the towel to the backboard, and manually support the patient's head in a neutral in-line position. An improperly fitted collar will do more harm than good.

Extrication from a Car Seat If you are at an automobile collision involving a child in a car seat, *you cannot use that car seat to stabilize the child for transport.* Car seats involved in crashes may have lost the integrity of the structure and may not provide protection to the child if another crash were to occur. Transfer the child to a backboard. If a child needs to be extricated from a car seat for treatment, follow the steps shown in EMT Skills 32-21.

EMT skills 32-1 Assessing Neurological, Motor, and Sensory Function

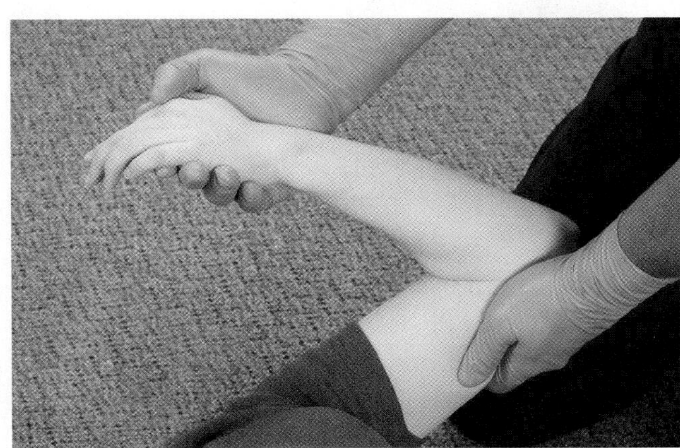

32-1A * Assess flexion.

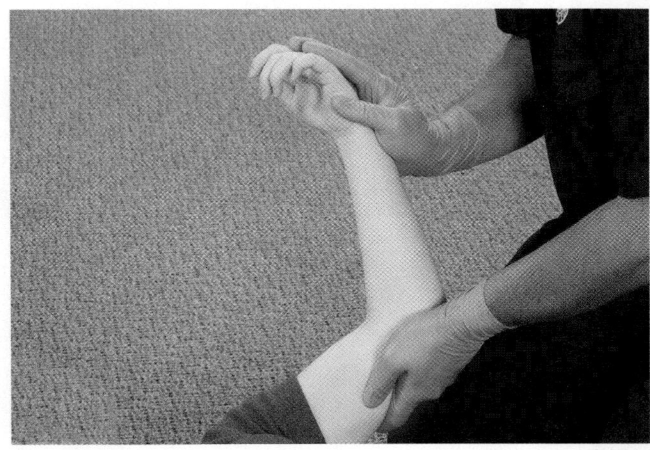

32-1B * Assess extension.

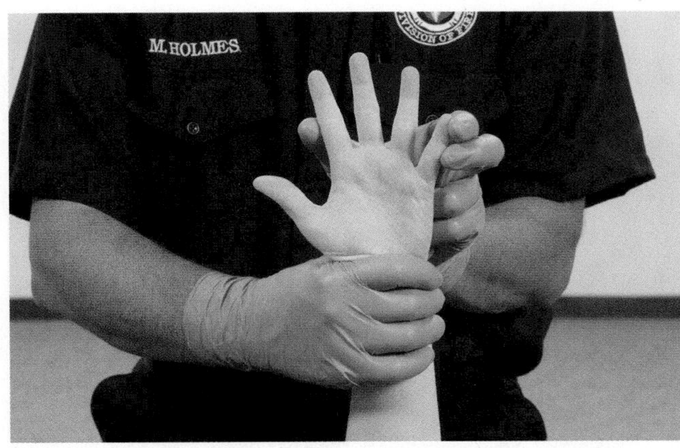

32-1C * Assess finger abduction.

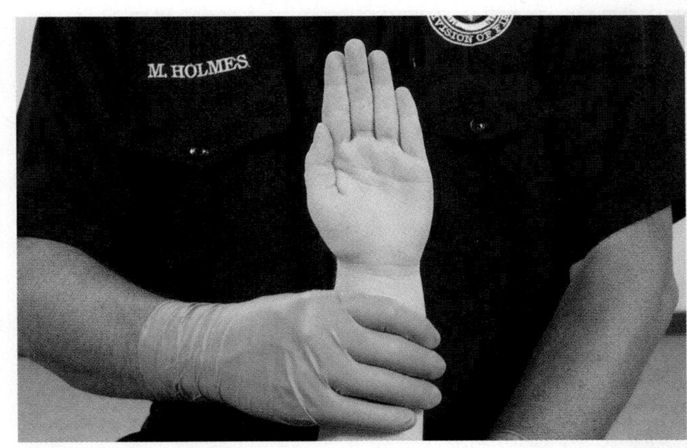

32-1D * Assess finger adduction.

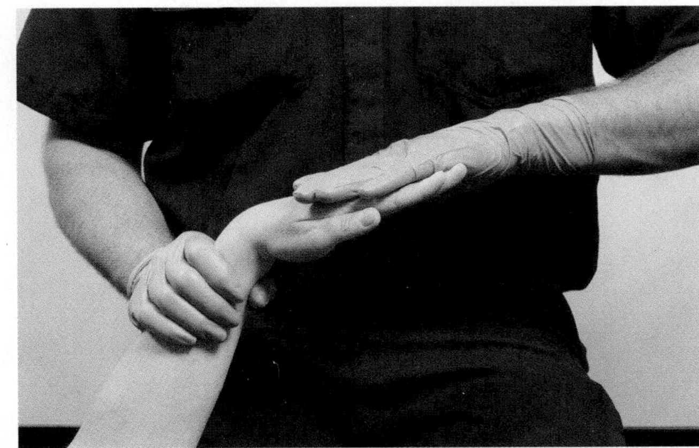

32-1E * Assess the wrist and hand.

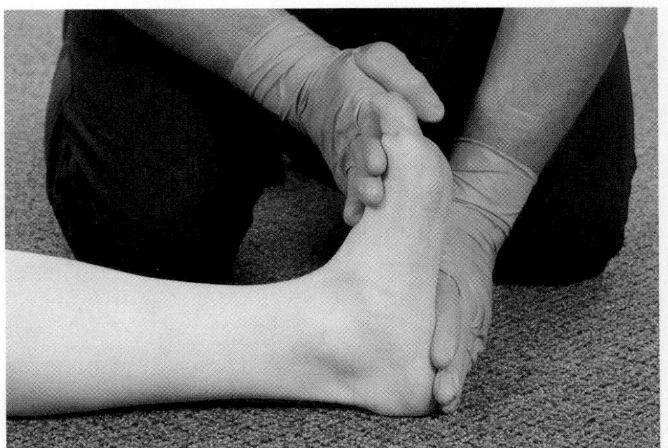

32-1F * Assess plantar flexion.

continued

Assessing Neurological, Motor, and Sensory Function
continued

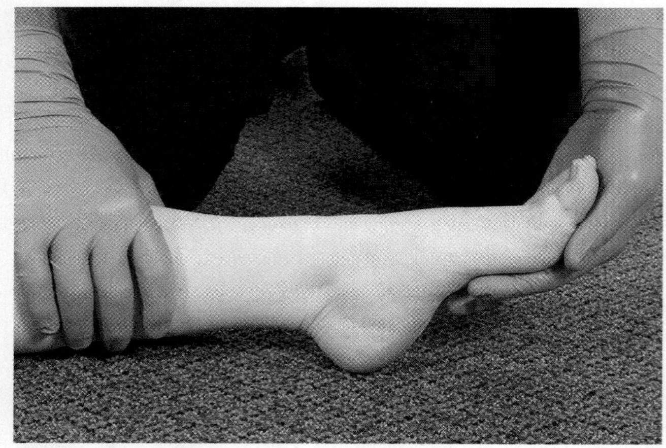

32-1G ✱ Assess dorsiflexion.

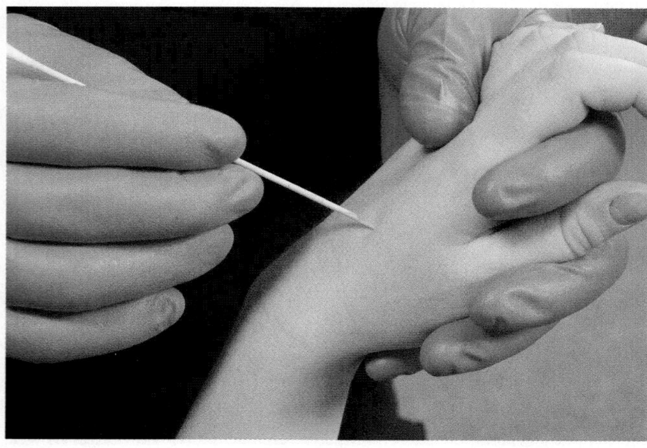

32-1H ✱ Assess pain response in the hand.

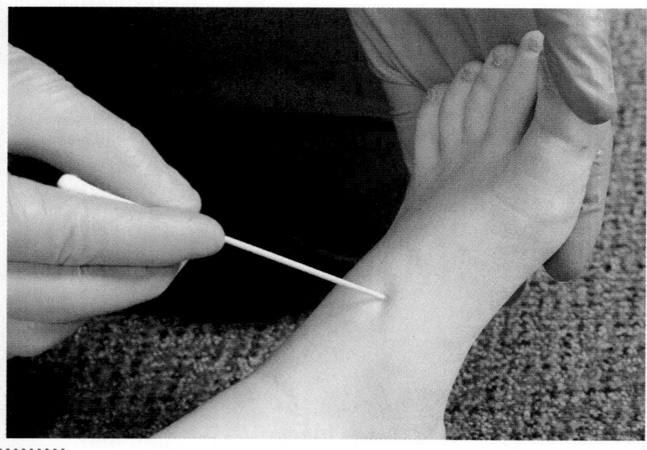

32-1I ✱ Assess pain response in the foot.

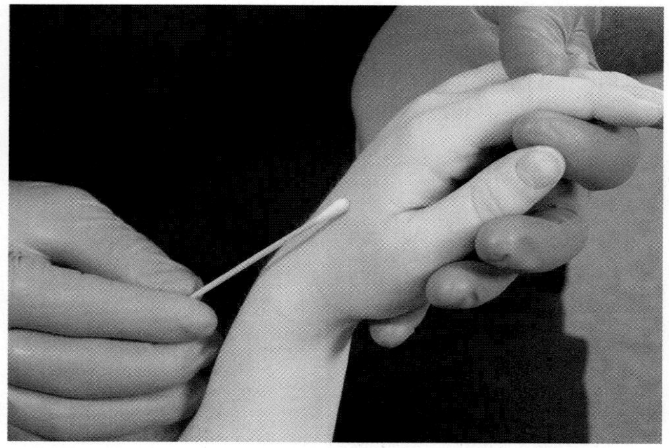

32-1J ✱ Assess light touch response in the hand.

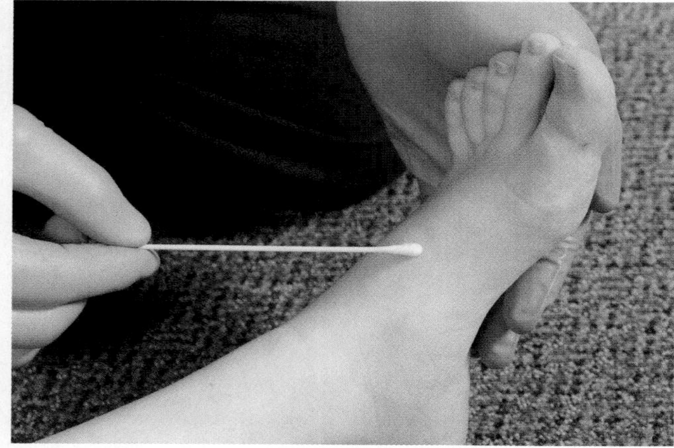

32-1K ✱ Assess light touch response in the foot.

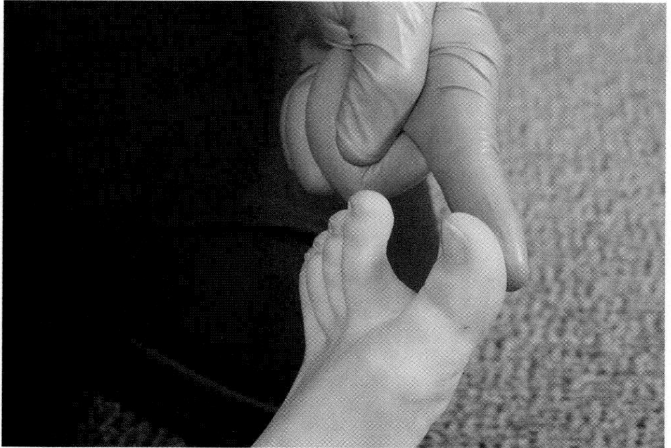

32-1L ✱ Assess flexion of the great toe on the same foot.

EMT skills 32-2 Establish Manual In-Line Stabilization

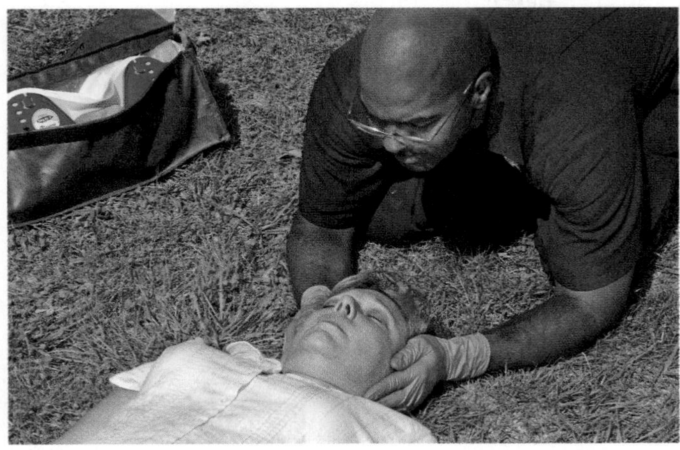

32-2A ✱ Properly position your hands.

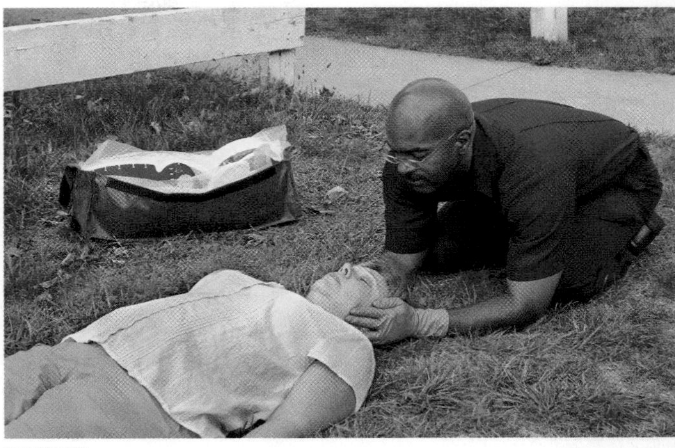

32-2B ✱ Keep the head in a neutral position and the nose in line with the patient's navel.

EMT skills 32-3 Cervical Spine Immobilization Collars

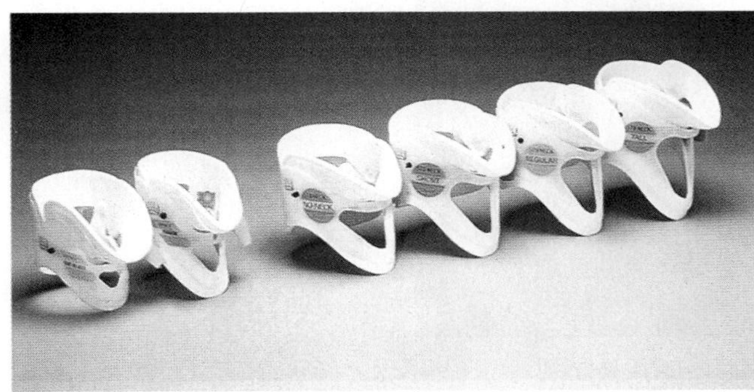

33-3A ✱ Stifneck cervical spine immobilization collars. (© Laerdal Medical Corporation)

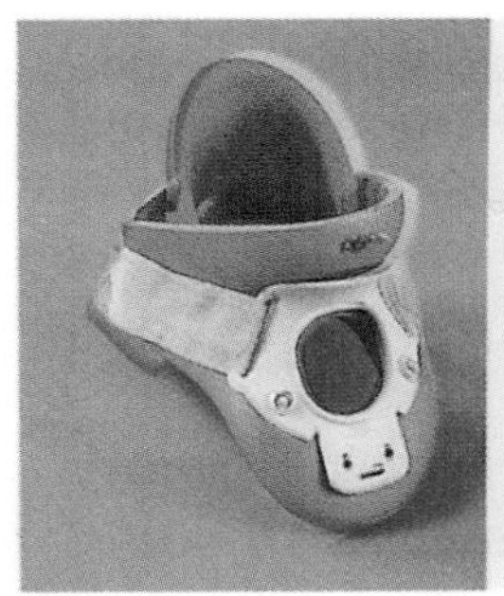

33-3C ✱ Philadelphia Cervical Collar assembled and disassembled. (© Philadelphia® Cervical Collar Co.)

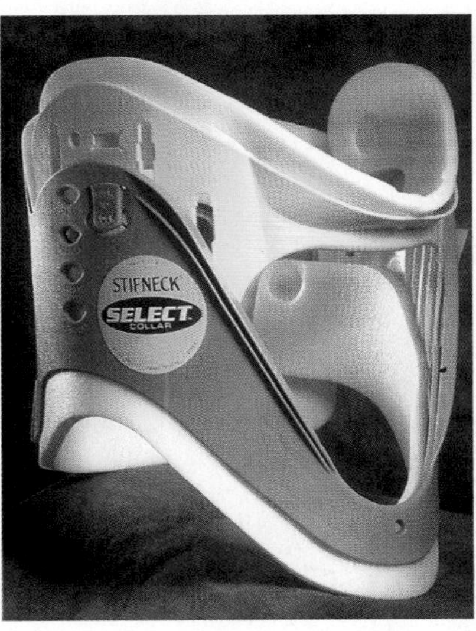

33-3B ✱ The Stifneck Select collar can be adjusted to fit all sizes. (© Laerdal Medical Corporation)

Sizing a Cervical Spine Immobilization Collar

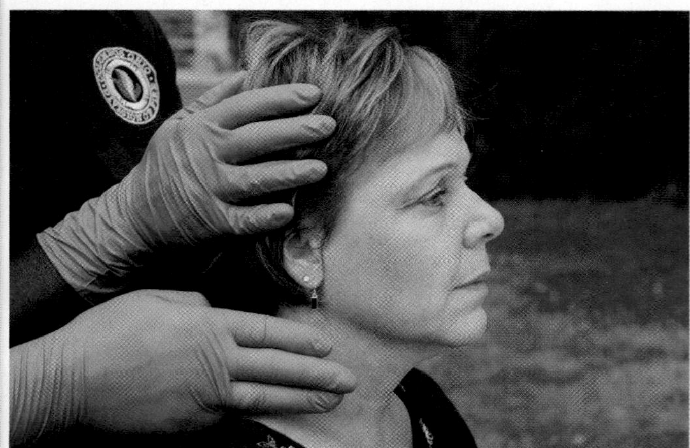

32-4A ✱ To size a cervical spine immobilization collar, first draw an imaginary line across the top of the shoulders and the bottom of the chin. Use your fingers to measure the distance from the shoulder to the chin.

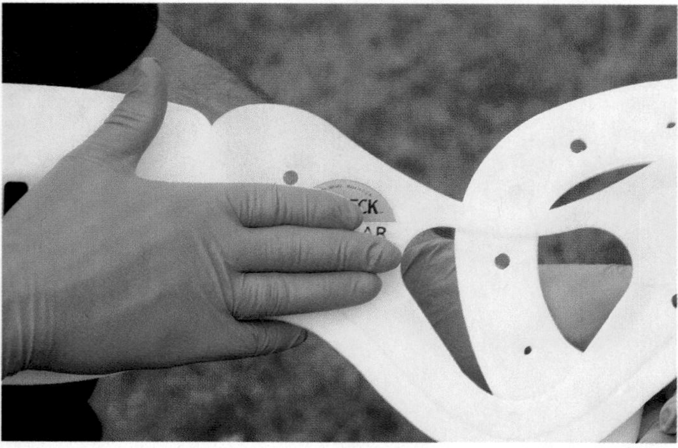

32-4B ✱ Check the collar you select. The distance between the sizing post (black fastener) and lower edge of the rigid plastic should match that of the number of stacked fingers previously measured against the patient's neck.

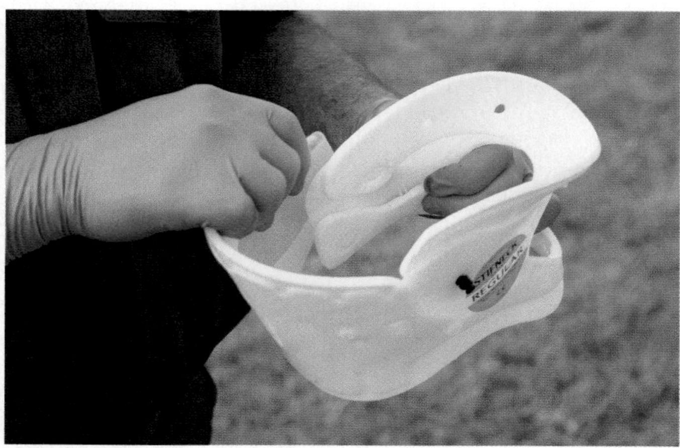

32-4C ✱ Assemble and preform the collar.

EMT skills 32-5 Applying a Cervical Spine Immobilization Collar to a Seated Patient

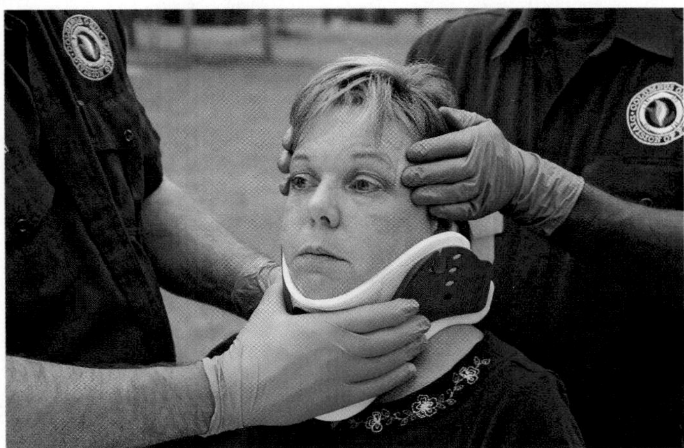

32-5A ✱ After selecting the proper size, slide the cervical spine immobilization collar up the chest wall. The chin must cover the central fastener in the chin piece.

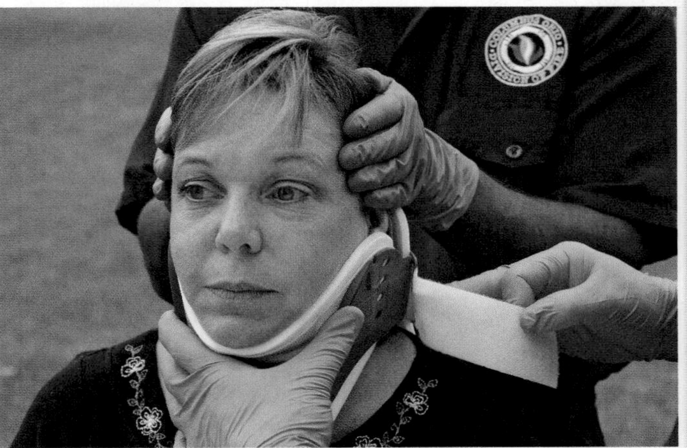

32-5B ✱ Bring the collar around the neck and secure the Velcro. Recheck the position of the patient's head and collar for proper alignment. Make sure the patient's chin covers the central fastener of the chin piece.

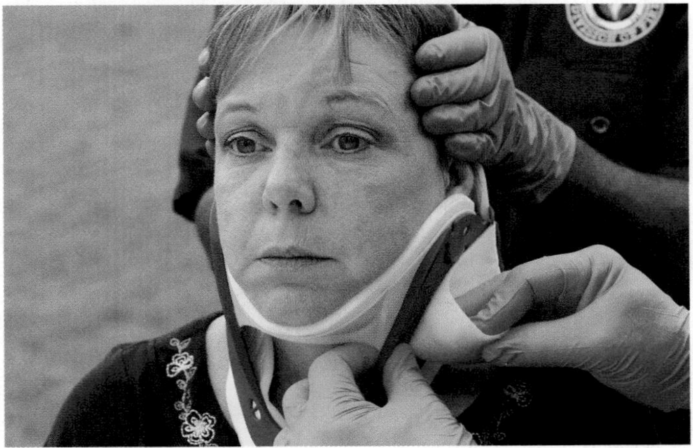

32-5C ✱ If the chin is not covering the fastener of the chin piece, readjust the collar by tightening the Velcro until a proper sizing is obtained. If further tightening will cause hyperextension of the patient's head, then select the next smaller size.

EMT skills 32-6 Applying a Cervical Spine Immobilization Collar to a Supine Patient

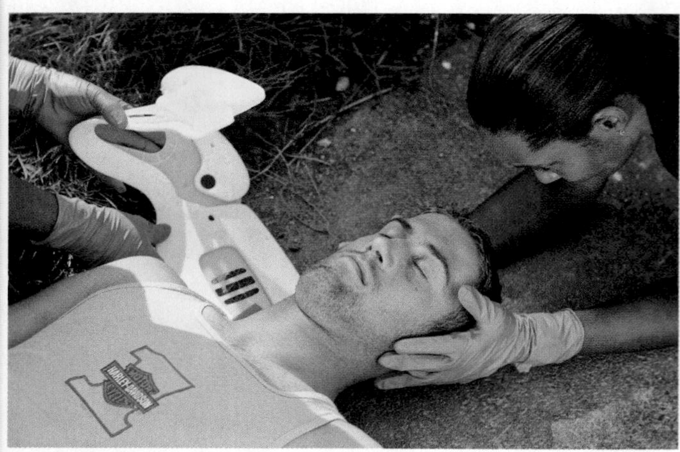

32-6A ✱ Slide the back portion of the cervical spine immobilization collar behind the patient's neck. Fold the loop Velcro inward on the foam padding.

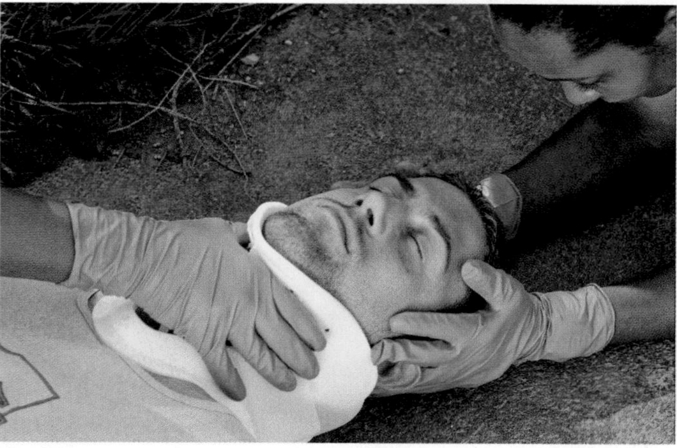

32-6B ✱ Position the collar so that the chin fits properly. Secure the collar by attaching the Velcro.

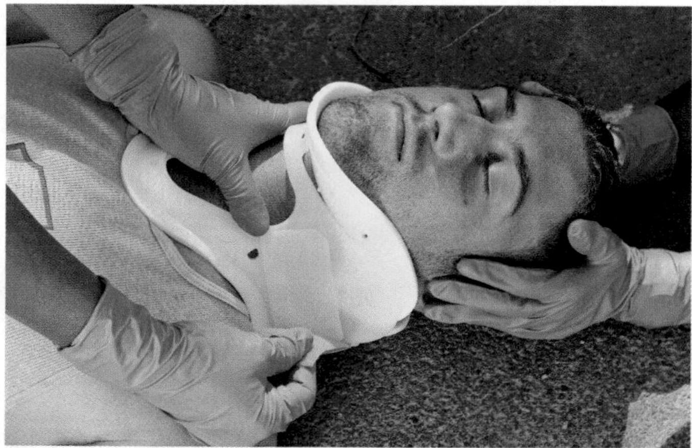

32-6C ✱ Hold the collar in place by grasping the trachea hole. Attach the loop Velcro so it mates with (and is parallel to) the hook Velcro.

EMT skills 32-7 Applying an Adjustable Collar to a Seated Patient

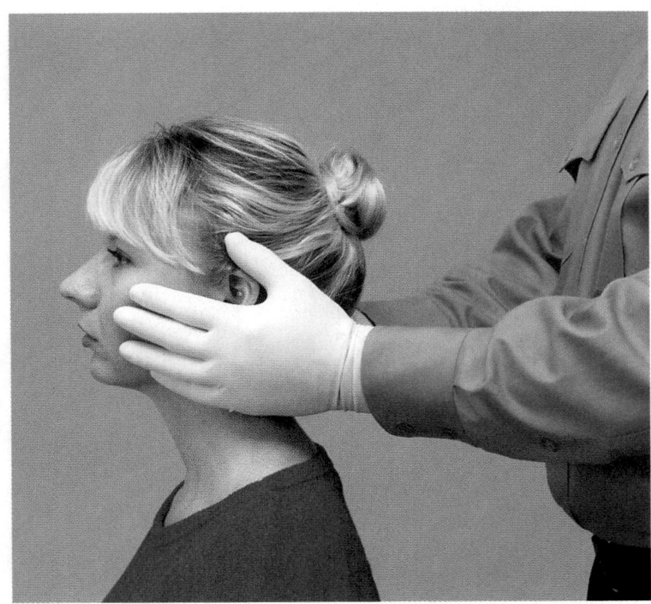

32-7A * Stabilize the head and neck from the rear.

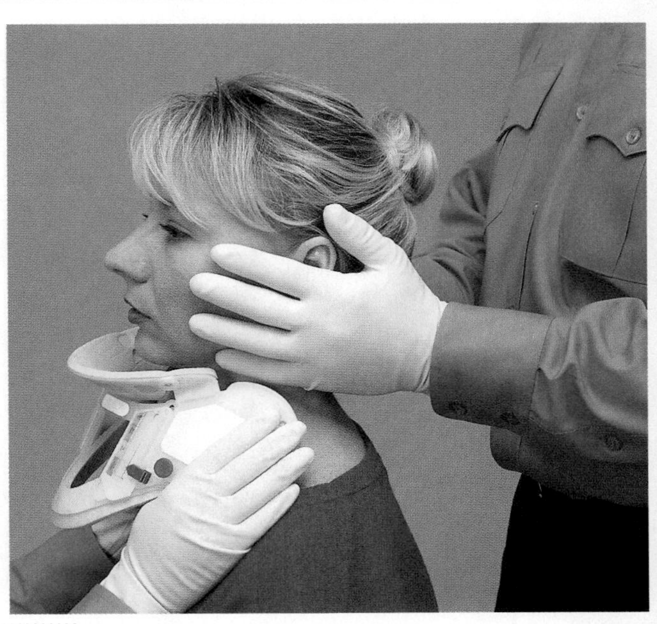

32-7B * Properly angle the collar for placement.

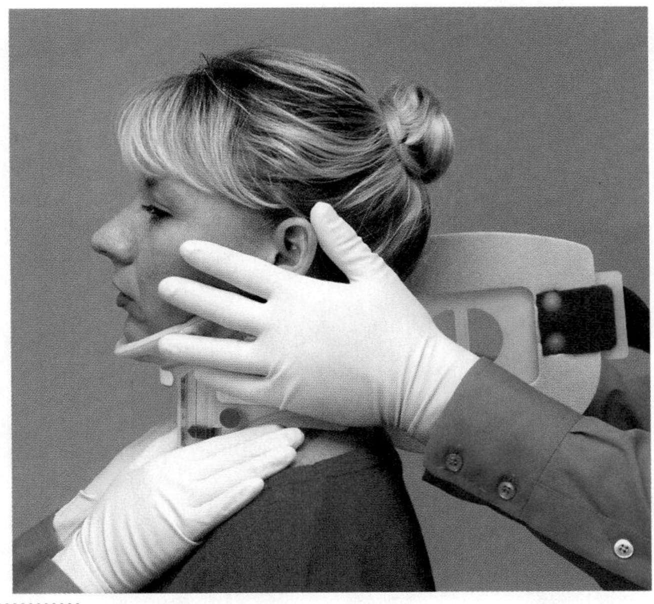

32-7C * Position the collar bottom.

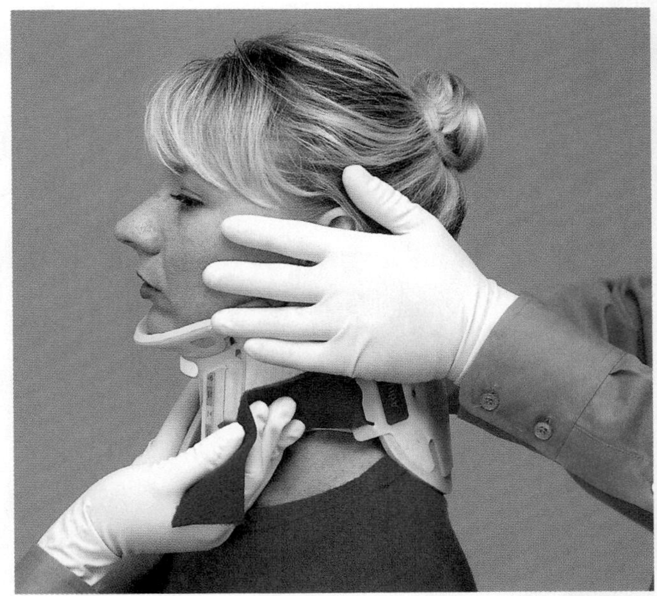

32-7D * Set the collar in place around the neck.

continued

EMT skills 32-7 Applying an Adjustable Collar to a Seated Patient *continued*

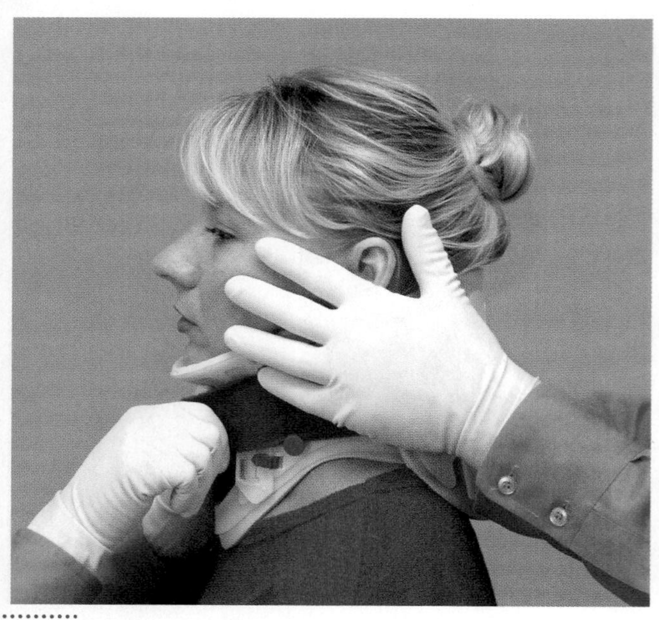

32-7E * Secure the collar.

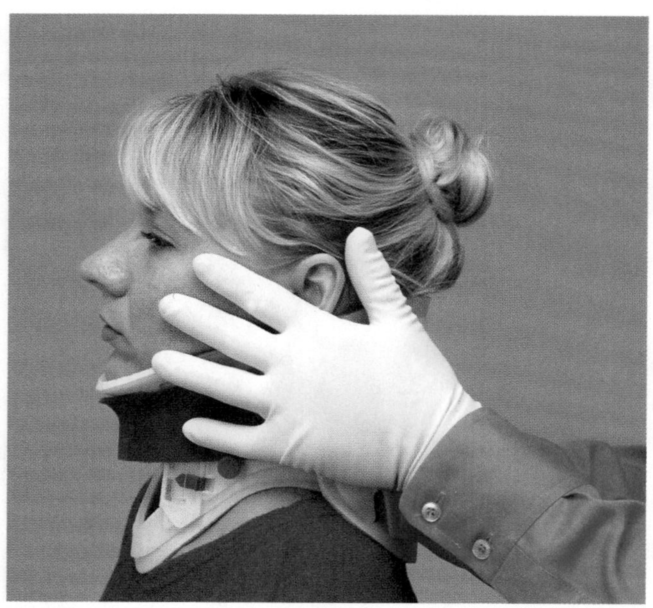

32-7F * Maintain manual stabilization of the head and neck.

EMT skills 32-8 Applying an Adjustable Collar to a Supine Patient

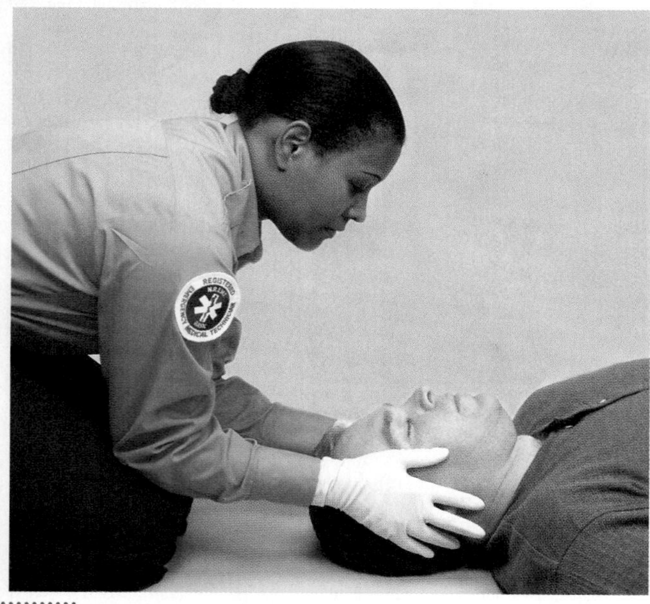

32-8A * Kneel at the patient's head and stabilize the head and neck.

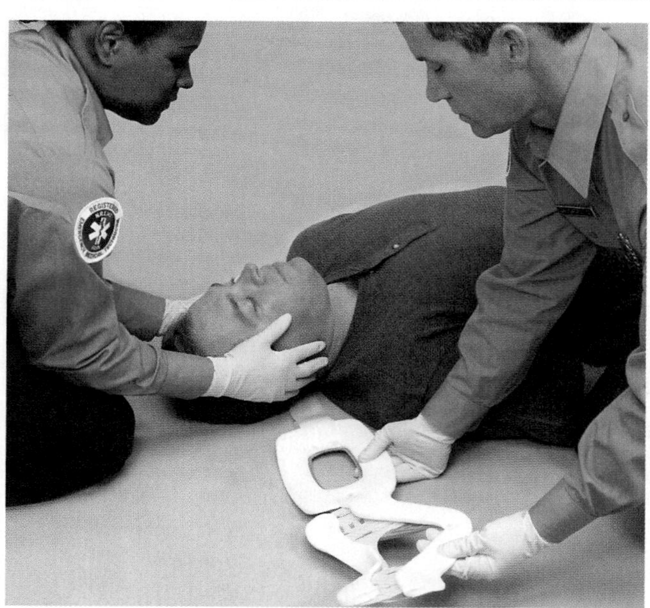

32-8B * Set the collar in place.

EMT skills 32-8 Applying an Adjustable Collar to a Supine Patient *continued*

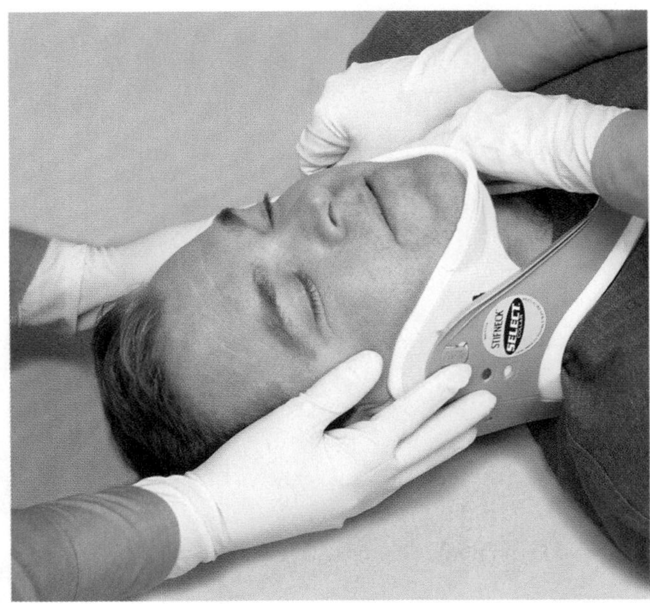

32-8C ✱ Secure the collar.

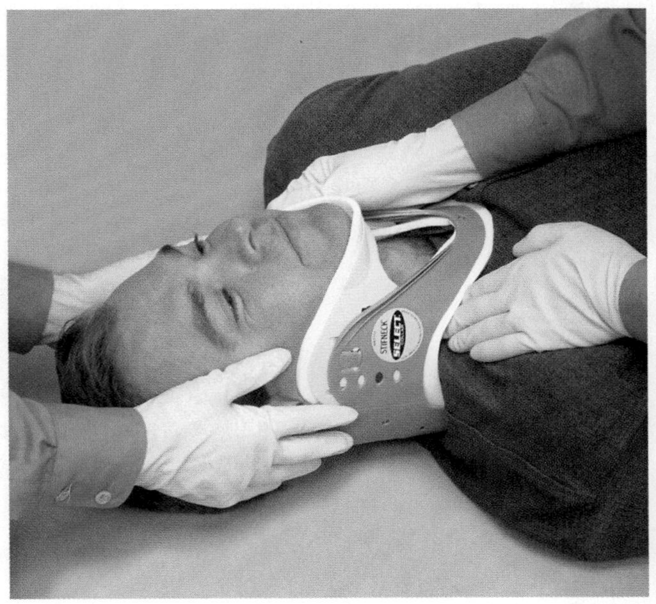

32-8D ✱ Continue to manually stabilize the head and neck.

EMT skills 32-9 Examples of Immobilization Devices

Always follow local protocol in purchasing and using immobilization devices.

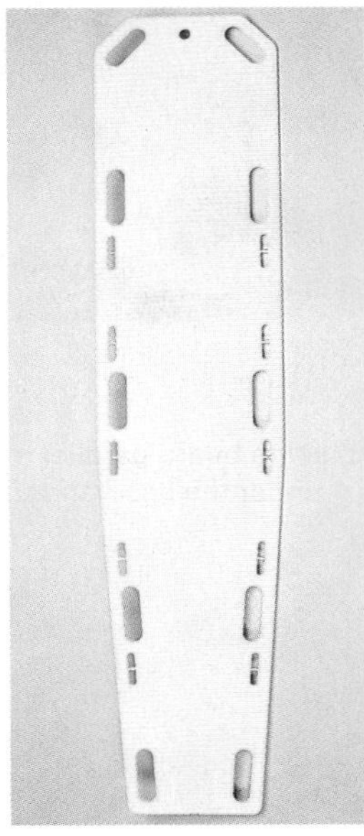

32-9A ✱ Composite backboard.

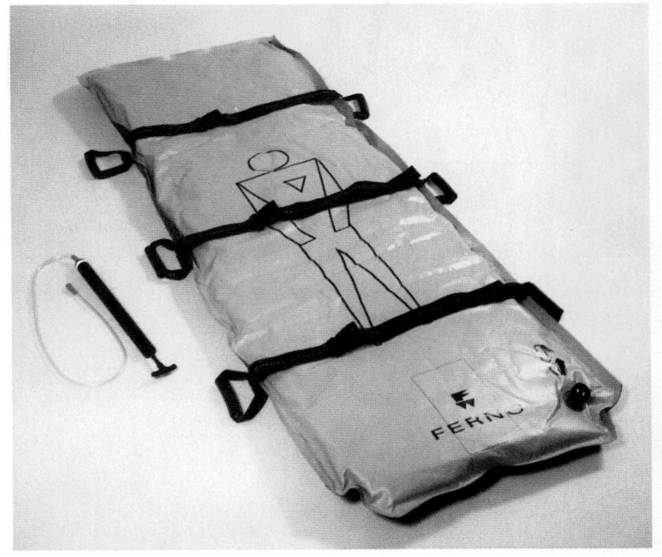

32-9B ✱ Full body vacuum splint. (© Ferno Corporation)

continued

EMT skills 32-9 Examples of Immobilization Devices *continued*

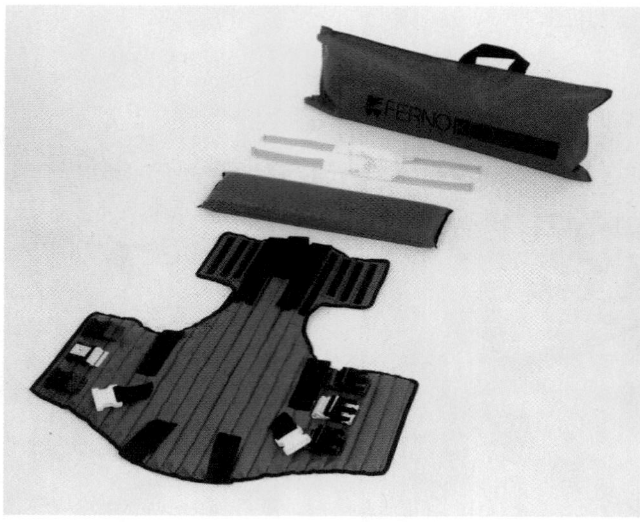

32-9C ✻ KED (Kendrick Extrication Device). (© Ferno Corporation)

EMT skills 32-10 Four-Rescuer Log Roll and Long Spine Board Immobilization

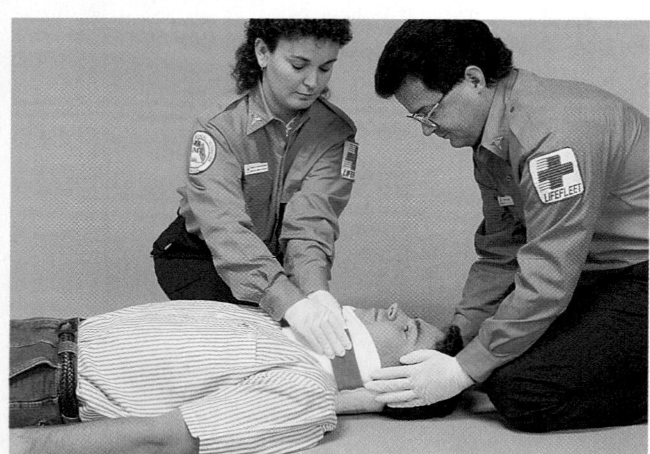

32-10A ✻ Establish and maintain in-line stabilization. Apply a rigid cervical spine immobilization collar.

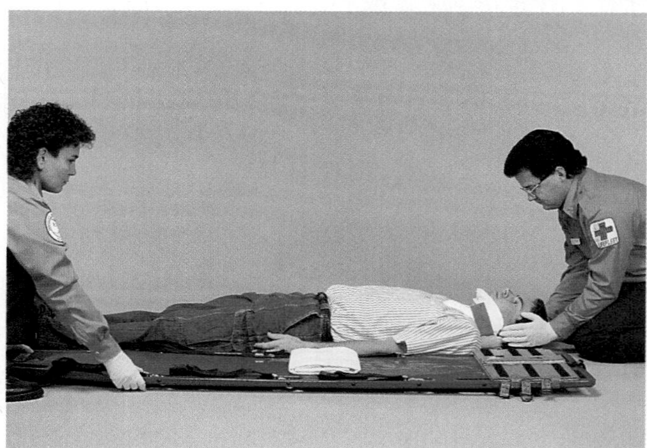

32-10B ✻ Place a long spine board parallel to the patient. If possible, pad the voids under the head and torso.

Four-Rescuer Log Roll and Long Spine Board Immobilization *continued*

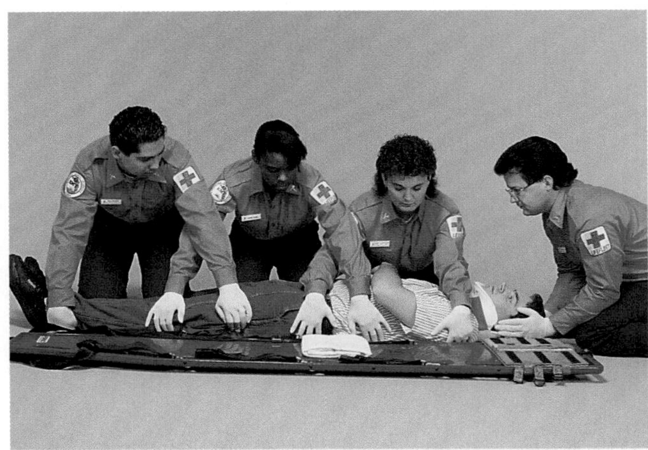

32-10C ✱ Three rescuers kneel at the patient's side opposite the board, leaving space to roll the patient toward them.

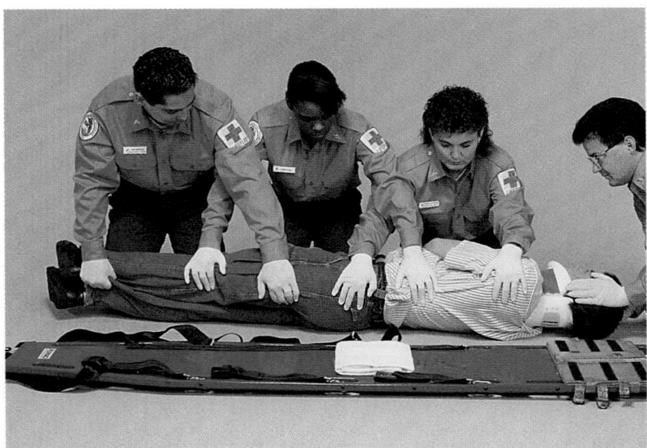

32-10D ✱ The EMT at the head directs the others to roll the patient as a unit onto his side. Assess the patient's posterior side.

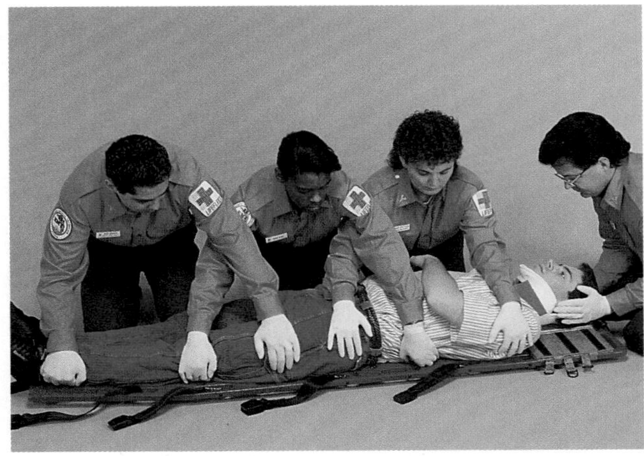

32-10E ✱ The EMT at the waist reaches over, grasps the spine board, and pulls it into position against the patient. (This can also be done by a fifth rescuer.) The EMT at the head instructs the rescuers to roll the patient onto the spine board.

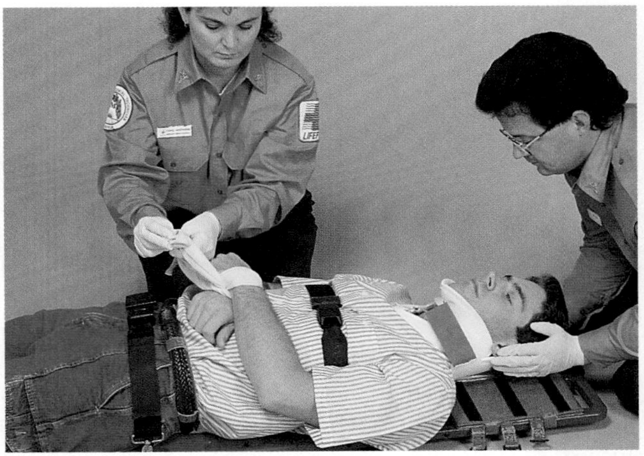

32-10F ✱ Secure the patient to the board with straps. Loosely tie the wrists together.

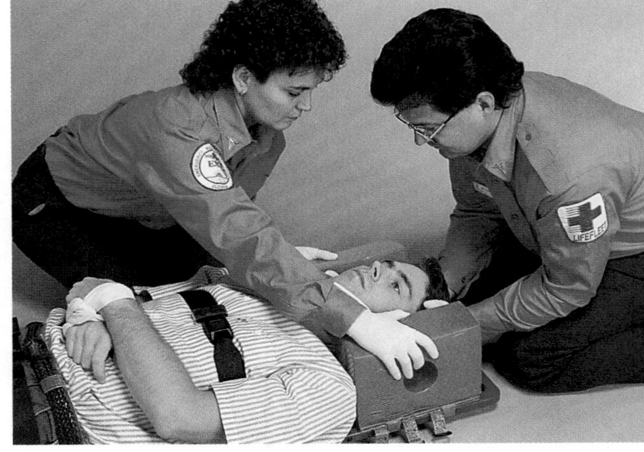

32-10G ✱ Using a head/cervical immobilizer, secure the patient's head to the spine board.

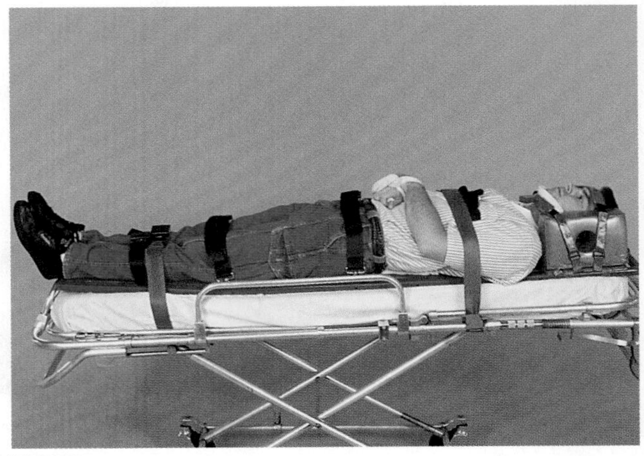

32-10H ✱ Transfer the patient and the spine board as a unit. Secure the patient and the spine board to the cot.

EMT skills 32-11 Immobilizing a Patient to a Long Board

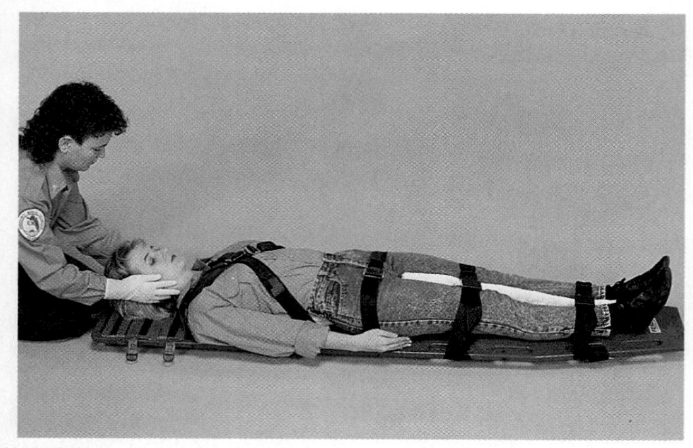

32-11A ✱ Apply straps to secure the patient to the backboard. Place one strap at the level of the chest, one at the hip, one above the knee, and another below the knee. Pad between the legs.

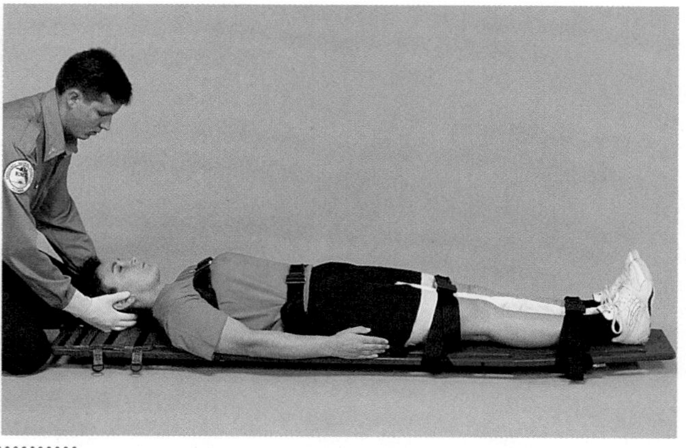

32-11B ✱ An "X" strap method secures the torso to the backboard. Also apply one strap at the hip, one above the knee, and one below the knee.

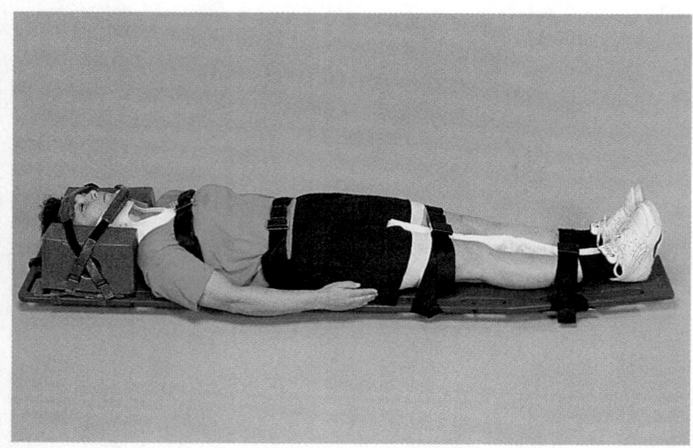

32-11C ✱ Secure the patient's head to the backboard with a head immobilization device.

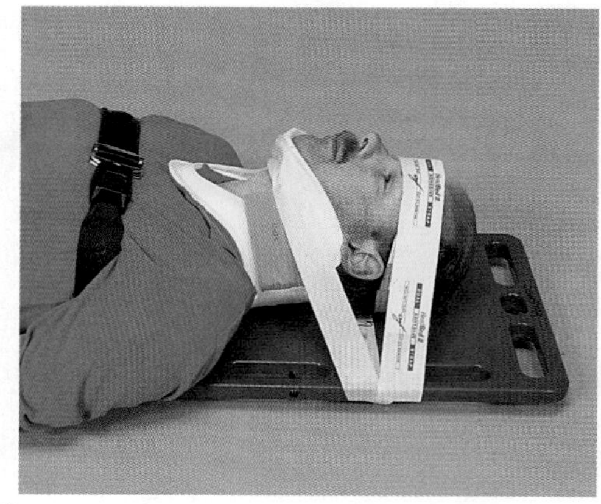

32-11D ✱ Disposable head immobilization device.

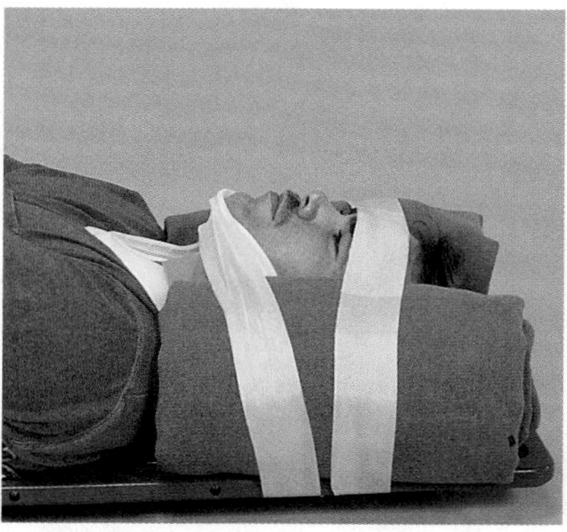

32-11E ✱ Blanket rolls and tape can be used.

EMT skills 32-12 Three-Rescuer Log Roll

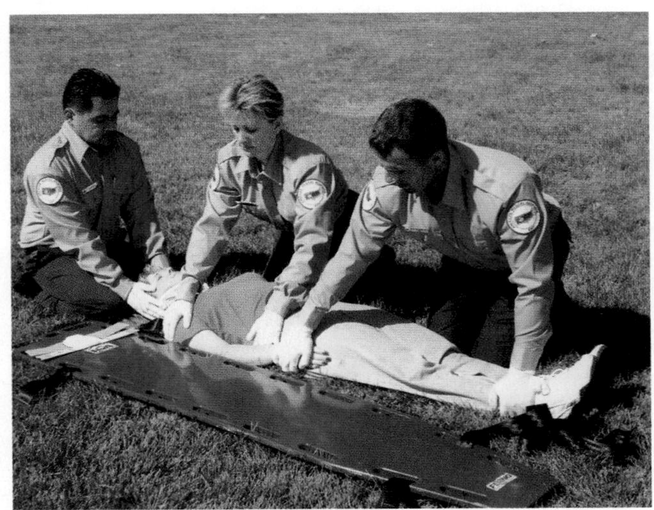

32-12A ✱ Maintain in-line spinal stabilization while preparing for the log roll.

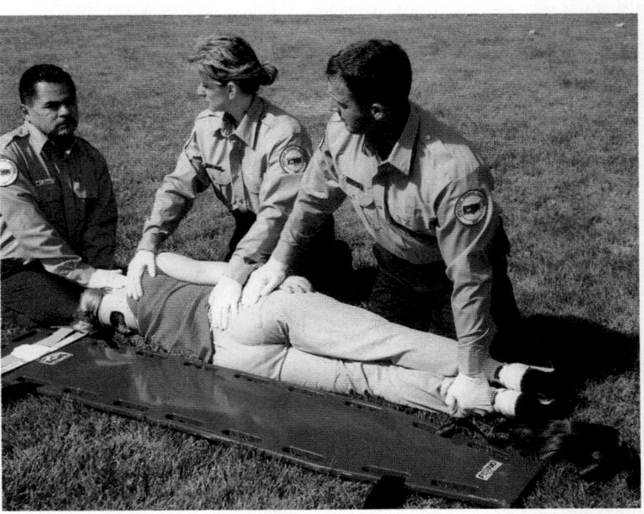

32-12B ✱ Roll the patient onto the side at command of the EMT maintaining stabilization. Inspect the back.

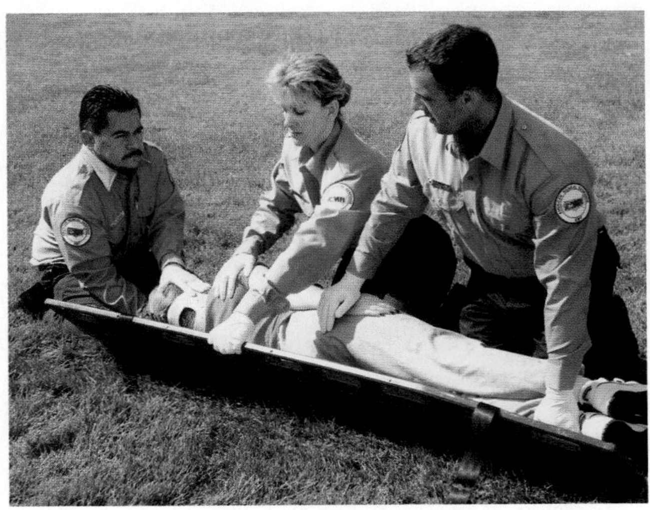

32-12C ✱ Move the spine board into place.

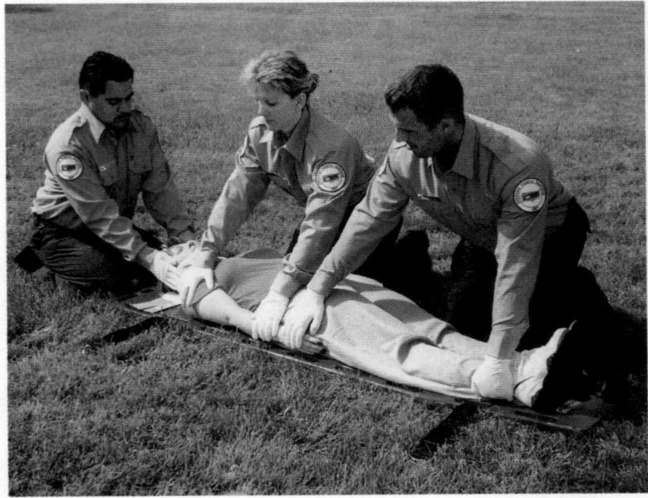

32-12D ✱ Lower the patient onto the spine board at command of the EMT maintaining in-line stabilization. Center the patient on the board.

EMT skills 32-13 Two-Rescuer Log Roll

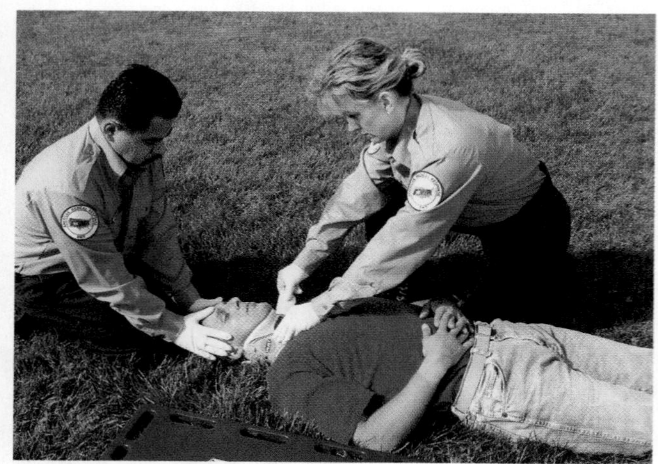

32-13A * Maintain an open airway and in-line spinal stabilization while applying a cervical spine immobilization collar.

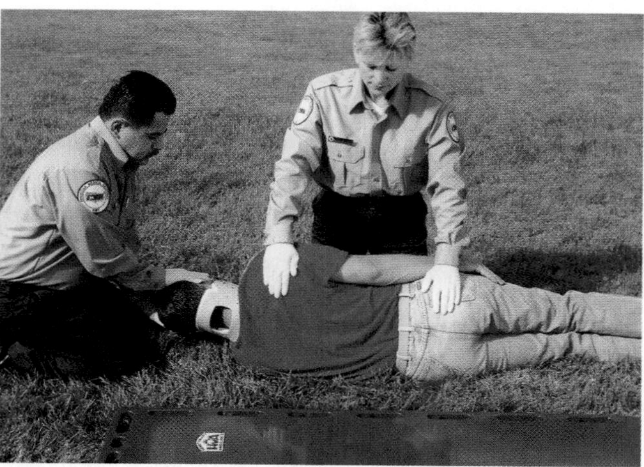

32-13B * Maintain in-line support while moving the patient onto the side.

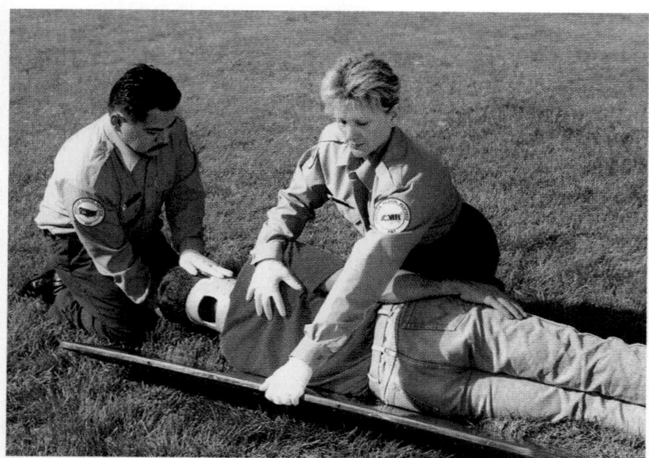

32-13C * Pull the board against the patient.

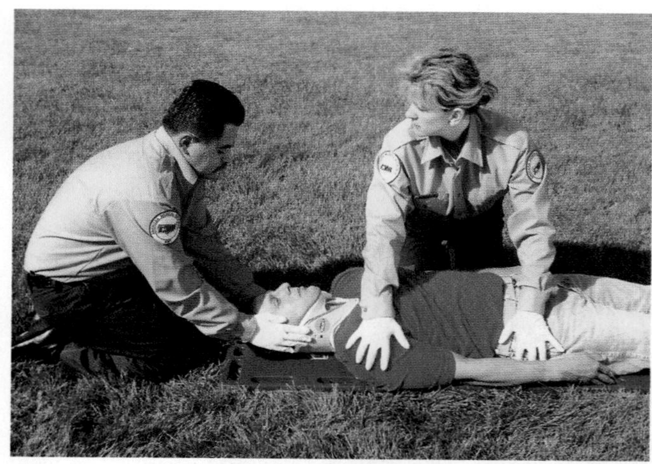

32-13D * Roll the patient gently onto the board and secure.

EMT skills 32-14 Immobilizing a Standing Patient—Three EMTS

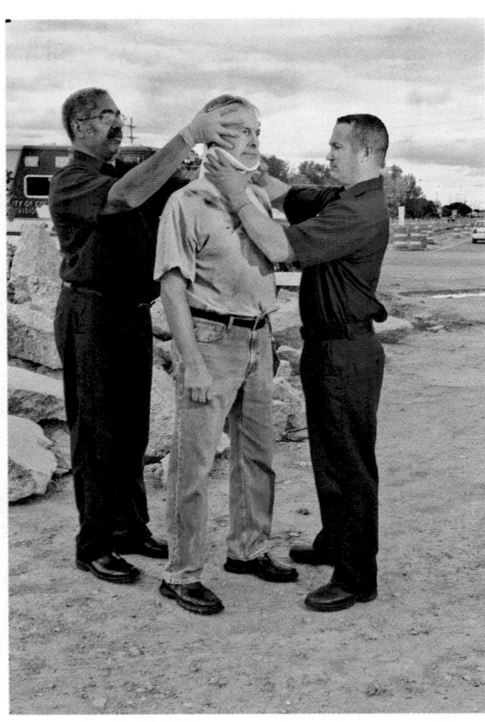

32-14A * Apply a cervical spine immobilization collar while in-line stabilization is being held.

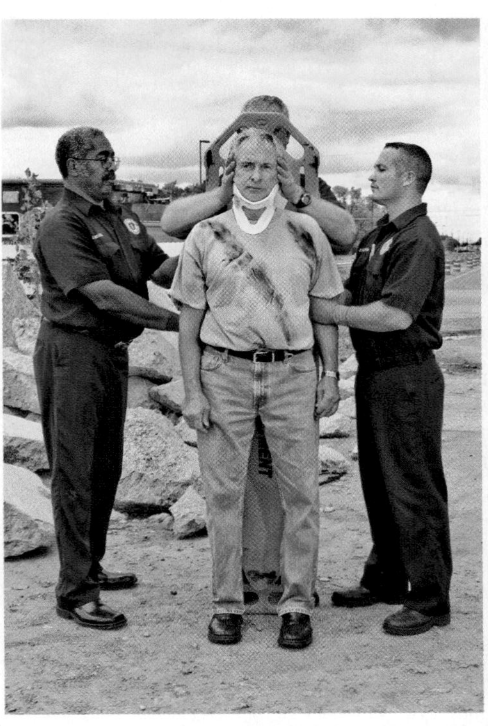

32-14B * Position the backboard behind the patient and align it properly. Check the position of the board from the front of the patient.

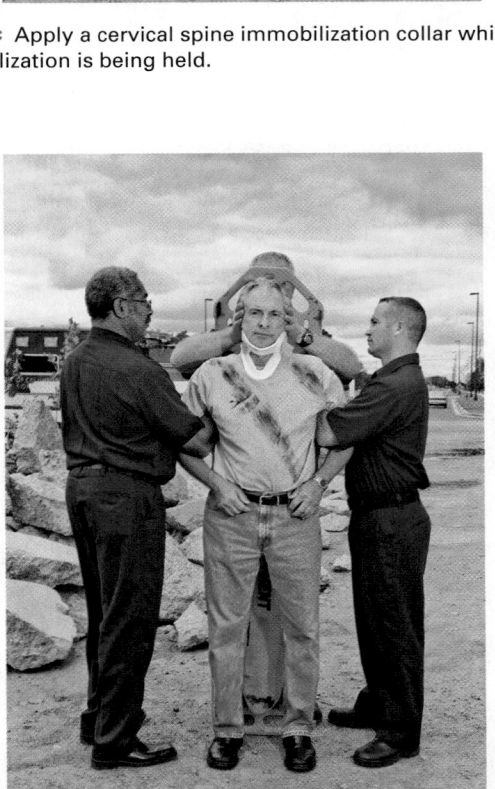

32-14C * The EMTs at the sides of the patient place their hands under each arm and grasp the next highest handhold. Their other hands grasp the elbows of the patient to provide additional stabilization on the board.

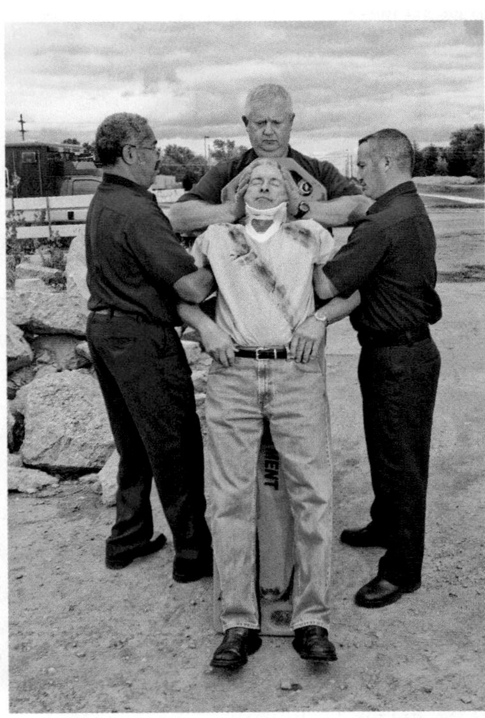

32-14D * Lower the patient to the ground. Continue holding in-line stabilization until the patient is completely immobilized to the backboard with a head/cervical immobilization device and straps.

EMT skills 32-15 Immobilizing a Standing Patient—Two EMTS

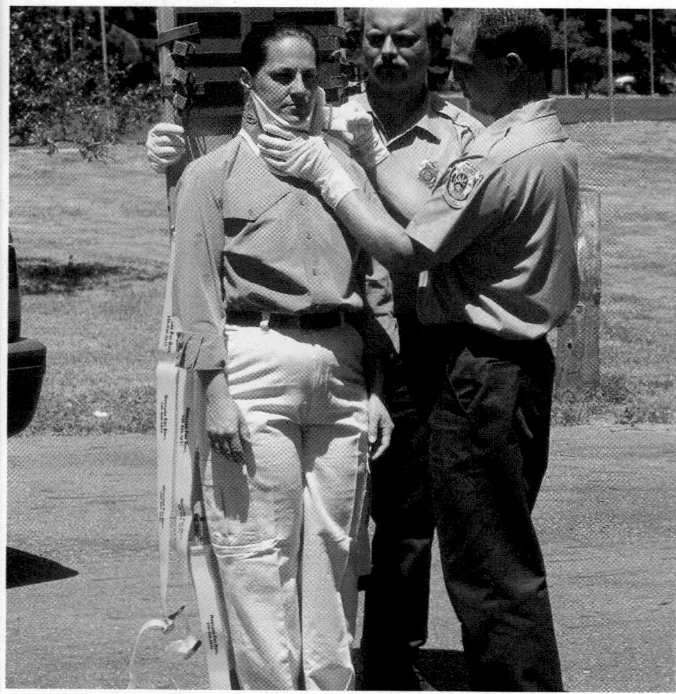

32-15A ✱ Apply a cervical spine immobilization collar and position the long board behind the patient.

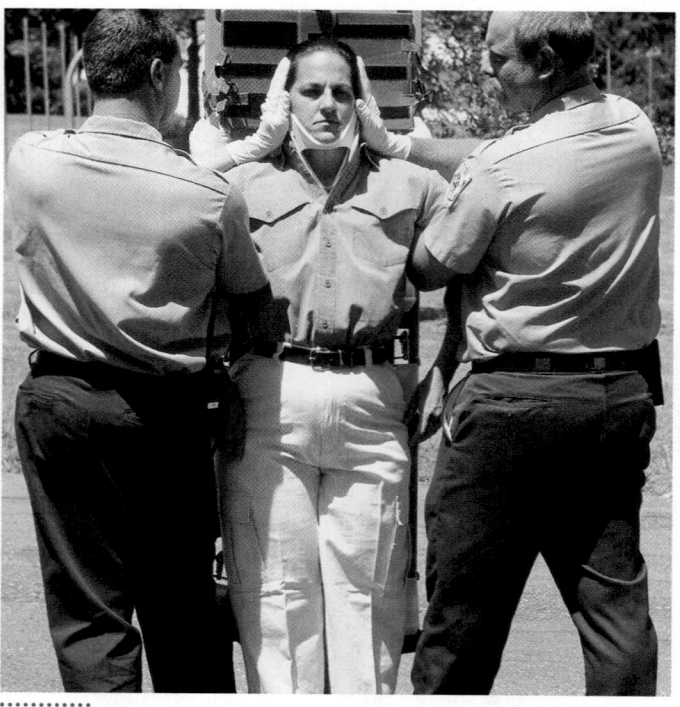

32-15B ✱ The EMTs on each side of the patient hold the long board in place and hold the patient's head in a neutral in-line position.

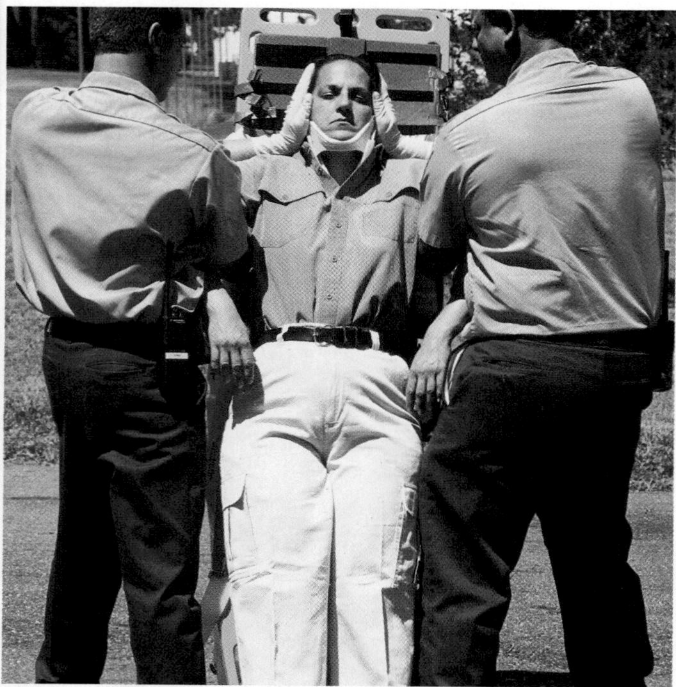

32-15C ✱ Each EMT then places the leg closest to the board behind it and lowers the board to the ground.

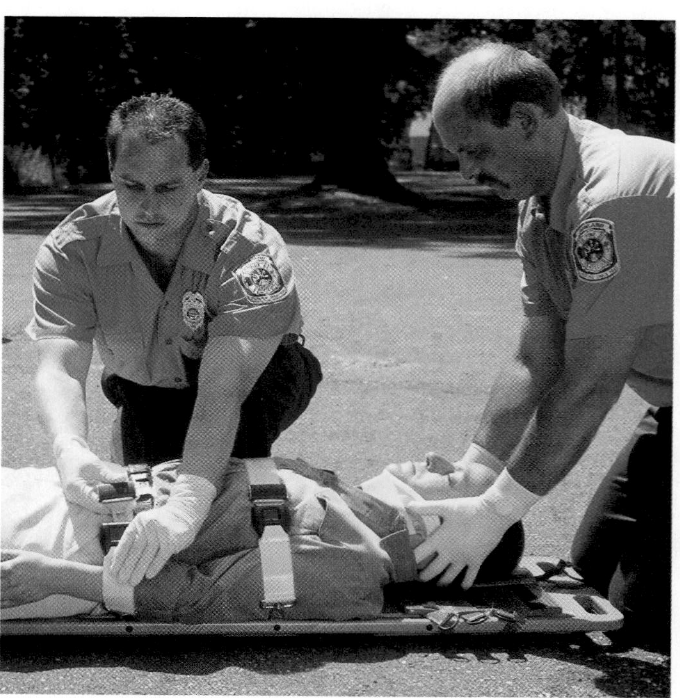

32-15D ✱ Once the patient is horizontal on the ground, one EMT takes over in-line stabilization until the patient is completely immobilized.

EMT skills 32-16 Immobilizing a Seated Patient with a Ferno K.E.D. Extrication Device

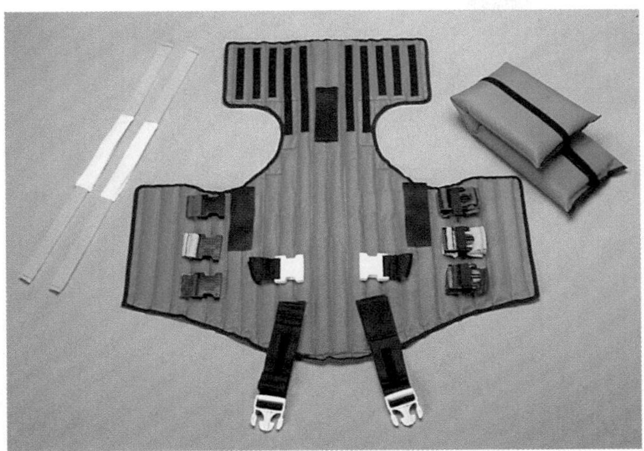

32-16A ✱ The Ferno Kendrick Extrication Device (K.E.D.). (© Ferno Corporation)

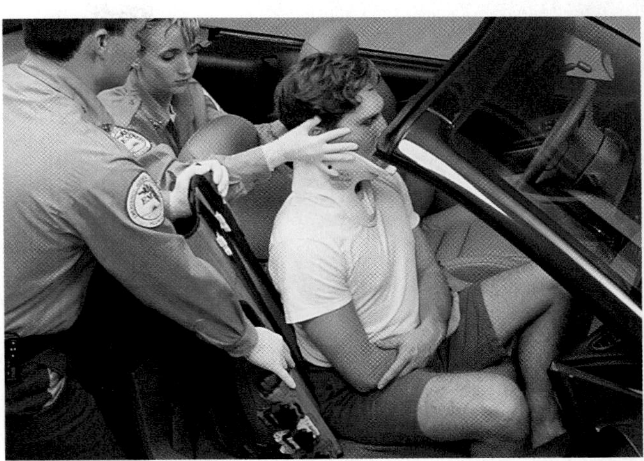

32-16B ✱ After a cervical spine immobilization collar has been applied, slip the K.E.D. behind the patient and center it.

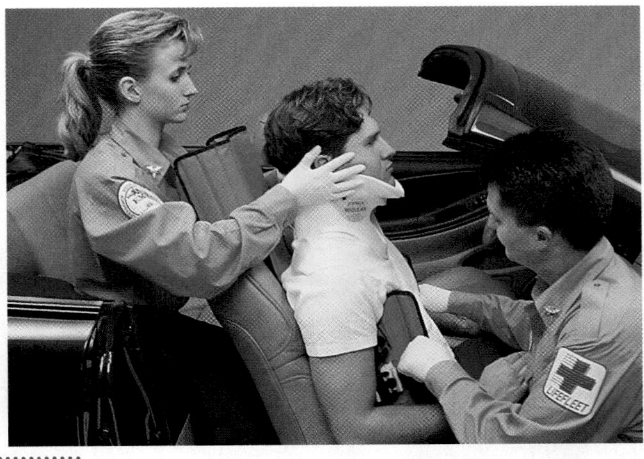

32-16C ✱ Properly align the device. Then wrap the vest around the patient's torso.

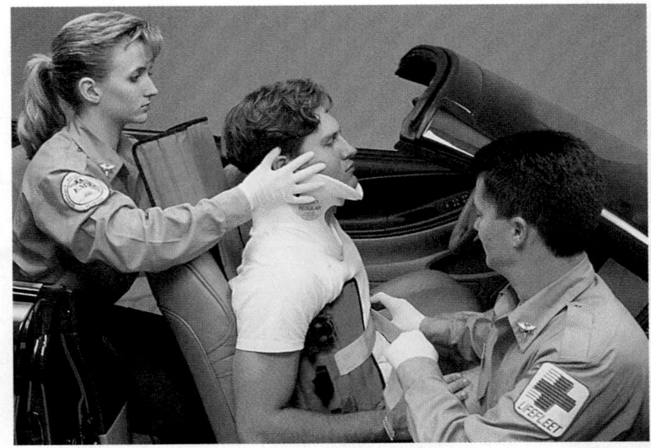

32-16D ✱ When the device is tucked well up into the armpits, secure the chest straps.

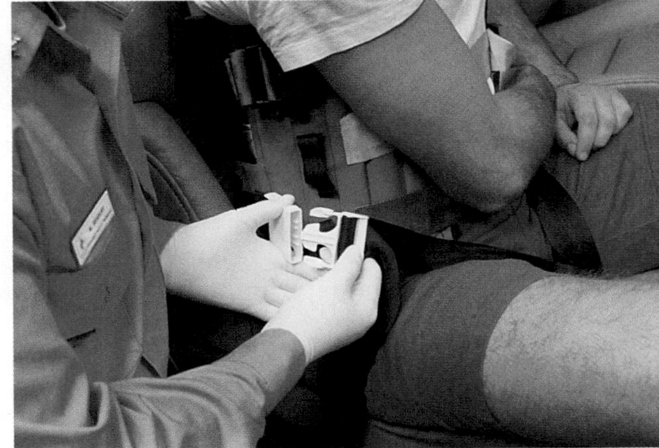

32-16E ✱ Secure the leg straps.

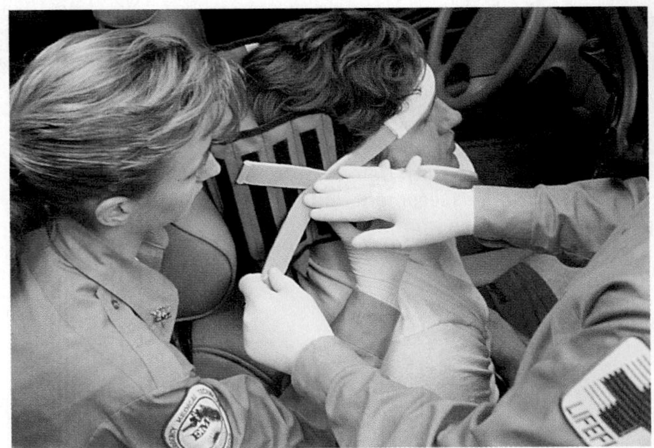

32-16F ✱ Secure the patient's head with the Velcro head straps.

continued

EMT skills 32-16 Immobilizing a Seated Patient with a Ferno K.E.D. Extrication Device *continued*

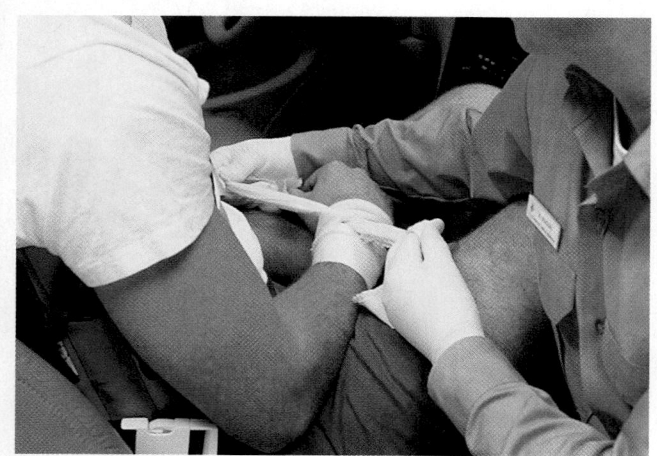

32-16G ✱ Tie the hands together.

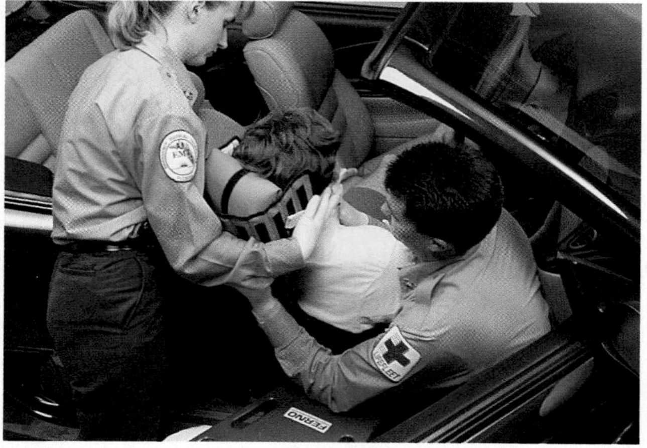

32-16H ✱ Pivot the patient onto the backboard while maintaining in-line stabilization.

EMT skills 32-17 Rapid Extrication

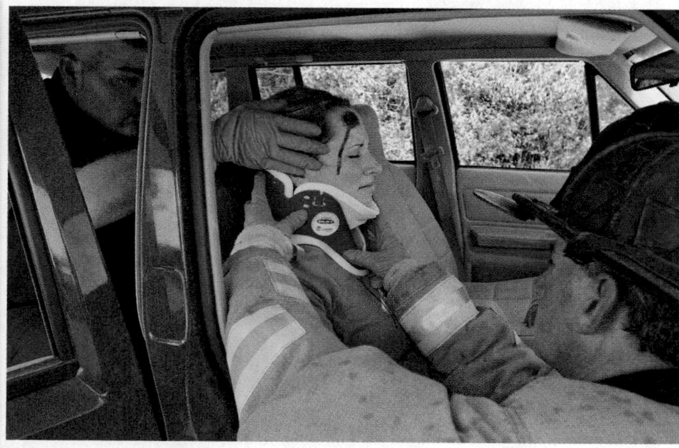

32-17A ✱ Bring the patient's head into a neutral in-line position. This is best achieved from behind or to the side of the patient. Perform a primary assessment and a rapid physical exam. Then apply a cervical spine immobilization collar.

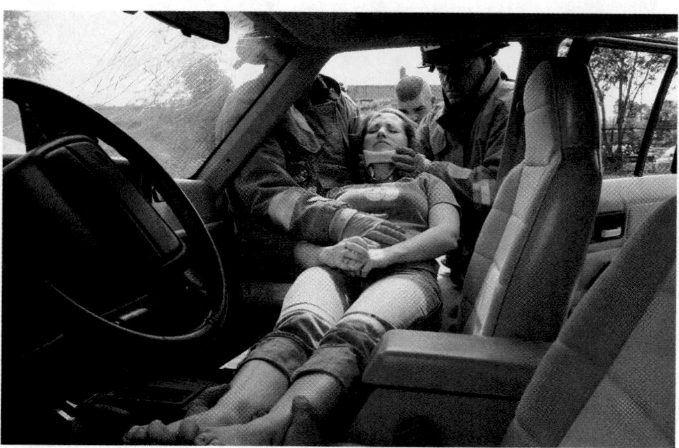

32-17B ✱ Support the patient's thorax. Rotate the patient until her back is facing the open car door. Bring the patient's legs and feet up onto the car seat.

32-17C ✱ Bring the board in line with the patient and against the buttocks. Stabilize the cot under the board. Begin to lower the patient onto the board.

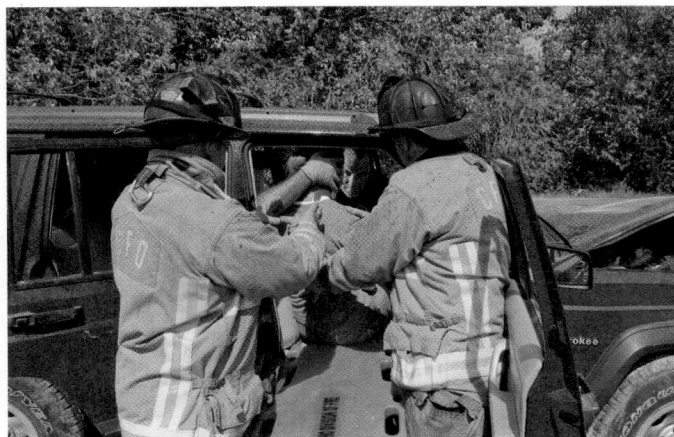

32-17D ✱ Lower the patient onto the board. Depending on the structure of the car, it may be necessary to change positions to maintain in-line stabilization while lowering the patient onto the board.

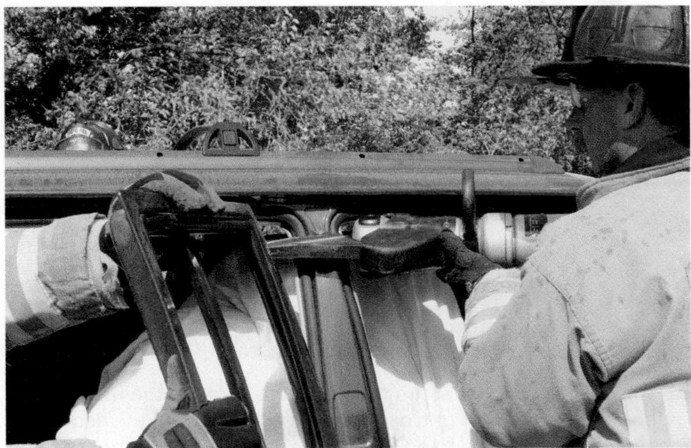

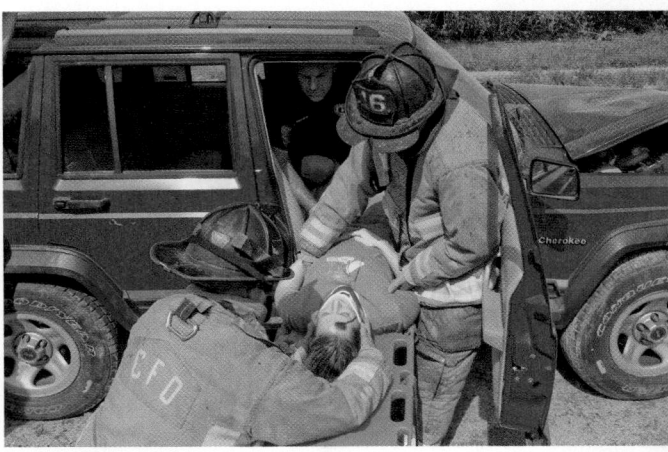

32-17E ✱ If the structural features of the vehicle, time, resources, and the patient's condition permit, it may be worthwhile to remove the roof before performing a rapid extrication.

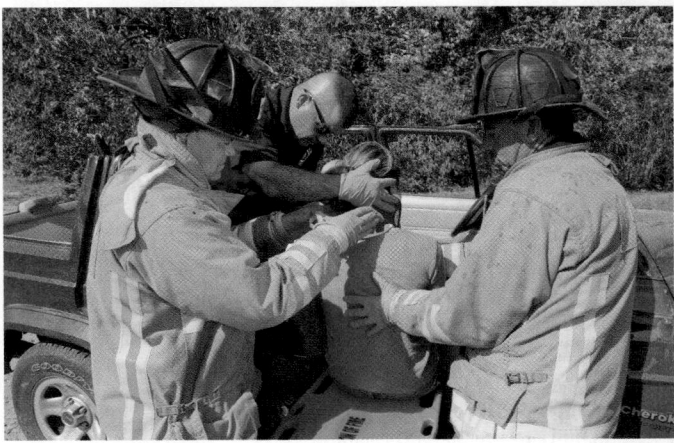

32-17F ✱ Depending on variables such as the vehicle's structure and the patient's condition, a rapid extrication may be performed more easily and safely if the roof has been removed.

Helmet Removal

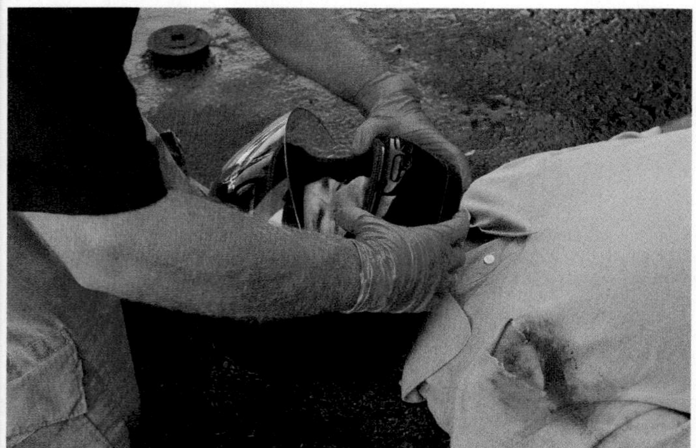

32-18A * One rescuer applies stabilization by placing hands on each side of the helmet with fingers on the patient's mandible to prevent movement.

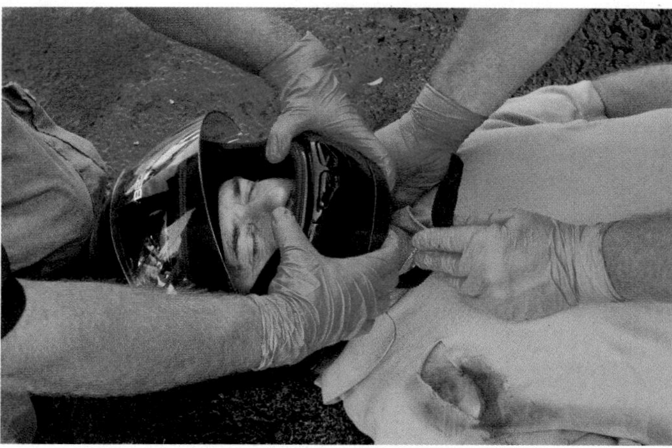

32-18B * A second rescuer places one hand on the mandible at the angle of the jaw.

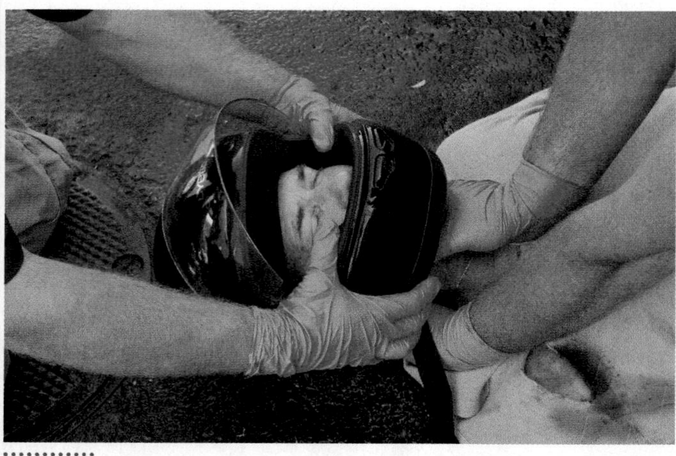

32-18C * With the other hand, the second rescuer holds the occipital region. This maneuver transfers the stabilization responsibility to the second rescuer.

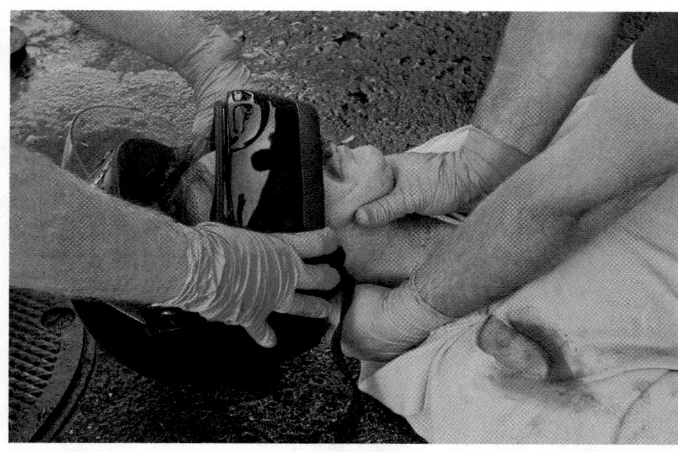

32-18D * The rescuer at the top begins to remove the helmet, pulling the sides apart to clear the ears and allowing the second rescuer to readjust his hand position around the mandible and under the occipital region.

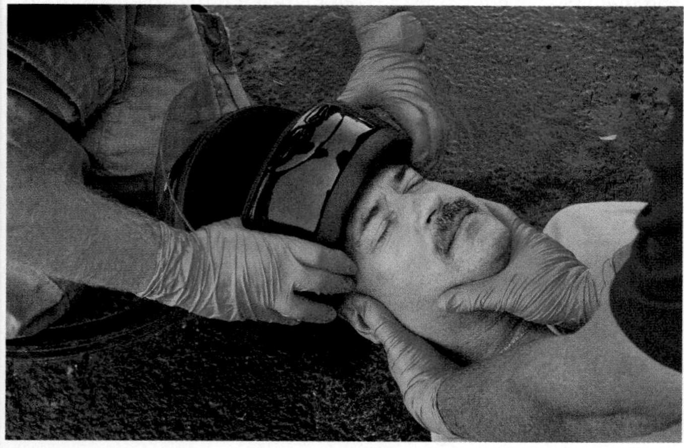

32-18E * Throughout the removal process, the second rescuer maintains in-line stabilization from below to prevent head tilt.

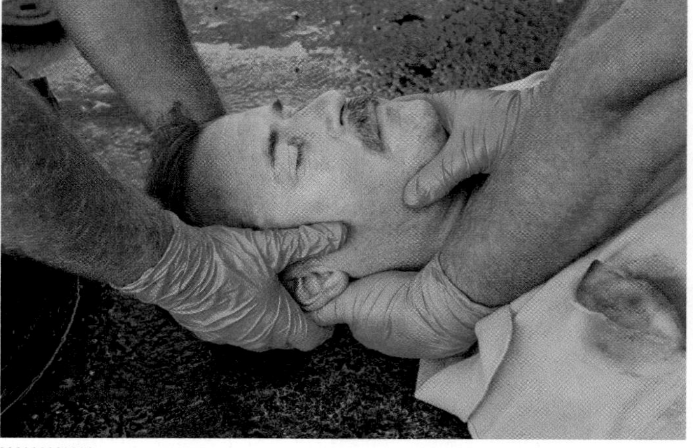

32-18F * After the helmet has been removed, the rescuer at the top replaces his hands on either side of the patient's head with palms over the ears, taking over stabilization.

EMT skills 32-18 Helmet Removal *continued*

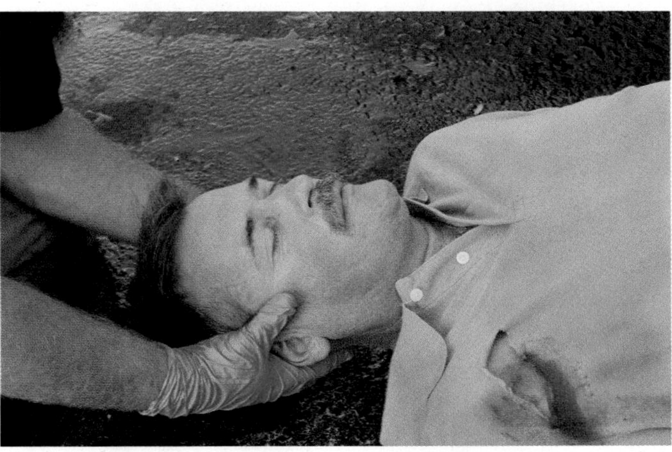

32-18G * Stabilization is maintained from above until a cervical spine immobilization collar is applied to the patient and complete immobilization to the backboard is achieved.

EMT skills 32-19 Helmet Removal—Alternative Method

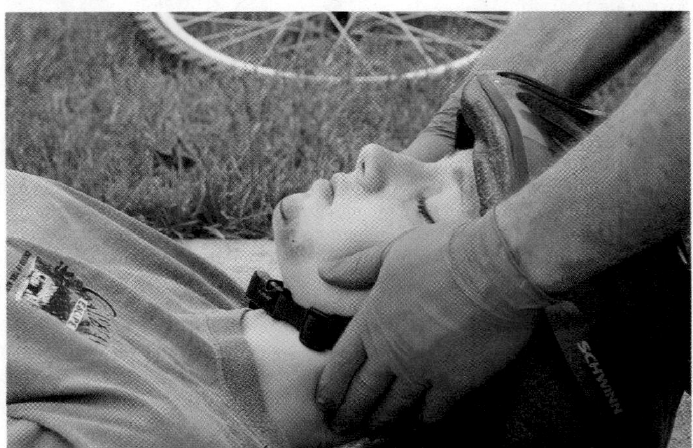

32-19A * Apply steady stabilization with the neck in neutral position.

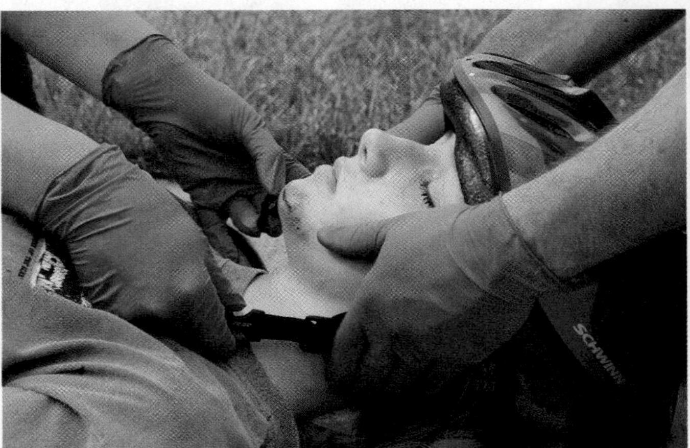

32-19B * Remove the chin strap.

continued

EMT skills 32-19 Helmet Removal—Alternative Method *continued*

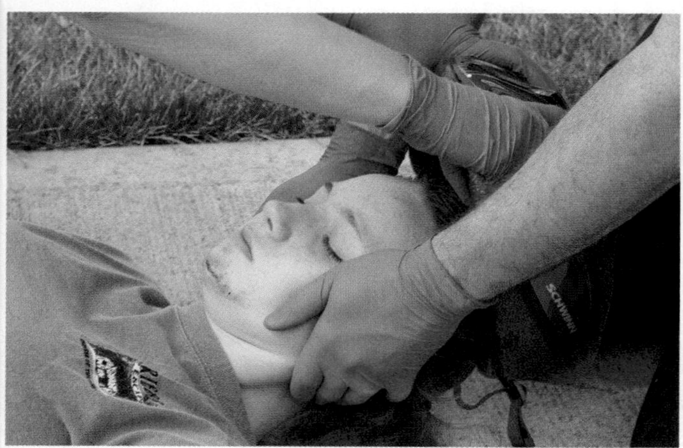

32-19C ✱ Remove the helmet by pulling out laterally on each side.

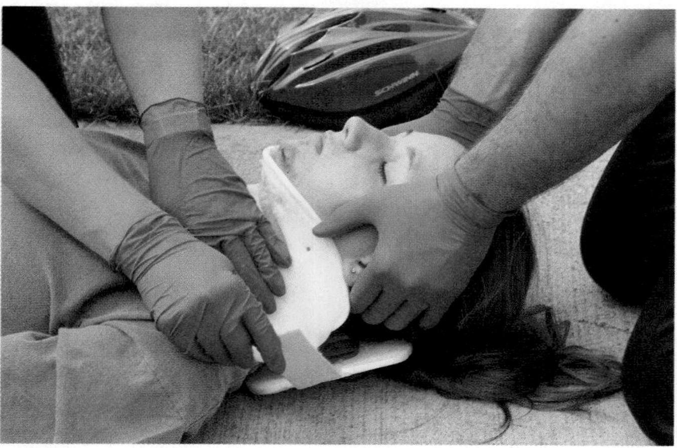

32-19D ✱ Apply a suitable cervical spine immobilization collar and secure the patient to a long board.

EMT skills 32-20 Immobilizing a Patient with a Football Helmet

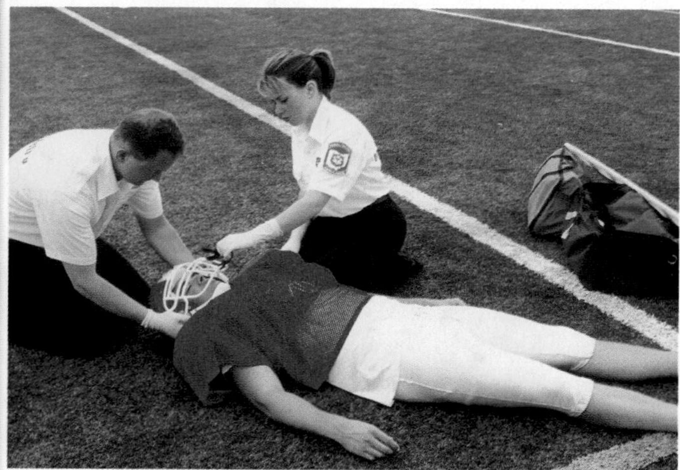

32-20A ✱ Take manual in-line stabilization and remove the mouthpiece.

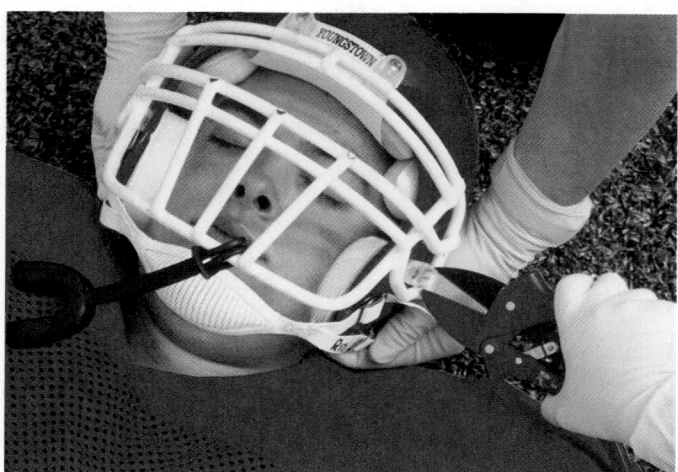

32-20B ✱ Cut the clips that secure the face mask.

EMT skills 32-20 Immobilizing a Patient with a Football Helmet *continued*

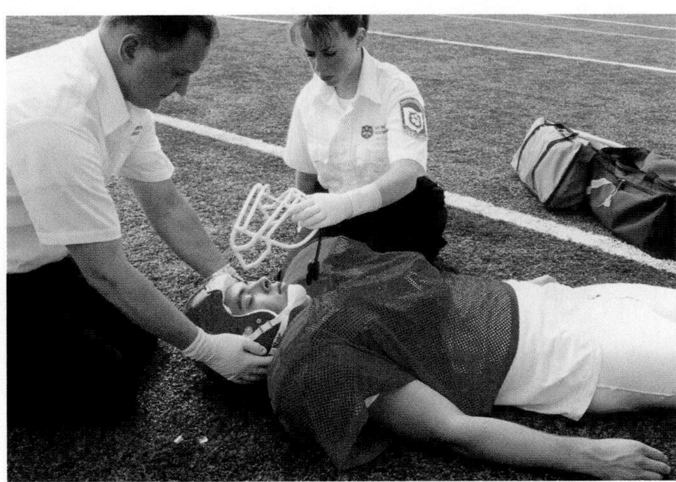

32-20C ✻ Remove the face mask by lifting it straight off the helmet.

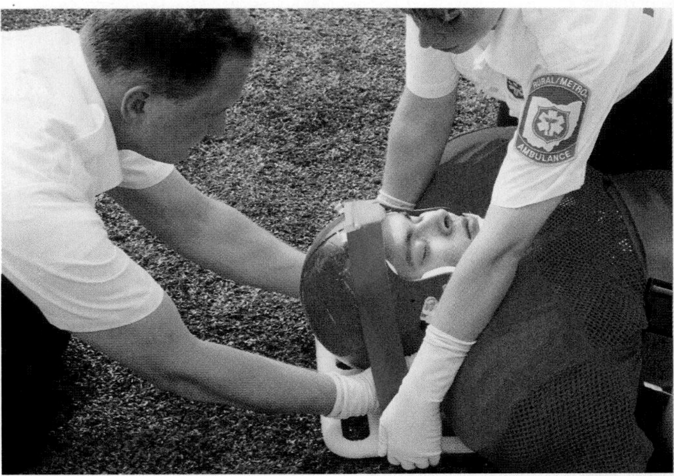

32-20D ✻ Immobilize the patient with straps and tape the helmet to the board last.

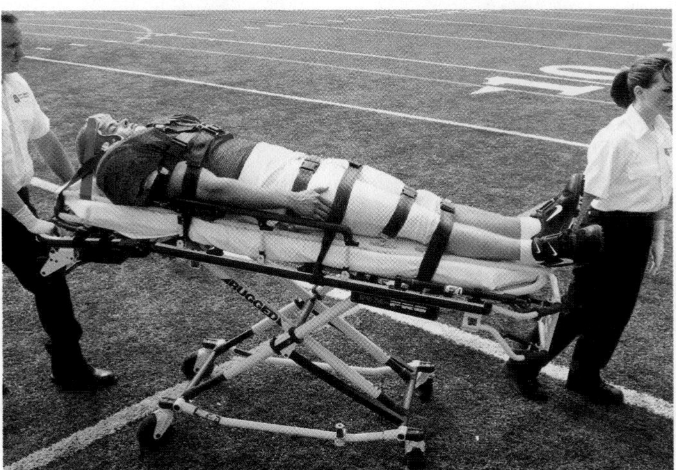

32-20E ✻ Transport the patient with the football equipment still in place.

EMT skills 32-21 Extrication from a Child Safety Seat

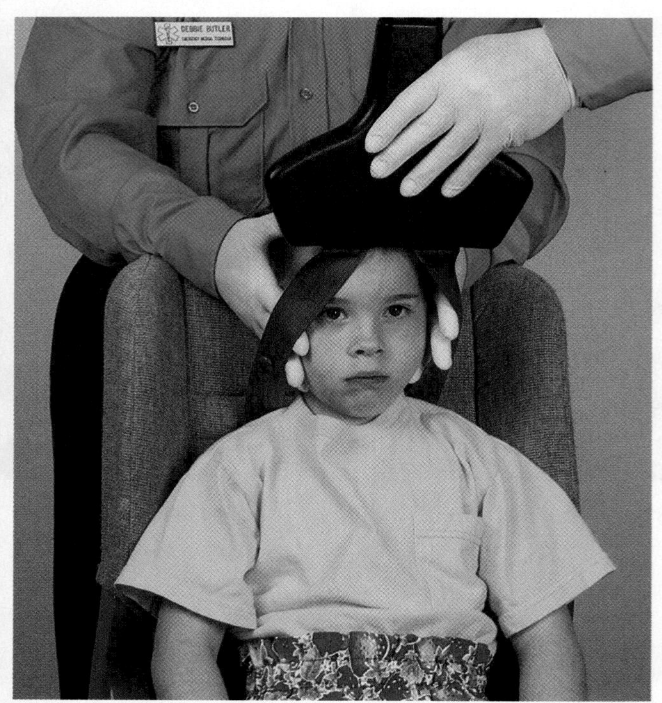

32-21A * EMT #1 stabilizes the car seat in an upright position and applies manual stabilization to the child's head and neck. EMT #2 prepares equipment, then loosens or cuts the seat straps and raises the front guard.

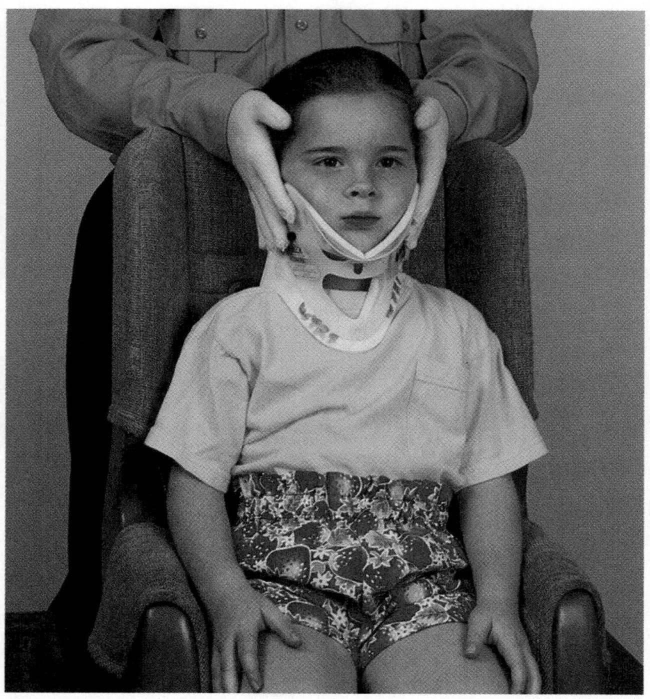

32-21B * A cervical collar is applied to the child as EMT #1 maintains manual stabilization of the head and neck.

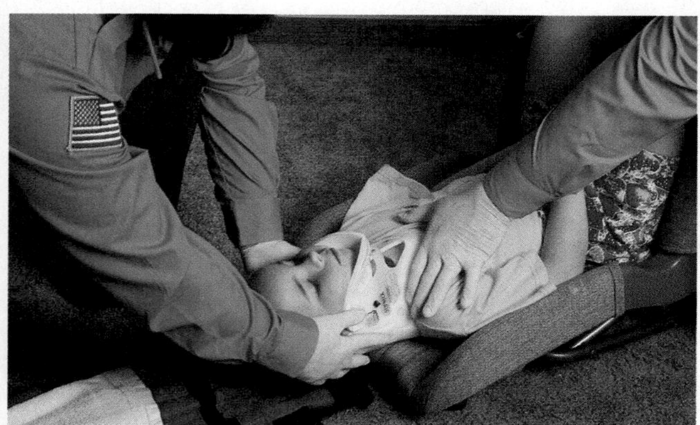

32-21C * As EMT #1 maintains manual stabilization, EMT #2 places the child safety seat on the center of a backboard and slowly tilts it into supine position. The EMTs are careful not to let the child slide out of the safety seat. For a child with a large head, place a towel under the area where the shoulders will eventually be placed on the board to prevent the child's head from tilting forward.

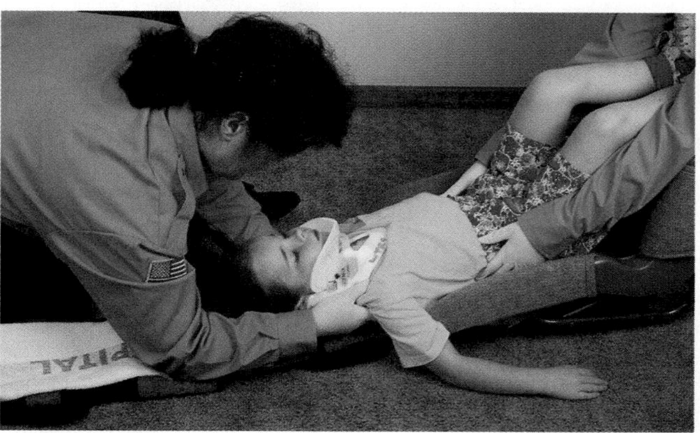

32-21D * EMT #1 maintains manual stabilization and calls for a coordinated long axis move onto the backboard.

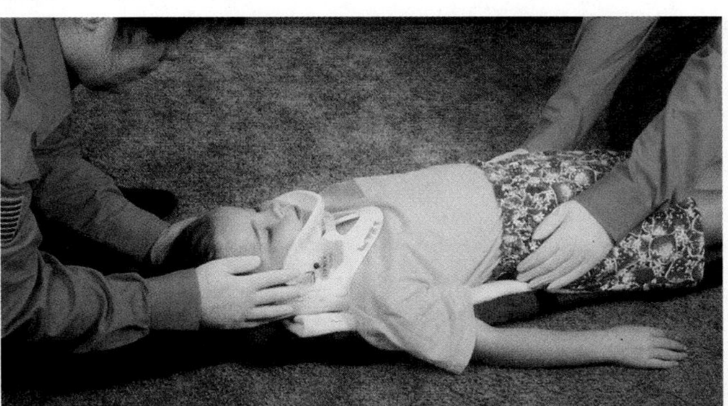

32-21E ✻ EMT #1 maintains manual stabilization as the move onto the board is completed with the child's shoulders over the folded towel.

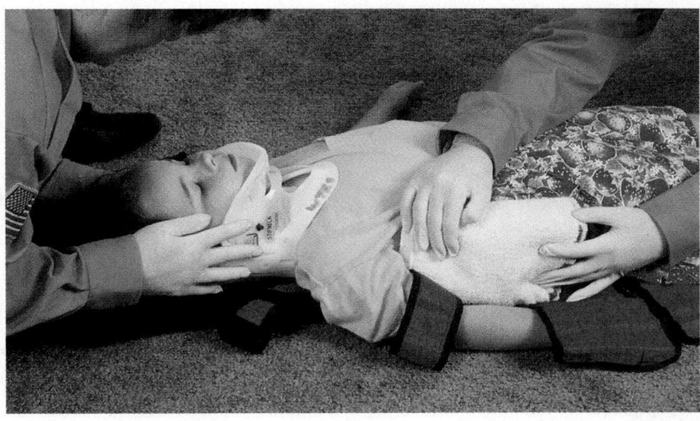

32-21F ✻ EMT #1 maintains manual stabilization as EMT #2 places rolled towels or blankets on both sides of the child.

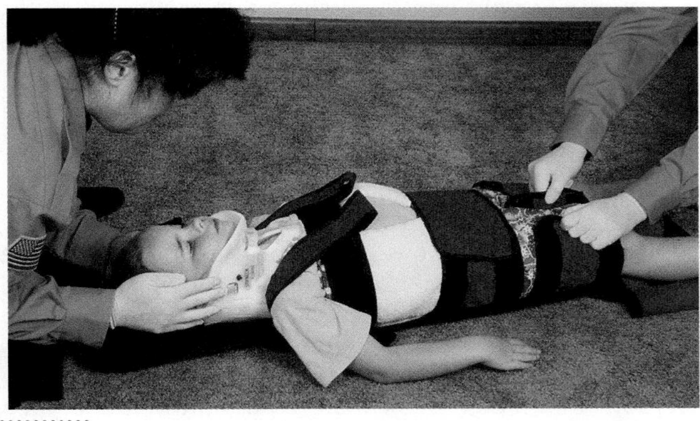

32-21G ✻ EMT #1 maintains manual stabilization as EMT #2 straps or tapes the child to the board at the level of the upper chest, pelvis, and lower legs. DO NOT STRAP ACROSS THE ABDOMEN.

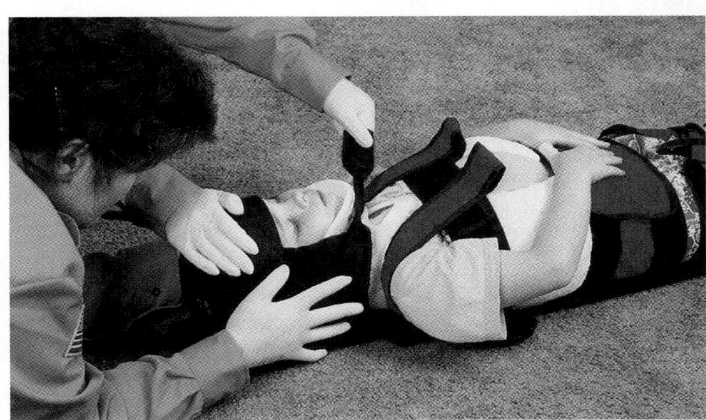

32-21H ✻ EMT #1 maintains manual stabilization as EMT #2 places rolled towels on both sides of the head, then tapes the head securely in place across the forehead and cervical collar. DO NOT TAPE ACROSS THE CHIN TO AVOID PRESSURE ON THE NECK.

CHAPTER REVIEW

SUMMARY

Spine injuries could lead to permanent damage to the spinal cord that results in paralysis and loss of sensation below the level of injury. Thus, it is imperative to assess for and manage the patient appropriately to reduce any risk of further injuring the spine or spinal cord. A patient may have a spinal column (vertebral) injury with no spinal cord involvement. Improper management by EMS could convert the spinal column injury into a spinal cord injury. If you have any suspicion that the patient has suffered a spinal injury, whether it is to the cord or to the column, take the necessary precautions and provide efficient and effective spinal immobilization.

A multitude of signs and symptoms may occur from a spine injury. An injury to the vertebrae will typically produce pain or tenderness along the spinal (vertebral) column. An injury to the spinal cord will usually produce motor or sensory deficits. Complications of spinal injury may include inadequate breathing effort, paralysis, and poor perfusion. Beware of confusing assessment findings, which may be an indication of an incomplete spinal cord injury.

Use the proper techniques and equipment to protect the spine and spinal cord from further injury. Complete spinal immobilization should be done on any patient suspected of having a spinal column or spinal cord injury.

CASE STUDY FOLLOW-UP

SCENE SIZE-UP

You are dispatched to a gymnastics meet for a 12-year-old girl who has fallen during the competition. As you arrive on the scene, you are directed into the gymnasium by an assistant. The lights are bright and the music is loud. You and your partner make your way around various pieces of gymnastics equipment to the far side of the gym, where a small group of girls, some in tears, are crowded around a young girl supine on the mat. Immediately above her are a set of uneven parallel bars at approximate heights of 10 and 6 feet. A woman, who identifies herself as the coach, is kneeling next to the girl and holding her head and body still. The coach says, "She missed a maneuver off the top bar. She fell and hit the bottom bar with the middle of her back, then landed head first on the floor."

PRIMARY ASSESSMENT

Recognizing the mechanism of injury, your partner immediately brings the patient's head and neck into a neutral position and establishes manual in-line spinal stabilization. You and your partner introduce yourselves and instruct the patient not to move. The young girl cries out, "My legs are numb and tingly! Am I going to be paralyzed?" You ask, "Can you tell me your name?" She says, "Carrie." "Well, Carrie," you say, "we're going to take good care of you and get you to the hospital where the doctors can figure out what's wrong and treat it."

Carrie's airway is patent and her breathing is rapid but adequate at a rate of approximately 28 per minute. Her radial pulse is strong and estimated at a rapid 125 per minute. Her skin is slightly cool to touch, slightly pale, and dry. You note, however, that the gymnasium temperature is relatively cool. You apply a pulse oximeter and obtain a reading of 98% on room air.

SECONDARY ASSESSMENT

You ask the coach if she actually saw the accident. You also ask if the patient attempted to get up or if she moved or was moved after the fall. The coach explains that she was standing next to Carrie when she fell. Because of how she landed, the coach immediately went to her side and instructed her to keep extremely still.

Because of the significant mechanism of injury, you proceed with a physical exam. Very gently, you assess the head and find a contusion along the scalp line above the right eye. You ask, "Carrie, does your neck or back hurt?" She cries, "I don't know. I just feel my legs are numb and tingly." As you carefully palpate her neck, Carrie complains of tenderness to the cervical region at about the level of the sixth vertebrae. You apply a cervical collar. The chest, abdomen, and pelvis have no signs of injury.

Following your inspection and palpation of her arms and determining that radial pulses are present bilaterally, you ask, "Can you move your hands just very slightly for me?" The patient complies and waves her hands slightly. You encourage her, "That's very good, Carrie." Keeping your hand out of her sight, you touch the little finger of her left hand and ask, "Can you tell me which hand and finger I'm touching?" Carrie replies, "My left hand, the pinkie." You touch her right hand and she again replies correctly. You then apply pinches to both hands and she identifies them correctly. Finally, you have her grip your fingers simultaneously and find the strength to be equal and strong in both upper extremities. Both radial pulses are strong.

You then inspect and carefully palpate the lower extremities for any signs of injury. The pedal pulses are present bilaterally. You instruct her to wave her foot very gently. She is able to move both feet. You touch the big toe on the right foot and ask, "Can you tell me which foot and toe I am touching?" She cries, "No!" Stabilizing the leg to avoid unsuspected and exaggerated movement, you pinch the top of the left foot. Carrie states, "I can feel that on my left foot." You repeat the same on the right foot and get a response to the pinch.

You enlist the help of the coach, who is familiar with log rolling, and instruct her to position herself at Carrie's feet. You position the backboard next to the patient. At the direction of your partner holding in-line stabilization at Carrie's head, you log roll her up and quickly assess her back, finding no deformities but some tenderness in the lumbar region. The backboard is positioned under her and she is rolled back onto it. A void behind the lumbar region is padded and straps are applied to the torso and legs and secured. A head/cervical immobilization device is applied and secured. Your partner releases manual in-line spinal stabilization and moves to the side to take the baseline vital signs. The blood pressure is 104/76 mmHg, the heart rate is 118 bpm, and the skin is slightly cool to touch, slightly pale, and dry. You obtain a history from the patient.

Carrie's parents have been notified by the gym staff. You and your partner meanwhile transfer Carrie to the ambulance and begin transport.

REASSESSMENT

During the reassessment, you re-evaluate the spinal immobilization. All straps are secure and all pads properly positioned. Carrie complains of some discomfort to her back but says it is from the hard backboard. You reassess her pulses and motor and sensory function in all the extremities and find no change. You reassess and record the vital signs.

Upon arrival at the emergency department, you help the hospital staff gently transfer the backboard to the emergency department bed. You provide an oral report regarding your findings. You briefly reassure Carrie then proceed to the EMS room to complete your prehospital care report as your partner restocks the ambulance. You finally notify dispatch that you are prepared for another call.

Later that day, on another call to the same hospital, you find time to check on Carrie's condition. The emergency medicine physician states that she suffered a spinal contusion and will completely recover. He praises the coach's work in keeping Carrie still until EMS arrived. He thanks you and your partner for the very detailed information provided both orally and in the prehospital care report regarding the scene characteristics and mechanism of injury. He also states, "Very nice immobilization job."

IN REVIEW

1. Describe the relationship between the spinal column and the spinal cord.
2. Name the most common mechanisms of spine injury.
3. List the signs and symptoms of potential spine injury.
4. Explain the types of stabilization and immobilization that must be applied in cases of suspected spine injury.
5. Describe how the airway is managed in a patient with suspected spine injury.
6. Explain the purpose and use of the cervical spine immobilization collar.
7. Explain how to assess motor and sensory function in a patient with suspected spine injury.
8. Explain the use of long and short spinal immobilization devices for seated patients with suspected spine injuries.
9. Under what circumstances is rapid extrication appropriate?
10. Under what circumstances should you leave a helmet in place in a patient with suspected spine injury?
11. Describe the patient presentation in a complete spinal cord injury.
12. Describe the patient presentation in an incomplete spinal cord injury.

CRITICAL THINKING

You arrive on the scene and find an elderly patient who is complaining of severe weakness to her upper extremities. She is alert and responding appropriately to your questions. Her respirations are 22 per minute with a good tidal volume. Her radial pulse is present at a rate of 92 bpm. Her skin is warm and dry. Her SpO_2 reading is 95% on room air. The patient states that she fell while coming down the stairs and struck her face on the floor. You note a contusion to the bottom of her chin. She is also complaining of pain to her neck and cervical region of the spine. She has a history of arthritis and atrial fibrillation. She takes Coumadin for the atrial fibrillation. She last ate approximately 20 minutes prior to her fall. She denies getting dizzy or light-headed or passing out. Her fall was caused by tripping over her slipper.

The patient's pupils are equal and reactive to light. Her anterior and posterior neck areas are tender. No deformities are noted. Her breath sounds are equal and clear bilaterally. Her abdomen is soft and nontender. Her pelvis is stable. Her radial pulses are present. She has severe weakness in the upper extremities, but she is moving her lower extremities with no problem. Her BP is 168/88 mmHg, HR 92 and irregular, R 22.

1. What initial emergency care would you provide to the patient?
2. What would you assess in your neurological exam on the patient?
3. Based on the presentation, what type of spinal cord injury do you suspect?
4. What other assessment findings would confirm the type of spinal injury suspected?
5. How would you manage the spinal injury?

EXPLORE PEARSON **mybradykit**™

Please go to **www.bradybooks.com** to access mykit for this text. You will find quizzes, critical thinking scenarios, weblinks, animations, and videos related to this chapter—and much more. Look for online information on spinal cord injuries as well as an animation on cervical injuries and application of a cervical collar.

Register your access code from the front of your book by going to **www.bradybooks.com** and selecting the mykit links.

CHAPTER 33

Eye, Face, and Neck Trauma

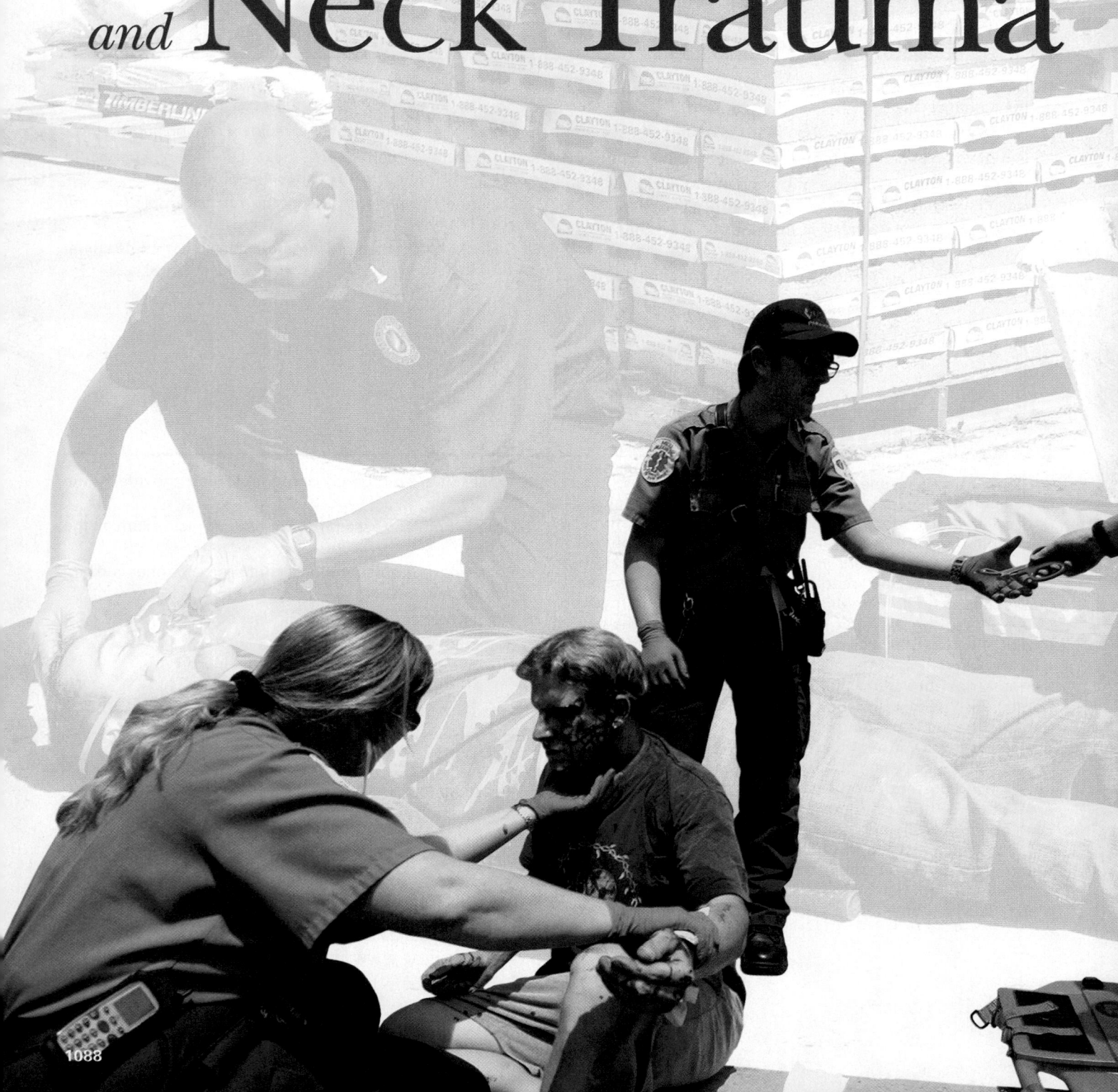

Navigation Guide

The following items provide an overview to the purpose and content of this chapter. The Standard and Competency are from the new National EMS Education Standards.

STANDARD **Trauma** (Content Area: Head, Facial, Neck, and Spine Trauma)

COMPETENCY Applies fundamental knowledge to provide basic emergency care and transportation based on assessment findings for an acutely injured patient.

OBJECTIVES: After reading this chapter, you should be able to:

33-1. Define key terms introduced in this chapter.
33-2. Describe the anatomy and function of the eye, face, and structures of the neck.
33-3. Discuss special considerations in the assessment and management of patients with injuries to the eye, face, and neck, including:
- **a.** Airway compromise
- **b.** Profuse bleeding
- **c.** Potential that injuries may be self-inflicted or due to violence
- **d.** Patient fears associated with these injuries

33-4. Discuss the assessment-based management of patients with injuries to the eye, face, and neck.
33-5. Demonstrate the assessment and management of specific injuries of the eye, including:
- **a.** Foreign body in the eye
- **b.** Injury of the orbit
- **c.** Injury to the eyelid
- **d.** Injuries to the globe of the eye
- **e.** Chemical burns to the eye
- **f.** Impaled objects in the eye
- **g.** Extruded eyeball

33-6. Explain the indications and procedure for removing contact lenses from an injured eye.
33-7. Demonstrate the assessment and management of specific injuries of the face, including:
- **a.** Facial fracture
- **b.** Avulsed tooth
- **c.** Impaled object in the cheek
- **d.** Injury to the nose
- **e.** Injury to the ear

33-8. Demonstrate the assessment and management of specific injuries of the neck, including:
- **a.** Penetrating injury to the neck
- **b.** Blunt injury to the neck

KEY TERMS: Page references indicate first major use in this chapter. For complete definitions, see the Glossary at the back of the book.

anterior chamber p. 1097
conjunctiva p. 1094
cornea p. 1095
diplopia p. 1095
eyelids p. 1094
globe p. 1094
iris p. 1098
mandible p. 1101
maxilla p. 1101
orbits p. 1094
pupil p. 1094
sclera p. 1099

MEDIA RESOURCES: Please go to www.bradybooks.com to access mykit for this text. You will find quizzes, critical thinking scenarios, weblinks, animations, and videos related to this chapter—and much more. Look for online information on eye and maxillofacial injuries.

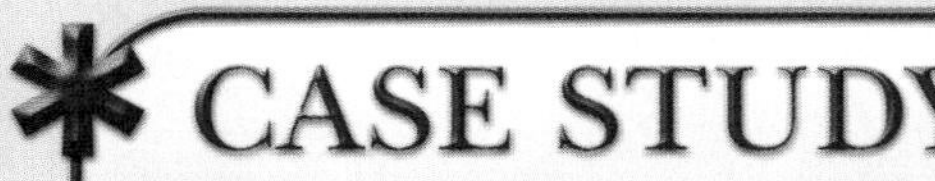

The Dispatch
EMS Unit 201—respond to 400 Mill Street—you have a 22-year-old male patient complaining of blindness and severe eye pain. Time out is 1345 hours.

Upon Arrival
As you pull into the patient's driveway, a neighbor greets you: "He's in the house!" Crossing the patient's driveway, you see battery jumper cables linking two

continued

Navigation Guide *continued*

cars together. Beneath the hood of one of the cars, you see powdery white battery acid sprayed across the engine. Once inside the patient's home, you hear someone screaming, "My eyes! My eyes! I can't see!"

How Would You Proceed to Assess and Care for This Patient?

During this chapter, you will learn special considerations of assessment and emergency care for a patient suffering eye, face, and neck injuries. Later, we will return to the case and apply the procedures learned.

Introduction

If you have ever experienced a serious eye, face, or neck injury, you can appreciate a patient's fear and panic associated with one of these emergencies. Aside from the pain, injuries to the eye cause emotional distress as the patient thinks about the possible loss of vision, and the patient who suffers a facial injury may fear permanent scarring or disfigurement. Neck injuries may lead to major bleeding, airway compromise, or permanent nerve damage.

As an EMT, you must remain aware that injuries to the eyes, face, or neck have a high probability of causing airway compromise, severe bleeding, and shock. Additionally, injury to the face and neck is likely to be associated with spinal injury. While caring for these sometimes dramatic or horrific injuries, you must always maintain a high index of suspicion for spinal injury and give first priority to care for life-threatening compromise of the airway and circulation.

Anatomy of the Eye, Face, and Neck

The Eye

The globe of the eye, or eyeball (Figure 33-1*), is a sphere approximately 1 inch in diameter. It is covered with a tough outer coat called the *sclera* (the exposed portion of the sclera is "the white of the eye"). The clear front portion of the eye, the *cornea,* covers the dark center, the *pupil,* and the colored portion, the *iris.* The cornea is the window through which light enters the eye. It is extremely sensitive and susceptible to injury. A superficial scratch or the smallest foreign object can cause extreme pain with redness and a flow of tears.

The pupil is the opening that expands or contracts to allow more or less light into the eye through the *lens,* just behind the pupil. The lens focuses light on the *retina,* or back of the eye. The inner surface of the eyelids and the

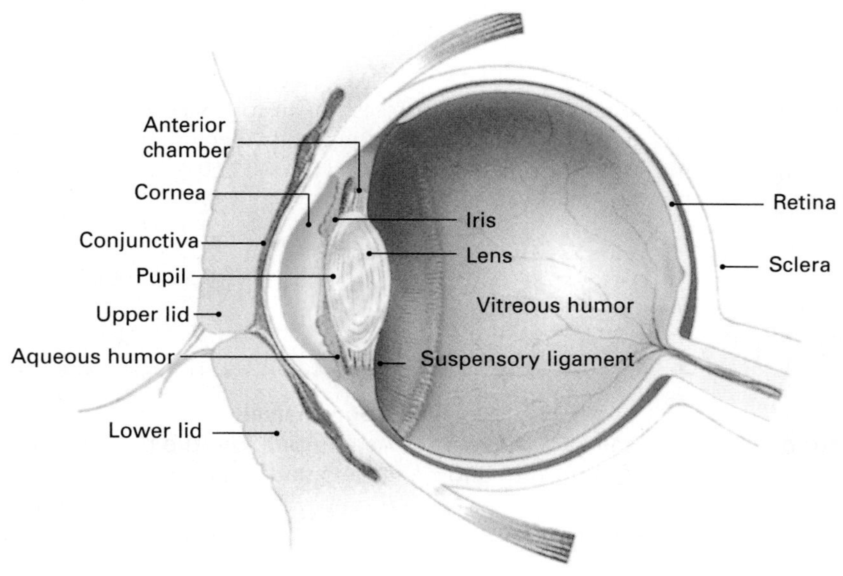

FIGURE 33-1 * The eye.

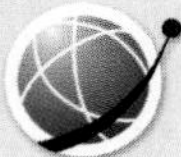

Media Resources

Go to www.bradybooks.com for mykit. Highlights:

- *Web Resource:* Jaw Fractures
- *Web Resource:* Orbital Fractures

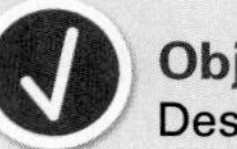

Objective 33-2

Describe the anatomy and function of the eye, face, and structures of the neck.

exposed portion of the sclera are lined with a paper-thin covering called the *conjunctiva*. The conjunctiva does not cover the cornea.

The interior of the eye contains the *anterior chamber* (front chamber), which is anterior to the iris and is filled with a watery fluid called the *aqueous humor*. Behind the lens is the large *vitreous body,* which is filled with a clear jelly called the *vitreous humor*. The bony structures of the skull that surround the eyes are called the *orbits,* or eye sockets.

All of the structures of the eyes, the muscles that hold the eyes in position, and the orbits of the eyes are susceptible to trauma ranging from minor abrasion and irritation, to impaled objects that invade the interior of the eye, to extrusions in which an eye is pulled out of its socket.

The Face

The bones of the skull and face were introduced in Chapter 7, "Anatomy, Physiology, and Medical Terminology." Collectively the skull is made up of 22 bones, 8 of which form the cranium and 14 that comprise the facial bones. Thirteen of these facial bones—the orbits of the eyes, the nasal bones, the zygomatic bones (cheekbones), and the maxillae (fused upper jawbones)—are immovable. One bone, the mandible (lower jaw), moves on hinged joints.

The face is extremely vascular (contains many blood vessels). Facial injuries, even otherwise minor ones, may bleed profusely. Blood and pieces of broken bone, teeth, and other tissues may cause airway compromise when the face is injured.

The facial bones are part of the skull. They provide minimal protection for the airway and allow points of attachment for the muscles that control facial expressions and the manipulation of food. Compromise of the facial structures (Figure 33-2∗) can cause a closed or an open brain injury with possible leakage of cerebrospinal fluid from the nose or ears. A mechanism of injury that causes trauma to the face is likely to have caused injury to the spine.

Understanding BODY PROCESSES

The facial structures are very vascular (contain many blood vessels) and are often injured with blunt and penetrating trauma to the anterior body. For this reason, the EMT should suspect and continuously assess the blunt anterior trauma patient for airway compromise. ■

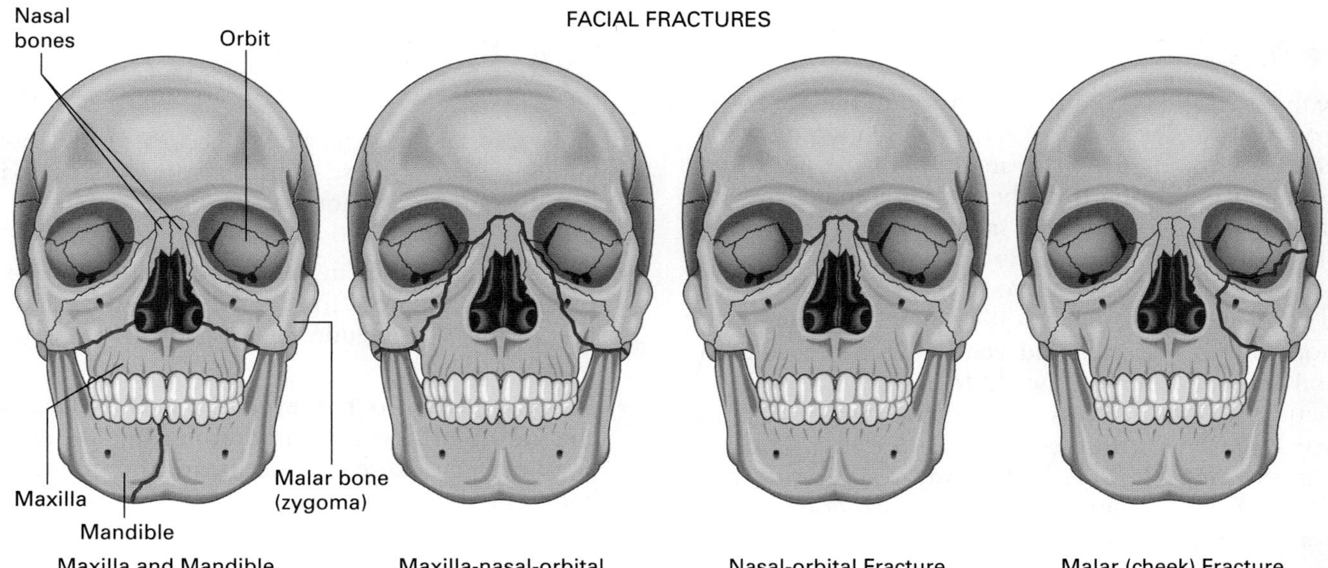

FIGURE 33-2 ∗ Facial fractures.

Key Points

The neck contains the major arteries and veins that carry blood to and from the head and major structures of the airway.

Objective 33-3

Discuss special considerations with injuries to the eye, face, and neck, including airway compromise, profuse bleeding, potentially violent or self-inflicted cause, and patient fears about the injury.

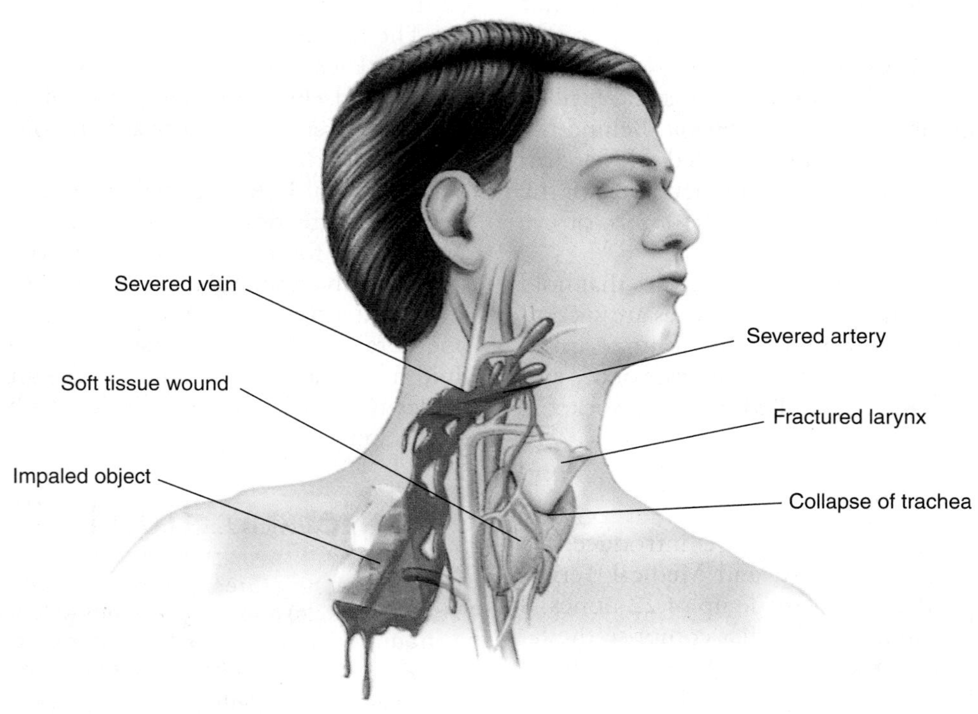

FIGURE 33-3 * Common neck and throat injuries.

The Neck

The major blood vessels and structures of the neck were introduced in Chapter 7, "Anatomy, Physiology, and Medical Terminology." The anatomy of the neck is of special concern to the EMT because it contains numerous vital structures in a very small space. Body systems represented within the neck include the cardiovascular, musculoskeletal, central nervous, respiratory, digestive, and endocrine. More specifically, the neck contains the major arteries (carotid) and veins (jugular) that carry blood to and from the head. It also contains major structures of the airway, including the trachea and the larynx. Injuries to the neck (Figure 33-3*) can cause life-threatening bleeding and airway compromise that can be difficult to control. Damage to structures of the airway is a serious life threat. The posterior neck contains the cervical spine, which houses and protects the proximal spinal cord. Any injury to the neck should automatically be assumed to have caused spinal injury.

Eye, Face, and Neck Injuries

The eyes, face, and neck may be subject to a wide variety of injuries. However, these injuries may present you with some challenges in common:

- **Eye, face, and neck injuries can hemorrhage profusely.** You will need to take the necessary Standard Precautions, to include gloves and protective eyewear.
- **Many injuries to the eyes, face, and neck are the result of assault.** In addition, injuries to the neck may be caused by accidental or intentional hanging.
- **You may need to treat emotional trauma as well as physical trauma.** The responsive patient who has suffered an eye injury fears blindness. A face injury arouses fear of permanent facial disfigurement or

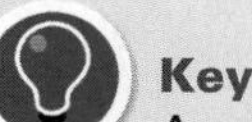

Key Points
Any patient with chemical burns to the eye, an impaled object in the eye, an extruded eyeball, respiratory distress, severe injuries to the face or neck, major bleeding, or airway compromise must be considered a high priority for immediate transport.

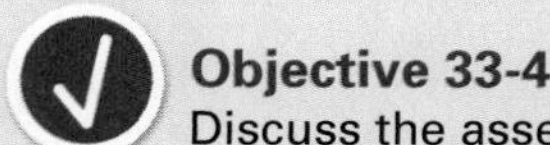

Objective 33-4
Discuss the assessment-based management of patients with injuries to the eye, face, and neck.

scarring. A neck injury may cause fear of immediate lethal bleeding or breathing difficulty. These patients, and their friends and family at the scene, may be emotionally distraught or panicked. You will need to display a calm and reassuring manner to gain the patient's confidence so you can begin care and treatment of the physical trauma.

Assessment-Based Approach: Eye, Face, and Neck Injuries

The assessment procedures and considerations described here will apply, overall, to the specific eye, face, and neck injuries described in the rest of this chapter.

Scene Size-Up

Because mechanism of injury will guide your treatment, you will want to think about the forces behind the injury as soon as you get the dispatcher's call. Soft tissue injury to the face and neck is common in trauma. Over half of the cases of facial trauma that present to the emergency department result from motor vehicle crashes, with assaults and sports-related injuries making up the majority of remaining cases.

During the scene size-up it may be difficult to gather information from the patient, because he is likely to be in a state of extreme pain and emotionally distraught. Try to determine the mechanism of injury or nature of the problem from bystanders, friends, or family. Make sure to protect your own safety and call for police backup if the mechanism of injury involves an assault.

Primary Assessment

While conducting your primary assessment, keep in mind that severe trauma to the face and neck can cause altered mental status, airway compromise, severe bleeding, and spinal injury. Establish manual in-line stabilization of the head and neck on first contact with the patient. Control major bleeding with direct pressure. Open the airway with a jaw-thrust maneuver and suction vomitus and other substances as needed. Consider advanced life support (ALS) backup, if available, since advanced airway procedures may be required. Provide oxygen at 15 lpm by nonrebreather mask if breathing is adequate; provide positive pressure ventilation with supplemental oxygen at a rate of 10–12 ventilations per minute if breathing is inadequate.

In making a priority decision, consider any patient with chemical burns to the eye, an impaled object in the eye, an extruded eyeball, respiratory distress, severe injuries to the face or neck, major bleeding, suspected spinal column or cord injury, or airway compromise to be a high priority for immediate transport with assessment and care continuing en route.

Secondary Assessment

Conduct a secondary assessment. Inspect and gently palpate for any sign of injury to the eye sockets or bones of the cheek, nose, or jaw. If the patient has suffered an eye injury, use a small penlight to examine the eyes. Never push directly on the eyes.

Record the vital signs and, in patients with severe bleeding, be prepared to treat for shock. Obtain a history. Particularly in the case of eye injuries where time could mean the difference between sight and loss of vision, ask the patient or bystanders questions regarding the events leading up to the injury.

Signs and symptoms of eye, face, and neck injuries, as well as emergency care steps, are detailed throughout this chapter within the sections on the particular injuries you will encounter.

Reassessment

Conduct a reassessment and check interventions. Monitor especially for deterioration of mental status, airway, or breathing. Conduct the reassessment every 5 minutes if the patient is unstable or every 15 minutes if the patient is stable.

Specific Injuries Involving the Eye, Face, and Neck

Injuries to the Eye

While usually not life threatening, an injury to the eye can take away the precious gift of sight. Time is a critical consideration in your treatment, particularly in cases such as chemical burns, impaled objects in the eye, or extruded eyeballs.

Key Terms

orbits the bony structures that surround the eyes; the eye sockets.

eyelids movable protective folds that can cover the eye.

Key Terms

conjunctiva the thin covering of the inner eyelids and exposed portion of the eye. Pl. conjunctivae.

globe the eyeball.

pupil the dark center of the eye; the opening that expands or contracts to take in more or less light.

Assessment and Care Guidelines

When you conduct the physical exam on a patient with an eye injury, assess the eyes separately and together with a small penlight (Figure 33-4a*) to evaluate:

- The **orbits** (eye sockets) for bruising, swelling, laceration, and tenderness
- The **eyelids** for bruising, swelling, and laceration
- The **conjunctivae** for redness, pus, and foreign bodies
- The **globes** for redness, abnormal coloring, and laceration
- The **pupils** for size, shape, equality, and reactivity to light

Additionally, ask the patient to follow your finger (Figure 33-4b*) as you move it left and right, up and down, to evaluate:

- *Eye movements in all directions* for abnormal gaze, paralysis of gaze, or pain on movement

Suspect significant damage if the patient has loss of vision that does not improve when he blinks, loses part of the field of vision, has severe pain in the eye, has double vision, or is unusually sensitive to light.

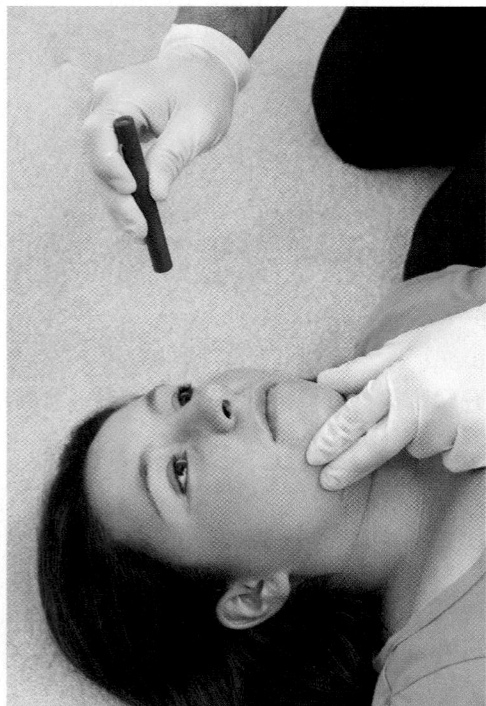

FIGURE 33-4a * Inspect the eyes for any abnormality.

Regardless of the injury, remember the following basic rules when giving emergency medical care for eye injuries:

- If the eye is swollen shut, avoid any unnecessary manipulation in examining the eye.
- Do not try to force the eyelid open unless you have to wash out chemicals.
- Consult medical direction or local protocol before irrigating. Some jurisdictions do not permit irrigating an injured eye, except in the case of a chemical burn.
- Do not put salve or medicine in an injured eye.
- Do not remove blood or blood clots from the eye. Sponge blood from the face to help keep the patient comfortable, but leave the eye alone.
- Have the patient lie down and keep quiet. Never let a patient with an eye injury walk without help, especially up or down stairs.
- Limit use of the uninjured eye. It is usually best to cover it along with the injured eye. Eyes move to-

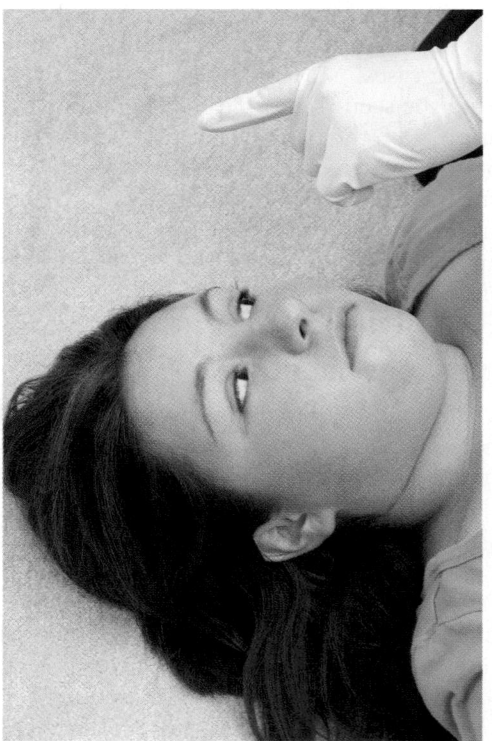

FIGURE 33-4b * Assess the patient's ability to move the eyes in any direction.

Objective 33-5
Demonstrate the assessment and management of specific injuries of the eye.

Key Terms
cornea the clear front portion of the eye that covers the pupil and the iris.
diplopia double vision.

gether, and if the patient is using the uninjured eye, chances are the injured eye is moving, too.

- Give the patient nothing by mouth in case general anesthesia is required at the hospital.
- Every patient with an eye injury must be transported for evaluation by a physician.
- Never apply direct pressure to an injured eye.
- If possible, bring the liquid or material to which the eye was exposed with the patient. If it is too dangerous or not possible to do so, clearly note the substance and ensure that the information is left with the receiving medical facility personnel.

Foreign Object in the Eye Foreign objects—such as particles of dirt, sand, cinders, coal dust, or fine pieces of metal—can be blown or driven into the eye and lodged there (Figure 33-5*). A flow of tears often washes out these substances before any harm is done. A patient with a foreign object in the eye will complain of feeling the object, and the globe will appear red. Determine if the patient or others made any attempt to remove the object, possibly causing abrasions to the **cornea**.

Generally, it is safer to transport the patient for further medical evaluation than to attempt to remove foreign particles from the eye in the field. You should attempt removal only of objects in the conjunctiva, not of those on the cornea or lodged in the globe.

If you need to remove a foreign particle from the conjunctiva, use the following techniques if permitted by medical direction or local protocol: If possible, flush the eye with clean water, holding the eyelids apart (Figure 33-6*). *Remember that some EMS systems do not recommend flushing the eye except in cases of chemical burns.*

If you cannot flush the eye, the removal technique depends on where the object is located. To remove an object from the white of the eye, pull down the lower lid while the patient looks up or pull up the upper lid while the patient looks down. Then remove the object with a piece of sterile gauze or a swab (Figure 33-7*).

If the object is under the upper lid, draw the upper lid down over the lower lid. As the upper lid returns to its normal position, the undersurfaces will be drawn over the lower lashes, possibly removing the object. If the object remains, grasp the lashes of the upper lid and turn the lid upward over a cotton swab or similar object. Carefully remove the object with the corner of a piece of sterile gauze or a swab (EMT Skills 33-1). If the object is under the lower lid, pull down the lid and remove the object with sterile gauze or a swab.

If a foreign object becomes lodged in the eyeball, do not attempt to disturb it. Place a bandage over both eyes and transport the patient as soon as possible.

Injury to the Orbits Trauma to the face may result in the fracture of one or several of the bones that form the orbits of the eyes (Figure 33-8*). If fracture of the orbits is suspected, establish and maintain spinal stabilization. Injuries serious enough to cause orbital fractures may also cause cervical spine trauma.

The signs and symptoms of orbital fracture include the following: **diplopia** (double vision); a marked decrease in vision; loss of sensation above the eyebrow, over the cheek, or in the upper lip; nasal discharge; tenderness to palpation; a bony "step-off" (defect in smooth contour of bone); or paralysis of upward gaze in the involved eye

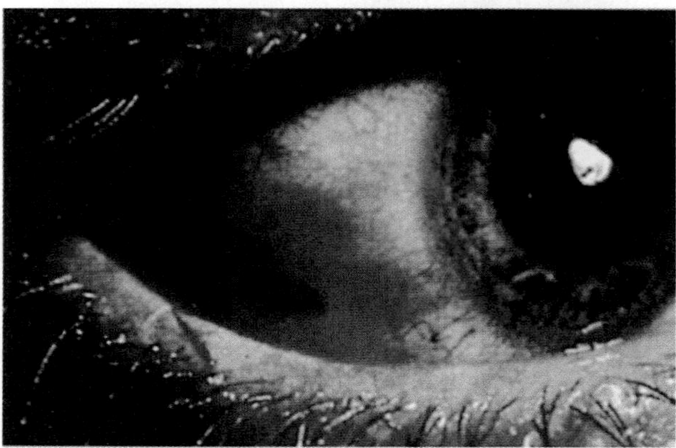

FIGURE 33-5 * Foreign object lodged in the eye.

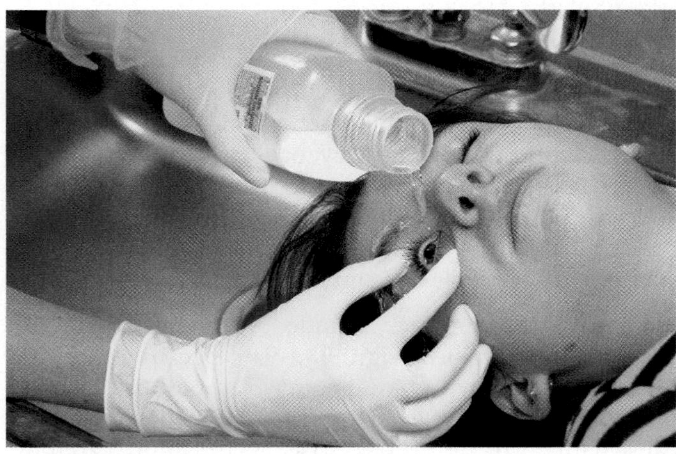

FIGURE 33-6 * Flushing a foreign particle from the eye.

Key Points
Generally, it is safer to transport the patient for further medical evaluation than to attempt to remove foreign particles from the eye in the field.

Key Points
Use light pressure from a dressing to control bleeding from a lid injury. Apply no pressure at all if the eyeball itself may be injured.

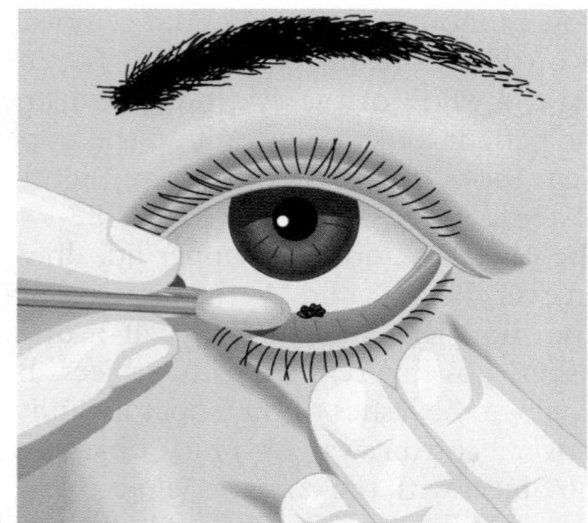

(a)

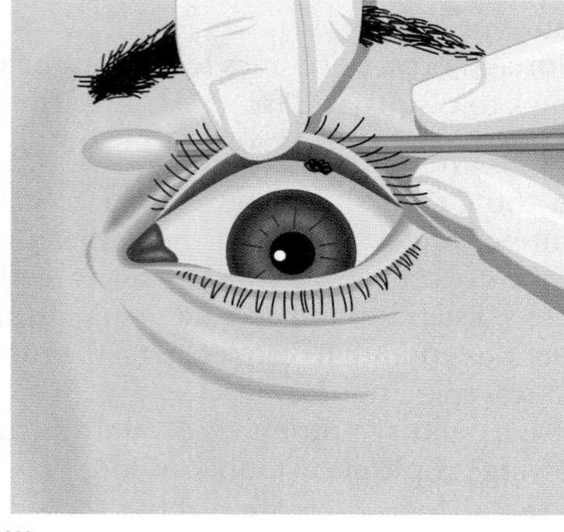

(b)

FIGURE 33-7 ✱ To remove particles from the white of the eye, **(a)** pull down the lower lid while the patient looks up or **(b)** pull up the upper lid while the patient looks down.

(the patient's eye will not be able to follow your finger upward).

Orbital fractures may require hospitalization and possible surgery. If the signs and symptoms lead you to suspect a possible orbital fracture, take the following emergency care steps: If the eyeball has not been injured, place cold packs over the injured eye to reduce swelling and transport the patient in a sitting position. If you suspect injury to the eyeball, avoid using cold packs and transport the patient in a supine position.

Lid Injury Lid injuries include bruising (black eyes), burns, and lacerations (Figure 33-9✱). Because the eyelid is richly supplied with blood vessels, lacerations can cause profuse bleeding. Anything that lacerates the lid can also cause damage to the eyeball, so assess the injury carefully. Inspect the area around the lid for evidence of injury.

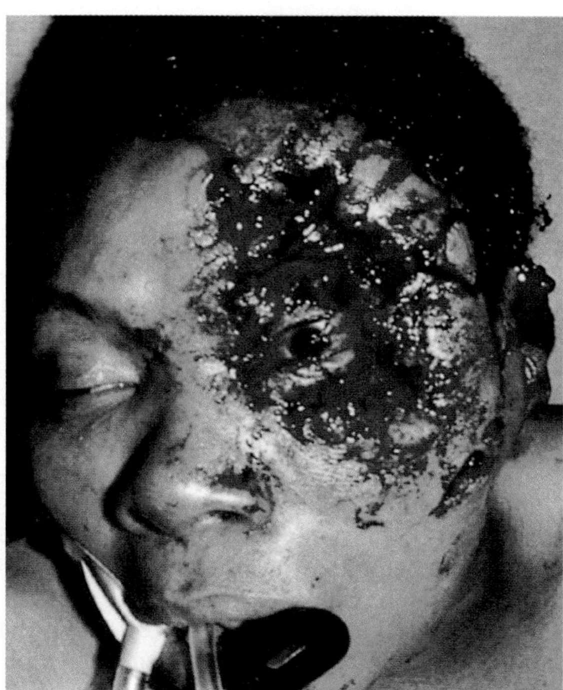

FIGURE 33-8 ✱ Eye orbit injury.

To treat a lid injury: Control bleeding with light pressure from a dressing; use no pressure at all if the eyeball itself may be injured. Cover the lid with sterile gauze soaked in saline to keep the wound from drying. Preserve any avulsed skin and transport it with the patient for pos-

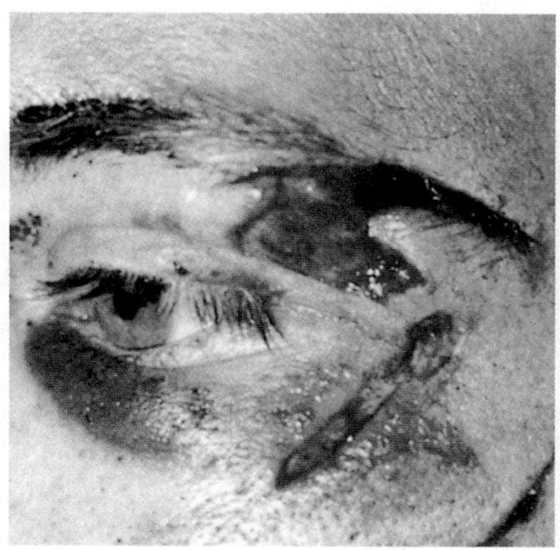

FIGURE 33-9 ✱ Eyelid injury.

sible grafting. If eyeball injury is not suspected, cover the injured lid with cold compresses to reduce swelling. Cover the uninjured eye with a bandage to decrease movement, and transport.

Injury to the Globe Injuries to the globe of the eye (Figure 33-10*) include bruising, lacerations, foreign objects, and abrasions. Overuse of contact lenses (even extended-wear lenses) can cause corneal abrasions, inflammation of the conjunctiva, and corneal ulcers. Deep lacerations and penetrating injuries can cut the cornea, causing the contents of the eyeball to spill out.

Some injuries to the globe—such as lacerations or embedded objects—are immediately apparent. Other signs and symptoms of injury to the globe may include a pear- or irregular-shaped eyeball and blood in the **anterior chamber** of the eye (a condition called *hyphema*). A high-speed activity such as grinding can lead to penetration of the globe with minimal external signs. Globe injuries should be treated with great caution.

Injuries to the globe are best treated at the hospital. In the field: Apply patches lightly to both eyes. Do not use a patch or any kind of pressure if you suspect a ruptured eyeball, since pressure can force the eye contents to leak out. Avoid the use of cold packs over the globe. If you apply an eye shield to the injured eye, be sure that it puts no pressure on the injury. Keep the patient supine, and transport.

Chemical Burn to the Eye A chemical burn to the eye (Figure 33-11*) represents a dire emergency. Permanent damage can occur within seconds, and the first 10 minutes of intervention following injury often determine the final outcome. *Burning and tissue damage will continue to occur as long as any substance is left in the eye, even if that substance is diluted.* If, during your scene size-up and primary assessment, you determine the mechanism of injury is a chemical to the eye, *you must begin treatment immediately!*

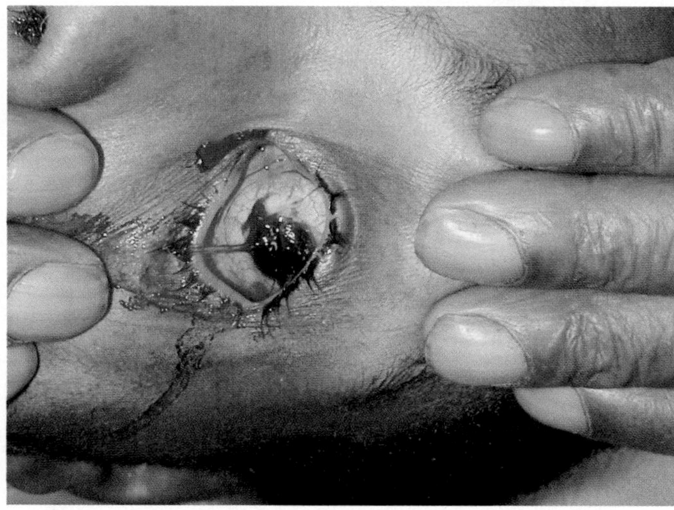

FIGURE 33-10 * Ruptured globe. The patient was using needle-nose pliers, which slipped, piercing the globe and causing blindness in that eye. (© Charles Stewart, MD, and Associates)

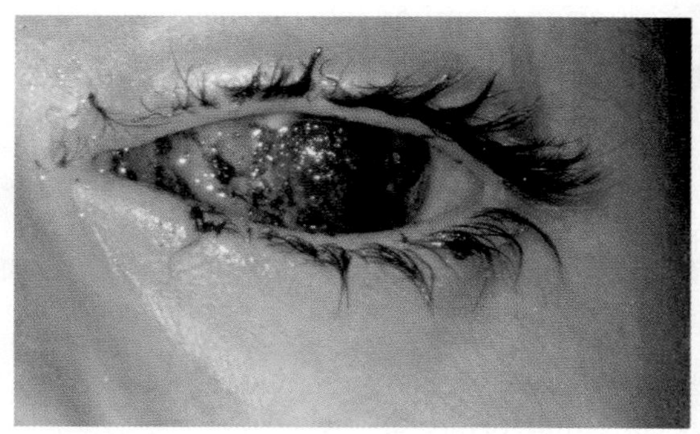

FIGURE 33-11 * Trauma to the corneas from hot sodium hydroxide. (Charles Stewart, MD and Associates)

The signs and symptoms of chemical burns to the eye include a history consistent with exposure; irritated, swollen eyelids; redness of the eye or red streaks across the surface of the eye; blurred or diminished vision; excruciating pain in the eyes; or irritated, burned skin around the eyes.

In all chemical burns of the eye, immediately begin irrigation with water or saline (Figure 33-12*). It need not be sterile, but it should be clean. Hold the eyelids open so all chemicals can be washed out from behind the lids. Continuously irrigate the eye for at least 20 minutes—or if the injury involves alkali, for at least an hour—or until arrival at the hospital. Use running water or continually pour the water or saline from the inside

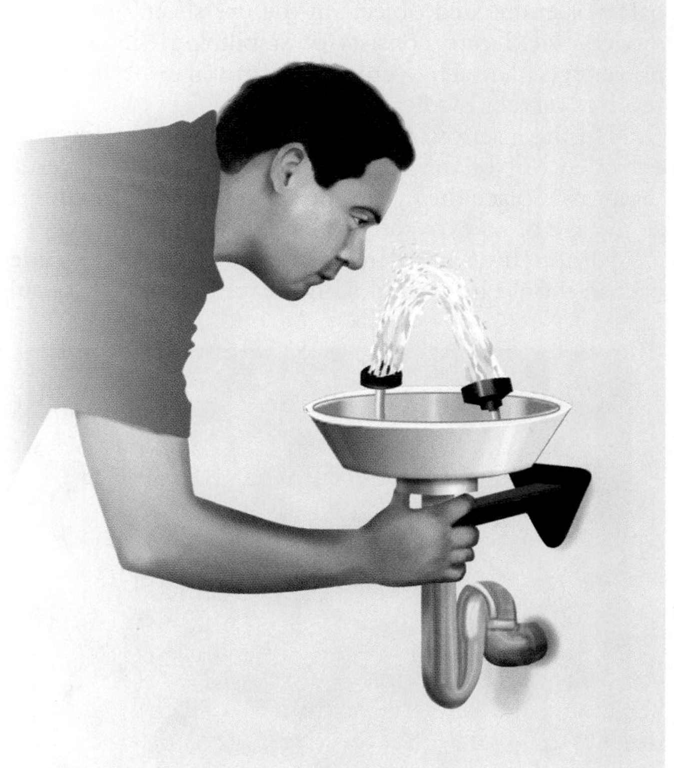

FIGURE 33-12 * Irrigate the chemical burn to the eye with large amounts of water.

Key Terms
anterior chamber the front chamber of the eye.

Thinking Critically
Your patient splashed drain cleaner into her eye. Her husband says, "Get her to the hospital now!" Her sister says, "No! Pour diluted vinegar into her eye!" What should you really do? Why?

Objective 33-6
Explain the indications and procedure for removing contact lenses from an injured eye.

Key Terms
iris colored portion of the eye around the pupil.
sclera coating of the eye; white of the eye.

corner, across the eyeball to the outside edge, taking care not to contaminate the uninjured eye. You may have to force the lids open, since the patient may be unable to do so because of pain. If available at the site, have the patient irrigate the eye(s) with an eye wash system. *Do not use any irrigants other than sterile saline available on the ambulance or clear water. Never irrigate the eye with any chemical antidote, including diluted vinegar, sodium bicarbonate, or alcohol—despite what any well-intentioned bystanders or family may want you to do.*

Contact lenses must be removed or flushed out. If left in, they will trap chemicals between the contact lens and the cornea (see the section on contact lens removal later). Remove any solid particles from the surface of the eye with a moistened cotton swab. Place the patient on his side on the stretcher, with a basin or towels under his head, and continue irrigation throughout transport.

Following irrigation, avoid contaminating your own eyes by washing your hands thoroughly and using a nail brush to clean under your fingernails.

Impaled Object in the Eye or Extruded Eyeball Impaled or embedded objects in the eye should not be removed. Field care consists of stabilizing the object to prevent accidental movement or removal until the patient receives further medical attention.

During a serious injury, the eyeball may be forced or extruded out of the socket (Figure 33-13*). Never attempt to replace the eye in the socket. An impaled object in the eye or an extruded eyeball is a true emergency.

Although an impaled object in the eye or extruded eyeball should be treated with great urgency, you should not manipulate the eye during treatment. Treatment for both is the same (EMT Skills 33-2): Place the patient supine and immobilize the head and spine. Encircle the eye and the impaled object or extruded eyeball with a gauze dressing or other suitable material, such as soft, sterile cloth. Do not apply pressure. You can cut a hole in a single bulky dressing to accommodate an impaled object. Place a metal shield, crushed paper cup, or cone over the impaled object or extruded eyeball. Do not use a Styrofoam cup, since it can crumble. The impaled object or eyeball should not touch the top or sides of the cup.

Hold the cup and dressing in place with a self-adhering bandage or roller bandage that covers both eyes. Do not wrap the bandage over the cup, which can push the cup down onto the impaled object or extruded eyeball. Make sure you bandage both eyes to prevent eye movement. If the patient is unresponsive, close the uninjured eye before bandaging to prevent drying, which can cause additional eye injury.

Give the patient nothing by mouth. Never leave the patient alone, and constantly provide verbal reassurance, because he might panic with both eyes covered. Transport immediately.

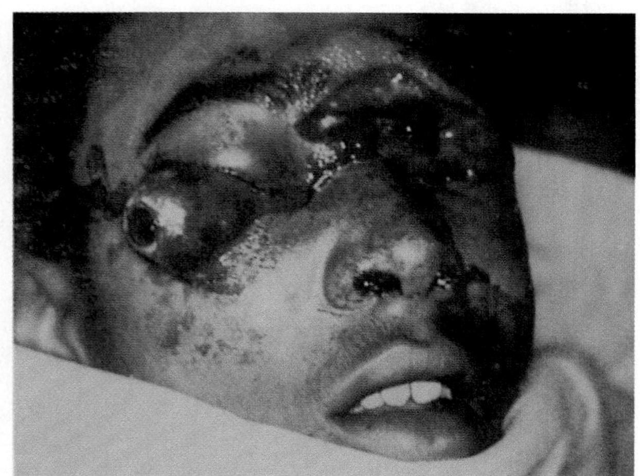

FIGURE 33-13 * Extruded eyeball.

Summary: Emergency Care—Eye Injuries

To review possible emergency care for eye injuries, see Figure 33-14*.

Removing Contact Lenses

Eye injuries are often further complicated by the presence of contact lenses. To detect lenses, shine a penlight into the eye at a slight angle. A soft lens will show up as a shadow on the outer portion of the eye, while a hard lens will show up as a shadow over the **iris**. Some patients wear a contact lens in only one eye, so do not dismiss the possibility of contact lenses after examining only one eye. Some patients, especially the elderly, wear both contact lenses and eyeglasses, so you also can't dismiss the possibility of contact lenses just because the patient is wearing eyeglasses.

When determining whether to remove contact lenses, seek medical direction and follow local protocol. Generally, you should remove contact lenses if:

- There has been a chemical burn to the eye.
- The patient is unresponsive and is wearing hard contact lenses, and transport time will be lengthy or delayed.

Emergency Care Protocol

EYE INJURY

1. Consider manual in-line stabilization based on mechanism of injury. Do not release it until the patient is immobilized onto a backboard.
2. Establish and maintain an open airway. Insert a nasopharyngeal or oropharyngeal airway if the patient is unresponsive and has no gag or cough reflex.
3. Suction secretions as necessary.
4. If breathing is inadequate, provide positive pressure ventilation with supplemental oxygen at a minimum rate of 10–12 ventilations/minute for an adult and 12–20 ventilations/minute for an infant or child.
5. If breathing is adequate, administer oxygen based on the SpO_2 reading and patient signs and symptoms. If the SpO_2 reading is greater than 95% and no signs or symptoms of hypoxia or respiratory distress are present, oxygen may not be necessary if the injury is isolated to the eye. If other injuries are present, or signs of hypoxia or respiratory distress are present, or the SpO_2 reading is less than 95%, place the patient on a nonrebreather mask at 15 lpm.
6. Control any major bleeding.
7. Place the patient in a supine position.
8. Treat the specific eye injury as follows:
   Foreign Object in Eye:
   If possible, transport the patient for further evaluation and removal of object by emergency department staff.
   Only attempt removal of objects in the conjunctiva.
   Do not attempt removal of objects on or lodged in the cornea.
   To remove a foreign object from the conjunctiva:
   Flush with water.
   If not successful and the object is under the upper lid, draw the upper lid down over the lower lid.
   If the object remains, lift the lid with a cotton swab or similar object and remove with a corner of the sterile gauze or swab.
   Orbital Injury:
   If the eyeball has not been injured, place ice packs over the injured eye.
   If the eyeball is injured, do not use cold packs. (Refer to the following information on management of a globe injury.)
   Lid Injury:
   Control bleeding with light pressure; do not use pressure if the eyeball is injured.
   Cover the lid with sterile gauze soaked in saline.
   Preserve avulsed skin and transport with the patient.
   If eyeball injury is not suspected, cover the lid with a cold compress.
   Patch both eyes.
   Injury to the Globe:
   Apply patches to both eyes.
   Do not apply any type of pressure.
   Apply an eye shield to the injured eye.
   Keep the patient supine.
   Chemical Burn to Eye:
   Begin irrigation with water or saline immediately and for at least 20 minutes or until arrival at the hospital.
   Do not contaminate the uninjured eye.
   Force the lids open if necessary to flush.
   Remove contact lenses.
   Remove solid particles from the eye surface with a moistened cotton swab.
   Continue to irrigate en route to the medical facility.
9. Immobilize the patient to a backboard if you suspect spine injury.
10. Transport.
11. Perform a reassessment every 5 minutes if unstable and every 15 minutes if stable.

FIGURE 33-14 ✱ Emergency care protocol: eye injury.

Generally, you should *not* remove contact lenses if:

- The eyeball is injured (other than a chemical burn).
- Transport time is short enough to allow emergency department personnel to remove the lenses.

Removing Soft Contact Lenses Even though they are designed for extended wear, soft contact lenses can cause damage if left in for a long time. Over time, they can gradually dehydrate and shrink, adhering to the cornea and making removal difficult.

Soft lenses are slightly larger than a dime and cover all of the cornea and some of the **sclera**. One way to remove them is to place several drops of saline on the lens, then gently lift the lens off the eye by pinching the lens between your thumb and index finger.

You can also remove soft lenses with the following method (Figure 33-15✱):

1. With your middle fingertip on the lower lid, pull the lid down.
2. Place your index fingertip on the lower edge of the lens, then slide the lens down to the sclera, or white of the eye.
3. Compress the lens gently between your thumb and index finger, allowing air to get underneath it, and remove it from the eye.

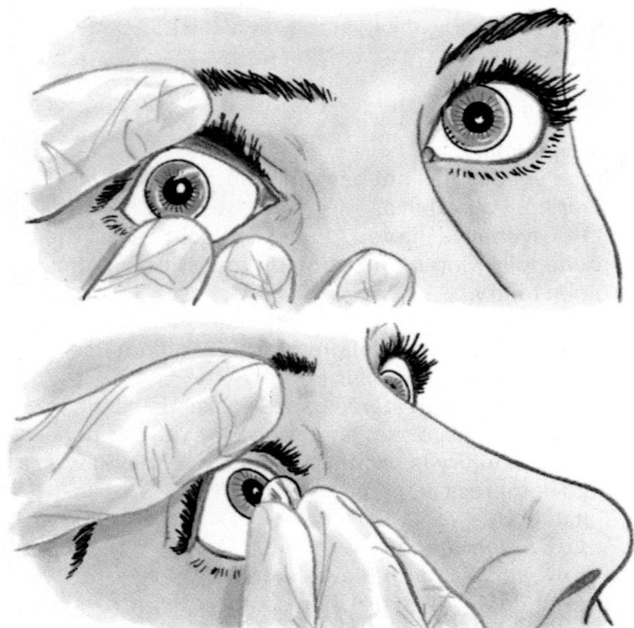

FIGURE 33-15 * Removing soft contact lenses.

4. If the lens has dehydrated on the eye, run sterile saline across the eye surface, slide the lens off the cornea, and pinch it up to remove it.
5. Store the removed soft contact lens in water or a saline solution.

Removing Hard Contact Lenses Even though soft contact lenses are much more popular, hard contact lenses are still in use. About the size of a shirt button, they fit over the cornea. To remove (Figure 33-16*):

1. Separate the eyelids.
2. Position the visible lens over the cornea by manipulating the eyelids.
3. Place your thumbs gently on the top and bottom eyelids, and open the eyelids wide.
4. Gently press the eyelids down and forward to the edges of the lens.
5. Press the lower eyelid slightly harder and move it under the bottom edge of the lens.
6. Moving the eyelids toward each other, slide the lens out between them.

You can also use a contact lens removal kit, which is commonly available on the ambulance. This is a kit that typically includes a small suction cup, affixed to a handle, which the EMT moistens with saline and uses to remove hard contact lenses. The kit also contains a portable lens case that you can put each contact lens in for safe transporting to the hospital (Figure 33-17*).

Injuries to the Face

The specialized structures of the face, prone to injury because of their location, can be permanently and irreversibly damaged (EMT Skills 33-3 and EMT Skills 33-4). Injuries to the face are quite common. Approximately 75 percent of all those involved in motor vehicle accidents sustain at least minor facial trauma. While some injuries to the face are minor, many such injuries are life threatening because they compromise the upper airway. In addition, many injuries of the face stem from impacts strong enough to cause cervical spine damage or skull fracture.

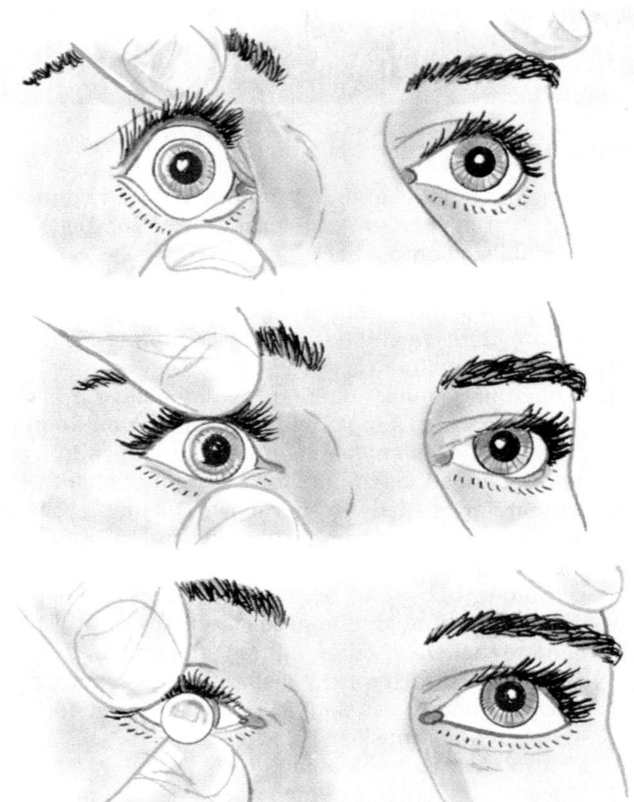

FIGURE 33-16 * Removing hard corneal contact lenses.

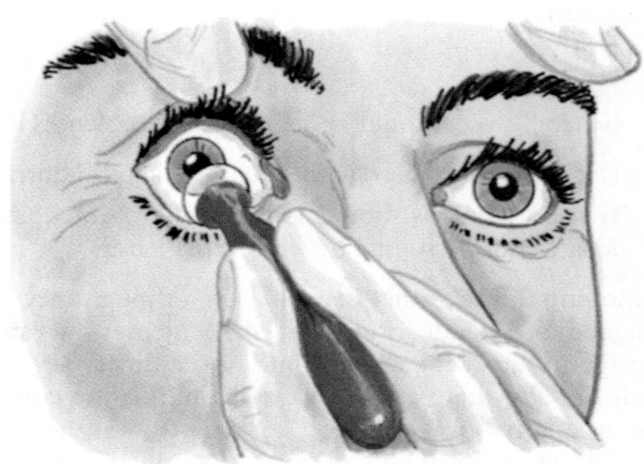

FIGURE 33-17 * Using a moistened suction cup to remove a hard contact lens.

Thinking Critically
A little league player standing too close to the batter's box was hit in the face, hard, when the batter swung at a pitch. Should you take spinal precautions in addition to controlling the bleeding? Why?

Key Terms
mandible the lower movable portion of the jaw.
maxilla the fixed upper portion of the jaw.

Objective 33-7
Demonstrate the assessment and management of specific injuries of the face.

Assessment and Care Guidelines

There are some special assessment considerations you should heed for injuries to the face, mouth, or jaw. During your scene size-up, it is important to consider the mechanism of facial injury. For example, during a head-on collision, did the patient's head strike the windshield? If so, what was the estimated speed of travel? In patients with trauma to the face, mouth, or jaw, you should suspect possible spinal cord injuries. Patients who sustain significant trauma to the face may also have fractures of the jaw and damage to or loss of teeth.

In any case of severe facial trauma, suspect cervical spine injury. Establish manual in-line stabilization of the spine on first contact with the patient and maintain it until the patient can be completely immobilized to a long backboard. An added benefit of cervical spine stabilization and immobilization is the stabilization of facial bones. During your primary assessment, immediately manage airway, breathing, and circulation problems. Be prepared to suction the immobilized patient. Severe trauma to the face may cause an altered mental status from possible head injury or hypoxia from airway compromise.

Understanding BODY PROCESSES

Facial injuries may need aggressive maneuvers to establish and maintain an airway. Since there is a high likelihood of head injury with facial trauma, hypoxia from an occluded airway could lead to severe secondary brain injury. ■

In patients with a significant mechanism of injury, conduct a secondary assessment. Inspect and palpate for evidence of trauma. When the **mandible** (lower jaw) is fractured, it is generally broken in at least two places and will be unstable. Bruising and swelling may be obvious. Fracture of the **maxilla** (upper jaw) is often accompanied by a black eye. The face may appear elongated, and the patient's bite will no longer be even. Again, swelling may be noticeable.

In the field, you do not need to diagnose whether a fracture has actually occurred. If the patient has any pain, swelling, deformity, crepitation, discoloration, or instability to the face, maxilla, or mandible—provide emergency care as follows:

1. Establish and maintain in-line spinal stabilization.
2. In establishing and maintaining a patent airway, do the following:
   - Inspect the mouth for small fragments of teeth or broken dentures, bits of bone, pieces of flesh, or foreign objects (such as pieces of broken glass). Pick them from the mouth or remove them with finger sweeps as thoroughly as possible.
   - If dentures are in the mouth and are secure and unbroken, leave them in place; they can help support the structures of the mouth. If dentures are broken or loose, remove them. Transport any dentures or pieces of dentures with the patient so the surgeon can use them to establish proper alignment when wiring the jaw.
   - In facial injury, the tongue may lose its support structure and may fall back, occluding the airway. Open the airway using a jaw-thrust maneuver and, if necessary, grasp the tongue to pull it forward. If possible, insert an oropharyngeal airway.
   - Suction any blood, vomitus, secretions, or small debris from the mouth and oropharynx throughout treatment and transport.
   - Request ALS backup, if needed and available, to provide advanced airway management.
3. Provide oxygen by nonrebreather mask at 15 lpm or, if breathing is inadequate, begin positive pressure ventilation with supplemental oxygen at a rate of 10–12 per minute in the adult and 12–20 per minute in an infant or child. It may be difficut to get a good mask seal with facial injuries.
4. Control severe bleeding. Several major arteries run through the face, and they can bleed profusely and rapidly enough to cause death if left unmanaged. Use direct pressure and pressure dressings. Apply pressure gently if you suspect fractured or shattered bones under the wound as pressure may further obstruct an already endangered airway.
5. If nerves, tendons, or blood vessels have been exposed, cover them with a moist, sterile dressing.
6. Treat for shock and transport. Consider ALS backup for airway compromise.

Avulsed Tooth If a tooth has been lost, try to find it. The tooth may be reimplanted. To treat for an avulsed tooth:

- Rinse the tooth with saline to gently remove any debris; never scrub the tooth. Transport the tooth in a cup of saline or wrapped in gauze soaked in sterile saline. *Seek medical direction. Follow local protocol.* Never wrap the tooth in dry gauze. Guard against the tooth drying out.

Thinking Critically
A patient with a facial injury has lost a tooth. Once you determine that the tooth isn't blocking his airway, should you ask someone to look for the tooth? Why or why not?

Key Points
Clear or bloody fluid draining from the ear can indicate a skull fracture. Place a loose, clean dressing across the ear, but do not exert pressure.

- Never handle the tooth by the root; there may still be ligament fibers attached that could enable successful reimplantation.
- If you cannot find teeth that have been knocked out, assume that the patient has swallowed or aspirated them.
- Control bleeding from the tooth socket with a gauze pad.

Injury to the Midface, Upper Jaw, or Lower Jaw Midface and jaw injuries (Figure 33-18∗) may be simple, such as undisplaced nasal fractures, or extensive, involving severe lacerations, bony fractures, and nerve damage. Such injuries can result from a blunt instrument, a blow from the fist, an automobile accident, or a gunshot.

The following are signs and symptoms of fracture or other severe trauma to the midface, upper jaw, and lower jaw:

- Numbness or pain
- Distortion of facial features
- Crepitation
- Irregularities in the facial bones that can be felt before swelling occurs
- Severe bruising and swelling; black eyes
- Distance between the eyes too wide or eyes not level
- Bleeding from the nose and mouth
- Diplopia (when the orbit is fractured)
- Limited jaw motion
- Palpable movement to the maxilla

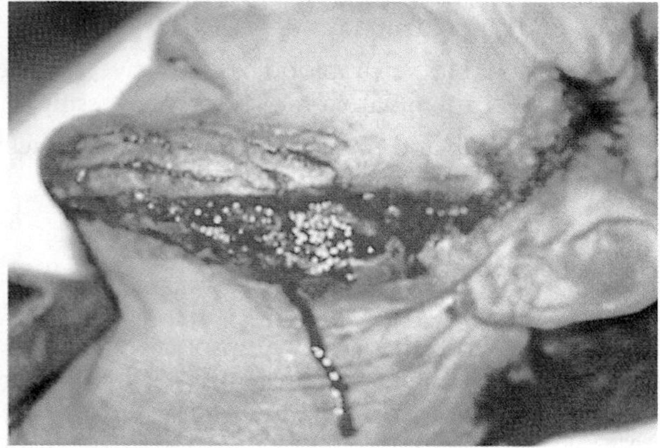

FIGURE 33-18 ∗ Soft tissue and bone injury to the mandible.

- Teeth not meeting normally
- Hematoma (collection of blood) under the tongue
- Limited jaw motion
- Mouth open or patient unable to open the mouth
- Saliva mixed with blood flowing from the mouth
- Drooling (pain prevents the patient from swallowing)
- Painful or difficult speech
- Missing, loosened, or uneven teeth (even if teeth are not missing, the patient may complain that teeth do not "fit together right")
- Pain around the ears

As emphasized earlier, you do not need to diagnose whether a facial fracture has actually occurred. If there is a significant mechanism of injury and any of the signs and symptoms just listed, treat as if a fracture has occurred. Your first priorities are establishing and maintaining spinal stabilization and a patent airway, supporting breathing as necessary, and controlling life-threatening bleeding. Request ALS backup if needed and available, because patients with severe facial trauma may be difficult to ventilate and require advanced airway procedures. Assess for spine injury, skull and/or brain injury, eye injury, and facial burns, which are commonly associated with facial injury.

Object Impaled in the Cheek If the patient has a foreign object impaled in the cheek, stabilize it with bulky dressings and transport the patient. If the object has penetrated all the way through the cheek and is loose—such that it may fall into the mouth, obstructing the airway—you need to remove it as follows:

1. Pull or push the object out of the cheek in the opposite direction to which it entered the cheek.
2. Pack dressing material between the patient's teeth and the wound. Leave some of the dressing outside the mouth and tape it there to prevent the patient from swallowing the dressing. Monitor closely to make sure the dressing doesn't become loose and compromise the airway.
3. Dress and bandage the outside of the wound to control bleeding.
4. Consider requesting ALS backup, as advanced airway procedures may be needed.
5. Suction the mouth and throat frequently throughout transport.

Objective 33-8
Demonstrate the assessment and management of specific injuries of the neck, including penetrating and blunt injury to the neck.

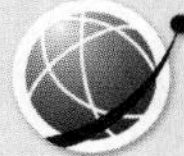

Media Resources
Go to www.bradybooks.com for mykit. Highlights:
- *Web Resource:* Eye Injuries

Injury to the Nose Soft tissue injuries to the nose should be assessed and cared for as you would other soft tissue injuries (EMT Skills 33-5). Take special care to maintain an open airway, and position the patient so that blood does not drain into the oropharynx or pharynx. Nasal fractures are the most common type of facial fracture because of the delicate structure of the nose. If a nasal fracture involves only the cartilaginous septum, it usually results in deformity, swelling, pain, and minor hemorrhage. If, however, the trauma is severe enough to break the underlying nasal bones and deeper nasal structures, such as the ethmoid bones, significant hemorrhaging can occur—especially if the vascular supply of the nasal turbinates is involved. In such cases, airway obstruction is of great concern. For information on the emergency medical care of nosebleeds, see Chapter 28, "Bleeding and Soft Tissue Trauma." Never pack the injured nose; clear or bloody fluids can indicate a skull fracture, and packing the nose can create dangerous pressure. Additional treatment includes the application of cold compresses to reduce swelling, and transport.

Foreign objects in the nose usually occur among small children. To treat, reassure and calm the child and parent, then transport the patient. Do not try to remove the object.

The most common signs and symptoms are swelling and deformity.

Injury to the Ear Cuts and lacerations of the ear are common (EMT Skills 33-6). Occasionally, a section of the ear may be severed. The pinna—the visible, exposed portion of the ear—is frequently traumatized with injuries to the head. Because of the limited blood supply to this cartilaginous framework of the external ear, it does not bleed significantly when injured. Assess and treat as for other soft tissue injuries. Save any avulsed parts; wrap avulsed parts in saline-soaked gauze, and transport with the patient. When dressing an injured ear, place part of the dressing between the ear and the side of the head. As a general rule, don't probe into the ear. Never pack the ear to stop bleeding from the ear canal. Clear or bloody fluid draining from the ear can indicate a skull fracture. Place a loose, clean dressing across the opening of the ear to absorb blood and fluids, but do not exert pressure to stop the bleeding.

Foreign objects in the external ear are a common problem among children. Do not attempt to remove the object. Instead, reassure the child and parent and transport the patient to the hospital.

Summary: Emergency Care—Facial Injuries

To review possible emergency care for facial injuries, see Figure 33-19*.

Injuries to the Neck

The neck can be injured by any blunt or penetrating trauma (EMT Skills 33-7). Common causes include hanging (accidental or intentional), impact with a steering wheel, knife wounds, gunshot wounds, or running or riding into a stretched wire or clothesline. In cases of accidental or intentional hanging, call law enforcement. If the neck is lacerated, bleeding from a major artery or vein can occur. Air may enter a lacerated vein. Other common consequences of neck injuries are a fractured larynx and a collapsed trachea. Do not overlook the possibility of a cervical spine injury.

Besides obvious lacerations or other wounds, signs and symptoms of an injured neck include the following:

- Obvious swelling, bruising, or hematoma formation
- Difficulty speaking
- Change in or loss of the voice
- Subcutaneous emphysema in the neck
- Airway obstruction that is not obviously due to other sources (such obstruction may be caused by swelling of the throat)
- Crepitation heard during speaking or breathing as air escapes from an injured larynx
- Displacement of the trachea to one side (also a sign of possible chest injury)

Maintaining an airway is extremely important in neck injuries, because—in addition to swelling or presence of damaged airway structures or debris such as bone fragments—blood will clot when it is exposed to air and can threaten the airway. Maintain a high index of suspicion for possible cervical spine injury.

To treat a neck injury, use proper Standard Precautions, establish and maintain in-line spinal stabilization, establish a patent airway, provide high-concentration oxygen or positive pressure ventilation with supplemental oxygen as necessary, control severe bleeding, treat for shock, and transport. Of special concern is a laceration of the jugular vein. Jugular vein laceration could permit development of an air embolism, because venous pressure drops below atmospheric pressure during deep inhalation if the patient is breathing spontaneously. In that cirumstance, the negative

Emergency Care Protocol

FACIAL INJURY

1. Establish manual in-line stabilization. Do not release it until the patient is immobilized onto the backboard.
2. Establish and maintain an open airway. Avoid using a nasopharyngeal airway if there is midface or nasal trauma.
3. Suction blood and secretions as necessary. Remove any broken teeth or loose bone fragments from the mouth.
4. If dentures are in the mouth and secure, leave them in place. If the dentures are loose, remove them.
5. If breathing is inadequate, provide positive pressure ventilation with supplemental oxygen at a minimum rate of 10–12 ventilations/minute for an adult and 12–20 ventilations/minute for an infant or child.
6. If breathing is adequate, administer oxygen based on the SpO_2 reading and patient signs and symptoms. If the SpO_2 reading is greater than 95% and no signs or symptoms of hypoxia or respiratory distress are present, oxygen may not be necessary if the injury is isolated to the soft tissue of the face. If massive facial injury, severe blood loss, head injury, spine injury, or multiple injuries are present, or signs of hypoxia or respiratory distress are present, or the SpO_2 reading is less than 95%, place the patient on a nonrebreather mask at 15 lpm.
7. Control any major bleeding.
8. Apply a moist sterile dressing to any exposed nerves, tendons, or blood vessels.
9. Treat specific injuries as follows:
   Avulsed Tooth:
   Rinse with saline; do not scrub or handle the tooth by the root.
   Place in a cup with sterile saline or wrap in gauze soaked in sterile saline.
   Do not wrap in dry gauze.
   Control the bleeding from the tooth socket with a gauze pad. Make sure that the pad does not work loose and become an airway obstruction.
   Foreign Object in Cheek:
   If the object did not penetrate completely through the cheek or is not loose, use bulky dressings to stabilize the object in place.
   If the object penetrated through to other side of the cheek and is loose, do the following:
   Push or pull the object out of the cheek in the same direction it entered.
   Pack with dressings between the teeth and wound; make sure dressings do not work loose and become an airway obstruction.
   Dress and bandage outside of wound.
   Suction blood as necessary.
   Injury to Nose:
   Manage as a soft tissue injury.
   Position the patient to allow blood to drain.
   Do not pack the nose.
   Transport if a foreign body is in the nose.
   Apply cold compresses if a nose fracture is suspected.
   Injury to Ear:
   Manage as a soft tissue injury.
   Save avulsed parts; wrap in saline-soaked gauze and transport with patient.
   Place part of dressing between the ear and side of head.
   Do not probe into the ear.
   Do not pack the ear.
   Place a loose dressing over the ear to absorb blood and fluid; do not apply pressure.
   Do not attempt to remove foreign objects in the ear.
10. Immobilize the patient to a backboard if you suspect spine injury.
11. Transport.
12. Perform a reassessment every 5 minutes if unstable and every 15 minutes if stable.

FIGURE 33-19 ✱ Emergency care protocol: facial injury.

pressure in the vein is likely to suck in air. For this reason, quick application of an occlusive dressing for this type of injury is necessary. Consider requesting ALS backup if advanced airway management is needed, especially with laryngeal or tracheal injuries.

If one of the major blood vessels of the neck is severed, follow the guidelines for care that were outlined in Chapter 28, "Bleeding and Soft Tissue Trauma," and summarized in EMT Skills 33-8. When treating bleeding wounds to the neck, never probe open wounds or use circumferential bandages, which can interfere with blood flow to the brain on the uninjured side of the neck and can also impair respiration.

Summary: Emergency Care—Neck Injuries

To review possible emergency care for neck injuries, see Figure 33-20✱.

Emergency Care Protocol

NECK INJURY

1. Establish manual in-line stabilization. Do not release it until the patient is immobilized onto a backboard.
2. Control any major bleeding from the neck by applying direct pressure.
3. Establish and maintain an open airway. Avoid using a nasopharyngeal airway if there is midface or nasal trauma.
4. Suction secretions as necessary.
5. If breathing is inadequate, provide positive pressure ventilation with supplemental oxygen at a minimum rate of 10–12 ventilations/minute for an adult and 12–20 ventilations/minute for an infant or child.
6. If breathing is adequate, the SpO_2 reading is greater than 95%, and no signs or symptoms of hypoxia or respiratory distress are present, oxygen may not be necessary if the injury is isolated to the soft tissue of the neck and no major bleeding is present. If severe blood loss, head injury, spine injury, or multiple injuries are present, or signs of hypoxia or respiratory distress are present, or the SpO_2 reading is less than 95%, place the patient on a nonrebreather mask at 15 lpm.
7. Apply a nonporous dressing taped on four sides.
8. Immobilize the patient to a backboard if you suspect spine injury.
9. Transport.
10. Perform a reassessment every 5 minutes if unstable and every 15 minutes if stable.

FIGURE 33-20 ✻ Emergency care protocol: neck injury.

EMT skills 33-1 Removal of Foreign Object—Upper Eyelid

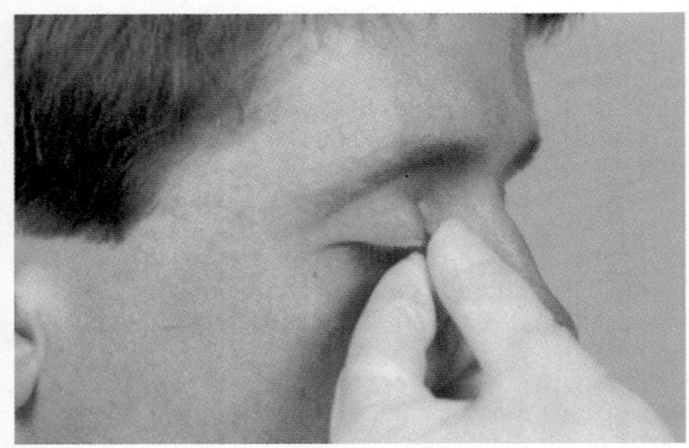

33-1A ✱ Grasp eyelashes between the thumb and forefinger and tell the patient to look downward.

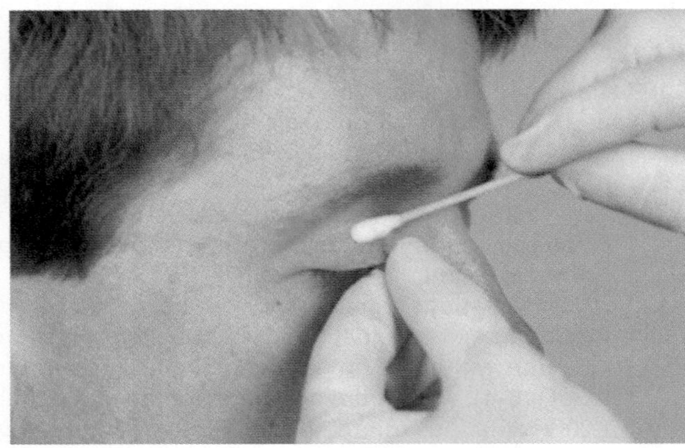

33-1B ✱ Place an applicator swab along the center of the upper eyelid.

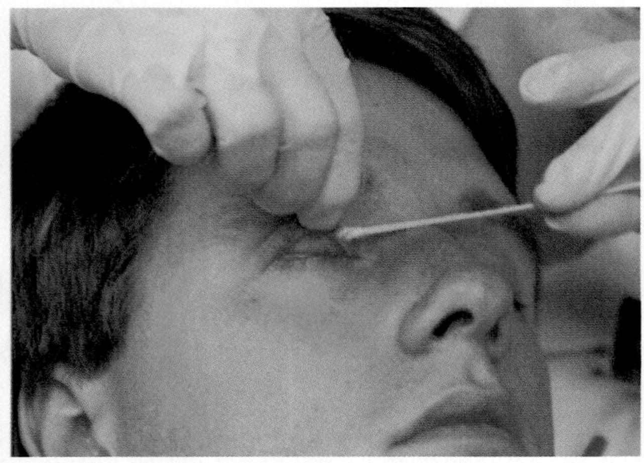

33-1C ✱ Pull the eyelid forward and upward over the applicator swab.

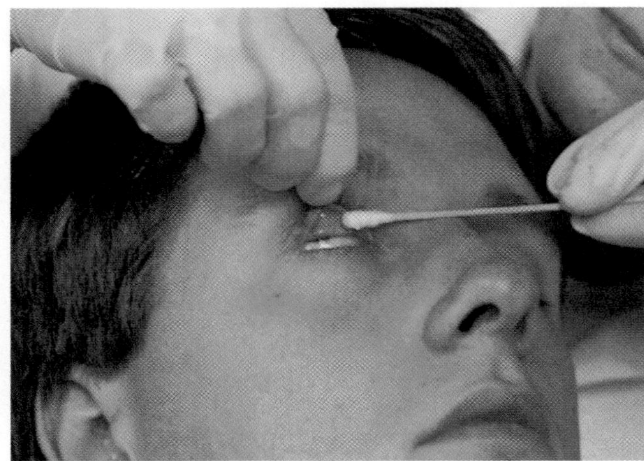

33-1D ✱ The undersurface of the eyelid is exposed and the foreign object can be gently removed with a sterile, moistened applicator swab.

EMT skills 33-2 Emergency Care—Impaled Object in the Eye

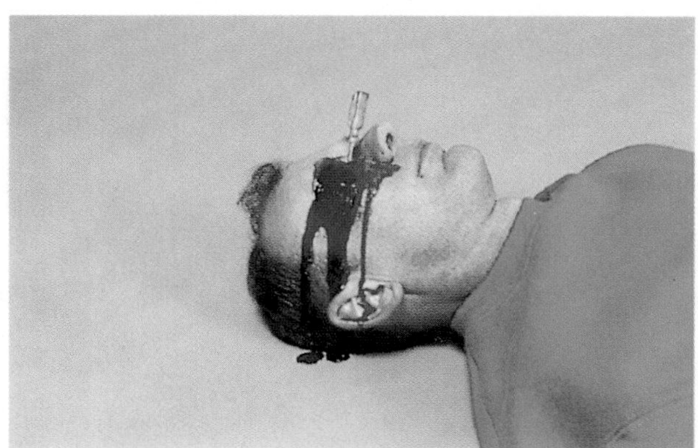

33-2A * Impaled object in the eye.

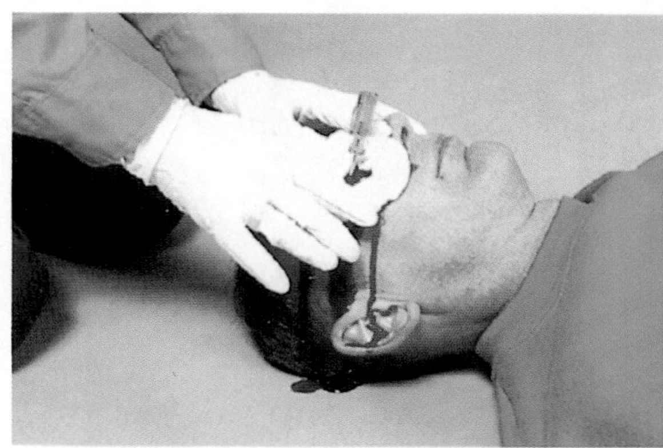

33-2B * Place padding around the object.

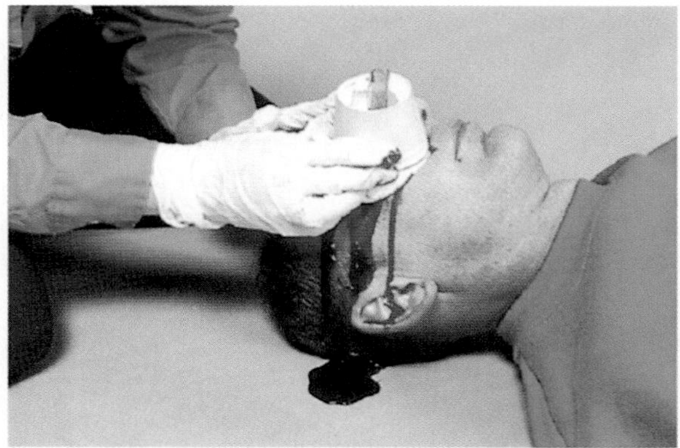

33-2C * Stabilize the impaled object with a cup.

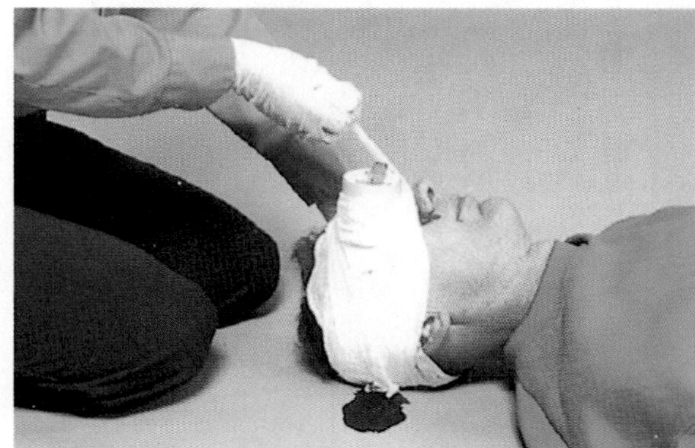

33-2D * Bandage the cup in place.

EMT skills 33-3 Injuries to the Face

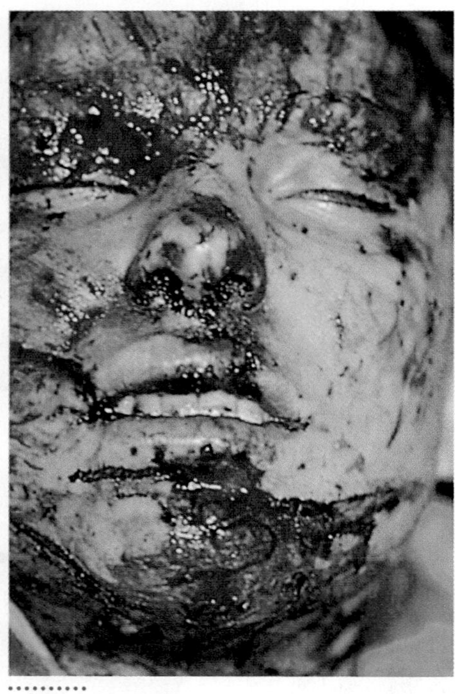

33-3A *

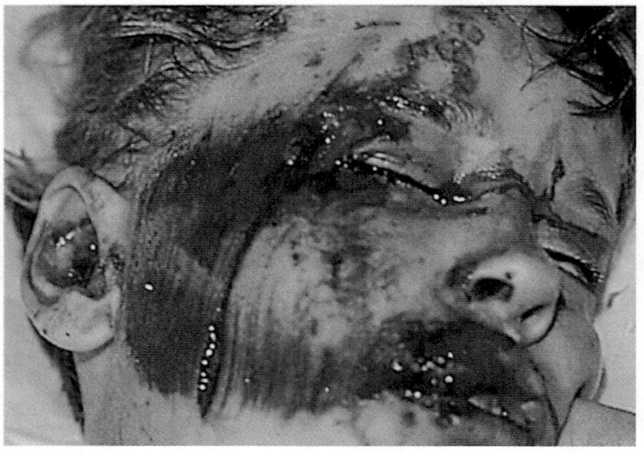

33-3B *

EMT skills 33-4 Injuries to the Mouth, Jaw, Cheek, and Chin

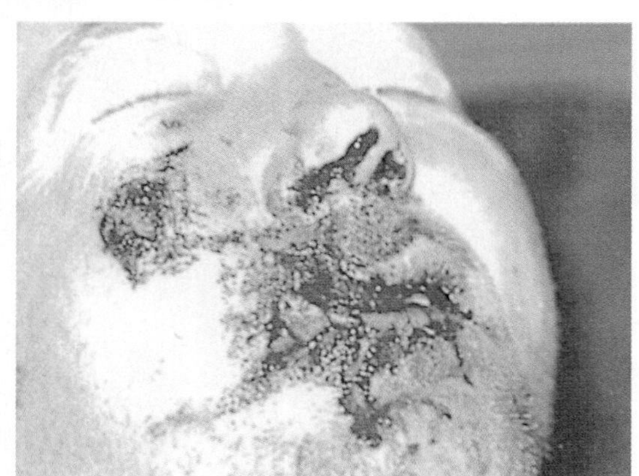

33-4A * Injuries to the mouth, jaw, cheek, and chin.

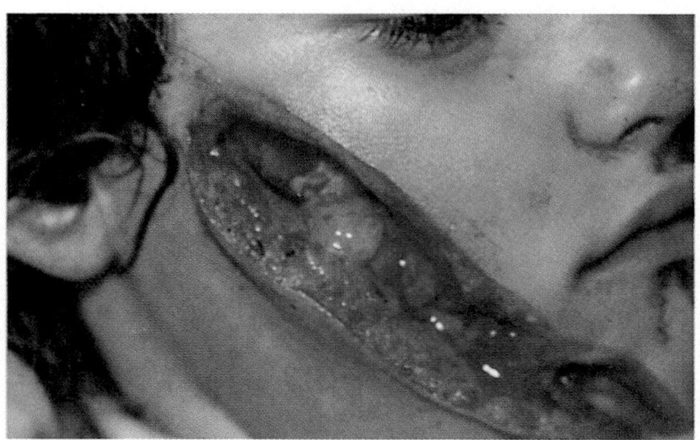

33-4B * Injuries to the jaw, cheek, and chin.

EMT skills 33-4 Injuries to the Mouth, Jaw, Cheek, and Chin *continued*

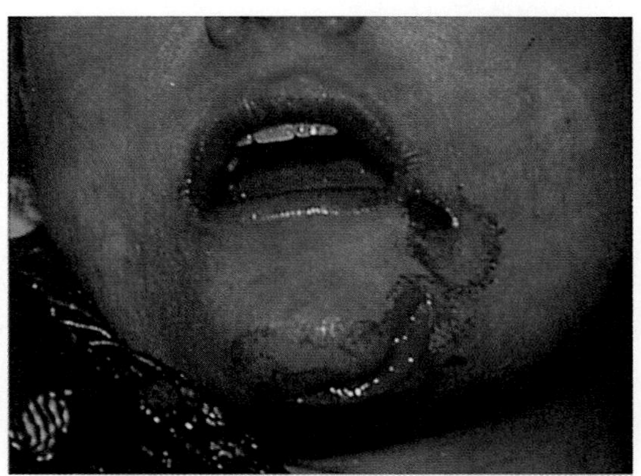

33-4C * Injuries to the mouth, cheek, and chin.

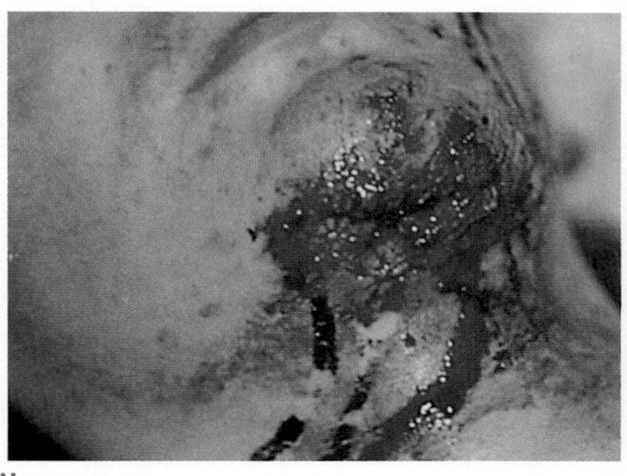

33-4D * Injuries to the chin.

EMT skills 33-5 Injuries to the Nose

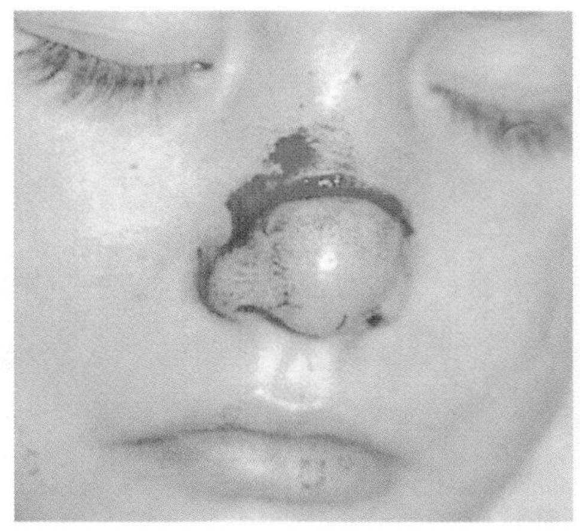

33-5A *

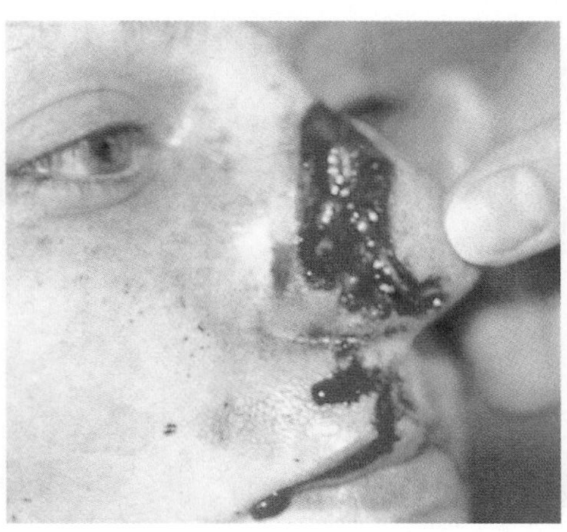

33-5B *

EMT skills 33-6 Injuries to the Ear

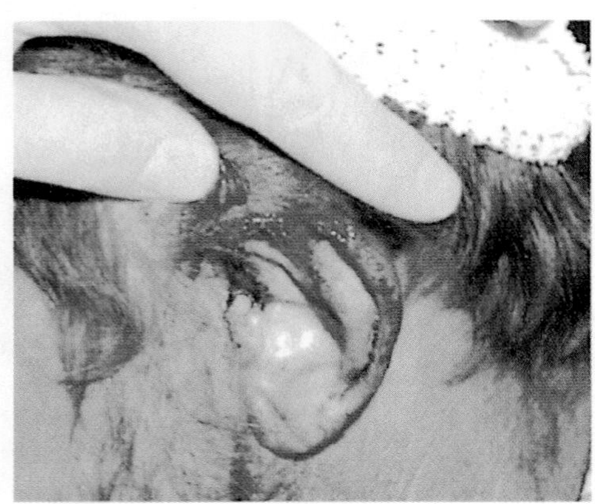
33-6A *

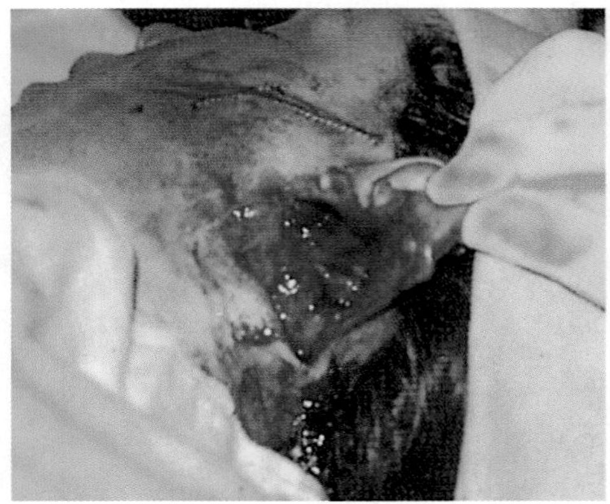
33-6B *

EMT skills 33-7 Injuries to the Neck

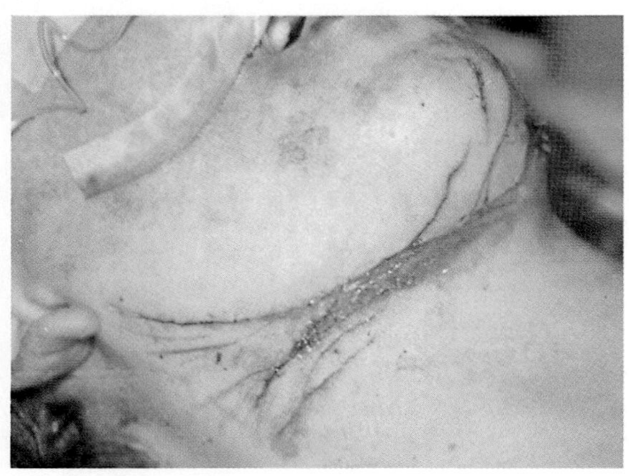
33-7A *

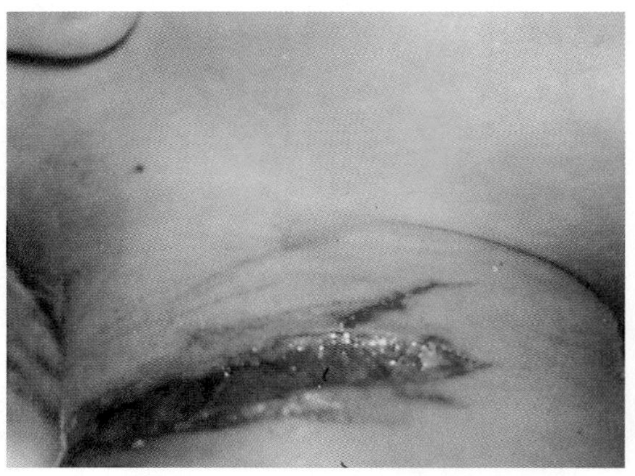
33-7B *

EMT skills 33-8 Emergency Care—Severed Blood Vessel of the Neck

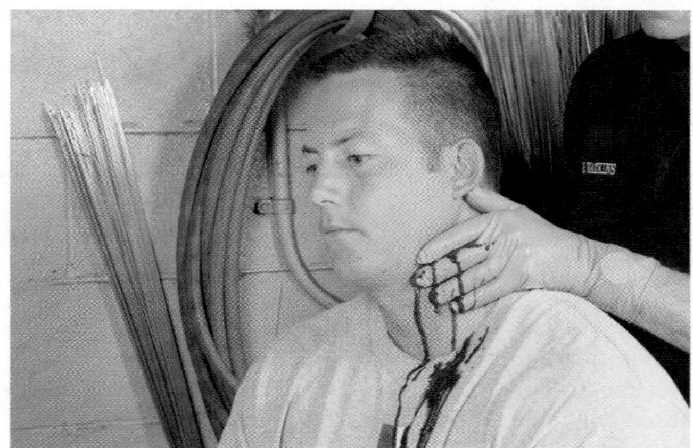

33-8A ✱ Place a gloved hand over the wound to control bleeding. Apply pressure to the carotid artery only if necessary to control bleeding. Never apply pressure to both sides of the neck at the same time.

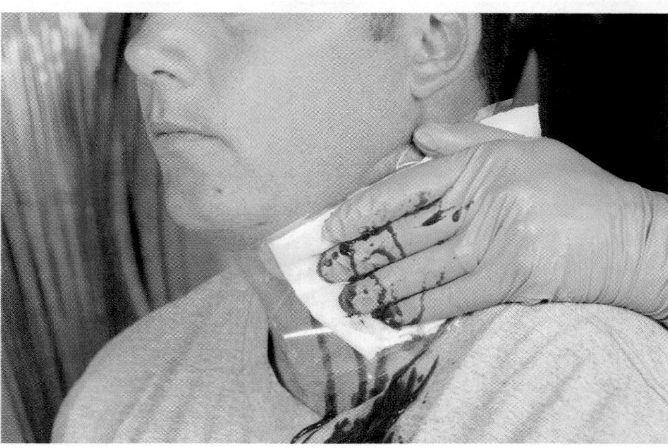

33-8B ✱ Apply an occlusive dressing, which should extend beyond all edges of the wound to avoid being sucked into the wound. Cover the occlusive dressing with a regular dressing. Apply only enough pressure to control the bleeding.

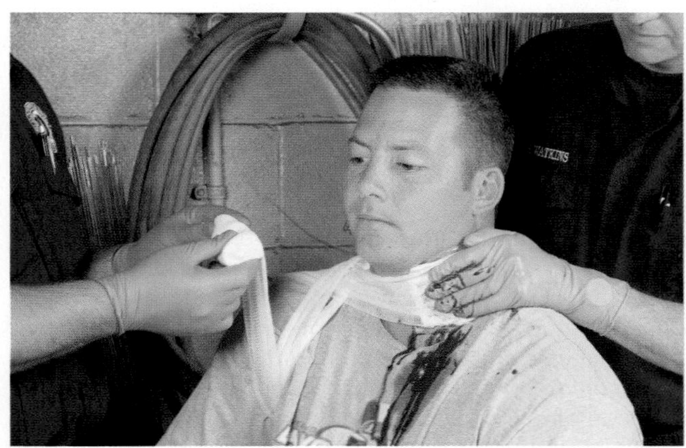

33-8C ✱ Once bleeding is controlled, apply a pressure dressing. A figure-eight bandage is wrapped over the dressing, across one shoulder, across the back, under the opposite armpit, and anchored at the shoulder.

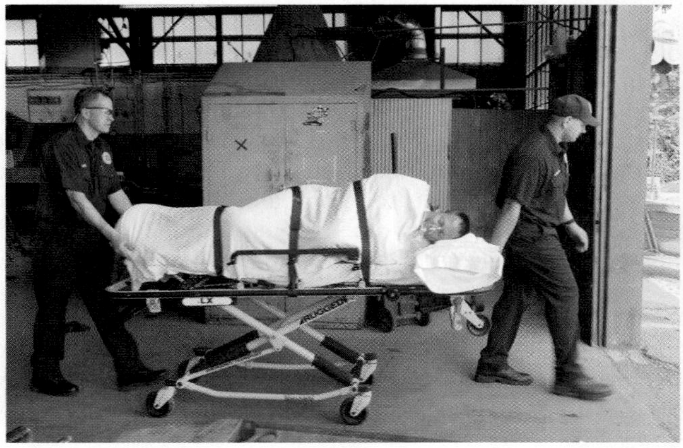

33-8D ✱ If spinal injury is not suspected, position the patient on his left side, head tilted downward. (If spinal injury is suspected and the patient is immobilized to a spine board, board and patient can be turned and tilted as a unit.) Continue administration of oxygen. Care for shock, and transport.

CHAPTER REVIEW

SUMMARY

During a career in EMS, the EMT will encounter many patients with significant injuries. Few of these will rival the potentially gruesome and clinically challenging patient with severe facial or neck trauma. Understanding the anatomy, physiology, injury presentation patterns, and management principles will allow the EMT to provide optimum emergency care to these patients and keep morbidity and mortality to a minimum. Even though most facial and neck trauma is not life threatening, there will be patients whose injuries require immediate intervention, because without it the likelihood of death or permanent disability is high. So long as the EMT follows a well-grounded assessment procedure and employs airway control, spinal immobilization, ventilatory support, and oxygenation as appropriate, along with soft tissue management—as described in this chapter—the patient will receive the best care possible.

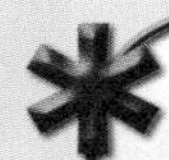

CASE STUDY FOLLOW-UP

SCENE SIZE-UP

You and your partner have been dispatched to a 22-year-old male patient complaining of blindness and severe eye pain. As you approach the patient's driveway, you see no safety hazards. Walking past two vehicles with jumper cables, you begin to think the mechanism of injury might be an exploding car battery. The sight of white battery acid sprayed across the car hood and a brief talk with a neighbor confirm your suspicion. The neighbor tells you the patient was smoking a cigarette over the car battery when there was a big explosion.

Once inside the patient's house, you find him running around the living room with a wet towel wrapped around his face. You try to calm him. He tells you his name is Hector Fernandez. He says he can't see, and it hurts "really bad."

PRIMARY ASSESSMENT

Since he is talking to you and answers questions appropriately, you determine that Hector's airway, breathing, and mental status are adequate. He denies breathing difficulty but tells you both eyes are extremely painful. Your general impression is that Hector seems alert and oriented, but he needs eye care immediately or he'll be in danger of losing his sight.

Quickly you walk the patient into the kitchen. You ask if he is wearing contact lenses. He says "no." You direct the patient to lean over the sink. Next you turn on the faucet and direct Hector to lean under it. You have him turn his head from side to side so that the water runs from the medial to the lateral side of each eye in turn.

SECONDARY ASSESSMENT

You are unable to conduct an exam of Hector's eyes while he is irrigating them at the kitchen sink, but your partner is able to take Hector's baseline vitals. He reports Hector's pulse at 120 bpm; blood pressure is 140/80 mmHg. His skin is warm and dry. His respirations are regular at 24 per minute. Meanwhile, you are able to gather a history from Hector who replies to your questions while continuing to keep his eyes under the running water. He describes the pain to his eyes as "about 7 or 8" on a scale of 1 to 10. He reports no known allergies and is not taking any medications or seeing a doctor for any medical problems. His last oral intake was lunch about an hour ago. Events leading to the present problem were, as described by the neighbor, an explosion of battery acid while he was working on his car.

While you are busy treating Hector's eyes, your partner conducts a secondary assessment to see if there were further injuries from the battery explosion. He does not find any further trauma. Medical direction instructs you to irrigate for a total of 20 minutes prior to transport and continue to irrigate en route.

After 20 minutes of irrigation with copious amounts of tap water, Hector's pain decreases. He says, "I can see, now—some." You place Hector on his side on the stretcher with a basin under his head. You continue irrigation with your ambulance's bottled water and transport.

REASSESSMENT

You perform a reassessment. Hector's vital signs are stable, and you reassess his eyesight to find that it continues to improve. Once at the hospital, you transfer Hector to the care of emergency department personnel, provide an oral report, complete your prehospital care report, and prepare the ambulance for return to service.

IN REVIEW

1. Describe the emergency care that may need to be undertaken during primary assessment of eye, face, or neck injuries.
2. Explain why, during the primary assessment, you should consider requesting advanced life support backup for injuries to the eyes, face, or neck.
3. Describe how to conduct the physical exam of a patient with an eye injury.
4. List the basic rules of emergency care for eye injuries.
5. Describe the emergency care steps for a patient with a foreign object (a) located on the white of the eye, (b) located under the upper eyelid, and (c) lodged in the eyeball.
6. Describe the emergency care steps for a patient with a chemical burn to the eye.
7. List the reasons for removing, and the reasons for not removing, contact lenses from a patient with an eye injury.
8. List the general emergency medical care guidelines for injuries to the face, mouth, and jaw.
9. Describe the care for a foreign object in the nose or ear.
10. In addition to obvious lacerations or wounds, list the signs and symptoms of neck injury.

CRITICAL THINKING

You are called one night for domestic violence. While en route, dispatch advises that the police are also en route and that you are to stage in the area until confirmation is received from the responding patrol officers that the scene is safe to enter. While you are staging, your partner quickly scans through the trauma bag to ensure that all supplies are there and that the oxygen level in the tank is good, since you have been running calls all day long. After about a 5-minute wait, you get the signal from dispatch that the police have entered the scene and it is now secure and safe for your entry. The police report that you have one male patient, 17 years of age, who was in an altercation with his stepfather.

Upon repositioning your ambulance outside the address and donning your protective equipment, you and your partner cautiously enter the scene. You first see the police with a handcuffed male adult, who they tell you reportedly attacked his stepson for coming home "drunk." The patient, a 17-year-old male, is found in the kitchen, where you see a moderate amount of blood splattered on the wall and countertop, and a bloodied handheld blender lying about 6 feet away. You stay away from the blender, as this is possible crime scene evidence that should not be disturbed.

During the primary assessment, you quickly discern that the patient is not alert or responding to verbal or painful stimuli and that there is an odor resembling alcohol about him. You also note extensive facial trauma, with his right eye almost completely extruded. The patient's nose is markedly deformed and displaced to the right, there is a large laceration to his upper lip bleeding briskly, and you can hear audible gurgling as the patient tries to breathe. You quickly glance at your partner to tell him to call for ALS backup, but you see him already lifting the portable radio to do so.

1. What is the most important initial step the EMT should perform in the management of this patient?
2. Briefly describe three different reasons that may explain why this patient is unresponsive.
3. If attempts at clearing the airway with suctioning fail, how else may the EMT ensure the adequacy of this patient's airway?
4. After treating all life threats, what would be the specific management for the eye injury?
5. What could be the advantage of calling ALS backup for this patient?

EXPLORE PEARSON **mybradykit**™

Please go to **www.bradybooks.com** to access mykit for this text. You will find quizzes, critical thinking scenarios, weblinks, animations, and videos related to this chapter—and much more. Look for online information on eye and maxilofacial injuries.

Register your access code from the front of your book by going to **www.bradybooks.com** and selecting the mykit links.

CHAPTER 34

Chest Trauma

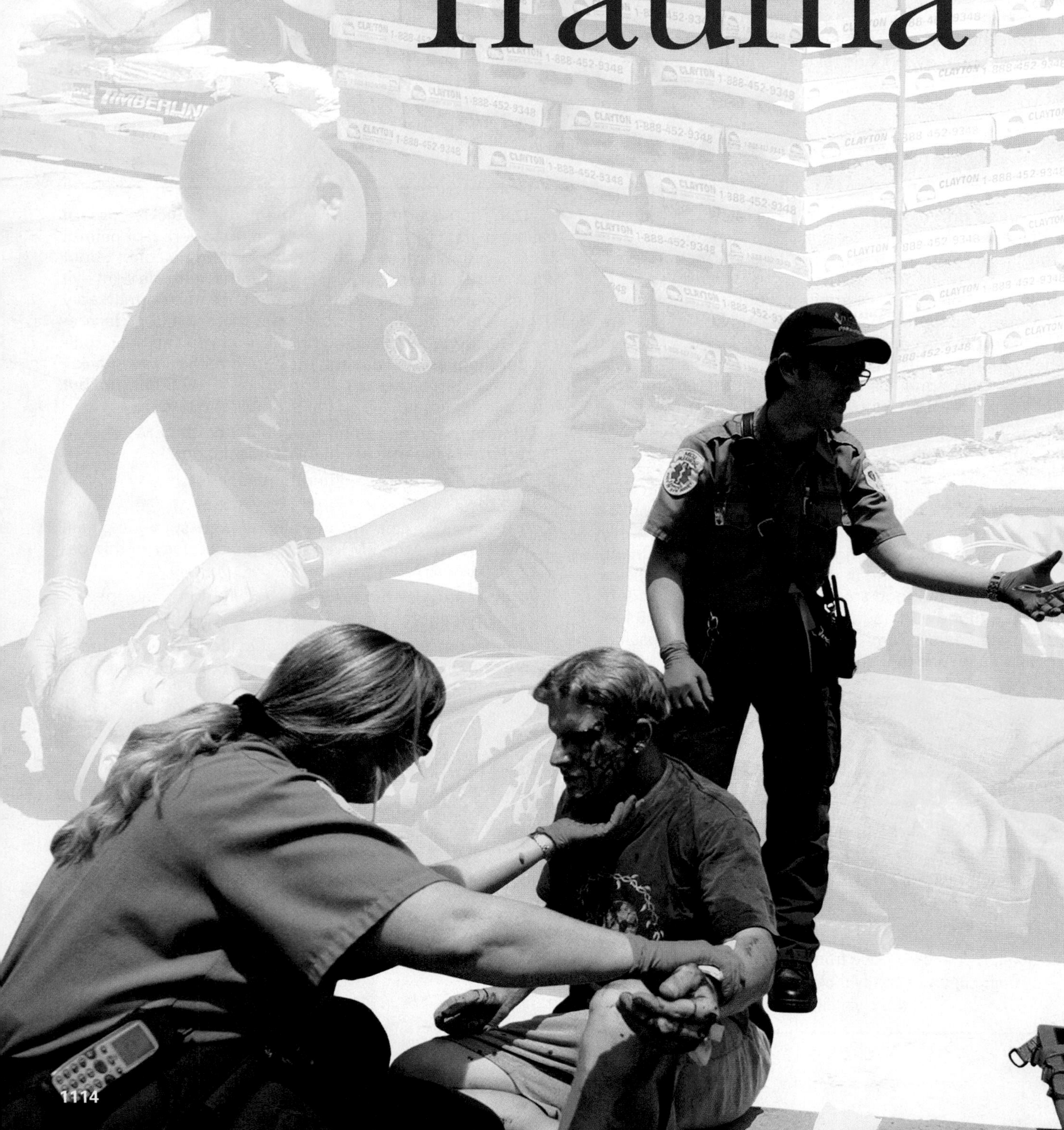

Navigation Guide

The following items provide an overview to the purpose and content of this chapter. The Standard and Competency are from the new National EMS Education Standards.

STANDARD **Trauma** (Content Area: Chest Trauma)

COMPETENCY Applies fundamental knowledge to provide basic emergency care and transportation based on assessment findings for an acutely injured patient.

OBJECTIVES: After reading this chapter, you should be able to:

34-1. Define key terms introduced in this chapter.
34-2. List the major structures of the thoracic cavity.
34-3. Define and list specific types of open chest injury.
34-4. Define and list specific types of closed chest injury.
34-5. Explain the pathophysiology of each of the following injuries:
- **a.** Flail segment
- **b.** Pulmonary contusion
- **c.** Open pneumothorax, tension pneumothorax, hemothorax
- **d.** Traumatic asphyxia
- **e.** Cardiac contusion
- **f.** Pericardial tamponade
- **g.** Rib injury

34-6. Discuss an assessment-based approach to manage patients with chest trauma.
34-7. Discuss the following aspects of chest trauma care:
- **a.** General emergency care for chest trauma
- **b.** Specific emergency care for an open chest wound
- **c.** Specific emergency care for a flail segment

KEY TERMS: Page references indicate first major use in this chapter. For complete definitions, see the Glossary at the back of the book.

cardiac contusion p. 1123
commotio cordis p. 1123
flail segment p. 1119
hemoptysis p. 1129
hemothorax p. 1122
open pneumothorax p. 1121
paradoxical movement p. 1119
pericardial tamponade p. 1123
pneumothorax p. 1117
pulmonary contusion p. 1120
sucking chest wound p. 1118
tension pneumothorax p. 1118
traumatic asphyxia p. 1122

MEDIA RESOURCES: Please go to www.bradybooks.com to access mykit for this text. You will find quizzes, critical thinking scenarios, weblinks, animations, and videos related to this chapter—and much more. Look for online information on pneumothorax and cardiac tamponade.

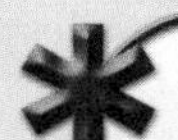

CASE STUDY

The Dispatch
EMS Unit 106—respond to the corner of Market Street and Breaden Avenue—you have a man down with an unknown problem—be advised that this was called in by a person driving by. Time out is 2206 hours.

Upon Arrival
As you and your partner are turning the corner onto Market Street, you note what appears to be a man lying in a prone position on the sidewalk. You pull up to the scene and turn on the driver-side scene lights. You look for any other people or activity. It is a cold night and the patient is dressed in a heavy overcoat.

You can hear him moaning as you step out of the ambulance. As you approach the patient, you say, "Sir, we are emergency medical technicians, and we are here to help you. Can you tell me if you are hurt or ill?" The patient responds with a moan.

How Would You Proceed to Assess and Care for This Patient?
During this chapter, you will learn about assessment and emergency medical care for patients suffering from chest trauma. Later, we will return to the case study and put in context some of the information you learned.

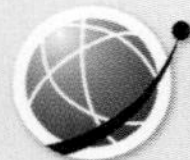

Media Resources
Go to www.bradybooks.com for mykit. Highlights:

- *Web Resource:* Rib Fractures and Flail Chest
- *Web Resource:* Pneumothorax

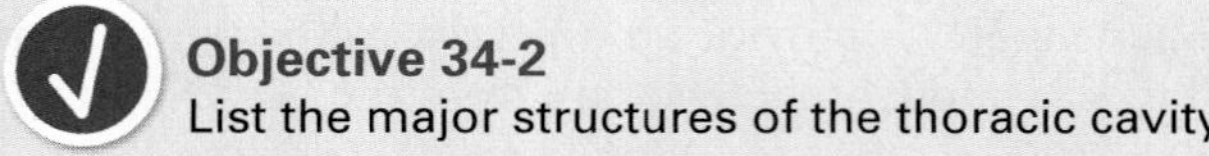

Objective 34-2
List the major structures of the thoracic cavity.

Introduction

Most injuries to the chest are not characterized by large, gaping wounds. Unlike some injuries to the extremities, they rarely involve bones protruding through the skin. Injuries to the chest, in fact, are often not very dramatic in appearance and can be easily overlooked in the physical assessment. The patient may actually complain of much more pain from injuries to bones and joints or from surface lacerations and abrasions. Initially, the patient may not even realize that he has a serious injury to the chest.

It is important to understand, however, that the chest contains vital organs, and injuries to the chest may be lethal. Chest injuries can cause a disturbance in respiration, oxygen exchange, and circulation and may produce severe internal bleeding and shock. Rely on the mechanism of injury, a high index of suspicion, and careful physical examination to determine and then care for life-threatening injuries to the chest.

The Chest

Anatomy of the Chest

Before you read this section on chest injuries, it may be helpful to review Chapter 7, "Anatomy, Physiology, and Medical Terminology," for descriptions of the structures and organs of the chest, as well as the anatomy and physiology of the circulatory and respiratory systems.

To recap briefly, the chest cavity is also known as the *thoracic cavity* (Figure 34-1*). It is surrounded by the ribs, which form a bony cage around the organs of the respiratory and circulatory systems. The thoracic cavity is bordered inferiorly by the *diaphragm,* which separates it from the abdominal cavity. A hollow area, the *mediastinum,* is located in the middle of the thoracic cavity between the right and left lungs. The mediastinum houses the *trachea* (conduit to the lungs), the *venae cavae* (the two great veins that collect blood from the upper and lower body and return it to the heart), the *aorta* (the great artery carrying blood from the heart to the body), the *esophagus* (the tubelike structure that connects the pharynx with the stomach), and the *heart.*

With this collection of vital organs, it is easy to see why injury to the chest can be life threatening.

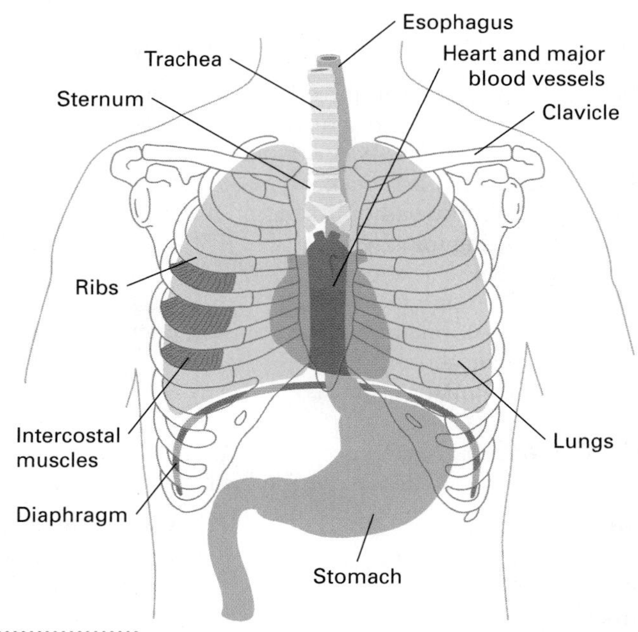

FIGURE 34-1 * The chest cavity.

The pleural lining of the thorax plays a major role in some types of chest injuries. The pleura consists of the *visceral pleura* and the *parietal pleura*. The visceral pleura is the innermost layer and is in contact with the lung. The parietal pleura is the outermost layer and is in contact with the thoracic wall. The two pleural layers are separated by serous fluid that provides lubrication to reduce the friction between them.

Between the pleural layers is a *potential space*. Because of the pull of the parietal pleura on the visceral pleura during inhalation, the pressure between the pleura is negative. It acts like a vacuum. As an example, a similar pull or vacuum would be created by placing a glass on a flat countertop surface with a film of water between the glass and the countertop and then pulling straight up on the glass. A vacuum is created between the glass and the countertop. The more forcefully you pull up on the glass

Understanding BODY PROCESSES

The constant pull or tug caused by the lung tissues' natural tendency to recoil and collapse creates the constant negative pressure inside the pleural space. ■

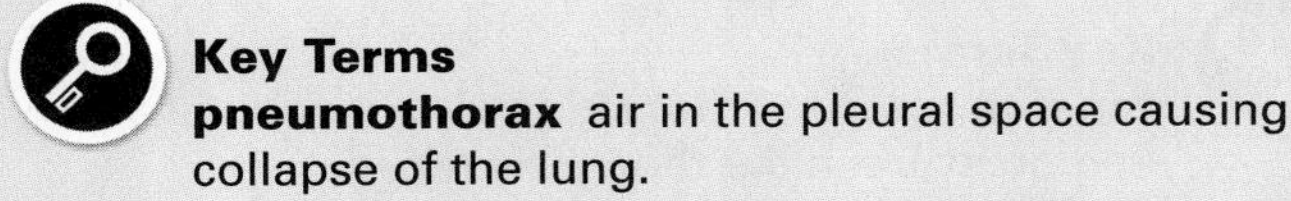

pneumothorax air in the pleural space causing collapse of the lung.

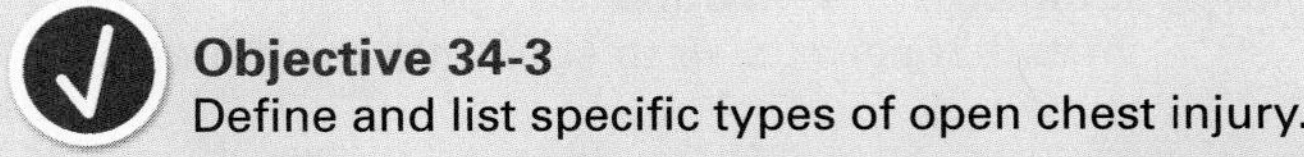

Define and list specific types of open chest injury.

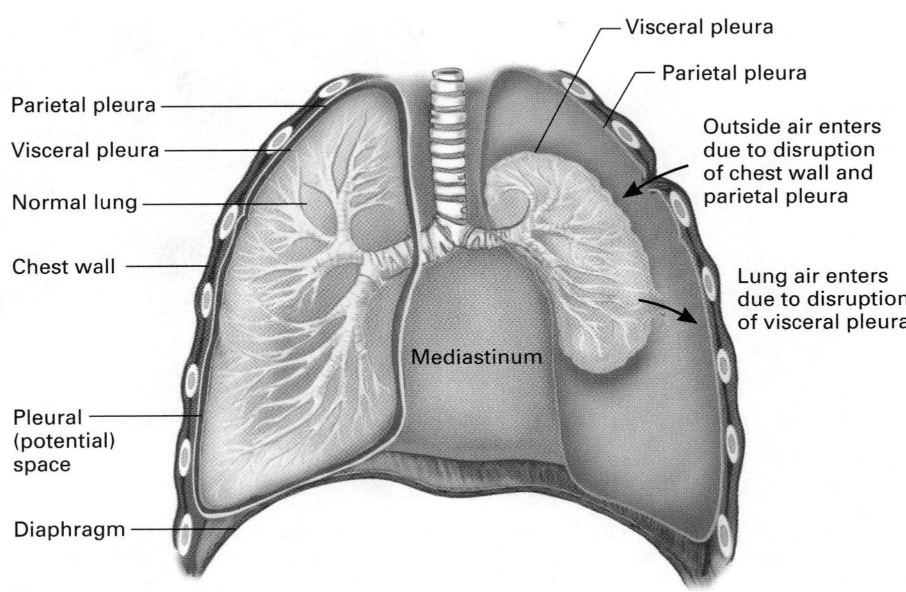

FIGURE 34-2 ✱ Normally, negative pressure acts like a vacuum, holding the visceral pleura that covers the lung to the parietal pleura that lines the chest wall and keeping the lung expanded. When either the lung and its visceral pleura are punctured or the chest wall and its parietal pleura are punctured, air enters the space between the pleura, creating positive pressure on the lung and causing it to collapse.

and try to separate it from the countertop, the greater the negative pressure that is created. Thus, each time the chest wall expands, the negative pressure or vacuum between the pleura increases.

If a puncture to the visceral pleura, the parietal pleura, or both pleura occurs, the seal is broken and air is sucked into the pleural space each time the chest wall expands. As the pleural space expands, it creates pressure on the lung and the lung collapses, leading to a **pneumothorax** (Figure 34-2✱). Since no gas exchange occurs outside of the alveoli, the air that flows into the pleural space is not contributing to gas exchange. As the lung continues to collapse, the gas exchange becomes more and more disturbed, and the patient becomes hypoxic.

This concept plays a major role in understanding chest injuries and open wounds to the chest. If an open wound to the chest is at least two-thirds the internal diameter of the trachea, a significant amount of air will be sucked into the open wound to the chest and into the pleural space, and not through the trachea and into the lungs. The normal adult trachea is about the size of a quarter. A hole about the size of a nickel would be a severe injury that would lead to a significant lung collapse.

General Categories of Chest Injuries

There are two general categories of chest injuries: open and closed. Closed injuries to the chest are the result of blunt trauma applied to the chest cavity, which can cause extensive damage to the ribs and internal organs. Blunt trauma is often associated with falls, automobile crashes, and blows to the chest.

Open Chest Injury

An open chest injury is the result of a penetrating chest wound caused by a knife, gunshot, or a wide variety of other objects such as ice picks, screwdrivers, letter openers, broken glass, nails, and car keys. A knife or similar object damages the tissues and organs along the path of penetration. A bullet, however, can make a tiny entrance wound to the chest in one area, ricochet around, and cause extensive internal damage throughout the chest cavity. It may create a second, or exit, wound, which is typically larger than the entrance wound if the bullet leaves the body (Figure 34-3✱). A bullet, because of its velocity, also causes cavitation—a

Key Terms
sucking chest wound an open wound to the chest that permits air to enter into the thoracic cavity.

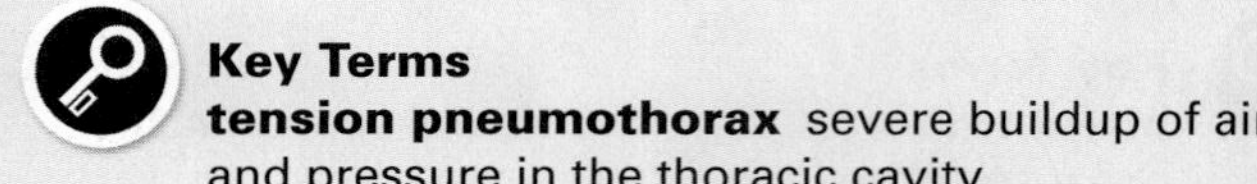

Key Terms
tension pneumothorax severe buildup of air and pressure in the thoracic cavity.

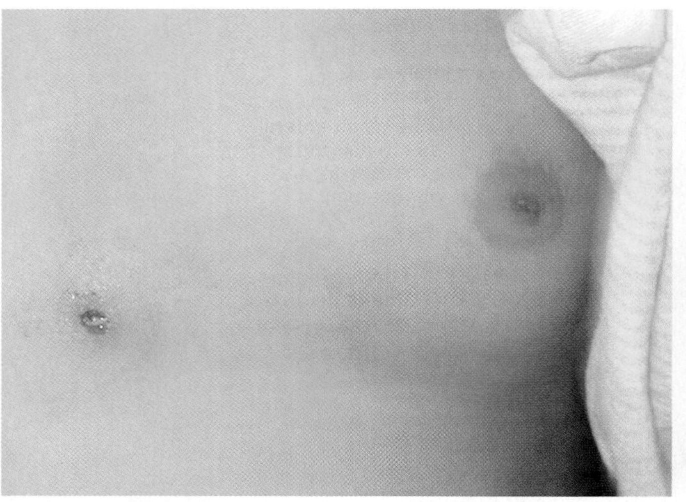

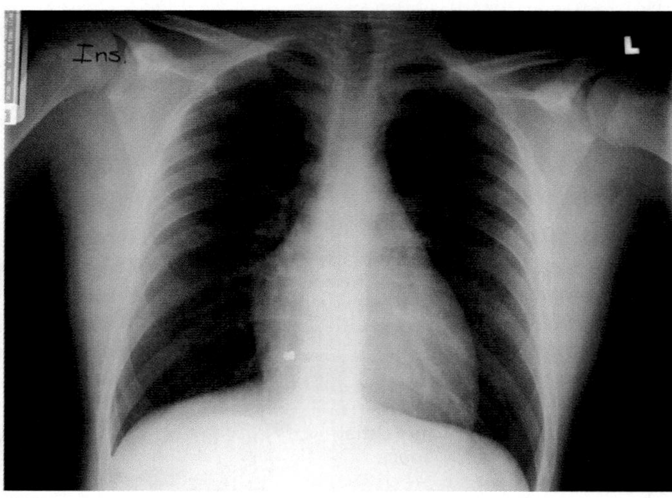

FIGURE 34-3 ✻ A pellet fired from an air gun creates an extremely small entrance wound. Although a pellet wound may be very small, a pellet can penetrate the thoracic cavity, ricochet around, and potentially cause lethal injuries. When you suspect trauma, you must expose and closely inspect the chest to avoid missing potentially lethal injuries. (Both photos: © Charles Stewart, MD, and Associates)

hollowing-out of tissues along the path of the bullet that is much greater in diameter than the bullet itself.

The heart is a special type of contractile muscle. It can be injured by both penetrating and blunt trauma: a knife or bullet, a fractured rib that slices into the heart or lung, or even the simple transmission of kinetic energy from a blow to the chest or impact with a steering wheel. Injury to the heart can lead to ineffective pumping or to severe blood loss.

The major vessels in the chest carry large amounts of blood, some at very high pressures, and if injured can result in immediate death.

The organs and structures responsible for breathing are also contained in the chest. Inhalation occurs when the muscles between the ribs, the *intercostal muscles,* pull the ribs upward to increase the size of the rib cage. The diaphragm contracts and moves slightly downward and flares the bottom portion of the ribs outward. This expands the space in the thoracic cavity, thus generating negative pressure, or a vacuum, which causes the lungs to inflate and "pull in" air from the atmosphere. Any gas will flow from a higher pressure to a lower pressure area. When the thoracic cavity expands and the lungs inflate, the pressure inside the lungs is lower than in the atmosphere and, as a consequence, atmospheric air flows into the airway and lungs. The reverse happens during exhalation when the intercostal muscles and diaphragm relax, the thoracic cavity gets smaller, and the pressure in the lungs becomes higher than in the atmosphere, so that air flows out of the lungs.

The ability of the lungs to inflate is seriously impeded when there is an open chest wound—when the chest wall is penetrated and air flows into the thoracic cavity around the lungs. As noted earlier, air in the chest cavity is called a *pneumothorax,* from *pneumo,* meaning "air," and *thorax,* meaning "chest." Pneumothorax can be caused even when there is no open wound to the chest: For example, a fractured rib can penetrate a lung, causing air to flow from the lung into the surrounding chest cavity, collapsing the lung. (Also see the following discussion of pneumothorax under "Specific Chest Injuries.")

An open chest wound can pull air into the thoracic cavity, sometimes with a noticeable sucking sound. This is referred to as a **sucking chest wound.** There are two problems in managing an open or sucking chest wound. One is preventing additional air from being sucked into the chest cavity, and the other is avoiding trapping the air that is already in the chest cavity.

Cover a sucking chest wound with your gloved hand on first identifying it, then apply a nonporous dressing and tape it on three sides. This will prevent both pulling in additional air and trapping air that is already in the cavity. (A **tension pneumothorax** that is caused by air leaking into the chest cavity from a damaged lung with *no* opening through the outer chest wall cannot be managed

Objective 34-4
Define and list specific types of closed chest injury.

Key Terms
flail segment two or more adjacent ribs that are fractured in two or more places and thus move independently from the rest of the rib cage.

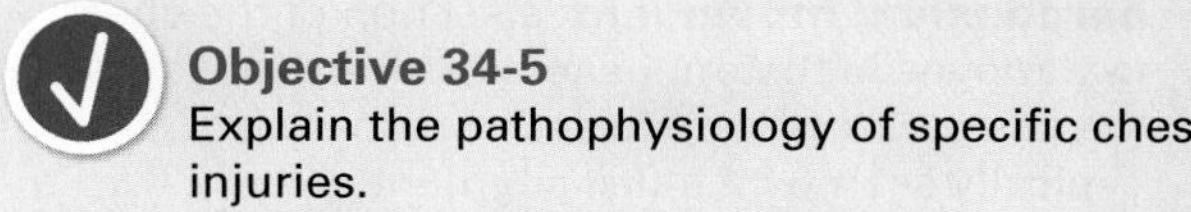
Objective 34-5
Explain the pathophysiology of specific chest injuries.

by EMTs in the prehospital setting. Early recognition and rapid transport is especially critical in this situation. See more about tension pneumothorax under "Specific Chest Injuries.")

Closed Chest Injury

A closed chest injury occurs when blunt trauma is applied to the chest but no open wound results. Injury to the lung, heart, great vessels (aorta and vena cava), respiratory tract, diaphragm, and esophagus can result from blunt trauma. A common life-threatening closed chest injury occurs when two or more adjacent ribs are broken in two or more places. This creates a segment of the chest that is unattached to the rest of the rib cage, an injury known as a **flail segment** (Figure 34-4*). A flail segment may also result from more than one rib being fractured and separated from the cartilage along the edge of the rib cage.

A large, unstable flail segment is life threatening because it interferes with proper expansion of the chest cavity, causing intrathoracic pressure changes and severe respiratory distress or inadequate respiration and rapid patient deterioration. Also, it is commonly associated with underlying lung injury.

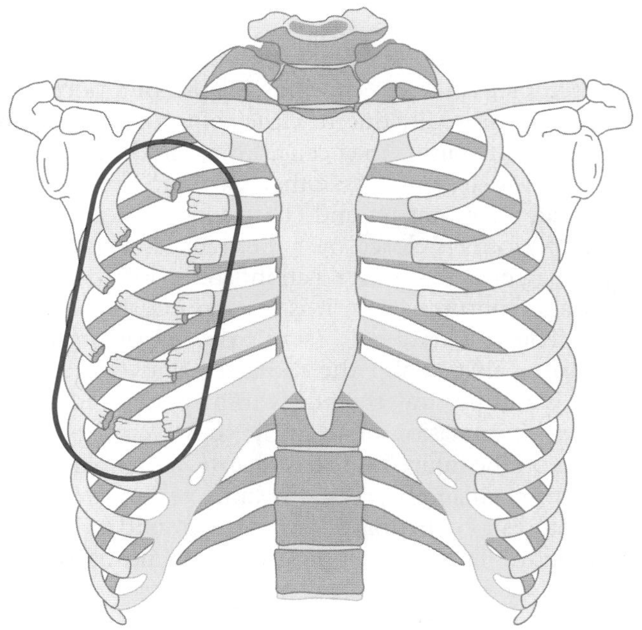

FIGURE 34-4 * Flail segment occurs when blunt trauma causes fracture of two or more ribs, each in two or more places.

Specific Chest Injuries

A variety of chest injuries can result from either penetrating or blunt trauma to the chest. Because these injuries can interfere with ventilation, oxygenation, or perfusion, they are considered to be, in most cases, life threatening.

Flail Segment

As already mentioned, a flail segment occurs when two or more consecutive ribs have been fractured in two or more places, producing a freely moving section of chest wall. During inhalation and exhalation, the flail segment displays **paradoxical movement;** that is, the flail segment moves in a direction opposite to the movement of the rest of the chest wall (Figure 34-5*).

The effects of pressure during inhalation and exhalation explain why paradoxical movement happens. Inhalation takes place when the chest expands, making pressure inside the chest less than the pressure outside the chest, which causes air to push in from outside the lungs. The pressure that pushes air into the expanded chest also pushes the flail segment inward. Exhalation takes place when the pressure inside the chest becomes greater than the pressure outside the chest, pushing air out of the lungs and decreasing the size of the chest. The pressure that pushes air out of the contracting chest also pushes the flail segment outward (Figure 34-6*). This is why a flail segment displays paradoxical movement, moving inward while the rest of the chest is moving outward, and moving outward when the rest of the chest is moving inward.

The flail segment requires immediate recognition and management, but the underlying contusion to the lung is a more serious injury, resulting from the blunt force applied to the chest. The flail segment will prevent the chest from generating the normal negative pressure necessary for inhalation. This may reduce the volume that can be breathed in, leading to hypoxia (oxygen deficiency) and poor oxygenation. With lung contusion, gas exchange between the alveoli and pulmonary capillaries is reduced, leading to hypoxemia.

Stabilization of the segment reduces the paradoxical movement and improves ventilation. Stabilization is achieved by splinting the flail segment. Because lung contusion and lung collapse are associated with a flail segment, positive pressure ventilation with supplemental oxygen is the ideal treatment. It expands the alveoli that are collapsed, greatly reducing the amount of hypoxia (oxygen deficiency) by forcing ventilation and increasing oxygenation.

Key Terms
paradoxical movement a section of the chest that moves in the opposite direction to the rest of the chest during the phases of respiration. Typically seen with a flail segment.

Key Terms
pulmonary contusion bleeding within the lung tissue that causes a disturbance in gas exchange between the alveoli and capillaries.

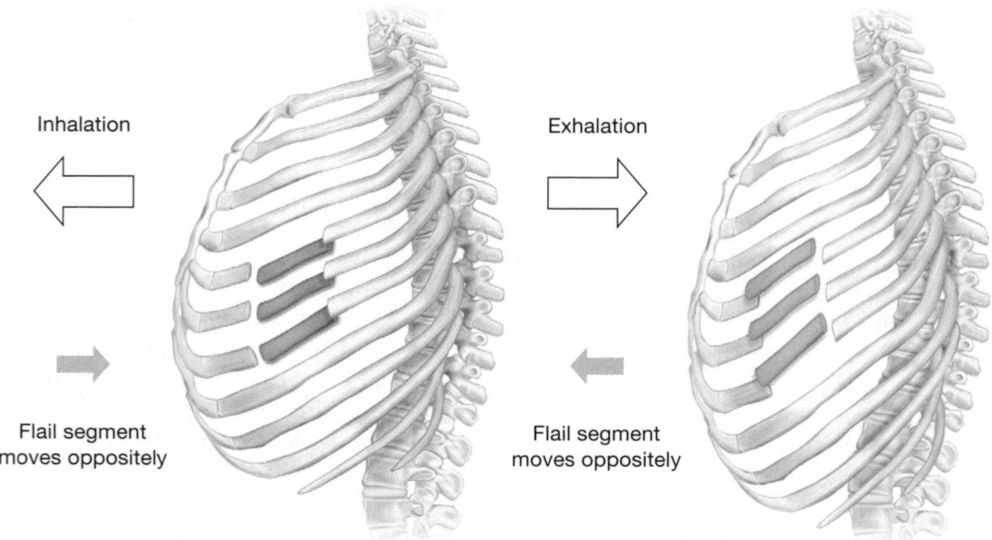

FIGURE 34-5 * Paradoxical movement.

ASSESSMENT Tips

Immediately after an injury, a flail segment may be stabilized by contraction of the intercostal muscles and may not initially produce dramatic paradoxical movement. However, as the muscles begin to fatigue, the stabilization provided will be reduced and obvious paradoxical movement may be seen. ■

Pulmonary Contusion

Pulmonary contusion (bleeding within the lung tissue) is often a serious consequence of a flail segment and can lead to death. Bleeding occurs in and around the alveoli and into the interstitial space that separates the alveoli and capillaries. This greatly reduces the exchange of oxygen and carbon dioxide, leading to severe hypoxia (oxygen deficiency) (Figure 34-7*).

A patient who has suffered a direct blow or any other blunt trauma to the chest should be suspected of having a pulmonary contusion. Such injuries are often seen in association with a flail chest.

The amount of respiratory distress depends on the amount of damaged lung tissue. Other signs and symptoms include dyspnea (shortness of breath), cyanosis, and signs of blunt trauma to the chest. Required emergency care for this condition is maximizing oxygenation by nonrebreather mask at 15 lpm for the patient who is breathing adequately or by positive pressure ventilation with supplemental oxygen for the patient breathing inadequately.

Pneumothorax

As noted earlier, a pneumothorax is the accumulation of air in the pleural cavity, causing collapse of a portion of the lung. It is usually due to either blunt or penetrating trauma. Blunt trauma may cause a fractured rib to penetrate the lung, leaving a hole that leaks air. The lung may rupture if, upon impact and chest compression, the patient's epiglottis is closed over the trachea. This causes a "paper-bag effect" similar to an inflated paper bag that is sealed and ruptures when it is compressed between the hands. The resultant hole in the visceral pleura of the lung allows air to enter the thoracic cavity. Penetrating trauma is another way the lung can be punctured.

The accumulation of air in the thoracic cavity causes the lung on the injured side to collapse, either partially or fully. This results in decreased volume within the alveoli, which causes a reduction of oxygen delivered to the cells of the body. Signs and symptoms of a pneumothorax include chest pain that worsens with deep inspiration, dyspnea (shortness of breath), tachypnea (faster than normal rate of breathing), and decreased or absent breath sounds on the affected side.

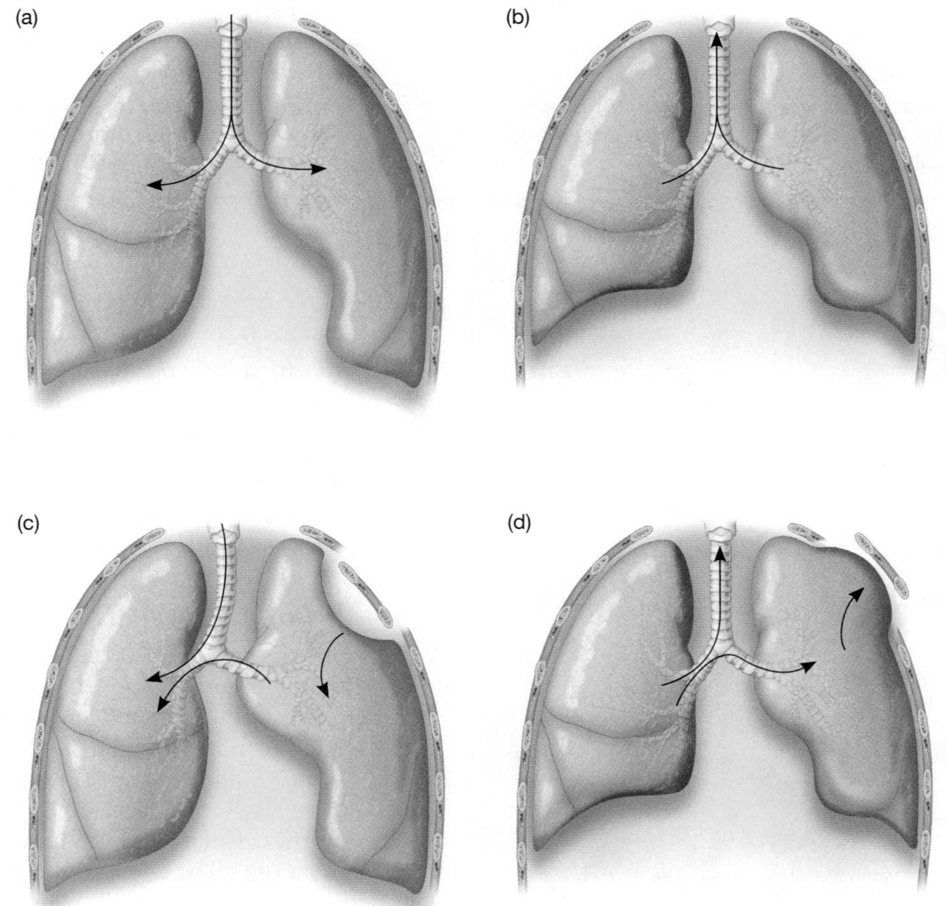

FIGURE 34-6 ✱ Normal versus paradoxical movement caused by flail segment. **(a)** Normal inhalation. **(b)** Normal exhalation. **(c)** Flail segment drawn inward as the rest of the lung expands with inhalation. **(d)** Flail segment pushed outward as the rest of the lung contracts with exhalation.

A patient may suffer a pneumothorax in the absence of blunt or penetrating trauma to the chest. This condition is called a spontaneous pneumothorax, because it occurs without an external cause. It usually is the result of a congenitally weak area on the surface of the lung (called a bleb), which ruptures and allows air to enter the thoracic cavity. Spontaneous pneumothorax is common among smokers and emphysema patients. A sudden onset of dyspnea (shortness of breath), respiratory distress, sharp chest pain, and absent breath sounds on one side are typical signs and symptoms.

ASSESSMENT Tips

A pneumothorax is primarily identified by decreased or absent breath sounds to the side of the chest where the lung is partially or totally collapsed. If the patient with a pneumothorax is in a seated position, gravity will cause the air in the pleural space to move upward, and the decreased breath sounds will be heard in the apex (top) of the lung first. ■

Open Pneumothorax

An **open pneumothorax** is a result of an open wound to the chest created by a penetrating object (Figure 34-8a✱). Air may be heard escaping or entering through the chest wound, creating a bubbling or sucking sound. An open pneumothorax is referred to as a "sucking chest wound," as discussed earlier in this chapter. The signs and symptoms of an open pneumothorax are the same as for a closed pneumothorax, with the exception of an open wound to the chest. You must immediately occlude an open wound to the chest. Initially seal it with your gloved hand and then with an occlusive dressing.

Tension Pneumothorax

A tension pneumothorax is an immediately life-threatening condition resulting from a pneumothorax that continues to trap air in the thoracic cavity with no relief or escape (Figure 34-8b✱). With each breath, a massive volume of air accumulates in the thoracic cavity on the injured side. This completely collapses the injured lung and begins to compress and shift the mediastinum over to the uninjured side. The uninjured lung, heart, and large veins are compressed,

Key Terms

open pneumothorax an open wound to the chest that allows air to enter the pleural space and cause lung collapse.

Key Terms

hemothorax blood in the pleural space, causing collapse of the lung.

traumatic asphyxia severe and sudden compression of the thorax that causes a rapid increase in pressure within the chest.

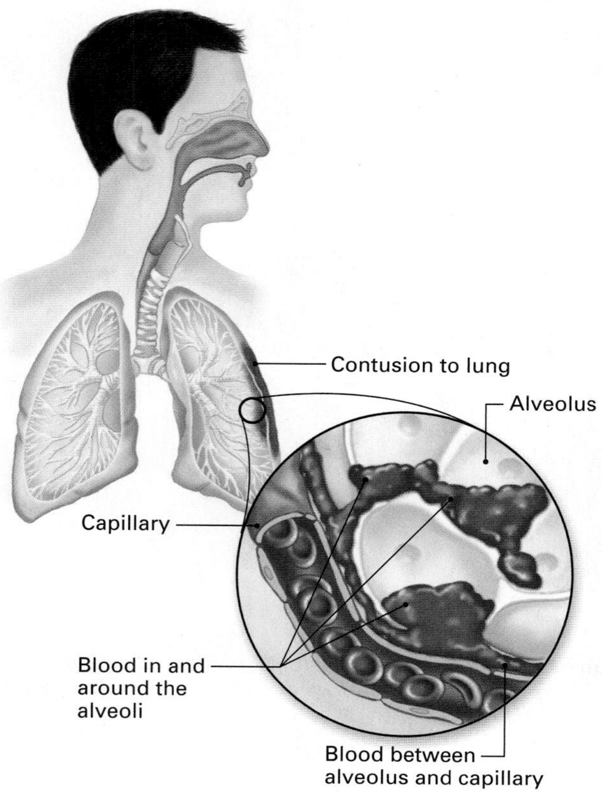

FIGURE 34-7 * When the lung is bruised (pulmonary contusion), there is bleeding into and around the alveoli and the space between the alveoli and the capillaries, greatly reducing the exchange of oxygen and carbon dioxide in the affected area.

leading to poor cardiac output, ineffective ventilation, inadequate oxygenation, and severe hypoxia. Death can occur rapidly.

Rapid deterioration, severe respiratory distress, signs of shock, and absent breath sounds on one side of the chest should alert you to a possible tension pneumothorax. Other signs and symptoms include cyanosis, unequal movement of the chest, distended neck veins, diminished breath sounds on the side opposite to the injury, and deviation of the trachea to the uninjured side. This condition may develop following the application of an occlusive dressing to an open chest wound. Alleviate the pressure by lifting the dressing and allowing air to escape during expiration, even if it is taped on only three sides. If you suspect a tension pneumothorax, rapid transport is critical.

Understanding BODY PROCESSES

In addition to collapsing the lung, a tension pneumothorax will shift the mediastinum and compress the vena cava, aorta, and heart, causing a decrease in the amount of blood being ejected from the left ventricle. The result is a decrease in blood pressure and perfusion. ■

Hemothorax

With a **hemothorax,** the thoracic cavity is filled with blood rather than air (*hemo* means "blood") (Figure 34-8c*). As the blood continues to collect, the lung is compressed. A hemopneumothorax, which is the collection of both blood and air (*hemo,* "blood"; *pneumo,* "air"), also may occur.

A hemothorax may be the result of blunt or penetrating trauma to the chest and may be associated with open or closed injuries. The bleeding usually originates from lacerated blood vessels in the chest wall or chest cavity caused by penetrating objects or fractured ribs. The patient can lose a significant amount of blood in the chest, which results in severe shock. Early signs and symptoms of hemothorax are usually the same as for shock. Signs and symptoms of respiratory distress develop late. Bleeding in and around the lung will commonly produce a pink or red frothy sputum when the patient coughs. Care is the same as for pneumothorax and shock.

Traumatic Asphyxia

Traumatic asphyxia is brought about when severe and sudden compression of the thorax causes a rapid increase in the pressure in the chest (Figure 34-8d*). The heart and lungs are usually severely compressed by the sternum and ribs, causing a backflow of blood out of the right ventricle and into the veins of the head, shoulders, and upper chest. The patient often looks as if he has been strangled.

The signs and symptoms of traumatic asphyxia include bluish or purple discoloration of the face, head, neck, and shoulders; jugular vein distention; bloodshot eyes that are protruding from the socket; cyanotic and swollen tongue and lips; and bleeding of the conjunctiva (area found under the lower eyelid). Provide emergency care for any wounds to the chest and for shock.

COMPLICATIONS OF CHEST INJURY

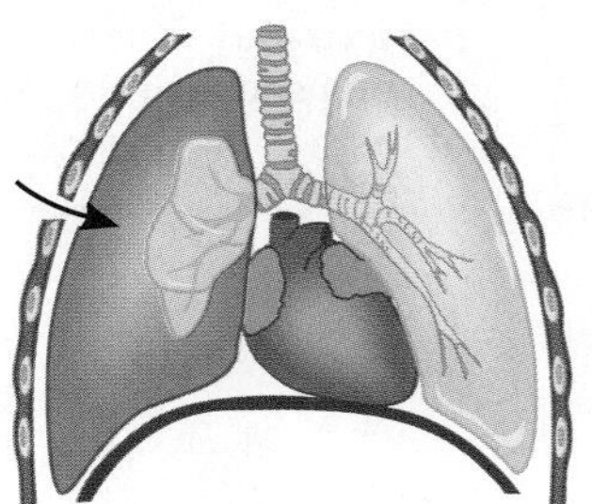

a. Air enters the chest cavity through an open chest wound or leaks from a lacerated lung. The lung cannot expand.

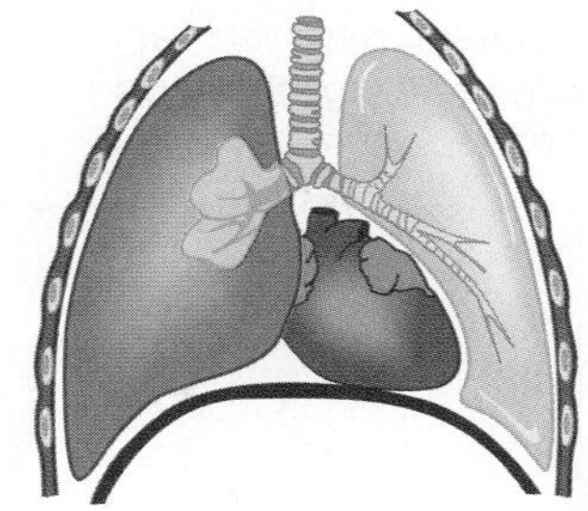

b. Air continuously fills pleural space, lung collapses, pressure rises, and the trapped air compresses the heart and other lung.

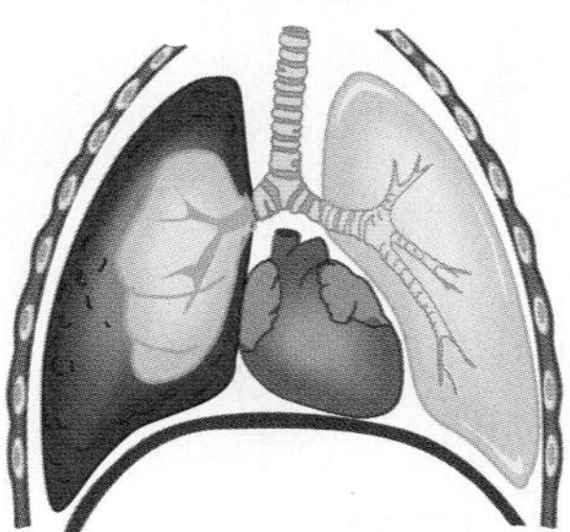

c. Blood leaks into the chest cavity from lacerated vessels or the lung itself and the lung compresses.

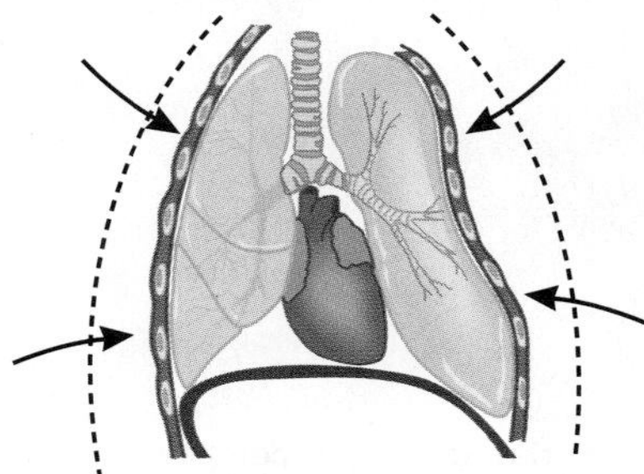

d. Severe chest compression puts pressure on heart and forces blood back into vein of the neck. It may cause severe lung damage.

FIGURE 34-8 ✻ Complications of chest injury include **(a)** open pneumothorax, **(b)** tension pneumothorax, **(c)** hemothorax, and **(d)** traumatic asphyxia.

Cardiac Contusion

Cardiac contusion is a common cardiac injury following severe blunt trauma to the chest. It occurs as the heart is violently compressed between the sternum and the spinal column (Figure 34-9a✻). An actual bruise may occur to the heart wall. The heart wall could be ruptured or a disturbance in its electrical conduction system may occur. The right ventricle, directly beneath the sternum, is the most likely area of the heart to be injured.

Signs and symptoms of cardiac contusion may include chest pain or chest discomfort; signs of blunt trauma to the chest, including bruises, swelling, crepitation (grating sensation), and deformity; tachycardia (faster than normal heart rate); and an irregular pulse. Prompt transport is required.

Cardiac arrest from blunt force applied to the precordial area of the chest (center of sternum) is a rare event. It is often seen in young males with no underlying cardiac disease during sporting events where a projectile such as a baseball strikes the patient in the center of the chest, causing ventricular fibrillation and cardiac arrest (sudden death). This condition is referred to as **commotio cordis.**

Pericardial Tamponade

Blunt or penetrating trauma may cause bleeding into the tough fibrous sac that surrounds the heart—the pericardial sac. Since this sac cannot expand outward very much with the filling blood, the result is inward compression of the heart (Figure 34-9b✻), which causes cardiac output to drop significantly and blood to back up in the venous system. This condition is known as **pericardial tamponade.** It is a life-threatening condition that requires prompt recognition and transport.

The most common cause of a pericardial tamponade is a penetrating wound to the heart from a knife or similar object. Bullets may also cause it, but more often a bullet wound directly to the heart causes immediate death.

The signs and symptoms of pericardial tamponade are similar to those of tension pneumothorax, except that breath sounds remain normal in pericardial tamponade because only the heart is involved and not the lungs. Signs and symptoms will progressively worsen as the pericardial sac fills with more blood. They include jugular vein distention; signs of shock (hypoperfusion); tachycardia, with

Key Terms

cardiac contusion a cardiac injury following severe blunt trauma to the chest where the heart is violently compressed between the sternum and spinal column, causing a bruise to the heart wall.

Key Terms

commotio cordis sudden cardiac arrest that results from a projectile, such as a baseball, striking the anterior chest.

pericardial tamponade blood or fluid filling the fibrous sac around the heart, causing compression of the heart.

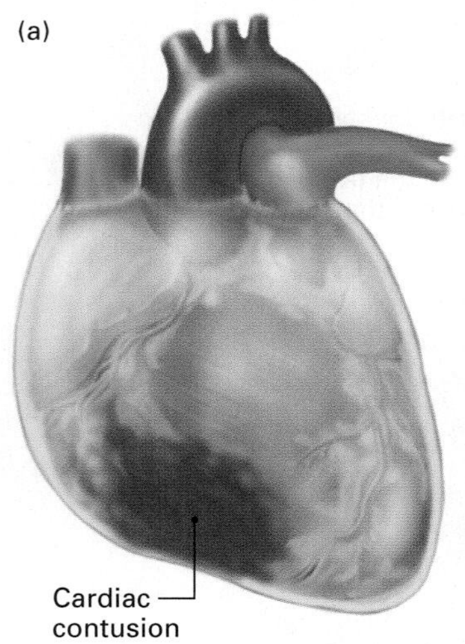

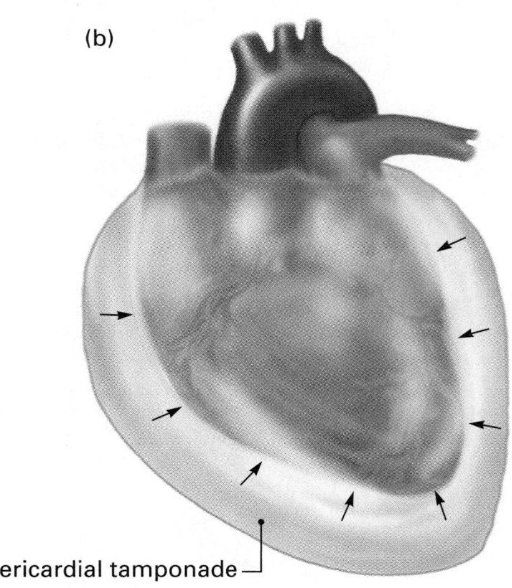

FIGURE 34-9 ✻ Traumatic cardiac injuries: **(a)** cardiac contusion; **(b)** pericardial tamponade.

a heart rate that is extremely high in severe cases; decreased blood pressure; narrow pulse pressure (less than 30 mmHg); and weak pulses, with radial pulses disappearing or diminishing during inhalation.

Rib Injury

While a fractured rib is not life threatening, it can cause life-threatening damage to other structures and organs. The most commonly fractured ribs are the third through the eighth. The most common site of fracture is on the lateral aspect of the chest. The intercostal artery or vein may be lacerated as a result of the fracture and cause bleeding into the chest cavity.

Rib fractures in children are less common because of a more resilient cartilage that does not break easily. The mechanism of injury should heighten your suspicion that chest injury may have occurred.

The most common signs and symptoms of rib injury include (Figure 34-10✻) pain, often excruciating, with movement and breathing; crepitation (grating sensation); tenderness upon palpation; deformity of the chest wall; inability to breathe deeply; coughing; and tachypnea (rapid breathing) that may be shallow.

If a simple rib fracture is suspected, the patient usually presents in the guarded position, holding his arm over the injured site. You can use the arm to splint the injury by placing it over the injury site and applying a sling and swathe to hold it in place (Figure 34-11✻). The patient could also be given a pillow to hold firmly over the injury in order to manually splint it. Do not completely wrap the chest or apply the swathe snugly. This would impede normal ventilation.

A patient who has suffered a chest injury may appear relatively well at first but can deteriorate suddenly and rapidly. The patient may not complain about a chest injury. In fact, the patient's chief complaint related to the chest may only be shortness of breath. It is your responsibility to suspect a potential chest injury based on mechanism of injury and a high index of suspicion, to adequately assess the patient, and to provide the necessary emergency medical care.

An open (sucking) chest wound and paradoxical movement (flail segment) are the two immediately life-threatening chest injuries that require management in the prehospital setting. Because they are life threatening, they must be managed immediately upon identification. Other injuries to the internal organs and structures of the chest cannot be directly treated in the field. Early recognition and rapid transport are critical.

Assessment-Based Approach: Chest Trauma

Scene Size-Up

Conducting a scene size-up to ensure your safety and that of your partner is especially important when the chest in-

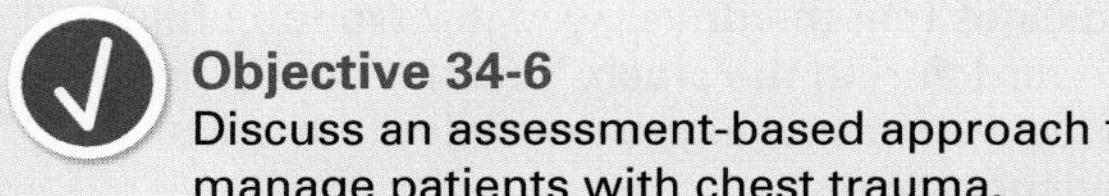

Objective 34-6
Discuss an assessment-based approach to manage patients with chest trauma.

Key Points
While waiting for the scene to be cleared of hazards, concentrate on the mechanism of injury. Scan the scene and ask bystanders to tell you what happened.

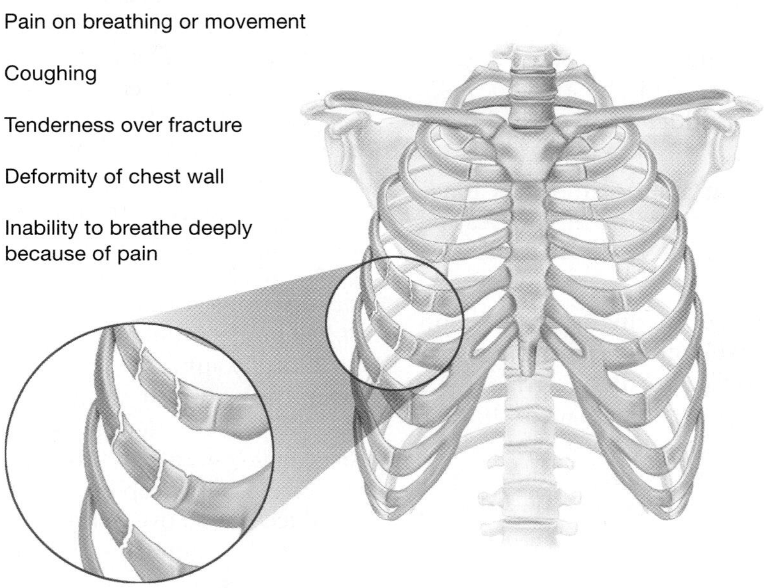

RIB INJURY
Pain on breathing or movement
Coughing
Tenderness over fracture
Deformity of chest wall
Inability to breathe deeply because of pain
If lung has been punctured, the patient may cough up frothy blood and feel a crackling sensation under the fingertips as you feel the area of the fracture (subcutaneous emphysema).

FIGURE 34-10 ✱ Rib injury.

jury was a result of violence with a knife or gun. When you arrive on the scene, a threat to your safety may still exist. *Do not enter the scene of a shooting or stabbing until the police secure it and tell you it is safe to enter.* Remember to take the necessary Standard Precautions. Since bleeding is often found with both blunt and penetrating injuries, it is necessary to be wearing gloves and eye protection before entering the scene.

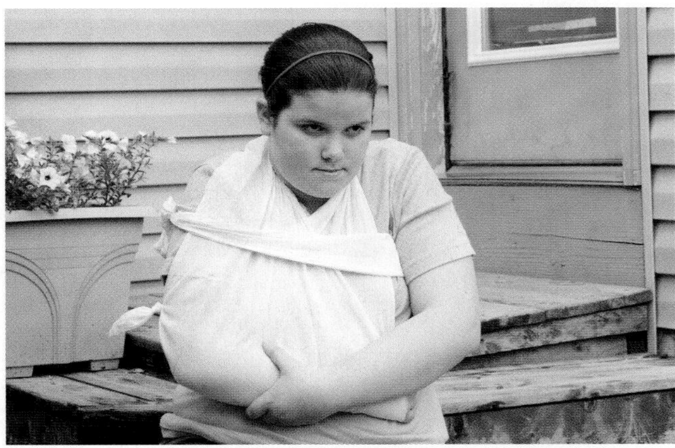

FIGURE 34-11 ✱ Apply a sling and swathe to stabilize the area of rib injury.

While the scene is being cleared of safety hazards, concentrate on the mechanism of injury. Ask bystanders to tell you what happened. Scan the scene. Blunt trauma commonly occurs in sports accidents, falls, blows to the chest during fights, and, most commonly, automobile crashes. Penetrating trauma most often is associated with violence.

As you consider the mechanism of injury, look for and note the following:

- **Was the patient involved in a sports accident?** Did the patient take a direct blow to the chest? A direct blow to the anterior chest by a football helmet, a line-drive baseball, a hockey puck, an elbow during a rebound in basketball, or other similar mechanisms can produce serious injury, including heart rhythm disturbance and sudden cardiac arrest.
- **Did the patient fall?** How far did the patient fall? How did he land? What did he hit on the way down? In what position was he found? What caused him to fall? What did he land on?

Key Points

A blow to the chest can be forceful enough to cause spine injury. If there is an index of suspicion for blunt trauma to the chest, establish spinal stabilization.

Thinking Critically

The deformed steering wheel in a collision vehicle indicates that the driver was thrown forcefully forward during the crash. You and your partner agree that he is a high priority for immediate transport. Why?

- **Was there a fight?** Was the patient punched or kicked in the chest? Were any weapons involved in the fight, such as a knife, gun, club, rocks, or bottles? Is there a bloody object found at the scene that could have penetrated the chest? Did the patient feel a sting or hear a pop and suddenly become short of breath?
- **Is there any evidence that a shooting took place?** Were gunshots heard? Are there spent shell casings on the ground? Did dispatch indicate that this was a shooting?
- **Was the patient involved in an auto collision?** How fast was the car traveling? Where is the impact to the vehicle (and therefore to the patient)? Is the steering wheel bent, broken, or damaged? Is there damage to the dashboard on the passenger side? Is there an impact mark to the windshield indicating the patient was violently thrown forward? Was the patient wearing a seat belt? Were both the shoulder and lap belts worn properly? Did the air bag deploy? Is there any protruding metal or object in the vehicle that may have penetrated the chest?
- **Was the patient crushed between two objects?** Was the patient possibly run over by a heavy object?
- **Was an explosion involved?** Blast injuries can cause blunt injury from the blast wave and penetrating injury from flying debris.

Primary Assessment

As soon as you have determined that the scene is safe, proceed with the primary assessment. If there is a significant mechanism of injury and a high index of suspicion for blunt trauma to the chest, establish and maintain in-line spinal stabilization. (A blow to the chest can be forceful enough to cause spine injury.) Form a general impression of the patient: Is the patient severely cyanotic? Does he appear to be in extreme respiratory distress? Is he breathing shallowly and rapidly? Is he holding his arms tightly against his chest to splint the movement? Does he appear to be in extreme pain? Are there any open wounds to the chest? Is the chest moving unevenly when he breathes?

Clothing can disguise a life-threatening sucking wound or flail segment. If the mechanism of injury indicates possible chest injury or the patient shows any signs of respiratory distress, *quickly expose the chest and examine it.* If you note an open wound to the anterior, lateral, or posterior chest, *immediately* seal it with a gloved hand. If there is paradoxical movement, *immediately* place a gloved hand over the flail segment to splint it in an inward position. The ideal treatment for a flail segment is positive pressure ventilation.

Continue with the primary assessment and determine the patient's mental status. An altered mental status or unresponsiveness may be an indication of severe hypoxia (oxygen deficiency) resulting from a significant chest injury. Visually inspect the airway in the patient with an altered mental status. Look for blood or other potential obstructions. Listen and feel for air movement. Because spinal injury should be suspected if the chest injury is due to blunt trauma, perform the jaw-thrust maneuver to open the airway, if necessary.

Note the patient's speech pattern. Does the patient speak a few words and then gasp for a breath? This would indicate severe respiratory distress. Many chest injuries produce ineffective ventilation. In some cases where the chest wall is injured and the ribs fractured, the pain is so severe that the patient purposely will breathe with extremely shallow, fast breaths in an attempt to reduce the pain. This can easily lead to hypoxia from inadequate breathing.

Carefully assess the breathing status. If breathing is adequate, administer oxygen with a nonrebreather mask at 15 lpm. If breathing is inadequate, immediately initiate positive pressure ventilation with supplemental oxygen (Figure 34-12∗).

If a tension pneumothorax exists, it will be increasingly difficult to ventilate the patient. (Expanding pressure in the chest cavity makes it increasingly difficult to

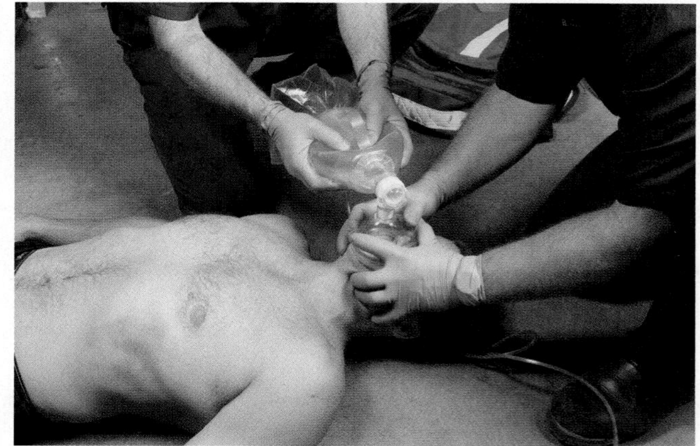

FIGURE 34-12 ∗ Provide positive pressure ventilation with supplemental oxygen if breathing is inadequate.

Thinking Critically

In the patient with suspected chest injury, you assess the neck for possible subcutaneous emphysema, jugular vein distention, and/or tracheal deviation. What might be the cause or causes of each of these signs?

Key Points

An open wound to the back or side of the chest is just as potentially lethal as one to the anterior chest. Immediately seal such a wound with your gloved hand.

inflate the lungs.) The pulses may be weak and fast if the injury is associated with bleeding in the chest or compression of the heart. Cyanosis is an indicator of poor oxygenation and ventilation. Pale skin may indicate early onset of hypoxia, blood loss, or poor pumping function of the heart. The skin may be moist and cool to the touch.

ASSESSMENT Tips

If the pulse becomes weak or absent during inhalation, it may indicate either a tension pneumothorax or pericardial tamponade (compression of the heart from blood or fluid in the pericardial sac). ■

All of these are indications of chest injury. The patient with a chest injury is considered a high priority because of the possibility of rapid deterioration, ineffective ventilation, and poor oxygenation. Immediate transport after the rapid trauma assessment, with assessment and care continuing en route, must be considered.

Note: If you suspect that the patient has been shot or stabbed, the patient complains of breathing difficulty, or the breathing rate or depth appears to be abnormal, it is vital that the patient is log rolled to assess the posterior body for another potentially life-threatening open (entrance or exit) wound.

Secondary Assessment

Perform a rapid secondary assessment. It is likely that other injuries exist, especially if the mechanism of injury suggests blunt trauma. Inspect and palpate for deformities, contusions, abrasions, punctures/penetrations, tenderness, lacerations, and instability.

Assess the breathing status. Cyanosis to the face, inside the mouth, or under the tongue indicates poor oxygenation. Be sure that the patient is on high-concentration oxygen or is being ventilated adequately. If the cyanosis is severe or progressively gets worse, re-evaluate the breathing status and consider positive pressure ventilation. Place the patient on a pulse oximeter, if available and if you are permitted to use the device.

Assess the neck for subcutaneous emphysema, jugular vein distention, and tracheal deviation. Air tends to flow upward; therefore, with chest injury *subcutaneous emphysema* (air trapped under the skin giving it a bubbly, inflated appearance and a crackling feel when palpated) is usually present in the upper chest and neck. *Jugular vein distention* is an indication of possible cardiac injury or tension pneumothorax. In a tension pneumothorax, the trachea will move toward the side of the uninjured lung (*tracheal deviation*). When assessing for tracheal deviation, it is necessary to palpate the trachea immediately above the suprasternal notch (indentation immediately above the sternum). Inspection of the trachea will rarely reveal the deviation; however, palpation may allow you to feel the abnormal shift prior to being able to see it. The buildup of pressure in a tension pneumothorax will also cause the heart and large vessels to be compressed, causing decreased blood flow to the heart and ineffective pumping, which produce signs and symptoms of shock (hypoperfusion). Jugular vein distention and tracheal deviation are very late signs of a tension pneumothorax. Signs and symptoms of respiratory distress are better indicators.

ASSESSMENT Tips

Watch the jugular veins during inhalation. If they engorge during inhalation, it may be a sign of a tension pneumothorax or pericardial tamponade. This engorgement is referred to as *Kussmaul sign.* ■

If a spinal injury is suspected, apply a cervical spine immobilization collar. Most immobilization collars have a large opening on the anterior side allowing for reassessment of the jugular veins and trachea. Do not release manual in-line stabilization until the patient is completely immobilized to a backboard.

If you have not already done so, expose the chest by cutting the clothing. Inspect the chest carefully and thoroughly for any open wounds. If you suspect a penetrating injury, log roll the patient and inspect the back for open wounds. Lift the arm and inspect the axillary (armpit) area. An open wound to the back or side of the chest is just as lethal as one to the anterior chest. If an open wound is found there, immediately seal it by placing a gloved hand over the wound. If paradoxical movement is noted, immediately stabilize the segment with your hand by applying inward pressure to the flail area.

One of the major complications associated with a flail segment is the inability of the patient to generate pressure changes in the chest necessary to adequately move air into the chest cavity. If the patient is exhibiting signs and symptoms of a flail segment with evidence of inadequate

Key Points
The most significant problem with a flail segment is potential contusion to the underlying lung area. This will interfere with gas exchange and lead to hypoxia.

Key Points
An increasing heart rate and decreasing blood pressure with increasing respiratory distress are ominous signs of severe chest injury.

breathing, the ideal treatment is to provide positive pressure ventilation. When positive pressure ventilation is delivered to the patient, the air being forced into the lungs overrides the inadequate movement of the chest to create a negative pressure to draw air into the lungs. In a sense, you are eliminating the need for the chest to create a negative pressure because you are delivering a positive pressure. Thus, you can effectively manage a flail segment through positive pressure ventilation. The most significant problem then associated with the flail segment is the potential contusion to the lung underlying the fracture. This will interfere with gas exchange and lead to hypoxia.

Look for retractions of the muscles, contusions, lacerations, or any other signs that blunt force may have been applied to the chest. Inspect the chest if the patient was a driver involved in an automobile crash. A bent or damaged steering wheel and positive markings on the patient's chest are indications of possible severe chest injury, especially if the driver was not wearing a seat belt. Air leaking from the respiratory tract or an injured lung may produce subcutaneous emphysema.

Palpate the chest, checking for symmetry (equal movement of both sides), paradoxical movement, swelling, and deformities. Fractures of the ribs may produce *crepitation* (a grating sound or sensation) and are usually accompanied by excruciating pain upon palpation. You will likely find that the patient with an injury to the chest wall or injury to the ribs will breathe shallowly and will place his arm over the injured area to guard and splint it during breathing (Figure 34-13∗).

Auscultate the breath sounds bilaterally. Determine if the breath sounds are clear and equal, decreased or absent on one side, or decreased or absent on both sides. Decreased or absent breath sounds may indicate a collapsed lung or air or blood in the thoracic cavity. The patient in severe pain from a chest wall injury may have decreased or absent breath sounds bilaterally, which may indicate that both lungs are collapsed. A tension pneumothorax usually produces absent breath sounds on the injured side and decreased breath sounds on the side of the uninjured lung. Closely re-evaluate the breathing status and determine if positive pressure ventilation should be initiated.

Inspect the abdomen for excessive muscle movement during breathing. This may be an indication of severe respiratory distress associated with a chest injury.

Assess the baseline vital signs. The blood pressure may be low because of either bleeding or compression of the heart. The breathing rate can be significantly increased. Pain associated with chest injury may cause the

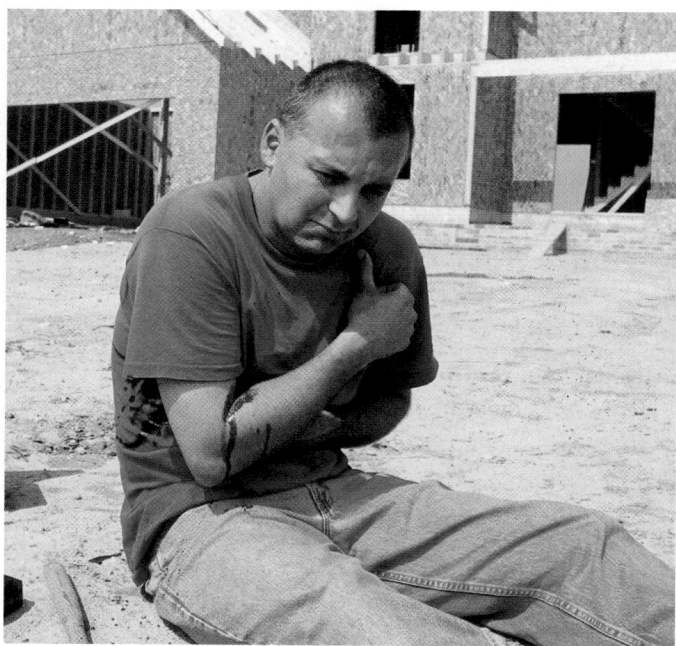

FIGURE 34-13 ∗ Typical "guarded" position of a patient with a rib injury.

patient's breathing to be very fast and shallow. The pulse is usually rapid and may be weak. The skin may appear cyanotic or pale, cool, and moist. The pulse oximetry may be less than 95% as a result of hypoxia associated with a chest injury. *An increasing heart rate and decreasing blood pressure associated with increasing respiratory distress is an ominous sign of severe chest injury. Immediate transport should be considered.*

ASSESSMENT Tips

A sudden drop in the systolic blood pressure by greater than 10 mmHg during inhalation may be another sign of a tension pneumothorax or pericardial tamponade. The drop in systolic blood pressure during inhalation is referred to as *pulsus paradoxus.* ■

Obtain a history from the responsive patient. If the patient is unresponsive or is unable to answer your questions, attempt to gather information from others at the scene.

Signs and Symptoms Certain signs and symptoms may occur in major open or closed chest trauma, many simultaneously. The major indications of chest trauma are:

Key Terms

hemoptysis coughing up blood or blood-stained sputum.

Objective 34-7

Discuss general emergency care for chest trauma and specific emergency care for an open chest wound and for a flail segment.

Key Points

Positive pressure ventilation may worsen a pneumothorax by forcing air out of the lung into the pleural space, further collapsing the lung. If ventilation must be provided, avoid forceful ventilations and continuously assess for deterioration of the patient's condition.

- Cyanosis to the fingernails or fingertips, lips, or face
- Dyspnea (shortness of breath)/difficulty in breathing
- Breathing rate that is faster (tachypnea) or slower (bradypnea) than normal and usually shallow
- Contusions, lacerations, punctures, swelling, or other obvious signs of trauma to the chest
- **Hemoptysis** (coughing up blood or blood-stained sputum)
- Signs of shock (decreasing blood pressure, narrowing pulse pressure, increasing heart rate, and pale, cool, and clammy skin)
- Tracheal deviation
- Paradoxical movement of a segment of the chest wall
- Open wound that may or may not produce a sucking sound
- Subcutaneous emphysema
- Jugular vein distention (JVD), especially during inhalation
- Absent or decreased breath sounds upon auscultation
- Pain at the injury site, especially pain that increases with inhalation and exhalation
- Failure of the chest to expand normally during inhalation
- Peripheral pulses that become extremely weak or become absent during inhalation
- A drop in systolic blood pressure of 10 mmHg or more during inhalation

Not all of these signs need to be present in order to suspect serious chest injury. Sometimes only subtle signs of pain or symptoms of slight breathing difficulty are present. Consideration of the mechanism of injury and signs of trauma to the chest cavity should heighten your suspicion that a serious chest injury has occurred. Remember that an altered mental status, alcohol intoxication, or head injury can decrease the patient's ability to complain of symptoms that might indicate chest injury.

General Emergency Medical Care—Chest Trauma

Chest injuries can be life threatening. Prompt recognition and emergency medical care is essential to the patient's survival. An open chest wound, a flail segment that produces paradoxical movement, and inadequate breathing are all conditions that must be managed immediately upon identification.

1. **Maintain an open airway.** Take in-line stabilization and open the airway, using a jaw-thrust maneuver if spinal injury is suspected. If the patient's condition continues to deteriorate, it may be necessary to insert a nasopharyngeal or oropharyngeal airway. Suction any secretions, blood, or vomitus. Remember that signs of inadequate breathing may occur from an occluded airway and not necessarily from a worsening chest injury. Continuously reassess the airway.
2. **Continue oxygen therapy.** Because most chest injuries produce disturbances in oxygen and carbon dioxide exchange in the lungs, the cells may not be receiving an adequate amount of oxygen. This leads to cellular hypoxia (oxygen deficiency). It is essential that a high concentration of oxygen is continuously administered to all patients with suspected chest injury via a nonrebreather mask at 15 lpm.
3. **Re-evaluate breathing status.** Chest injuries can cause sudden and rapid deterioration. You should carefully and continuously reassess the breathing status and circulation. If at any time signs of inadequate breathing appear, immediately begin positive pressure ventilation with supplemental oxygen.

   Keep in mind that providing positive pressure ventilation may actually worsen a pneumothorax by forcing air out of the lung through the visceral pleura and into the pleural space. This will increase the air in the pleural space and cause the lung to collapse more. Even though this is a complication associated with ventilation of a patient with a chest injury, if the breathing is inadequate you have no choice but to provide positive pressure ventilation. Be vigilant and continuously assess for deterioration of the patient, worsening cyanosis, and increases in resistance noted by more difficulty when squeezing the bag of the bag-valve-mask device. Do not provide forceful ventilations. A pneumothorax can be converted into a tension pneumothorax by ventilating a patient. Consider ALS backup or immediate transport.
4. **Stabilize an impaled object in place.** If an impaled object is found, do not remove it. Stabilize the object with bulky gauze and bandages to prevent excessive movement.
5. **Completely immobilize the patient if spinal injury is suspected.** A cervical spine immobilization collar

must be applied and the patient must be immobilized to a backboard with straps and a head immobilization device.

6. **Treat the patient for shock (hypoperfusion) if signs and symptoms are present.** Many chest injuries involve blood loss or cardiac compromise from compression of the heart.

Emergency Medical Care—Open Chest Wound

The open chest wound is an immediately life-threatening emergency that can lead to rapid deterioration and death if not managed properly. Emergency medical care includes the general care we have just detailed, plus the following:

1. **Immediately seal the open wound with your gloved hand.** Do not delay in order to find a dressing.
2. **Apply an occlusive dressing to seal the wound** (not a regular porous dressing, which would allow air to enter easily). Plastic wrap from an oxygen mask, the wrap covering an intravenous fluid bag, or Vaseline gauze may be used. The occlusive dressing should be a few inches wider than the wound. Place it over the entire wound and tape it on three sides (Figure 34-14*). During inhalation, the dressing is sucked up against the wound, preventing air from entering. The side that is not taped allows for air that has built up in the thoracic cavity to escape during exhalation (Figure 34-15*). An alternative method is to tape the dressing on four sides and occasionally lift a corner during expiration to relieve any pressure. Paramedics and some Advanced EMTs are able to decompress the chest to relieve the trapped air using an over-the-catheter needle. A valve may be connected to prevent air from being drawn into the catheter. The Asherman Chest Seal (ACS) is a commercially available self-adhesive translucent occlusive dressing that covers the open chest wound and has a built-in one-way flutter valve to allow air to be relieved during exhalation (Figure 34-16*).
3. **Continuously assess the patient's respiratory status.** If the patient's condition begins to deteriorate and you notice more severe signs and symptoms of respiratory distress along with signs of shock, a tension pneumothorax may be developing. The occlusive dressing, even if taped on only three sides, may have become obstructed by trauma or clotted blood, preventing air from exiting the open wound in the chest, or air may be entering the thoracic cavity from a hole in the lung. The following signs and symptoms

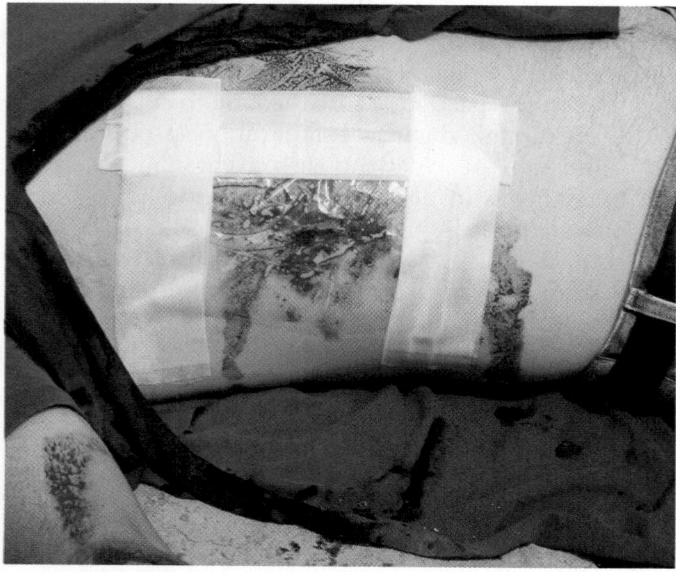

FIGURE 34-14 * For an open chest wound, position a nonporous occlusive dressing directly on the chest wall. Tape it on three sides.

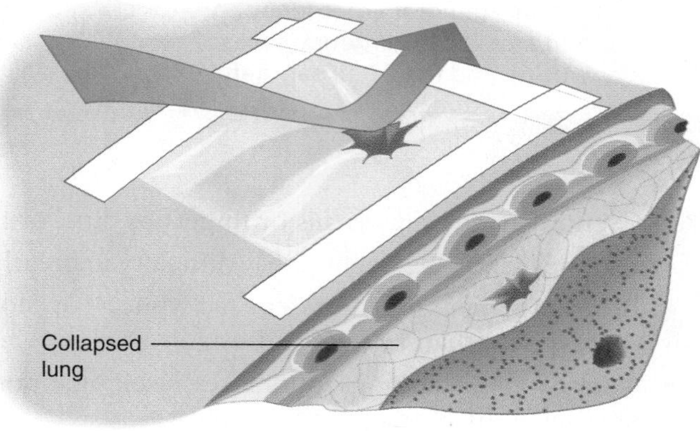

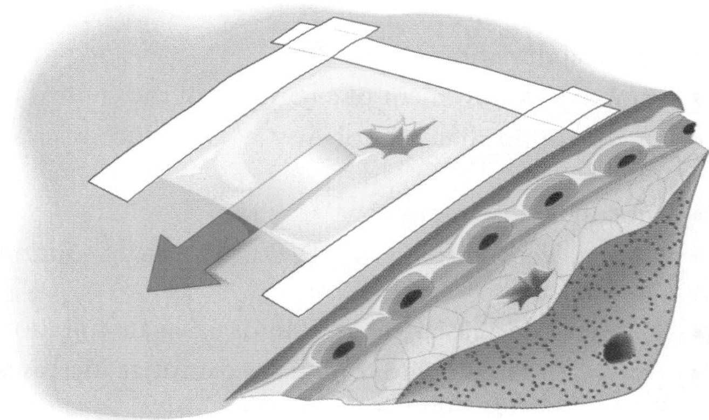

Expiration allows trapped air to escape through untaped section of dressing

FIGURE 34-15 * By taping the occlusive dressing on three sides, you create a flutter valve that helps to prevent tension pneumothorax.

Thinking Critically

You have placed an occlusive dressing over the patient's open chest wound. Subsequently, the patient begins to show signs of breathing difficulty. You lift a corner of the dressing for a few moments. Why?

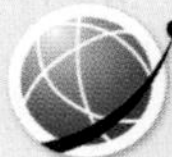

Media Resources

Go to www.bradybooks.com for mykit. Highlights:

- *Web Resource:* Pulmonary Contusions
- *Web Resource:* Cardiac Tamponade

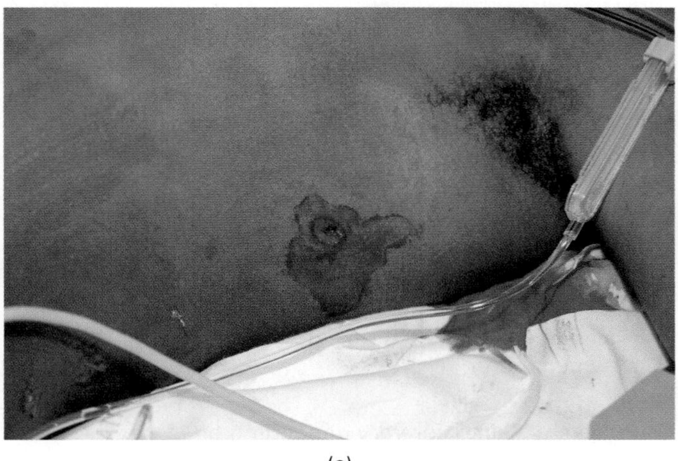

(a)

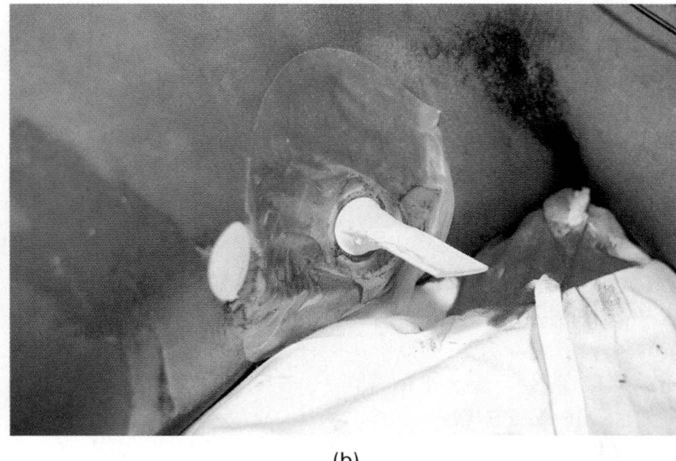

(b)

FIGURE 34-16 ✻ **(a)** A gunshot wound to the chest. **(b)** An Asherman Chest Seal (ACS) covers the wound and allows accumulated air to be relieved during exhalation. (Both photos: © Edward T. Dickinson, MD)

indicate a complication associated with the sealed wound and a developing tension pneumothorax. *The first three are the most important to recognize:*

- *Difficulty breathing, with increased respiratory distress and dyspnea (shortness of breath)*
- *Tachypnea (breathing rate faster than normal)*
- *Severely decreased or absent breath sounds on the injured side*
- Cyanosis
- Tachycardia (heart rate faster than normal)
- Decreasing blood pressure with a narrowing pulse pressure
- Jugular vein distention (late sign)
- Tracheal deviation (late sign)
- Unequal movement of the chest wall (the injured side remains hyperinflated and will not move equally with the uninjured side)
- Extreme anxiety and apprehension
- Increased resistance to positive pressure ventilation

If these signs and symptoms develop after the occlusive dressing has been applied, you must lift a corner of the dressing for a few seconds to allow the air to escape during expiration. A rush of air may be heard or felt, and immediate relief of the signs and symptoms of severe compromise should occur. Reseal the wound with the occlusive dressing. It may be necessary to repeat this procedure several times.

Emergency Medical Care—Flail Segment

Paradoxical movement of a flail segment should be initially splinted in an inward position by placing your hand over the unstable flail segment (EMT Skills 34-1A). If the patient is breathing inadequately, initiate positive pressure ventilation during the primary assessment. Paradoxical movement can also be stabilized by placing bulky dressings, a pillow, or towels over the unstable segment (EMT Skills 34-1B), or by securing the patient's arm to his body (EMT Skills 34-1C).

Reassessment

During the reassessment, evaluate the effectiveness of your treatment and assess for further deterioration of the patient's condition. Signs and symptoms of increasing breathing difficulty, decreasing mental status, decreasing breath sounds, worsening cyanosis, and shock should prompt you to re-evaluate your treatment and to repeat the rapid secondary assessment, looking for signs of injury that might have been missed initially. It may be necessary to reconsider the need to provide positive pressure ventilation if it has not already been initiated. Look for signs of a developing tension pneumothorax. If an occlusive dressing is in place, lift it to relieve any pressure that has potentially built up.

Reassess and record the baseline vital signs. A decreasing blood pressure, increasing heart rate, increasing respiratory rate, and cyanotic, cool, moist skin may indicate a worsening chest injury or shock from blood loss.

Summary: Assessment and Care—Chest Trauma

To review possible assessment findings and emergency care for chest injuries, see Figures 34-17* and 34-18*.

ASSESSMENT Tips

The diaphragm, which separates the thoracic and abdominal cavities, is located approximately at the level of the nipple line. Injuries below the nipple line are likely abdominal and not thoracic, depending on the phase of respiration when the injury occurred. ■

Assessment Summary

CHEST TRAUMA

The following findings may be associated with a chest injury.

SCENE SIZE-UP

Pay particular attention to your own safety. Look for:
- Mechanism of injury
- Automobile crash, bent steering wheel
- Sports accident, especially blow to chest as from football helmet, baseball
- Fall
- Gunshot wound
- Fight, especially with blow to chest
- Crush injury
- Explosion

Primary Assessment

General Impression
- Severe cyanosis
- Extreme respiratory distress
- Patient splinting chest with arm
- Obvious open wound to chest
- Uneven chest wall movement
- Speech pattern: gasping for breath between words

Mental Status
- Alert to unresponsive, based on type and degree of injury
- Unresponsiveness or decreasing mental status associated with hypoxia and hypoperfusion

Airway
- Assume airway is closed if patient has an altered mental status

Breathing
- May be absent, inadequate, or normal
- May be very shallow if ribs are injured
- May be labored

Circulation
- Pulse and skin color vary depending on injury
- Pulse may be normal
- Pulse is increased if hypoxia, blood loss, or tension pneumothorax
- Skin may be normal if minor chest injury
- Cyanosis if perfusion disturbance or hypoxia

Status: Priority patient if any chest injury

Secondary Assessment

Physical Exam

Head:
- Cyanotic tongue, oral mucous membranes, and face
- Assess neck for subcutaneous emphysema
- Jugular venous distention and tracheal deviation (late signs of tension pneumothorax)
- Neck veins that become engorged during inhalation—Kussmaul sign indicating a tension pneumothorax or pericardial tamponade

Chest:
- Evidence of blunt trauma to chest: contusions, lacerations
- Penetrating trauma to chest: knife, gunshot wounds (look for exit wound)
- Retractions of suprasternal notch, supraclavicular spaces, lateral neck
- Palpate for symmetry, deformities, crepitation, pain
- Paradoxical movement (indicates flail segment; minimal paradoxical movement may be noted early in flail segment because of muscle splinting, but will become more prominent as the intercostal muscles fatigue)
- Breath sounds diminished or absent on one side or both

FIGURE 34-17a * Assessment summary: chest trauma.

Assessment Summary

Abdomen:
- Excessive movement during breathing (indicates severe respiratory distress)

Extremities:
- Weak peripheral pulses (may indicate a tension pneumothorax or poor perfusion)
- Pulse that weakens with inspiration (may indicate a tension pneumothorax)

Posterior Body:
- Inspect for entrance and exit wounds
- Evidence of blunt trauma

Baseline Vital Signs
- BP: normal; may be low if severe hypoxia, blood loss, tension pneumothorax, or cardiac tamponade
- HR: normal, or tachycardia from severe hypoxia, blood loss, tension pneumothorax, or cardiac tamponade
- Pulses may become weak or absent during inhalation indicating a tension pneumothorax or pericardial tamponade
- RR: normal, irregular, decreased, absent, or labored
- Skin: normal; may be pale, cool, clammy if severe hypoxia, blood loss, tension pneumothorax, or cardiac tamponade
- Pupils: equal and reactive, may be sluggish to respond to light
- SpO_2: <95% if gas exchange is affected

History
- Dyspnea
- Coughing up frothy blood
- Pain at site of injury
- Cyanosis
- Obvious trauma to chest
- Shock
- Decreasing blood pressure with increasing pulse that becomes weaker
- Tracheal deviation and distended neck veins
- Paradoxical movement of chest
- Absent or decreased chest sounds
- Failure of chest to rise with inhalation

FIGURE 34-17a ✱ Assessment summary: chest trauma. *continued*

Emergency Care Protocol

CHEST TRAUMA

1. Establish manual in-line stabilization. Do not release it until the patient is immobilized onto a backboard.
2. If you find an obvious open wound to the chest during the general impression, place a gloved hand over the wound until it can be covered with a nonporous dressing taped on three sides.
3. Establish and maintain an open airway. Insert a nasopharyngeal or oropharyngeal airway if the patient is unresponsive and has no gag or cough reflex.
4. Suction secretions as necessary.
5. If breathing is inadequate, provide positive pressure ventilation with supplemental oxygen at a rate of 10–12 ventilations/minute for an adult and 12–20 ventilations/minute for an infant or child.
6. If breathing is adequate, administer oxygen by nonrebreather mask at 15 lpm for chest trauma, because of the potential for gas exchange disturbances and hypoxia.
7. Control any major bleeding.
8. Treat the specific condition or wound:
   Impaled Object:
   Stabilize the impaled object in place.
   Open Chest Wound:
   Place a gloved hand over the wound immediately.
   Apply an occlusive, or nonporous, dressing taped on three sides.
   Flail Segment (Paradoxical Chest Wall Movement):
   If inadequate breathing, begin positive pressure ventilation, which will splint the segment internally.
   Place a gloved hand over the segment, then stabilize with a blanket, pillow, bulky dressing, or the patient's own arm.
9. Treat for shock.
10. Immobilize to a backboard if you suspect spine injury.
11. Transport. Consider ALS backup.
12. Perform a reassessment every 5 minutes if unstable and every 15 minutes if stable.
13. If an open chest wound is occluded with a dressing and the patient suddenly begins to deteriorate, lift the dressing off the wound during exhalation to relieve trapped air, then reapply the dressing.

FIGURE 34-17b ✱ Emergency care protocol: chest trauma.

Emergency Care Algorithm: **Chest Trauma**

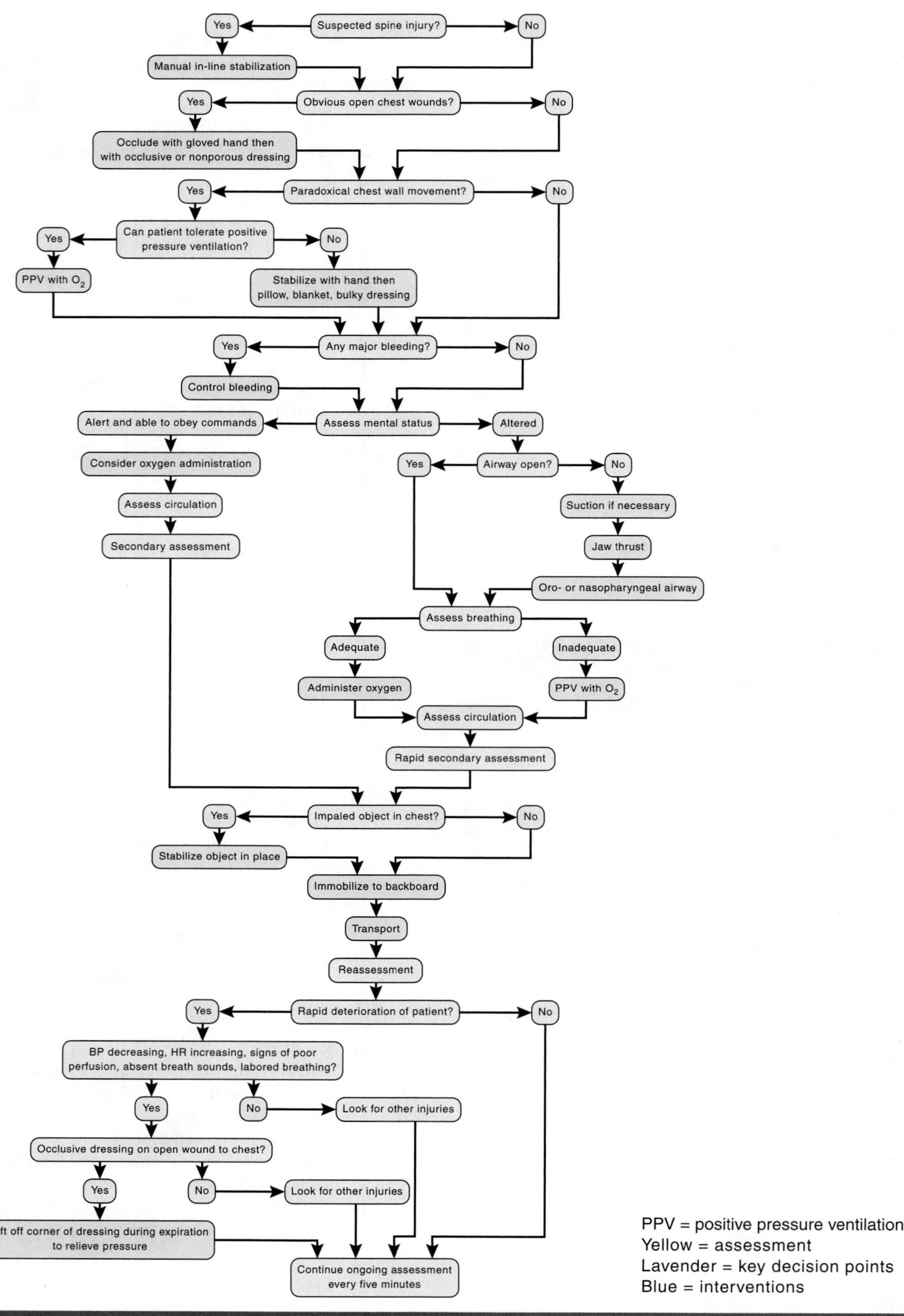

FIGURE 34-18 ✱ Emergency care algorithm: chest trauma.

EMT skills 34-1 Stabilizing a Flail Segment

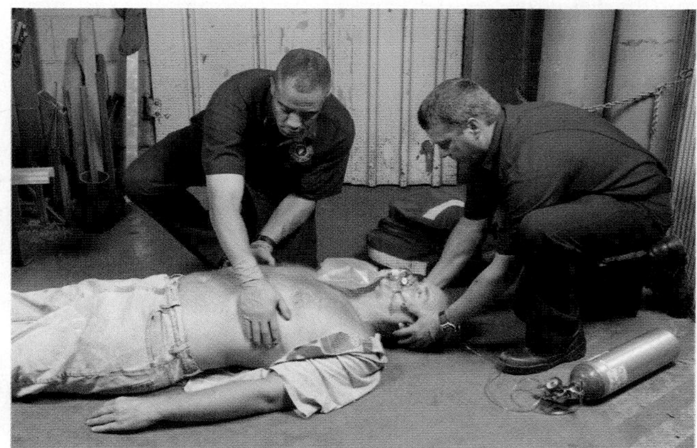

34-1A ✱ Initially stabilize the flail segment with your gloved hand.

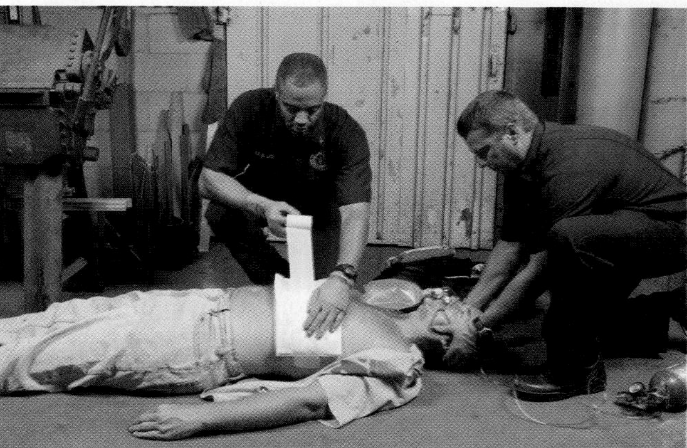

34-1B ✱ Stabilize the flail segment by applying a bulky dressing or clean towel to the chest.

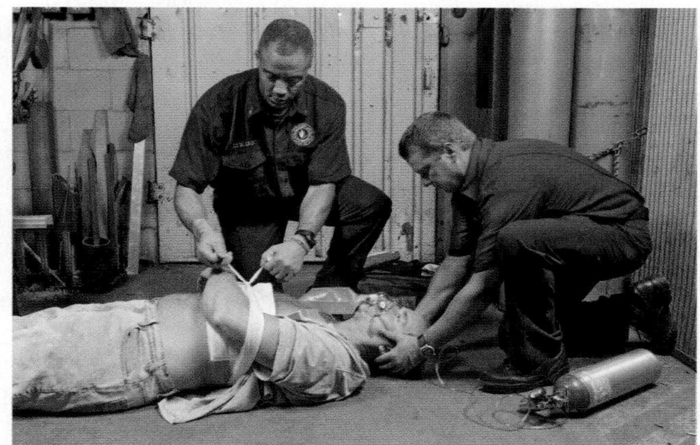

34-1C ✱ The patient's arm can be used to help splint the flail segment.

CHAPTER REVIEW

SUMMARY

Chest injuries may be life threatening. Chest injuries could lead to severe respiratory compromise and poor ventilation and oxygenation status. They also could be a source of serious bleeding. An open wound to the chest, tension pneumothorax, and flail segment must be recognized and managed during the primary assessment. All open wounds to the chest must be covered with an occlusive dressing taped on three sides. A flail segment must be stabilized to prevent exaggerated movement of the free-floating segment during ventilation.

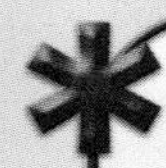

CASE STUDY FOLLOW-UP

SCENE SIZE-UP

You have been dispatched to a street corner for a man down. As you drive up to the scene, no bystanders appear to be present. It is dark outside, so you turn on the scene lights and carefully assess for hazards. None are observed so you and your partner exit the ambulance. However, you still have your guard up. As you approach the patient, you note that he is lying in a prone position on the sidewalk. He is dressed in a heavy overcoat, and he is moaning. No visible blood is noted. You and your partner tell the patient you are emergency medical technicians and are there to help. The patient responds with a moan.

PRIMARY ASSESSMENT

Because you are unaware of the mechanism of injury or nature of the illness, your partner establishes in-line spinal stabilization. You log roll the patient as a unit with spinal precautions being maintained. You ask, "Sir, are you hurt or ill?" The patient only responds with a moan. There still does not appear to be any visible injury or bleeding anywhere to the body. The airway is open and clear of any secretions or vomitus. The breathing is rapid and shallow at a rate of approximately 40 per minute. You prepare the bag-valve-mask device and instruct your partner to begin ventilating with supplemental oxygen. He kneels at the head of the patient, holding in-line stabilization with his upper legs. The radial pulse is weak and very rapid. The skin is cool, moist, and pale. You identify this patient as a high priority.

SECONDARY ASSESSMENT

In-line spinal stabilization is maintained by your partner as he continues to ventilate the patient with a bag-valve-mask device. The patient is still responding to verbal commands only with moans. There is no evidence of trauma to the head. The pupils are equal and reactive, but sluggish to respond. The jugular veins are flat and the trachea is midline. You quickly expose the chest and find what appears to be a small-caliber gunshot wound to the right anterior aspect of the chest at about the third intercostal space on the midclavicular line. A bubbly crackle is heard when the patient inhales spontaneously. You immediately place your gloved hand over the wound. You then apply the plastic wrap from the oxygen tubing over the wound and tape it on three sides.

You log roll the patient and closely inspect the back for an exit wound and find none. You also assess the axillary region for any other wounds to the chest. Auscultation of the lungs reveals significantly decreased breath sounds to the right and good breath sounds on the left. There is no evidence of any wounds or trauma to the abdomen or pelvis. Palpation of the abdomen does not elicit a moan or other pain response. The extremities are quickly inspected. Pedal pulses are absent and the radial pulses are extremely weak and fast. A pinch to the extremities causes the patient to moan.

The carotid pulse is 138 beats per minute. The spontaneous respiratory rate is 35 per minute and shallow. The blood pressure is 80/60 mmHg. The skin is cyanotic, pale, cool, and moist. The pulse oximeter will not provide a reading because of the poor perfusion status. A history is unobtainable.

You apply a cervical spine immobilization collar and immobilize the patient to a backboard with straps and a head immobilization device. You place the patient in the back of the ambulance and transport rapidly.

REASSESSMENT

En route to the hospital, the mental status remains unchanged. You insert a nasopharyngeal airway and reassess ventilation. Positive pressure ventilation is continued with supplemental oxygen. The pulse rate has decreased slightly to 130 per minute. The cyanosis has subsided slightly. The skin remains pale, cool, and moist. You record the vital signs.

Suddenly you notice that it is becoming extremely difficult to ventilate the patient. The heart rate has increased to 148 per minute and the skin is becoming severely cyanotic. You immediately lift the corner of the occlusive dressing off the wound and note the sound of air escaping. Almost immediately the patient's condition improves and you replace the dressing. You contact the hospital and give a report.

Upon arrival at the hospital, you give an oral report to the physician who is waiting for you at the door. The patient is transferred to the hospital bed in the trauma room. While your partner cleans the ambulance and gathers the necessary supplies, you complete the prehospital care report. You check on the patient prior to leaving and are told by the physician that he is now in surgery. His prognosis is unknown. You clear the hospital and mark back in service.

IN REVIEW

1. Identify and describe the two general categories of injuries to the chest.
2. List the signs and symptoms associated with major chest trauma.
3. Describe the general guidelines for emergency medical care of trauma to the chest.
4. Describe additional emergency medical care required for (a) an impaled object to the chest, (b) an open wound to the chest, and (c) a flail segment (paradoxical movement).
5. Describe the difference between pneumothorax, open pneumothorax, hemothorax, and tension pneumothorax.

CRITICAL THINKING

You arrive on the scene and find the driver of a vehicle that was in a frontal collision with another vehicle. The patient was not wearing his seat belt. The air bag deployed during the crash. The patient is responding to verbal stimuli with moans. He is breathing at 34 times per minute with a shallow chest rise. His radial pulse is 124 bpm and is barely palpable. The skin is pale, cool, and clammy. During the rapid secondary assessment, you note a large contusion to his left upper chest. Upon inhalation, that portion of the left upper chest moves inward. He moans loudly when his chest is palpated. His pedal pulses are absent. His blood pressure is 72/64 mmHg, HR 124 bpm, R 34 with poor chest rise, and the SpO_2 is not obtainable because of a continuous error reading.

1. What emergency care would you provide in the primary assessment?
2. What signs and symptoms in this patient are indicators of shock?
3. What type of chest injury is the patient suffering from?
4. How would you manage the chest injury?
5. What overall emergency care would you provide?

PEARSON

EXPLORE mybradykit™

Please go to **www.bradybooks.com** to access mykit for this text. You will find quizzes, critical thinking scenarios, weblinks, animations, and videos related to this chapter—and much more. Look for online information on pneumothorax and cardiac tamponade.

Register your access code from the front of your book by going to **www.bradybooks.com** and selecting the mykit links.

CHAPTER 35

Abdominal and Genitourinary Trauma

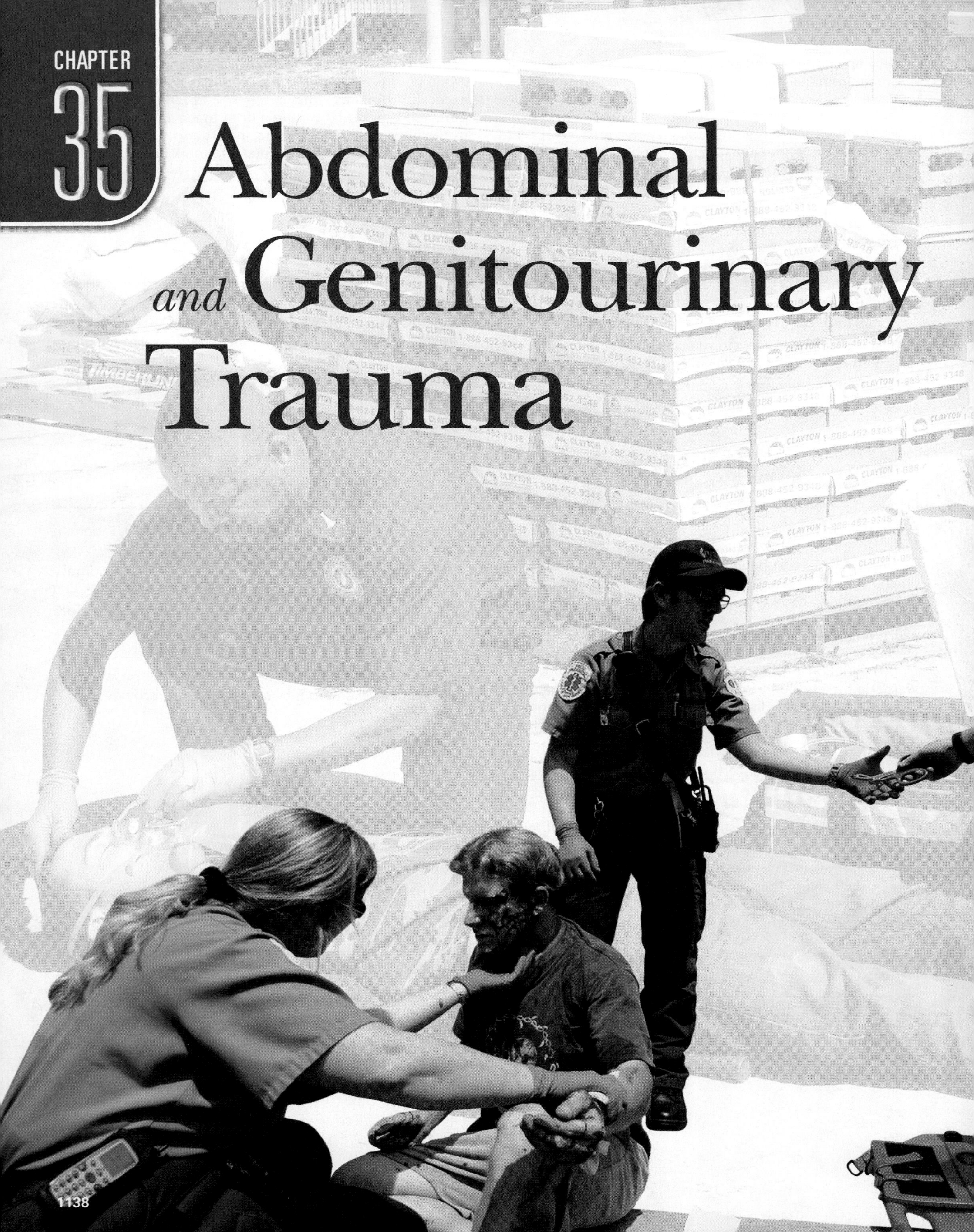

Navigation Guide

The following items provide an overview to the purpose and content of this chapter. The Standard and Competency are from the new National EMS Education Standards.

STANDARD **Trauma** (Content Area: Abdominal and Genitourinary Trauma)

COMPETENCY Applies fundamental knowledge to provide basic emergency care and transportation based on assessment findings for an acutely injured patient.

OBJECTIVES: After reading this chapter, you should be able to:

35-1. Define key terms introduced in this chapter.
35-2. Describe the anatomy of the abdominal cavity and its contents.
35-3. Differentiate hollow and solid organs and vascular structures in the abdomen.
35-4. Give examples of both blunt and penetrating mechanisms of abdominal trauma and discuss the potential for severe internal bleeding.
35-5. Discuss an assessment-based approach to management of the patient with open and closed abdominal injury, including evisceration and impaled objects.
35-6. Recognize signs and symptoms associated with injuries to the abdomen.
35-7. Explain the general emergency medical care for abdominal trauma.
35-8. Explain the emergency medical care for abdominal evisceration.
35-9. Explain the special considerations in management of trauma to the male and female genitalia.

KEY TERMS: Page references indicate first major use in this chapter. For complete definitions, see the Glossary at the back of the book.

abdominal evisceration p. 1141
Kehr sign p. 1141
peritoneal cavity p. 1140
peritonitis p. 1140
retroperitoneal cavity p. 1140

MEDIA RESOURCES: Please go to www.bradybooks.com to access mykit for this text. You will find quizzes, critical thinking scenarios, weblinks, animations, and videos related to this chapter—and much more. Look for online information on penetrating abdominal trauma.

CASE STUDY

The Dispatch

EMS Unit 14—respond to May's Coffee Shop at 154 Bayside Village for a man who was struck by a car while jogging—time out is 0740 hours.

Upon Arrival

While still en route, you get gloves and eye protection ready for both you and your partner. When your partner pulls up to the diner's parking lot, you spot the police unit. The police officer affirms that there is only one patient as you and your partner exit the unit and move toward him. The jogger is lying supine on the sidewalk, holding his abdomen and moaning in pain.

How Would You Assess and Care for This Patient?

During this chapter, you will learn about assessment and emergency medical care for patients suffering from abdominal and genitourinary injuries. Later, we will return to the case study and put in context some of the information you learned.

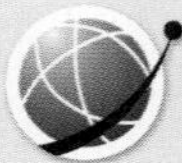

Media Resource
Go to www.bradybooks.com for mykit. Highlights:
- *Web Resource:* Penetrating Abdominal Trauma

Objectives 35-2 and 35-3
Describe the anatomy of the abdomen including hollow and solid organs and vascular structures.

Key Terms
peritoneal space the anterior abdominal cavity that houses the majority of the abdominal organs.
retroperitoneal cavity the space located behind the peritoneal cavity.

Introduction

Abdominal trauma is typically considered a critical injury because of the potential for severe bleeding and development of hemorrhagic shock. The abdomen contains vascular solid organs that have a tendency to bleed extensively, hollow organs that contain substances that can be spewed out and cause severe damage or infection, and vascular structures that can result in severe hemorrhage and blood loss if injured.

The key to assessment and management of abdominal trauma is to recognize that a potential abdominal injury has occurred and to understand the need for immediate emergency care and transport. It is not the role of the EMT to identify the specific organ that has been injured. The emergency care of the patient will not change based on what organ is bleeding or injured; however, the patient presentation might change. Pay close attention to the various signs and symptoms the patient may exhibit when an abdominal organ has been injured in order to recognize the condition as early as possible.

The urinary structures and organs are located in the abdominal cavity and will be included in the discussion of trauma to the abdominal organs. Genital trauma is primarily an external soft tissue injury that can lead to severe blood loss. Because the external genitalia are not contained within the abdominal cavity, this topic is discussed separately later in the chapter.

The Abdomen

Anatomy of the Abdominal Cavity

Before reading further, you may find it helpful to review Chapter 7, "Anatomy, Physiology, and Medical Terminology," for a description of the abdominal cavity and the organs it contains. A brief description follows.

The abdominal cavity contains the major organs of the digestive, urinary, and endocrine systems. The abdomen is separated from the chest cavity superiorly by the diaphragm. The inferior border is the heavy, bony pelvic ring. Tough, thick, flat muscles form the bulk of the anterior border along with the lower portion of the rib cage. Posteriorly, the spinal column and strong muscles provide protection.

The abdominal cavity is lined by a two-layer, sheath-like membrane called the *peritoneum*. The innermost lining—the *visceral peritoneum*—adheres to and supports the organs. The *parietal peritoneum* is the outer lining that adheres to the walls of the abdominal cavity. Between the two layers is a small amount of fluid that serves as a lubricant to reduce friction when the surfaces rub over each other. The potential space between the visceral and parietal peritonea is called the **peritoneal space.** Some organs in the posterior abdominal cavity lie partially or completely outside of the peritoneum. They are said to be *retroperitoneal,* or located in the **retroperitoneal cavity.** Organs contained within the retroperitoneal space are the duodenum, pancreas, inferior vena cava, aorta, kidneys, and ureters.

Understanding BODY PROCESSES

The peritoneal lining has very sensitive nerves that produce severe, constant pain when irritated by substances leaking into the abdominal (peritoneal) cavity. ■

Types of Abdominal Organs and Structures

The abdomen contains vascular structures as well as solid and hollow organs. It is important to understand the differences between these types of organs and structures because they cause various signs and symptoms when injured.

Hollow Organs Hollow organs contained within the abdominal cavity include the following:

- Stomach
- Gallbladder
- Urinary bladder
- Ureters
- Internal urethra
- Fallopian tubes
- Small intestine
- Large intestine

Hollow organs are not as vascular as solid organs, but they typically contain a substance. Thus, if ruptured or lacerated they do not bleed very much, but they spill their contents into the abdominal cavity, causing an irritation and inflammation of the peritoneal lining known as **peritonitis.** The leaking contents might include gastric juices from the stomach, highly acidic and partially digested food from the upper small intestine, bacteria from the large intestine, or urine from the bladder. If the sub-

Key Terms

peritonitis irritation and inflammation of the abdominal lining.

Kehr sign severe shoulder pain referred from a hemorrhaging injury within the abdominal cavity.

Key Terms

abdominal evisceration abdominal organ protrusion through an open wound.

Objective 35-4

Discuss blunt and penetrating mechanisms of abdominal trauma and potential internal bleeding.

stance leaking out of the organ is acidic or contains irritating substances, it will typically cause immediate and excruciating pain. Leakage of bacteria does not usually produce immediate pain; however, as the peritoneal lining becomes infected the patient will begin complaining of pain. This delay in onset of pain may take several hours. The patient could have an injury to an abdominal organ but yet not complain of severe pain while on the scene. Meanwhile, leakage of bacterial substances could lead to severe and life-threatening infection.

Solid Organs Solid organs within the abdominal cavity include the following:

- Liver
- Spleen
- Pancreas
- Kidneys

Solid organs usually contain a rich blood supply. A solid organ may bleed into the capsule that surrounds it for some time before the capsule ruptures and allows the blood to spill into the abdominal cavity. The major complication associated with the laceration or tearing of a solid organ is major bleeding and severe shock. In a patient who presents with evidence of abdominal trauma, look for signs and symptoms of hemorrhagic shock. Blood is not very irritating to the peritoneal lining and may not cause severe abdominal pain, even though the patient may be bleeding severely. However, the blood may irritate the diaphragm and cause referred pain to the shoulder. This referred pain to the shoulder is called **Kehr sign**.

Vascular Structures Vascular structures that lie partially within the abdominal cavity include the following:

- Abdominal aorta
- Inferior vena cava

In addition to the abdominal aorta and inferior vena cava, there are many large arteries and veins that supply the abdominal organs. All of these vascular structures are primarily stationary, are very large, and carry large amounts of blood. If lacerated, ruptured, or torn, the aorta or vena cava will bleed massively and rapidly lead to severe hemorrhagic shock and death. The signs and symptoms associated with a major abdominal vascular injury are those of hemorrhagic shock. This patient may deteriorate very quickly while on scene and en route to the medical facility.

Additional Structures

The Diaphragm The diaphragm is not an organ but a muscle that separates the thoracic and abdominal cavities. The diaphragm forms the upper border of the abdominal cavity and lower border of the thoracic cavity. During exhalation, the diaphragm would be located at approximately the level of the fourth or fifth intercostal space, which is at the nipple line. During inhalation, the diaphragm moves lower by as much as 3 inches.

The diaphragm could be injured from a penetrating injury or from a severe blunt force applied to the abdomen. The diaphragm is responsible for approximately 60 to 70 percent of the effort to breathe; therefore, injury to the diaphragm will likely cause respiratory distress. If the diaphragm injury is severe, the abdominal contents may enter the thoracic cavity. In this case, the breath sounds would be decreased on the side of the injured diaphragm.

ASSESSMENT Tips

The diaphragm, which separates the thoracic and abdominal cavities, is located approximately at the level of the nipple line during exhalation, lower during inhalation. Injuries below the nipple line are likely abdominal and not thoracic, depending on the phase of respiration when the injury occurred. ■

The Abdominal Wall An **abdominal evisceration** occurs when an open wound through the abdominal wall allows abdominal contents, usually the small intestine, to protrude and be exposed. Protect the exposed organs from further injury or contamination. Do not attempt to replace the organs. Specific management of an abdominal evisceration is discussed later in the chapter.

Abdominal Injuries

Abdominal injuries are caused by either blunt trauma or penetrating trauma. The mechanisms of injury are similar to those of chest injury. Blunt trauma to the abdomen is especially lethal because of the large number of organs that can be affected.

Injuries to the abdomen are classified as either open or closed. Open injuries result from penetrating trauma from bullets, knives, ice picks, sharp metal, broken glass, screwdrivers, and other sharp objects (Figure 35-1*).

Key Points

Open abdominal wounds are dramatic and easy to find, but closed abdominal injuries could be much more dangerous.

Objective 35-5

Discuss an assessment-based approach to management of the patient with open and closed abdominal injury, including evisceration and impaled objects.

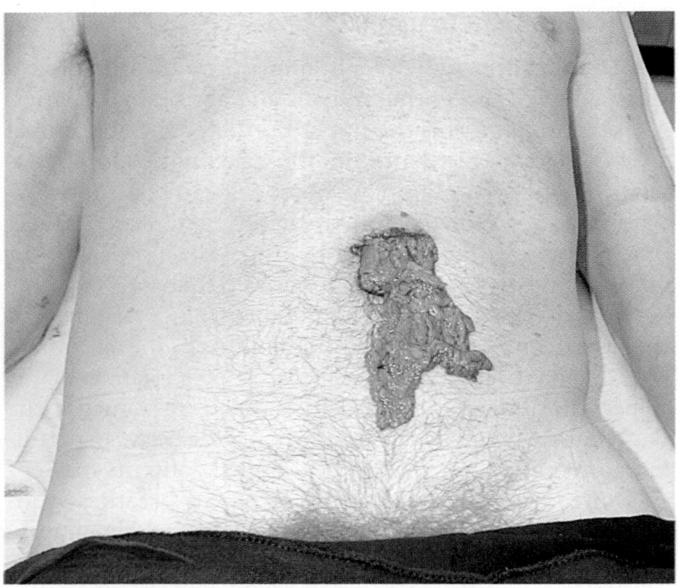

FIGURE 35-1 ✱ This patient was using a screwdriver to repair equipment that had been left running. The equipment "bucked," driving the screwdriver into his abdomen, causing evisceration. (© Charles Stewart, MD, and Associates)

Bullets, once they enter the body, can involve almost any organ or structure. If the patient is shot in the abdomen, the bullet could have entered the chest, fractured the pelvis, or lodged in the spinal column. The entrance wound may be to the anterior abdomen and the exit wound to the posterior thorax. The patient may have been shot in the chest, with the bullet traveling through the diaphragm and into the abdomen. With any gunshot wound, be highly suspicious that other organs, bones, and vessels have also been injured. Always search for an exit wound. If you focus on just the entrance wound, you could easily miss the potentially life-threatening exit wound.

Open wounds to the abdomen are much more dramatic and easier to find upon assessment than closed wounds. For example, a severe form of an open wound to the abdomen is an evisceration, in which organs are protruding through the skin. However, closed abdominal wounds could be much more dangerous. Blunt trauma applied to the abdomen can crush, tear, or rupture a large number of organs, causing severe internal bleeding. You must look at the mechanism of injury and physical assessment findings, as well as maintain a high index of suspicion that a closed abdominal injury exists.

Assessment-Based Approach: Abdominal Trauma

Assessment of the patient with a suspected abdominal injury is geared to identifying that a potential injury exists and not toward identifying the particular organ that has been injured. Consider the mechanism of injury, patient complaints, signs, and symptoms.

Scene Size-Up

The scene size-up can provide clues as to whether the trauma was caused by blunt or penetrating forces. Once you have ensured your own safety, scan the scene and develop suspicions of what may have caused the injury. Look for evidence of knives, guns, sharp metal, and other objects that may have penetrated the body. Ask the police or any bystanders at the scene if a gun was involved or if gunshots were heard. If the penetrating object is located, estimate the length and width (stabbing) or caliber (gunshot). This may be important information for the physician. However, do not spend valuable time looking for a weapon and trying to identify its characteristics.

Remember: Do not expect abdominal wounds to be obvious if the patient is clothed. Suspicion of a penetrating wound should prompt you to expose and inspect the entire body for open wounds.

Blunt trauma is associated with motor vehicle crashes, falls, pedestrian–vehicle collisions, motorcycle collisions, assaults, heavy objects thrown at or falling on the patient, and crushing injuries from machinery or other heavy equipment. The motor vehicle collision is by far the most common cause of blunt trauma to the abdomen. Attempt to determine the following when a motor vehicle collision is involved:

- Type of vehicle
- Approximate speed the vehicle was traveling (fast, slow, stationary)
- Type of collision and point(s) of impact
- Whether the patient was the driver, a passenger, or a pedestrian
- Where the patient is found and his position
- Whether the patient was thrown from the vehicle
- Impact marks to the windshield, steering wheel, and dashboard
- Whether a seat belt was used (If so, try to determine if both the shoulder and lap belts were properly positioned.)

Key Points

Abdominal wounds will probably not be obvious if the patient is clothed. Expose and inspect the entire body for wounds.

Key Points

Abdominal injuries may produce only subtle signs and symptoms, and the patient's response to pain may be reduced. Base your index of suspicion for abdominal trauma on the mechanism of injury.

Abdominal injuries may produce only subtle signs and symptoms, so you must base your suspicions on the mechanism of injury. Also, alcohol intoxication, head injury, and the influence of other drugs and substances may reduce the patient's response to pain.

Primary Assessment

As you approach the patient, begin to form a general impression as the first step of the primary assessment. Typically, you will find the patient with an abdominal injury lying extremely still with knees flexed up toward the chest (Figure 35-2*). This is done to decrease the tension on the abdominal muscles and reduce the abdominal pain. The patient may be moaning and complaining of severe pain. If you suspect spinal injury, establish in-line spinal stabilization.

Ensure an open airway and adequate breathing. Inspect the airway for evidence of bloody vomitus that may be associated with the injury and suction if necessary. Deliver oxygen by a nonrebreather mask at 15 lpm if breathing is adequate. If performing positive pressure ventilation, be sure supplemental oxygen is connected to the ventilation device. Assess circulation. The radial pulse may be weak or absent as a result of associated bleeding. The heart rate is typically increased beyond the normal limit. The skin may be pale, moist, and cool. These are all signs of shock, which indicates a severe abdominal injury and blood loss, and criteria to establish the patient as a priority for immediate transport.

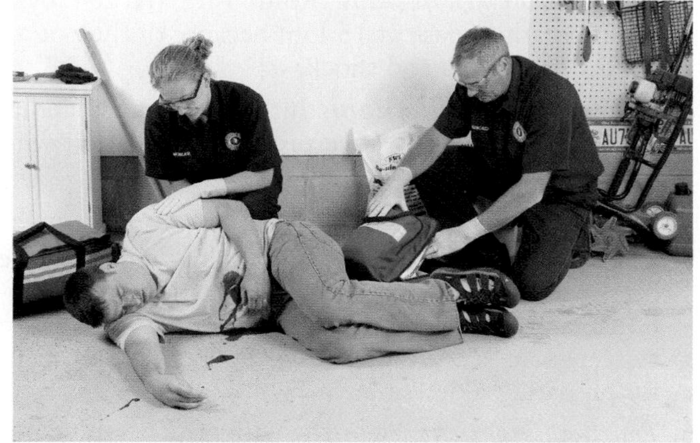

FIGURE 35-2 * Patients with abdominal injuries often lie with legs drawn up in the fetal position.

Secondary Assessment

During your secondary assessment, consider the patient's complaints and the mechanism of injury. Whether the injury is due to blunt or penetrating trauma, it is essential that you expose the entire body and perform a rapid secondary assessment to identify other potential injuries. Since abdominal injuries can produce severe pain, the patient may not complain of any other injuries. If you allow yourself to develop tunnel vision and not inspect other areas of the body, you can easily miss life-threatening injuries. First inspect the head, neck, and chest. If the patient has been shot in the abdomen, examine the chest for a possible exit wound or another gunshot wound. Remember that because of the excursion of the diaphragm during breathing, the boundary between abdomen and chest varies.

Apply a cervical spine immobilization collar if a spinal injury is suspected. Do not release manual in-line spinal stabilization until the patient is completely immobilized to a backboard.

Inspect the abdomen. Look for contusions, lacerations, abrasions, and punctures. Determine if the abdomen appears to be distended. (If it is, several liters of blood may have been lost into the abdominal cavity. It takes 1 to 2 liters of blood to expand the abdominal girth by 1 inch.) Inspect around the umbilicus (navel) and the flank areas for discoloration and bruising, which also indicate that bleeding is occurring inside the abdomen. This is a late sign and may be an indication that the patient had been bleeding for some time before contacting EMS. Look for bruising over the lower abdomen that could be caused by an improperly worn lap belt if the patient was involved in a motor vehicle collision.

Inspect and provide emergency medical care for any abdominal evisceration. Then palpate the abdomen, starting from the point farthest away from the pain. Note any tenderness or masses. If the patient has a decreased mental status, watch the face for a grimace as you palpate. The abdomen may be rigid from contraction of the abdominal muscles. The patient may be voluntarily contracting the muscles to guard against pain during your assessment, or the muscles may be involuntarily contracted by a reflex.

Assess the extremities for injury. Check and compare the strength of the pulses of both the upper and lower extremities. Abdominal aortic injury may cause the pulses of the lower extremities to be weaker than the upper extremities or even absent. If no pedal (foot) pulses are found, check for popliteal (back of the knee) or femoral

Objective 35-6
Recognize signs and symptoms associated with injuries to the abdomen.

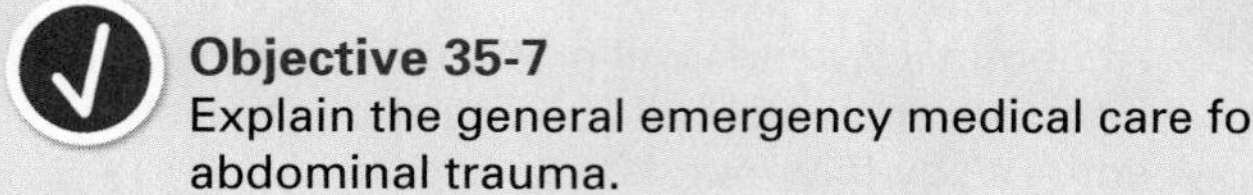

Objective 35-7
Explain the general emergency medical care for abdominal trauma.

(thigh) pulses. These should be equal to or stronger than the radial pulse, even in hemorrhagic shock. Keep in mind that blood loss and shock will reduce the pulse strength in the most distal pulses. Also assess motor and sensory function.

Log roll the patient and inspect the entire back and lumbar region for any signs of trauma. If the patient is suspected of having a spinal injury, log roll the patient onto a backboard at this time.

Assess baseline vital signs, especially for indications of blood loss and shock. A low blood pressure, tachycardia, or pale, cool, and moist skin are indicators that the patient is in shock. The breathing rate is typically fast and shallow in abdominal injuries because of the increase in pain associated with deep breathing.

From the responsive patient, obtain a history. The abdominal pain can be evaluated using the OPQRST mnemonic to help you. If the patient is unresponsive, ascertain as much information as possible from any bystanders at the scene. The signs and symptoms and events prior to the injury are extremely important points of information to gather.

Signs and Symptoms Patients with abdominal injury may exhibit the following signs and symptoms:

- Contusions, abrasions, lacerations, punctures, or other signs of blunt or penetrating trauma
- Pain that may initially be mild, then worsening
- Tenderness on palpation to areas other than the site of injury
- Rigid abdominal muscles
- Lying with legs drawn up to the chest in an attempt to reduce the pain
- Distended abdomen
- Discoloration around the umbilicus or to the flank (late finding)
- Rapid, shallow breathing
- Signs of hemorrhagic shock (decreasing blood pressure, narrowing pulse pressure, increasing heart rate, and increasing respiratory rate)
- Nausea and vomiting (may contain blood)
- Abdominal cramping possibly present
- Pain that radiates to either shoulder from irritation of the diaphragm (Kehr sign)
- Weakness

A mechanism of injury involving either blunt or penetrating trauma, early signs and symptoms of hemorrhagic shock, shallow and rapid respirations, and abdominal pain and rigidity are all significant and early signs of a serious abdominal injury. Any patient who complains of abdominal pain should be taken seriously and assessed carefully.

General Emergency Medical Care—Abdominal Trauma

Emergency medical care is basically the same for both open and closed abdominal injuries: aggressive management of the airway, breathing, oxygenation, and circulation. Since you are limited in the emergency medical care you can provide for abdominal injury, early recognition and prompt transport is a key element.

1. *Maintain an open airway and appropriate spinal protection.* Reassess the airway continuously. The patient may suddenly vomit, which can easily occlude the airway. Suction any vomitus, blood, or other secretions from the mouth. If the condition continues to deteriorate, it may be necessary to perform a jaw-thrust maneuver and to insert an oropharyngeal or nasopharyngeal airway. If the abdominal trauma is associated with a gunshot wound to the abdomen, in-line spinal stabilization must be established because of the possibility of the patient having suffered a spinal column injury from the bullet. The airway must be opened using a jaw-thrust maneuver. The patient must be completely immobilized before moving him to the ambulance.
2. *Continue oxygen therapy.* Administer oxygen by a nonrebreather mask at 15 lpm because of the potential for blood loss and shock.
3. *Reassess the breathing status.* If the breathing becomes inadequate, begin positive pressure ventilation with supplemental oxygen.
4. *Treat for hemorrhagic shock.*
5. *Control any external bleeding.* Apply a dry, sterile dressing to open wounds to the abdomen, the exception being an abdominal evisceration. In case of an evisceration, see the guidelines in the next segment for preparing a dressing.
6. *Position the patient.* Place the patient in a supine position with legs flexed at the knees (legs brought up toward the chest) if no injury to the lower extremi-

Thinking Critically
Your patient fell from a ladder while making a roof repair and landed face down, doubled over onto a sawhorse. He is moaning and holding his stomach. His wife says, "I gave him some tea and toast before you got here. I thought he'd feel better if he ate something." Why was feeding the patient a bad idea? What should you do about it now?

Objective 35-8
Explain the emergency medical care for abdominal evisceration.

Objective 35-9
Explain the special considerations in management of trauma to the male and female genitalia.

ties, hips, pelvis, or spine is suspected. Remember not to give anything by mouth, even if the patient complains of thirst. Do not allow the patient to eat or drink any amount of food or liquid. If spinal injury is suspected, immobilize the patient to a backboard.

Understanding BODY PROCESSES

Patients with abdominal injuries are not allowed to eat or drink any fluid in case they may need to have emergency surgery. The food or drink could cause them to vomit after receiving the anesthesia, risking aspiration. ■

7. *Stabilize an impaled object.* Do not remove it. Dress the wound around the impaled object to control the bleeding. Stabilize the object with bulky dressings and bandages to prevent movement.
8. *Apply the pneumatic antishock garment (PASG), if indicated and allowed by local protocol.*
9. *Transport as quickly as possible.*

Emergency Medical Care—Abdominal Evisceration

A large open wound to the abdomen may allow organs to protrude. Do not touch or attempt to replace the protruding organs. In caring for an evisceration, follow the general guidelines already discussed for abdominal injury, except dress the evisceration in the following way (EMT Skills 35-1A to 35-1C):

1. *Expose the wound.* Cut away clothing, if necessary. Do not touch or attempt to replace any of the organs.
2. *Position the patient* on his back and flex the legs up toward the chest if spinal injury is not suspected.
3. *Prepare a clean, sterile dressing* by soaking it with saline or sterile water. Apply the dressing over the protruding organs. Do not use absorbent cotton or any other material that might cling to the organs when wet, such as paper towels or toilet tissue.
4. *Cover the moist dressing with an occlusive dressing* to retain moisture and warmth. Plastic wrap will do. Avoid the use of aluminum foil, if possible, since it may lacerate the protruding organs. Secure the dressing in place with tape, cravats, or a bandage.
5. *Administer high-concentration oxygen. Be prepared to treat for shock.*

En route to the hospital, perform a reassessment. During the reassessment, monitor the patient for further deterioration. The reassessment may indicate if your emergency medical care has been effective. Reassess and record vital signs, paying particular attention to signs of hemorrhagic shock. Monitor for an increasing heart rate, decreasing blood pressure, narrow pulse pressure, decreasing level of consciousness, and pale, cool, moist skin. If you note deterioration, re-evaluate the priority status of the patient and expedite transport.

Reassessment

During the reassessment en route, evaluate the effectiveness of your treatment and assess for further deterioration of the patient's condition, repeating appropriate elements of the primary and secondary assessments. Reassess vital signs, and observe especially for indications of the presence or worsening of blood loss and shock: deteriorating mental status, falling blood pressure, tachycardia, or pale, cool, moist skin. Recall that a rapid, shallow breathing rate is typical with abdominal injuries from associated pain, so continue to administer oxygen.

Summary: Assessment and Care—Abdominal Trauma

To review possible assessment findings and emergency care for abdominal injuries, see Figures 35-3a*, 35-3b*, and 35-4*.

Genital Trauma

While injuries to the genitalia are rarely life threatening, they are typically extremely painful and could be quite embarrassing for the patient.

- *Injuries to the male genitalia* include lacerations, abrasions, avulsions, penetrations, amputations, and contusions. They usually produce excruciating pain and cause great concern to the patient. The penis is very vascular and can bleed excessively. An injury to the penis or scrotum should be treated as a soft tissue injury, which can be controlled with direct pressure.

Assessment Summary

ABDOMINAL TRAUMA

The following findings may be associated with an abdominal trauma.

SCENE SIZE-UP

Pay particular attention to your own safety. Look for:
- Mechanism of injury
- Automobile crash, bent steering wheel
- Sports accident, especially blow to abdomen
- Gunshot wound
- Stab wound
- Fight, especially with hard, direct blow to abdomen
- Crush injury
- Explosion

Primary Assessment

General Impression
- Patient lying very still with knees flexed up toward chest
- Obvious open wound to abdomen
- Severe abdominal pain

Mental Status
- Alert to unresponsive, based on type and degree of injury
- Unresponsiveness or decreasing mental status associated with hemorrhagic shock and poor cerebral perfusion

Airway
- Assume airway is obstructed if patient has altered mental status

Breathing
- Normal
- May be fast and shallow because of pain associated with breathing
- Labored breathing may be present if diaphragm is injured

Circulation
- Pulse and skin color vary depending on injury
- Pulse is increased in shock state and in association with severe pain
- Skin will be pale, cool, and clammy in shock state

Priority Status: Priority patient if abdominal trauma is associated with severe pain or signs and symptoms of hemorrhagic shock

Secondary Assessment

Physical Exam

Head:
- Pale oral mucous membranes in shock state
- Pupils may be sluggish to respond in shock state

Chest:
- Decreased breath sounds bilaterally if breathing is shallow because of pain

Abdomen:
- Contusions, lacerations, punctures, abrasions, or other evidence of trauma
- Inspect for distention
- Discoloration around umbilicus and in flank areas (late sign of intra-abdominal bleeding)
- Inspect for abdominal evisceration
- Palpate for rigidity and guarding
- Pain on palpation
- Palpate for masses

Extremities:
- Weak peripheral pulses indicating poor perfusion
- Difference in strength of pulses in upper and lower extremities indicating possible aortic injury

Posterior Body:
- Evidence of blunt or penetrating trauma

Baseline Vital Signs
- BP: may be low because of blood loss
- HR: tachycardia from severe pain and blood loss
- RR: normal; may be increased because of pain, or labored if diaphragm injured
- Skin: pale, cool, clammy if blood loss and shock
- Pupils: may be sluggish to respond to light because of poor perfusion
- SpO_2: reading may not be obtained if shock is present

FIGURE 35-3a ✱ Assessment summary: abdominal trauma.

Media Resources
Go to www.bradybooks.com for mykit. Highlights:
- *Web Resource:* Genital Trauma

Emergency Care Protocol

ABDOMINAL TRAUMA

1. Establish manual in-line stabilization. Do not release it until the patient is immobilized onto a backboard.
2. Establish and maintain an open airway. Insert a nasopharyngeal or oropharyngeal airway if the patient is unresponsive and has no gag or cough reflex.
3. Suction secretions as necessary.
4. If breathing is inadequate, provide positive pressure ventilation with supplemental oxygen at a rate of 10–12 ventilations/minute for an adult and 12–20 ventilations/minute for an infant or child.
5. If breathing is adequate, administer oxygen by nonrebreather mask at 15 lpm.
6. Control any major bleeding.
7. Treat the specific condition or wound:
   Impaled Object:
   Stabilize the impaled object in place.
   Abdominal Evisceration:
   Place a moist, sterile dressing over the entire wound, overlapping by 2 inches.
   Apply an occlusive dressing taped on all four sides.
   Flex knees up toward the chest.
   Open Wound to Abdomen:
   Apply a dressing over the wound.
8. Treat for shock. Consider application of the pneumatic antishock garment (PASG) if intra-abdominal hemorrhage is suspected with severe hypotension or if retroperitoneal hemorrhage is suspected with hypotension.
9. Immobilize to a backboard if you suspect spine injury.
10. Transport.
11. Perform a reassessment every 5 minutes if unstable and every 15 minutes if stable.

FIGURE 35-3b ✱ Emergency care protocol: abdominal trauma.

Cold compresses may be applied to the scrotum to reduce the pain and swelling associated with injury. If the penis has been avulsed or amputated, apply direct pressure to control the bleeding. If the amputated or avulsed part is located, wrap it in a sterile dressing moistened with sterile saline, place it in a plastic bag, and keep it cool by placing the bag on a cold pack or ice that has been wrapped in a towel. Provide oxygen at 15 lpm by nonrebreather mask, carefully assess for signs and symptoms of shock, and transport the patient with any amputated parts.

- *Injuries to the female genitalia* can occur from straddle injuries, sexual assault, blunt trauma, abortion attempts, lacerations following childbirth, and foreign bodies inserted into the vagina. Because a large number of nerves are located in this area, injuries usually produce excruciating pain and cause great concern to the patient. The female genital area is very vascular and can bleed profusely. Control any bleeding with direct pressure, using moistened compresses such as a sterile sanitary napkin. Never pack or place dressings inside the vagina. Carefully assess for signs and symptoms of shock, provide oxygen at 15 lpm by nonrebreather mask, and transport.

Emergency Care Algorithm: **Abdominal Trauma**

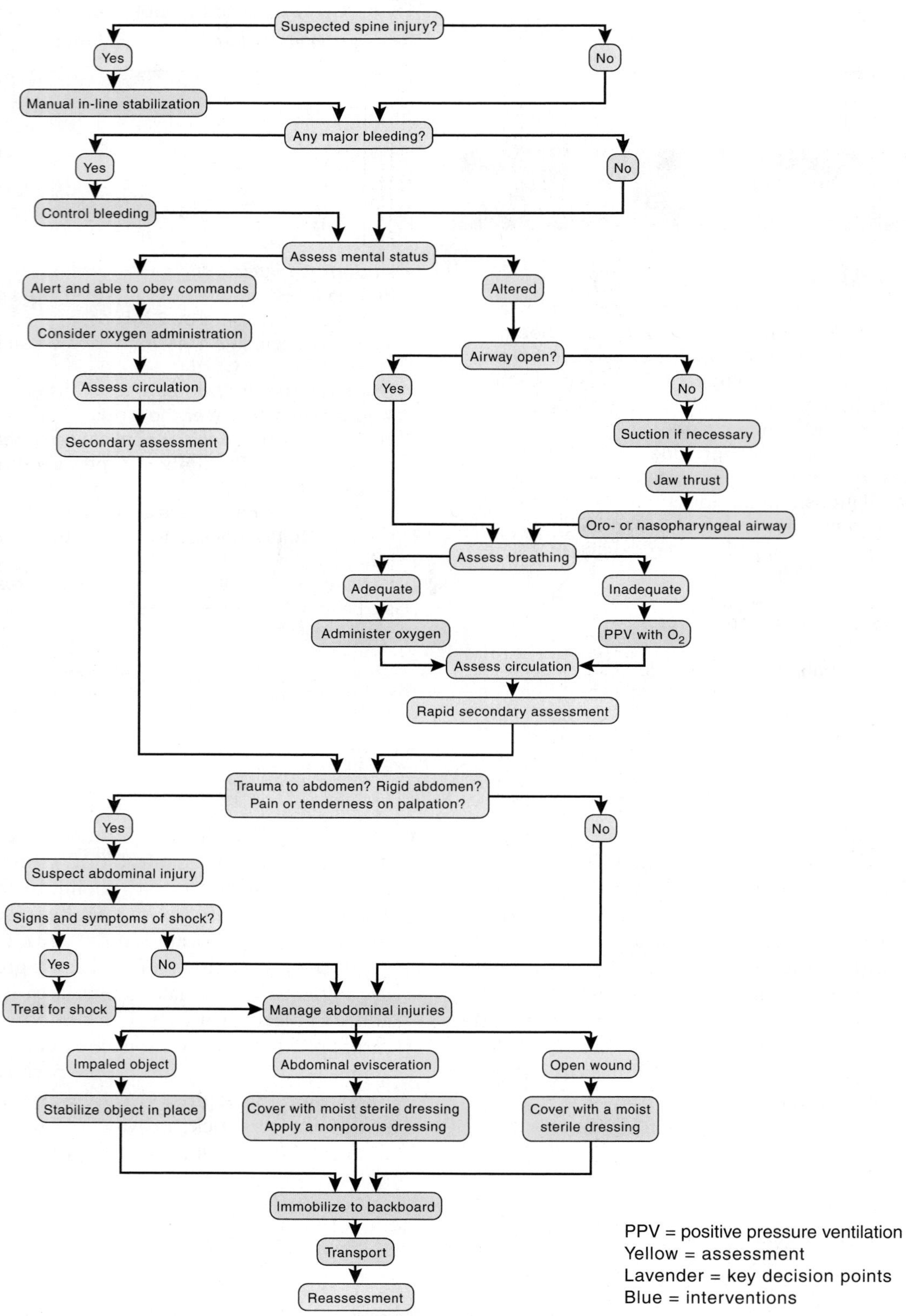

FIGURE 35-4 ✱ Emergency care algorithm: abdominal trauma.

Dressing an Abdominal Evisceration

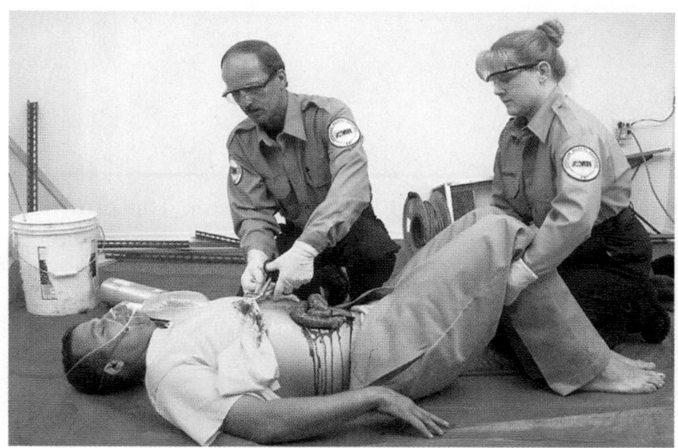

35-1A ✱ Cut away clothing from the wound and support the knees in a flexed position.

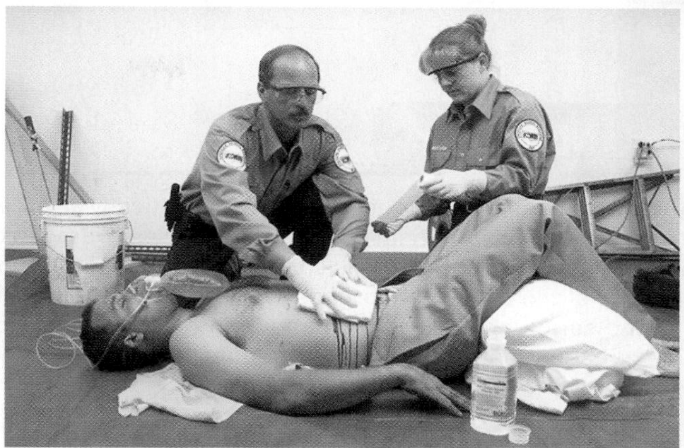

35-1B ✱ Place a premoistened dressing over the wound (follow local protocol) and gently tape it in place. Do not attempt to replace intestines within the abdomen.

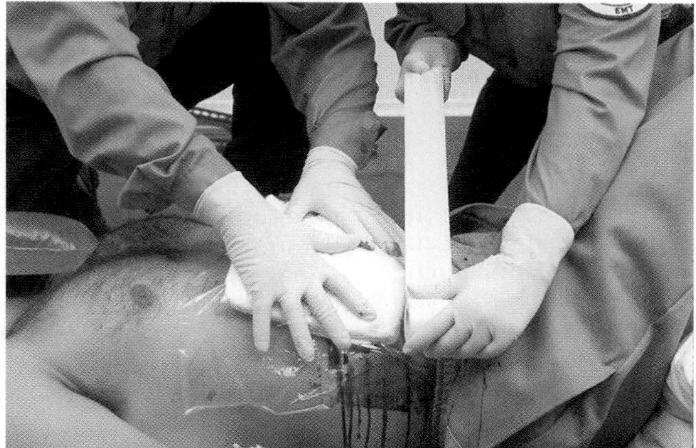

35-1C ✱ Apply an occlusive covering (follow local protocol). Tape it loosely to keep the dressing moist.

CHAPTER REVIEW

SUMMARY

Abdominal injuries may not present as dramatically as other injuries; however, the main concern is possible severe internal bleeding and hemorrhagic shock. Laceration or rupture of many of the abdominal organs can lead to severe bleeding and serious blood loss. An abdominal evisceration occurs when a portion of an abdominal organ protrudes through the open wound in the abdomen. The protruding organ must be covered by a moist, sterile dressing and then sealed with an occlusive dressing to hold in the moisture and heat.

Male and female genitalia injuries are managed as soft tissue injuries. These injuries are rarely life threatening.

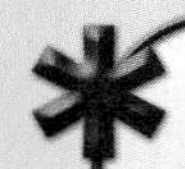

CASE STUDY FOLLOW-UP

SCENE SIZE-UP

You and your partner are at the scene of a patient struck by a car while jogging. A male patient, who introduces himself as Harvey Young, is lying supine on the sidewalk and holding his abdomen. The police have indicated that he is the only patient.

PRIMARY ASSESSMENT

Your partner immediately takes manual in-line spinal stabilization. The patient is alert, responsive, and complaining of severe abdominal pain. He is talking with you, so you know his airway is open. His breathing appears to be adequate but is rapid. His skin is pale, cool, and clammy and his radial pulse is weak and rapid. You apply a nonrebreather mask at 15 lpm.

You decide that the patient is exhibiting signs and symptoms of hemorrhagic shock; therefore, he is a priority transport. You quickly cut the clothes away from the patient to completely expose him to conduct a rapid secondary assessment.

SECONDARY ASSESSMENT

Mr. Young tells you he was jogging down the street when a car "came out of nowhere." He explains that the car swerved but still hit him as he turned to try to get out of the way. Most of the impact was to his abdomen.

You begin the rapid secondary assessment looking for any other life-threatening injuries. He has multiple contusions and abrasions to the body. The pupils are equal and reactive to light. There is no blood or cerebral spinal fluid leaking from the nose, mouth, or ears. You do not find any evidence of trauma to the head or neck. The jugular veins are flat and the trachea is midline. You do not note any subcutaneous emphysema on palpation. Upon inspection of the chest, you do note some minor contusions and abrasions. The patient does not complain of any pain on palpation nor do you find any abnormalities. The breath sounds are equal and clear bilaterally. You note a large contusion to the left upper quadrant. Upon palpation, the patient complains of severe pain to the left upper quadrant. The abdomen is rigid. The pelvis is stable when palpated. You note contusions and abrasions to extremities; however, no deformity, pain, angulation, discoloration, or edema is found. The pulses are weak and rapid in all four extremities. The skin is pale, cool, and clammy. You log roll the patient and find minor contusions and abrasions to the posterior body. You place the patient onto the backboard.

As your partner completes the immobilization, you take the patient's vital signs, which are: pulse 126 bpm; blood pressure 102/78 mmHg; respirations 26; skin pale, cool, and clammy. Immediately after the immobilization is complete, you begin rapid transport to the trauma center.

En route you obtain a brief history. Mr. Young reports that he has no known allergies, takes no medications on a daily basis, and has no other medical problems or history. He last had a drink of water before jogging.

REASSESSMENT

While you are en route to the hospital, you conduct a reassessment. You contact the hospital and provide an oral report. Upon arrival, you give the triage nurse a brief report and he has you transfer Mr. Young to a trauma room. You then begin your documentation of the call as your partner readies the ambulance for the next patient.

Later in the week you find out from the triage nurse that Harvey Young ruptured his spleen and required surgery. He is expected to make a full recovery.

IN REVIEW

1. List the signs and symptoms associated with trauma to the abdomen.
2. Describe the general guidelines for emergency medical care of both open and closed abdominal injuries.
3. Describe emergency medical care for an abdominal evisceration.
4. Describe the general emergency care for injuries to the male or female genitalia.

CRITICAL THINKING

You arrive on the scene in a residential neighborhood and find a 48-year-old male patient lying on his right side on the garage floor. You see large pools of blood on the floor. You note a circular saw with blood on it and some wood on the floor also. The patient's eyes are open and he is moaning in pain. The patient states he was cutting some wood when the saw kicked back and struck him in the abdomen. The patient's respirations are 38 and shallow. His radial pulse is present but weak. His skin is pale, cool, and clammy. His heart rate is 126 bpm. After exposing the patient, you note a large, gaping laceration to the abdomen with what appears to be a portion of the small intestine protruding through the wound.

1. What immediate emergency care would you provide for the patient?
2. How would you manage the protruding abdominal organs?
3. What do the vital signs indicate?
4. How would you position the patient for transport?

EXPLORE PEARSON **mybradykit**™

Please go to **www.bradybooks.com** to access mykit for this text. You will find quizzes, critical thinking scenarios, weblinks, animations, and videos related to this chapter—and much more. Look for online information on penetrating abdominal trauma.

Register your access code from the front of your book by going to **www.bradybooks.com** and selecting the mykit links.

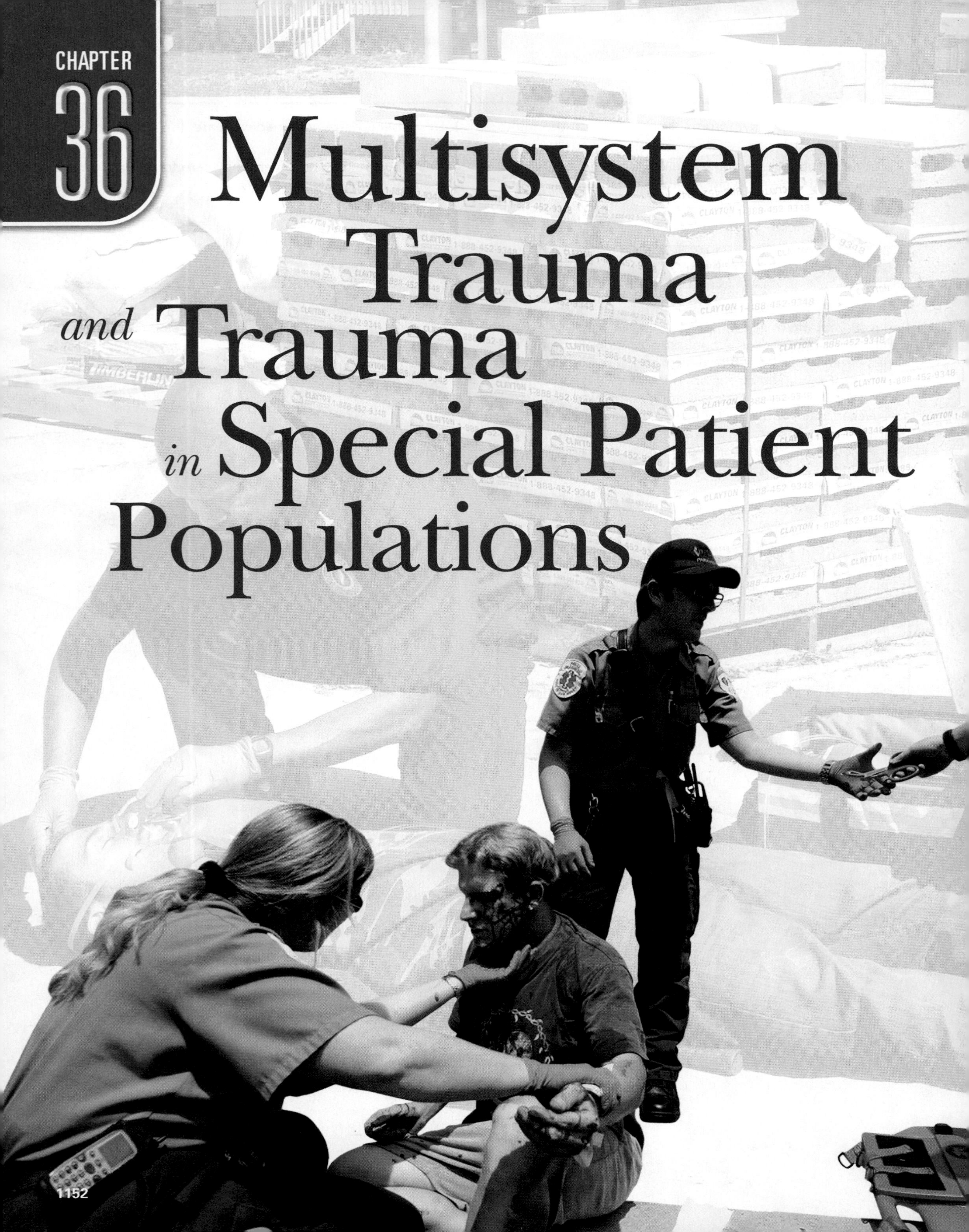

CHAPTER 36

Multisystem Trauma *and* Trauma *in* Special Patient Populations

Navigation Guide

The following items provide an overview to the purpose and content of this chapter. The Standard and Competency are from the new National EMS Education Standards.

STANDARD **Trauma** (Content Area: Multisystem Trauma; Special Considerations in Trauma)

COMPETENCY Applies fundamental knowledge to provide basic emergency care and transportation based on assessment findings for an acutely injured patient.

OBJECTIVES: After reading this chapter, you should be able to:

36-1. Define key terms introduced in this chapter.
36-2. Discuss the increased morbidity and mortality associated with multisystem trauma.
36-3. Describe the importance of the golden principles of prehospital multisystem trauma assessment, care, and transport.
36-4. Summarize anatomical and physiological changes of pregnancy that create special considerations in assessing and managing, and transporting pregnant trauma patients.
36-5. Describe the relationship of maternal injuries to fetal distress and death.
36-6. Summarize anatomical and physiological changes in children that create special considerations in assessing and managing, and transporting pediatric trauma patients.
36-7. Summarize anatomical and physiological changes in the elderly that create special considerations in assessing and managing, and transporting geriatric trauma patients.
36-8. Discuss special considerations in assessing, managing, and transporting cognitively impaired trauma patients.
36-9. Discuss the assessment-based approach to multisystem trauma and trauma in special patient populations.

KEY TERMS: Page references indicate first major use in this chapter. For complete definitions, see the Glossary at the back of the book.

abruptio placentae p. 1157
multisystem trauma p. 1154

MEDIA RESOURCES: Please go to www.bradybooks.com to access mykit for this text. You will find quizzes, critical thinking scenarios, weblinks, animations, and videos related to this chapter—and much more. Look for online information on pediatric and geriatric trauma.

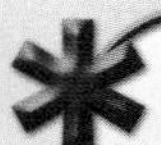

CASE STUDY

The Dispatch
EMS Unit 43—proceed to 587 Biltmore Lane—you have a 30-year-old patient who fell. Time out is 1730 hours.

Upon Arrival
As you arrive on the scene at a single-family residence, you are met by four small children screaming and crying. You approach the residence and hear a voice yell "Help me!" from inside. The children run past you into the house and lead you to the stairwell. There, you see an obviously pregnant woman lying on the floor at the base of the stairs next to a pile of laundry.

How Would You Proceed to Assess and Care for This Patient?
In this chapter, you will learn about special considerations when caring for specific trauma populations. Later, we will return to the case study and apply the principles learned.

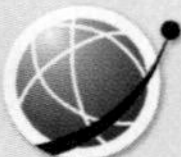

Media Resources

Go to www.bradybooks.com for mykit. Highlights:

- *Web Resource:* Pediatric Trauma Considerations
- *Web Resource:* Geriatric Trauma Considerations

Objective 36-2
Discuss the increased morbidity and mortality associated with multisystem trauma.

Objective 36-3
Describe the importance of the golden principles of prehospital multisystem trauma assessment, care, and transport.

Introduction

In previous chapters you have learned how to properly assess and manage an adult trauma patient. However, not every trauma patient is the same. Some trauma patients have multiple body systems that have been injured, which makes their assessment and care more challenging. Other patients may be part of a special population such as pregnant women, children, elderly adults, and people with cognitive impairments that can also require additional assessment and management skills. If the patient is part of a special population, the EMTs should be able to incorporate their knowledge about that particular type of patient into their assessment and emergency care.

Multisystem Trauma

Traumatic injuries pose some of the greatest challenges to the EMT. With trauma, patients are subjected to significant forces that increase their risk for injuries to multiple organs within the body at the same time. Almost all trauma affects more than one body system. Typically a patient is considered to have **multisystem trauma** when more than one major system is involved. For example, a patient with multisystem trauma might have head and spinal injuries, chest and abdominal injuries, or chest and multiple extremity injuries. As an EMT, you should suspect multisystem trauma in any patient who has been subjected to a significant external force.

Multisystem trauma has a high incidence of morbidity and mortality. Trauma is the leading cause of death for young people 1 to 37 years of age. Because multiple organ systems are involved, numerous injuries and their complications should be anticipated by the EMT. The signs and symptoms associated with the injuries will vary based on the body systems that are affected. The emergency care that you will need to provide will also depend on the systems and injuries sustained by the patient (Figure 36-1*). It is important to note that patients with multisystem trauma are at a greater risk of developing shock than trauma patients whose injuries affect only one system.

The definitive care for a patient with multisystem trauma may be surgery, which obviously cannot be performed in the prehospital environment. As an EMT, you are often the first member of a team of medical professionals who will assess and treat these patients. Once you have taken the patient to the hospital, the hospital staff and trauma team will continue to manage the patient's care. Often a team of physicians, including specialists such as neurosurgeons, thoracic surgeons, and orthopedic surgeons, are needed to properly treat the patient's injuries.

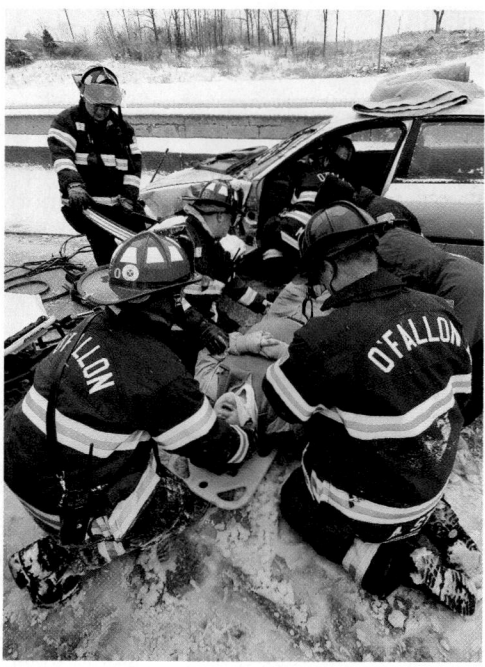

FIGURE 36-1 * Emergency care of the multisystem trauma patient will depend on the systems and injuries sustained by the patient. (© Ray Kemp/911 Imaging)

Golden Principles of Prehospital Multisystem Trauma Care

The following are golden principles for prehospital multisystem trauma care. Keep these principles in mind when you manage a patient with multisystem trauma:

- **Ensure safety of the rescue personnel and the patient.** Your personal safety is most important and should be maintained when you arrive on the scene and throughout your patient's care. Remember that an injured EMT cannot provide care to others. Be sure to assess your environment and look for possible hazards that could put you or others at risk. Some of these dangers include passing automobiles, hazardous materials, hostile environments, unsecured

Key Terms
multisystem trauma trauma in which more than one major body system is involved.

Thinking Critically
You arrive at the scene of a car-tree collision to find the belted-in driver screaming, "Help me!" while someone who may have been a passenger is sitting quietly against the tree. The driver should obviously be attended to first—true or false? Explain your reasoning.

crime scenes, and suicidal patients who may become homicidal.

- **Determine additional resources needed.** After arriving on the scene, determine if you need additional resources. Because multisystem trauma can result from various causes, the additional resources required might vary. The use of advanced life support (ALS) intercept and air medical resources for a multisystem trauma patient should be seriously considered. Know your local protocols and procedures for requesting these resources.
- **Understand kinematics.** Knowing the mechanism of injury can help the EMT anticipate what injuries the patient may have. Multisystem trauma can result from blunt trauma, penetrating trauma, motor vehicle collisions, blast injuries, deceleration injuries, or any other type or combination of mechanisms. As an EMT, always maintain a high index of suspicion that multiple systems are involved when you approach any trauma patient. Sometimes an obvious injury is not the one that has the most potential for harm. Do not develop "tunnel vision" by focusing on patients who complain and are screaming for your help. Other, quiet patients on the scene may be hypoxic or may have internal bleeding that has resulted in an altered level of consciousness and may not be able to call out for help.
- **Identify and manage life threats.** Airway, ventilation, and oxygenation are key to the successful management of a multisystem trauma patient. Each multisystem trauma patient should be assessed and that patient's specific emergency care needs identified. For example, you should control arterial bleeding as soon as you find it, even if that precedes airway and ventilation assessment. A large amount of emergency care for the multisystem trauma patient can be provided en route to the receiving facility.
- **Manage the airway while maintaining cervical spinal stabilization.** Because multisystem trauma patients may have suffered a spinal injury, always establish and maintain spinal stabilization. Inspect for possible airway obstructions and apply suction if necessary. Open the airway using the jaw thrust. The airway of the patient must remain open and clear throughout the duration of your care.
- **Support ventilation and oxygenation.** Determine if your patient is breathing adequately based on the rate and tidal volume. If the ventilation is inadequate, provide positive pressure ventilation. Patients with a low minute volume will need assisted ventilations. Administering high-concentration oxygen is necessary in the multisystem trauma patient to saturate the hemoglobin with as much oxygen as possible and to attempt to maintain delivery of oxygen to the cells. The patient's oxygen saturation should be maintained greater than 95% at all times and should be monitored by pulse oximetry.
- **Control external hemorrhage and treat for shock.** Cellular oxygenation is impaired when a patient is bleeding profusely. The loss of hemoglobin reduces the ability of the blood to carry and deliver oxygen to the cells. This leads to cellular hypoxia and anaerobic metabolism. Because of this, it is necessary to stop major external hemorrhage rapidly. If the bleeding cannot be controlled by direct pressure, consider the use of a tourniquet. Multisystem trauma patients are at risk for developing shock. If any signs and symptoms of shock are present, initiate emergency care for shock (see Chapter 15, "Shock and Resuscitation"). Maintain a normal body temperature and prevent hypothermia by covering the trauma patient with blankets.
- **Perform a secondary assessment and obtain a medical history.** After treating immediate life threats, perform a rapid secondary assessment to identify any additional injures that could potentially be life threatening. This is very important, especially when you are trying to determine if multiple body systems may have been injured. The signs and symptoms discovered during your assessment will vary according to the organs and systems that are involved and must be treated appropriately. Try to obtain a medical history from the patient or bystanders. Keep in mind that the traumatic injuries may have resulted because of an underlying medical condition. Also, underlying medical conditions and medications can alter the body's ability to respond appropriately to the injury and blood loss. As an example, a patient who is taking beta blockers or calcium channel blockers will present with a heart rate that may appear within normal limits but does not correspond with other presenting signs and symptoms of shock and blood loss.
- **Splint musculoskeletal injuries and maintain spinal immobilization on a long spine board.** Multisystem trauma patients may be found standing, sitting, prone, or supine when you arrive on the

Key Points
Whether the trauma patient is found standing, sitting, prone, or supine, cervical spine stabilization must be maintained at all times.

Objective 36-4
Summarize anatomical and physiological changes of pregnancy that create special considerations in assessing and managing, and transporting pregnant trauma patients.

scene. All of these patients require cervical spine stabilization that must be maintained at all times. Proper cervical spine stabilization, log rolling techniques, and use of a backboard by the EMT can help protect the spinal cord and prevent additional injuries. Any musculoskeletal injuries should be splinted en route if the patient is unstable. The backboard acts like a splint and provides minimal stabilization until time and patient condition permit further fracture care. Splinting fractures at the scene for a multisystem trauma patient will delay transport, something that should not occur in trauma patients. Splinting possible fractures en route, however, may help minimize blood loss, minimize neurovascular damage, and prevent closed fractures from becoming open ones.

- **Make transport decisions.** Rapid extrication and rapid transport of the critically injured multisystem trauma patients is essential. The on-scene time is critical and should not be prolonged. The on-scene time is considered part of the platinum 10 minutes and the golden period between injury and definitive care at the hospital, a time span that should not be exceeded and should be minimized if possible. It is critical that you know your local trauma system capabilities and transport your patient to the closest appropriate facility. Notify the hospital as early as possible so they can prepare for the patient's arrival. Many of these patients require surgery for their injuries.

Trauma in Special Patient Populations

Trauma can occur in all populations. Some patients—like pregnant women, children, elderly adults, or patients who are cognitively impaired—require additional assessment considerations and some modifications in treatment for their traumatic injuries. Identifying and treating life-threatening injuries is a priority in all of these special patient populations.

Trauma in Pregnant Patients

Trauma occurs in approximately 6 to 7 percent of all pregnancies and is the leading cause of death for pregnant women. Pregnant patients can sustain all types of trauma and are especially susceptible to physical abuse and falls (Figure 36-2*). Motor vehicle crashes account for about half of all injuries sustained during pregnancy.

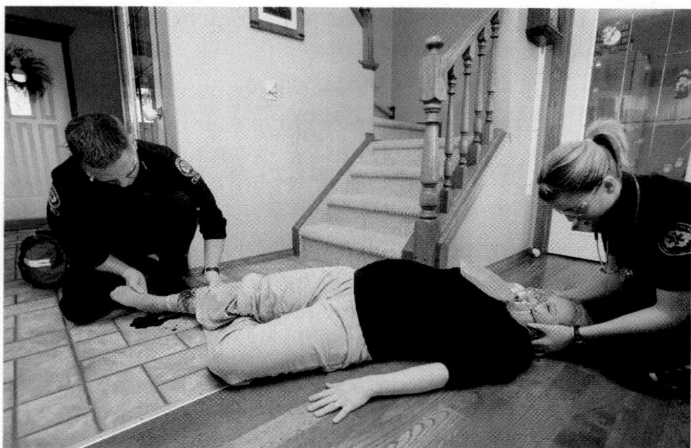

FIGURE 36-2 * Pregnant women may sustain all types of trauma and are especially susceptible to physical abuse and falls.

There are two patients when you deal with a pregnant trauma patient: the mother and the fetus. The number of weeks the patient has been pregnant and the size of the fetus are important to the fetus's chance of survival. Because it is difficult to assess the fetus, it is important to treat the mother aggressively, especially if there is severe trauma. All pregnant women who have suffered an injury should be evaluated by a physician in the emergency department.

Anatomical and Physiological Considerations in the Pregnant Trauma Patient

A woman's body changes during pregnancy, and these changes may influence the patient's presentation. One of the most important changes is a gradual increase in the total blood volume of about 50 percent in the pregnant patient. The mother will have a 10–15 bpm increase in her heart rate during the third trimester. The pregnant woman's uterus also becomes more vascular and helps to supply the increased oxygen demand and consumption the fetus needs to survive. All of these changes can make the pregnant patient more susceptible to shock.

The pregnant woman's diaphragm elevates, making her susceptible to developing a tension pneumothorax. She might have an altered perception of pain in the abdomen because her abdominal viscera are pushed up-

Key Points
A pregnant woman has a greatly increased blood volume and an increased need for oxygen to sustain the fetus. These conditions make her especially susceptible to shock when she is injured.

Objective 36-5
Describe the relationship of maternal injuries to fetal distress and death.

Key Terms
abruptio placentae the separation of the placenta from the uterine wall.

ward. Gastric motility decreases in the pregnant patient, which increases her risk of vomiting and aspiration. Her uterus grows throughout the pregnancy and rises out of the pelvis, making injury to it more likely than when she is not pregnant. The pregnant woman's bladder is displaced into the abdominal cavity, which places it at greater risk for traumatic injury. The pregnant woman's renal blood flow is also increased. Her pelvic joints are loosened and her center of gravity changes, both of which can make her prone to accidents and falls.

Fetus size during the third trimester can affect the patient's venous return. If a pregnant patient is lying flat on her back, it can result in supine hypotensive syndrome, which can be managed by tilting the backboard to the left.

Assessment Considerations in the Pregnant Trauma Patient

Trauma to a pregnant woman, whether severe or minor, can have significant effects on the health of the fetus. It is estimated that 1 to 3 percent of minor traumas involving pregnant women result in fetal loss. The more severe the injury to the mother, the greater the chances of fetal injury. Fetal death rates are nine times higher than maternal death rates following trauma. The most common problem caused by maternal trauma is uterine contractions that may progress into labor. You must assess for crowning or bleeding in these trauma patients.

Abruptio placentae, or the separation of the placenta from the uterine wall, can also result from a traumatic injury (see Chapter 37, "Obstetrics and Care of the Newborn"). It is most common when the patient has suffered blunt trauma. Abdominal pain and vaginal bleeding are often present with this condition and pose a high risk of fetal and maternal death. Fetal injury and death can also result from penetrating trauma. Because the patient's uterus has grown in size, it can help shield the mother against some abdominal injuries; however, it puts the fetus at greater risk for injury. For example, stab wounds to the uterus can produce 93 percent morbidity to the fetus.

Motor vehicle crashes account for a large number of maternal and traumatic injuries. Pregnant patients wearing their seat belts properly are more likely to have a favorable outcome when involved in a crash than those who don't wear seat belts. The unbelted pregnant crash victim is twice as likely to have vaginal bleeding or to give birth, and fetal death is three to four times more likely. Uterine rupture is a rare event that sometimes occurs when the woman's pelvis strikes the uterus in a vehicular crash. It can result in maternal and fetal death.

Fetal distress can also be caused by hypoxia or hypovolemic shock, which can result from any traumatic injury. Shock and internal blood loss in a third-trimester patient may be difficult to detect. Because of the cardiovascular changes in the pregnant patient, the signs of maternal hypotension resulting from traumatic bleeding may be delayed or masked. You must anticipate shock and not rely solely on vital sign changes to manage the patient aggressively. Shock is a frequent cause of death to both the fetus and the mother.

It is estimated that 41 percent of fetuses die when the mother suffers a life-threatening injury. A traumatic maternal cardiac arrest poses a significant risk to the fetus. A pulseless woman in the third trimester should be transported to the nearest appropriate medical facility for attempted resuscitation of the mother and fetus unless instructed otherwise by medical direction. Although the chance of the fetus surviving maternal cardiac arrest is poor, it still may be possible. Make sure you know and follow your protocols regarding this type of scenario.

Management Considerations for the Pregnant Trauma Patient

Most of the emergency care for a pregnant trauma patient is the same as for nonpregnant trauma patients and obstetric emergencies. Some additional management considerations for a pregnant trauma are:

- Full spinal immobilization is required for pregnant patients suspected of having spinal injury; however, you will need to tilt the long spine board to the left if the patient is in her third trimester or obviously pregnant. This will help prevent supine hypotensive syndrome. The pregnant patient should remain on her left side throughout transport.
- Airway, ventilation, and oxygenation are critical to the pregnant trauma patient. You should anticipate vomiting and have suction readily available. Assess if the patient is breathing adequately and if bilateral breath sounds are present. Assist the patient's ventilations if they are inadequate. Administer oxygen by nonrebreather mask if the breathing is adequate or via the bag-valve mask in the patient with inadequate breathing. Administer supplemental oxygen to maintain the SpO_2 reading as high as possible. Attempt to achieve 100% oxygen concentration delivery. The

Key Points
The most common problem in maternal trauma is uterine contractions that may progress into labor. Continually monitor the patient with this possibility in mind.

Objective 36-6
Summarize anatomical and physiological changes in children that create special considerations in assessing and managing, and transporting pediatric trauma patients.

fetus is vulnerable to any reduction in oxygen and can become severely hypoxic before the pregnant patient shows signs of hypoxia.

- Assess the patient's circulation and check for major bleeding. If vaginal bleeding is present, absorb the blood flow with a pad and do not pack the vagina. Anticipate, prevent, and treat shock.
- Perform a visual exam at the vaginal opening to assess for crowning or bleeding. Remember that you have two patients. If labor occurs as a result of the trauma, you will want additional resources to help you manage both the mother and the newborn.
- Consider ALS intercept or air medical transport for major traumas involving pregnant patients. Follow your local protocol. Inform the trauma center as soon as possible that the patient involved in the trauma is pregnant. This will allow the receiving facility time to assemble a trauma team and other necessary resources to manage the fetus.
- The best method to care for the fetus is by anticipating injuries and shock and aggressively managing the mother.

Trauma in Pediatric Patients

Pediatric patients are frequently victims of major and minor trauma. Children may experience traumatic injuries from drowning, burns, falls, penetrating trauma, motor vehicle crashes, abuse, pedestrian versus vehicle collisions, as well as any other traumatic mechanism (Figure 36-3*). See Chapter 38, "Pediatrics," for more information on assessment and emergency care of the pediatric trauma patient.

Half of all deaths in children ages 1 to 14 are the result of trauma. Motor vehicle collisions account for the majority of traumatic injuries as well as almost half of the traumatic deaths. Improper car seat usage or placement can greatly contribute to the injuries sustained by pediatric patients involved in motor vehicle collisions.

Children are at risk of being abused by adults and older children. Child abuse accounts for approximately 25 to 35 percent of pediatric trauma deaths. It also can result in significant injuries and impairments. Some findings that may prompt you to suspect abuse include:

- Bruises or burns in unusual shapes and locations
- An injury that doesn't seem to correlate with the cause provided

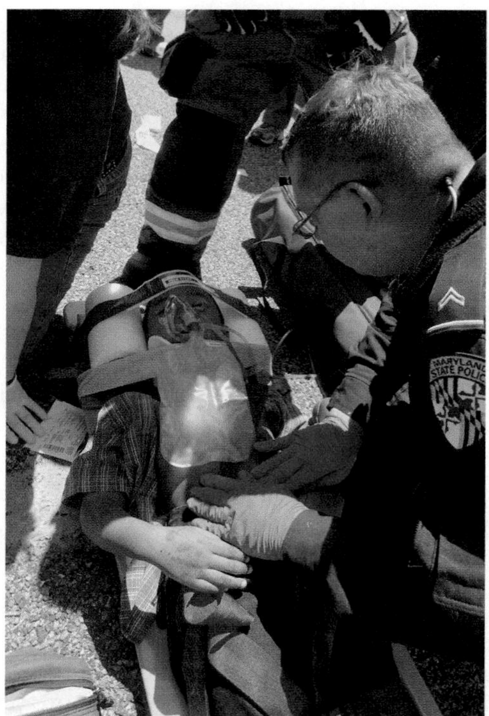

FIGURE 36-3 * Children are frequently victims of major and minor trauma. (© Mark C. Ide)

- More injuries than usual for a child that same age
- Multiple injuries in various healing stages

Shaken baby syndrome is one of many causes of brain injury. Other injuries can also result in life-threatening emergencies for abused children.

Trauma involving a pediatric patient is one of the most difficult types of calls for EMTs to respond to. Knowing that the young patient has endured a traumatic injury can be especially stressful for you as well as for the family and bystanders. It is important to act professionally, competently, and compassionately throughout the call, remembering that the assessment and care you provide to these patients directly impact their outcomes.

Anatomical and Physiological Considerations in the Pediatric Trauma Patient

Pediatric patients have anatomical and physiological characteristics that play a significant role in trauma assessment and management. Traumatic forces are more widely dis-

Key Points
Half of all deaths in children ages 1 to 14 are from trauma, and 25 to 35 percent of those deaths are caused by abuse. Be aware of the signs of abuse and report any suspicions according to your local and state guidelines.

Key Points
Subtle changes in heart rate, blood pressure, or perfusion status may indicate cardiorespiratory failure in the pediatric patient.

tributed in pediatric patients than in adults, and this makes them more prone to suffering multisystem trauma. The child's body surface area is greater than an adult's and, therefore, can lose heat faster. Pediatric patients have heavy heads and weak neck muscles that increase their risk of head and cervical spinal injuries. Their internal organ placement makes them more susceptible to injuries to the spleen and liver.

Infants and children have greater chest wall flexibility than adults, which can allow for injuries with few external signs of trauma. You must look closely for signs and symptoms of a flail chest in pediatric trauma patients, and maintain a high index of suspicion that severe underlying trauma exists. The growth plates in children are not fully developed, and trauma to these plates may impact the bones' normal growth. Children also have higher energy requirements and can fatigue faster than adults.

Assessment Considerations in the Pediatric Trauma Patient

Children respond differently to injury than adults. Their physiological response and vital signs are influenced by their age and the severity of their injury.

The pediatric assessment triangle developed by the American Academy of Pediatrics (Figure 36-4*) can help you form a general impression. The triangle is composed of three sides: appearance, work of breathing, and circulation to skin. The appearance side refers to the child's overall mental status, body position, and muscle tone. The work of breathing side relates to the visual effort of breathing and any audible sounds associated with the patient's respiration. The circulation side is assessed through the patient's skin color. See Chapter 38, "Pediatrics," for a full discussion of the pediatric assessment triangle and forming a general impression of the pediatric patient.

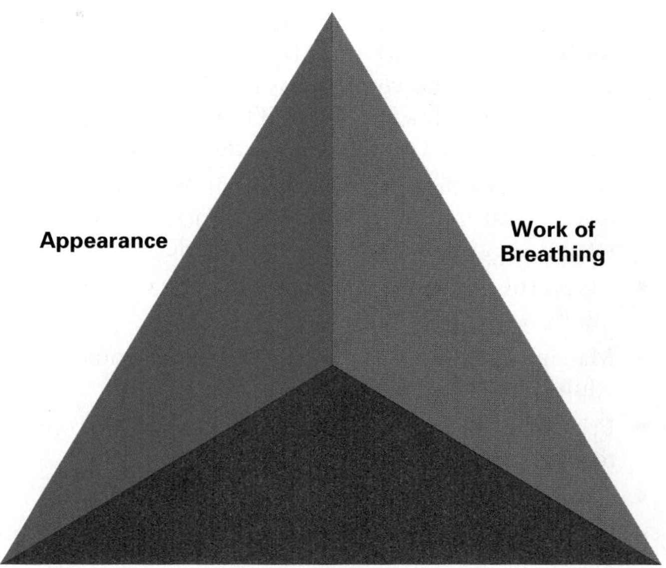

FIGURE 36-4 * The pediatric assessment triangle can help you form a general impression. (Used with permission of the American Academy of Pediatrics)

A patent airway, adequate ventilation, oxygenation, and circulation are essential to the pediatric trauma patient. Any diaphragmatic impairment can compromise the patient's ventilation. Inspect for accessory muscle use, which is more prominent during respiratory distress. Adequate oxygenation does not reflect sufficient ventilation. Therefore, the rate and quality of the patient's ventilations must be assessed.

Subtle changes in the pediatric trauma patient's heart rate, blood pressure, or perfusion status may indicate cardiorespiratory failure. A slow pulse rate in these patients may indicate hypoxia, which is not tolerated well by a child. The brachial pulse should be assessed in an infant less than 1 year of age. Remember that normal blood pressures may be present in pediatric patients with compensated shock. Blood pressure readings are unreliable in children 3 years of age or less. Because of these characteristics, you should rely on other signs and symptoms such as skin color, temperature, and condition; mental status; and capillary refill to assess the pediatric patient's perfusion status.

Management Considerations for the Pediatric Trauma Patient

Most of the management for a pediatric trauma patient is the same as for adults. Some management considerations for a pediatric trauma patient are:

- Spinal immobilization is required for suspected spinal injuries and should be maintained throughout care. Pad beneath the child who is less than 8 years of age from the shoulders to the hips during cervical spine immobilization to prevent flexion of the neck.
- Open the airway and assess for any possible obstructions from injury, teeth, blood, or vomitus. Gurgling or stridor may indicate an upper airway obstruction.

Key Points
The risk of death and significant injury in the elderly is greater than for younger patients. Falls are the most common cause of injury in the elderly.

Objective 36-7
Summarize anatomical and physiological changes in the elderly that create special considerations in assessing and managing, and transporting geriatric trauma patients.

- Assess the breathing rate and tidal volume. Look at both the chest and the abdomen when doing so. Carefully provide ventilations if either the rate or the tidal volume is inadequate or if bradycardia is present. Pediatric trauma patients can fatigue very quickly.
- Administer a high concentration of oxygen and monitor the saturation via the SpO_2 monitor. Keep the saturation as close to 100% as possible.
- Assess the circulation and control any external bleeding by direct pressure.
- Manage hypovolemia and shock as you would for an adult.
- Prevent hypothermia. These patients are susceptible to heat loss.
- Transport to an appropriate facility.
- Continually reassess the pediatric trauma patient.

Trauma in Geriatric Patients

Geriatric or elderly patients account for 10 to 14 percent of all trauma patients. The risk of death and significant injury in the elderly is greater than for younger patients. Falls, most of which occur at home, are the most common cause of injury in the elderly and account for 40 percent of all elderly traumas. As many as one quarter of these falls are the result of medical conditions such as strokes, syncope, and hypovolemia. The most common injury associated with elderly falls is fractures. Loss of strength, sensory impairment, and medical illnesses increase the risk of falls in this population. All elderly traumas should be investigated as to the reason for the fall. See Chapter 39, "Geriatrics," for more information on assessment and emergency care for the geriatric patient.

Burns, penetrating trauma, pedestrian versus vehicle collisions, vehicle crashes, and elder abuse can also cause traumatic injuries in elderly patients. Motor vehicle collisions are the second most common cause of trauma in the elderly (Figure 36-5*). Older drivers are more likely to be killed or injured in these accidents than younger drivers. Most crashes involving the elderly occur during the day and close to their home. Auto versus pedestrian accidents are the third most common injury in this age group and carry the highest fatality rate. Poor eyesight and hearing, decreased mobility, and longer reaction times make elderly patients more susceptible to motor vehicle collisions and pedestrian accidents than their younger counterparts.

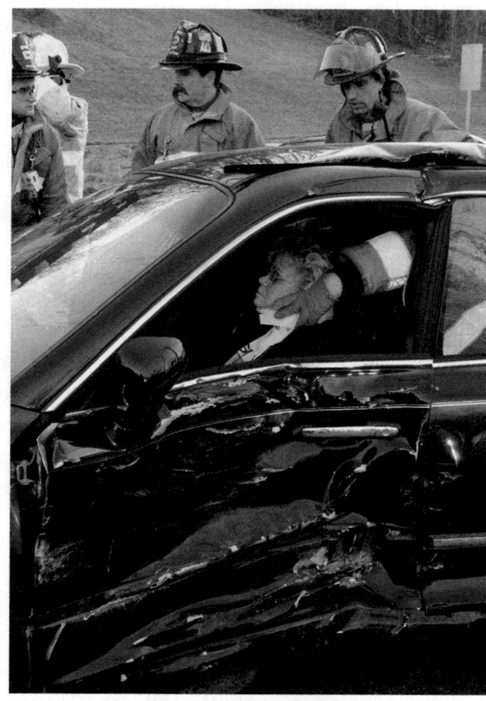

FIGURE 36-5 * Motor vehicle collisions are the second most common cause of trauma in the elderly—second only to falls. (© Mark C. Ide)

Anatomical and Physiological Considerations in the Geriatric Trauma Patient

Physiological changes are a natural part of aging; however, such changes in the pulmonary, cardiovascular, neurological, and musculoskeletal systems make older patients more susceptible to trauma. Circulation changes can lead to the inability to maintain vital signs during hemorrhage; for example, the elderly trauma patient's blood pressure drops sooner than a younger adult's. With aging, the brain shrinks, which can lead to a higher risk of cerebral bleeding following head trauma. Skeletal changes can cause curvature of the upper spine that may require padding during supine spinal immobilization.

Geriatric patients are more susceptible to injury than other adults, even in cases of minor trauma. As noted in Chapter 30, "Musculoskeletal Trauma," many elderly patients have osteoporosis, a medical condition characterized by weakening of the bone tissue, which places these patients at increased risk for fractures and other injuries, even with minor traumatic force or no traumatic force at

Key Points
Do not attribute an elderly trauma patient's altered mental status to age; instead, suspect a head injury.

Objective 36-8
Discuss special considerations in assessing, managing, and transporting cognitively impaired trauma patients.

all. Minor chest trauma can cause lung injury. Decreased muscle size in the abdomen may mask abdominal trauma in the elderly. Thinner skin in the elderly results in more easily inflicted soft tissue injuries.

Assessment Considerations in the Geriatric Trauma Patient

Elderly patients have a decreased ability to respond to trauma when compared to a younger patient. Pre-existing medical conditions may affect the traumatic injuries sustained and influence the patient's outcome. Multiple medications are more common in this age group and may also affect the patient assessment and outcome. Medications can especially affect the patient's vital signs and blood-clotting capabilities.

As with other trauma patients, an altered mental status in the elderly trauma patient may indicate a severe injury. You should not attribute a patient's altered mental status to age and should suspect a head injury. Many elderly patients use dentures, which may cause an airway obstruction in the trauma patient. Elderly patients have a decrease in their cough reflex and may require suctioning. Chest wall injuries may quickly lead to respiratory failure in this population. You should monitor the elderly trauma patient's oxygenation, using pulse oximetry. Elderly patients who were hypertensive prior to an injury may have normal blood pressures when they are in shock. Pelvic and hip fractures are common in this population.

Management Considerations for the Geriatric Trauma Patient

The management for an elderly trauma patient is similar to that provided to other adults. However, you should understand how the changes in the patient may impact the patient's presentation and outcome prior to the injury. Some management considerations for elderly trauma patients include the following:

- Spinal immobilization is required for suspected spinal injuries and should be maintained throughout care. Add padding around the spaces in the back if necessary.
- Open and maintain a clear airway. Suctioning is important in the elderly due to a decreased cough reflex.
- Provide and support ventilation as needed. Administer high-concentration oxygen and use pulse oximetry to monitor the patient's oxygen saturation.
- Prevent hypothermia.
- Splint factures. Remember that traction splints are not used to treat hip fractures.
- Provide rapid transport to the closest appropriate facility. The American College of Surgeons recommends that all trauma patients older than 55 years of age be taken to trauma centers.

Trauma in Cognitively Impaired Patients

Cognitively impaired patients are more susceptible to trauma than patients who do not have cognitive impairment. Some of the conditions that may result in cognitive impairments are vascular dementia, autistic disorders, brain injuries, strokes, Alzheimer disease, and Down syndrome (Figure 36-6*). Many other causes of cognitive impairments exist that may affect your patient's assessment and treatment.

It can be difficult to recognize patients with cognitive impairment when you begin your assessment. Some patients have no physical signs of their mental condition. They may be confused or unresponsive, making assessment of their condition difficult. Never assume that the altered mental status of your trauma patient is due to a previous cognitive impairment or medical condition. Always maintain a high index of suspicion that your patient may have suffered a traumatic head injury.

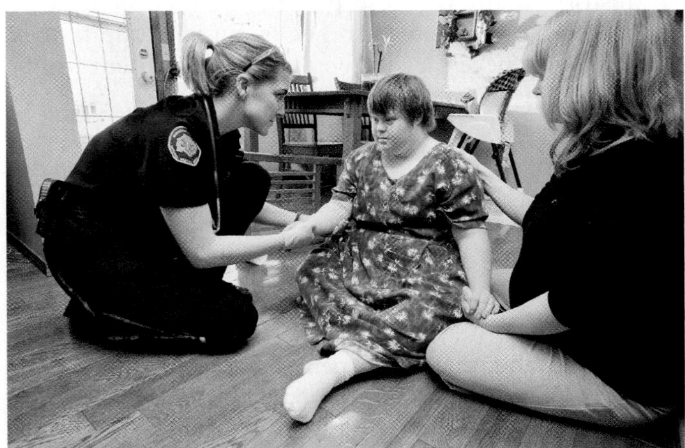

FIGURE 36-6 * A Down syndrome patient may have a mild-to-moderate developmental impairment. You may have to rely on a parent or other caregiver to help reassure the patient and to provide information about the patient's history.

Thinking Critically
Your patient is lying on the garage floor, bleeding, while his mother holds his hand. You ask him what happened and where he hurts. His answers are halting and vague. You don't know if he is cognitively impaired or may have a head injury. How should you continue obtaining the history?

Objective 36-9
Discuss the assessment-based approach to multisystem trauma and trauma in special patient populations.

Anatomical and Physiological Considerations in the Cognitively Impaired Trauma Patient

The anatomical and physiological considerations related to a cognitively impaired trauma patient depend on the underlying cause of each individual's impairment. Many patients have sensory loss related to aging and disease. This may increase their risk of injury and can alter their response to an injury. Some patients with dementia experience cardiovascular changes that make them prone to injury. Other patients have a loss in musculoskeletal strength due to aging or impairment that can lead to falls and other injuries. Memory loss from Alzheimer disease or other cognitive impairments will alter the patient assessment.

Assessment Considerations in the Cognitively Impaired Trauma Patient

Include the following considerations in your assessment of a cognitively impaired trauma patient:

- Patients with cognitive impairments are poor historians; that is, they are not good at recalling or relating their past medical history or events of the trauma. You should address them with respect and initially approach them in the same fashion as you would any other patient; however, you will often have to rely on others to provide information about the patient's past history. Many of these patients may be bedridden, under nursing home care, or living in group homes. It may be necessary for you to obtain consent from a legal guardian or parent to provide them care (see Chapter 3, "Medical, Legal, and Ethical Issues").
- The psychological implications of trauma may be different in this population. Many of these patients may not know what is happening even before the trauma. They may be confused or upset. The traumatic event may make it more difficult for them to communicate and cooperate with you.
- Understand that their pain perception may be altered. This may affect some of the responses that would normally be associated with injury.
- The trauma assessment will provide the most pertinent information about your patient. Because many of these patients will not be able to tell you what is wrong, it is important that you constantly re-evaluate them.
- Always maintain a high level of suspicion that your patient's presenting signs and symptoms have resulted from trauma. Do what is in the best interest of the patient, and treat as if the patient has a head injury.

Management Considerations for the Cognitively Impaired Trauma Patient

Cognitively impaired trauma patients need special care. The following are a few management considerations for this population, in addition to your normal trauma care:

- It is often necessary to involve the patient's caregivers in emergency treatment. Like children, these patients may be more cooperative if a trusted caregiver is present. These caregivers may be able to provide you with important information about the patient's conditions.
- Err on the side of caution and do what is in the best interest of the patient. Manage the patient as if he has a head injury.

Assessment-Based Approach: Multisystem Trauma and Trauma in Special Patient Populations

You have studied many of the elements of assessment that apply to multisystem trauma and trauma in special populations in earlier chapters. The primary goal for all of these patients is to identify and manage life-threatening injuries. We review and develop these assessment elements on the following pages, taking into consideration some adjustments for these special populations.

Scene Size-Up

Because traumatic injuries can occur from so many different mechanisms, ensuring a scene that is safe for you and others is of utmost importance. Look for a possible mechanism of injury and maintain a high index of suspicion that more than one major body system is affected in your patient. Identify if your patient belongs to any special populations and use your knowledge about that population throughout your assessment. Unresponsiveness

Thinking Critically
Your patient fell about 20 feet to the ground and is breathing irregularly. An EMT trainee riding with your crew volunteers to perform a head-tilt, chin-lift to align the patient's airway. How should you respond to this suggestion?

Key Points
Be aware that patients who belong to special populations may not complain of pain or other symptoms of trauma as you would normally expect.

or altered mental status, especially in trauma patients, should always suggest the possibility of head injury. Never assume that mental status changes in a trauma patient are due to drug or alcohol intoxication or previous medical conditions.

Primary Assessment

When performing the primary assessment on a trauma patient, you should suspect a cervical spine injury. Forces applied to the head may have been strong enough to injure the cervical spine as well, especially in pediatric patients. Be aware that other traumatic forces may have caused additional spinal injuries. Manual in-line stabilization of the spine should be your first step and should be maintained throughout your care.

Assess your patient's mental status, using the AVPU mnemonic. Utilize tools such as the Glasgow Coma Scale and the pediatric assessment triangle to provide additional information about the patient's mental status. This will provide a baseline when you reassess your patient. If the patient has an altered mental status, note what type of stimuli, if any, the patient responds to.

Establish an airway, using a jaw-thrust maneuver, while holding in-line spinal stabilization. Ensure that the airway is free from obstructions like blood, vomit, or dentures. Suction the airway if necessary. Remember that elderly and pregnant patients may vomit easily.

Maintain the patient's airway and assess the breathing rate and quality. Provide oxygen by nonrebreather mask at 15 lpm if breathing is adequate in the multisystem trauma patient or in those presenting with signs of hypoxia, respiratory distress, or poor perfusion. If the patient's breathing is inadequate, provide positive pressure ventilations via bag-valve mask with supplemental oxygen. Determine the appropriate ventilation rate based on the patient's age. If the pediatric patient is bradycardic, you should provide assisted ventilations. Monitor the patient's oxygenation via pulse oximetry. A pregnant trauma patient's SpO_2 should be maintained at close to 100% at all times.

Assess the patient's circulatory status and check the pulse. In infants, check the brachial pulse. In children, remember that the capillary refill and skin condition will provide valuable information about your patient's condition. Look for major bleeding and control it with direct pressure. To control major vaginal bleeding in a pregnant patient you should use a pad and never pack the vagina.

Secondary Assessment

When dealing with trauma patients who belong to special populations, perform a rapid secondary assessment to identify signs of trauma and injuries to the body. When multiple body systems are involved in the trauma, the patient is more likely to have an unfavorable outcome. It is important to note that patients in these special populations may not complain of pain or other symptoms of trauma as you would normally expect. The patient's age, physiological changes, medical conditions, and cognitive abilities may influence his responses to both you and the assessment.

Following the rapid secondary assessment, check vital signs and obtain a history. If the patient is alert and oriented, you or your partner might decide that one of you will gather the history while the other performs the rapid trauma assessment and obtains vitals.

Physical Exam

Perform a rapid physical exam. Keep in mind that multiple systems may be affected by the trauma. If your patient is pregnant, you have two patients to consider.

Vital Signs

Check and record vital signs every 5 minutes, staying alert to any changes. The normal vital signs are based on the patient's age (see Chapter 9, "Life Span Development"). Remember that in pregnant women and the elderly you may have what appear to be normal vital signs, even though your patient is in shock. Even the slightest changes in a pediatric trauma patient's vital signs may indicate impending cardiorespiratory failure and must be managed aggressively.

History

The history can provide vital information about the mechanism of injury. Patients, especially children, those with cognitive impairments, or those with an altered mental status, may not be able to provide you with the information you need. You may have to obtain this information from others at the scene. The following are some questions that are relevant when assessing special trauma populations:

- When and how did the incident occur?
- What is the patient's chief complaint?

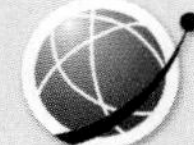

Media Resources
Go to www.bradybooks.com for mykit. Highlight:
- *Animation:* Multiple System Injuries in Front End Collisions

- Does the patient have any signs or symptoms associated with the trauma?
- Is the patient pregnant? If so, how far along is she? Is there any vaginal bleeding or crowning?
- How old is the patient?
- Does the patient take any medications? Is the patient allergic to anything?
- What is the patient's medical history? Is there a history of previous trauma or a cognitive impairment?

Signs and Symptoms

Signs and symptoms will vary based on the patient and the trauma. Special trauma patients may not respond to injury the same way that another trauma patient would. Document any signs and symptoms accurately.

Emergency Medical Care

Consider and apply the following to your trauma patient's care:

1. *Take Standard Precautions.*
2. *Establish and maintain manual in-line spinal stabilization.*
   - Maintain neutral positioning of the head and neck manually, even after a cervical collar is applied, until the patient is completely immobilized to a backboard.
   - If the patient is pregnant and in her third trimester, tilt the backboard to the left.
   - If the patient is a child (typically less than 8 years of age), pad beneath the child from the shoulders to the hips during cervical immobilization to prevent flexion of the neck.
   - If the patient is elderly, add padding around the spaces in the back if necessary.
3. *Maintain a patent airway, and adequate breathing and oxygenation.*
   - Use a jaw thrust to open the airway.
   - Remove any foreign bodies from the mouth, and suction blood and mucus.
   - Protect against aspiration by having suction available at all times and by being prepared to roll the secured patient to clear the airway.
   - Administer oxygen by nonrebreather mask at 15 lpm if breathing is adequate, or positive pressure ventilation based on the patient's age with supplemental oxygen if it is inadequate. Maintain the SpO_2 reading at 100% if the patient is pregnant.
4. *Monitor the airway, breathing, pulse, and mental status for deterioration.* Any patient who deteriorates must be transported immediately.
   - Remember, bradycardia in the pediatric patient requires ventilation.
5. *Control bleeding.*
   - If the pregnant patient is bleeding from the vagina, use a pad to collect the blood flow.
   - If major bleeding is not stopped with direct pressure, consider the use of a tourniquet.
6. *Treat for shock.*
   - Cover any special population trauma patient with blankets to prevent hypothermia.
7. *Identify any other injuries and treat them appropriately.*
   - A lot of treatment can be performed en route to the receiving facility if you have a critical patient.
   - Make sure that you splint injuries appropriately.
8. *Transport immediately.*
   - Notify the receiving facility specifically what type of trauma patient you are bringing to their facility.
   - Consider the use of ALS intercept or air medical transport for these patients. Follow your local protocol.

Reassessment

Provide reassessment during transport, paying close attention to the mental status, airway, breathing, and circulation of all these patients. Repeat the vitals every 5 minutes.

CHAPTER REVIEW

SUMMARY

As an EMT, you should suspect multisystem trauma in any patient who has been subjected to a significant external force. In many traumas, more than one body system has been affected, which can affect the patient's presentation and injuries. When this occurs, the EMT must identify what life threats exist and utilize golden principles of trauma care to help manage them appropriately.

Special populations of patients, such as pregnant women, elderly patients, children, and patients with cognitive impairments, require additional assessment and management considerations when they are involved in trauma. The EMT must identify the special needs of these trauma patients and incorporate knowledge of these patients into the care provided. These populations are more susceptible to injury than others and often have worse outcomes when compared to other trauma patients. Some of the injuries sustained by special trauma patients are influenced by the anatomical and physiological changes these patients experience. It is important for the EMT to know what changes are to be expected and to use that knowledge to help anticipate and manage the injuries that these patients may have.

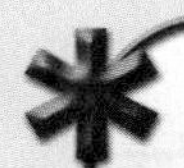

CASE STUDY FOLLOW-UP

SCENE SIZE-UP

You have been dispatched to a 30-year-old female patient who fell. As you arrive on the scene of a single-family residence, you are met by four small children screaming and crying. You look around to ensure the scene is safe, and you do not see anything that would suggest it is not. As you and your partner approach the residence with your equipment in hand, you hear a woman yell "Help me!" from inside. The children run past you into the house and lead you to the stairwell. There, you see an obviously pregnant woman lying at the base of the stairs on the floor next to a pile of laundry. You notice a couple of toys on the floor between you and your patient. You remove the toys from the stairwell and proceed to your patient who is lying supine on the floor.

PRIMARY ASSESSMENT

You immediately establish in-line spinal stabilization and ask the woman her name and what happened. She replies that she is Hope Miller and that she tripped on a toy when she was carrying the laundry downstairs to the washer. She states that she is 7 months pregnant and is now bleeding and having contractions. Her airway is open and clear. She is breathing 23 times a minute with an adequate tidal volume. Your partner places her on a nonrebreather mask with supplemental oxygen and the pulse oximeter to monitor the SpO_2. You feel her pulse and note that it is 120 beats per minute and thready. You identify that she does have some vaginal bleeding, but crowning is not present. You place a pad next to the vagina to absorb the blood flow. You suspect this patient may be in shock.

SECONDARY ASSESSMENT

Your partner performs a rapid trauma assessment and takes vital signs. Vital signs are blood pressure 100/62 mmHg, pulse 120 bpm, and respirations 23 per minute. Lungs are clear and equal bilaterally. In addition to the vaginal bleeding and contractions (which are strong and about 10 minutes apart), she has neck pain, abdominal pain and tenderness, and pain and swelling to the right side of her face. There are no signs of injury to the rest of her body.

In the meantime, you obtain a history from Mrs. Miller. It reveals that she has been pregnant five times and has four living children. She has never had any complications with her pregnancies and has been receiving prenatal care. She does not take any medications outside of prenatal vitamins, and she is allergic to penicillin.

Once the exam and history findings are recorded, you and your partner prepare the patient for rapid transport. You apply a cervical spine immobilization collar and log roll her onto a backboard. When immobilization is complete, you tilt the backboard to the left side and treat her for shock. You call the trauma center in advance so they can prepare for your patient's arrival.

With Mrs. Miller's permission, the children are left with a neighbor who has come to the home to see if she can help. Mrs. Miller is taken to the ambulance and rapidly transported to the receiving trauma facility.

REASSESSMENT

En route to the hospital, you monitor Mrs. Miller's airway, breathing, circulation, and level of responsiveness. You reassess her vitals every 5 minutes throughout the transport. You also continue to document her contractions and the number of pads that she saturates with blood.

During transport, you note no change in Mrs. Miller's condition. You apply an ice pack to her swollen right cheek. At the emergency department, she is transferred to the trauma team staff. You and your partner complete a prehospital care report and prepare the ambulance for another call.

IN REVIEW

1. List three principles associated with multisystem trauma care.
2. Describe how to manage a third-trimester pregnant patient who has been injured.
3. Identify three anatomical or physiological changes that may influence an elderly trauma patient's care.
4. List three causes of cognitive impairments.
5. Describe how a cognitive impairment may affect your assessment of a trauma patient.
6. Explain why normal vital signs may appear when pregnant women or elderly patients are in shock.
7. List three injuries that pediatric patients are more susceptible to than adults.
8. Describe how an elderly trauma patient's past medical history and medications may influence your assessment.

CRITICAL THINKING

You arrive on the scene of a nursing home and find a 93-year-old male patient who fell out of his wheelchair after he won a bingo game in the recreation area. The patient is lying prone on the cement floor with obvious bleeding from his face and mouth. The patient moans as you approach him but does not respond verbally to any of your questions. His respirations are irregular at a rate of approximately 28 per minute with minimal chest rise and fall. Your partner indicates the radial pulse is strong and the heart rate is 96 bpm. The nursing staff states he has a history of myocardial infarctions, congestive heart failure, lordosis, osteoporosis, and two strokes. They give you a medication list, tell you that he is to be transported to the local emergency department, and then leave.

1. What immediate emergency care would you provide for the patient?
2. Do you consider this patient to be a high priority? Why?
3. What additional assessment and management considerations do you have for this patient based on his age?
4. What role do you believe his past history may have on his current condition?

PEARSON

EXPLORE mybradykit™

Please go to **www.bradybooks.com** to access mykit for this text. You will find quizzes, critical thinking scenarios, weblinks, animations, and videos related to this chapter—and much more. Look for online information on pediatric and geriatric trauma.

Register your access code from the front of your book by going to **www.bradybooks.com** and selecting the mykit links.

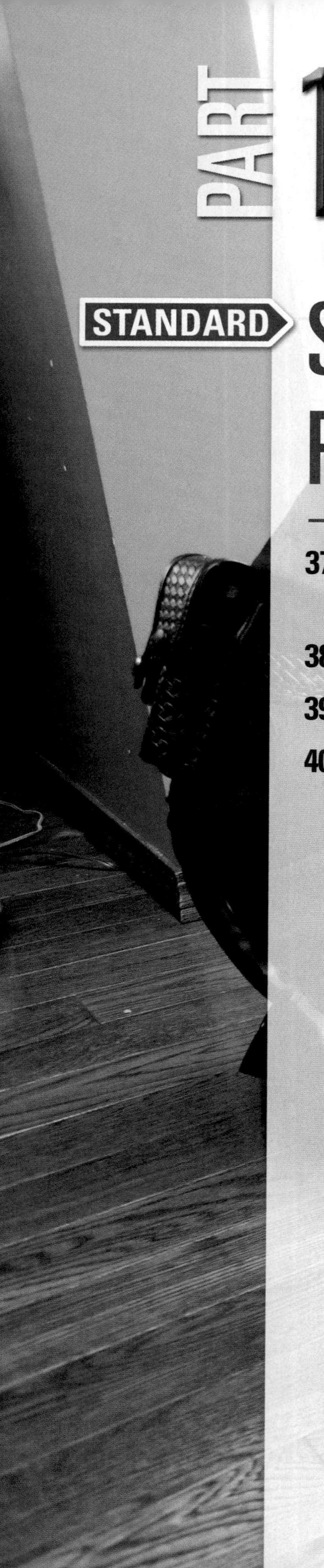

PART 11

STANDARD

Special Patient Populations

COMPETENCY

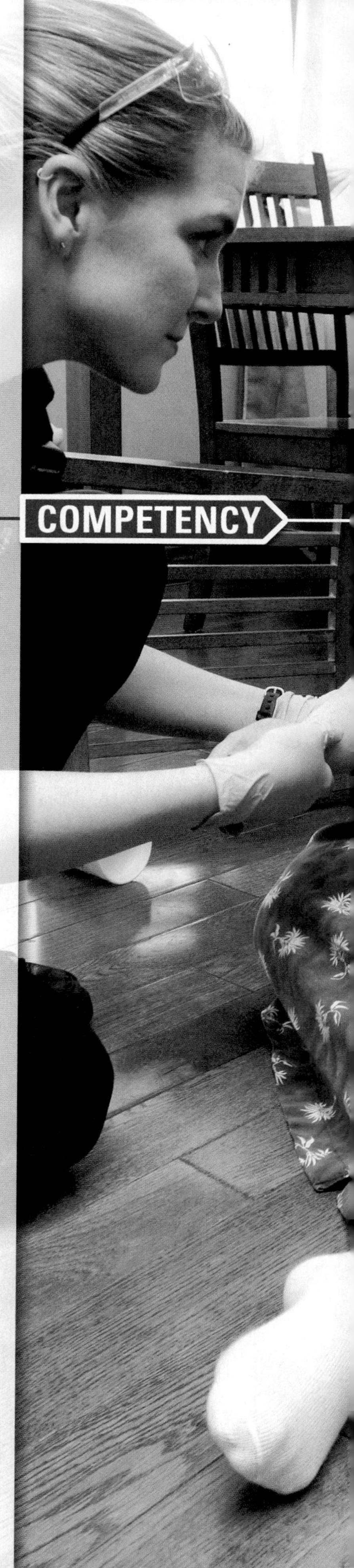

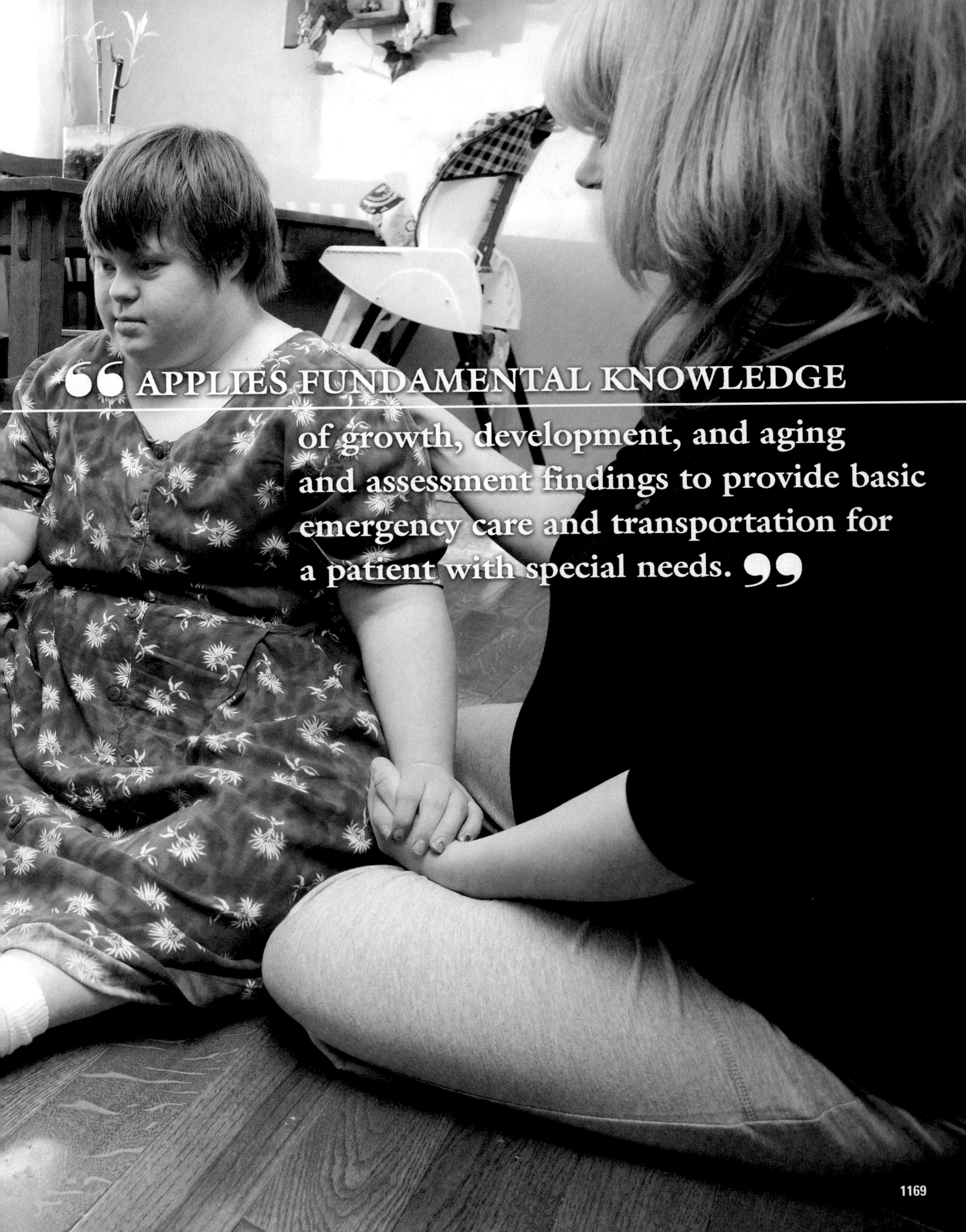

"APPLIES FUNDAMENTAL KNOWLEDGE of growth, development, and aging and assessment findings to provide basic emergency care and transportation for a patient with special needs."

CHAPTER 37 Obstetrics and Care of the Newborn

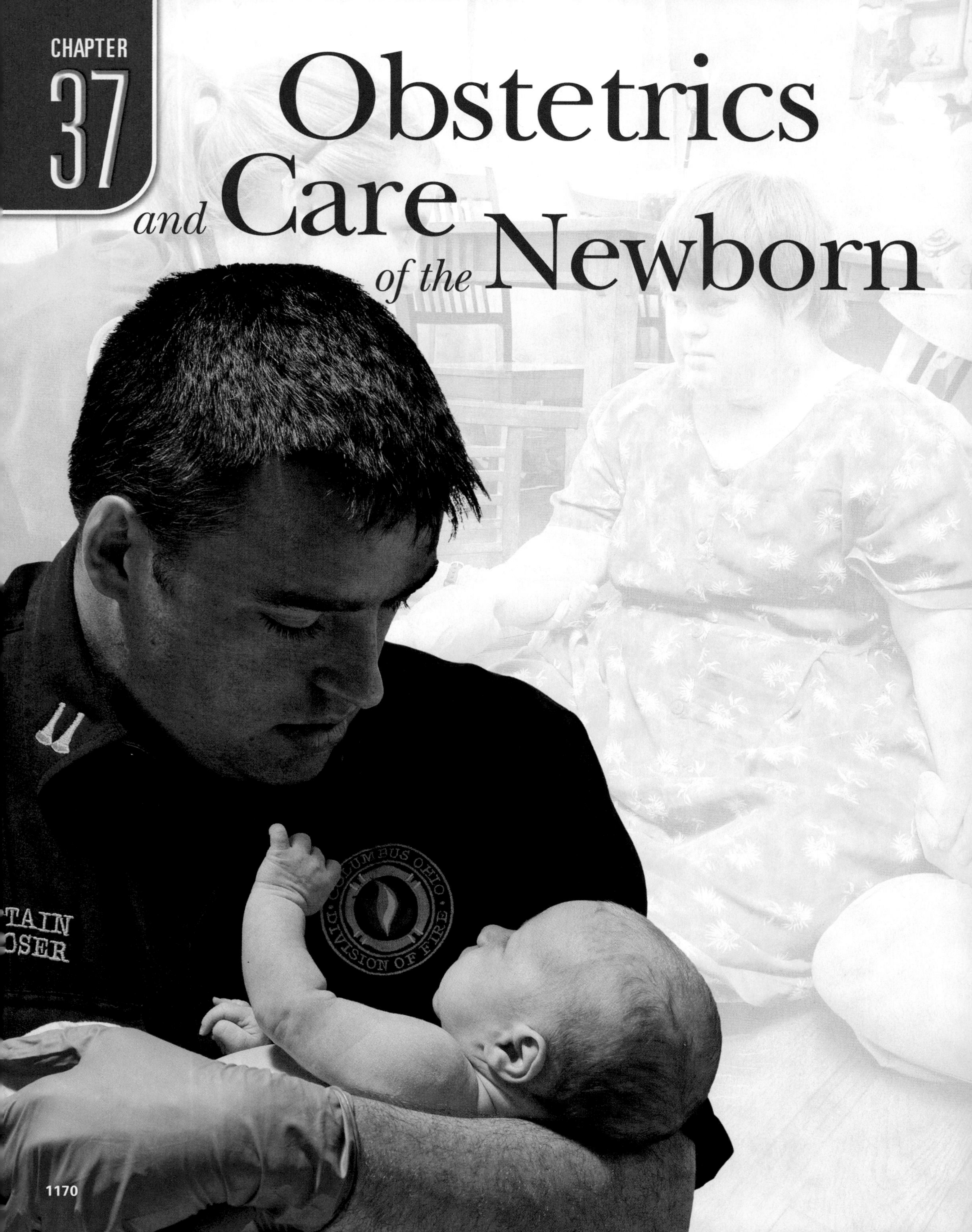

Navigation Guide

The following items provide an overview to the purpose and content of this chapter. The Standard and Competency are from the new National EMS Education Standards.

STANDARD **Special Patient Populations** (Content Area: Obstetrics; Neonatal Care)

COMPETENCY Applies fundamental knowledge of growth, development, and aging and assessment findings to provide basic emergency care and transportation for a patient with special needs.

OBJECTIVES: After reading this chapter, you should be able to:

37-1. Define key terms introduced in this chapter.

37-2. Describe the anatomy of pregnancy, the menstrual cycle, and the prenatal period.

37-3. Describe physiological changes in pregnancy, including changes to the following systems:
- **a.** Reproductive
- **b.** Respiratory
- **c.** Cardiovascular
- **d.** Gastrointestinal
- **e.** Urinary
- **f.** Musculoskeletal

37-4. Describe the pathophysiology, assessment, and emergency care of patients with antepartum emergencies, including:
- **a.** Spontaneous abortion
- **b.** Placenta previa
- **c.** Abruptio placentae
- **d.** Ruptured uterus
- **e.** Ectopic pregnancy
- **f.** Preeclampsia/eclampsia
- **g.** Pregnancy-induced hypertension
- **h.** Supine hypotensive syndrome

37-5. Describe the assessment-based approach to antepartum emergencies.

37-6. Describe the stages of labor.

37-7. Describe the assessment-based approach to a patient in active labor with normal delivery.

37-8. Describe the steps of assisting with a normal prehospital obstetric delivery.

37-9. Discuss reassessment of the postpartum patient for blood loss.

37-10. Describe the assessment-based approach to a patient in active labor with abnormal delivery.

37-11. Take steps to manage abnormal prehospital obstetric deliveries, including:
- **a.** Prolapsed umbilical cord
- **b.** Breech and limb presentations
- **c.** Multiple births
- **d.** Meconium staining
- **e.** Premature birth
- **f.** Post-term pregnancy
- **g.** Precipitous delivery
- **h.** Shoulder dystocia
- **i.** Preterm labor
- **j.** Premature rupture of membranes

37-12. Take steps to manage postpartum complications, including:
- **a.** Postpartum hemorrhage
- **b.** Embolism

37-13. Demonstrate the steps of assessing and managing the newborn, including:
- **a.** Initial care, including drying, wrapping, suctioning, and positioning
- **b.** Apgar scoring and stimulation to breathe if necessary
- **c.** Apgar scoring

37-14. Recognize signs that indicate the need for neonatal resuscitation.

37-15. Apply the concepts of the neonatal resuscitation pyramid to the care of neonates in need of resuscitative measures.

KEY TERMS: Page references indicate first major use in this chapter. For complete definitions, see the Glossary at the back of the book.

afterbirth p. 1174
amniotic sac p. 1174
antepartum p. 1176
bloody show p. 1173
breech birth p. 1193
cervix p. 1173
crowning p. 1189
fallopian tubes p. 1172
fetus p. 1173
intrapartum p. 1193
labor p. 1185
limb presentation p. 1194
meconium staining p. 1196
miscarriage p. 1176
multiple birth p. 1195
neonate p. 1189
nuchal cord p. 1191
obstetric p. 1181
ovaries p. 1172
perineum p. 1188
placenta p. 1174
postmaturity syndrome p. 1196
postpartum p. 1198
postpartum hemorrhage p. 1198
postterm pregnancy p. 1196
precipitous delivery p. 1196

continued

Navigation Guide *continued*

MEDIA RESOURCES: Please go to www.bradybooks.com to access mykit for this text. You will find quizzes, critical thinking scenarios, weblinks, animations, and videos related to this chapter—and much more. Look for online information on pregnancy, labor, and delivery.

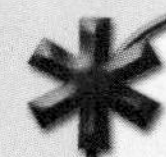

CASE STUDY

The Dispatch

EMS Unit 118—respond to Taggert's Laundromat on West Martin Street—a 30-year-old female in labor. Time out is 1926 hours.

Upon Arrival

Upon arrival, a man runs out of the laundromat and tells you, "There is some woman in there about to have a baby. Boy, is she screaming!" You and your partner proceed into the laundromat to find a female sitting on the floor in the corner, her anxious husband holding her hand. As you approach her, she says in a gasping breath, "I think the baby is coming."

How Would You Proceed?

During this chapter, you will learn how to recognize and provide emergency medical care for obstetric and gynecologic emergencies. Later, we will return to the case study and put in context some of the information you learned.

Introduction

Childbirth is a normal, natural process that is typically conducted in the hospital. However, the EMT may need to perform the delivery of a baby in the prehospital setting.

Care of patients experiencing an emergency involving the reproductive organs is not a common event. However, you must be prepared to deal with these emergencies in a professional, effective, and compassionate way. Review assessment and emergency medical care procedures for these types of emergencies as often as you can.

Anatomy and Physiology of the Obstetric Patient

Anatomy of Pregnancy

You may want to review the material on the reproductive system in Chapter 7, "Anatomy, Physiology, and Medical Terminology." A general description of the major organs and structures involved in pregnancy (Figure 37-1*) follows.

The **ovaries** are the female gonads or sex glands. There are two ovaries, one on each side of the uterus, in the upper portion of the pelvic cavity. The ovaries are responsible for secreting the hormones estrogen and progesterone and for development and release of the mature egg necessary for reproduction. The mature egg that is released from the ovary each month is referred to as the ovum. Estrogen and progesterone are hormones that prepare the uterus for implantation of a fertilized ovum and maintain the uterus during pregnancy.

The two **fallopian tubes**, also known as uterine tubes, are thin flexible structures that extend from the uterus to the ovaries. The end near the ovary is funnel shaped with fingerlike projections. This end is not directly connected to the ovary and is open to the abdominal cavity. The opposite end is connected to the uterus. Upon ovulation, the ovum is released from the ovary and received in the funnel-shaped end of the fallopian tube. Fertilization of the ovum with sperm typically occurs in the distal third of the fallopian tube. The ovum, whether fertilized or not, is transported down the fallopian tube

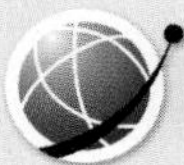

Media Resources
Go to www.bradybooks.com for mykit. Highlights:

- *Web Resource:* Pregnancy, Labor, and Delivery
- *Web Resource:* Vaginal Bleeding During Pregnancy

Objective 37-2
Describe the anatomy of pregnancy, the menstrual cycle, and the prenatal period.

Key Terms
ovaries the female gonads or sex glands.

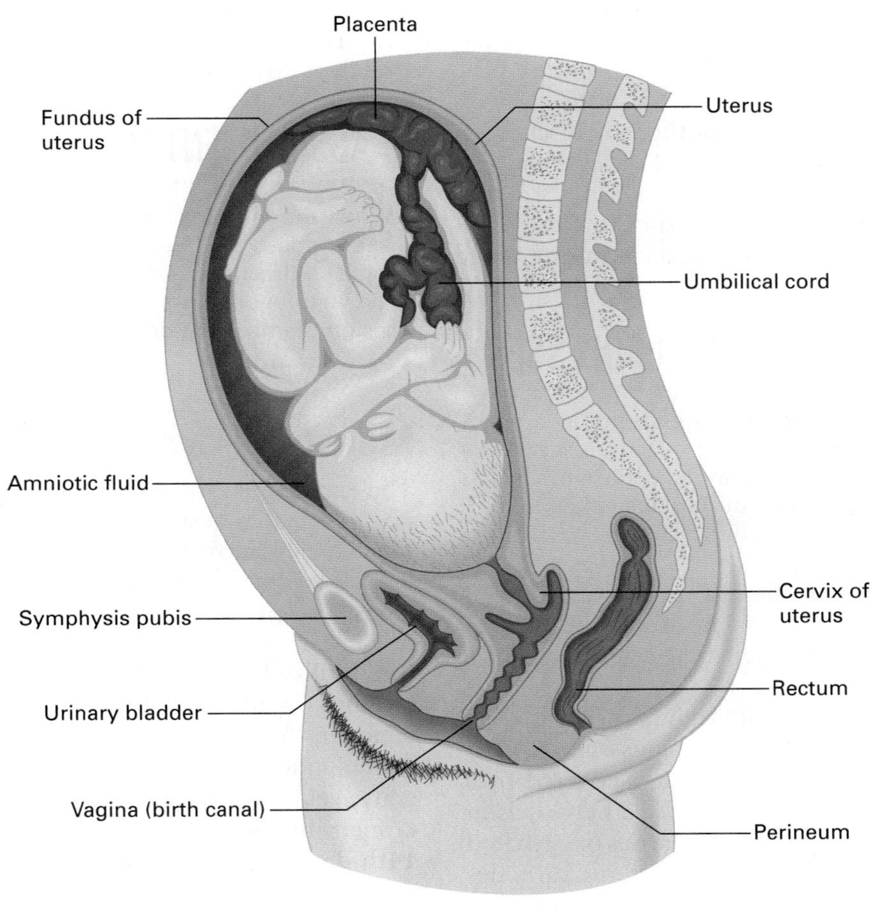

FIGURE 37-1 ✱ Anatomy of pregnancy.

by peristalsis (wavelike movement from muscular contraction) and into the uterus.

The **uterus** is the pear-shaped organ that contains the developing **fetus,** the unborn infant. Its special arrangement of smooth muscle and blood vessels allows for great expansion during pregnancy and forcible contractions during labor and delivery. The uterus also is capable of rapid contractions after delivery, which help to tone up the uterus, constrict blood vessels, and prevent hemorrhage. The top portion of the uterus is referred to as the *fundus,* the middle portion is the *body* or *corpus,* and the narrow tapered neck is the *cervix.* The uterine wall is made up of three layers: endometrium, myometrium, and perimetrium. The endometrium is the innermost lining. Each month, estrogen and progesterone build up the lining for implantation of a fertilized ovum. If the ovum is not fertilized or does not implant, the lining is shed during the menstrual period. The myometrium is the thick middle layer of smooth muscle. The smooth muscle contracts from the fundus downward during labor to expel the fetus. The perimetrium is a serous membrane that partially covers the corpus of the uterus.

The **cervix** connects with the vagina. The cervix contains a plug of mucus that seals the uterine opening, preventing contamination from entering the uterus. The plug is discharged when the cervix starts to dilate, or open, and appears as pink-tinged mucus in the vaginal discharge. The expulsion of the plug signals the first stage of labor and is known as the **bloody show.**

Key Terms

fallopian tubes thin, flexible structures that extend from the uterus to the ovaries.

uterus organ in which a child develops from fertilized egg until birth.

fetus child from the third month of pregnancy to birth; prior to that time it is called an embryo.

Key Terms

cervix the neck of the uterus.

bloody show the mucus and blood that are expelled from the vagina as labor begins.

placenta the fetal organ through which the fetus exchanges nourishment and waste products during pregnancy.

The **placenta,** also known as the "organ of pregnancy," is a disk-shaped inner lining of the uterus that begins to develop after the ovum is fertilized and attaches itself to the uterine wall. Rich in blood vessels, the placenta is the sole organ through which the fetus receives oxygen and nourishment from the mother and discharges carbon dioxide and waste products. The exchange is made between the mother's and infant's bloodstreams within the placenta; however, the blood of the fetus and the blood of the mother do not mix, except during birth or miscarriage.

Understanding BODY PROCESSES

The normal implantation site for the placenta is superior and posterior within the fundus of the uterus. An abnormal site of implantation may lead to complications later in the pregnancy and during delivery. ■

After the infant is born, the placenta separates from the uterine wall and is delivered as the **afterbirth.** It usually weighs about a pound, or generally one-sixth of the infant's weight.

The **umbilical cord** is the unborn infant's lifeline, attaching the fetus to the placenta. It contains one vein and two arteries in a spiral arrangement that is covered by a protective substance called *Wharton jelly.* The vessels in the umbilical cord are unique: the vein carries oxygenated blood and nutrients to the fetus, and the arteries carry deoxygenated blood and waste products back to the placenta. The structure of the cord—and the blood traveling through it—keep it from kinking. When the infant is born, the umbilical cord resembles a sturdy rope about 22 inches long and 1 inch in diameter.

The **amniotic sac,** sometimes referred to as the *bag of waters,* is filled with the amniotic fluid in which the infant floats, insulating and protecting it throughout the pregnancy. The amount of amniotic fluid varies from 500 to 1,000 milliliters. At the onset of labor, the sac usually tears. This "rupturing of the bag of waters" is one of the first indications to the pregnant mother that her labor is starting. The amniotic fluid helps to lubricate the birth canal and remove any bacteria. During labor, part of the amniotic sac is forced ahead of the infant, serving as a resilient wedge to help dilate the cervix.

The lower part of the birth canal is called the **vagina.** About 8 to 12 centimeters in length, the vagina originates at the cervix of the uterus and extends through to an external opening of the body. During pregnancy, the vagina undergoes changes that prepare it for passage of the infant. The smooth muscle layer of the vagina allows it to stretch gently to accommodate the infant during delivery.

ASSESSMENT Tips

When the fetus has moved down into the vagina, the head causes the vaginal walls to bulge, especially during a contraction, and the top of the head will appear at the vaginal opening. This is known as *crowning* and is a sign of imminent delivery. ■

Menstrual Cycle

The female goes through a monthly menstrual cycle that is controlled by estrogen and progesterone. The menstrual cycle lasts from 24 to 35 days with an average of 28 days. The first day of the menstrual cycle begins with menstruation. Menstruation is the sloughing of the endometrial tissue that was preparing for implantation of the fertilized ovum. Menstruation is marked by vaginal bleeding of about 60 to 80 mL over 3 to 5 days. Contained in the blood is tissue and mucus that was built up in the endometrium. Once menstruation is over, estrogen levels increase and again begin to prepare the endometrium for implantation of a fertilized ovum. On the 14th day of the cycle, ovulation occurs and the mature ovum is released from the ovary. The ovum descends through the fallopian tube within the next 5 to 7 days. If it is fertilized, it implants itself in the prepared endometrial lining of the uterus. If it is not fertilized, it is discharged with the outer layer of endometrial tissue during menstruation, which occurs 14 days after ovulation.

Prenatal Period

Ovulation is the release of the mature ovum from the ovary. The ovum is picked up by the fallopian tube and moves down toward the uterus. The fertilized egg implants in the wall of the uterus and the pregnancy begins. Approximately 3 weeks after implantation of the fertilized egg on the uterine wall, the placenta develops.

During the pregnancy, the stages of development of the baby are known by different terms. The first 14 days after conception are called the pre-embryonic stage. The embryonic stage is from day 15 to 8 weeks. The fetal

Key Terms

afterbirth the placenta and other tissues that are expelled immediately after the birth of a child.

umbilical cord an extension of the placenta through which the fetus receives nourishment.

amniotic sac membrane that forms the sac that holds the fetus suspended in amniotic fluid.

Key Terms

vagina the passageway through which the fetus is delivered. The lower part of the birth canal.

Objective 37-3

Describe physiological changes in pregnancy, including changes to specific body systems.

stage begins at 8 weeks and ends with delivery of the baby, which is termed a *neonate*. Pregnancy is also referred to as *gestation*. Gestational age refers to the age of the fetus in weeks from the time of fertilization of the ovum through delivery. As an example, you might refer to a fetus in a pregnant patient in her 36th week of pregnancy as being in the 36th week of gestation. If a physician or nurse were to ask "What is the gestational age of the fetus?" it is the same as the number of weeks of fetal growth during the pregnancy.

A full-term pregnancy lasts approximately 280 days from the first day of the last normal menstrual cycle. Each 3-month period of the approximately 9-month pregnancy is referred to as a *trimester*. Thus, months 1 through 3 (weeks 1 to 12) are the first trimester, months 4 through 6 (weeks 13 to 27) are the second trimester, and months 7 through 9 (weeks 28 to 40) are the third trimester. Most emergencies that you will deal with occur during the first or third trimester. However, a patient can experience some of these emergencies during the second trimester.

Physiological Changes in Pregnancy

Many physiological changes occur in pregnancy. Most are due to alterations in the circulating hormones, expanding of the uterus, and the increased metabolic demands on the mother. These physiological changes, grouped by body system, can be summarized as follows:

Reproductive System

- The prepregnant uterus weighs about 2 ounces and holds about 10 mL. At the end of pregnancy the uterus weighs more than 2 pounds and holds 5,000 mL.
- The pregnant uterus is extremely vascular and contains about one-sixth of the total blood volume of the mother.
- A mucous plug forms in the opening to the cervix (os) to protect the fetus from infection.
- The breasts enlarge and become more nodular in preparation for lactation (milk production).

Respiratory System

- Oxygen demand of the mother increases.
- The respiratory tract resistance decreases as a result of hormones causing smooth muscle dilation.
- The tidal volume increases by 40 percent.
- The respiratory rate increases only slightly.
- There is an increase in oxygen consumption of approximately 20 percent.

Cardiovascular System

- Cardiac output increases.
- Maternal blood volume increases by 45 percent. There is also an increase in red blood cell (RBC) content and plasma; however, the plasma volume increase is greater than the RBCs, causing a relative anemia. The pregnant patient is given iron supplements to increase oxygen binding on the RBC. This blood volume increase delays the signs and symptoms of shock in the pregnant patient, as discussed in Chapter 36, "Multisystem Trauma and Trauma in Special Patient Populations."
- The maternal heart rate increases by 10 to 15 bpm.
- Blood pressure decreases slightly during the first and second trimester and returns to normal during the third trimester.

Gastrointestinal System

- Nausea and vomiting commonly occur during the first trimester as a result of hormone changes and the change in the need for carbohydrates.
- Bloating and constipation may occur from a decrease in peristalsis in the gastrointestinal tract.

Urinary System

- Renal blood flow increases.
- Glomerular filtration increases by approximately 50 percent during the second trimester and remains elevated.
- The urinary bladder is displaced superiorly and anteriorly, increasing the risk of injury.
- An increase in urinary frequency is common in the first and third trimester due to compression of the bladder by the uterus.

Musculoskeletal System

- The pelvic joints loosen as a result of hormone changes.
- There is a change in the center of gravity for the mother caused by the heavy uterus. The patient compensates and therefore often experiences lower back pain.

Objective 37-4
Describe the pathophysiology, assessment, and emergency care of patients with specific antepartum emergencies.

Key Terms
antepartum the period of pregnancy prior to the onset of labor.

Key Terms
spontaneous abortion without apparent cause, the termination of a pregnancy before the fetus reaches the stage of viability, generally before the 20th week of pregnancy. Also called **miscarriage.**

Antepartum (Predelivery) Emergencies

Antepartum emergencies are those that occur in the pregnant patient prior to the onset of labor. These complications often involve the potential for severe hemorrhage and fetal death. The following are specific antepartum emergencies you may encounter in a pregnant patient.

Antepartum Conditions Causing Hemorrhage

Hemorrhage is one of the leading causes of death in the pregnant patient. The uterus during pregnancy is very vascular; thus, it is prone to severe bleeding if injured. Uterine bleeding may or may not be associated with vaginal bleeding, depending on the site of bleeding and the position of the fetus. If bleeding occurs behind the placenta where the margins of the placenta are intact, there will be no vaginal bleeding, even though the patient may lose a significant amount of blood and present in hypovolemic shock. If the margin of the placenta is torn away from the uterine wall, the patient will likely present with vaginal bleeding. If the uterine bleeding occurs late in pregnancy, the fetus may be engaged low in the pelvis and vaginal canal, which would block external blood flow. Vaginal bleeding may sometimes occur late in the pregnancy, with or without pain. If the bleeding is excessive, it can be a life-threatening emergency for the mother and fetus. The bleeding may be due to spontaneous abortion, placenta previa, abruptio placentae, ruptured uterus, or an ectopic pregnancy. Be especially alert to the early signs and symptoms of shock (hypoperfusion).

Spontaneous Abortion

A **spontaneous abortion,** or **miscarriage,** may occur for any number of reasons and is defined as delivery of the fetus and placenta before the fetus is viable (before it can live on its own). Viability is usually considered to begin after the 20th week of pregnancy. Approximately 80 percent of spontaneous abortions occur prior to the 12th week of gestation, which is during the first trimester of pregnancy.

Pathophysiology Spontaneous abortion occurs in 15 to 20 percent of all recognized pregnancies. The cause is usually genetic (50 percent of cases), or it may be caused by a uterine abnormality, infection, drugs, or maternal disease. Cramping and vaginal bleeding are usually present at 8 to 12 weeks of gestation.

The patient history is extremely important in spontaneous abortion. Ask the patient about uterine cramping and vaginal bleeding. Do not mistake a spontaneous abortion for a heavy period.

Assessment The signs and symptoms of a possible spontaneous abortion include:

- Cramplike lower abdominal pain similar to labor
- Moderate to severe vaginal bleeding, which may be bright or dark red
- Passage of tissue or blood clots

An elective abortion is different from a spontaneous abortion. The spontaneous abortion is a naturally occurring expulsion of the fetus that is generally related to a genetic abnormality. An elective abortion is the termination of the pregnancy upon request of the mother in a medical setting.

Understanding BODY PROCESSES

Any tissue that is retained within the uterus following a spontaneous abortion may lead to severe bleeding and infection. Transport any patient with a suspected spontaneous abortion. ■

Emergency Care In addition to the general guidelines for emergency medical care described later for antepartum emergencies, ask when the patient's last menstrual period began. Provide emotional support to the mother and the members of her family throughout treatment and transport. Intense grief over loss of the pregnancy is normal and expected in both parents.

ASSESSMENT Tips

Some patients may mistake the vaginal bleeding and abdominal cramping from a spontaneous abortion for a menstrual period. Ask the patient about other early signs of pregnancy. ■

Key Points
Vaginal bleeding sometimes occurs late in pregnancy, with or without pain. If excessive, the bleeding can be life-threatening to mother and fetus.

Key Points
Late-term vaginal bleeding may be due to spontaneous abortion, placenta previa, abruptio placentae, ruptured uterus, or ectopic pregnancy.

Placenta Previa

Placenta previa, which occurs in about 1 in 250 births, is a major cause of third-trimester bleeding.

Pathophysiology Placenta previa is associated with abnormal implantation of the placenta over or near the opening of the cervix (the os) (Figure 37-2*). The placenta is normally implanted in the fundus (top portion) of the uterus and posteriorly. When the fetus changes position in the uterus, or the cervix begins to efface (thin) and dilate, the placenta is prematurely torn away from the lower portion of the uterine wall. This results in bleeding, which can be excessive because of the rich blood supply. The bleeding is not associated with any abnormal uterine contraction or abnormal pain.

There are three types of placenta previa:

- **Total.** In a total placenta previa, the placenta completely covers the os. This blocks the birth canal and can prevent delivery of the baby. As the cervix dilates and effaces, significant bleeding may occur.
- **Partial.** In a partial placenta previa, the placenta covers the os of the cervix partially, but not completely. As with the total placenta previa, the partial placenta previa may obstruct delivery of the baby.
- **Marginal.** In a marginal placenta previa, the placenta is implanted near the neck of the cervix. When the cervix effaces and dilates, it may cause the placenta to partially tear.

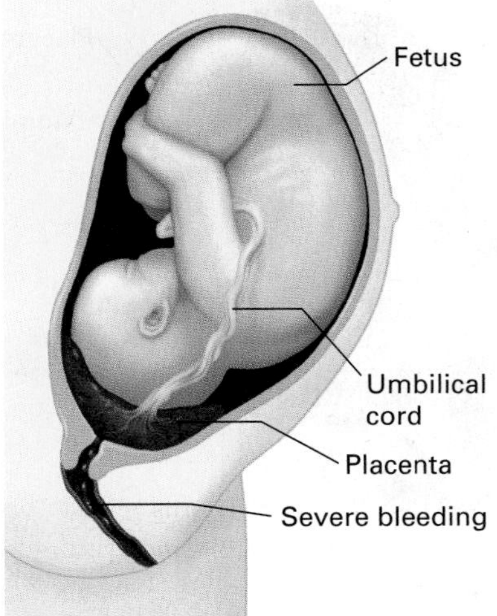

FIGURE 37-2 * Placenta previa.

Predisposing factors for a placenta previa are:

- Multiparity (more than two deliveries)
- Rapid succession of pregnancies
- Greater than 35 years of age
- Previous placenta previa
- History of early vaginal bleeding
- Bleeding immediately after intercourse

Assessment The hallmark sign of placenta previa is third-trimester vaginal bleeding that is painless. The uterus typically remains soft and nontender on palpation. It was once thought that the bleeding with placenta previa was characteristically bright red; however, it is now understood that the color of the blood does not differentiate between placenta previa and other conditions. The bleeding may be bright, dark, or an intermediate color. In addition to the vaginal bleeding, also look for signs of hypovolemic shock.

Emergency Medical Care Follow the same guidelines as for any antepartum emergency, which will be discussed later. Your major concern is blood loss for the mother and hypoxia and distress for the fetus. Administer oxygen via a nonrebreather mask at 15 lpm. Treat for shock. Transport immediately.

Abruptio Placentae

An abruptio placentae is the abnormal separation of the placenta from the uterine wall prior to birth of the baby. It occurs in approximately 1 in 120 births.

Pathophysiology Small arteries located in the lining between the placenta and uterus are prone to rupture. When they rupture and bleed, the accumulating blood begins to tear and separate the placenta from the uterine wall (Figure 37-3*). As the bleeding continues, the placenta continues to tear away from the uterine wall.

Separation of the placenta causes two major problems:

- Poor gas, nutrient, and waste exchange between the fetus and the placenta
- Severe maternal blood loss

There are two types of abruption:

- **Complete.** In a complete abruption, the placenta completely separates from the uterine wall. A complete abruptio placentae carries a 100 percent fetal mortality rate.

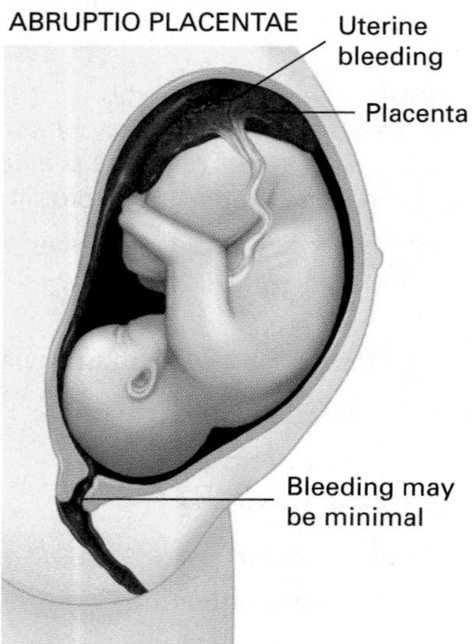

FIGURE 37-3 ✱ Abruptio placentae.

- **Partial.** In a partial abruptio placentae, the placenta is partially torn from the uterine wall. Because it remains partially attached, it is associated with a 30–60 percent, rather than a total, fetal mortality rate.

The predisposing factors for an abruptio placentae are:

- Hypertension
- Use of cocaine or other vasoactive drugs
- Preeclampsia
- Multiparity (several births)
- Previous abruption
- Smoking
- Short umbilical cord
- Premature rupture of the amniotic sac
- Diabetes mellitus

Assessment The signs and symptoms associated with an abruptio placentae are as follows:

- Vaginal bleeding is associated with constant abdominal pain (the hallmark sign).
- Abdominal pain due to muscle spasm of the uterus may be mild, sharp, or acute.
- Pain may be found in the lower back.
- Uterine contractions are usually present.
- Abdomen is tender on palpation.
- Bleeding can be dark red or bright red; however, the color of the blood does not differentiate the condition from others.
- Vaginal bleeding may be severe, minimal, or absent depending on the location of the head of the fetus.
- Signs and symptoms of hypovolemic shock are present.

If the head of the fetus is already in the birth canal, it will block the bleeding from escaping through the vaginal canal. Therefore, you may find a patient with a complete abruption, who has severe bleeding from separation of the placenta from the uterus but has no vaginal bleeding. The patient could be in severe hypovolemic shock with no external bleeding. Thus, the amount of vaginal bleeding does not directly correlate with the amount of internal bleeding the mother is experiencing. It has been reported that 2,500 mL of blood can be concealed in the uterus. Maternal blood loss and resulting hypovolemia and fetal distress and death are the problems associated with abruptio placentae.

ASSESSMENT Tips

Because the head of the fetus may be blocking a large amount of blood flow from the vaginal opening, use the clinical signs and symptoms of shock to gauge the severity of blood loss. ■

Emergency Medical Care The emergency medical care for the patient suffering from an abruptio placentae is the same as in the placenta previa. The primary treatment is to administer oxygen, treat for shock, and provide immediate transport.

Ruptured Uterus

Pathophysiology As the uterus enlarges during pregnancy, the uterine wall becomes extremely thin, especially around the cervix. This can lead to a spontaneous or traumatic rupture of the uterine wall, thereby releasing the fetus into the abdominal cavity (Figure 37-4✱). Mortality to the mother from a ruptured uterus is usually 5–20 percent; infant mortality is over 50 percent. A ruptured uterus requires immediate surgery.

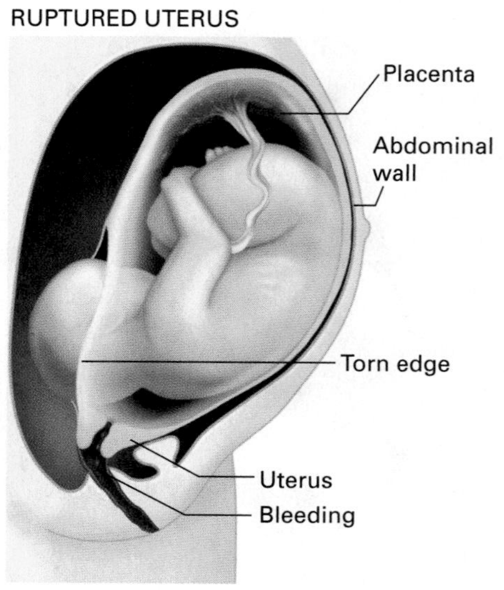

FIGURE 37-4 ✱ Ruptured uterus.

Assessment The following history and assessment findings should alert you to this emergency:

- History of previous uterine rupture
- History or findings of abdominal trauma
- History of a large fetus
- Having borne more than two children
- History of prolonged and difficult labor (which may force a large infant out through the uterine wall)
- History of prior cesarean section or uterine surgery
- A tearing or shearing sensation in the abdomen
- Constant and severe abdominal pain
- Nausea
- Signs and symptoms of shock (hypoperfusion)
- Vaginal bleeding (typically minor bleeding, but could be heavy)
- Cessation of noticeable uterine contractions
- Ability to palpate the infant in the abdominal cavity

Emergency Medical Care For treatment follow the general guidelines for emergency medical care of a predelivery emergency. Administer oxygen at 15 lpm by nonrebreather mask and provide immediate transport.

Ectopic Pregnancy

Pathophysiology In a normal pregnancy the ovum, or egg, is implanted in the uterus. In an ectopic pregnancy (Figure 37-5*), the egg is implanted outside the uterus in one of the following locations: in a fallopian tube (approximately 90 percent), on the abdominal peritoneal covering, on the outside wall of the uterus, on an ovary, or on the cervix. The placenta eventually invades surrounding tissue and, unable to accommodate the growing embryo, the tissue ultimately ruptures. Ectopic pregnancy is the third leading cause of maternal death, responsible for 6 percent of maternal mortality. Ectopic pregnancy occurs in 2 percent of all pregnancies and is most common in women 25 to 34 years of age.

The predisposing factors for an ectopic pregnancy are:

- Previous ectopic pregnancies
- Pelvic inflammatory disease (PID)
- Adhesions from surgery
- Tubal surgery, including elective tubal ligation

Assessment The following history and assessment findings should alert you to an ectopic pregnancy:

- Dull, aching-type pain that is poorly localized and becomes sudden, sharp, or "knifelike" abdominal pain, localized on one side of the lower quadrants
- Shoulder pain from blood in the abdominal cavity that irritates the diaphragm
- Vaginal bleeding that may be heavy, light, or absent
- Lower abdominal pain, possibly radiating to one or both shoulders
- Tender, bloated abdomen
- A palpable mass in the abdomen (either the embryo or a blood clot)—very rare
- Weakness or dizziness when sitting or standing
- Decreased blood pressure
- Increased pulse rate
- Signs of shock (hypoperfusion)
- Discoloration around the navel, if the rupture occurred hours earlier
- Urge to defecate

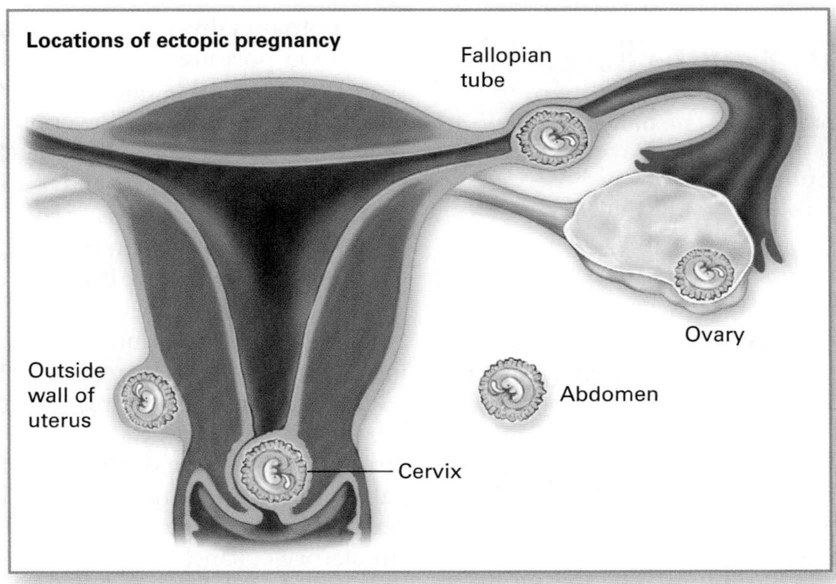

FIGURE 37-5 * Ectopic pregnancy.

Key Points
Seizures during pregnancy can be life-threatening to mother and fetus. Provide emergency care as for any seizure patient and transport the patient in as calm and quiet a manner as possible.

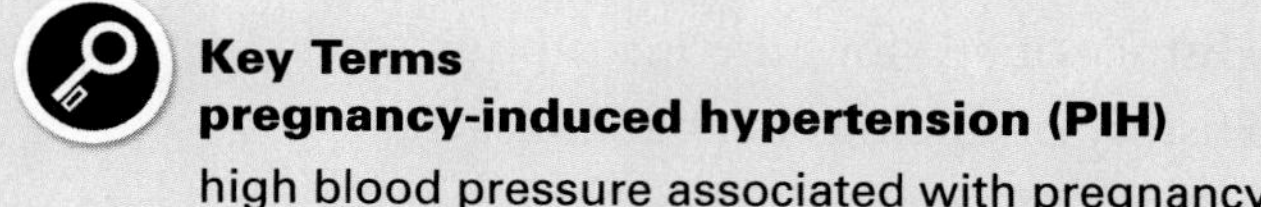

Key Terms
pregnancy-induced hypertension (PIH)
high blood pressure associated with pregnancy.

The site of implantation in the fallopian tube determines the length of time before the patient will experience pain or other associated symptoms and before rupture may occur. Rupture may occur from 2 to 12 weeks after fertilization. Most commonly, the rupture will occur in 5 to 9 weeks.

Emergency Medical Care Follow the general guidelines for emergency medical care of a predelivery emergency. Treat the patient for shock (hypoperfusion), administer oxygen at 15 lpm by nonrebreather mask, constantly reassess vital signs, and provide immediate transport.

Antepartum Seizures and Blood Pressure Disturbances

Seizures During Pregnancy

Seizures during pregnancy can be a life-threatening emergency for the mother and the fetus. Provide emergency medical care the same as for any seizure patient. It is especially important to protect the pregnant patient from injuring herself. Transport the patient on her left side. Since light, noise, and movement can set off seizures in some conditions associated with pregnancy, transport the patient in as calm and quiet a manner as possible. Seizures may be associated with eclampsia.

Understanding BODY PROCESSES

Prolonged seizures can produce a state of hypoxia (low oxygen) and hypercarbia (high carbon dioxide), affecting not only the mother but also the fetus. ■

Preeclampsia/Eclampsia

Preeclampsia, once known as toxemia during pregnancy, is a common condition, affecting about 1 in 20 pregnant women.

Pathophysiology Preeclampsia occurs most frequently in the last trimester and is most likely to affect women in their 20s who are pregnant for the first time. Women with a history of diabetes, heart disease, kidney problems, or high blood pressure are at the greatest risk, as are those whose mothers or sisters have had preeclampsia. Eclampsia is a more severe form of preeclampsia and includes coma or seizures. The exact cause of preeclampsia and eclampsia is not clearly understood. One theory is that a disorder of the placenta causes the vessels throughout the body to spasm, leading to a reduction in blood flow to organs.

Assessment Preeclampsia is characterized by high blood pressure and swelling in the extremities. History and assessment findings also include the following:

- History of hypertension, diabetes, kidney (renal) disease, liver (hepatic) disease, or heart disease
- No previous pregnancies
- History of poor nutrition
- Sudden weight gain (2 pounds a week or more)
- Altered mental status
- Abdominal pain
- Blurred vision or spots before the eyes
- Excessive swelling of the face, fingers, legs, or feet
- Decreased urine output
- Severe, persistent headache
- Persistent vomiting
- Elevated blood pressure usually greater than 140/90 mmHg or a systolic increase of over 30 mmHg and/or a diastolic increase of over 15 mmHg of prepregnancy pressure

Pregnancy-induced hypertension (PIH) is defined as a blood pressure in a pregnant woman that is greater than 140/90 mmHg on two or more occasions at 6 hours apart. If the patient has a lower blood pressure prior to the pregnancy, an increase in the systolic blood pressure of greater than 30 mmHg and a diastolic blood pressure greater than 15 mmHg is used to define the condition. When edema and protein in the urine are found with the elevated blood pressure, it is defined as preeclampsia.

Preeclampsia is characterized by high blood pressure, swelling, headaches, and visual disturbances. Eclampsia includes the signs and symptoms of preeclampsia with the addition of life-threatening seizures or coma. During a seizure, the placenta can separate from the uterine wall (abruption), causing death of the fetus and severe maternal hemorrhage. Death of the mother can also result from cerebral hemorrhage, respiratory arrest, kidney failure, or circulatory collapse.

Emergency Medical Care For treatment, follow the general guidelines for emergency medical care of a prede-

Key Terms
supine hypotensive syndrome inadequate return of venous blood to the heart, reduced cardiac output, and lowered blood pressure resulting from pressure on the inferior vena cava by the uterus and fetus when a patient in late pregnancy is supine.

Key Terms
obstetric having to do with pregnancy or childbirth.

Objective 37-5
Describe the assessment-based approach to antepartum emergencies.

ASSESSMENT Tips

The cause of preeclampsia is unknown; however, it is thought to be a result of vasospasm increasing the mother's blood pressure and decreasing blood flow to the fetus. Preeclampsia typically occurs in the last 10 weeks of pregnancy or during labor or within the first 48 hours after delivery. Eclampsia (seizure or coma) is often preceded by visual disturbances, such as seeing spots or flashing lights. Epigastric pain or right upper quadrant pain also often indicates an impending eclamptic seizure. ■

livery emergency. Administer oxygen at 15 lpm by nonrebreather mask, and keep suction close at hand. If a seizure begins, you may need to provide positive pressure ventilation during the seizure to prevent oxygen deprivation. Since light, noise, and movement can set off seizures in patients with preeclampsia, transport the patient in as calm and quiet a manner as possible.

Supine Hypotensive Syndrome

Pathophysiology **Supine hypotensive syndrome** is typically a third-trimester complication that occurs when the weight of the fetus compresses the inferior vena cava when the patient is in a supine position. This reduces the blood flow to the right atrium, which decreases the preload. The decrease in preload reduces the stroke volume and in turn reduces the cardiac output. The decrease in cardiac output reduces the systolic blood pressure and perfusion.

Assessment The patient commonly complains of dizziness or light-headedness when in a supine position. In severe cases, the patient may experience a decrease in blood pressure, tachycardia, and pale, cool, clammy skin. It is extremely important to assess the patient for blood loss.

Emergency Medical Care To avoid supine hypotensive syndrome, the patient should be placed in a sitting position, if appropriate, or lying on her left side, or supine with the right hip elevated, which takes the uterus off the vena cava. (It has traditionally been thought that it is necessary to place the patient on her left side to relieve the pressure on the vessel, since the inferior vena cava is located more on the right side of the body. However, it has been shown that placing the patient on either side is actually enough to relieve the pressure and reverse the supine hypotensive syndrome.) With the weight of the fetus removed from the inferior vena cava, there is an increased venous return to the right atrium, which increases preload, stroke volume, cardiac output, systolic blood pressure, and perfusion.

Assessment-Based Approach: Antepartum (Predelivery) Emergency

Scene Size-Up

Information provided by the dispatcher may be the first indication that the patient is experiencing a potential **obstetric** emergency (an emergency having to do with pregnancy or childbirth). However, the stress and anxiety of the emergency may prevent the patient from relaying information accurately. Your scene size-up is very important in this situation. As a general rule, any women of childbearing age (about 12 to 50 years old) could potentially be experiencing an obstetric emergency. Use a high index of suspicion when assessing such a patient.

Primary Assessment

After taking Standard Precautions and making sure the scene is safe, perform an initial assessment, including the mental status, airway, breathing, and circulation of the patient. Use the same assessment and treatment techniques as for a patient who is not pregnant.

Secondary Assessment

Use SAMPLE questions including the OPQRST mnemonic to gather a quick history. Some patients may not realize that they are pregnant and experiencing an obstetric emergency. In this case, information collected in the history should provide the best evidence that the patient may be pregnant.

Include the following questions as appropriate:

- Have you ever been pregnant before?
  - If so, how many pregnancies?
  - How many pregnancies resulted in live births?
  - Were the births vaginal or by cesarean section?
  - Any complications with any of the births?

When reporting this information to the hospital, you should use the terms *gravida* and *para*. *Gravida* refers to pregnancy. When a Roman numeral is added after gravida,

Key Points
To avoid supine hypotensive syndrome, place the pregnant patient on either side.

Key Points
Constant abdominal pain that does not subside between contractions may indicate uterine rupture.

it indicates the number of pregnancies. For example, a gravida I is a patient who is pregnant for the first time. This is also referred to as a *primigravida*. A patient who is pregnant for the third time is reported as a gravida III.

Para refers to a woman who has given birth. Para I would indicate a mother who gave birth for the first time or once to one or more children. Para III would indicate a mother who has given birth three times. If the first-time mother delivers twins, she would be gravida I, para I, because para refers to the number of delivery events and not to the number of children. A *primipara* is a mother who gave birth for the first time. Para is not used until after the birth has occurred.

- Are you experiencing any pain or discomfort?
  - What is the quality of the pain (dull, crampy, sharp, and so forth)?
  - How intense is the pain?
  - Did the pain have a sudden or a gradual onset?
  - Does the pain radiate?
  - Can you point to the pain with one finger?
  - Is the pain constant? Does it come in regular or irregular intervals?
  - What is the duration of the pain or cramps?
  - How often do the cramps occur?
  - Are you nauseated? Have you thrown up?
  - Is the pain related to a menstrual cycle or sexual intercourse?

Understanding BODY PROCESSES

A sudden onset of intense, sharp, constant abdominal pain during delivery that does not subside between contractions may be an indication that the uterus has ruptured or was torn during the labor process, which will result in severe bleeding from the uterus and hypovolemia. ■

- When was your last menstrual period?
  - Date?
  - Was the volume and color of blood normal?
  - Have there been any episodes of bleeding between menstrual periods?
  - Have your periods been regular?
- Have you missed a menstrual period?
  - Is there any chance of pregnancy?
  - Is there any breast tenderness, an increase in urination, fatigue, nausea, or vomiting? (All are early indicators of pregnancy.)
- Have you had any unusual vaginal discharge?
  - What color was it?
  - Did it have an abnormal or foul odor?
  - How much was discharged?
- When (if patient knows she is pregnant) is your due date?
  - Have you had any prenatal care?
  - How many pregnancies have you had?
  - How many children do you have?
  - Did you have any complications with previous pregnancies?

Examine the abdominal region. Look for any abnormal distention or signs of injury. Palpation can help to determine the location of the pain as well as identify if there is any abdominal guarding, tenderness, or abnormal masses. If there is abdominal pain, consider conditions related to an acute abdomen.

Also obtain a set of baseline vital signs.

Signs and Symptoms Pregnancy is a normal process that is usually event free. However, problems may occur, such as spontaneous abortion, abruptio placentae, placenta previa, preeclampsia or eclampsia, other causes of vaginal bleeding not associated with the birth, or trauma.

In general, a pregnant patient may be experiencing an *antepartum* emergency if she presents with one or more of the following:

- Abdominal pain, nausea, vomiting
- Vaginal bleeding, passage of tissue
- Weakness, dizziness
- Altered mental status
- Seizures
- Excessive swelling of the face and/or extremities
- Abdominal trauma
- Shock (hypoperfusion)
- Elevated blood pressure (hypertension)

Note: Pregnancy may mask early signs and symptoms of shock (hypoperfusion). The initial indications may be subtle or even absent. This is because a woman's blood volume is normally increased during pregnancy, which will mask a fall in blood pressure associated with shock. Also, the mother's body will shunt blood away from the fetus and redirect it back to the vital organs of the mother. So even though the mother seems well, the fetus could be in extreme distress. Any pregnant patient who is

Thinking Critically
An EMT concludes that her pregnant patient cannot be in shock because her blood pressure is normal. Is she right or wrong? Why?

Key Points
CPR started immediately or within a few minutes on a pregnant patient who has died in an accident may save the life of the infant.

currently experiencing, or experienced prior to your arrival, some type of abnormality (pain, discomfort, or bleeding) needs to be seen by a physician.

Emergency Medical Care

In general, provide the pregnant patient with the same emergency medical care you would provide to any patient with the same signs and symptoms.

However, for the pregnant patient who is in the third trimester, take precautions against supine hypotensive syndrome. If there is bleeding, the hypotension will be worsened. Watch for lower-than-expected blood pressure readings. Be alert for syncope (fainting).

Understanding BODY PROCESSES

As the cardiac output decreases during supine hypotensive syndrome, the perfusion of the brain also decreases. This produces the symptoms of lightheadedness, dizziness, or actual fainting that occur with the patient in the supine position. Typical syncope or fainting occurs with the patient in a standing or seated position (in fact, typical fainting will self-correct once the patient is supine)—in contrast to fainting from supine hypotensive syndrome. ■

General guidelines for emergency medical care of a predelivery emergency include the following:

1. **Ensure adequate airway, breathing, oxygenation, and circulation.** Administer oxygen at 15 lpm by nonrebreather mask. (Note: In general, the pregnant patient and fetus consume a greater amount of oxygen than a nonpregnant patient. Provide oxygen to any pregnant patient to help ensure fetal oxygenation, or provide positive pressure ventilation with supplemental oxygen if breathing is inadequate.)
2. **Care for bleeding from the vagina.** If there is vaginal bleeding, place a sanitary pad over the vaginal opening. Never pack the vagina in an attempt to control bleeding. Never touch the vaginal area or insert your fingers into the vagina. If the pad becomes soaked with blood, replace it. Save and transport with the patient any passed tissue or any evidence of blood loss (such as bloody sheets, towels, sanitary pads, or underwear).

ASSESSMENT Tips

Most sanitary pads hold approximately 20–30 mL of blood. Ask the patient how often she has changed the pad to gauge the severity of the bleeding. However, keep in mind that the best method to estimate the extent of blood loss is by the patient's clinical signs and symptoms. ■

3. **Treat for shock (hypoperfusion), if indicated.**
4. **Provide emergency medical care as you would for the nonpregnant patient based on any other signs and symptoms.**
5. **Transport the patient on her left side.** If she is on a backboard, tilt the board to the left.

Reassessment

Perform a reassessment en route to the hospital. Repeat the primary assessment. Repeat vital signs. Check any interventions, being especially careful about oxygen mask fit and adequate flow of oxygen. Be attentive for and treat any signs of developing shock (hypoperfusion). If the patient is stable, repeat reassessment every 15 minutes, if unstable every 5 minutes.

Note: If a pregnant patient dies in or as a result of an accident, CPR started immediately or within the first few minutes may save the life of the infant by continuing the oxygenation and circulation of the mother's blood. If you do begin CPR, it must be continued throughout transport and until you reach the medical facility where the infant may be delivered surgically. The key to saving the infant is to prevent the mother's condition from deteriorating in the field. That is, protect the airway; support breathing, oxygenation, and blood pressure; transport rapidly; and notify the receiving facility as soon as possible. Vigorous resuscitation of a mother to save a fetus is acceptable even if you believe that the mother will not be successfully resuscitated.

Summary: Assessment and Care—Antepartum (Predelivery) Emergency

To review possible assessment findings and emergency care for an antepartum obstetric emergency, see Figures 37-6∗ and 37-7∗.

Assessment Summary

ANTEPARTUM (PREDELIVERY) OBSTETRIC EMERGENCY

The following findings may be associated with an antepartum (predelivery) obstetric emergency.

SCENE SIZE-UP

Pay particular attention to your own safety. Look for:
- Mechanism of injury
- Blood in toilet or around patient
- Bleeding from the vagina
- Bloody tissue or blood clots

Primary Assessment

General Impression
- Does patient appear to be pregnant?
- Posture: lying still with knees to chest indicates severe abdominal pain, or supine
- Any evidence of seizure activity?
- Is umbilical cord or fetal body part other than the head present at vaginal opening?

Mental Status
- Alert to unresponsive based on condition and potential blood loss

Airway
- Potentially closed airway if mental status is altered

Breathing
- Increased if associated with anxiety, pain, or blood loss

Circulation
- Heart rate may be increased
- Peripheral pulses may be weak or absent associated with blood loss
- Skin may be cool, clammy, and pale

Status: Priority patient if associated with shock, significant vaginal bleeding, or abnormal presenting part

Secondary Assessment

History

Signs and symptoms:
- Abdominal pain, may be crampy
- Vaginal bleeding, may be profuse or minimal, dark or bright red
- Weakness, dizziness
- Seizure activity
- Peripheral edema
- Signs and symptoms of shock
- Fainting while lying supine (supine hypotensive syndrome)

History:
- What is the onset, provocation, quality, radiation, severity, and duration of the pain?
- When was your last menstrual period?
- Have you missed a menstrual period?
- Have you had any unusual vaginal discharge?
- When is your due date?
- Have you had previous problems with pregnancies?
- Have you been seeing a physician for this pregnancy?
- Do you get dizzy or faint while lying flat on your back? (supine hypotensive syndrome)

Physical Exam

Head, neck, and face:
- Edema to face and neck (may indicate preeclampsia)

Abdomen/genitalia:
- Large, palpable masses
- Is the abdomen/uterus rigid, soft, or tender?
- Any evidence of crowning or abnormal presenting part?
- Any passed tissue from the vagina?
- Vaginal bleeding, dark or bright red, may or may not be associated with pain

Extremities:
- Edema to hands and feet (may indicate preeclampsia)

Baseline Vital Signs
- BP: may be normal, decreased in shock, or increased in preeclampsia
- HR: may be normal or increased in shock
- RR: may be normal or increased
- Skin: may be normal or pale, cool, and clammy in shock
- Pupils: may be dilated and sluggish
- SpO_2: 95% or greater if no excessive bleeding is associated with the emergency

FIGURE 37-6a ✻ Assessment summary: predelivery obstetric emergency.

Key Terms

labor the physiological process by which the fetus is expelled from the uterus into the vagina and then to the outside of the body.

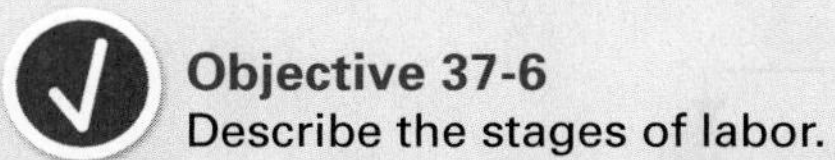

Objective 37-6
Describe the stages of labor.

Emergency Care Protocol

ANTEPARTUM (PREDELIVERY) OBSTETRIC EMERGENCY

1. Establish and maintain an open airway; insert a nasopharyngeal or oropharyngeal airway if the patient is unresponsive and has no gag or cough reflex.
2. Suction secretions as necessary.
3. If breathing is inadequate, provide positive pressure ventilation with supplemental oxygen at a rate of 10–12 ventilations/minute.
4. If breathing is adequate, administer oxygen by nonrebreather mask at 15 lpm to maximize oxygenation of the fetus, regardless of the maternal SpO_2 reading.
5. If the patient is pregnant, check for crowning or an abnormal presenting part. If crowning is present, go to the protocol on "Active Labor and Delivery." If an abnormal presenting part is found, such as a prolapsed cord, hand, or foot, perform the following:
   a. Position patient in knee-chest position or elevate buttocks using pillows.
   b. If umbilical cord is prolapsed, insert gloved hand into vagina and push presenting part of fetus away from cord.
   c. Cover presenting part with a sterile moist dressing.
   d. Rapidly transport patient and notify receiving facility of patient's condition.
6. If vaginal bleeding is present, place a sanitary napkin over the vaginal opening. Do not insert anything into or pack the vagina.
7. Position the patient on her left side to prevent or manage supine hypotensive syndrome. If the patient is immobilized on a backboard, tilt the right side of the board to the left.
8. Transport.
9. Perform a reassessment every 5 minutes if unstable, every 15 minutes if stable.

FIGURE 37-6b * Emergency care protocol: predelivery obstetric emergency.

Labor and Normal Delivery

Labor

Labor is the term used to describe the process of birth. It consists of contractions of the uterine wall, which expel the fetus and the placenta out of the uterus and vagina. Normal labor can be divided into three stages—*dilation, expulsion,* and *placental* (Figure 37-8*). The length of each stage varies in different women and under different circumstances.

Toward the end of a full-term pregnancy, in the third trimester, the fetus moves into a head-down position. When the head descends through the broad upper inlet of the mother's pelvis, the uterus moves downward and forward. Mothers can feel the difference and say that the infant has "dropped." This position is the one most common for the infant's passage through the cervix to the vagina.

First Stage: Dilation

The first stage of labor is from the beginning of true labor (contractions) to complete cervical dilation. During this first and longest stage, the cervix becomes fully dilated at 10 cm, which allows the infant's head to progress from the body of the uterus to the birth canal. Through uterine contractions, the cervix gradually dilates (stretches) and effaces (thins) until the opening is large enough to allow the infant to pass through.

The contractions usually begin as an aching sensation in the small of the back. Within a short time, the contractions become cramplike pains in the lower abdomen. These recur at regular intervals, each one lasting about 30 to 60 seconds. At first, the contractions occur about 10 to 20 minutes apart and are not very severe. They may even stop completely for a while and then start again. Appearance of the plug of mucus (the bloody show) may occur before or during this stage of labor. Also before or during this stage, the amniotic sac may rupture, resulting in a brief flow of fluid from the vagina.

Stage one may continue for as long as 18 hours or more for a woman having her first child. Most typical for the first-time mother is 8–10 hours for this first stage of labor. Women who have had a child before may experience only 5–7 hours of first-stage labor. The dilation stage ends when contractions are at regular 3- to 4-minute intervals, last at least 60 seconds each, and feel very intense.

Emergency Care Algorithm: Antepartum (Predelivery) Obstetric Emergency

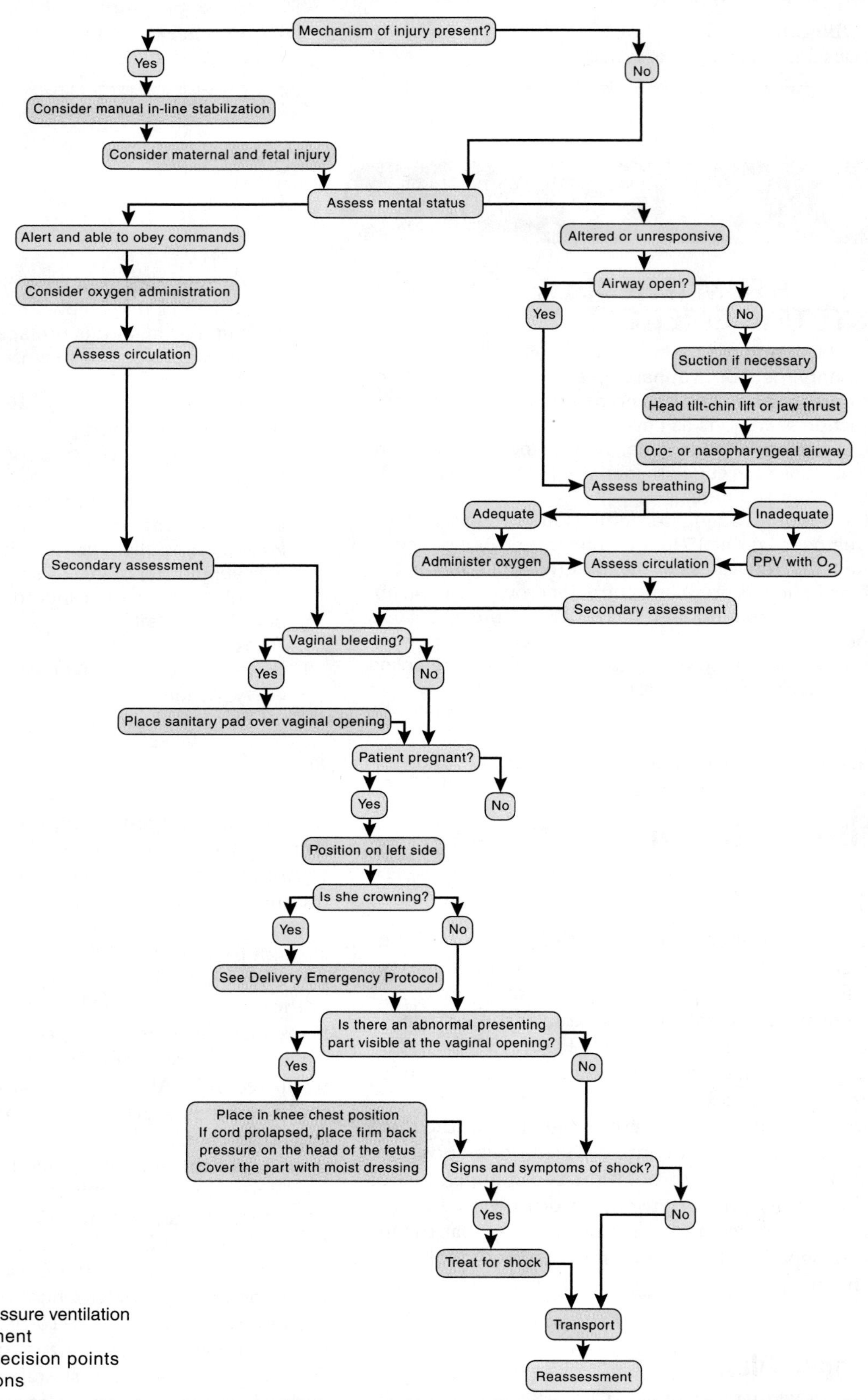

PPV = positive pressure ventilation
Yellow = assessment
Lavender = key decision points
Blue = interventions

FIGURE 37-7 ✱ Emergency care algorithm: antepartum (predelivery) obstetric emergency.

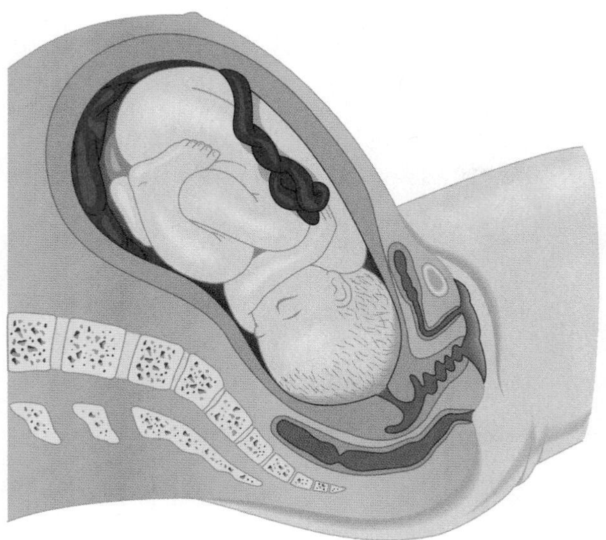
FIRST STAGE:
First uterine contraction to dilation of cervix

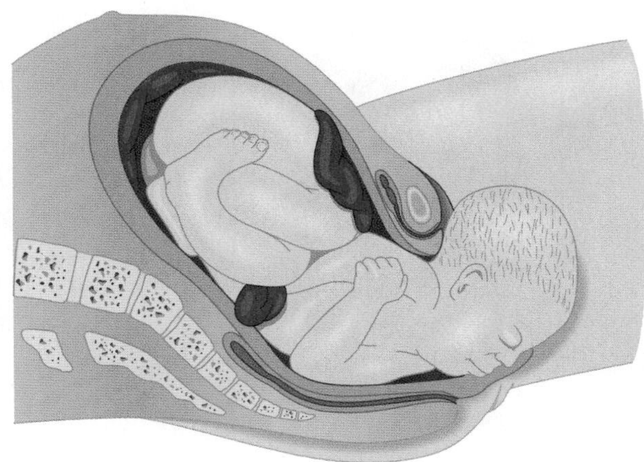
SECOND STAGE:
Birth of baby or expulsion

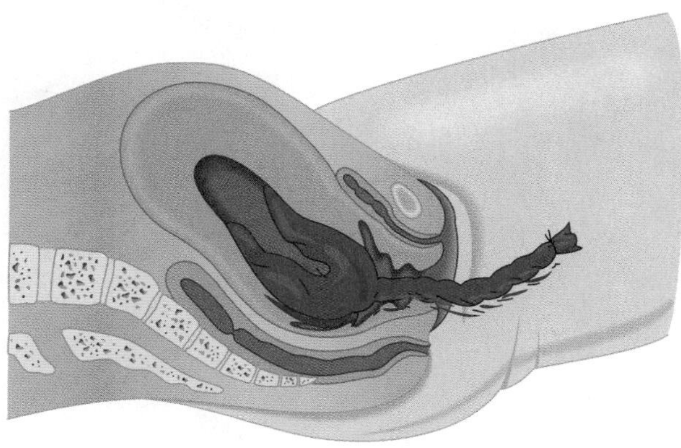
THIRD STAGE:
Delivery of placenta

FIGURE 37-8 ✱ Stages of labor.

Braxton-Hicks Contractions Braxton-Hicks contractions, often referred to as false labor, are painless, short-duration, irregular contractions that may occur as early as the 13th week of gestation. These contractions are thought to be a conditioning process for the uterus in preparation for the actual labor. It is also thought that Braxton-Hicks contractions improve placental blood flow. There is no cervical dilation or effacement with the contractions. Prior to true labor, the Braxton-Hicks contractions may become more frequent and intense; however, they typically remain irregular. There is no way to absolutely differentiate Braxton-Hicks from true labor in the prehospital setting; thus, any patient with contractions should be transported.

ASSESSMENT Tips

Contractions that follow a pattern of greater intensity, longer duration, and a shortening interval between them indicate true labor. ■

Second Stage: Expulsion

The second stage of labor begins with complete cervical dilation and ends with the delivery of the baby. During this stage, the infant moves through the vagina (the birth canal) and is born (Figure 37-9✱). Contractions are closer together—2 to 3 minutes apart—and last longer—60 to 90 seconds each. As the infant moves downward, the mother experiences considerable pressure in her rectum, much like the feeling of a bowel movement. When the mother has this sensation, it is usually an indication that delivery is imminent. The mother often complains of the feeling that she needs to defecate.

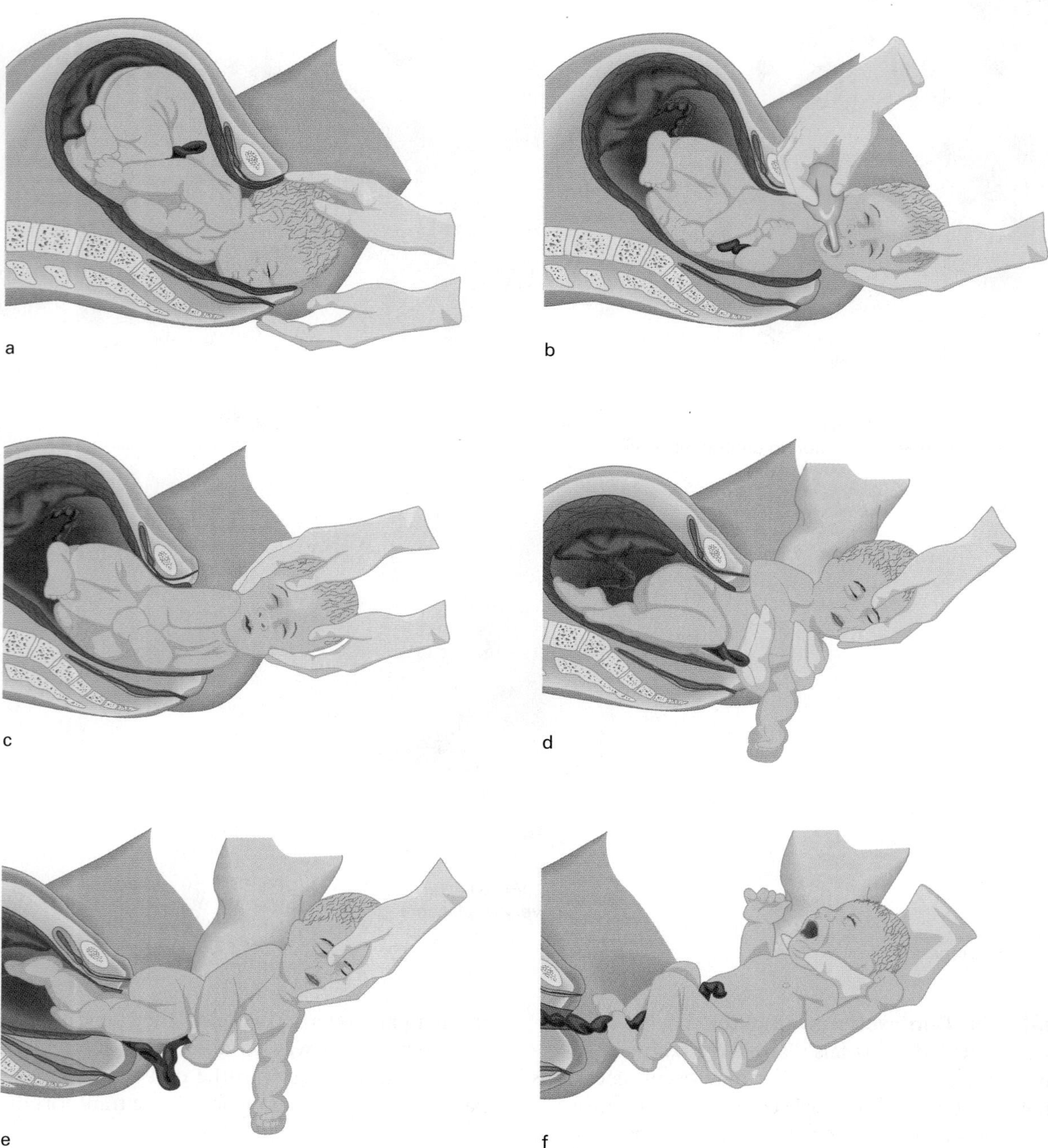

FIGURE 37-9 ✱ **(a)** The fetus moves down through the birth canal. **(b)** Suction the nose and mouth immediately upon delivery of the head. **(c)** Support the head to prevent an explosive delivery. **(d)** Deliver each shoulder. **(e)** Support the infant with both hands. **(f)** Keep the infant at or above the level of the vagina until the umbilical cord is cut.

ASSESSMENT Tips

The feeling of the urge to defecate during labor is a result of the pressure being placed on the rectum. This is another sign of imminent delivery. ■

The tightening and bearing-down sensations will become stronger and more frequent. The mother will have an uncontrollable urge to push down, which she may do. The mother may experience low back pain. There probably will be more bloody discharge from the vagina at this point. The **perineum,** the area of skin between the vagina and the anus, bulges significantly—a sign of impending birth.

Key Terms

perineum the area of skin between a female's vagina and anus.

crowning the stage in delivery when the fetal head presents at the vagina.

Objective 37-7

Describe the assessment-based approach to a patient in active labor with normal delivery.

Key Terms

neonate an infant from birth to discharge from the hospital.

Understanding BODY PROCESSES

The perineum is primarily skin, muscle, and other soft tissue that may be traumatically torn during a field delivery. ■

Soon after, the infant's head appears at the opening of the birth canal. This is called **crowning.** At this point, the mother should be coached to push with each contraction. The shoulders and the rest of the infant's body follow. For the patient in whom this is the first delivery, the second stage typically will last 50–60 minutes. In the patient who has delivered more than two children, the second stage may last only 20–30 minutes.

ASSESSMENT Tips

The top of the head is the presenting part in a normal delivery, called a *cephalic delivery.* The face will be positioned downward. ■

Third Stage: Placental

The third stage of labor begins following the delivery of the baby and ends with the expulsion of the placenta. During this stage, the placenta separates from the uterine wall and is expelled from the uterus. The placenta is usually delivered 5–20 minutes following the birth of the baby. The mother will continue to have contractions, even though not as severe, until the placenta is expelled. The signs that the delivery of the placenta is imminent are (1) there is a sudden increase in bleeding from the vagina, (2) the uterus becomes smaller in size, (3) the umbilical cord begins to lengthen, and (4) the mother has an urge to push. Never tug or pull on the umbilical cord in an attempt to facilitate delivery of the placenta.

Understanding BODY PROCESSES

Pulling or tugging on the umbilical cord in an attempt to deliver the placenta may cause the uterus to invert. If inverted, the uterus will not be able to contract and tone up effectively. This will lead to serious hemorrhage. ■

Assessment-Based Approach: Active Labor and Normal Delivery

Scene Size-Up, Primary Assessment, and Secondary Assessment

For a woman in labor or having a normal delivery, the scene size-up, primary assessment, and secondary assessment are essentially the same as you would provide in an antepartum (predelivery) emergency, as just described. If you determine that the patient is in active labor (review the stages of labor described earlier in the chapter), your assessment and treatment goals will focus on assisting the mother with delivery and providing initial care to the **neonate** (the newborn infant).

As a general rule, it is best to transport a mother in labor so that the delivery can take place at a hospital. However, if delivery is imminent, you will need to prepare to assist in the delivery at the scene. In order to determine if you should transport or commit to a delivery on scene, answer the following questions:

- How many times has the patient been pregnant?
- Is this the patient's first delivery? If not, how many deliveries has she experienced?
- How long has the patient been pregnant?
- Has there been any bleeding or discharge (bloody show or amniotic fluid)?
- Are there any contractions or pain present?
- What is the frequency and duration of contractions?
- Is crowning occurring with contractions?
- Does the patient feel the need to push?
- Does the patient feel as if she is having a bowel movement with increasing pressure in the vaginal area?
- Is the abdomen (uterus) hard upon palpation?

Note: There are three cases in which you must assist in the delivery of the infant: if you have no suitable transportation; if the hospital or physician cannot be reached due to bad weather, a natural disaster, or some other kind of catastrophe; or if delivery is imminent. The answers to the preceding questions can help you determine if delivery is about to happen. Also see the following signs and symptoms for indications that delivery is imminent.

Thinking Critically

Your pregnant patient is experiencing intense contractions 2 minutes apart. Should you transport her to the hospital for delivery, or should you prepare to deliver the infant at the scene? What is the basis for your decision?

Objective 37-8

Describe the steps of assisting with a normal prehospital obstetric delivery.

Signs and Symptoms Delivery can probably be expected within a few minutes, if the following signs and symptoms are present:

- Crowning has occurred.
- Contractions are 2 minutes apart or closer, and they are intense and last from 60 to 90 seconds.
- The patient feels the infant's head moving down the birth canal (sensation of the urge to defecate).
- The patient has a strong urge to push.
- The patient's abdomen is very hard.

If birth is imminent with crowning, contact medical direction for a decision to commit to delivery on site. If delivery does not occur within 10 minutes, contact medical direction for permission to transport. If you determine that you must assist in the delivery of the infant, remember:

- Take all appropriate Standard Precautions, including gloves, gown, and eye protection.
- Do not touch the patient's vaginal area, except during delivery and in the presence of your partner.
- Do not allow the patient to use the bathroom. If the patient does move her bowels or urinate, replace soiled linens with clean ones.
- Do not hold the mother's legs together. Do not do anything to attempt to delay or restrain the delivery, unless it is an abnormal delivery, which is discussed in a later section.
- Use a sterile obstetrics (OB) kit. Recommended equipment includes (Figure 37-10*):
  - Surgical scissors or scalpel (for cutting the umbilical cord)
  - Cord clamps or cord ties
  - Umbilical tape or sterilized cord
  - Bulb syringe
  - Towels, five or more
  - Gauze sponges, 2 × 10
  - Sterile gloves
  - One infant blanket
  - Individually wrapped sanitary napkins, three or more
  - Large plastic bag, at least one
  - Germicidal wipes

If you are to assist the mother in delivery, stay calm and explain to her that you are trained to help. As much as possible, ensure the mother's comfort, modesty, and peace of mind. Try to limit distractions and onlookers. Most importantly, recognize your own limitations. If you get into a situation you cannot handle, call medical direction for help and permission to transport.

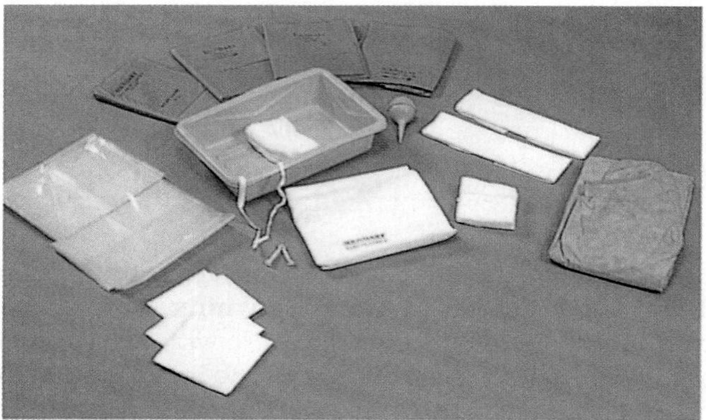

FIGURE 37-10 * Disposable obstetrics (OB) kit.

Emergency Medical Care

Take all appropriate Standard Precautions. Wear protective gloves, gown, and eye protection. The amount of blood and body fluid exposure during delivery is usually significant. Handle blood- and fluid-soaked dressings, pads, and linens carefully, and bag them in moisture-proof bags to prevent leakage. Seal and label the bags.

Emergency medical care of the patient in active labor for a normal delivery (EMT Skills 37-1) is as follows:

1. **Position the patient.** Have the patient lie on a firm surface with her knees drawn up and spread apart. Elevate the patient's buttocks several inches with a folded blanket, sheet, towels, or other clean objects. The patient's feet should be flat on the surface beneath her, which will help her brace herself. She should be several feet in from the edge of the surface to help provide extra support for the slippery infant as it is born. Support the mother's head, neck, and shoulders with pillows or folded blankets so she does not feel like she is slipping "downhill."
2. **Create a sterile field around the vaginal opening if time permits.** Use sheets from the OB kit, sterile towels, or paper barriers. Remove the patient's clothing or push it up above her waist. Place one sheet under the woman's hips, unfolding it toward her feet, and another sheet over her abdomen and legs. Place your OB kit or equipment close enough

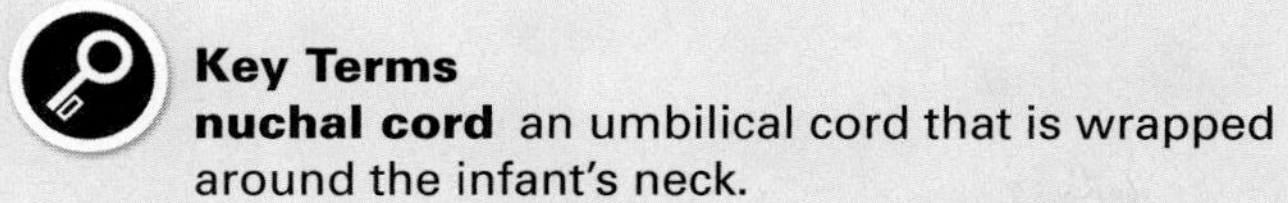
Key Terms
nuchal cord an umbilical cord that is wrapped around the infant's neck.

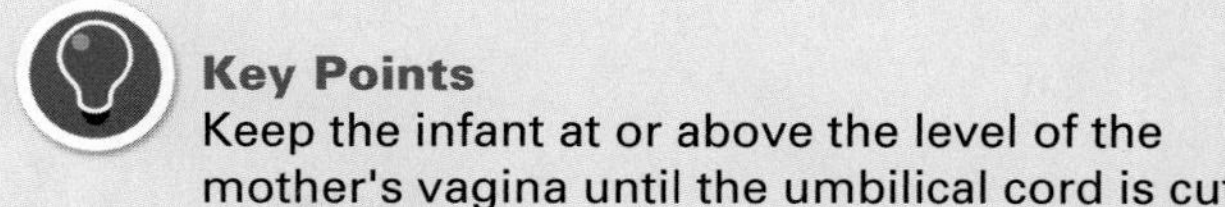
Key Points
Keep the infant at or above the level of the mother's vagina until the umbilical cord is cut.

to reach, but away from the birth canal so it will not be contaminated by the vaginal discharge, blood, and amniotic fluid.

3. **Monitor the patient for vomiting.** Have your partner or a close family member stay at the patient's head. If she vomits, this person can be ready to turn her head to one side and clean out her mouth manually or with suction.
4. **Continually assess for crowning.** The vaginal wall and perineum will bulge with each contraction. The top of the head will appear at the vaginal opening.

ASSESSMENT Tips

If crowning is occurring, then the head suddenly disappears, and the mother begins to complain of sharp, intense, constant abdominal pain, suspect a possible uterine rupture. If the uterus ruptures during delivery, the fetus might be expelled into the abdominal cavity. ■

5. **Place your gloved fingers on the bony part of the infant's skull when it crowns.** Exert very gentle pressure to prevent an explosive delivery. Avoid touching and exerting pressure on the infant's face and on any soft spot (fontanelle) on the head. With a sterile dressing, exert gentle pressure horizontally across the perineum to reduce the risk of traumatic tears.
6. **Tear the amniotic sac if it is not already ruptured.** Use your fingers to rupture the sac, and then push it away from the infant's head and face as they appear.
7. **Determine the position of the umbilical cord.** As the infant's head is delivered, determine if the umbilical cord is around the infant's neck. If so, this is referred to as a **nuchal cord**. A nuchal cord must be managed immediately as it is found. Use two fingers to slip the cord over the infant's shoulder. If you cannot move the cord, place two clamps 2–3 inches apart and cut between the clamps. Remove the cord from around the neck.
8. **Suction fluids from the infant's airway.** As soon as the head is delivered, support it with one hand and first suction the mouth and then the nostrils two or three times each with a bulb syringe, or until clear of fluid and secretions. Suction the mouth first to avoid stimulating aspiration of any fluid still in the mouth or pharynx. Make sure you compress the bulb syringe before you bring it to the infant's face. Insert the tip of the compressed bulb 1–1.5 inches into the infant's mouth, slowly releasing the bulb to allow mucus and fluids to be drawn into the syringe. Avoid touching the back of the mouth. Remove the syringe, then discharge the contents onto a towel, and repeat. Use the same procedure to suction each nostril. Note any dark greenish substance (meconium) in the amniotic fluid or on the baby or in the airway.
9. **As the torso and full body are expelled, support the newborn with both hands.** Never pull the infant from the vagina. The newborn will be slippery with a whitish, cheeselike substance (vernix caseosa) over its body. However, do not put your fingers in the infant's armpit; pressure there can damage nerve centers. Receive the newborn in a clean or sterile towel to help you hold it safely.
10. **Grasp the feet as they are born.** Do not pull on the umbilical cord as you lift or receive the infant.
11. **Clean the newborn's mouth and nose.** Wipe blood and mucus from the infant's mouth and nose with sterile gauze. Then suction the mouth and nose again. The infant will probably cry almost immediately, if not already doing so.
12. **Dry, wrap, warm, and position the infant.** Dry the infant with towels. Remove the wet towels well away from the infant's body to avoid inadvertent cooling. Place the infant in a warm, dry blanket and on its back or side with the neck in a neutral or slightly extended position. A towel could be placed under the small of the back of the mother to warm the area during the delivery. Once the neonate is delivered and dried, remove the towel from under the mother and wrap it around the infant to provide warmth and insulation. Keep the infant at or above the level of the mother's vagina until the umbilical cord is cut.
13. **Assign your partner to monitor and complete initial care of the newborn.** You should complete emergency medical care of the mother.
14. **Clamp, tie, and cut the umbilical cord as pulsations cease (Figure 37-11*).** Place two clamps or ties on the cord about 3 inches apart. The first clamp should be approximately four finger widths (6 inches) from the infant's abdomen. Use sterile surgical scissors or a scalpel to cut the cord between the two clamps. Periodically check the end of the cord for bleeding, and

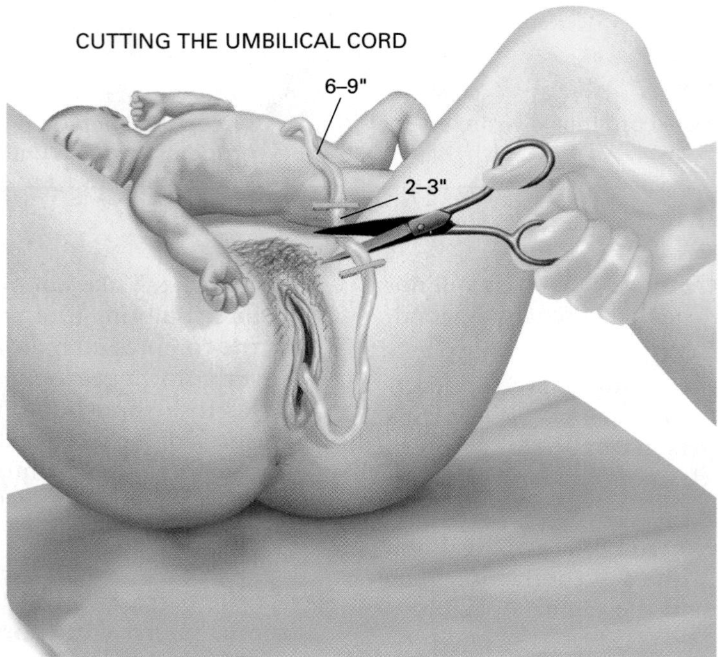

FIGURE 37-11 * Cutting the umbilical cord.

control any that may occur by placing another clamp or tie proximal to the one you have already placed on the cord.

15. **Observe for delivery of the placenta.** While preparing the mother and infant for transport, continue to watch for delivery of the placenta. It usually is delivered within 10 minutes of the infant, and almost always within 20 minutes. When the placenta appears at the vagina, grasp it gently. Never pull. Instead, slowly and gently guide the placenta and the attached membranes from the vagina. Do not delay transport while waiting for the delivery of the placenta.

Understanding BODY PROCESSES

A piece of placenta that is retained within the uterus may cause the mother to continue to bleed. ■

16. **Transport the delivered placenta.** When the placenta has completely delivered, place it in the plastic bag contained within the OB kit for transport to the hospital. A physician will examine it to confirm that delivery was complete. Be sure to turn off the air conditioning in the back of the ambulance so you don't cause the infant to become hypothermic during transport.
17. **Place one or two sanitary pads over the vaginal opening.** When covering the vaginal opening, inspect the perineum (the area between the vaginal opening and the anus). This area is frequently torn during the delivery. If it is bleeding, apply sterile dressings and direct pressure to control the bleeding. Then lower the patient's legs and help her hold them together. Elevate her feet if necessary.
18. **Record the time of delivery and transport the mother, infant, and placenta to the hospital.** Keep mother and infant warm. Transport gently.

Note that there will be vaginal bleeding after delivery. Up to 500 mL of blood loss is normal and well tolerated by the mother. However, if blood loss appears to be excessive, provide oxygen to the mother and massage the uterus as follows. Massage helps to stimulate contractions, which decrease the uterine size and help to stop bleeding.

1. **Place the medial edge of one hand (fingers extended) horizontally across the abdomen, just above the symphysis pubis.** This will help prevent the uterus from prolapsing with the massage.
2. **Cup your other hand around the uterus.** Use a kneading or circular motion to massage the area. It should feel like a hard grapefruit.
3. **Allow the infant to suckle on the mother's breast.** This will release oxytocin, a naturally occurring hormone that causes the uterus to contract.

Understanding BODY PROCESSES

Oxytocin is a naturally occurring hormone that is released from the posterior pituitary gland. It causes the smooth muscle of the uterus to contract and tone up. Toning the uterine muscle will cause the vessels to constrict, and the bleeding will cease. ■

Objective 37-9
Discuss reassessment of the postpartum patient for blood loss.

Objectives 37-10 and 37-11
Describe the assessment- based approach to a patient in active labor with abnormal delivery and the management of specific abnormal deliveries.

Key Terms

intrapartum the period of time from the onset of labor to delivery of the infant.

prolapsed cord when the umbilical cord, rather than the head of the fetus, is the first part to protrude from the vagina.

4. **If bleeding continues to appear to be excessive, check your massage technique, continue massage, and transport immediately.**

Reassessment

During the reassessment, regardless of the estimated amount of blood loss after delivery, if the mother appears to be suffering shock (hypoperfusion), treat and transport immediately. You can initiate uterine massage during transport.

Abnormal Delivery

Assessment-Based Approach: Active Labor with Abnormal Delivery

Scene Size-Up, Primary Assessment, and Secondary Assessment

Just as you would perform a scene size-up, primary assessment, and secondary assessment on a patient having a normal delivery, so would you assess a patient who is experiencing a delivery emergency.

Signs and Symptoms In general, you can recognize an abnormal delivery emergency by observing one or more of the following signs or symptoms:

- Any fetal presentation other than the normal crowning of the fetus head
- Abnormal color or smell of the amniotic fluid
- Labor before 38 weeks of pregnancy
- Recurrence of contractions after the first infant is born (indicating multiple births)

Emergency Medical Care and Reassessment

In general, emergency medical care of the mother and newborn is similar to that of a normal delivery. Exceptions are outlined as follows and include an emphasis on immediate transport, administration of high-concentration oxygen, and continuous monitoring of vital signs during the reassessment.

Intrapartum Emergencies

An **intrapartum** emergency is one that occurs during the period from the onset of labor to the actual delivery of the neonate. There are several conditions that may lead to an abnormal delivery. In almost all of these conditions, delivery is not possible. A continued attempt at delivery puts the pregnant patient and fetus at great risk for injury or even death. Thus, immediate transport is a key in the emergency care of abnormal delivery emergencies.

Prolapsed Cord

After the amniotic sac ruptures, the umbilical cord, rather than the head, may be the first part presenting at the vaginal opening. This is called a **prolapsed cord** (Figure 37-12∗). In this situation the umbilical cord may get compressed against the walls of the vagina and the bony pelvis by the pressure of the infant's head or buttocks. As a result the infant's supply of oxygenated blood can be cut off. This is a true emergency. Predisposing factors include prematurity, multiple births, and premature rupture of the amniotic sac.

For a prolapsed cord, follow these guidelines:

1. Instruct the patient **NOT** to push to avoid additional compression of the umbilical cord. During the contractions, instruct the patient to "pant like a dog" to prevent her from contracting her abdominal muscles and pushing. It is important that you coach the patient during the contractions because her natural urge is to push.
2. Position the patient on the stretcher in a "knee-chest" position (kneeling and bent forward, face down, head down, chest to knees) with the stretcher in a Trendelenburg position if possible.
3. Insert a sterile, gloved hand into the vagina, and gently push the presenting part of the fetus, head or buttocks, up, back, or away from the pulsating cord. (Note: This is the one time it is permissible to insert your hands into the mother's vagina.) Do *not* try to push the cord back into the vagina. *Follow local protocol and seek medical direction.*
4. Cover the umbilical cord with a sterile dressing moistened with a sterile saline solution.
5. Transport the patient rapidly while maintaining pressure on the head or buttocks to keep pressure off the cord, and monitor pulsations in the cord. (Pulsations should be present.)

Breech Birth

A **breech birth** presentation is one in which the fetal buttocks or lower extremities are low in the uterus and are the first to be delivered (Figure 37-13∗). Delivery may be

Key Terms
breech birth a common abnormality of delivery in which the fetal buttocks or lower extremities are low in the uterus and are the first to be delivered.

Key Terms
limb presentation when an arm or leg is the first fetal part to protrude from the vaginal opening.

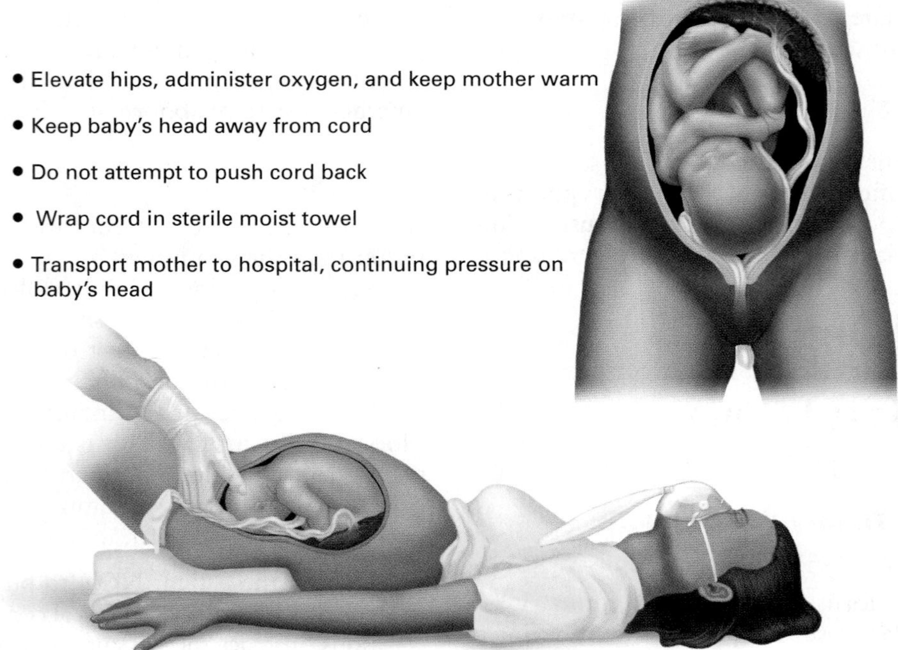

• Elevate hips, administer oxygen, and keep mother warm
• Keep baby's head away from cord
• Do not attempt to push cord back
• Wrap cord in sterile moist towel
• Transport mother to hospital, continuing pressure on baby's head

FIGURE 37-12 ✻ Prolapsed cord.

prolonged for these newborns, who are at great risk of delivery trauma. The mother is also at risk for delivery trauma. There is an increased risk of a prolapsed cord, compression of the cord, or an anoxic insult during delivery where oxygenation is cut off to the fetus. Transport immediately upon recognition of a breech presentation. Administer oxygen to the mother, and keep the mother in a supine head-down position with her pelvis elevated so gravity will discourage the movement of the fetus into the birth canal.

A breech delivery is best managed in the hospital. You should not attempt to deliver a breech presentation in the field. However, if the delivery is unavoidable, perform the following emergency care:

1. Position the mother with her buttocks at the edge of a firm surface or bed.
2. Have her hold her legs in a flexed position.
3. As the infant delivers, do not pull on the legs, but support them.
4. Allow the entire body to be delivered as you simply support it. Continue with care for the neonate as in the normal delivery.

A complication of breech delivery is that the body is delivered but the head cannot be delivered. If this occurs, insert your index and middle gloved fingers into the vagina, forming a "V" along the vaginal wall with the baby's nose and mouth between the fingers. Push against the vaginal wall to create a space for respiration. Immediately transport while maintaining this position.

Understanding BODY PROCESSES

Breech presentations are often associated with premature births, placenta previa, multiple births, and uterus and fetal abnormalities. ■

Limb Presentation

When one arm or one leg is the first to protrude from the birth canal, it is considered a **limb presentation** (Figure 37-14✻). Under no circumstances would you attempt a field delivery of a limb presentation. Transport immediately, because a cesarean section will be re-

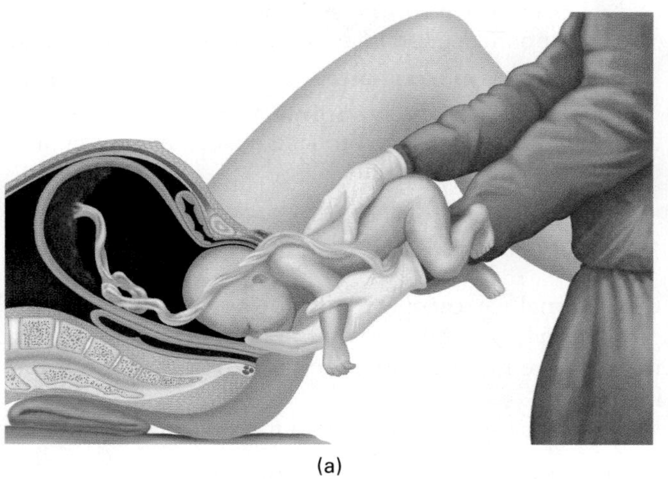

(a)

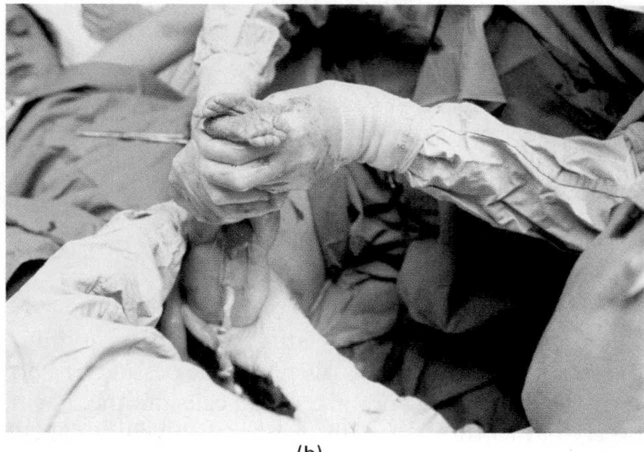

(b)

FIGURE 37-13 * **(a)** Establish an airway during a prolonged breech delivery. **(b)** Breech delivery. (Eddie Lawrence/Photo Researchers, Inc.)

quired to deliver the fetus. Administer oxygen to the mother, and place the mother in a knee-chest position with her pelvis elevated. Never pull on the infant by its arm or leg and, again, never attempt delivery in this situation. Have the mother pant if she has the urge to push with contractions.

Understanding BODY PROCESSES

Limb presentation is most often seen when the fetus is lying transversely across the uterus. Touching the presenting limb may stimulate the fetus to gasp for a breath and aspirate amniotic fluid. ■

Multiple Births

In a **multiple birth** (twins, triplets, and so on) each infant may have its own placenta or the infants may share a placenta. Even if the mother is unaware that she is carrying more than one infant, you should be prepared for a multiple birth if one or more of the following is observed:

- The abdomen is still very large after one infant is delivered.
- Uterine contractions continue to be extremely strong after delivering the first infant.
- Uterine contractions begin again about 10 minutes after one infant has been delivered.
- The infant's size is small in proportion to the size of the mother's abdomen.

Follow the general guidelines for emergency medical care in a normal delivery, with the following exceptions: Be prepared to care for more than one infant. Call for assistance. Note that about one-third of the deliveries of the second infant will be breech, so assess carefully and take immediate action. If the second infant is not breech, handle the delivery as you would for a single infant. Expect and manage hemorrhage following the second birth. If the second infant has not delivered within 10 minutes of the first, transport the mother and the first infant to the hospital for delivery of the second infant. Multiple-birth babies have a tendency to be low birth weight and may require additional resuscitation.

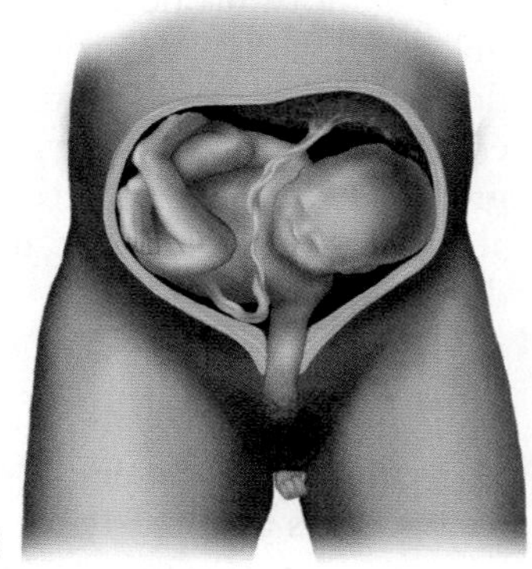

(a)

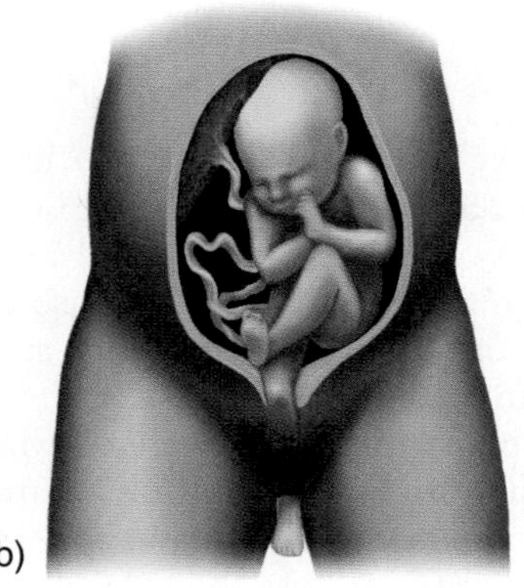

(b)

FIGURE 37-14 * Limb presentations: **(a)** arm, **(b)** leg.

Key Terms

multiple birth delivery of more than one baby during a single birth such as twins or triplets.

meconium staining a greenish or brownish yellow staining of the amniotic fluid, caused by a fetal bowel movement resulting from distress.

Key Terms

premature infant an infant weighing less than 5 pounds, or an infant born before the 38th week.

postterm pregnancy gestation beyond 42 weeks.

postmaturity syndrome when gestation beyond 42 weeks leads to reduced oxygen and nutrient delivery to the fetus.

Meconium

During a difficult labor the fetus may undergo significant distress. One result of this distress is the passing of a bowel movement in the amniotic fluid, causing the normally clear fluid to turn greenish or brownish yellow. This coloring is called **meconium staining.** It is an indication that the fetus experienced a hypoxic event. If the infant aspirates into its lungs any of the meconium-stained fluid, infection and aspiration pneumonia can result. Meconium staining is most often seen in breech births. If meconium is present, aggressively suction the airway until clear to avoid aspiration.

Understanding BODY PROCESSES

When the fetus becomes hypoxic, the digestive tract increases movement (peristalsis) and the anal sphincter relaxes, causing the meconium to be released into the amniotic fluid. In a breech delivery, the uterus contracts against the fetus's head and stimulates the parasympathetic nervous system, which increases the peristalsis in the intestines, making meconium staining more likely to occur. Typically, the thicker and darker the color of the meconium the higher the risk for more fetal problems. ■

If you observe meconium staining of the amniotic fluid, suction the infant's mouth and nose as soon as the head emerges from the birth canal. *Do not stimulate the infant before you suction its mouth and nose.* The most critical aspect of treatment for meconium staining is to clear the mouth and nose before the infant takes its first breath. Transport the infant as soon as possible, maintaining the airway and supporting ventilation, if necessary, throughout transport.

Premature Birth

An infant weighing less than 5 pounds, or an infant born before its 38th week of development, is defined as a **premature infant** and requires special care. Because of their underdevelopment, premature babies are more susceptible to hypothermia and respiratory distress.

You can generally tell by appearance whether an infant is premature. A premature infant is thinner and smaller, and its skin has a reddened and wrinkled appearance. There will be a single crease across the sole of the foot, there will be fuzzy scalp hair that is very fine, and the external ear cartilage will not be fully developed. A premature infant, because of its incomplete development, may require more vigorous resuscitation than a full-term infant.

Provide this additional care for a premature infant:

1. Be sure to dry the infant thoroughly and avoid heat loss. Keep the infant warm by using warmed blankets or a plastic bubble-bag swaddle, making sure that the head is covered but the face is unobstructed.
2. Use gentle suction with a bulb syringe to keep the infant's nose and mouth clear of fluid.
3. Prevent bleeding from the umbilical cord. A premature infant cannot tolerate losing even the smallest amount of blood.
4. Administer supplemental oxygen by blowing oxygen across the infant's face, with the end of the oxygen tube approximately 1 inch above the infant's mouth and nose. Never blow the oxygen directly into the face. Support ventilation if breathing is inadequate.
5. Premature babies are highly susceptible to infection. Prevent contamination and do not let anyone breathe into the infant's face.
6. Wrap the infant securely to keep it warm, and heat the vehicle during transport.

Postterm Pregnancy

In **postterm pregnancy** the gestation of the fetus extends beyond 42 weeks. Postterm pregnancy causes **postmaturity syndrome**, a deterioration of conditions necessary to support the well-being of the fetus. At 42 weeks, the placenta begins to decline, leading to a decrease in oxygenation and nutrient delivery to the fetus from decreased placental blood flow. The postmature baby is more prone to insufficient oxygen and nutrient delivery, hypoxia, a hardened skull that causes a more difficult delivery, and the presence of meconium from increased bowel maturity. The postmature fetus is at greater risk for intrapartum hypoxia because of the inability of the placenta to meet the demands of the fetus during labor.

Precipitous Delivery

A **precipitous delivery** is one in which the birth of the fetus occurs after less than 3 hours of labor. Precipitous delivery is most often seen in patients who have delivered several children (multipara). Since the delivery occurs so

Key Terms

precipitous delivery birth of the fetus after less than 3 hours of labor.

shoulder dystocia when the fetal head delivers but the shoulders are too large to deliver.

Key Terms

preterm labor labor that occurs after the 20th but prior to the 37th week.

premature rupture of membranes (PROM) spontaneous rupture of the amniotic sac prior to true labor and before the end of the 37th week.

rapidly, there is an increased risk of trauma to the fetus, trauma to the mother, and tearing of the umbilical cord. The delivery would be conducted in the same manner as any other; however, it may occur rapidly and without much warning. The care for the neonate is the same as in a normal delivery.

Shoulder Dystocia

A **shoulder dystocia** is when the fetal shoulders are larger than the fetal head. The head delivers, but then it retracts back into the vagina because the shoulders are caught between the symphysis pubis and the sacrum (Figure 37-15✱). The retraction into the vagina is referred to as a "turtle sign." It occurs in larger birth-weight babies, as seen in diabetic mothers and those who are past their due dates. If a shoulder dystocia occurs, do not pull on the head of the fetus in an attempt to deliver. Transport immediately. Have the mother pant to reduce the force and pressure of contractions. Place the mother on her back with her knees drawn up as close to her chest as possible. This is known as the McRobert position (Figure 37-16✱). This maneuver moves the symphysis pubis anteriorly and superiorly and drops the sacrum, creating a larger opening for delivery of the shoulders.

Preterm Labor

Preterm labor, also known as premature labor, occurs after the 20th but prior to the 37th week of gestation. This is a different condition from preterm birth. *Preterm labor* refers specifically to the onset of labor. It does not always lead to birth of the baby if the labor can be stopped. A mother with a history of preterm labor is usually placed on bed rest during the pregnancy. Preterm labor carries a higher incidence of abnormal presentations of the fetus during delivery. Cocaine and other drugs are known to induce labor. If you suspect preterm labor, keep the mother calm and do not allow her to push. Place the patient on oxygen. Consider calling an advanced life support unit.

Premature Rupture of Membranes

Premature rupture of membranes (PROM) is the spontaneous premature rupture of the amniotic sac prior to the onset of true labor and before the end of the 37th week of gestation. Although this is not an emergency, there is an increased risk of infection of the uterus and its contents. Amniotic fluid acts as a lubricant during delivery; thus, premature rupture of the amniotic sac prevents adequate lubrication of the vaginal canal at the time of birth, which may lead to a more difficult delivery.

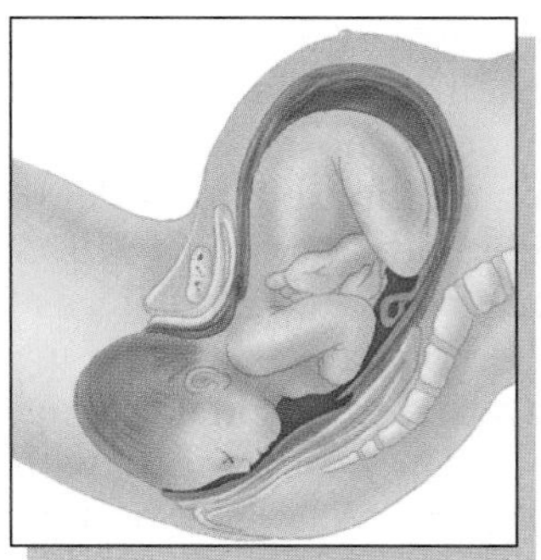

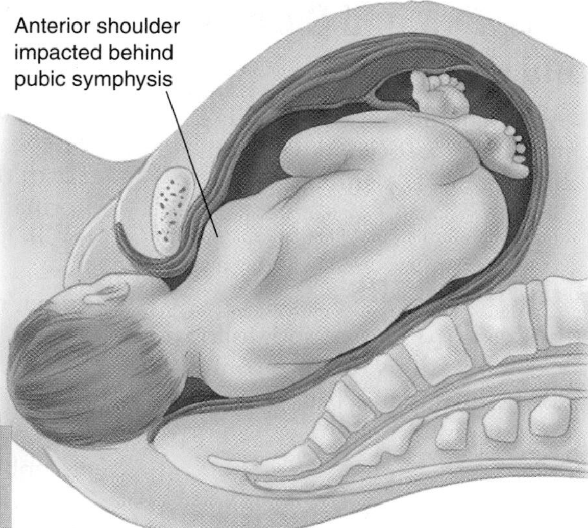

Dangers Include:
- Entrapment of cord
- Inability of child's chest to expand properly
- Severe brain damage or death if child is not delivered within minutes

FIGURE 37-15 ✱ Shoulder dystocia.

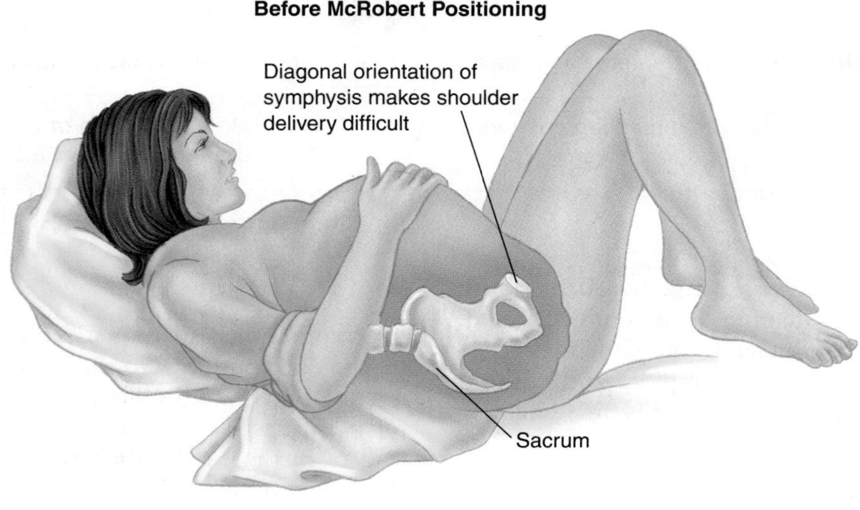

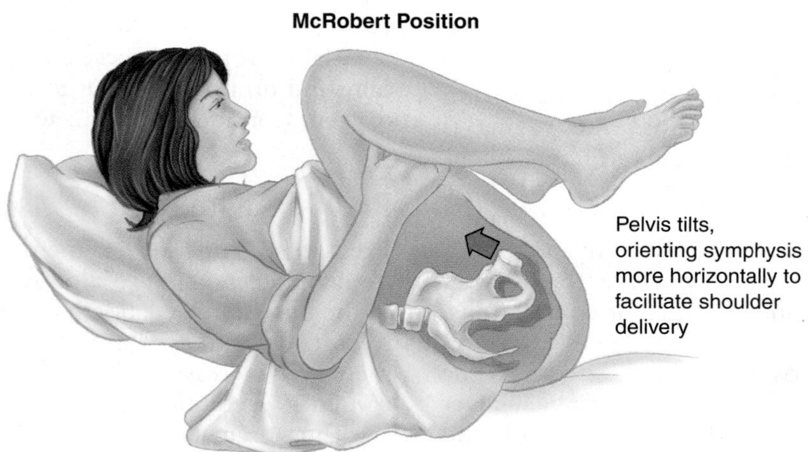

FIGURE 37-16 ✻ The McRobert maneuver for shoulder dystocia.

Summary: Assessment and Care—Active Labor and Delivery

To review possible assessment findings and emergency care for an obstetric emergency associated with active labor and delivery, see Figures 37-17✻ and 37-18✻.

Postpartum Complications

The term **postpartum** refers to the period following delivery. Postpartum complications involve only the mother. Hemorrhage is the most dangerous of the postpartum conditions.

Postpartum Hemorrhage

Postpartum hemorrhage is defined as the loss of greater than 500 mL of blood following delivery. The most common cause of postpartum hemorrhage is failure of the uterus to regain its muscle tone (uterine atony). Postpartum hemorrhage is most common in multigravida patients following multiple births or delivery of a large baby. Prolonged labor and precipitous delivery can lead to failure of the uterus to tone. If the uterus fails to return to a normal size, hemorrhage can occur up to 2 weeks after the delivery. In the prehospital setting, hemorrhage following delivery can be managed with oxygen therapy, fundal massage, and immediate transport.

Embolism

The pregnant or postpartum patient is at greater risk for an embolism because of the increased blood volume and coagulation properties of the blood. Clot formation in the venous system can lead to a pulmonary embolism. The patient with a pulmonary embolism may present with shortness of breath, syncope, tachycardia, sharp

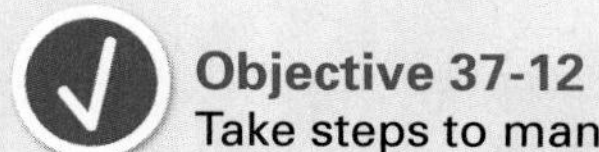

Objective 37-12
Take steps to manage postpartum complications, including postpartum hemorrhage and embolism.

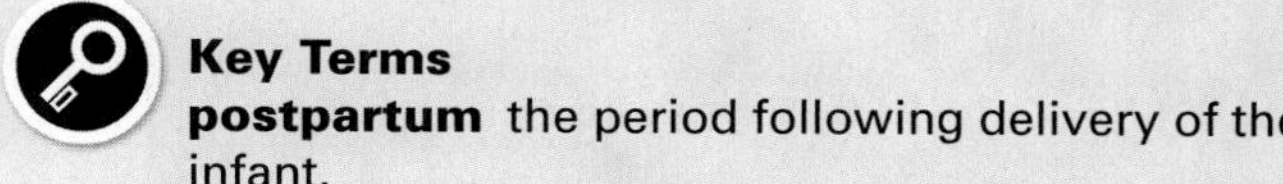

Key Terms
postpartum the period following delivery of the infant.

postpartum hemorrhage the loss of greater than 500 mL of blood following delivery.

chest pain, hypotension, cyanosis, and pale, cool, clammy skin. Amniotic fluid embolism (AFE) may occur when amniotic fluid, fetal cells, hair or other material enter the mother's circulation. The condition, which is not completely understood, may be more associated with an anaphylactic reaction and can lead to cardiopulmonary compromise. Your emergency care for embolism or AFE will focus on ensuring adequate ventilation and maximizing oxygenation. Provide oxygen via a nonrebreather mask at 15 lpm. If the patient's breathing becomes inadequate, begin positive pressure ventilation with supplemental oxygen connected to the ventilation device.

Assessment Summary

OBSTETRIC EMERGENCY—ACTIVE LABOR AND DELIVERY

The following findings may be associated with an obstetric emergency occurring during active labor or delivery.

SCENE SIZE-UP

Pay particular attention to your own safety. Look for:
- Mechanism of injury
- Blood in toilet or around patient
- Bleeding from vagina
- Bloody tissue or blood clots
- Fetus protruding from vagina
- Mucus discharged, tinged with blood
- Amniotic fluid
- Meconium staining

Primary Assessment

General Impression
- Does the patient appear to be in a full-term pregnancy?
- Posture: lying still with knees to chest indicates severe abdominal pain, or supine
- Any evidence of seizure activity?
- Is the umbilical cord or fetal body part other than the head present at the vaginal opening?
- Does the patient appear to be having contractions that are intense, regular, frequent, and with a duration of about 60 seconds?

Mental Status
- Alert

Airway
- Open and usually not obstructed

Breathing
- Increased due to pain

Circulation
- Heart rate may be increased

Status: Priority patient if associated with shock, significant vaginal bleeding, or abnormal presenting part, or if greater than 10 minutes is spent attempting to perform delivery

Secondary Assessment

History
Signs and symptoms:
- Abdominal pain due to contractions

True labor contractions:	Regular Occur at about *2- to 3-minute intervals* Last about 30–90 seconds Are intense
False labor (Braxton-Hicks) contractions:	Irregular Interval time varies Duration varies Intensity varies May be relieved by walking

- Vaginal discharge of amniotic fluid, clear with yellowish tint
- Crowning

continued

FIGURE 37-17a ✱ Assessment summary: obstetric emergency—active labor and delivery.

Assessment Summary

Question:

Onset, provocation/palliation, quality, radiation, severity, and duration of pain
When was your last menstrual period?
Have you had any unusual vaginal discharge or bleeding?
When is your due date?
Have you had previous problems with pregnancies?
Have you been seeing a physician for this pregnancy?
Is this your first delivery?
Do you feel as if you are having a bowel movement?

Physical Exam

Abdomen/Genitalia:

Obvious protruded abdomen
Evidence of crowning or abnormal presenting part?
Any passed tissue from the vagina?
Vaginal bleeding, dark or bright red, may or may not be associated with pain
Amniotic fluid present
Meconium staining to amniotic fluid

Baseline Vital Signs

BP: may be normal or increased
HR: may be normal or increased
RR: may be normal or increased
Skin: normal
Pupils: normal size, equal, and reactive to light
SpO_2: $> 95\%$

FIGURE 37-17a ✱ Assessment summary: obstetric emergency—active labor and delivery. *continued*

Emergency Care Protocol

OBSTETRIC EMERGENCY—ACTIVE LABOR AND DELIVERY

1. Place the patient supine with knees drawn up and check for crowning.
2. If crowning is occurring; contractions are 2 minutes apart, intense, and lasting 30–90 seconds; and the mother has the urge to push, prepare to deliver.
3. Check for crowning or an abnormal presenting part. If an abnormal presenting part is found, such as a prolapsed cord, hand, or foot, perform the following:
   a. Position patient in knee-chest position on a stretcher that is in a Trendelenburg position.
   b. If umbilical cord is prolapsed, insert gloved hand into vagina and push presenting part of fetus away from cord.
   c. Cover presenting part with a sterile moist dressing.
   d. Rapidly transport patient and notify receiving facility of patient's condition.

   If the fetal head is crowning, proceed with delivery as described in steps 4–13.
4. Prepare the OB kit and create a sterile field around the vaginal opening.
5. If the amniotic sac is still intact, rupture it with your fingers and tear it away from the infant's face.
6. As the head and neck are delivered, inspect to determine if the umbilical cord is wrapped around the infant's neck (nuchal cord). If it is, do the following:
   a. Slip cord over infant's head.
   b. If cord cannot be slipped over head, immediately clamp cord in two places and cut between clamps.
7. Suction the mouth and nose as the head is delivered.
8. Continue with delivery until the entire body is expelled.
9. Keep the infant level with the mother. See "Emergency Care Protocol: Newborn Infant."
10. Place an umbilical clamp or tie about 6 inches from the newborn's abdomen and a second one about 3 inches from the first. Cut the cord.
11. Deliver the placenta. If greater than 10 minutes is spent waiting for placental delivery, transport.
12. Apply a sanitary napkin over the vaginal opening.
13. Perform a reassessment every 5 minutes if unstable, every 15 minutes if stable.

FIGURE 37-17b ✱ Emergency care protocol: obstetric emergency—active labor and delivery.

Emergency Care Algorithm: Obstetric Emergency—Active Labor and Delivery

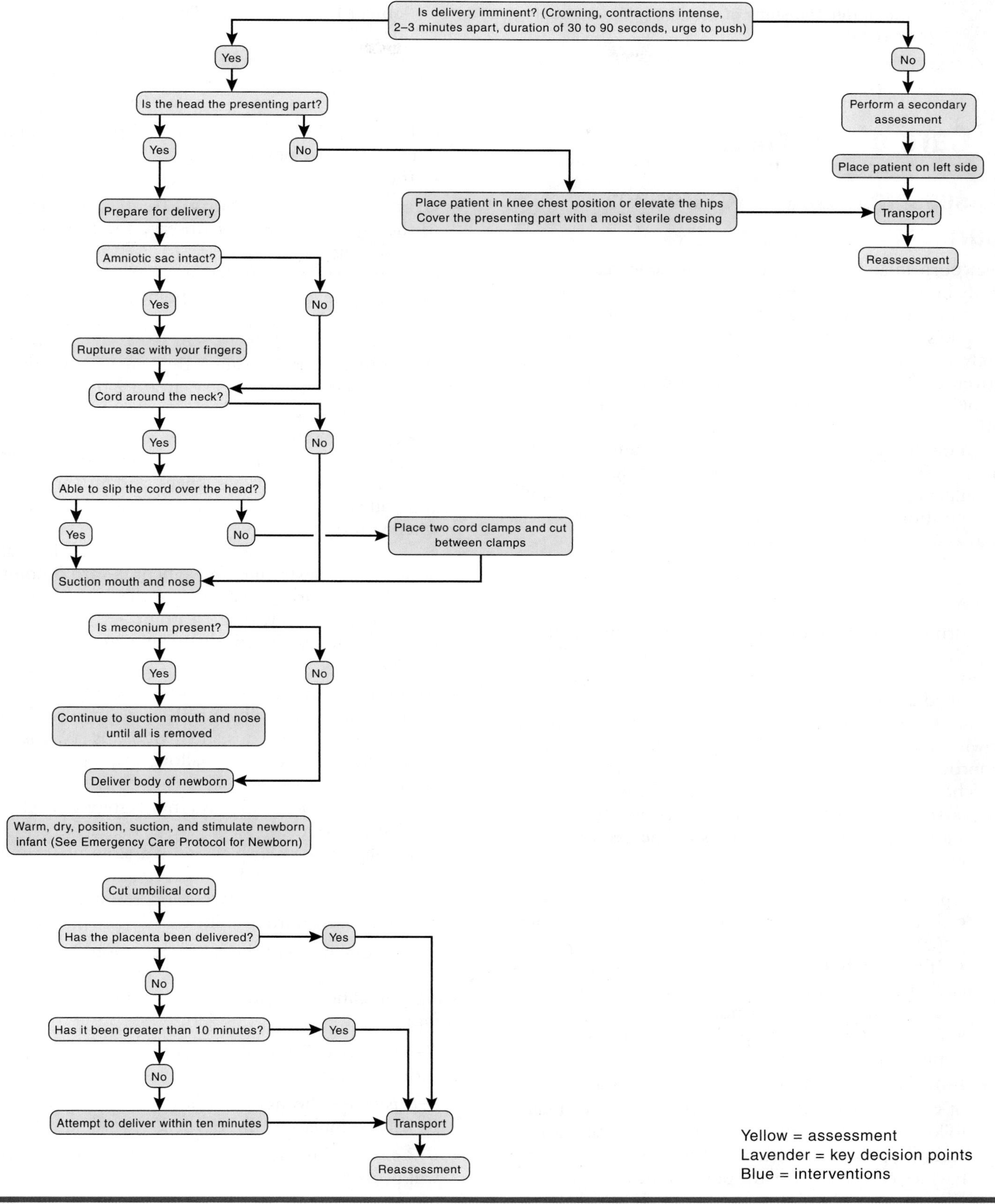

FIGURE 37-18 ✻ Emergency care algorithm: obstetric emergency—active labor and delivery.

Key Points
Apgar scoring can provide an overall indication of the baby's condition. Determine the score at 60 seconds after birth and again in 4 minutes to obtain 1-minute and 5-minute scores following birth.

Objective 37-13
Demonstrate the steps of assessing and managing the newborn.

Care of the Newborn

Assessment-Based Approach: Care of the Newborn

Newborn infants, also referred to as neonates, can lose body heat quickly. Protecting them against heat loss preserves their energy and avoids the complex problem that hospitals face in trying to rewarm a cold infant. Immediately dry the infant. Be sure to dry the head well, and cover it. Then wrap the newborn in a blanket or a plastic bubble-bag swaddle. Repeat suctioning to make sure the infant's mouth and nostrils are clear. Position the newborn on his back or side with the neck slightly extended in a sniffing position. Place some padding under the shoulders to maintain the head and neck in a slight sniffing position. Do not hyperextend or flex the neck; this may cause airway obstruction.

Assessment

Perform a thorough assessment of the infant. You can use the Apgar scoring system to get a good overall indication of the baby's condition. The score should be determined at 60 seconds after birth, and then repeated in 4 minutes to obtain a 1-minute and a 5-minute score following birth. A change in the Apgar score may indicate improvement (higher score), worsening (lower score), or no change. To assess the newborn using the Apgar scoring system, you can use the letters in Apgar as a mnemonic to remember the parts of the assessment, as follows:

- **Appearance.**
  - If the skin of the newborn's entire body is blue (cyanotic) or pale, award 0 points.
  - If the newborn has blue hands and feet with pink skin at the core of the body (a condition called acrocyanosis), award 1 point.
  - If the skin of the extremities as well as the trunk is pink, award 2 points.
- **Pulse.** Heart rate is one of the most important signs of whether oxygen is reaching the newborn's tissues following birth. Count the heart rate for at least 30 seconds, preferably with a stethoscope. If you do not have a stethoscope, feel the pulse of the umbilical cord where it joins the abdomen or at the brachial artery.
  - If no pulse is present, award 0 points.
  - If the heart rate is under 100 (also a serious finding), award 1 point.
  - If the heart rate is over 100, award 2 points.
- **Grimace (reflex irritability).** Gently flick the soles of the newborn's feet, or observe the facial expressions during suctioning.
  - If the newborn displays no reflexive activity to your stimulation, award 0 points.
  - If the newborn displays only some facial grimace, award 1 point.
  - If your stimulation causes the newborn to grimace and cough, sneeze, or cry, award 2 points.
- **Activity.** This score refers to extremity reflexes/movement, or the degree of flexion of the arms and legs and the resistance to straightening them. The normal newborn's elbows, knees, and hips are flexed, and you should encounter some degree of resistance when you try to extend them.
  - If during your assessment the newborn is limp and displays no extremity movement, award 0 points.
  - If the newborn only displays some flexion without active movement, award 1 point.
  - If the newborn is actively moving around, award 2 points.
- **Respiration.** Another important assessment sign is the newborn's breathing effort. The newborn should have regular respirations and a vigorous cry. Distress is indicated by irregular, shallow, gasping, or absent respirations.
  - If the newborn displays no respiratory effort, award 0 points.
  - If the newborn displays only a slow or irregular breathing effort with a weak cry, award 1 point.
  - If the newborn displays good respirations and a strong cry, award 2 points.

At the conclusion of the assessment, you should have a numeric value that ranges from 0 to 10. Use the following guidelines to determine the significance of your finding:

- *7–10 points*—The newborn should be active and vigorous. Provide routine care.
- *4–6 points*—The newborn is moderately depressed. Provide stimulation and oxygen.
- *0–3 points*—The newborn is severely depressed. You will probably need to provide extensive care including oxygen with bag-valve-mask ventilations and CPR, as described later.

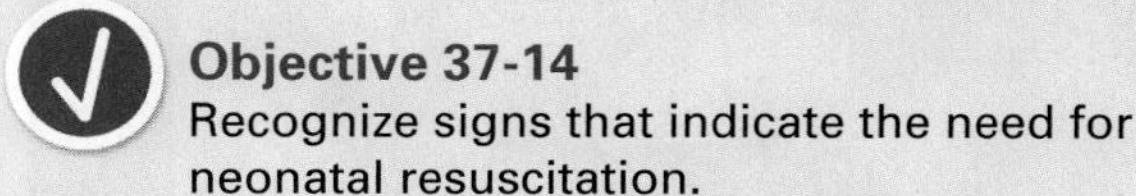

Objective 37-14
Recognize signs that indicate the need for neonatal resuscitation.

Objective 37-15
Apply the concepts of the neonatal resuscitation pyramid to the care of neonates in need of resuscitative measures.

Be sure to stimulate the newborn if he is still not breathing adequately. You can stimulate respirations by gently flicking the soles of the feet or by rubbing the back in a circular motion with three fingers (Figure 37-19*). En route to the hospital, provide continual assessment for the newborn. Pay particular attention to body temperature; airway, breathing, and oxygenation status; heart rate; color; and activity level. Contact medical direction to update them on the mother's and newborn's condition.

Signs and Symptoms Most newborns require no resuscitation beyond temperature maintenance, mild stimulation, and suctioning. Of those who require additional resuscitation, most need oxygen or bag-valve-mask ventilations. A minority of newborns are so depressed that they will also need chest compressions or resuscitative medications.

Certain physical abnormalities, medical complications, or even distressed deliveries can lead to a severely depressed newborn in need of immediate and aggressive treatment. The signs of a severely depressed newborn are:

- Respiratory rate over 60 per minute
- Diminished breath sounds
- Heart rate over 180 per minute or under 100 per minute
- Obvious signs of trauma from the delivery process
- Poor or absent skeletal muscle tone
- Respiratory arrest, or severe distress
- Heavy meconium staining of amniotic fluid
- Weak pulses
- Cyanotic body (core and extremities)
- Poor peripheral perfusion
- Lack of or poor response to stimulation
- Apgar score under 4

Emergency Medical Care

If one or more of the preceding signs are noted during your assessment following birth, you should gather the necessary equipment for neonatal resuscitation. It is important to remember that newborns cannot tolerate even brief periods of inadequate oxygenation without serious effects. *The establishment and maintenance of an adequate airway, ventilation, and oxygenation is "cornerstone" treatment for any newborn infant.*

Most newborns do not require aggressive treatment. Approximately 80 percent require no resuscitation beyond keeping them warm and suctioning the airway. If their responses are slightly depressed, most will respond to blow-by oxygen or to bag-valve-mask ventilations with supplemental oxygen. A small number may require chest compressions, and an even smaller number may require the medications or intubation that an advanced life support team can provide. The relative frequency of need for resuscitative measures is often shown as an

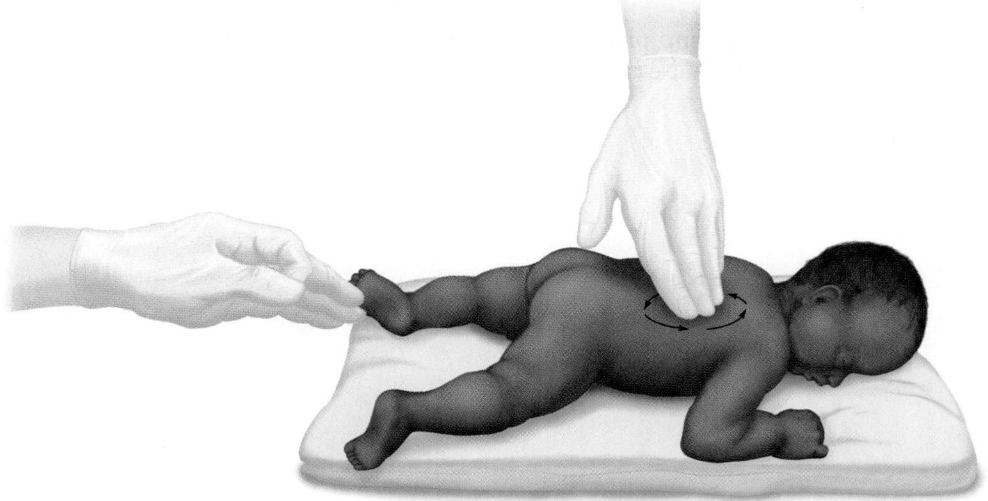

FIGURE 37-19 * Stimulate the infant who is not breathing by flicking the soles of the feet or by rubbing the back.

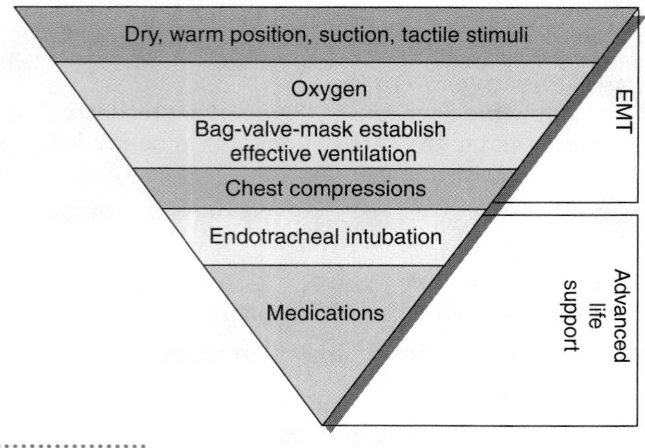

FIGURE 37-20 ✱ The inverted pyramid for neonatal resuscitation shows that the majority of newborns will respond to simple routines of care; only a few will require aggressive resuscitation.

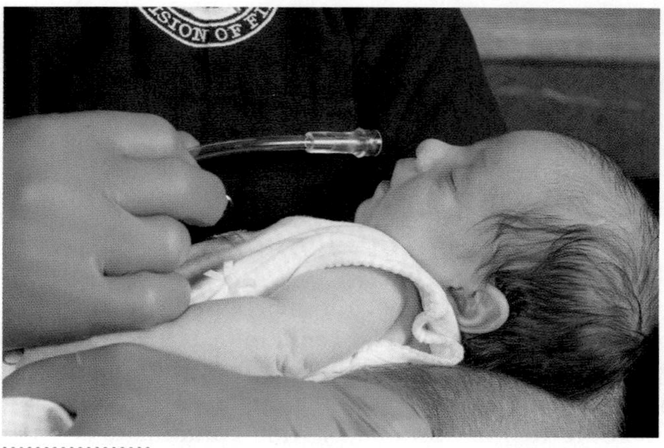

FIGURE 37-21 ✱ Blow-by administration of oxygen to a newborn.

inverted pyramid with the simple care most newborns require at the top (Figure 37-20✱).

Based on the signs and symptoms, you should provide the following treatment:

1. If the infant has bluish discoloration (cyanosis) of the skin, but has spontaneous breathing and an adequate heart rate (greater than 100 per minute), you should provide blow-by oxygen. Hold the tube 1 inch from the nose and mouth and direct the oxygen flow, at 5 lpm or greater, across the mouth and nose (Figure 37-21✱). Make sure the infant is kept warm and the airway remains clear.
2. Provide ventilations by bag-valve mask with supplemental oxygen at the rate of 40–60 per minute (EMT Skills 37-2A) if the newborn displays any of the following:
   - The infant's breathing is shallow, slow, gasping, or absent following brief stimulation.
   - The infant's heart rate is less than 100 beats per minute.
   - The infant's core body remains cyanotic (blue) despite provision of blow-by oxygen.

   Maintain a tight face mask seal, and provide the ventilations with just enough force to raise the infant's chest. Reassess after 30 seconds of ventilation. If the breathing has not improved and the heart rate is less than 100/minute, continue ventilations and reassess every 30 seconds. If ventilation is required for more than 2 minutes and the infant's stomach becomes distended and impedes ventilation, it may be necessary to insert a gastric tube to relieve the distention.
3. If, despite adequate ventilations, the infant's heart rate drops to less than 60 beats per minute, continue ventilations and begin chest compressions.

Circle the torso with your fingers and place both thumbs on the lower third of the infant's sternum. If the infant is very small, you may need to overlap the thumbs. If the infant is very large, compress the sternum with the ring and middle fingers one finger's depth below the nipple line. Compress the chest approximately one-third the depth of the chest at 120 compressions per minute (EMT Skills 37-2B). Deliver a 3:1 ratio of compressions to ventilations.

Summary: Care of the Newborn

To review emergency care for the newborn, see Figures 37-22✱ and 37-23✱.

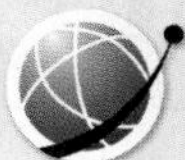

Media Resources
Go to www.bradybooks.com mykit. Highlights:

- *Video:* Childbirth
- *Video:* Preeclampsia

Emergency Care Protocol

NEWBORN INFANT

1. If meconium is present, aggressively suction the airway until clear.
2. Dry the newborn with towels.
3. Wrap the newborn in warm towels or blankets. Be sure to cover the head and prevent hypothermia.
4. Position the newborn on his back, or in a lateral recumbent position if there is a large amount of secretions. Slightly extend the neck in a sniffing position. Place a small pad under the shoulders to maintain the airway position. Do not hyperextend or flex the neck.
5. Stimulate the newborn by rubbing his back or flicking the soles of the feet if breathing or activity is inadequate.
6. Perform an Apgar score 1 minute after birth.
7. If breathing is inadequate, perform positive pressure ventilation (PPV) with supplemental oxygen for 30 seconds to 1 minute. Then reassess. Continue PPV as necessary.
8. Assess pulse.
   - *If heart rate is greater than 100/minute,* assess color (see step 9).
   - *If heart rate is less than 100/minute but greater than 60/minute,* begin PPV with oxygen at 40–60 ventilations per minute for 30 seconds to 1 minute. Then reassess heart rate. If heart rate remains less than 100/minute, continue PPV with oxygen until rate exceeds 100/minute.
   - *If heart rate drops to less than 60/minute,* perform aggressive ventilation and begin chest compressions to a depth of one-third the depth of the chest at a rate of 120/minute and a ratio of 3:1 chest compressions to ventilations.
   - *If at any time heart rate drops below 60/minute,* begin chest compressions and continue PPV.
9. Assess color. If the body is cyanotic but breathing is adequate and heart rate is greater than 100/minute, administer blow-by oxygen at 5 lpm or greater until color improves. If heart rate is less than 100/minute, return to step 8.
10. Continue to reassess the airway, suctioning secretions, and reassess breathing, heart rate, and skin color. Ensure the infant is dry, wrapped, and warm.
11. Perform another Apgar score 5 minutes after birth
12. Transport.

FIGURE 37-22 ✻ Emergency care protocol: newborn infant.

Emergency Care Algorithm: Newborn Care and Resuscitation

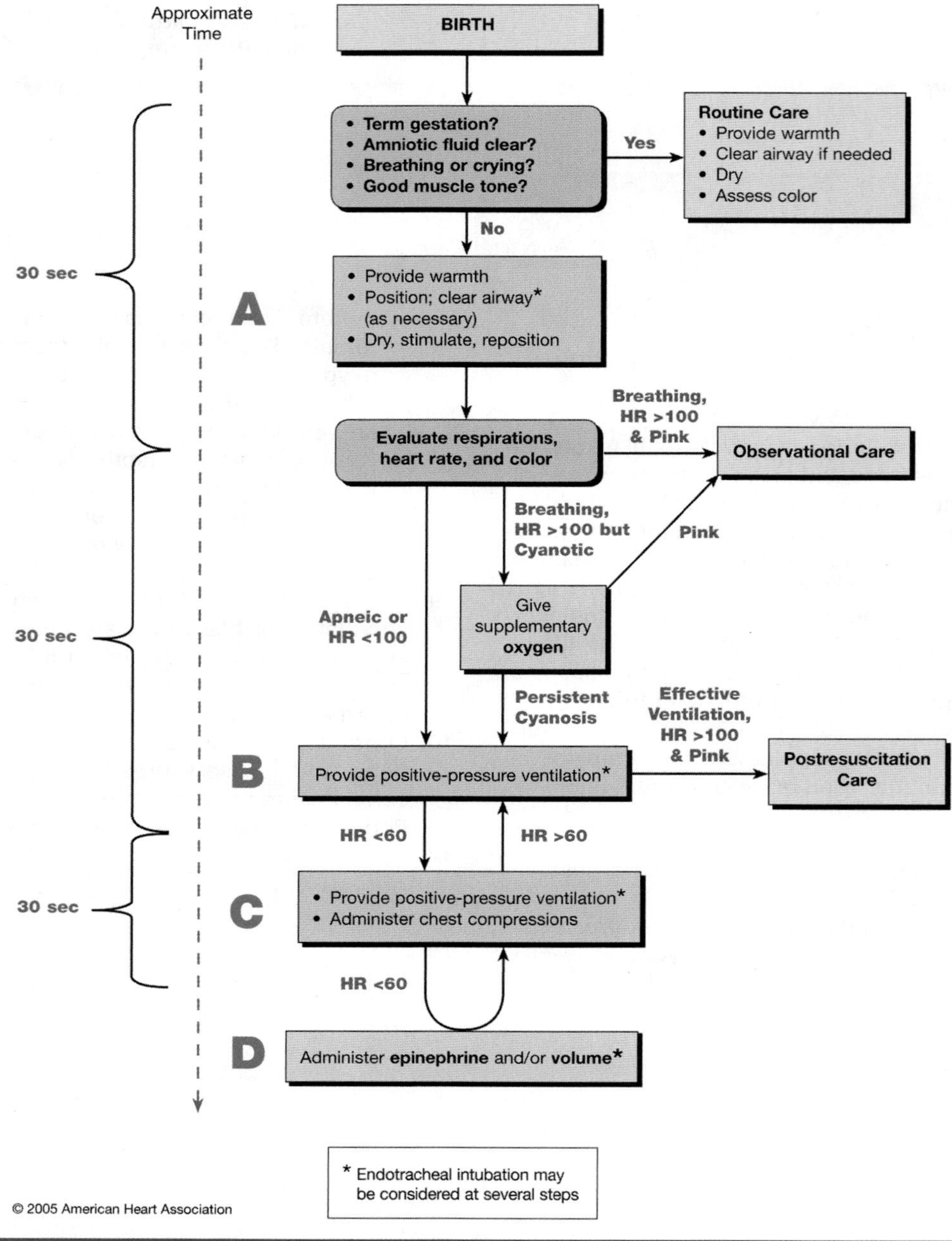

FIGURE 37-23 ✻ Emergency care algorithm: newborn care and resuscitation. Reproduced with permission from "2005 American Heart Association Guidelines for Cardiopulmonary Resuscitation and Emergency Care," *Circulation 2005*, Volume 112, IV-189. © 2005 American Heart Association.

EMT skills 37-1 Childbirth

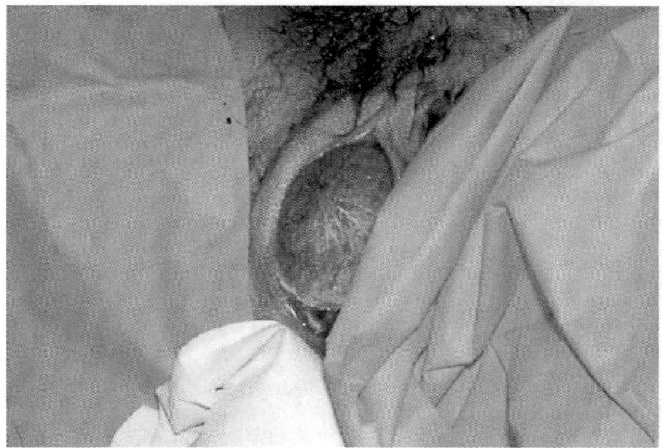

37-1A ✱ Crowning.

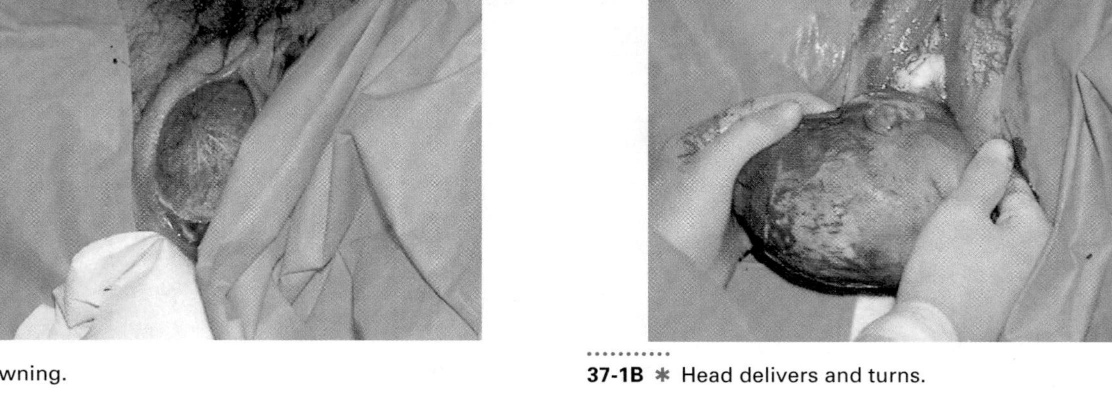

37-1B ✱ Head delivers and turns.

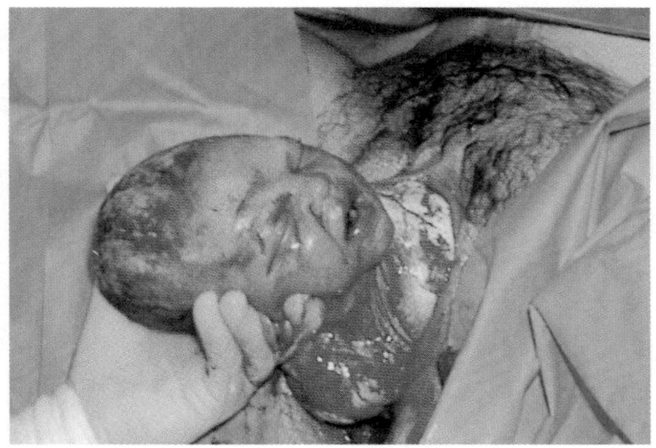

37-1C ✱ Shoulders deliver.

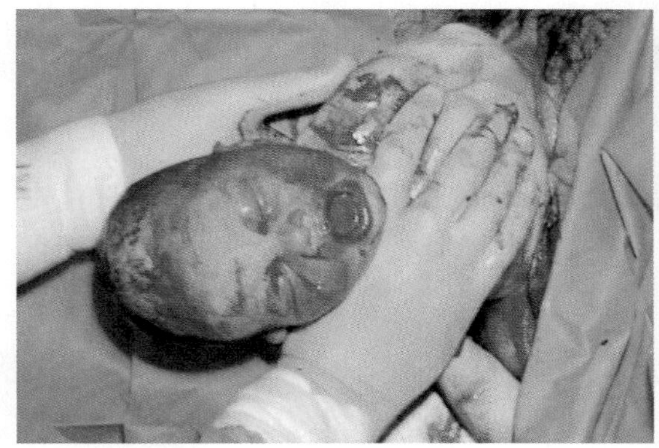

37-1D ✱ Chest delivers.

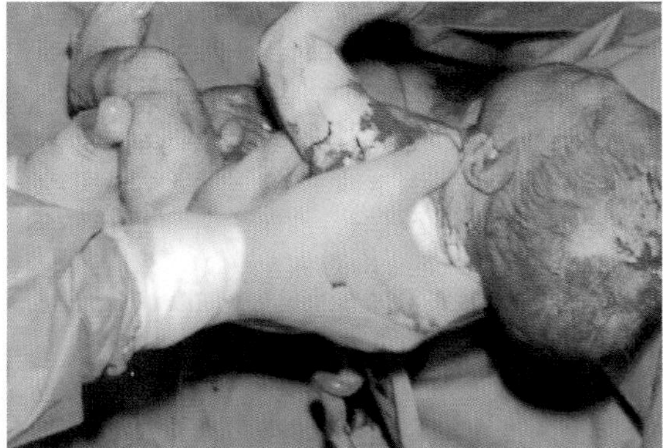

37-1E ✱ Infant delivered.

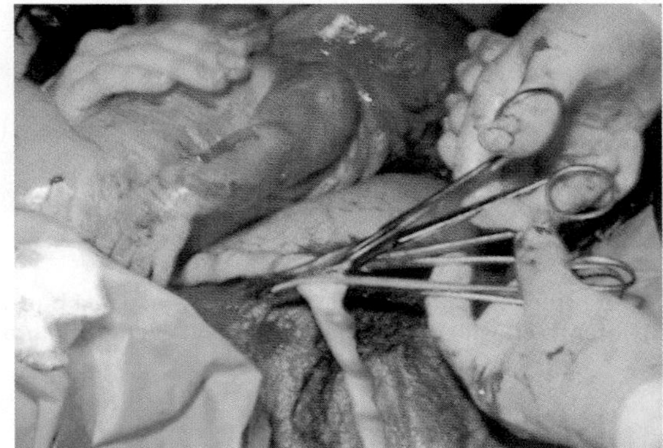

37-1F ✱ Cutting of cord.

continued

EMT skills 37-1 Childbirth *continued*

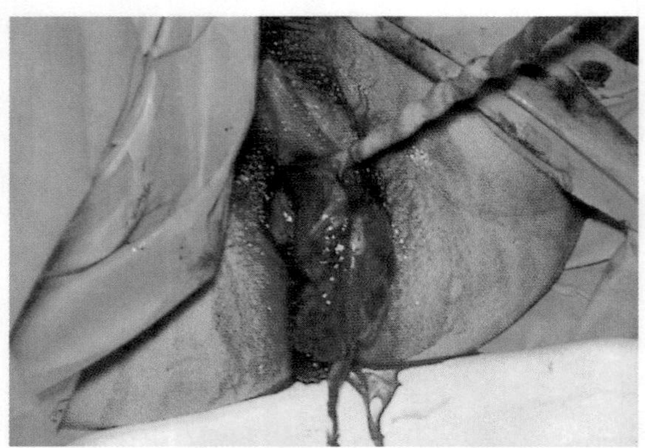

37-1G ✱ Placenta begins delivery.

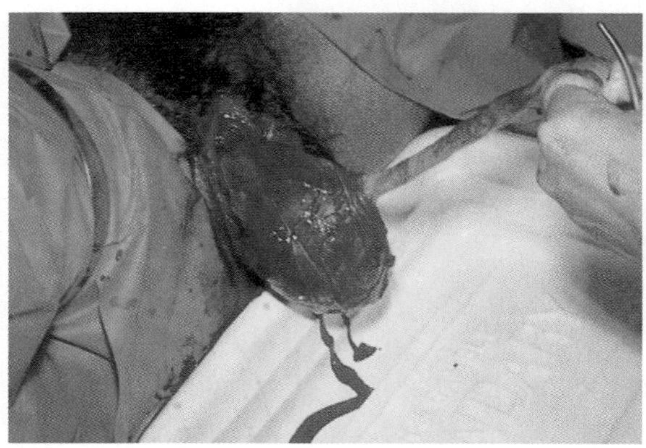

37-1H ✱ Placenta delivers.

EMT skills 37-2 Neonatal Resuscitation

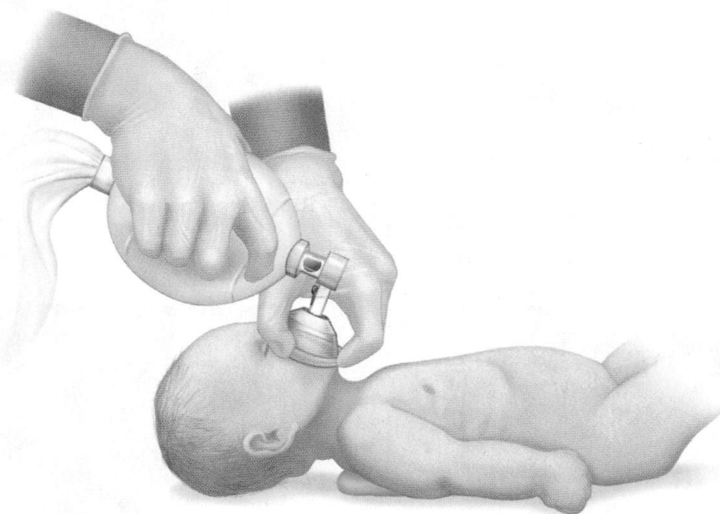

37-2A ✱ To provide positive pressure ventilation, use a bag-valve mask. Maintain a good mask seal. Ventilate with just enough force to raise the infant's chest. Ventilate at a rate of 40–60 per minute for 30 seconds. Then reassess.

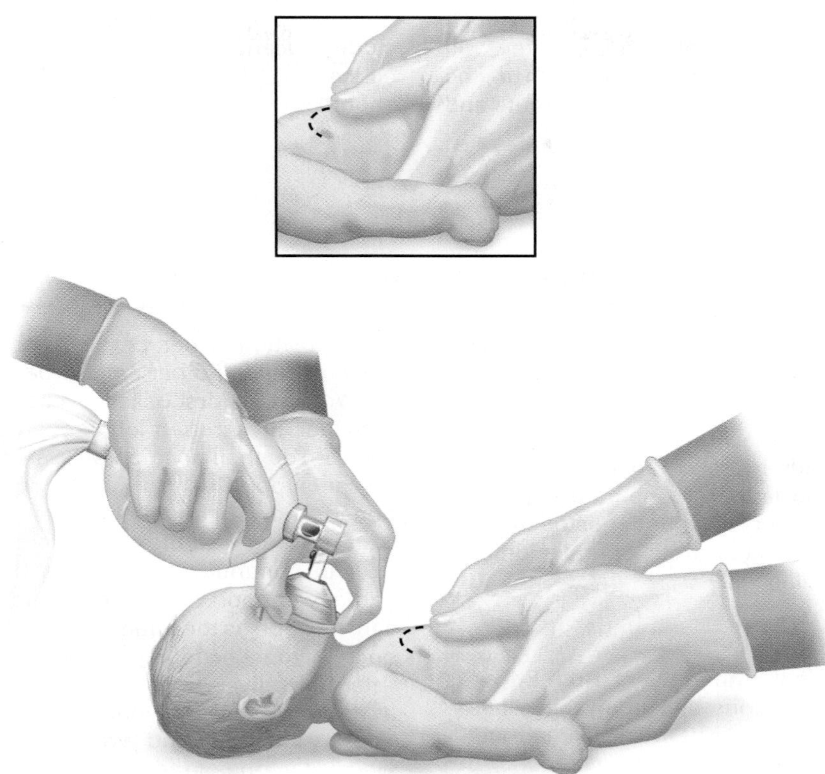

37-2B * To provide chest compressions, circle the torso with the fingers and place both thumbs on the lower third of the infant's sternum. If the infant is very small, you may need to overlap the thumbs. If the infant is very large, compress the sternum with the ring and middle fingers placed one finger's depth below the nipple line. Compress the chest one-third the depth of the chest at the rate of 120 per minute and a ratio of 3:1 compressions to ventilations.

CHAPTER REVIEW

SUMMARY

The uterus is the primary organ of pregnancy. It is composed of smooth muscle and has the ability to stretch drastically to house the growing fetus and other fluid and tissues and also to contract forcefully to expel the fetus during labor. The uterus is a very vascular organ and will bleed heavily if ruptured or torn. There are three stages of labor: dilation, expulsion, and placental. The duration of the stages of labor varies, depending on the number of pregnancies and births of the mother.

When assessing an obstetric or gynecologic patient, in addition to the typical history questions, it is important to gather information about the menstrual cycle. This may provide some clues as to the condition the patient may be experiencing—especially whether the patient may be pregnant.

Predelivery emergencies may include spontaneous abortion, seizures, vaginal bleeding, and trauma. Supine hypotensive syndrome is a concern in any patient in her third trimester, thus it is important to transport any pregnant patient in the third trimester with her hip elevated to take the weight of the fetus off the inferior vena cava.

Delivery is best achieved in the hospital. If delivery is imminent, you may need to proceed with the delivery process in the field. Be sure to take the necessary Standard Precautions. Prepare the mother, have your obstetric kit readily available, and proceed with the delivery. Pay particular attention to clearing the neonate's nose and mouth, drying him, and keeping him warm. Some neonates may need stimulation, blow-by oxygen, and ventilation. Very few will need chest compressions and medications. Once the neonate is delivered, perform an Apgar score 1 minute and 5 minutes after birth.

You may encounter abnormal deliveries in the prehospital setting to include a prolapsed cord, breech birth, limb presentation, multiple births, meconium, and premature births. Be sure to understand the emergency care for each of these conditions. Other predelivery emergencies may include placenta previa, abruptio placentae, preeclampsia, eclampsia, ruptured uterus, Braxton-Hicks contractions, shoulder dystocia, and precipitous delivery.

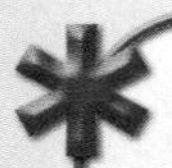

CASE STUDY FOLLOW-UP

SCENE SIZE-UP

You have been dispatched to the scene of a 30-year-old female experiencing active labor. She and her husband tell you that she was having contractions earlier that day, but they were short and slightly irregular, so she figured she would have time to get her laundry done before going to the hospital. Meanwhile, your partner has enlisted the help of some bystanders to bring in the stretcher and additional equipment from the ambulance.

PRIMARY ASSESSMENT

Your general impression is that the patient, Ruth Baker, is experiencing uterine contractions and is in active labor. From the appearance of her slacks, it looks as if her water has already broken. You start to ask her questions, but every time she tries to answer you, her husband, Randy, cuts her off and finishes answering. Seeing this, your partner takes him aside and begins to question him about events prior to the emergency. This allows you to direct your attention to the patient.

You determine that she is alert and oriented with a patent airway and adequate breathing. Her pulse is strong and regular, and her skin is warm and slightly sweaty. There is no evidence of bleeding so far. At this time you apply the pulse oximeter. It provides a reading of 98%. You choose to place the patient on a nasal cannula at 4 lpm in case you have to perform a delivery.

SECONDARY ASSESSMENT

During your history, you learn that this is Mrs. Baker's third child and the other pregnancies progressed without any complications. You ask her about her due date, and she tells you, "Not for 2 more weeks." The police have arrived and, at your request, they disperse the crowd so that you can continue the assessment with some privacy. Currently, contractions are occurring every 2 minutes, with a 50-second duration.

The patient cries out, "I think the baby is coming." You rapidly perform a visual inspection of the perineum and identify crowning, with the head bulging out further with each contraction. You also notice that the amniotic fluid appears to be clear.

At this point you advise the patient that delivery will take place here, and you ask her not to bear down until you have positioned her properly. Your partner notifies dispatch to send another unit for backup.

You move Mrs. Baker to a supine position on the floor with her hips raised off the ground with some folded sheets. You then position Mr. Baker behind his wife so that he can support her during the delivery. Once she is positioned, and your equipment is ready, you encourage her to start pushing with the next contraction.

You continually support the infant during delivery, and verbally support Mrs. Baker to help her relax as best she can. As soon as the infant's head is born, you are very thorough in your suctioning of the newborn's mouth and nose. After full delivery of the infant, you clamp and cut the cord as appropriate while your partner begins to dry the infant. You dry the baby and wrap it in towels your partner has warmed in one of the laundromat dryers.

Your initial Apgar score of the newborn boy is 7, and after brief stimulation, the respiratory rate increases to 46 per minute with an adequate depth. The infant starts to cry and is more vigorous in muscular activity. Since there is some cyanosis to the core and extremities, you provide blow-by oxygen.

REASSESSMENT

You place both the mother and the child in the back of your ambulance. The father sits up front. Your partner has turned up the heat to be sure your two patients are warm enough. You ask Joe Garwood, an EMT from the backup unit, to accompany you to the hospital to care for the mother while you focus your attention on the newborn. En route, the mother continues to have some minor vaginal bleeding and then delivers the placenta, which Joe places in a container for the emergency department staff. He then goes on to perform a uterine massage and bleeding soon stops.

The mother, although tired from the birthing process, is in good spirits and has no unusual complaint or distress. Her mental status is normal, vitals are stable, and she spends the rest of the trip thinking about the possible names for a boy that she and her husband have been discussing.

You repeat the Apgar score a second time and the newborn scores a 10. The baby has "pinked up" so that his color is now normal at the core and the extremities. His respirations are adequate at a rate of 48 per minute, and the heart rate is 146 and regular. The infant is actively moving around and has a good, strong cry. You notify the hospital of the condition of the mother and newborn and arrive 10 minutes later.

After transferring care to the emergency department staff, you complete your prehospital care report and head back to the ambulance to get it ready for the next call. On your way out of the hospital, you stop to congratulate the new father and learn from him that the newborn will be named Jacob Allen Baker.

IN REVIEW

1. List the signs and symptoms that would indicate a predelivery emergency, and describe the general guidelines for emergency medical care.
2. Describe signs that would indicate an imminent delivery.
3. Describe how to properly position a mother in active labor and how to create a sterile field around the vaginal opening.
4. Describe the emergency medical care for a patient in active labor for a normal delivery.
5. Describe how you would recognize an abnormal delivery.
6. Describe the specific steps you would take to provide emergency medical care for (a) a prolapsed cord, (b) a breech birth or limb presentation, (c) a multiple birth, (d) meconium staining, and (e) a premature birth.
7. Describe the initial care that is required for the majority (80 percent) of newborns that do not require aggressive resuscitation.
8. Describe the indications and procedures for neonatal resuscitation.

CRITICAL THINKING

You arrive on the scene and find a 23-year-old female patient complaining of contractions. She is obviously pregnant. She states she is due in 2 weeks. She is alert but uncomfortable. Her respirations are 24 per minute. Her radial pulse is 128 per minute and her skin is warm and slightly moist. She indicates the contractions began in the middle of the night, about 6 hours ago, and have progressively worsened in intensity and increased in duration. The contractions are also more frequent. This is her first pregnancy. She has no allergies, is on a beta_2 agonist metered-dose inhaler, and has a history of asthma. Her last oral intake was approximately 2 hours ago when she had two pieces of toast and some juice. She has been lying in bed because of the discomfort. She states that when she lies on her back she feels very light-headed. Her blood pressure is 108/62 mmHg and her SpO_2 is 98% on room air. Upon inspection, you note the vaginal walls and perineum are bulging and the infant's head is present at the vaginal opening. You note the sheets are soaked in fluid, and there is a light green tarry substance in the fluid.

1. What signs would lead you to believe the labor is true labor and not Braxton-Hicks?
2. Why is she experiencing light-headedness?
3. How would you proceed with the emergency care of the patient?
4. What signs are indicative of imminent delivery?
5. What is the significance of the green substance in the fluid on the sheets?

PEARSON

EXPLORE mybradykit™

Please go to **www.bradybooks.com** to access mykit for this text. You will find quizzes, critical thinking scenarios, weblinks, animations, and videos related to this chapter—and much more. Look for online information on pregnancy, labor, and delivery.

Register your access code from the front of your book by going to **www.bradybooks.com** and selecting the mykit links.

CHAPTER 38

Pediatrics

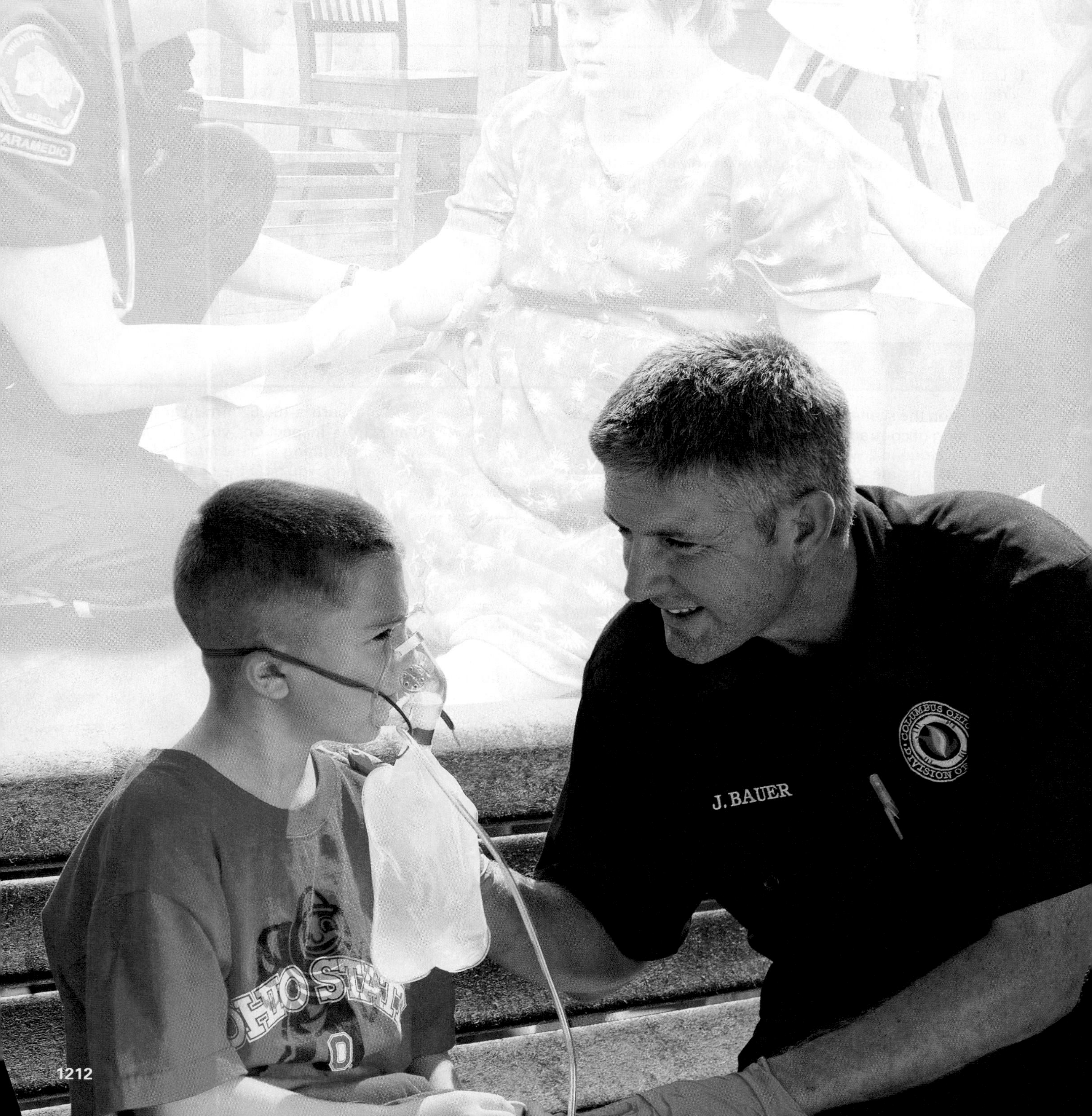

Navigation Guide

The following items provide an overview to the purpose and content of this chapter. The Standard and Competency are from the new National EMS Education Standards.

STANDARD **Special Patient Populations** (Content Area: Pediatrics)

COMPETENCY Applies fundamental knowledge of growth, development, and aging and assessment findings to provide basic emergency care and transportation for a patient with special needs.

OBJECTIVES: After reading this chapter, you should be able to:

38-1. Define key terms introduced in this chapter.

38-2. Explain the special considerations in dealing with the caregiver of a sick or injured child.

38-3. Describe the major developmental characteristics and modifications of patient assessment and management techniques recommended for patients in each of the following age groups:
- **a.** Neonates
- **b.** Infants
- **c.** Toddlers
- **d.** Preschoolers
- **e.** School-age children
- **f.** Adolescents

38-4. Describe the major anatomical and physiological differences in children with regard to the following:
- **a.** Airway
- **b.** Head
- **c.** Chest and lungs
- **d.** Respiratory system
- **e.** Cardiovascular system
- **f.** Abdomen
- **g.** Extremities
- **h.** Metabolic rate
- **i.** Skin and body surface area

38-5. Discuss the normal vital signs for children in various age groups.

38-6. Use the Pediatric Assessment Triangle (PAT) to determine a pediatric patient's status.

38-7. Discuss special considerations for the following elements of the pediatric secondary assessment:
- **a.** Physical exam
- **b.** Vital sign assessment
- **c.** History taking

38-8. Recognize signs of respiratory distress, respiratory failure, and respiratory arrest in pediatric patients.

38-9. Discuss the guidelines for emergency care of the following:
- **a.** Respiratory emergencies
- **b.** Foreign body airway obstruction

38-10. Describe the presentation and emergency medical care for pediatric patients with the following conditions:
- **a.** Croup
- **b.** Epiglottitis
- **c.** Asthma
- **d.** Bronchiolitis
- **e.** Pneumonia
- **f.** Congenital heart disease
- **g.** Shock
- **h.** Cardiac arrest

38-11. Explain the assessment steps and emergency care protocol for a respiratory or cardiopulmonary emergency in the pediatric patient.

38-12. Describe the presentation and emergency medical care for pediatric patients with the following conditions:
- **a.** Seizures, including status epilepticus
- **b.** Altered mental status
- **c.** Drowning
- **d.** Fever
- **e.** Meningitis
- **f.** Gastrointestinal disorders
- **g.** Poisoning
- **h.** Apparent life-threatening emergencies (ALTE)
- **i.** Sudden infant death syndrome (SIDS)

38-13. Describe special considerations in the scene size-up, emergency medical care, and assisting family members in case of suspected SIDS and the importance of the presence of parents during pediatric resuscitation.

38-14. Integrate consideration of a pediatric patient's size and anatomy into the assessment of mechanisms of injury.

38-15. Demonstrate removal of a pediatric patient from a child car seat.

38-16. Demonstrate proper spinal immobilization of a pediatric patient.

38-17. Explain the importance of injury prevention programs to reduce pediatric injuries and deaths.

38-18. Discuss the purpose of the federal Emergency Medical Services for Children (EMSC) program and the concept of family-centered care.

38-19. Discuss factors that can increase EMS providers' stress on pediatric calls and ways of managing the stress that may be associated with a pediatric call.

continued

KEY TERMS: Page references indicate first major use in this chapter. For complete definitions, see the Glossary at the back of the book.

MEDIA RESOURCES: Please go to www.bradybooks.com to access mykit for this text. You will find quizzes, critical thinking scenarios, weblinks, animations, and videos related to this chapter—and much more. Look for online information on infant dehydration, child maltreatment, and child behavior disorders.

CASE STUDY

The Dispatch

EMS Unit 101—respond to 24313 South Avenue for an 11-month-old infant—unknown medical emergency. Time out is 1651 hours.

Upon Arrival

As you turn onto the busy street, you see a man frantically waving at you and pointing to the residence. You position your ambulance in front of the house, out of traffic flow. The man, who you assume to be the infant's father, is almost in tears as he says to you, "Oh god—please hurry, something is wrong with Jason. I don't think he's breathing." Almost simultaneously, the mother bursts out of the front door running toward you, carrying an infant in her arms. She runs to you, crying, and thrusts the infant into your arms. Every fiber in your body tightens as you realize the infant is blue, limp, and not breathing.

How Would You Proceed to Assess and Care for This Patient?

During this chapter, you will learn about special assessment and emergency care considerations when dealing with pediatric patients. Later, we will return to the case and apply the procedures learned.

Introduction

Nearly 45,000 children die in the United States each year. Approximately one in four children will sustain an injury during their childhood that requires medical attention. Trauma is the leading cause of fatal injuries in children under the age of 14, particularly motor vehicle crashes, drowning, burns, poisonings, and falls. Of medical problems, respiratory problems are the most serious.

If asked, experienced EMS providers would probably concur that dealing with infants and children is one of the most (if not the most) stressful situations they encounter. This is mainly due to the relative infrequency of dealing with pediatric patients, the particularities of assessment and treatment, and having to deal with the emotions of the pediatric patient and the distressed parents as well as their own feelings. In spite of the stress of pediatric calls, however, as an EMT you must be able to keep your emotions from interfering with the task at hand: assessing and treating the young patient.

While your assessment approach to the ill or injured child will be somewhat different from your approach to an adult, the basic treatment goals are the same. Most of the emergency care will focus on managing the airway, ventilation, oxygenation, and circulation. The difference from treating adults is that, for most conditions in the pediatric patient, the time to intervention is an even more critical factor in the morbidity and mortality of the condition.

Dealing with Caregivers

When a child is critically ill or injured, you may have more than one person to care for. The parent or other caregiver may also need attention. Some caregivers are calm, cooperative, and even helpful (especially if they are experienced).

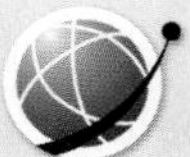

Media Resources
Go to www.bradybooks.com for mykit. Highlights:

- *Web Resource:* Shaken Baby Syndrome
- *Web Resource:* Infant Dehydration
- *Web Resource:* Maternal and Child Health Bureau

Objective 38-2
Explain the special considerations in dealing with the caregiver of a sick or injured child.

Objective 38-3
Describe the major developmental characteristics and modifications of patient assessment and management for various age groups.

Others may be perceived by the EMT as a hindrance. It is not uncommon for a caregiver to be upset, to cry, to blame himself, or to get mad at someone—even you. You need to listen carefully and remain nonjudgmental. While taking the history and inquiring about the circumstances of the event, let caregivers verbalize their emotions. Conclude with something brief and supportive like, "Thanks for telling me this. We'll do the very best we can for Susie." Remember that calm, supportive interaction with the child's family is in the child's best interest: calm caregivers = a calm child; agitated caregivers = an agitated child.

Emotionally distressed caregivers need to see that you are competent, calm, and confident. Do not allow yourself to display doubt or indecision, which would certainly reduce their confidence in you.

In addition to the guilt, anger, concern, and apprehension that caregivers may be feeling, be aware that caregivers may not understand emergency medical procedures. Keep the caregiver informed about what you are doing and about the condition of the child. Usually it is best to keep your language jargon free, but use your judgment. Some caregivers, especially if they are professionals or highly educated, may feel more reassured if you use technical terminology. Do not lie to the caregiver. If the child is very seriously injured, do not say "Everything will be OK." A false reassurance like this is not only unethical, it will make matters worse when the true condition of the child is revealed.

You will probably need to question the caregivers and other witnesses to get a history of the incident. Ask the caregivers how the child normally acts and whether a particular characteristic you may discover during assessment is normal for this child. While caregivers typically don't have medical training, they are experts on what is normal for their child; listen to what they say. If possible, enlist their help in treating the child—allowing them to hold the child, when appropriate, or assist in administering oxygen. This approach allows the caregivers to feel that they are participants in their child's care, not just bystanders.

Dealing with the Child

Developmental Characteristics

What you can expect from a pediatric patient depends to some degree on age. Many growth and development considerations come into play. Children can be classified in the following age groups:

Neonate—a child from birth to 1 month of age
Infant—a child from 1 month to 1 year of age
Toddler—a child between 1 and 3 years of age
Preschooler—a child between 3 and 6 years of age
School-age child—a child between 6 and 12 years of age
Adolescent—a child between 12 and 18 years of age

The reason for becoming familiar with this classification is simple. Each age group has specific emotional and physical characteristics that may complicate assessment and treatment. Of course the children within each age group are not all alike, but knowing the general characteristics of the group can help you to develop a strategy for assessment and care.

Be aware, however, that pain is difficult to assess in most of these age groups. Young children often lack the body awareness and vocabulary to describe the location and nature of the pain they are experiencing. Pain, especially when accompanied by bleeding, is usually so frightening that they cannot separate the emotional component from the physical. Ask the caregivers, if possible, how the child usually responds to pain to get some idea of how typical the reactions are. It is important to realize that all patients feel pain, even the neonate and young infant. Be considerate when providing emergency care to all age groups when pain is or may be involved.

Neonates (Newborn to One Month of Age)

Newborn babies are totally dependent on others for their survival. Although neonates are a subgroup of infants, the first month of life is a very different time as far as growth and development are concerned. Birth defects (or congenital anomalies) and unintentional injuries are common causes of emergencies in this age group.

Infants (1 Month to 1 Year of Age)

Up to 6 months, babies will usually let you undress them, lay them on a warm, flat surface, and touch them with warm hands and equipment (stethoscope, splints, and so on) (Figure 38-1*). Infants can recognize their caregiver's face and voice and are emotionally tied to that person. Older infants (>6 months) will be distressed and almost always cry if separated from their caregiver, a response commonly referred to as "stranger anxiety." Complete your

Key Points
As for adults, emergency care for children will focus on the airway, ventilation, oxygenation, and circulation, but the time to intervention is an even more critical factor for children.

Key Terms
neonate an infant from birth to 1 month of age.

Key Points
When a child is critically ill or injured, the parent or other caregiver may also need attention.

Key Terms
infant a child from 1 month to 1 year old.
toddler a child 1 to 3 years of age.

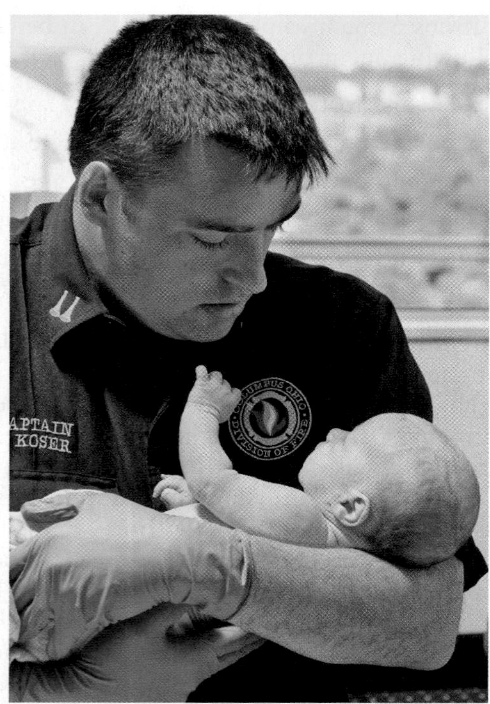

FIGURE 38-1 ✱ Up to 6 months of age, babies are usually not afraid to let the EMT handle them.

scene size-up and primary assessment as thoroughly as possible while you view the infant from across the room. Then, if possible, allow a familiar person to hold the baby while you complete your examination unless the infant is critically injured or ill. Your assessment should start with the feet or the trunk and end with the head if the infant is not critically ill or injured. Initial stimulation around the highly sensitive area of the face will frighten infants and small children and may precipitate extreme anxiety and crying.

Toddlers (1 to 3 Years of Age)

Toddlers may be more challenging to assess than infants and neonates. They have numerous "do not like . . ." considerations that will challenge your skills:

- They do not like to be touched, so limit your touch to necessary assessment and management needs.
- They do not like to be separated from their caregiver. If possible, the caregiver should be present and in view of the toddler at all times (Figure 38-2✱).
- They do not like having their clothing removed. You should therefore remove the clothing (as necessary), examine, and replace the clothing. (It's a good idea to enlist the help of the caregivers in this.)
- They do not like having an oxygen mask over their face. To them it is frightening and noisy, and they will resist it. (Alternative methods of oxygen administration are discussed later in this chapter.)
- They do not like needles, they fear pain, and they may actually believe that the injury or illness they have is a punishment. It is not uncommon to have an injured, crying child apologize for being hurt.

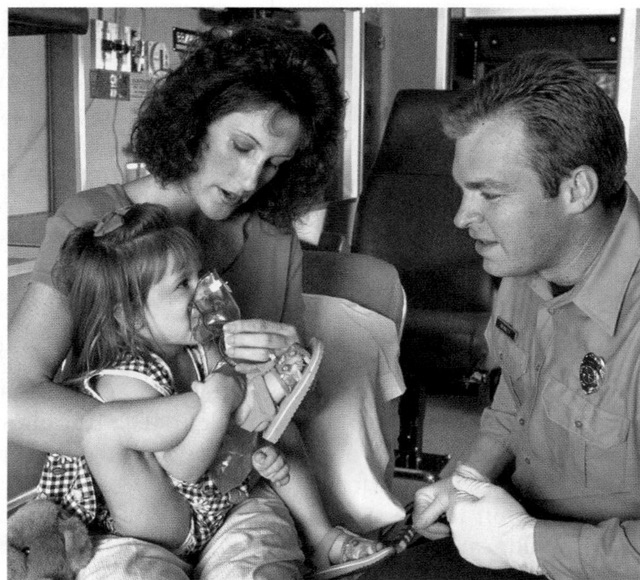
FIGURE 38-2 ✱ Toddlers do not like to be separated from their caregiver.

Remain calm, speak soothingly, and try to distract the child with a favorite toy or somehow engage his interest. Decide which parts of the physical assessment are essential and get through them as best you can. Also, try using a toe-to-head or trunk-to-head approach when performing your secondary assessment for the stable toddler. Since this group is often reliant on security objects such as a stuffed toy or blanket, try to allow the toddler to take this object with him.

Sometimes reducing the number of ways you are assessing the anxious child can help—look but don't touch, touch but don't look, talk but don't look or touch, and so on. Hypersensitive, anxious children or children in pain may be able to handle only one modality (tactile, visual, or auditory) at a time, and reducing the number of modalities you use at different times in your assessment can help

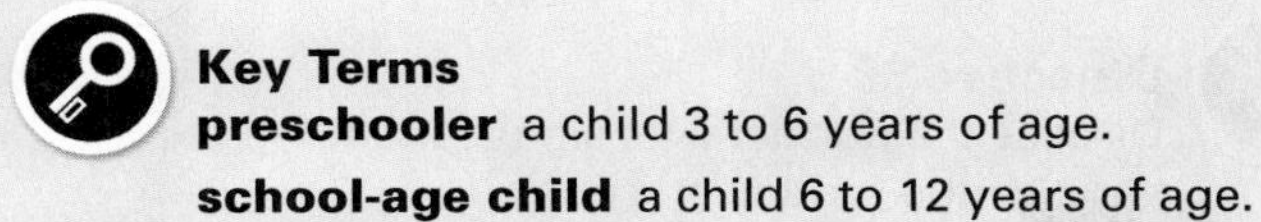
Key Terms
preschooler a child 3 to 6 years of age.
school-age child a child 6 to 12 years of age.

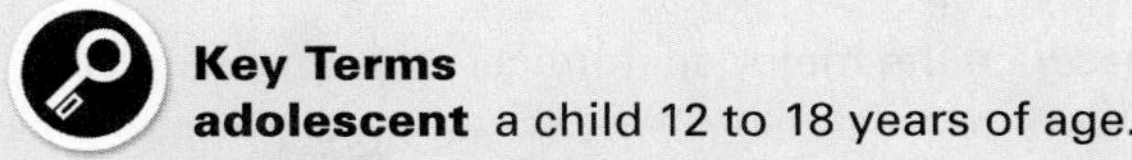
Key Terms
adolescent a child 12 to 18 years of age.

ease their anxiety. For instance, listening to the chest with your stethoscope but not looking directly at or talking to the child can help. Respect their "space" and think of your exam as an intrusion. Earn their respect and they will engage you and even help you; if you disrespect the child, watch out—the "terrible twos" are called that for a reason.

Preschoolers (3 to 6 Years of Age)

Children in this age group have concrete thinking and interpret literally what they hear. At the same time, they have vivid imaginations and are able to dramatize events. They still believe that an illness or injury is their own fault and will view it as punishment. They are modest, resisting your attempt to unclothe them for assessment. While their vocabulary is larger, they may still confuse common words. You should explain medical procedures slowly and in simple terms they can understand: "Now I'm going to press on your tummy to see if everything's okay. Tell me if it hurts." Or, "Now I'm going to shine my light in your eyes." Allow the child to see your equipment in full view before you use it, if possible, and let the child touch the stethoscope or other equipment. Put it first on the child's leg or the caregiver's hand so that the preschooler can see it is not threatening. If you use a stethoscope with a rubber ring on the diaphragm, it will not be as cold.

Have a caregiver present, if possible. Have the caregiver hold the child in his lap if the child is not critically ill or injured. Otherwise, the child will almost certainly squirm, thrash, and even try to run away. If necessary, set a few ground rules: "It's okay to cry. I know this hurts. But biting and kicking are not okay."

Children these ages are aware of death and are afraid of pain, blood, and permanent injuries. They also fear loss of body integrity. Be tactful and direct in dealing with physical fears. Cover bleeding injuries as soon as possible. Explain the obvious: "Your arm is hurt, but it can be fixed. We'll take you to the hospital where they can help fix you." Be sensitive to a child who is toilet trained and becomes overwhelmed by a bowel or bladder accident brought on by the illness or injury. Let the child hold his security object.

School-Age Children (6 to 12 Years of Age)

Usually children from age 6 on are more cooperative, even curious. They are able to rationalize. This age group can be the easiest to manage, because most school-age children have an understanding of what EMS is about.

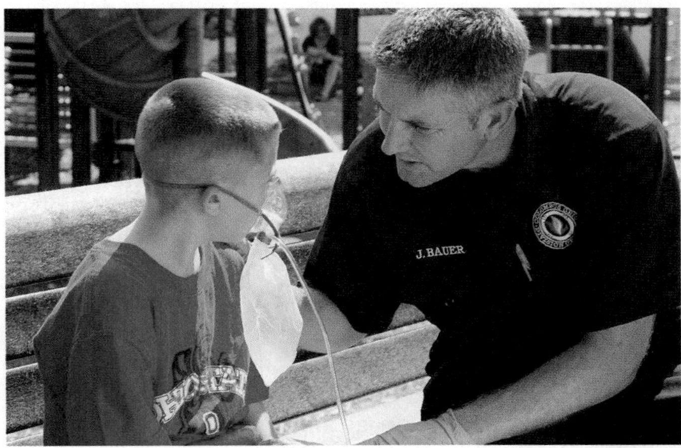
J. BAUER

FIGURE 38-3 * School-age children like to be informed about what is going on.

They understand that you are there to help them. They also have a simple understanding of their body. It is easy to engage their interest in the procedures or your equipment. They will be fascinated by the contents of each cabinet in the ambulance. However, keep in mind that an illness or injury may cause children to regress emotionally. A 6-year-old may throw a temper tantrum like a 2-year-old after an injury. On the other hand, the child may act exceptionally mature. Maturity levels are highly individualized and variable at this age.

Honesty is very important with school-age children. Treat them with respect and try to make them partners in their care. Information is reassuring to them and may need to be repeated until they understand, so explain each procedure in detail using appropriate language (Figure 38-3*). Concerns about death and disability emerge at this age.

Children this age and even younger know that they need to take care of what they are wearing and sometimes get very anxious if you cut their clothes. Modesty and body image also are issues at this age. Explain gently but firmly, "I need to cut this sleeve off so that I can look at your arm." Be aware that pain, the sight of blood, permanent injuries, and disfigurement are still real fears for them. Take advantage of their increased vocabulary skills by explaining their physical injuries.

Adolescents (12 to 18 Years of Age)

Adolescents use concrete thinking but are developing their abstract thinking skills. Children in this age group

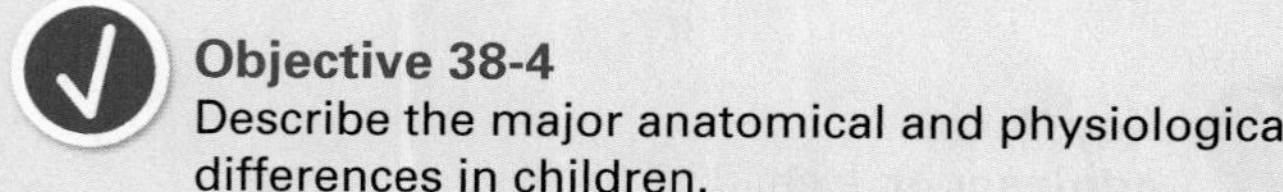
Objective 38-4
Describe the major anatomical and physiological differences in children.

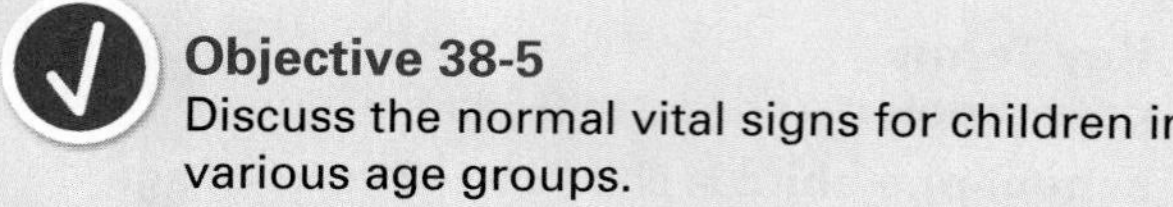
Objective 38-5
Discuss the normal vital signs for children in various age groups.

generally believe that nothing bad can happen to them or, in other words, that they are invincible. They may take risks that lead to trauma. However, if injured or ill, they will still fear the possibility of disability and disfigurement.

Some experts suggest using a relaxed, rather than a professional, approach when performing a history and secondary assessment—especially if the situation involves conflict with an authority figure such as a teacher, police officer, or caregiver. If the adolescent is critically ill or injured, a rapid and systematic approach to assessment and emergency care is necessary.

Asking the same questions to the adolescent when he is alone with you may generate very different answers than when he is with an authority figure. Smile, speak softly, and speak slowly. If the adolescent trusts you, he will be more likely to give you truthful information. Most adolescents, either patients or their peers, will be reluctant to disclose information about their sexual history, drug use, personal habits, and illegal activities; ask for only the information that you need, and explain why you need it. Sometimes the presence of a peer, caregiver, or close friend is both physically and emotionally reassuring. Acknowledge the patient's friends, and allow them to help by notifying caregivers, holding equipment, and so on. You may need to explain to the patient that it is all right to react to pain, since you need to know what hurts.

Adolescents are preoccupied by their bodies and extremely concerned about modesty. An injury intensifies this preoccupation. They may ask about their greatest fears—for example, whether a facial cut will leave a scar or whether a broken leg signals the end of their basketball career. Be honest—up to a point. If available, have a same-sex provider conduct examinations of the genital area. Such exams are rarely necessary in the prehospital setting, generally required only when there is severe bleeding from the genital area. When it is necessary, if at all possible save this exam for last.

Occasionally you may encounter an adolescent who appears to be overreacting to the illness or injury. This age group is capable of hysterical reaction and may become involved in "mass hysteria." Be tolerant of this reaction and try not to get caught up in it or become angry.

Anatomical and Physiological Differences

As mentioned earlier, most emergencies involving children are managed similarly to those involving adults experiencing the same emergency. However, there are certain modifications you may need to make based on the anatomical and physiological development of children. For the average, normally developing child, the following considerations are appropriate. For an infant or child with special health care needs, the anatomical and physiological differences may be quite different from the norm and using the caretaker to help with the assessment is critical. When you are treating a child, be aware of some of the following special conditions and situations. Also be aware that the most significant of these differences typically concern the airway (Figure 38-4*). There are various charts that identify ranges of normal vital signs for pediatric patients. A rough estimate of a normal heart rate, respiratory rate, and systolic blood pressure is listed in Table 38-1. Pediatric blood pressures will be discussed in greater detail later in the chapter.

Airway

- *Infants have proportionally larger tongues* than adults as compared to the size of the mouth. You need to carefully assess the airway in a child with an altered mental status because it is easy for his airway to become occluded by his tongue. Also, the larger tongue leaves little room for airway swelling.
- *The diameter of a newborn's trachea is only about 4 to 5 mm, or about one-third the diameter of a dime, or the size of a straw,* compared to 20 mm for the adult trachea. Injury and inflammation to the trachea (caused by inhaling steam or toxic fumes, for example) can cause life-threatening airway swelling not only faster but with less exposure to the fumes/gas/steam than in an adult.
- *The pediatric trachea is much more pliable than the adult trachea* because children's tracheal rings are underdeveloped (with the exception of the first tracheal ring). The increased pliability of the trachea may lead to complete or partial occlusion of the airway when the neck is hyperextended or hyperflexed or when infants are working hard to breathe.
- *Pressure on the soft tissue under the chin can easily cause the tongue to be displaced* back into the pharynx, leading to an airway obstruction. Pressure on the soft tissue may occur during the chin-lift or jaw-thrust maneuver when opening or maintaining an airway.
- *Newborns and infants are obligate nose breathers.* That is, they prefer to breathe through their nose and not

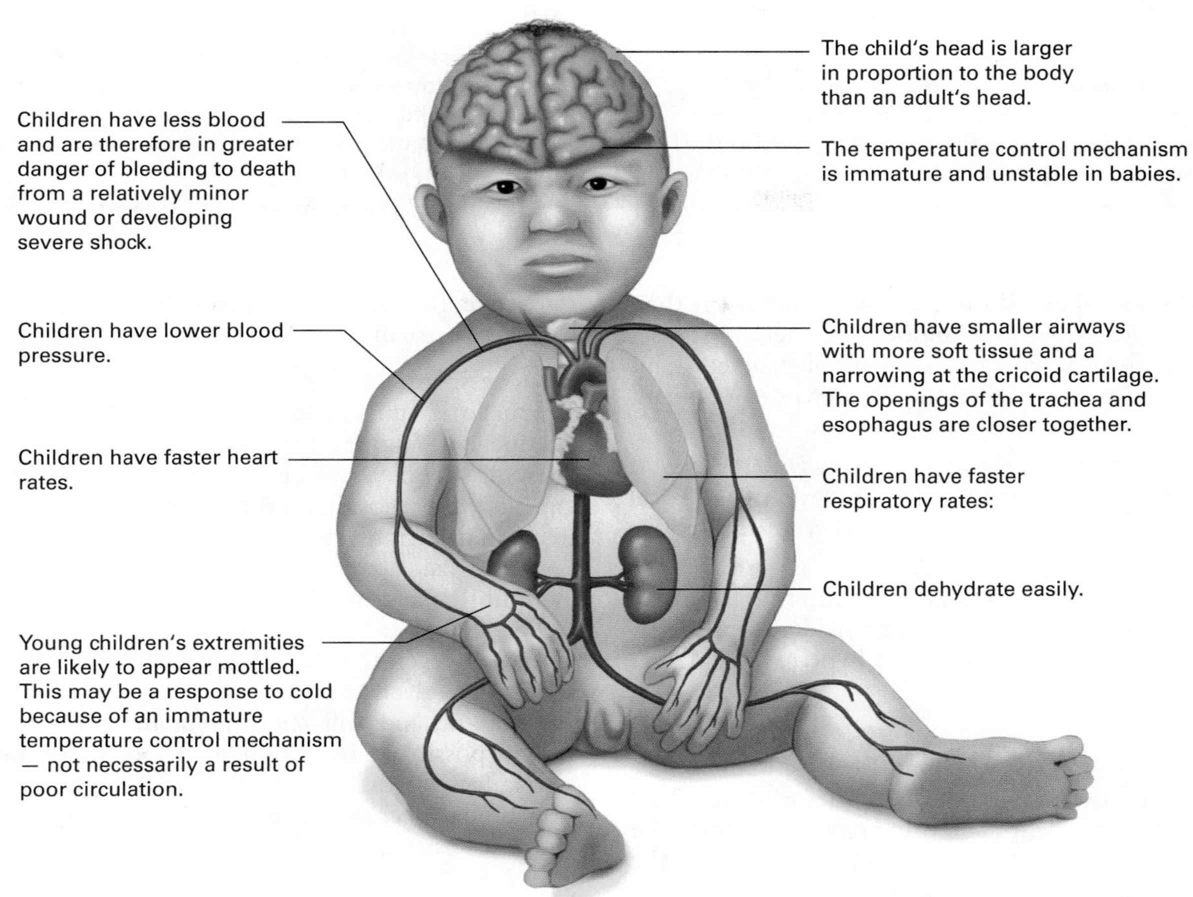

The child's head is larger in proportion to the body than an adult's head.
The temperature control mechanism is immature and unstable in babies.
Children have less blood and are therefore in greater danger of bleeding to death from a relatively minor wound or developing severe shock.
Children have lower blood pressure.
Children have smaller airways with more soft tissue and a narrowing at the cricoid cartilage. The openings of the trachea and esophagus are closer together.
Children have faster heart rates.
Children have faster respiratory rates:
Children dehydrate easily.
Young children's extremities are likely to appear mottled. This may be a response to cold because of an immature temperature control mechanism — not necessarily a result of poor circulation.

FIGURE 38-4 ✱ Anatomical and physiological considerations in the infant and child.

TABLE 38-1 Estimated Normal Pediatric Heart Rate, Respiratory Rate, and Systolic Blood Pressure

Age	Heart Rate	Respiratory Rate
Newborn to 1 year	140 bpm	40/minute
1 year to 4 years	120 bpm	30/minute
4 years to 12 years	100 bpm	20/minute
Older than 12 years	80 bpm	15/minute
Age	**Systolic Blood Pressure**	
Newborn to 1 month	60 mmHg	
1 month to 1 year	70 mmHg	
1 year to 10 years	Lower limit of normal: 70 mmHg + (2 × years of age) Median normal: 80 mmHg + (2 × years of age) Upper limit of normal: 90 mmHg + (2 × years of age)	
Older than 10 years	90 mmHg	

Note: The *diastolic* BP for 1 year to 10 years of age can be calculated as 2/3 the *systolic* BP estimated by the formulas given above.

Source: Adapted from Inaba, A.S. (2002). A simple way to remember pediatric vital signs. *Contemporary Pediatrics, 19,*16.

Key Terms

fontanelle the "soft spot" on the top of an infant's head where the bony plates of the skull have not yet fused together.

Key Points

Assessment of the fontanelle is difficult to perform and not very accurate. To identify a possible increase in intracranial pressure it is much more important to recognize a decreased mental status.

their mouth. They do not automatically open their mouth when secretions, blood, or other substances obstruct their nose. If the nares are obstructed or inflamed because of infection, the newborn or infant can easily develop respiratory distress.

- *The smallest area of the upper airway is at the level of the cricoid cartilage* and not at the level of the vocal cords as seen in the adult. This is true until about 6 years of age.
- *The epiglottis is much higher in the airway* than in an adult. This may lead to a higher incidence of aspiration, especially when the neck is hyperextended.

Head

- *Children's heads are proportionally larger than adults'.* This predisposes them to head injuries when involved in falls, auto accidents, and other types of trauma. The large occiput (back) of the child's head causes the neck to flex forward if the child is supine on a flat surface. To prevent this during immobilization, the EMT should place a small amount of padding under the shoulders to maintain neutral alignment of the airway and cervical spine (Figure 38-5*). Until a child's body proportionately catches up with the head at approximately 8 or 9 years of age, padding is necessary. Adult dimensions are reached at about age 10.
- *Infants younger than 6–7 months old typically cannot fully support their own heads.* Always support a baby's head when you pick him up.
- *Infants have a "soft spot" on the head* from incomplete closure of the skeletal plates that make up the skull. Typically, the anterior soft spot (anterior **fontanelle**) closes between 12 and 18 months of age. The posterior soft spot (posterior fontanelle) closes by 2 months of age. Be careful when handling an infant not to press on or poke into the fontanelle.

Assessment of the fontanelle—to determine if the fontanelle is sunken, indicating dehydration, or if the fontanelle is bulging, indicating increased pressure within the skull—is not very accurate and may be difficult to perform in the prehospital setting. To identify a possible increase in intracranial pressure, it is much more important to recognize a decreased mental status. (It is often thought that because the skull is not completely fused together, an infant can tolerate higher intracranial pressures. However, if the swelling is acute—that is, with a rapid onset, over hours to days—the dura will not allow the swelling and will result in brain compression.) To identify possible dehydration, it is more important to recognize tachycardia and mottling as well as the caregiver reporting a decrease in tear production and urination (fewer wet diapers).

Chest and Lungs

- *The child's ribs are much more pliable than the adult's.* This means that the rib cage cannot protect the internal organs as effectively. While this flexibility decreases the likelihood of rib fractures, it increases the likelihood of internal organ damage with blunt trauma to the chest.
- *The child's ribs are more horizontal than they are rounded.* The horizontal nature of the ribs allows very little leverage to increase the anterior and posterior diameter of the chest. This prevents the degree of lift that is necessary for an attempt to increase the volume of air within the chest. Thus, the child must rely much more on the diaphragm to compensate for changes in demands on breathing.

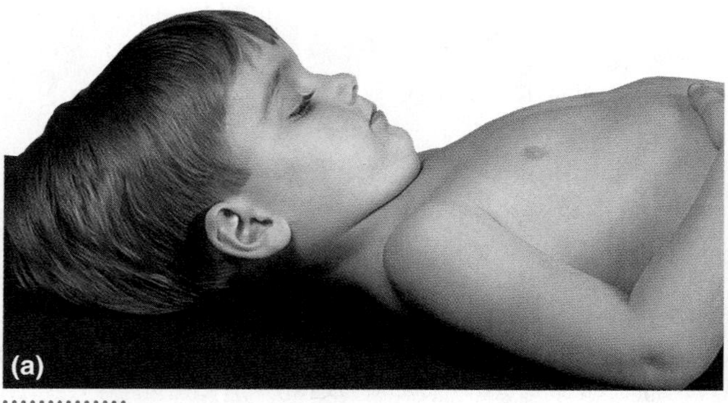

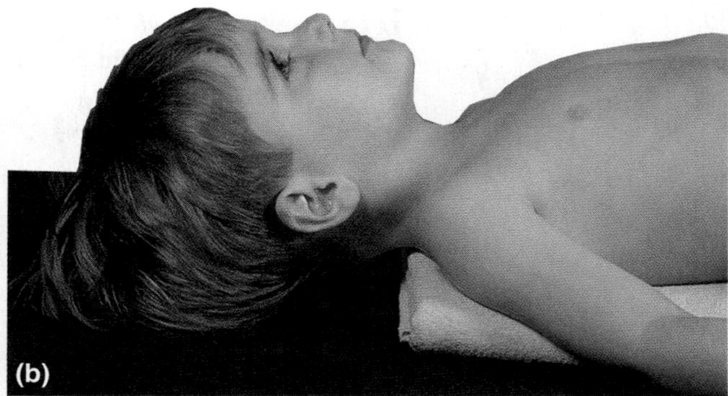

FIGURE 38-5 * **(a)** When a child is supine, the head tilts forward. **(b)** Pad behind the shoulders to maintain airway alignment.

- *Lung tissue is much more fragile,* which may lead to a higher incidence of pulmonary contusion with blunt trauma to the chest.
- *The chest will move minimally with respiration* in the healthy child, because of the immaturity of the ribs and flexibility of the rib cage. *It is normal for the abdomen to rise with inhalation and the abdomen to fall with exhalation.*
- *The chest muscles are underdeveloped and used more as accessory muscles* in infants and young children. This leads to early retractions in respiratory distress. Intercostal muscle retractions (between the ribs) will be seen in mild respiratory distress. Suprasternal (above the sternum), supraclavicular (above the clavicles), and sternal retractions would indicate a more severe respiratory distress.

The combination of the compliant chest wall, smaller airways, and diaphragm dependence means that infants' lungs are prone to collapse. Since infections can cause both airway swelling and increased secretions in the airways and lungs, infants typically "grunt" to try to keep their airways and lung units open. They do this by closing off their vocal cords ("laryngeal braking") and bearing down abdominally at the end of inspiration to try to restore or maintain a positive pressure in their lungs to prevent collapse. Try it and see how long you can do it yourself; it's exhausting.

Respiratory System

- *The breathing is inadequate once the respiratory rate reaches 60 breaths per minute or greater in children.* If the respiratory rate begins to decrease, it may be an indication of respiratory failure.

  Infants may have episodes of apnea in response to stress. Parents may report that their infant stopped breathing for a short period of time and turned blue. This is a very concerning sign and should prompt a rapid transport.
- *Infants and children less than 5 years of age will breathe at a rate two to three times faster than the adult patient.* The breaths are also shallower than in the adult, since less volume and pressure are required to ventilate the lungs.

  The muscles of the diaphragm in the infant are prone to fatigue. Since this is the primary muscle of respiration, working to breathe is very costly. The oxygen consumed by the infant who is working to breathe may not be there to supply other organ function. Typically this infant is too lethargic or tired to respond appropriately. This lack of "attitude" or normal behavior signifies a very ill infant who needs advanced care immediately.

Cardiovascular System

- *The heart rate increases in response to fear, fever, anxiety, hypoxia, activity, and hypovolemia.*
- *In infants and children, bradycardia is a late response to hypoxia. In newborns, bradycardia is the initial response to hypoxia.*
- *Infants and children have a smaller circulating blood volume than adults* because of their smaller size. This means you must stop any bleeding as quickly as possible, since what would be a comparatively small blood loss in an adult would be a major hemorrhage for a child.
- *Hypotension will not usually develop in infants and children until greater than 30 percent of the blood volume has been lost. The onset of hypotension is sudden once the compensation falls.*
- *Infants and young children have a limited ability to increase the strength of cardiac contraction.* When adults experience cardiovascular compromise, they compensate by increasing the heart rate and the strength of the cardiac contraction and through vasoconstriction. The infant or child does not have the ability to compensate by increasing the strength of cardiac contraction. The pediatric patient's cardiac compensation primarily consists of changes in the heart rate and an increase in the degree of peripheral vasoconstriction—increasing systemic vascular resistance—as evidenced by mottling of the skin and cool extremities. As with the adult patient, the pediatric patient's blood pressure is based on cardiac output and systemic vascular resistance ($BP = CO \times SVR$).

Abdomen

- *The child's abdominal musculature is less well developed than the adult's,* increasing the likelihood of internal organ damage with blunt trauma to the abdomen.
- *Until the child reaches puberty, the liver and spleen are more exposed and less protected* by the ribs in the abdominal cavity. This offers less protection to the organs against injury.

Extremities

- *The bones of the extremities in a child fracture more often by bending and splintering* (referred to as a greenstick fracture).
- *The infant and young child's motor development occurs from the head to the toes.* The head is one of the first things the infant can control. The lack of coordination leads to frequent injury from falls.

Metabolic Rate

- *Infants and children have a much faster metabolic rate, even at rest.* The cells in their bodies use oxygen and glucose from the bloodstream two to three times faster than in adults, and periods of apnea (absence of breathing), hypoventilation (depressed breathing), or poor oxygenation can be more dangerous. Central nervous system damage can occur more quickly, with

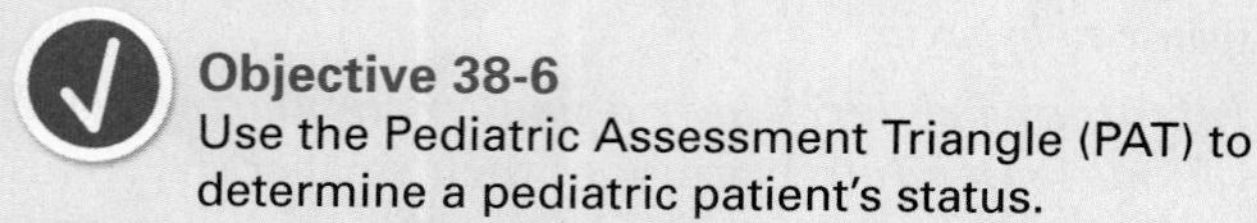

Objective 38-6
Use the Pediatric Assessment Triangle (PAT) to determine a pediatric patient's status.

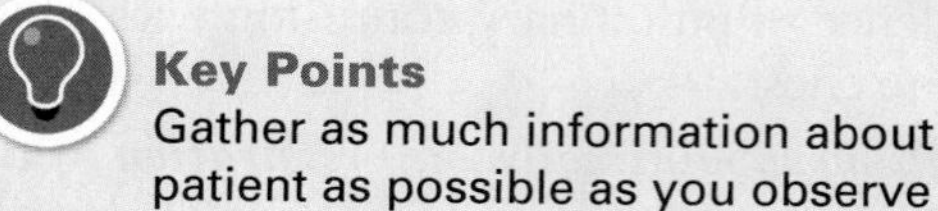

Key Points
Gather as much information about the young patient as possible as you observe him from across the room.

more serious injuries affecting respiratory function, resulting in poor ventilation and/or oxygenation. This explains why the pediatric patient exhibits signs and symptoms of carbon monoxide poisoning earlier than the adult patient.

- *Pediatric patients are at a significant risk for the development of acute hypoglycemia* because of any of these: (1) poor glucose stores, (2) inability to stimulate the release of glucose stores from an immature liver, (3) an increased metabolic rate, resulting in the utilization of large quantities of glucose, or (4) a known history of diabetes. Indications of hypoglycemia in the pediatric patient may include twitching, seizures, limpness, eye rolling, apnea, or irregular respirations. The onset of the signs and symptoms of hypoglycemia is rapid and, as a result, requires rapid intervention to prevent cerebral injury.

Skin and Body Surface Area

- *A child's skin surface is large compared to his body mass,* making children more susceptible to hypothermia in cold environments. You should take great care in protecting the young patient from extremes in the environment.
- *The skin is thinner and much more delicate than in an adult.* There is much less subcutaneous tissue. Less subcutaneous tissue along with a poorly developed hypothalamus leads to temperature regulation problems and hypothermia in newborns. The lack of subcutaneous tissue also leads to a higher incidence of hypothermia in infants and young children.

Assessment-Based Approach to Pediatric Emergencies

Scene Size-Up

The first component of the assessment process is the scene size-up. As with the adult patient, take the necessary Standard Precautions prior to assessment. The scene size-up can provide many clues to the nature of the emergency, the initial status of the infant or child, and obstacles that may hamper extrication to the ambulance. Determine if the pediatric patient is a medical or trauma patient, if there is only one patient, and if any additional resources are needed at the scene.

Determine if the scene is safe for you to enter. The EMT may believe that because the call involves a child there will be no threat to EMS providers (as compared to a bar fight, auto accident, or unknown medical emergency). Never get a false sense of security that the scene will be safe. The child may be a victim of violence that is ongoing or can erupt again, adults at the scene may be prone to hysterical or violent responses because of the stress of the emergency, or the child may have fallen victim to a poison or hazardous substance that can also affect EMS workers and others at the scene. Keep in mind that safety is a dynamic condition that must be constantly considered while you are at the scene.

Primary Assessment

The key to pediatric assessment is the quick identification and management of immediate life threats. This is even more true for pediatric than for adult patients, because children can deteriorate very quickly.

The components and flow of the primary assessment for the pediatric patient are:

- Forming a general impression using the Pediatric Assessment Triangle (PAT)
- Assessing the level of consciousness (AVPU)
- Airway assessment
- Breathing assessment
- Circulatory assessment
- Priority determination

Pediatric Assessment Triangle (PAT)

Remember that infants and young children may not have the mental capabilities to recognize or understand why someone unknown to them (the EMT) is coming toward them intently. You may scare them to a point where they become agitated, cry, and resist your assessment efforts. Therefore, your primary assessment should begin "at the doorway." You should gather as much information about the young patient as possible as you observe him from across the room, while he is interacting with his caregiver and environment and has possibly not yet noticed or reacted to your presence.

This assessment of the patient's general condition, done in only a few moments as you scan the environment, should be guided by the parameters of the Pediatric Assessment Triangle.

The Pediatric Assessment Triangle (PAT), which was developed by the American Academy of Pediatrics, is integrated into the general impression portion of the primary assessment for the pediatric patient. The PAT evaluation tool is used to quickly identify a "sick" child in order to provide immediate intervention during the primary assessment. The PAT is a visual assessment that you make as you approach the child and without using any palpation or auscultation.

This tool can quickly provide valuable information about the child's condition while exhausting little time and with minimal contact that might upset the child and alter vital signs and other critical findings. Time is critical with pediatric patients, and the PAT is effective in identifying, *at the start of the assessment process*, a child who requires immediate intervention. (Naturally, if you see signs of impending respiratory arrest or other life-threatening conditions, you will begin treatment immediately.) Further assessment will be done as you progress through the primary assessment of the airway, ventilation, oxygenation, and circulation status.

The three sides of the Pediatric Assessment Triangle (PAT) (Figure 38-6*) represent the three most critical parameters of the general impression:

- *Appearance*
- *Work of breathing*
- *Circulation to skin*

The following are characteristics to assess under each PAT category:

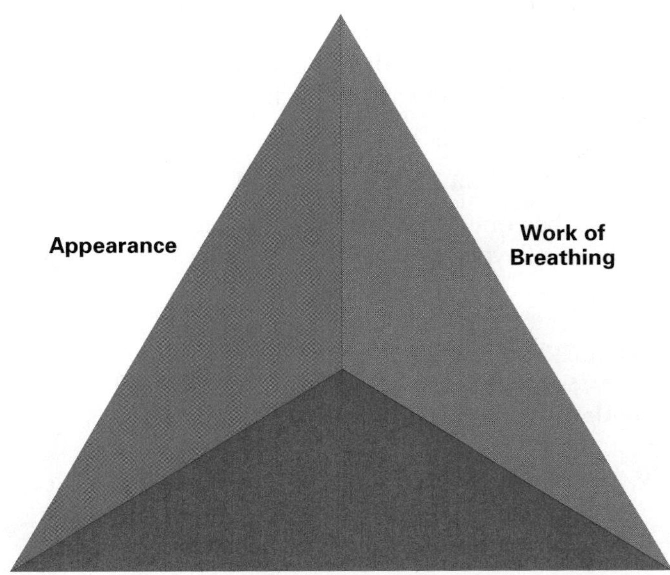

FIGURE 38-6 * The Pediatric Assessment Triangle (PAT). (Used with permission of the American Academy of Pediatrics)

Appearance

- **Tone.** Assess for muscle tone, movement of child, resistance to examination, limpness, listlessness, and flaccidity.
- **Interactivity and irritability.** Assess for alertness; reactivity to an object, sound, or person; grasp and play with a toy or exam equipment; and disinterest in the environment and people at the scene.
- **Consolability.** Assess for the child's ability to be consoled by the parent or primary caregiver.
- **Look or gaze.** Assess for a fix or gaze on a face, a glassy-eyed stare, or the look as if "nobody is home."
- **Speech or cry.** Assess for the strength of crying, sound of the crying, or speech pattern and content in older children.

These characteristics to assess for on the appearance side of the triangle can be remembered by using the mnemonic TICLS (pronounced "tickles"). If the child has good muscle tone, is interacting appropriately with the environment, is not irritable, can be consoled, responds to stimuli and people, and has a normal cry, he can be assumed to have a "normal" appearance. This typically indicates an adequate airway, ventilation, oxygenation, and brain perfusion.

Irritability is typically one of the first signs of poor brain perfusion. The irritability will often lead to lethargy and then unresponsiveness. If the child is sleeping and wakes to a stimulus, becomes irritable and shakes, and reverts immediately to sleep when the stimulus is removed, you should suspect poor brain perfusion. A high-pitched cry is associated with brain injury. The glassy-eyed look is often seen in brain injury or infection.

Work of Breathing

- Abnormal sounds—stridor, grunting, snoring, wheezing, hoarseness
- Abnormal posture or position—sniffing, tripod position, refusal to lie down
- Retractions
- Nasal flaring
- Head bobbing

Listen for abnormal airway sounds without a stethoscope and from a distance. Once the child begins to cry, the assessment of breathing becomes more difficult. Grunting typically indicates collapsing bronchioles or fluid-filled alveoli. Stridor is indicative of upper airway edema or partial obstruction. Muffled speech or hoarseness also typically indicates swelling to the laryngeal tissue. Listen to determine if wheezing is occurring in both the inspiratory and expiratory phases of breathing. In an airway obstruction the child typically assumes a sniffing position. The tripod position is assumed by the child in order to fully use the accessory muscles in respiratory distress or failure. Retractions indicate accessory muscle use and an increase in the work of breathing. Remember, abdominal breathing in young infants is typically normal; however, seesaw breathing (in which extreme respiratory effort draws the chest inward and forces the abdomen outward) is always abnormal. Nasal flaring with head bobbing indicates a significant increase in work of breathing. Rapid breathing with no increase in work of breathing may be an indication of compensatory or decompensatory shock. Irregular respirations are often associated with an increase in intracranial pressure.

When the child transitions from respiratory distress to respiratory failure, you might find that the work of breathing and the respiratory rate both decrease. If the decrease in work of breathing and respiratory rate is due to effective emergency care, you would expect to see an improvement in the appearance side of the triangle. However, if the decrease in work of breathing and respiratory rate is due to exhaustion and respiratory failure, you would expect to see a deterioration in the appearance side of the triangle.

Circulation to Skin

- Pallor—Assess skin and mucous membranes
- Mottling
- Cyanosis
- Petechiae—Assess for small pinpoint hemorrhages to the skin

Assess the skin visually. Pale skin with tachycardia indicates compensated shock. As the perfusion further deteriorates (shock develops), the skin will become mottled, which is an ominous sign. Cyanosis usually indicates respiratory failure or decompensated shock. Cyanosis may be seen in children with congenital heart defects and chronic cardiac or pulmonary disease.

Pediatric Assessment Triangle Application and Interpretation Use the PAT—your observations of the overall appearance, work of breathing, and circulation to skin—to form a general impression as to whether this is a "well" versus a "sick" child. Does the patient:

- Display normal behavior for his age (as discussed earlier)?
- Move about spontaneously? (or) seem lethargic?
- Appear attentive and recognize the parents or caregivers?
- Maintain any eye contact (appropriate for the patient's age)?
- Seem easily consoled by the parents or caregiver? (or) seem inconsolable?
- Respond to the parent or caregiver calling him? (or) respond inappropriately? (or) not respond at all?

A relatively "well" baby will be interactive with both the caregiver and the environment, be actively moving, have good color, and have a good, strong cry. Although noisy and upsetting at times, a crying baby is (at least) a breathing baby. A "sick" baby at first sight will be limp or flaccid, have a weak or absent cry, not interact with the environment or parents, possibly have poor skin color, and not seem to notice your approach.

The following conditions will present with these normal and abnormal PAT findings:

- **Respiratory distress.** Normal appearance, abnormal work of breathing, and normal circulation to skin
- **Respiratory failure.** Abnormal appearance, abnormal work of breathing, and normal or abnormal circulation to skin
- **Compensated shock.** Normal appearance, normal work of breathing, and abnormal circulation to skin
- **Decompensated shock.** Abnormal appearance, normal to abnormal work of breathing, and abnormal circulation to skin
- **Poor brain perfusion or brain injury.** Abnormal appearance, abnormal work of breathing, and abnormal circulation to skin
- **Cardiopulmonary failure.** Abnormal appearance, abnormal to absent work of breathing, and abnormal circulation to skin

After forming the general impression using the PAT, proceed with the remainder of the primary assessment by assessing level of consciousness, airway, breathing, and circulation.

Assessing the Level of Consciousness (AVPU)

Following the general impression using the PAT, you must assess the child's level of consciousness (EMT Skills 38-1A). The simplest method for determining the level of consciousness in a pediatric patient is the AVPU scale (Table 38-2). It is a variation of the adult AVPU scale.

Airway Assessment

The number one cause of death in children is hypoxia. One cause of hypoxia is an obstructed airway. When open-

TABLE 38-2 AVPU Scale in the Pediatric Patient

A (Alert)	Infant or child is curious, alert, and awake.
V (Verbal response)	Infant or child turns head to sounds.
P (Painful response)	Infant or child moans or cries to pain.
U (Unresponsive)	Infant or child does not respond or displays no activity.

ing and assessing the airway, keep the pediatric anatomical and physiological differences in mind (EMT Skills 38-1B).

Breathing Assessment

In adults, we often evaluate respiratory rates for 15 seconds and multiply those rates by 4. However, normal respirations in an infant can be irregular. The variability of respiration rates in infants may not produce an accurate rate when only observed for 15 seconds. For this reason, respiratory rates should be assessed over a minimum of 30 seconds but ideally over 60 seconds.

It is also important to note that the normal variable rate of respiration in infants may include cessation in breathing for up to a maximum of 20 seconds. Any cessation in breathing for greater than 10 seconds, however, should be considered abnormal and require intervention. True apnea is defined as cessation of breathing for 15 seconds or longer, but many pediatric experts will not wait for that duration to diagnose respiratory failure in the very young infant.

As with the adult, tidal volume must also be assessed to determine if the breathing is adequate. Inspect for chest rise and listen for air movement. If the respiratory rate or tidal volume is inadequate, begin positive pressure ventilation with supplemental oxygen connected to the ventilation device.

During your primary assessment, you should be acutely aware of alterations in the respiratory effort (EMT Skills 38-1C). Respirations can be counted by watching the chest rise or by placing your hand on the patient's abdomen. Adequate breathing can be assessed by watching for rise and fall of the chest at the child's clavicles. Assess the abdomen for rise and fall, since young children use the abdominal muscles to breathe. Because the clavicles are the highest point of the chest (and the last to fill with air), movement there signifies good expansion of the lung.

Because of the importance of the respiratory system in successful management of the infant or child, be alert for the following as clues to the infant or child's airway and respiratory status: rapid breathing, noisy breathing, and diminished breathing.

- **Rapid breathing.** As a general rule, children breathe faster than adults. The key to recognizing rapid breathing is to be familiar with normal ranges of respirations (25–30 per minute in an infant; 15–30 per minute in a child) and to repeat assessment of respiratory rate frequently, each time counting the rate over a complete minute. In cases of rapid breathing (tachypnea) look for breathing through the mouth, flaring of the nostrils, retractions, and/or the use of accessory muscles. Also check for cyanosis around the mouth and changes in mental status. Possible causes of rapid breathing are:
  - Oxygen deficiency (hypoxia)
  - Head injury
  - Lung infection
  - Fever, which raises the metabolic rate, increasing the need for oxygen
  - Diabetes, when glucose levels get very high
  - Aspirin overdoses and other forms of poisoning
  - Stress, pain, or fear
  - Shock
- **Noisy breathing.** Children may breathe more loudly than adults through the nose and, occasionally, through the mouth because of anatomical differences. Check with a caregiver if you hear an unusual sound to determine whether it is normal. When assessing breath sounds with a stethoscope, listen along both midaxillary lines (below the armpits). This is necessary since breath sounds typically transmit easily from one side of the child's small chest to the other. Listening midaxillary or down the back will reduce the amount of sound you are hearing that is transmitted from the opposite side. The following is a checklist of sounds characteristically produced by certain problems:
  - *Coughing, gagging, or gasping* will be violent when the child breathes in a foreign body or body secretions, creating a partial blockage of the airway. (If blockage is complete, however, there will be no cough or gasp.)
  - *Crackles* (sometimes called rales), sounds that resemble the noise of rolling a few strands of hair near the ear, are commonly heard on listening to chest sounds when certain respiratory diseases have caused fluid to accumulate in and around the alveoli.
  - *Wheezing* is caused by air moving at a high rate through narrowed bronchioles during exhalation, is more "musical" than crackles, and may sometimes be a whistle. Wheezing sounds are caused by medical emergencies that cause narrowing of the lower airway (or bronchospasm) and can also be caused by aspiration of blood, vomitus, or foreign objects. Wheezing is usually only heard on exhalation.

ASSESSMENT Tips

If wheezing in a sick child resolves without any medication administration, this should concern you. It often implies that the child, instead of getting better, has actually worsened and is no longer moving enough air to create the wheezing sound. ■

  - *Stridor* (as discussed earlier) is a harsh, high-pitched sound that occurs typically during inspiration. It results from severe obstruction in the upper airway, as in the case of swelling to the larynx. Because stridor occurs only with upper airway problems, if it is absent, the cause is more likely to be an emergency involving the lower portions of the airway.
- **Diminished breathing.** When something (blood, fluid, or air) prevents the lungs from inflating, there is a loss of breath sounds. The causes of diminished

breathing can include obstruction, medical problems, or traumatic injuries like a pneumothorax (air in the chest cavity, collapsing one or both lungs). Consider providing positive pressure ventilation to the infant or child if breath sounds are not obvious.

Circulatory Assessment

Like pediatric respiratory rates, pediatric heart rates are variable. Pulse points are the same in children as they are in adults, but there are some differences in the way these pulses are evaluated. In small children, it is recommended that peripheral pulses be obtained at the brachial artery (inside of the bicep) (EMT Skills 38-1D). Central pulses may be obtained at either the carotid or the femoral artery (EMT Skills 38-1E). In the older child, check the radial pulse (EMT Skills 38-1F). Compare the strength of the central (carotid or femoral) pulse to the strength of the peripheral pulse (EMT Skills 38-1G). If no pulses can be palpated, the EMS provider should consider auscultating the heart with a stethoscope. If a heartbeat can be heard, the child likely has a pulse, but the presence of a pulse does not mean that there is adequate perfusion.

Capillary refill time is typically quite an accurate measurement in children and is considered to be reliable in most cases. Healthy children do not have the vascular disease that many adults do, so the child's capillary blood flow is very responsive. However, just as in the adult patient, environmental factors such as cold ambient temperatures can influence pediatric capillary refill times. For this reason, capillary refill time should be assessed closer to the core in areas like the kneecap or forearm (EMT Skills 38-2A to 38-2D). Normal capillary refill time is under 1–2 seconds. You must evaluate the pulses, skin, blood pressure, urine output, and mental status to determine if hypoperfusion and shock exist. Capillary refill alone cannot provide conclusive evidence of hypoperfusion and shock, but it is one of the best measures we have available.

Other circulation assessment parameters include the following:

- Pulse rate and strength—Infants and children maintain cardiac output by adjusting the heart rate. Although there can be many reasons for tachycardia in the child (e.g., fever, pain, hypoxia, anxiety), you cannot exclude a compensated shock state and must assume the potential for decompensation when tachycardia is present.
- Strength of peripheral versus central pulses—Weak or absent peripheral pulses typically indicate poor perfusion status, a decrease in cardiac output, and shock.

ASSESSMENT Tips

Weak or absent peripheral pulses typically indicate poor perfusion status or a decrease in cardiac output. Shock must be suspected in this case. ■

- Warmth and color of the hands and feet.
- Urinary output—A sign of the adequacy of kidney perfusion (ask if there have been more or fewer diaper changes than normal).
- Mental status—Poor mental status may indicate poor cerebral perfusion and may be another indication of shock.

Priority Determination

From the information you have gathered thus far, you need to make a determination (based on your scene size-up and primary assessment, including your general impression using the Pediatric Assessment Triangle, whether the patient should be a priority for immediate transport. *Any patient with signs and symptoms of early respiratory distress, decompensated respiratory failure, respiratory arrest, or poor perfusion should be considered a priority patient.*

Secondary Assessment

For the secondary assessment, follow the guidelines from the earlier section "Dealing with the Child" as well as the tips for examining infants and children listed in Table 38-3, adapting them to the patient's age and condition. If it is a medical emergency, gather the history first, then perform the physical exam including baseline vital signs. If it is a trauma emergency, perform the physical exam and gather vital signs before obtaining the history. If two EMTs are working together, some of these steps can be performed simultaneously.

Complete the history, using the OPQRST mnemonic if pain is identified during your assessment. If the developmental age of the patient allows, the EMT should gather this history from the patient and confirm it with the bystanders or caretaker; if not, question the family or bystanders. While gathering the history, find out if any care or treatment has been rendered already and, if so, whether it was effective. Remember to ask if all shots and immunizations are up to date.

When performing the physical exam on an infant or young child, you should follow a toe-to-head or trunk-to-head approach. This means you will assess the extremities and core of the patient's body prior to the head. Although this is age- and situation-dependent, it allows you to gather the most physical exam information while, at the same time, increasing the infant's or child's anxiety level as little as possible. If the child is older or is unresponsive, you can follow the traditional head-to-toe assessment format performed in the adult patient to identify any life threats as early as possible (EMT Skills 38-3A to 38-3M).

If this is a medical problem and the patient is responsive, you may perform a focused medical assessment, concentrating on the areas related to the problem. If trauma is suspected or the patient is unresponsive or unable to

Objective 38-7
Discuss special considerations for the pediatric physical exam, vital sign assessment, and history taking.

TABLE 38-3 Ten Tips for Examining Infants and Children

When examining an infant or child . . .

1. If possible, have only one EMT deal with the infant or child. This reduces the fear the patient may experience by being assessed by two unknown individuals.
2. Get down to the child's eye level. Towering above an infant or child will only increase his fear and anxiety. Sit down next to the child whenever possible.
3. With children under school age, start the assessment with your hands and save stethoscopes, blood pressure cuffs, and scissors until you have developed some trust with the child. Keep the most painful parts of the examination for the end.
4. Speak in a calm, quiet voice and maintain eye contact as much as possible. Even infants will respond to a calm voice, and an apparently unresponsive child may actually hear much of what you say.
5. Never become impatient or lose your temper. This will just ignite the patient's temper. Switch off with a partner or take a brief time-out for yourself, if you need to.
6. Avoid questions that require "yes" or "no" answers. Given the choice, a child will almost always say "no" when asked if you can do something to him. Instead, ask questions in this format: "Would you like your mother to take off your shirt, or may I do it?" Giving the child a choice also empowers him in what may be a very scary situation.
7. Involve the caregivers (or a familiar person) as much as possible during care and transport. If the child sees his caretaker respecting and trusting you, he is much more likely to do the same.
8. Be honest. For instance, you might say, "It will hurt when I touch you here, but it will only last a moment. If you feel like crying, it's okay." Children can tolerate some pain if they are prepared for it and are given adequate support.
9. Ask children for their help and assure them that they are doing a good job. Have toys, stickers, or other "rewards" to console and encourage a child.
10. Be gentle. Use all appropriate measures to reduce the amount of pain that a child must endure. If you must restrain a child, be sure that it is absolutely necessary. Use only the minimum degree of restraint to be safe and allow you to provide good care. As a general rule, "humane" (soft) restraints are much better than "mechanical" ones.

communicate clearly, perform a complete rapid secondary assessment. Since injuries present the same in adults and children, you will be looking for the same indicators of injury. Assess each anatomical area and body system.

Special Considerations for the Physical Exam

The same anatomical regions and body systems are assessed in the secondary assessment of the pediatric patient as in the adult. However, the steps may be altered, depending on the age of the child and his condition. Some of these accommodations were previously mentioned, such as doing a toe-to-head assessment on the pediatric patient. Other special pediatric considerations are discussed in the next sections.

Pediatric Glasgow Coma Scale (PGCS)

The standard Glasgow Coma Scale (GCS), used to determine and quantify the level of consciousness in adults, must be modified for the noncommunicative child. For this purpose, the Pediatric Glasgow Coma Scale (PGCS) has been developed (see Table 38-4).

Assessing Lung Sounds

One of the most common techniques for assessing the lungs is auscultation. Auscultating lung sounds in a child should ideally be conducted in a relatively quiet environment and should take into consideration that the child has a small and thin chest wall. Lung sounds should be auscultated in the midaxillary region (below the armpits) to ensure that referred breath sounds are not heard. Referred breath

TABLE 38-4 The Pediatric Glasgow Coma Scale

	> 1 Year	< 1 Year	
Eye opening	4 Spontaneous	Spontaneous	
	3 To verbal command	To shout	
	2 To pain	To pain	
	1 No response	No response	
	> 1 Year	**< 1 Year**	
Best motor response	6 Obeys		
	5 Localizes pain	Localizes pain	
	4 Flexion-withdrawal	Flexion-withdrawal	
	3 Flexion-abnormal (decorticate rigidity)	Flexion-abnormal (decorticate rigidity)	
	2 Extension (decerebrate rigidity)	Extension (decerebrate rigidity)	
	1 No response	No response	
	5 Years	**2–5 Years**	**0–23 Months**
Best verbal response	5 Oriented and converses	Appropriate words and phrases	Smiles, coos, cries appropriately
	4 Disoriented and converses	Inappropriate words	Cries
	3 Inappropriate words	Cries and/or screams	Inappropriate crying and/or screaming
	2 Incomprehensible sounds	Grunts	Grunts
	1 No response	No response	No response

sounds are sounds that can be transmitted from one side of the chest to another. Hearing referred breath sounds in children is possible because the child's thin chest wall is capable of transmitting sounds easily.

Pulse Oximetry

The use of pulse oximetry in children is highly recommended and often very reliable. Just as with vital signs, pulse oximetry readings can be monitored over time to detect worsening or improvement of the patient's condition after interventions. Be cautious about using pulse oximetry for anything other than noting trends in the patient's condition. Rely on the entire patient presentation and not just a single SpO_2 reading when doing your assessment.

A pulse oximetry reading of greater than 95% is generally adequate. If a child cannot maintain a saturation above 95% on room air, the child will require supplemental oxygen. If the child's saturation remains below 95% on a nonrebreather mask, this is an indication that the child is experiencing consistent hypoxia and probably a ventilation or oxygenation compromise. If the child were removed from the nonrebreather mask, it is likely that the SpO_2 reading would deteriorate further. Closely and continuously assess the child's mental status as well as the respiratory effort, rate, and depth.

If the child deteriorates to respiratory failure, immediately begin positive pressure ventilation with supplemental oxygen connected to the ventilation device. A child may still be sick despite an adequate pulse oximetry reading. Treat the patient, not the SpO_2 reading, especially in children with congenital heart problems. If the child looks sick, he likely is sick and requires intervention.

Pulse oximetry has limitations. As a result of shock or hypothermia, peripheral perfusion may be diminished, resulting in low or absent saturation readings. Movement, a constant issue with children, ambient light, and nail polish can also lead to poor readings.

Other Physical Exam Considerations

Other special considerations for the physical exam include the following:

- Infants and many children are unable to cough "productively," especially when they are quite sick or tired from an increased work of breathing.
- Look at the interest of the child in the situation to determine the mental status and level of orientation. The greater the interest, the better the mental status. When an infant is very irritable and cannot be comforted by the parent or caregiver, it may be an indication of an altered mental status. Rely on the parent or caregiver to provide information about the child's normal alertness and activity level.
- Hoarseness can indicate a partial upper airway obstruction. Moaning may indicate shock or a decreased

mental status. An increase in intracranial pressure may produce a high-pitched cry in the infant.

- An anxious child with nasal flaring who is very focused on his breathing is probably in respiratory distress.
- Grunting may indicate severe respiratory distress. By grunting, the infant or child prematurely closes the epiglottis over the glottic opening. This traps air inside the terminal bronchioles and alveoli, not allowing the structures to collapse. If the airways did collapse after each exhalation, the next inhalation—which must move air through the bronchioles and into the alveoli—would require much more effort and the infant or child would fatigue rapidly from the increased work of breathing. Thus grunting is an attempt to keep the airway structures open and make the next breath the infant or child takes less work. Grunting is typically seen with labored breathing. A child in respiratory distress who is no longer grunting is in impending respiratory failure and must be transported immediately.
- Obtain the respiratory rate prior to examining the child, since your touching the child will cause anxiety and an increase in the respiratory rate.
- The heart rate normally increases when the child takes in a breath and decreases with exhalation.
- The blood pressure cuff must cover at least two-thirds the circumference of the arm and two-thirds the width (length of the bone). The blood pressure can be taken at the upper arm, lower arm, or thigh. Use the blood pressure cuff where it fits. In children less than 3 years of age, the blood pressure is difficult to assess and is often not accurate. Rely on the quality and rate of the pulses, comparison of the strength of the central and peripheral pulses, and skin temperature, color, and condition as well as mental status and capillary refill to assess cardiovascular status in children less than 3 years of age.
- To estimate the normal systolic blood pressure in a child who is 1 to 10 years of age, take 80 + (2 × age in years) for the median average systolic blood pressure limit. The diastolic pressure should be approximately two-thirds of the systolic pressure.
- Hypotension (low blood pressure) indicating shock would be a systolic blood pressure less than 60 mmHg in a newborn (neonate 0–28 days), less than 70 mmHg in an infant (1–12 months), less than 70 + (2 × age in years) in a 1- to 10-year-old child, and less than 90 mmHg in a child older than 10 years.
- To estimate the upper limit of a normal systolic blood pressure for a child between 1 and 10 years of age, you would take 90 + (2 × years in age). See Table 38-5.
- Children 3 years of age and older will obey your commands to move fingers, squeeze fingers, wiggle toes, or push up against your hands when you are doing the neurological exam. It is easiest to make the assessment into a game to gain the most cooperation from the child.

TABLE 38-5 Evaluating Blood Pressure in the Pediatric Patient

Neonate	Systolic BP less than 60 mmHg is considered hypotensive
Infant	Systolic BP less than 70 mmHg is considered hypotensive
Child 1 to 10 years of age	Upper limit of normal for systolic BP = 90 + (2 × age in years)
	Median systolic BP = 80 + (2 × age in years)
	Lower limit of normal systolic BP = 70 + (2 × years in age)
	Diastolic BP is 2/3 the systolic BP
Child older than 10 years	Systolic BP less than 90 mmHg is considered hypotensive

If the child is not cooperating and is crying, look at the quality (strong and full or weak and shallow) of the cry; inspect for the presence of tears in the eyes (no tears may indicate severe dehydration); assess the color, temperature, and condition of the skin; auscultate the breath sounds in between the cries when the child gasps for a breath; and inspect the face for symmetry (equality on both sides).

Special Considerations for Assessing the Vital Signs

As you go on to assess the baseline vital signs in infants and children, you should be aware that, outside of heart and respiratory rates, vital signs play only a limited role in your determination of the patient's overall status. Instead, pay more attention to the general impression you developed of the child's appearance of "sickness" or "wellness." Infants and children have excellent compensatory mechanisms that delay deterioration. It is only after the exhaustion of these mechanisms that you may see indicative changes in the vital signs. By then, the changes may occur very quickly, and the child's condition typically deteriorates rapidly. Here are some special considerations for assessing the vitals:

- **Respirations.** Obtain the respiratory rate at regular intervals, based on techniques and normal ranges discussed earlier.
- **Pulse.** It is very difficult to feel a carotid pulse in infants and toddlers. To assess circulation, use the radial pulse in a child and the brachial pulse in an infant. (Review EMT Skills 38-1D.) Still another alternative is the femoral pulse near the crease between the pelvis and thigh in an infant. (Review EMT Skills 38-1E.)

  Another means of assessing heart rate is by auscultation of the apical pulse (at the apex of the heart). To locate it, place your hand over the fourth or fifth intercostal space on the left midclavicular line. Place your stethoscope here and count each "lub-dub" as one beat. This method will provide you with a heart rate, but it is not a measure of perfusion.

To evaluate circulation status you will want to compare central or core pulses with peripheral pulses. The farther away from the heart the peripheral pulse can be detected, the better the perfusion status. Another technique is to manually compare core and peripheral skin temperatures at the time of the pulse check. As overall perfusion decreases, the peripheral extremities will be significantly cooler than the central areas.

- **Skin.** Check skin color (e.g., pink, blue, flushed, yellow), relative temperature (the back of your hand on the patient's forehead or abdomen), and condition (dry or sweaty). Capillary refill can also be assessed.
- **Pupils.** Check for size, equality, and reactivity of pupils by shining your penlight into the eyes, especially if trauma is suspected or the patient is unresponsive. Note the extraocular movements of the eyes; they should be symmetric and smooth.
- **Blood Pressure.** Do not attempt to take the blood pressure of a child under the age of 3 years. Instead, rely on other indicators of perfusion discussed earlier. In children over age 3, be sure that you check the blood pressure with a correct-size cuff; it should cover about two-thirds of the upper arm. Do not take a blood pressure if the appropriate equipment is not available.

Special Considerations for Taking a History

History taking requires a different approach in the child than in the adult. Some valuable information may be learned from the child who provides his own history information. Additional valuable information may be gained by watching the child's reactions and activities. A history should be sought from the parent or primary caregiver until the child reaches 4 years of age. At this point, the child should be able to provide the history information relevant to the complaint or injury (Figure 38-7*). The following are special considerations when obtaining a history in a child:

- Children usually seek out the parent or caregiver for reassurance. If the child has a normal mental status but appears to not seek out the parents or caregiver when injured, consider the possibility of child abuse.
- If no life threats are present, try to gain the child's trust by allowing the child to become more familiar with you. You may use a teddy bear or doll to gain the child's trust. If the child has critical injuries or is seriously ill, however, do not waste time trying to gain trust.

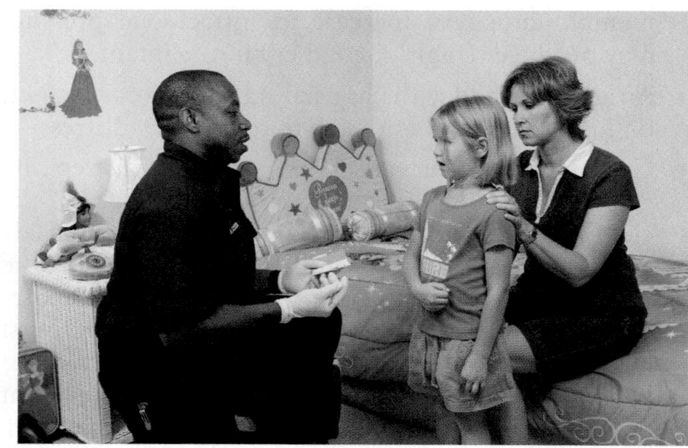

FIGURE 38-7 * After age 4, the child should be able to provide history information about the complaint or injury.

- Use a reassuring and calm voice when speaking to the child. Include the child in the conversation with the parent or caregiver, especially if the child is 4 years of age or older.
- Get down to the eye level of the child. This will reduce the "authoritarian" posture you may present when you are so much bigger than the child and make the child more comfortable and willing to provide information. Smile frequently and do not stare. Staring will threaten the child.
- Avoid rapid-fire "yes" and "no" questions. Ask the following types of open-ended questions: What happened? Are you feeling any pain? What does the pain feel like?
- Avoid certain words that increase the anxiety of the child such as *cut* (cutting implies pain, as in cutting off an arm); *take* (implies that you are taking something away, as in taking a blood pressure; say "measure" instead of "take"); or *bleeding* (children think that they will lose all of their blood).
- Keep the child with the parent during the assessment, if at all possible. This will typically reduce apprehension and may prevent the child from crying during the exam.
- Perform the secondary assessment from the feet to the head. Usually, once you start assessing the head and face the child becomes frightened and cries.
- Do not explain things too far in advance. This will cause confusion and will not be understood by the child. Explain things one step at a time.
- Let the child handle the stethoscope, penlight, blood pressure cuff, or other equipment before you use it. This will reduce the child's fear and anxiety of what the device is used for and if it will hurt.

Reassessment

The reassessment must be performed on all patients to continuously monitor for changes in mental status,

Objective 38-8
Recognize signs of respiratory distress, respiratory failure, and respiratory arrest in pediatric patients.

Key Points
Failure to properly assess, establish, and maintain the airway, ventilatory, or oxygenation status will defeat any other or subsequent treatment.

Key Terms
early respiratory distress increased respiratory effort caused by impaired respiratory function.

compensated respiratory distress *see* early respiratory distress.

airway, breathing, and circulation status (watch any patient with respiratory distress for the development of respiratory failure; remember that compensatory mechanisms fail rapidly and without warning). Also assess and record the vital signs and check interventions. Repeat the reassessment at least every 3–5 minutes or as frequently as possible for the pediatric patient with any airway or cardiopulmonary compromise. Communicate your findings and treatment to the receiving medical facility.

Airway and Respiratory Problems in Pediatric Patients

If *anything* should be emphasized when dealing with the assessment and treatment of infants or children, it is the assessment, establishment, and maintenance of the airway and respiratory function. The primary goal in treating any infant or child patient is the anticipation and recognition of respiratory problems, and to support any function that is compromised or lost. *Failure to properly assess, establish, and maintain the airway, ventilatory, or oxygenation status will defeat any other or subsequent treatment, without exception!* Make no mistakes regarding this aspect of prehospital care.

The respiratory system is responsible for providing the body with fresh oxygen for the blood as well as removing carbon dioxide and other wastes. Unfortunately, failure of this system is relatively common in pediatric patients. Failure of respiratory function can rapidly lead to cardiac arrest. In fact, *while cardiovascular disease is the leading medical cause of cardiac arrest in the adult, the leading medical cause of cardiac arrest in the infant or child patient is failure of the respiratory system.*

Compensatory mechanisms, which attempt to maintain normal physiological functioning, often run at maximum in infants and children until total exhaustion occurs, leading to rapid respiratory deterioration and cardiac arrest. Even when the primary assessment of the respiratory status appears normal, you should maintain a high index of suspicion regarding the patency of the airway and adequacy of respiratory function. Even if it seems obvious that the patient is suffering from some other form of life threat (e.g., severe hemorrhage, head injury), do not drop your guard concerning proper airway management and oxygenation.

Determining the origin of the respiratory dysfunction may not be possible in the prehospital setting, but such a determination is not necessary to initiate appropriate treatment. Focus your attention on the presenting signs and symptoms of respiratory dysfunction (the indications that there is respiratory dysfunction, without regard to what may have caused it) and provide emergency care.

It is important to recognize the difference between upper airway obstruction (from a foreign body) and obstruction caused by a respiratory infection. The methods for removing a foreign body from a pediatric patient's airway could be deadly if applied to a patient with a condition such as epiglottitis. Any attempt to put an object, such as your fingers or suction equipment, into the throat of a child with epiglottitis can cause fatal swelling or spasm. As a result of national immunization programs, the incidence of epiglottitis is now relatively low, but the fact remains that many conditions affect children differently from the way they affect adults—and the child's inability to compensate is directly related to his anatomical and physiological immaturity.

Early Respiratory Distress

If the infant or child displays the signs in the following list, but still maintains an adequate respiratory depth and rate, the patient is said to be in **early respiratory distress**, otherwise known as **compensated respiratory distress** (Figure 38-8*). *The patient in early respiratory distress is still in serious trouble. The patient can progress from early (compensated) respiratory distress to decompensated respiratory failure and respiratory arrest in minutes.* As the name implies, the infant or child is in distress but is able to compensate and his breathing has not yet failed. His respiratory rate and tidal volume are still adequate to meet his requirements. Therefore, the patient could be

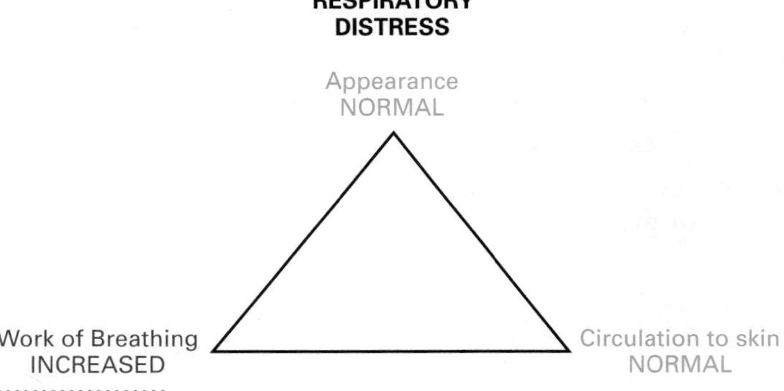

FIGURE 38-8 * Findings for a child in respiratory distress.

Key Points
The pediatric patient in early respiratory distress can progress to respiratory failure and respiratory arrest in minutes. Your ability to recognize and manage early respiratory distress is critical.

Key Terms
decompensated respiratory failure when the respiratory compensatory mechanisms have begun to fail and respiration becomes inadequate.

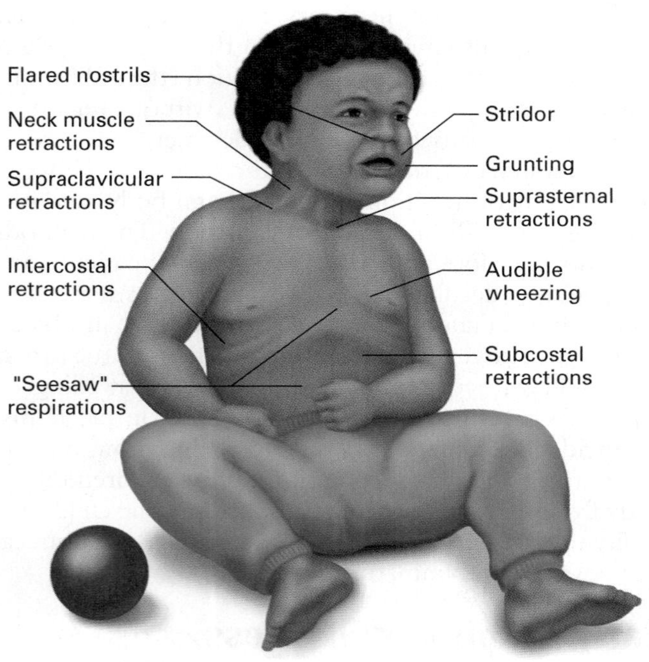

FIGURE 38-9 * Signs of early respiratory distress.

placed on a high concentration of oxygen, but assisted ventilations are not necessary because the breathing rate and tidal volume remain adequate. The following are signs of early respiratory distress (Figure 38-9*):

- An increase in respiratory rate above the normal rate for the child's age
- Nasal flaring
- Intercostal retractions on inspiration (retractions of the tissues and muscle between the ribs)
- Supraclavicular and subcostal retractions on inspiration (retractions of the tissues above the clavicles and beneath the margin of the ribs)
- Neck muscle use
- Audible breathing noises such as stridor, wheezing, or grunting
- Seesaw respirations
- An alert or easily arousable child demonstrating behavior that reflects some energy reserve, or "attitude"

If these signs are present, provide oxygen (by methods that will be described in the "Emergency Care" sections of this chapter) and prompt transport to the hospital (Figure 38-10*). If at any time the respiratory rate or the tidal volume becomes inadequate, the patient has progressed from compensated respiratory distress to decompensated respiratory failure. This patient requires immediate ventilation with a bag-valve-mask device or other acceptable ventilation device and supplemental oxygen as tolerated.

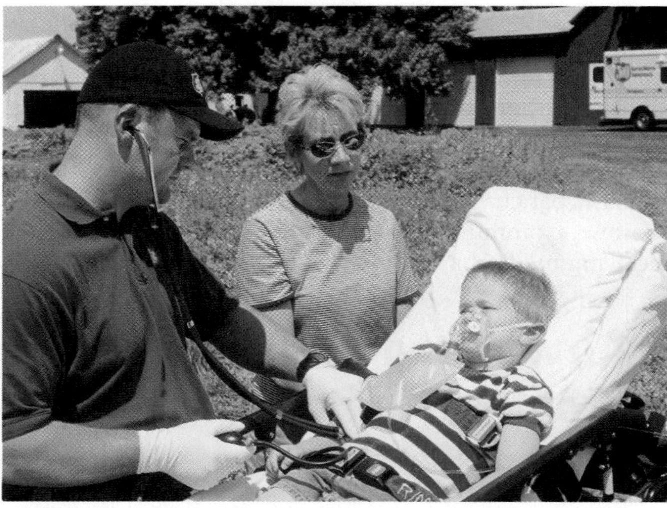

FIGURE 38-10 * If signs of early respiratory distress are present, provide oxygen and prompt transport to the hospital.

Decompensated Respiratory Failure

The EMT may also encounter an infant or child in **decompensated respiratory failure** (Figure 38-11*). As the name implies, the infant or child is failing to compen-

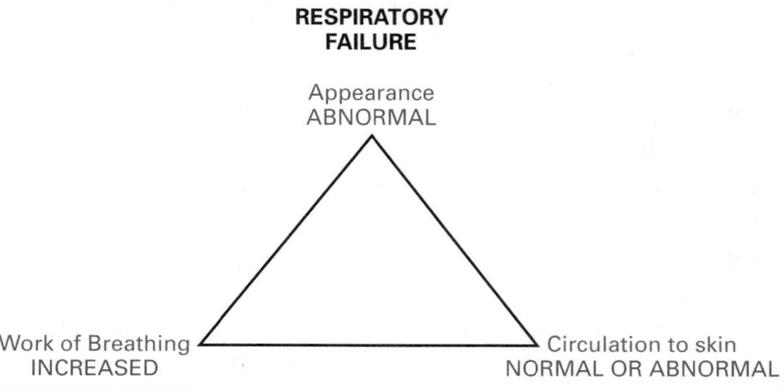

FIGURE 38-11 * Findings for a child in decompensated respiratory failure.

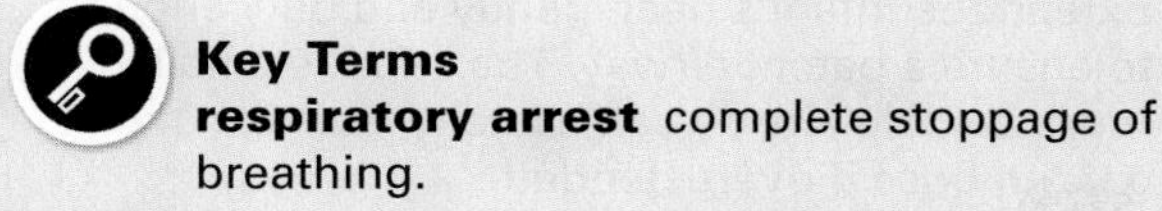

Key Terms
respiratory arrest complete stoppage of breathing.

Key Points
Since children often place things in their mouths, keep a high index of suspicion for an obstructed airway in infants and children.

sate for the impaired respiratory condition and is unable to maintain adequate breathing. Either the respiratory rate or the tidal volume is inadequate and the infant or child requires immediate intervention, which may include suctioning the upper airway, repositioning, high-concentration oxygen, delivery of nebulized therapies, or even ventilation with a bag-valve-mask or other ventilation device. Supplemental oxygen must be delivered via the ventilation device. Decompensated respiratory failure is characterized by the signs of early respiratory distress (compensated respiratory failure) that were previously listed, plus any of the following:

- Respiratory rate over 60 per minute
- Cyanosis (blue color)
- Decreased muscle tone
- Severe use of accessory muscles to aid in respirations
- Poor peripheral perfusion
- Altered mental status (in relation to the patient's developmental stage)
- Grunting (may also be present in early respiratory distress)
- Head bobbing

If these signs are present, provide positive pressure ventilation with a bag-valve-mask device or other acceptable ventilation device and supplemental oxygen and immediately transport to the hospital.

Respiratory Arrest

Respiratory arrest (Figure 38-12*) occurs when the compensatory mechanisms designed to maintain oxygenation of the blood have failed. Indications of respiratory arrest include the following:

- Respiratory rate less than 10 per minute (or absent breathing)
- Irregular or gasping respirations
- Limp muscle tone
- Unresponsiveness
- Slower than normal or absent heart rate
- Weak or absent peripheral pulses
- Hypotension (low blood pressure) in patients over 3 years of age

Remember, cardiopulmonary arrest in children is usually preceded by the progressive failure of the respiratory system. If any of the conditions listed here are present, the patient should be treated aggressively with oxygenation and positive pressure ventilation, and transported immediately to the hospital.

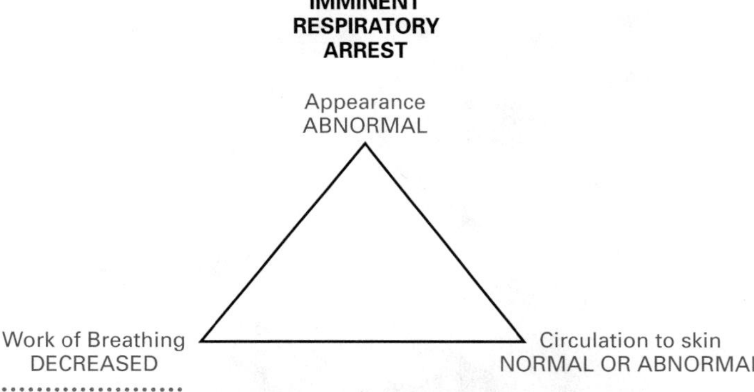

FIGURE 38-12 * Findings for a child in imminent respiratory arrest.

Airway Obstruction

The patient may also present with some type of airway obstruction, since children often place things in their mouths. Keep a high index of suspicion for an obstructed airway in infants and children, because by the time you arrive they may be in a stage of compensated or decompensated respiratory failure—possibly even respiratory arrest.

As a general rule, the presentation and treatment goals of a choking infant or child mirror those of an adult. The difference, however, is how you attempt to relieve a complete obstruction.

In a *partial airway obstruction,* some air is still getting past the obstruction. The following are indications of a partial airway obstruction:

- The patient may still be alert and pink, with peripheral perfusion.
- The skin may be normal or slightly pale with peripheral perfusion present.
- Stridor may be present (an inspiratory, high-pitched sound indicative of blockage around the level of the vocal cords).
- Retractions of intercostal, supraclavicular, and subcostal tissues may be present.
- Possible crowing or other noisy respirations may be heard.
- The patient may be crying.
- A forceful cough may still be present.

Objective 38-9
Discuss the guidelines for emergency care of respiratory emergencies and foreign body airway obstruction.

Key Points
Extend the infant's head gently and only enough to ensure a patent airway. The infant's smaller, more flexible airway can actually kink like a garden hose if overextended.

If the patient displays the signs just listed and still maintains an adequate respiratory volume, general treatment principles include allowing the patient to assume a position of comfort (except do not lay the patient down). Enlist the help of the parents or caregivers while you administer oxygen. Encourage the patient to cough if a tangible obstruction is present. Limit your exam so as not to further agitate the patient, and transport immediately.

Indications of a *complete airway obstruction* include:

- No crying or talking
- Ineffective or absent cough
- Altered mental status, including possible loss of responsiveness
- Cyanosis probable

ASSESSMENT Tips

If a child becomes cyanotic, he has experienced profound hypoxia and is in significant trouble. ■

If the patient is displaying the signs just listed and is not maintaining an adequate respiratory volume, and if there are no indications of a medical condition that might be causing the obstruction, general treatment procedures should be based on foreign body airway obstruction procedures for an infant or child. These will be discussed later under "Emergency Medical Care—Foreign Body Airway Obstruction." Treatment for specific medical conditions, some of which may cause airway obstruction, will be discussed in the next sections.

Signs and Symptoms

Signs and symptoms of a respiratory emergency require your immediate intervention, whether or not you know the exact cause of the condition. The next two sections discuss emergency medical care for respiratory emergencies in general and emergency medical care for foreign body airway obstruction.

Emergency Medical Care—Respiratory Emergencies

When any of the signs of a respiratory emergency are present, provide care as described next. For more detail on these techniques, including adaptations for infants and children, review Chapter 10, "Airway Management, Artificial Ventilation, and Oxygenation."

1. **Establish and maintain a patent airway.** If no cervical spine injury is suspected, perform the head-tilt, chin-lift maneuver, but with caution. Since the infant's airway is much smaller and more flexible, excessive hyperextension of the head can result in the airway "kinking" (like a garden hose), actually resulting in airway occlusion. Extend the head only enough to ensure a patent airway; once that point is reached, stop (Figure 38-13*). When performing a chin lift, little or no pressure should be applied to

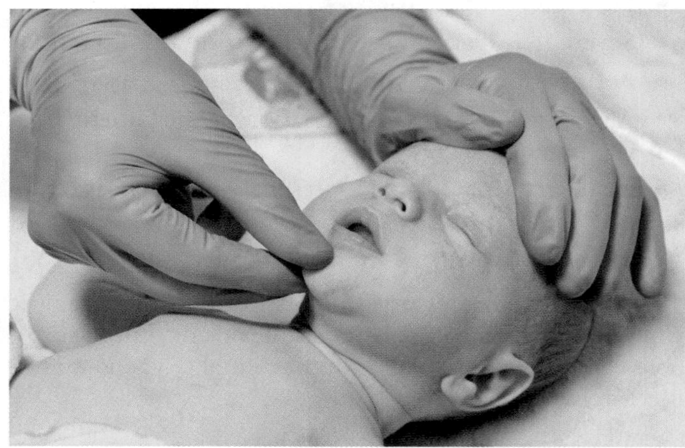

FIGURE 38-13a * Head-tilt, chin-lift maneuver in an infant. Avoid overextension.

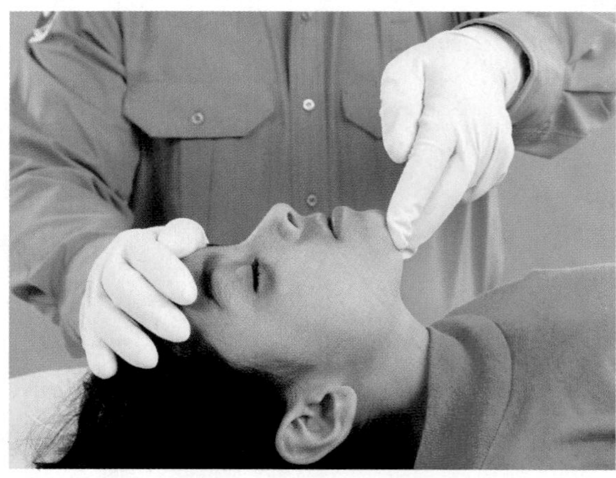

FIGURE 38-13b * Head-tilt, chin-lift maneuver in a child.

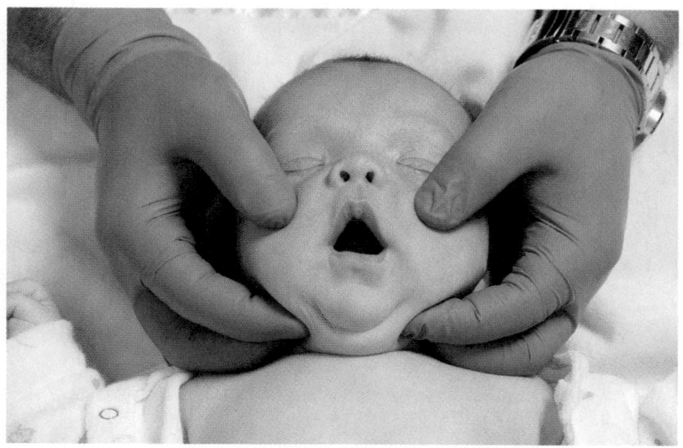

FIGURE 38-14a ✱ Jaw-thrust maneuver in an infant.

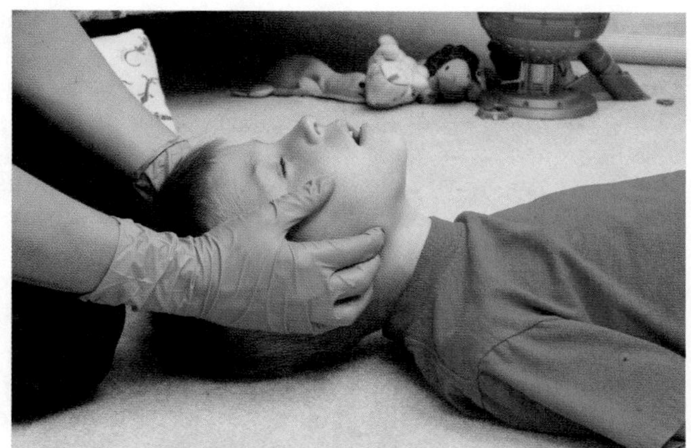

FIGURE 38-14b ✱ Jaw-thrust maneuver in a child.

the soft tissue under the chin, which will occlude, rather than open, the airway. In pediatric patients with possible spine injury, you should perform a manual jaw-thrust technique to help establish the airway (Figure 38-14✱).

2. **Suction any secretions, vomitus, or blood.** The suctioning process temporarily prevents air from being breathed into the lungs. When suctioning an infant or child, do not suction any longer than 3–5 seconds at a time, so as not to promote hypoxia. Use appropriately sized equipment (Figure 38-15✱). Be careful not to damage tissues while inserting and moving the suctioning device in the mouth. If the patient is responsive and has a gag reflex, be careful not to suction deeply enough to cause the patient to vomit.
3. **If you need to assist ventilations, maintain a patent airway with an oropharyngeal or nasopharyngeal airway.** Use an oropharyngeal airway (EMT Skills 38-4A to 38-4D) if the child is unresponsive and there is no gag reflex. Use a nasopharyngeal airway (EMT Skills 38-5A to 38-5C) if the patient cannot tolerate an oral airway. However, nasopharyngeal airways should be avoided in patients

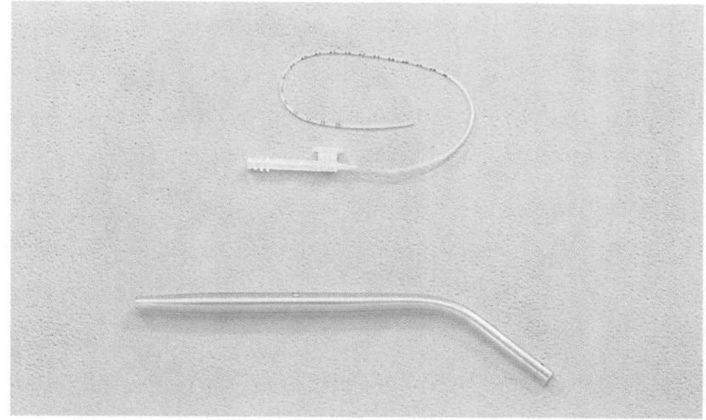

FIGURE 38-15 ✱ Pediatric-size suction catheters. Top: soft suction catheter. Bottom: rigid or hard suction catheter.

with possible head trauma. Since children are prone to having adenoidal hypertrophy, nasopharyngeal airways can "core out" adenoidal tissue resulting in significant upper airway bleeding that is very difficult to control. In general, nasopharyngeal airways should be avoided in children and especially in infants whose nares are so small in diameter that the airway resistance created by the very small diameter of the nasopharyngeal airway is too great to make breathing through it effective.
4. **Initiate positive pressure ventilation.** If the infant or child is in decompensated respiratory failure or respiratory arrest—that is, with inadequate breathing or not breathing—you should start positive pressure ventilation using a bag-valve-mask device or a pocket mask. Supplemental oxygen must be attached to the ventilation device as soon as possible.

   When using a mouth-to-mask device, use a one-way valve to prevent disease transmission. If using a bag-valve-mask device, be sure to use an appropriate-sized bag. Infants and children need a respiratory tidal volume of approximately 6–8 mL/kg. Therefore, bag-valve-mask devices for a full-term newborn, infant, or child should have a minimum volume of 450–500 mL. The bag-valve mask should be no larger than 250 mL for a neonate. Select an appropriate-sized mask that fits over the bridge of the nose and into the cleft above the chin (Figure 38-16✱). Ensure a good mask seal by using one or two hands to hold the mask to the face (Figure 38-17✱). A two-handed seal is preferred to ensure delivery of an adequate tidal volume. Although this might require a second rescuer, it is truly a lifesaving skill that depends on a good seal and just enough manual compression of the bag to make the chest rise.

   The infant or child patient should be ventilated at a rate of 20–25 per minute. Breathe into the pocket mask or squeeze the bag-valve-mask device slowly and evenly to ensure adequate chest rise. If regurgitation is a problem, applying cricoid pressure may help prevent it.

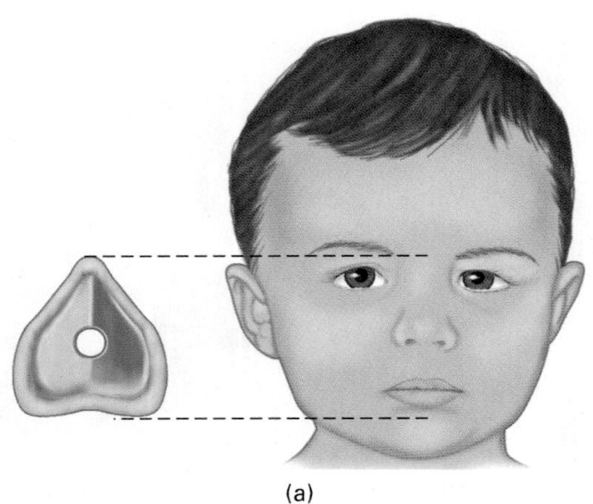

(a)

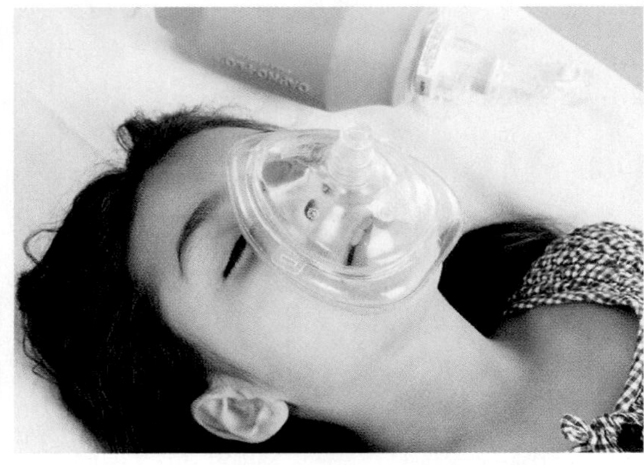

(b)

FIGURE 38-16 ✱ Correct placement of a properly sized mask is necessary to ensure a good mask seal. **(a)** Correct placement of the mask. **(b)** The mask placed on a child.

5. **Maintain oxygen therapy.** If the patient is breathing adequately but has other signs of early respiratory distress, administer oxygen at 15 lpm via a nonrebreather mask (Figure 38-18a✱). If the patient will not tolerate the mask, try a "blow-by" method. Push the oxygen tubing through a hole created in the bottom of a disposable cup (not Styrofoam, which flakes), and hold it near the patient's mouth. This may be less frightening to younger patients, who may be curious and interested in the cup (Figure 38-18b✱). You may also hold the end of the oxygen tubing close to the patient's face to administer the oxygen. The child may feel less anxious if the parent, other relative, or caregiver holds the tubing near his face. In general, you can use the following guidelines for ventilation and oxygenation:

   Provide oxygen at 15 lpm via a nonrebreather mask to all infants and children who:
   - Have indications of early respiratory distress but still have an adequate respiratory effort

   Provide bag-valve-mask ventilation with supplemental oxygen attached to the device for all infants and children who:
   - Have respiratory distress and altered mental status
   - Have cyanosis present despite oxygen via a nonrebreather mask
   - Display respiratory distress with poor muscle tone
   - Are in respiratory failure or in respiratory arrest
6. **Position the patient.** Patients who are in mild respiratory distress will probably prefer to be sitting in the lap of the caregiver. If the patient is unresponsive, place him in a lateral recumbent position to help prevent aspiration, and have suction available. If the patient requires ventilation, he must be kept in a supine position.

(a)

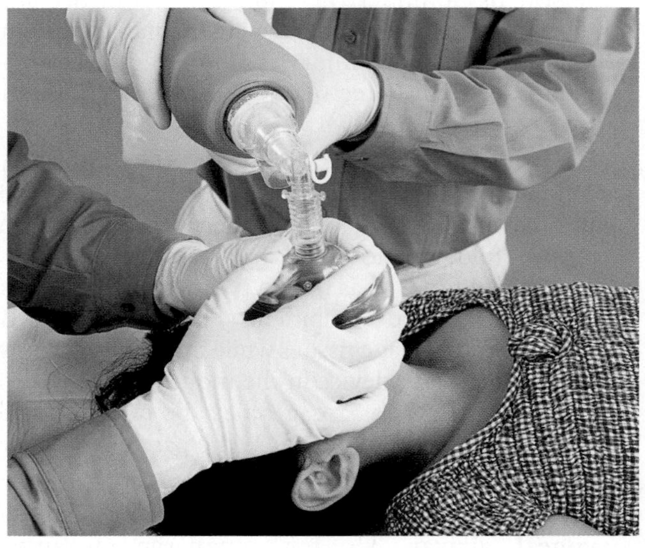

(b)

FIGURE 38-17 ✱ Ensure a good mask seal by using proper hand placement. **(a)** For a one-handed technique, place the middle, ring, and little finger of your nondominant hand along the jaw in an "E" or "3"shape. (Avoid pressing the soft tissues under the chin, which may cause airway occlusion.) Place the thumb and index finger on the mask in a "C" shape, thumb over the bridge of the nose and index finger over the anterior jaw. **(b)** For a two-handed technique, position yourself behind the patient's head and apply the same "E-C" or "3-C" position as described for the one-handed technique, but with the two hands on opposite sides of the mask.

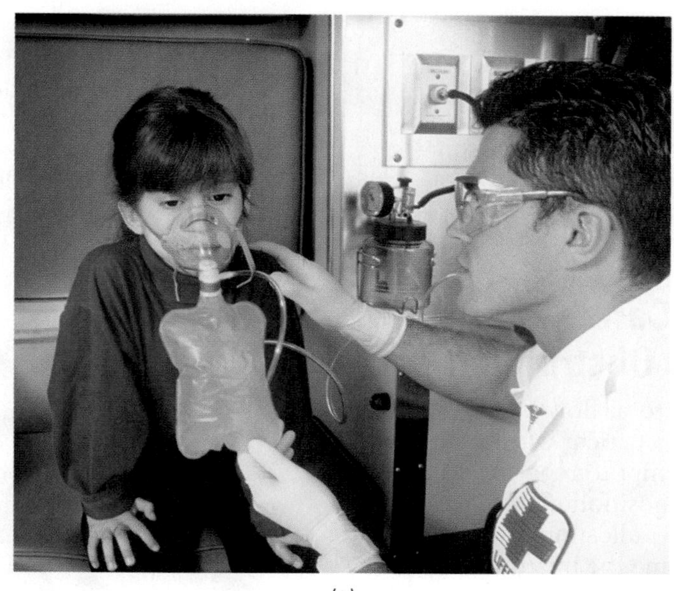

(a)

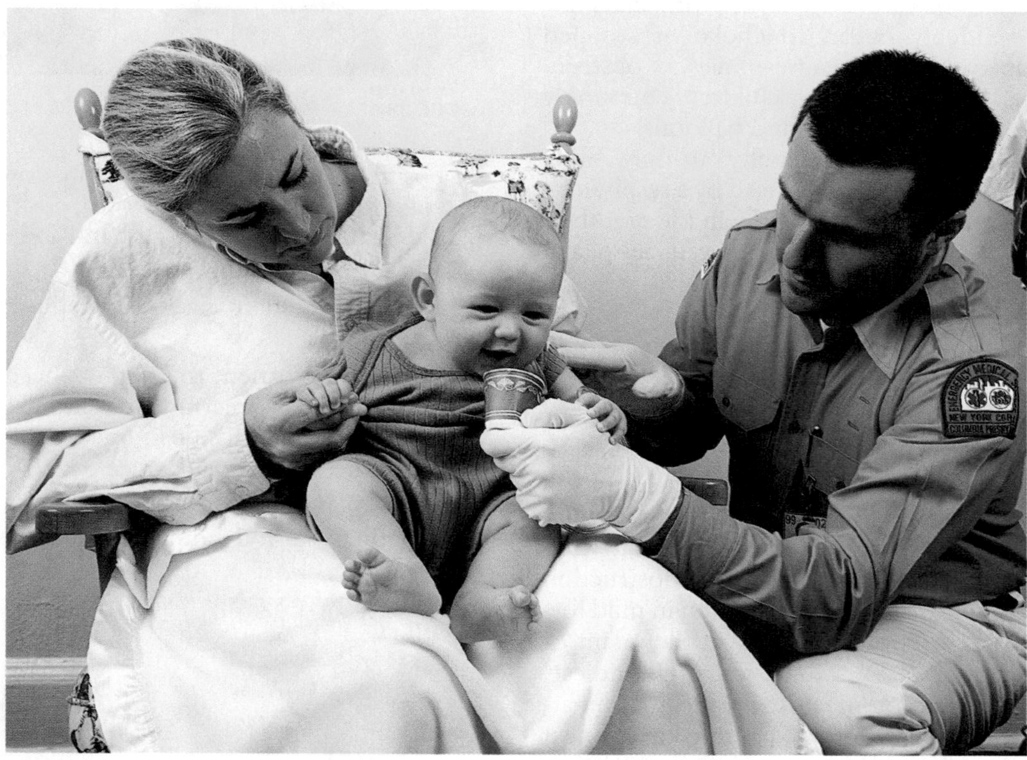

(b)

FIGURE 38-18 ✻ To administer oxygen **(a)** a nonrebreather mask is appropriate for a child; **(b)** the blow-by method, using oxygen tubing and a paper cup, is appropriate for an infant or for a child who will not tolerate a mask.

It may be necessary to immobilize the infant or child to prevent possible aggravation of an existing spine injury. Any pediatric patient with an altered mental status, and no caregiver who is able to give you a history that would rule out trauma, should be immobilized as well. The key in immobilizing the infant or child patient is to place a folded towel (or similar item) beneath the shoulder blades to keep the head from flexing forward. More information about immobilizing an infant or child is provided later in the chapter.

7. **Transport.** Any pediatric patient with a respiratory complaint, or with evidence of respiratory distress, needs to be transported to an appropriate medical facility for further evaluation, preferably a children's hospital or a hospital with specialized pediatric practitioners.

Thinking Critically

You feel a high resistance to airflow as you attempt to ventilate your 2-year-old patient. Repositioning does not improve flow. The child does not appear to be ill. What do you assume is the problem and what should you do about it?

Thinking Critically

Your 5-year-old patient's mother says she thinks he is choking on something. You can tell that he is moving some air, because he is coughing and crying weakly. What should you do?

Emergency Medical Care—Foreign Body Airway Obstruction

If you notice a high resistance to airflow after initiating positive pressure ventilation on a patient with respiratory failure or respiratory arrest, attempt to reposition the airway and reventilate. If, after repositioning, the airway is still not patent, and there are no indications that the child is suffering from an illness, assume the infant or child has an airway obstructed by a foreign body—especially if the child was observed to be eating or playing with small objects and then suddenly began to choke or stopped breathing. The most common cause of airway obstruction in infants is liquids, whereas children commonly choke on small objects, food, toys, and balloons.

Perform the next steps immediately, but only if you are sure that the obstruction is not caused by a respiratory disease. Remember that putting anything in the mouth of a pediatric patient with respiratory disease can cause fatal swelling or spasms of the airway.

Infant or Child with a Mild Foreign Body Airway Obstruction

In a mild foreign body airway obstruction, the infant (less than 1 year of age) or child (over 1 year of age) will still be able to cough and make sounds. He will be moving air. In this case, you should allow the infant or child to continue to cough in an attempt to remove the obstruction on his own. **Do not** perform any intervention in mild foreign body airway obstruction. However, if the infant or child can no longer make any sounds or cough, indicating a severe obstruction, you must react quickly in an attempt to remove the obstruction, as described in the next section. You must constantly and closely assess the infant or child with a mild obstruction for signs of a developing severe obstruction. You can provide blow-by oxygen to the infant or oxygen by nonrebreather mask to the child with a mild obstruction.

Infant with a Severe Foreign Body Airway Obstruction

If the infant (less than 1 year of age) is unable to cough or make any sounds, a severe foreign body airway obstruction is suspected. You must intervene immediately in an attempt to remove the obstruction. Perform the following steps.

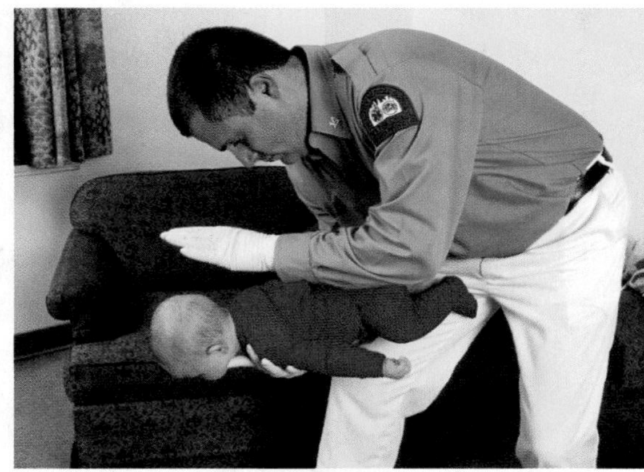

FIGURE 38-19 * Position the infant to deliver back slaps.

1. Position the patient prone (belly down, back up) on your forearm in a head-down position, supporting the infant's head with your hand and supporting your arm on your thigh (Figure 38-19*).
2. Deliver five sharp back slaps (blows) between the shoulder blades.
3. Transfer the patient to a supine, head-down position on your other forearm, and deliver five chest thrusts using two fingertips positioned one finger width beneath the nipple line (Figure 38-20*).
4. Continue to repeat the steps en route until the obstruction is dislodged, the infant becomes unrespon-

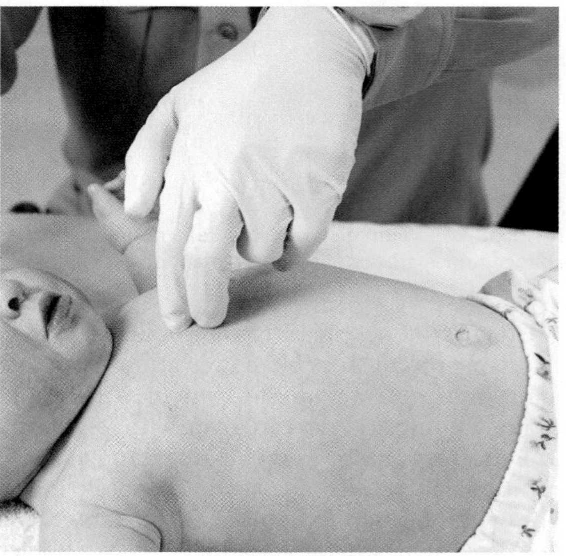

FIGURE 38-20 * Position the infant to deliver chest thrusts.

sive, or you arrive at the medical facility. Consider ALS backup. If the infant becomes unresponsive, go to the steps on relieving an airway obstruction in an unresponsive infant.

Unresponsive Infant with a Foreign Body Airway Obstruction

If the infant (less than 1 year of age) is unresponsive and a foreign body airway obstruction is suspected, or if the infant with a mild or severe foreign body airway obstruction becomes unresponsive during your treatment, immediately perform the following steps.

1. Open the airway, using a head-tilt, chin-lift maneuver.
2. Open the mouth and look for the foreign body. If the foreign body is seen in the oropharynx, attempt to remove it (Figure 38-21∗). Do not perform blind finger sweeps. Doing so may push the obstruction farther down the pharynx or may damage the oropharynx.
3. Provide two ventilations over a 1-second period.
4. Using the same landmarks and techniques as for CPR, provide 30 chest compressions at a rate of 100 per minute.
5. After the chest compressions, look in the mouth for the obstruction. If it can be seen in the oropharynx, attempt to remove it.
6. Provide two ventilations followed by another set of 30 compressions.
7. Continue this sequence until the foreign body is removed. The patient should be transported without delay. Connect oxygen to the bag-valve-mask device via a reservoir to deliver the highest possible concentration of oxygen.
8. If the foreign body cannot be visualized and/or removed, continue chest compressions and attempted ventilations.

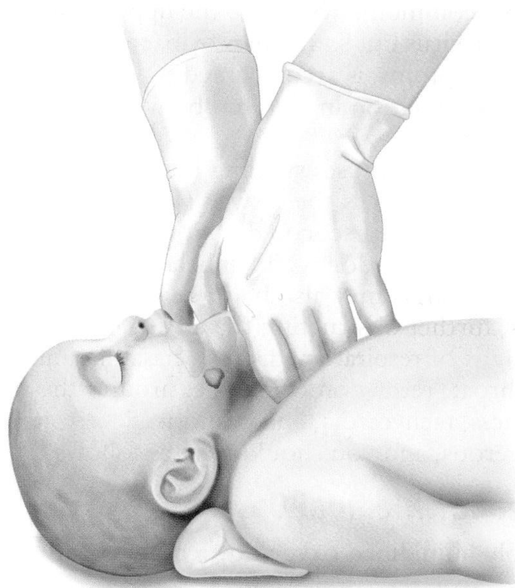

FIGURE 38-21 ∗ Use the finger sweep only when the foreign body is visible.

Child with a Severe Foreign Body Airway Obstruction

If the patient is older than 1 year of age, has a severe foreign body airway obstruction, and is no longer able to cough or make sounds, perform subdiaphragmatic abdominal thrusts (the Heimlich maneuver) as follows:

1. Assure the patient that you are there to help.
2. Position yourself behind the child, and reach your arms around his abdomen (Figure 38-22∗).
3. Locate the navel and place the thumb side of one clenched fist midway between the navel and the xiphoid process (cartilage below the sternum).
4. Wrap the other hand over the clenched hand.
5. Deliver five abdominal thrusts inward and upward, at a 45-degree angle toward the head.
6. Continue to deliver sequential series of five abdominal thrusts until the object is dislodged, you arrive at the medical facility, or the patient becomes unresponsive.

Unresponsive Child with a Foreign Body Airway Obstruction

If the child (over 1 year of age) is unresponsive and a foreign body airway obstruction is suspected, or if the child

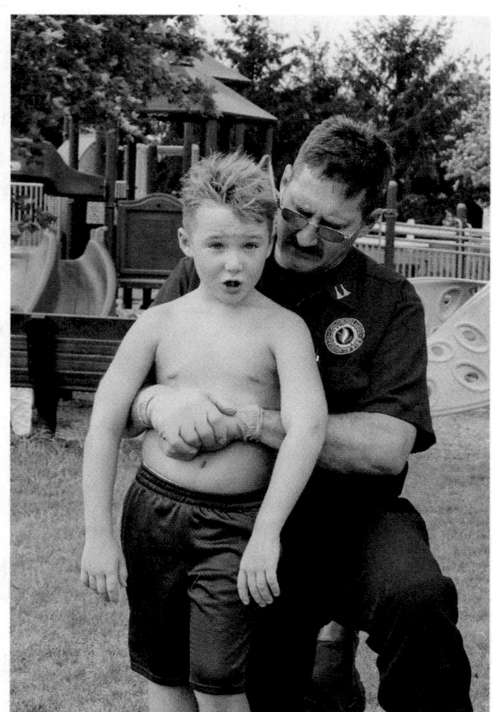

FIGURE 38-22 ∗ Abdominal thrusts on a choking but responsive child.

Key Points
If the foreign body cannot be visualized or removed, continue chest compressions and attempted ventilations.

Objective 38-10
Describe the presentation and emergency medical care for pediatric patients with specific respiratory and cardiopulmonary conditions.

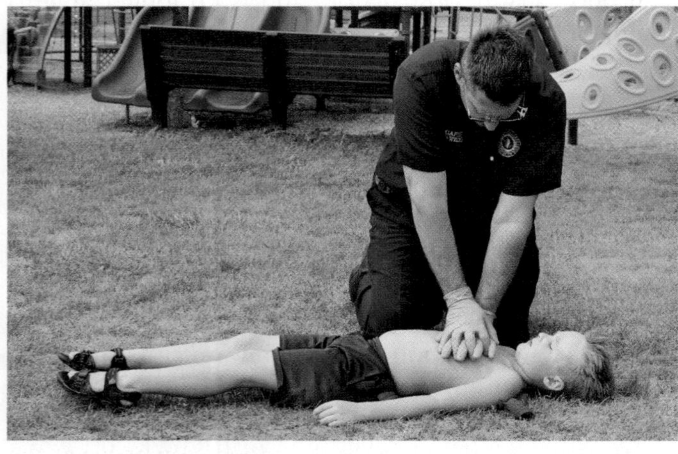

(a)

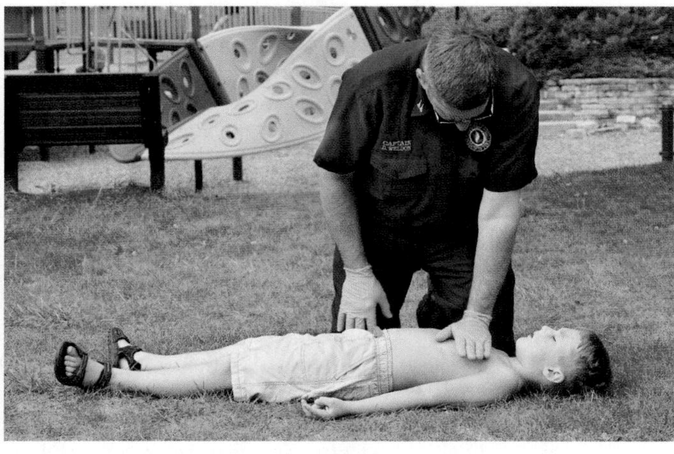

(b)

FIGURE 38-23 ✱ Chest compressions on a child who is unresponsive. **(a)** For an older child, place one hand on top of the other. **(b)** For a younger child, delivering the compressions with one hand may be safer.

with a mild or severe foreign body airway obstruction becomes unresponsive during your treatment, immediately perform the following steps:

1. Open the airway, using a head-tilt, chin-lift maneuver.
2. Open the mouth and look for the foreign body. If the foreign body is seen in the oropharynx, attempt to remove it. Do not perform blind finger sweeps. Doing so may push the obstruction farther down the pharynx or may damage the oropharynx.
3. Provide two ventilations over a 1-second period.
4. Using the same landmarks and techniques as for CPR, provide 30 chest compressions at a rate of 100 per minute (Figure 38-23✱).
5. After the chest compressions, look in the mouth for the obstruction. If it can be seen in the oropharynx, attempt to remove it.
6. Provide two ventilations followed by another set of 30 compressions.
7. Continue this sequence until the foreign body is removed. The patient should be transported without delay. Be sure to connect oxygen to the bag-valve-mask device via a reservoir to deliver the highest possible concentration of oxygen.
8. If the foreign body cannot be visualized and/or removed, continue chest compressions and attempted ventilations.

Specific Pediatric Respiratory and Cardiopulmonary Conditions

Croup

Croup is a common infection of the upper airway, usually caused by a virus but sometimes by bacteria. It has a slow onset of symptoms, is accompanied by a low-grade fever, and is most common in children between 6 months and 4 years of age.

The infection causes swelling beneath the glottis and progressively narrows the airway (Figure 38-24✱). The child is typically hoarse, coughs with a harsh "seal bark," and produces stridor with inhalation. High-pitched squeaking sounds may also be present. As the condition worsens, further obstructing the airway, you will see the classic signs of respiratory distress: nasal flaring, tugging at the throat, retraction of muscles around the rib cage, restlessness, tachycardia, and cyanosis. Severe attacks can be dangerous, and you should treat as follows.

Emergency Medical Care

1. Apply humidified oxygen by a nonrebreather mask.
2. Keep the patient in a position of comfort, either propped up or in a caregiver's arms.

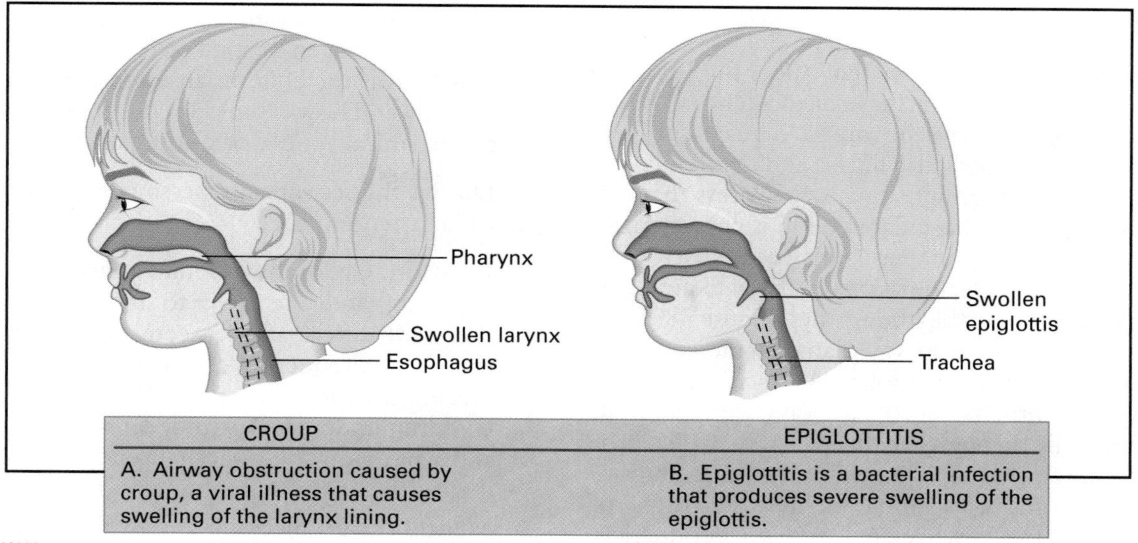

FIGURE 38-24 * Croup and epiglottis.

3. Transport the patient to the hospital with as little disturbance as possible. In severe cases, consider ALS.
4. Be aware that cool night air may reduce the swelling in the airway, bringing relief. You may need to explain the original signs to emergency department personnel if the patient appears much better after transport.

Epiglottitis

A condition that resembles croup, epiglottitis is caused by a bacterial infection that inflames and causes swelling of the epiglottis (review Figure 38-24). *Epiglottitis is life threatening; if left untreated it has a 50 percent mortality rate. The onset is usually rapid and is accompanied by a high temperature.*

Epiglottitis has been traditionally referred to as a disease of children between the ages of 2 and 7 years. This is no longer necessarily the case. There has been vast progress in the reduction of epiglottitis since the mid-1980s, and this is primarily attributed to the introduction of the Hib (*Haemophilus influenzae* type B) vaccine. The majority of epiglottitis cases were previously caused by Hib. As a result of the Hib vaccine, epiglottitis is currently being seen more in young adults than in children. The exception to this rule is in those areas where immunizations are not commonplace and where agents causing the disease are different, for example strep.

Signs and symptoms are:

- Pain on swallowing
- High fever (102°F–104°F) and a "toxic" ill-appearing child
- Drooling (because it is painful to swallow)
- Mouth breathing
- Changes in voice quality and pain upon speaking
- Sitting up and leaning forward (tripod position)
- Chin and neck thrust outward
- Inspiratory stridor
- Respiratory distress
- A strikingly still appearance as the attack worsens

Emergency Medical Care

1. Do not place anything in the child's mouth since this can increase swelling of the epiglottis and cause laryngospasm that can completely block the airway. Nothing in the mouth means no oropharyngeal airway, no suctioning equipment, and no fingers—unless the patient becomes completely unresponsive is not moving any air.
2. Allow the child to assume a position of comfort (usually sitting upright, leaning forward).
3. Provide oxygen at 15 lpm by a nonrebreather mask. Provide blow-by oxygen if the child does not tolerate the mask. Be careful that it does not cause irritation or coughing. If the child's airway is completely obstructed, provide bag-valve-mask ventilations with supplemental oxygen, forcing oxygen past the swollen epiglottis and spasmed larynx.
4. Consider ALS backup if it does not delay transport. Patients with epiglottitis may need endotracheal intubation or a surgical airway, and this should be done in a controlled setting such as an emergency department or operating room by skilled personnel.
5. Transport.

Asthma

Some of the pulmonary diseases that affect the pediatric population have begun to decrease in incidence. Unfortunately, other diseases have begun to increase substantially, leading to more pediatric illness and death.

Asthma is a long-term inflammatory process that targets the lower airways. This inflammation is characterized by increased production of mucus and an acute narrowing of the airways through inflammation of airway tissue, leading to edema (swelling) within the airways (Figure 38-25✱).

The narrowing of the airway diameter increases airway resistance in the bronchioles. As the bronchiolar smooth muscle contracts and the airways are narrowed, air moves forcefully through the tiny passages, which produces the wheezing that is heard upon auscultation. Common symptoms of asthma include shortness of breath, chest tightness, wheezing, and nonproductive, "tight" coughing. For a more detailed discussion of asthma signs, symptoms, and emergency medical care, see Chapter 16, "Respiratory Emergencies."

Get the patient's history from the caregivers by asking the following questions:

- How long has the child been wheezing?
- How much fluid has he taken during this period?
- Has he had a recent cold or other infection, particularly one involving the respiratory tract?
- Has he had any medication for this attack? What is it? When? How much? (It is especially important to ask about metered-dose inhalers.) Does he take steroids? When was the last dose of these medications?
- Does he have any known allergies to drugs, foods, pollens, or other inhalants?
- Has he visited an emergency department recently? Has he ever been hospitalized for an acute asthmatic attack? Was the child in an intensive care unit? How recently and how often? Has the patient ever required a mechanical ventilator during an attack?

During the secondary assessment of the patient, pay particular attention to:

- **Position.** Children with mild attacks of asthma often appear agitated and prefer to sit, but will lie still. Children with severe attacks seem exhausted and unable to move. Frequently they prefer to lean forward, bracing themselves on their elbows (tripod position). Children under the age of 2 often show no agitation and will lie on their backs, even when this increases their difficulty in breathing.
- **Mental status.** Sleepiness and changes in mental status are progressively more serious signs of hypoxia, acidosis, and retention of carbon dioxide.
- **Vital signs.** As an attack worsens, the pulse grows faster and weaker. Blood pressure may fall. Bradycardia (slower-than-normal heart rate) is an ominous sign of impending respiratory and potential cardiac arrest.
- **Skin color and condition.** Pinch the skin to look for evidence of dehydration ("tenting"). Check for cyanosis of the tongue and mucous membranes, suggesting hypoxia. Usually these children have some degree of dehydration from poor oral intake, severe coughing that might stimulate vomiting, and increased insensible losses from rapid respirations.
- **Respirations.** A mild to moderate attack of asthma is characterized by loud breathing sounds, loud wheezes, and occasional crackles. As the attack wors-

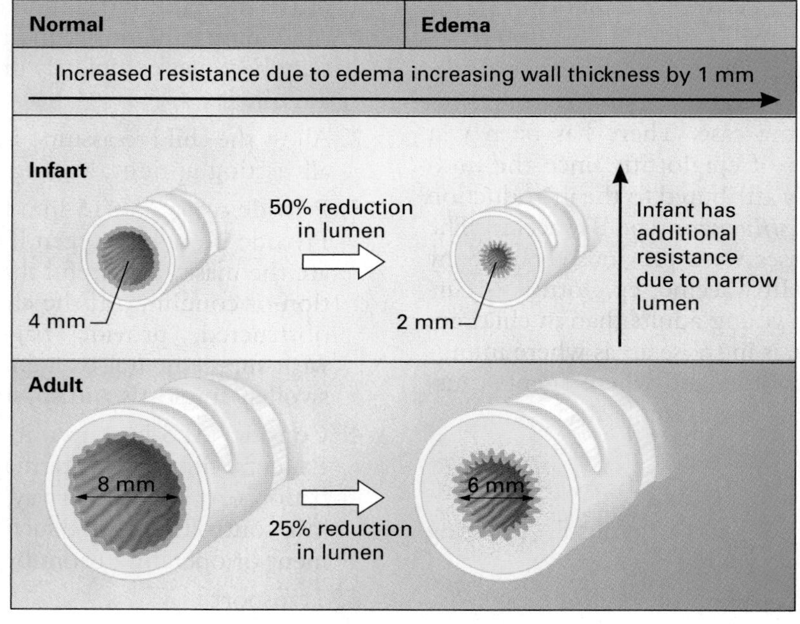

FIGURE 38-25 ✱ Effects of edema on airway resistance in the infant compared to the adult.

Key Points

A severe asthma attack that cannot be controlled with medication is extremely serious. Consider ALS backup.

Key Points

A finding in pneumonia specific to children is a tendency to lie on the side with knees drawn up to the chest to minimize pleuritic pain and improve ventilation.

ens, the breath sounds become less audible and are completely absent in a severe attack. Auscultate the entire chest, since localized wheezes suggest a foreign body obstruction, whereas asthma causes generalized wheezes.

Emergency Medical Care

Because of the emotional component of asthma (stress makes it worse), try to be as calm and reassuring as possible and follow these treatment steps (but move somewhat quickly because definitive treatment is available at the hospital).

1. Apply humidified oxygen at 15 lpm by nonrebreather mask. Assist ventilations if breathing is not adequate.
2. Allow the child to assume a position of comfort.
3. If the child has a prescribed inhaler, follow the same emergency care procedures for administration of the medication via metered-dose inhaler as for the adult. (Review Chapter 16, "Respiratory Emergencies," for information on prescribed inhalers.) Consult medical direction for permission to administer it.
4. Usually, you will need to transport the patient for further care.

Note: A severe attack that cannot be managed with medication is called status asthmaticus and is extremely serious. Consider ALS backup, if available.

Bronchiolitis

Bronchiolitis, which is easily confused with asthma, is caused when the mucosal layer within the bronchioles in the lungs becomes inflamed by a viral infection. During exhalation, the child will wheeze loudly. He will also have other signs similar to those of asthma. Bronchiolitis typically occurs in children less than 2 years of age. The younger the age, the more severe the symptoms such that infants with the disease typically require hospitalization and, often, mechanical ventilation. To prehospital care providers, the best known infectious form of bronchiolitis is respiratory syncytial virus (RSV). Symptoms of bronchiolitis include a low-grade fever, tachycardia and/or tachypnea (rapid heart rate and rapid breathing), shortness of breath, chest tightness, wheezing, and coughing.

Collect the same history and perform the same assessment as you would for asthma.

Emergency Medical Care

Generally speaking, management of bronchiolitis is almost identical to that for other types of respiratory distress:

1. Apply humidified oxygen at 15 lpm by nonrebreather mask, and assist breathing as necessary.
2. Let the child assume a position of comfort or place him in a Fowler position with his neck slightly extended if this position is more comfortable.
3. Monitor the pulse rate and mental status while you transport the child to the hospital.

Pneumonia

Pneumonia is estimated to cause approximately 4 million deaths among children worldwide. In the United States from 1939–1996, mortality caused by pneumonia in children declined by 97 percent. This decline is most likely attributable to the introduction of antibiotics, vaccines, improvements in medical care, and the expansion of medical insurance coverage for children. Pneumonia is a bacterial, viral, mycoplasmal, and fungal infection of the lung. It accounts for an extremely high amount of morbidity and is the sixth leading cause of death in the United States.

Viral pneumonia usually results from spread of infection along the airways resulting in airway obstruction from swelling, abnormal secretions, and cellular debris. The small diameter of airways in young infants makes them particularly susceptible to severe infection. Viral infection of the respiratory tract can also predispose to secondary bacterial infection by disturbing normal immune system response mechanisms.

When bacterial infection is established in the lung, the extent of injury is dependent on the particular bacteria. The end result, however, is typically the same: cellular destruction and an inflammatory response in the airways. As the infection progresses, cellular debris, inflammatory cells, and mucus cause airway obstruction and ultimately respiratory compromise.

Common symptoms of pneumonia include shortness of breath, chest tightness, diminished breath sounds, and dry, hacking, productive-sounding cough. A finding in pneumonia that is specific to the pediatric population is a tendency for the child to lie on his side with his knees drawn up to the chest to minimize pleuritic pain and improve ventilation. For a more detailed discussion of pneumonia signs, symptoms, and

Key Points
When pneumonia is suspected, apply humidified oxygen, allow the child to assume a position of comfort, and transport for further care.

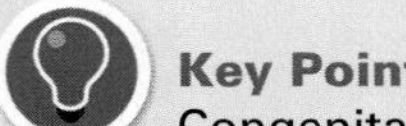

Key Points
Congenital heart defects are responsible for more deaths in the first year of life than any other birth defects.

emergency medical care, see Chapter 16, "Respiratory Emergencies."

Obtain the history from the caregivers by asking:

- How long has the child been ill?
- How much fluid has he taken during this period?
- Has he had a recent cold or other infection, particularly one involving the respiratory tract?
- Has he had any treatment for this current illness? What is it? When?
- Has he had a fever?

During the physical exam of the patient, pay particular attention to:

- **Position.** Children with pneumonia may lie on their side with their knees drawn up to the chest. Children with severe respiratory distress seem exhausted and unable to move. Frequently they prefer to lean forward, bracing themselves on their elbows (tripod position). Children under the age of 2 often show no agitation and will lie on their backs, even when this increases their difficulty in breathing.
- **Mental status.** Drowsiness and intermittent periods of restlessness are commonly associated with pneumonia.
- **Vital signs.** As the disease progresses, the pulse grows faster and weaker. Blood pressure may fall. Bradycardia (slower-than-normal heart rate) is an ominous sign of impending respiratory and potential cardiac arrest. Children with bacterial pneumonia are at high risk for developing sepsis and septic shock. Monitor the SpO_2 very carefully.
- **Skin color and condition.** Pinch the skin to look for evidence of dehydration ("tenting"). Check for cyanosis of the tongue and mucous membranes, suggesting hypoxia.
- **Respirations.** A mild to moderate exacerbation is characterized by diminished breathing sounds, and may occasionally include wheezes and/or crackles.

Emergency Medical Care

1. Apply humidified oxygen at 15 lpm by nonrebreather mask. Assist ventilations if breathing is not adequate.
2. Allow the child to assume a position of comfort.
3. Usually, you will need to transport the patient for further care.

Congenital Heart Disease (CHD)

Congenital heart defects are responsible for more deaths in the first year of life than any other birth defects, according to the National Institutes of Health. The initial presentation of the infant with CHD can be inconsistent, looking like respiratory distress, infection, failure to thrive, and shock. The presenting symptoms of CHD in the infant or child are (1) inadequate pulmonary blood flow resulting in cyanosis and hypoxia; (2) excessive pulmonary blood flow resulting in congestive heart failure, hypoperfusion, and systemic shock; or (3) respiratory distress with or without cyanosis or shock. Since the defect can be due to abnormal valves, vessels, or chambers, diagnosing the defect is less important than recognizing the abnormality on assessment, initiating emergency care, and transporting rapidly to an appropriate medical facility.

Emergency Medical Care

1. *Ensure an open airway and provide oxygen* at 15 lpm by nonrebreather mask.
2. *Provide positive pressure ventilation via bag-valve mask with supplemental oxygen connected to the ventilation device if breathing is inadequate.*
3. *Support the cardiovascular system as necessary. Consider ALS support.*

Shock

Severe shock in children is unusual because their blood vessels constrict efficiently, which helps to maintain blood pressure but only for so long. When adverse conditions are not corrected in a timely fashion and the conditions leading to shock continue, the blood pressure will eventually drop. It will usually drop rapidly and eventually precipitate cardiac arrest. Remember, that cardiopulmonary arrest is typically due to either respiratory failure or shock.

Newborns have been known to go into shock from loss of body heat. They have immature thermoregulatory systems and cannot shiver or warm themselves through muscular activity. Their skin surface area is large in relation to their body weight, which increases their rate of heat loss.

Shock can also be precipitated by certain medical problems that can cause the same response in adults. Hypovolemic, obstructive, distributive, and cardiogenic causes of shock are also experienced by the pediatric patient. Common findings include diarrhea and dehydration,

SIGNS OF SHOCK (HYPOPERFUSION) IN A CHILD

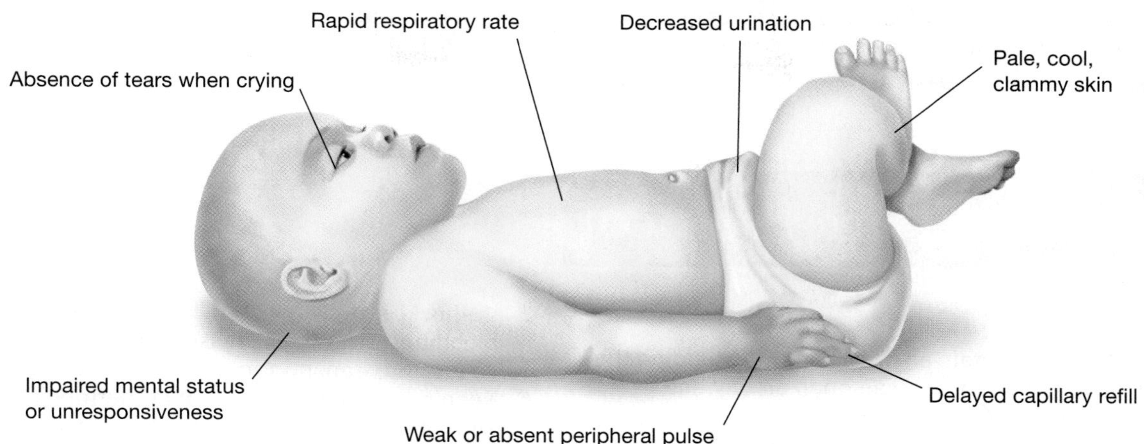

FIGURE 38-26 ✱ Signs of shock (hypoperfusion) in a child.

trauma, vomiting, blood loss, infection, and abdominal injuries. Less common causes of shock are allergic reactions, poisoning, or cardiac events. Refer to Chapter 15, "Shock and Resuscitation," for a review of shock.

The goal of treatment is to correct any abnormalities that may compound the hypoperfusion state (e.g., hypoxia, continued blood loss).

Signs of shock include rapid respiratory rate; pale, cool, clammy skin; mottling; decreased mental status; prolonged capillary refill; and weak or absent peripheral pulses (see Figure 38-26✱ and Table 38-6). The onset of these signs in children may be sudden, occurring quickly as their compensatory mechanisms become exhausted and fail. This means that when pediatric patients deteriorate because of hypoperfusion, they deteriorate faster and more severely than adults.

Emergency Medical Care

1. *Ensure an open airway and provide oxygen* at 15 lpm by nonrebreather mask.
   Call for ALS intercept if available.
2. *Provide positive pressure ventilation via bag-valve mask with supplemental oxygen connected to the ventilation device if breathing is inadequate.*
3. *Control any bleeding* if present.
4. *Place the patient in a supine position.*
5. *Keep the patient warm and as calm as possible.* If the patient is a newborn, preheat an isolette or your ambulance to at least 98°F (36.5°C) for full-term babies. If you do not have an isolette, wrap the baby in warm blankets (prewarmed, if possible), then aluminum

TABLE 38-6 Pulses and Capillary Refill as Indicators of Compensated and Decompensated Shock

Indicator		Normal	Sign of Compensated Shock	Sign of Decompensated Shock
Pulses				
Peripheral pulse: adequate	Central pulse: adequate	X		
Peripheral pulse: weak or absent	Central pulse: adequate		X	
Peripheral pulse: absent	Central pulse: weak or absent			X
Capillary refill				
Normal (≤ 2 seconds)		X		
Delayed (2–4 seconds)			X	
Absent (> 4 seconds)				X

Key Points
Almost all cardiac arrests in children result from airway obstruction or respiratory distress leading to respiratory arrest. Most other cases of pediatric cardiac arrest result from shock.

Key Points
Your goal for the cardiac arrest patient is to keep the brain viable.

Emergency Care Protocol

PEDIATRIC SHOCK

1. Establish and maintain an open airway, extending the head only enough to allow an open airway and avoid hyperextension.
2. Suction secretions no longer than 3–5 seconds each time.
3. Provide positive pressure ventilation with supplemental oxygen connected to the ventilation device at a rate of 12–20 ventilations/minute if breathing is inadequate.
4. If breathing is adequate, administer oxygen via nonrebreather mask at 15 lpm; consider blow-by oxygen in infants and very young children.
5. If shock is due to blood loss, control any external bleeding with direct pressure. If internal bleeding is suspected, transport immediately and expeditiously.
6. Keep the patient warm. If hypothermia is suspected, wrap the patient in warm blankets and place the ambulance heater on high. Cover the infant or child's head. (Note: All patients in shock should be kept warm.)
7. Consider calling advanced life support.
8. Expedite transport.
9. Perform a reassessment every 5 minutes.

FIGURE 38-27 ∗ Emergency care protocol: pediatric shock.

foil, to preserve body heat. Be sure that the baby's head (but not the baby's face) is covered.

6. *Transport* to the emergency department quickly.

To review emergency care for hypoperfusion in the infant or child, see Figure 38-27∗.

Cardiac Arrest

Although cardiac arrest is not a respiratory problem per se, it is a very real concern if the patient's respiratory status deteriorates. Almost all cardiac arrests in children result from airway obstruction or respiratory distress leading to respiratory arrest; most of the remaining are caused by shock (hypoperfusion). It is extremely important to aggressively manage both respiratory problems and shock before they progress to cardiac arrest. Provide positive pressure ventilations if breathing is inadequate or signs of respiratory failure are present. Chest compressions should be started if the heart rate drops below 60 beats per minute and signs of poor perfusion are evident.

Signs of cardiac arrest in a child are:

- Unresponsiveness
- Gasping or no respiratory sounds
- No audible heart sounds
- Chest that is not moving
- Pallor or cyanosis
- Absent pulse (assess the brachial pulse in the infant, the carotid pulse in the child over 1 year of age)

Your goal is to keep the brain viable. Standing orders that provide you with orderly direction of treatment, easy access to paramedic backup, and continuous assessment are important. Unless too much time has elapsed between the arrest and initiation of artificial ventilation, the child may recover with minimal or no neurological deficit—even following comparatively long periods of arrest.

Emergency Medical Care

Key components of management include the following steps:

1. Provide positive pressure ventilation with supplemental oxygen.
2. Perform CPR effectively with minimal interruption. The automated external defibrillator (AED) should be applied to a child 1 year of age or older. Pediatric AEDs may be applied to children less than 1 year of age. Follow your local protocol. An AED that is capable of delivering an energy level suitable for children up to 8 years of age through a dose-attenuating system, typically pediatric pads and cables, should be

Key Points

Management for cardiac arrest includes positive pressure ventilation with supplemental oxygen, CPR and, if the patient is older than 1 year, AED, ALS backup, and transport to a facility with cardiac arrest treatment capability.

Objective 38-11

Explain the assessment steps and emergency care protocol for a respiratory or cardiopulmonary emergency in the pediatric patient.

used. If a dose-attenuating system is not available, an adult AED should be applied, regardless of the child's age. An adult AED is used for children older than 8 years of age. If an AED is applied, the protocol for use should only employ a single shock followed by 2 minutes of CPR prior to reanalysis of the rhythm.

3. Call for ALS backup.
4. Transport rapidly to the closest medical facility capable of handling a patient in cardiac arrest.

For a review of artificial ventilation and CPR techniques, see Appendix 1, "Basic Cardiac Life Support."

Summary: Pediatric Respiratory and Cardiopulmonary Emergencies

To review possible assessment findings and emergency care for respiratory or cardiopulmonary emergencies in the infant or child, see Figures 38-28∗ and 38-29∗.

Assessment Summary

RESPIRATORY OR CARDIO-PULMONARY EMERGENCY IN THE PEDIATRIC PATIENT

The following findings may be associated with an airway or cardiopulmonary emergency in the infant or child.

SCENE SIZE-UP

Ensure your own safety. Look for:

Mechanism of injury; toxic inhalation or hazardous materials; patient in a confined space; evidence of poisoning; metered-dose inhalers or nebulizers

Primary Assessment

General Impression

Pediatric Assessment Triangle:

- **Appearance**
- **Work of breathing**
- **Circulation to skin**

Is the child "sick" or "well"? Displaying normal behavior for his age? Moving spontaneously or lethargic or flaccid? Maintaining eye contact?

If older than 2 months, does he recognize his parents? Respond when the parent calls his name?

Is he sitting up, leaning forward, neck jutting out, drooling?

Mental Status (depending on age of patient)

Alert to unresponsive; decreasing mental status; increased anxiety; disorientation; restlessness

Seizure activity; weak or absent cry

Does not react with environment

Does not seem to notice your presence

Cannot be consoled by parent

Airway

Occluded by tongue, secretions, blood, or vomitus

Signs of laryngeal edema (stridor, crowing)

Swollen tongue; drooling

Harsh cough that sounds like a "barking seal"

Breathing

Tachypnea (>50 respirations/minute in an infant and >30 respirations/minute in a child)

Inadequate ventilation

Wheezing; crackles

Mouth breathing; accessory muscle use; nasal flaring

Coughing, gagging, or gasping

Circulation

Weak central or peripheral pulses; tachycardia; bradycardia

Red, warm, and dry skin

Pale, cool, clammy skin; cyanosis

Capillary refill that is delayed >2 seconds with other findings of hypoperfusion

Status: Priority patient if showing signs and symptoms of respiratory arrest, respiratory failure, or respiratory distress

continued

FIGURE 38-28a ∗ Assessment summary: respiratory or cardiopulmonary emergencies in the pediatric patient.

Objective 38-12
Describe the presentation and emergency medical care for pediatric patients with specific medical conditions.

Assessment Summary

Secondary Assessment

Physical Exam

Head, neck, and face:
- Edema to face, hands, neck, and lips
- Hives; itching
- Warm, tingling feeling
- Difficulty in swallowing
- Itchy and watery eyes
- Runny or stuffy nose
- Coughed-up mucus
- Headache
- Stiff neck
- Bulging anterior fontanelle (infants <1 year)
- Neck jutted out and drooling
- Evidence of trauma to the head, neck, or face

Chest:
- Retractions; accessory muscle use
- Wheezing in all lung lobes; crackles
- Evidence of trauma to the chest

Abdomen:
- Nausea/vomiting
- Abdominal cramping
- Diarrhea; loss of bowel control
- Excessive abdominal muscle use
- Evidence of trauma to abdomen

Extremities:
- Warm, tingling feeling in hands and feet
- Itching, especially hands and feet
- Edema to hands and feet
- Cool, pale, cyanotic hands and feet
- Red, warm, dry skin
- Weak or absent peripheral pulses
- Poor skin turgor
- Rashes, petechiae, bruising

History

Signs/symptoms of early respiratory distress:
- Tachypnea
- Nasal flaring
- Retractions
- Stridor, wheezing, or grunting
- "Seesaw" respirations

Signs/symptoms of decompensated respiratory failure:
- Tachypnea >60/minute
- Cyanosis
- Decreased muscle tone
- Poor peripheral perfusion
- Altered mental status
- Grunting
- Head-bobbing

Signs of respiratory arrest:
- Respiratory rate less than 10/minute
- Irregular respirations
- Flaccid (limp) muscles
- Unresponsiveness
- Bradycardia
- Weak or absent peripheral pulses
- Hypotension

Baseline Vital Signs

- BP: Take BP in children >3 years of age; BP may be decreased with severe respiratory failure
- HR: tachycardia with weak peripheral pulses that may progress to bradycardia
- RR: tachypnea; may have wheezing and labored breathing; bradypnea is sign of impending respiratory failure and respiratory arrest
- Skin: usually pale, cool, clammy, and cyanotic; may be red, warm, dry; hives, itching if allergic reaction
- Pupils: normal to dilated; sluggish to respond to light
- SpO_2: less than 95%

FIGURE 38-28a ✱ Assessment summary: respiratory or cardiopulmonary emergencies in the pediatric patient. *continued*

Other Pediatric Medical Conditions and Emergencies

The previous section dealt primarily with respiratory and cardiac emergencies in infants and children. In particular, airway and respiratory emergencies can be life threatening and are associated with many other emergencies in the pediatric patient. Regardless of the type of medical emergency, maintaining an airway and adequate breathing and oxygenation are the primary goals. The general principles and steps of assessment—scene size-up, primary assessment, secondary assessment, and reassessment—are the same no matter what medical emergency precipitates the call.

Emergency Care Protocol

RESPIRATORY OR CARDIOPULMONARY EMERGENCY IN THE PEDIATRIC PATIENT

1. Establish and maintain an open airway, extending head only enough to allow an open airway and avoid hyperextension.
2. If severe (not coughing or not making sounds) or foreign body airway obstruction is suspected, perform the following:

   Infant (<1 year of age):
   a. Position supine.
   b. Deliver five back slaps (blows).
   c. Deliver five chest thrusts.
   d. Assess inside mouth; finger sweep only if object is visualized.
   e. Begin immediate transport if airway is not cleared.
   f. Continue until obstruction is dislodged.

   Responsive child with severe foreign body airway obstruction:
   a. Deliver five abdominal thrusts.
   b. Repeat twice until obstruction is dislodged or child becomes unresponsive.
   c. Begin immediate transport; continue abdominal thrusts en route.

   Unresponsive infant or child with severe foreign body airway obstruction:
   a. Open the mouth and inspect for an obstruction. If at any time it is seen in the oropharynx, remove it. Do not perform blind finger sweeps.
   b. Deliver two ventilations.
   c. Perform 30 chest compressions.
   d. Inspect inside the mouth prior to delivering the next two ventilations. If the obstruction is seen in the oropharynx, remove it.
   e. Begin immediate transport; continue with the CPR en route.
3. If the infant or child has a mild foreign body airway obstruction, apply a nonrebreather mask, allow the patient to assume a position of comfort, and encourage the patient to cough forcefully; do not delay transport; continue en route.
4. Suction secretions no longer than 3–5 seconds each time.
5. Provide positive pressure ventilation with supplemental oxygen via reservoir at a rate of 12–20 ventilations/minute if:
   Respiratory failure
   Respiratory arrest
   Inadequate breathing
   Respiratory distress and altered mental status
   Cyanosis is present despite oxygen delivery by nonrebreather mask
   Respiratory distress with poor muscle tone
6. If breathing is adequate, administer oxygen via nonrebreather mask at 15 lpm; consider blow-by oxygen in infants and very young children.
7. If signs and symptoms of allergic reaction and respiratory distress and/or hypotension, and with permission from medical direction, administer epinephrine by patient-prescribed auto-injector: **epinephrine pediatric dose: 0.15 mg** up to 66 lb. If the child's weight is greater than 66 lb, an adult (0.30 mg) auto-injector should be used.
8. If signs and symptoms of respiratory distress and wheezing and if the patient has a prescribed metered-dose inhaler, and with permission from medical direction, administer the MDI.
9. Consider calling advanced life support.
10. Expedite transport.
11. Perform a reassessment every 5 minutes.

FIGURE 38-28b ✱ Emergency care protocol: respiratory or cardiopulmonary emergency in the pediatric patient.

On the following pages, additional pediatric medical emergencies are discussed with general principles of assessment and care with special application to each type of emergency.

Seizures

Seizures in infants and children may be caused by any condition that would also produce seizures in adults: epilepsy, head injury, meningitis, oxygen deficiency, drug overdose, electrolyte abnormalities, brain tumors, and low blood sugar (hypoglycemia). However, adults seldom have febrile seizures (seizures caused by fever), but children may. The risk of seizures is high among children up to age 2, and approximately 3–5 percent of all children in the United States will have experienced a febrile seizure by the time they reach their 5th birthday. Although these childhood seizures may be frightening, they generally have no permanent adverse effects and usually do not predict the development of epilepsy in the child unless there is a family history of epilepsy and the seizure is particularly prolonged or difficult to control.

Assessment Considerations

During the "generalized, tonic-clonic" seizure, the child's arms and legs may become rigid, the back arches, the muscles may twitch or jerk in spasm, the eyes roll up and become fixed, the pupils dilate, and the breathing is often irregular or ineffective. The patient may lose bladder and

Emergency Care Algorithm: Respiratory or Cardiopulmonary Emergency in the Pediatric Patient

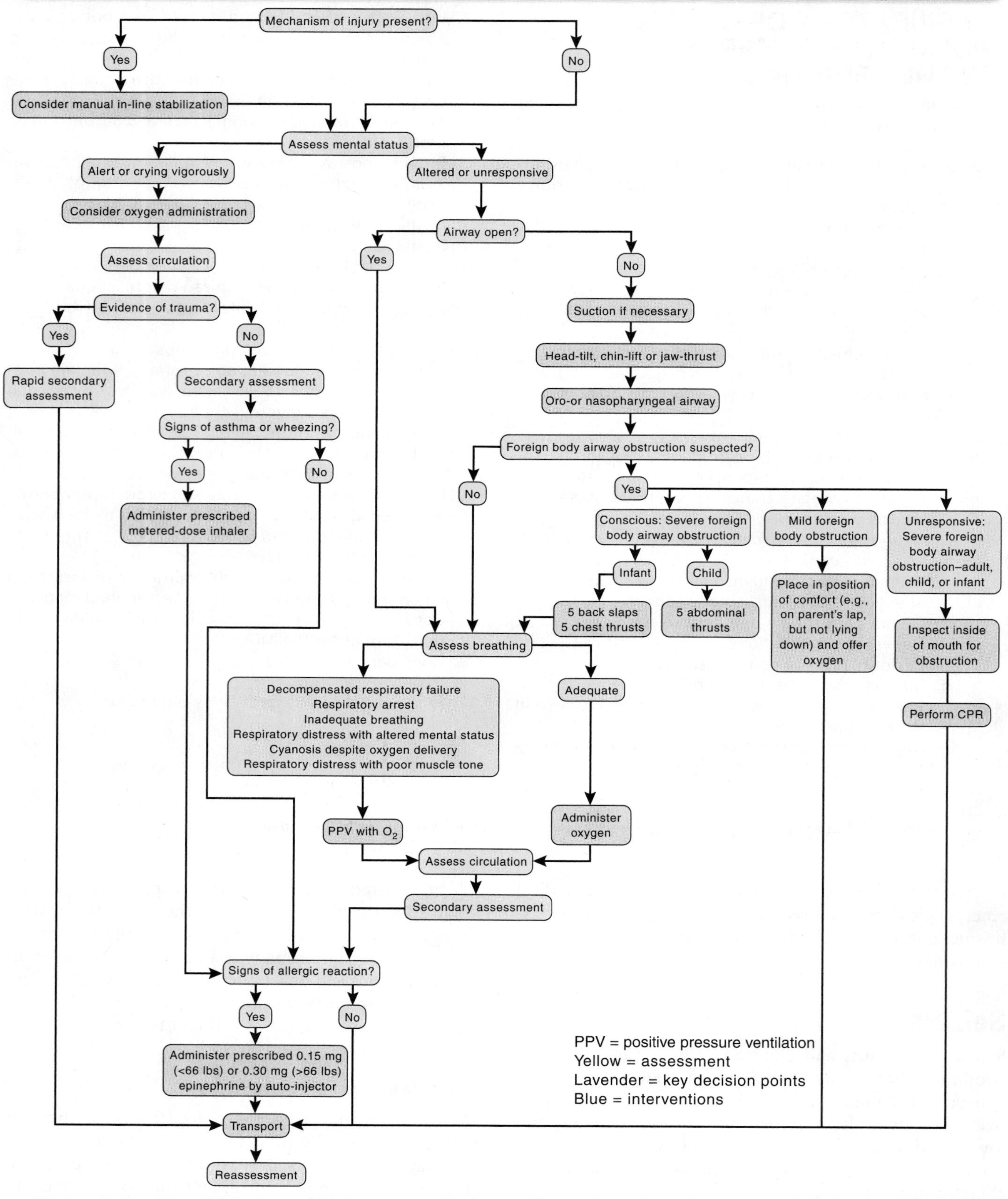

FIGURE 38-29 ✱ Emergency care algorithm: respiratory or cardiopulmonary emergency in the pediatric patient.

bowel control and will be completely unresponsive. If the seizure lasts long enough, the skin can turn cyanotic from ineffective respirations. The muscle spasms may prevent the child from swallowing effectively. Hence, excessive saliva coming from the mouth is a common finding (saliva production is also more copious during the seizure). If saliva is trapped in the throat, the child will make a gurgling sound with respirations.

EMS providers may have difficulty differentiating a syncopal episode from a seizure in the pediatric population. The key difference between a seizure and another loss of consciousness is that the activity in a seizure will not alter or cease in response to your (or the parent's) interventions. Remembering AVPU, the actively seizing patient will have no response to painful stimuli, whereas many other conditions causing an alteration in consciousness will have some, albeit a nonspecific, response to painful stimuli. As an EMS provider, you may find yourself responding to the scene of an unresponsive child. Given the high stress associated with pediatric medical emergencies, a good history of events can be difficult to obtain.

Incontinence is an uncommon finding in the patient who experienced a syncopal episode, whereas incontinence is common in seizure activity. This finding is not reliable in a diaper-dependent child since it is difficult to determine the time the diaper was soiled in relationship to the physiological event. Syncope does not present with any history of tonic-clonic activity and typically occurs with generalized symptomatology. In contrast, a seizure patient will often have a recent history of generalized tonic-clonic activity or localized, focal motor activity. However, some patients with syncope may have activity during the event that is described as seizure-like.

Determining the duration of loss of consciousness may help to establish if the etiology is related to syncope or seizures. In a syncopal event, the child generally has a relatively short duration (less than 5 minutes) of unconsciousness in contrast to a relatively longer duration (greater than 5 minutes) in a seizure.

While obtaining the history, ascertain whether the child has had prior seizures and, if so, find out whether this is the child's normal seizure pattern. Determine whether the child has taken his antiseizure medications, if any have been prescribed.

Emergency Medical Care

A single seizure is usually self-limiting, ends within minutes, is generalized in nature (all muscles involved), and does not recur. If the child has a single seizure, maintain an airway and be sure that he does not injure himself. Transport as soon as possible after the single seizure.

1. *Ensure the airway is open.*
2. *Position the patient on his side* if there is no possibility of spine trauma, and make sure he cannot strike any nearby objects and injure himself.
3. *Be prepared to suction.* Do not insert a hard suction catheter into the oropharynx of an actively seizing patient.
4. *Provide oxygen or ventilate as appropriate.* Provide oxygen at 15 lpm by nonrebreather mask or, if inadequate breathing is present, provide positive pressure ventilation with supplemental oxygen connected to the ventilation device.
5. *Transport.* Although brief seizures are generally not harmful, there may be a more dangerous underlying condition.

If seizures last longer than 5 minutes or recur without a recovery period, this is a condition called *status epilepticus,* which is a *true medical emergency.* Provide positive pressure ventilation with supplemental oxygen during a prolonged seizure, if possible. After the seizure has ended, it may still be necessary to provide positive pressure ventilation. Provide rapid transport to the hospital, paying particular attention to maintaining the airway and protecting the patient from injury.

To review emergency care for seizures in the infant or child, see Figure 38-30∗.

Altered Mental Status

An altered mental status can be the reason for the emergency call (mother informs you the baby "just isn't acting right") or a sign or a result of the initial reason for the emergency call (a patient with a diabetic condition who becomes unresponsive) (Figure 38-31∗). It is most important to assess and treat any life threat to the airway, breathing, oxygenation, or circulation associated with the altered mental status. Your pediatric patient could have an altered mental status for the same reason an adult patient would, such as hypoglycemia, poisoning, post seizure, or severe blood infection. If your protocol permits, assess the blood glucose in any patient presenting with an altered mental status. Note that if the altered mental status is associated with poor brain perfusion or brain injury, all three PAT findings—appearance, work of breathing, and circulation to skin—may be abnormal.

Assessment Considerations

The child's level of maturity will greatly influence the format of your assessment of mental status. If using AVPU or the Glasgow Coma Scale, you will need to modify them for a child. Review Table 38-4 for the Pediatric Glasgow Coma Scale (PGCS). Ask the child simple questions. If the child appears to be lethargic, inconsolable, or agitated, ask the caregivers if this is a typical or an unusual response.

To assess the unresponsive infant or child, shout to elicit a response to verbal stimulus. Inflict a pinch to see if the child will respond to pain. *Never shake an infant or child for any reason.*

Emergency Care Protocol

PEDIATRIC SEIZURES

1. Establish and maintain an open airway, extending the head only enough to allow an open airway and avoid hyperextension.
2. Protect the infant or child from injuring himself; place him on his left side.
3. Suction secretions no longer than 3–5 seconds each time.
4. Provide positive pressure ventilation with supplemental oxygen via reservoir at a rate of 12–20 ventilations/minute if breathing is inadequate.
5. If breathing is adequate, administer oxygen via nonrebreather mask at 15 lpm; consider blow-by oxygen in infants and very young children.
6. Check the blood glucose level, if your protocol permits.
7. Expedite transport in any of the following situations:
   a. Epileptic seizures lasting > 5 minutes
   b. Two or more epileptic seizures without a period of consciousness between them
   c. Febrile seizures lasting > 15 minutes
   d. Seizure from any other cause (e.g., hypoxia, head injury)
8. Consider calling advanced life support.
9. Expedite transport.
10. Perform a reassessment every 5 minutes.

FIGURE 38-30 ✱ Emergency care protocol: pediatric seizures.

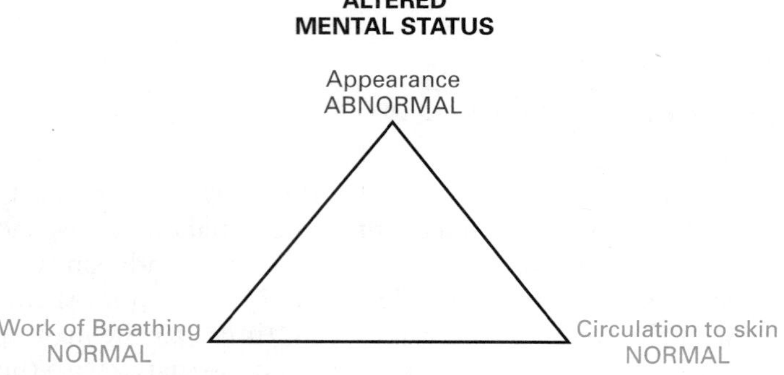

FIGURE 38-31 ✱ Findings in the pediatric patient with altered mental status.

Emergency Medical Care

Treatment of a pediatric patient with an altered mental status is aimed at managing life threats such as airway compromise. Treatment procedures include the following:

1. *Ensure patency of the airway,* using manual and mechanical airway procedures as appropriate.
2. *Be prepared to suction the airway.*
3. *Administer oxygen at 15 lpm or positive pressure ventilation with supplemental oxygen,* as needed.
4. *Expedite transport.* A pediatric patient with an altered mental status is always a high priority.

To review emergency care for an altered mental status in the infant or child, see Figure 38-32✱.

Drowning

Drowning can occur in any amount of water—from the ocean, to the bathtub, to a bucket. The main cause of death in infants or children who are submerged is not the aspiration of fluid (although it can occur in some patients). Rather, it is the hypoxia that occurs secondary to glottic closure reflex, which occurs when the water comes in contact with the glottic opening. The majority of deaths are "dry drownings" where the person dies from suffocation and fluid does not enter the lungs.

Assessment Considerations

When confronted with a drowning emergency, you need to be aware of the possibility of trauma and/or hypothermia. Infants and children are especially prone to hypothermia. In any drowning emergency, you should also be alert for secondary drowning syndrome, a deterioration that takes place after normal breathing is restored—from minutes to hours after the event. For a more detailed discussion of drowning and other water emergencies, see Chapter 25 "Submersion Incidents".

Emergency Medical Care

In the case of a cold-water drowning, you should be particularly aggressive and persistent about resuscitating a pediatric patient. In response to the cold water, the mammalian dive reflex, which is pronounced in children, may slow blood perfusion and metabolism. This means that the residual oxygen in the blood will last longer for the brain to consume. Numerous cases of "saves" have been reported even after prolonged submersion in cold water (30 minutes or more). It is controversial whether these saves are made possible by the mammalian dive reflex or the cold water. If you are unclear about the length of time under water, always give the patient the benefit of the doubt and initiate resuscitation.

Emergency Care Protocol

PEDIATRIC ALTERED MENTAL STATUS

1. Establish and maintain an open airway, extending the head only enough to allow an open airway and avoid hyperextension.
2. Suction secretions no longer than 3–5 seconds each time.
3. Provide positive pressure ventilation with supplemental oxygen at a rate of 12–20 ventilations/minute if breathing is inadequate.
4. If breathing is adequate, administer oxygen via nonrebreather mask at 15 lpm; consider blow-by oxygen in infants and very young children.
5. Check the blood glucose level, if your protocol permits.
6. If signs and symptoms of hypoglycemia are present and the child is a known diabetic on medication for the condition, consider oral glucose if the child is able to swallow and medical direction approves.
7. Consider calling advanced life support.
8. Expedite transport.
9. Perform a reassessment every 5 minutes.

FIGURE 38-32 ✱ Emergency care protocol: pediatric altered mental status.

1. *Remove the patient from the water.* Be sure that the person who rescues the patient is properly trained and equipped for water rescue. Remove clothing and provide passive warming with blankets and a warm environment in the ambulance.
2. *Assume that a spinal injury has occurred and provide full immobilization* while establishing an airway.
3. *Clear the airway, and provide positive pressure ventilation via a bag-valve mask with supplemental oxygen connected to the ventilation device if breathing is inadequate or absent.*
4. *Check circulation. Provide CPR as needed. Attach the AED.* If hypothermia is suspected, deliver only one defibrillation.
5. *Maintain the treatment en route, and monitor the airway closely for regurgitation and aspiration. Have suction readily available.*

To review emergency care for drowning in the infant or child, see Figure 38-33✱.

Fever

Fevers in children of 104°F–105°F are concerning. Causes of high temperature include infection (such as meningitis) and heat exposure (from being left in a hot car, for instance).

Assessment Considerations

The degree of temperature is not always of the greatest concern, but how quickly the temperature "spikes." If the temperature rises rapidly, a febrile seizure (a seizure caused by a high body temperature) may result. Not all high temperatures produce seizures.

Emergency Care Protocol

PEDIATRIC DROWNING

1. Remove the infant or child from the water. If diving was involved in children or adolescents, consider in-line spinal stabilization and complete spinal immobilization.
2. Establish and maintain an open airway, extending the head only enough to allow an open airway and avoid hyperextension.
3. Suction secretions no longer than 3–5 seconds each time.
4. Provide positive pressure ventilation with supplemental oxygen connected to the ventilation device at a rate of 12–20 ventilations/minute if breathing is inadequate.
5. Perform chest compressions if no pulse is present. Apply the AED if the child is greater than 1 year of age. Contact medical direction otherwise for orders. If hypothermia is suspected, deliver only one defibrillation.
6. If breathing is adequate, administer oxygen via nonrebreather mask at 15 lpm; consider blow-by oxygen in infants and very young children.
7. If hypothermia is suspected, remove wet clothing, wrap the patient in warm blankets, and place the ambulance heater on high. Cover the infant or child's head.
8. Consider calling advanced life support.
9. Expedite transport.
10. Perform a reassessment every 5 minutes.

FIGURE 38-33 ✱ Emergency care protocol: pediatric drowning.

Emergency Care Protocol

PEDIATRIC FEVER

1. Establish and maintain an open airway, extending the head only enough to allow an open airway and avoid hyperextension.
2. Suction secretions no longer than 3–5 seconds each time.
3. Provide positive pressure ventilation with supplemental oxygen via reservoir at 12–20 ventilations/minute if breathing is inadequate.
4. If breathing is adequate, administer oxygen via nonrebreather mask at 15 lpm; consider blow-by oxygen in infants and very young children.
5. Febrile seizures > 15 minutes are a dire emergency and require expeditious transport and consideration for advanced life support.
6. Consider calling advanced life support.
7. Transport.
8. Perform a reassessment every 5 minutes.

FIGURE 38-34 ✻ Emergency care protocol: pediatric fever.

In addition to seizures, another common result of fever is dehydration caused by the increased insensible (evaporative) loss of fluids and electrolytes, especially if fever has been present for some time. Signs and symptoms include nausea, loss of appetite, vomiting, and possible fainting. A dehydrated child's pulse will be weak and rapid, the skin pale, the eyes sunken, and the mucous membranes dry and parched. When you pinch the skin, it might stay "tented." Dehydration in the infant may also result in a sunken fontanelle. The caregiver may indicate a decrease in frequency of urination by reporting fewer diaper changes than usual.

Emergency Medical Care

Lower the body temperature based only on local protocol, administer oxygen at 15 lpm via a nonrebreather mask, and remove excess layers of clothing.

If the elevated core body temperature is a result of exposure to a hot environment, conduct cooling if the core temperature is excessive. Remove the child from the hot environment and avoid extreme cooling and shivering while cooling. Sponge the child's skin with tepid water. Transport the patient and remain alert for seizures. If cooling is done, it should be performed in a slow, controlled manner unless the child has a temperature over 106.9°F. If a child with an elevated core body temperature is cooled too quickly, the brain will be overstimulated and the child may seize.

To review emergency care for fever in the infant or child, see Figure 38-34✻.

Meningitis

In meningitis, the lining of the brain and spinal cord (the meninges) are infected by either bacteria or viruses. These infections can be rapidly fatal, so they must be assessed promptly and treated in a timely and appropriate manner. Fever in a child younger than 3 months should be considered meningitis until proven otherwise.

Assessment Considerations

Signs and symptoms of meningitis in children include recent ear or respiratory tract infection, high fever, lethargy, irritability, or vomiting. They generally do not have headaches or stiff necks but are lethargic and will not eat. The fontanelle may be bulging unless the child is dehydrated. Movement is painful so the caretakers may report that "he cries every time we pick him up." Rash may or may not be present.

Emergency Medical Care

If you suspect meningitis, you should wear a mask, gloves, and possibly a gown. Complete the assessment rapidly and transport to the hospital. If the child is in shock (hypoperfusion), provide oxygen at 15 lpm by nonrebreather mask.

Gastrointestinal Disorders

Diarrhea, which is characterized by frequent and watery bowel movements, is often caused by gastrointestinal infections, although it can also come from other illnesses or changes in diet. The most common cause of diarrhea in children is an infection of the gastrointestinal tract, also known as gastroenteritis, and is a leading cause of dehydration in young children.

Appendicitis is an inflammation of the vermiform appendix, most commonly seen in young adults. Acute appendicitis is the most common surgical emergency you will encounter in the field, mostly in older children and young adults. In the majority of cases, acute appendicitis is caused by an obstruction of the appendix by fecal material. Once the appendix becomes obstructed, it becomes inflamed and can lose its blood supply. The loss of blood flow to the appendix results in tissue hypoxia and, eventually, tissue death. As the appendix dies, its walls weaken and may rupture, spilling infectious contents into the peritoneal cavity.

Assessment Considerations

Appendicitis commonly presents with diffuse, crampy pain surrounding the umbilicus. Other symptoms may include nausea and vomiting and sometimes a low-grade fever. As the infection worsens, the pain may become localized to the right lower quadrant, but not always. Once the appendix actually ruptures, the pain again becomes diffuse and the patient can become critically ill with septic shock and signs of hypoperfusion.

Emergency Medical Care

For acute abdominal pain where appendicitis is suspected, provide oxygen by nonrebreather mask or blow-by, as appropriate to the age of the child. Place the patient in a position of comfort, usually with knees flexed. If the patient is vomiting, place him on his side. Transport without delay.

Poisoning

Poisonings constitute a large number of emergency runs for pediatric patients. Because of children's inquisitive nature, they are always moving about and getting into things. Recent scientific studies have suggested that the greatest incidence of poisonings occurs in children between 1 and 2 years of age. Poisonings in children less than 4 years of age account for approximately 46 percent of all poison exposures.

Assessment Considerations

For these patients, a thorough secondary assessment is critically important. Because poisons can enter the body through numerous routes (ingestion, inhalation, absorption, injection), it is important to gather as much information as possible about the type of overdose prior to transporting the patient to the hospital.

For specifics on assessment and management, see Chapter 22, "Toxicologic Emergencies."

Emergency Medical Care

Emergency treatment of poisoned patients is geared toward the effects of the poisoning on the patient, rather than treating the specific type of poisoning. General emergency care for a pediatric patient suffering from a poisoning is as follows.

If the Patient Is Alert

1. *Contact medical direction or the local poison control center.* You may be instructed to administer activated charcoal if a poison was ingested; however, activated charcoal is not effective in most situations, so it is unlikely that you will ever administer it. The dose of activated charcoal given is 1 gram/kg of body weight. Follow your local protocol, online medical direction, or the poison control center's advice on the use of activated charcoal.
2. *Provide positive pressure ventilation by bag-valve mask* if the respiratory rate or tidal volume is inadequate. If breathing is adequate, administer oxygen based on the SpO_2 reading and patient signs and symptoms. If the SpO_2 reading is greater than 95% and no signs or symptoms of hypoxia or respiratory distress are present, oxygen may not be necessary. In this case, you may choose to apply a nasal cannula at 2–4 lpm. If signs of hypoxia or respiratory distress are present, or the SpO_2 reading is less than 95%, or the poisoning is by inhalation, place the patient on a nonrebreather mask at 15 lpm.
3. *Transport* any patient who was poisoned. Conduct a reassessment en route, closely monitoring for a change in mental status or for airway or breathing compromise. If possible, transport any medication or substance of the type that was ingested along with the patient.

If the Patient Is Initially Unresponsive or Becomes Unresponsive en Route

1. *Establish and maintain an open airway,* and be prepared to suction.
2. *Provide oxygen at 15 lpm by nonrebreather mask; provide positive pressure ventilation via a bag-valve-mask device with supplemental oxygen connected to the reservoir if breathing is inadequate.*
3. *Expedite transport.*
4. *Perform a rapid secondary assessment* to identify or rule out trauma as a cause of the altered mental status. Check blood glucose level, if your protocol permits.

To review emergency care for poisoning in the infant or child, see Figure 38-35∗.

Apparent Life-Threatening Events

In 1986 the National Institutes of Health and Consensus Development Conference on Infantile Apnea and Home Monitoring defined an apparent life-threatening event (ALTE) as: "an episode that is frightening to the observer and that is characterized by some combination of apnea (central or occasionally obstructive), color change (usually cyanotic or pale but occasionally erythematous or plethoric), marked change in muscle tone (usually marked limpness), choking, or gagging. In some cases, the observer fears that the infant has died." This is relevant to EMS because EMS units are often called for these episodes to evaluate the infant.

Assessment Considerations

An ALTE may include a combination of symptoms (often transient) affecting infants, including:

- Apnea
- Skin color change

Key Terms

sudden infant death syndrome (SIDS) the sudden and unexpected death of an infant or young child in which an autopsy fails to identify the cause of death.

Objective 38-13

Describe special considerations in the scene size-up, emergency medical care, and assisting family members in case of suspected SIDS and the importance of the presence of parents during pediatric resuscitation.

Emergency Care Protocol

PEDIATRIC POISONING

1. Extend the head only enough to allow an open airway; avoid hyperextension.
2. Suction secretions no longer than 3–5 seconds each time.
3. Provide positive pressure ventilation with supplemental oxygen at a rate of 12–20 ventilations/minute if breathing is inadequate.
4. If breathing is adequate, administer oxygen via nonrebreather mask at 15 lpm; consider blow-by oxygen in infants and very young children.
5. Treat the specific poisoning:

   Ingestion

   If you are instructed to administer activated charcoal and the patient is alert and able to swallow, give at 1 g/kg (12.5–25 grams). Activated charcoal is contraindicated in the following:
   - Altered mental status
   - Ingestion of acids or alkalis
   - Patient who is unable to swallow

   Inhalation

   Remove from toxic environment. Maximize oxygenation by nonrebreather mask at 15 lpm if breathing adequately or by positive pressure ventilation if breathing inadequately.

   Absorption

   Flush with water for 20 minutes at the scene. If eyes are involved, continue to flush en route.

   Injection

   Carefully monitor airway and breathing. If allergic reaction, and with order from medical direction, consider administration of epinephrine by auto-injector at 0.15 mg if the child weighs less than 66 lb. If the child's weight is greater than 66 lb, an adult (0.3 mg) auto-injector should be used. Apply a constricting band proximal to site of bite or injection.
6. Consider calling advanced life support.
7. Expedite transport.
8. Perform a reassessment every 5 minutes.

FIGURE 38-35 ✱ Emergency care protocol: pediatric poisoning.

- Changes in muscle tone
- Unexplained choking or gagging

Emergency Medical Care

If called for an infant exhibiting any of these transient signs, immediately transport to a medical facility for further evaluation.

Sudden Infant Death Syndrome

Sudden infant death syndrome (SIDS), commonly known as "crib death," is defined as the sudden and unexpected death of an infant (under 1 year of age) in which an autopsy fails to identify the cause of death. It is the leading cause of death among infants between 1 month and 1 year of age, with a peak incidence at 2 to 4 months. SIDS is a postmortem diagnosis, not one that can be made in the field. While the facts behind SIDS will be outlined here, *do not make a firm diagnosis to a family member.*

To date, no reliable ways to predict or prevent SIDS are known. The etiology of SIDS remains unknown. It almost always occurs while the baby is sleeping. The typical SIDS case involves an apparently healthy infant, frequently with a history of having been born premature, who suddenly dies during a sleep period in his crib. No illness need be present, though the baby may have had recent cold symptoms. There is usually no indication of struggle. Sometimes, though, the child has obviously changed position near the time of death. Risk factors include sleeping in a prone (belly down) position, sleeping on a soft surface, and secondhand smoke.

There is much confusion about SIDS among both the general public and the medical profession. Not until recently has serious medical research on SIDS been conducted. However, its exact cause is still unknown.

Assessment Considerations

SIDS cannot be diagnosed in the field. When you arrive in response to the emergency call, you will find the patient in cardiac arrest and you will proceed with care as you would for any patient in this condition. Do not delay resuscitation (as described in the next section) but, as practical, obtain a brief history of the infant and observe the surroundings, including:

- Physical appearance of the infant
- Position of the infant in the crib
- Physical appearance of the crib
- Presence of objects in the crib
- Unusual or dangerous items in the room (such as plastic bags)
- Appearance of the room/house
- Presence of medication, even if it is for adults
- Circumstances concerning discovery of the unresponsive child
- Time the infant was put to bed or fell asleep
- Problems at birth
- General health
- Any recent illnesses
- Date and result of last physical exam

Since this may be a potential crime scene rather than a medical case of SIDS, be very careful not to convey by the wording of your questions or your manner any suspicion that the parents or caretakers may be responsible for the child's condition.

Emergency Medical Care

When you find an infant in respiratory and cardiac arrest—a condition for which SIDS is only one of many possible causes—proceed as follows:

1. *Immediately try to resuscitate.* Attempt aggressive resuscitation of the infant. The exceptions are rigor mortis (when joints become rigid) and dependent lividity (discoloration created by gravity causing the blood to pool in the lowest body areas). If the patient displays rigor mortis or lividity, he should be left in the position found and local authorities should be called according to local protocol.
2. *Encourage the caregivers to talk and tell their story.*
3. *Do not provide false reassurances.*
4. *Transport* the infant to the hospital. Tell the caregivers where you are taking the child and provide clear directions about how to get there. Encourage them to have someone else drive them, and remind them to arrange for care of any siblings.
5. *Deliver the infant into the hands of the emergency department staff.* Be careful of what you say to your colleagues at the hospital. Casual comments such as "smothered" or "injured" may be overheard by the family and cause unnecessary emotional distress. Never say anything that the family may overhear that makes them feel they are to blame or are being blamed for the infant's death.

To review emergency care for sudden infant death syndrome, see Figure 38-36✱.

Aiding Family Members in SIDS Emergencies

The reactions of family members to the SIDS incident will be varied. One of the most common immediate reactions of caregivers to SIDS is shock and disbelief. This may cause family members to become immobilized—incapable of making decisions. Or it may cause them to act as if they are cold and unfeeling. It is not that they do not care, just that they are having a hard time facing reality.

Emergency Care Protocol

SUDDEN INFANT DEATH SYNDROME

1. If rigor mortis and dependent lividity are present, do not attempt to resuscitate. Turn your attention to supporting the parents.
2. Attempt resuscitation if any chance of survival exists:
   a. Establish and maintain an open airway, extending the head only enough to allow an open airway and avoid hyperextension.
   b. Suction secretions.
   c. Provide positive pressure ventilation with supplemental oxygen connected to the ventilation device at 12–20 ventilations/minute and chest compressions at a rate of at least 100/minute.
   d. Consider calling advanced life support.
   e. Expedite transport.
   f. Perform a reassessment every 5 minutes.
3. Care for the caregivers or parents.
   a. Encourage them to talk and tell their story.
   b. Do not provide false reassurances.
   c. Avoid any statements that might place blame on the caregiver or parents.
4. If resuscitation is not attempted, contact the coroner or follow your local protocol regarding moving the infant for transport.

FIGURE 38-36 ✱ Emergency care protocol: sudden infant death syndrome.

Key Points

Do not dismiss the caregivers in a SIDS emergency because they are not patients in the traditional sense. Small caring gestures and offers of assistance are very important.

Objective 38-14

Integrate consideration of a pediatric patient's size and anatomy into the assessment of mechanisms of injury.

It may be difficult for you to deal with extreme reactions. Some caregivers may physically act out their emotions, resulting in hysteria, crying, or wailing. Caregivers may be confused and overwhelmed with guilt feelings, unfairly venting their anger and frustration on each other—or on you.

Do not dismiss the caregivers because they are not the patients in the traditional sense of the word. The tendency is to ignore the mother's barrage of questions concerning her child, and to tell her politely to go away. While you are there to give medical care and not to become personally "involved," you must understand that these caregivers and family members need your care also. Small, often nonverbal, gestures on your part are very important. By simply sitting with the caregivers, you are showing them that someone cares. Offer to be of assistance to them—to make phone calls or to get them coffee. A sympathetic ear may be all they need.

Don't neglect your own emotional turmoil. After a SIDS call, it is common for rescuers to experience anxiety, guilt, or anger. Ignoring your emotions will not cause them to go away. You should talk out your feelings with colleagues, friends, or your partner or spouse.

Presence of Parents During Pediatric Resuscitation

Several scientific studies conducted within the recent past suggest that the presence of parents during resuscitation is beneficial to both children and the parents. When a child died during resuscitation, parents in one study stated that they felt more accepting of the death if they were able to be with the child at the time of death. Children who survived appeared to be more cooperative and accepting of procedures when their parents were present. The studies also found that there were minimal negative effects on the success rates of clinicians who performed the interventions.

▶ Pediatric Trauma

Trauma is the leading cause of death in children from ages 1 to 14. Each year, thousands of children die from unintentional injury and more are permanently disabled. Fifty percent of deaths from trauma occur within the first hour after an injury. The primary killer of American children is the automobile; however, children may experience trauma while riding bicycles, all-terrain vehicles, and motorcycles; while climbing trees; as pedestrians; during recreational activities; and even from homicide and suicide.

Despite highly effective injury prevention strategies (car seats and other child passenger restraint systems, seat belts, helmets, and educational programs for children and caretakers alike), these preventable injuries and deaths still occur at alarmingly high rates. To quote the former U.S. Surgeon General C. Everett Koop, MD, himself a pediatric surgeon, "If a disease were killing our children in the proportions that injuries are, people would be outraged and demand that this killer be stopped."

Blunt trauma is the most common injury in children. Quite frequently, a child will be severely injured but display no early, obvious signs. (Review Chapter 27, "Trauma Overview: The Trauma Patient and the Trauma System.") At the scene, try to reconstruct the incident and understand the mechanism of injury.

When assessing mechanism of injury during the scene size-up, look at not only the vehicle (or other object) that caused the trauma, but also the size of the patient in relation to what he came into contact with. The following are mechanisms of injury and the common patterns of injury to expect in infants and children:

- Unrestrained children in cars will probably suffer head and neck injuries because the child's head is proportionally larger than the adult's, and it is likely to come into contact with the interior of the car (e.g., the dashboard). Child passengers in the front seat may suffer face, neck, or chest injuries from deployment of a passenger-side air bag.
- Restrained passengers will probably suffer abdominal and/or lumbar injuries from the stress applied by the seat belt during the accident. This is especially true if the child was improperly restrained in the automobile.
- If the child was struck while riding a bike, he is likely to sustain head injuries, spinal injuries, and abdominal injuries because these areas of the body are typically near the same height as the bumper and hood of a car.
- If the young patient was struck by a car while walking, one should suspect the high likelihood of some or all of the three elements of the Waddell triad: head injuries, chest/abdominal injuries, and lower extremity injuries. A quick estimation of the patient's pain site as well as the height of the bumper and hood on the car can help localize where the patient suffered trauma.
- If the patient was diving into water or fell from a height, suspect head and spinal injuries.

Key Points
Regardless of injury, the treatment emphasis for the pediatric trauma patient is always airway, breathing, circulatory management, and spinal immobilization.

Thinking Critically
Your young trauma patient has a reddened area over her ribs and she says they feel sore, but no ribs seem to be broken. Should you conclude that she has not been seriously injured? Why or why not?

- If the mechanism of injury involved burns, be aware that the burns may be more severe to the infant or child because his skin is not as thick or durable as an adult's. The inhalation of smoke, toxic fumes, or superheated air during a fire can cause airway swelling more rapidly and severely than in adults.
- Sports injuries typically involve injuries to the head and neck.
- Unfortunately, child abuse is another cause of trauma. Child abuse is discussed later in the chapter.

Trauma and the Pediatric Anatomy

A full discussion of trauma is presented in Chapters 27 to 36; the following is a brief overview of injuries as they relate to the infant or child patient. Remember that the treatment emphasis (regardless of injury) will always be airway, breathing, and circulatory management and consideration of spinal immobilization.

Assessment Considerations

Because of differences in infant and child anatomy, as compared to adult anatomy, there are some special considerations for the assessment of the infant or child trauma patient. Some of these considerations for injuries to the head, chest, abdomen, and extremities are discussed next.

Head Head injuries are common in children because of the relatively larger size of the child's head compared to the body (Figure 38-37∗). The weight of the head will carry it forward in advance of the body. Often in trauma the head is the first thing to strike an object. Common findings of head injury include:

- Nausea and vomiting; altered mental status
- Respiratory arrest (common to serious head injuries)
- Facial and scalp injuries (in infants and children, blood loss can be profound enough to cause hypoperfusion)

The most common cause of hypoxia in the unresponsive patient with a head injury is the tongue obstructing the airway. Therefore, an important consideration in the primary assessment is the airway.

Shock is not typically one of the signs of a closed head injury. If signs of shock are present with a closed head injury, you should suspect that other injuries (e.g., internal injuries) are more likely causing the shock.

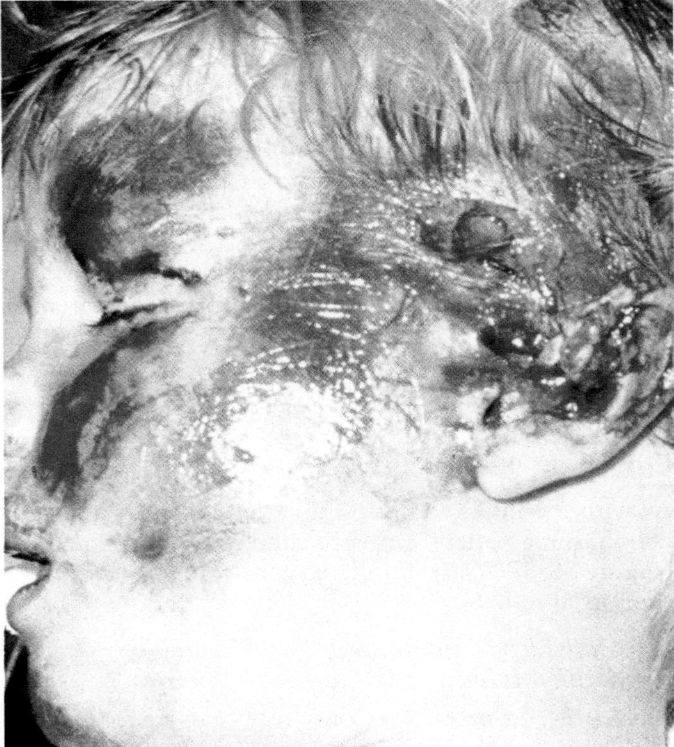

FIGURE 38-37 ∗ Head injuries are common in children because of the relatively large size of the child's head.

Chest Infants and children have ribs that are more pliable than adult ribs. This means that the young patient is less likely to suffer rib fractures, but is more likely to sustain internal damage (lung injury, heart wall injury) because the ribs do not protect these structures very well from forces applied to the chest. Even when you see minimal signs of external trauma, still suspect serious intrathoracic injuries.

Abdomen The abdominal muscles are not as developed in the child as in the adult, so they cannot offer as much protection from blunt trauma. If you have a patient who is deteriorating rapidly without external signs of injury, suspect hidden injuries of the abdomen. Consider any trauma to the abdomen as a serious injury, and transport the patient immediately.

Extremities The presentation of injuries to the extremities is the same for infants, children, and adults, and assessment and treatment of them is essentially the same. However, you should be sure to use the appropriately

Key Points
If the car seat a child is found in was involved in a crash, do not use it to transport the child.

Objective 38-15
Demonstrate removal of a pediatric patient from a child car seat.

sized immobilization equipment rather than trying to "makeshift" an adult device to fit an infant or child.

Burns Infants and children under the age of 5 years suffer more severe consequences from burns than do older children and adults. They are more at risk for hypothermia, fluid loss, and other effects, partly because of their greater skin surface in relation to body mass. In a trauma emergency that involves burns, remember to cover the burn with a dry, sterile burn dressing and keep the patient warm. If the burns meet the criteria for burn center admission in your area, transport to that facility. Review the special segments on infants and children in Chapter 29, "Burns."

Emergency Medical Care—Pediatric Trauma

As with an adult, the priorities in treating an infant or child trauma patient center around airway management (Figure 38-38✱), breathing, oxygenation, and circulatory support as follows:

1. *Establish and maintain in-line spine stabilization and the airway,* using a jaw thrust.
2. *Suction as necessary.* Constantly reassess for hemorrhage into the mouth.
3. *Provide oxygen at 15 lpm by nonrebreather mask if ventilations are adequate, or initiate positive pressure ventilation with supplemental oxygen connected to the ventilation device if breathing is inadequate.*
4. *Provide complete spinal immobilization* (a discussion of infant/child immobilization is given later in this chapter). Never use sandbags as a means to secure the head to a long spinal board. If it ever becomes necessary to roll the backboard with the patient secured (for vomiting), the heavy sandbags will put unnecessary pressure on the head.
5. *Transport* to a hospital. See Figure 38-39✱ for criteria that may require transport to a trauma center. Pediatric emergencies often involve charged emotions. Remember that the safety of everyone is crucial during transport. All passengers should be properly restrained, the use of lights and sirens should be limited, and safe driving practices should be adhered to.

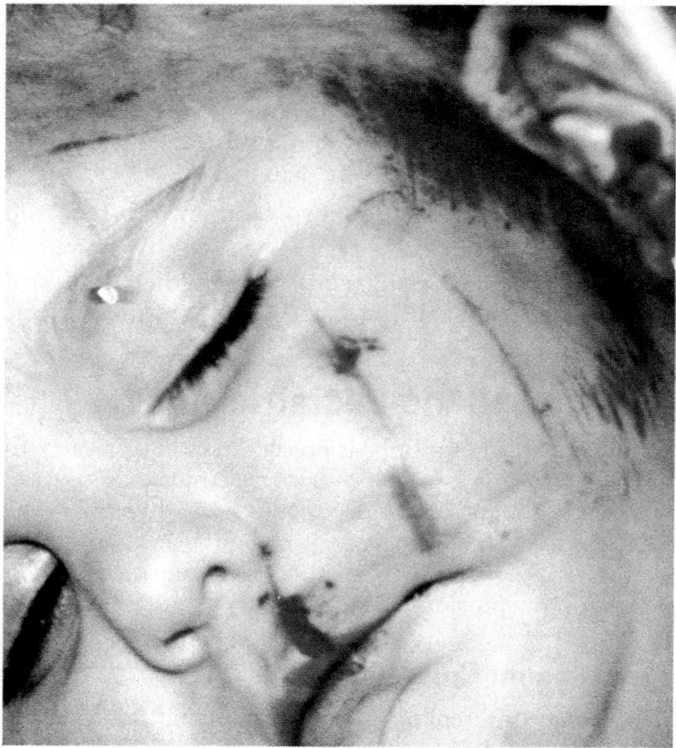

FIGURE 38-38 ✱ Be aware that children with facial injuries are especially vulnerable to airway compromise.

Infant and Child Car Seats in Trauma

Because of child-restraint laws in many states, you will encounter an increasing number of children involved in motor vehicle crashes who are in child safety seats. These seats, if properly installed, are designed to hold a child in place during impact, particularly from head-on or rear-end collisions. Their effectiveness in broadside or rotating crashes is not yet clear. A survey of caretakers by the National SafeKids Campaign found that more than half of all children are either buckled incorrectly into child safety seats or don't use restraints at all. The most common mistakes caregivers make include choosing an inappropriate seat size for the child, improperly threading the safety belt through the seat, and failing to make the safety strap fit snugly enough.

Removing the Infant or Child from a Car Seat

If the car seat the child was in was involved in a motor vehicle crash, do not use it to transport the child. Once a car seat has been involved in a crash, the structural integrity is in question. The child must be removed from

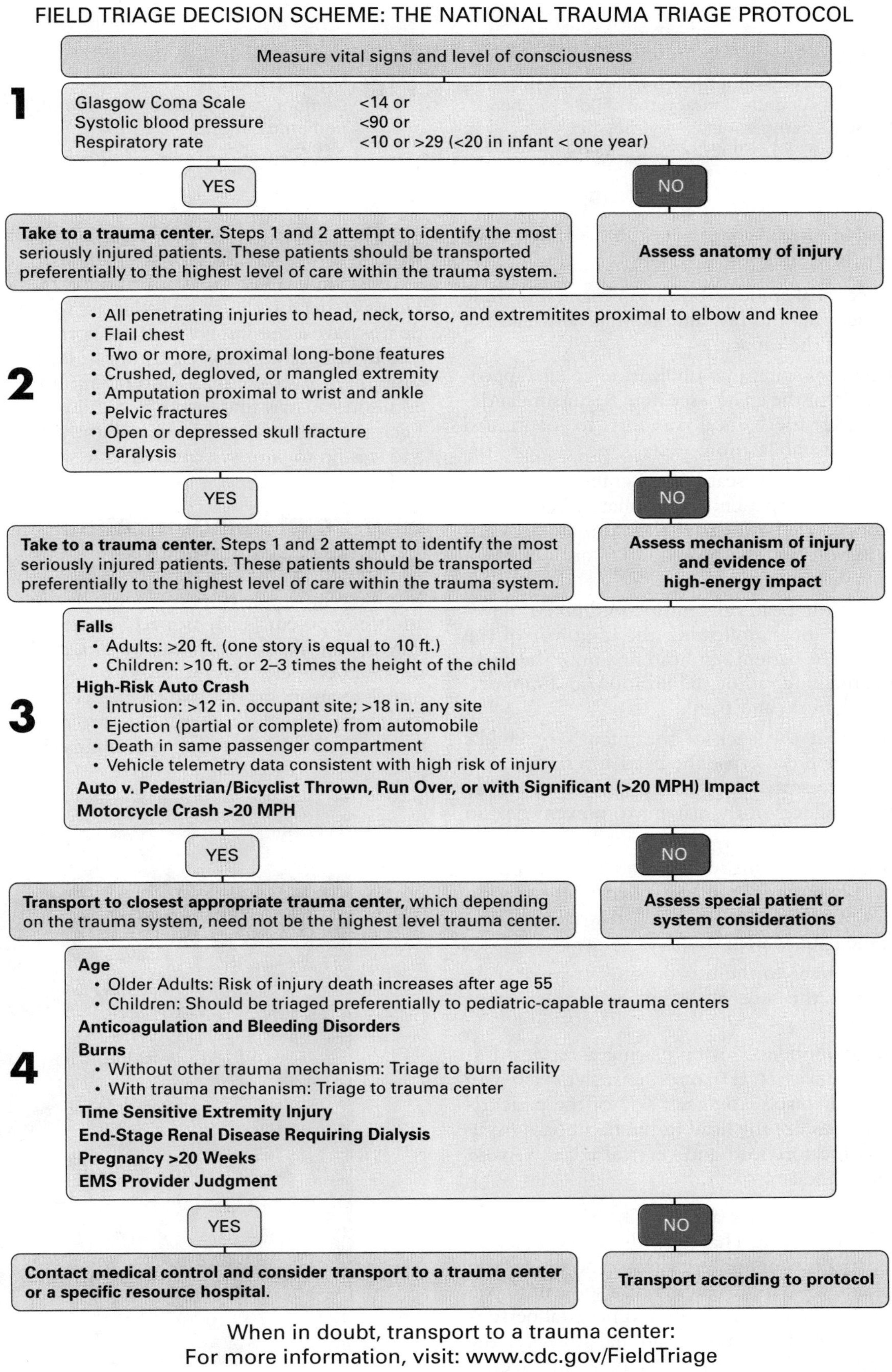

FIELD TRIAGE DECISION SCHEME: THE NATIONAL TRAUMA TRIAGE PROTOCOL

Measure vital signs and level of consciousness

1

Glasgow Coma Scale	<14 or
Systolic blood pressure	<90 or
Respiratory rate	<10 or >29 (<20 in infant < one year)

YES: **Take to a trauma center.** Steps 1 and 2 attempt to identify the most seriously injured patients. These patients should be transported preferentially to the highest level of care within the trauma system.

NO: **Assess anatomy of injury**

2

- All penetrating injuries to head, neck, torso, and extremitites proximal to elbow and knee
- Flail chest
- Two or more, proximal long-bone features
- Crushed, degloved, or mangled extremity
- Amputation proximal to wrist and ankle
- Pelvic fractures
- Open or depressed skull fracture
- Paralysis

YES: **Take to a trauma center.** Steps 1 and 2 attempt to identify the most seriously injured patients. These patients should be transported preferentially to the highest level of care within the trauma system.

NO: **Assess mechanism of injury and evidence of high-energy impact**

3

Falls
- Adults: >20 ft. (one story is equal to 10 ft.)
- Children: >10 ft. or 2–3 times the height of the child

High-Risk Auto Crash
- Intrusion: >12 in. occupant site; >18 in. any site
- Ejection (partial or complete) from automobile
- Death in same passenger compartment
- Vehicle telemetry data consistent with high risk of injury

Auto v. Pedestrian/Bicyclist Thrown, Run Over, or with Significant (>20 MPH) Impact

Motorcycle Crash >20 MPH

YES: **Transport to closest appropriate trauma center,** which depending on the trauma system, need not be the highest level trauma center.

NO: **Assess special patient or system considerations**

4

Age
- Older Adults: Risk of injury death increases after age 55
- Children: Should be triaged preferentially to pediatric-capable trauma centers

Anticoagulation and Bleeding Disorders

Burns
- Without other trauma mechanism: Triage to burn facility
- With trauma mechanism: Triage to trauma center

Time Sensitive Extremity Injury

End-Stage Renal Disease Requiring Dialysis

Pregnancy >20 Weeks

EMS Provider Judgment

YES: **Contact medical control and consider transport to a trauma center or a specific resource hospital.**

NO: **Transport according to protocol**

When in doubt, transport to a trauma center:
For more information, visit: www.cdc.gov/FieldTriage

FIGURE 38-39 ✱ Field Triage Decision Scheme: The National Trauma Triage Protocol.

Key Points
Almost any child under age 5 will resist being restrained. A gentle hand on the child's forehead or having a caregiver close by may help.

Objective 38-16
Demonstrate proper spinal immobilization of a pediatric patient.

the car seat and immobilized on a backboard. If that is the case, follow these guidelines:

1. Establish cervical spine stabilization manually, while your partner cuts the restraining straps and lifts the front guard of the car seat.
2. Apply a cervical spine immobilization collar (appropriately sized for the child—see item 8), or similar device, to offer mechanical support to continued manual in-line stabilization.
3. Position the entire car seat in the center of the backboard to which the patient will ultimately be secured. With a coordinated effort, tilt the car seat backward until resting on the backboard. Take care not to let the patient slide out.
4. The EMT at the head calls for a coordinated movement of the patient, following the long axis of the body, sliding the patient out head first onto the backboard, maintaining in-line stabilization, and supporting the head, neck, and trunk.
5. Remember that the back of the infant's or child's head is large and can cause the head and neck to flex forward. If necessary, place a small, folded towel beneath the shoulders of the patient to prevent flexion of the head and neck.
6. While you maintain manual in-line spinal stabilization, have your partner place rolled-up towels on both sides of the patient to help pad spaces prior to securing the patient with straps.
7. Secure the patient to the board using straps or wide tape. Position the securing straps across the chest, hips, and legs.
8. Finish the immobilization by placing a cervical immobilization device (CID), or other such device (you can use rolled towels), on each side of the patient's head. Finally, secure the head to the backboard using tape across the forehead and cervical collar. (Avoid taping across the chin.)

Almost any child under age 5 will resist being restrained. Sometimes laying a hand gently on the forehead will keep the patient from fighting against the straps. You may have to manually stabilize the cervical spine until you arrive at the emergency department and hospital personnel take over. To minimize the emotional stress for the child, have a caregiver close enough to maintain eye contact with, talk to, and touch the child.

There are a number of pediatric immobilization devices on the market today. The "baby size" cervical collars are designed to fit a child at or about 24 months of age. Don't try to force a larger collar on a small child. If you do not have a cervical collar of the correct size, improvise one by rolling up a towel, taping it, laying it in a horseshoe shape over the neck, and taping down the ends. In addition you may find specialized child-size immobilizers. Each manufacturer produces a slightly different product and it is up to your system to decide which type to use.

Four-Point Immobilization of an Infant or Child

If some very simple rules of immobilization are followed, adult equipment (such as a KED—Kendrick Extrication Device—or like product) can be modified to immobilize the child properly (Figure 38-40✱). When you must immobilize an infant or child to a stretcher, be aware that most straps attached to stretchers are designed to accommodate an adult. One way to accommodate children and

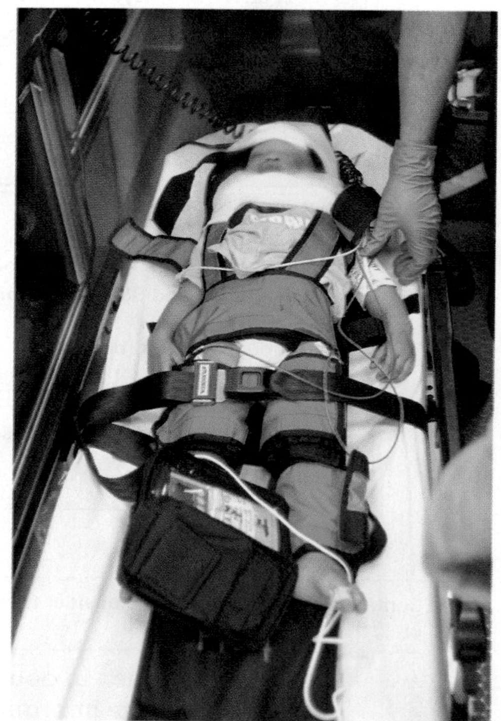

FIGURE 38-40 ✱ Child fully immobilized. (© Mark C. Ide)

Objective 38-17
Explain the importance of injury prevention programs to reduce pediatric injuries and deaths.

Key Terms
abuse causing deliberate harm to another person.
physical abuse causing deliberate physical injury or harm.
neglect the provision of insufficient attention or respect to someone who has a claim to that attention.

Emergency Care Protocol

PEDIATRIC TRAUMA

1. Establish and maintain in-line spine stabilization and open the airway, using a jaw-thrust maneuver.
2. Suction secretions no longer than 3–5 seconds each time.
3. Provide positive pressure ventilation with supplemental oxygen connected to the ventilation device at a rate of 12–20 ventilations/minute if breathing is inadequate.
4. If breathing is adequate, administer oxygen via nonrebreather mask at 15 lpm; consider blow-by oxygen in infants and very young children.
5. Occlude any open wounds to the chest with a nonporous dressing taped on three sides.
6. Manage abdominal evisceration by applying a moist sterile dressing to exposed organs, covered by a nonporous dressing secured in place.
7. If spinal injury is suspected, completely immobilize the patient to a long board.
8. Consider calling advanced life support.
9. If a pelvic injury is suspected and the patient has abdominal pain, apply the pneumatic antishock garment according to local protocol.
10. Expedite transport.
11. Splint fractures and dress wounds.
12. Perform a reassessment every 5 minutes.

FIGURE 38-41 * Emergency care protocol: pediatric trauma.

infants is to use a four-point safety harness, as shown in EMT Skills 38-6A to 38-6C.

Injury Prevention

Because injury is the leading cause of death and disability in children and adolescents, there must be an intentional process for identifying and preventing pediatric injuries. The term *injury* is not synonymous with *accident*. Unlike an accident, a childhood injury is an understandable, predictable, and preventable occurrence.

Pediatric injury prevention is one of the most important and challenging aspects of child health care. Young children inherently lack mature decision-making skills to protect themselves from injury, while some older children and adolescents engage in risky behaviors. No child is immune to all dangers that pose a threat to his health and safety. Statistics show that preventable childhood injuries account for 44 percent of all deaths in individuals between the ages of 1 and 19 years. In 2002, unintentional injury resulted in the death of 20,000 children, adolescents, and young adults. Rates and statistics cited here are mainly from the American Academy of Pediatrics (AAP) Policy Statements, pediatric medical journals, and the AAP publication *Injury Prevention and Control for Children and Youth*.

Injury prevention must be of paramount concern to EMS providers. Common injury prevention strategies currently employed by EMS providers across the United States include child safety seat education and inspections, fire safety programs, and community CPR training, among others. As an EMS provider, you should identify and engage in injury prevention programs within your local jurisdiction.

To review emergency care for trauma in the infant or child, see Figure 38-41*.

Child Abuse and Neglect

The estimated number of children who are abused or neglected in the United States is staggering. Estimates range between 500,000 and 4 million cases annually, with thousands of abused children dying. In fact, child **abuse** is the only major cause of infant and child death that has increased in the last 30 years.

Physical abuse takes place when improper or excessive action is taken so as to injure or cause harm. **Neglect** is the provision of inadequate attention or respect to someone who has a claim to that attention. The adult (usually a caregiver) who abuses a child often behaves in an evasive manner, volunteering little information or giving contradictory information about what happened to the child. The caregiver may show outright hostility toward the child or toward another caregiver in the household and rarely shows any guilt. The abused child will usually show fear when asked to describe how the injury occurred.

In many cases, a child will be the victim of a combination of physical, emotional, and sexual abuse and neglect. General indicators of abuse and neglect include (EMT Skills 38-7A to 38-7J):

- Multiple abrasions, lacerations, incisions, bruises, or broken bones
- Multiple injuries or bruises in various stages of healing
- Injuries on both the front and back or on both sides of the child's body
- Unusual wounds (such as cigarette burns or from a belt buckle)
- A fearful child
- Injuries to the genitals
- Injuries, often lethal, to the brain or spinal cord that occur when the infant or child is violently shaken (known as "shaken baby syndrome")
- Situations in which the injuries do not match the mechanism of injury described by the caregivers or the patient
- Lack of adult supervision
- Untreated chronic illnesses (e.g., no medication for a child with asthma)
- Malnourishment and unsafe living environment
- Delay in reporting injuries
- Implausible explanations (e.g., 6-month-old infant pulled boiling water onto himself)

Accidental bruises are often found on the lower arms, knees, shins, iliac crests, and forehead, and under the chin. "Suspicious" bruises are found on the buttocks, genitalia, thighs, ears, side of face, trunk, and upper arms.

Emergency Medical Care Guidelines for Child Abuse

You should be familiar with several important guidelines when called to a possible child abuse situation. While the following care steps assume that a caregiver is the abuser, remember that a child may also be abused by a relative, sibling, or neighbor.

- **Gaining entry.** If the call came from outside the family, the caregivers may resist, and entry should be handled by the police. If you are asked to help the child, calm the caregivers and indicate that you are there to help and render emergency care to the child. Speak in a low, firm voice. If the scene is, or becomes, dangerous, request law enforcement to be dispatched.
- **Dealing with the child.** Speak softly and call the child by his first name. Do not ask the child to tell what happened while he is still in the crisis environment, with the possible abuser still present.
- **Examining the child.** If you have reason to suspect abuse, perform a head-to-toe (toe-to-head or trunk-to-head for an infant or toddler) rapid trauma assessment for evidence of and clues to internal injury. Look carefully for signs of head trauma, closely examining the ears and nose for blood or cerebrospinal fluid and the eyes for pupillary changes. Conduct the examination in a matter-of-fact fashion, and keep your suspicions to yourself. Since this is likely a crime scene, also note all that you have observed at the scene (e.g., condition of the home; any objects that might have been used to hurt the child, such as a belt or straps).
- **Dealing with the caregivers.** After administering emergency care, tell the caregivers that the child should be taken to the hospital for further care. In a separate room from the child, ask the caregivers to describe how the injury occurred. (This will permit the hospital staff, social service workers, or others later to compare the child's account with that of the caregivers.) *Do not question the caregivers about abuse, or act accusatory in any way. This is inappropriate and will only delay transport.* Simply gather information concerning the injuries as you would for any other problem.
- **Transporting the child.** Do not allow the child to be left alone with the suspected abuser. This may provide the opportunity for further abuse or intimidation.
- **Providing documentation.** When you reach the hospital, privately convey your suspicions and findings to the physician. Know your state's reporting laws for child abuse but also know that federally you are a mandated reporter of any *suspected* child abuse—you need not be able to prove it, only suspect it—and failure to report is punishable. Document everything, but be objective, not subjective. It is not your role to write "The patient was abused," which is a judgment. Rather, by your accurate, objective, and detailed description of the injuries and history, the person reading the run report will come to this conclusion. Record all of your findings regarding the assessment, the conditions of the home, the behavior of the caregivers, and so on. Make drawings of injury patterns or locations of injuries. Maintain total confidentiality regarding the incident; do not share it with your family or friends.

It is critical that you be aware of the reporting laws in your state and the reporting protocols for your EMS system. Aspects of the law to know are:

Key Points
Child abuse cases are especially painful for EMS providers. Without divulging particulars of the case, be sure to talk out your feelings with someone you trust.

Objective 38-18
Discuss the purpose of the federal Emergency Medical Services for Children (EMSC) program and the concept of family-centered care.

Emergency Care Protocol

PEDIATRIC ABUSE AND NEGLECT

1. Consider calling law enforcement to gain entry or if the scene becomes unstable or dangerous.
2. Establish and maintain an open airway, extending the head only enough to allow an open airway and avoid hyperextension. If spinal injury is suspected, provide in-line spine stabilization and perform a jaw-thrust maneuver.
3. Suction secretions no longer than 3–5 seconds each time.
4. Provide positive pressure ventilation with supplemental oxygen connected to the ventilation device at a rate of 12–20 ventilations/minute if breathing is inadequate.
5. If breathing is adequate, administer oxygen via nonrebreather mask at 15 lpm; consider blow-by oxygen in infants and very young children.
6. Manage immediately life-threatening wounds.
7. If spinal injury is suspected, completely immobilize the patient to a long board.
8. Consider calling advanced life support if a priority patient.
9. Expedite transport.
10. Splint fractures and dress wounds.
11. Perform a reassessment every 5 minutes.
12. Special considerations when dealing with child abuse and neglect:
    a. Speak softly and call the child by his first name.
    b. Do not ask the child to re-create the situation or answer questions while still in the abusive environment.
    c. Your main goal is to conduct an assessment and treat the injured infant or child. You are not there to investigate a crime; however, note and report objectively what was observed at the scene.
    d. Do not question the caregivers about the abuse, but ask what happened.
    e. Do not let the child be left alone with the suspected or possible abuser.
    f. Provide accurate and objective documentation in the EMS report.
    g. Report your suspicions to receiving staff.

FIGURE 38-42 ✱ Emergency care protocol: pediatric abuse and neglect.

- Who must report the abuse
- What types of abuse and neglect must be reported
- To whom the reports are to be made
- What information a reporter must give
- What immunity the reporter is granted
- Criminal penalties for failing to report

Child abuse cases are particularly painful for EMS providers. Be sure you talk out your feelings with someone you can trust (making sure not to divulge particulars of the case). Feelings of anger, revulsion, frustration, and helplessness are normal. In most instances, there is no perfect solution, whether the child remains in the home or is placed elsewhere. Yet, an EMT's skillful interviewing and reporting can make a positive difference, even in bad situations.

To review emergency care for abuse and neglect in the infant or child, see Figure 38-42✱.

Special Care Considerations

Emergency Medical Services for Children (EMSC)

The federal Emergency Medical Services for Children (EMSC) program is designed to ensure that all children and adolescents, no matter where they live, attend school, or travel, have access to and receive appropriate care in a health emergency. The program is jointly administered by the Maternal and Child Health Bureau of the U.S. Department of Health and Human Services Health Resources and Services Administration and the National Highway Traffic Safety Administration of the U.S. Department of Transportation. Since its establishment in 1984, the EMSC program has provided grant funding to all 50 states, the District of Columbia, and five U.S. territories.

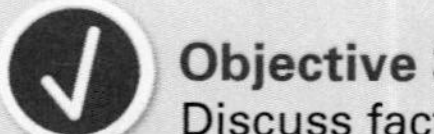

Objective 38-19
Discuss factors that can increase EMS providers' stress on pediatric calls and ways of managing the stress that may be associated with a pediatric call.

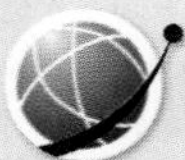

Media Resources
Go to www.bradybooks.com for mykit. Highlights:

- *Web Resource:* Child Maltreatment
- *Web Resource:* Child Behavior Disorders

Family-Centered Care

The concept of family-centered care was introduced in 1987 as a component of former U.S. Surgeon General C. Everett Koop's initiative for family-centered, community-based, coordinated care for children with special health care needs and their families. Family-centered care suggests that health care providers acknowledge and make use of the family's knowledge of their family member's condition and make use of the family's abilities to communicate with their family member. Although the concept of family-centered care is not new, it is new to EMS as an initiative championed by the EMSC program.

A major principle of family-centered care is the need for a comprehensive understanding of normal growth and development, which will enable the EMS provider to better anticipate the physiological and emotional needs of the child who is affected by illness or injury. Additionally, family-centered care advocates open communication with family members throughout the assessment and management of the child.

Taking Care of Yourself

Taking care of a critically ill or injured child is one of the most challenging facets of an EMS career. The death of a child has a profound effect on every one of us. Almost half of the children in the United States who die from unintentional injuries are pronounced dead either at the scene or in the emergency department. EMTs who treat infants or children commonly experience stress and anxiety from:

- Lack of experience in treating children (from the relative infrequency of treating children)
- Fear of failure
- Identifying patients with their own children (e.g., "This could be my daughter . . .")

To help alleviate stress:

- Understand that much of what you learned about adults does apply to children; typically it is not what you do but how you do it that varies when your patient is an infant or child.
- Learn skills and practice using equipment with and examining children; the best defense against anxiety is preparation, practice, and more practice.
- Focus on the task at hand while treating infants and children. In other words, temporarily separate how you feel from what you must do.

As a professional EMT, you will need to control your emotions so that you can render the best possible assistance to your patient and be supportive of other victims. But after the incident is over, you still need to deal with those feelings. Most EMS systems have ready access to mental health services that can help defuse the stress that certain events can create. Use them. If not, find a trusted friend who will listen to you and allow you to talk about the EMS field.

EMT skills 38-1 Pediatric Primary Assessment

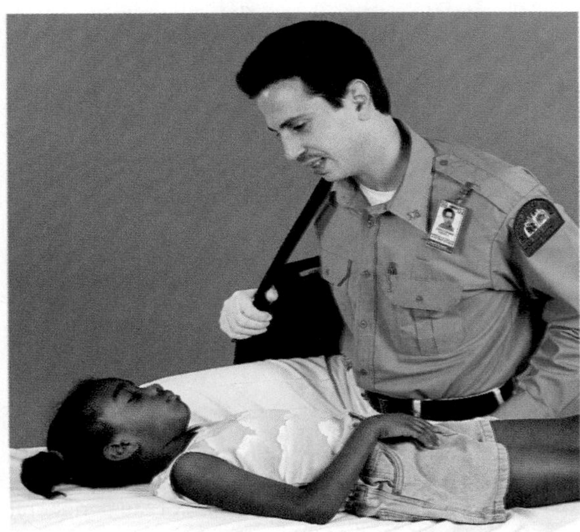

38-1A * Assess mental status using the AVPU method.

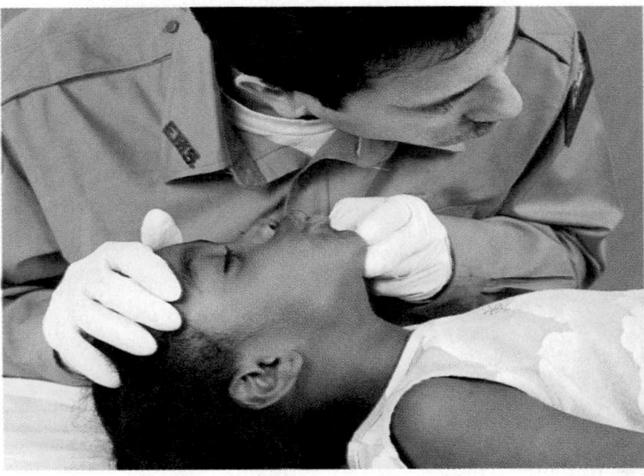

38-1B * Ensure an open airway. Listen for abnormal sounds that may indicate a need for suctioning.

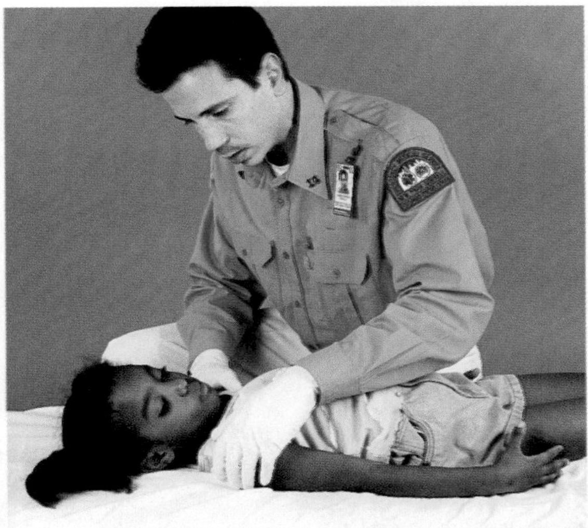

38-1C * Assess breathing. Listen for noisy breathing. Assess for diminished breathing.

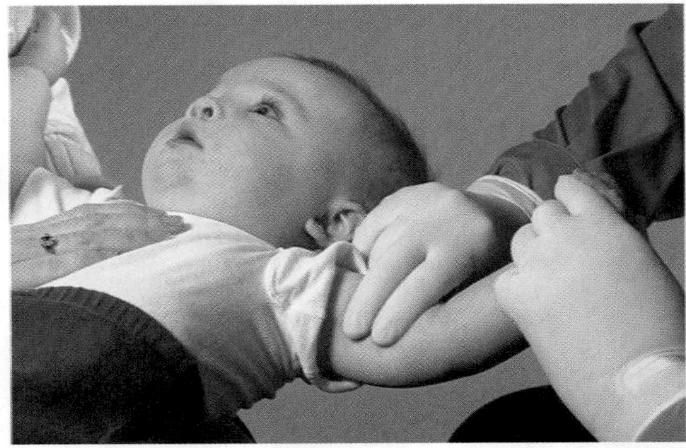

38-1D * Assess the strength of the peripheral pulse. In an infant, check the brachial pulse.

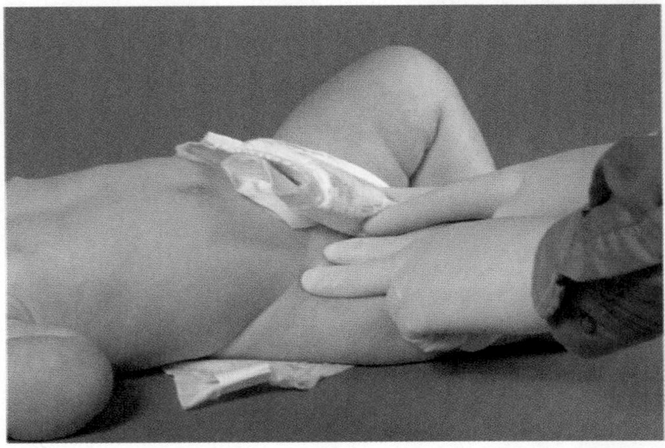

38-1E * Assess the strength of the central pulse. In an infant, check the femoral pulse. Locate this pulse by identifying the midpoint of an imaginary line extending from the anterior superior iliac spine to the symphysis pubis, then moving your fingertip about one to two finger breadths inferior.

continued

EMT skills 38-1 Pediatric Primary Assessment *continued*

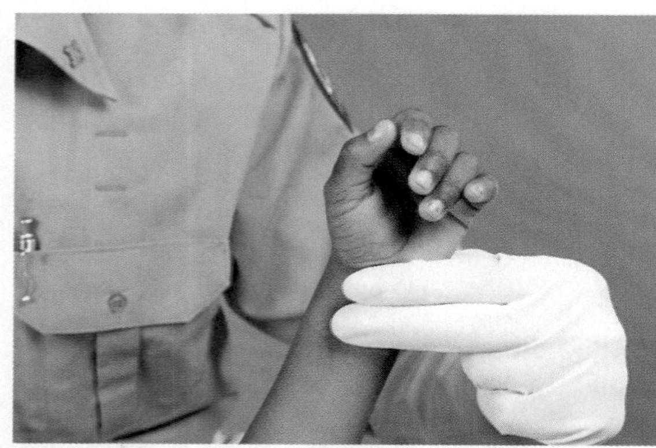

38-1F * In a child, check the radial pulse.

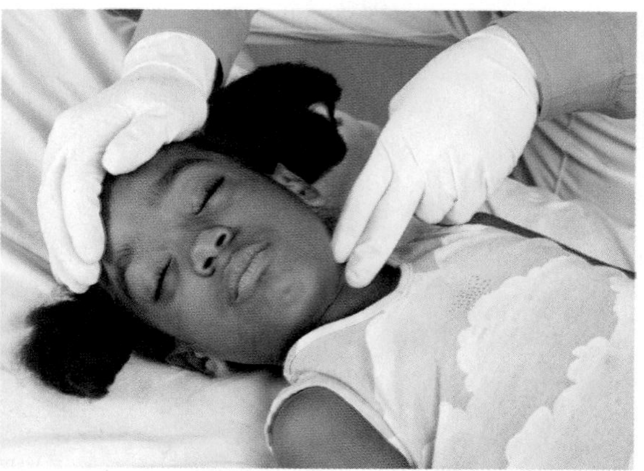

38-1G * To assess the strength of the central pulse in an older child, check the carotid pulse. Compare the strength of the central pulse to the previously determined strength of the peripheral pulse.

EMT skills 38-2 Checking Capillary Refill

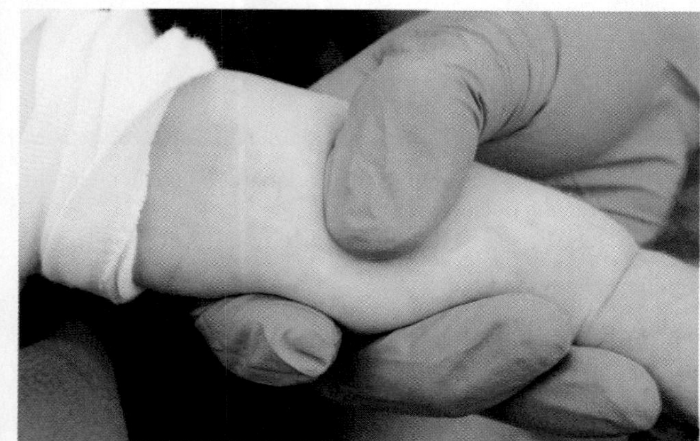

38-2A * Press the patient's forearm. (© Daniel Limmer)

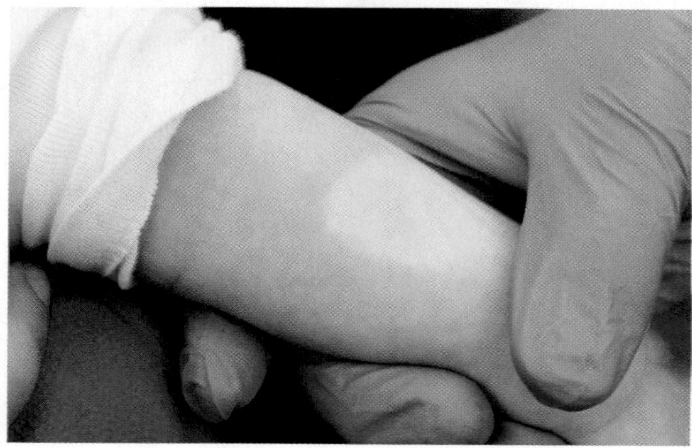

38-2B * Note how long the skin remains blanched after release. (© Daniel Limmer)

EMT skills 38-2 Checking Capillary Refill *continued*

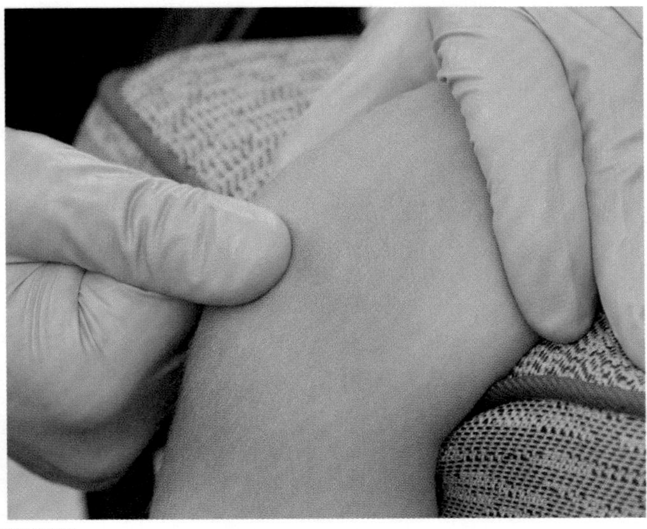

38-2C ✱ Alternatively, press the patient's kneecap.

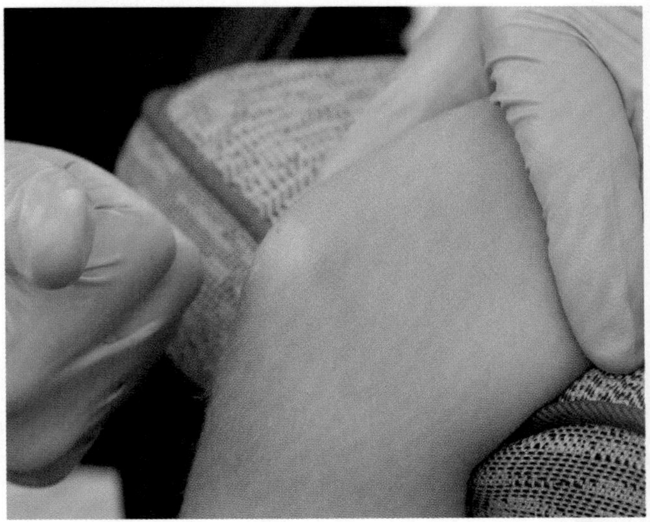

38-2D ✱ Note how long the skin remains blanched after release.

EMT skills 38-3 The Pediatric Physical Exam

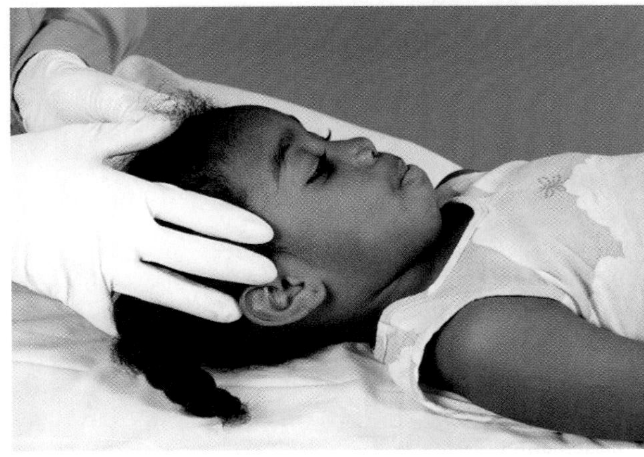

38-3A ✱ Examine the head. Look for bruising or blood or clear fluid draining from the nose or ears. Palpate gently for soft or spongy areas, skull irregularities, or crepitus (feeling of grinding bone fragments). In infants, check the fontanelle.

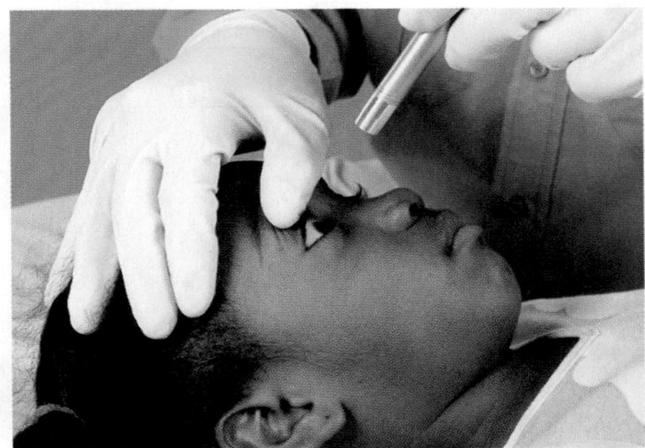

38-3B ✱ Check the eyes. The pupils should be equal in size and reactive to light.

continued

The Pediatric Physical Exam *continued*

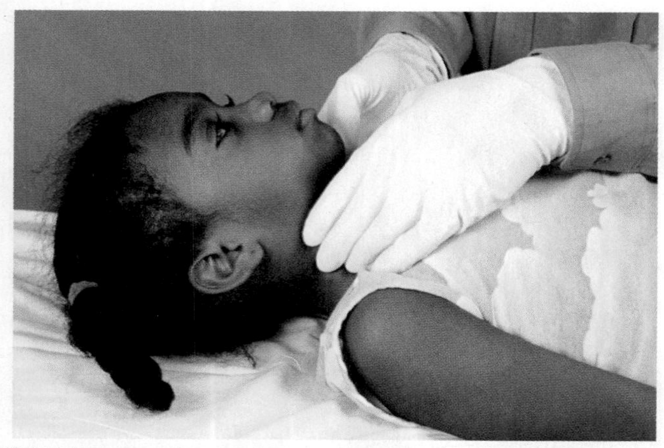

38-3C ✱ Examine the neck. Check for the position of the trachea, swollen neck veins, stiffness, tenderness, or crepitus.

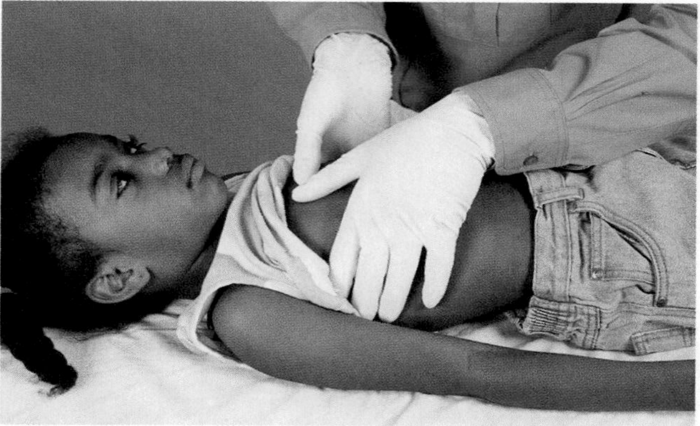

38-3D ✱ Examine the chest. Check for bruising, crepitus, and equal chest rise and fall. Watch for signs of breathing difficulty.

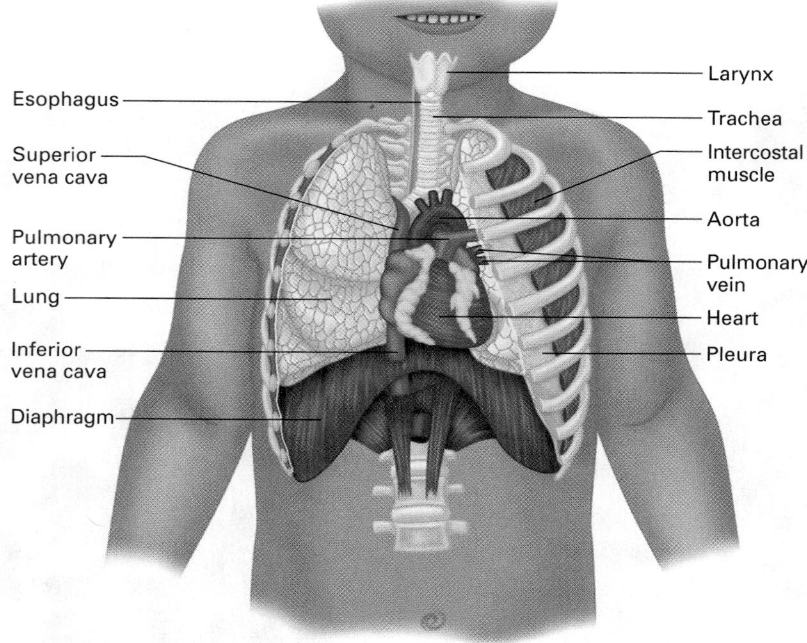

38-3E ✱ While examining the chest, be aware of the contents of the thorax.

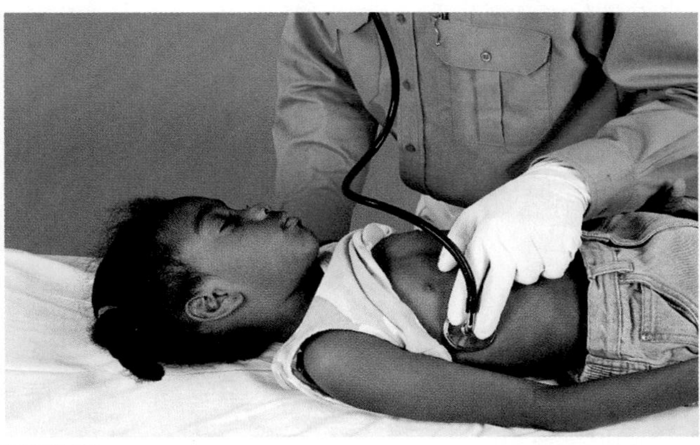

38-3F ✱ Auscultate for breath sounds over all lung fields.

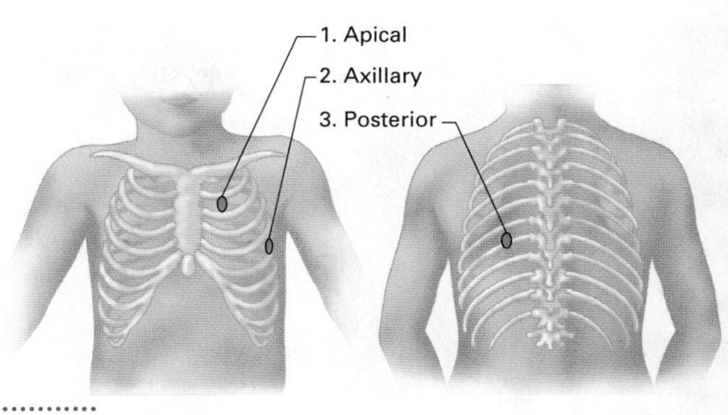

38-3G ✱ Auscultation sites.

38-3H ✱ Examine the abdomen. Check for bruising, tenderness, or guarding. Look for swelling that may indicate swallowed air.

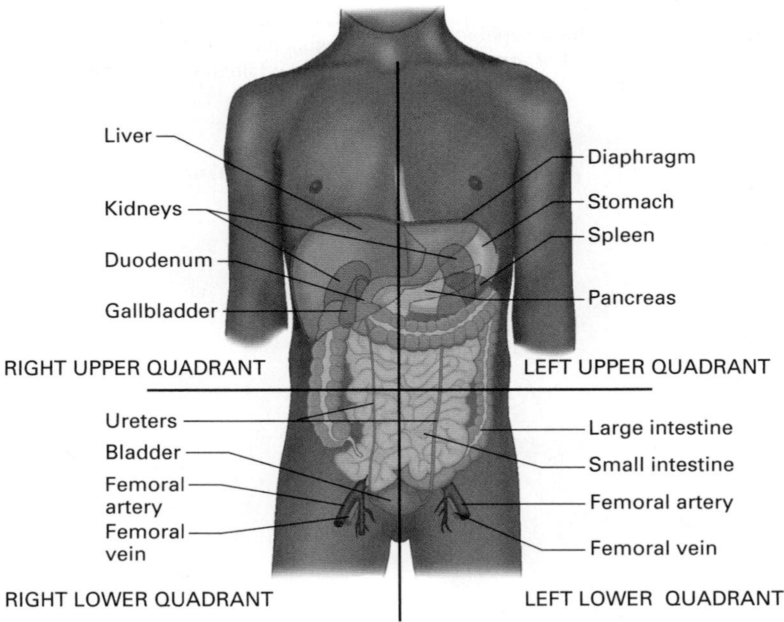

38-3I ✱ Divide the abdomen into quadrants and examine each one while remembering which organs are located in each quadrant.

continued

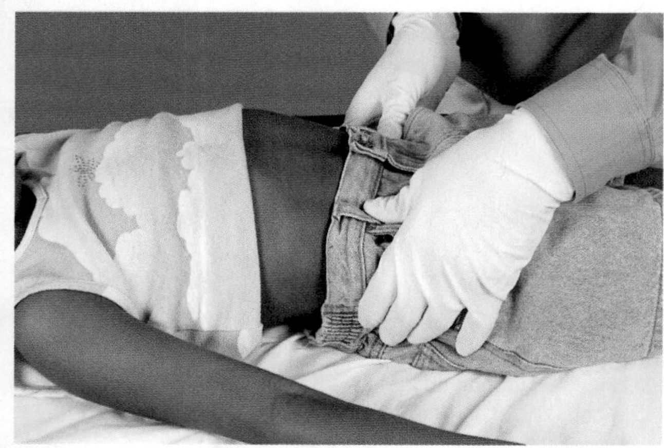

38-3J ✱ Examine the pelvis for tenderness, swelling, bruising, or crepitus.

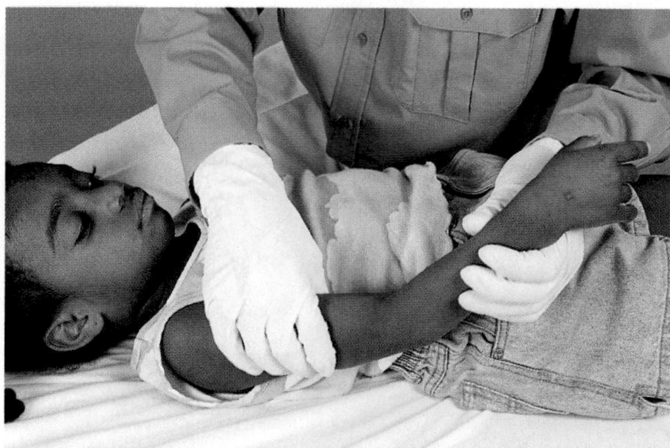

38-3K ✱ Examine the extremities. Evaluate pulses, sensation, and warmth. Look for unequal movement.

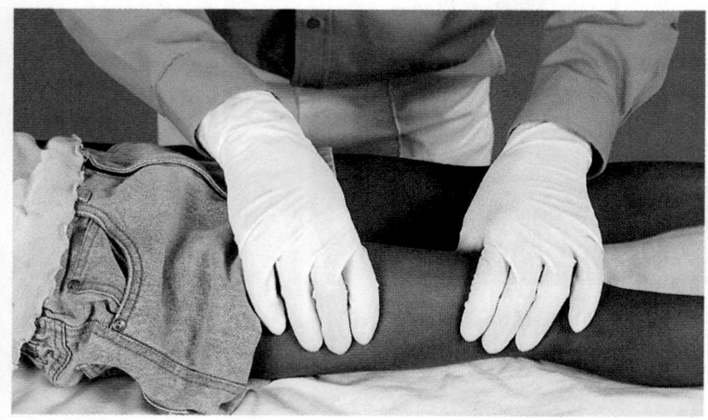

38-3L ✱ If there is unequal movement in the extremities, immobilize the spine and the affected extremity. Check capillary refill and peripheral pulses and compare with the other arm or leg, both before and after immobilizing an extremity.

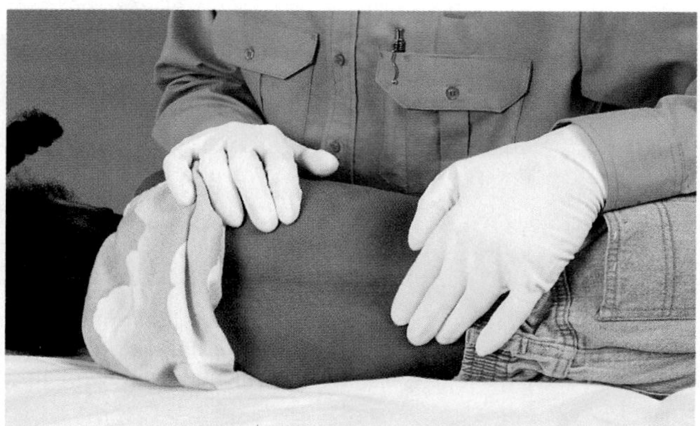

38-3M ✱ Examine the back. Assess for tenderness, bruising, and crepitus. If the child requires immobilization, the back can be checked while the child is being log rolled onto the spine board.

Oropharyngeal Airway

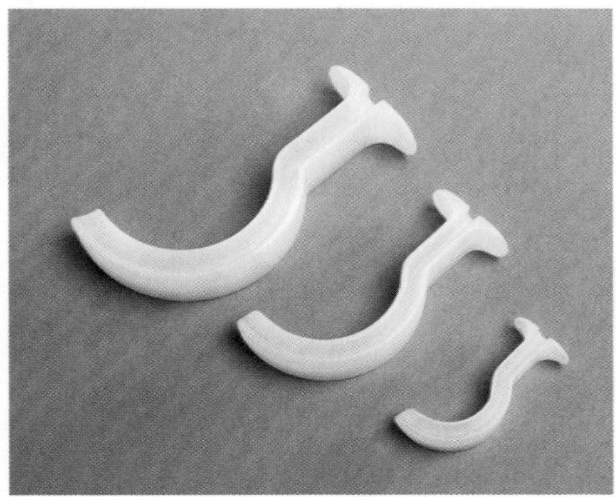

38-4A * A variety of oropharyngeal airways.

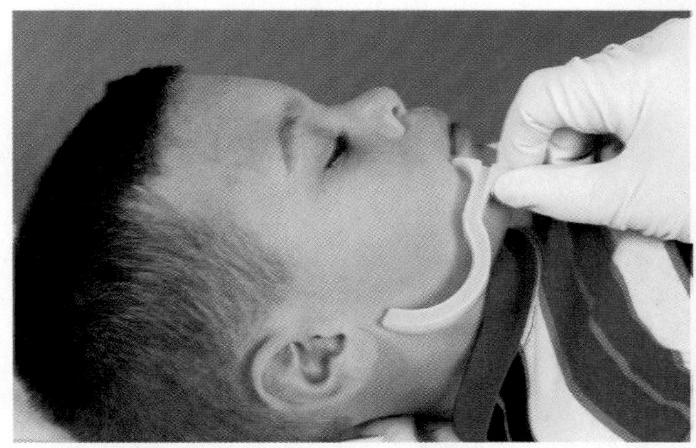

38-4B * Sizing an oropharyngeal airway.

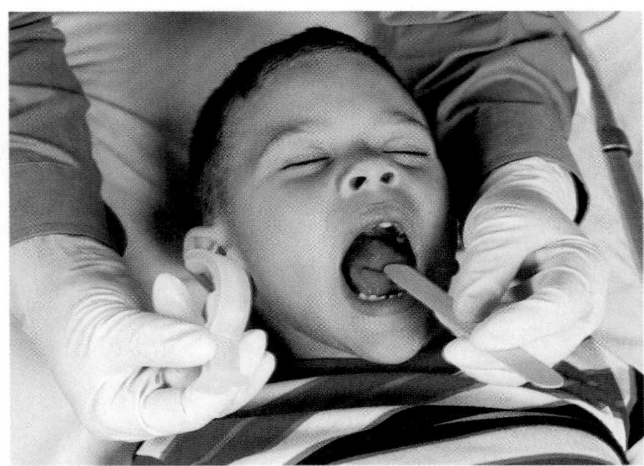

38-4C * Inserting an oropharyngeal airway, using a tongue depressor for insertion in a pediatric patient.

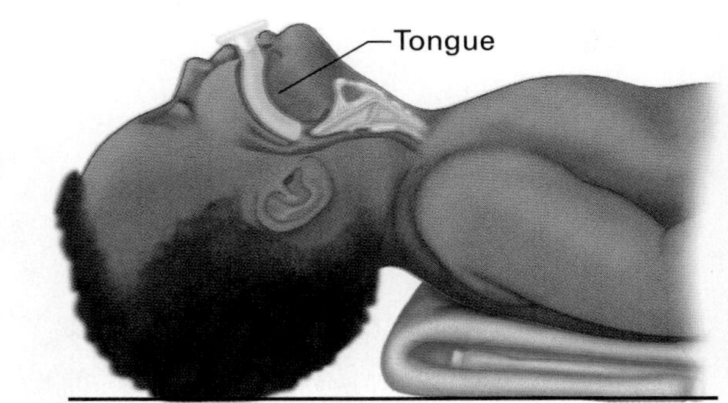

38-4D * An oropharyngeal airway in place.

EMT skills 38-5 Nasopharyngeal Airway

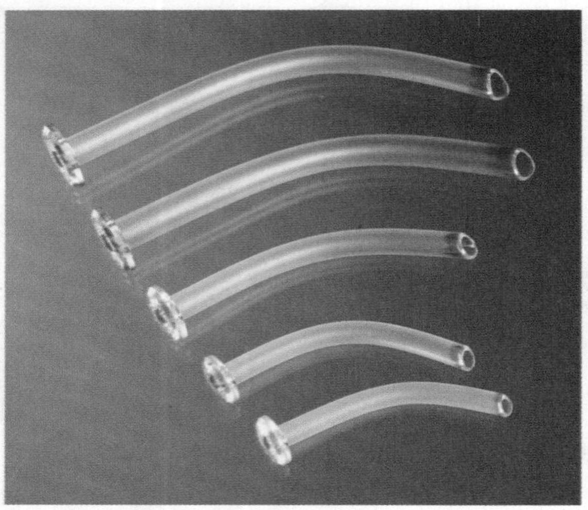

38-5A ✱ Nasopharyngeal airways in a variety of pediatric and adult sizes.

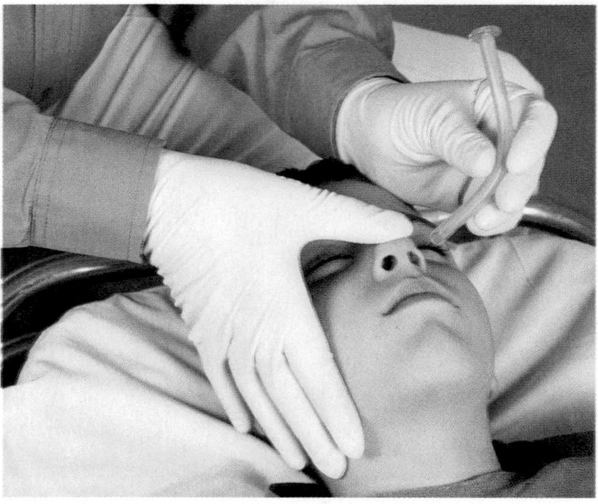

38-5B ✱ Retract the tip of the nose prior to inserting the nasopharyngeal airway into the nare.

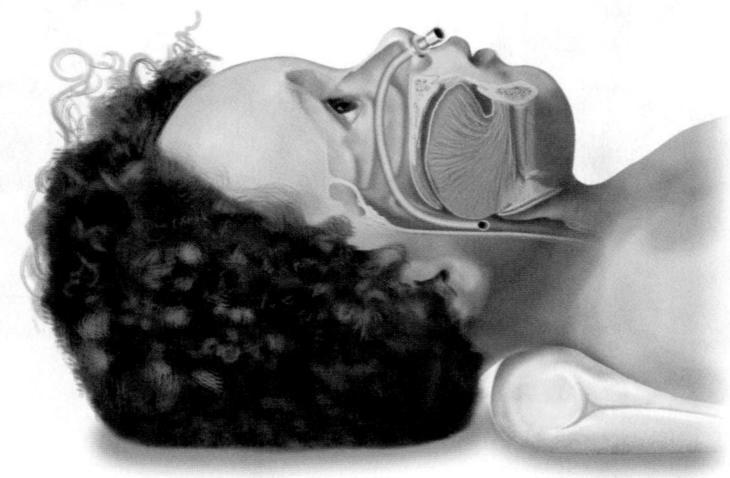

38-5C ✱ A nasopharyngeal airway in place.

EMT skills 38-6 A Pediatric Immobilization System

Before moving the patient to the pediatric immobilization sleeve and backboard, an appropriate-sized cervical collar should be applied. After application of the cervical collar, in-line stabilization of the head should be maintained until the entire body, including the head, is secured to the device. In addition to the cervical collar and manual stabilization, head blocks should be placed on both sides of the patient's head, as shown in these photos.

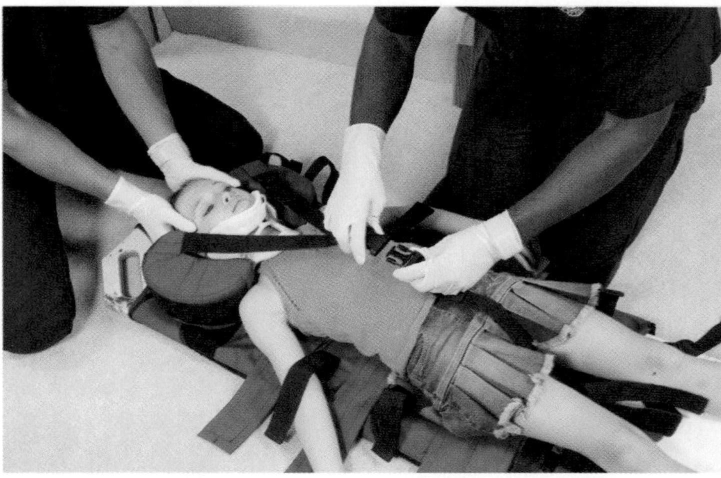

38-6A * While maintaining manual in-line stabilization, attach the three-point safety harness and adjust it for proper length.

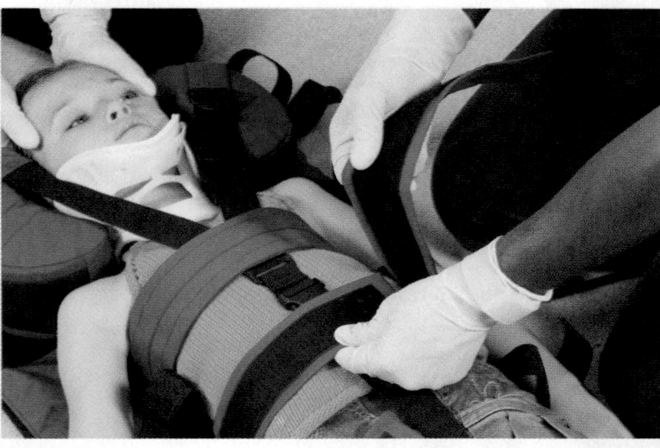

38-6B * Secure the three body straps across the patient at the chest, waist, and above the knees.

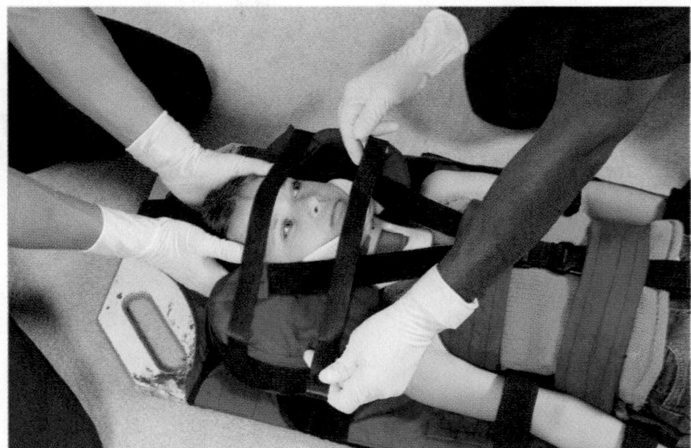

38-6C * Secure the arms and legs, using the extremity straps. Place straps across the forehead and chin to securely affix the patient's head to the pediatric sleeve.

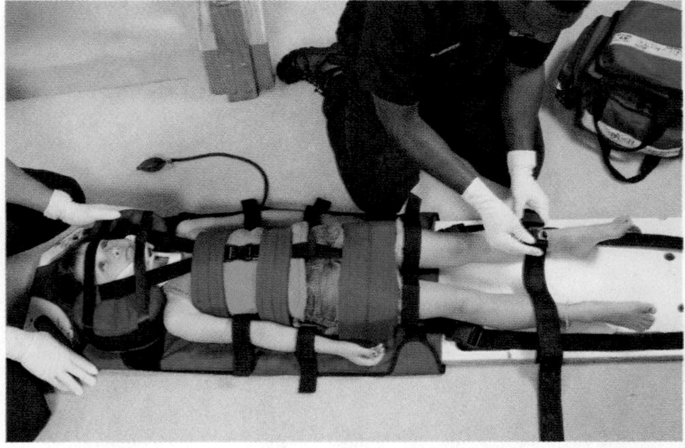

38-6D * The patient is now completely immobilized to the device. Secure the patient's legs to the backboard, using a backboard strap.

Note: The air pressure control bulb shown in photo D inflates a bladder within the device that pads voids between the patient and the pediatric sleeve. In younger patients with larger heads, the bladder should be inflated as needed to maintain the spine and the airway in a neutral position.

continued

EMT skills 36-6 A Pediatric Immobilization System *continued*

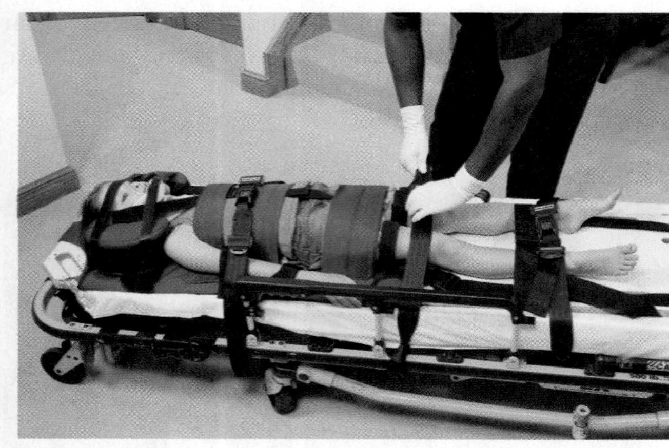

38-6E ✻ The completely immobilized patient secured to the cot.

Note: Always follow local protocols when performing this, or any, procedure.

EMT skills 38-7 Child Abuse and Neglect

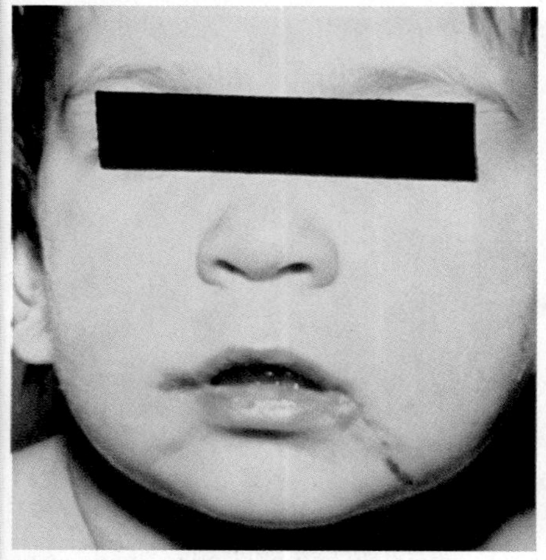

38-7A ✻ Bruising to the mouth.
(© Robert A. Felter, MD)

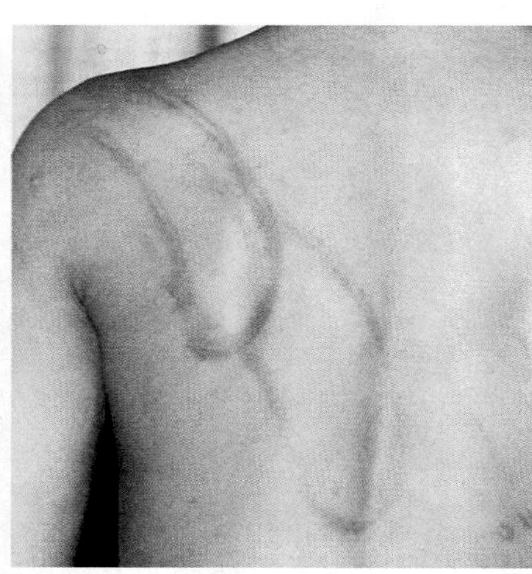

38-7B ✻ Cord bruise to the back.
(© Robert A. Felter, MD)

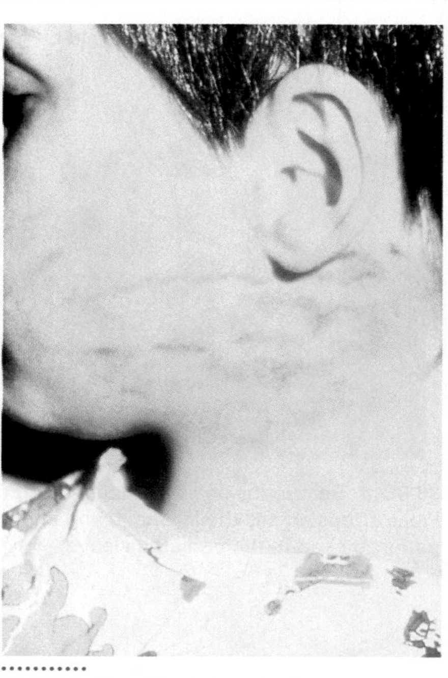

38-7C ✻ Hand bruise to the face.
(© Robert A. Felter, MD)

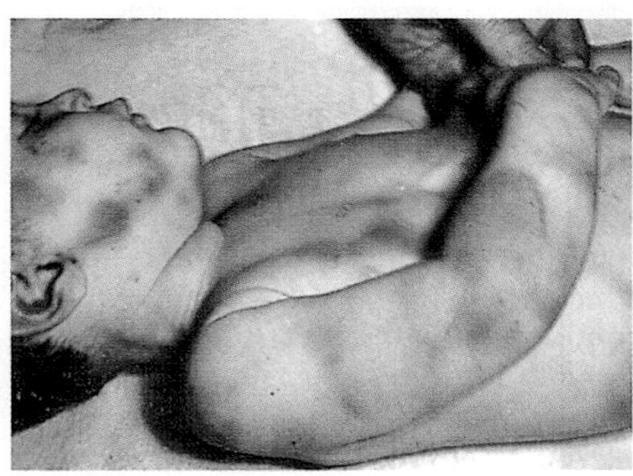
38-7D ✱ Death from multiple injuries.

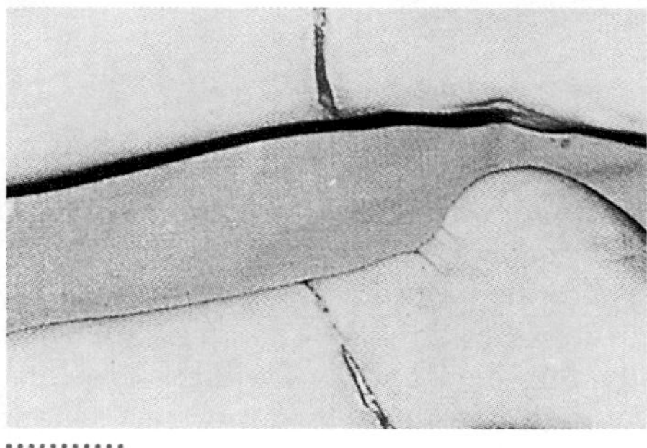
38-7E ✱ Restraining by tying.

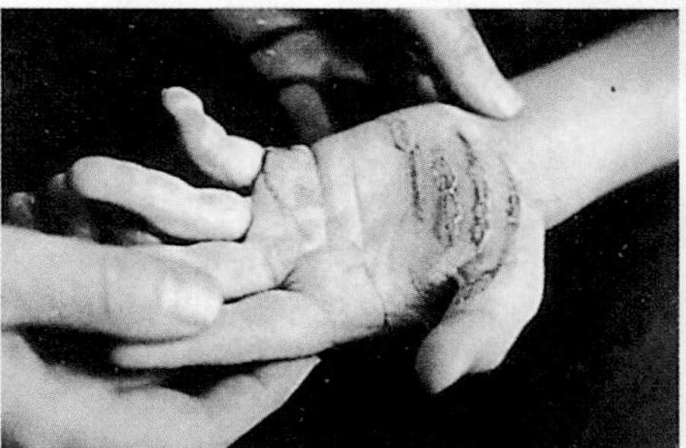
38-7F ✱ Stove burn to the hand.

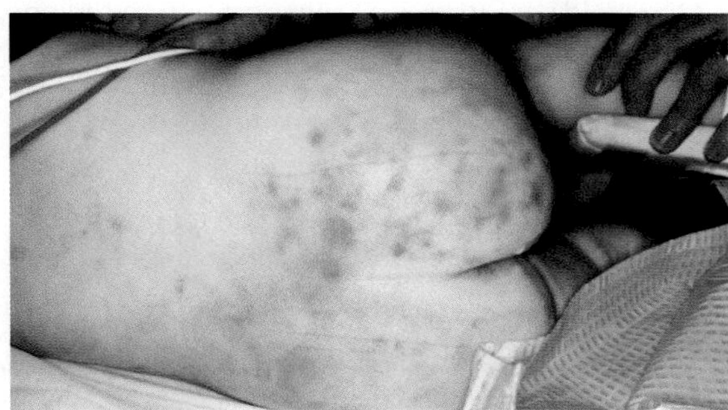
38-7G ✱ Bruises to the buttocks. (© Robert A. Felter, MD)

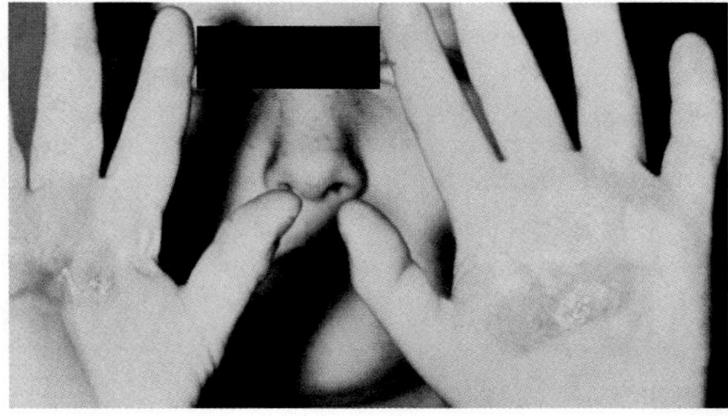
38-7H ✱ Cigarette burns to the hands. (© Robert A. Felter, MD)

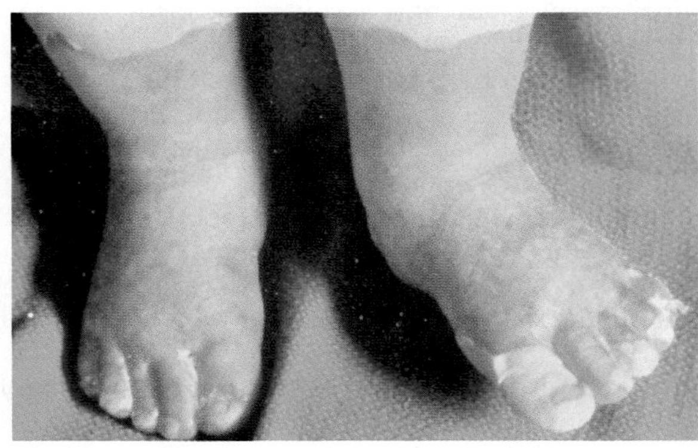
38-7I ✱ "Stocking" burns to the feet. (© Robert A. Felter, MD)

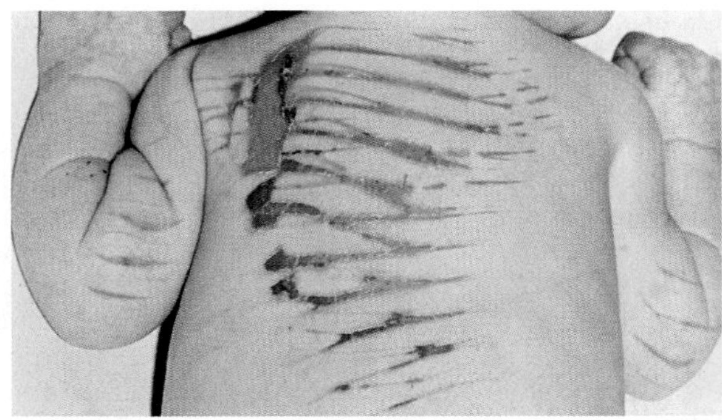
38-7J ✱ Cigarette lighter burns to the back. (© Robert A. Felter, MD)

CHAPTER REVIEW

SUMMARY

There are two major differences between caring for an adult patient and caring for an infant or child: (1) with pediatric patients you must usually also deal with their parents or other caregivers and (2) you must consider the developmental characteristics of pediatric patients and their anatomical and physiological differences from adults. A rapid general impression of the pediatric patient can be made "from the doorway" by using the pediatric assessment triangle to evaluate the infant or child's appearance, work of breathing, and circulation.

The primary goal in treating any infant or child is to anticipate and recognize respiratory problems and to immediately support any respiratory function that is compromised or lost. Failure to do so will defeat any other or subsequent treatment.

You must also be prepared to assess and provide emergency medical care for other medical problems common to infants and children, including seizures, altered mental status, poisonings, fever, shock (hypoperfusion), and drowning. A particularly difficult situation is SIDS, or the sudden death of an infant from an unidentified cause. SIDS cannot be diagnosed in the field, and you must immediately attempt resuscitation and transport the infant to the emergency department.

Trauma is the leading cause of death in children ages 1 to 14. Differences in the pediatric anatomy must be considered, especially with head, chest, abdominal, and extremity injuries. In cases where you suspect child abuse, your job is to treat the child's injuries and transport him to the hospital, to objectively document your findings and care, and to report any suspicion of abuse to the proper authorities according to the laws of your state.

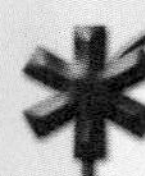

CASE STUDY FOLLOW-UP

SCENE SIZE-UP

You have been dispatched to an 11-month-old infant with an unknown medical problem. Having parked your ambulance out of the flow of traffic, you have almost no time for further scene size-up as the parents come running out of the house and thrust an infant into your arms, exclaiming, "Oh, help! Help! Jason's not breathing!"

PRIMARY ASSESSMENT

As soon as you see the infant, you identify cyanosis, flaccid muscles, and an absence of any response to the environment. It is obvious that this child is terribly ill, with ominous signs of respiratory arrest. As you immediately attempt to open the airway and assess for respirations, your EMT partner takes the parents and directs the mother to the passenger side of the ambulance, with the father to follow in a private vehicle to the hospital.

With little Jason in your arms, you rapidly proceed into the back of the ambulance. Your immediate opening of the airway did not result in spontaneous respirations. The mother cries from the front of the unit, "What's wrong with my baby!"

After confirming breathlessness, you attempt to provide positive pressure ventilation without success. You reposition Jason's airway and attempt ventilation again. Still no success. Your partner starts the unit moving to the hospital. Jason's color worsens.

SECONDARY ASSESSMENT

Since Jason is still suffering from a life threat, you have not proceeded to the secondary assessment. However, your partner quickly asks Jason's mother if he had shown any signs of illness. She shouts back to you, "He was absolutely fine." Because Jason's mother says he was not ill (which tends to indicate the problem is not related to a respiratory disease), and because repositioning the airway was unsuccessful, you now assume that Jason's airway is obstructed by a foreign body.

You lay Jason on a backboard, open his mouth, and look inside for evidence of an obstruction. Finding none, you position his airway and attempt to deliver two ventilations by bag-valve-mask device. You then deliver 30 compressions. You inspect inside the mouth prior to delivering the next two ventilations. This time, when you look into Jason's mouth, you see what looks like a peanut in the back of his throat. You quickly turn him on his side to remove it.

Jason is still not breathing so you insert an oropharyngeal airway and continue to provide positive pressure ventilations using a bag-valve mask with oxygen attached. This time, you are able to make Jason's chest rise with each ventilation, so you know that you have succeeded in unblocking his airway. You continue ventilations at 20 breaths per minute while assessing the pulse. The brachial pulse is currently 110/minute, and peripheral perfusion seems sluggish. His SpO_2 reading is 84% but increasing. Through her tears, the mother states that Jason was alone in the living room when he pulled himself up against a coffee table that had snacks in a bowl. When she returned into the living room, she says he was "just lying on the floor, gazing up, not moving—that's when I called."

REASSESSMENT

You are still about 4 minutes away from the hospital when you notice that Jason's color has changed from blue to a normal pink. His muscle tone has returned, and he is moving around actively. You stop the ventilations and assess Jason's spontaneous respiratory effort. You find it to be at a rate of 30 per minute and with a normal depth. Jason starts crying as you now apply oxygen at 15 lpm via a nonrebreather mask. You've never been so happy to hear a crying baby before! Jason's mother starts crying all over again when she hears him—this time tears of joy. Peripheral perfusion has returned to normal by the time you arrive at the hospital.

You communicate your assessment and treatment to the receiving facility and complete the appropriate paperwork. Before leaving the hospital, you stop in Jason's room and find him to be alert and responsive to his surroundings. Both parents start crying again when they see you. The mother hugs you and your partner and the father slaps you hard on the back as they thank you for saving their son's life.

You and your partner give each other a couple of happy grins as you mark back in service, prepared for the next call.

IN REVIEW

1. Describe differences in anatomy and physiology of the infant and child as compared to the adult patient.
2. Differentiate between early (compensated) respiratory distress and decompensated respiratory failure.
3. List the signs of an obstructed airway.
4. Describe the methods of determining end organ perfusion in the infant and child patient.
5. List the common causes of seizures in the infant and child patient and describe the management of seizures for the pediatric patient.
6. Describe the patterns of injury most likely to occur when pediatric patients are victims of trauma.
7. List the indicators of possible child abuse and neglect.
8. Discuss ways the EMT can deal with the emotional consequences of a difficult infant or child transport.

CRITICAL THINKING

You arrive on the scene at a residence and are directed to the second-floor bedroom by a male who is frantic. He indicates he is the father of a 2-year-old child who is really sick. He tells you that his wife placed the child in the bathtub and left for a couple of minutes to answer the phone. When she returned, the baby was submerged in the water. As you enter the bedroom, you note that the toddler is cyanotic and is limp. You yell the child's name and then squeeze the trapezius muscle but receive no response to either. The carotid pulse is absent and there is no ventilation evident.

1. What emergency care would you immediately provide for the toddler?
2. What special anatomical characteristics would you consider when establishing an airway and ventilating the toddler as compared to the adult?
3. How would you perform CPR on this toddler?
4. Would you apply the AED? If so, what special considerations must you contemplate when using the AED on a 2-year-old?

CHAPTER 39

Geriatrics

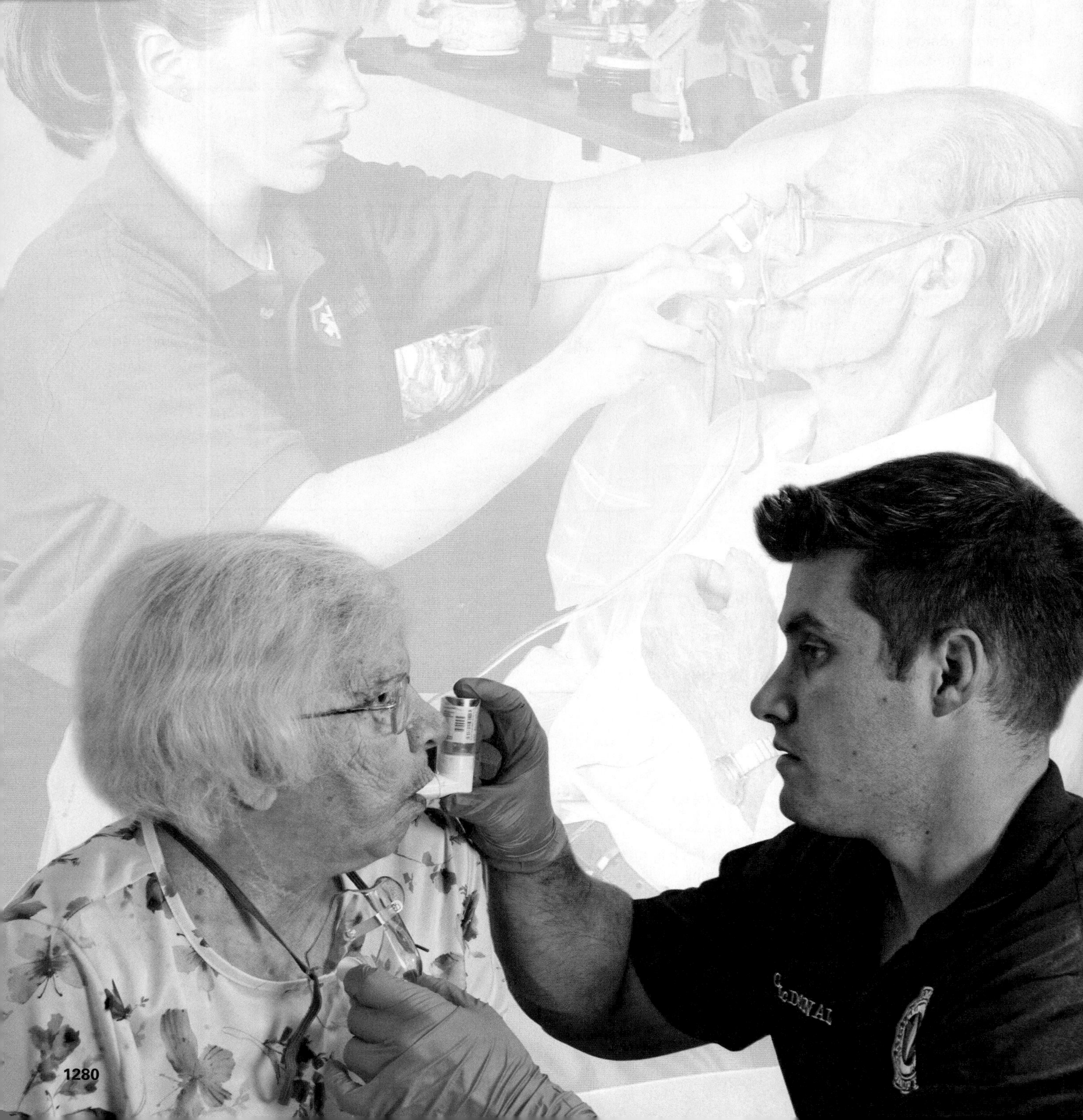

Navigation Guide

The following items provide an overview to the purpose and content of this chapter. The Standard and Competency are from the new National EMS Education Standards.

STANDARD **Special Patient Populations** (Content Area: Geriatrics)

COMPETENCY Applies fundamental knowledge of growth, development, aging, and assessment findings to provide basic emergency care and transportation for a patient with special needs.

OBJECTIVES: After reading this chapter, you should be able to:

39-1. Define key terms introduced in this chapter.

39-2. Summarize age-related anatomical and physiological changes for each of the following systems:

- **a.** Cardiovascular
- **b.** Respiratory
- **c.** Neurological
- **d.** Gastrointestinal
- **e.** Endocrine
- **f.** Musculoskeletal
- **g.** Renal

39-3. Discuss characteristic findings and emergency care steps for common medical emergencies in the elderly population, including:

- **a.** Myocardial infarction
- **b.** Congestive heart failure
- **c.** Pulmonary edema
- **d.** Pulmonary embolism
- **e.** Pneumonia
- **f.** Stroke
- **g.** Chronic obstructive pulmonary disease
- **h.** Stroke and transient ischemic attack
- **i.** Seizure
- **j.** Syncope
- **k.** Hyperosmolar hyperglycemic nonketotic syndrome (HHNS)
- **l.** Drug toxicity
- **m.** Dementia and delirium
- **n.** Alzheimer disease
- **o.** Trauma or shock
- **p.** Gastrointestinal bleeding
- **q.** Environmental emergencies
- **r.** Abuse

39-4. Describe modifications that may be necessary to effectively assess and treat geriatric patients.

KEY TERMS: Page references indicate first major use in this chapter. For complete definitions, see the Glossary at the back of the book.

acute p. 1282
ageism p. 1297
Alzheimer disease p. 1295
arteriosclerosis p. 1284
aspiration pneumonia p. 1291
cardiac hypertrophy p. 1283
chronic p. 1282
chronic obstructive pulmonary disease (COPD) p. 1291
congestive heart failure (CHF) p. 1289
delirium p. 1294
dementia p. 1294
drug toxicity p. 1294
dysrhythmias p. 1284
hyperthermia p. 1297
hypothermia p. 1297
intracranial pressure (ICP) p. 1292
kyphosis p. 1287
neuropathy p. 1286
osteoporosis p. 1287
pneumonia p. 1291
pulmonary edema p. 1290
pulmonary embolism p. 1290
seizure p. 1293
silent heart attack p. 1288
stenosis p. 1282
stroke p. 1292
syncope p. 1293
transient ischemic attack (TIA) p. 1293

MEDIA RESOURCES: Please go to www.bradybooks.com to access mykit for this text. You will find quizzes, critical thinking scenarios, weblinks, animations, and videos related to this chapter—and much more. Look for online information on hypertension and healthy aging.

continued

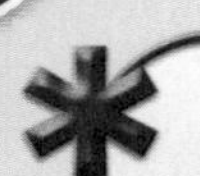

Navigation Guide *continued*

CASE STUDY

The Dispatch

EMS Unit 102—respond to 1793 Aberdeen Avenue for a 72-year-old female with respiratory distress. Time out is 0813 hours.

Upon Arrival

As you arrive, you are met by an elderly male. He identifies himself as Harold Vaughn, the patient's husband. He tells you he called for his wife, Madeline. "She hasn't been feeling well for the last 3 or 4 days. Yesterday she started having trouble catching her breath."

Mr. Vaughn asks you to "please hurry" as you gather the equipment from the ambulance. He leads you to the back bedroom of the house where you find an elderly female sitting upright in bed, her back propped against several pillows. She smiles weakly at you when you speak to her, and then she places her hand behind her ear as if to say, "Speak louder, I can't hear you."

How Would You Proceed to Assess and Care for This Patient?

During this chapter, you will learn about physiological changes, special assessment concerns, and emergency care considerations for geriatric patients. Later, we will return to the case and apply the procedures learned.

Introduction

In the United States, people over age 65 are the fastest growing segment of the population. In fact, the majority of EMS calls involve geriatric patients. Therefore, it is important that you understand the characteristics of geriatric patients and how to tailor your assessment to their special needs.

Geriatric patients differ from their younger counterparts. The elderly are at greater risk for nearly all types of injuries and illnesses. They present with different signs and symptoms because of the changing physiology of the geriatric body system. Additionally, the geriatric patient often has one or more coexisting long-term conditions that may require multiple medications. All of these factors can mask or change the presentation of the current emergency problem.

Effects of Aging on Body Systems

The human body changes with age. As a person ages, there are changes in cellular, organ, and system functioning. This change in physiology—which typically starts around age 30—is a normal part of aging. Although people may try to slow the aging process by diet, exercise, health care, and so on, it cannot be stopped entirely.

One trend, however, is that people are living longer with **chronic** (long-term or progressing gradually) illnesses. This means that the elderly are likely to constitute a larger percentage of an EMT's patient volume. Most elderly patients will have not one but a combination of different disease processes in varying stages of development.

The aging body has fewer reserves with which to combat diseases, and this ultimately contributes to the incidence of **acute** (severe, with rapid onset) medical and traumatic emergencies. However, although illness is common among the elderly, it is not an inevitable part of aging.

It is important that you understand and recognize changes in geriatric body systems so that you can provide appropriate care for elderly patients (Figure 39-1∗). The physiological changes discussed on the following pages result from the normal aging process, not from disease progression. However, any disease or injury the patient experiences will only worsen—or be made worse by—these changes.

The Cardiovascular System

With age, degenerative processes affect the ability of the heart to pump blood. Calcium is progressively deposited in areas of deterioration, especially around the valves of the heart. Damage to the valves of the heart from this degeneration can result in a variety of problems. One problem is **stenosis** (narrowing) of the valve opening. When this occurs it restricts the flow of blood through the

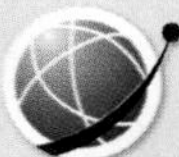

Media Resources

Go to www.bradybooks.com for mykit. Highlights:

- *Web Resource:* Aging Hearts and Arteries
- *Web Resource:* Balance Problems in the Elderly
- *Web Resource:* Hypertension

Objective 39-2

Summarize age-related anatomical and physiological changes for specific body systems.

Key Terms

chronic long term, progressing gradually.

acute with rapid onset.

CHANGES IN THE BODY SYSTEMS OF THE ELDERLY

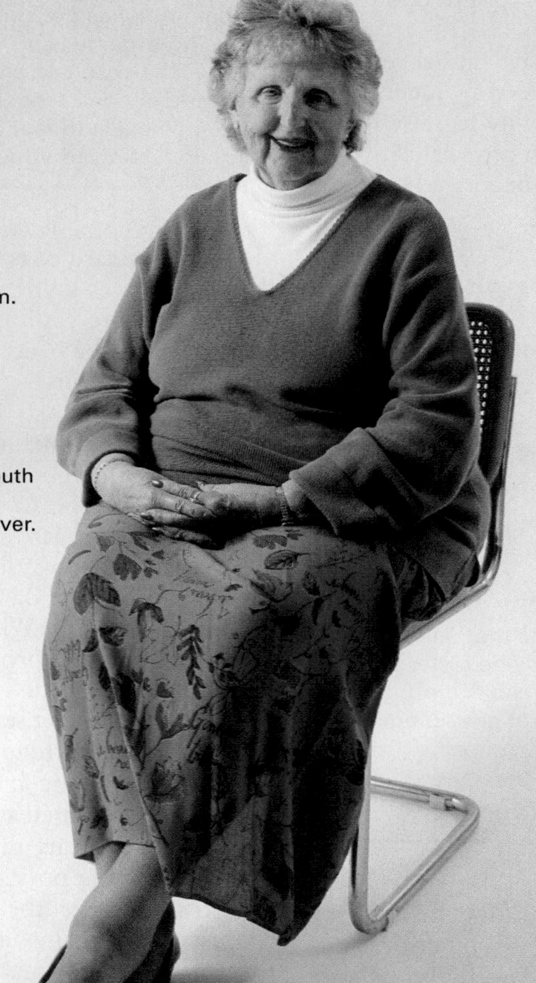
Neurological System
• Brain changes with age.
• Clinical depression common.
• Altered mental status common.
Cardiovascular System
• Hypertension common.
• Changes in heart rate and rhythm.
Gastrointestinal System
• Constipation common.
• Deterioration of structures in mouth common.
• General decline in efficiency of liver.
• Impaired swallowing.
• Malnutrition as result of deterioration of small intestine.
Musculoskeletal System
• Osteoporosis common.
• Osteoarthritis common.
Respiratory System
• Cough power is diminished.
• Increased tendency for infection.
• Less air and less exchange of gases due to general decline.
Renal System
• Drug toxicity problems common.
• General decline in efficiency.
Skin
• Perspires less.
• Tears more easily.
• Heals slowly.
Immune System
• Fever often absent.
• Lessened ability to fight disease.

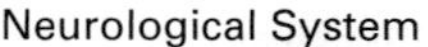

FIGURE 39-1 ✱ Changes in the body systems of the elderly.

heart. In extreme cases it may reduce blood flow through the heart to the point where the heart cannot meet the demands of the body, causing deterioration of the patient. Another problem with valve damage is regurgitation (backward flow of blood). If a valve can no longer seal correctly, blood may be forced back through it. This is more common with the bicuspid than with the tricuspid valve. When this occurs, blood regurgitates into the left atrium, which can cause a backup of blood into the lungs, resulting in pulmonary edema.

With age, fibrous tissue begins to replace muscle tissue throughout the cardiovascular system. The walls of the heart become generally thickened without any increase in the size of the atrial or ventricular chambers. This thickening of the heart walls is known as **cardiac hypertrophy**. It causes a decrease in the stroke volume of the heart (because the heart is unable to hold as much blood), resulting in less blood being ejected from the heart with each contraction and a consequent decrease in cardiac output, which is defined as the amount of blood

Key Terms
stenosis constriction or narrowing of a passage or opening such as heart valves.

cardiac hypertrophy increased size of the heart from thickening of the heart wall.

Key Terms
dysrhythmias irregular myocardial contractions from electrical disturbances in the heart.

arteriosclerosis loss of vascular wall elasticity from thickening and hardening.

ejected from the heart over a minute's time. This decreases the efficiency of the body's compensatory mechanisms in the face of stress that may be brought about by illness or injury.

Although older patients generally have higher resting heart rates than younger people, necessary to meet normal demands, older hearts have less ability to raise their rate to meet an increased demand from physical activity, stress, or illness. This contributes to a decreased cardiac output in the older patient.

Understanding BODY PROCESSES

As the heart grows older, there are fewer electrical conducting cells ("pacemaker cells"). This causes the heart to be unable to elevate its rate significantly when heightened cardiac output is required. ■

ASSESSMENT Tips

The decrease of pacemaker cells means that, although the older patient's resting heart rate may be faster than in a younger patient, his heart cannot achieve a maximum heart rate, even during moments of physiological stress from conditions such as infection, shock, or respiratory distress that would raise the heart rate in a younger person. ■

Other contributors to the deterioration of cardiac output in the geriatric patient, which can be critical or even fatal at times, are **dysrhythmias.** Dysrhythmias are irregular contractions of the myocardium secondary to electrical disturbances in the heart.

Understanding BODY PROCESSES

Just as all other muscles in the body contract in response to an electrical impulse, the heart muscle contracts in response to electrical impulses created by the conduction system of the heart. With aging, there can be a general deterioration in the heart's conduction system, resulting in the inability of the heart to initiate and propagate a normal impulse. ■

ASSESSMENT Tips

When the heart's conduction system begins to fail, causing a decreasing ability to generate a normal impulse, the result is an irregularity in the heart's rate, rhythm, or contraction force. All of these can cause the patient's pulse to feel weak, irregular, or, in the case of certain fatal dysrhythmias, absent. ■

Another cardiovascular change as the body ages is that the arteries lose their elasticity (their ability to constrict and dilate easily), which creates greater resistance against which the heart must pump to maintain adequate blood flow through the vascular system. Widespread hardening of the arteries, or **arteriosclerosis,** tends to occur with age, which causes the arteries to become stiff and leads to further increases in the pressure the heart must pump against. Compounding the stiffness of the arteries is a drop in baroreceptor sensitivity. (Baroreceptors are specialized "pressure sensors" in the aortic arch and the carotid bodies. Baroreceptors serve only to monitor the blood pressure. When a rise or drop in pressure occurs, baroreceptors provide this information to the brain stem so that corrective measures can be taken.) With a drop in baroreceptor sensitivity, it becomes harder for the geriatric patient to regulate his blood pressure. This often leads to orthostatic hypotension, or postural hypotension, which is defined as a drop in systolic pressure and elevation in the heart rate when the patient goes from a lying to standing position.

To summarize, the aging heart grows weaker even as it must pump against a higher resistance in the arteries, there may be abnormal heart rates or rhythms because of the degeneration of the conduction system, the systolic blood pressure may start to rise because of increased arterial resistance to blood flow, and the blood vessels will not react as fast (or as efficiently) in response to stimulation from the central nervous system, which compromises blood pressure regulation during times of stress or emergency.

The Respiratory System

Almost every component of the respiratory system experiences some type of deterioration over time. These changes in the aging respiratory system occur mainly as a result of alterations in the respiratory muscles and in the elasticity and recoil of the thorax. Specifically, there is a decrease in the size and strength of the muscles used for respiration, and calcium deposits begin to form where the ribs join the sternum, causing the rib cage to become less pliable. The average person continues to generate new alveoli until the age of 20. In the elderly, there is a decline in diffusion of oxygen and carbon dioxide across the alveolar membrane as alveolar surfaces progressively decrease. Chemoreceptors located in the aortic arch, in the carotid bodies, and on the surface of the brain stem that monitor the levels of carbon dioxide and oxygen in the blood become less sensitive over time. This results in a relative inability to detect oxygen depletion (hypoxia) or increased carbon dioxide levels (hypercapnia) in the blood and tissues.

Another change is in the airflow in and out of the lungs. In a younger person, the smaller airways (bronchioles) are supported by smooth muscle, which allows them to keep their open shape so that oxygen is easily inhaled with each incoming breath and carbon dioxide is easily exhaled with each exiting breath. With aging, there is a decrease in both the number and strength of these smooth muscle fibers that support the smaller airways. The result is turbulent airflow, which diminishes airflow to the terminal alveoli during inspiration and may also result in air trapping during exhalation. Airflow velocity through the airways slowly starts to diminish after the age of 30, and is accentuated by pathological diseases such as chronic obstructive pulmonary disease. These factors are further exaggerated with the heightened respiratory activity needed during episodes of stress, shock, or pulmonary conditions such as pneumonia.

The ability of the lungs to inhibit or resist disease and infection is also diminished with age. The cough reflex, which helps eliminate inhaled particles from the airway, may not trigger as readily, and because of the weakening of muscles, the coughing that does occur may be less forceful. The hairlike projections (cilia) that line the airway and help remove foreign particles trapped in the mucous lining are less able to move the material up and out of the airway. The nose and breathing passages secrete less of an antibody substance into the mucus that protects the body from viruses. Thus, the elderly are more susceptible to pneumonia and other types of lung infections. Dehydration, common in the elderly, increases the tendency for respiratory infection.

The net effect of these respiratory system changes in an elderly patient is that the body is less able to detect hypoxia or hypercapnia, less air enters and exits the lungs, less gas exchange occurs, the lung tissue loses its elasticity, and many of the muscles used in breathing lose their strength and coordination.

The Neurological System

The neurological (nervous) system also becomes impaired by the normal effects of aging. There is an actual decrease in the mass and weight of the brain and a resulting increase in the amount of cerebral spinal fluid (CSF) that occupies the extra space in the skull. As brain neurons degenerate, waste products can collect in tissues, causing abnormal structures called plaques and tangles to form. As these changes from atrophy, plaques, and tangles take place, the overall ability of the brain to operate as it did when younger becomes increasingly impaired.

Nerve cells (neurons) begin to degenerate and die as early as the mid-20s, and over time this impedes the ability of the body to adapt rapidly to changes within and outside of the body. Nerve cell degeneration is responsible for the slowing of reflexes. The elderly have a harder time perceiving or sensing their body position, resulting in their becoming less steady on their feet. The combination of neurological degeneration and changes in the musculoskeletal system make it easy to understand why falls are so prevalent and serious in the geriatric population. Sight diminishes (especially at night). Although hearing loss is not inevitable, the ability to discern higher-frequency sounds may slowly be lost. Also, the geriatric patient may have difficulty in differentiating close from background noise. The illnesses and injuries that result from neurological deterioration over time can be some of the most devastating and costly to the geriatric patient.

The ability of the elderly brain to control many of the body's processes becomes less efficient. Because of changes that occur in the brain stem and other regulatory centers of the brain, the ability to perceive hunger and thirst is altered. The ability of the brain to monitor and regulate vital functions such as the rate and depth of breathing, heart rate, blood pressure, and core body temperature can become deranged and not operate with the same efficiency during stressful times as in the younger patient.

Sensory perception tends to diminish over time, including everyday senses such as auditory, visual, olfactory (smell), touch, pain, hot and cold sensations, and body position. For example, there is diminishment in visual acuity (the ability to see clearly) and visual accommodation (the ability to adjust the lens of the eye to maintain clear vision on objects of varying distances). The deterioration of these visual capabilities can contribute to accidental trauma from falls and contribute to the inability to see medications clearly enough to ensure proper dosage. As part of the eyesight deterioration, there is a drop in the ability to discriminate color and progressive impairment to see clearly when it is darker in a room or outside. Diminished tear production leads to eye irritation from inadequate moisture. The disease processes listed next also compromise the elderly patient's ability to see clearly:

- *Cataracts* are a clouding of the lens of the eye. The clouding (sometimes referred to as opacity) can be slight, causing some visual disturbance, or significant, severely obstructing light from entering the eye. If sufficient light cannot pass into the eye for focusing

Key Points
Deteriorating vision can contribute to accidental trauma.

Key Terms
neuropathy any disease of the nerves. *Peripheral neuropathy* involves weakness, numbness, tingling, or other neuropathic symptoms in the extremities.

on the retina, then it becomes difficult or impossible to see clearly.

- *Glaucoma,* which is the second leading cause of blindness in the United States, is a disease process in which increased intraocular pressure damages the optic nerve and inhibits the ability of the eye to transmit visual information properly.
- *Macular degeneration* typically occurs in older adults and affects the ability to see objects in the center of the visual field. This makes activities like reading or recognizing a person's face difficult or impossible. Sometimes, however, there may be enough peripheral vision left intact that the person can still carry on with most activities of daily life.
- *Retinal detachment* is a condition where the retina (the light-sensitive portion of the posterior eye) becomes detached from the supportive tissue behind it. The retina converts light images to nerve impulses for transmission via the optic nerve to the brain, but when it becomes detached it can no longer do so. Retinal detachment may be local or complete, causing visual disturbances up to and including blindness.

ASSESSMENT Tips

Neurological changes, especially diminished vision and hearing, separately or in combination, can easily result in falls, automobile crashes, and other causes of injury. ■

Although many people experience hearing loss from exposure to loud noise over time, there may also be some natural degeneration of a person's ability to hear with aging. The effect of aging on hearing is known as presbycusis, or age-related hearing loss. It is described as progressive, bilateral, and symmetrical hearing loss. The hearing loss is most marked at higher frequencies. If hearing loss becomes severe enough that it inhibits communication, the patient may need a hearing aid (or sometimes hearing aids for both ears). When communicating with a patient who needs a hearing aid, ensure that the patient is wearing it and that it is turned on. Do not talk loudly when communicating with a person with a hearing aid, as it may cause what is heard to be distorted and difficult to understand.

Another neurological disorder is **neuropathy,** which is any derangement or abnormal function of the motor, sensory, and autonomic nerve tracts. It could be diffuse, involving multiple neurons and nerve tracts that affect many parts of the body, or focal neurons that affect a single, specific nerve and part of the body. Generally, its findings include pain, numbness, tingling, swelling, muscle weakness, or even absent pain perception. This can further complicate the presentation of findings characteristic to a particular problem. For example, recall how diabetic patients may not experience the pain from a myocardial infarction because of the neuropathy that develops secondary to long-term diabetes. This patient may not realize he is having a heart attack because he doesn't feel the characteristic pain. Many diabetics are especially prone to developing peripheral neuropathy, which affects the extremities, especially the hands and feet.

The Gastrointestinal System

Changes in the gastrointestinal system contribute to various medical conditions, including malnutrition. A reduction in the senses of taste and smell results in decreased food enjoyment (possibly causing the person to stop eating regularly). Deterioration of structures in the mouth and periodontal disease can cause loss of gum tissue and consequent tooth loss. There is a drop in salivary flow from degeneration of the salivary glands. The smooth muscle contractions of the esophagus decrease, and the opening between the esophagus and the stomach loses tone, which can result in chronic heartburn as gastric acid enters the esophagus from the stomach. There is also a decrease in the amount of hydrochloric acid secreted into the stomach. This contributes to less efficient breaking down of food prior to its entering the small intestine.

With age, the liver decreases in size, weight, and function, which decreases hepatic enzymes, causing a loss in the liver's ability to aid in digestion and to metabolize certain drugs. These effects are further hampered by the reduction in blood flow that occurs over time to the liver.

Smooth muscle contractions (peristalsis) throughout the gastrointestinal tract are slowed, so it takes longer for food to move through the system. As a result of degeneration of the lining of the small intestine, nutrients are not as readily absorbed, further contributing to malnutrition. Fecal impaction and constipation are common because smooth muscle contractions of the large intestine diminish. In some, degeneration of the rectal sphincter muscle can cause loss of bowel control.

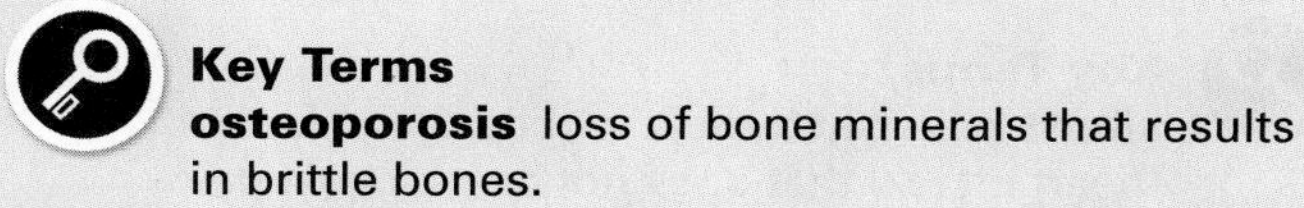

Key Terms
osteoporosis loss of bone minerals that results in brittle bones.

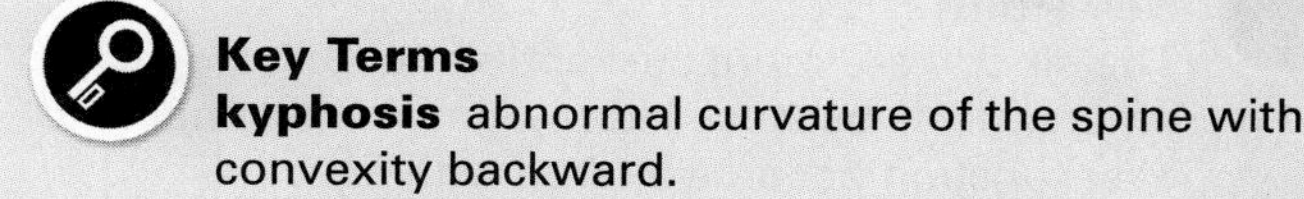

Key Terms
kyphosis abnormal curvature of the spine with convexity backward.

The Endocrine System

The progression of age-related changes to the endocrine system is unique. For most people, the changes in the endocrine system have no noticeable effect on overall health. The changes may, however, increase the risk of some health problems. For example, changes in insulin effectiveness increase the risk of type 2 diabetes.

Both hormone levels and target organ response are altered in the aging endocrine system. There can be an increase in the levels of hormones that increase blood pressure (vasopressor hormones such as norepinephrine and vasopressin), which contributes to development of hypertension (high blood pressure). The levels of certain hormones that help regulate the body's fluid balance (such as renin and aldosterone) become deranged and contribute to fluid imbalance, which has further effects on blood pressure. A decrease in target organ response to beta (sympathetic) stimulation in the heart and vascular smooth muscle is caused by diminishment in receptor cell sensitivity. The net effects of these endocrine changes are seen in the clinical syndromes of hypertension and orthostatic hypotension that are characteristic of the elderly.

In addition, aging produces mild carbohydrate intolerance and a minimal increase in fasting blood glucose levels, caused by a drop in receptor cell responsiveness to insulin. Atrial natriuretic hormone (ANH) from atrial muscle tissue helps to regulate water, sodium, potassium, and fat. The serum level of this hormone is typically increased in the elderly and contributes to fluid imbalance. Aging also decreases the metabolism of thyroxine, a hormone that influences metabolic activity of the body. With a drop in the secretion of thyroxine, there is also a decrease in its conversion into triiodothyronine, the most powerful thyroid hormone, which affects almost every process in the body, including body temperature, growth, and heart rate.

Collectively, changes to the endocrine system may cause elevation of blood sugar levels (especially after eating a large meal), alteration of the blood pressure (resulting in high or low blood pressure), and fluid imbalance (resulting in either fluid retention or dehydration).

The Musculoskeletal System

The most significant musculoskeletal change resulting from aging is a loss of minerals in the bones, which is known as **osteoporosis.** This makes the bones more brittle and susceptible to fractures and slows the healing process. The osteoporosis itself is less a problem than the possible resulting bone injury or immobility, which can lead to illness and death.

The disks located between the vertebrae of the spine start to narrow, which causes the characteristic curvature of the spine, seen in two out of every three elderly patients, known as **kyphosis.** This curvature is seen along the entire spine but is usually most pronounced in the thoracic vertebrae and can complicate spinal immobilization. It may be necessary to place additional padding under the patient to fill voids and create effective immobilization (EMT Skills 39-1).

Joints begin to lose their flexibility with aging. There is a thinning of the cartilage that covers the articular surfaces where joints meet, and the synovial fluid that surrounds these joints starts to thicken. The ligaments that provide joints with stability start to weaken as well. The effects are diminished range of joint motion, possible pain with movement, and increased risk of joint injury. Complicating this is the general and progressive loss of skeletal muscle mass. The elderly are more prone to falls because of general weakness, worsening balance, and a loss in joint mobility. Because of the changes in bone structure, these falls commonly result in skeletal fractures that take longer to heal than in younger people and that may also cause other medical emergencies.

The Renal System

The normal aging process also affects the renal system (kidneys). The kidneys become smaller in size and weight because of a loss of the functional parts of the kidney, the nephrons. The loss of nephrons can reduce the actual weight of the kidneys by about one-third of their normal weight. The effect is a decrease in the surface area of the kidney available to filter blood. The arterial system supplying the kidneys is also subject to the changes in the cardiovascular system, which results in a drop in renal blood flow. In combination, these changes result in a lesser amount of blood per minute passing through the kidneys for filtration, in addition to the decrease in available filtration surface area.

Since the kidneys play a vital role in fluid and electrolyte balance, kidney malfunction or injury typically leads to a secondary disturbance in fluid balance and electrolyte distribution. Since many drugs (including antibiotics) are filtered out by the kidneys, it is common for the elderly to suffer from drug toxicity if they take too much medication or take it too frequently. The geriatric renal system may be functional enough to meet the demands

Key Points
The elderly are more susceptible to toxicologic emergencies because kidney, gastrointestinal, and liver function become altered with age.

Objective 39-3
Discuss characteristic findings and emergency care steps for common medical emergencies in the elderly population.

Key Terms
silent heart attack a myocardial infarction (heart attack) that does not cause chest pain.

of the body on a day-to-day basis, but as a result of acute illness or injury the elderly patient's renal system may fail.

ASSESSMENT Tips

Because of the diminished kidney function, altered gastrointestinal absorption, and altered liver function, elderly patients are more susceptible to toxicologic emergencies. Other factors that may place the elderly patient at an even greater risk of a toxicologic emergency include poor eyesight, medication noncompliance, polypharmacy, and poor motor skills. ■

The Integumentary System

Aging results in tremendous changes in the integumentary system (the skin). The skin becomes thinner from a deterioration of the subcutaneous layer, and there is less attachment tissue between the dermis (inner layer) and epidermis (outer layer). An elderly person's skin is much more prone to injury than the younger person's skin. Replacement cells are produced less rapidly, so wounds heal more slowly and skin is slow to replace itself. Less perspiration is produced, and the sense of touch is dulled. As the skin breaks down, there is a tendency for sores and tearing injuries to occur. This diminishes the effectiveness of the skin as a protective barrier in keeping microorganisms out of the body.

▶ Special Geriatric Assessment Findings

Because of the general decline in virtually every body system of the geriatric patient, the elderly are prone to certain traumatic and medical emergencies that can cause rapid deterioration. As stated earlier, aging may change the individual's response to illness and injury. Pain may be diminished or absent, and consequently the patient or EMT may underestimate the severity of the patient's condition. It is important that the EMT recognize these emergencies and provide appropriate emergency care. Having an understanding of what is occurring physiologically in these emergencies will help in recognizing and providing prompt, appropriate care. Be alert for the findings discussed on the following pages as you assess patients over the age of 65. As you read about these conditions, refer to Table 39-1 for special considerations regarding such medical conditions in the elderly.

Assessment Finding: Chest Pain or Absence of Chest Pain

Heart Attack (Myocardial Infarction)

A lack of oxygen and other nutrients to the heart typically produces chest discomfort in a younger person. In contrast, as a result of decreased pain perception, geriatric patients may experience what is known as a **silent heart attack.** The elderly heart attack patient may have no, or very little, chest discomfort. Instead, the geriatric patient suffering a heart attack will usually present with general complaints such as weakness, fatigue, confusion, dizziness, nausea/vomiting, abdominal pain, and syncope. Trouble breathing is also a common initial complaint. Although one-third of elderly heart attack patients never experience pain, aching shoulders and indigestion are common.

The patient who chronically experiences chest pain may take nitroglycerin for the problem, so finding nitroglycerin medication at the scene will clue you in to a patient's history of heart problems. If the patient does take nitroglycerin, you may be able to assist in the administration of it with permission from medical direction (Figure 39-2*). (Refer to Chapter 17, "Cardiovascular Emergencies," for a thorough discussion of nitroglycerin.)

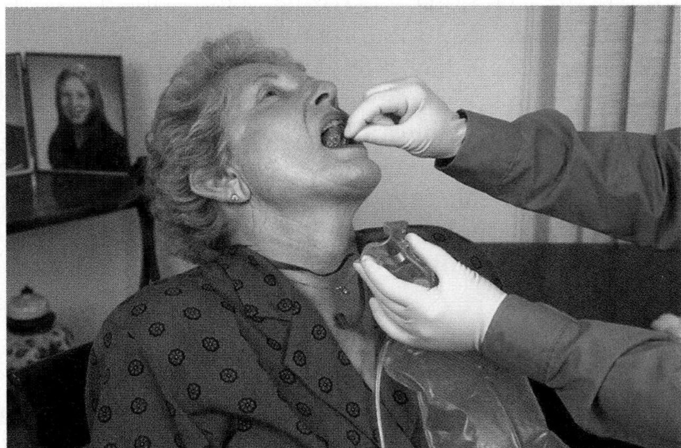

FIGURE 39-2 * With permission from medical direction, you may be able to assist the patient suffering from chest pain in taking prescribed nitroglycerin.

Key Terms

congestive heart failure (CHF) disease in which the heart cannot pump blood effectively.

TABLE 39-1 Special Considerations in Medical Conditions in the Elderly

Acute coronary syndromes, including heart attack (myocardial infarction)	Approximately one-third of patients over 75 years of age exhibit symptoms of coronary artery disease. Close to half of males and one-third of females over 74 years of age will suffer an unrecognized heart attack (myocardial infarction).
	Incidence of chest pain decreases with age. The most common signs or symptoms are syncope (fainting), confusion, and dyspnea (shortness of breath).
Pneumonia	Elderly patients with pneumonia commonly do not present with classic signs and symptoms. Cough is a common complaint, except with those, often in nursing homes, who can't complain because of an altered mental status. In those patients, altered mental status is the predominant sign.
	Other signs of pneumonia may be falls or a rapid decline in the patient's ability to do normal daily activities.
	More than half of patients may not have a fever (are afebrile) with the pneumonia.
	Increased respiratory rate (tachypnea) is almost always present in pneumonia.
	Crackles may not be heard when the chest is auscultated because the elderly patient may not cooperate and take deep breaths when requested during the physical exam.
Pulmonary embolism	Approximately 90 percent of emboli originate from deep vein clots in the lower extremities and near vessels in the pelvis.
	Elderly patients are more prone to pulmonary emboli because of immobility or reduced activity, congestive heart failure, tumors, and surgery.
	The most common signs and symptoms are shortness of breath (dyspnea), chest pain, and cough. Some elderly patients will not complain of any of the three most common complaints and may only present with confusion. Also look for rapid respiratory rate (tachypnea) and rapid heart rate (tachycardia).
Stroke	Headache, including migraine, is less common in the elderly; therefore, headache may be a significant finding in the elderly.
	Head pain may indicate bleeding within the brain or skull, tumors, infection, herpes zoster (skin lesions, "shingles"), or metabolic disorders.

Emergency care steps for a suspected heart attack—whether or not the patient's symptoms include chest pain—are to administer high-concentration oxygen, administer nitroglycerin as appropriate in consultation with medical direction, and transport the patient expeditiously (but cautiously) to the hospital.

Congestive Heart Failure

Congestive heart failure (CHF) is another type of emergency seen typically in the geriatric patient (see Chapter 17, "Cardiovascular Emergencies"). It can be a chronic condition that the patient may tell you about during your history taking, or it may have an acute onset and be the cause for the elderly person summoning EMS.

Even though CHF is primarily caused by a cardiac disease, it can present differently than a heart attack. It is caused by a heart that becomes weakened over time as a result of the changes in aging, as well as hypertension, arteriosclerotic disease, dysrhythmias (abnormal heart rhythms), and heart valve damage. As a result of these changes, the heart can no longer pump as effectively, and blood begins to cause a "backup" in the peripheral blood vessels and the vessels in the lungs. This causes fluid to leak out of the vessels. Assessment findings characteristic to CHF include edema in the extremities, jugular vein distention, altered mental status, fatigue, rales or crackling upon auscultation, possible wheezing, dyspnea, orthopnea, tachypnea, chest pain, and anxiety. Emergency care steps for CHF include administering high-concentration oxygen, placing the patient in a Fowler position, and expediting transport. Be sure to watch for inadequate breathing, and be prepared to ventilate.

Assessment Finding: Shortness of Breath (Dyspnea)

Respiratory distress can result from a number of conditions occurring in the geriatric patient. It can be the primary symptom of a pulmonary problem, or it can be a symptom secondary to failure of a different body system (CHF, for example, can cause difficulty in breathing). Difficulty breathing or "shortness of breath" (dyspnea) is one of the more common complaints noted in the elderly (see Chapter 16, "Respiratory Emergencies"). The elderly already have diminished respiratory function. Any additional burden can easily overwhelm the respiratory system and lead to inadequate breathing. The four most common causes of shortness of breath are pulmonary edema, pulmonary embolism, pneumonia, and chronic obstructive pulmonary disease (Figure 39-3*).

Pulmonary Edema

Pulmonary edema, or fluid in the lungs, can have a gradual or sudden onset and can result in death if proper emergency care is not provided. Pulmonary edema typically results from the failure of the heart's pumping function. Causes include CHF, heart attack, dysrhythmia, or valve damage. The left ventricle starts to eject less blood than the right (the ventricles should eject the same amount of blood simultaneously) resulting in excessive pressure in the vessels in the lungs. Fluid begins to "leak" into the space between the alveoli and the capillaries, causing pulmonary edema, which results in inadequate gas exchange and respiratory distress.

Assessment findings include severe respiratory distress especially when lying down (orthopnea), altered mental status, coughing with possibly blood-tinged sputum, and other signs of CHF. As with CHF, emergency care includes administering oxygen at 15 lpm by nonrebreather mask, placing the patient in a Fowler position, monitoring for inadequate breathing, and transporting expeditiously. It may be necessary to perform positive pressure ventilation in severe cases.

Pulmonary Embolism

Pulmonary embolism, or blockage in the arteries of the lungs, is a respiratory emergency seen more frequently in elderly than in younger patients. Pulmonary embolism may present with a sudden onset of dyspnea, in conjunction with chest discomfort that is localized and does not radiate (there may also be back or shoulder pain), weakness, or possibly syncope. The patient may also be anxious. This emergency usually occurs when a blood clot (embolism) breaks free from veins of the lower extremities or pelvis and is transported back through the right side of the heart. The clot eventually lodges somewhere in the arteries of the lungs.

This results in poor oxygen and carbon dioxide gas exchange in the alveoli because the clot is preventing blood from flowing through the capillaries. The inadequate exchange of oxygen and carbon dioxide results in respiratory distress. The degree of respiratory distress depends on the size of the blood clot. With large clots the

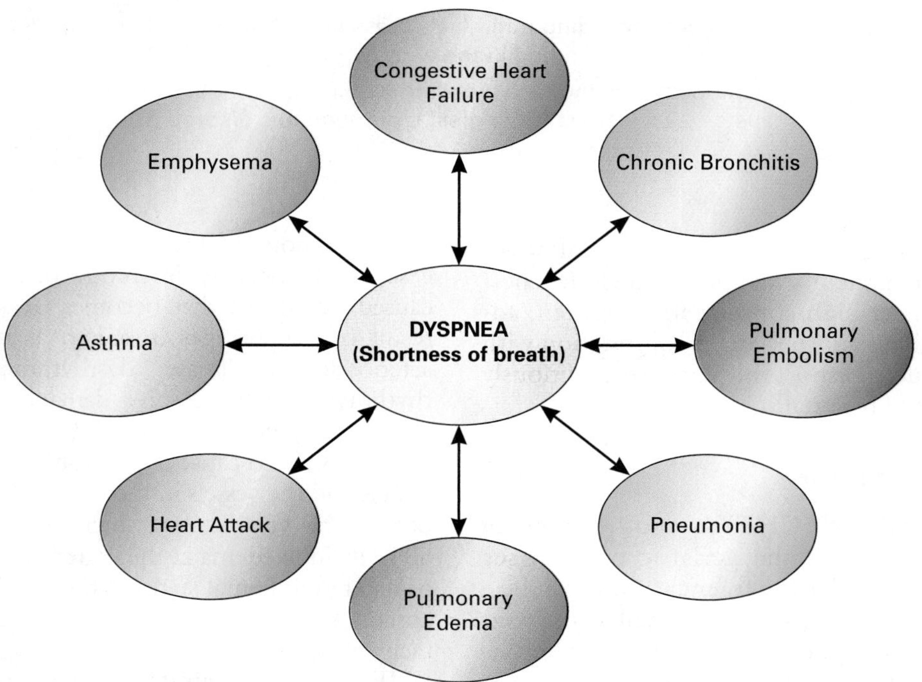

FIGURE 39-3 * Common causes of dyspnea (shortness of breath) in the elderly patient.

Key Terms

pulmonary edema fluid in the lungs.

pulmonary embolism blockage in the arteries of the lungs.

pneumonia infection of the lungs, usually from a bacterium or virus.

Key Terms

aspiration pneumonia lung inflammation from aspiration of vomitus or foreign matter.

chronic obstructive pulmonary disease (COPD) pulmonary diseases such as emphysema or chronic bronchitis.

blood cannot make it from the right side of the heart to the left, and hypotension ensues. The EMT may also notice localized wheezing to one of the lungs, and with blockage the pulse oximeter may drop dangerously low.

If a large embolism occludes more than half of the pulmonary circulation, it can rapidly cause death.

Predisposing factors to a pulmonary embolism include aging, smoking, cancer, fractures of large bones, major surgery, existing cardiovascular disease, prolonged bed rest, and trauma. Emergency care includes administering oxygen and monitoring for inadequate breathing. Provide positive pressure ventilation, if necessary, and transport the patient rapidly to the hospital with ALS intercept.

Pneumonia

Pneumonia is an infection of the lungs caused by a bacterium, virus, or other pathogen. It is common in the elderly because of a diminished ability of the respiratory system to fight off infections. Of special concern is **aspiration pneumonia,** which often results from accidental aspiration of food or vomitus into the lungs. That is why preventing aspiration of foreign material is so important in the maintenance of the geriatric airway.

Pneumonia has a tendency to strike when multiple risk factors are present. Some of these include advancing age, being bedridden at home or institutionalized, immune system compromise, a history of other pulmonary diseases (for example, chronic obstructive pulmonary disease), cancer, and a history of inhaled toxins.

The elderly pneumonia patient may be insensitive to the subtle pain from pneumonia and may not exhibit the classic signs and symptoms of pneumonia that would appear in a younger patient (high fever, chills, chest pain, coughing up bloody sputum). In the elderly, watch for increased respiration rate, progressive worsening of dyspnea, dyspnea with exertion, congestion with or without fever and chills, a cough with some sputum production, possible wheezing, and other findings of malaise (nausea, vomiting, musculoskeletal pain, weakness, and weight loss). The patient may also display an altered mental status. In severe cases of pneumonia, the patient may be found to be breathing inadequately, hypotension could occur, dehydration could be present, percussion of the chest may produce dull sounds, and increased vocal fremitus (also known as tactile fremitus) may be present.

Emergency care is primarily supportive and includes maintaining the patient's airway, administering high-concentration oxygen, and transporting the patient in a Fowler position or a position of comfort. If breathing becomes inadequate, provide oxygen via positive pressure ventilation.

Chronic Obstructive Pulmonary Disease

Chronic obstructive pulmonary disease (COPD) is actually a disease complex that includes a number of individual pulmonary disease processes (principally chronic bronchitis and emphysema) that result from the gradual deterioration of the pulmonary structures. (Refer to Chapter 16, "Respiratory Emergencies," for a discussion of COPD.) The effects of COPD cause a disturbance in gas exchange in the lungs.

The EMT will typically encounter the elderly COPD patient complaining of respiratory distress and will observe the patient using accessory muscles when breathing. Upon arrival at the scene, the EMT may find the patient already on oxygen from a home oxygen unit (Figure 39-4*). Emergency care includes the administration of oxygen at 15 lpm by nonrebreather mask. The EMT may also help relieve the respiratory distress, after consultation with

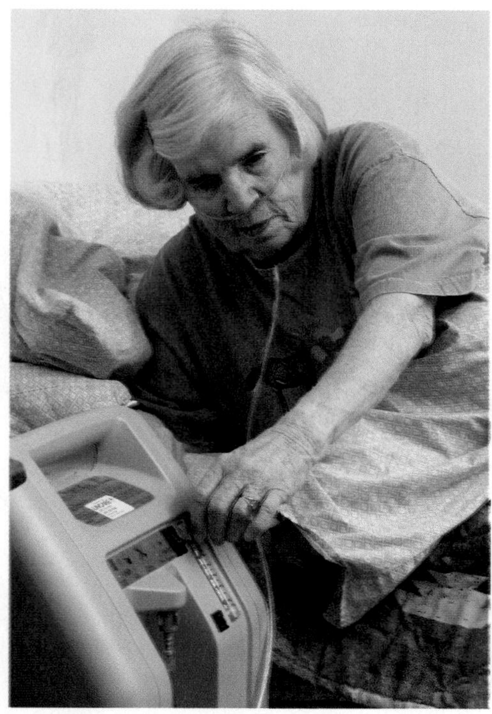

FIGURE 39-4 * The COPD patient may use a nasal cannula with a home oxygen unit. (© Michal Heron)

medical direction, by assisting the patient with administering his prescribed metered-dose inhaler.

Transport the patient in a position of comfort, which will usually be a Fowler (sitting) position. Since the COPD patient can become easily fatigued from the effort of breathing, monitor the patient closely for signs of inadequate breathing. If breathing becomes inadequate, provide positive pressure ventilation with supplemental oxygen.

Assessment Finding: Altered Mental Status

You will encounter many elderly patients who are alert and who respond appropriately to you and to their environment. Some, however, will be unable to remember details, whereas others may be routinely confused or totally unresponsive. The geriatric person presenting with altered mental status may be one of the most challenging patients you will encounter. There can be a variety of causes of altered mental status (Figure 39-5✱). The patient may have an altered mental status from some chronic condition (such as Alzheimer disease), from an acute onset of the primary emergency (such as stroke), as a sign of an underlying medical illness (for example, poor perfusion of the brain when the volume of blood is depleted by severe bleeding), or even from the effect of prescription drugs.

Never assume that a patient's altered mental status is normal for him or that it is "what happens when you get old" and risk missing an important sign of injury or illness. As you assess the patient, attempt to determine if the patient's mental status is normal for him or if it represents a significant change. (Family members or others who know the patient may be able to supply this information.) Remember also that the noise of radios, a siren, strange voices, or a different environment may add to the patient's confusion. Attempt to explain or reduce the noise.

While the management principles remain essentially the same regardless of the cause of the altered mental status, an understanding of common underlying causes will assist you in knowing what to look for during scene size-up and in formulating questions to ask the patient, friends, or bystanders during history taking. Following are certain types of emergencies that can cause altered mental status in an elderly patient.

Stroke

Stroke is a common reason for altered mental status in the elderly patient (see Chapter 18, "Altered Mental Status, Stroke, and Headache"). A stroke occurs when a blood vessel in the brain becomes blocked by a clot, obstructing blood flow, or ruptures and allows blood to accumulate in the brain tissue. Since the skull does not expand, the pressure within the brain (**intracranial pressure,** or **ICP**) sharply increases, while the nerve cells in the brain start to die or malfunction from the pressure. The level of carbon dioxide in the brain increases, which causes cerebral vessels to dilate and further increases the ICP.

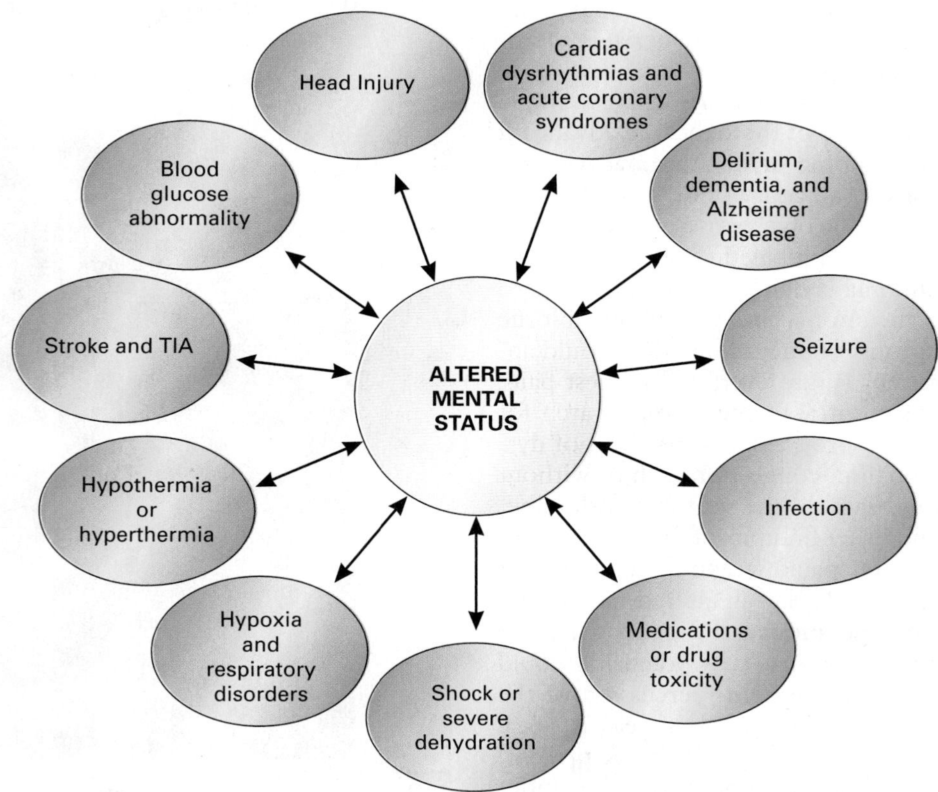

FIGURE 39-5 ✱ Common causes of altered mental status in the elderly patient.

Key Terms

stroke a sudden disruption in blood flow to the brain that results in brain cell damage.

intracranial pressure (ICP) the amount of pressure within the skull.

transient ischemic attack (TIA) strokelike symptoms that disappear within 24 hours.

Key Terms

seizure a sudden and temporary alteration in the mental status caused by massive electrical discharge in a group of nerve cells in the brain.

syncope brief unresponsiveness from lack of blood flow to the brain; fainting.

The extent and location of the stroke affects the severity of the altered mental status. The patient could be simply slightly disoriented or totally unresponsive. A massive stroke can lead to death within minutes. Aside from altered mental status, you may also find the following signs and symptoms:

- Inequality of pupils
- Slurred speech or abnormal speech patterns
- Headache
- Memory disorders
- Alterations in the respiratory pattern
- A rapid, or abnormally slow, heart rate
- High systolic pressure (hypertension), which gradually becomes normal or hypotensive
- Possible seizures
- Nausea or vomiting
- Muscle weakness or paralysis (usually to one side of the body)
- Sensory loss

Key emergency care for a stroke centers around recognition, aggressive oxygenation, and ventilation. Your emergency care steps for stroke should include protecting the airway and suctioning as necessary to prevent aspiration. You will transport the patient in a Fowler position, if possible, or a lateral recumbent (recovery) position if he is unresponsive and there is no suspicion of trauma.

Transient Ischemic Attack

Transient ischemic attack (TIA), or "mini stroke," is similar in presentation to a stroke, but the signs and symptoms are completely reversed within 24 hours of onset, usually sooner. No permanent neurological dysfunction occurs with a TIA. A TIA is caused when blood supply to an area of the brain is temporarily occluded, causing a malfunction of brain tissue that is not being perfused. The malfunctioning brain tissue can cause the same signs and symptoms as stroke. Treatment steps are the same as those discussed for stroke.

Seizure

Seizure, a sudden and temporary alteration in the mental status caused by massive electrical discharge in a group of nerve cells in the brain, is another cause of disorientation in the elderly. (Refer to Chapter 19, "Seizures and Syncope," for a full explanation.) You may encounter the patient while he is actively seizing, or after the seizure is over and the person is still unresponsive or slow to respond (the postictal state, or recovery period). Common causes of seizures in the elderly include cardiac arrest, low blood sugar, tumors, head trauma, stroke/TIA, infections, or electrolyte imbalance from kidney problems.

Treating an elderly seizure patient is the same as treating the younger seizure patient. Do not physically restrain the patient while he is actively seizing. Monitor the airway and suction as necessary (patients often vomit during seizures). Administer oxygen at 15 lpm by nonrebreather mask if breathing is adequate, or provide positive pressure ventilation if breathing is inadequate. Place the patient in a recovery position to help prevent aspiration if he is unresponsive and if trauma is not suspected.

Syncope

Syncope (fainting) is a common emergency for the elderly patient. Syncope is a temporary loss of responsiveness that usually reverses once the patient is lying down. Caused by a reduced blood flow to the brain, it can be a sign of a number of underlying diseases as well as a side effect of medications or even a reaction to strong emotion. Emergency care steps in treating a syncopal episode include ensuring an adequate airway, providing high-concentration oxygen by a nonrebreather mask or with positive pressure ventilation, if necessary, and placing the patient in a recovery position to prevent aspiration if he is still unresponsive. If the patient suffered a fall in conjunction with the syncopal episode, he should be fully immobilized as a precautionary measure.

Hyperosmolar Hyperglycemic Nonketotic Syndrome

Hyperosmolar hyperglycemic nonketotic syndrome (HHNS) is a diabetic complication that is more common to the elderly patient with diabetes mellitus (see Chapter 20, "Acute Diabetic Emergencies"). HHNS is a condition where the blood glucose level elevates because of inadequate insulin secretion or action on target cells, but enough insulin is secreted to keep mass amounts of fat from being metabolized for energy. This limits the amount of ketone bodies that are formed. The glucose level does raise high enough to cause excessive urination from osmotic diuresis, which in turn causes severe dehydration.

The elderly patient with HHNS will most likely present with an altered mental status, typically with a gradual onset (possibly progressing over a day or two), a possible history of diabetes, and an elevated blood glucose level. Other associated findings are:

- Polydipsia (excessive thirst)
- Polyuria (excessive urination)
- Dry oral mucous membranes
- Dizziness
- Confusion
- Seizures

During your assessment of the elderly patient with HHNS, you may note signs and symptoms of significant dehydration. The mucous membranes will likely be dry, the tongue furrowed, the skin dry, and the heart rate elevated. The most important findings consistent with this emergency are an altered mental status of gradual onset and an elevated blood glucose level. There may or may not be a history of diabetes. This may be the first indication of a diabetic condition in the patient. Check the blood glucose level in any patient who presents with signs of excessive urination, thirst, or dehydration regardless of history. Management will include positioning to protect the airway, supplemental oxygen, positive pressure ventilation if the patient is breathing inadequately, circulatory support, and consideration of an ALS intercept during transport to the hospital.

Drug Toxicity

Drug toxicity, or an adverse or toxic reaction to a drug or drugs, is a condition for which the elderly patient is more at risk than the younger patient (see Chapter 22, "Toxicologic Emergencies"). The geriatric population takes approximately one-third of all prescription medications. They also buy the greatest number of over-the-counter medications (Figure 39-6✱). Since they tend to have a number of coexisting diseases, they are at greater risk for drug interaction from prescription medications.

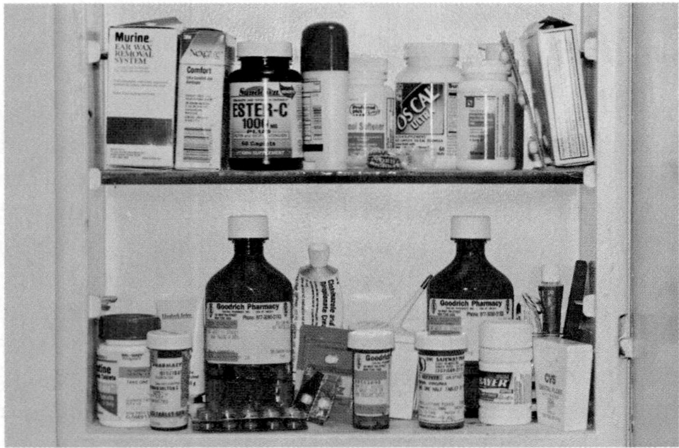

FIGURE 39-6 ✱ Drug toxicity may result from too many drugs or drugs taken incorrectly. (© Michal Heron)

Certain medications (taken individually or in conjunction with others) have a tendency to alter the patient's mental status, cause a syncopal episode, or even cause total unresponsiveness. Drug toxicity may also be caused by an error in dosing: the elderly person may take a wrong dose because of poor eyesight, confusion, forgetfulness, or a tendency to take the medication after it is no longer needed.

Treatment for a patient suffering from drug toxicity is based on figuring out how the drug is affecting the patient's airway, breathing, and circulation status—not what drug caused the problems. Thus, key treatment includes airway maintenance, oxygenation, and prevention of aspiration. If possible, take all medications found on the patient or at the scene (prescription and nonprescription) to the hospital with the patient.

Dementia and Delirium

Dementia is a condition resulting from the malfunctioning of normal brain activity. It is a chronic, irreversible condition that can be severely worsened by infection, medication change, trauma, or another acute condition. It is normal for the mental processes to undergo changes as a person ages, but approximately 15 percent of those over the age of 65 develop severe dementia, which results in profound disturbances in mental functioning. The characteristic results of dementia are chronic changes in cognition, including loss of short-term memory; decline in intellectual abilities; and decline in judgment, math ability, and abstract thought. The patient with dementia may present as angry. It is important to remember that the anger is not directed at the EMT; rather it is a product of the disease process.

Dementia may be caused by medications, especially analgesics, sedatives, tranquilizers, and those taken to reduce blood pressure or ease the symptoms of Parkinson disease. Other common causes of dementia in the elderly include Alzheimer disease, strokes, brain trauma and tumors, visual and auditory problems, endocrine and metabolic disorders, heart disease, constipation, urinary retention, infection, depression, alcohol use, chronic pain, certain workplace exposures, and other underlying diseases such as Huntington chorea.

Management of the patient with dementia is supportive in nature, and includes oxygen, positioning, and transport to the hospital with reassessments to ensure patient stability. While this seems straightforward, problems may arise in the management of a patient with dementia because of the altered mental functioning. For example, the patient may be uncertain of what the actual complaint is, or may simply be a poor historian and not be able to adequately verbalize the signs or symptoms. These patients may not be able to follow your simple commands, and coupled with the anxiety they may experience as you take them out of their known home environment or as you treat them, their anger may escalate into physical aggression.

Delirium can also result in an alteration in mental status, but unlike dementia—which is a chronic condition—

Key Terms
drug toxicity adverse or toxic reaction to a drug or drugs.

dementia chronic malfunctioning of normal cerebral processes.

Key Terms
delirium sudden onset of illusions, disjointed thoughts, incoherent speech, and increased or decreased psychomotor activity.

Alzheimer disease disease characterized by cerebral function loss.

delirium presents with a more recent and sudden onset. Delirium is often described by family members as starting abruptly, and it may present with delusions. The patient may have a history consistent with a delirium episode that can include intoxication or withdrawal from alcohol, sedative use, infectious medical conditions, dehydration, fever, stroke, blood sugar level abnormality, a psychiatric disorder, malnutrition, hypoxia, endocrine disorders, or even environmental emergencies. During your assessment of the patient with delirium, you may note the following findings: faster onset, disjointed (nonsensical) thought processes, incoherent speech, declines in mental status, and increased or decreased psychomotor activity.

Delirium is not an emergency in itself; rather, it is indicative of a significant disturbance in some body system (e.g., renal failure or hepatic failure). The additional physical findings (vitals, breath sounds, pupils, motor, and so on) will reflect the underlying pathology that is causing the delirium. The best way to differentiate delirium from dementia is to ask a family member or the primary care provider about the patient's mental status an hour ago or even on the previous day. A history consistent with a recent onset signals delirium. If the change in mental status has progressed over a long period, or if the condition has been present for a number of years, it signals dementia. Management of delirium, as for dementia, is primarily supportive in nature and includes oxygen, patient positioning, protection from injury, and transportation to the hospital. Remember though, if the delirium is caused by a reversible cause the EMT can treat (for example, low blood sugar), provide specific management for that condition.

Alzheimer Disease

Alzheimer disease is believed to affect more than 2 million Americans and to be responsible for more than 100,000 deaths each year in the United States. The disease does not directly cause death, but it can cause patients to stop eating, become immobile, and eventually be subject to numerous infections. It is thought to be the most common cause of dementia in the elderly. While its cause is presently unknown, it is believed to be a disease of the nerve cells in which brain cells degenerate and die. Alzheimer disease is both progressive and global in nature, involving the central nervous system. Although it is commonly a disease of the elderly, it can affect people as young as age 40.

The signs and symptoms of Alzheimer disease mimic those of many other conditions. (The presence of Alzheimer disease can be determined definitively only on examination of the brain during autopsy.) The disease causes confusion, emotional depression, irritability, and violence between lucid intervals. There is a progressive loss of appetite and a decreasing ability of the patient to care for his own needs. Eventually, the patient does not recognize loved ones; in late stages, the patient becomes childlike. Alzheimer disease patients often attempt or commit suicide.

The treatment of patients suffering from Alzheimer disease or any other form of dementia requires special compassion from the EMT. Naturally, you must take necessary actions to establish and maintain the airway, breathing, and circulatory systems. But often you will be transporting these patients in a nonemergency setting. You may find the patient very uncooperative, even combative, with biting, spitting, and punching at times. Remember that the uncooperativeness and aggression are symptoms of the disease, not conscious acts of aggression against you personally. You may also find yourself informing the patient of the same thing over and over because his mind may not be able to process, let alone remember, what you are saying. Do not take the patient's actions or words personally.

Assessment Finding: Signs of Trauma or Shock

Trauma is one of the leading causes of death in the geriatric population. The type of trauma seen most frequently in the elderly is blunt trauma from falls, motor vehicle crashes, and pedestrians struck by automobiles. There are numerous reasons for this, including:

- Altered mental status from a variety of conditions
- Slower reflexes
- Failing eyesight and hearing
- Medication effects
- Activities that exceed physical limitations
- Arthritis
- Blood vessels that are less elastic and more subject to injury
- Fragile tissues1297, brittle bones, and stiffer joints
- General loss in muscle tone and strength

Falls are responsible for half of all accidental deaths in the elderly and are a common cause of head injuries. There are sometimes environmental reasons why the elderly fall. These may include stairways without handrails, slippery bathtubs, loose rugs, steep steps, or improperly fitting footwear. There are also a number of medical reasons why the elderly fall. The most common are dizziness, side effects from medications, heart rhythm problems, spinal weakness, syncope, transient ischemic attacks, low blood pressure, internal bleeding, and poor vision.

Many elderly people who fall do not develop life-threatening injuries and do not die as a result of the fall. But certain injuries are common among those who fall. Make sure you assess for a hip fracture, head injuries, chest and abdominal injuries, spinal fractures, and fractures of the hand, wrist, forearm, or shoulder (caused by falling on an outstretched hand).

Head injuries are harder to detect in the elderly. As mentioned previously, the brain shrinks in size during the aging process. Even though there is additional cerebrospinal fluid surrounding the smaller brain, there is still more space in which the brain can swell or blood can accumulate in response to injury. Signs of brain injury in an older person may take days or weeks to develop, and the patient may have forgotten the initial injury by the time the signs and symptoms develop.

Regardless of the type of injury incurred, whenever you assess an elderly fall patient, you should determine if the fall was preceded by dizziness, faintness, or palpitations, indicating a potential medical emergency, or if it resulted from slipping or tripping on something.

The effects of years of disease processes sharply diminish the ability of the geriatric body to handle the stress of trauma. Because the heart and the arteries of an elderly person don't respond well, shock progresses much more rapidly in the elderly than in any other age group. Loss of even a small amount of blood can drive an elderly person into shock. The compensatory mechanisms do not function nearly as effectively nor last as long, and the organs cannot tolerate periods of hypoperfusion (see Chapter 15, "Shock and Resuscitation").

Treatment of geriatric trauma must be executed expeditiously. Stabilize the spine during the primary assessment, always administer high-concentration oxygen, and provide positive pressure ventilation if the patient is breathing inadequately. Regard any signs of poor perfusion (such as pale skin, tachycardia, disorientation, hypotension, or increased respiratory rate) as signs of serious trauma and transport the patient as rapidly as possible.

Assessment Finding: Gastrointestinal Bleeding

Gastrointestinal (GI) bleeding is a rather common and potentially life-threatening emergency in the elderly. GI bleeding may occur anywhere along the digestive tract from the mouth to the anus and may be obvious or may be occult (hidden). While GI bleeding is a sign that some disease of the gastrointestinal tract is present, it is not a disease itself. Bleeding may come from the upper GI tract or the lower GI tract as a result of an ulcerative disease, inflammation, infection, or obstruction. The most common finding with any abdominal pathology is abdominal pain. The type, location, presentation, history of the pain, and associated complaints will help isolate the type and source of bleeding.

Being able to recognize that GI bleeding is present is more important to the EMT for managing it appropriately than diagnosing exactly where along the digestive tract the bleed is originating or what is causing it. Findings that support the field impression of GI bleeding in an elderly patient include the following:

- Hematemesis (vomiting blood)
- Hematochezia (red undigested blood in bowel movement)
- Melena (dark tarry bowel movement, indicative of digested blood)
- Dyspepsia (indigestion)
- Hepatomegaly (enlarged liver)
- Jaundice (yellowing of sclera and skin, indicative of liver problems)
- Constipation or diarrhea
- Agitation
- Dizziness
- Inability to find a comfortable position

While these findings are consistent with GI disorders, a geriatric patient may also present with significant signs of shock, which can result from even a small amount of blood loss because of aging compensatory mechanisms. Since the liver is often involved in chronic disease, there may also be peripheral, sacral, and periorbital edema from venous congestion. Other findings may include a low-grade fever, respiratory distress, and vital sign changes.

Your approach and assessment should be similar to any assessment format for the geriatric patient. Focus on ensuring a patent airway, and provide manual or mechanical airway assistance if the patient is unable to protect the airway himself, possibly because of a depressed mental status. If the breathing is adequate, provide supplemental oxygen; if breathing is inadequate, the oxygen should be provided via positive pressure ventilation. Keep the patient in a recovery position if he is conscious, or supine if he is unresponsive or if you are maintaining the airway and/or breathing. In a conscious patient, if the blood pressure is 10 mmHg lower when the patient is standing as compared to lying supine, consider it a positive sign for volume depletion. Summon ALS intercept while you expedite transport to the hospital.

Assessment Finding: Environmental Temperature Extremes

The effects of the aging process leave the elderly at greater risk of experiencing an emergency as a result of changes in the environmental temperature. The ability of the body to create heat when cold, or to dissipate heat when hot, may

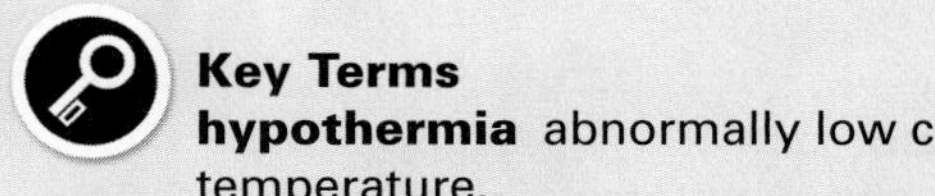

Key Terms

hypothermia abnormally low core body temperature.

hyperthermia abnormally high core body temperature.

Objective 39-4

Describe modifications that may be necessary to effectively assess and treat geriatric patients.

Key Terms

ageism stereotyping or discrimination against old people.

be impaired not only from the aging process but from certain diseases and medications the patient may be taking. Whenever you enter the scene of a geriatric emergency, you should be acutely aware of any extremes in the ambient air temperature to which the patient has been subjected. Even a temperature that seems only moderately warm or cool to you may be intolerable to the elderly person.

A body temperature less than 35°C (95°F), or **hypothermia,** is of special concern in an elderly patient. A number of factors make the elderly more prone to hypothermia. These factors include a smaller insulating layer of fat, reduced muscle mass, the body's metabolic rate slowing with age, impaired reflexes, decreasing blood flow (especially to the extremities), and a reduced shivering response. Living on a fixed income may result in being unable to keep the home adequately heated. Because of physical impairments, the elderly may not be able to move around much, so they get colder much more easily. Also, certain medications may make the elderly patient prone to hypothermia.

Treatment includes protecting the airway and maintaining normal breathing and circulatory status. Not only should you remove the patient from the cold environment, but you should also remove any wet clothes and insulate the patient in a dry blanket. Use caution when handling a severely hypothermic patient as excessive handling or moving may put the patient into a lethal heart rhythm.

Equally serious is the elderly patient suffering from a heat-related disorder or an increased body temperature (**hyperthermia**). The geriatric patient's core temperature can increase more rapidly than the younger patient's, and the length of time exposed to the environmental extreme should be taken into consideration when preparing to treat the patient. To institute prehospital cooling of a hyperthermic geriatric patient, you would follow the same guidelines as for treating a younger patient. A complete discussion of the prehospital treatment for hypothermia and hyperthermia can be found in Chapter 24, "Environmental Emergencies."

Assessment Finding: Geriatric Abuse

Abuse of the elderly occurs in some care centers and other institutions, but it also happens in the home. Any elderly person is especially at risk if he is cared for by someone who is under stress from other sources. Abuse of the elderly can be physical, financial, or mental (usually involving threats or insults). At highest risk are those elderly who are bedridden, demented, incontinent, or frail, or who have disturbed sleep patterns.

Signs of abuse can include bruises, bite marks, bleeding beneath the scalp (indicative of hair-pulling), lacerations on the face, trauma to the ears, broken bones, deformities of the chest, cigarette burns, and rope marks. If you suspect abuse, pay particular attention to inconsistencies when you get your history from the patient and from the provider or family. Your priority is to provide emergency care for the injuries. Do not confront the family or care provider with your suspicion of abuse. Instead, you should make your suspicion known to the receiving hospital's staff so that they may follow up with the appropriate authorities. Follow local protocols or state laws regarding reporting of suspected abuse.

Assessment-Based Approach: Geriatric Patients

Since geriatric patients are among the patients the EMT will encounter most frequently, you should understand some of the historical, environmental, and social factors that impact the elderly. First, the number of elderly in the United States is growing rapidly. Current statistics show that the number of people over the age of 65 has boomed over the last century and that the number of people over the age of 85 is actually growing faster than the number over age 65. Many have special health care needs that should always be treated with the utmost respect and compassion.

The EMT should always consider it an honor to help care for a geriatric patient in need. The compassion and attitude shown to the geriatric patient should reflect this. Always consider approaching the geriatric patient with the same degree of concern and consideration that you would show a pediatric patient. Additionally, avoid any of the purposeful or accidental stereotyping of **ageism.** Ageism occurs when a person either knowingly or unknowingly discriminates against people who are old. Derogatory terms such as "old geezer" or "gomer" are extremely unprofessional. Even addressing the elderly person as "dear," "honey," or "pops," or calling him by his first name without having permission to do so are forms of ageism and should be avoided. Consider for a moment the amount of the history retained by the elderly. An elderly patient nearing his 90th birthday will have lived through the Great Depression, two World Wars, numerous military conflicts (i.e., Korea and Vietnam), the

Thinking Critically

Your elderly patient is refusing transport. His daughter takes you aside and says, "He's afraid if he goes to the hospital he'll never come home. And he can't afford a hospital stay." You feel the patient needs to go to the hospital. How can you try to persuade him?

Key Points

The signs and symptoms of specific diseases and conditions may be masked by or confused with the physiological changes of aging.

Cold War with the Soviets, the Civil Rights Movement, space flight, the computer age, and more currently the turmoil in the Middle East. They have witnessed what most EMT students have only read about in school. They have earned the respect of a nation, and should receive nothing less from the EMT.

Other considerations with the geriatric population are their social issues. Probably the two greatest are isolation and marital status. With advancing age comes the loss of many friends and family near their own age. This isolates the elderly from the rest of society as their social network decreases. Contributing to this and compounding it greatly is the loss of a spouse. Pinched finances are also a common issue facing the geriatric population. Unless a great deal of financial planning was done at an earlier age, many elderly patients find themselves on a fixed income of governmental support that often does not meet their economic needs. Too often, the elderly patient may have to choose between paying for rent, food, or the medications needed to treat chronic conditions.

ASSESSMENT Tips

The financial straits in which many elderly patients find themselves may be manifested by a reluctance to go to the hospital for fear of the ambulance and hospital bills that will be incurred. ■

Many geriatric patients may be found living in independent or dependent living arrangements. Independent living is when an elderly person lives in his own home, tending to his own needs. Independent living is also when the geriatric patient lives in a "gated" adult community, senior apartments, or independent living in congregate housing. While this type of independence is valued by most elderly people, it is not always possible. Many geriatric patients live with family members who care for them. Other geriatric patients have a high degree of independence but, because of a chronic condition or disability, they live in some type of assisted living facility where there is 24-hour supervision and access to a health care professional should a problem arise. Living arrangements of this nature include residential care, boarding homes, or the traditional "nursing home." A patient with Alzheimer disease may reside in an Alzheimer care facility. In instances of terminal illness that can no longer be managed by medicine, the elderly may be found at home where they receive palliative care through a hospice care program.

One consistent feature of almost all these living arrangements is that the EMT may be delayed in getting to the patient's side by the locked doors of care facilities, privacy gates in adult communities, or simply waiting for the patient's primary care provider to arrive and give the patient's medical and physical history. Attempt to obtain as much information as possible from the patient himself. If this is impossible because of the patient's mental state, the EMT can still initiate the physical exam while awaiting the medical history from the appropriate primary care provider.

An important concern of many elderly is advance directives. Advance directives are designed to express the patient's wishes as to the care he will receive should he experience a significant change in his health. For example, an elderly person with incurable cancer may have had advance directives prepared on his behalf should he later experience another significant health crisis. Since the depth and breadth of advance directives vary from state to state, it is up to the EMT to become familiar with how they are handled in his particular state and EMS system.

The leading causes of illness and death in the geriatric population—starting with the highest-frequency cause and listing downward from there—are heart disease, cancer, stroke, chronic obstructive pulmonary disease, pneumonia, diabetes, trauma (e.g., fractures, falls), and misuse of drugs. The signs and symptoms of any of these problems may be masked by, or confused with, the physiological changes of aging. You may wonder if a sign or symptom is the result of a present illness or injury, or the result of the normal aging process.

Also, as a result of the normal aging process, the response to illness is altered. Many medical problems present with different signs and symptoms in the elderly than in the general population. For example, a lack of chest pain in a geriatric patient who is experiencing a heart attack is common.

In general, the geriatric patient needs to be assessed and treated carefully. Any delay in recognizing health care needs and providing care may have devastating, irreversible consequences. Especially at risk are those elderly people who:

- Live alone
- Are incontinent
- Are immobile
- Have been recently hospitalized
- Have been recently bereaved
- Have an altered mental status

Scene Size-Up

Begin the scene size-up by determining if there are any safety hazards to yourself, your crew, your patient, or bystanders. As always, you should approach the patient with Standard Precautions taken. Since tuberculosis is prevalent in nursing homes and other extended-care facilities, wear a HEPA mask when you encounter a patient with signs or symptoms of a respiratory disorder (such as a cough and, perhaps, blood-tinged sputum) in such a facility. Elderly patients often have a depressed immune system. If the EMT has a simple cold or flu, it would be very easy to pass this accidentally to the elderly patient, with potentially disastrous effects. It is always warranted that the EMT wear gloves, but it is also advised to don a protective mask if you fear you may have a cold or flu that could be passed to your patient. The best advice in this situation is simply to not function as an EMT while you are recovering from an illness.

Since many elderly live on fixed incomes, it is not uncommon to find an elderly patient inside a house without proper heating during the winter or cooling in the summer. Remember to assess the environmental temperature (even if it means taking your arm out of your jacket in the wintertime to determine room temperature). Since the elderly patient has deteriorating compensatory mechanisms, the body's response to environmental extremes of temperature will be diminished, potentially leading to cold- or heat-related emergencies more rapidly than in a younger person.

When the elderly patient shares living quarters, or lives in an extended-care facility, numerous patients may be victim to an environmental emergency (e.g., temperature extremes, toxic fumes). Determine if any additional patients are present and call for additional resources, if necessary.

Part of the scene size-up is determining whether the patient is suffering from trauma or a medical problem. Be alert to the fact that the cause of the emergency may be more complex than is first apparent. For example, since the geriatric patient may have numerous chronic diseases, an unresponsive patient (seemingly a medical emergency) may actually be unresponsive because he failed to eat a meal, which caused a diabetic reaction, which caused him to fall from a chair, which resulted in a head injury that is now presenting with delayed symptoms—a combined medical and trauma emergency.

There may be reliable family members or bystanders who witnessed or are aware of what happened to the patient. However, while you may make a preliminary determination of the nature of the problem during the scene size-up, maintain a high index of suspicion. Look for clues to chronic or acute conditions (Table 39-2).

Be ready to change your focus of care as you gather additional information during the primary and secondary assessments.

Primary Assessment

In performing the primary assessment, keep in mind the following special considerations for the geriatric patient (Table 39-3):

- **Mental status.** The geriatric patient's mental status may be influenced by a chronic illness, the present illness or injury, prescription drugs he is taking, or relative familiarity with his surroundings. The purpose of assessing the mental status is to determine a baseline level of consciousness and the possible need for airway protection and ventilatory assistance. It is important to ask family or caregivers to describe the

TABLE 39-2 Clues to Illness Found in the Scene Size-Up

Clues	May Indicate
Bucket next to bed	The patient suffers from nausea and vomiting.
Hospital bed	The patient has no or limited mobility and a pre-existing chronic illness.
Nebulizer setup	Patient has a chronic respiratory disease process.
Oxygen tank setup or oxygen concentrator	Patient has a chronic respiratory or cardiac disease.
Medications found at the scene	A clue as to the patient's preexisting condition(s).
Washcloth on the patient's forehead or near the patient	Patient has a severe headache or fever.
Patient in nightclothes in the middle of the afternoon	The patient has been sick all day.
Tripod position	The patient has significant respiratory distress.
Patient propped up on pillows	The patient has difficulty breathing when lying flat, commonly because of congestive heart failure.
A hot room temperature in the summer months	A possible heat emergency caused by dehydration or hyperthermia (elevated core body temperature).
A cold room temperature in the winter months	A possible cold emergency, hypothermia (decreased core body temperature).

TABLE 39-3 Special Considerations in the Primary Assessment of the Geriatric Patient

Chief complaint	The elderly patient may not complain of pain because of a pre-existing central nervous system condition, such as stroke. However, any complaint of pain in the elderly must be taken seriously.
	Some elderly patients will not experience pain when suffering a serious condition, such as a heart attack, because of a disease process that affects the nerve endings. This is common in diabetic patients.
	Prickling and burning-type pain is usually caused by a condition affecting the superficial structures of the body, whereas an aching-type pain usually indicates an organ is involved in the condition.
	Changes in the peripheral nerves in the skin can affect the elderly patient's ability to distinguish between hot and cold.
	A sudden loss of vision in one eye is not normal in the elderly and normally indicates a retinal artery occlusion or retinal detachment.
	Depression in the elderly is a serious complaint and must be managed properly. A depression state may cause the patient to not report or to minimize significant symptoms. There is a high rate of suicide among the elderly.
	Alcohol abuse is more common in the elderly. Keep a higher index of suspicion and look for evidence of alcohol abuse in the scene size-up.
	Side effects of medications or interactions with other medications may cause the presenting signs and symptoms.
	Fainting may be a serious complaint associated with conditions affecting the brain, lungs, heart, or circulatory system such as heart attack, pneumonia, blocked pulmonary artery (pulmonary embolism), shock, head injury or stroke, or congestive heart failure.
Mental status	Hypoxia causes agitation and aggression. High levels of carbon dioxide cause confusion and disorientation.
	A sudden onset of an altered mental status is not a normal part of aging and is not considered to be dementia. It is usually an indication of a serious illness or injury.
	Altered mental status may be due to inadequate perfusion to the brain, hypoxia in the brain, dehydration, electrolyte disturbances, change in the blood glucose level, infection, cold emergency (hypothermia), stroke, head injury, tumors, drugs, or alcohol intoxication.
Airway	A reduction in the patient's reflexes may cause a high incidence of choking and aspiration of food or other substances.
	Cervical arthritis may make performing an effective head-tilt, chin-lift maneuver difficult because of the stiffness of the neck structures. A jaw-thrust maneuver may provide a better manual airway.
	Loose dentures may cause an airway obstruction. If the dentures are loose or poorly fitted, remove them. If the dentures are well fitted and snug in place, do not remove them. In a patient without dentures or teeth, it is much more difficult to get an effective mask seal if ventilation needs to be performed.
Breathing	Elderly patients have higher resting respiratory rates. A resting respiratory rate greater than 20 per minute may be completely normal.
	Elderly patients have lower tidal volumes. This can lead to early onset of hypoxia.
	Retractions are less likely to occur in the elderly because of the less elastic and compliant chest wall muscles.
Circulation	Elderly patients have higher resting heart rates, typically greater than 90 beats per minute unless they are on beta blockers.
	An irregularly irregular pulse (no regular rhythm or pattern) may be normal in an elderly patient.
Skin	The skin will normally appear to be dry and less elastic. Assessment of skin turgor in the elderly is not a reliable test of skin hydration. Inspect the inside of the mouth or under the lower eyelid to check for hydration status.
	Cold skin may indicate hypothermia, even when the elderly patient is found in his or her home. This is referred to as "urban hypothermia." A reduction in subcutaneous fat and skin vessel response may cause the body core temperature to decrease faster.
	Fever is less common in the elderly patient, even with serious infections.
	Hot skin may indicate a heat emergency, such as heat stroke. Elderly patients are more prone to heat emergencies because of their inability to dilate the vessels to assist in cooling the body.

Thinking Critically
An elderly patient is answering your questions so slowly you are becoming impatient. What might be the reason or reasons for his slowness? How can you best deal with the situation?

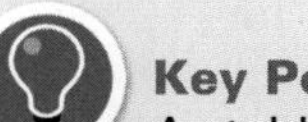

Key Points
A stable patient is one with an intact airway and adequate breathing, circulation, and mental status who requires minimal support during the primary assessment. An unstable patient is one who presents with abnormalities in any of these categories.

patient's normal mental status. One of the best assessment tools when determining the patient's mental status is patience on the EMT's part. Not only will geriatric patients normally process information more slowly than their younger counterparts, the stress and confusion of an emergency may slow them even more.

ASSESSMENT Tips

Give the geriatric patient time to formulate a response to your questioning, rather than simply dismissing the failure to answer immediately as a form of altered mental status. ■

- **Airway and breathing.** The elderly patient's diminished gag reflex makes him vulnerable to aspiration of fluids and food or other solids, which can be fatal. Therefore, monitoring the elderly patient's airway is especially important.

  Also pay close attention to breathing patterns. If a geriatric patient is suffering acute respiratory distress, the muscles of respiration may fatigue and fail more rapidly than in a younger person. This can cause inadequate breathing (hypoventilation), which the geriatric patient tolerates even less than a younger patient. (Although it is normal for hypoxia, or oxygen deprivation, to cause an increase in respiratory rate, don't get a false sense of security if the geriatric patient's rate starts to slow. This may actually indicate respiratory failure rather than improved oxygenation.) *Be prepared to initiate positive pressure ventilation.*
- **Circulation.** Assess central and peripheral pulses, noting the rate, strength, and rhythm. Your initial pulse check should include an assessment of the radial pulse. However, since the geriatric patient is predisposed to peripheral vascular diseases, the radial pulse may be markedly diminished or absent. This is not necessarily an abnormal sign; just be sure to check other pulses if the radial pulse is weak or absent.

  Although it is natural for the pulse rate of an elderly patient to be slightly higher at rest than a younger person's, you should note any irregularity to the rhythm. This could be from the degenerative processes that affect the conduction system of the heart or from a drug (or drugs) that the patient is taking. Nonetheless, an acute onset of an irregular pulse should be considered an abnormality that necessitates emergency department evaluation.
- **Skin condition and temperature.** When assessing the skin, remember that the geriatric body does not display the same signs and symptoms of dehydration as in the younger patient. Since the geriatric patient has, overall, a lower amount of body water, and because of the changes in the skin from aging, dry-looking skin may be normal. If you suspect dehydration, the best way to assess for it is to look at the mucous membranes of the eyes and in the mouth. Normal hydration status will show them to be moist. A dehydrated patient will have a dry mouth, the tongue may be furrowed, the eyes may appear to be "sunken" into the orbits, and the membranes around the eyes will also appear dry. It is no longer advised to check for "skin tenting" as an assessment for dehydration in the geriatric patient since almost all will display tenting. This is usually secondary to skin elasticity degeneration and a loss of subcutaneous fat rather than from significant dehydration.

  Equally important is skin temperature. The geriatric patient has a depressed response to infection. Whereas you may feel unusually warm skin from a fever in a young patient, you may not feel warm skin in a geriatric patient even if he does have an infection (e.g., pneumonia, upper respiratory infection). The temperature-regulating mechanism may be depressed, leading to minimal or absent fever or even hypothermia with severe infection. (Again, this contributes to the geriatric patient's susceptibility to temperature-related emergencies.)

  Like the pediatric patient, you can quickly categorize the elderly patient as "stable," implying no life threats, or "unstable," indicating that a life threat is present. Categorizing the patient as stable or unstable is relatively easy. The patient with an intact airway and adequate breathing, circulation, and mental status who requires minimal support during the primary assessment is considered stable. Conversely, the patient who presents with any disturbance or abnormality to the airway, breathing, circulation, and mental status is identified as unstable.

  If there is any question as to whether the patient is stable or unstable, err on the side to benefit the patient and manage him as unstable. Be extremely alert to the stable patient who can deteriorate rapidly into an unstable patient. As you progress through your secondary assessment you may change the patient's status. For example, you may have completed a primary assessment in a patient with a complaint of vomiting up blood and have not identified any abnormality. The heart rate is slightly elevated, but you think it might be attributed to anxiety associated with the situation. As you assess the abdomen you find rigidity and tenderness. This finding would cause you to change the patient's status from stable to unstable.

The following points can help you identify which category the geriatric patient should be assigned to:

- **Stable.** An elderly patient who is alert and has an open airway, adequate breathing, signs of good peripheral perfusion, and a strong peripheral pulse is categorized as stable.
- **Unstable.** An elderly patient with an acute change in mental status, an obstructed airway, inadequate breathing, or signs of poor perfusion is categorized as unstable and is in need of immediate emergency care during the primary assessment. Note that *any one* of these conditions is enough to place the patient in the unstable category.

Secondary Assessment

Gather the history and conduct your physical exam based on the patient's mechanism of injury (if trauma) or chief complaint (if medical). When interviewing a geriatric patient, you may encounter characteristic challenges resulting from the general depression of the sensory organs (especially failing eyesight and diminished hearing). These special considerations are discussed next with suggestions on how best to communicate to ensure a reliable history:

- **Diminished sight or blindness.** You can expect increased patient anxiety because of an inability to see surroundings, coupled with an inability to exert control over the situation. You must talk calmly and be positioned so that the patient can best see you if he has any sight at all (Figure 39-7*). Explain your procedures carefully. If the patient has eyeglasses, make sure he is wearing them. The elderly patient may have cataracts or glaucoma and be less able to tolerate bright lights and glare. These conditions contribute to diminished sight or blindness and can easily heighten your patient's anxiety.
- **Diminished hearing or deafness.** Many elderly people cannot hear high-frequency (or pitch) speech, especially consonants. Obtaining a history can be difficult if the patient cannot understand questions. Do not assume that the patient is deaf without first inquiring with the family or bystanders. The majority of geriatric patients still have intact hearing.

  If the patient is wearing a hearing aid, make sure that it is turned on. Do not shout, as it distorts sounds if the patient has some hearing, and it does not help if the patient is deaf. However, increasing the volume of your voice (rather than the pitch) may help with the hearing-impaired patient. You may also try placing your stethoscope earpieces in the patient's ears and speaking into the diaphragm. If the patient can lip-read, speak slowly and directly toward the patient. Note-writing may help, too. Whenever possible, verify the history with a reliable relative or friend, or seek assistance from these individuals in communicating with the patient.

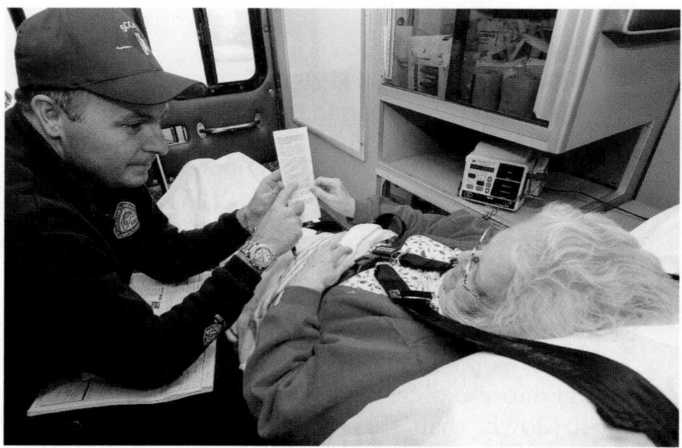

FIGURE 39-7 * Position yourself so that the geriatric patient can clearly see you when you are speaking. (© Ray Kemp/911 Imaging)

For the Geriatric Trauma Patient

Note the mechanism of injury if possible trauma is involved. Just as with younger patients, the elderly can be involved in car accidents, falls from ladders or rooftops, falls down stairs, assaults, and so on. In fact, the elderly are at a greater risk for experiencing a traumatic injury (primarily from falls) (Figure 39-8*) because of a variety of factors, which we discuss later in the chapter. Situations that may be minor in other age groups may require aggressive care in the elderly.

The geriatric trauma patient, if responsive, may not indicate that the pain he is experiencing is severe. This may be a function of the aging process. The elderly patient may have a decreased sensitivity to pain; therefore, the severity of pain is unreliable as an indicator of the seriousness of the injury. *You should maintain a high index of suspicion and treat any complaint of pain as a symptom of a serious injury.*

Examine the head, neck, chest, abdomen, pelvis, extremities, and posterior body. Inspect and palpate for any evidence of trauma. See Chapter 36, "Multisystem Trauma and Trauma in Special Patient Populations," for more information on trauma in the elderly.

While completing the secondary assessment, you will also assess and record baseline vital signs (Table 39-4) and obtain a history from the patient if he is responsive,

Key Points
The geriatric patient may have one or more chronic diseases or may be taking multiple medications that mask or alter signs and symptoms and make it difficult to determine the chief complaint.

Key Points
Talk to the patient about the emergency rather than talking about the patient to others.

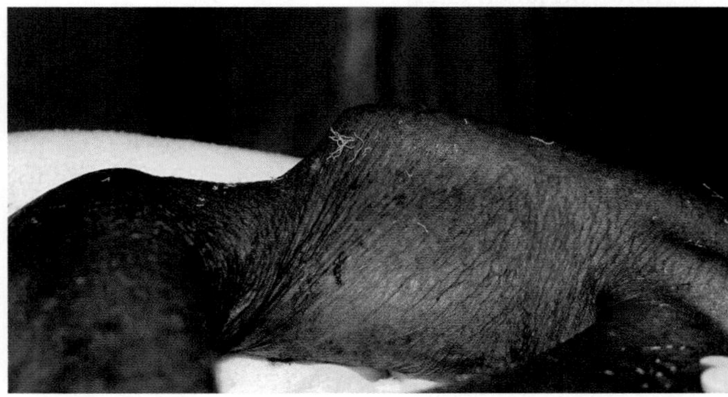

FIGURE 39-8 ✻ Broken right femur in an 80-year-old man from a fall on the boardwalk. (© Maria A. H. Lyle)

or from family and bystanders. Special considerations for obtaining a history from the geriatric patient are detailed in the following section.

Remember, the elderly deteriorate much more rapidly than do young people, especially following trauma. A minor problem may become a major one in a short period of time. To properly treat the geriatric patient, you need to perform an entire physical examination.

TABLE 39-4 Special Considerations in Vital Signs of the Elderly

- *The resting respiratory rate* is normally higher in the elderly.
- *The resting heart rate* is normally greater than 90 bpm.
- *The skin* is normally dry and less elastic.
- *Fever* is less common in the elderly, even when a serious infectious disease is present.
- *The systolic blood pressure* will increase in the elderly patient, making systolic hypertension more common. The hypertension may give a false reading in the patient who has lost blood or who is dehydrated; however, the blood pressure will fall quickly since the patient cannot compensate well.
- *The pupils* are more sluggish to respond to light as a result of the normal aging process. The pupils may be distorted (not round) because of cataract surgery or other conditions. Eye drops that the patient may be taking for conditions such as glaucoma may cause the pupils to dilate and not react normally to light.

For the Geriatric Medical Patient

While the mechanism of injury in a geriatric trauma patient may be easy to determine, discerning a chief complaint in a medical emergency may be more difficult. The geriatric patient may have one or more chronic diseases or medications, which can mask or alter the presentation of signs and symptoms; the elderly patient may not be a reliable source of information for exactly the same reasons.

Because of the aging process, the patient's memory, hearing, sight, and orientation may be diminished. This can challenge your ability, or even the patient's ability, to determine the chief complaint (what prompted the present emergency call). For example, a geriatric patient may report experiencing a headache or neck pain but forget that he fell yesterday. Compounding this, the geriatric patient typically does not have a single chief complaint. Rather, the EMT may find that geriatric patients present with various forms and combinations of pain, fatigue, weakness, discomfort, and so on. The EMT must diligently assess the geriatric patient so that it is possible to delineate normal findings from those caused by chronic or acute illness or injury.

Yet you should remember that not all geriatric patients are deaf or blind, or have a diminished mental status. While these problems may be more common among the elderly than among the young, they are not the rule. The best way to destroy the patient–provider relationship is to assume that the patient has diminished hearing, sight, or mental capabilities.

Approach the geriatric patient with concern and compassion and *talk to* the patient about the emergency (Figure 39-9✻) rather than *talking about* the patient to others, unless unavoidable. If you have some doubts about whether the patient can grasp what you are saying, you may want to make sure, subtly of course, that a family member or bystander also is hearing and noting the information. The bottom line is, don't assume the elderly patient has diminished capabilities until you have evidence (through your assessment) of it.

Remember that the geriatric patient may not report everything that is wrong. One reason is that the older patient doesn't perceive pain or discomfort as readily as the younger patient. This may lead him to delay the call for an ambulance until the situation becomes critical. Or the geriatric patient may attribute his ailment to "just old

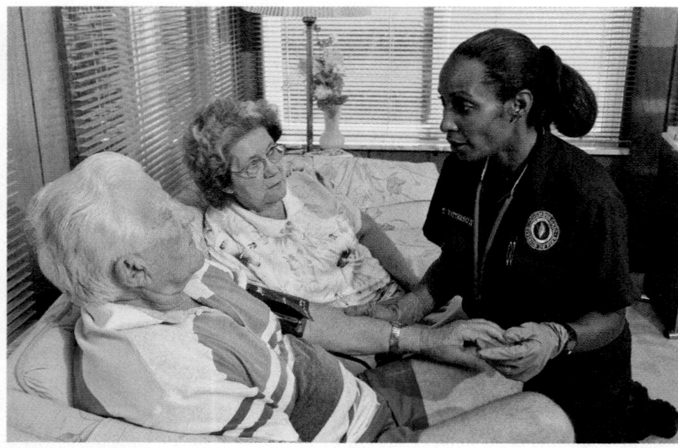

FIGURE 39-9 ∗ If possible, talk to the geriatric patient rather than talking about the patient to others.

age" when, really, there is a serious emergency progressing. Sometimes patients minimize their symptoms because they fear losing their independence if admitted to the hospital. (Their perception may be that old people go to the hospital to die or, at the least, to be moved on to a nursing home instead of being allowed to come home.) The EMT should exercise extreme caution, and use thorough history and physical assessment skills to ensure that there are no other life-threatening conditions the patient is suffering from.

In obtaining the history and conducting the physical examination of the geriatric medical patient, remember the following points:

- The patient may become fatigued easily.
- You should clearly explain what you are going to do before examining the elderly patient.
- The patient may minimize or deny symptoms because he fears being bedridden or institutionalized or losing his self-sufficiency.
- Peripheral pulses may be difficult to evaluate.
- You must distinguish signs and symptoms of chronic problems or natural aging processes from the signs and symptoms of acute problems:
  - Loss of skin elasticity and mouth breathing may give the false appearance of dehydration.
  - Edema (swelling) may be caused by varicose veins, inactivity, and position rather than heart failure.

Since you should anticipate that the elderly patient may not report or fully report all complaints, elicit as much information as you can by asking questions such as these:

- Have you had any trouble breathing?
- Have you had a cough lately? (If so, have you been coughing up anything like mucus or blood?)
- Have you had any chest pain?
- Did you get dizzy? (If so, what were you doing when this occurred?)
- Have you fainted?
- Have you had any headaches lately?
- Have you been eating and drinking normally?
- Have there been any changes in your bowel or bladder habits?
- Have you fallen lately?

As discussed previously, it is best to address the elderly patient as "Mr." or "Mrs." or "Miss," as appropriate. Despite current misconceptions, the geriatric patient is not "set at ease" when an unknown EMT arrives on the scene and talks to him as if they have been friends for years. It is inappropriate to address the elderly patient by his first name or a nickname and contributes to ageism stereotyping. The only exception is if the elderly patient voluntarily tells you otherwise.

As you begin the physical exam, you will notice that the geriatric patient is typically dressed in layers of clothing, since the ability of the elderly to regulate body temperature is usually impaired. This makes performing a physical exam more difficult since the manipulation necessary to remove the patient's clothing can easily fatigue the patient. In fact, it may be tempting just to skip the physical exam rather than take the time to remove clothing. This could, however, be fatal if you miss a life-threatening injury or problem because you chose not to perform a complete physical exam.

If the patient is unresponsive or has an altered mental status because of the medical emergency, perform a physical assessment of the head, neck, chest, abdomen, pelvis, extremities, and posterior body to find and treat any life threats that may be causing the alteration in mental status. Scan the scene for any clues to the patient's problem (medicine bottles, mechanism of injury, environmental extremes, and so on). It is important to collect and transport the patient's medications. Finally, assess and record baseline vital signs.

As with geriatric trauma patients, you will perform a secondary exam on geriatric medical patients whether they are alert, have an altered mental status, or are unresponsive. Even the mentally competent geriatric patient may not give reliable information—for reasons discussed earlier—so the physical exam will better enable you to assess for injuries, or signs of injury, or other medical abnormalities.

Emergency Medical Care and Reassessment

A geriatric patient can deteriorate rapidly. It is critically important to anticipate problems and to continuously reassess the patient. In the geriatric patient, the injury or failure of one body system can rapidly cause the failure of

Key Points

A geriatric patient can deteriorate rapidly, so it is important to anticipate problems and continually reassess the patient.

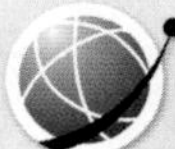

Media Resources

Go to www.bradybooks.com for mykit. Highlights:

- *Web Resource:* Frailty and Aging
- *Web Resource:* Healthy Aging

others. Key considerations and emergency care steps for the geriatric patient are:

1. **Maintain a patent airway.** Geriatric patients often wear dentures, and if these dentures become dislodged, they can create an airway obstruction. Look in the mouth to determine if the dentures (or any other foreign object or substance) is blocking the airway. If necessary, suction and clear the airway immediately before assessing the breathing status. If the neck is stiff and not flexible enough to perform a head-tilt, chin-lift maneuver, perform a jaw thrust to establish a patent airway.
2. **Insert an airway.** The geriatric patient's mental status is subject to rapid deterioration. If the patient is unable to maintain his own airway as a result of injury or altered mental status, insert an oropharyngeal airway. If the patient cannot tolerate an oropharyngeal airway, insert a nasopharyngeal airway.
3. **Assess and be prepared to assist ventilations.** It is vitally important to assess the geriatric patient's rate and depth of respirations. Because of the general decline in respiratory muscle strength, a minor chest injury or lung disorder can easily put the patient into respiratory failure unless proper care is initiated. If the rate or depth is inadequate, positive pressure ventilation should be initiated immediately. Be careful not to ventilate the patient with excessive pressure or volumes, which could cause lung injury. Although loose dentures could cause an airway obstruction, if they are still firmly seated in the elderly patient in need of positive pressure ventilation it may be advisable to leave them in place. The dentures will help support the soft tissues around the mouth on which the mask of the ventilation device will be seated.
4. **Establish and maintain oxygen therapy.** As with all patients, be sure to provide supplemental oxygen with positive pressure ventilation if the patient's breathing is inadequate. If breathing is adequate, administer oxygen based on the SpO_2 reading and patient signs and symptoms. If the SpO_2 reading is greater than 95% and no signs or symptoms of hypoxia, poor perfusion, or respiratory distress are present, oxygen may not be necessary. In this case, you may choose to apply a nasal cannula at 2 to 4 lpm. If signs of hypoxia, poor perfusion, or respiratory distress are present, or the SpO_2 reading is less than 95%, place the patient on a nonrebreather mask at 15 lpm.
5. **Position the patient.** Exercise extreme caution when preparing the patient for transport, based on the type of emergency as outlined in the following guidelines:
   - If the emergency is medical in nature and the patient is alert and able to protect his own airway, place the patient in a position that is comfortable for him. This is typically a Fowler (sitting-up) position.
   - If the patient has an altered mental status and is unable to protect his own airway, he should be placed in a left lateral recumbent position (recovery position) to avoid aspiration.
   - If spinal injury is suspected, the patient needs immediate manual stabilization of the spine during primary assessment, followed by immobilization to a long backboard. One limitation, however, is the geriatric patient with severe curvature of the spine caused by kyphosis. The patient with severe kyphosis could actually be injured if forced to be immobilized in the same fashion as a younger person. You may need to be creative and construct the cervical immobilization devices out of blankets to accommodate the curvature of the spine.
   - If the patient is unresponsive, assume a possible cervical spine injury and immobilize the patient fully as a precautionary measure.
6. **Transport.** Reassess the patient en route to the hospital, remembering that the geriatric patient's condition can rapidly deteriorate without warning.

In order to ensure appropriate care, re-evaluate the geriatric patient frequently. The length of time spent with the patient or the condition of the patient will assist in establishing how often to repeat the reassessment phase. Repeat and record the assessment at least every 15 minutes for a stable patient. If the patient is unstable, repeat and record at a minimum of every 5 minutes.

Overall, successful assessment and treatment of a geriatric patient will depend in a large part upon your approach, demeanor, and attitude. It can be extremely stressful to the elderly patient if you immediately start "pulling out equipment and doing things" without first gaining the patient's cooperation. Your goal is to help lower the patient's anxiety, not increase it. Remember, what you do as an EMT on a regular basis (assessments, treatment, and so on) becomes routine to you. In contrast, this may be the first experience with EMS and emergency care for the patient, who has no idea what to expect. You need to explain everything that you are doing.

EMT skills 39-1 Immobilizing a Patient with Kyphosis

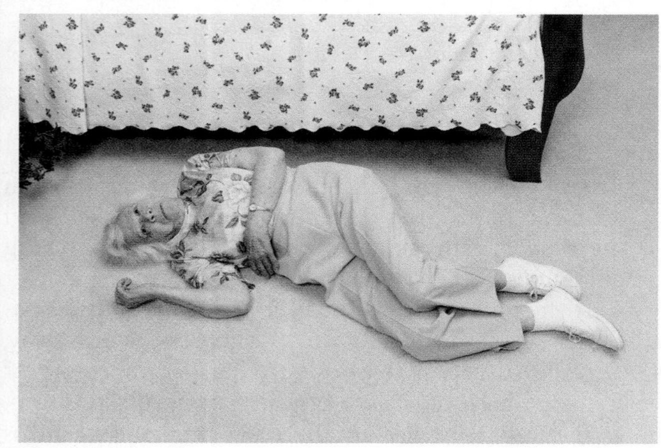

39-1A * Patient with kyphosis who has suffered a fall.

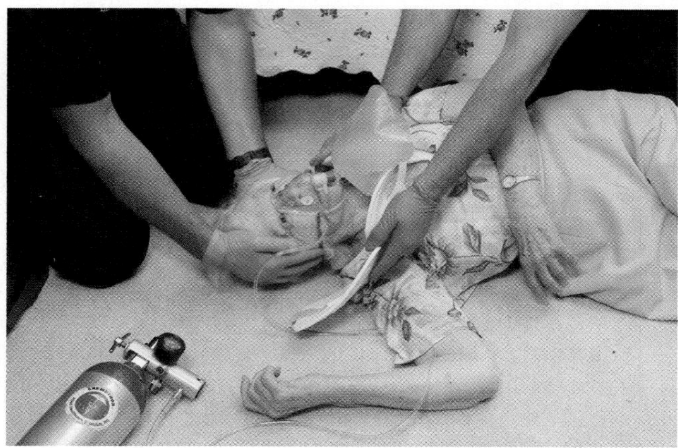

39-1B * One EMT holds manual stabilization as a second EMT applies a cervical collar.

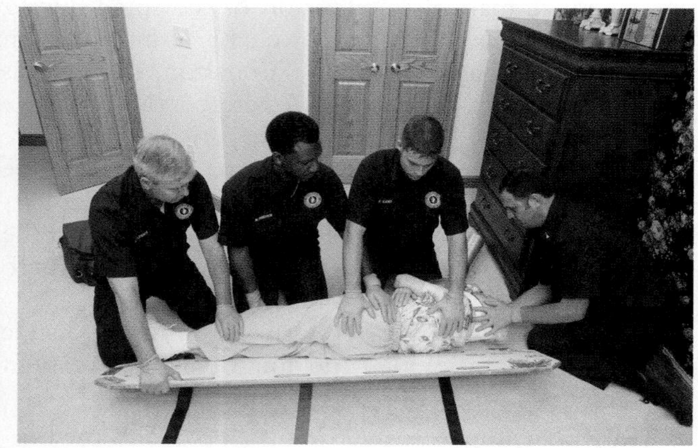

39-1C * Three EMTs log roll the patient onto a backboard.

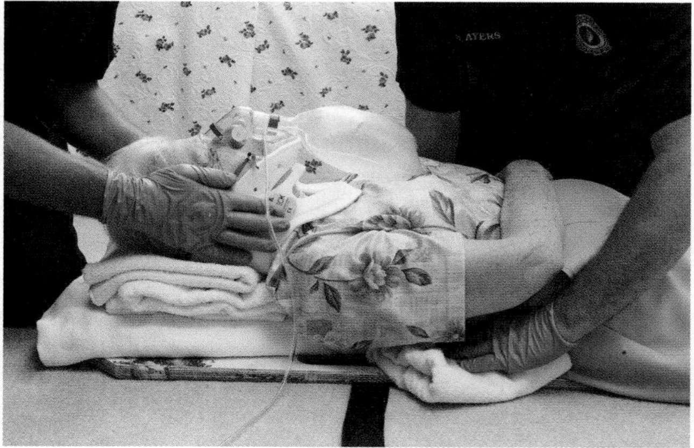

39-1D * EMTs apply padding to make the patient comfortable on the backboard.

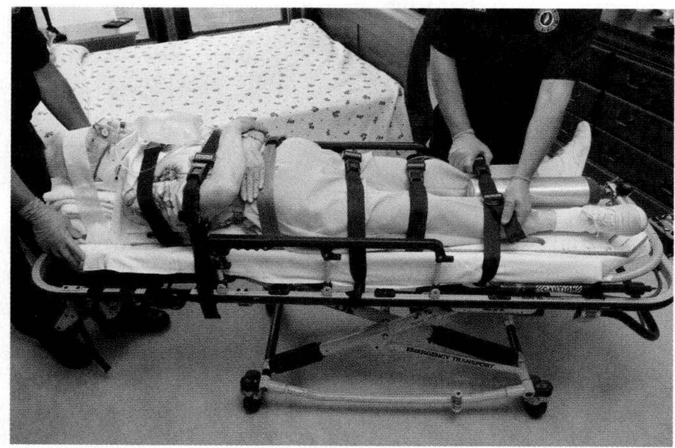

39-1E * The patient is fully immobilized to the backboard.

CHAPTER REVIEW

SUMMARY

As people age, they experience many changes to body systems, including the cardiovascular, respiratory, musculoskeletal, neurological, gastrointestinal, renal, endocrine, and integumentary systems. Assessment findings in the elderly often associated with these body systems include chest pain (or absence of chest pain in conditions where it might be expected), shortness of breath, altered mental status, and abdominal pain. Other common findings in the elderly include trauma, environmental temperature extremes, and, sadly, geriatric abuse. In addition to understanding findings commonly associated with various body systems, it is also important to understand the social and financial considerations that many elderly persons experience. Always remember to treat elderly patients with the respect they have earned.

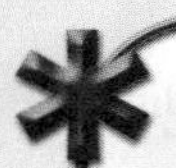

CASE STUDY FOLLOW-UP

SCENE SIZE-UP

You have been dispatched to the scene of a 72-year-old female patient complaining of difficulty in breathing. While you are walking into the house, the patient's husband, Mr. Vaughn, tells you that the patient has not been feeling well over the past few days and that yesterday she started having trouble "catching her breath." You note no particular hazards to yourself or your partner and do not see any obstacles that would make the extrication difficult. As you enter the bedroom, you note that the patient is sitting up in bed, wearing her nightgown, and you notice a bottle of nighttime cold medicine on her nightstand.

PRIMARY ASSESSMENT

When you introduce yourself, Mrs. Vaughn makes a motion indicating that she cannot hear you. You repeat your statement a little louder, but she still cannot hear you. You ask her husband if she has any hearing impairments, and he says that she is deaf in one ear and uses a hearing aid in the other. After assisting her in placing her hearing aid, you begin to ask her questions.

By her responses, you determine that Mrs. Vaughn is conscious with an open airway and is exchanging air adequately. She tells you that she has some trouble taking deep breaths. You immediately apply high-concentration oxygen via a nonrebreather mask at 15 lpm. Her radial pulse is present and strong with an approximate rate of 100 per minute. Her skin is warm, and she appears slightly flushed in color. Despite the fact that Mrs. Vaughn displays only minor respiratory distress at this time, because of her age you decide to treat her as a priority patient. Your partner leaves to get the stretcher while you continue with the history and physical exam.

SECONDARY ASSESSMENT

While waiting for your partner to return with the stretcher, you obtain more information regarding the respiratory distress complaint. In answer to the OPQRST questions, Mrs. Vaughn tells you that she was almost over a cold when she started to experience some trouble breathing and a cough, which started yesterday. She complains of no other discomfort and denies any dizziness, nausea or vomiting, chest pain, or abdominal pain. On a scale of 1 to 10, she calls her breathing discomfort "about 5." Mrs. Vaughn adds that she just took her temperature and found it to be only slightly elevated at 99.2°F.

As you continue to obtain the history, you find that the patient is not allergic to any medications and does not take prescribed medicine for high blood pressure or any other condition, although she states that she has a medical history of hypertension and arthritis. She has not had anything to eat or drink since last night when she started to feel worse. She reports no events that brought on the breathing difficulty other than the cough and cold.

During your secondary assessment exam, you determine that the patient has moist mucous membranes and her pupils are equal and reactive to light. You note no jugular vein distention. Breath sounds reveal crackles to the right and left lung fields. The patient is not using any accessory muscles to aid respirations. You assess baseline vitals and find the blood pressure to be 130/88, the heart rate is 96 and regular, and the respirations are somewhat rapid at 30 times a minute. The skin is warm and still slightly flushed. The pulse oximeter SpO_2 reading is 92%.

You place her on the stretcher in a Fowler position, which helps her to breathe, and start moving her to the ambulance. While en route to the hospital, you complete your assessment and determine that there are no visible or palpable areas of injury to the head, neck, torso, or extremities, nor indications of elder abuse. You ask her if she has experienced any injuries recently, and she denies this.

REASSESSMENT

You reassess the patient every 15 minutes. Mrs. Vaughn states that the oxygen must be working, because she feels much better and her respiratory distress is diminishing. You notify the receiving physician of your findings, and emergency care thus far. Reassessment of the vital signs reveals a pressure of 126/86, the breathing is regular at a normal rate of 20 per minute, and the pulse is 78 per minute. The SpO_2 reading on the pulse oximeter has increased to 96% while Mrs. Vaughn is on the nonrebreather mask. After you arrive at the hospital, you give your verbal report, write the prehospital care report, and prepare the ambulance for another trip.

On the way out of the hospital, you check in on Mrs. Vaughn, and she tells you that the doctor said that she has pneumonia and will be starting antibiotics. As you leave, you recall that even though she did not display the "classic" signs of pneumonia as seen in younger patients, such as high fever, chills, and chest pain, she did display signs classic to the elderly patient with pneumonia: increasing breathing difficulty, rapid respirations, and a cough. You remember that the differences are due to physiological changes as a result of aging.

IN REVIEW

1. A 79-year-old male patient is crossing the street to get his mail when he is struck by a vehicle traveling at 45 miles per hour. Discuss the changes in the following body systems from the normal aging process that would increase his susceptibility to injury and the aftereffects of injury: cardiovascular system, respiratory system, and musculoskeletal system.
2. Describe communication challenges caused by sensory degeneration in an elderly patient, and outline strategies for overcoming these challenges.
3. List questions you should ask the elderly patient in order to help obtain an accurate history.
4. Explain the reasons why a secondary assessment should always be performed on all geriatric patients, whether trauma or medical, unresponsive or alert.
5. Give emergency care guidelines for positioning and packaging the following geriatric patients: the alert medical patient, the patient with altered mental status, and the patient with suspected spinal injury. Also explain procedures for immobilizing a patient with spinal curvature.
6. Discuss how an assessment finding of denial of chest pain in the geriatric patient differs from the same finding in a younger adult patient.
7. List factors that make the elderly more likely to fall.
8. List at least five possible causes of, and discuss special treatment considerations for, altered mental status in the geriatric patient.
9. Explain why geriatric patients are predisposed to environmental heat or cold emergencies.
10. List signs and symptoms of geriatric abuse and discuss emergency care procedures when there is a high index of suspicion for geriatric abuse.

CRITICAL THINKING

You respond to a nursing home for an 82-year-old female patient. On your arrival, the staff indicates that the patient's mental status has deteriorated over a period of several days. They indicate that she is normally awake and alert; however, she is usually disoriented, especially at night. As you enter the room, you find the patient lying supine in bed with her head propped up on two pillows. You hear an obvious snoring sound with each respiration. She responds to a trapezius pinch with moans. Her respiratory rate is 22/minute. Her radial pulse is present at a rate of 92 bpm. The skin is warm and dry. She has a history of type 2 diabetes mellitus and takes an oral hypoglycemic agent. Her blood pressure is 178/72 mmHg and the SpO_2 reading is 95% on room air. Her blood glucose is 98 mg/dL.

1. What action would you immediately take to manage this patient's airway?
2. What other emergency care would you provide in the primary assessment?
3. What is your interpretation of the SpO_2 reading?
4. What is your interpretation of the blood glucose reading?
5. What conditions might cause this patient to experience an altered mental status?

PEARSON

EXPLORE mybradykit™

Please go to **www.bradybooks.com** to access mykit for this text. You will find quizzes, critical thinking scenarios, weblinks, animations, and videos related to this chapter—and much more. Look for online information on hypertension and healthy aging.

Register your access code from the front of your book by going to **www.bradybooks.com** and selecting the mykit links.

CHAPTER 40

Patients with Special Challenges

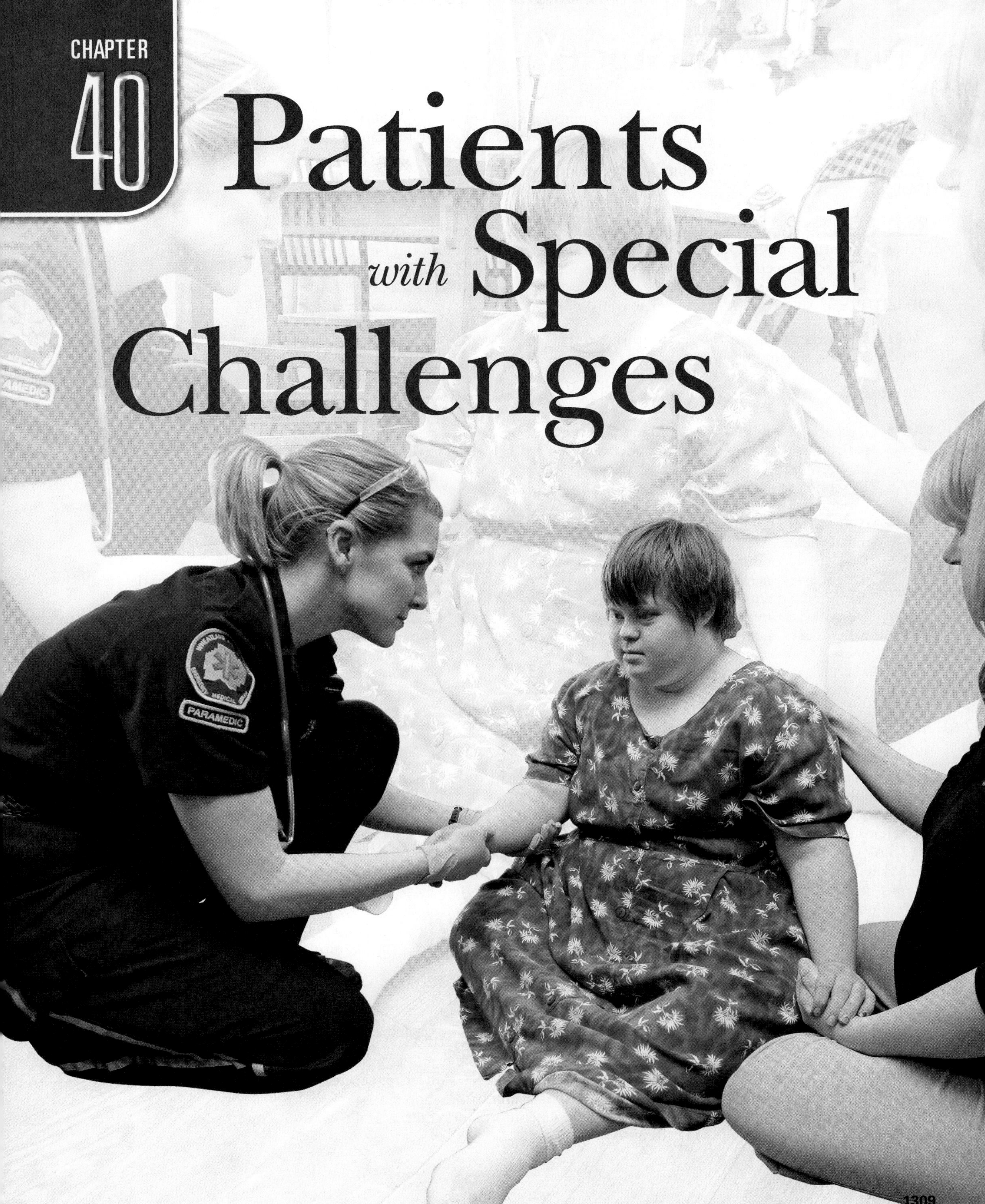

Navigation Guide

The following items provide an overview to the purpose and content of this chapter. The Standard and Competency are from the new National EMS Education Standards.

STANDARD **Special Patient Populations** (Content Area: Patients with Special Challenges)

COMPETENCY Applies fundamental knowledge of growth, development, aging, and assessment findings to provide basic emergency care and transportation for a patient with special needs.

OBJECTIVES: After reading this chapter, you should be able to:

40-1. Define key terms introduced in this chapter.
40-2. Explain the importance of understanding the care of patients with special challenges.
40-3. Give examples of special challenges and their causes.
40-4. Describe accommodations and modifications to patient assessment and management required for patients with sensory impairments.
40-5. Describe accommodations and modifications to patient assessment and management required for patients with cognitive and emotional impairments.
40-6. Describe accommodations and modifications to patient assessment and management required for paralyzed patients.
40-7. Describe accommodations and modifications to patient assessment and management required for obese patients.
40-8. Describe accommodations and modifications to patient assessment and management required for homeless or poor patients.
40-9. Describe accommodations and modifications to patient assessment and management required for abused patients.
40-10. Describe accommodations and modifications to patient assessment and management required for patients who are dependent on the following types of technology:
  a. Airway and respiratory devices
  b. Vascular devices
  c. Renal dialysis
  d. Gastrointestinal and genitourinary devices
  e. Intraventricular shunts
40-11. Describe accommodations and modifications to patient assessment and management required for patients who are terminally ill and describe the philosophy of hospice care.

KEY TERMS: Page references indicate first major use in this chapter. For complete definitions, see the Glossary at the back of the book.

acute renal failure (ARF) p. 1334
apnea monitor p. 1326
bariatrics p. 1317
bilevel positive airway pressure (BiPAP) p. 1328
birth defects p. 1314
cataract p. 1312
central intravenous catheter p. 1333
child abuse p. 1322
chronic kidney disease (CKD) p. 1334
chronic renal failure (CRF) p. 1334
continuous positive airway pressure (CPAP) p. 1328
diabetic retinopathy p. 1312
dialysis p. 1334
dialysis shunt p. 1334
dysarthria p. 1313
elder abuse p. 1323
enteral feeding p. 1336
glaucoma p. 1312
hospice p. 1340
intraventricular shunt p. 1339
medical oxygen p. 1325
ostomy bag p. 1336
paraplegic p. 1316
pulse oximeter p. 1327
quadriplegic p. 1317
stoma p. 1327
surgically implanted medication delivery devices p. 1333
terminally ill p. 1340
totally implantable venous access system (TIVAS) p. 1333
tracheostomy p. 1327
urinary catheter p. 1337
vascular access device (VAD) p. 1332

MEDIA RESOURCES: Please go to www.bradybooks.com to access mykit for this text. You will find quizzes, critical thinking scenarios, weblinks, animations, and videos related to this chapter—and much more. Look for online information on cerebral palsy, paraplegia, and performing a tracheostomy.

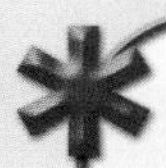

CASE STUDY

The Dispatch

EMS Unit 114—proceed to 86 Skyline Drive—you have a 2-year-old male patient who, family states, is lethargic. Be advised, parents state the patient had a "ventricular shunt" replaced about a week ago. Time out is 1132 hours.

On Arrival

You safely park the ambulance on the side of the street and keep your emergency lights illuminated. You exit the ambulance with your partner and look around at the quiet, mature neighborhood while you don your gloves. As you approach the house, a woman who turns out to be Mrs. Davidson comes out the front door and says, "It's my son, Bryan. He's been sleeping more lately, which hasn't been bothering me, but today I can't get him to wake up." She adds, "He really hasn't been quite the same since they replaced the shunt in his brain last week." You proceed into the house and find the patient lying supine in bed, with no outward signs of acute distress, lying there just as if he were peacefully asleep.

How Would You Proceed to Assess and Care for This Patient?

During this chapter, you will learn about assessment and emergency care for a patient with a "special challenge." Later, we will return to the case and apply the procedures learned.

Introduction

Because of changes in medicine and lifestyle, the life span of Americans is increasing. Another positive outcome of these changes is the compression of morbidity that many individuals now enjoy—that is, maximizing the number of healthy years in one's life while simultaneously minimizing the number of years of disease or disability at the end of life.

Despite these improvements in life span and length of healthy years, there are still people born with congenital defects and those who suffer significant trauma or endure illnesses that leave chronic residual deficits. Nevertheless, advances in medical care and medical technology are allowing people with certain deficits to live at home (either independently or with family) who formerly could only have been properly cared for in an extended-care facility. Deficits that today can be compensated by medicine and technology may be as minimal and common as a hearing impairment that can be ameliorated with hearing aids and communication-assist devices or as severe as a loss of the ability to breathe spontaneously that requires dependence on a mechanical ventilator.

During your career in EMS, you will certainly encounter patients who have special medical challenges or who are dependent on medical technologies to live. When a pre-existing condition worsens, a medical device fails, or the patient experiences an emergency not related to his special challenge, EMS is usually the first called on to intervene. The challenge to the EMT is determining how to properly assess, manage, and transport a patient with a special challenge—especially if there is medical equipment or other conditions that complicate the situation—while focusing on and treating the complaint that prompted the call for help.

This chapter introduces some of the special challenges you may find in patients you are called to assist and provides guidelines on how to recognize and accommodate these special conditions in order to provide the best possible care.

Estimating the number of people in the United States with some type of disability is next to impossible since there is no common registry for these people, nor is there a unified definition of what a "special needs" or "specially challenged" patient is. While it *is* known that over 8 million such patients receive health care from professional providers, it is estimated that millions of others receive their care from family members or other volunteers.

As already mentioned, with the aid of medicine, medical technology, and medical equipment, many people with special challenges are now living at home rather than in an extended-care facility. Although the person's primary care provider or providers are usually well versed in the equipment or technology being used, they may not be as well trained in what to do if that equipment fails or if the patient's status begins to deteriorate. Situations like these require sensitivity on the part of the EMS provider. Even if the patient's condition is terminal and death is expected soon, emotions can run high and easily overwhelm the capabilities of the family when the person deteriorates. Recognize that this may happen and do not allow yourself to get caught up in the emotional turmoil. Maintain your professional demeanor and focus on what you can do to help.

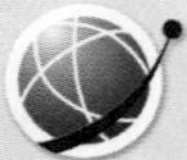

Media Resources

Go to www.bradybooks.com for mykit. Highlights:

- *Web Resource:* Cerebral Palsy
- *Web Resource:* Paraplegia
- *Web Resource:* Fact Sheet About the Homeless

Objective 40-2
Explain the importance of understanding the care of patients with special challenges.

Objective 40-3
Give examples of special challenges and their causes.

A person may be receiving care at home for any of a multitude of reasons. Perhaps his condition is not severe enough to warrant admission to a hospital or rehabilitation center. Perhaps the patient's status or condition is expected to improve over time and he wants to be with his family. Some patients have conditions that will not improve, but they want to live at home and, with the help of medical technology, they can do so with some degree of normality.

While it is impossible to discuss everything that you may encounter regarding patients with special challenges, this chapter is intended to provide you with the fundamental knowledge required to meet the needs of these patients. After completing your EMT class, however, it becomes your responsibility as an EMT to stay abreast of current home health care trends and equipment commonly found in use by these patients.

▶ Recognizing the Patient with Special Challenges

Any number of medical or traumatic conditions can cause loss of function to a body system. As noted earlier, these changes can be mild (such as hearing loss) or substantial (such as inability to breathe spontaneously). For example, a patient may be born with a birth defect that renders him incapable of communicating with you. There may be a number of lost functions as well. For example, a patient who had experienced a stroke may be paralyzed on one side of the body and unable to feed himself normally; so in addition to accommodations for the muscular paralysis, you may find that a special feeding tube has been inserted through the patient's abdominal wall.

Impairments may result from aging, birth defects, chronic illnesses, traumas, abuse, neglect, and other causes. Following are some of the more common causes for these challenges.

▶ Sensory Impairments

A sensory impairment might involve hearing, vision, or speech. This may lead to difficulty in the patient communicating with you or you communicating with the patient. You must be resourceful when dealing with patients with these disabilities in order to provide effective emergency care.

Hearing Impairment

Hearing impairment occurs when there is a loss or diminishment in the person's ability to hear sounds. This becomes especially problematic when the hearing loss is significant enough to hamper normal verbal communication. *Deafness* is a term that is commonly used to describe the inability to hear. Deafness may involve both ears or just one ear, and the patient may be partially deaf or totally deaf.

Vision Impairment

Just as there are multiple causes for deafness, there are also multiple causes for visual impairments, which can be loosely categorized into three etiologies: loss from disease, loss from injury, and loss from degenerative disorders.

Certain diseases, such as **glaucoma**, result in an abnormal increase in intraocular pressure that damages the optic nerve, resulting in peripheral vision loss and eventual blindness. Patients with diabetes mellitus may become blind from **diabetic retinopathy**, which occurs when the long-term effects of their disease damage the small blood vessels of the eye. Injury to the eye can be caused by puncture or penetration injuries, blunt trauma to the face, or chemical and thermal burns. This type of vision loss is usually acute but may not be permanent, depending on the degree of trauma endured by the eye and associated structures. With aging there may be some degeneration of the eyeball, the optic nerve, the optic nerve pathways, or all three. **Cataracts** are a condition in which the lens of the eye becomes cloudy from pathologic changes within the lens itself. Cataracts cause the pupil of the eye to look cloudy on assessment, and over time the patient experiences a diminishment in visual acuity to the point where he may not be able to carry on with activities of daily living.

Vision loss may have an acute onset or a slow onset. It may affect one eye or both eyes. It may affect just a certain field of vision in the patient (for example, peripheral vision or central vision). Some types of vision loss are reversible, while others are progressive and permanent. It is important to understand common etiologies of vision loss, so that you can determine if vision loss in a patient is the result of a chronic disability or a new finding from some acute illness or injury that you are there to treat.

Objective 40-4
Describe accommodations and modifications required for patients with sensory impairments.

Key Terms
glaucoma abnormal increase in intraocular pressure that damages the optic nerve.

Key Terms
diabetic retinopathy damage to the small blood vessels of the eye from effects of diabetes

cataract clouding of the lens of the eye from pathologic changes within the lens.

dysarthria defective speech caused by impairment of the tongue or other muscles.

Speech Impairment

Communicating with the patient is of utmost importance. There are times when the patient is unresponsive and communication is impossible, but that is not the norm. In the majority of patient contacts you will have during your career, the patient will be able to communicate. However, that does not mean that there is always *effective* communication. Communication can become deranged by four basic types of speech impairments: articulation disorders, voice production disorders, language disorders, and fluency disorders.

With articulation disorders caused by impairment of the tongue or other muscles needed for speech, called **dysarthria**, the patient cannot pronounce words correctly. Improper articulation can result from learning words incorrectly or from a hearing impairment. It may also be manifested in a patient with damage to the nerve tracts that coordinate the brain with the larynx, mouth, or lips.

Voice production disorders occur when there is damage to the larynx, vocal cords, or related supporting structures from illness or injury. The patient may attempt verbal communication, but the sounds he produces may be abnormally harsh, hoarse, or of an unusual pitch, or have nasal distortion that makes his speech difficult to understand.

Language disorders occur when the patient displays an impaired or absent ability to understand the spoken word. This can result from congenital problems in children, hearing deficits, or inadequate language stimulation in early life. In later life, language disorders can occur as a result of a stroke, head trauma, brain tumor, or even significant emotional distress.

Fluency disorders present as "stuttering" speech patterns. Although the exact cause for this disorder is not fully understood, the patient struggles with pronouncing words fluidly. The resulting speech pattern has sounds or syllables that are repeated. Communication may be possible, but stuttering typically lengthens the interview process as the patient struggles to provide answers.

Accommodations for Patients with Sensory Impairments

The hearing-impaired patient may have a hearing aid. If so, try to ensure it is on and working properly before you try to communicate with the patient. Many hearing-impaired patients lip-read, so always try to position yourself so your face is in clear view and the area is adequately lit. It may be necessary to communicate in writing if vital information is unobtainable through oral communication. If the patient is able to sign, it may be necessary to have a family member or other person at the scene who knows sign language to act as an interpreter.

For the visually impaired patient, be sure to speak clearly, since the patient may not be able to see your lips, and always explain what you are going to do before you do it (Figure 40-1*). Some visually impaired patients use a service dog. This may become an issue with the patient when making the decision to transport. The patient may insist on taking the service dog to the medical facility. You will have to follow your local protocol and service policies and procedures. It may be necessary for you to act as the patient's guide. Most often the visually impaired patient will want to take your arm or place his hand on your shoulder for guidance.

In any situation of speech impairment, whether from a congenital defect or from an acute process, ask questions in a way that allows the patient to answer in as few words as possible. Do not attempt to finish the patient's words or statements for him; this typically frustrates the patient and tends to worsen the speech impairment. Remember that a speech impairment does not equal inadequate intelligence. Allow the patient the time to respond to your questions, and only utilize the family or other communication techniques (e.g., writing responses or

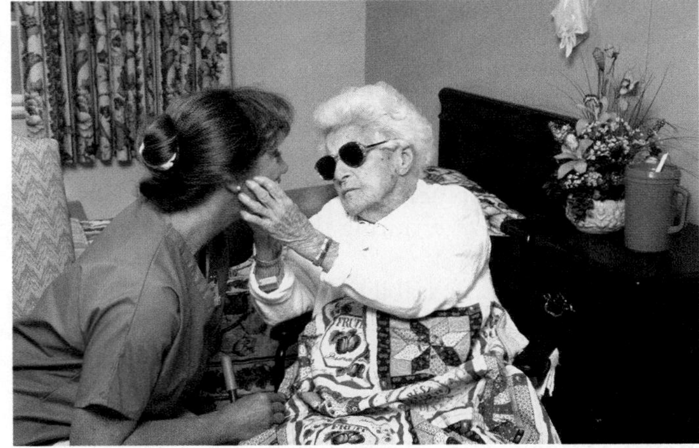

FIGURE 40-1 * For the visually impaired patient, speak clearly and always explain what you are going to do.

Objective 40-5
Describe accommodations and modifications required for patients with cognitive and emotional impairments.

Key Terms
birth defect a variation from normal structure or function that is present at birth.

Key Points
When a patient appears to have some cognitive impairment, family members or caregivers may help by telling you if today's behavior is or is not normal for this patient.

using hand gestures) when verbal communication has failed. Never pretend that you understood something the patient said when in fact you didn't. You may miss an important piece of information that would have an impact on how you treat the patient.

Cognitive and Emotional Impairments

Mental or Emotional Impairments

As discussed in the behavioral emergency chapter, mental and emotional illnesses can present as a unique challenge to the EMT. The impairment that the patient demonstrates may range from being so mild it's almost imperceptible to being significant. For example, a patient with a psychosis in which he struggles with interpreting reality may be incapable of communicating effectively with you. A patient with an extreme emotional dysfunction such as depression or anxiety may be so mentally and emotionally impaired that he is unable to focus on your questions or respond appropriately. For a more detailed discussion of mental and emotional problems and how to deal with them, review Chapter 26, "Behavioral Emergencies."

Developmental Disabilities

Developmental disabilities are conditions that interfere with how a body part or system operates. They typically are present at birth (**birth defects**), although they may not be diagnosed until later in life. Many times the developmental disability involves the brain and causes an inability to learn at a normal rate. The problem may not be noted until the child fails to reach certain developmental milestones. Developmental disabilities can occur as a result of trauma *in utero*, during the birth process, or at any time after birth.

Developmental disabilities may involve the brain, spinal cord, nervous system, and endocrine system. In addition to a negative impact on intelligence and the ability to learn, they may cause problems such as speech impediments, behavioral disorders, language difficulties, and movement disorders. Disabilities that commonly affect the nervous and/or endocrine systems are Down syndrome (Figure 40-2*), fragile X syndrome, autism, fetal alcohol syndrome, phenylketonuria (PKU), hypothyroidism, and Rett syndrome.

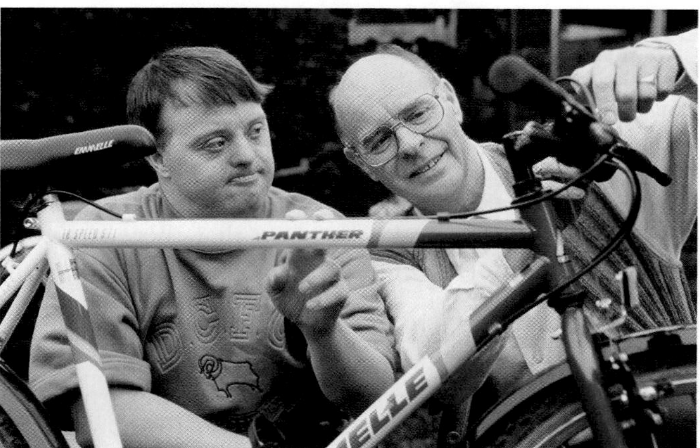

FIGURE 40-2 * Persons with Down syndrome may have numerous disabilities but can participate in normal activities with help from family and friends. (© J.B.S.I./Custom Medical Stock Photography)

Accommodations for Patients with Mental, Emotional, or Developmental Impairments

Treat this patient with respect as you would any other patient. Unless the patient you are caring for is found in some type of medical, specialized residential, or group home, it may be difficult to recognize some of these disorders if the symptoms are mild. If this is the case, then rarely are there significant problems in gathering a history or completing your physical exam. If, however, during your assessment of the patient you start to discern some developmental or cognitive problems, you may need to rely on the patient's primary care provider (family or professional) for your information.

Often, care providers can tell you specifically what is wrong with the patient because of their experience with him (e.g., "He's not laughing like he used to . . ." or "She normally watches TV, but for the last day she's been sleeping all the time and is barely eating"). Use these descriptions as clues to a diminishment in the patient's mental status or other condition when trying to obtain the chief complaint. You may also need to rely on the care

Key Points
Although patients may display significant cognitive or verbal disabilities, they are often sensitive to body language and tone of voice.

Thinking Critically
Your patient has cerebral palsy and impaired speech. Should you assume she is mentally retarded? Why or why not?

provider in obtaining the patient's history and information about any care that has been provided relative to today's emergency.

When caring for a patient with developmental disorders, provide clear explanations to assist the patient in understanding the situation and what is occurring during the emergency care and transport.

ASSESSMENT Tips

Although some impairment may be obvious when you first encounter the patient, others, such as hearing and vision impairments, may not be as readily evident. Always approach the patient as if all sensory abilities are intact, but remain alert for evidence that the patient may have some type of deficit. However, don't assume he will have a deficit just because of his age. ■

Although patients may display significant cognitive or verbal disabilities, they are often sensitive to body language and tone of voice. They can often recognize anger, disrespect, or carelessness as easily as other people, and their response to it may be anger, frustration, or even swinging their fists at the care providers. This will only complicate your assessment and management and may raise your stress level which will, in turn, heighten the patient's.

Keep in mind that many patients with disabilities have been taught to be wary of strangers, and they may become frightened by you, your uniform, your equipment, your cot, and your ambulance. It is important to gain trust with the patient from the outset. Make it clear that you are there to help, and enlist the support of the care provider or another person the patient trusts. These patients may not understand, or even remember, that you are there to help them. Avoid loud noises or extreme changes in lighting when caring for the patient, and consider keeping the primary care provider within eyesight of the patient during transport to the hospital. At the hospital, the primary care provider needs to be nearby in order to answer questions the emergency department staff may have.

Brain-Injured Patients

Previously traumatized patients can be another type of patient with special challenges. Trauma to the brain at any age can result in permanent damage as evidenced by changes in cognition, learning abilities, emotional abilities, and/or use of muscles. Causes can include infant abuse, meningitis, encephalitis, and head injury.

Cerebral palsy is an umbrella term for motor impairments that result from brain abnormalities that arise early in development. Although there are different types and degrees of impairment, most people with cerebral palsy demonstrate difficulties in controlling muscle function and may demonstrate muscular stiffness and joint contractures. You may also see wringing of the hands, and some patients may not be able to swallow normally so they tend to drool. Facial grimacing may be noted as well. Although many people with cerebral palsy have some degree of mental retardation, others are highly intelligent. In some, muscular control difficulties and speech impairments are mild. Many patients with cerebral palsy have difficulties communicating verbally, but these patients have probably developed some mode of communication that their care providers will be aware of.

Understanding BODY PROCESSES

Brain dysfunction from head trauma is a debilitating injury that usually leaves the patient permanently dependent on outsiders for medical care. The dysfunction of the brain from the injury may result in problems in breathing, heart rate, and blood pressure regulation. ■

Brain trauma can easily result in a multitude of residual disabilities. The disability may be mild, such as changes in speech pattern or mild cognitive changes, or may be so severe that the patient is unresponsive to external stimuli and dependent on ventilators for breathing, feeding tubes for nutrition, and care providers for day-to-day washing, turning, and bedding changes. Most patients with previous head injury lie somewhere between those two extremes.

Accommodations for Brain-Injured Patients

Beyond their current chief complaint, patients with a history of brain trauma will display abnormalities based on the site of injury. The presenting signs and symptoms you note must be categorized as either a "chronic" finding (a residual effect of the trauma) or an "acute" finding (a recent change to a body system that is in need of diagnosis).

Key Terms
paraplegic paralized from the waist down.

Thinking Critically
Your paralyzed patient is totally reliant on her wheelchair but rules forbid transporting a wheelchair in the ambulance. How would you handle this situation?

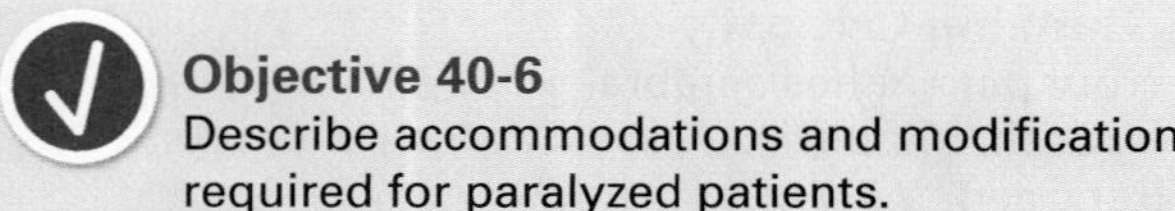
Objective 40-6
Describe accommodations and modifications required for paralyzed patients.

Gathering a history in these patients will reveal the type of injury sustained earlier and will help identify the changes in the patient's current condition as either chronic or acute. You should also be methodical when completing your primary and secondary physical assessments.

Brain injury patients may use a large amount of medical technology in order to survive (e.g., pumps, ventilators, catheters), and the EMT must be aware of and manage this equipment during patient transfer. Because of their reliance on medical equipment in the severest of brain injuries, these patients are more likely to develop upper respiratory infections or even pneumonia, to have infected sites where tubes or lines are inserted into the body, to experience problems with nutrition regulation, and to develop bed sores at pressure points of the body.

The care you render for this patient will depend on the condition(s) for which you were summoned. Above all, remember to maintain a patent airway, ensure adequate breathing, and keep peripheral perfusion intact. Consider summoning ALS for a patient who is critically unstable or deteriorating.

ASSESSMENT Tips

Patients with pre-existing brain trauma may range anywhere from being awake and oriented, to confused, to combative, to unresponsive. It is important to accurately determine their baseline mental state and whether their current status is normal for them. ■

Paralysis

It is not uncommon for EMS, summoned to the scene of an accident, to find a patient who has sustained an injury that has resulted in paralysis, or the complete loss of muscle function to one or more groups of muscles. Similarly, it's not uncommon when summoned to a medical emergency to find a patient experiencing a stroke who has paralysis to one side of his body. What may be uncommon, however, is being summoned to a patient complaining of respiratory distress or chest pain to find that this patient is also paralyzed from some previous traumatic event or medical condition. In this situation, you will have to make necessary accommodations for the patient's pre-existing paralysis while concurrently treating him for the complaint that occasioned the call to EMS.

Understanding BODY PROCESSES

A patient who is paralyzed or has significant muscular weakness will be unable to perform many activities of daily living and will be dependent on others to provide care. In addition, ongoing muscle weakness and paralysis may lead to breathing inadequacy and reliance on a mechanical ventilator. ■

Patients who are paralyzed are susceptible to multiple additional problems. For example, if the paralysis involves the respiratory muscles, the patient may be ventilator dependent. Such patients have frequent respiratory infections because of their inability to cough and clear inhaled debris from their airway. They may also be susceptible to urinary tract infections. (Totally paralyzed patients are routinely catheterized.) Because many of these patients are bedridden and unable to turn themselves from side to side, they may develop pressure necrosis (bed sores) over bony areas of the body. If there is a feeding tube inserted (as will be discussed later), the insertion site may become infected or the tube may become occluded. Secondary emergencies from feeding tube problems can include blood sepsis, dyspnea, chest pain, open soft tissue deterioration, and a myriad of other problems.

Accommodations for Paralyzed Patients

Accommodations that need to be made for a paralyzed patient will depend on the degree of paralysis. If just one extremity is paralyzed from some pre-existing event, chances are the patient will still be able to lead a nearly normal life, so there would be nothing too unusual that the EMT would have to manage. If a patient is **paraplegic**, he will display paralysis from the waist down. He may be found in a wheelchair, and so long as there is no cognitive decline, he should be able to communicate with you normally. Your assessment and management will be almost identical to that for any other patient; the only real concern is moving the patient from his bed or wheelchair onto your cot. Many paralyzed patients will want you to take their wheelchair to the hospital. This is often not allowed by the EMS agency because ambulances do not have the mounting hardware needed to properly secure the wheelchair in case of a sudden stop or ambulance crash. Coordinate with the family or primary care pro-

Key Terms
quadriplegic paralyzed from the neck down.

Key Points
Always look to see if the paralyzed patient has a urinary catheter in place before you move him.

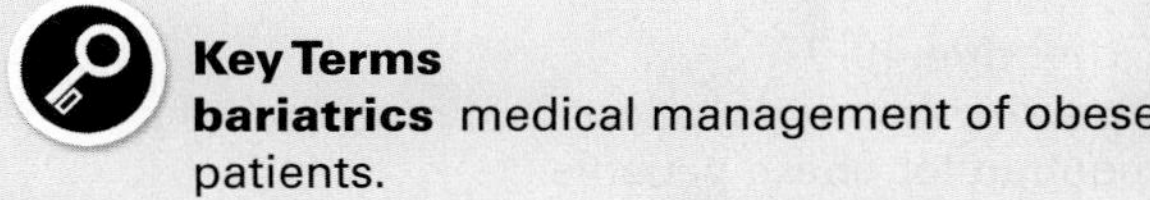

vider to ensure assisting devices the patient relies on (e.g., wheelchairs, canes) are taken to the hospital by someone else (Figure 40-3*).

If a patient is paralyzed to all four extremities, he is said to be **quadriplegic**. If the patient with quadriplegia has had a spinal injury in the vicinity of C3–C5, or if he is suffering from a neuromuscular disease, he may be unable to breathe adequately on his own. In this case, the patient will be ventilator dependent and will likely have an airway tube placed into the trachea near the base of the neck anteriorly. When you are dealing with a home ventilator, keep the settings the same as they were when you arrived. Keep suction nearby in case the breathing tube that the ventilator is attached to becomes occluded. (There will be more information on dealing with ventilators and stomas later in the chapter.) Keep a bag-valve unit nearby as well in case a problem occurs with the home ventilator.

Always look to see if the patient has a urinary catheter in place before you move the patient. You do not want to accidentally pull the catheter out of the urethra during patient movement. Never place the urinary collection bag at a level above the insertion site or at the same level as the insertion. Doing so may cause urine to flow back into the patient or may inhibit drainage from the urinary bladder, increasing the risk of urinary tract infection. Ensure that any feeding tubes or colostomy bags (to be discussed later) are properly secured.

Remain alert to the patient's needs and to the medical equipment used to keep the patient alive. Be careful

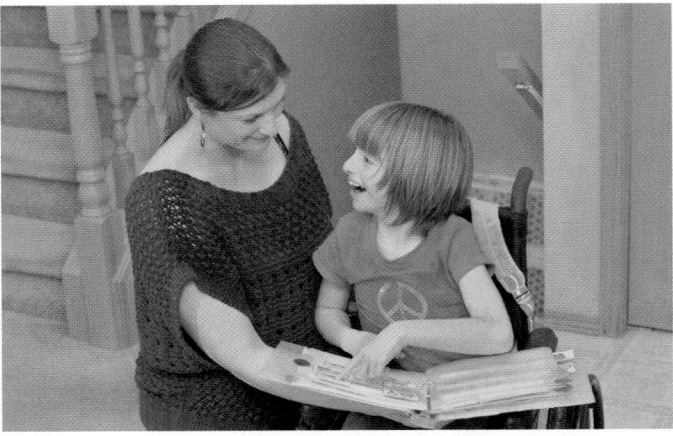

FIGURE 40-3 * Patients with paralysis or muscle weakness may want you to arrange for transport of their assisting devices, such as wheelchairs or canes, to the hospital.

while moving the patient to ensure that no care or medical equipment is accidentally disabled. Many times, the family members or primary care providers can offer suggestions about how to best move the patient, given all this technology. If they offer a suggestion, it is usually wise to heed it.

There is a lot to take care of with paralyzed patients. Do not allow these necessary tasks to distract you from the fact that you were probably called for some other emergency that you must concurrently attend to.

Obesity

Bariatrics is the branch of medicine that deals with the management of obese patients. There is much concern about obesity in the United States. In fact, escalating rates of adult and childhood obesity are one of the nation's leading health problems. According to the Centers for Disease Control, in 2009 approximately one-third of adult Americans were obese, while nearly 70 percent of adults were either obese or overweight. A person who weighs any amount over his ideal weight is considered to be overweight. Traditionally, a person who is 20 percent or more over his ideal weight is considered to be obese. Some obese patients are considered to be morbidly obese. Morbid obesity has multiple definitions. Commonly accepted definitions are that a morbidly obese person weighs 50 to 100 percent more than his ideal weight or is more than 100 pounds over his ideal weight.

Obesity is the second leading cause of preventable death today, second only to smoking. More than $80 billion in public and private health care money is spent each year to combat obesity and its associated disease states. Of great concern is the increase of obesity in children and the consequent multiple risk factors for additional disease over their lifetime. Obesity is associated with coronary heart disease, type 2 diabetes, immobility, sleep apnea, and hypertension, all of which can reduce the life span if no corrective measures are taken (Table 40-1).

Understanding BODY PROCESSES

Obesity places great demands on the body's systems. Over time, this heightened demand can lead to serious medical conditions such as high blood pressure, sleep apnea, diabetes, and cardiovascular disease.

Objective 40-7
Describe accommodations and modifications required for obese patients.

Key Points
When an obese patient is placed in a supine position, excess adipose tissue can exert pressure on airway structures and may even totally occlude the airway.

TABLE 40-1 Effects of Excess Weight on Body Systems

System	Disease State
Cardiovascular	Hypertension, coronary artery disease, congestive heart failure, stroke
Respiratory	Obstructive sleep apnea, asthma, chronic obstructive pulmonary disease
Endocrine and reproductive	Diabetes mellitus, infertility, birth defects, menstrual disorders
Gastrointestinal	Esophageal reflux, liver disease
Musculoskeletal	Osteoarthritis, gout, back injuries, immobility
Psychological	Depression, suicide

As rates of overweight, obesity, and morbid obesity continue to climb, EMS crews are encountering these patients more often. It is likely that you will be treating one or more patients within your community who weigh in excess of 500 pounds.

Obesity can occur for a number of reasons. While the short explanation is that the patient is consuming more calories than he is burning (i.e., overeating with a sedentary lifestyle), obesity can also be caused by physiological problems. For example, a patient with hypothyroidism may have a lowered metabolic rate, which means he burns calories more slowly. Some medications, such as CNS depressants and anticonvulsant medications, can lower the metabolic rate and contribute to weight gain. Genetic factors have been cited as contributing to obesity in certain people. It has also been noted that obese people tend to form relationships with each other, and their children are often obese as well, whether from genetics, predisposition, or lifestyle.

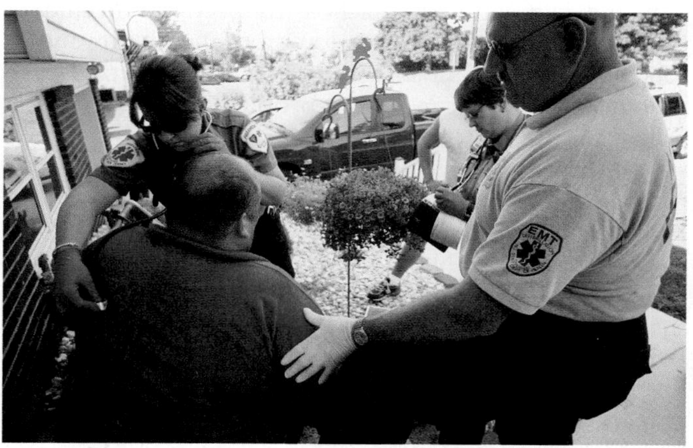

FIGURE 40-4 * Assessment and care of the obese patient follows a normal format, but modifications may be required because of the patient's size. (© Mark C. Ide)

Accommodations for Obese Patients

When an emergency occurs, assessment of the obese patient follows a normal assessment format, but modifications may be needed because of the patient's size (Figure 40-4*). Often, obese patients have "extra" skin and adipose tissue around the face, chin, and neck, and on the posterior surface of the upper thorax. When the patient is standing or sitting upright, the extra tissue usually doesn't interfere with normal respiratory function; however, when placed in a supine position, problems can develop. Extra adipose tissue in the cheeks, lower jaw, and anterior neck places pressure on the tongue and airway structures, causing closure. Airway complications may arise from the "fat pad" or "buffalo hump" sometimes seen between the patient's shoulder blades that further inhibits airway patency.

Airway occlusion can be prevented by proper positioning of the patient. If the patient is conscious, allow him to assume a position of comfort—usually sitting upright or in a slightly reclined position. If the patient is unable to protect his own airway, ensure that the airway is maintained in a neutral position to allow airflow. A technique that is often overlooked is positioning the obese patient with multiple towels or bath blankets under the shoulder blades and behind the neck (if no cervical injury is suspected) to provide cervical extension. To displace the tongue mechanically, use an oral or nasal pharyngeal airway. Remember that the oral airway can stimulate vomiting in a patient with an intact gag reflex. In that case, use a nasal pharyngeal airway. You may need to per-

Thinking Critically
Placing an obese patient supine or lower than a semi-Fowler position may impact how well the patient can breathe. Why? Other than positioning the patient correctly, how and why should this fact affect your management of the patient?

Objective 40-8
Describe accommodations and modifications required for homeless or poor patients.

form a modified jaw thrust to move the jaw and tongue forward and prevent a partial airway obstruction.

Once the airway is ensured, turn your attention to oxygenating and ventilating the patient. Spontaneous breathing in this patient may be impaired by his body size when he is in a semireclined or supine position. In these positions, the posterior thoracic wall has limited mobility and the anterior thoracic wall is weighed down by the patient's own adipose tissue. Rapid fatigue of the respiratory muscles may occur. In an attempt to compensate for decreased respiratory effort, the patient's respiratory rate may be elevated, but with tachypnea comes hypopnea (shallow breathing). You must *always* remember that a breathing patient does not necessarily equal an adequately breathing patient. Along with the rate of ventilation, you must be astute in assessing the depth of ventilation. If the patient needs ventilatory assistance or requires mechanical ventilation, the patient's size must be taken into account. It is significantly more difficult to ventilate a patient weighing 380 lb than a patient weighing 180 lb.

ASSESSMENT Tips

How the obese patient is positioned on the cot for transport may have a significant impact on how well he can breathe. Try to keep the patient upright or lowered to no more than a semi-Fowler position, and diligently monitor the airway and breathing status. ■

After the airway is secured and oxygenation and ventilation have been established, a rapid circulatory assessment can be performed. One of the first signs of inadequate circulation and perfusion is a change in mentation. Alterations in heart rate (tachycardia or bradycardia) and blood pressure (hypotension or hypertension) can influence the patient's mental status. Treat these abnormalities in accord with your protocol.

The extra weight is problematic when it comes to lifting and moving the obese patient. Beyond enlisting the help of additional personnel to move the patient to the portable cot (one of the greatest injuries to health care providers everywhere is back injuries from lifting), the patient's weight may exceed the structural limitation of the cot. Cot manufacturers now design "bariatric devices," which include special cots (able to hold greater weight) and bariatric loading devices such as special ramps and winches that interface with specially designed ambulance cot-locking systems (Figure 40-5*).

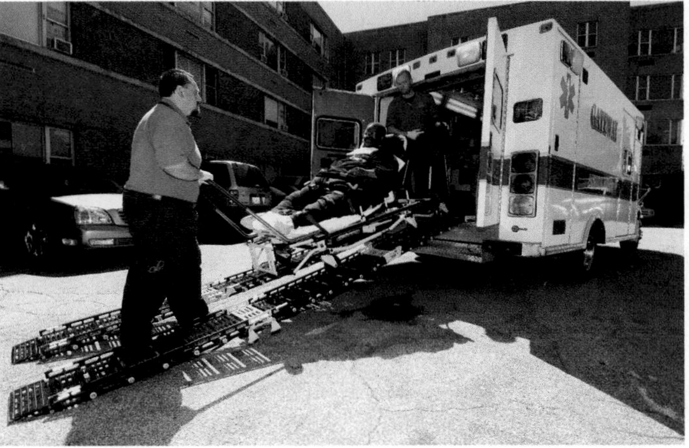

FIGURE 40-5 * Bariatric devices include special cots designed to support the greater weight of an obese patient and loading devices such as ramps and winches that interface with specially designed ambulance cot-locking systems. (© Ray Kemp/911 Imaging)

During transport, continue assessment and management according to the patient's needs. When you notify the receiving facility about this patient, let them know that they will need to prepare their special stretcher and that help may be needed for patient off-loading.

Homelessness and Poverty

During a "single point" assessment that was made in January of 2007, the U.S. Department of Housing and Urban Development (HUD) reported that there were almost 700,000 people in the United States that met the definition for homelessness. Worldwide, this number is estimated to exceed 100 million people. HUD defines chronically homeless as "an unaccompanied homeless individual with a disabling condition who has either been continuously homeless for a year or more, or has had at least four episodes of homelessness in the past three years."

Several factors contribute to a person becoming homeless, or as said in legal circumstances, having "no fixed abode" (NFA). These factors include:

- Poverty (from unemployment or underemployment)
- Substance abuse

- Lack of affordable housing
- Mental illness
- Prison release back into society
- Domestic violence
- Mortgage foreclosures and forced evictions
- Natural disaster

Homeless people, because they do not have a safe and suitable home, typically face social disadvantages and reduced access to services provided by both public and private entities. In fact, services that could be available to them may be denied because they cannot document their date of birth or address. Because of the inability to protect their personal items, documents like identification and birth certificates are lost, stolen, or destroyed. Trying to obtain replacements is difficult because either they lack the money for required replacement fees or they don't have an address for the documents to be mailed to.

Many times, a homeless person is so focused on surviving day to day that he is unable to devote time or resources to activities that would help get him off the streets. The following are examples of disadvantages and reduced access to services that homeless people must endure:

- Increased risk of violence and abuse
- Increased risk of illness/disease
- Discrimination from others (perception that they are "crazy" or "lazy")
- Reduced access to health care
- Limited or no access to education
- Limited or no access to modern communications (telephone, Internet)
- Not seen as suitable for employment purposes

Because of the lack of a permanent residence or place for storage of their possessions, the homeless have to cart their belongings with them from place to place, for example in bags or shopping carts. When an emergency arises, there is no "address" for you to respond to. Often you'll be summoned to street corners, alleys, or phone booths when an emergency involves a homeless person (Figure 40-6*). The following are types of locations where homeless people may find refuge:

- Abandoned or condemned buildings
- Public places such as parks, train or bus stations, airports, college campuses
- Vehicles (their own or abandoned)
- Outdoors in improvised shacks or on the ground with sleeping bags
- In an unoccupied house (without the owner's knowledge or permission)
- Homeless shelters (usually sponsored by churches or community agencies)

Because of their exposure to the environment and lack of preventive care or any medical care when minor injuries or illnesses arise, the homeless person is at risk for even greater emergencies. Ongoing conditions such as poor nutrition, environmental exposure (heat and cold extremes, rain or snow), lack of access to medication, and vulnerability to violent acts leave them at risk for cardiac, pulmonary, vascular, and traumatic emergencies.

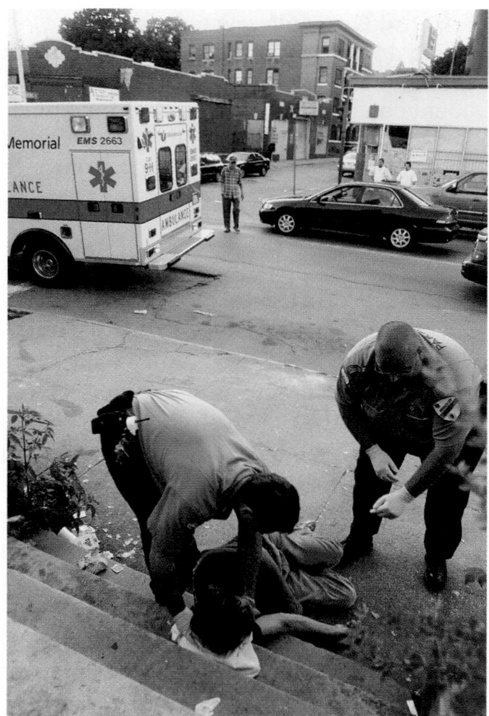

FIGURE 40-6 * EMS is often summoned to street corners and other public places to care for a homeless patient. (© Mark C. Ide)

Most of the time homelessness and poverty go hand in hand. Many of the concerns for homeless patients hold true for impoverished patients and vice versa. Presently in the United States, there are 36.5 million people (about 1 in 8 Americans) who fall below the official poverty threshold. Almost 10 percent of the people below the poverty level are older than 65. Also, a family that is above the poverty level does not necessarily have the financial resources to take care of all their household needs (e.g., food, medical bills, clothing, rent, or mortgage payments).

Like the homeless, people who fall below the poverty level are at greater risk for illness and injury, partly from their environment and partly from the lack of primary medical care, screening, and treatment needed to prevent the advanced development of disease (Figure 40-7*). For example, you may be caring for a patient with respiratory distress who claims he has never had a pulmonary problem; in fact, however, he may never have been screened for chronic obstructive pulmonary disease (COPD) because of a lack of normal medical care. The first time this patient presents to you with dyspnea may well be his first indication of deterioration since developing the disease. While you should always listen to what the patient tells you, do not disregard physical assessment findings that tell you a different story. Patients who live at or near the

Key Points
Some patients will resist transport because they cannot afford the ambulance or hospital fee. Be familiar with services in your community that can provide medical or financial aid to those who need it and know how to recommend or to help put patients in touch with such services.

Objective 40-9
Describe accommodations and modifications required for abused patients.

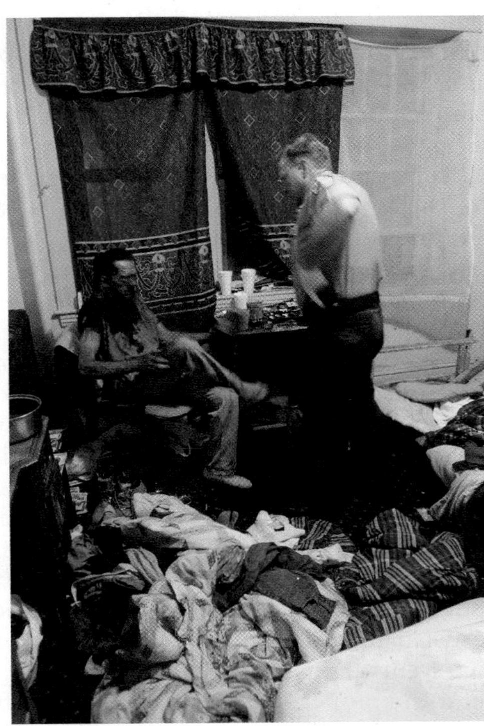

FIGURE 40-7 ✻ People who fall below the poverty level are at great risk for illness and injury from the environment they are in and the lack of resources to seek primary medical care. (© Mark C. Ide)

poverty level are more likely to be subject to accidental trauma, physical abuse, or crimes and to develop chronic medical conditions (e.g., heart disease, lung disease, hypertension, diabetes) and yet have limited access to health care. All too often, impoverished people have to choose between buying medications for themselves and buying food for the family or paying the heating bill.

Accommodations for Patients Who Are Homeless or Poor

The health of a person living in the United States is strongly correlated with the income of that person (or family). The poor or homeless are less healthy than those who are financially better off. Regardless of how you measure it—by mortality, the incidence of diseases, or the frequency of mental health issues—people lower on the economic ladder suffer from higher rates of illness and death.

Statistics show that over 90 percent of Americans will, at some time, live below the poverty level for at least a year and will face the challenges just discussed. In making special accommodations for these patients, perhaps one of the best things you can do is *not* be judgmental. Homeless and impoverished people are well aware of their surroundings and their lack of monetary resources. They do not need someone telling them that they "need a job" or "could have prevented this." The patient has summoned EMS because he is in a situation that he cannot handle on his own, and he should be treated with the same respect and compassion as any patient who may have access to more services. You are as much an advocate for this patient and his needs as you are a skilled provider delivering emergency care. Remember, you're treating the patient *because he needs your help*, not because he has a bank account.

In the absence of a specific mental, emotional, or physical disability (such as those already discussed in this chapter, all of which are more prevalent in this patient category), your assessment and management of the patient will not vary much from that provided to other patients with similar complaints. One concern you may hear from the patient is that he does not have the money to pay for the ambulance or hospital bill. In this situation, explain to the patient that almost all heath care providers offer a certain degree of reduced cost or free medical care. Become familiar with hospitals and services in your community that provide medical care, shelter, food, or other services to families (or individuals) in need.

ASSESSMENT Tips

If you spend any amount of time in EMS, you will undoubtedly encounter homeless people. Your duty to assess and care for these patients is the same as for patients who are not as disadvantaged. ■

▶ Abuse

Abuse and neglect have many definitions and can present in numerous ways, but consistent features include any action or failure to act that results in unreasonable suffering, harm, or misery to a person, whether physical or mental. Although commonly thought of as affecting children or the economically disadvantaged, abuse transcends all age, gender, race, and socioeconomic groups. In addition to child abuse, common categories include elder abuse and partner abuse.

The actual incidence of abuse is hard to estimate because it is greatly underreported. Many times, especially when the abused person lives with the abuser, the victim is unable to report the situation to the authorities because of physical or mental conditions that prohibit a call for help. The abused person may be dependent on the person perpetrating the abuse and may feel unable to survive independently or may feel that there will be repercussions if a call for help is made. The abused person may also believe that the abuser will stop the abuse, which abusers commonly promise.

Despite these obstacles, some numbers do exist to help describe the magnitude of this problem. Consider the following:

- Over 3 million children annually are found to be victims of abuse, most commonly from their parents.
- Adult Protective Services (APS) nationwide, as reported by the National Center for Elder Abuse, indicated there were over 560,000 reports of elder abuse in a 2006 study.
- Between 3 and 4 million people annually, primarily women, are victims of spouse or partner abuse.

The factors that contribute to the underreporting of abuse also contribute to delays in actually receiving help. Often the victim of abuse will report it only as a desperate act after years of silence. All too often, EMS will be the first to the victim of abuse. Although it is not the EMT's role to confront the abuser in the absence of police being on scene, it *is* your responsibility to make notifications of any suspicion of abuse to the proper authorities according to your state's guidelines.

Child Abuse

Child abuse occurs when a child (from newborn to 18 years of age in most states) falls victim to abuse or neglect. Child abuse is the only major cause of infant and child death to increase in the last 30 years. The abuser is not necessarily the parent; it can be a babysitter, foster parent, sibling, stepsibling, stepparent, or anyone else that is responsible for the child's care. Child abuse could range from actual physical and emotional harm to the neglect of the body's basic needs. Generally speaking, child abuse falls into three categories: physical abuse (which can include neglect), emotional abuse, and sexual abuse (Figure 40-8*).

Physical abuse occurs when improper or excessive action is taken so as to injure or cause harm. Neglect is the provision of inadequate attention or respect to someone who has a claim to that attention. Emotional abuse, according to the American Medical Association (AMA), occurs when "a child is regularly threatened, yelled at, humiliated, ignored, blamed or otherwise emotionally mistreated." This type of abuse could be manifested as making fun of the child, constantly finding fault with the child, or even name calling. The result is often serious behavioral, cognitive, emotional, or mental disorders that plague the child for the rest of his life. Emotional abuse is often the most difficult to prove because of the lack of outward physical signs. Sexual abuse is said to occur when a child is subject to an older child or adult's advances that have a sexual nature. It can include both contact and noncontact events. Exposing oneself to a child, pressuring a child for improper body contact, or outright genital contact all are considered to be sexual abuse. Most

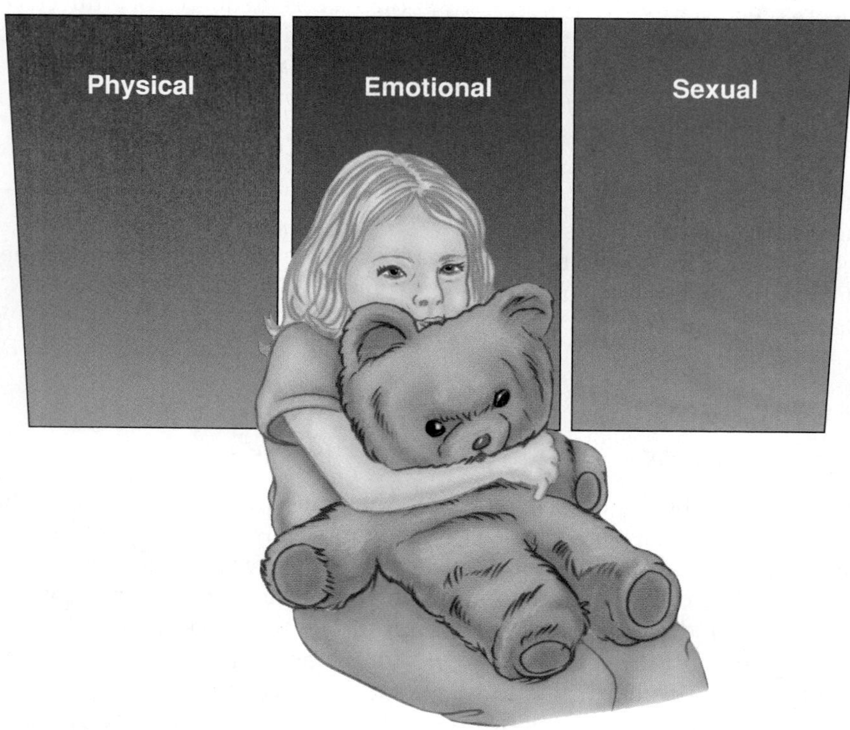

FIGURE 40-8 * Child abuse comes in many forms.

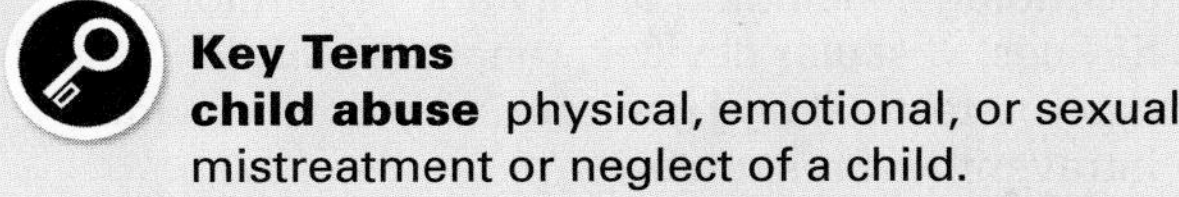

Key Terms
child abuse physical, emotional, or sexual mistreatment or neglect of a child.

Key Terms
elder abuse neglect or physical, sexual, financial, or emotional/mental mistreatment of an elderly person.

abusers know the child they abuse and many are related to the child.

The adult (usually a caregiver) who abuses a child often behaves in an evasive manner, volunteering little information or giving contradictory information about what has happened to the child. The caregiver may show outright hostility toward the child or toward another caregiver in the household and rarely evidences any guilt. The abused child will usually show fear when asked to describe how the injury occurred. In situations of emotional abuse, the EMT may note the child has improper coping or socialization skills for his age or for the situation. Chapter 38, "Pediatrics," has more information regarding this topic.

Elder Abuse

Elder abuse may occur in care centers and other medical institutions, but it also happens at home. Any elderly person is especially at risk if he is cared for by someone who is under stress from other sources. Abuse of the elderly can occur in many forms similar to pediatric abuse, and includes neglect, physical abuse, sexual abuse, financial abuse, or emotional/mental abuse. At highest risk are those elderly who are bedridden, demented, incontinent, or frail, or who have disturbed sleep patterns. The most common type of elder abuse is to elderly females who live with a son.

Geriatric neglect is similar to pediatric neglect. It is the withholding of attention or medical care by a care provider that the victim is entitled to. This type of neglect could occur passively or actively, the difference being the intent of the care provider. In situations of active neglect, there is an intentional failure of the care provider to meet his obligations to the elderly victim. With passive neglect, the failure is said to occur unintentionally and is often the result of the care provider feeling overwhelmed by the needed tasks or that the care provider simply does not know or understand the care or interventions that the patient needs. Regardless of reason, this type of neglect could be manifested as failing to provide adequate nutrition or hydration, failing to provide medications or accessing medical services when warranted, failing to care for personal hygiene, or even the development of bed sores because the care provider does not turn the patient as needed to prevent the breakdown and deterioration of the skin.

Physical abuse can involve hitting, unnecessary restraining, shaking, or shoving an elderly patient. Because of the elderly person's frailty, the injuries incurred from these attacks can be significant (Figure 40-9*). Sexual abuse is said to occur when there are unwanted or unwarranted advances of a sexual nature (either through body contact or exposure) that the older person does not consent to or is incapable of giving consent to. The EMT may note signs of soft tissue trauma around or near the genital region in situations of sexual abuse. Financial abuse consists of the care provider exploiting the material possessions, property, credit, or monetary assets of the elderly patient for personal gain. With emotional or mental abuse, there is an infliction of psychological distress or mental harm to the elderly patient through verbal assaults, verbal insults, ignoring the elderly patient, or threats of physical harm. Chapter 39, "Geriatrics," contains additional information on this subject.

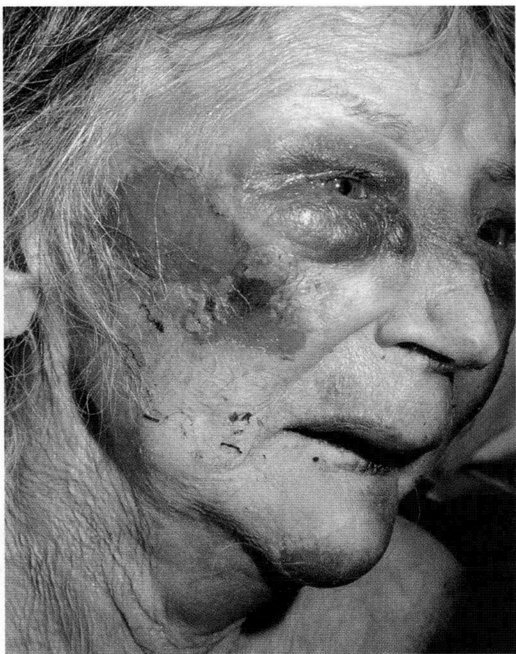

FIGURE 40-9 * Physical abuse of an elderly person can have dire consequences because of the patient's frailty.

ASSESSMENT Tips

Many indications, both physical and emotional, that the EMT will encounter can point to abuse. Your primary role is to provide assessment and care for the patient. Do not try to investigate the suspicion of abuse or attempt to confront the alleged abuser. However, do report your findings to the medical staff and provide thorough and objective documentation in your prehospital care report. ■

Objective 40-10

Describe accommodations and modifications required for patients who are dependent on technology, including airway and respiratory devices, vascular devices, renal dialysis, gastrointestinal and genitourinary devices, and intraventricular shunts.

Key Points

Do not confront family members or care providers if you suspect abuse. Treat the patient's injuries and report your suspicions to the hospital staff or according to your local protocols.

Accommodations for Victims of Abuse

Detecting either pediatric or elder abuse can be challenging. Sorting out what could have been an accident rather than a purposeful action (i.e., abuse) may be difficult. The EMT can't automatically assume that a fall was accidental just because elderly patients fall a lot. Similarly, the EMT can't assume that soft tissue trauma to a child's face is accidental just because children are more active outdoors or more likely to have a fight at school. Although EMTs should assume that the findings of trauma are "innocent" initially, they cannot ignore the fact that pediatric and geriatric abuse occurs daily. The EMT should always hope for the best, but be prepared for the worst with these age populations.

Signs of abuse to either pediatrics or geriatrics can be physical: bruises, bite marks, bleeding beneath the scalp (indicative of hair-pulling), lacerations on the face, trauma to the ears, broken bones, deformities of the chest, cigarette burns, rope marks, genital trauma, or scalding burns. The signs can be emotional: depression, fear, improper or inadequate coping strategies, or even an inappropriate mental status for the patient's age or physical condition. If you suspect any type of abuse, pay particular attention to inconsistencies when you get a history from the patient and from the provider or family. In children, consider developmental capabilities when obtaining a history. For example, it would be difficult to believe that a 6-month-old pulled scalding water onto himself.

Your priority is to provide emergency care for the injuries. The treatment of soft tissue injuries, burns, or musculoskeletal injuries should follow the same assessment and treatment guidelines as discussed elsewhere in this text. Remember to place great emphasis on the airway and respiratory components with pediatric patients. With geriatric patients, remember that any kind of trauma is usually worse in this patient population because of their frail bodies and poor-to-depressed compensatory mechanisms. The geriatric patient may rapidly deteriorate from a physical insult caused by the abuse. For victims of emotional abuse, always use a safe and reassuring tone in your voice and through your actions. The abused patient is not likely to trust someone coming from the outside, so the EMT's "people skills" are especially important here.

Do not confront the family or care provider with your suspicion of abuse. Instead, if you suspect either pediatric or elder abuse, you should make your suspicion known to the receiving hospital's staff so that they can follow up with the appropriate authorities. Also ensure, in your documentation for a suspected victim of abuse, that you remain absolutely objective in describing your findings. Do not document that you believe the patient is being abused; rather describe the patient's environmental conditions, family, and physical findings exactly as they are. If the conditions are such that you suspect abuse, chances are your documentation will reflect the same and provide other health care providers with the documentation they need to investigate your suspicions further. Your documentation will likely be very closely scrutinized by many agencies and individuals if abuse is suspected. Follow local protocols or state laws regarding reporting of suspected abuse. Your ability as an EMT to recognize the findings of abuse and to initiate the appropriate medical/legal response will provide a healing for the patient that will go far beyond the care you provided for any injuries the patient sustained that day.

Technology Dependence

There was a time when the patient would remain hospitalized to receive ongoing treatment until the injury/illness that he was suffering from had been treated to the greatest extent possible. The result was prolonged hospital stays with the expenditure of significant health care dollars.

This practice began to change in the latter half of the twentieth century because of governmental and insurance initiatives designed to curb rising health care costs. Concurrently, there has been the development of medications and medical technology designed to help sustain life in the home setting. Consequently, there has been a shifting of patients from an in-hospital setting for ongoing medical care to the home setting. The result has been a dramatic increase in the number of health care providers who function outside the hospital, usually in the patient's home, as well as a large increase in the use of medical technology in the home setting for patients who rely on it for survival. Studies indicate that over 8 million people in the United States receive some type of professional health care at home, with millions of other patients receiving ongoing care from family members, friends, or other volunteers.

While some medical equipment is designed to enhance the quality of life and allow patient independence (e.g., feeding tubes or urinary catheters), some medical equipment found in the home setting actually sustains life (e.g., mechanical ventilators). You must remain abreast of trends in home-based medical technology. It is now common for the EMT to be summoned to the home of a patient where the medical equipment has failed, or where the patient's clinical status has changed to the point where the medical equipment can no longer provide the needed support, or where the patient who is dependent on the medical equipment has suffered some other emergency that exceeds the primary care provider's ability to manage the situation. You must be able to determine what the medical device is supposed to be doing for the patient, how critical its function is to patient survival, and what type of impact the device has, if any, on other medical or traumatic emergencies the patient may suffer. Often you will need to depend on the primary health care providers for information about the equipment the patient is reliant on prior to initiating any care (Figure 40-10*).

For the discussion in this chapter, we categorize the most common medical equipment as airway and respiratory devices, vascular access devices, dialysis shunts, gastrourinary support devices, and intraventricular shunts. It is impossible to cover all types and makes of medical technology used in the home, so as you approach the technology-dependent patient you should ask yourself the following questions to help determine the best course of action for ongoing assessment and care:

1. *Where would I get the best information regarding this piece of equipment?*
2. *What does this device do for the patient?*
3. *Can I replicate its function should the device fail?*
4. *Will this equipment have an effect on how I assess the patient, or on the findings I may discover?*
5. *Has this problem ever occurred previously, and if so, what fixed it?*
6. *Has anyone attempted to remediate the problem?*
7. *Are there specific considerations I need to make when deciding how to best prepare the patient for movement and transport the patient?*

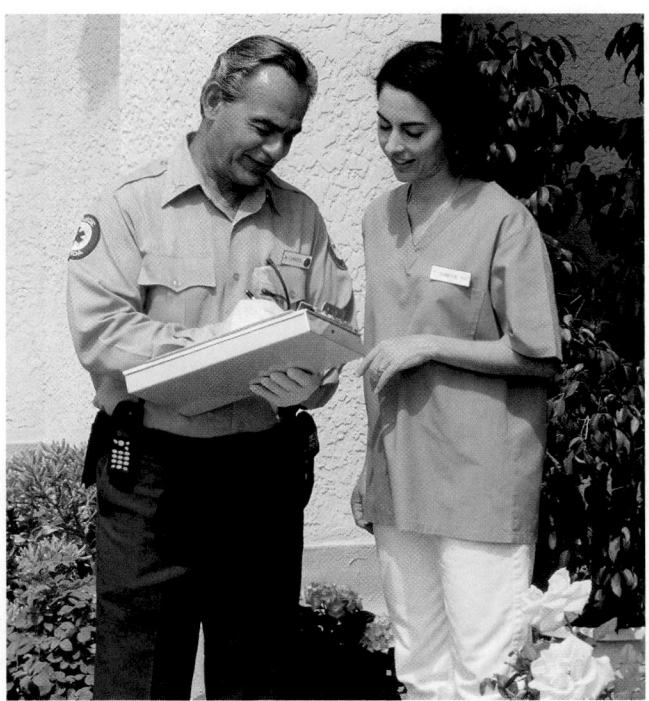

FIGURE 40-10 * The patient's primary health care provider can usually provide information about the equipment the patient relies on.

Although much of the equipment you will see in patients' homes is similar to what you would see in a hospital setting, there is usually a difference in the size and the complexity of the device. Try not to become overwhelmed with the medical equipment, but realize that since the patient is dependent on this equipment, his clinical status is probably already diminished and he may decompensate faster than other patients. Constantly assess the patient and be prepared to intervene should deterioration occur. In emergencies, keep your approach to the patient simple, focusing on the following tasks:

- Keep the airway open and patent.
- Ensure good ventilations with supplemental oxygen.
- Intervene as needed to support any lost function to the circulatory system.

If, at a minimum, you provide this care, you will ensure the patient the best chance for survival regardless of the immediate emergency and the patient's dependence on medical technology.

Airway and Respiratory Devices

These are devices that support the most vital of body functions: airway, ventilation, and oxygenation. Equipment that will be discussed relates to use of medical oxygen in the home, apnea monitors, pulse oximetry, tracheostomy tubes, and respiratory devices (continuous positive airway pressure and mechanical ventilators).

Medical Oxygen

The use of **medical oxygen** has been increasing over the past several decades with the advent of better portable devices for oxygen delivery as well as better diagnostic procedures for determining its need. The use of oxygen in the home significantly increases the quality of life and life span of those who need it. Oxygen use in the home is easy to manage, with most problems able to be corrected by the patients themselves.

Home oxygen equipment is similar to the oxygen equipment you would use on the ambulance. For example, there is an oxygen source (compressed liquid or an oxygen concentrator machine), a flow regulator, oxygen

Key Terms
medical oxygen oxygen administered as a medication or to support or enhance a patient's oxygenation.

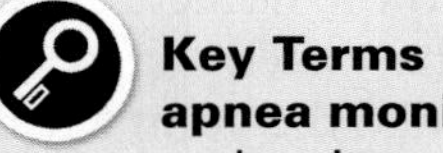

Key Terms
apnea monitor device that monitors breathing and emits a warning signal if breathing stops.

supply tubing attached to the oxygenation adjunct such as a nasal cannula, and an in-line system for humidifying the oxygen. It is often easy to determine if the patient is on oxygen at home because you will see a sign indicating oxygen use as you approach the front door or the patient's bedroom, or you will see the oxygen supply tubing extending from the oxygen source to the patient.

While the EMT uses oxygen that is compressed in a tank, oxygen may be provided somewhat differently in the home setting. Three sources of oxygen for patients at home are:

- **Oxygen cylinder.** This design is similar to, if not exactly like, what the EMT is already accustomed to. The oxygen is compressed in a tank, just like on the ambulance, and it is adjusted by a flowmeter and administered to the patient via an oxygenation adjunct (for example, a nasal cannula).
- **Oxygen concentrator.** This medical device extracts oxygen from the ambient environment and then supplies it to the patient. Because of the oxygen extraction limits of the machine, the flow commonly delivered is less than 6 lpm.
- **Liquid oxygen.** Liquid oxygen is atmospheric oxygen that has been cooled to –183°C and then stored under pressure in a container (similar in structure to a thermos). In liquid form, it can be stored for long periods, which makes this storage system especially attractive to patients who are chronically dependent on oxygen. (One liter of liquid oxygen will produce 860 liters of gas.) There will usually be a larger liquid oxygen storage unit in the home that is used to refill small portable oxygen containers the patient can carry, allowing mobility not possible with other oxygen sources like a tank or concentrator.

As already noted, few problems arise from the oxygen systems themselves, and if a problem does arise, it is usually remediated by the patient or primary care providers (Table 40-2). Usually the problems that require EMS involve some equipment failure in which the system stops providing oxygen. The EMT can easily correct this situation. Another situation in which EMS may be summoned is if the patient's condition changes or worsens, and the amount of oxygen he is receiving at home for his chronic condition is no longer sufficient. (For example, a patient with COPD may develop pneumonia and start to complain of dyspnea.) In these situations, administer oxygen according to the same protocols as for any other patient with respiratory distress who is in need of oxygen.

Apnea Monitors

An **apnea monitor** is designed to constantly monitor the patient's breathing and emit a warning signal should breathing cease. Some are also designed to monitor heart rate, since changes in the heart rate may signal failure of the respiratory system. This type of equipment is commonly found in the home with an infant, especially a newborn infant who was born prematurely. These devices emit a loud piercing sound to signal a problem, and often emit a series of beeps indicating how long the machine has been alerting should the care providers be out of hearing range when the signal starts. For example, the device may emit one beep as an initial warning, then progress to two beeps as time elapses, and then three beeps, and so on.

TABLE 40-2 Common Technical Problems with Oxygen Systems

Problem	Possible Cause	Corrective Action
Oxygen not flowing freely	Faulty tubing	Check for obstruction or replace tubing.
	Dirty or plugged humidifier	Remove from oxygen supply, clean, and refill with sterile water or replace with prefilled bottle.
Buzzer goes off on oxygen concentrator	Unit unplugged	Check plug.
	Power failure	Check fuses, circuit breaker, or, in cases of power outages, use backup oxygen tank until power is restored. (Or call EMS as necessary to make use of oxygen administration from the ambulance or at the hospital.)
Oxygen tank empties too quickly or hisses	Leak in tank	Open all windows, extinguish all flames, and summon help from the fire department, EMS, and/or supplier.

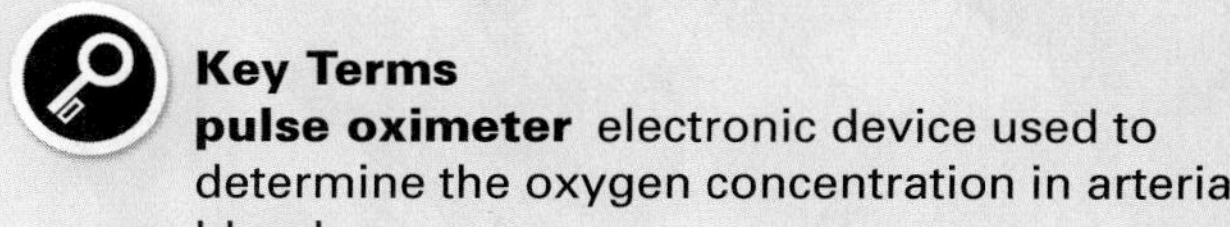

Key Terms
pulse oximeter electronic device used to determine the oxygen concentration in arterial blood.

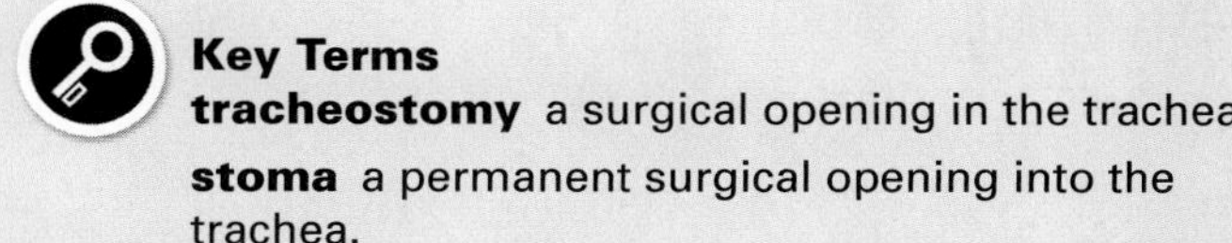

Key Terms
tracheostomy a surgical opening in the trachea.
stoma a permanent surgical opening into the trachea.

Try to ascertain from the primary care provider how long the machine was alerting a problem prior to EMS arrival. Also ascertain what type of interventions the care provider has done prior to your arrival. Commonly the parents or care providers for neonates who need this equipment are taught basic airway and ventilation skills to use in an emergency. Remember to be thoughtful of the care providers. When the parents have an infant with medical problems and an emergency occurs, it can be an extremely frightening experience.

When you are summoned to the home of a patient with this technology, you should perform your normal scene size-up and primary assessment. Since the apnea monitor is designed to signal a respiratory problem, be especially diligent in your assessment of the patient's respiratory rate and tidal volume. Apnea can also be a sign of a very serious infection in an infant. If you find that the patient is breathing adequately, it may be from some intervention provided by the parents, an incorrect alarm triggered by the machine, or the resumption of spontaneous breathing by the infant. In any instance, do not try to "diagnose" what is wrong with the apnea monitor. Instead provide oxygen to the infant and transport him to the hospital for evaluation. If the patient is found to be apneic or breathing inadequately, provide airway control and positive pressure ventilation with supplemental oxygen while you transport the infant to the hospital.

Pulse Oximetry

The **pulse oximeter** is a medical monitoring adjunct that the EMT is already familiar with. It is not only a device that EMTs can use to monitor oxygen saturation in patients, it can also be used as a monitoring device in the home. Often pulse oximetry is done in conjunction with apnea monitoring for newborn infants. Other common reasons for pulse oximetry in the home include the following:

- A patient with chronic pulmonary disease who needs to adjust oxygen intake to maintain a certain level of blood oxygen saturation
- Medical need to keep oxygen saturation within a specific therapeutic range
- Need to monitor oxygen needs in a patient who has a fluctuating oxygen demand (for example, during feeding, sleeping, or movement)

If a patient has continuous pulse oximetry monitoring at home, he is likely to have an acute or chronic pulmonary condition. This is important to note, because pre-existing pulmonary conditions may rapidly deteriorate into respiratory distress or arrest, either from the original disturbance or from failure of some other body system. Often the patient with this type of home technology will have complaints that center around the pulmonary system. Be sure to determine from either the patient or care provider what the oxygen saturation trends were prior to arrival and what interventions, if any, were done (e.g., patient positioning, use of home oxygen). Even if the pulse oximeter the patient is using is portable, you should use your own pulse oximeter in assessing the patient. This will help to ensure that the reading you get is accurate, since your equipment on the ambulance may undergo more rigorous biomedical compliance procedures than a home unit.

Tracheostomy Tubes

A **tracheostomy** is performed when it becomes necessary to open a new airway in patients with certain medical or traumatic conditions. It is a surgical opening made through the neck and into the trachea to provide an alternative route for air to move into and out of the body, bypassing the mouth and nose. The site for this surgical opening is usually the inferior trachea, somewhere near the second through fourth tracheal ring anteriorly. A tracheostomy may be performed as a temporary measure, or it can be a permanent opening. If the opening is to be permanent, it is referred to as a **stoma**.

A tracheostomy is commonly provided for patients who have either long-term upper airway problems or medical conditions that result in long-term dependence on a mechanical ventilation. Patients who have sustained blunt or penetrating trauma to the larynx, epiglottis, or other upper airway structures that result in permanent airway damage may need a tracheostomy. Additionally, tracheotomies are sometimes performed on patients who have cancer of the larynx or neck with resulting long-term structural damage to the original airway structures. Patients with neuromuscular disorders, congenital deformities, coma, spinal cord injuries, or other conditions that affect the ability to breathe usually have a tracheostomy tube that is inserted into the stoma to keep the opening patent.

A tracheostomy tube placed in the stoma of an infant commonly has just a single lumen because of the small size of the trachea. For older children and adults, there is an outer cannula and an inner cannula (Figure 40-11∗). The outer cannula keeps the stoma open and is held in place

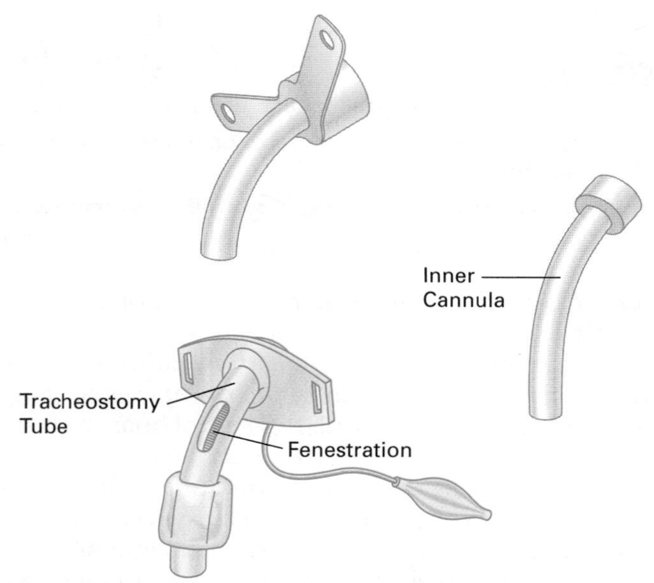

FIGURE 40-11 ✱ A tracheostomy tube for older children and adults has an outer cannula and an inner cannula.

by a Velcro strap or twill tape around the neck. The inner cannula is smaller in diameter and slides into the outer cannula. The distal end of the inner cannula has a low-pressure cuff (similar to that of an endotracheal tube) that when inflated helps to hold it in place and create a good seal against the walls of the trachea. The proximal end of the tracheostomy tube has an adapter that will fit a standard bag-valve-mask or flow-restricted, oxygen-powered ventilation device should positive pressure be needed.

A patient with a tracheostomy tube may or may not be able to speak, depending on the condition of the upper airway structures (larynx and vocal cords). If these structures are still intact, the patient can plug the tracheostomy with a finger, which directs the exhaled air through the vocal cords to permit speech. If these structures are damaged or have been surgically removed, normal speech will be impossible. To compensate for this, the patient may have a device shaped like a small flashlight that, when held up to the neck and activated, will produce a vibration sound the patient learns to manipulate by changing the shape of his mouth. This allows verbal communication to happen, but you may have difficulty initially trying to understand the words. In the absence of any form of spoken communication, you will need to use hand gestures or writing to communicate with the patient.

Emergencies that concern a patient with a tracheostomy tube usually involve one of two things. First, the tube itself may have become plugged by mucus. Since the upper airway is bypassed by the tube, the normal functions of the upper airway such as filtering and humidification of inspired air are lost, and as a result the tracheostomy tube needs regular suctioning. Second, the inner cannula of the tube could have become dislodged from movement or may have become occluded by a foreign body. Less common emergencies that pertain to the tracheostomy tube include infection or bleeding at the

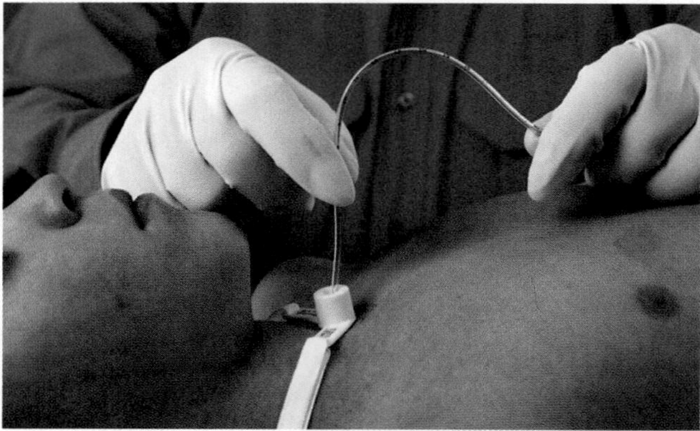

FIGURE 40-12 ✱ Use a soft suction catheter to clear blood or secretions from the tracheostomy tube.

insertion site. During your assessment of a patient with an emergency pertaining to a tracheostomy tube, you must rapidly determine if the problem is that of airway occlusion or (if the patient is also ventilator dependent) if the ventilator is malfunctioning.

If the tube is partially or totally occluded from bleeding or heavy secretions, use a whistle-tip (soft) suction catheter to clear the airway (Figure 40-12✱). Measure the depth of insertion for the suction catheter by comparing it to the tracheostomy tube obturator. (The obturator is a blunt-tipped plug that fits inside the tracheostomy tube during the insertion process and is then removed after successful placement. It can usually be found with the patient's other tracheostomy supplies.) If the obturator cannot be found quickly, gently insert the catheter tip until mild resistance is met. Apply suction and slowly withdraw the catheter while twisting it between your fingers. Do not suction for longer than 10–15 seconds in an adult, and 5 seconds in a pediatric patient at once. Oxygenate your patient between suctioning attempts, and rinse out the lumen of the suction catheter with sterile water between attempts.

Manipulation of a tracheostomy tube may be outside the EMT's protocol, so make certain that you are allowed to perform these interventions before doing so. The primary care provider, if available, is probably the most skilled in tracheal suctioning for this patient, so try to enlist the care provider's help.

If you find the tracheostomy tube to be patent, the problem may be with the patient's ventilator. This emergency will be discussed later in this chapter, but the short answer is to remove the ventilator circuit and provide positive pressure ventilation by attaching your bag-valve-mask device directly to the tracheostomy tube's external fitting.

CPAP and BiPAP

Both **continuous positive airway pressure (CPAP)** and **bilevel positive airway pressure (BiPAP)** machines are designed to provide a therapeutic back-pressure during

Key Terms
continuous positive airway pressure (CPAP) device that provides a constant level of back pressure during inhalation and exhalation to keep bronchioles open and improve ventilation and oxygenation.

Key Terms
bilevel positive airway pressure (BiPAP) device that provides back pressure, higher during inhalation and lower during exhalation, to keep bronchioles open and improve ventilation and oxygenation.

respiration via an airway circuit attached to a mask that covers the mouth and/or nose. While the CPAP device provides a constant pressure during the ventilatory cycle, the BiPAP machine provides a higher pressure during inhalation and a lower pressure during exhalation. The primary therapeutic goal of either device is to keep the bronchioles open during exhalation, which improves both oxygenation and ventilation and also decreases the work of breathing. Some CPAP and BiPAP machines also allow the administration of oxygen during their use.

Understanding BODY PROCESSES

When there is damage to the lower airway structures from disease, it is difficult for the airways to remain open. The use of CPAP or BiPAP will help keep these smaller airways stented open so that better ventilation can be achieved. ■

This equipment is commonly used in patients diagnosed with COPD or sleep apnea. A prehospital CPAP device is commercially available and is used in many EMS systems for patients suffering from respiratory distress with a history and clinical presentation consistent with COPD or congestive heart failure (CHF). Local protocols may allow its use in other clinical situations.

Emergencies related to a CPAP or BiPAP machine are rare. During your assessment of a patient who uses a CPAP or BiPAP machine for sleep apnea, you will likely learn that EMS was summoned not for an emergency related to the device but rather for a respiratory distress complaint arising from the patient's chronic pulmonary condition or some other medical emergency. This is because CPAP or BiPAP is used during sleep, and while the patient is awake he is not dependent on the device. During your assessment and management of this patient, you may utilize a CPAP machine if your protocol allows and the patient meets your inclusion criteria. If, however, you are assessing and treating a patient for some complaint and he also concurrently uses a CPAP or BiPAP while sleeping, you may want to transport the device to the hospital with the patient and be sure to alert the receiving facility of the patient's need for it during sleep.

Home Mechanical Ventilators

A home mechanical ventilator is designed to assist a patient with breathing who cannot breathe adequately on his own. The patient may have any one of several reasons to be dependent on a ventilator. Causes typically center around the brain's inability to initiate a spontaneous breath, a structural defect to the thorax or lungs that prohibits or greatly diminishes normal gas exchange, or a neuromuscular disease that renders the respiratory muscles of the body useless. Causes may also include history of a debilitating stroke, brain damage following head trauma, or long-term pulmonary problems (e.g., COPD, lung cancer). Commonly, you will learn the reason for the patient's ventilator dependency while you are ascertaining his medical history.

There are two types of mechanical ventilators: negative pressure and positive pressure. Negative pressure ventilators, such as the "iron lung," encircle the patient's chest and generate a negative pressure around the thoracic cage. The negative pressure draws the rib cage out, which creates a negative intrathoracic pressure that causes air to be drawn into the lungs. These devices are rarely used in the home setting because newer and better technology is available. Today, the devices commonly encountered are positive pressure ventilators. With these devices, air from the ventilator is pushed into the patient's lungs, much as when an EMT squeezes a bag-valve-mask device in order to force air into the lungs during artificial ventilation. Exhalation ensues when the positive pressure stops and the chest wall and lungs recoil.

Home ventilation units come in various sizes. The small, newer devices can be similar in size to a laptop computer, weighing just pounds. Some ventilators are larger, and may weigh up to 20 pounds or more. There are several ventilators available for use in the home or extended-care facility, and they can vary significantly in cost and sophistication. Regardless of size, they are generally designed for convenience and ease of use by the patient or the patient's primary care provider.

Home ventilation units typically have two or three controls: one for the ventilatory rate, one for adjusting the size of each breath (tidal volume), and in some cases one control that adjusts the amount of oxygen that is provided during ventilation. Tidal volume in most is adjustable, while the ventilatory rate and oxygen supply, if provided, may be either fixed or adjustable. The ventilator attaches to the patient by large-diameter tubing that is referred to as the ventilator circuit. The vent circuit attaches to the tracheostomy tube placed in the patient's trachea (Figure 40-13*). The proximal end of the tracheostomy tube has a standard 15/22 mm adapter on it, so any type of ventilatory device (bag-valve mask, flow-restricted,

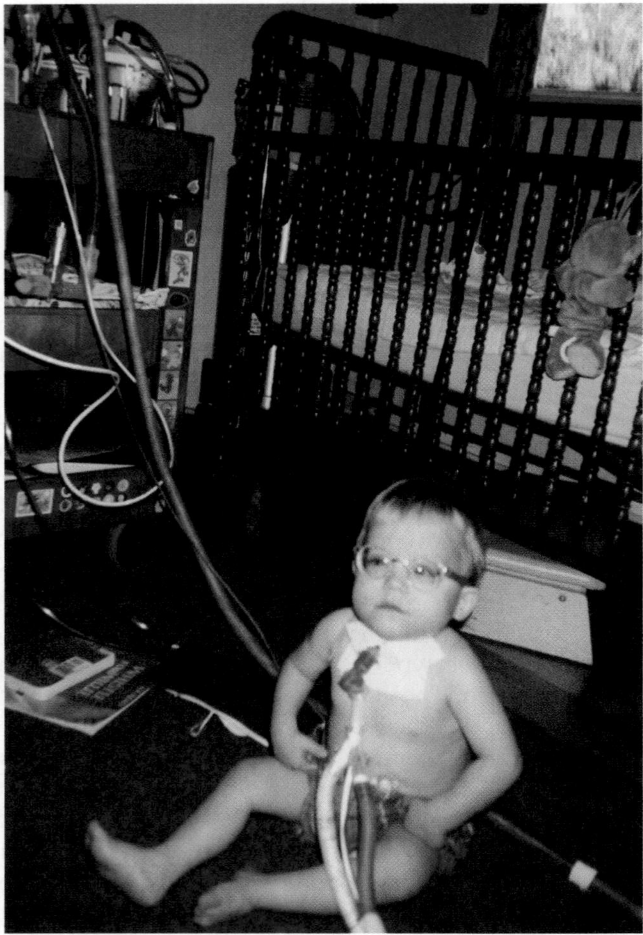

FIGURE 40-13 ✻ The tubing from the home ventilator attaches to the patient's tracheostomy tube.

oxygen-powered device, or mechanical ventilator) can be operated through the same ventilation port.

Ventilators may have several alarms to alert the care provider if the ventilator is not functioning properly. In fact, one of the alarms going off may be the reason EMS is summoned. Because of variances among these devices, the particular ventilator your patient uses may or may not have the following alarms:

- **High-pressure alarm.** A high-pressure alarm is activated when the pressure needed to cause lung inflation exceeds the present value. The cause can be increased airway resistance, such as increased secretions occluding the tracheostomy tube, kinking of the ventilator circuit, movement of the tracheostomy tube, bronchospasms, or the patient coughing during inspiration. The alarm can also be triggered by decreased lung compliance. Causes for decreased lung compliance include the development of a pneumothorax, progressive pneumonia, development of acute pulmonary edema, or even alveolar collapse (atelectasis).
- **Low-pressure alarm.** The low-pressure alarm is usually set to activate when the tidal volume falls 50–100 mL below the set tidal volume.This usually indicates a problem in the breathing circuit, such as a disconnected segment or a leak in the cuff of the tracheostomy tube.
- **Apnea alarm.** Some patients who have a vent may still have some respiratory effort, but it is inadequate to sustain life. Their home ventilator may be set up to not trigger a breath until the patient starts to breathe in. In these models, the apnea alarm sounds when the patient stops breathing. Causes are usually physiological and include decreased mental status, overmedication, and respiratory muscle fatigue.
- **Low FiO_2.** A low FiO_2 alarm will occur when the oxygen source is disconnected or depleted.

When approaching the patient with a ventilator emergency, be aware that the alarms going off may have been caused by a change in the patient's clinical condition, not necessarily by ventilator malfunction. Although the ventilator may fail because of electrical supply interruption, failure of some internal component of the ventilator, or even a problem with the ventilator circuit, the *real* problem your patient is experiencing may not be the ventilator's fault at all. A change in the patient's clinical status, for example, could make the ventilator malfunction. If the high-pressure alarm goes off, it could be from tracheostomy tube occlusion resulting from mucus buildup, or from the development of a spontaneous pneumothorax causing an increase in airway pressure. Another example could be the patient who also uses a pulse oximeter for whom the low saturation alarm may alert, which could be from a malfunctioning ventilator but could also be from hypoxia related to pneumonia, lung collapse, or even a heart attack.

Do not assume that if the ventilator starts to alarm, the remedy is to disconnect it and use a bag-valve mask. Although it may seem logical to simply disconnect the mechanical ventilator and bag the patient manually, if the inadequate breathing is from a change in the patient's status (e.g., pneumothorax, airway occlusion), ventilating him manually will provide no more help than the mechanical ventilator could supply. Always troubleshoot the ventilator *and* the patient.

ASSESSMENT Tips

When dealing with a patient who has a malfunctioning ventilator, pay close attention to the quality of breath sounds and chest rise and fall during manual ventilation. Be sure not to overventilate or underventilate the patient. ■

Accommodations for Patients with Airway or Respiratory Devices

You may not always know that the patient is reliant on airway- or respiratory-assist technology prior to your arrival on the scene. That depends on what the caller told dispatch. You must be prepared to interact with this type of equipment at a moment's notice. Your assessment of the patient will not change drastically despite the presence of this technology. Since this equipment is being used to support or replace a lost function of the body, you will automatically assess its adequacy in supporting that lost function while you perform your usual primary assessment, history, and physical exam.

Most likely, the complaint received by dispatch will be one of the following: airway occlusion, respiratory distress, altered mental status, ventilator/CPAP alarm, or low pulse oximeter finding. In most emergencies like these, the primary care provider has been taught by the medical equipment company to alert EMS when certain aspects of the device fail to function properly. Although the problem may turn out to be a false alarm, you must be ready to take over should some piece of technology fail.

Dispatch may be able to tell you the type of medical technology the patient uses. This will allow you to start planning your approach to the patient while you are en route. On arrival, do not be complacent and neglect to perform a scene size-up for your own safety. Information gained during the scene size-up will also let you know if you need to summon additional backup to help move the patient and his equipment from their current location to the ambulance.

The primary assessment should be conducted in the same sequence for a patient with airway or ventilatory devices as for those without such devices. Form your general impression as you approach the patient. While you are completing your primary assessment, talk to the patient's primary health care provider to determine the history and recent status of the patient, if possible. After evaluating the patient's mental status, focus on the airway. If the patient has an anatomically intact and patent upper airway, you will move to the assessment of breathing. If the upper airway is occluded, you will follow the steps for airway clearance as discussed in previous chapters.

If you find the patient has a tracheostomy tube, you will need to rapidly assess it for patency. If it is blocked by mucus or fluid, it must be immediately cleared or the patient will continue to deteriorate into cardiac arrest (just like any patient with an airway occlusion). If there is a primary care provider immediately available with experience in suctioning the tracheostomy, enlist that person's help. If this is not an option, and if your protocol allows, select a soft or flexible suction catheter and insert it carefully into the tracheostomy tube. Remember that the trachea is considered to be a sterile field, so if at all possible use a sterile technique for suctioning with sterile gloves. Try not to insert the suction catheter farther than the length of the inner cannula of the tracheostomy. Measure the suction catheter against the obturator used for the insertion process (which, as noted earlier, is usually found with the patient's other airway supplies). If the obturator cannot be located, insert the suction catheter carefully until you meet resistance.

Once the catheter is placed, apply suction (–80 to –120 cm H_2O) while you withdraw the catheter. Rolling the catheter between your fingers during extraction will provide better clearing of the mucus or fluid. Suction for only 10–15 seconds in an adult and only 5 seconds in a child. The tracheal stimulation from your suction catheter will probably cause the patient to cough, sometimes forcefully. Although this is to be expected, the coughing may cause mucus or fluid to be blown out of the opening. Be sure to wear the necessary protective equipment so that your eyes and face are not exposed.

After each episode of suctioning, rinse out the suction catheter with sterile water. If the tracheostomy tube blockage appears to be from dislodgment rather than fluid or mucus plugging, removing it may be the only option available to restore a patent airway. Remember that the adult tracheostomy has an inner cannula with a distal cuff. This cuff needs to be deflated with a 10 mL syringe prior to removal. After removal, the airway can be suctioned as needed and then re-evaluated. Removal of the inner cannula should only be performed by the primary care provider if that person is capable of doing so, or by an ALS provider. Once the airway is patent again, only then should you focus on the next step of the primary assessment, breathing.

Determination of adequate breathing should be performed in the same manner as for any patient who is spontaneously breathing. If the spontaneously breathing patient is found to have inadequate ventilations, positive pressure ventilation with oxygen should be provided, just as it would for any other patient.

If the patient uses a CPAP machine at night, more than likely he will be awake while in your presence and not need the CPAP machine. In fact, medical emergencies related to the CPAP are uncommon. If problems arise with CPAP, it is usually handled by the company or provider that services the unit for the patient (if it's mechanical), or the patient's respiratory therapist if the problem relates to difficulty in use of the device. If, however, the patient is experiencing some medical or traumatic emergency independent of the CPAP machine, you should treat the patient as appropriate and may wish to take the CPAP unit to the hospital with the patient in case he is admitted and needs the device during sleep.

A patient who is dependent on a mehanical ventilator is a slightly different situation. If on arrival you find the patient to be breathing inadequately with the device (as evidenced by minimal chest movement and diminished to absent breath sounds in the bases of the lungs), you must rapidly determine if the inadequate breathing is secondary to airway occlusion, ventilatory circuit occlusion or kinking, mechanical failure of the ventilator, or a change in the patient's clinical status that has rendered the ventilator ineffective.

First remove the ventilator circuit, place a bag-valve mask on the 15/22 mm adapter of the tracheostomy tube, and attempt one or two ventilations (Figure 40-14*).

Thinking Critically
If a patient's ventilator is not working and you can't fix it, what care should you provide between home and hospital?

Key Terms
vascular access device (VAD) a medical device that is used when a patient is in need of ongoing intravenous medications.

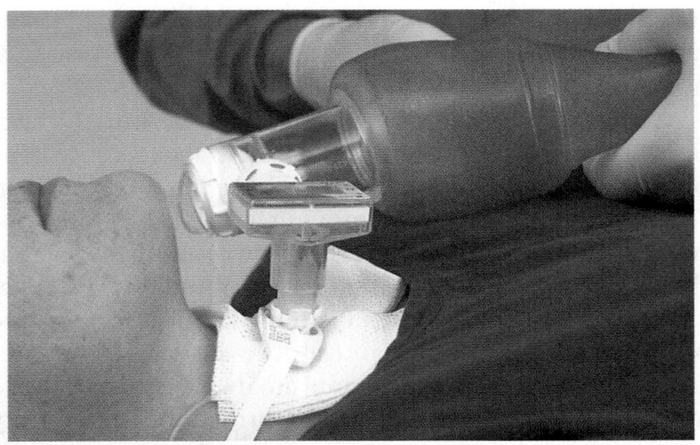

FIGURE 40-14 ✻ You can ventilate a patient with a tracheostomy by attaching the bag-valve device to the tracheostomy tube's 15/22 mm adapter.

If the ventilations *do go in easily* and you see chest wall movement, the problem is likely either ventilator failure or a problem with the ventilation circuit. If that is the case and you can fix the problem with the ventilator, or if your protocol allows you to adjust the ventilator's settings (rate and tidal volume) to meet the patient's needs, the ventilator may be reapplied during transport to the hospital.

If you *do not* see immediate rise and fall of the chest, the bag-valve mask is hard to squeeze, and/or you don't hear alveolar breath sounds, the problem may lie with the patient. First reassess the airway as described earlier and clear it as appropriate, then reattempt ventilation. If there is still a problem, assess for clinical findings such as bronchoconstriction, pneumothorax, tension pneumothorax, or severe pneumonia. Provide management as appropriate for the offending problem as discussed in previous chapters, contact ALS, and continue with manual ventilations while en route to the hospital.

Once the airway and breathing components are ensured or restored, next focus on the circulatory assessment. Assess the heart rate and skin characteristics to rapidly gauge the patient's perfusion status. Provide management as appropriate for disturbances in the circulatory system.

The patient should be considered unstable and rapidly transported if there is some acute lost function to the airway, breathing, or circulatory components that the EMT must support during transport. The patient should be considered potentially unstable if there was a mechanical malfunction or clinical change that precipitated a critical intervention by the EMT but now the current status is seemingly stable. Finally, the patient should be considered stable if there was no acute loss of function, no critical interventions were warranted, and the patient is receiving primarily supportive care while en route to the hospital for evaluation.

Regardless of the interventions provided by the EMT for the patient who has a ventilator or CPAP emergency, special considerations will need to be made in transporting the patient to the hospital. If the ventilator is still operating normally for the patient, you may want to use the bag-valve mask to ventilate the patient carefully while you move him to the ambulance. Once inside the ambulance, plug the patient's ventilator into the onboard inverter and place it back on the patient. If the ventilator is no longer functioning, you may still wish to take it to the hospital with the patient and explain any problems with the device to the receiving facility staff. Remain flexible in your approach, management, and transfer of the patient with airway or ventilatory equipment.

One final concern with airway and ventilatory devices is how you document your findings and care. A significant percentage of claims and lawsuits that are filed against prehospital providers involve inadequate patient ventilation. It is critical that you document in medically correct and legally sufficient terms exactly what was done in managing the patient's airway and ventilation. Such documentation can save you from a claim or lawsuit being filed or, in the unfortunate event that one is filed, can help you to prevail.

Vascular Access Devices

A **vascular access device (VAD)** is a medical device that is used when a patient is in need of ongoing intravenous medications. Usually these devices are placed in patients who need medication for longer than 7 to 10 days, but they may be used on a longer-term basis as well. The type of device and duration of its use are largely dependent on the disease process and medical needs of the patient. Over half a million devices of this nature are placed annually, typically in patients who require ongoing chemotherapy, peritoneal dialysis, hemodialysis, total parenteral nutrition (TPN), or antibiotic therapy. Although the EMT does not access a VAD for medication administration, a knowledge of their presence, basic function, and how to care for them during assessment and transport is important (Figure 40-15✻).

Key Terms
central intravenous catheter a catheter that is designed to deliver medication into the central circulation of the body.

Key Terms
surgically implanted medication delivery devices medication administration devices surgically placed beneath the skin outside the rib cage. Also called a **totally implantable venous access system (TIVAS).**

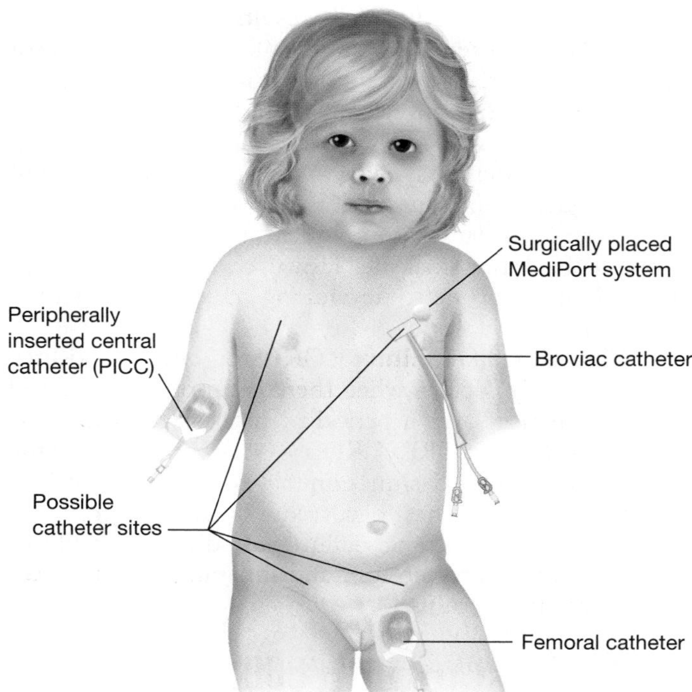

FIGURE 40-15 * Vascular access devices include central IV catheters such as a PICC line, central venous lines such as the Broviac catheter, and implanted ports such as the MediPort system.

Understanding BODY PROCESSES

Sometimes a medication that is needed to manage a patient's condition must be administered often or, because of the drug's action, must be administered into a large central vein. Placement of a venous access device allows this to be done outside the hospital setting. ■

Central Intravenous Catheters

A **central intravenous catheter** is placed while the patient is in the hospital and is designed to deliver medication into the central circulation of the body. Generally speaking, these VADs have a long, thin hollow tube (catheter) that is inserted into a vein of the arm or neck, or the subclavian vein just below the clavicle. The tip of the catheter is threaded into a large blood vessel of the chest, and provides a simple and painless means for the administration of medications or nutrients. These devices are somewhat similar to peripheral IV catheters that the EMT may be more familiar with when working in an ALS system, but central catheters can stay in place for several weeks or months at a time. One common type you may encounter is a *peripherally inserted central catheter (PICC)* line. This device is often inserted into the patient's arm at the antecubital fossa and from there is threaded into the body until the tip lies in the central circulation.

Central Venous Lines

Another type of VAD is the *central venous line.* You will notice the proximal port(s) secured to the anterior chest, just below the clavicle. Several types of central venous lines exist, including *Broviac, Groshong,* and *Hickman.* The portion of the device remaining outside the body typically has a medication port similar to a traditional intravenous port. They are commonly sutured to the skin to help them remain properly placed.

Implanted Ports

You may also encounter **surgically implanted medication delivery devices**, known also as a **totally implantable venous access system (TIVAS)**, that are commonly referred to as an "implanted port." These medication administration devices are surgically placed beneath the skin, but outside the rib cage. Known as *Port-A-Cath, MediPort, Microport, Bardport, Passport,* or *Infuse-a-Port*, these disk-shaped devices can be easily palpated beneath the surface of the skin after they are placed. They are typically embedded into the upper chest on the right side.

Accommodations for Patients with Vascular Access Devices

VADs are not without problems. Since they involve a catheter inserted into the central circulation of the body, the catheter may become obstructed by clot formation at the tip. An associated emergency could be a thrombus that forms on the catheter but then breaks off and lodges elsewhere in the body. (This problem is more likely if the patient is physically inactive.) The person with a VAD may also be placed on systemic anticoagulant therapy, which renders the patient more susceptible to bleeding

Key Points
Keep the insertion site of a VAD dry and covered with a sterile dressing while you are caring for the patient. Note any signs of infection at the insertion site.

Key Terms
acute renal failure (ARF) a rapid loss of renal function that results in poor urine production and disturbance of electrolyte and fluid balances.

chronic renal failure (CRF) progressive loss of kidney function over a period of months to years. Also called **chronic kidney disease (CKD)**.

disorders. Gastrointestinal bleeding, strokes, and bruising are most commonly seen.

Another complication you should be aware of is the risk of accidental air embolism. VADs can allow air to directly enter the core circulation. If this happens, it is a dire medical emergency that can result in death of the patient if a significant amount of air makes its way into the body. You may need to respond for a patient who suddenly complains of dyspnea (but has clear lung sounds), has a severe headache, complains of sudden sharp chest pain, or displays an altered mental status. If the patient has a VAD in place, suspect an accidental air embolism as a potential cause of the condition.

ASSESSMENT Tips

If a patient has a VAD that has an external port for medication administration, always inspect the site for bleeding or infection. Also note the depth of insertion and document this on your prehospital care report. If a problem arises with the depth of insertion, it should be made clear that the EMT was not responsible for causing either withdrawal or deeper insertion of the device. ■

During your care for the patient, keep the insertion site of the VAD dry and covered with a sterile dressing. Notice during your assessment if there is any redness, tenderness, warm skin, or purulent discharge at the site that may indicate an infection. (A patient may quickly become septic from a severe blood infection as a result of insertion site infection.) Also look for any bleeding at the insertion site as tension or tugging on the external portion of the VAD may cause it to dislodge. If this occurs, cover the site with a bulky sterile dressing and maintain pressure on the site.

Renal Failure and Dialysis

Under normal circumstances, the kidneys function to remove waste products in the bloodstream, and maintain water balance as well as regulate many electrolytes in the body. However, this function can become impaired by many causes, a condition that is generically called renal failure.

Acute renal failure (ARF) is said to occur when there is a rapid loss of renal function that results in poor urine production, electrolyte disturbance, and fluid balance disturbance. ARF usually results from either a sudden cessation of renal blood flow (from vascular and/or direct kidney trauma or poor cardiac output) or from some type of toxic overload in the bloodstream (e.g., drug abuse or overdose, antibiotics, chemotherapy). Although the patient may need ongoing hospital treatment until normal kidney function is restored, ARF can often be reversed if treated promptly and the patient can continue to lead a normal life. However, these patients are typically more prone to developing renal failure again in the future.

Chronic renal failure (CRF) or **chronic kidney disease (CKD)** occurs when there is a progressive loss of kidney function over a period of months to years. The clinical findings of CRF/CKD are often insidious and the diagnosis of kidney dysfunction may not be made until irreparable damage has occurred. The most common causes for chronic renal failure are diabetes mellitus, long-standing hypertension, and inflammation or infection to the glomerulus.

Understanding BODY PROCESSES

The functional unit of the kidney is the glomerulus. The blood that passes through it is filtered, and water and electrolyte balance is maintained. If too many glomeruli are damaged, this function is lost and must then be supplemented by a machine. ■

Dialysis is a medical procedure designed to support the lost function of the kidneys, although total replacement of all renal functions is not possible. Dialysis removes the buildup of toxins that occurs when the kidneys can no longer filter these toxins out. *Hemodialysis* is the type of dialysis in which blood is extracted from the body and sent through a machine called a dialyzer. The dialyzer filters the blood from the body through a membrane that also uses a dialysate fluid to help cleanse the blood. Following the cleansing process, the blood is returned to the body. The process takes anywhere from 2 to 5 hours. Dialysis typically occurs in a dialysis center, and must be repeated two to three times per week.

Peritoneal dialysis is done in the home or the extended-care facility. With this type of dialysis (which the EMT is more likely to encounter), dialysate fluid is introduced into a port that leads into the peritoneal cavity. The fluid then surrounds the intestines where it interacts with the body to remove waste products. After a

Key Terms

dialysis medical procedure designed to support lost function of the kidneys.

dialysis shunt a joining of arterial and venous systems in such a way that the repeated needlesticks for dialysis cause a minimal damage to the body.

Thinking Critically

You are called to a dialysis center where a patient is experiencing symptoms of a cardiac emergency. Your partner says, "Let's get him off that dialysis machine so we can assess him." Is this the right first step? Why or why not?

ASSESSMENT Tips

As an EMT, you may occasionally be called to a dialysis center for a patient with a medical emergency. Be sure to find out from the health care staff if the patient had completed his dialysis session, and if there is any known "volume overload" or "volume deficit."

An important consideration when dealing with patients who receive regular hemodialysis for renal failure is their **dialysis shunt.** A dialysis shunt is a generic term for one of three different ways to join the arterial and venous systems together (*arteriovenous* or*AV*) in such a way that the repeated needlesticks required to take and return blood to the body several times a week cause a minimal amount of damage to the body. An *AV shunt* is used on short-term hemodialysis patients or on patients who have recently started dialysis (Figure 40-16✻). Either an *AV fistula* or an *AV graft* is used for long-term dialysis patients. An AV fistula typically results in a visible or palpable "bump" immediately under the surface of the skin. Similar to a fistula, a graft will result in a visible and palpable mass beneath the surface of the skin. In addition, an AV graft often will have a soft vibration (called a thrill) with gentle palpation as a result of the blood passing through it. ■

specific amount of time, the fluid is removed from the abdominal cavity and replaced with fresh fluid. Since this form of dialysis is not as effective as hemodialysis, it must be repeated several times a day. However, because of current technology, the procedure is relatively easy for the patient to do without assistance and allows the patient greater freedom in daily activities, since he is not bound to making several long appointments a week at the dialysis center.

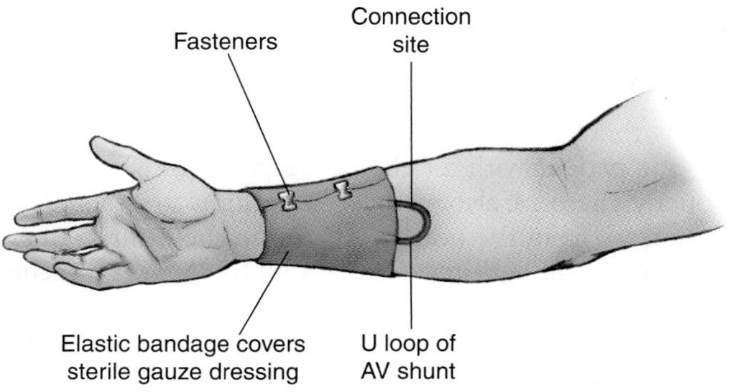

FIGURE 40-16 ✻ An AV shunt for short-term use may consist of an external loop that connects an artery and a vein. For longer-term use, AV grafts and fistulas are formed beneath the patient's skin.

Accommodations for Patients on Dialysis

If a patient is receiving dialysis at a facility and an emergency occurs (whether related to the dialysis or not), a couple of important considerations exist. First, if the patient is still attached to the dialysis machine, do not attempt to remove the patient prematurely. The removal of the patient from the dialysis machine should only occur under the supervision of the dialysis center staff. Multiple complications such as volume overload, hemorrhage, or volume depletion could occur and complicate matters even more.

After the patient is removed from the machine, your assessment and management of the patient should follow steps already mentioned, given the presenting problem. One consideration that must be followed regards the dialysis shunt. You should never attempt to obtain a blood pressure in any extremity that has an AV shunt, AV fistula, or AV graft. The surgical procedures used to create the shunt can be significantly or irreparably damaged by the application and inflation of a blood pressure cuff. Always use an extremity that does not have an AV shunt.

You must also be aware that the AV shunt, if damaged, can bleed excessively. The bleeding could be external, with significant amounts lost rapidly, or internal, with the formation of a large hematoma beneath the surface of the skin. In either instance, you should apply direct pressure to the site to help control the bleed, treat for shock (administer high-concentration oxygen and keep the patient warm), and expedite transport to the hospital. Do not release your direct pressure until told to do so by the receiving physician.

Emergencies with peritoneal dialysis are usually not as severe and typically involve either a displaced catheter, inflammation at the catheter insertion site, or infection of the peritoneal space (peritonitis). The patient will probably complain of abdominal pain, there may be signs of infection at the insertion site for the catheter, and he may have missed one or more sessions of peritoneal dialysis. Management includes keeping the catheter insertion site clean and dry, supporting any lost function that may be present, and transporting the patient to the hospital for evaluation by the receiving physician.

Key Terms
enteral feeding provision of nutrition through a tube inserted through the nose, the mouth, or a surgical opening in the abdomen into the gastrointestinal system.

Key Terms
ostomy bag a pouch or bag that is attached outside the body to collect feces that are removed from the body through an opening in the abdominal wall.

Gastrointestinal and Genitourinary Devices

Certain medical problems that occur to the gastrointestinal or genitourinary systems of the body may result in reliance on medical devices to supplement lost functions of these systems. Devices such as feeding tubes for nutritional support or external collection bags for bowel and/or bladder emptying may be encountered in chronically ill patients at home or in extended-care facilities. How the EMT should interact with these devices depends on the reason EMS was summoned. EMS may be summoned because of some other emergency the patient is experiencing (for example, a heart attack or stroke) or because of some disturbance in the normal functioning of these devices. Since these devices are so common in patients with chronic or debilitating conditions, the EMT should remain abreast of this medical technology.

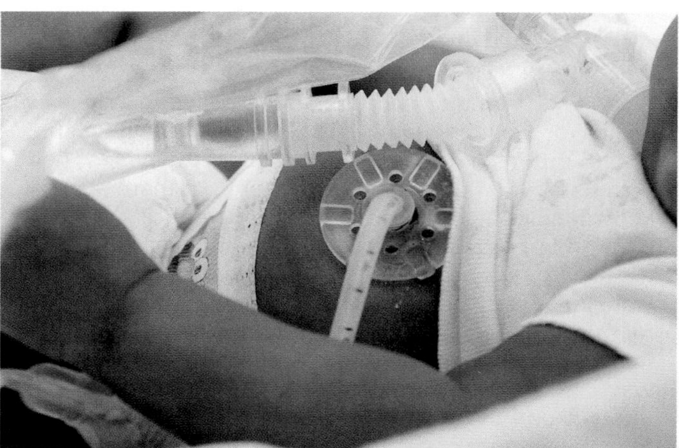

FIGURE 40-17 ✱ For long-term nutritional support, a feeding tube may be surgically inserted through the abdominal wall and directly into the gastrointestinal system. (© Ray Kemp/911 Imaging)

Feeding Tubes

Feeding tubes are medical devices that provide nutrition to patients who cannot chew or swallow because of medical or traumatic conditions resulting in paralysis or unconsciousness. Patients who receive their nourishment this way are said to be receiving **enteral feeding**, or tube feeding. The device is typically a flexible tube that is long and small in diameter. It is named according to the site of insertion. If it is inserted through the nose and ends in the stomach, it's termed a *nasogastric tube*, or *NG tube*. If the tube is inserted through the mouth and ends up in the stomach, it's called an *orogastric tube*, or *OG tube*.

Nasogastric tubes are more commonly seen by the EMT because ALS and emergency department providers will place an NG tube so they can decompress the stomach if there is excessive air accumulation. NG tubes may also be placed so that ingested toxins can be suctioned out (in cases of accidental or purposeful overdoses). Lastly, they can be used for short-term nutritional support.

Orogastric tubes are slightly larger than nasogastric tubes but serve basically the same purposes (nutrition, decompression, and suctioning out the stomach). Some orogastric tubes end with the tip located in either the duodenum or jejunum.

When long-term nutritional support is warranted, a tube may be surgically inserted through the abdominal wall and directly into the GI system (Figure 40-17✱). The procedure that places a gastric tube into the abdomen is termed *gastrostomy*. A gastrostomy is performed for patients in need of long-term nutritional support from a variety of conditions, such as Alzheimer disease, severe mental retardation, or significant brain injury from head trauma or debilitating stroke.

Many types of gastric tubes may be used, and although they all serve the same basic function, they may be placed in different areas of the small intestine. A *gastric tube (G tube)* is a feeding tube that is placed through the abdominal wall with the tip residing in the stomach. A *jejunal tube (J tube)* is another type of feeding tube that is inserted through the gastric wall with the tip placed in the jejunum.

Ostomy Bags

Just as there are special tubes and procedures to ensure that the patient with a debilitating problem is nourished properly, there are also medical procedures that help to remove feces from the body by directing them through the abdominal wall and into a pouch or bag that is attached outside the body. These are referred to as **ostomy bags** or ostomy pouches. This procedure may be done on a temporary or a long-term basis and is used in patients with Crohn disease, ulcerative colitis, colon cancer, or diverticulitis. During this procedure, a surgical opening is made through the abdominal wall, and a section of the bowel is

> **Key Terms**
> **urinary catheter** a device that is used to divert urine out of the bladder.

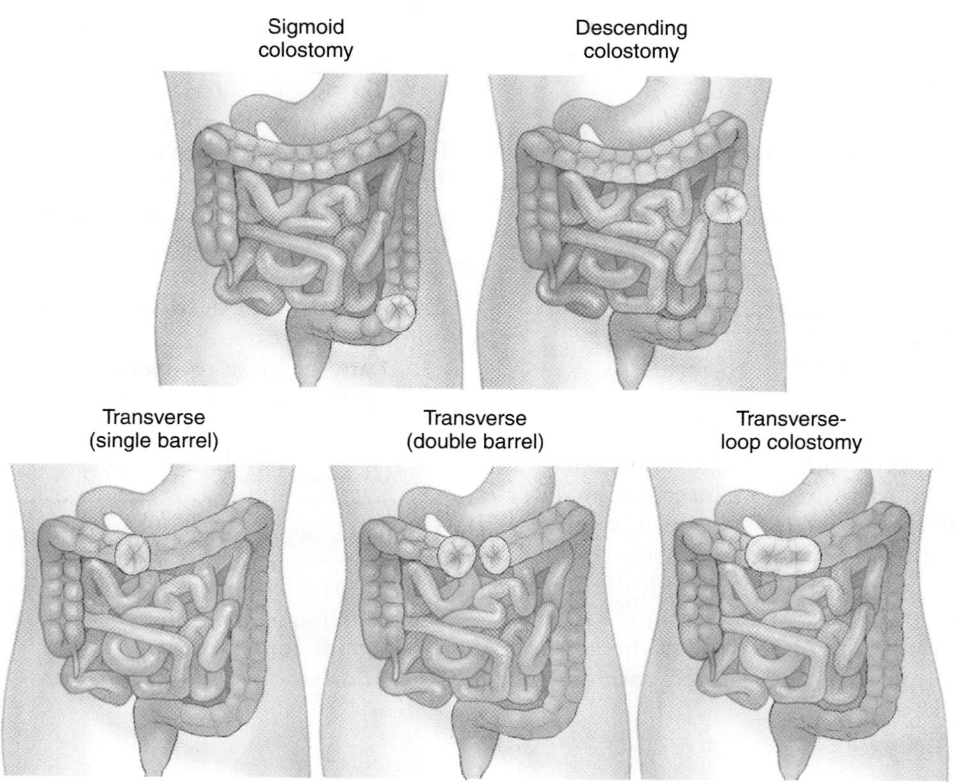

FIGURE 40-18 ✱ Ostomy stomas may be found at various abdominal locations.

diverted through this opening so that the flow of fecal material can be directed outside the body (Figure 40-18✱).

Urinary Tract Devices

A **urinary catheter** is a device that is used to divert urine out of the bladder when there is some type of urinary tract dysfunction. The least invasive of these is called a *Texas catheter* (or condom catheter), because it attaches to the external male urethra in the same manner as a prophylactic condom would (Figure 40-19a✱). At the tip of the condom, a catheter is attached that directs the flow of urine into a collection bag. This type of urinary catheter is often used when the patient can still expel urine from the bladder but cannot control when this happens.

There are also internal catheters that are threaded into the urethra (indwelling with the tip entering into the urinary bladder). The most common type is a *Foley catheter*, and this is the most common type used for a patient with a urinary tract dysfunction. Once placed in the urethra of the male or female, a small balloon positioned at the tip of the device is inflated to help keep the tip within the urinary bladder (Figure 40-19b✱). These devices are tolerated well, are used for long periods of time, and are commonly seen in home health care settings, hospitals, and extended-care facilities. As the urine drains from the catheter, it flows into a collection bag that can be emptied when needed.

A less common type of urinary catheter that you may encounter is the *suprapubic catheter.* This type of catheter is surgically inserted through the abdominal wall just superior to the symphysis pubis and into the urinary bladder. It also drains the urine into an external collection bag and is used when there is some problem with the external genitalia that precludes insertion of a Foley catheter.

You may encounter a patient who has a *urostomy.* This procedure is performed when the urinary bladder is unable to collect urine. In this procedure, the urinary tract is surgically diverted through a stoma created in the abdominal wall where a collection bag is attached.

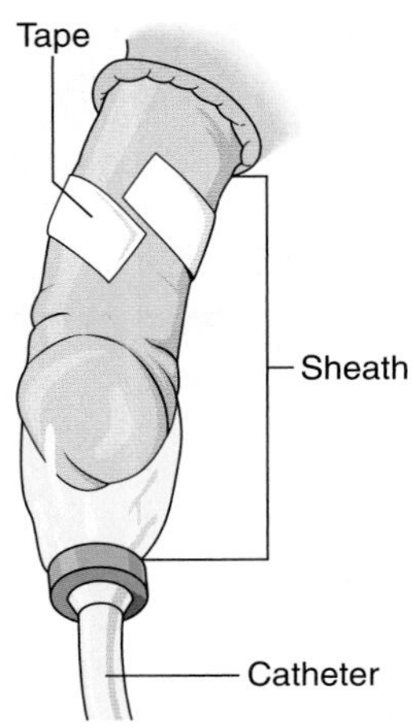

FIGURE 40-19a ✱ An external urinary catheter.

Accommodations for Patients with Gastrointestinal and Genitourinary Devices

Most problems that occur with gastrointestinal and genitourinary (GI/GU) devices are from insertion site infection, device malfunctions from misplacement, or obstruction. The nutrition that is administered through a feeding tube is usually thick and may block the feeding tube. In other situations, the primary care provider must crush medications and administer them through the feeding tube. If the pills are not crushed enough, they may block the feeding tube. Dislodgment occurs when there is accidental tugging on the device (for example, when the patient is being moved or rolled over). It may also happen if the patient has an altered mental status and pulls at the device. Indwelling catheters are prone to infection because they provide a portal of entry for bacteria. In some settings, the primary care provider may not clean and care for the site as well as necessary, also fostering the development of a urinary tract infection (UTI). UTIs may be identified by lower abdominal pain and cloudy, blood-tinged, or "tea-colored" urine.

The surgical sites where feeding tubes enter or ostomy bags exit the abdominal wall are also prone to infections from improper or insufficient care and cleaning. Like feeding tubes, ostomy bags may become obstructed. This may be due to the consistency of fecal material, and the digestive enzymes in the bowel may start to break down the skin surrounding the stoma if the infection goes unnoticed for too long or if the patient is immunosuppressed.

If any of these problems are identified, it is beyond the EMT's scope of practice to correct the situation. If

ASSESSMENT Tips

If during inspection of a GI/GU device it appears that the device has shifted or become misplaced, do not attempt to correct the situation yourself. Secure the device in the location found and transport the patient to the hospital while monitoring the site. ■

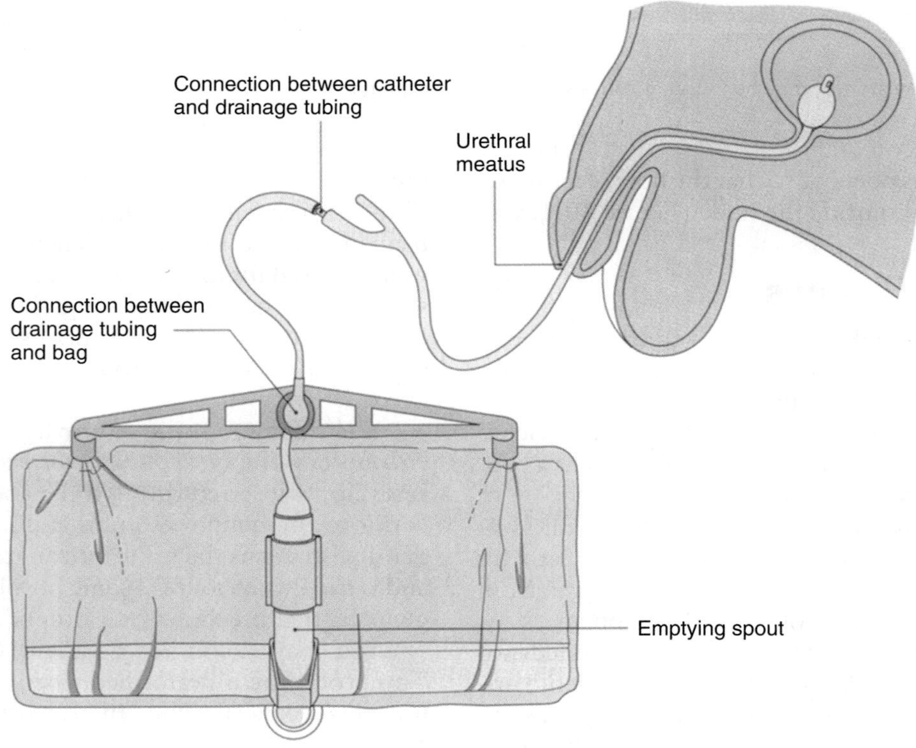

FIGURE 40-19b ✱ An internal urinary catheter with balloon.

Key Points

When called to a patient who has a GI/GU device, determine if the emergency involves malfunction of the device or a problem unrelated to the device. Do not try to fix a device malfunction, but transport the patient with the device to the hospital.

Key Terms

intraventricular shunt a tube surgically placed in a ventricle of the brain that extends to a blood vessel in the neck, the heart, the abdomen, or an external collector to drain excess cerebrospinal fluid from the brain and keep intracranial pressure at an acceptable level.

EMS was summoned because of a malfunction of a GI/GU device, the patient will need transport to the hospital along with his medical device for evaluation and repair.

If EMS is summoned for some other traumatic or medical emergency, you should perform your assessment and treatment in the same manner as for any other patient with a similar problem. Just be cautious when moving the patient with these types of medical devices, because they may easily become dislodged. One special note: If the patient has a urinary catheter, it is a good idea to drain the collection bag prior to transport, taking note of the volume of urine removed and any irregularities in color or odor. This information should be shared with the receiving medical facility staff and documented on your prehospital care report. Never place the urinary collection bag between the patient's legs or on his stomach while during transportation. The collection bag needs to be positioned below the urethra so that gravity will cause the urine to flow into the collection bag and not flow back into the urinary bladder.

Intraventricular Shunts

Certain patients, mainly pediatrics, may have a medical illness or anatomical defect that results in either the overproduction of cerebrospinal fluid (CSF) in the brain, inadequate reabsorption of CSF, or irregular flow of CSF through the ventricles and/or meningeal layers of the brain. When excess CSF accumulates, the patient is said to have *hydrocephalus*. Regardless of the reason for the hydrocephalus, excess CSF within the cranial vault is bad. Since the skull is a fixed size and cannot expand to accommodate the extra fluid, the pressure within the skull (intracranial pressure, or ICP) builds, which can result in compression of brain tissue. To alleviate the rising ICP, a long, hollow tubelike device called an **intraventricular shunt** is surgically placed. It originates within a ventricle of the brain and extends to a blood vessel in the neck, the heart, the pleural space, or the abdomen to drain excess CSF and keep the ICP at an acceptable level. In some patients, you may also find a reservoir on the side of the skull, placed beneath the scalp, that collects the excess CSF for testing purposes (Figure 40-20*).

Intraventricular shunts cause emergencies only about 30 percent of the time with only 5 percent being serious. Most common problems include infection, shunt occlusion, and subdural bleeding. Since the shunt is placed within the brain and extends to a distal site (neck, heart, abdomen, or external collection reservoir), there is always a chance for infection. With infection, the patient may present with feelings of malaise, fever, and headaches. If the shunt drains into an external reservoir there may be signs of local skin infection where the tube exits the body. In severe cases, or in situations where the patient is immunosuppressed, a local infection involving the shunt may result in a systemic blood infection (sepsis). Another infection that may occur secondary to the device is meningitis, or an inflammation of the meningeal layers. A patient with meningitis will typically complain of general malaise, headaches, and fever. This patient may also display a fine rash over the body's surface and have neck stiffness or pain.

The intraventricular shunt may become occluded. The obstruction may occur because of the body trying to block off the shunt, because one of the two ends has become dislodged and can no longer allow CSF to flow out, or because of a physical obstruction within the shunt itself. When this occurs, excess CSF will accumulate in the brain and start to raise ICP to potentially dangerous levels. With slight elevations in the ICP, the patient may complain of headaches, vertigo, nausea, and weakness. As ICP continues to rise, more significant findings of brain compression include vomiting, changes in mental status, sensory/motor dysfunctions, seizures, and respiratory depression. If the ICP becomes so high that the brain stem starts to herniate through the base of the skull, the patient may display increased blood pressure, unresponsiveness, and pupillary changes.

Accommodations for Patients with Intraventricular Shunts

Although hydrocephalus is more common in infants, adults may develop it also. The speed with which the patient's symptoms develop as it relates to the intraventricular shunt depends on the type of problem. Infection usually takes a few days to develop, so symptoms will be more subtle in their onset. If the shunt causes bleeding beneath the outer meningeal layer (subdural bleed), the findings may also develop over a short course of time. If the etiology is occlusion of the shunt, the speed with which CSF accumulates and pressure builds will directly impact the clinical deterioration of the patient.

Key Points

If the patient with an intraventricular shunt is experiencing an altered mental status, gear treatment to supporting depressed or lost functions, especially airway ventilation, and oxygenation. Initiate rapid transport.

Objective 40-11

Describe accommodations and modifications required for patients who are terminally ill and describe the philosophy of hospice care.

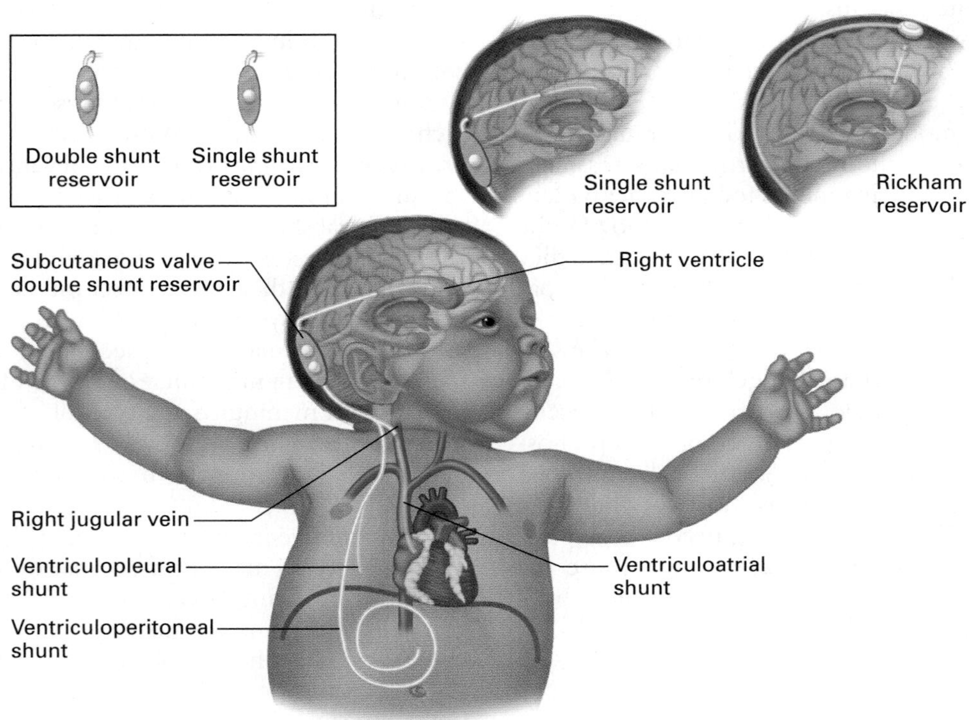

FIGURE 40-20 ✱ Intraventricular shunts allow excess cerebrospinal fluid to drain from the brain to a site in the neck, heart, pleural space, or abdomen, or into a reservoir beneath the scalp.

Commonly, the initial complaint seen with intraventricular shunt emergencies is confusion, difficulty with simple tasks, and headaches. As the problem continues, symptoms will worsen. The treatment is geared to supporting depressed or lost functions. First, manage the airway. Be alert for occlusion by the tongue if the mental status is diminished. If the breathing is found to be inadequate, provide positive pressure ventilation with oxygen. Keeping the patient in a lateral recumbent position will help maintain the airway. Rapidly transport the patient to the hospital. If the patient is a high priority, contact ALS to either meet you on-scene or intercept with you en route to the hospital.

▸ Terminally Ill Patients

Terminally ill patients have a disease process that is realistically expected to result in death, despite current medical treatment designed to halt or reverse the condition. *Terminal illness* is the medical term used to describe the actual disease process that results in the progressive deterioration causing death. Although the life expectancy of a terminally ill patient is generally considered to be 6 months or less, the estimate made by the patient's physician is not usually exact. In other words, a terminally ill patient may die of the disease process in less than 6 months or live beyond the 6-month estimate. Despite this, it is believed by both the physician and the patient that the course of the disease will certainly result in death.

Given the definition of terminal illness, there is no cure for the disease, but patients may still pursue medical interventions or therapies that minimize pain or discomfort during this final stage of their life. The term *palliative care* is used to describe medical interventions centered on reducing the severity of disease symptoms (not on reversing progression of the disease).

Hospice is a philosophy of care that is aimed at providing palliation of symptoms for the patients and sup-

Key Terms

terminally ill condition of an individual with a disease that is realistically expected to result in the death of the patient, despite medical treatment.

hospice a philosophy of care aimed at relief of symptoms for patients and support for their families during late stages of a terminal condition.

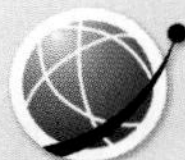

Media Resources

Go to www.bradybooks.com for mykit. Highlights:

- *Web Resource:* Health Care for Minority Populations
- *Web Resource:* Intimate Partner Violence
- *Web Resource:* Tracheostomy

port for their families. Commonly, patients who receive hospice care do so during the terminal stages of the following conditions:

- Cancer
- AIDS
- Alzheimer disease
- Cystic fibrosis
- Congestive heart failure
- COPD

These programs seek to alleviate symptoms, manage pain or discomfort, and provide a certain degree of control to the patients and their families during the final stage of life. Although hospice programs primarily work with the elderly, services are also provided to children with terminal diseases.

Accommodations for Terminally Ill Patients

The benefit of hospice programs is that they aim to make the final stages of one's life as comfortable as possible while preparing the family for the inevitable. This, however, does not mean that the EMT will not be faced with a difficult situation. For example, a family member or primary care provider may summon EMS when the patient nears death rather than contacting the hospice provider as instructed. Although rare, the patient's feelings or the family's feelings may change with the realization that death is imminent. It is important for the EMT to provide emotional support to both the patient and the family during this time and to determine clearly their intentions. The EMT will need to communicate with the patient's hospice program provider if the hospice does not already have a care provider at the patient's side to help determine the best course of action. Remember, the desire of the patient to not receive resuscitation does not mean the patient does not desire or need comfort care. If you transport the patient who is in a hospice program to the hospital, you should make all efforts needed to minimize additional discomfort or pain during transport as well as provide emotional support and reassurance.

ASSESSMENT Tips

It is not uncommon to encounter a hospice patient at the end of life who has accepted that death is imminent while the family is more frightened or in denial than the patient. Your emotional support to these families can be just as valuable as the palliative care you may be providing to the patient. ■

Not all patients who have a terminal illness receive hospice care, and the EMT cannot make an assumption one way or the other. You will need to communicate with the patient, the family, or the primary care provider about any advance directives that may be in place in the absence of a hospice program. Although this discussion often clarifies what you should do regarding resuscitation in the event of arrest, it does *not* mean that you need not provide comfort care and emotional support. In these situations, your ability to be compassionate far outweighs your clinical skills.

CHAPTER REVIEW

SUMMARY

During your career as an EMT, you will encounter patients with a variety of challenges, such as hearing or sight impaired, obesity, poverty, and homelessness. You must understand the special characteristics of these patients and variations in assessment findings and emergency care.

Home medical devices are becoming more commonplace. Primary care providers who are responsible for these patients are also becoming more knowledgeable about how to handle such devices. Never discount the intelligence of primary care providers. Use them as a valuable resource during your assessment and management of the patient.

Remember the reason that you are summoned to a patient who relies on any of these devices, and intervene with the equipment only if you identify a malfunction. Usually, your intervention will involve either shutting off or removing the medical device (especially those that provide nutrition, ongoing medication, or mechanical ventilation) if you are comfortable and knowledgeable about how to do so. Again, ask family members or the primary care provider for assistance if needed. The failure of medical equipment that replaces the airway and ventilations can easily result in death of the patient. In such a case, intervene quickly and support lost function while transporting the patient to the hospital.

Finally, do not become overwhelmed with the multitude or complexity of medical devices the patient may be using. Analyze each piece, ask questions, and intervene only when it is obvious that the equipment is malfunctioning and is detrimental to the patient's condition. Summon ALS early as needed, communicate with the receiving hospital early so they can prepare for your arrival, and carefully document all findings, care rendered, and medical equipment used on your prehospital care report.

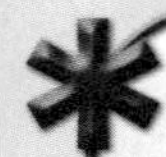

CASE STUDY FOLLOW-UP

SCENE SIZE-UP

You have been dispatched to the home of a 2-year-old male patient who has a diminished orientation according to the patient's mother. After ensuring scene safety you enter the home and are directed into the young boy's room. When you walk in you see a child lying in bed, wearing pajamas, covered with his blanket, and seemingly sleeping. The mother tells you that the boy has a "shunt in his brain" that was replaced just a week earlier. The history, according to the mother, is that the child's orientation had been diminishing and he had started to develop a fever.

PRIMARY ASSESSMENT

Your general impression is that the patient appears to be sleeping quietly in bed. As you approach him, you address him by his name but get no response. You call his name louder but he still does not open his eyes. As your partner goes around to the other side of the bed, you apply a light noxious stimulus with a trapezius pinch. The boy moans and his eyes flutter, but he does not wake up or move his extremities. You pinch again a little harder, and this time the boy's arm moves as if to try to push your hand away.

You listen to his airway and hear no sonorous or gurgling sounds. The rise and fall of his chest is normal, but the rate seems quick. You can palpate both central and peripheral pulses. They are strong and regular. The rate feels to be about 120 per minute. The skin is very warm to the touch and moist. Since the child's mental status appears to be altered but the airway and ventilations are currently adequate, your partner places a nonrebreather mask at 15 lpm. You categorize the patient as potentially unstable because of the diminished mental status.

SECONDARY ASSESSMENT

Since this change in mental status is not normal for this child, nor normal for a 2-year-old boy, you elect to perform a thorough but rapid secondary assessment. His pupils are equal and respond to light. Slight jugular vein distention is noted in the neck, but the child is lying supine. You can palpate the shunt that courses under the skin of the neck. The breath sounds are equal bilaterally. His abdomen is soft and no tenderness is noted. You find good pulses in all extremities, but he is tachycardic. You find no evidence of trauma anywhere on the body. You find no medical alert identification tag.

The patient's blood pressure is 94/54 mmHg. His heart rate is 118 per minute. Respirations are 26 per minute and of normal depth. His skin color is flushed, very warm to the touch, and moist. His SpO_2 reading was 98% on room air, and now it reads 100%. You record the vital signs.

During the secondary assessment, you gather a history. On questioning the mother, you learn that the patient has had an intraventricular shunt placed for "quite a while now" for "excessive water in the brain." You recognize this as probably the medical condition known as hydrocephalus. She further adds that his shunt was just replaced about a week ago because of his growing bigger, but ever since then his mental status has been gradually diminishing to the point where it is now. As you learn more about the patient's medications and allergies, your partner readies the cot. You carefully pick up the young child and carry him into the living room where the cot has been prepared. After properly securing him to the cot and ensuring the oxygen is still flowing normally, you begin transport to the hospital some 25 minutes away and contact your dispatch for an ALS intercept.

REASSESSMENT

En route to the hospital you continue to evaluate the patient's vital functions. His airway remains intact, breathing is still adequate, and his peripheral perfusion is normal. There has been no significant change in his mental status or vital signs during the transport. After reassessing the vitals, you document them on your computerized prehospital care report. The pulse oximeter is still reading 99 to 100%. ALS intercept occurs about 10 minutes out from the hospital and you resume transport to the hospital. En route, you converse with the ALS provider and you both conclude that either the patient is developing an infection in the brain secondary to the shunt placement, or perhaps the shunt is occluded and pressure in the brain is starting to rise.

As you arrive at the hospital, you prepare the patient for movement out of the ambulance. The patient's mental status has not changed; he still responds to deep noxious stimuli with purposeful motion. Vitals are stable and there has been no change in the patient's vital functions. You give the hospital an oral report of the patient's condition and help transfer him to the hospital bed. You complete your prehospital care report, restock the ambulance, and prepare for another call.

IN REVIEW

1. Identify and describe sensory problems commonly encountered in the prehospital environment.
2. Name some common emergencies the obese patient may suffer that would require EMS help.
3. Describe the medical care warranted for a patient with an occluded tracheostomy tube.
4. Explain why airway management is a major concern in the patient with a severe brain injury.
5. What are the most common reasons for a mechanical ventilator to fail?
6. Why might a patient have a VAD placed?
7. A CPAP machine would be used by what type of patient?
8. Describe alternative ways of ventilating a patient whose mechanical ventilator has failed.
9. Discuss the types and purposes of GI/GU devices commonly encountered.
10. If a patient has an intraventricular shunt placed, how might the patient present if it becomes occluded and stops draining excess CSF?

CRITICAL THINKING

You respond to a call for an unknown emergency at a residential address. On arrival at the scene, you are directed to a 68-year-old female in her bedroom, lying supine in a hospital bed. A loud beeping is coming from a mechanical ventilator sitting on a table beside the patient's bed. The ventilator is attached to a tracheostomy tube placed in her trachea. She is not alert, and you hear rattling sounds of mucus congestion coming from the ventilator circuit. The red light that is illuminated on the ventilator is signaling a high-pressure alarm. The distressed family on scene tells you quickly that the patient just came home from the hospital the day before. She was in the hospital because of a massive stroke and was placed on the ventilator there. She was brought home so the family could provide ongoing care, rather than placing her in a geriatric facility. The family, however, is not very familiar with the mechanical ventilator and became scared when it started to alarm.

1. What emergency care would you provide during the primary assessment?
2. Based on the signs, what condition do you suspect the patient is experiencing?
3. What in your opinion is causing the ventilator to alarm?
4. What type of care would you provide to this patient to support lost function?
5. Should this patient be transported to the hospital, and if so, why?

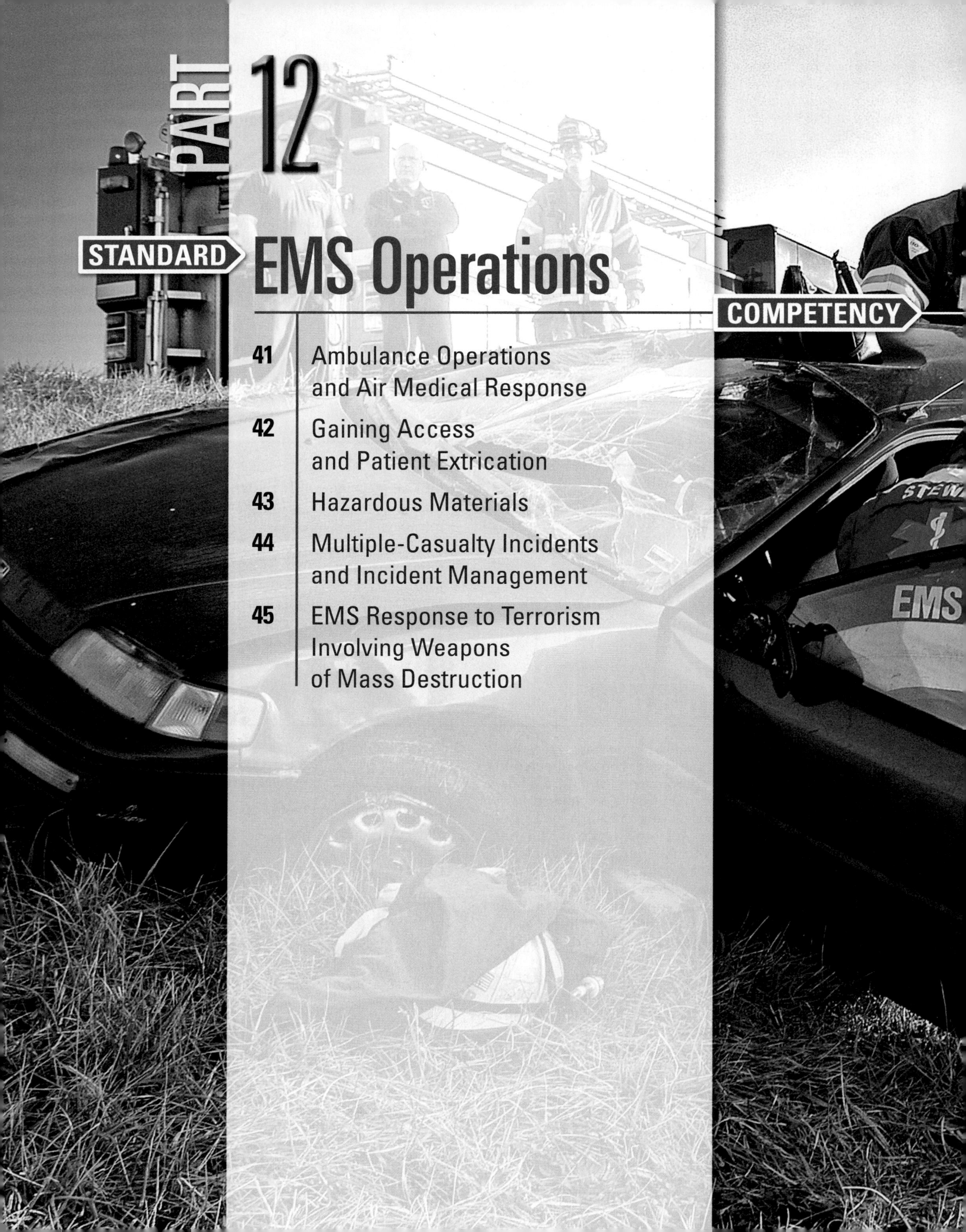

PART 12

STANDARD

EMS Operations

COMPETENCY

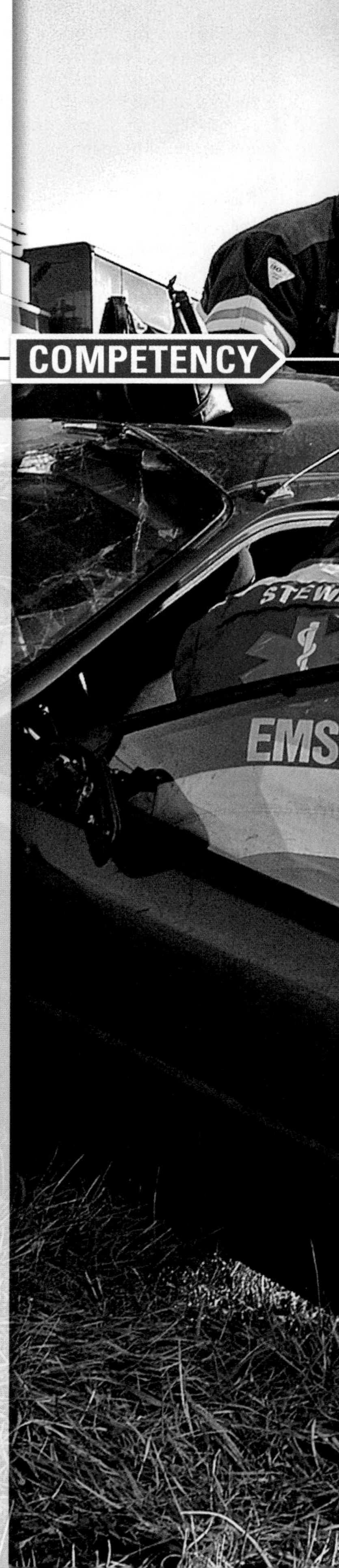

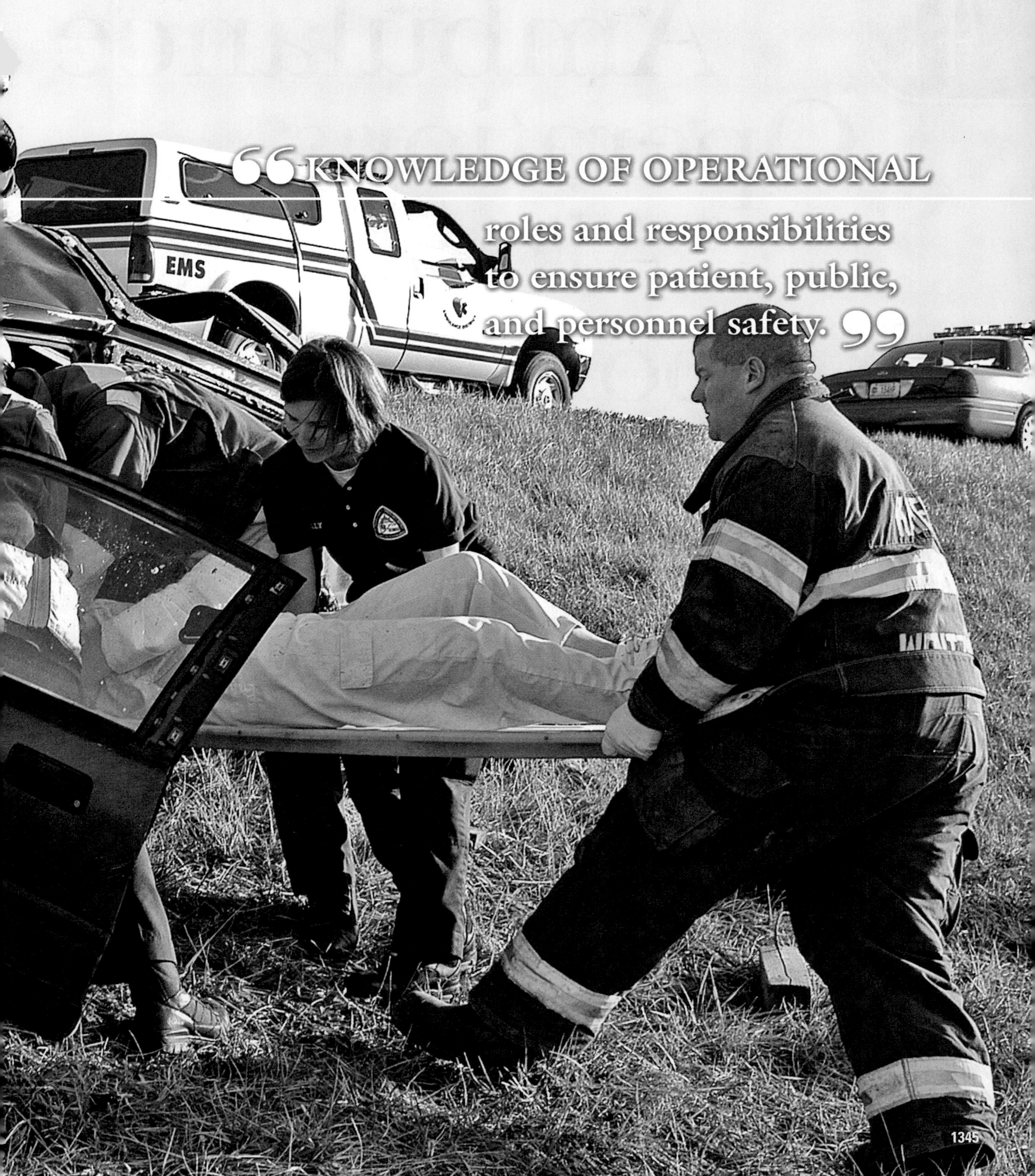

"KNOWLEDGE OF OPERATIONAL roles and responsibilities to ensure patient, public, and personnel safety."

CHAPTER 41

Ambulance Operations *and* Air Medical Response

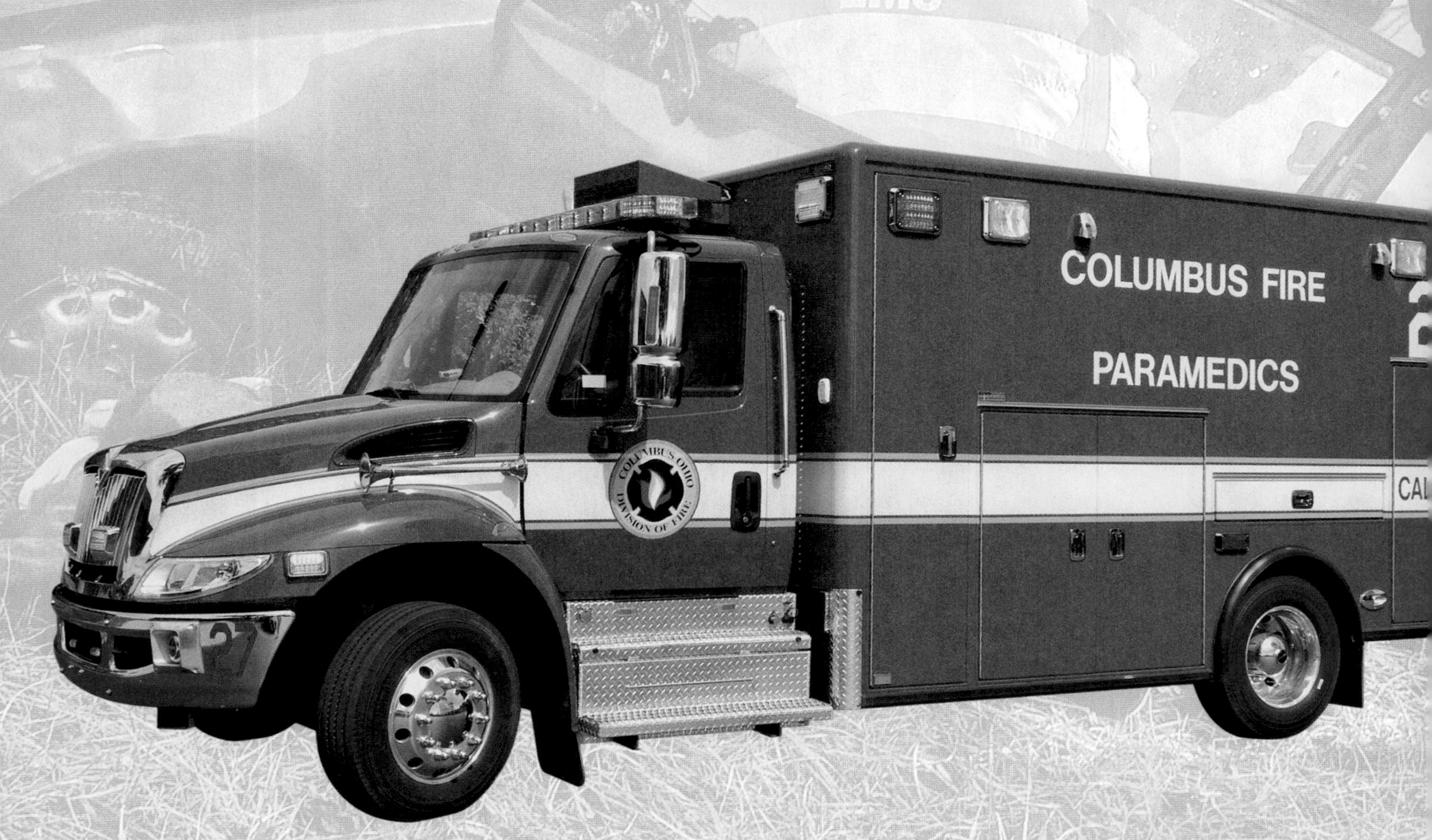

Navigation Guide

The following items provide an overview to the purpose and content of this chapter. The Standard and Competency are from the new National EMS Education Standards.

STANDARD **EMS Operations** (Content Area: Principles of Safely Operating a Ground Ambulance; Air Medical)

COMPETENCY Applies knowledge of operational roles and responsibilities to ensure patient, public, and personnel safety.

OBJECTIVES: After reading this chapter, you should be able to:

41-1. Describe the privileges afforded to EMTs operating emergency vehicles and the precautions that must be observed while using these privileges.
41-2. Give examples of habits and behaviors that improve driving safety.
41-3. Discuss factors that can affect your ability to maintain control while driving an ambulance.
41-4. Explain precautions that should be taken when driving an ambulance in inclement weather.
41-5. Explain precautions that should be taken when driving an ambulance at night.
41-6. Describe the appropriate use of emergency warning devices, such as lights and sirens.
41-7. Describe the safety precautions to be taken when working at scenes on and near roadways.
41-8. Give examples of the EMT's responsibilities during each of the major phases of an ambulance call.
41-9. Describe post-run actions that should be taken to reduce the spread of infection to you, your coworkers, and patients.
41-10. Discuss situations in which air medical transport should be considered, potential disadvantages of air medical transport, and guidelines for setting up a landing zone.
41-11. Describe the recommendations of the National Association of Emergency Medical Technicians with respect to EMT security and safety.
41-12. Explain precautions to avoid exposing yourself or others to increased levels of carbon monoxide associated with ambulance operations.

MEDIA RESOURCES: Please go to www.bradybooks.com to access mykit for this text. You will find quizzes, critical thinking scenarios, weblinks, animations, and videos related to this chapter—and much more. Look for online information on safe driving tips and on the FACE Program.

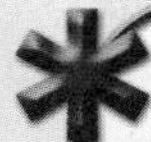

CASE STUDY

The Dispatch

Medic One—respond to the rest area at Interstate 80 and the Black Canyon Exit. You have a 33-year-old female patient with labor pains. Time out is 1511 hours.

En Route

You move quickly to your vehicle. Your partner is driving. You fasten your seat belt. The garage door opens. The engine starts. Your vehicle moves slowly and then picks up speed. Additional patient information from dispatch crackles over the radio. It's difficult to hear. You inhale deeply and tell yourself, "Relax." You are prepared. You begin to picture in your mind what you need to do and how you should perform throughout the ambulance call.

This chapter will provide you with information on how to prepare yourself, your equipment, medical supplies, and your vehicle for an ambulance run. Later, we will return to the case study and apply the steps learned.

Introduction

The ambulance is the vehicle that brings care to the patient in times of emergency and transports the patient to a medical receiving facility for follow-up care. It is a crucial part of the EMS system.

An ambulance should be a place of comfort and support to patients suffering from life-threatening problems. It should not pose additional hazards to them. But statistics tell a different story: There are approximately 5,000 ambulance crashes each year in the United States. On average, there is one fatality each week from an ambulance crash and many more serious injuries.

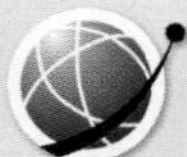

Media Resources
Go to www.bradybooks.com for mykit. Highlights:

- *Web Resource:* Safe Driving Tips
- *Video:* Body Substance Isolation and Equipment

Objective 41-1
Describe the privileges afforded to emergency vehicles and the precautions these privileges entail.

Key Points
At no time is it justified to operate an ambulance in a manner that jeopardizes anyone else.

To keep from adding to these statistics, the EMT must learn to drive an ambulance skillfully and safely. The process takes time; however, the regulations and guidelines can be learned before getting behind the wheel. This chapter describes how to operate an ambulance safely. It also details other procedures to help ensure the most efficient operation of a properly equipped ambulance.

Driving the Ambulance

As an EMT, you have the responsibility for getting an ambulance safely to the scene of an emergency and transporting patients safely in it to medical care. To drive an ambulance well, you need a combination of the right knowledge, skills, and attitude.

Laws, Regulations, and Ordinances

As an ambulance operator, you should be familiar with the laws and regulations that apply on both the state and local levels and consistently obey them. You have certain privileges under the law as the operator of an emergency vehicle, as do the operators of police vehicles and fire apparatus. At no time is it justified to operate an ambulance in a manner that jeopardizes anyone else. Remember that your first duty to your patient is to arrive at the scene—safely! After that, you must get your patient to definitive care carefully and safely.

While statutes in each state vary slightly, most states give you the privilege, with proper precautions, to do the following while driving the ambulance to an emergency:

- Exceed the speed limit posted for the area as long as you are not endangering lives or property.
- Drive the wrong way down a one-way street or drive down the opposite side of the road.
- Turn in any direction at any intersection.
- Park anywhere as long as you do not endanger lives or property.
- Leave the ambulance standing in the middle of a street or intersection.
- Cautiously proceed through a red light or red flashing signal.
- Pass other vehicles in no-passing zones.

In passing, you must first signal, ensure that the way is clear, and avoid endangering life and property by driving with due regard for the safety of others.

By law, you must meet several qualifications before you can exercise these privileges:

- You must have a valid driver's license. Most states mandate that you attend an approved driving course.
- You must be responding to an emergency of a serious nature.
- You must use warning devices—emergency lights, horns, and sirens—so that other vehicles on the road will be aware of you and have a chance to yield. You must use these devices in the manner prescribed by law.
- *You must exercise due regard for the safety of others.* You may cautiously move through a red light, but you must slow down while entering the intersection so that all traffic can stop to allow you to pass. You may park your ambulance anywhere to care for a patient, but you must not park it just over the crest of a hill on a busy highway unless you post flares and get a police officer or a volunteer to divert traffic out of your lane, and you must use good roadway safety practices, which are discussed later in the chapter. *The law states that if you do not exercise due regard for the safety of others, you are liable for the consequences.*
- Many EMS systems provide additional guidance. For instance, some specify that your top speed cannot be more than 10 miles per hour over the speed of traffic, which may or may not be the posted speed. This allows the emergency vehicle to overtake other moving traffic but promotes safer driving. In some areas, ambulances entering an intersection against the light must come to a complete stop before proceeding.

Be sure that you know the general vehicle code, the regulations for emergency vehicles, and your agency code. Also, know the qualifications in your state for operating an ambulance and be sure that you can qualify. Several states require special licenses and/or special training for ambulance operators.

Driving Excellence

An excellent ambulance operator understands the capabilities and limitations of his vehicle, evaluates weather and road conditions quickly and accurately, appraises and

Objective 41-3
Discuss factors that can affect ability to maintain control while driving an ambulance.

Objective 41-2
Give examples of habits and behaviors that improve driving safety.

Key Points
A number of factors other than speed affect your ability to control the ambulance.

responds to traffic conditions quickly and appropriately, and minimizes risk and discomfort to other members of the crew and to the patient. Notice that fast, dramatic driving is not part of the definition.

Basics of Good Driving

Always wear seat belts when you drive the ambulance. Make sure other team members wear theirs as well.

Hold the steering wheel with both hands at all times. One hand should be in the 9 o'clock and the other in the 3 o'clock position. In turning, one hand pulls while the other slides, paralleling the pulling hand's position. Neither hand should pass the 12 or 6 o'clock positions to prevent them from becoming tangled. When you reach these limits, the opposite hand begins to grip the wheel and the first hand slides.

You need to practice enough with your ambulance that you are familiar with how it accelerates and decelerates, the kind of space it requires for its fenders and bumpers, how it brakes, and how it corners.

When driving an ambulance, you must recognize and respond to changes in weather and in road conditions. Adjust your speed to allow for decreased visibility at night and in fog and road handling during rain, snow, and ice storms.

During transport, select the route best suited for safe travel—this is not necessarily the shortest route. Avoid schools, railroad crossings, detours, construction sites, bridges, tunnels, and similar trouble areas whenever you can, even if it means driving a few extra miles. If you are unfamiliar with the roads in your city or area, get a detailed local map and study it. Patrolling will help you get a feel for topography. Keep informed about roads undergoing repair or new building sites, and avoid them when you can. Select an alternative route during rush-hour traffic. If you are responding to a traffic collision that can back up traffic on a busy highway, select an alternative route to avoid being caught in the traffic jam.

Maintain a safe following distance. Use headlights to improve your vehicle's visibility. Exercise caution when using red lights and the siren.

Maintaining Control

For vehicle control, remember the rule about speed: Go the posted limit unless the situation is critical. Speed can complicate patient care by providing a rougher ride, decrease ambulance stability, and risk the safety of everyone in the ambulance (Figure 41-1*).

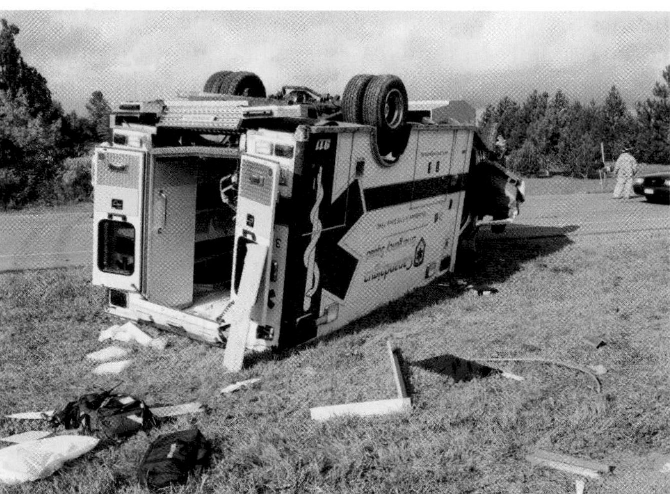

FIGURE 41-1 * A number of factors can cause an operator to lose control of the ambulance. (Courtesy Canandaigua Fire and Rescue)

A number of factors other than speed affect your ability to control the ambulance, and you need to be alert to them to stay in constant control as you drive.

Braking Sudden braking may result in loss of control. In older ambulances without antilock braking systems, the brakes will cause wheels to lock, and you may skid dangerously. In these vehicles, you should pump your brakes slowly and smoothly. Newer ambulances typically have an antilock braking system in which the brakes should be applied firmly and steadily, not pumped. Never brake on a curve. Brake when going into the curve and gradually accelerate when going out. When decelerating, rest your foot lightly on the brake. Your stopping distance is the time it takes you to react plus your braking time.

Driver Distractions When driving an ambulance, it is important to minimize distractions as much as possible. Always remember that those driving the vehicles around you may be distracted by cell phone use, loud music, conversations, eating and drinking, or a number of other things. When you are driving an ambulance, you are subject to all of these same distractions, as well as additional ones such as global positioning systems, mobile computers, mobile radios, and the operation of the lights and siren. Particularly when driving in an emergency situation, you must focus your attention on the road. Your primary goal is to arrive safely at your destination.

Driving Alone When transporting a patient to the hospital, you must operate the vehicle without any support

Thinking Critically

You are transporting a critical patient to the hospital, knowing that time is of the essence for this patient, when you see the gates coming down at the railroad grade crossing. What should you do? (Discuss what the alternatives might be if there is such a crossing in your service area.)

Key Points

When a school bus is stopped with red lights flashing, always be prepared for the possibility that a child will dart out to cross the road to or from the bus.

from other crew members, who will be in the patient compartment. In these cases, maintain focus on the safe operation of the ambulance and the safe transportation of your crew and patient. Do not allow yourself to be distracted by operation of the lights and siren, communications equipment, global positioning systems, or other activities within the ambulance.

Fatigue Driving while fatigued greatly increases the risk of an accident. Proper rest and nutrition can decrease this risk. When on duty, you must be physically prepared for any driving situations that may arise.

Railroads You may encounter a railroad crossing and have to wait for a long train to crawl along the tracks. Keep calm and monitor the patient. If there is simply no way to get around the train, such as an underpass or overpass within a reasonable distance, wait it out instead of trying inappropriate stunts. Plan an alternative route when you can.

School Buses Be especially alert when approaching a stopped school bus with its red lights flashing. You must always be prepared for the possibility that a child will dart out across the road heading to or from the bus. Laws regarding ambulances and school buses vary from state to state. In some, an ambulance must come to a full stop and remain stopped until signaled ahead by the bus driver. Follow your state law.

Bridges and Tunnels There is little room for passing on bridges or in tunnels. If you are in heavily congested traffic near a bridge or tunnel, consider an alternative route. If there is none, try to get control of the situation before you enter the bridge or tunnel. Remember that you probably will not be able to pass, so go with the flow of traffic at a safe speed until you emerge. Also be sure the height of the bridge or tunnel will accommodate the height of the ambulance.

Day of the Week You can expect less traffic on weekends than on workdays in most areas. Traffic around shopping centers is heaviest on Saturdays, to and from resort areas on Fridays and Sundays, and on commuter routes or in urban and industrialized areas on Monday through Friday. Keep in mind what kind of traffic you are likely to encounter and, when possible, adjust your route accordingly.

Time of Day Rush-hour traffic is more congested in most urban centers than rural areas, so plan accordingly. Watch for school zones and industrial plant shift changes.

Road Surface Always be on the lookout for potholes and bumps. Your goal is to give your patient the smoothest ride possible. The two inner lanes on a four-lane highway are generally the smoothest. At times, it may be necessary to drive the ambulance on unpaved roadways in order to get to the scene of an emergency. In these situations, decrease speed and exercise increased caution.

Backing Up Many ambulance collisions occur when the ambulance is backing up. Use all resources (e.g., mirrors, EMT in the rear of the ambulance) and back up slowly and carefully.

Higher Speeds At higher speeds, be alert to the following:

- Be especially careful on curves that lead into population pockets (a town or school), curves that lead to intersections, and curves that crest hills. Practice negotiating curves in the ambulance during the early mornings when there is little traffic. Get a good idea of what speed you need to get around the curve safely.
- Brake to the proper speed before you enter a curve. Enter the curve at the outside (or the "high" part), and start turning as early as possible. Go only as fast as feels comfortable while in the curve. Do not accelerate or brake in the curve—the scrubbing action of the tires will slow the ambulance down sufficiently. It is dangerous to brake after you have entered the curve, so make sure that you decelerate to a safe speed before entering.
- Accelerate carefully and gradually as you leave the curve. Too quick an acceleration can cause you to lose control.
- Keep your exit from the curve slow and steady.
- When going down a long hill, use a lower gear instead of riding your brake to maintain control.
- Always use a smooth braking motion. Your stopping distance increases dramatically as your speed increases; allow for it.

Aggressive Drivers It is important to remember that driving an ambulance does not necessarily change the habits of other drivers on the roadways. Aggressive drivers, in particular, can pose a significant increased risk to you and your vehicle. If you notice another vehicle weaving in and out of traffic, speeding, or otherwise driving in an aggressive or erratic manner, exercise extreme caution when approaching or passing that vehicle. Aggressive drivers are often distracted and may not even notice the presence of the ambulance. When in doubt, it is always

Key Points
Always approach an intersection with caution, even when you have the green light. Watch for other motorists who may be running the red light and for pedestrians. Maintain a safe distance from any emergency vehicle that may be in front of you.

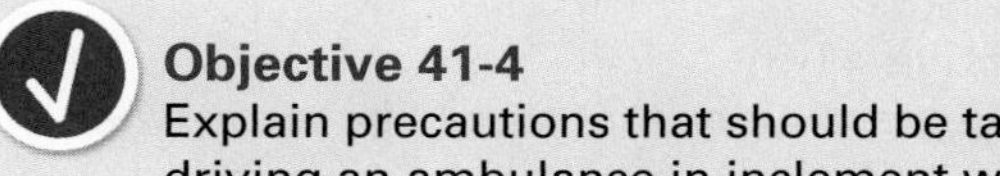

Objective 41-4
Explain precautions that should be taken when driving an ambulance in inclement weather.

best to slow down, assess the situation, and choose the safest method for continuing to your destination, even if that means choosing a different route of travel to avoid dangerous roadway situations.

Escorts Using a police or other emergency vehicle escort en route to a response or the hospital should be a last resort. It is dangerous, not only to the escort, but also to the EMT driver, to the patient in the ambulance, and to others on the road. All hazards associated with ambulance driving are doubled when an escort is involved, because you are the second vehicle through an intersection and motorists may expect only one.

Use an escort only if you are unfamiliar with how to get to the hospital or if you do not think that you can find the patient's location. Allow for a safe distance between the escort vehicle and your ambulance.

Intersection Collisions The most common collisions in which ambulances are involved are those at intersections. There are three main causes of intersection collisions:

- A motorist approaches the intersection just as the light is changing; he does not want to sit through the red light, so he sails through the intersection. Always slow down at each intersection to make sure that it is clear. If you are crossing against the light, come to a complete stop and proceed only when all traffic is clear or appropriately stopped.
- There are two emergency vehicles when motorists expect only one. Maintain a safe distance between your vehicle and the emergency vehicle in front of you, but follow closely enough so that the motorist can see both of you in the same glance. Do not use the same siren mode on both vehicles. Whenever you are using the emergency privileges that allow you to suspend traffic regulations, always use your flashers and siren for the fullest possible warning to the public. In some states, use of your siren when you are driving in the emergency mode is mandated by law.
- Vehicles waiting at an intersection may block your view of pedestrians in the crosswalk. Again, slow down and anticipate people in the crosswalk. Come to a complete stop if you are unsure if pedestrians are entering the intersection.

Driving in Inclement Weather

Bad weather affects your ability to control your ambulance. Stopping on wet pavement takes approximately twice the distance as stopping on dry pavement. On ice or sleet, it takes you five times the distance to stop. Leave adequate space between you and the vehicle in front of you in any kind of weather. Utilize the following precautions for specific weather situations.

Rainy or Wet Weather About six times more people are killed on wet roads than on snowy and icy roads combined. Roads are most slippery as a rainstorm begins. When the road is wet, your vehicle can hydroplane—that is, the front tires literally lift so that the vehicle is riding on a film of water rather than on the pavement itself. Hydroplaning can begin at speeds as low as 35 miles per hour if the tires are worn. Do the following when driving on wet roads:

- Keep your mirrors cleared of water.
- Avoid sudden braking and sudden moves of the steering wheel.
- If you are about to go through a large standing puddle, slow down and turn on your wipers before you hit the water. As you leave the water, tap the brake lightly a few times to dry it out. If the ambulance pulls to one side, pump the brake slowly and smoothly to dry the brake out.
- If you begin to hydroplane, hold the wheel steady, take your foot from the accelerator, and gently pump the brake. If you turn the wheel from side to side, or jam on the brake, you will probably skid.

Winter Driving Sleet, freezing rain, packed snow, and ice decrease visibility and increase skidding. Powder snow and gusty winds can create a total whiteout with zero visibility for several hundred yards. To ensure safety, do the following:

- Make sure that your engine is tuned, your heater and defroster are in good working order, and your battery is charged.
- Carry emergency weather equipment—chains, a shovel, sand, booster cables, and a towing device.
- Equip the ambulance with studded snow tires if you can. Chains are the best insurance against skidding. Follow local and state protocols and laws.
- Stay aware of the temperature. Wet ice and freezing rain, the most hazardous road conditions, occur between 28°F and 40°F. Bridges and overpasses freeze sooner than road surfaces.
- Avoid sudden movements of the steering wheel and sudden braking.

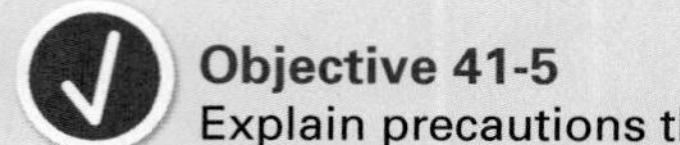

Objective 41-5
Explain precautions that should be taken when driving an ambulance at night.

Key Points
The acuity of night vision varies widely among individuals.

Fog, Mist, Dust Storms, Smog When visibility is poor, do the following:

- Slow down but avoid decelerating suddenly.
- Watch the road ahead and behind carefully for other cars that are traveling slowly.
- Turn on your lights, regardless of the time of day, and use your wipers. (Never use the high beams on your headlights. The reflection of the high beams from the fog will actually reduce your ability to see.) Even if the lights do not improve your ability to see ahead, they will make it possible for other motorists to see you better.
- If you are traveling 15 miles per hour or more below the speed limit, use four-way flashers. (These may not be legal in some states.) Use the four-way flashers if you pull off the road and stop.
- Use the defroster to keep as much fog as possible off the inside of the windshield.
- If you need to slow down, tap your brake pedal several times so that the flash of your brake lights will warn motorists behind you.
- Fog can occur suddenly, and patches of greater density may appear. Vehicles in front may brake suddenly or come to a complete stop when encountering a thicker patch of fog. Be alert for vehicles in front of you.

Driving at Night

While only about one-third of all collisions occur at night, more than half of the fatalities from collisions stem from nighttime driving. In fact, based on miles driven, there are two and a half times more fatal collisions at night than during the day (Figure 41-2*). This is because less light is available and vision is restricted. Night vision varies considerably among people. Older people generally cannot see well in the dark, and eyestrain can substantially reduce night vision. Bright light, such as lightning or high-beam headlights, can cause temporary blindness at night.

Headlights on low beams illuminate the roadside for about 150 feet. On high beams, visibility will be 350–400 feet. At 55 miles per hour, it takes 4.5 seconds to cover 350 feet. For night driving, control speed so that your stopping range is within headlight range.

To improve your visibility and the ability of others to see you, do the following:

- Make sure that your ambulance has quartz-halogen headlights, which provide much more light to the road.

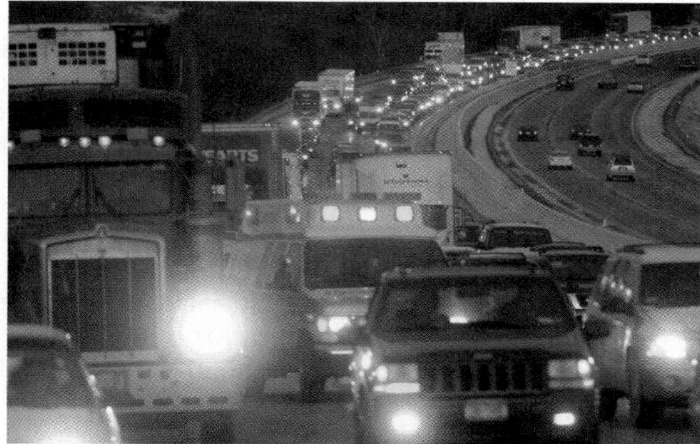

FIGURE 41-2 * Take extra care when driving at night. (© Mark C. Ide)

- Have your headlights on whenever you are traveling in an emergency.
- Keep your headlights clean and properly aimed. Check them each day before your shift begins. If the weather is bad, especially if there is sleet or snow, stop as necessary during your shift to clean debris off your headlights.
- Replace burned-out bulbs immediately.
- Dim your high beams within 500 feet of an approaching vehicle or within 300 feet of a vehicle in front of you.
- Never stare into the high beams of another car; guide your ambulance by watching the right edge of the road.
- Do not flick your high beams up and down to remind another driver to dim his brights—it can blind him temporarily.
- Never use high beams when going into a curve.
- Keep your windshield clean, inside and out. Keep a bottle of windshield or glass cleaner in the ambulance for mirrors and interior windshields.
- Keep your instrument panels dim.
- Keep your eyes moving; avoid focusing on any one object.
- If the washing solution under your hood does not leave the glass clean after ten wiper cycles, replace the blades or use a stronger concentration of washing fluid.
- Be sure that you are rested before you begin a night driving shift. Between 11:00 P.M. and 3:00 A.M., be par-

Thinking Critically

When you are driving your own vehicle, how do you generally react to warning signals from an ambulance? What reactions have you observed from other drivers? Why do you think individuals might react differently to warning signals?

Objective 41-6

Describe the appropriate use of emergency warning devices, such as lights and sirens.

ticularly alert for intoxicated or drowsy drivers. If you notice erratic speeds, weaving across lines, or delayed starts at intersections, use extreme care in passing.

▶ Warning Devices

Ambulances are equipped with a variety of warning devices. The use of these devices may save some time when responding to a call or when transporting a patient to definitive care. However, they may also increase the risk to ambulance personnel, patients, and the general public. Always take the increased risk of warning device usage into consideration, and weigh it against the benefit of saving a few minutes in transit time. Most agencies, and many counties and states, have specific protocols for use of these devices. Remember that they are only a means of requesting the right of way from others on the road and do not give the ambulance any special rights or guarantee of clear traffic. Due regard for the safety of others must still be exercised at all times, particularly when using warning devices. Following are some general guidelines and suggestions for the use of warning devices.

Colors and Markings

Ambulance colors and markings are an aid to traffic safety and reduce the need for excessive dependence on lights and sirens. An early U.S. Department of Transportation (DOT)/EMS study, "Ambulance Design Criteria" by the National Academy of Sciences, recommended a nationwide system of specific colors and markings. Later, the General Services Administration and DOT developed and published federal specifications for ambulances (1974:KKK-1822). The colors and markings are typically designed to provide quick identification that the vehicle is an ambulance and also to maximize visibility in traffic (Figure 41-3*).

The standard color is white; the markings are an orange stripe running around the body, blue lettering, and the "Star of Life" symbol. It is recommended that any added lettering be kept below the orange stripe so as not to distract from the basic markings. For maximum effectiveness, these standard colors and markings should not be duplicated on vehicles that are not ambulances.

Warning Lights and Emergency Lights

Activate emergency lights on the ambulance at all times when responding to an emergency call. Lights should be used even when you are not using the siren. You should also turn on your headlights during the daytime—in some situations, the warning lights on top of the vehicle are not noticeable because they blend in with traffic lights, signs, Christmas decorations, building colors, and tail lights of vehicles traveling in the opposite direction.

Placement of the ambulance emergency lights on the vehicle is very important. They should be high enough to cast a beam above the traffic. Lower lights are needed to be visible in the rearview mirror of the car ahead of you.

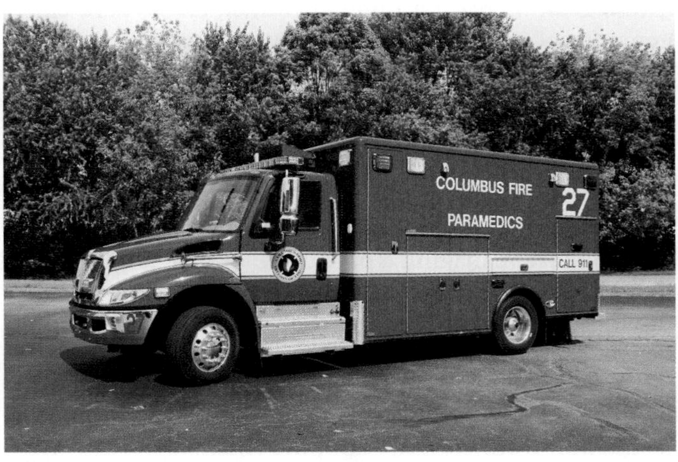

(a)

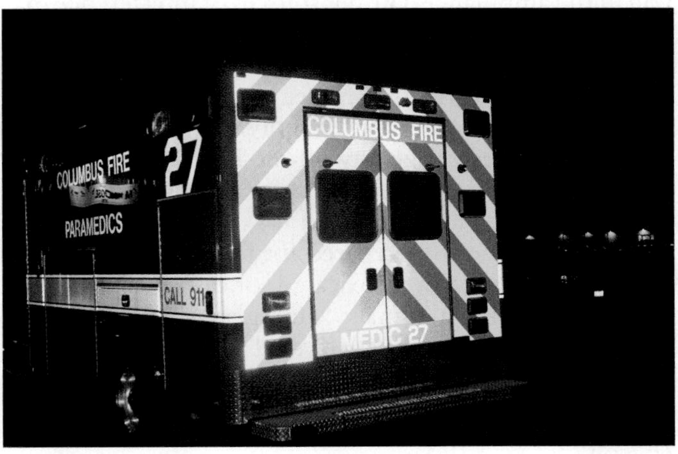

(b)

FIGURE 41-3 * **(a)** Colors and markings are typically designed to provide quick identification that the vehicle is an ambulance and **(b)** to maximize visibility in traffic.

Key Points
Working in or near moving traffic poses a high risk. EMS personnel must set up an environment to protect themselves, and wear high-visibility apparel, when working on or near a roadway.

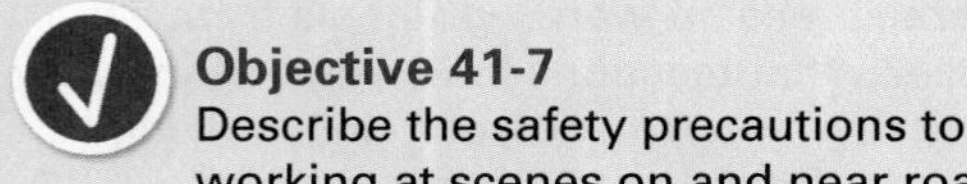

Objective 41-7
Describe the safety precautions to be taken when working at scenes on and near roadways.

When an ambulance has strobe lights, use them with emergency lights that flash or revolve with a longer duration. White lights can be seen from a longer distance than red or blue, especially at sunrise or sunset. They can also be seen more effectively when wet streets are reflecting.

Headlights are a part of the emergency lighting system and should be on whenever you are traveling in an emergency. Specially wired headlights that flash alternately are also effective in gaining attention. (These are not legal in some states—check local protocol.) You can use a spotlight to get the attention of a driver who has not noticed you, but do not panic him. Quickly flash the light across the driver's rearview mirror so that it gets his attention but is gone before he looks in the mirror. The glare could blind him or oncoming traffic, so be careful.

Use only minimal lighting during heavy fog or when you are parked. Use your emergency lights only when needed, such as when the patient's condition requires rapid transport.

Using Your Siren

Even if you are operating your flashing lights and sirens, do not assume that drivers are aware of you unless they look up to check their interior rearview mirror, look to the left to check the exterior rearview mirror, pull over, or stop.

The insulation in newer automobiles can reduce the interior decibel level of an approaching siren by 35–40 percent when parked. In motion, the noise of the motor, air-conditioner/heater, and radio in the automobile may make the siren completely inaudible. (This also applies to you in the ambulance!) Other sources of interference may be conversation, pelting rain, dense shrubbery or trees, buildings, and thunder. If the driver is wearing headphones, talking on a cell phone, inattentive, or hearing-disabled, your problem is even more severe. Some drivers may not even recognize a two-tone Klaxon as a siren.

Never pull directly behind a car and blast your siren. The driver may panic and slam on the brakes or swerve into another lane. Be prepared for the irrational maneuvers of inexperienced, intoxicated, or disoriented drivers.

Since the siren signals "emergency," it can create emotional stress (as well as physical stress from the noise level) for your patient. This is another reason for using your siren sparingly. Always let your patient know before you activate the siren.

Be aware of the siren's effect on you. Even if you can normally drive your own car or the ambulance flawlessly, the siren can have a bizarre effect on your ability to drive the ambulance safely. Studies have shown that ambulance operators tend to increase their speed about 15 miles per hour when the siren is going—an increase that sometimes takes them out of the limits of safe speeds. Some drivers are easily hypnotized by the siren and are unable to negotiate curves, turns, and obstacles; this hypnotic trance makes it seem as though the siren itself were controlling the vehicle. The siren can also prevent you from hearing sirens or horns of other emergency vehicles responding to the same or other incidents.

Follow your state laws and local protocols regarding siren use.

Using Your Air Horn

Avoid overuse of the air horn, but consider it when you need to clear traffic quickly. You can use the air horn with or without the siren, depending on your state law and local protocol. Do not sound your horn when you are close to other vehicles—it may frighten a driver and cause him to slam on the brakes or swerve. (The air horn may, however, be used safely much closer to other cars than may your siren.) Do not assume that other drivers can hear or will heed your horn.

Roadway Incident Scene Safety

There is an increasing number of incidents where emergency response personnel are severely injured or killed while attending to patients on a roadway. These incidents occur not only on freeways and highways with fast moving traffic but also on residential and city streets. You expose yourself to a high risk when you are working in or near moving traffic. EMS personnel must set up an environment so that they are best protected from injury whenever they are managing a patient on or near a roadway.

The same characteristics that make drivers hazardous to you while you are driving the ambulance on an emergency response also make them a hazard while you are on the scene in moving traffic. Factors such as vision impairment, inexperienced drivers, loud music, cell phone use, distraction from conversation, inclement weather, intoxication, medical conditions that impair reflexes, and high speed can make these drivers and vehicles a significant threat to you on the scene of a roadway incident. Nighttime incidents are even more hazardous because of the reduction in visibility and a reduction in the reaction time of drivers.

High-Visibility Apparel

A recently approved federal law requires all EMTs and other rescue personnel responding to accidents or other emergencies on or near a roadway to wear approved high-visibility apparel in an attempt to reduce the incidence of injury to emergency responders.

The American National Standards Institute (ANSI) and International Safety Equipment Association (ISEA) created the standard ANSI/ISEA 107-2004, American National Standard for High-Visibility Safety Apparel and Headwear. Three classes of garments were established:

- **Class 1.** Designed for workers in parking lots and other areas with traffic flow moving at less than 25 mph
- **Class 2.** Designed for personnel whose attention is diverted from traffic or where the traffic flow is moving at 25 mph or greater
- **Class 3.** Designed for personnel whose work greatly diverts their attention from the roadway and where they are at serious risk from hazards created by moving vehicles

The ANSI/ISEA 207-2006 American National Standard for High-Visibility Public Safety Vests (PSV) was approved to increase the visibility of emergency personnel on the roadway and to reduce the incidence of roadway hazards. The newer standard made significant changes to standard class garments to accommodate the public safety responder. The PSV has the same retro-reflective material as the Class 2 vest and nearly the same amount of fluorescent material. The PSV includes breakaway features, specific vest dimensions to allow for fit over turnout gear, and color-specific markings to allow for differentiation between law enforcement, fire, and EMS personnel.

Currently, the Code of Federal Regulations requires all emergency personnel who are exposed to traffic within the right-of-way of a highway that receives federal funding to wear high-visibility safety apparel that meets the Class 2 or 3 standards of ANSI/ISEA 107-2004 or the Public Safety Vest standard ANSI/ISEA 207-2006.

Safety Benchmarks

According to the University of Extrication *Safe Parking Standard Operating Procedures* by Ron Brown, there are certain safety procedures, or "safety benchmarks," that you can practice at the scene of a roadway incident to lessen your chances of becoming a casualty of the scene. They are:

- **Do not trust approaching traffic.** Approaching traffic may not be aware of the scene ahead or may be distracted and not paying attention to any warning lights, cones, or other markers.
- **Do not turn your back to approaching traffic.** Always position yourself so that you can see oncoming traffic when walking to and from the scene or while working on scene. If that is not possible, use a spotter to continuously monitor the traffic and notify you immediately of any unsafe or irregular traffic flow.
- **Position the first arriving emergency vehicle to create a block and a physical barrier between upstream traffic and the scene.** Using a vehicle as a block will provide some protection to those working on the scene. The wheels of the vehicle should be turned away from the scene. Block at least one additional lane and block the most critical lane or the lane in which there is the highest volume of traffic. Ambulances should be positioned so that personnel are protected when loading the patient. Park the ambulance in the safe zone of other blocking vehicles, and face the loading area away from the closet lane of traffic. Load patients only while in a protected zone area.
- **Wear appropriate personal protective equipment and ANSI high-visibility vests.** Federal law requires EMTs to wear approved high-visibility vests. By doing so, you will be more visible to oncoming traffic and better protected.
- **At nighttime, turn off vision-impairing lights, including headlights and spotlights, on emergency vehicles that are positioned to oncoming traffic.** The high-visibility lights, especially white lights, may blind or confuse oncoming traffic.
- **Use other emergency vehicles, such as police and fire apparatus, to initially slow down and redirect the flow of traffic.** When arriving on the scene of an incident that potentially involves critically injured or ill patients, there may not be enough time to set up traffic control devices to slow down and redirect the flow of traffic. Emergency vehicles could be positioned to do so until other units and personnel arrive on the scene to provide better traffic flow control.
- **Use advance warning signs and other traffic control measures upstream of the scene to reduce the speed of the oncoming traffic.** Advance warning signs and other traffic control devices should be used to slow the speed of traffic approaching the scene.
- **Use traffic cones for traffic control.** Traffic cones can be used to alert motorists and divert the flow of traffic away from the scene.
- **Assign a person to monitor oncoming traffic.** Assign an emergency responder to monitor the oncoming traffic and to immediately sound an alarm to notify you of any motorist who deviates from the traffic control measures.
- **Uphill/upwind.** When approaching an unknown roadway incident that may involve hazardous materials,

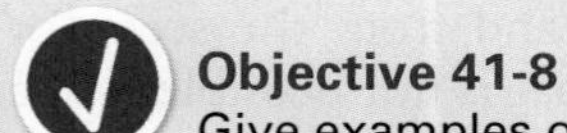

Objective 41-8
Give examples of the EMT's responsibilities during each of the major phases of an ambulance call.

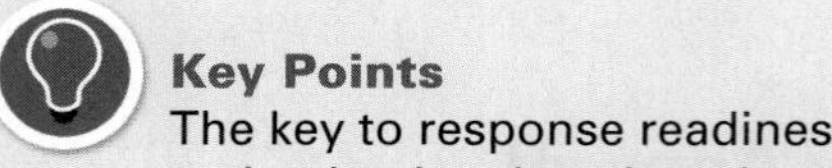

Key Points
The key to response readiness is a properly maintained and equipped ambulance.

it is always best to place your vehicle uphill and upwind from the scene to avoid potential contamination from leaking or airborne chemical or other hazards.

By taking some traffic control measures to protect yourself, your partner, the patients, and other personnel at the scene of a roadway incident, you may prevent an injury or death.

Phases of an Ambulance Call

The major phases of an ambulance call are:

1. Daily prerun vehicle and equipment preparation
2. Dispatch
3. En route to the scene
4. At the scene
5. En route to the receiving facility
6. At the receiving facility
7. En route to the station
8. Post run

Daily Prerun Preparation

The key to response readiness is a properly maintained and equipped ambulance. Having a vehicle ready to respond at all times and in all conditions and equipped with all necessary supplies will ensure that you can reach, care for, and transport your patients.

Ambulance Maintenance

Basic ambulance maintenance should include oil and filter changes, transmission and differential checks, wheel bearing check, brake check, and tie rod end inspection.

A comprehensive and regularly scheduled preventive vehicle maintenance schedule is essential. Benefits of a professional vehicle maintenance and inspection schedule include:

- Decreased vehicle downtime
- Improved response times to the scene
- Safer emergency and nonemergency responses
- Improved transport times to the medical facility
- Safer patient transports to the medical facility

You should know and practice your service's policies and procedures for reporting and correcting vehicle problems. Do not be afraid to take personal responsibility for ensuring that your vehicle is fit for duty. Remember, proper care for your ambulance is part of proper care for your patients and helps to ensure the safety of you and your crew.

Daily Inspection of Vehicle

Inspect the vehicle systems daily (EMT Skills 41-1). Most ambulance systems have a checklist of the items to be checked, which will typically include the items listed in Table 41-1.

TABLE 41-1 Daily Ambulance Inspection

Items Typically Included in a Daily Ambulance Inspection Checklist
Fuel
Oil
Fluid circulation system
Batteries
Brakes
Tires and wheels
Shoreline power connectors
Headlights
Brake lights
Turn signals
Emergency lights
Wipers
Horn
Siren
Windows
Door closing and latching devices
Power systems
Air-conditioning, heating, and ventilation systems
Radiator hoses and fan belts
Seat belts
Dash lights
Radio
Supplies
Interior and exterior cleanliness

Your service should have a clear protocol for reporting problems with vehicles, taking them out of service if they are deemed unsafe, and performing regular service and maintenance. Legally, you may be within your rights to refuse to use a vehicle that you have reason to believe is unsafe; and incidentally, you may be legally liable for damage caused by a malfunctioning ambulance if you are aware of the problem.

Ambulance Equipment

Your ambulance must contain supplies and equipment for handling medical emergencies, injuries, extrications, and childbirth. Supplies and equipment should be checked each day and restocked, cleaned, or maintained after each run. Table 41-2 lists supplies and equipment as identified in the EMT curriculum. All equipment and supplies located in the ambulance must be properly secured to prevent them from becoming projectiles and endangering personnel and patients. This applies to equipment within the cab area, as well as the rear compartment and cabinets.

Personnel

A properly equipped and maintained ambulance is important to emergency prehospital care. Properly trained personnel to operate the ambulance and make optimum use of its equipment are even more important. Staffing requirements for ambulances vary among states and localities. In some states, one EMT in the patient compartment is considered the minimum standard; however, two are preferred in some situations involving critically injured or ill patients. Follow your state laws and local protocols about staffing.

TABLE 41-2 Basic Ambulance Supplies

Medical Supplies
Basic supplies
Patient transfer equipment
Airways
Suction equipment
Artificial (positive pressure) ventilation devices
Oxygen inhalation equipment
Automated external defibrillator (AED)
Basic wound care supplies
Splinting supplies
Childbirth supplies
Medications
Nonmedical Supplies
Personal protective equipment (Standard Precautions)
High-visibility safety vests
Preplanned routes, comprehensive street maps

Dispatch

A message from the communications center will start you on your run. The communications component of the EMS system has been discussed in greater detail in Chapter 5, "Communication." The call taker will usually have performed the first assessment of the situation when receiving a call. The dispatcher should provide you with the following information:

- Location of the call
- Nature of the call
- Name, location, and callback number of the caller
- Location of the patient or patients at the scene
- Number of patients (if more than one) and the severity of the problem
- Any other special problems or circumstances that may be pertinent

Write this information down so you can refer to it. Use it to prepare yourself physically and mentally for the call. Ask the dispatcher to repeat or restate information if anything is unclear.

En Route to the Scene

Your ambulance is checked and ready to respond. The vehicle's medical and nonmedical equipment and supplies are clean and operational. You receive a call. Follow these guidelines on your way to the scene:

- Before departure, quickly check the vehicle to make sure outside compartment doors are closed and secure, external shoreline cords are disconnected, and any jump kits are retrieved and properly stowed.
- Fasten your seat belt and ensure that the seat belts of all other people in the ambulance are fastened.
- Write down information from the dispatcher on a notepad.
- Confirm the following dispatch information:
  - Location of the call
  - Nature of the call
  - Location of the patient or patients
  - Number of patients and the severity of the problem
  - Any other special conditions or problems
  - If any other units are en route
- Listen for status reports from other units on the scene.
- Think about what equipment you will want to take into the scene.
- Remain relaxed, yet focused. (Studies indicate that fewer than half of all ambulance runs are requested as emergencies. Only half of those are true emergencies, with less than 5 percent being life threatening.)
- Drive responsibly, maintaining a 3- to 4-second following distance between your ambulance and the vehicle directly ahead of you.

- Determine what the responsibilities of team members will be before arriving on the scene, and make sure those responsibilities are clear.
- Call for advanced life support, if necessary.

At the Scene

Follow these guidelines while at the scene:

- Notify dispatch of arrival on scene.
- Park the ambulance in the safest place that will allow you to load the patient and later depart from the scene, taking into consideration the traffic, the roadway, and any known hazards. Follow local ordinances regarding the use of warning signals and devices at the scene (Figure 41-4*).
- Perform a full 360-degree scene survey, paying particular attention to any downed electrical lines, leaking fuels or fluids from accident vehicles, smoke or fire, broken glass, trapped or ejected patients, mechanism of injury, and other indicators of increased risk to you, your crew, or your patients. Review the procedures discussed in Chapter 12, "Scene Size-Up."
- If other emergency vehicles are on scene and are positioned to block the scene, park in front of or behind a collision, but never alongside it. If no other vehicles are on scene, position the ambulance to provide a safety zone. On a narrow, no-parking road, take up the entire road so that no one will try to squeeze past you. Park in a driveway or on the shoulder of the road whenever possible. Stay a minimum of 100 feet from wreckage or a burning vehicle and 2,000 feet from a hazardous materials spill, ideally uphill and upwind (Figure 41-5*). Come to a complete stop. Set the parking brake prior to placing the transmission in the "park" position.
- Prior to exiting the ambulance, put on an approved high-visibility safety vest if you will be working on or near a highway or other roadway.
- Take the necessary Standard Precautions. Determine if you will need eye protection, gloves, mask, and gown before making patient contact.
- Determine if it is safe to approach the patient. Identify and control hazards. If the scene is unsafe, make it safe or do not enter until the scene is secure for you, incoming units, any bystanders, and your patient. Review the procedures discussed in Chapter 12, "Scene Size-Up."
- If a mechanical failure occurs or you need backup equipment or personnel to help, call the dispatcher immediately.
- Although your dispatcher has told you what to expect, be prepared to shift your perspective quickly. You may encounter an entirely different situation or incident. Remain calm and poised. Unruffled management of the unexpected emergency is part of your job.
- Carefully observe the complete incident or situation as you approach. Look for children, curiosity seekers, or patients who may have wandered away from the scene. Decide if the patient may require immediate movement because of hazardous conditions.
- Determine the patient's mechanism of injury. Follow guidelines from Chapter 12, "Scene Size-Up," Chapter 13, "Patient Assessment," and Chapter 27, "Trauma Overview: The Trauma Patient and the Trauma System."
- Determine the total number of patients. Initiate multiple-casualty-incident response if necessary, following the procedures described in Chapter 44, "Multiple-Casualty Incidents and Incident Management." Do this before making patient contact. You are less likely to call for help once you begin intense patient care and treatment. If necessary, begin patient triage.
- Determine your priority of care. Your approach to medical and trauma patients during your primary assessment should be organized. Keep the goal of prompt transport foremost in your mind.
- For motor vehicle crashes, carefully gain access to the patient or patients and extricate them safely. Proper procedures to follow are discussed in Chapter 42, "Gaining Access and Patient Extrication."
- Take the time needed to properly splint and immobilize injured extremities before you move the patient, unless he is unstable and determined to be a high priority for immediate transport. Proper spinal immobilization is critical to appropriate patient care. Review the procedures discussed in Chapter 30, "Musculoskeletal Trauma," and Chapter 32, "Spinal Column and Spinal Cord Trauma."
- Carefully remove the patient from any wreckage and move him to the ambulance, choosing methods of moving the patient based on his illness or injury. Follow the patient lifting and moving principles and procedures you learned in Chapter 6, "Lifting and Moving Patients," and Chapter 32, "Spinal Column and Spinal Cord Trauma."
- Transfer the patient to the waiting ambulance. Keep him warm, and watch for any changes in his condition. Make sure the patient is securely strapped on the wheeled stretcher with spinal immobilization performed as necessary. Lock the stretcher securely in place within the ambulance.

En Route to the Receiving Facility

Once you are ready to transport your patient to the appropriate medical facility, follow these guidelines (EMT Skills 41-2):

- Prior to leaving the scene, ensure that all hazards have been controlled, pick up and dispose of equipment properly, and turn the scene over to the appropriate

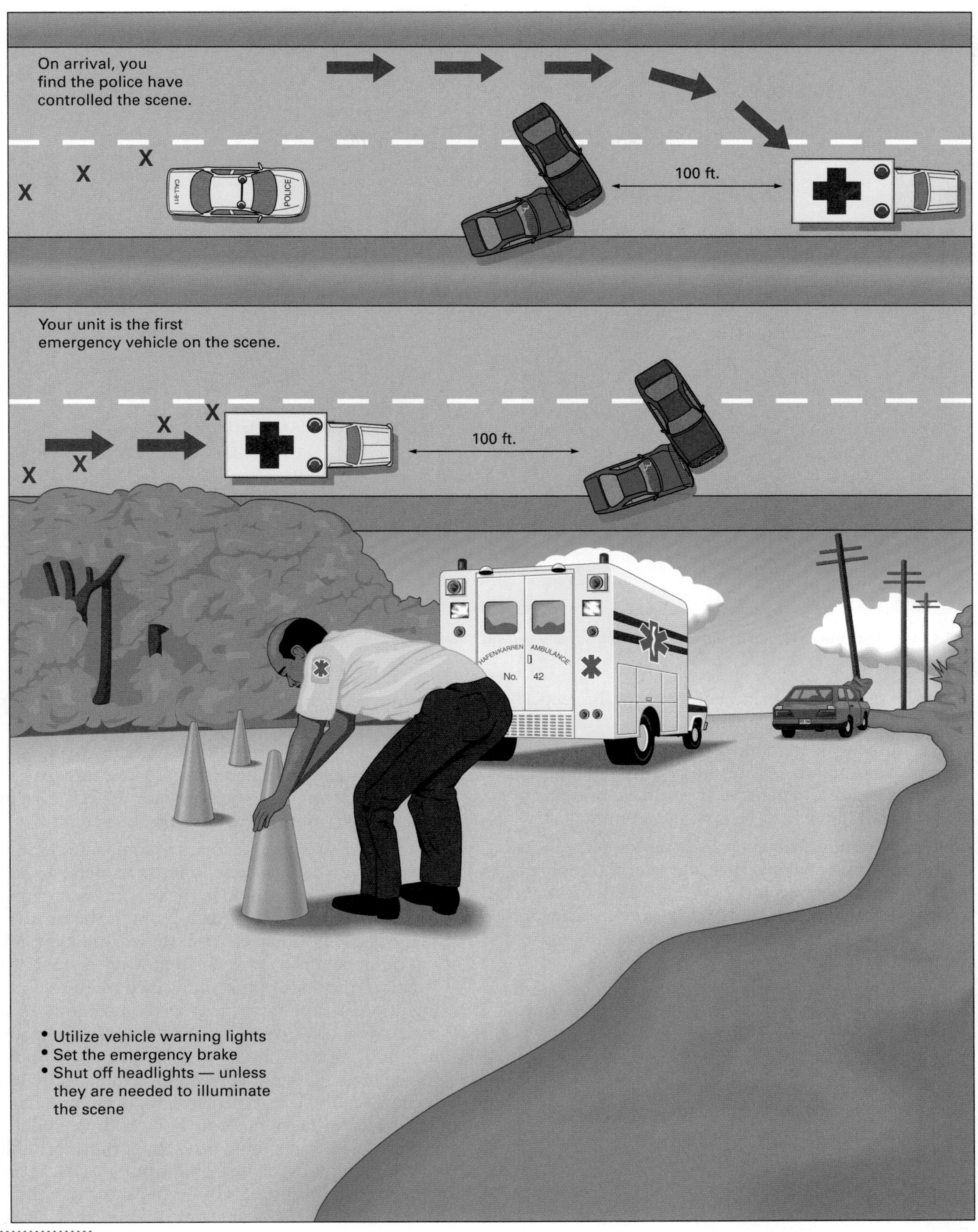
On arrival, you find the police have controlled the scene.
100 ft.
CALL-911
POLICE
Your unit is the first emergency vehicle on the scene.
100 ft.
HAFEN/KARREN AMBULANCE
No. 42
• Utilize vehicle warning lights
• Set the emergency brake
• Shut off headlights — unless they are needed to illuminate the scene

FIGURE 41-4 ✱ Safety at the scene.

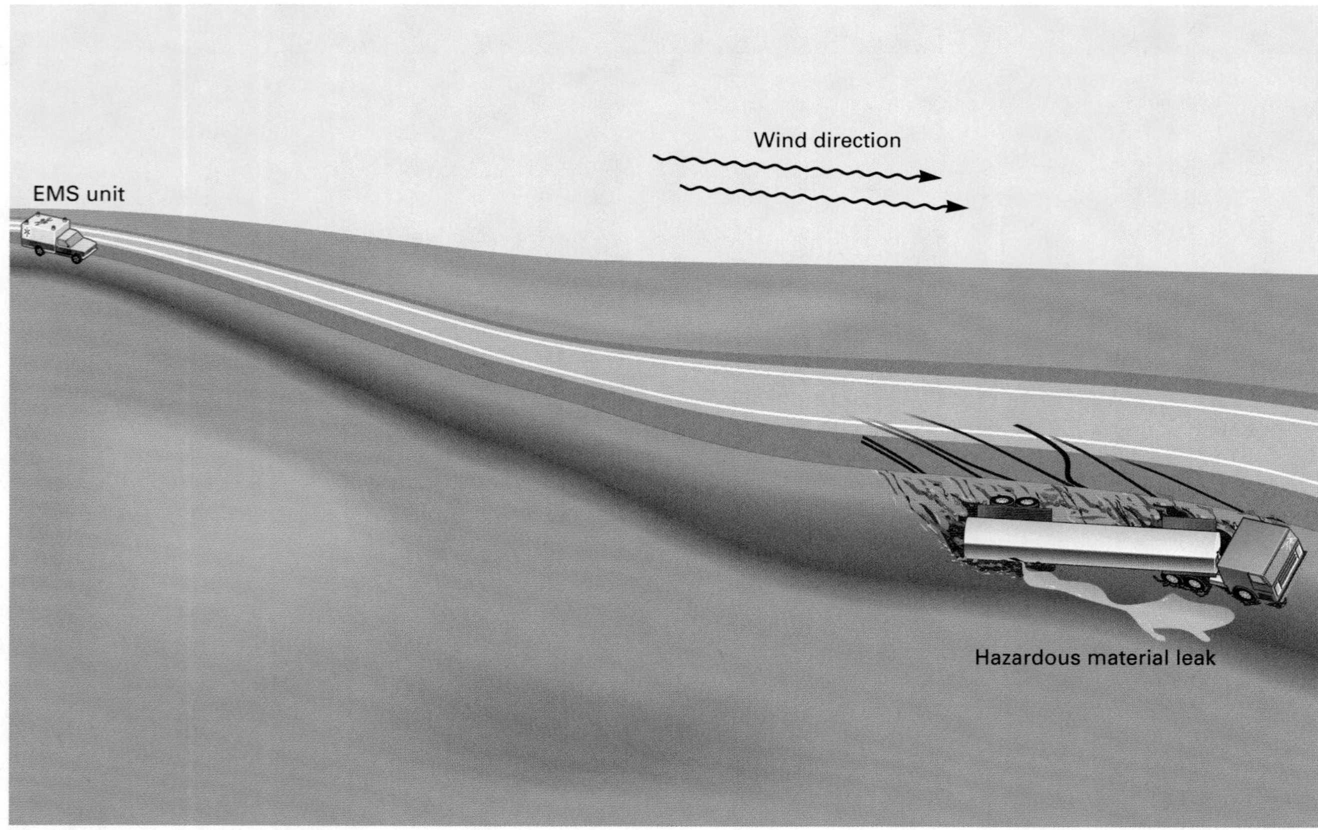

FIGURE 41-5 * Park the EMS unit uphill and upwind from any leaking hazardous materials.

agency if required (e.g., law enforcement, fire department, or highway department).

- Make sure your patient is settled and securely strapped to the cot before moving the ambulance. Calmly reassure the patient. If you have not already done so, tell him where he is being taken.
- Before departure, the vehicle driver should quickly check the unit, making sure the outside compartment doors are closed and secure. All equipment and supplies should be appropriately secured within the cab, rear compartment, and cabinets prior to departing for the hospital.
- All personnel riding in the vehicle should be properly seated and secured with safety belts, including those attending to the patient.
- Prior to departing, determine the necessity of using lights and sirens during the transport. Keep in mind the increased risk to the ambulance and its occupants when warning devices are used, and weigh this against the patient's condition and need for rapid intervention at the receiving facility.
- Begin your reassessment. This includes a reassessment of the patient's mental status, airway, and breathing, and the recording of vital signs. Conduct a reassessment at least every 15 minutes for a stable patient, every 5 minutes for an unstable patient.
- Notify dispatch that you are en route to the hospital. Follow local protocols regarding transmission of additional patient information.
- Check any patient interventions. Make sure oxygen is delivered at the correct flow rate. Check dressings and splints. Continue to reassure the patient.
- If a patient's relative or friend accompanies him, follow local guidelines as to where this person should sit. Allow the companion in the patient compartment only if local protocols permit it and if the relative or friend is in emotional control. If the patient is a child, it is often helpful to have a parent with you. Safety restraint in the back of the ambulance when transporting more than one patient or companions of the patient is a major concern. Any patient or companion in the ambulance must be in a safety restraint, including children. It is not an acceptable practice to place the child in the lap of the parent or primary caregiver and strap both to the cot. For children under 40 pounds, a car seat should be used for transport unless the child requires full immobilization to a backboard. Follow your local protocol on transport of children, one or more patients, and companions, paying particular attention to safety restraint.
- Focus on the patient. Reassure him as often as you can. Take advantage of brief stops to monitor blood

Thinking Critically
At the emergency department you look for someone to take over care of your patient. Your unit is needed back in service, so you are impatient. A woman approaches wearing a smock like the nurses usually wear. Should you leave your patient with her?

Key Points
Begin preparation for return to service as soon as possible.

pressure. Treat each patient like an individual, not a "case." Gentleness, listening, answering questions honestly, and providing as much explanation as the patient wants will make a world of emotional difference—for him and for you.

- The driver should drive prudently, use only the necessary speed, and obey all regulations to keep the patient as comfortable as possible during the trip.
- If you are the EMT with the patient, you should keep the driver informed of the patient's condition. Instruct him to slow down or take a different route if the patient is uncomfortable from the speed and bouncing.
- During your reassessment, if the patient's condition worsens and it becomes urgent to reach the hospital immediately, tell your driver so he can proceed as quickly as possible.
- Notify the receiving medical facility as soon as your patient's condition permits you to call in a report. Sometimes this may not be possible. In those situations where the patient's condition demands your full attention, request that your partner notify the hospital. Refer to Chapter 5, "Communication," to review the information that should be radioed to the receiving facility.
- Continue to reassess your patient's condition and notify the receiving facility if that condition deteriorates.

At the Receiving Facility

Once you arrive at the receiving facility, you should follow these guidelines:

- Notify dispatch of your arrival at the medical facility.
- You must make an official transfer of care to an appropriate health care provider at the receiving facility. As you make the transfer of care, continue to concentrate your care on the patient. If the receiving facility is crowded, continue to care for your patient until you can officially transfer your patient care responsibility to qualified personnel. Never leave the patient unattended or make a transfer of care to an unqualified individual!
- When you are able, transfer all records and information about the patient to appropriate emergency department personnel.
- To ensure proper continuity of care, a complete oral report should be given to emergency department personnel at the patient's bedside. You should summarize the information given over the radio:
  - Introduce the patient by name (if known).
  - Repeat the patient's chief complaint.
  - Provide additional vital signs taken en route.
  - Report any history not given previously.
  - Report any additional treatment you provided.
- If requested, assist emergency department personnel in lifting and moving the patient to a hospital gurney or bed.
- Make sure that any valuables or personal effects belonging to the patient are also transferred, and indicate this on your report.
- Once you have released your patient to the care of emergency department personnel, exchange any linens, spine boards, and other equipment you may have to leave at the hospital.
- Complete the prehospital care report before you leave the hospital. Leave a copy at the emergency department. Follow local protocol if your system also requires you to leave a copy of your written report with the patient.
- Before you leave, ask hospital personnel if you are needed further. You may need to transfer the patient to another medical facility or return the patient home if his condition is not serious enough to warrant hospital admission.

En Route to the Station or Response Area

Begin preparation for return to service as soon as possible. Follow these guidelines for returning to the station or your response area:

- At the hospital, clean and inspect your ambulance, patient care equipment, reusable supplies, and patient care compartment before notifying dispatch of your availability. During particularly busy shifts, this can be difficult. Always follow your agency's biohazard disposal procedures. Dispose of any contaminated linen. Disinfect any reusable patient care equipment. These steps are essential for the safety and health of you and your patients. After some calls, the ambulance requires extensive cleaning, disinfecting, and restocking. It may

Objective 41-9
Describe post-run actions that should be taken to reduce the spread of infection to you, your coworkers, and patients.

Key Points
Always follow infection control procedures. Dispose of sharps. Wash hands. Clean/disinfect/sterilize contaminated equipment. Launder soiled clothing and linens. Safely dispose of infectious wastes.

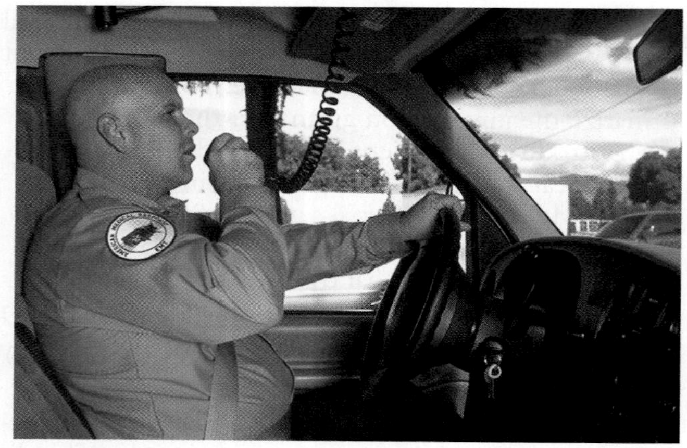

FIGURE 41-6 ✱ Advise dispatch when you are returning to the station or your response area.

be necessary to go "out of service" and return to the station to clean, disinfect, and restock the ambulance.

- Wash your hands.
- Radio the dispatcher that you are returning to the station or your response area (Figure 41-6✱).
- Buckle your seat belt, then proceed to the station or your response area in a safe, cautious manner.
- Refuel according to local protocol.

Post Run

Follow these guidelines after the run (EMT Skills 41-3):

- Fill out and file any reports as required by local protocol. Do not postpone this activity.
- After each run, check fuel; fill the fuel tank when necessary.
- Complete an inventory of equipment and supplies. Replace what you used during the run, and complete the cleaning and disinfection of nondisposable equipment used.
- Change soiled uniforms.
- Notify dispatch you are in service, available for calls.

Infection Control Procedures

To prevent the spread of infection, follow the procedures outlined next as you ready your unit and yourself for return to service.

Dispose of Sharps Make sure that needles, blades, and all other disposable sharp items have been placed in clearly labeled, puncture-resistant containers for disposal. (This should have been done immediately after use throughout the call.)

Wash Hands Use ordinary soap and water to wash your hands at the end of the run and after all cleaning procedures have been completed. (You should also have washed your hands immediately after each contact with a potentially contaminated patient or item.) Use waterless antiseptic hand cleaner if ordinary washing facilities are not available. As soon as you are able, wash your hands thoroughly with soap and water.

Clean, Disinfect, or Sterilize Contaminated Equipment Use proper procedures to clean (wipe up), disinfect (kill some microbes on), or sterilize (kill all microbes on) contaminated reusable patient care equipment or any items that have or will come in contact with patients. (Review cleaning, disinfecting, and sterilization in Chapter 2, "Workforce Safety and Wellness of the EMT.")

1. **First, clean up visible spills of blood, vomitus, or other body fluids.** Put on protective gloves (use gloves that are heavy enough to resist puncture from sharp edges or while scrubbing). Wear appropriate face and eye protection if you anticipate splashing. If there is a great amount of blood in the area, wear impervious shoe coverings. Use disposable towels or use other materials that can be placed in a plastic bag of contaminated laundry after use. After removal of visible material, decontaminate surfaces with a germicide or a 1:100 or 1:10 solution of household bleach and water (see guidelines that follow). Use clean towels with germicide to wipe the area. Let the area air dry. After the area has been decontaminated, place shoe coverings, gloves, and other contaminated items in a sealed plastic bag for disposal.
2. **Then disinfect reusable patient care equipment.**

For disinfecting surfaces and equipment, choose an appropriate level of disinfection or sterilization as outlined next. Some judgment about the level of disinfection or sterilization required must be exercised:

- **Use low-level disinfection for routine housekeeping on environmental surfaces such as**

Key Points
Use appropriate levels of disinfection: Low for routine housekeeping, intermediate for surfaces that contact intact skin, and high for instruments that contact mucous membranes. Sterilize invasive equipment.

Objective 41-10
Discuss situations in which air medical transport should be considered, potential disadvantages of air medical transport, and guidelines for setting up a landing zone.

floors, ambulance seats, and countertops when there is no visible blood and contamination by body fluids or exposure to tuberculosis is not suspected. Use a 1:100 solution of household bleach and water or an EPA-registered "hospital disinfectant" chemical germicide with no claim on the label for tuberculocidal activity. These disinfectants will destroy some viruses, most bacteria, and some fungi but not *Mycobacterium tuberculosis* or bacterial spores.

- **Use intermediate-level disinfection for surfaces that come into contact with intact skin, such as stethoscopes, blood pressure cuffs, or splints.** Use a 1:10 solution of household bleach and water or an EPA-registered "hospital disinfectant" chemical germicide with a claim on the label that it is tuberculocidal. These disinfectants will destroy *Mycobacterium tuberculosis*, most viruses, vegetative bacteria, and most fungi, but not bacterial spores.
- **Use high-level disinfection for reusable instruments that come into contact with mucous membranes, such as laryngoscopes, blades, and handles.** Use either hot water pasteurization (80°C–100°C for 30 minutes) or immerse in an EPA-registered chemical sterilant for 10–45 minutes (follow the instructions specific to the sterilant). This method will destroy *Mycobacterium tuberculosis*, most viruses, vegetative bacteria, and most fungi, but not bacterial spores.
- **Sterilize equipment that will be used invasively.** Immerse in an EPA-registered chemical sterilant for 6–10 hours (only if a heat sterilization process is not available) or expose to steam (autoclave), gas, or dry heat sterilization. This method will destroy all forms of microbial life. It is used primarily in hospitals rather than in prehospital settings. When possible, disposable items are preferred to avoid the need to disinfect or sterilize and to prevent transmission of disease to other patients.

Launder Soiled Clothing and Linens The risk of disease transmission from soiled clothing or linen is minimal. However, follow these recommendations:

- Handle soiled laundry as little as possible. Always wear protective gloves when doing so.
- Bag soiled items in clearly marked biohazard bags to prevent leaking or contamination of other clothing, persons, or equipment.
- Wash in normal laundry cycles with regular detergent according to the recommendations of the washing machine manufacturer.
- Wear gloves when bagging and placing contaminated clothing into washing machines.
- Launder uniforms according to the label instructions.

Dispose of Infectious Wastes Place all infectious wastes in clearly labeled and sealed biohazard bags for disposal according to your local protocols.

Air Medical Transport

Many medical personnel involved in helicopter rescue consider a helicopter to be not just transport but an extension of the emergency department (Figures 41-7a and 41-7b*). Fixed wing aircraft (airplanes) may be used where transport distances are long.

When to Request Air Medical Transport

Follow local protocols or seek on-line medical consultation when you think air medical transport may be needed.

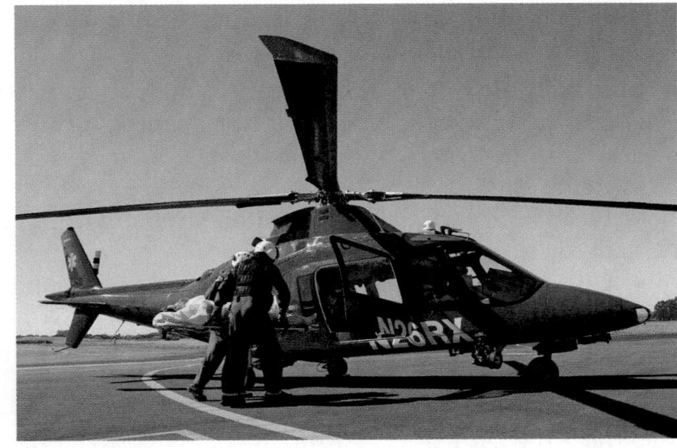

FIGURE 41-7a * Loading the patient into the helicopter.

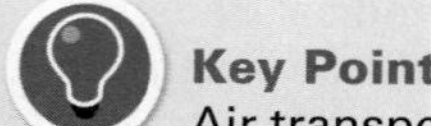

Key Points
Air transport should be considered using both operational and medical guidelines.

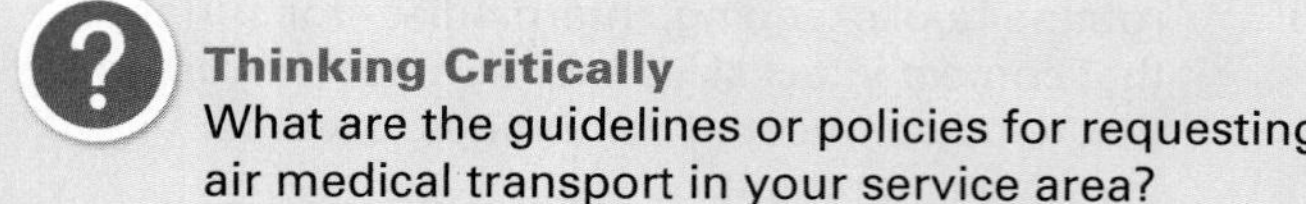

Thinking Critically
What are the guidelines or policies for requesting air medical transport in your service area?

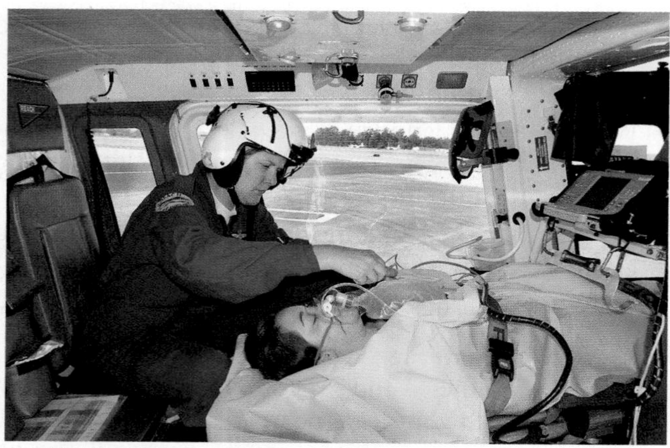

FIGURE 41-7b * The patient inside the helicopter.

Air transport should be considered according to the following general guidelines:

- **Operational guidelines.**
  - The patient needs to be transported to a trauma center or other specialty care facility that is distant from his present location.
  - A high-priority patient is entrapped and a prolonged extrication is expected.
  - Air transport will clearly save time over ground transport in a time-critical patient.
  - The patient is in a remote area that cannot be reached by ground vehicles.
  - Ground ambulance transport is blocked.
  - The air transport crew possesses specialty medical skills, supplies, or equipment not available with the ground ambulance.
- **Medical guidelines.** The patient is a high priority for air transport where the patient has a time-critical illness or injury, such as the following:
  - Acute stroke
  - Head injury with altered mental status and signs of herniation
  - Chest or abdominal trauma with signs of respiratory distress or shock
  - Serious mechanism of injury with unstable primary assessment findings or unstable vital signs
  - Penetrating injury to the body cavity with unstable primary assessment findings

Some air medical services may also provide aerial support to search and rescue operations. Consult with your regional air medical services to find out if they provide this service.

Requesting Air Medical Transport

In many cases, local and state guidelines exist regarding the use of air medical transport and may even provide specific criteria for when it can be used. Some city, county, or regional ordinances may require that the fire department be present when landing a helicopter. Make sure that you are familiar with any guidelines or policies in your area.

When calling for a helicopter transport, you should be prepared to provide the following information:

- Your name
- Department name
- Callback number
- Nature of the incident
- Exact location of the incident (landmarks and crossroads or GPS coordinates are helpful)
- Radio frequency you use, so that you can communicate with the helicopter or plane
- Exact location of the landing zone and surrounding hazards

Additional Considerations for Air Medical Transport

When considering the use of air medical transportation, you should also consider some of the potential disadvantages:

- **Weather/environmental limitations.** Inclement weather, such as snow, rain, fog, or heavy winds, may prevent helicopters from being able to fly. Establish communications with the air medical service's dispatch to determine flight capability during bad weather.
- **Altitude limitations.** Patients with certain medical conditions and injuries, such as lung trauma or certain diving injuries, may not be good candidates for the increased altitude associated with air transport.
- **Airspeed limitations.** In windy conditions, air travel may actually take longer than travel by ground. Con-

sult with the air medical service's dispatch center to help determine feasibility of air transport.

- **Aircraft cabin size.** The space inside a helicopter's cabin is often quite small, depending upon the type of aircraft. Obese patients, or those with extensive deformities or large impaled objects, may not be suitable for air transport because of these space restrictions.
- **Terrain.** Irregular terrain may make it difficult to locate a safe landing area for a helicopter. When this occurs, ground transport or rendezvous with the helicopter at a predetermined approved helipad or landing zone may be considered.
- **Cost.** Aircraft are quite expensive to operate, and requests for their use should only be made when the benefit to the patient is likely to outweigh the risk and additional cost. Under no circumstances, however, should access to air medical transport be denied based upon a perceived ability to pay.
- **Patient preparation.** Because of the small cabin size of many helicopters, it is necessary to ensure that splinting, proper immobilization, and complete assessments are performed prior to loading into the aircraft. The EMT can help to expedite patient transport by ensuring that these procedures are complete prior to transfer of care to the air medical crew.
- **Noise-limited assessment.** Noise within the aircraft will limit your ability to conduct a thorough assessment of the patient, especially when hearing is necessary as in monitoring breath sounds or auscultating blood pressure.

Setting Up a Landing Zone

In setting up a landing zone for a helicopter, keep these guidelines in mind:

- Make sure that the landing area is clear of obstructions. This area should ideally be a flat square with 60-foot sides by day for a small helicopter, but larger—about 100-foot sides—by night. If the helicopter is medium or large in size, it will need about double that area. Pick up loose debris that might blow up into the rotor system. Choose a landing site at least 150 feet away from collision vehicles, if possible, so that noise and rotor wash will not be a problem for rescuers. Contact your local service for landing zone requirements and safety specifications.
- If the landing site is a divided highway, stop the traffic going in both directions, even though the aircraft will land on only one side of the highway.
- Consider the wind direction. Helicopters take off and land into the wind by preference, rather than making vertical descents and ascents. Establish radio communications with the incoming flight crew and warn them of any power lines, poles, antennas, trees, or other obstructions.
- Mark each corner of the landing area with a highly visible device: a flag or surveyor's tapes by day and a flashing or rotating light at night. Use flares by day or night but only if there is no danger of fire. A beam of light should not be directed upward.
- Put a fifth warning device on the upwind side to designate the wind direction.
- If conditions are dusty or dry enough to create a fire hazard, have the area wet down, if possible.
- Keep the patient and crew clear of the air downwash area. Spectators should be at least 200 feet away. EMT personnel should be at least 100 feet away during landing.
- Assign one person to guide the pilot in. He should wear eye and ear protection and should stand near the wind direction marker with his back to the wind, facing the touchdown area, arms raised overhead to indicate the landing direction (Figure 41-8*).
- Give primary care to the patient and follow exactly the instructions of the pilot or crew members relating to the craft's operation. Never try to open a door or approach the tail of the aircraft without instructions and approval from the pilot and crew.
- Be extremely cautious about the rotor blades. Remember that the tips can dip as low as 4 feet above the ground. Always crouch when approaching or leaving the helicopter (Figure 41-9a*), and approach or leave only at the pilot's direction.
- Never approach a helicopter until the pilot indicates it is safe. Never approach from behind the pilot. The pilot cannot see behind the craft, the tail rotor is spinning very quickly, and the pilot sometimes needs to move the tail boom without warning. If you have to go from one side to another, always cross in front of the craft, never behind it or underneath it.
- Secure all loose items so that nothing will blow into the rotor blades when you are approaching or leaving a helicopter.
- No one should smoke within 50 feet of the aircraft.
- If the helicopter has to land on an incline, always approach from the downhill side, never from the uphill side (Figure 41-9b*).
- Never point spotlights up at a helicopter that is on its final approach at night.
- In certain cases, a rendezvous with the helicopter may be arranged at a predesignated helipad. The advantage of helipads, such as those found at most hospitals, is that the site is already correctly designed for optimal landing of the aircraft. Terrain, size, markings, wind direction, and lighting are typically not concerns for the EMT on the ground in these cases.

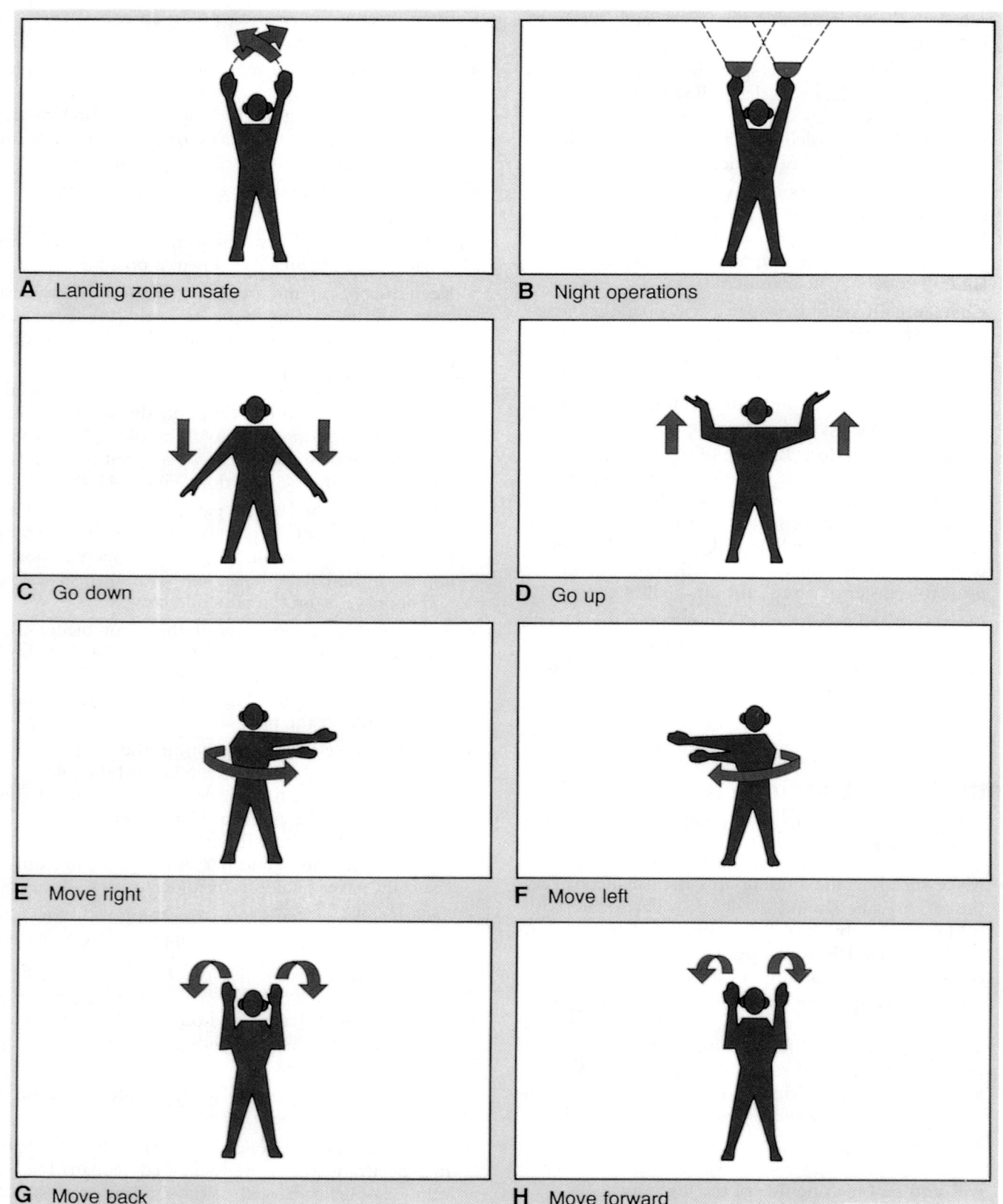

FIGURE 41-8 ✱ Guiding the helicopter pilot in.

Objective 41-11
Describe the recommendations of the National Association of Emergency Medical Technicians with respect to EMT security and safety.

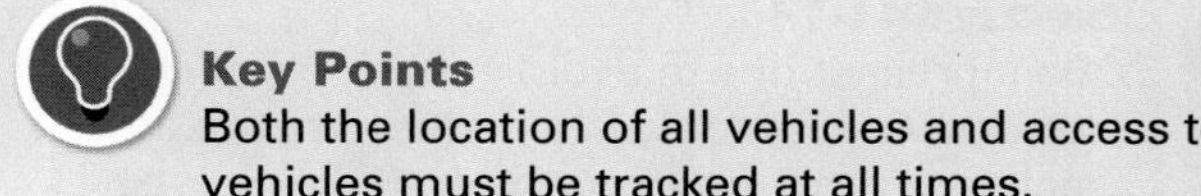

Key Points
Both the location of all vehicles and access to vehicles must be tracked at all times.

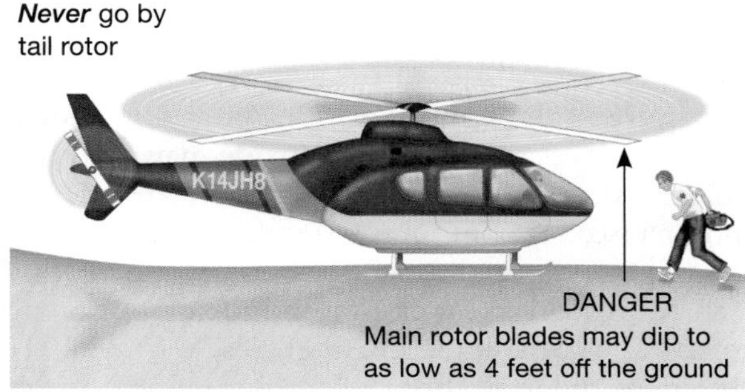
Never go by
tail rotor
K14JH8
DANGER
Main rotor blades may dip to
as low as 4 feet off the ground

FIGURE 41-9a ✱ Always crouch when approaching or leaving a helicopter.

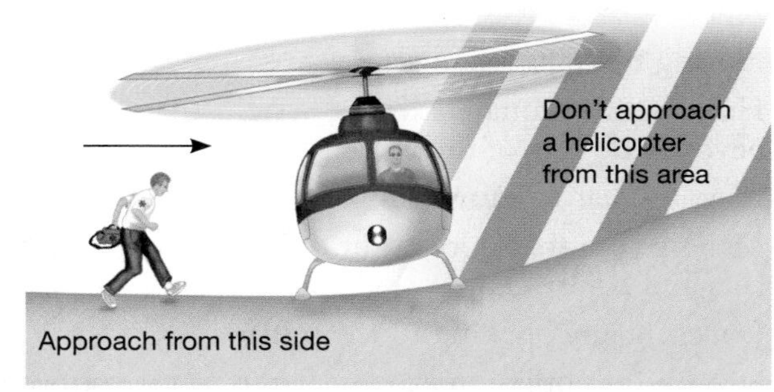
Don't approach
a helicopter
from this area
Approach from this side

FIGURE 41-9b ✱ Approach a helicopter from downhill.

Security and Safety

Operational Security Measures

The National Association of Emergency Medical Technicians (NAEMT) has established recommended guidelines to ensure better operational safety and security measures to avoid the possible use of emergency service vehicles in domestic terrorist attacks and to reduce the risk of an EMS vehicle being stolen or used in a manner that is not intended. The following are the recommended security measures:

Personnel

- Security briefings should be conducted at the beginning of each shift regarding any possible threats to the EMS crews or service. These briefings may be conducted as meetings, information sheets, postings, or supervisor briefings at the beginning of each shift.
- EMS crews should have the opportunity to be well informed and take part in the development of operational security measures and situation awareness. A greater degree of understanding by the field personnel is necessary.

Vehicle

- All EMS vehicles must be tracked at all times. That includes vehicles that are in service, out of service being repaired, and off service. It also includes reserve units and those units that are no longer in service and will be salvaged.
- EMS vehicles should never be left running or unattended with the keys in the ignition or in the vehicle.

Tracking of Vehicle Access

- Authorized persons must secure all off-service vehicles at stations or other locations to eliminate access and use by unauthorized persons. Random and routine vehicle audits should be conducted.
- A comprehensive key log must be kept to account for all keys that may allow for entry into restricted stations and areas in which a person may gain access to an EMS vehicle. If keys are not accounted for, measures should be taken to correct the security breach.
- Ensure that security measures are strongly enforced when the EMS vehicle is off the EMS premises for repairs or other work conducted by repair or installation facilities. These should include securing the vehicle indoors overnight when the facility is not open, not leaving the keys in the vehicle or in a place where there is easy access, not allowing the vehicle to leave the premises for any unauthorized travel when being repaired, and reporting any unusual interest by an individual related to an EMS vehicle.
- Any vehicles that are no longer in service but are to be sold to persons or organizations other than another bona fide EMS organization and those vehicles that are to be salvaged must have all EMS markings completely removed or destroyed by stripping, grinding, or painting. Any emergency lights or other warning devices should be uninstalled.

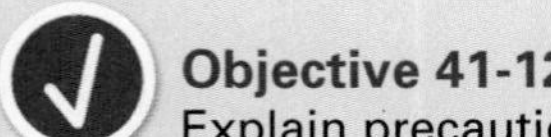

Objective 41-12
Explain precautions to avoid exposing yourself or others to increased levels of carbon monoxide associated with ambulance operations.

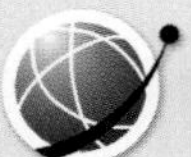

Media Resources
Go to www.bradybooks.com for mykit. Highlights:
- *Web Resource:* American Ambulance Association
- *Web Resource:* The FACE Program

Uniforms and Identification Items

- EMS patches and identification cards or badges must be safeguarded against access or distribution to unauthorized individuals.
- Identification cards or badges should be counterfeit resistant and include a photo of the authorized EMS member.
- Uniform stores must verify the identification of any individual seeking to purchase any EMS uniform or identification articles. The EMS agency should provide identification credentials to anyone who is to purchase EMS uniforms or identification items. A check should be made against a database of authorized purchasers of these types of items.

Carbon Monoxide in Ambulances

Another emergency situation that you may encounter while driving an older model ambulance is the buildup of carbon monoxide gas. Carbon monoxide (CO) is colorless, odorless, tasteless, and deadly. If an ambulance is not properly cared for, a CO level that is harmful to injured or ill patients and even to emergency personnel may build up. Any amount of CO over 10 parts per million above the ambient CO level in the air may be dangerous. Excessive amounts of CO may come from:

- The vehicle's own exhaust gases
- Supplemental equipment that is powered by gasoline or liquid petroleum gas
- The exhaust gases of vehicles parked next to or traveling by the ambulance
- Greater outside air pressure, which forces the CO into the ambulance

Be aware of the symptoms of carbon monoxide poisoning. Low levels of carbon monoxide may cause yawning, dizziness, dimmed vision, headache, irregular heart rhythm, nausea, or vomiting. Extended exposure or high concentrations can lead to seizures, coma, and death. Review the information on carbon monoxide poisoning in Chapter 22, "Toxicologic Emergencies."

If any of the indications of carbon monoxide occur, remove the patient from the ambulance and administer oxygen by nonrebreather mask. Resuscitate the patient, if necessary.

Prevent CO poisoning by:

- Having frequent engine tune-ups
- Having an adequate exhaust system that discharges beyond the side of the vehicle
- Keeping rear windows shut
- Making sure that doors shut tightly with proper gaskets and adjustments
- Covering any opening to the outside
- Not using ventilation exhaust fans or static roof vents
- Keeping the heater or air-conditioner on (They create continuous positive interior pressure.)
- Not using supplemental equipment that is powered by gasoline or liquid petroleum gas inside the ambulance

A bright light or water spray under pressure will help you identify possible spots where CO can enter. CO testers for the inside of ambulances are available. There are also color-change CO monitors that stick to the sun visor or dash and audible CO alarms.

EMT skills 41-1 Elements of the Daily Vehicle Inspection

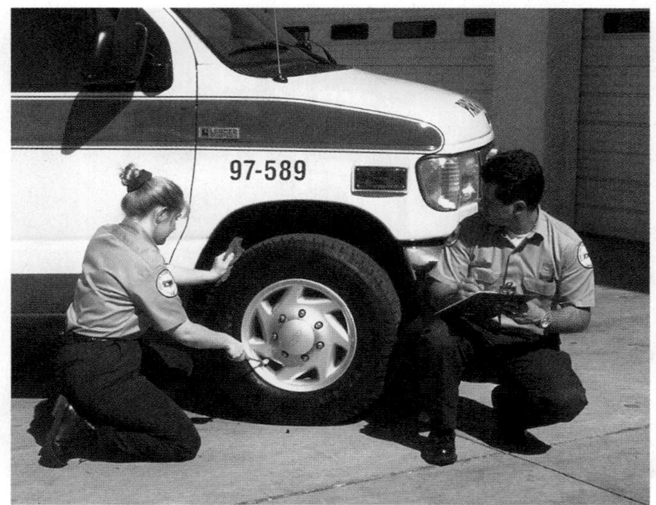

41-1A ✱ Check tires for inflation, wear, or danger spots.

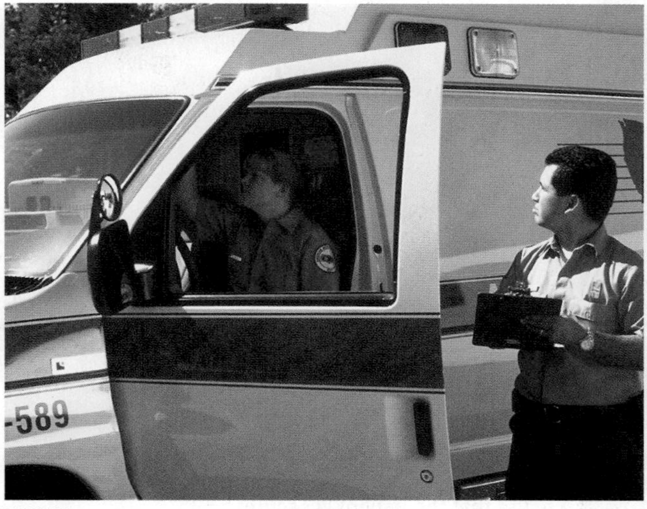

41-1B ✱ Make sure all lights are functional.

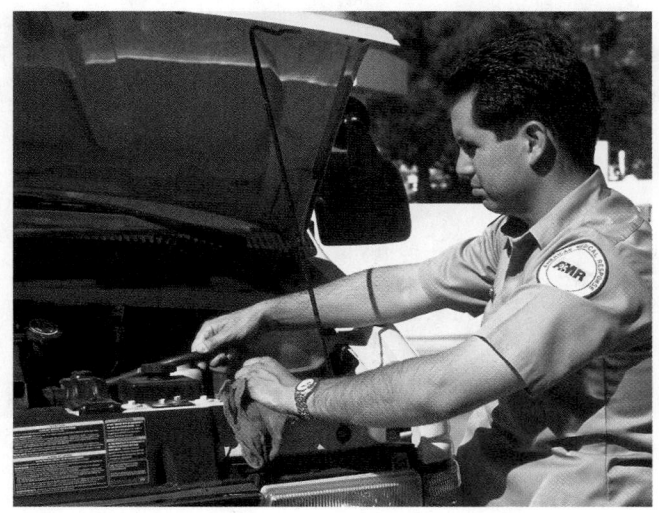

41-1C ✱ Check all belts and hoses.

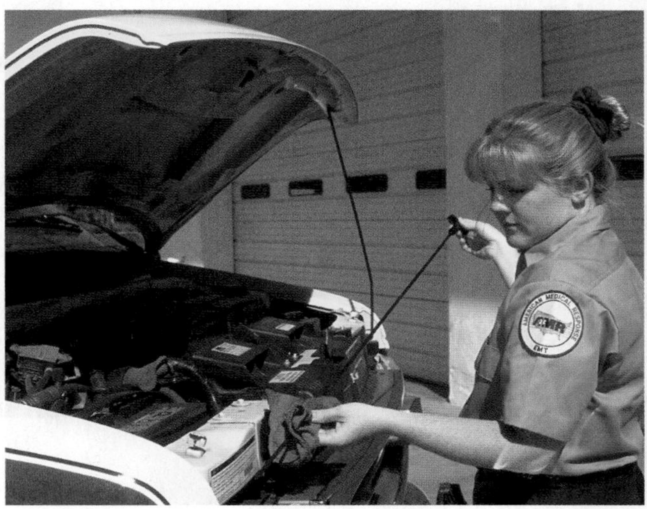

41-1D ✱ Check all fluid levels and keep them up.

En Route to the Receiving Facility

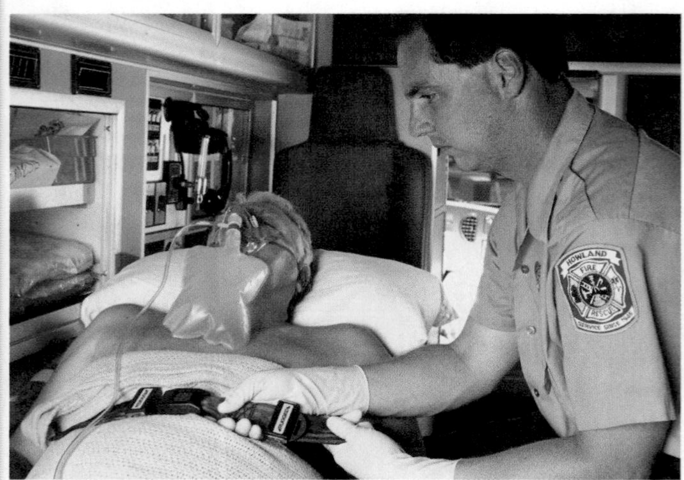

41-2A * Ensure that the patient is secure.

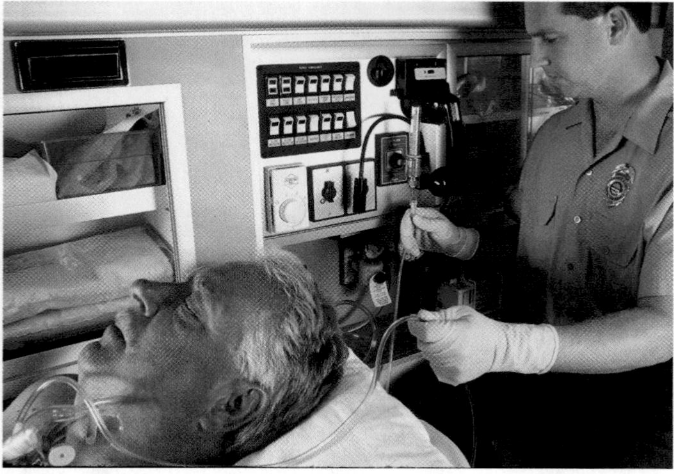

41-2B * Change to on-board oxygen.

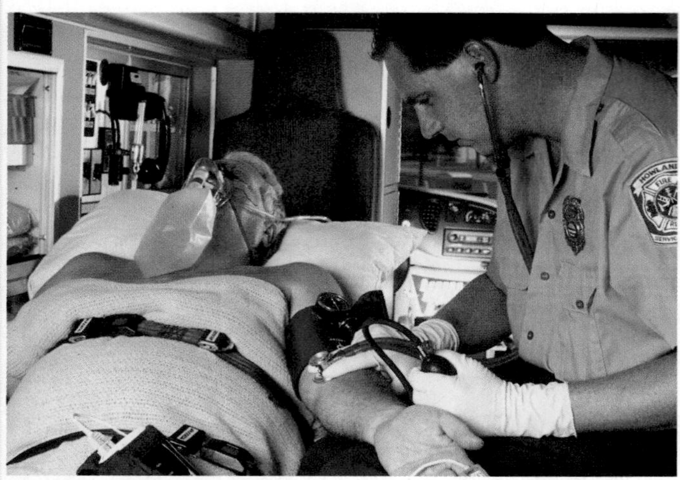

41-2C * Perform reassessment.

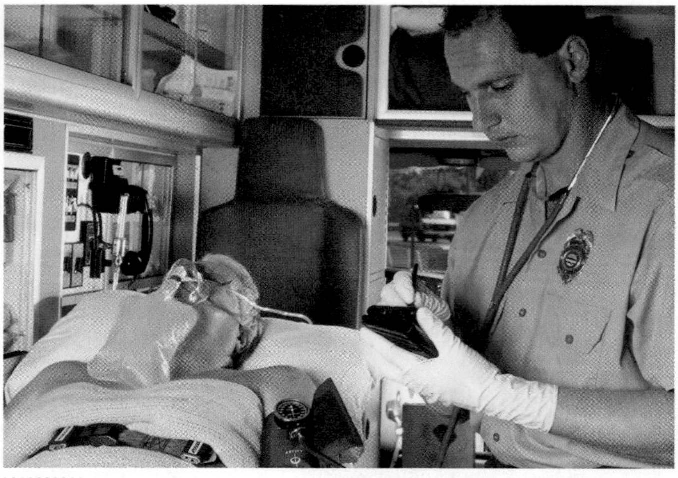

41-2D * Document your history and other assessment findings.

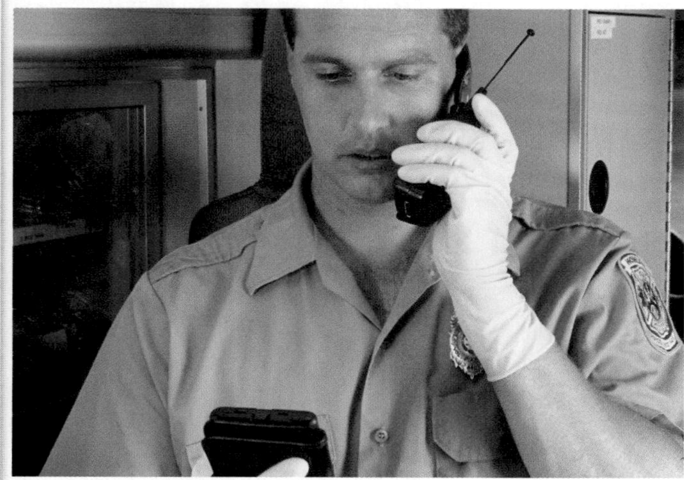

41-2E * Communicate with medical direction and the receiving medical facility.

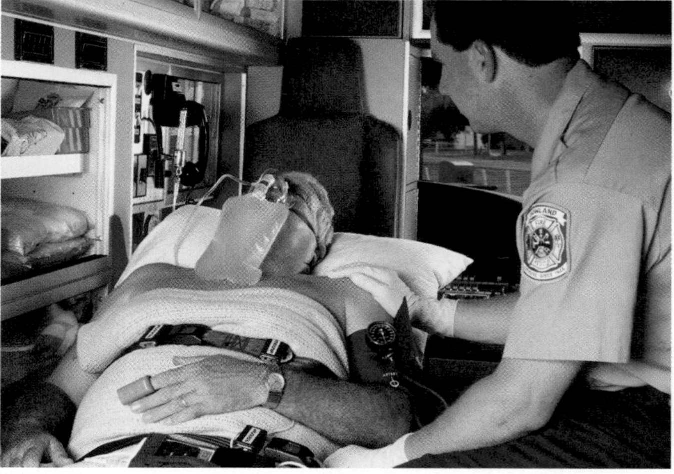

41-2F * Make the patient comfortable and reassure him.

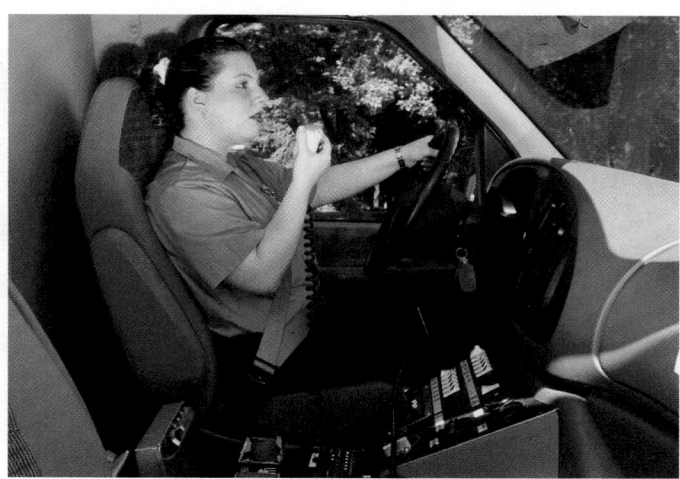

41-2G ✱ Notify dispatch when you are en route and when you have arrived at the receiving medical facility.

EMT skills 41-3 Post Run

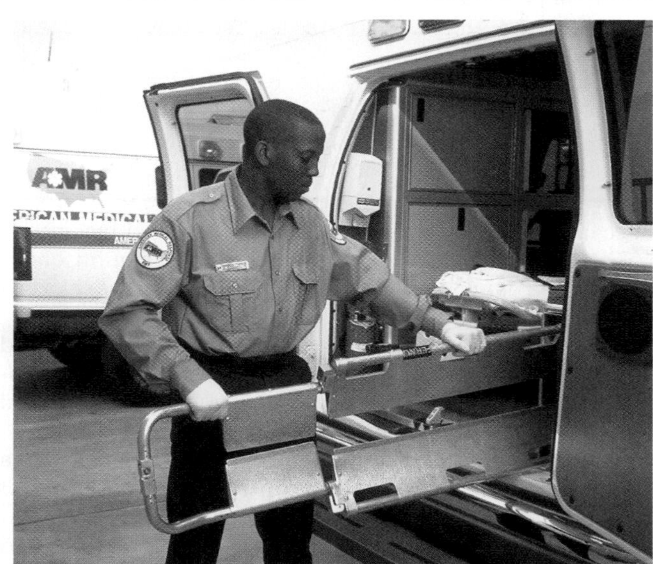

41-3A ✱ Put all equipment in its proper place.

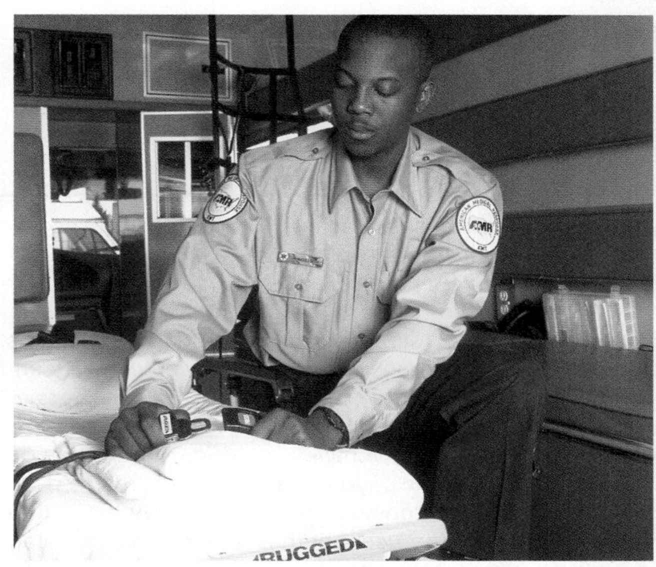

41-3B ✱ Make up the wheeled stretcher and lock it in place.

continued

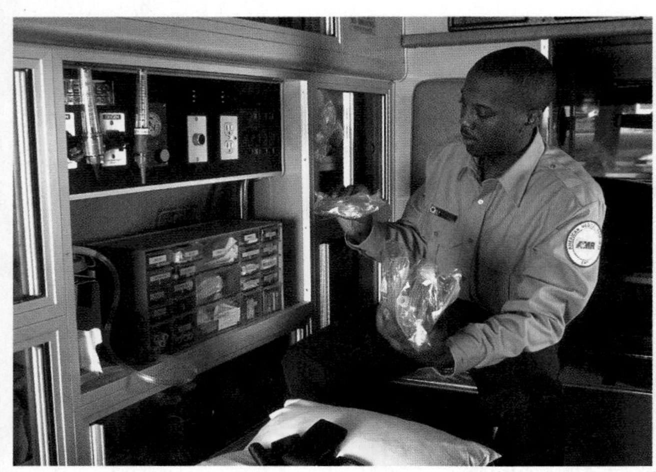

41-3C ✻ Complete an inventory of equipment and supplies. Replace necessary equipment so that the ambulance is fully stocked.

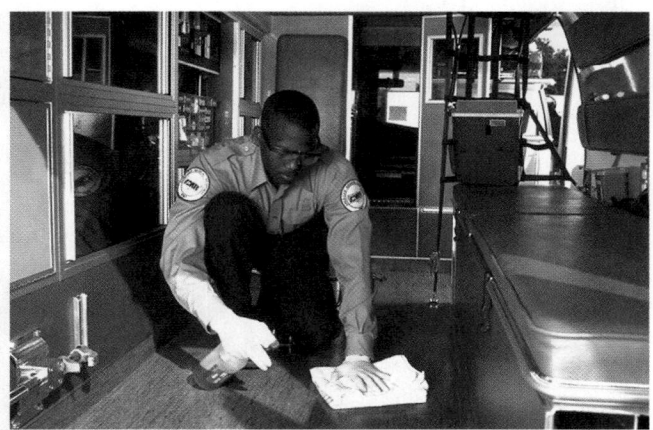

41-3D ✻ Clean and disinfect the patient compartment.

CHAPTER REVIEW

SUMMARY

A large number of crashes each year involve ambulances in which EMTs, patients, and others are severely injured or killed. Ambulance operation is a serious matter. When operating an ambulance, obey all laws, regulations, and ordinances as well as your standard operating procedures, policies, and local protocols. Always drive defensively and maintain complete control of the ambulance. Consider and anticipate changes in road conditions, weather conditions, and movements by other vehicles in traffic. The warning devices are to notify traffic of your approach and you must use them only for that purpose. Although you may have all of the warning devices in use, another driver may not recognize your approach, especially from behind. Be prepared for sudden and erratic movements by startled, distracted, or impaired drivers.

Ambulance operation usually follows a standard sequence of phases: prerun preparation, dispatch, en route to the scene, at the scene, en route to the medical facility, arrival at the medical facility, en route to the station or response area, and post run. Always exercise the highest degree of competency and professionalism in each phase.

Air medical transport is sometimes needed to respond to and transport critically injured or ill patients to the medical facility. Follow your protocols for requesting air medical transport and what information to provide once they have been notified. On-scene emergency personnel must set up a landing zone that allows the helicopter to land and take off safely.

Emergency personnel have been severely injured and even killed while working in or near moving traffic. Exercise safety precautions to limit your exposure to traffic and make yourself very visible. Always remain alert and attentive to oncoming traffic. Use emergency vehicles to block and protect yourself and others who are at the scene.

CASE STUDY FOLLOW-UP

EN ROUTE TO THE SCENE

You've been dispatched to a 33-year-old female patient with labor pains at a highway rest area. You remember that during the patient compartment check you made sure the OB kit was stocked. As your partner drives, you look at your notepad and reconfirm the location of the call. You request a further update from dispatch on the nature of the call. "The mother believes she will have the baby before you arrive!" Emergency Medical Responders at the location give you a report on the radio: "It's a girl!"

AT THE SCENE

You notify dispatch when you reach the rest area. While looking through your vehicle's front window, you begin the scene size-up. Your partner sets the parking brake and then puts the transmission in park. The vehicle is parked so you won't have to back into traffic when leaving. The scene is safe. You put on your personal protective gear, turn on the patient compartment heat, and grab the OB kit. You take a deep breath and try to relax.

The Emergency Medical Responders tell you the patient's name is Karen Austin and direct you to the sleeper cab of a semi-tractor trailer. You in fact have two patients, mother and child. You begin your primary assessment of the mother and baby. After providing initial OB care and treatment, you prepare them for transport. Both are covered with warm blankets and loaded into your warmed ambulance. The truck driver tells you he's Tom Austin, the father, and wants to ride along. You say okay, but politely advise him that your agency requires that he ride in the front seat of the ambulance. You ask an Emergency Medical Responder for assistance en route to the receiving facility. She gladly agrees and jumps in the back.

EN ROUTE TO THE RECEIVING FACILITY

In the patient compartment, you complete your secondary assessment. Prior to leaving the scene, your partner makes sure all equipment and vehicle compartments are secure. He asks for assistance from a police officer in stopping traffic. He then notifies dispatch he is en route to the hospital with two patients. You calmly inform the mother where she will be transported. She is settled, and the baby is resting comfortably.

You are still 30 minutes away from the nearest medical facility. You begin your reassessment. You reassess the mother's and child's mental status, airway, breathing, and circulation, and all of your medical interventions. You then tell your partner and the father that the mother and baby are doing fine. Your partner decides to continue driving at the posted speed limit. You radio a report on the condition of your two patients to the receiving facility.

AT THE RECEIVING FACILITY

As you arrive at the facility, your partner notifies dispatch. You are greeted at the door by emergency department staff. Mother and baby are immediately wheeled into a patient room. You continue to make sure they are kept warm. Next, you provide your oral report to both the emergency physician and the nurse.

Meanwhile, your partner has already started to clean and prepare the vehicle for your next run. After transferring the care of your patients to the hospital staff, you ask your partner if he wants help in resupplying the ambulance. He tells you to go ahead and write the prehospital care report while he gets clean linens and disinfects the cot.

You finish your report and leave a copy with the patient's records. Your partner advises you the unit has been cleaned and resupplied. You ask emergency department personnel if they need any further information. They say thanks but everything seems all right. "Good job," they tell you.

EN ROUTE TO THE STATION

Your partner has already disposed of contaminated linen and supplies. The vehicle and reusable supplies have been disinfected according to your agency's protocol. Both of you remembered to wash your hands. You advise dispatch you are available for another call and are returning to the station. You and your partner buckle your seat belts and decide to refuel.

POST RUN

Once at the station, you recheck your supplies and finish cleaning the patient compartment floor. Also, you decide to wash the vehicle's exterior. Your station phone rings. It's Tom Austin calling from the hospital. The baby's name is Sandra. You contact dispatch and let them know.

IN REVIEW

1. List some of the privileges that may be granted to an ambulance operator. List the qualifications necessary for using these privileges.
2. Explain when an ambulance operator should use a police escort.
3. List the major causes of intersection collisions.
4. Explain the problems use of a siren can pose for ambulance safety.
5. List the phases of an ambulance run.
6. List information an ambulance crew should receive from dispatch before beginning a run.
7. Describe the procedures you should follow in turning a patient over to a receiving facility.
8. Explain when cleaning and restocking of an ambulance after a run should begin, and why.
9. List the infection control procedures that should be followed.
10. Explain how you should mark a landing area for air ambulance use.

CRITICAL THINKING

You are dispatched to respond to a motor vehicle crash on a highway. It is raining lightly and the roadways are very slippery. You are informed by dispatch that the crash involves two vehicles with four patients. The police are on the scene and indicate that the patients appear to be critically injured. You know this highway to be very busy, especially at this time of day.

1. What emergency vehicle driving practices would you use to ensure a safe response to the scene?
2. What other resources may you request to respond to the scene?
3. What specific steps would you take to improve your safety while on the scene of the crash?
4. What personal protective equipment should you wear while on scene?
5. If a helicopter is requested, how would you prepare a landing zone?

PEARSON

EXPLORE mybradykit™

Please go to **www.bradybooks.com** to access mykit for this text. You will find quizzes, critical thinking scenarios, weblinks, animations, and videos related to this chapter—and much more. Look for online information on safe driving tips and the FACE program.

Register your access code from the front of your book by going to **www.bradybooks.com** and selecting the mykit links.

CHAPTER 42

Gaining Access and Patient Extrication

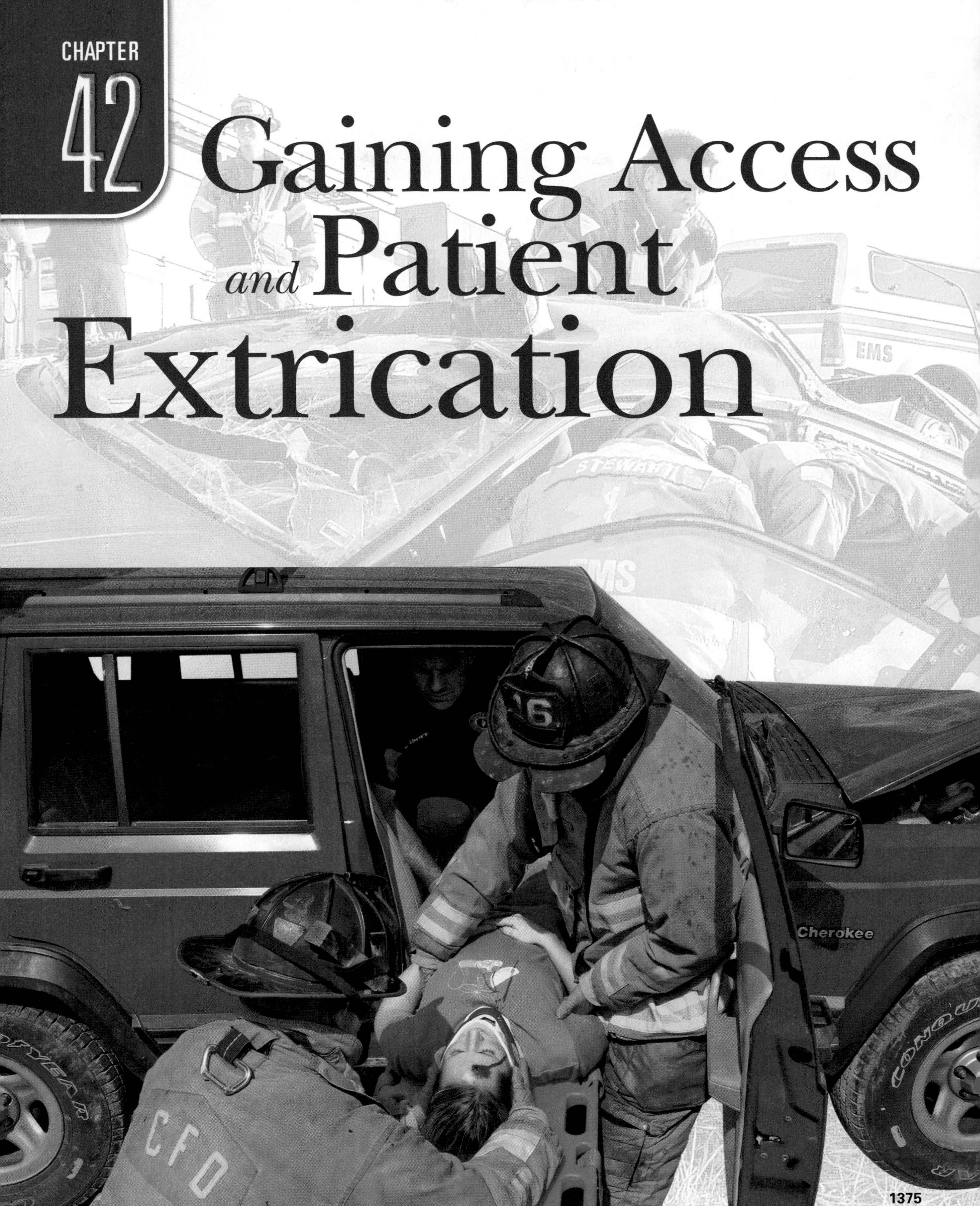

Navigation Guide

The following items provide an overview to the purpose and content of this chapter. The Standard and Competency are from the new National EMS Education Standards.

STANDARD **EMS Operations** (Content Area: Vehicle Extrication)

COMPETENCY Applies knowledge of operational roles and responsibilities to ensure patient, public, and personnel safety.

OBJECTIVES: After reading this chapter, you should be able to:

42-1. Define key terms introduced in this chapter.
42-2. Explain elements of dispatch information, including location and whether it is a motor vehicle collision or other type of emergency, that would indicate possible obstacles to patient access, extrication, and care, and discuss how you can plan for such situations.
42-3. Use scene size-up findings to anticipate and prepare for the following:
  a. Potential problems in accessing patients
  b. Need for additional resources
  c. Appropriate personal protective equipment
  d. Appropriate measures to improve scene safety
  e. Location of all patients
  f. Vehicle safety in a collision situation
42-4. Explain actions that may be required to gain residential access.
42-5. Explain actions that may be required to gain motor vehicle access, including the concepts of simple and complex access.
42-6. Describe the role of the EMT and basic considerations for caring for a patient entrapped in a vehicle.
42-7. Describe equipment and methods for stabilizing an upright vehicle, a vehicle on its side, and a vehicle on its roof.
42-8. Describe various methods of accessing, disentangling, and extricating a patient entrapped in a vehicle.

KEY TERMS: Page references indicate first major use in this chapter. For complete definitions, see the Glossary at the back of the book.

complex access p. 1383
simple access p. 1383

MEDIA RESOURCES: Please go to www.bradybooks.com to access mykit for this text. You will find quizzes, critical thinking scenarios, weblinks, animations, and videos related to this chapter—and much more. Look for online information on air bags and air medical services. You will also find a video on rapid extrication.

CASE STUDY

The Dispatch

EMS Unit 204—respond to Solzman Road just north of Pin Oak Court—vehicle crash with reported multiple injuries and entrapment. Time out is 2337 hours.

Upon Arrival

You find a small red vehicle sitting nose to nose with a large dump truck. The front of the automobile has collapsed and is underneath the front axle of the truck. The front bumper of the truck is even with the windshield of the automobile. You can see two motionless young people in the front seat of the car with a considerable amount of blood coming from multiple facial lacerations. The dash is crushed down onto the patients, pinning them in the vehicle.

How Would You Proceed?

During this chapter, you will learn about your role as an EMT in patient rescue situations. Later, we will return to the case study and put in context some of the information you learned.

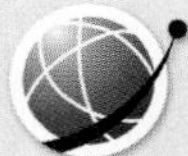

Media Resources
Go to www.bradybooks.com for mykit. Highlights:

- *Web Resource:* Airbags During Emergencies
- *Video:* Rapid Extrication

Objective 42-2
Explain elements of dispatch information that would indicate possible obstacles to patient access, extrication, and care, and discuss how you can plan for such situations.

Introduction

By far the most common rescue situations encountered by the EMT are motor vehicle crashes. The National Highway Traffic Safety Administration (NHTSA) reports that 2,491,000 people were injured and 41,059 were killed in motor vehicle crashes in the United States in 2007. Patient rescue begins with the scene size-up. It includes stabilization of the scene as well as stabilization of the vehicle, gaining access, and safely extricating, packaging, and moving the patient. During the entire process, it is necessary to ensure the safety of the patient, bystanders, your partner, yourself, and any other emergency personnel on the scene.

Access and extrication are also issues at scenes other than vehicle crashes. Usually, you will find your patients in safe, easily accessible locations where gaining access requires no more than a knock on a door. However, there will be occasions when advanced rescue techniques must be used to get to and help a patient—for example, on a remote mountainside, from a raging river, or from entrapment under machinery or a collapsed building.

Obviously you cannot receive advanced rescue training from this or any other EMT text. You can, however, become familiar with the situations in which patients are found and the roles you can play in rescue. The primary role of the EMT in a rescue situation is gaining access to the patient as quickly as can be safely accomplished to perform patient assessment and emergency care, even as the rescue operation proceeds. In some situations, it may be necessary that you perform simple extrication to remove the patient from the vehicle. More complex extrication situations require advanced training and tools. Your two major priorities in a rescue situation are (1) to keep yourself and your partner safe and (2) to prevent further harm to the patient.

Planning Ahead

Dispatch

As soon as you receive the call from dispatch, you must evaluate whether there are obstacles to patient access and extrication—in other words, whether the situation requires special rescue procedures. Begin with these questions:

- Is the patient ill or injured?
- What is the mechanism of injury?
- What is the location of the incident?
- What time of day is it?
- What is the weather?
- Is there a report of entrapment?
- Is there a report of a leak or a spill?

Most illnesses occur at home and offer little challenge to access and extrication other than an occasional locked door or protective pet dog. However, an incident involving trauma may offer considerable challenge. A trauma patient may be found anywhere under any circumstances. Based on the dispatch information, the EMT can begin to plan for access and extrication problems.

Location

Consider the location of the incident. For example, on a call to a fall in a parking lot at the local mall you may encounter heavy traffic. A cardiac emergency may be easy to handle at a residence, but on the 16th green of the local golf course or in the stands at the high school football game, it can be difficult. Access to a home may be easier than access to an industrial site.

Know your territory. Look around your community and begin to identify locations and occupations that may present access difficulties for EMS personnel. For example:

- Utility employees work above and below ground.
- Construction workers work everywhere from ditches to rooftops and around heavy equipment.
- Painters work off ladders and scaffolding, which may be placed on soft, unstable ground.
- Antennas and water towers need periodic maintenance.
- Industrial sites offer all these potential risks and problems and more.
- Some intersections are well known for serious collisions.

Excluding motor vehicle collisions, most injuries are the result of gravity. People either fall or something falls on them. Consider all the things that can fall on people—for example, a car on top of the weekend mechanic, a tree

Key Points
Excluding motor vehicle collisions, most injuries are the result of gravity. People either fall or something falls on them.

Objective 42-3
Use scene size-up findings to anticipate and prepare for access problems, need for additional resources, appropriate personal protective equipment and scene safety measures, location of all patients, and vehicle safety in a collision situation.

after a sudden storm, construction material at a new building site, or a few tons of dirt from a cave-in of a ditch or excavation.

People can crawl, climb, and walk to many locations that your ambulance and wheeled stretchers cannot traverse. Be prepared. Have strategies for gaining access in mind, and know the types of specialized rescue teams available through your system.

Motor Vehicle Collisions

Motor vehicle collisions present the most frequent rescue problems. Consider factors such as location and time of day to begin to mentally weigh the odds of patient entrapment and difficult access.

The numbers of accidents are greater during high traffic times, but with more traffic come slower speeds and less chance of entrapment and serious injuries. As traffic thins, speeds increase and so do the number of entrapments, serious injuries, and fatalities. A collision on a freeway holds a greater chance of entrapment than a collision in a parking lot.

The majority of examples discussed in this chapter concern vehicle collisions, because they are the rescue situation you will most commonly encounter as an EMT.

▶ Sizing Up the Scene

Expect the unexpected. Do not rely solely on the information received from dispatch. It can be sketchy or inaccurate. Know your territory, and stay alert for potential hazards. For example, when responding in industrial areas or to motor vehicle collisions involving common carriers and other commercial vehicles, stay alert for potential hazardous materials spills and releases. They present special challenges. Be sure your ambulance is equipped with binoculars, so you can assess the scene from a safe distance and position.

Scene size-up is a continual process. Even after you reach your patient, stay alert for changes in your surroundings. Wrecked vehicles can catch fire, an unsteady power line may fall, or the overturned container may begin to leak. Every scene is dynamic and must be approached cautiously and continually reviewed until it is stabilized.

Perform a 360-Degree Assessment

Once you are on the scene, perform a 360-degree assessment. You should perform this assessment prior to exiting the ambulance, if at all possible. However, to effectively perform the 360-degree assessment you must look at the front of the vehicle, at both sides, and at the rear. Also, inspect above and below the vehicle. The entire time, you will assess for potential hazards to yourself, your partner, other emergency personnel, the patient, and bystanders. Potential hazards include downed electrical wires; leaking fuels or fluids; smoke or fire coming from the vehicle or near or around the vehicle; and broken glass, jagged metal, and other sharp objects. While performing the 360-degree assessment, also attempt to identify trapped or ejected patients and potential mechanisms of injury.

Evaluate the Need for Additional Resources

Based on the initial information provided by the caller, the communications officer may have already dispatched additional resources to the scene, such as police for traffic control and crash investigation or the fire department or rescue services for extrication. Once on the scene, you may identify the need for other resources, such as the electric company for downed wires or the hazardous materials team for crashes involving hazardous cargo or spills. Consider the need for the following additional resources when responding to and assessing the scene:

- Extrication team or equipment
- Fire suppression
- Law enforcement
- Hazardous material team
- Utility company (electric, natural gas)
- Air medical evacuation
- Swift water rescue if vehicle is trapped in fast moving water

Personal Protective Equipment

The scene of a typical motor vehicle collision or other rescue situation is inherently hazardous. Materials such as shattered glass, sharp metal, flammable liquids, battery acid, and blood are commonplace. *Proper protective cloth-*

Thinking Critically
Arriving on the scene of a collision, you see shattered glass, twisted metal, a dark liquid flowing out from under one of the wrecked cars, patients trapped inside. What personal protective equipment will you need for this situation?

Thinking Critically
You are first on scene at a collision. From the ambulance, you can see that power lines are down across the hood of the vehicle. A driver and passenger are inside. What should you do?

ing and equipment must be used at every incident when such hazards are or may be present.

The safety of any rescuer must never be jeopardized. Rescuers must always wear the level of protection needed for their particular role in the rescue process. The minimum level of protection for the EMT includes eye protection, disposable gloves, and any additional protection necessary to prevent direct contact with any blood or body fluid.

A major hazard to EMTs at vehicle crashes is being struck by a passing vehicle. Any time you are working on or near a roadway, it is necessary to wear a high-visibility safety vest to lessen your chances of becoming a victim yourself.

Your everyday work uniforms do not provide much protection from the glass and sharp objects usually present at collisions and other rescue scenes. Protective coveralls, for example, may protect you from a patient's body fluids, but they may not protect you from hidden or flying debris. If you need to enter a wrecked vehicle to provide patient care, wear the appropriate protective clothing.

Full turnout gear, including coat, brightly colored and highly visible vest, bunker pants, and steel-toed boots, is required for personnel involved in the patient extrication process. Head protection, such as a standard fire helmet, will protect your head from impact. The ear flaps and a wide brim will help protect you from shattering glass and falling debris. In addition to goggles or safety glasses, the helmet's face shield offers protection for the face and eyes. Heavy leather gloves worn over disposable gloves will help protect your hands from both sharp objects and body fluids.

Know your local protocols and standard operating policies, which may dictate additional precautions.

Scene Safety

As stated earlier, *your safety is always the highest priority in any emergency.* Focus on risk analysis, not risk taking. Never commit yourself to a situation that is not completely secure. Although it may be difficult to remember at times, the biggest difference between you and the average person is your training. Do not compound the emergency or risk other rescuers' lives by becoming part of the problem.

If you are the first to arrive at the scene of an emergency, you are responsible for scene size-up and scene stabilization until police, fire, and other rescue personnel arrive. The list of hazards that you may encounter at motor vehicle collisions and other emergencies is much too lengthy to address in this chapter. However, common hazards include electrical lines and traffic. Unique hazards when you are working inside or around the vehicle include alternative-fueled vehicles, undeployed safety devices, energy-absorbing bumpers, and hazardous materials. Refer to Chapter 41, "Ambulance Operations and Air Medical Response," for safety methods to protect yourself when you are on scene in or near moving traffic. Also refer to Chapter 43, "Hazardous Materials," for risks to and responsibilities of the EMT when hazardous materials are involved.

Electrical Lines

Hazards commonly found at collision scenes are downed electrical lines and damaged poles holding electrical lines and equipment. *Always assume a downed power line is electrically alive.* If you see that electrical lines are down near or in contact with the vehicle, the area must be secured to avoid accidental contact.

Often, the electrical distribution equipment supplying the power to the lines will have automatic resets. This is a method the power companies use to restore power when something such as a fallen tree branch causes a temporary short. When the power is automatically restored to the downed line, it can cause the line to whip and arc. Therefore, if a line is down and broken 75 feet from the pole, the area to be secured should be greater than 75 feet in all directions from the pole. If the power lines are in contact with the vehicle, *stay away.* Request special assistance from your local electric service company.

If patients are still in the vehicle, shout or communicate with them over your unit's public address (PA) system. Advise them that the electric company is en route. Tell them to stay inside the vehicle, which is safer than attempting to get out. If patients were to climb out of the automobile, the electricity could pass from the vehicle and through them to the ground even before a foot touches the ground. Vehicle tires provide some insulation between the vehicle and the ground, but discourage the patients from touching any metal within the vehicle.

If the situation is immediately threatening to life, or if the electric company is unable to respond, rescue personnel specially trained in handling electrical emergencies may move the downed line using special equipment and techniques designed for that purpose. In the case of fire, the patients may have to be told to jump clear of the vehicle with their feet together, avoiding contact with the car and the ground at the same time. The proper way to move away from downed power lines is to shuffle away with small steps, keeping the feet together and on the ground at all times. (When separated feet touch the ground, a circuit is created—up one leg, through the body, and down the other leg—so feet must be kept together.)

Control Traffic Flow

Traffic must be controlled for scene safety. In most parts of the country, directing traffic is primarily the responsibility of the police. However, if this job falls to rescue personnel in your area, or if you must control traffic before the police arrive, special prior training in traffic direction and control is necessary. If the police are not on the scene, designate a person specifically to be responsible for traffic control to ensure that traffic is constantly being managed during the extrication.

In general, the safest method for traffic control at a serious vehicle collision is to stop all traffic and reroute it to different roads. This is not only for the safety of patients and bystanders but also for the safety of rescuers at the scene. If the regular flow of traffic must be channeled around the scene, it should be routed at least 50 feet from the wrecked cars (Figures 42-1a to 42-1d*).

Even specially trained personnel must take extreme care when directing traffic away from an accident scene. Use fire apparatus and other emergency response vehicles as blockers to provide a safety zone. Position the ambulance so that the patient loading doors are angled away from the moving traffic. Always face the oncoming traffic and be attentive to erratic vehicle movement by drivers. Additional rescue personnel and warning devices such as flares, chemical lights, or reflective cones are needed. Watch for fluids spilled on the roadway, and do not place flares where they might contact or become contacted by a fluid spill. All those who are working in or near the traffic should wear adequate reflective clothing or high-visibility vests so that they can be clearly seen. Visual signals must be clear, so that approaching drivers can quickly understand exactly what they are being asked to do. *Flares or cones should begin far enough from the scene so that a car can safely stop before it hits the scene, even if the driver did not notice the flares or cones from a distance.*

Another consideration in vehicle positioning is substances leaking from a vehicle involved in a crash. Park the ambulance upwind to avoid being affected or overcome by potentially hazardous fumes. Also park the ambulance uphill if a potentially hazardous liquid is leaking from a vehicle so that the liquid will flow away from the ambulance.

Posted speed (mph)	Stopping distance for that speed		Posted speed (in feet)		Distance of the farthest warning device
20 mph	50 feet	+	20 feet	=	70 feet
30 mph	75 feet	+	30 feet	=	105 feet
40 mph	125 feet	+	40 feet	=	165 feet
50 mph	175 feet	+	50 feet	=	225 feet
60 mph	275 feet	+	60 feet	=	335 feet
70 mph	375 feet	+	70 feet	=	445 feet

FIGURE 42-1a * Flares are positioned according to a formula that includes the stopping distance for the posted speed plus a margin of safety.

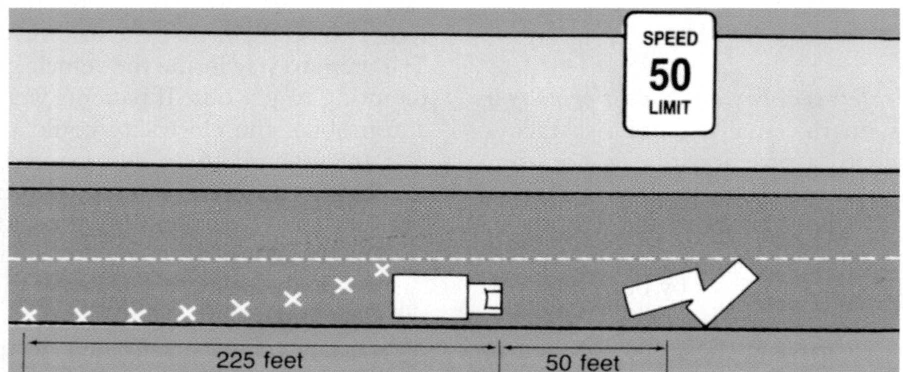

FIGURE 42-1b * Flares positioned on a straight road. Approaching vehicles are moved into the correct lane before they reach the edge of the danger zone.

Thinking Critically
Your crew is called to work a collision on the shoulder of a busy roadway. What methods can be used to protect emergency workers from being struck by passing traffic?

Key Points
Be aware of additional hazards that may be present at a collision scene, such as high-voltage batteries and cables in hybrid vehicles, high-pressure fuel containers in alternative-fuel vehicles, undeployed air bags, and energy-absorbing bumpers.

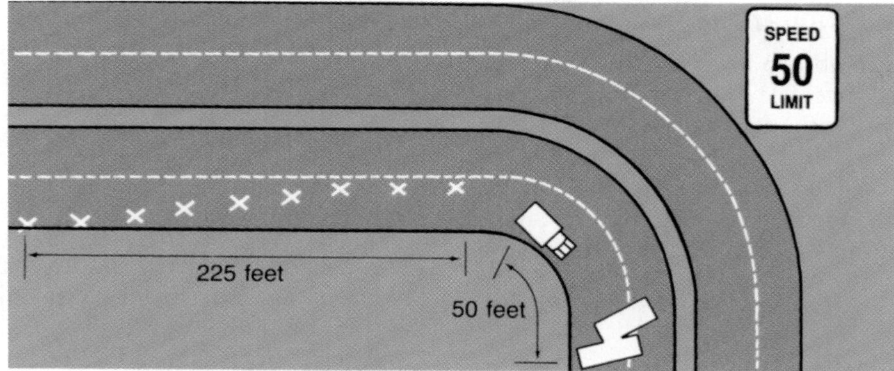

FIGURE 42-1c * Flares positioned ahead of a curved section of road. The start of the curve is considered to be the edge of the danger zone.

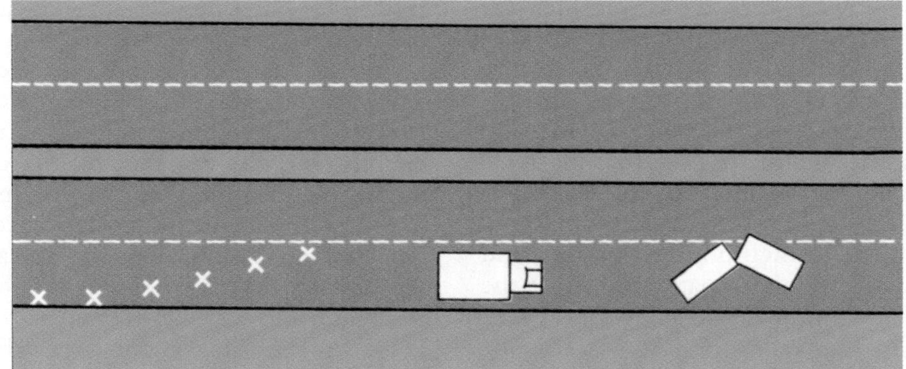

FIGURE 42-1d * Flares positioned on a hill. The flares slow approaching vehicles and make them turn into the correct lane before they reach the top of the hill.

Alternative-Fueled Vehicle Systems

Alternative-fueled vehicle systems are gaining much popularity as gasoline prices rise and people become more environmentally conscientious. Hybrid vehicles use a combination of gasoline and electricity to power the vehicle. High-voltage batteries and cables are used as an alternative fuel source. This poses a risk of electric shock to the rescuer if an electric discharge occurs or if the high-voltage cables are breached.

Vehicles may use other alternative fuels, such as natural gas or hydrogen. These fuels are stored in high-pressure containers that could pose a significant risk if a fire were involved or if the container were to be accidentally punctured during the extrication process.

Undeployed Air Bags

Air bag systems have evolved over the years from a single driver-side air bag to multiple air bags placed throughout the vehicle. Undeployed air bags pose a safety risk to rescuers who enter the vehicle to assess, treat, or extricate the patient. Air bags are deployed with significant force by a controlled explosion from a canister device. If a rescuer is positioned in front of an undeployed air bag that suddenly deploys, the force of the air bag striking the rescuer could severely or mortally injure him. It is necessary to deactivate air bags before any type of extrication to avoid accidental deployment. Deactivation is usually done by simply disconnecting the car's battery cables.

Key Points
When disconnecting a car battery, always remove the negative cable first. Removing the positive cable first can result in a spark that ignites a fire or an explosion.

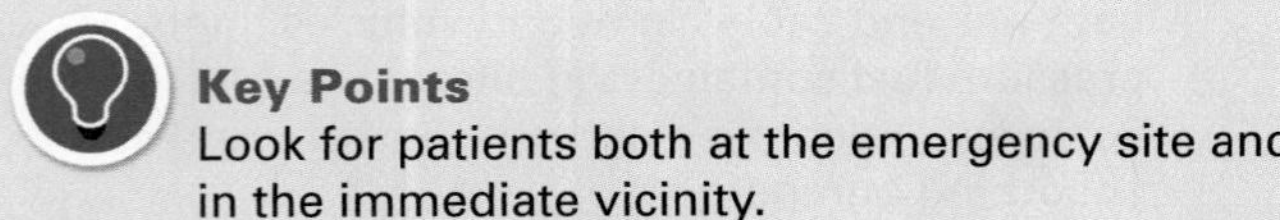

Key Points
Look for patients both at the emergency site and in the immediate vicinity.

Energy-Absorbing Bumpers

Bumpers are designed to absorb low-velocity impacts to the front and rear of the vehicle. These bumpers, commonly referred to as "five-mile-per-hour bumpers," use a piston-type system to absorb the impact of the collision. If the piston is pushed inward it is considered to be "loaded." If a rescuer happens to be standing in front of the bumper when it springs back outward, it may cause serious injury.

Locate All Patients

Most incidents involve a single patient who is easily accessible. Always locate that patient before attempting to gain access. By doing so you will prevent further injury. For example, you can make sure the patient is protected with a blanket before a rescue team breaks a car windshield for emergency extrication. You may also be able to check if an injured or ill patient is behind a bedroom door before the rescue team forces it open.

Some incidents involve more than one patient, and they are not always easy to identify or find. In explosions, building collapses, trench or confined-space rescues, and hazardous materials incidents it is often difficult to locate patients. That is also true in high-impact, rollover, and off-road vehicle collisions. Look for patients both at the site of the emergency and in the immediate vicinity. Unrestrained automobile occupants, for instance, can be thrown great distances and hidden by uneven terrain, darkness, vegetation, and debris.

Look for clues to "missing" patients. Get information from witnesses and patients about others who may be hurt at the scene. An empty child's car seat or a small sweater and coat in the backseat may be an indication that a child was involved in the incident. If in doubt, have the police contact relatives in an attempt to learn who might have been in the vehicle. Also ask bystanders if a patient walked away from the scene or if a passerby took a patient away. Before leaving the scene, a thorough search of the area for all victims must be conducted by emergency personnel. You may arrive on the scene to find no obvious crash or emergency at all. Take the time to look for signs that a vehicle might have left the road, for example, skid marks or damaged guard rails. (In one real-life incident, a car went off a freeway and under a chain-link fence without damaging or even displacing the fence!)

It can be frustrating to wait in a safe area while specialized rescue teams locate, extricate, and deliver patients to you. Realize that in difficult and complex rescue situations, a team effort is required to successfully perform a rescue. Follow directions from the scene commander, and provide emergency medical care to patients as necessary and as possible.

Vehicle Safety

If a fire engine company is not yet on the scene, remove the fire extinguisher from your vehicle and place it near the collision in case of fire.

After all hazards are addressed and the scene is secure, the vehicles involved must be properly stabilized for the safety of everyone at the scene. A vehicle is considered stable when it is in a secured position and can no longer move, rock, or bounce. Remember, even vehicles found on all four wheels and on a level surface need to be stabilized to minimize movement. This can be done by placing stabilizing chocks under the vehicle and deflating the tires.

If necessary, there are steps you can take to stabilize a vehicle without using special equipment. For example, if the vehicle is upright, resting on all four wheels, and safe to approach, you can shut off the engine. Then set the parking brake, and shift the automatic transmission to "park" or the manual transmission to any gear. Also employ cribbing and chocking for stabilization by placing firm objects such as a spare tire, pieces of wood, or logs in front of and behind a wheel to minimize vehicle movement. These steps usually will prevent a vehicle from rolling until rescue crews can properly and completely stabilize it.

Although rescue personnel may determine it to be necessary to disconnect the vehicle's battery, the majority of electric current and associated hazards can be eliminated by simply turning the ignition off. Before disconnecting power, attempts should be made to lower the power windows, unlock power door locks, and move the power seat to a position that provides the greatest patient access.

If it is necessary to disconnect the car battery, the engine compartment must be accessed. Cut or use a wrench to remove the negative battery cable first. Remove the positive cable last. *Note: If the positive cable is removed first, a spark may occur that could ignite acid fumes from the battery or gasoline spilled from the accident.*

If you determine that the vehicle is in an unstable and unsafe position and you cannot stabilize it with available equipment, do not enter it and do not put any weight in or on it. Wait for additional rescue personnel to properly stabilize the vehicle. (More information on vehicle stabilization is provided later in the chapter.)

Key Term

simple access a way to gain access to a patient that does not require specialized tools.

complex access a way to gain access to a patient that requires the use of tools and specialized equipment.

Objective 42-4
Explain actions that may be required to gain residential access.

Objective 42-5
Explain actions that may be required to gain motor vehicle access.

Gaining Access

There are two basic ways a rescuer can gain access to a patient. **Simple access** is access in which tools are not required. **Complex access** requires the use of tools and specialized equipment.

Fortunately, most incidents do not present access problems. However, when confronted with one, you must quickly evaluate the situation and decide if a simple or complex access procedure is necessary. If complex access is required, it is best to call for rescuers who have had specialized training. (Specialized training programs available for complex access include trench, high angle, and basic vehicle rescue.)

Residential Access

To gain access to a residence when the door is locked, first walk around the house to check for open windows or doors. Attempt to locate the patient by shouting through doors and windows and looking in windows. If you are able to converse with the patient, ask if a neighbor has a key. If you cannot speak to the patient, ask neighbors if they have a key or if they know someone who does.

You can evaluate the need for a rapid, forced entry based on dispatch information, what you observe at the scene, and your conversation with the patient. If you need to forcefully enter the scene (break into the house or apartment), have the police and fire department dispatched. If possible, wait for their arrival.

The easiest and least costly method of forceful entry usually is breaking a window. Breaking a pane of glass in or next to a door may permit you to reach in and unlock the door. Kicking the door in is not recommended, since you may be injured and it can cause costly structural damage. It is also more difficult to secure the residence afterward.

After police and fire personnel are on the scene, proceed with a forceful entry as follows:

1. Check all windows and doors for one that is unlocked or open. At the same time, look and shout through each window to try to locate the patient and check for hazards.
2. If a window is open but blocked by a screen, cut through the screen.
3. If you must break a window, choose a room in which there are no patients and a window through which you can see what is on the other side. Locate the smallest and least expensive window that will still allow you access.
4. If the patient is awake and responsive, inform him of what you are going to do.
5. Wear eye protection, heavy work gloves, and a coat.
6. Stand alongside the window to be broken (Figure 42-2*).
7. Using an object like a flashlight or a tire iron, grasp one end firmly and strike the top corner of the pane nearest you. Do not reach above your head.
8. Clear the broken pieces of glass out of the frame before reaching in to unlock the window or door.

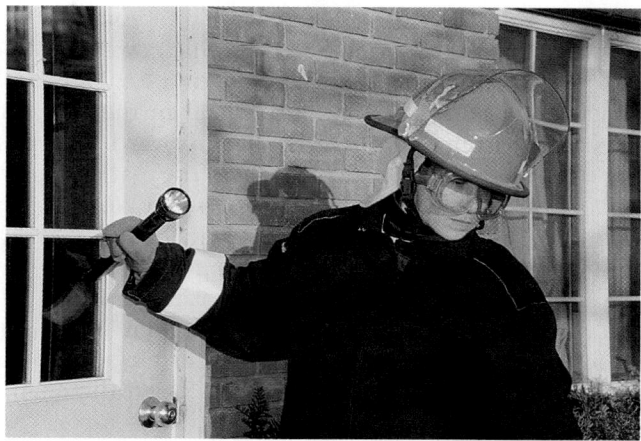

FIGURE 42-2 * The easiest and least costly method of gaining access to a patient inside a locked house usually is by breaking a window.

People are becoming more security conscious. In many urban areas and areas of high crime, for example, people often cover windows and doors with security bars. As a result, it is difficult to force entry into many homes and apartments. Specialized rescue techniques and tools are constantly being developed and refined. It is best to call on rescue companies within the fire department or other emergency services to gain access in these situations.

Motor Vehicle Access

By far, the most common access problems encountered by the EMT involve motor vehicle collisions. Throughout the process of gaining access, your main function is

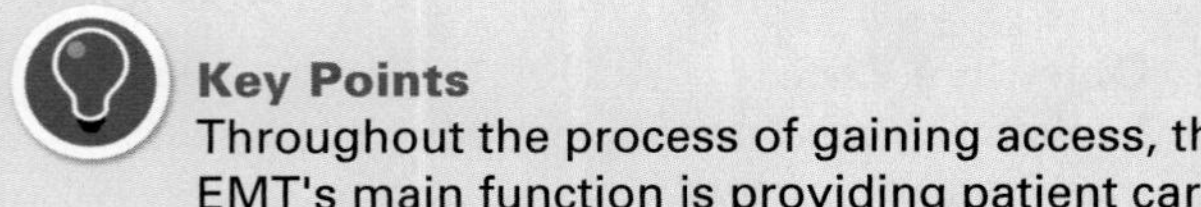

Key Points
Throughout the process of gaining access, the EMT's main function is providing patient care.

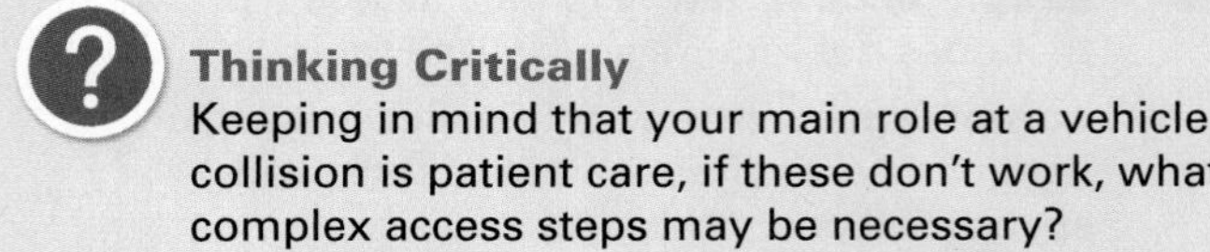

Thinking Critically
Keeping in mind that your main role at a vehicle collision is patient care, if these don't work, what complex access steps may be necessary?

patient care. Once the scene is secure and you have decided that it is safe to approach the vehicle, walk around it once to identify mechanisms of injury, and approach facing the patient. (If you approach from the side, the patient may attempt to turn his head toward you, possibly aggravating a spinal injury.) If the patient is responsive, look directly into his eyes while you tell him not to move his head or neck. Tell the patient everything you and other rescuers are going to do before you do it. Until you gain access to the patient and are able to stabilize the cervical spine, remind him repeatedly not to move. Tell the patient that focusing on any object directly in front of him will help lessen the chance of neck movement.

Simple Access

The door is always the simple access of choice because it is the largest uncomplicated opening into the passenger compartment of a car. Always start by testing the door handle to see if it will open. If the doors are locked, reach in any open window to unlock one of them. If all windows are intact and rolled up, say to one of the patients: "Without moving your head or neck, try to unlock a door or lower the window." Be sure to state the instruction not to move the head or neck first. If you wait until the end of your request, he may move and injure himself further in his eagerness to help.

Complex Access

If none of these methods of gaining access work, the quickest means of gaining access is by breaking a window. The side windows in a modern automobile are made of tempered safety glass that will break into rounded pieces rather than sharp shards. (The windshield and back window are made of a different kind of safety glass with a layer of plastic between layers of glass.) When breaking windows or using rescue tools near patients or rescuers, cover them with a heavy blanket or tarp whenever possible.

To break a window in an automobile, tell the patient what you are going to do. Then:

1. Wear personal protective equipment. Heavy gloves and eye protection are necessary.
2. Locate the window farthest from the patient and, if time allows, cover it with contact paper or strips of broad tape to prevent the shattered glass from flying in on the patient. Or, if possible, cover the patient or have the patient cover himself before you break the glass—a procedure that is less time-consuming than taping the window.
3. Place a sharp tool such as a screwdriver, center punch, or other commercial window shattering device against a lower corner of the window and strike the tool with a hammer. Hold the tool with your hand resting against the car so your hand will not go through the window when it breaks. Rescue personnel often carry a spring-loaded punch. Available at most hardware stores, this tool can easily be carried in a pocket or equipment holster. It is used in much the same way as just described except that, when you place it against the lower corner of a tempered safety-glass window, you simply push until the spring causes the tip to punch, or you pull back on the spring and suddenly release the spring for the tip to punch and break the glass. Again, you must take care to avoid pushing your hand through the window. The spring punch model shown in EMT Skills 42-1 prevents the hand of the rescuer from pushing through the broken glass. In older model cars, a makeshift tool that can be used in an emergency is the car's whip antenna. Snap off the antenna and hold it at one end along the metal of the door frame just below the window, allowing the opposite tip to touch the corner of the glass. Pull the tip away from the glass, causing the antenna to bow. When released, the tip of the antenna will strike the glass with enough force to shatter the window.
4. Carefully remove the broken glass, starting at the top and continuing until all has been removed. Broken correctly, although completely shattered, most tempered safety glass will remain in place even if it was not taped.
5. Attempt to unlock the door. If unsuccessful, cover the door edge with a blanket or tarp before crawling into the vehicle to gain access to your patient.

Other complex access methods require much more specialized training and equipment and will be discussed later in the chapter.

Once you gain access, evaluate the patient's condition. At that time make the decision to perform rapid or normal extrication (as explained in Chapter 32, "Spinal Column and Spinal Cord Trauma").

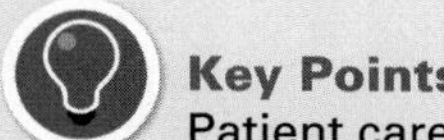

Key Points
Patient care always precedes removal from the vehicle unless delaying removal would endanger lives.

Objective 42-6
Describe the role of the EMT and basic considerations for caring for a patient entrapped in a vehicle.

Extrication

The purpose of extrication is to remove the patient as rapidly and safely as possible from wreckage—most commonly the wreckage of a vehicle collision—in which he is entrapped.

The Role of the EMT

The fundamental components of extrication include scene size-up, stabilization, gaining access, disentanglement, and patient removal. The role of the EMT in vehicle stabilization and patient extrication is that of patient care provider. The EMT may be responsible for gaining simple access to the patient prior to the rescue team's arrival. However, in some cases, access to the patient is delayed because of the inability to gain simple access or because the vehicle is deemed to be unstable. Once specialized rescue personnel assure you that the vehicle is stable and the scene is safe to enter, you may approach the patient to perform an assessment and administer emergency medical care.

Note: Patient care always precedes removal from the vehicle unless delaying removal would endanger the life of the patient, EMS personnel, or other rescuers.

While always bearing in mind that your responsibility is seeing to the welfare of the patient, work with other rescuers. Cooperate in every way possible with personnel who are working to disentangle the patient. Help them make certain that the patient is removed from the vehicle in a way that minimizes risk of further injury.

In some EMS systems, EMS providers are both emergency medical care providers and rescuers. In those systems, a chain of command should be established to ensure patient care priorities.

Caring for the Patient

As in any emergency, your first priority is always your own safety. (You are no good to the patient if you become another casualty.) Be sure the scene is safe, the vehicle is stable, and you are wearing the appropriate personal protective equipment before you try to reach the patient.

Basic considerations when dealing with a patient entrapped in a vehicle include the following:

- Maintain manual spinal stabilization at all times during the extrication process.
- Perform a primary assessment and manage any immediate life threats.
- Perform a controlled rapid extrication of the patient.
- Remove the vehicle from around the patient and not the patient from around the vehicle, if possible.
- Use adequate personnel.
- Use the path of least resistance that provides the least chance of further injury to the patient.

After gaining safe access to the patient, provide the same care you would provide to any trauma patient. Stabilize the cervical spine, complete the primary assessment, and provide critical interventions. Be sure you have, or have called for, sufficient personnel to help you provide proper care and to help you protect the patient from hazards.

Once you have access to the patient, establish a rapport. Remain with the patient throughout the rescue. Along with assessment, stabilization, and resuscitation efforts, you are responsible for assisting the patient through the extrication process and preparing him mentally and physically for disentanglement from the wreckage. Communicate with the patient and keep him informed of your actions and the actions of the rescue team. This communication is necessary for the safety of both you and the patient. Often, two EMTs need to be inside the vehicle during the extrication process—one to maintain manual in-line spinal stabilization and inform the patient of the actions of the rescue team, and another to assess the patient's condition and treat potentially serious injuries.

Before a forcible rescue is initiated, its effect on the patient must be analyzed. The usual approach to rescue is to remove the vehicle from around the patient. However, when the condition of the patient or the scene dictates speed, the parts of the vehicle that will allow for rapid extrication while protecting the patient's cervical spine should be removed first.

Use heavy blankets, a tarp, or a salvage cover to protect yourself, the patient, and other EMTs from the glass and flying debris that commonly result from disentanglement operations. During some extrication procedures, it may be necessary to place a solid object such as a backboard between the tool activity area and the patient.

Continually monitor the patient's condition and position in relation to the extrication tools and procedures.

Thinking Critically
Keeping in mind that your main role at a vehicle collision is patient care, if access to the patient is blocked, what additional actions might the EMT crew take?

Objective 42-7
Describe equipment and methods for stabilizing an upright vehicle, a vehicle on its side, and a vehicle on its roof.

If there is a potential problem, relay this information to the person in charge of the extrication team. If the patient's condition begins to deteriorate or otherwise becomes unstable, advise the rescue crew. They will change the approach to the incident and get the patient out as quickly as possible.

The patient entrapped by a vehicle collision is often in a highly agitated state. He will not be emotionally capable of handling the noise and confusion often associated with extrications and rescues. Even with a diminished level of responsiveness, the patient will be very frightened and may even attempt to move or crawl out of the vehicle.

To avoid this, it is very important that you prepare the patient for the rescue operation. Make him aware of the amount of time that the disentanglement might take and why it is necessary. Explain the activities, movements, and associated noises that will be encountered during the extrication process. Give the patient the opportunity to have some control over the process. For example, when the rescue crew asks you if you are ready for them to do a particular function, such as remove the door, check with the patient. Asking if he is ready to have the door or dash removed provides him with a feeling of control. If properly prepared, the patient will readily agree with each step of the extrication.

Stabilize and, if possible, immobilize the spine securely before you remove the patient from the vehicle by normal or rapid extrication procedures. The only exception to this rule is when there is an immediate threat to your patient's life or your own, such as fire, that requires an urgent move without spinal protection.

Specialized Stabilization, Extrication, and Disentanglement Techniques

Stabilizing a Vehicle

Vehicle stabilization is carried out by specialized personnel using equipment such as wood cribbing and wedges, step chocks, air bags, hydraulic tools and rams, come-alongs, jacks, chains, and winches (Table 42-1).

Upright Vehicle

The way to properly stabilize an upright vehicle is to immobilize the suspension. The first step in this process is to position plastic step chocks under the vehicle parallel

TABLE 42-1 Common Equipment Used for Vehicle Stabilization

Type	Description and Use
Air bag	A rubber bag, found in various shapes and sizes, that, when inflated with air, has great lifting ability.
Come-along	A ratcheting cable device used to pull in a straight direction.
Cribbing	4 × 4 or 2 × 4 blocks of hardwood cut to approximately 18-inch-long sections.
Hydraulic cutter	A hydraulic power tool used to cut metal.
Hydraulic ram	A hydraulic power tool used to push or pull in a straight direction.
Hydraulic spreader	A hydraulic power tool used to open, spread, and separate items such as vehicle doors.
Jack	A manual device used much as a ram would be used.
Step chock	A set of several 2 × 6 blocks of hardwood cut to varying lengths and secured together to form "steps." Plastic step chocks are premanufactured, faster to deploy, lighter than wood, and resistant to most of the fluids spilled at motor vehicle collisions.
Wedge	A 4 × 4 piece of cribbing tapered to an edge at one end.
Winch	A powered cable reel usually electrically or hydraulically driven and mounted to a truck, which is used to pull.

Key Points

Stabilization of an upright vehicle or of a vehicle on its side or on its roof is carried out by specially trained personnel.

Objective 42-8

Describe various methods of accessing, disentangling, and extricating a patient entrapped in a vehicle.

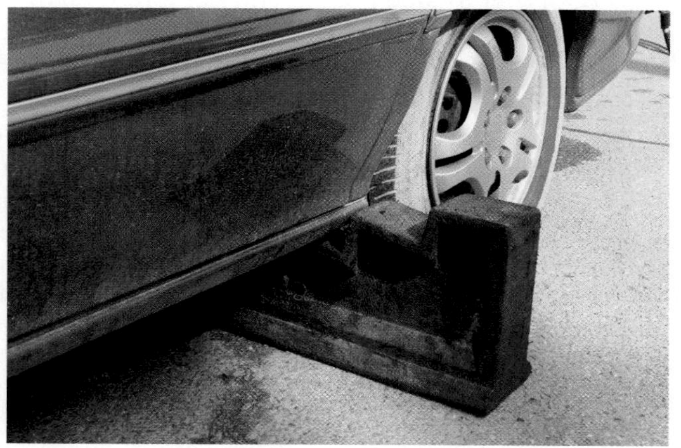

FIGURE 42-3 ✱ Plastic step chocks, as seen here, are strong and light and can be easily cleaned.

to each wheel (Figure 42-3✱). Plastic chocks are lighter than wood chocks and are resistant to most of the fluids spilled at motor vehicle crashes. The chocks can be pushed in until they touch the undercarriage. The vehicle should not be lifted to place the chocks. If step chocks are unavailable, a box crib with wedges can function in much the same manner. Either procedure will prevent the vehicle from rocking.

The air should then be removed from the tires. A quick and easy way to deflate tires is to pull out the tire's valve stems, using a pair of pliers. This will allow the air to escape from the tires, neutralizing the vehicle's suspension and virtually eliminating any movement. Sometimes, however, it may be desirable to be able to replace the air in the tires. If this is the case, air can be removed using a deflation tool or a valve stem removal tool. Valve stems would be cut and tires would be sliced only when it is absolutely necessary to use these methods to release the air.

Vehicle on Its Side

A vehicle on its side is inherently unstable and particularly dangerous to EMS personnel. Never attempt to enter such a vehicle before it is stabilized. A vehicle on its side is likely to roll onto its roof, thereby aggravating a patient's existing injuries and posing a severe risk of injury to rescuers both in and around the vehicle.

The first step in stabilizing this vehicle, when the equipment is available, is to attach a stabilizing pole, pulling device, cable, or chain from the undercarriage of the car to another vehicle or strong immovable object. Rescuers would then crib the length of the vehicle's side where it has contact with the ground. Every void between the ground and the vehicle should be filled with box cribbing and wedges to minimize movement. The 12- to 18-inch space between the top of the door frame along the roof line and the ground should also be filled.

If additional support is needed on either side of the vehicle to prevent rollover, rescue struts can be placed from the ground to the undercarriage or roof (EMT Skills 42-2). If these struts are unavailable, 3- to 6-foot pieces of 4 × 4 cribbing can be used instead.

Vehicle on Its Roof

A vehicle that has landed on its roof usually is in one of two conditions. It will either be held up by its roof posts or, if one or more posts collapse, it may be resting on the hood, trunk lid, or both.

Since the roof posts are not designed to support the weight of the vehicle, the vehicle must be stabilized before you can get to the patient. Whether the posts have collapsed or not, the weight of the vehicle must be taken off the posts. This can be accomplished by building a box crib under the hood and trunk and using wedges to remove any remaining space.

Air bags under either the front or the rear of the vehicle can also be used to stabilize the vehicle. Low-pressure bags may be used by themselves because of their greater lift height. If high-pressure air bags are used, a box crib should be built to within a couple of inches of the surface of the vehicle. Rescuers would then slide the air bag into that space. When the air bag is inflated and one end of the vehicle begins to lift, the other end will settle onto the box crib and the weight of the vehicle will be totally removed from the roof posts.

Remember, even if the vehicle seems stable initially, opening or removing doors during patient extrication will reduce the strength of the post. Without proper stabilization, that could lead to collapse.

Extricating a Patient

Patient disentanglement is carried out by specialized personnel. The primary goal is to remove the vehicle from around the patient, thus ensuring that the patient's injuries are not aggravated. Key factors in meeting that goal are that all personnel are familiar with extrication procedures and the incident command system (see Chapter 44, "Multiple-Casualty Incidents and Incident Management") and that all personnel can communicate with other members of the rescue team.

The most common tool used in vehicle extrication and patient disentanglement is the power hydraulic tool. This tool, along with various attachments, can be used to spread, push, cut, and pull. The power hydraulic rescue tool creates tremendous forces from several thousand pounds of force to well in excess of 20,000 pounds. In order to prevent injury to rescuers and patients, it should be continually monitored for safety during use.

"Rip and Blitz" Disentanglement

A sequence of patient extrication called the "rip and blitz" is illustrated in EMT Skills 42-3. This is just one of a number of specialized procedures that can be carried out by highly trained and qualified personnel. The vehicle is cut from around the patient, minimizing movement and protecting the patient and rescuers at all times. An EMT is inside the vehicle with the patient, maintaining spine stabilization and continually reassessing the patient's condition during the entire procedure until the patient is removed from the wreckage. The sequence is as follows:

1. An EMT enters the vehicle and establishes and maintains stabilization of the cervical spine as rescue personnel begin to stabilize the vehicle by placing chocks under the wheels (EMT Skills 42-3A and 42-3B).
2. Most electrical hazards can be avoided by simply turning off the ignition. To thoroughly minimize all risks, the battery cables should be disconnected or cut, always the negative terminal first, then the positive. This will reduce the risk of post-crash fire or unexpected air bag deployment. As an added precaution, the patient should be covered with a fire-retardant blanket (EMT Skills 42-3C).
3. Hydraulic spreaders are used to "pop" the rear door. Then the post between the front and rear sections of the passenger compartment—the B post—should be cut. A strap or rope should be attached to the rear door. As the cutter finishes the cut to the bottom of the B post, another rescuer uses a hydraulic ram or spreader to "rip" open the doors (EMT Skills 42-3D to 42-3G). (Keep in mind that the A posts are the front posts supporting the car roof. The B posts are the middle posts. C posts are at the rear.)
4. Next, the roof should be removed. The hydraulic cutters or a Sawzall (reciprocating saw) is used to cut both the A and C posts and the opposite-side B post, and a glass-cutting saw or Sawzall is used to cut across the bottom of the windshield. Care must be taken not to penetrate the passenger compartment with the cutting tool any farther than necessary. During the cutting process, one of the rescuers must monitor and control the cutting from a vantage point inside the vehicle. Hydraulic cutters then cut the roof from the vehicle (EMT Skills 42-3H and 42-3I).
5. "Jacking the dash" or performing a "dash roll" is very important when a patient is trapped by the dashboard. A relief cut should be made where the rocker panel meets the bottom of the A post. Hydraulic spreaders can then be used to push the dash off the patient. Some hydraulic spreaders have a spreading force of over 37,000 pounds and can spread up to 40 inches (EMT Skills 42-3J). Be sure to continually reexamine the patient's position during this procedure to avoid causing further injury.
6. As previously stated, the whole purpose of cutting the vehicle from around the patient is to protect the patient from further injury of both the cervical spine and the lower spine. The proper way to remove an injured patient from a damaged vehicle is vertically, or in line with the spine. Having a patient, especially one complaining of pain, "spin" or rotate his body onto a backboard is unacceptable (EMT Skills 42-3K).

Side-Impact or Head Protection Air Bags

Special consideration must be given when cutting any posts in vehicles that have side-impact or head protection systems. These deployment systems may utilize high-pressure stored-gas cylinders to deploy the air bags, which can cause serious injuries to rescue personnel or patients if they are punctured by cutting tools.

Other Methods of Access and Disentanglement

Other methods commonly used for access and disentanglement are described in the next sections.

Door Removal Sometimes all that needs to be done to access patients at a vehicle collision is opening or removing a door. Always check all doors and confirm that none are able to be opened normally prior to forcing entry.

A rescuer can force or "pop" a door with manual pry tools, hydraulic spreaders, and air chisels. Remember to protect yourself and the patient from flying debris by covering yourselves with a blanket during the procedure. If possible, place a solid object such as a spine board between the tool activity area and the patient. Keep the patient advised of reasons for the noise and any movement that may be encountered.

The front doors are most easily opened by prying at the latch site on the B post. All glass should be broken and removed on the side of the vehicle to be opened.

Often, when using hydraulic spreaders, there is not enough of a gap to fit the tip of the tool in near the latch. The rescuer must begin by widening the gap with a thinner hand pry tool (halligan or hux bar). Another method of widening the gap is by placing the tips of the partially

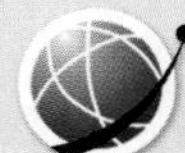

Media Resources
Go to www.bradybooks.com for mykit. Highlights:

- *Web Resource Traffic Safety During an Emergency*
- *Web Resource Air Medical Services*

opened hydraulic spreader vertically in the window opening of the door and forcibly enlarging this opening, which will cause the gap near the latch to widen. If the patient position allows clear access to the inside of the door, a third method is to place the partially opened tool over the door with one arm of the tool on each side of the door 6–12 inches from the latch. As the arms of the spreader begin to close, pinching the door, the gap near the latch will widen.

Once an opening has been created, the hydraulic spreader will be placed in the gap directly above or below the latch and begin to spread the arms. As long as the metal does not begin to rip, the rescuer should continue to spread the arms. If the metal begins to rip, the rescuer will stop, close the tool as needed, and get another grip nearer the latch.

Once open, the door may need to be removed completely to facilitate patient removal. With the proper technique, the hinges may be cut to remove the door completely. If this is not possible, the door may be removed by placing the tips of the spreader near each hinge and spreading the arms until the hinge fails. When any item is completely separated from the vehicle, such as when you remove the door, the object may suddenly be propelled several feet. This movement can be controlled but not prevented. Care must be taken to secure the object so it will not strike anyone when it becomes detached.

Windshield Removal and Roof Rolling Although it is usually preferable to totally remove the roof from a damaged vehicle, occasionally it might be decided to just "flap the roof" (displace the roof and windshield of the vehicle) to facilitate patient removal. Since this procedure involves maneuvers close to the patient, it is very important that you and the patient are well protected from the tools and flying debris.

Before the rescuers displace the roof, the windshield must first be separated from the vehicle. Depending on the type of mounting found, either the mounting or the windshield is cut. Rubber mounts can often be cut with a razor knife and the windshield removed intact. Sometimes the windshield will be cut as described earlier in the "Rip and Blitz Disentanglement" section.

Next, the A posts and B posts must be cut. Normally, either a hack saw, air cutting tool, or hydraulic cutting tool is used. Care must be taken to cut the A posts as close to the dash and the B posts as close to the door as possible. This will increase patient accessibility and minimize potential injury from the remaining post stubs. The roof is then creased just in front of the C posts using a long pry bar, pike pole, or other similar item. The roof can be grasped near the A post on each side and folded up and back toward the trunk.

After the roof is displaced, the stubs of the posts must be covered with duct tape or pieces of old 2½ fire hose to protect the patient and rescuers from any exposed sharp metal.

Special Disentanglement Procedures

No two vehicle extrications are exactly alike. Some can be quite complex. Very often, improvisation and common sense must prevail.

One complication occurs when a patient's foot is caught under the brake pedal. In this situation, a rope pulling device or portable hydraulic tool can be used to force the pedal sideways around the steering column to free the extremity. This procedure involves using tools in very close proximity to the patient, who may have an injury to the trapped part that is causing considerable pain. Therefore, disentanglement must be accomplished with utmost care so as not to disturb the injury. Often the rescuer can simply grab the brake pedal with a hand and pull firmly upward away from the floor, lifting it enough to free the foot.

A patient also may be trapped in a way that requires the seat to be moved or removed, such as a patient in the backseat of a two-door vehicle or a patient with a leg trapped under the seat. Disentanglement may be accomplished by using the seat adjustment lever to gently move the seat. If greater movement is needed, it can be done slowly by using hand tools to remove the nuts securing the seat or quickly by forcing the seat using portable rams or spreaders or a come-along. If the seat is forced, the patient will receive a considerable jolt. If injuries dictate that such movement may be harmful, other options must be considered.

Extricating a patient who is trapped in a vehicle on its side involves some different techniques. Rapid access and removal are important because the patient in a vehicle on its side may be experiencing a tremendous gravitational pull on the spine. Access to the patient may be gained by removing the rear window. The best way to extricate the patient is to cut the upper posts of the vehicle and fold the roof down (EMT Skills 42-4).

Once the patient has been disentangled, you will remove him from the wreckage using normal or rapid extrication procedures as discussed in Chapter 32, "Spinal Column and Spinal Cord Trauma."

EMT skills 42-1 Breaking an Automobile Window

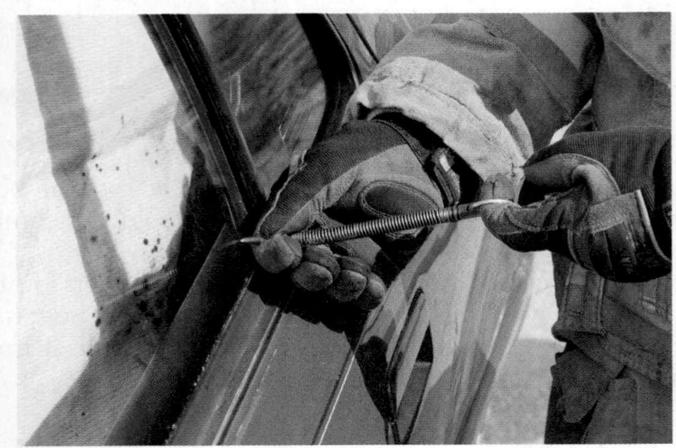

42-1A ✻ Position the punch in the corner of the side window and pull back on the spring.

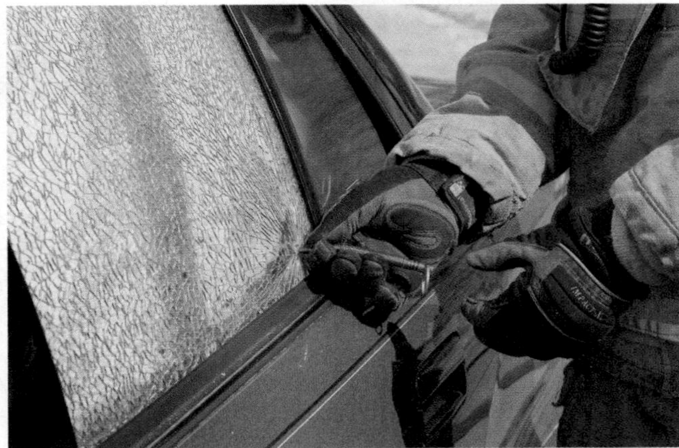

42-1B ✻ Keeping the tip of the punch in place, let go of the spring to shatter the window.

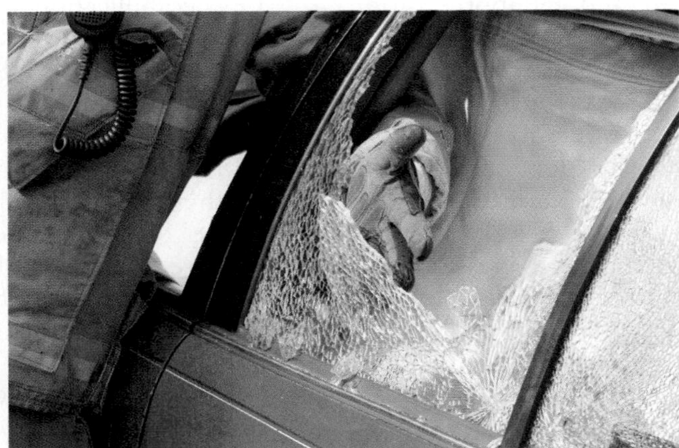

42-1C ✻ Starting at the top of the window, carefully push the broken glass away from the interior of the vehicle.

EMT skills 42-2 Stabilizing a Vehicle on Its Side

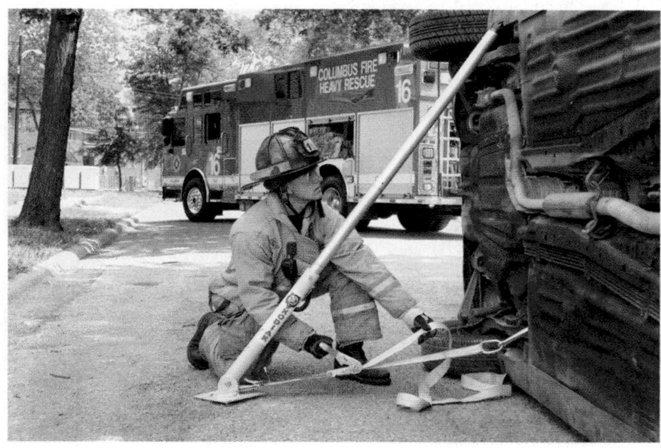

42-2A ✻ Rescue struts can be used to prevent a vehicle on its side from rolling over onto its top or back onto its wheels.

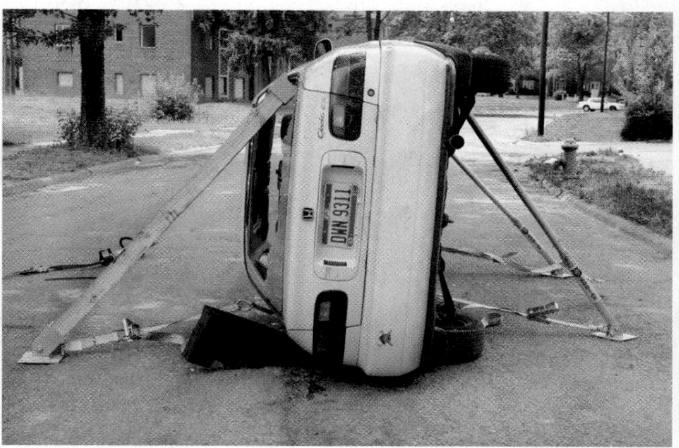

42-2B ✻ For extra safety, rescue struts can be placed against both the underside and the top of a vehicle on its side.

EMT skills 42-3 Extricating an Entangled Patient

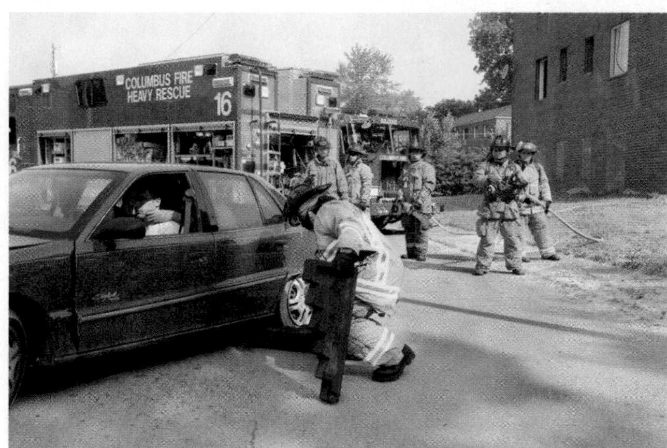

42-3A ✻ While the EMT maintains spine stabilization from inside, rescue personnel will begin to stabilize the vehicle.

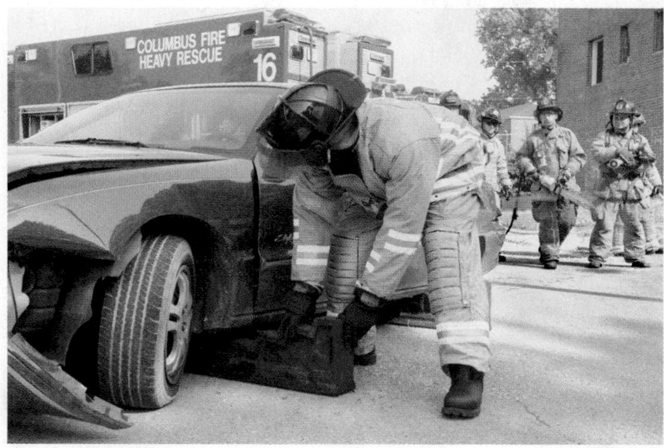

42-3B ✻ The first step in stabilizing the vehicle is to place chocks under the vehicle. Chocks should be pushed in until they touch the undercarriage; the vehicle should not be lifted up to fit the chocks into place.

continued

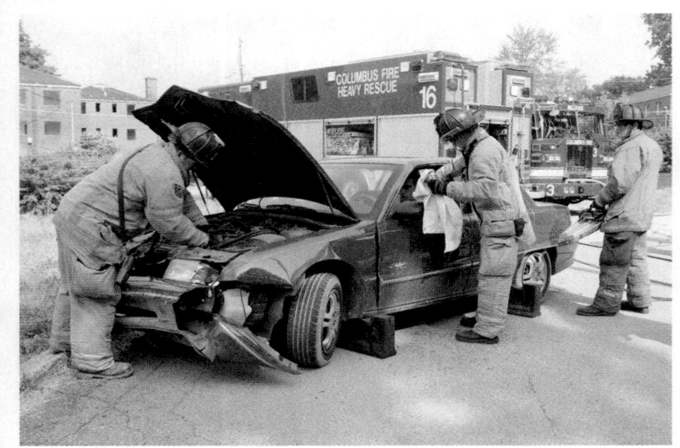

42-3C ✱ The patient should be covered with a fire-retardant blanket. The air should be released from the tires and the battery should be disconnected. Always disconnect the negative terminal first.

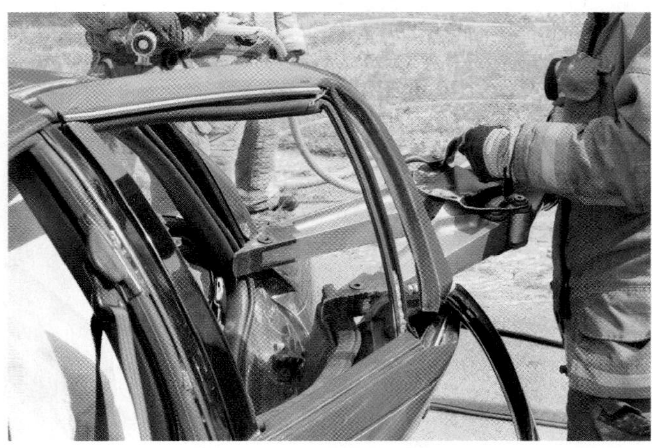

42-3D ✱ Hydraulic spreaders are used to "pop" open the rear door.

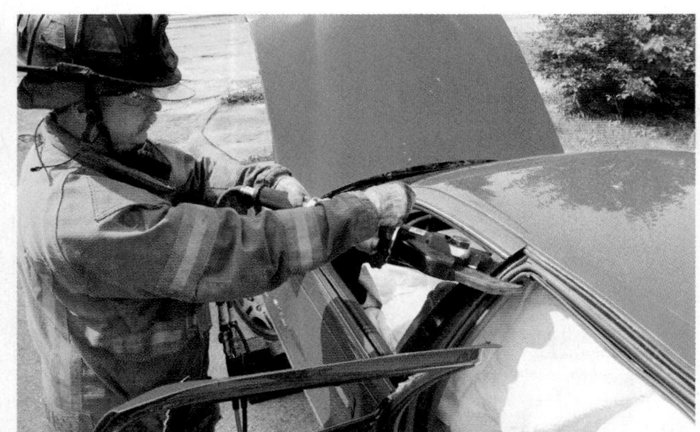

42-3E ✱ Cut the B post at the top by the roof.

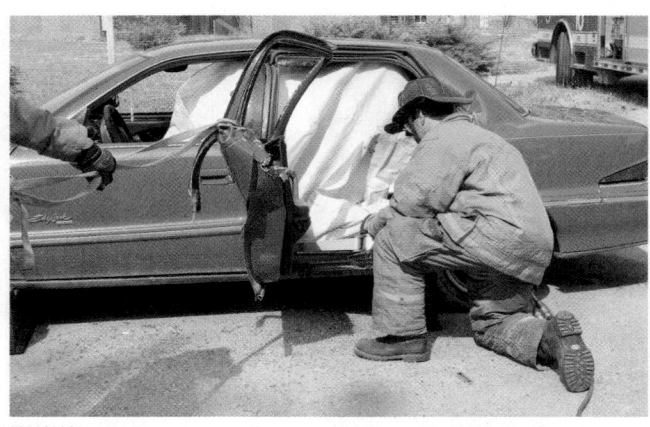

42-3F ✱ Cut the B post at the bottom by the floor.

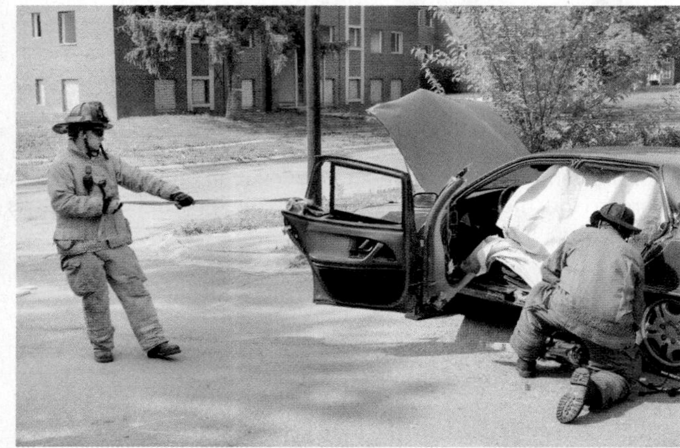

42-3G ✱ Using a hydraulic ram or spreaders, "rip" the B post while pulling the doors open on the front hinges.

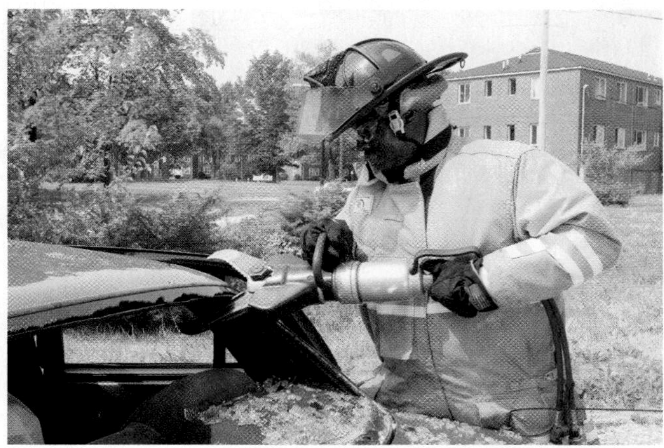

42-3H ✱ Hydraulic cutters are used to cut the roof from a vehicle.

EMT skills 42-3 Extricating an Entangled Patient *continued*

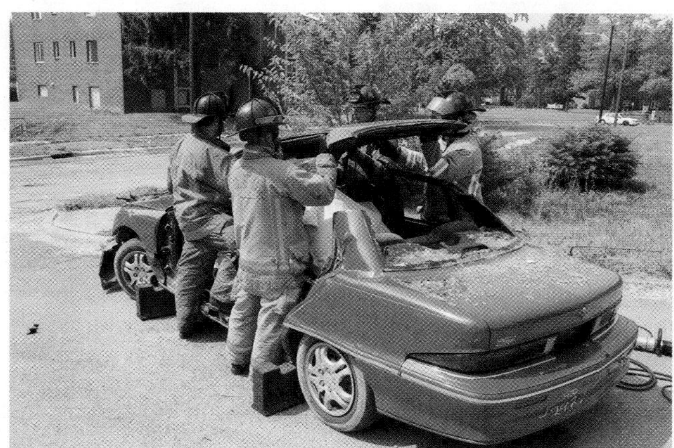

42-3I ✻ Use as many people as necessary to safely lift the roof up and away from the vehicle.

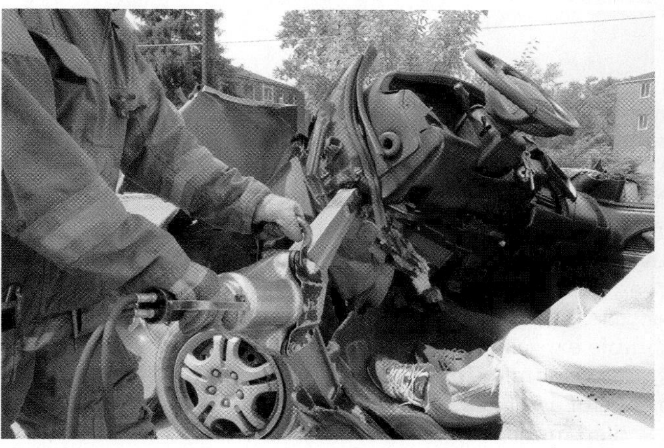

42-3J ✻ Hydraulic spreaders are used to free the patient from entrapment by the dashboard.

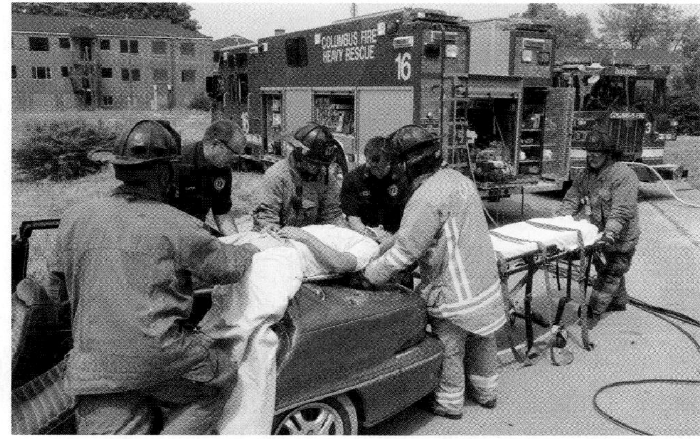

42-3K ✻ To prevent further injury to the patient, it is best to remove him vertically out of the vehicle.

EMT skills 42-4 Extricating a Patient from a Vehicle on Its Side

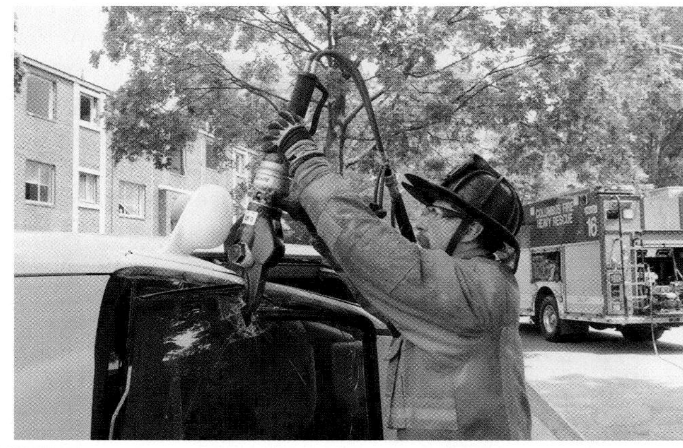

42-4A ✻ To extricate a patient from a vehicle on its side, first cut the upper posts using a hydraulic cutter or other cutting tool. The windshield should also be cut.

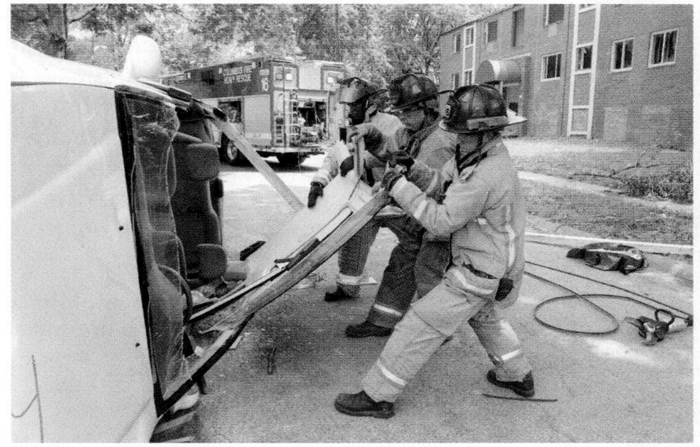

42-4B ✻ Then fold the roof down to provide an adequate space from which to remove the patient.

CHAPTER REVIEW

SUMMARY

Motor vehicle collisions account for the majority of incidents where an EMT must gain access to the patient. However, some medical patients may be in a confined area or in their own locked home to which the EMT would need to gain access. Extrication is the removal of a patient. You perform simple extrication every time you remove a patient from his home. Complex extrication is most often required at the scene of a vehicle collision when the patient is entrapped in tangled metal.

It is imperative that EMTs wear the proper personal protective equipment at the scene, to include high-visibility vests, while working on or near the roadway. If jagged metal and glass are present, EMS personnel should wear full turnout gear. Be sure to consider safety hazards such as downed electrical lines, traffic, and unstable vehicles. Also, it is necessary to locate all patients at the scene. Pay attention to scene clues that may indicate additional patients who are not immediately present or visible.

It may be necessary to gain immediate access to the patient to initiate emergency care. In a vehicle collision, this may be done by simply opening a door or shattering a window. Explain to the patient what you are doing. Once you have gained access to the patient, shift your attention to providing emergency care. The fire department may need to perform complex extrication maneuvers to remove you and the patient from the vehicle. Protect the patient and communicate with the extrication team to ensure that no further harm is done to the patient.

At times it may be necessary to gain access to a patient in a home behind a locked door. Contact the police or fire department and wait for their arrival, if possible, prior to gaining access. If you need to gain entry yourself, you may be able to shatter a small window in a door near the lock mechanism, then simply reach in, disengage the lock, and open the door. Do not kick in doors, since this may cause injury to you and excessive and unnecessary property damage.

CASE STUDY FOLLOW-UP

SCENE SIZE-UP

You have been dispatched to a motor vehicle collision between a large dump truck and a small passenger vehicle. You see from your unit that this is a complex rescue situation. You have multiple patients with potentially life-threatening injuries. They are entrapped in the wreckage of what was, minutes before, a bright red sports car.

There are no other emergency personnel immediately responding, so you call for rescue crews and an additional ambulance for each additional patient. Before exiting the unit, you size up the scene, identifying real and potential hazards. You make a mental note of all necessary precautions—including personal protective clothing and equipment—to protect yourself, bystanders, and the patients from further injury.

You position your vehicle 100 feet from the wreckage—the minimum safe distance since there are no electrical lines down or other visible hazards—to provide easy access to your equipment while being out of the way of rescue operations. You review what you and your partner need to do:

- If the patient access is prevented or hampered, attempt to assess the patients' condition based on the findings of whatever portion of the primary assessment you can perform.
- If you can, establish and maintain an airway, stabilize the cervical spine, and control any serious bleeding from outside the vehicle.
- Provide direction to other responding units as to what the situation is and what you need from them.
- Once the rescue crews arrive and the scene is secure, the incident commander and rescue crews will assess the situation and direct you in your assignment.
- If the incident requires complex rescue operations, a team approach using an incident command system with one commander is vital for success.
- Your attention should be given not only to the patients in the sports car. The driver of the truck may also be injured and many potential hazards must not be overlooked.

You and your partner arrive back at the station and discuss the extrication among a group of rescuers who were at the scene. It was a difficult experience for everyone. You were there when the teenager in the passenger side of the sports car died, well before extrication was completed and in spite of all your attempts to keep him alive. You know that the driver of the car, also a teenager, died in the ambulance after prolonged extrication and emergency medical procedures. Neither of the teenagers was wearing a seat belt. Both of them had been drinking. You are grateful to learn that the truck driver will recover.

The same questions are on the minds of everyone in the room. Is there anything we could have done better or faster? Is there any way we could have saved those kids' lives? As you, your partner, and the other rescuers defuse while discussing the call, you feel reasonably reassured that you did everything you could. And you and the rescue crew have worked out some refinements in procedure that might make the next rescue a little faster, safer, and more effective.

IN REVIEW

1. Name your first priority in this and any other type of emergency situation.
2. Describe the role of the EMT in vehicle stabilization and patient extrication.
3. Identify the first step you should take upon arriving at the site of a motor vehicle collision.
4. Explain how you can locate all the patients involved in an emergency such as a motor vehicle collision.
5. Explain why it is important to approach a motor vehicle collision from the front.
6. Identify which process comes first—patient care or patient extrication—and describe the exceptions.
7. Describe how you can protect the patient from further physical injury during extrication.
8. Describe the minimum level of personal protective equipment required at a motor vehicle collision site.
9. Describe the steps that may be taken after you identify downed electrical lines at the scene.
10. Describe a "stable" vehicle. Then name some simple steps that you can take to stabilize a vehicle in danger of rolling until rescue crews can properly and completely stabilize it.

CRITICAL THINKING

You arrive on the scene and find a vehicle that struck a pole in a head-on crash. The driver of the vehicle is not alert and is not responding when you call to him. The windows are all up and the doors are not opening.

1. Do you need to gain immediate access to the patient or should you wait for the extrication crew to arrive?
2. What methods could be used to gain immediate access to the patient?
3. Once access has been gained, what is your primary role?
4. How can you assist the extrication crew while providing care to the patient?

PEARSON

EXPLORE mybradykit™

Please go to **www.bradybooks.com** to access mykit for this text. You will find quizzes, critical thinking scenarios, weblinks, animations, and videos related to this chapter—and much more. Look for online information on air bags and air medical devices as well as a video on rapid extrication.

Register your access code from the front of your book by going to **www.bradybooks.com** and selecting the mykit links.

CHAPTER 43

Hazardous Materials

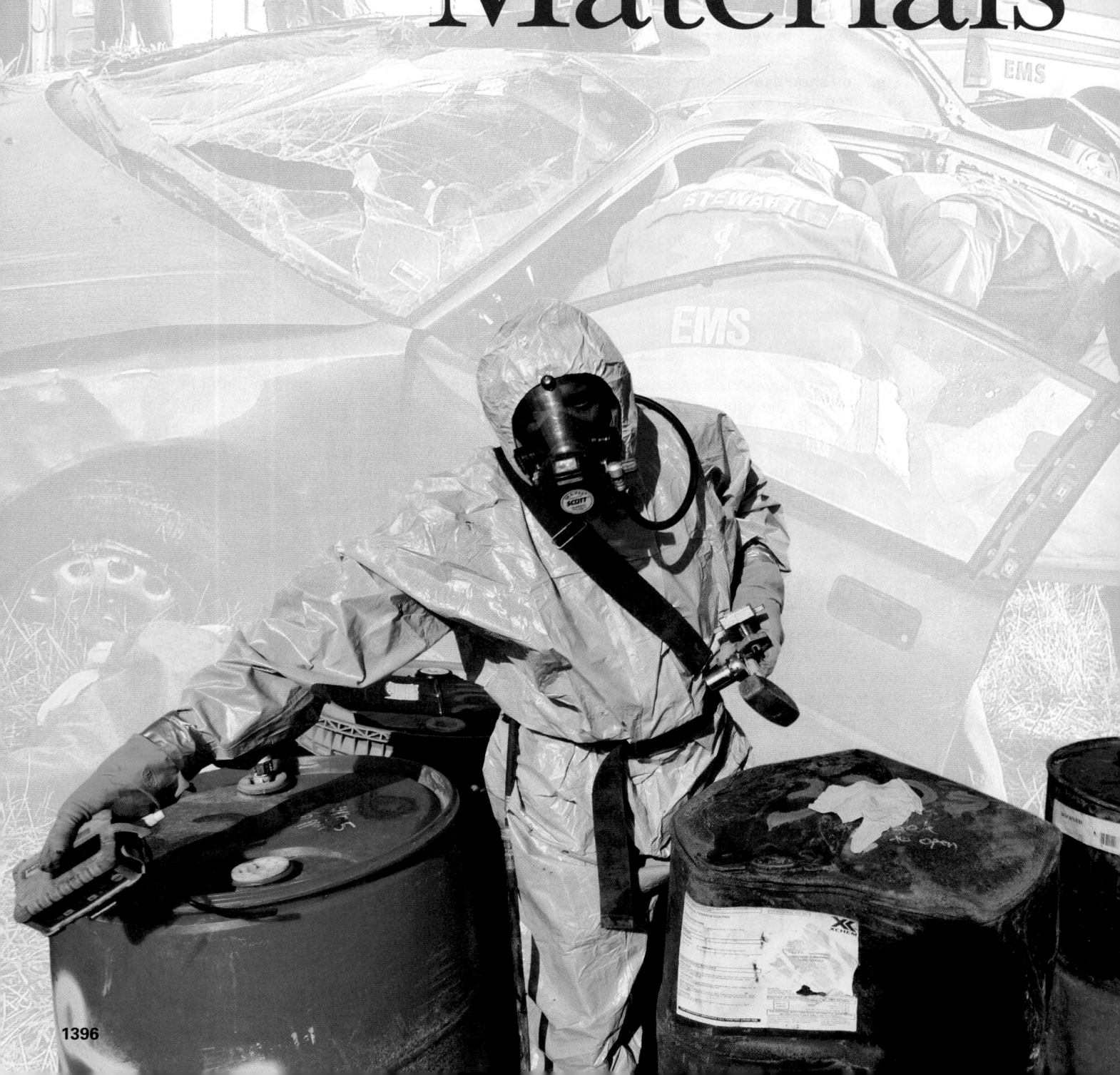

Navigation Guide

The following items provide an overview to the purpose and content of this chapter. The Standard and Competency are from the new National EMS Education Standards.

STANDARD **EMS Operations** (Content Area: Hazardous Materials)

COMPETENCY Applies knowledge of operational roles and responsibilities to ensure patient, public, and personnel safety.

OBJECTIVES: After reading this chapter, you should be able to:

43-1. Define key terms introduced in this chapter.
43-2. Explain the U.S. Department of Transportation placard system and the National Fire Protection Association symbols for identifying hazardous materials.
43-3. Explain the purpose of shipping papers and material safety data sheets.
43-4. List sensory indications that a hazardous materials situation may exist.
43-5. Identify resources that can be used in the identification and management of hazardous materials incidents.
43-6. Differentiate between the levels of hazardous materials training identified by the Occupational Safety and Health Administration.
43-7. Explain the general rules of hazardous materials rescue.
43-8. Discuss the components of hazardous materials incident management, including:
- **a.** Preincident planning
- **b.** Considerations in implementing the plan
- **c.** Establishing safety zones
- **d.** Emergency procedures, including decontamination, that should take place in each zone

43-9. Describe special considerations in responding to and managing patients exposed to or contaminated with radiation.
43-10. Differentiate between radiation sickness, radiation injury, and radiation poisoning.
43-11. List factors that determine the amount of risk posed to patients and rescuers by a source of radiation.
43-12. Describe the importance of being knowledgeable about terrorist attacks involving weapons of mass destruction.

KEY TERMS: Page references indicate first major use in this chapter. For complete definitions, see the Glossary at the back of the book.

cold zone p. 1408
hazardous material p. 1398
hot zone p. 1408
safety zones p. 1407
warm zone p. 1408

MEDIA RESOURCES: Please go to www.bradybooks.com to access mykt for this text. You will find quizzes, critical thinking scenarios, weblinks, animations, and videos related to this chapter—and much more. Look for online information on managing acute chemical exposures and radiation emergencies.

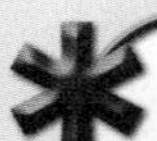

CASE STUDY

The Dispatch

EMS Unit 101—proceed to the intersection of Route 46 West and Baldwin Road—you have a collision involving a truck and passenger vehicle. No patient information is available. Time out is 1452 hours.

Upon Arrival

As soon as you near the collision site, you spot police rerouting traffic. They have cordoned off the scene. Up ahead on the west side of 46 you can just see a passenger vehicle in front of a large tanker truck on the shoulder of the highway.

How Would You Proceed?

During this chapter, you will learn special considerations related to hazardous materials emergencies. Later, we will return to the case and apply the procedures learned.

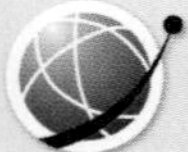

Media Resources
Go to www.bradybooks.com for mykit. Highlights:
- *Web Resource:* Hazardous Materials
- *Web Resource:* Emergency Response Guidebook
- *Web Resource:* Managing Acute Chemical Exposures

Key Terms
hazardous material material that poses a threat or unreasonable risk to life, health, or property.

Objectives 43-2 and 43-3
Explain various systems and symbols for identifying hazardous materials.

Introduction

Billions of tons of hazardous materials are manufactured in the United States annually. More than 800,000 shipments transport more than 4 billion tons of hazardous materials within this country every year, including explosives, compressed and poisonous gases, flammable liquids and solids, oxidizers (substances that give off oxygen and stimulate combustion of organic matter), corrosives, and radioactive materials. Hazardous materials spills and other accidents are common problems (Figure 43-1∗).

The EMT is not required to deal directly with hazardous materials. That takes specialized training. It is, however, important for you to know how to recognize and react to a hazardous materials emergency.

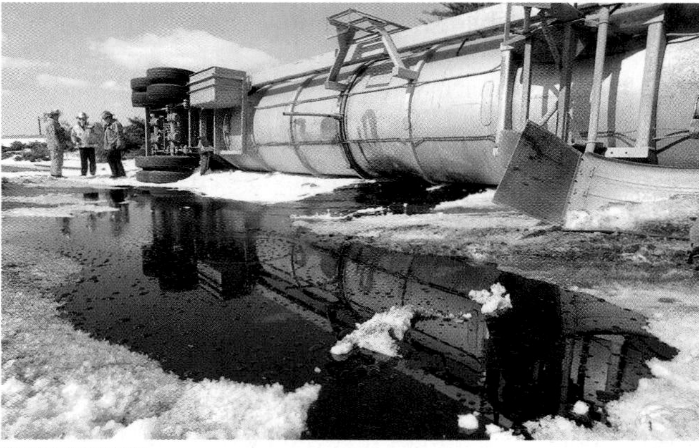

FIGURE 43-1 ∗ Hazardous materials spills and other accidents are common problems. (© Mark C. Ide)

Identifying Hazardous Materials

What Is a Hazardous Material?

A **hazardous material** is defined as one that in any quantity poses a threat or unreasonable risk to life, health, or property if not properly controlled during manufacture, processing, packaging, handling, storage, transportation, use, and disposal (Table 43-1). Hazardous materials include chemicals, wastes, and other dangerous products. The principal dangers hazardous materials present are toxicity, flammability, and reactivity.

Hazardous materials can asphyxiate, irritate, increase the risk of cancer, act as nerve or liver poisons, or cause loss of coordination or altered mental status. They can cause skin irritation, burns, respiratory distress, nausea and vomiting, tingling or numbness of the extremities, and blurred or double vision. The acronym *TRACEM* can be used to remember the types of damage that can be caused by hazardous materials: thermal, radiological, asphyxiation, chemical, etiological, and mechanical (Table 43-2). The amount of damage depends on the dose, concentration, route of exposure, and amount of time the patient is exposed.

Accidental exposure to hazardous materials can be limited to a few victims, but an accident also can cause widespread destruction and loss of life. Therefore, the primary concern in any hazardous materials emergency is safety of the rescuer, the patient, and the public.

Placards and Shipping Papers

U.S. Department of Transportation (DOT) regulations require vehicles containing hazardous materials to be marked with specific hazard labels or placards (Figures 43-2∗ and 43-3∗). A vehicle driver must have shipping papers, which identify the exact substance, quantity, origin, and destination.

A placard is a four-sided, diamond-shaped sign used to designate hazardous materials in transit on roadways. The placard contains important information that can aid the EMT in determining the best course of action. Often, a placard will display a four-digit UN number (United Nations identification number) that can be used to identify the hazardous material. The color of a placard also indicates what class of hazard is contained within. A legend that indicates whether the material is flammable, radioactive, explosive, or poisonous is also commonly displayed.

The National Fire Protection Association (NFPA) has adopted an internationally recognized diamond-shaped symbol, which is divided into four smaller diamonds (Figure 43-4a∗), for use in marking hazardous materials located at fixed facilities. This system—the NFPA 704 system—identifies potential danger with the use of background colors and numbers ranging from 0 to 4. The blue diamond is a gauge of health hazard; the red, fire hazard; and the yellow, reactivity hazard. The white diamond is used for symbols that indicate additional

TABLE 43-1 Hazardous Materials

Classification	Examples	Route of Exposure	Signs and Symptoms	BLS Treatment
1. Explosives	TNT Ammunition Fireworks Black powder	Skin and eyes Inhalation Ingestion Absorption	CARDIOVASCULAR Circulatory collapse and dysrhythmia RESPIRATORY Tachypnea and dyspnea GASTROINTESTINAL Nausea, vomiting, and diarrhea CNS Headache, dizziness, stupor, and coma EYES Chemical conjunctivitis SKIN Dermatitis and skin eruptions	*Airway: Consider tracheal intubation Oxygen at 15 lpm by nonrebreather mask Monitor for shock Flush skin Flush eyes 8 oz of water if ingested
2. Toxic and flammable gases	Chlorine Ammonia Nitrogen Carbon dioxide Acetylene Propane Butane Hydrogen	Skin and eyes Inhalation	CARDIOVASCULAR Circulatory collapse and dysrhythmia RESPIRATORY Tachypnea and dyspnea, respiratory failure, pulmonary edema GASTROINTESTINAL Nausea, vomiting, and diarrhea; irritated mucous membranes CNS Headache, dizziness, seizures, stupor, and coma EYES Chemical conjunctivitis SKIN Dermatitis and skin eruptions	*Airway: Consider tracheal intubation Oxygen at 15 lpm by nonrebreather mask Monitor for shock Flush skin Flush eyes Treat pulmonary edema Anticipate seizures Treat burns and frostbite
3. Flammable (F) and combustible (C) liquids	Gasoline (F) Acetone (F) Diesel (C) Brake fluid (C) Oil (C)	Skin and eyes Inhalation Ingestion Absorption	CARDIOVASCULAR Dysrhythmia and tachycardia RESPIRATORY Tachypnea and dyspnea, upper respiratory, and rapid pulmonary edema GASTROINTESTINAL Nausea, vomiting, and diarrhea; irritated mucous membranes CNS Headache, dizziness, seizures, stupor, and coma EYES Chemical conjunctivitis and cyanosis SKIN Dermatitis, irritation, and cyanosis	*Airway: Consider tracheal intubation Oxygen at 15 lpm by nonrebreather mask Monitor for shock Flush skin Flush eyes Treat pulmonary edema Anticipate seizures 8 oz. of water if ingested Treat burns Avoid vomit contact

*This patient may require advanced airway management and assisted ventilation.

continued

TABLE 43-1 Hazardous Materials *continued*

Classification	Examples	Route of Exposure	Signs and Symptoms	BLS Treatment
4. Flammable solids, dangerous when wet, spontaneously combustible	Phosphorus Magnesium Titanium Lithium Calcium resinate	Skin and eyes Inhalation Ingestion Absorption	CARDIOVASCULAR Dysrhythmia or shock RESPIRATORY Tachypnea and dyspnea, upper respiratory, and rapid pulmonary edema GASTROINTESTINAL Nausea, vomiting, abdominal pain, garlic odor CNS Headache, dizziness, fatigue, and seizures EYES Conjunctivitis and injury SKIN Chemical burns and jaundice	*Airway: Consider tracheal intubation Oxygen at 15 lpm by nonrebreather mask Monitor for shock Flush skin Flush eyes Treat pulmonary edema Anticipate seizures 8 oz of water if ingested Treat burns Avoid vomit contact
5. Oxidizing substances and organic peroxides	Lithium peroxide Calcium chlorite Pool chlorine	Skin and eyes Inhalation Ingestion	CARDIOVASCULAR Hypovolemic shock, rapid weak pulse RESPIRATORY Acute pulmonary edema, asphyxia, chemical pneumonia, and upper airway obstruction GASTROINTESTINAL Acute toxicity, nausea, vomiting, and diarrhea CNS Hypoxia, stupor, lethargy, and coma EYES Conjunctivitis and blindness SKIN Chemical burns, full and partial thickness	*Airway: Consider tracheal intubation Oxygen at 15 lpm by nonrebreather mask Monitor for shock Flush skin Flush eyes Treat pulmonary edema Anticipate seizures 8 oz of water if ingested Treat burns Avoid vomit contact
6. Toxic and infectious substances	Cyanide Arsenic Phosgene Insecticides Pesticides	Skin and eyes Inhalation Ingestion Absorption	CARDIOVASCULAR Cardiovascular collapse and dysrhythmia RESPIRATORY Acute pulmonary edema, asphyxia, chemical pneumonia, and upper airway obstruction GASTROINTESTINAL Nausea, vomiting, diarrhea, and abdominal pain	*Airway: Consider tracheal intubation Oxygen at 15 lpm by nonrebreather mask Monitor for shock Flush skin Flush eyes Treat pulmonary edema

*This patient may require advanced airway management and assisted ventilation.

TABLE 43-1 Hazardous Materials ***continued***

Classification	Examples	Route of Exposure	Signs and Symptoms	BLS Treatment
			CNS Coma, depression, and seizures	Anticipate seizures
			EYES Conjunctivitis and burns	8 oz of water if ingested Treat burns
			SKIN Chemical burns, flushing	Avoid vomit contact
7. Radioactive materials	Plutonium Cobalt Uranium 235	Skin and eyes Inhalation	CARDIOVASCULAR Tachycardia	*Airway: Consider tracheal intubation
		Ingestion Absorption	RESPIRATORY Dyspnea and cough with irritation and edema to the nose, mouth, and throat	Oxygen at 15 lpm by nonrebreather mask Monitor for shock
			GASTROINTESTINAL Nausea, vomiting, and diarrhea	Flush skin
			CNS Altered mental status, coma, headache, lethargy, tremors, and seizures	Flush eyes Treat pulmonary edema Anticipate seizures
			EYES Conjunctivitis, lacrimation	8 oz of water if ingested Treat burns
			SKIN Chemical burns, irritation	Avoid vomit contact
8. Corrosive substances	Hydrochloric acid Sulfuric acid Caustic	Skin and eyes Inhalation	CARDIOVASCULAR Tachycardia and shock	*Airway: Consider tracheal intubation
		Ingestion Absorption	RESPIRATORY Dyspnea and cough, burns, and edema to the nose, mouth, and throat	Oxygen at 15 lpm by nonrebreather mask Monitor for shock
			GASTROINTESTINAL Nausea, vomiting, and diarrhea, abdominal pain, mouth burns, stomach and esophagus	Flush skin Flush eyes Treat pulmonary edema
			CNS Altered mental status, coma, headache, lethargy, tremors, and seizures	Anticipate seizures 8 oz of water if ingested
			EYES Conjunctivitis and lacrimation	Treat burns Avoid vomit contact
			SKIN Dermatitis and skin eruptions	Do not induce vomiting

*This patient may require advanced airway management and assisted ventilation.

Key Points
Use the acronym *TRACEM* to remember the types of damage that can be caused by hazardous materials: thermal, radiological, asphyxiation, chemical, etiological, and mechanical.

Objective 43-4
List sensory indications that a hazardous materials situation may exist.

TABLE 43-2 TRACEM: Types of Damage from Hazardous Materials

T	**T**hermal: Heat sources, burning, radiant heat
R	**R**adiological: Nuclear fuels and by-products, nuclear bombs
A	**A**sphyxiation: Lack of O_2 due to chemical vapors, heavy gases
C	**C**hemical: Toxic or corrosive chemicals
E	**E**tiological: Biological hazards
M	**M**echanical: Trauma from bullets, shrapnel, and so on

information, such as radioactivity, oxidation, need for protective equipment, and so on. For example, a symbol that has a 1 in the blue diamond and a 4 in the red diamond would indicate a material that presents a relatively low health hazard but is extremely flammable. For another example of NFPA 704 labeling, see Figure 43-4b✱.

Shipping papers and material safety data sheets (Figure 43-5✱) are also important. If you can find them, shipping papers will have the name of the substance, the classification (such as flammable or explosive), and the four-digit UN identification number. With few exceptions, shipping papers are required to be in the cab of a motor vehicle, in the possession of a train crew member in the engine or caboose, in a holder on the bridge of a water vessel, or in the aircraft pilot's possession.

Using Your Senses

Another (but the least reliable) way to determine the presence of hazardous materials at the scene of an accident is to use your senses. Quickly scan the scene looking for signs of potential hazardous materials such as signs restricting entry, storage tanks, or containers with placards (Figure 43-6✱). A number of visual clues can indicate the probable presence of a hazardous material:

- Smoking or self-igniting materials
- Extraordinary fire conditions

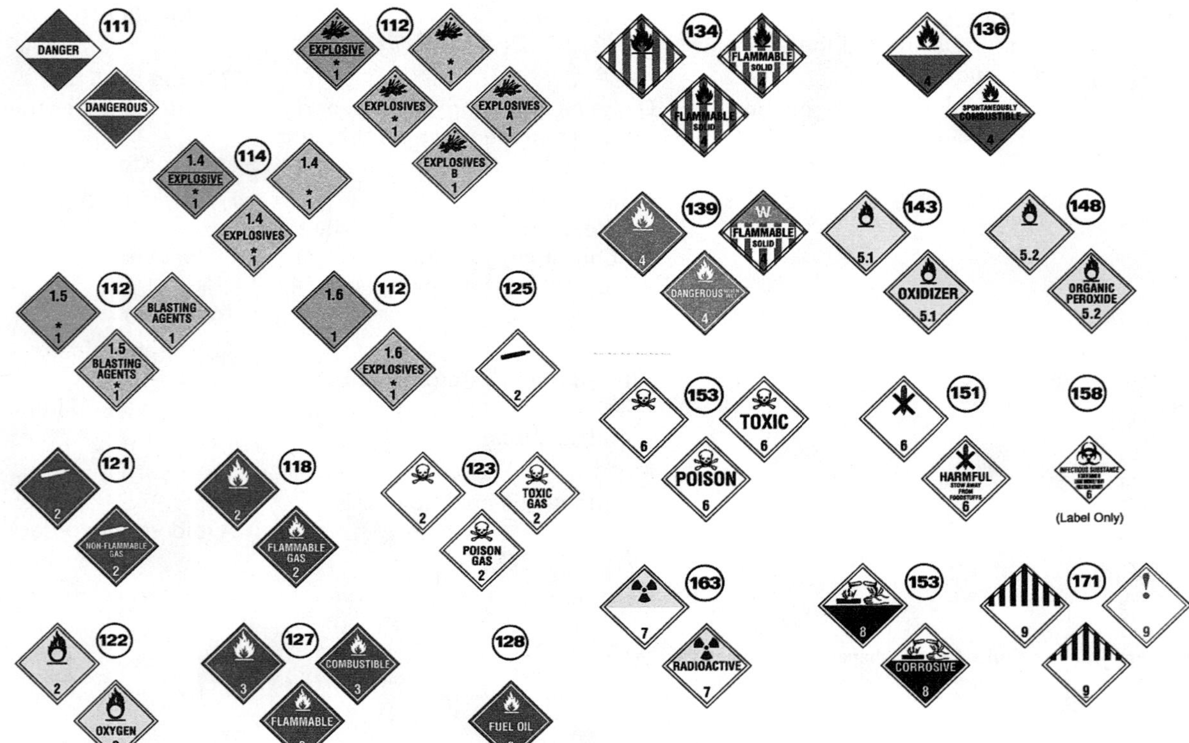

FIGURE 43-2 ✱ The U.S. Department of Transportation requires packages, storage containers, and vehicles containing hazardous materials to be marked with specific hazard labels.

Key Points
Never rely on your senses alone. You may not be able to see or smell the hazardous material.

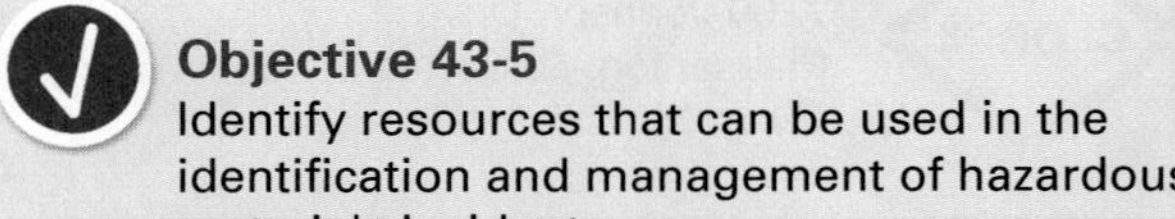

Objective 43-5
Identify resources that can be used in the identification and management of hazardous materials incidents.

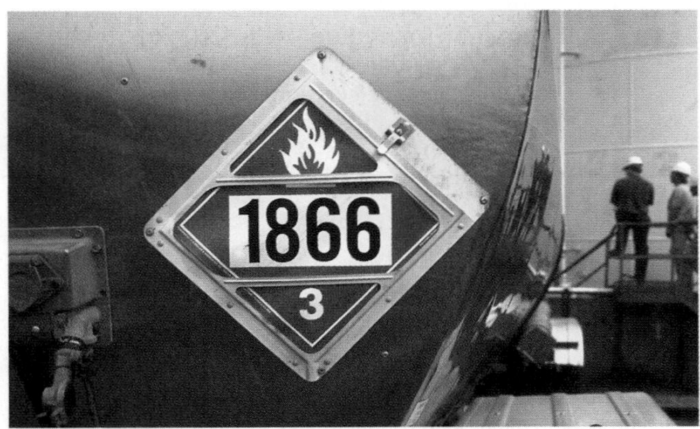

FIGURE 43-3 ✻ Any tank, vehicle, train, or ship that carries hazardous materials must have a placard that identifies the substance.

- Boiling or spattering of materials that have not been heated
- Wavy or unusually colored vapors over a container of liquid material
- Characteristically colored vapor clouds
- Frost near a container leak (indicative of liquid coolants)
- Unusual condition of containers (peeling or discoloration of finishes, unexpected deterioration, deformity, or the unexpected operation of pressure-relief valves)

Remember: You may not be able to see or smell the hazardous material. Some are odorless and colorless, while others have anesthetic properties and will deaden your senses. Never rely on your senses alone—sight, smell, taste, or touch—to detect a hazardous material. Always assume that the area surrounding a spill or leak is dangerous.

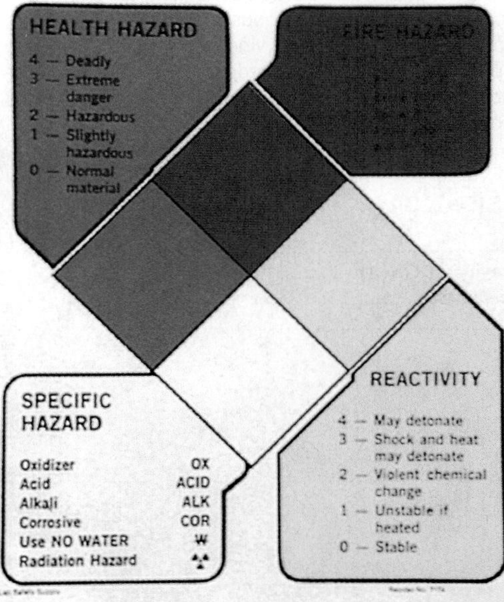

FIGURE 43-4a ✻ NFPA 704 hazardous materials classification.

Resources

Several resources can assist you in proper identification of hazardous materials emergencies. They include printed materials, the American Chemistry Council (www.americanchemistry.com), and state and local agencies including specialized "hazmat" teams. Poison control centers also provide resources.

One concise print reference is a guidebook published by the U.S. Department of Transportation, Transport Canada, and the Secretariat of Communications and Transportation of Mexico called the *Emergency Response Guidebook*. The *Emergency Response Guidebook* is updated

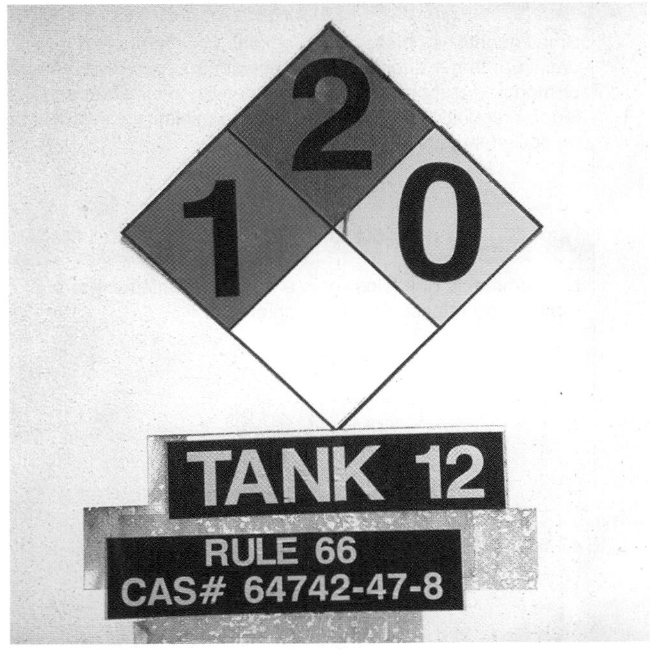

FIGURE 43-4b ✻ NFPA 704 labeling on a tank.

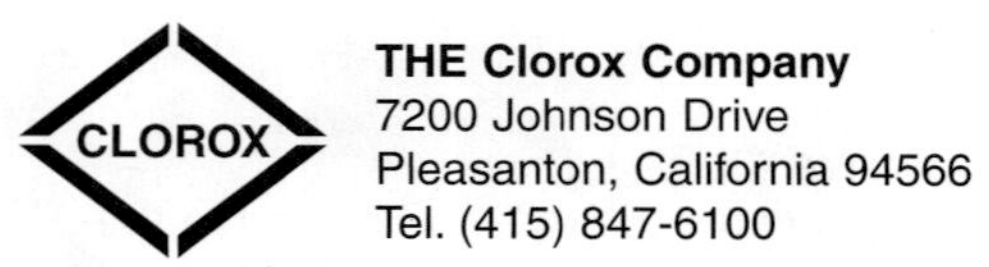

THE Clorox Company
7200 Johnson Drive
Pleasanton, California 94566
Tel. (415) 847-6100

Material Safety Data Sheets

Health	2+
Flammability	0
Reactivity	1
Personal Protection	B

I – CHEMICAL IDENTIFICATION

Name	regular Clorox Bleach	CAS No.	N/A
Description	clear, light yellow liquid with chlorine odor	RTECs No.	N/A

Other Designations
EPA Reg. No. 5813-1
Sodium hypochlorite solution
Liquid chlorine bleach
Clorox Liquid Bleach

Manufacturer
The Clorox Company
1221 Broadway
Oakland, CA 94612

Emergency Procedure
- Notify your supervisor
- Call your local poison control center OR
- Rocky Mountain Poison Center (303)573-1014

II – HEALTH HAZARD DATA

- Causes severe but temporary eye injury. May irritate skin. May cause nausea and vomiting if ingested. Exposure to vapor or mist may irritate nose, throat and lungs. The following medical conditions may be aggravated by exposure to high concentrations of vapor or mist: heart conditions or chronic respiratory problems such as asthma, chronic bronchitis or obstructive lung disease. Under normal consumer use conditions the likelihood of any adverse health effects are low. FIRST AID: EYE CONTACT: Immediately flush eyes with plenty of water. If irritation persists, see a doctor. SKIN CONTACT: Remove contaminated clothing. Wash area with water. INGESTION: Drink a glassful of water and call a physician. INHALATION: If breathing problems develop remove to fresh air.

III – HAZARDOUS INGREDIENTS

Ingredients	Concentration	Worker Exposure Limit
Sodium hypochlorite CAS# 7681-52-9	5.25%	not established

None of the ingredients in this product are on the IARC, NTP or OSHA carcinogen list. Occasional clinical reports suggest a low potential for sensitization upon exaggerated exposure to sodium hypochlorite if skin damage (e.g., irritation) occurs during exposure. Routine clinical tests conducted on intact skin with Clorox Liquid Bleach found no sensitization in the test subjects.

IV – SPECIAL PROTECTION INFORMATION

Hygienic Practices: Wear safety glasses. With repeated or prolonged use, wear gloves.

Engineering Controls: Use general ventilation to minimize exposure to vapor or mist.

Work Practices: Avoid eye and skin contact and inhalation of vapor or mist.

V – SPECIAL PRECAUTIONS

Keep out of reach of children. Do not get in eyes or on skin. Wash thoroughly with soap and water after handling. Do not mix with other household chemicals such as toilet bowl cleaners, rust removers, vinegar, acid or ammonia containing products. Store in a cool, dry place. Do not reuse empty container; rinse container and put in trash container.

VI – SPILL OR LEAK PROCEDURES

Small quantities of less than 5 gallons may be flushed down drain. For larger quantities wipe up with an absorbent material or mop and dispose of in accordance with local, state and federal regulations. Dilute with water to minimize oxidizing effect on spilled surface.

VII – REACTIVITY DATA

Stable under normal use and storage conditions. Strong oxidizing agent. Reacts with other household chemicals such as toilet bowl cleaners, rust removers, vinegar, acids or ammonia containing products to produce hazardous gases, such as chlorine and other chlorinated species. Prolonged contact with metal may cause pitting or discoloration.

VIII – FIRE AND EXPLOSION DATA

Not flammable or explosive. In a fire, cool containers to prevent rupture and release of sodium chlorate.

IX – PHYSICAL DATA

Boiling point.................................212°F/100°C (decomposes)
Specific Gravity (H_2O = 1).............1.085
Solubility in Water.........................complete
pH...11.4

FIGURE 43-5 ✱ A material safety data sheet.

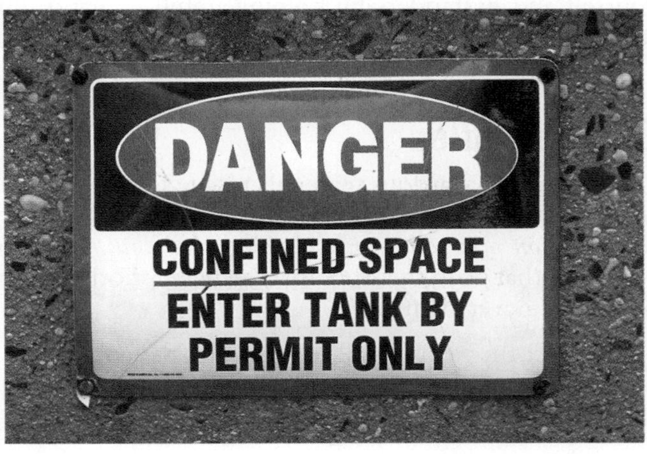

a

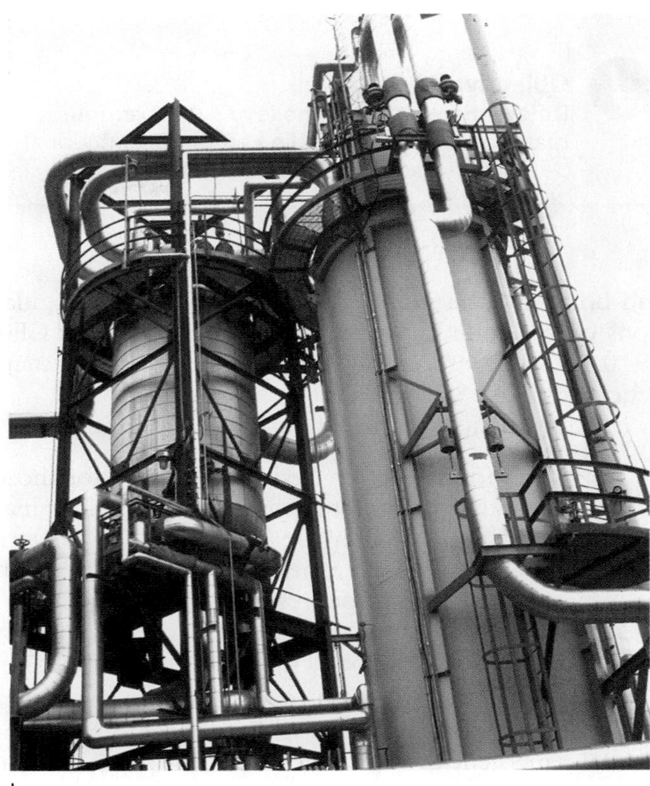

b

FIGURE 43-6 * Look for clues to potential hazardous materials, such as **(a)** signs and **(b)** storage tanks.

every 4 years in an effort to keep current with new transportation hazards. Compact enough to be carried with your usual equipment and supplies, the book lists more than a thousand hazardous materials, each with a four-digit UN identification number cross-referenced to complete emergency instructions. Hazardous materials emergency response information is also available electronically and in handheld PDAs. Other print materials are also available.

CHEMTREC (Chemical Transportation Emergency Center) is a public service division of the Chemical Manufacturer's Association and another important resource. Officials at CHEMTREC can answer any question and advise you on how to handle any emergency involving hazardous materials. They will even locate the shipper of the hazardous materials for appropriate follow-up. You can reach the CHEMTREC emergency response line around the clock, 7 days a week, by calling their toll-free number at 1-800-424-9300.

Chemtel, Inc. is another emergency response communications service that can be reached at 1-800-255-3924 in the United States and Canada. For calls outside the United States or Canada or for collect calls, the number is 1-813-979-0626. These resources and others, along with their phone numbers, can be found in the front section of the *Emergency Response Guidebook*. Also, your regional poison control center is a good source of information for hazardous materials incidents.

When contacting an organization, be prepared to provide the following information:

- Your name, callback number, and fax number
- Nature and location of product
- UN identification number or name of product(s)
- Name of carrier, shipper, manufacturer, consignee, and point of origin
- Type of container and size (rail, truck, housed open)
- Quantity of material
- Local weather conditions
- Number of injuries and/or exposures
- Emergency services that are present or are responding

Accidents involving hazardous materials often occur at inconvenient locations, making communication difficult. It is critical that you make every effort to keep a phone line open.

Training Required by Law

Because of the frequency and potential impact of hazardous materials emergencies, two federal agencies—the Occupational Safety and Health Administration (OSHA) and the Environmental Protection Agency (EPA)—have developed regulations to enhance the safety of rescuers

Objective 43-6
Differentiate between the levels of hazardous materials training identified by the Occupational Safety and Health Administration.

Objective 43-7
Explain the general rules of hazardous materials rescue.

Key Points
Avoid risking your life or your health if the only threat is to the environment.

and bring about a more effective response. The regulations can be found in the OSHA publication "29 CFR 1910.120—Hazardous Waste Operations and Emergency Response Standards."

The regulations identify four levels of training:

- **First Responder Awareness.** This level is for those who are likely to witness or discover a hazardous materials emergency. They are trained to recognize a problem but are not expected to take any action other than call for proper resources and prevent others from entering the scene. This level of training is commonly required for all operating EMTs.
- **First Responder Operations.** This level of training is for those who initially respond to hazardous materials emergencies to protect people, property, and the environment. They are trained in the use of specialized personal protective equipment and help to stop the emergency from spreading.
- **Hazardous Materials Technician.** This extensive level of training is for rescuers who actually plug, patch, or stop the release of a hazardous material.
- **Hazardous Materials Specialist.** Rescuers with this training have advanced knowledge and skills. They provide command and support activities at the site of a hazardous materials emergency.

Employers are responsible for determining and documenting the appropriate level of training for each employee. Because training addressed by OSHA usually has a fire-service focus, the National Fire Protection Association has published Standard 473, which deals with competencies for EMS personnel at hazardous materials emergencies. Refer to the OSHA and NFPA standards for more information on training requirements. Most EMTs are trained to the First Responder Awareness level.

Guidelines for Hazardous Materials Rescues

Note: Never attempt a hazardous materials rescue unless you have had the necessary specialized training (to the hazardous materials technician level or better) and have had the proper training in the use of self-contained breathing apparatus (SCBA) and chemical protective clothing. If you have had no training, radio immediately for help. While you are waiting for help to arrive, protect yourself and bystanders by keeping uphill, upwind, upstream, and away from the danger.

General Rules

One rule of a hazardous materials rescue is to *avoid contact with any unidentified material, regardless of the level of protection offered by your clothing and equipment.* In achieving that goal, there are three general priorities in an order that never changes:

1. Protect the safety of all rescuers and patients.
2. Provide patient care.
3. Decontaminate clothing, equipment, and the vehicle.

Another rule of hazardous materials rescue is to *avoid risking your life or your health if the only threat is to the environment.* In other words, if victims are not involved, do not enter the scene. Let specially trained environmental workers clean up the hazard.

At the First Responder Awareness level of training, your actions at a hazardous materials incident should include the ability to *recognize* that a hazardous materials incident has occurred, *avoid* contact with the hazardous substance, *isolate* the area, and *notify* the appropriate authorities or response agencies. These actions can be easily remembered using the acronym *RAIN* (Table 43-3).

Simply cordon off the area and evacuate bystanders. Even if there are patients involved, this is one situation in which you should not automatically begin rescue work. Generally accepted guidelines call for you to weigh the emergency according to your best judgment, determining whether the risk to rescuers is justified by the lives that can be saved. Consider the difficulty of the rescue,

TABLE 43-3 RAIN: Awareness-Level Responsibilities at a Hazardous Materials Incident

R	*Recognize* that a hazardous materials incident has occurred.
A	*Avoid* contact with the hazardous substance.
I	*Isolate* the area.
N	*Notify* the appropriate authorities or response agencies.

Objective 43-8
Discuss the components of hazardous materials incident management, including planning, plan implementation, safety zone establishment, and safety zone procedures.

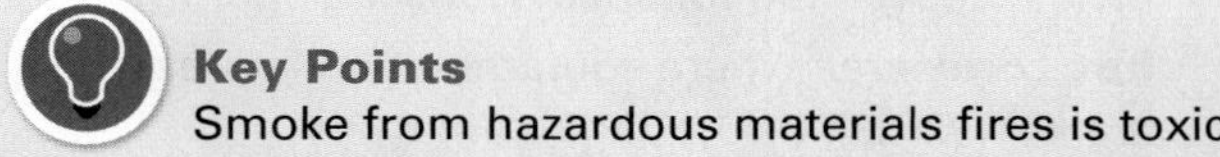

Key Points
Smoke from hazardous materials fires is toxic.

the flammability of materials, the possibility of explosion, any time or distance constraints, available escape routes, and the probability of patients surviving if they receive medical care. If you decide to begin rescue operations, act quickly—time is critical, but do not work so quickly that you endanger yourself or others or make patient injuries worse. The *Emergency Response Guidebook* can be of great assistance in your decision-making process.

As a first course of action, secure the scene and limit the exposure of rescuers and bystanders. Then make sure there is enough additional equipment, trained personnel, and whatever else you might need to handle the emergency effectively. Finally, make sure that every rescuer who enters the scene has adequate protective equipment: a positive pressure SCBA and a full suit of appropriate chemical protective clothing, at least two layers of gloves, boots, helmet, eye protection (preferably full-face protection), and lifelines (EMT Skills 43-1). Use wide duct tape to seal off the protective suits at the wrists, ankles, neck, and other gaps or openings. You will need specialized suits if you are working in high temperatures or areas where you could be splashed with corrosive chemicals. Only responders trained to the First Responder Operations level or above should ever consider entering a dangerous hazardous materials scene.

Incident Management

Preincident Planning

The most essential part of hazardous materials rescue is effective preincident planning. Before a hazardous materials emergency ever develops, all agencies that would probably be involved in a rescue need to know how various forces will be mobilized to handle the emergency.

Generally, you should prepare for the worst possible scenario. That way, the community will be capable of handling any emergency that arises. Your plan should be specifically tailored to the individual circumstances in the community. However, the following should be included:

- One command officer, who is responsible for all rescue decisions, should be appointed. All rescuers should be aware of who the command officer is. If the command officer hands over the decision-making power to someone else, all rescuers should be notified of the change in command.
- There should be a clear chain of command from each rescuer to the command officer.
- There should be an established system of communications used throughout the emergency. The system should be one all rescuers are informed about, know how to use, and have access to.
- Receiving facilities should be predesignated. Choose facilities that are capable of handling large numbers of patients, have surgical capacity, and, if possible, have established decontamination procedures.

Implementing the Plan

The first priority in implementing a plan is to immediately establish an incident command system and a command post from which orders are given and to which information is directed. Then—to identify the best plan of action under the circumstances as quickly as possible—get the following information:

- Nature of the problem
- Identification of the hazardous material or materials involved
- The type and condition of containers
- Existing weather conditions
- Whether there is presence of fire
- Time that has elapsed since the emergency occurred
- What has already been done by people at the scene
- The number of patients
- The danger of victimizing more people

Smoke from hazardous materials fires presents an environmental hazard. It carries toxins and particles of hazardous materials through the air, widening the area of contamination. This "secondhand smoke" not only threatens the immediate safety of patients and rescuers, it also threatens long-term health, in some cases increasing risk of cancer and chronic effects involving the brain, liver, lungs, and kidneys.

Unless you are a trained firefighter, do not attempt to extinguish the fires yourself. Hazardous materials fires often require special techniques. (For example, some cannot be extinguished with water; in fact, water would make them worse.)

Establishing Safety Zones

As an early priority at the scene of any hazardous materials emergency, **safety zones** are established in which rescue operations and a specific sequence of decontamination

Key Terms

safety zones areas surrounding a hazardous materials accident, such as hot, warm, and cold zones, designated for specific rescue operations.

hot zone area where contamination is present, generally adjacent to the accident site.

Key Terms

warm zone area adjacent to the hot zone, where life-saving care is performed.

cold zone area adjacent to the warm zone, where normal treatment is performed.

procedures take place. Some EMS areas use the circular model for depicting safety zones (Figure 43-7*). Remember: You may not be able to see or smell the hazardous material. Always assume that the area surrounding a spill or leak is dangerous and avoid entry unless you are wearing appropriate protective gear.

As an EMT, when decontaminating a patient, follow steps 1–9 of the decontamination procedure (Figure 43-8*) the same as rescuers. After step 4, if the patient is experiencing life-threatening illness or injury, move the patient to the ambulance and transport immediately. Do not complete steps 5–9 in this case.

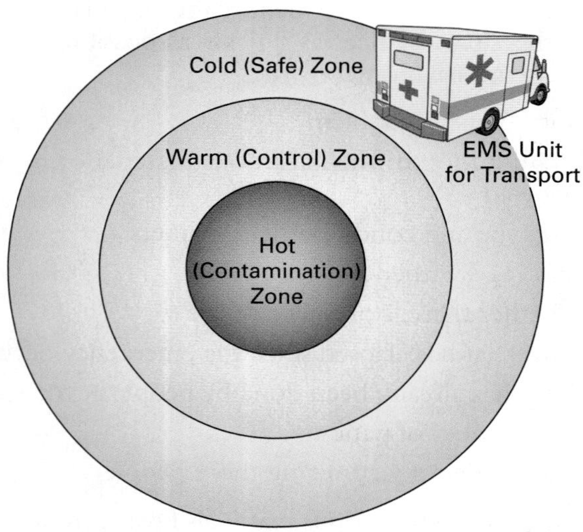

Hot (Contamination) Zone

Contamination is actually present.
Personnel must wear appropriate protective gear.
Number of rescuers limited to those absolutely necessary.
Bystanders never allowed.

Warm (Control) Zone

Area surrounding the contamination zone.
Vital to preventing spread of contamination.
Personnel must wear appropriate protective gear.
Lifesaving emergency care is performed.

Cold (Safe) Zone

Normal triage, stabilization, and treatment performed.
Rescuers must shed contaminated gear before entering the cold zone.

FIGURE 43-7 * Establishing safety control zones at the site of a hazardous materials emergency.

Hot Zone The **hot zone,** also known as the exclusion zone, is where contamination may actually be present. It generally is the area that is immediately adjacent to the accident site and where contamination can still occur. To help limit the spread of contamination, a single point at which all rescue personnel enter and exit the hot zone is established. An emergency exit is designated to be used in case the scene deteriorates rapidly (in case of an explosion, for example). Never smoke, eat, or drink in the hot zone, because you would risk inhaling or ingesting the hazardous material.

The hot zone should be restricted. Only as many trained rescuers as absolutely necessary should enter it. In areas with a specialized hazmat team, only members of that team should enter the hot zone. Bystanders should never be allowed in the hot zone. If necessary, cordon off the whole area and appoint people to keep bystanders away.

The only work done in the hot zone is hazard assessment, control of the release or hazard, and rescue performed by trained personnel who are wearing appropriate protective equipment.

Warm Zone The **warm zone,** also known as the contamination reduction zone, is immediately adjacent to the hot zone. While the hazardous materials may not actually be in the warm zone, there is still danger of contamination from the patients and rescue personnel who have exited the hot zone. For that reason, *all personnel in the warm zone must wear appropriate protective gear.*

The warm zone is vital in preventing the spread of contamination. All supplies used in the warm zone must remain there until fully decontaminated. All water used in this area must also be contained here. Rescue work done in the warm zone consists of lifesaving emergency care, such as airway management and immobilization. All initial decontamination efforts take place within the warm zone.

Cold Zone The **cold zone,** also known as the support zone, is immediately adjacent to the warm zone. Before entering the cold zone from the warm zone, rescuers should shed all contaminated protective gear and patients should be as fully decontaminated as possible. By design, the cold zone should not contain any contamination, but since contamination can still enter the cold zone, you should continue to exercise caution and take measures to protect your equipment and vehicle.

By the time patients enter the cold zone, life-threatening problems should have been initially managed. Continue emergency care. Triage patients to

NINE-STEP DECON PROCEDURE*

CLEAN SIDE

← DIRECTION OF TRAVEL

CONTAMINATED SIDE

		ENTER HERE
Lay out plastic to contain the contamination. It should be about 12–15 feet wide. Length can vary depending on space available. Personnel enter decon area and drop tools and monitors on the plastic. Move to Step 2.	1	1 TOOL DROP AREA
Position decon pools. Use one to wash gross contaminates off with brushes, soap, and water. Place a portable shower in the second pool to rinse off as much contamination as possible. Dilution is conducted inside the pool and diked area. All rescuers are still wearing suits and SCBA. Move to Step 3.	2	2 DECON WASH POOL DECON RINSE POOL WITH SHOWER
Open the chemical suit and remove the SCBA. Place them on the contaminated side. If the rescuer is returning to the incident, replace the SCBA cylinder, question the rescuer to establish that health conditions are OK, and close the suit. The rescuer should re-enter using the contaminated side. Move to Step 4.	3	3 SCBA REMOVAL OR REPLACEMENT
		REENTRY RETURN
Remove protective clothing and place on the contaminated side. Move to Step 5 or transport personnel to a fixed decon facility during inclement weather.	4	4 PROTECTIVE CLOTHING REMOVAL
	TRANSPORT IF NEEDED	
Remove all personal clothing and isolate items on the contaminated side. Bag all personal items. Move to Step 6.	5	5 PERSONAL CLOTHING REMOVAL
Shower and care for personal hygiene using soap and sponges. Dry off and bag cleaning items for disposal, including clothing, sponges, towels, etc. Move to Step 7.	6	6 PERSONAL HYGIENE & SHOWER
Personnel put on clean clothes or paper garments. Move to Step 8.	7	7 APPLY CLEAN CLOTHES
Personnel receive EMS medical evaluation, including ECG, and treatment as necessary. Rehabilitation includes cooling off and replacing fluids. Move to Step 9.	8	8 REHABILITATION AND EMS MEDICAL EVALUATION INCLUDING ECG
Identify personnel and complete exposure records. Transport personnel to hospital, if needed, or to a fixed decon facility for Steps 5 through 9.	9	9 DOCUMENTATION & EXPOSURE REPORT WRITING

During inclement weather, Steps 5–9 may be moved to a fixed decon facility.

During inclement weather, Steps 5–9 may be moved to a fixed decon facility.

*Written by Kenneth Bouvier, NREMT-P, Hazardous Materials Specialist, New Orleans, Louisiana.

FIGURE 43-8 * Nine-step decontamination procedure.

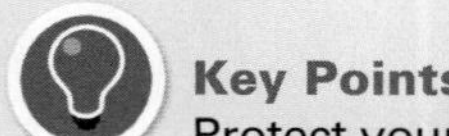

Key Points
Protect your equipment and vehicle during transport of hazmat patients, even if they have been decontaminated. Leave all clothing and equipment used in the hot or warm zones at the scene.

Key Points
Contamination occurs most easily in areas of the body where skin is thin or usually moist such as under the arms and in the groin.

determine the order of care, perform necessary treatment, and stabilize patients prior to transport (see Chapter 44, "Multiple-Casualty Incidents and Incident Management").

Emergency Procedures

Anyone entering the warm zone or the hot zone must be properly trained and wearing appropriate protective equipment. The type of protective equipment needed is dictated by the type of hazardous material being dealt with and the rescue scene itself.

Initial (gross) decontamination should be performed at the entry to the warm zone. The patient should be removed from the actual accident site while any necessary management of immediate life threats is performed. Initial decontamination always involves the use of copious amounts of water, and may also include the use of a simple soap. The patient's clothing, tools, and equipment should be left in the hot zone.

A primary assessment of patients is also performed in the warm zone. Protective equipment must be worn in the warm zone. Once the immediate life threats are managed, complete decontamination is performed. Following thorough decontamination in the warm zone, a physical assessment is performed. Treat the patient's major injuries, immobilize the spine as appropriate, splint where needed, and move the patient to the cold zone.

All of the protective equipment is removed before entering the cold zone. In the cold zone, take a set of vital signs and history and prepare the patient for transport.

Take precautions to protect your equipment and vehicle during transport, since there may still be some contamination on the patient. Prior to transport, cover the benches, floor, and other exposed areas of your vehicle with thick plastic sheeting. Secure the sheeting with duct tape. Patients should be fully decontaminated before being placed into a helicopter. A contaminated patient in such a closed, tight space could affect the breathing or vision of the air transportation team, resulting in a crash. Contamination of an aircraft can take it out of service for several days.

All clothing and equipment used in the hot or warm zones must be left at the scene so it can be properly contained. Any contaminated equipment or clothing must be sealed in plastic bags or in metal containers with tightly fitting lids. All corpses at the scene need to be decontaminated fully before being transported to a morgue. This must be performed by appropriately trained rescuers.

If you are accidentally exposed to hazardous materials during the rescue, decontaminate yourself thoroughly (Figure 43-9*). Contamination occurs most easily in areas of your body where skin is thin or usually moist such as under the arms and in the groin. Wash with mild detergent, such as Dawn or a similar grease-cutting detergent, or with green soap and plenty of running water. Green soap is preferred for hazmat decontamination because it is known to be nonreactive and does not contain additional chemicals such as perfumes or stabilizers that can interact with hazardous substances. Irrigate exposed skin for at least 20 minutes or until any localized burning or discomfort stops. Seek medical attention, document the emergency, and report it to your employer.

All rescuers should have a thorough medical examination and medical surveillance to treat any exposure-related injuries or illnesses. Some do not manifest for hours or even days after exposure. Following a hazardous materials emergency, watch yourself for signs of exposure. Seek medical help immediately if you develop

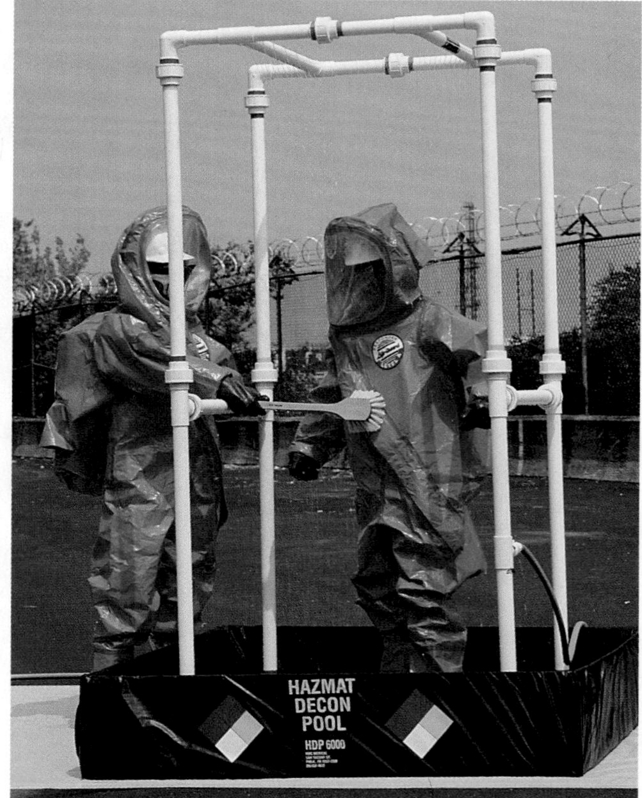

FIGURE 43-9 * Rescuer in decontamination process.

Thinking Critically
You start feeling nauseated and dizzy. A coworker says, "Maybe it's from that hazmat scene we were at last week. You should get that checked out." You shake your head. "No, that was days ago. I'm sure it's just the flu." Who is right, you or your coworker? Why?

Objective 43-9
Describe special considerations in responding to and managing patients exposed to or contaminated with radiation.

headache; nausea or vomiting; abdominal cramps or diarrhea; difficulty breathing; dizziness; lack of coordination; blurred vision; excessive salivation; irritation of the skin, eyes, nose, throat, or respiratory tract; or any other unusual symptoms.

Following rescue, decontaminate your equipment and vehicle by washing them thoroughly inside and out. Caution: If you fail to clean them thoroughly, the result may be chronic chemical exposure. The clothing under your protective gear also needs decontamination. However, do not take clothing home to launder, since it may contaminate your family and the general sewer system.

Radiation Emergencies

Exposure and Contamination

In a radiation accident, the patient may suffer from exposure, contamination, or both. Exposure occurs when the patient is in the presence of radioactive material without any of the radioactive material actually touching his clothing or body. The exposure he receives may be harmful to him, but the patient does not become radioactive and does not pose any threat to rescue personnel. (Remember, however, that the source of the radioactivity may pose a threat to rescuers who come close enough to it.)

Contamination occurs when the patient has come into direct contact with the source of radioactivity or with radioactive gases, liquids, or particles. The radioactive material is present on the patient's clothes or skin, which poses a hazard for the rescuer as well as the patient. The contaminated patient is considered a risk to emergency personnel.

Guidelines for Radiation Emergencies

Remember two major principles about radiation-related accidents: (1) *protect yourself and others from contamination as your first priority and* (2) *no EMT should ever attempt to decontaminate a radiation patient.* If you suspect a patient is contaminated by radiation, you have two choices:

- *Wait for a Radiation Safety Officer (RSO),* an expert specifically trained under federal government provisions to handle such situations. The RSO in your area is probably employed by the county or state health department and will respond to the scene when possible.
- If an RSO cannot come to the site, you can transport the patient to the hospital for decontamination by experts there. To transport, place the patient in a body bag up to the neck, cover the hair completely with a cap or towel, and use disposable wipes to clean the face. Put the disposable wipes in a plastic bag, seal it, and take it to the hospital with you.

Time is the critical factor in managing radiation emergencies. Trained personnel should remove the patient from the source of radiation as quickly as possible before you begin emergency care. Increase distance between yourself and the source of radiation. Depending on the type of radiation, provide shielding between the patient and the source of radiation. Alpha rays can be stopped by clothing. Beta rays can be stopped by aluminum or like materials. Gamma rays require lead shielding.

Procedures for Radiation Emergencies

Limit your stay in a contaminated area to as little time as possible. Keep as far away from the source as you can and involve as few rescuers as possible. (Exposure to radiation is cumulative and is determined by an inverse square relationship. That is, if you are twice as close, you will receive four times the exposure. If you move twice as far away, you cut your exposure by four times.)

Remember the priorities for hazardous materials emergencies listed earlier in this chapter: *(1) protect the safety of all rescuers and patients; (2) provide patient care; and (3) decontaminate clothing, equipment, and the vehicle.* Keeping these priorities in mind, follow the guidelines for scene safety, patient care, and personal decontamination that are outlined next.

Scene Safety First establish scene safety. Follow these guidelines:

1. As you approach the accident scene in your vehicle, visually survey the area for the radiation symbol on the sides of vehicles, machinery, or containers involved (Figure 43-10*). Determine the location of a possible source of radiation. Be alert for the presence of other hazardous materials as well. If you determine that radiation is a possibility, park your vehicle upwind of the accident to reduce the chance of radiation particles being blown to your location. Do not park near any liquid spills or near any transport vehicle that may be leaking. Do not park near any container that might have been cracked or damaged in the accident.

Thinking Critically

At a radiation accident, the rescue teams are short-handed. As an experienced EMT, you volunteer to help with decontaminating patients as they are brought out of the accident scene. Is this a good idea? Why or why not?

Key Points

In radiation emergencies, your priorities are (1) safety of rescuers and patients, (2) patient care, and (3) decontamination procedures.

Objective 43-10

Differentiate between radiation sickness, radiation injury, and radiation poisoning.

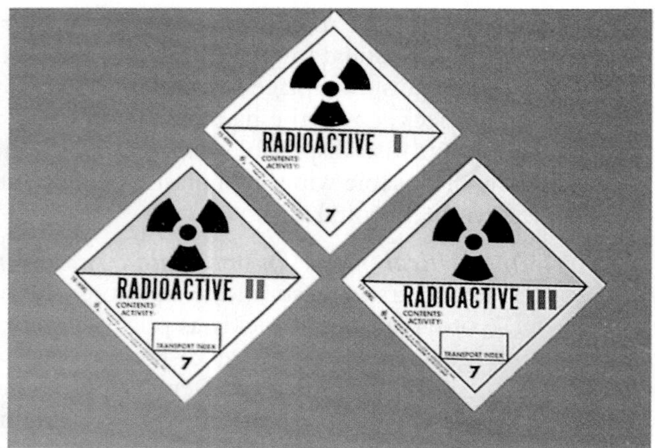

FIGURE 43-10 * Radiation hazard labels.

2. As soon as you suspect radiation and before you enter the suspected area of contamination, and if trained to an appropriate level, put on a positive pressure self-contained breathing apparatus plus protective clothing. Leave no skin or hair exposed. Wear several layers if you can, with an outer layer of tightly woven protective clothing. Seal all openings with duct tape. Wear two pairs of protective gloves under a pair of heavy work gloves. Wear a pair of shoes covered by two pairs of paper shoe covers under a pair of heavy rubber boots.

Personal Protection Protecting yourself from exposure to radiation includes consideration of the following factors:

- **Time.** The less time spent near the radiation source, the less radiation exposure.
- **Distance.** The farther you are from the radiation source, the lower the radiation dose.
- **Shielding.** The denser the material between you and the radiation source, the greater the protection. SCBA and protective clothing or simple examination gloves may be all that is required to adequately shield yourself from the radiation. In some cases, lead shields are required. Increasing the time and distance factors can reduce the amount of shielding needed.
- **Quantity.** Decreasing the amount of radioactive material in the area will decrease exposure. Remove the patient from the radioactive material or remove the radioactive material from the patient.

Patient Care Emergency care for a patient with radiation exposure must center on the patient's immediate life threats and injuries and not on the radiation itself. Remove the patient from the source of radiation as quickly as possible. Conduct a primary assessment and a secondary assessment and manage injuries or medical conditions as you normally would. Consult with medical direction and the poison control center when radioactive contamination is a concern.

Personal Decontamination After providing the necessary patient care, transport, and transfer of the patient to the hospital, turn your attention to your own personal decontamination. Report and document your exposure to the radiation source and follow the recommendations of the hospital or local protocol for personal decontamination.

Vehicle/Equipment Decontamination Any equipment that you used to care for the patient—including blankets, towels, bandages, cots, stretchers, or equipment used in transportation—must be checked for radiation contamination before it can be used again. Authorities at the hospital or medical center can arrange for an equipment check.

The vehicle used to transport the patient needs to be washed inside and out before it is placed back in service. Any radioactive dust must be removed from the vehicle. Pay special attention to the tires and other contact points. You may need to use a commercial decontamination solution on your equipment (never use one on the skin). Follow local protocol.

If equipment or tools cannot be completely decontaminated, they will need to be disposed of. Signs of incomplete decontamination include debris adhering to the equipment, discoloration, corrosion, and stains.

Problems Caused by Radiation

Radiation is a general term that describes energy transmission. There are three general kinds of problems caused by radiation: radiation sickness, radiation injury, and radiation poisoning.

Radiation sickness is caused by exposure to large amounts of radiation. Symptoms start anywhere from a few hours to days following exposure to the radiation and, depending on the dose, can last anywhere from a few days to 7 or 8 weeks. In fact, the amount of time between radiation exposure and the onset of symptoms is a relatively reliable indicator of how much radiation a person

Objective 43-11
List factors that determine the risk posed to patients and rescuers by a source of radiation.

Objective 43-12
Describe the importance of knowledge regarding terrorist attacks with weapons of mass destruction.

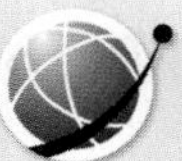

Media Resources
Go to www.bradybooks.com for mykit. Highlights:

- *Web Resource:* CHEMTREC
- *Web Resource:* Radiation Emergencies

has absorbed. Common signs and symptoms include nausea and vomiting, diarrhea, hemorrhage, weight loss, appetite loss, malaise, fever, and sores in the throat and mouth. Radiation sickness also affects the immune system, lowering resistance to disease and infection.

Radiation injury is a local injury that is generally caused by exposure to large amounts of less penetrating particles, such as beta particles. General signs and symptoms include hair loss, skin burns (Figure 43-11∗), and generalized skin lesions.

Radiation poisoning occurs when the patient has been exposed to dangerous amounts of internal radiation. The result is a host of serious diseases, including cancer and anemia.

While a victim of a radiation accident is not "contagious" or infectious and generally will not endanger a rescuer, you are at risk of becoming contaminated if the patient still has radiation particles on his skin or clothing. Always put on full protective gear as soon as you recognize a radiation accident.

Protection from Radiation

As you approach the scene of an accident, protect yourself and other rescuers if you know ahead of time that radiation sources are present. Immediately contact the Radiation Safety Officer or Emergency Management Agency within your jurisdiction.

The following factors determine the amount of radiation damage that you may sustain during a rescue if an unshielded radiation source is present in the vicinity:

- The amount and type of personal shielding you use
- The strength of the radiation source
- Your distance from the radiation source
- The type of radiation
- How long you are exposed
- How much of your body is exposed

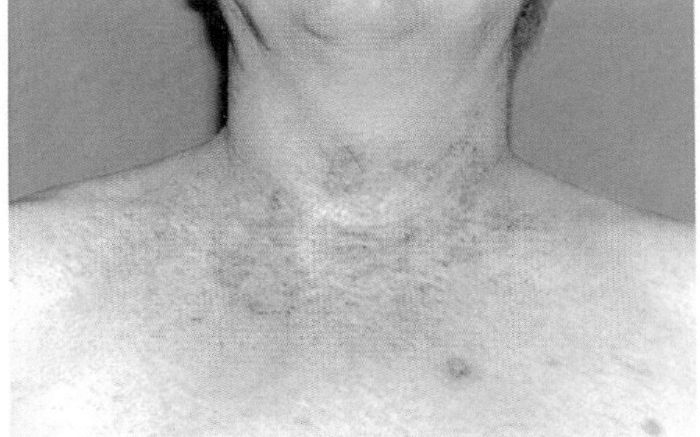

FIGURE 43-11 ∗ Radiation burn.

You can reduce your risk. The best approach is to divide the rescue work among many rescuers, with teams composed of as few rescuers as possible. The Federal Nuclear Regulatory Commission recommends that an individual in an emergency situation, while engaged in activities deemed necessary for the preservation of life, be exposed to no more than a one-time whole-body dose of 25 roentgens. This means that if the Geiger counter at the patient's location indicates 50 roentgens per hour, then a new team of rescuers should move in and relieve the first team after 30 minutes.

Another approach to reducing risk is to shield the radiation source itself (not you or the patient). For example, the best protection against gamma rays (one type of radiation that is extremely dangerous) is lead, preferably 1–2 inches thick. If lead is not available, any material that has thick mass (such as bricks, concrete, or several feet of dirt) will do.

Know your community's plan for hazardous materials emergencies. Know how to reach your Radiation Safety Officer. Always wear your protective gear, including a self-contained breathing apparatus, as soon as you suspect the involvement of radiation. Never smoke in an area where radiation has contaminated the air, and do not eat food that comes from a contamination site. (Smoking and eating are the two most common ways to become internally contaminated.)

Terrorist Attacks Involving Weapons of Mass Destruction

The threat of a terrorist attack has heightened the awareness of a need to better prepare EMTs to respond to incidents involving weapons of mass destruction (WMD) including nuclear devices, biological agents, and chemicals. The more common chemicals that could be used by a terrorist are listed in Class 2 Toxic and Flammable Gases, Class 6 Toxic and Infectious Substances, or Class 7 Radioactive Materials (review Table 43-1). It is recommended that EMTs and other EMS personnel enroll in a counterterrorism class. See also Chapter 45, "EMS Response to Terrorism Involving Weapons of Mass Destruction."

Hazardous Materials Protective Equipment

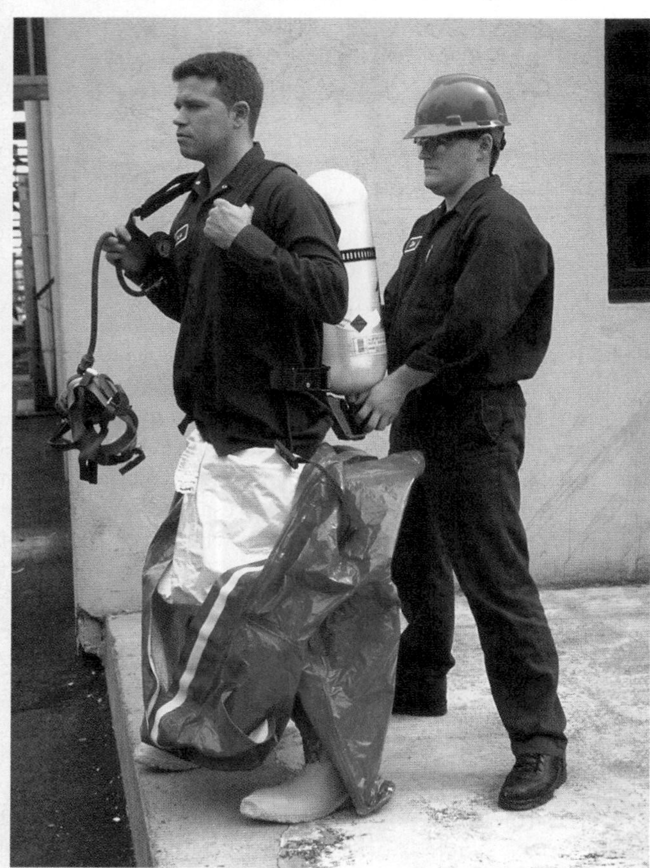

43-1A * Assisting with a self-contained breathing apparatus (SCBA).

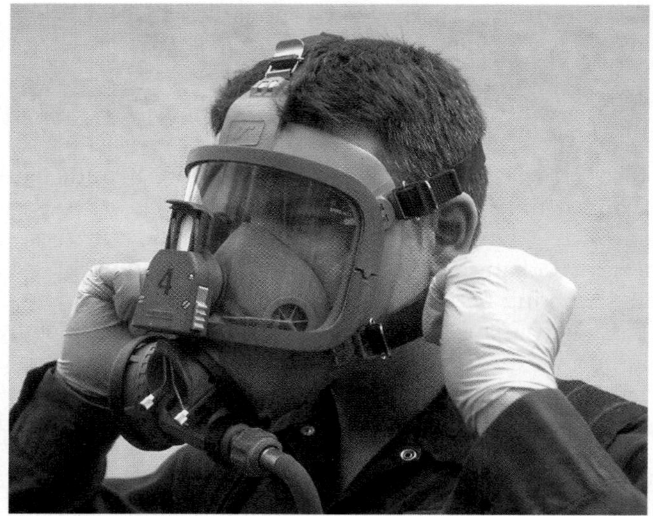

43-1B * An airtight seal must be achieved when putting on the mask.

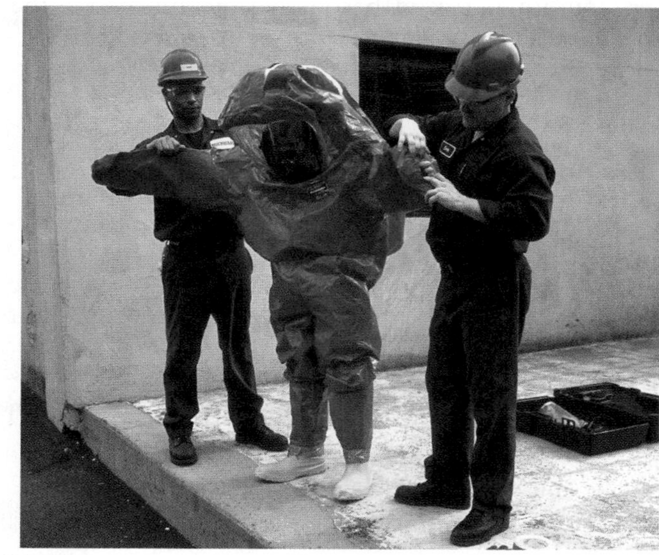

43-1C * The hazmat suit must be sealed at the wrists and ankles.

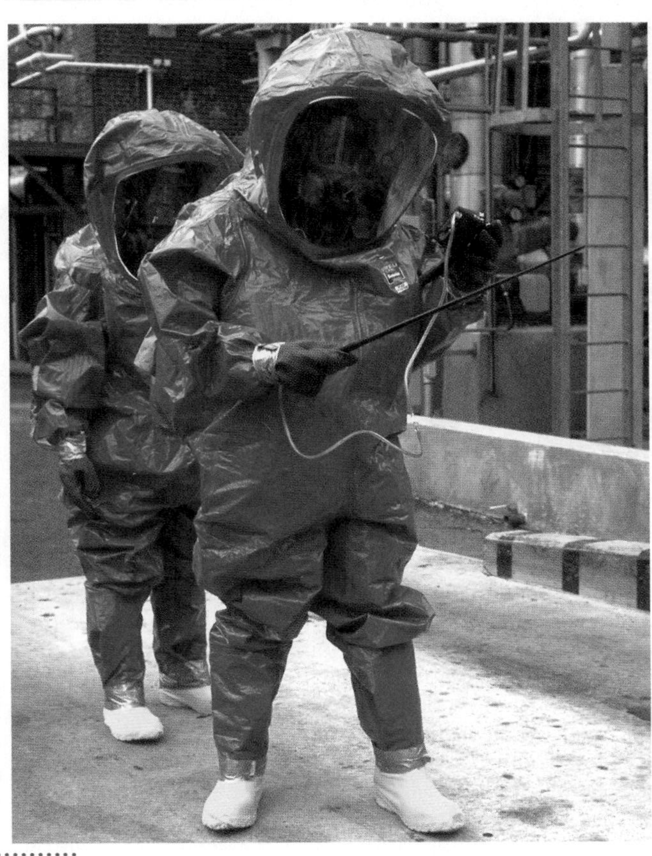

43-1D ✱ Hazmat team, fully suited.

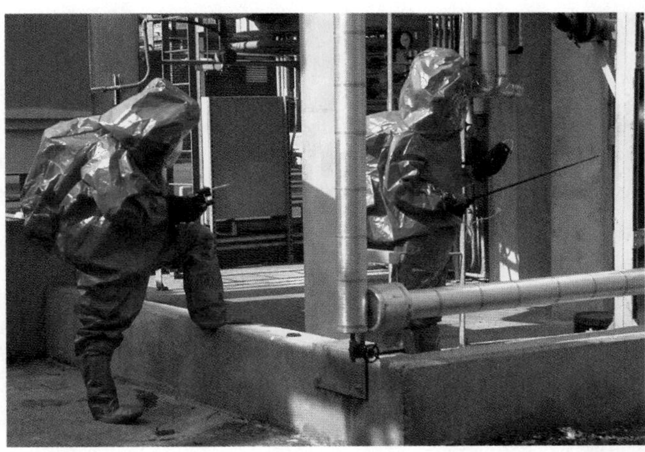

43-1E ✱ Using sensors to detect hazardous materials.

CHAPTER REVIEW

SUMMARY

A hazardous material is a substance that in any quantity can pose a threat or risk to life, health, or property. Hazardous material is identified by placards and shipping papers. Do not use your senses in an attempt to identify the hazardous material since some may be odorless and colorless. There are several resources available to responding emergency personnel to assist in the identification of the hazardous material and to determine the threat to life, health, and property. It is important that emergency responders are trained at some level of hazardous material response. Most EMS personnel are trained to the First Responder Awareness level. This primarily is designed to provide information to keep the EMS personnel safe at the scene. Awareness-level responders should always adhere to the RAIN principles (recognize, avoid, isolate, notify).

General priorities of hazardous materials scene management are to protect the safety of rescuers and patients; provide patient care; and decontaminate clothing, equipment, and the vehicle. Preincident planning is a key in getting all of the responding emergency personnel to work together effectively.

Three zones must be established at the scene: hot zone, warm zone, and cold zone. Only those with specialized protective equipment are allowed in the hot or warm zone. EMTs without specific hazardous materials operations or technician training must stay in the cold zone. The patient will be delivered to you in the cold zone once decontamination has occurred.

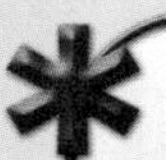

CASE STUDY FOLLOW-UP

SCENE SIZE-UP

You have been dispatched to a multiple-vehicle accident involving a tanker truck and passenger vehicle. In addition to the injuries to the patients caused by the impact, you realize that the tanker may pose a possible hazardous materials emergency. As your partner decides on a safe place to park—uphill, upwind, and away from the potential danger—you pull out your *Emergency Response Guidebook*.

From your present safe position, you note the size and shape of the tank and, with binoculars, search for some form of identification. You finally recognize one—a "Flammable Liquid" placard. Using your guidebook, you find that danger can come from fire or explosion and you realize that everyone at the scene needs to make sure they don't accidentally start one with an open flame, heat, or sparks. Continuing to size up the scene, you look for signs of damage to the container. You spot a small leak and vapors.

You report to incident command. Just as you exit your vehicle, the fire department arrives and begins to set up an entry and decontamination area.

PRIMARY ASSESSMENT

You observe the patients as they begin to walk toward the EMS unit. Your general impression is of a male and female in their 40s, neither of whom looks very steady. They were exposed to the vapors, so they are probably dizzy.

Over the loudspeaker, incident command instructs the patients to stop where they are. Their clothes are contaminated, and they must strip. They don't need much convincing. They can smell the vapors. The patients are soon in the decontamination area being washed down, with rescuers holding manual in-line stabilization.

Once the patients have been decontaminated and are in clean clothes, you and your partner complete the primary assessment while an Emergency Medical Responder continues to hold manual in-line stabilization. Both patients are talking coherently and so you conclude that they are alert and have open airways. Their breathing rates are slightly rapid but adequate. Pulses for both are present, strong, regular, and slightly rapid. Skin color, temperature, and condition are normal. There is no bleeding. You provide both patients oxygen by nonrebreather mask at 15 lpm. You conclude that neither patient is a high priority for immediate transport and you can continue with the secondary assessment at the scene.

SECONDARY ASSESSMENT

You and your partner perform a secondary assessment on both patients. Neither appears to have been injured, but since the mechanism of injury was significant (the collision with the truck), you apply cervical spine immobilization collars and immobilize each patient to a long spine board. You take vital signs—all are within normal ranges for both patients—and gather a history. The only symptom either patient reports is dizziness. Neither reports any allergies. The female is taking no medications; the male is taking a medication for high blood pressure. Neither has any pertinent past medical history except for the blood pressure problem. Their last meal was lunch at a fast food restaurant just before the collision. Events leading to the present problem are obvious to all.

Another ambulance arrives at the scene. Both ambulance crews cover the stretchers and other items in the ambulance with thick plastic. Each patient is loaded onto a plastic-covered wheeled stretcher and transferred to one of the ambulances for transport.

REASSESSMENT

Since your patient is stable, a reassessment is needed only every 15 minutes. Transport time is relatively short, so you have time to perform only one reassessment en route. You repeat the primary assessment, the secondary assessment, and vital signs measurements. You check that the patient is still securely immobilized and that oxygen is flowing adequately. You arrive at the hospital without any change in the patient's condition. You and your partner transfer the patient to the care of the emergency department personnel, complete your oral and written reports, and then proceed to decontaminate yourselves and the ambulance.

IN REVIEW

1. List clues that tell you a hazardous material may be present at an accident scene.
2. Name the first thing an EMT should do after recognizing that hazardous materials might be involved in an accident.
3. Explain what qualifies the EMT to attempt a hazardous materials rescue.
4. List specific actions you can take to protect bystanders.
5. If you have had no specialized training, explain what you should do while waiting for expert help to arrive.
6. List the resources available to the EMT at the site of a hazardous materials emergency.
7. Explain what you can do to protect yourself, others, and your vehicle from contamination.
8. List the "safety zones" and describe what work should be done in each.
9. List the information that is necessary for trained personnel to decide on a course of action at a hazardous materials emergency.
10. Name the required elements of an incident management plan.

CRITICAL THINKING

You are called to the scene for a factory worker who has collapsed in a storage area. As you arrive on the scene, the foreman tells you that the storage facility contains a large number of hazardous chemicals in containers. He states that a leaking chemical container was found in the storage area. He is not sure if the patient was exposed to a leaking chemical or if he suffered some other medical problem. As you look around the corner, you note the patient is not moving and is lying in a prone position. No odors or vapors are noted in the area.

1. What would be your first action?
2. How would you manage the scene?
3. Would you call for any additional resources? If so, who?
4. When would you begin your emergency care for the patient?

EXPLORE PEARSON **mybradykit**™

Please go to **www.bradybooks.com** to access mykit for this text. You will find quizzes, critical thinking scenarios, weblinks, animations, and videos related to this chapter—and much more. Look for online information on managing acute chemical exposures and radiation emergencies.

Register your access code from the front of your book by going to **www.bradybooks.com** and selecting the mykit links.

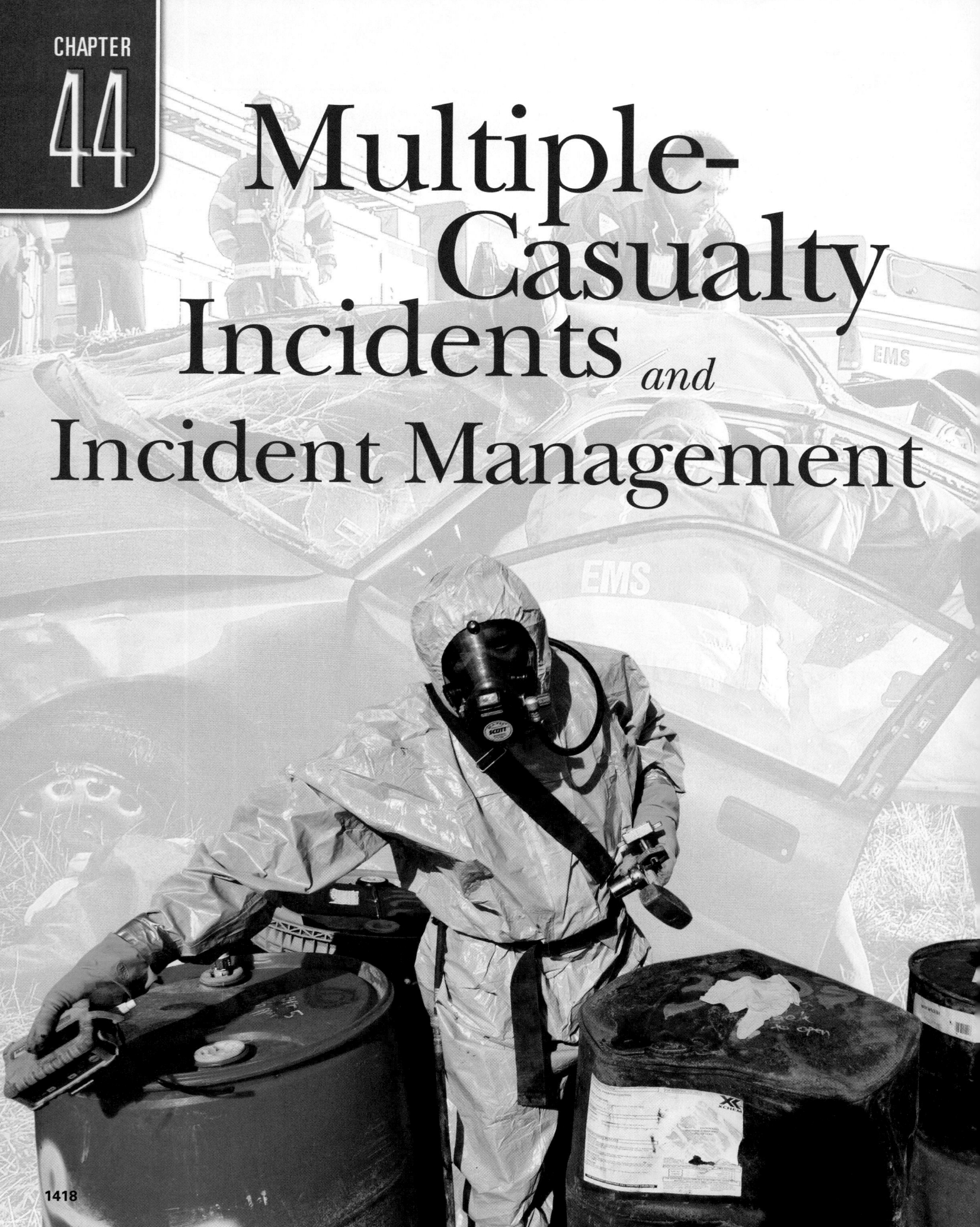

CHAPTER 44

Multiple-Casualty Incidents *and* Incident Management

Navigation Guide

The following items provide an overview to the purpose and content of this chapter. The Standard and Competency are from the new National EMS Education Standards.

STANDARD **EMS Operations** (Content Area: Multiple-Casualty Incidents)

COMPETENCY Applies knowledge of operational roles and responsibilities to ensure patient, public, and personnel safety.

OBJECTIVES: After reading this chapter, you should be able to:

44-1. Define key terms introduced in this chapter.
44-2. List situations that might result in multiple trauma casualties and situations that might result in multiple medical casualties.
44-3. List aspects important to effective management of an MCI.
44-4. Explain the purposes for establishment of the National Incident Management System (NIMS).
44-5. Describe the purposes and desirable features of the incident command system (ICS).
44-6. Identify responsibilities that may be assigned to EMS (units that might be established) at a multiple-casualty incident.
44-7. Describe the principles of a triage system.
44-8. Describe and contrast primary triage with secondary triage.
44-9. Given a scenario with multiple patients, categorize patients according to a color-coded triage system.
44-10. Explain the principles and assessment categories used in START triage.
44-11. Explain why JumpSTART was developed for triage of pediatric patients, contrast JumpSTART with START, and explain how to identify a "child" for triage purposes at the scene of an MCI.
44-12. Explain the important principles of a patient-tagging system to be used during triage.
44-13. Explain the interrelationship of triage and treatment within the treatment unit at an MCI.
44-14. Discuss the logistics of staging and transport at an MCI.
44-15. Discuss common issues with communications in MCI and disaster situations.
44-16. List measures that can be taken to reduce rescuer stress during and after an MCI response.
44-17. Describe requirements of effective disaster assistance.
44-18. Anticipate psychological reactions of disaster victims and describe ways in which EMS providers can assist disaster survivors.

KEY TERMS: Page references indicate first major use in this chapter. For complete definitions, see the Glossary at the back of the book.

disaster p. 1435
incident command system (ICS) p. 1421
incident commander p. 1421
multiple-casualty incident (MCI) p. 1420
National Incident Management System (NIMS) p. 1420
primary triage p. 1425
secondary triage p. 1425
staging unit p. 1432
transport unit p. 1433
treatment unit p. 1431
triage p. 1425
triage unit p. 1425

MEDIA RESOURCES: Please go to www.bradybooks.com to access mykit for this text. You will find quizzes, critical thinking scenarios, weblinks, animations, and videos related to this chapter—and much more. Look for online information on resources for emergency workers and on START. You will also find a video about responding to children during disasters.

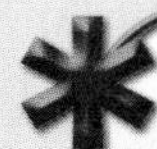

CASE STUDY

The Dispatch
EMS Unit 105—respond to the Firebird Raceway—we have reports that two race cars have crashed through a fence into a bleacher full of people. Initial reports indicate as many as 10 dead and 40 critical injuries. Time out is 1612 hours.

Upon Arrival
While en route to the scene, you request dispatch to activate the multiple-casualty incident plan. Dispatch advises you they are contacting appropriate emergency response agencies from the call-up list and that area hospitals have been notified.

continued

Upon arrival, you see two demolished vehicles in the midst of a collapsed bleacher. Bystanders are helping the injured. People scream for your help. You estimate there are at least 50 injuries. Since you are the senior EMT, according to your multiple-casualty incident plan you are the incident manager for EMS operations.

How Would You Begin Your Assessment and Emergency Care in This Multiple-Casualty Incident? *During this chapter, you will learn about the roles and responsibilities of an EMT during a multiple-casualty incident. Later we will return to the case study and apply the principles you have learned.*

Introduction

This chapter provides an overview of how to organize and provide emergency medical care when there is an event that involves a number of patients: a multiple-casualty incident, or MCI. The number of patients required to declare an MCI varies on the jurisdiction and the availability of resources. MCIs may range from a vehicle collision with several injured passengers to a major disaster such as a hurricane, flood, earthquake, bombing, building collapse, or airliner crash. For a more advanced understanding of MCIs and disaster response, you must regularly practice your community's MCI or disaster response plan.

In this chapter you will learn the fundamentals of MCI response, but these fundamentals must be adapted to your own region. You will learn about the incident management system, EMS units, triage, components of a disaster response plan, and—most importantly—how to get the right patient to the right hospital in the right amount of time.

Multiple-Casualty Incidents

A **multiple-casualty incident (MCI)**—sometimes called a *mass casualty incident* or a *multiple-casualty situation (MCS)*—is any event that places excessive demands on personnel and equipment. Typically, an MCI involves three or more patients. A multiple-patient incident with three patients may be routine in a large metropolitan area, but three critically injured patients can quickly overwhelm a small community or rural area with limited resources and personnel.

Motor vehicle crashes, gang-related violence, or apartment fires are just some of the situations in which you may encounter multiple patients. But MCIs do not always involve trauma patients. Your MCI plan should prepare you to manage the multiple-patient incident involving food poisoning, toxic gas inhalation, and in some parts of the nation, refugee influx.

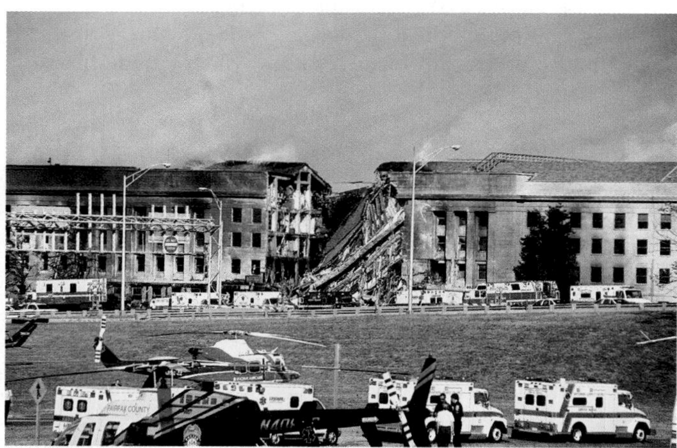

FIGURE 44-1 ∗ Many resources were required at the scene of the terrorist-hijacked plane crash at the Pentagon, September 11, 2001. (© Rob Crandall/Image Works)

In any MCI, the key to effective emergency care is to call for plenty of help early (Figure 44-1∗). Make sure that you call for enough, or more than enough, rescuers with advanced lifesaving skills as soon as you encounter the incident. Remember: *It's better to call too many rescuers than too few.*

Getting help, however, is only one aspect of managing the multiple-casualty incident. Effective management of MCIs consists of getting enough help, positioning vehicles properly, giving appropriate emergency medical care, transporting patients efficiently, and providing follow-up care at receiving facilities.

National Incident Management System

In February 2003, President George W. Bush signed Homeland Security Presidential Directive #5 (HSPD5), which authorized the Secretary of Homeland Security to develop and administer the **National Incident Management System (NIMS).** NIMS provides for a consistent

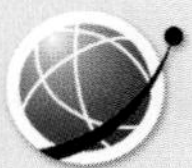

Media Resources

Go to www.bradybooks.com for mykit. Highlights:

- *Web Resource:* Mass Casualty Information
- *Web Resource:* NIMS Resource Center
- *Web Resource:* START

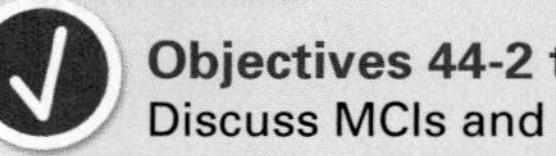

Objectives 44-2 to 44-4

Discuss MCIs and NIMS.

Key Terms

multiple-casualty incident (MCI) an event that places excessive demands on EMS.

National Incident Management System (NIMS) national MCI management system.

approach to managing disasters by all responders to the incident that may include emergency response personnel and local, state, and federal government agencies and employees. The incident command system (ICS), which provides a standardized approach of management for mass casualty incidents, is a subset of the NIMS.

NIMS provides for two main components: flexibility and standardization. These two components are the keys to managing any disaster and ensuring cooperation and operability between various agencies. Every agency that may respond to a disaster was required to become NIMS-compliant through the completion of training in basic incident command systems and the National Incident Management System by September 2006. This training is intended to ensure that all responders comprehend and employ the same terminology and have a standardized knowledge of the incident command system. However, this is only the beginning of NIMS compliance. Agencies and responders must also participate in preparedness standardization. The components of preparedness standardization are planning, training, mutual aid agreements, and preparedness exercises involving multiple response agencies. Preparedness standardization is intended to lessen the confusion as to who is in charge in multiple-casualty incidents, to facilitate the building of working interdepartmental relationships, and to provide responders experience in the incident management system.

These are the building blocks that provide a strong foundation for effective management of a multiple-casualty incident or a disaster. Relationships built during training and preparedness exercises assist in eliminating unrealistic expectations of responders and agencies. (After-action reviews following Hurricane Katrina [Figure 44-2*]—which devastated New Orleans and the Gulf Coast in 2005—revealed that, when everything else seemed to fail, the relationships that had been developed during the preparedness phase did work to the advantage of the responders and agencies. These relationships led to resolutions of issues that were initially not apparent.) Completing training exercises in a controlled environment provides experience to responders and leads to the certification and qualification that is necessary to manage a disaster or multiple-casualty situation. The training exercises help identify and resolve problems with the disaster and multiple-casualty plans before an event actually occurs.

NIMS is the template—the gold standard—in incident management systems and command. When implemented, it helps prevent disaster response and management from becoming their own disaster and allows responders to do the greatest good for the greatest number of people affected by the incident.

Incident Command System

The **incident command system (ICS)** is an incident management concept that has become the standard for on-scene management of disasters and multiple-casualty incidents. As a standardized command system used among all of the responding agencies, ICS allows flexibility within the structure of the system to meet the needs of the incident regardless of the complexity and type of incident. The purpose of ICS is to use best management practices to ensure:

- The safety of the emergency responders and others
- The achievement of tactical objectives
- The efficient use of resources

Features of ICS that make it a desirable and effective system are as follows:

- *Common terminology is used, including standardization of titles for facilities and positions. Plain English is used for all communication.* Codes or agency-specific jargon has been eliminated. This lessens confusion and promotes straightforward communication among responders and agencies.
- *Common designations are assigned to all organizational resources including personnel, facilities, equipment, and supplies* to avoid confusion and increase operational effectiveness between responders and agencies.
- *Manageable spans of control are used* to maintain control of the incident.
- *Incident facilities are identified by common terminology with specific activities and functions performed at each facility. Also identified are which members of the ICS can be found at each facility.* Incident facilities include the incident command post, staging areas, base camp, helibase, and helispots. Only the facilities needed to manage the incident will be established.
- *Distinct titles are used.* Only the **incident commander** is called "commander" (Figure 44-3*). Section leaders or heads are called "chiefs." The incident commander is responsible for coordinating all aspects of the incident. The incident commander must have the necessary training, experience, and expertise to serve in this

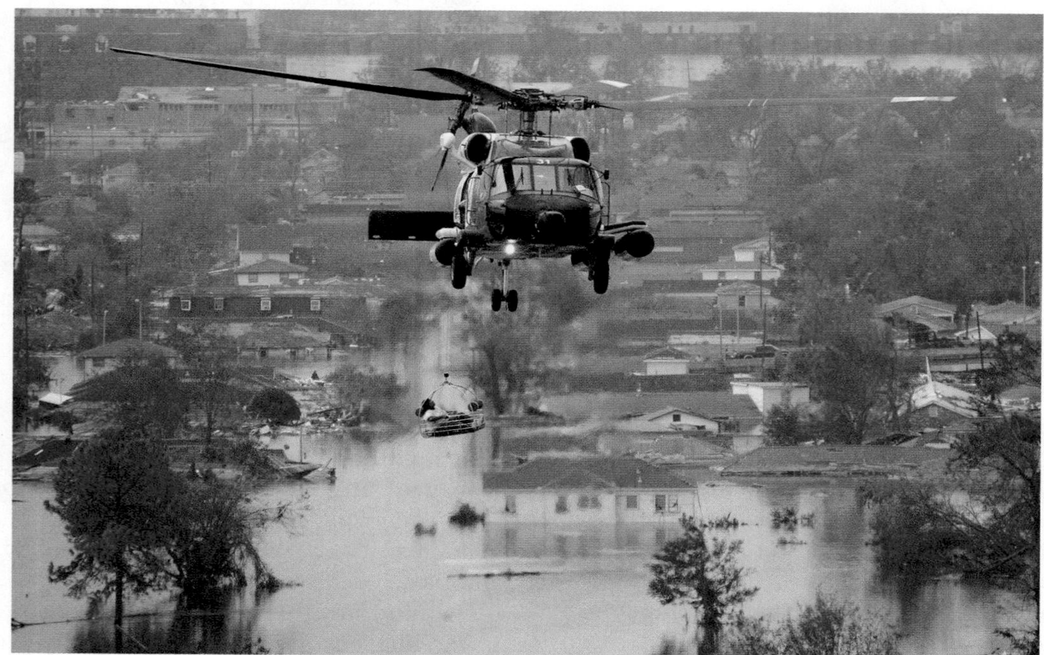

(a)

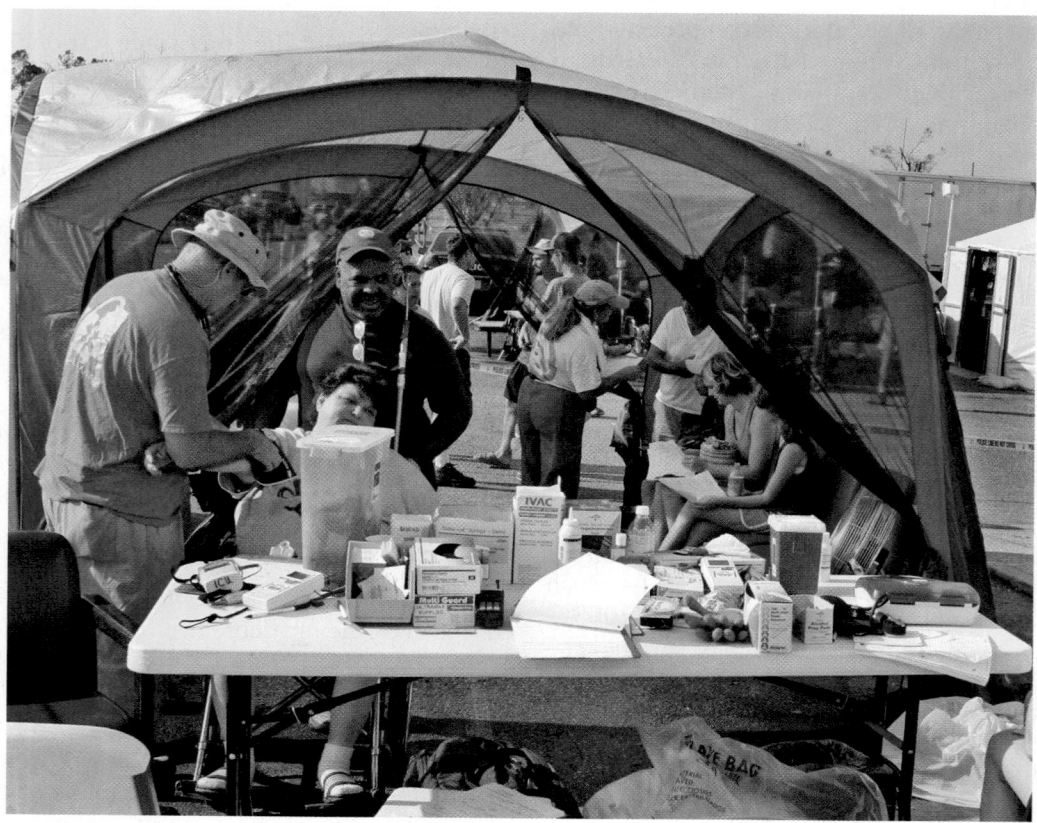

(b)

FIGURE 44-2 ✱ Relationships developed during the preparedness phase of NIMS worked to the advantage of responders and agencies in the aftermath of Hurricane Katrina, 2005: **(a)** a helicopter rescue above flooded streets; **(b)** disaster triage and treatment. (Photo a: © AP Photo/Vincent LaForet/POOL; photo b: © AP Photo/Dennis Paquin)

Objective 44-5
Describe the purposes and desirable features of the incident command system (ICS).

Key Terms
incident command system (ICS) the incident management concept that has become the standard for on-scene management of MCIs.

Key Terms
incident commander the person who is responsible for coordinating all aspects of a disaster or multiple-casualty incident.

Objective 44-6
Identify responsibilities that may be assigned to EMS at a multiple-casualty incident.

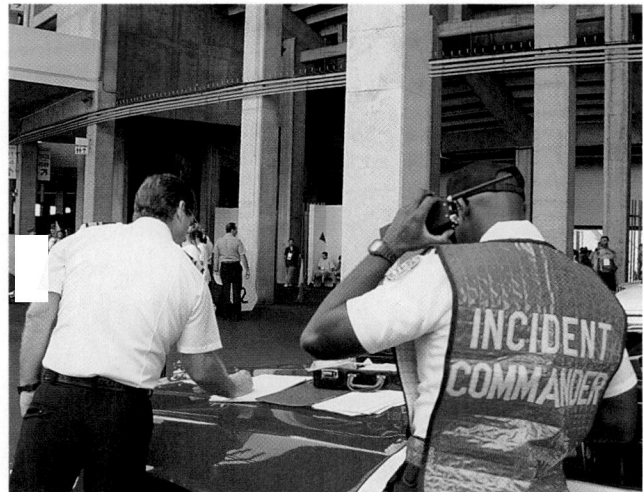

FIGURE 44-3 ✱ The incident commander directs the response and coordinates resources at a multiple-casualty incident.

capacity. The highest ranking officer is not always the incident commander. With standard terminology, it is clearly understood what position each person holds and what duties he is expected to perform.

- *Incident action plans (IAPs) identify the objectives to be accomplished during the incident.* IAPs are used to issue assignments, plans, procedures, and protocols. The results of the objectives are documented and reported so that they can be used in further planning.
- *An integrated communications approach is organized* so that information can be transferred within the command structure and outside of the command structure.
- *Accountability applies at all levels and within all functional areas.* Knowing in advance who is accountable to whom provides an orderly chain of command and makes it easier for responders to check in, regardless of their home agency. Each responder is assigned to only one designated supervisor, the person to whom that responder is accountable.

The incident command system has several designated sections. They are:

- Command
- Finance/administration
- Logistics
- Operations
- Planning

Incident command is typically assumed by the most experienced and senior member of the first emergency service arriving on the scene. Thus, it may be the most senior EMT on the EMS unit that is initially assuming incident command. Incident command can be transferred to the most qualified individual; however, this transfer must be done in a highly organized and informed manner.

Upon arrival at the scene, the initial action of scene size-up and triage may be conducted until additional resources arrive. When additional resources arrive, the incident commander will begin to organize and delegate the responsibilities of the various established branches depending on the scale of the multiple-casualty incident. In a unified command structure, police, fire, and EMS would each be represented and would establish one unified command. Each service would then likely be established under the operations section and retain its autonomy. The unified incident commanders of the three agencies would work together in one command post to solve problems and direct the management of the incident.

The incident commander can choose to establish a number of branches within the structure. These branches are managed by branch directors, who report to a section chief. As an example, the EMS branch director would be responsible for managing all triage, treatment, and transportation of patients within his operation. He would report to the operations chief, who in turn would report to the incident commander. In a large-scale multiple-casualty incident, the EMS branch director would typically assign a unit leader referred to as the leader or supervisor to the triage unit, treatment unit, transport unit, staging unit, and morgue unit (Figure 44-4✱). Each unit may also be referred to as an area, sector, or section. Each leader would supervise the activity within his unit to ensure effective and efficient management of patients and casualties. As an EMT working in any of these areas, you would report to the unit leader, who reports to the EMS branch director.

The responsibilities of the EMS units might include:

- **Triage unit.** This unit sorts patients by criticality and assigns priorities for emergency care and transport.
- **Treatment unit.** Emergency care is provided to patients in this unit. This is done based on the priority assigned to the patient by the triage unit.
- **Transport unit.** In this unit, patients are moved to ambulances or helicopters for transportation to a medical facility, and communications are organized to notify the receiving medical facilities.

Key Points
As a responding EMT you will report to the incident commander and wait for an assignment.

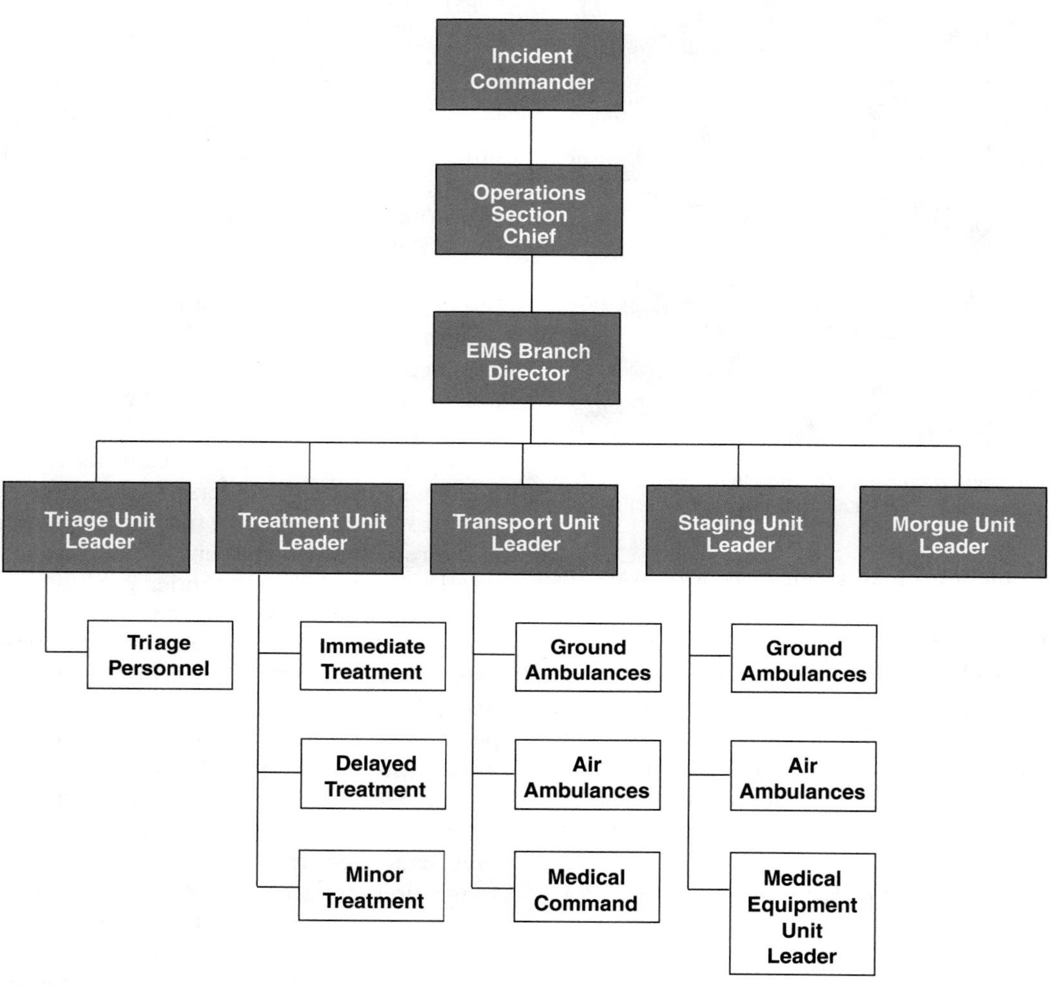

FIGURE 44-4 ✱ EMS branch organization for a major incident.

- **Staging unit.** Ambulances, helicopters, and additional equipment are held in this area until they are assigned to a particular task. Sometimes a *supply unit* is established as part of or separately from the staging unit to gather and distribute supplies and equipment required by all units.
- **Morgue unit.** Deceased casualties are moved to this unit where they are held and processed.

As a responding EMT, you will report to the incident commander and wait for an assignment. You would likely be assigned to the operations section that deals with emergency care of the patients. If qualified, you may be assigned as a section chief or a unit leader. In a smaller-scale incident, the command structure for EMS would typically include the incident commander, the operations section chief, and the triage, treatment, and transport unit leaders (Figure 44-5✱).

Objectives 44-7 and 44-8
Describe the principles of triage and contrast primary with secondary triage.

Objective 44-9
Given a scenario with multiple patients, categorize patients according to a color-coded triage system.

Key Terms
triage sorting patients to determine order of care. **Primary triage** occurs immediately on arrival of EMS. In the **triage unit,** patients are reevaluated during **secondary triage.**

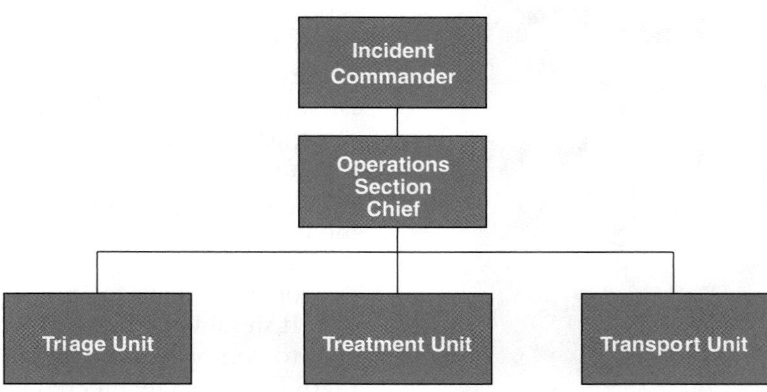

FIGURE 44-5 * Basic ICS organization for a small- to medium-sized incident.

Triage

During the early phases of an MCI, you may be directed to assist in triage. **Triage** is a system used for sorting patients to determine the order in which they will receive medical care or transportation to definitive care. Basically, triage determines which persons need immediate emergency care in order to survive their injuries, which patients will live with a delay in emergency medical care, and which patients will die regardless of the emergency care provided. Triage is one of the first functions performed at the scene of a multiple-casualty incident and has a direct effect on all other aspects of the operation (Figure 44-6*).

Primary and Secondary Triage

There are typically two phases or types of triage that are conducted at the scene of a multiple-casualty incident. **Primary triage** occurs immediately upon the arrival of the first EMS crew.

This triage is usually conducted at the actual site of the incident, provided the scene is safe. For example, primary triage in the case of a bus rollover would be conducted inside the vehicle, provided the bus is properly stabilized and free of safety hazards. The primary triage is done quickly and provides a basic categorization of the severity of the patients involved in the incident. The patients are usually tagged as red, yellow, green, or black with colored ribbon or tape for easy recognition by rescue crews for removal of patients according to priority. The person performing primary triage is also responsible for providing an initial report back to the EMS commander, who may be one of the first-arriving EMTs acting in the position at this time, regarding the estimated number of patients and resources needed at the scene.

The universally recognized triage categorizations by color are:

Color	Category	Priority Status
Red	Immediate care and transport necessary	Priority 1 (P-1)
Yellow	Delayed emergency care and transport	Priority 2 (P-2)
Green	Minor injuries and ambulatory patients	Priority 3 (P-3)
Black	Deceased or fatal injuries	Priority 4 (P-4)

Once the patients are moved from the scene to the **triage unit,** the secondary triage occurs. The **secondary triage** is designed to re-evaluate the patient categorization, during which the patient may be upgraded to a higher priority, downgraded to a lower priority, or kept at the same priority status. This occurs as the patient is brought into the triage unit and the triage unit leader performs the reassessment of the patient to categorize him for treatment and transport. During the treatment phase, the patient is retriaged and may be recategorized as a higher or lower priority.

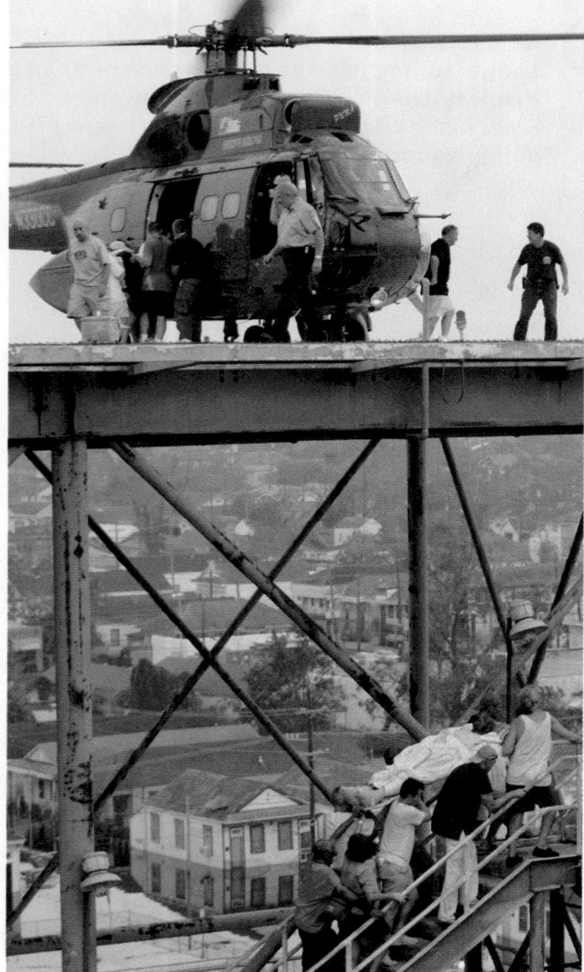

(a)

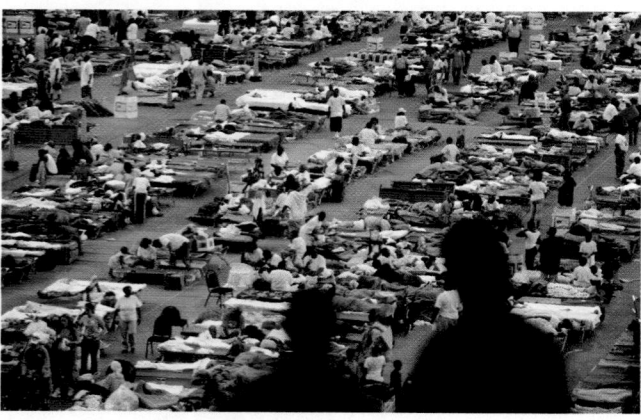

(b)

FIGURE 44-6 ✱ **(a)** Hurricane Katrina victims evacuated from New Orleans, September 2005. **(b)** Triage sector at the Houston Astrodome where up to 16,000 evacuees stayed. (Photo a: © Brad Loper/Dallas Morning News/Corbis; photo b: © Carlos Barria/ Reuters/Corbis)

Typically, the most knowledgeable and experienced EMT arriving on the scene will perform the initial triage of the patients; however, all EMS personnel must be trained to triage patients at a multiple-casualty incident. All EMS units must carry the necessary triage equipment to allow for prompt recognition of priority status of patients.

START Triage System

A widely accepted and used triage system is the START (simple triage and rapid transport) system. The Newport Beach Fire and Marine Department and Hoag Memorial Hospital in Newport Beach, California, developed START. It is an easy triage system to use and allows for rapid categorization of patients into the priority categories for further assessment, treatment, and transport (Figure 44-7✱). START is recommended for adults and can also be used for children who are older than 8 years of age and greater than 100 pounds in weight. Your first assessment that falls into the "immediate" category should cause you to stop triage, tag the patient as "red," and have the patient moved to the triage unit.

The START triage is performed primarily to initially categorize patients for priority movement to the triage unit. It should not take you more than 30 seconds per patient to complete. The three basic categories assessed in START, easily remembered by the mnemonic RPM, are:

- Respiratory status
- Perfusion status
- Mental status

Ability to Walk (Ambulatory or "Walking Wounded")

Upon initial triage, any patients who are already up walking around the scene and those who indicate that they are able to get up and walk should be collected and moved to a safe area. Any patient who is able to walk, despite the injuries he has suffered, is considered to be a lower priority initially and is tagged "green." A green tag, ribbon, tape, or other identifier is placed on each ambulatory patient. These patients are then moved to one site and confined there. Do not allow them to continue to walk around the scene. These patients will be reevaluated in the triage unit but will be the last to be treated in the treatment unit and moved from the scene to the hospital.

Respirations

Begin assessing the nonwalking patients by looking, listening, and feeling for respiratory effort. If the patient is breathing and the respiratory rate is greater than 30 respirations per minute, tag the patient as "red" and move on to the next patient. If the respirations are less than 30 per minute, move on to assess perfusion. If there are no respirations present upon assessment, open the airway. Upon opening the airway, if the patient begins to breathe, determine the respiratory rate. If the respiratory

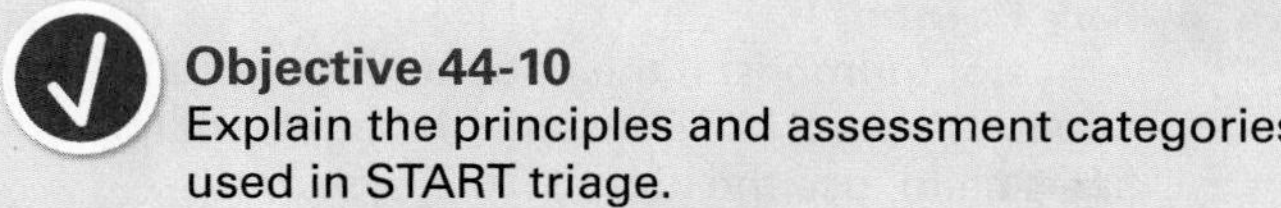

Objective 44-10
Explain the principles and assessment categories used in START triage.

Key Points
START is recommended for adults and can be used on children who are greater than 8 years old and weigh more than 100 pounds. It should be completed in no more than 30 seconds.

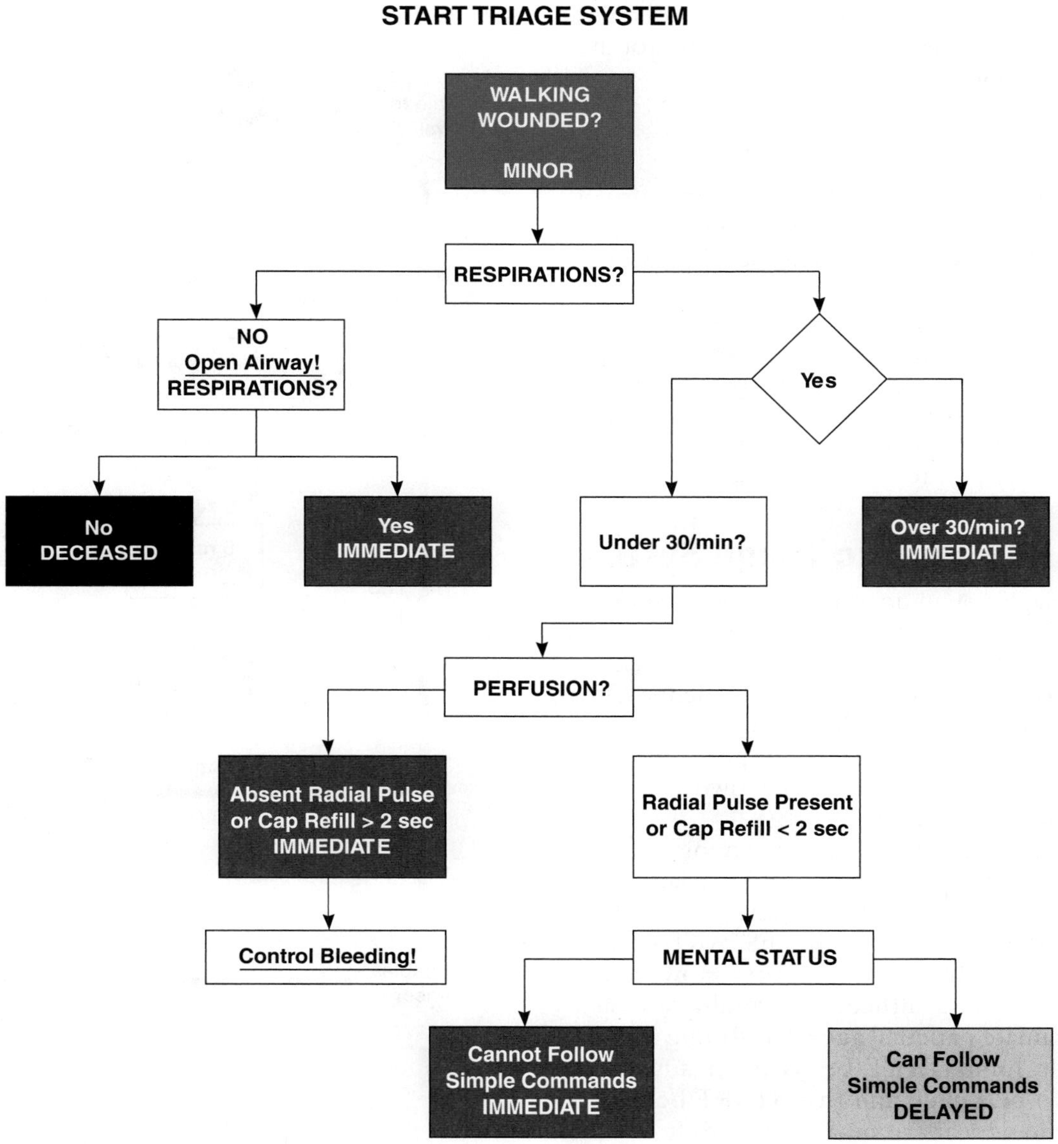

START TRIAGE SYSTEM

WALKING WOUNDED?
MINOR

RESPIRATIONS?

NO
Open Airway!
RESPIRATIONS?

No
DECEASED

Yes
IMMEDIATE

Yes

Under 30/min?

Over 30/min?
IMMEDIATE

PERFUSION?

Absent Radial Pulse
or Cap Refill > 2 sec
IMMEDIATE

Control Bleeding!

Radial Pulse Present
or Cap Refill < 2 sec

MENTAL STATUS

Cannot Follow
Simple Commands
IMMEDIATE

Can Follow
Simple Commands
DELAYED

FIGURE 44-7 ✱ The START system.

rate is greater than 30 per minute, tag "red" and move on. If the patient's respirations are less than 30 per minute, and he is breathing, assess his perfusion status. If the respirations are shallow or inadequate and require assistance, tag "red" and move on to the next patient. If you open the airway in the patient who is not breathing and he has no respiratory effort, tag the patient as "black" (deceased) and move on to the next patient.

Perfusion

Perfusion status is determined by assessing the capillary refill and radial pulse. If the capillary refill is less than 2 seconds and the radial pulse is present, go to the neurological assessment. If the capillary refill is greater than 2 seconds or the radial pulse is absent, tag the patient "red" and move on to the next patient. Keep in mind that a 2-second capillary refill time is subject to many factors,

Objective 44-11
Explain why JumpSTART was developed for triage of pediatric patients, contrast JumpSTART with START, and explain how to identify a "child" for triage purposes at the scene of an MCI.

Key Points
A rule of thumb is: if the patient looks like an adult, use the START system. If the patient looks like a child, use the jumpSTART system.

including age, sex, and environmental considerations; therefore, the radial pulse may be a better indicator in assessment of perfusion.

Mental Status

The last component to assess is the mental or neurological status of the patient. At this point, if you are assessing the neurological status of the patient, he will have had a respiratory rate less than 30 per minute with adequate respirations, a radial pulse, and a capillary refill of less than 2 seconds. Ask the patient to squeeze your fingers. If the patient obeys your command, tag him "yellow" and move on to the next patient. If the patient is not alert, does not obey your commands, or is unresponsive, tag him "red" and move on to the next patient.

JumpSTART Pediatric Triage System

The START triage system does not take into account the physiological differences between adult patients and young children. Therefore, the START triage system may be applied erroneously to these young patients. Often, the EMT may overtriage a child patient, expending an unnecessary amount of time triaging or providing extensive initial care because of the EMT's own insecurities when dealing with pediatric patients.

In order to facilitate triage in young children, Dr. Lou Romig developed JumpSTART, a triage system specifically for pediatric patients (Figure 44-8∗). Previously, it was suggested that the JumpSTART triage be used only for children ages 1–8 years. However, because it is stressful and difficult at a multiple-casualty incident to estimate patients' ages, Dr. Romig now recommends that JumpSTART be used on any patient who appears to be a child and that START be used on any patient who appears to be a young adult or older. The lower end of the age range is used to capture those children who are usually able to walk. Infants (less than 12 months) have significant physiological variations in vital signs; therefore, the JumpSTART system is not designed for them.

Infants less than 1 year of age could be triaged using JumpSTART; however, more screening may be necessary. If all of the criteria point to the "delay" category, and there are no obvious external injuries, the infant may be categorized as "ambulatory." If the patient looks like a young adult, use the START system. If the patient looks like a child, use JumpSTART.

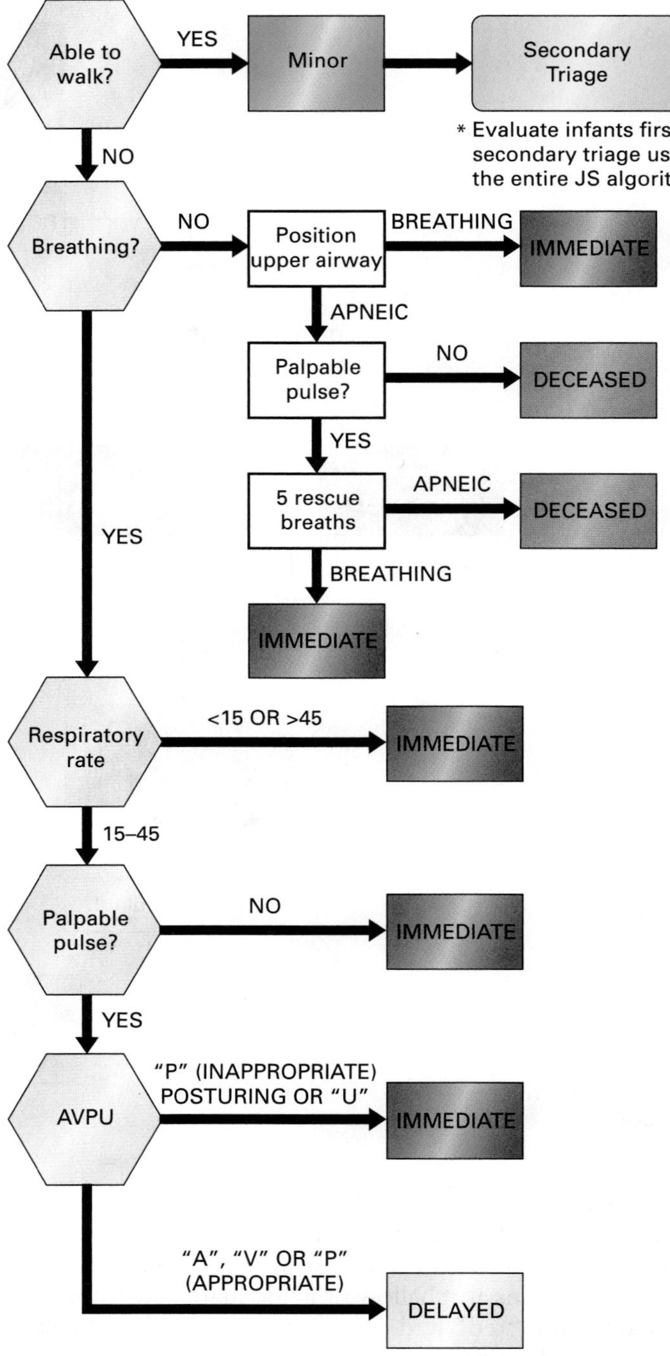

FIGURE 44-8 ∗ The JumpSTART system. (© Lou Romig, MD, FAAP, FACEP, 2002)

Key Points
Ventilation is briefly provided as the "jumpstart" for the child, because in children cardiac arrest usually results from respiratory arrest.

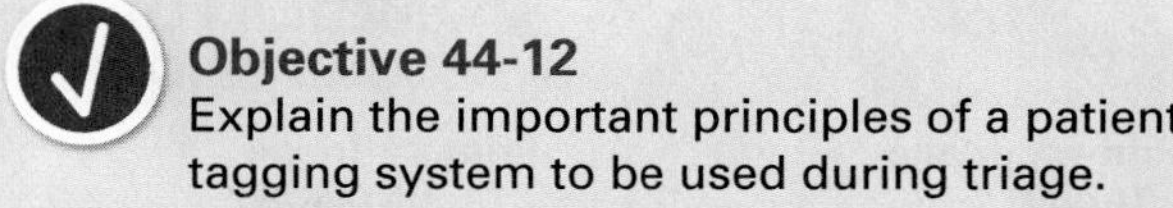

Objective 44-12
Explain the important principles of a patient-tagging system to be used during triage.

The reason for the use of JumpSTART in pediatric patients is primarily some physiological differences in young children as compared to adults. In the adult patient, respiratory failure due to a traumatic event usually occurs after severe blood loss with circulatory failure or severe head injury. Thus, an adult patient in respiratory arrest has more than likely suffered a significant amount of cardiac damage from hypoperfusion and hypoxia that makes his condition beyond saving.

In a child, it is usually the opposite. The child will typically go into respiratory arrest, followed by circulatory failure and cardiac arrest. Respiratory arrest in a young child may occur rapidly after shorter periods of hypoxia. The child could be apneic (not breathing) and the pulse could be present because the child has not yet become extremely hypoxic. During this period, opening the airway and providing ventilation to the child may stimulate spontaneous ventilation until more emergency care can be provided. This brief provision of ventilation to the child is considered the "jumpstart" for the child to start breathing on his own.

JumpSTART uses the same categories as START. You would assess the following:

- Respiratory status
- Perfusion status
- Mental status

The JumpSTART triage system should take no more than 15 seconds to perform on each pediatric patient.

JumpSTART Ambulatory Assessment

Any patient who is walking around the scene should be directed or escorted to the "green" area for secondary triage. Children who are developmentally unable to walk and are still at the scene will be screened using the JumpSTART system. If they do not meet any of the "immediate" criteria, they should be tagged as "green" and moved to that area for further assessment and treatment.

Children with special needs should be considered the same as the developmentally unable to walk and should be triaged at the scene the same as the very young child who can't walk yet.

JumpSTART Breathing Assessment

If the child is breathing, assess the respiratory rate. If the breathing is between 15 and 45 breaths per minute, assess the pulse. If the patient is breathing spontaneously and the breathing rate is less than 15 per minute, greater than 45 per minute, or irregular, tag the patient "red" and move on to the next patient. If there is no breathing or it is very irregular, open the airway using a manual maneuver. If the airway maneuver causes the patient to begin to breathe spontaneously, tag the patient "red" and move on to another patient. If there is no breathing after opening the airway, check for a peripheral pulse. If the pulse is absent, tag the patient "black" and move on to another patient. If a pulse is present after opening the airway and finding no breathing, provide 15 seconds of mouth-to-mask ventilation (about five breaths). If the patient remains apneic (no breathing), tag the patient as "black" and move on to another patient. If breathing is restored after the "jumpstart," tag the patient "red" and move on to the next patient.

JumpSTART Perfusion Assessment

If the peripheral pulse is palpable, assess the mental status. If no peripheral pulse is present, tag the patient "red" and move on to the next patient. The pulse should be checked in the least injured extremity. Capillary refill assessment is not performed.

JumpSTART Mental Status Assessment

Conduct a quick assessment of AVPU. If the child is alert, responds to voice, or responds to pain by localizing it, withdrawing from it, or trying to push it away, the patient is tagged "yellow" and placed in the delayed category. If the child is unresponsive to all stimuli or responds to pain with incomprehensible sounds or inappropriate movement (does not localize pain, or no purposeful flexion or extension), tag the child "red" and move on to the next patient.

Patient Tagging

Patient tagging or identification (Figures 44-9∗ and 44-10∗) is critical to the successful initial triage of every patient. Tagging the sick or injured helps arriving EMTs quickly and efficiently identify treatment priorities. The tagging system should be easy to understand, standardized, and easily affixed to the patient:

- **Highest Priority/Red/Immediate.** The highest-level priority, "red," is assigned to patients with the

(RED) HIGHEST OR FIRST PRIORITY	(YELLOW) MEDIUM OR SECOND PRIORITY	(GREEN) LOWEST OR THIRD PRIORITY	(BLACK) NO PRIORITY OR DECEASED
Primary Triage (Adult) • Breathing spontaneously after opening the airway • Respiratory rate > 30/minute • Capillary refill > 2 seconds • Doesn't obey commands **(Pediatric)** • Breathing after opening airway and after 5 rescue breaths • Respiratory rate < 15 or > 45/minute • No palpable pulse • Inappropriate posturing or unresponsive	**Primary Triage (Adult)** • Unable to walk • Respiratory rate < 30/minute • Capillary refill < 2 seconds • Obeys commands **(Pediatric)** • Unable to walk, if age-appropriate • Respiratory rate > 15 or < 45/minute • Palpable pulse • Alert or responds to verbal or painful stimuli	**Primary Triage (Adult)** • Able to walk • **(Pediatric)** Able to walk, if age-appropriate	**Primary Triage (Adult & Pediatric)** • No breathing
Secondary Triage • Airway and breathing difficulties • Uncontrolled or severe bleeding • Decreased mental status • Severe medical problems: poisoning, diabetic and cardiac emergencies, etc. • Severe burns • Shock (hypoperfusion)	**Secondary Triage** • Burns without airway problems • Major or multiple bone or joint injuries • Back injuries with or without spinal cord damage	**Secondary Triage** • Minor burns • Minor bone or joint injuries • Minor soft tissue injuries	**Secondary Triage** • Obviously dead • Will not survive

FIGURE 44-9 ✻ Triage summary.

most critical injuries who may be able to survive the incident with quick treatment and transport. Notice that most of the red category abnormalities are correlated with the primary assessment. The red category is the same as the START/JumpSTART "immediate" category.

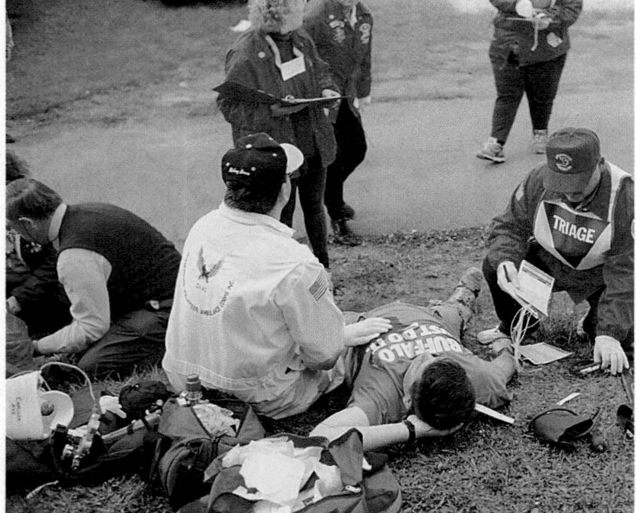

FIGURE 44-10 ✻ Triage tagging is essential in multiple-casualty situations.

- **Second Priority/Yellow/Delayed.** The second-level priority, or "yellow," is assigned to patients who are suffering severe injuries; however, some delay in treatment should still provide the patient a good chance of survival. The yellow category's abnormalities would more closely correlate with those findings and life threats identified in the rapid trauma assessment. The yellow category is the same as the START/JumpSTART "delayed" category.
- **Lowest Priority/Green/Minor.** The lowest-level priority, or "green," is assigned to injuries in which delay in treatment will not reduce the patient's chance of survival. Fractures and soft tissue injuries without life-threatening bleeding commonly fall into this category. The green category is the same as the START/JumpSTART "minor" category.
- **Black/Deceased.** The final category, "black," is reserved for those patients who will not survive, even with treatment, or who are already dead. For example, a patient who has suffered a massive head injury with brain matter oozing from an open wound to the head has suffered a fatal wound and will not survive. It

Thinking Critically

Why is a patient in cardiac arrest not categorized as a "red," high-priority patient?

Objective 44-13

Explain the interrelationship of triage and treatment within the treatment unit at an MCI.

Key Terms

treatment unit unit responsible for collecting and treating patients in a centralized treatment area.

makes no sense to expend resources on a patient who has no chance of survival. The START/JumpSTART "deceased" category correlates to the black category.

During an MCI, emergency personnel may respond from many miles and across many jurisdictions. If patients are to receive definitive care and transportation, then EMS personnel must have a universally understood triage identification tag system (Figure 44-11*).

The issue in triage and multiple-casualty incidents is to maximize the limited resources to do the most good for the most people. That is why patients in cardiac arrest at a mass casualty are immediately tagged as "black" or deceased. Realistically, it would require three EMTs to attempt to resuscitate a cardiac arrest patient. It makes no sense to use those three EMTs on a patient whose chance of survival is extremely low while neglecting others who could be effectively treated by those same three EMTs.

Treatment

A **treatment unit** or area (Figure 44-12*) should be designated close to the area where ambulances arrive. It should be on high ground and, if possible, covered and lighted. It should be safe from falling debris, a safe distance from the incident, and clearly marked. Use a tall flag if you have one. Depending on the size and scope of the MCI, it may be necessary to have more than one treatment unit.

Patients should be moved from the triage unit to the treatment unit in order of their priority. Immobilize all patients before moving them, if necessary, and place them in rows according to their triage category.

Remember that triage is ongoing. Many patients' categories will change as their conditions improve or deteriorate.

Treat only salvageable patients. If color-coded triage tags, cards, or ribbons are used, the same colors should

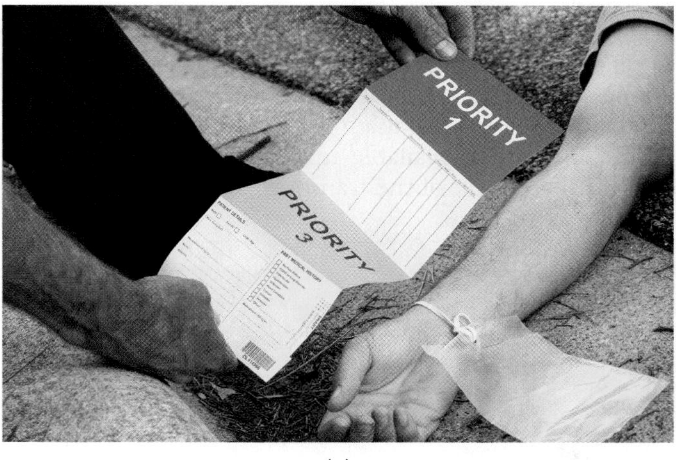

(a)

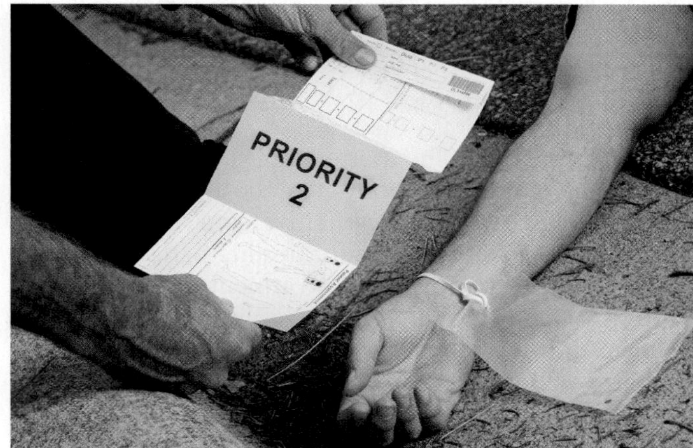

(b)

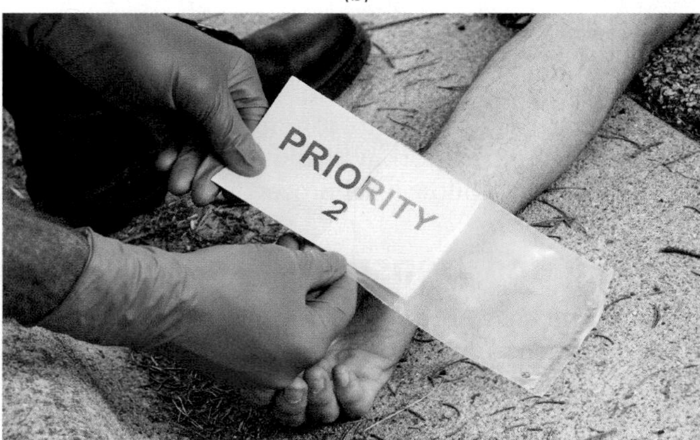

(c)

FIGURE 44-11 * EMS personnel must have a universally understood triage identification tag system as shown in photos **(a)**, **(b)**, and **(c)**.

Objective 44-14
Discuss the logistics of staging and transport at an MCI.

Key Terms
staging unit unit that monitors, inventories, and directs available ambulances to the treatment unit.

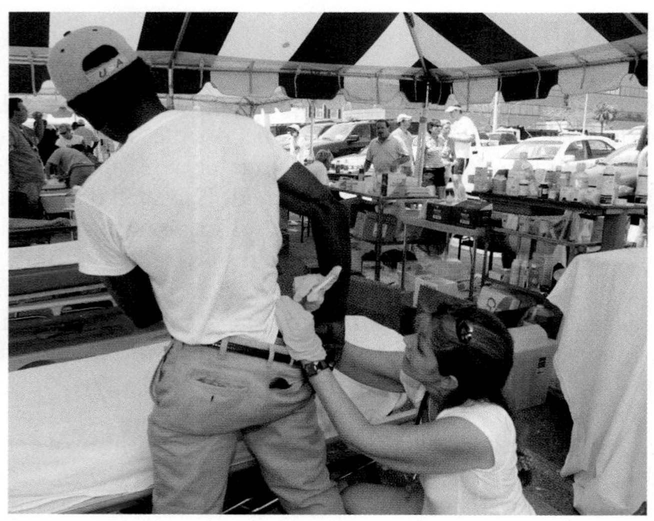

(a)

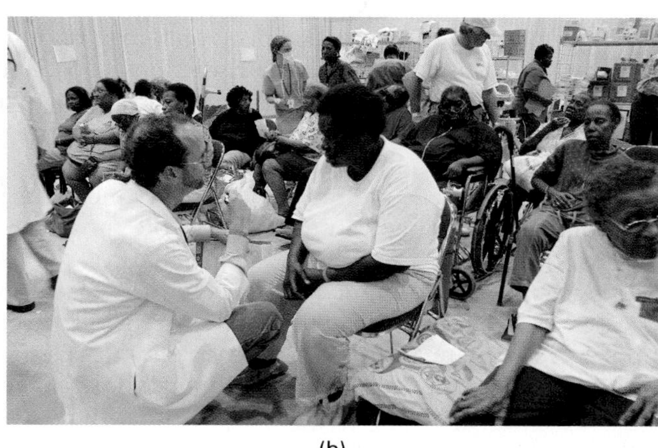

(b)

FIGURE 44-12 ✱ Treatment units responding to the 2005 Gulf Coast hurricane disasters: **(a)** Biloxi, Mississippi; **(b)** Houston Astrodome. (Photo a: © Barry Williams/Getty Images; photo b: © David Portnoy/Getty Images)

be used on color-coded flags that are erected at the triage units. Position patients in rows as they await treatment.

Since the dead are the last to be transported, establish a morgue unit. The morgue unit leader would coordinate the removal of bodies to the morgue with the coroner's office or its representative. You should become familiar with your local plan for dealing with the dead.

If you are working in the treatment unit, a key concept to remember is to provide only necessary care to manage non-life-threatening injuries. For example, immobilize patients to long boards instead of trying to splint each individual extremity injury. Give a patient who is able a 4 × 4 dressing and ask him to apply direct pressure to a bleeding wound—his own or someone else's. Once the highest-priority patients have been stabilized, move to the second-priority patients.

The triage, treatment, and transport unit leaders should remain in constant communication with each other regarding transport availability and needs. Become familiar with and follow local protocol.

Staging and Transport

Once patients have been properly assessed and cared for in the treatment unit, the triage process continues. Working closely together, the treatment, staging, and transport unit leaders make decisions regarding patient transport priorities.

To begin the process of transporting priority patients to the appropriate medical facility, a **staging unit** (Figure 44-13✱) is set up. A staging unit leader monitors, inventories, and directs available ambulances to the treatment unit at the request of the transport unit leader.

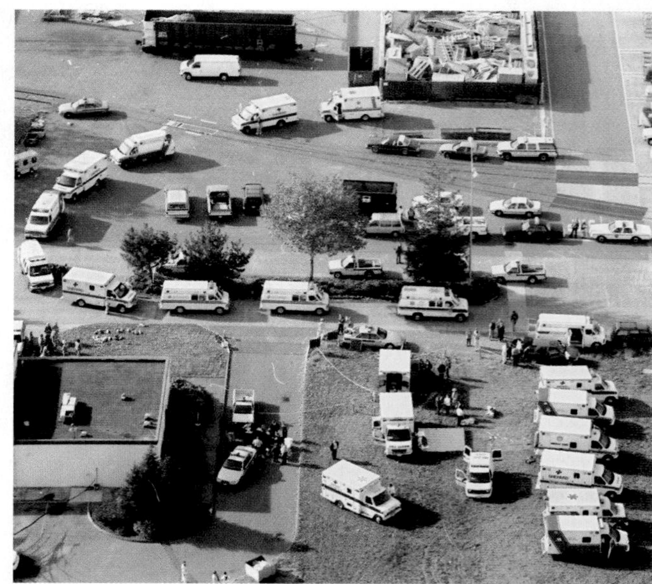

FIGURE 44-13 ✱ Staging sector at a multiple-casualty incident. (© Benjamin Benschneider/THE SEATTLE TIMES)

Key Terms
transport unit unit that coordinates patient transportation with the triage and staging units and receiving hospitals.

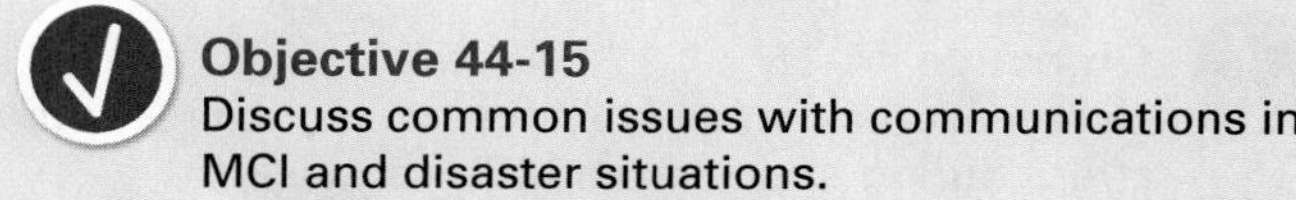

Objective 44-15
Discuss common issues with communications in MCI and disaster situations.

The **transport unit** leader ensures that ambulances are accessible and that transportation does not occur without the direction of the incident commander or operations section chief. The transport unit leader also coordinates patient transportation with the triage unit leader and communicates with the hospitals involved. The transport unit leader must consider the following when making decisions on where to transport each patient:

- Distribution of patients to each medical facility
- Surge capacity of each hospital or medical facility
- Need for transport to a specialty medical facility such as burn unit or pediatric emergency department
- Need for constant coordination and communication

To effectively transport patients of a multiple-casualty incident:

- As the highest-priority patients are stabilized (airway managed, life-threatening bleeding controlled), begin transport. Before and during transport, one or two triage leaders (depending on the number of patients) should move along the rows constantly, monitoring patients for a change in status.
- High-priority patients should be transported first, immediately after treatment; these serious patients should be evenly distributed among available hospitals.
- Before leaving the incident, EMTs should receive specific instructions from the transport unit leader or staging unit leader on how to leave the area (preferred route) and to which hospital to take the patients.
- If the routing in the area is complex, the staging leader should provide EMTs with marked maps to the appropriate hospital.
- As each ambulance leaves, the transport unit leader should radio the hospital that the ambulance is en route, briefly describing the injuries involved and giving an estimated time of arrival. Individual EMTs should not try to communicate with the hospital unless an emergency develops during transport. Individual ambulance communication will jam lines and cause confusion.
- When the only patients left at the site are ambulatory, consider loading them onto a bus that has been brought to the site for this purpose. Five to ten personnel carrying essential equipment (oxygen masks, suction equipment, emergency kits, and portable radio) should board the bus, and a fully equipped ambulance with its crew should lead the bus slowly and safely to an outlying hospital that has little or no patient load. If a patient on the bus suddenly deteriorates during the trip to the hospital, EMTs on board can handle the situation and, if necessary, call for intercept by another ambulance.

Communications

Effective communication between emergency responders is one of the most difficult aspects of a multiple-casualty incident. As an EMT, you can expect a variety of MCI communication difficulties. Upon your arrival at the scene of an MCI, oral communications between emergency responders may initially appear chaotic. Tasks are not always clear, and duties may not have been assigned.

Once an incident command system and mobile command center are established, the state of confusion will diminish. Throughout an MCI, you may also find radio communications of any kind difficult. Communication "dead spots," frequency unavailability, and channel gridlock are a few of the more common radio communications problems you will encounter. These kinds of difficulties are mentioned to prepare you for the "real world" of patient care during an MCI. Don't let communication difficulties distract you from your patient care. Plain English should be used in all communications at a multiple-casualty incident to avoid any miscommunication.

Follow-Through

When all patients have been moved from the incident scene, emergency personnel should go to hospitals to assist hospital personnel. However, the incident manager and an assistant should remain at the scene to supervise cleanup and complete restoration.

Once you arrive at the hospital, instructions for care and treatment will come from the facility's incident manager. Depending on the size and nature of the MCI, some facilities may need your help, while other hospitals may have enough personnel to manage the MCI without your assistance. If your services are not needed, you should prepare your vehicle and equipment for other EMS calls. Update your dispatch center regarding your status and availability for response to additional calls.

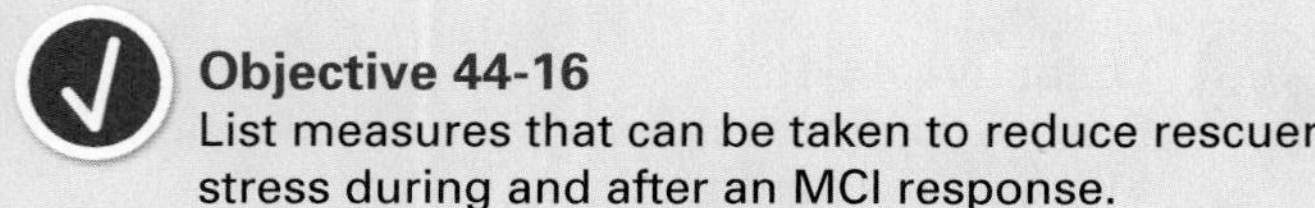

Objective 44-16
List measures that can be taken to reduce rescuer stress during and after an MCI response.

Reducing Posttraumatic and Cumulative Stress

Psychological stress is acute at the scene of a multiple-casualty incident. Rescuers, too, react to disaster, often the same way patients do. Common are fears regarding personal safety, crying, anger, guilt, numbness, preoccupation with death, frustration, fatigue, and burnout. Approximately two-thirds of all rescuers suffer long-term reactions. Most rescuer reactions peak within about 1 week and then diminish. Approximately half of rescuers have recurrent dreams and repeated recollections of the disaster for weeks or months afterward. In some cases, the rescuer may not react at all, then react weeks or months later. Methods to reduce emergency personnel stress should be a part of the postincident standard operating procedures.

Any rescuer who breaks down or becomes hysterical during the incident operation should be removed immediately to a hospital; a rescuer who is injured or becomes ill during rescue operations should be treated immediately and transported so that other rescuers can continue their work.

To reduce stress on yourself and other rescue personnel who report to you:

- Try not to get overwhelmed by the immensity of the incident. Carefully evaluate injuries and determine which patients should be cared for first. Then set about administering the aid, caring for patients one by one. This will help you maintain some calm and feel that you are making progress.
- As each rescue worker reports to the staffing area for assignment, he should be instructed to rest at regular intervals, maybe as often as once every 1 to 2 hours (Figure 44-14✱). Follow local protocol. During rest periods, the rescuer should return to the staffing area (preferably an area that is away from the hub of the disaster), sit or lie down, have something to eat or drink, and relax as much as possible.
- If rest periods are effectively rotated, there will always be enough rescue workers to carry on disaster assistance, and the entire team will be rested and relieved periodically.
- Make sure that each rescue worker is fully aware of his exact assignment. Have a well-designed plan that enables you to fully utilize your personnel, and clearly explain to each worker what his responsibility is.

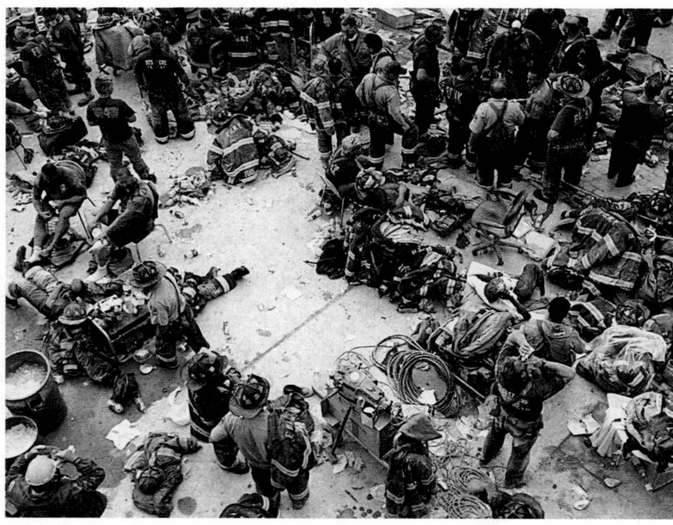

FIGURE 44-14 ✱ Firefighters and rescue workers take a break in a rehab unit near "Ground Zero," New York City, September 12, 2001. (© Tim Fadek/Gamma)

- Several workers in the staffing area should circulate among the rescue workers and watch for signs of physical exhaustion or stress. If one of the workers appears to be having problems, he should immediately be required to return to the staffing area and rest for a longer period than usual. After resting, a less stressful task should be assigned, possibly in another area of the disaster site.
- Make sure that rescue workers are assigned to tasks appropriate for their skills and experience. If there is a question about whether a certain worker can manage a task, don't take the chance.
- Provide plenty of nourishing food and beverages; encourage rescue workers to eat and drink whenever necessary to keep up their strength.
- Encourage rescue workers to talk among themselves; talking helps relieve stress. This is a form of defusing that may be helpful at the scene of the incident to reduce stress. Discourage light-hearted conversation and joking, however—some patients as well as workers may be offended by it, increasing the stress level at the scene.
- Make sure that rescuers have the opportunity to talk with trained counselors after the incident. If your team has access to organized stress debriefing processes, make sure that all rescuers who worked on the disaster take advantage of this process.

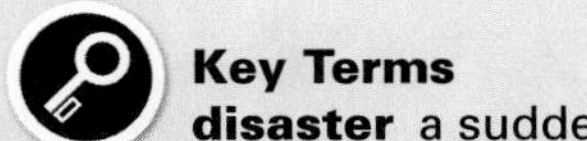

Key Terms
disaster a sudden catastrophic event that overwhelms natural order and causes great loss of property and/or life.

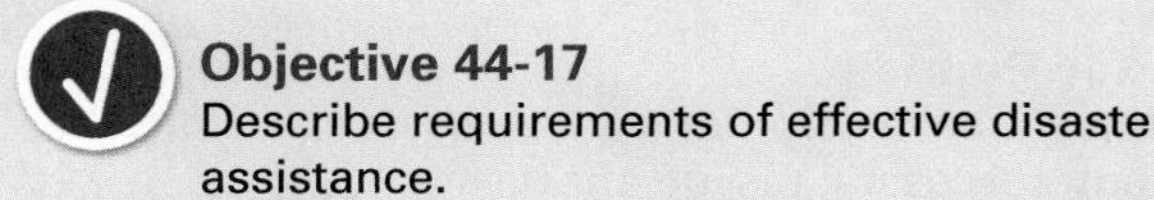

Objective 44-17
Describe requirements of effective disaster assistance.

Disaster Management

In general, a **disaster** is a sudden catastrophic event that overwhelms natural order and causes great loss of property or life.

In a disaster, there is a great disparity between casualties and resources. It exceeds the capabilities of available management resources and may disrupt the community, the medical establishment, or both. It may be designated a disaster because of the overwhelming number of patients involved, or because just a few patients are so severely injured.

Disasters may be natural—such as hurricanes, earthquakes, floods, and tornadoes—or man-made—such as airline crashes, fires, toxic gas leaks, and nuclear accidents. The National Incident Management System and incident command systems apply to natural disasters.

Requirements of Effective Disaster Assistance

You think, "It can't happen to me!" Yet, disasters do happen. Effective disaster assistance begins with emergency responders promoting the need for individual and community disaster preparedness. In general, effective disaster assistance requires:

- Preparation of the entire community; community members at large trained in basic life-supporting first aid and simple rescue procedures
- Careful preplanning
- The ability to quickly implement a plan
- Effective communications among responders
- The application of triage skills
- The ability to organize quickly and utilize fully all emergency personnel
- The ability to adapt the plan to meet special conditions, such as inclement weather or isolated locations
- A contingency plan that provides for shelter and transportation of people in an entire area, such as an entire community or county
- Doing the greatest good for the greatest number
- A plan that avoids simply relocating the disaster from the scene to the local hospital

Warning and Evacuation

In some cases, such as a hurricane or tornado, you may learn that a disaster is approaching and may have time to evacuate local residents. If you can conduct an orderly evacuation, you can prevent further injury, preserve life, and possibly protect property.

Relocation should, as much as possible, keep people in their natural social groupings. Make every effort to provide home-based relocation instead of relocating people to hospitals and clinics if they are not injured.

Alerts for the evacuation must be repeated often and with clarity. You must convince people that a disaster is really about to occur and that there is a substantial threat to their safety. At a minimum, the evacuation and warning message must contain the following information:

- The nature of the disaster and its estimated time of impact on the area; if possible, a description of the expected severity
- Safe routes to take out of the area
- Appropriate destinations for those who evacuate, indicating where food and shelter will be available

Use whatever means you have available to spread the message frequently and with urgency—by radio, television, roving police cars with loudspeakers, public address systems in buildings, and short-wave radios. Make sure that each message contains all pertinent details concerning the nature and impact of the disaster, how people should evacuate, which routes are safest, and where people should meet for assistance after evacuation.

Disaster Communications Systems

Critical to any successful rescue effort is an efficient communications system that includes a backup system in case the primary system fails. The specific system that you choose will depend on your area and requirements, but the following general guidelines apply to any disaster communications system:

- Establish details of the system ahead of time. The communications network should be a part of your disaster drill. Decide what radio frequency and kind of system you want, who will be responsible for operating it, and what equipment will be used.
- Appoint only one person at the scene of the disaster who will communicate to those outside the disaster

Key Points
An effective communications system is critical to any successful rescue effort.

Objective 44-18
Anticipate psychological reactions of disaster victims and describe ways in which EMS providers can assist disaster survivors.

area. It is usually best to use the disaster control chief. That person should be aware at all times of what is going on and can be a source of reliable information to the outside.

- The person who is designated to communicate should stay in touch with local hospitals and rescue units who may be called on to respond to the disaster. Make sure ahead of time that the person will have access to appropriate equipment to keep in touch with the outside.
- Area-wide communications are vital. They give people warning of an impending disaster and help people receive information regarding the status of family members, friends, and the community as a whole.
- Since it may be impossible to restore immediate telephone service to an area, establish a central location where people can register concerning their whereabouts, safety, health status, and so on.
- Make sure that information regarding road conditions, alternative routes, and closed roads is constantly monitored and communicated, especially in the case of a weather-related disaster.
- Constantly monitor and link all hospitals, trauma centers, and clinics in the area so that you can determine which can receive more patients and when those patients can be transported to the specific facility. The status of hospitals will change constantly throughout and after the disaster; therefore, keep communications open.
- Do not allow emergency vehicle operators or EMTs who are en route to the hospital to communicate via radio to the hospital unless an emergency occurs en route. The person designated to take care of communications will contact the appropriate hospital as the ambulance leaves the disaster scene.
- If the disaster area is large, individual rescue workers should be equipped with portable radios so they can communicate with their commands.
- Include a recorder or some other device that will allow you to record and later reassess crucial communications.

The Psychological Impact of Disasters

Faced with the grim physical injuries that can accompany a disaster, it is difficult to remember that the psychological injuries can be severe—even among those not physically injured. The overwhelming reaction to disaster is a reaction to the loss of either life or property.

Almost all people experience fear; many also feel shaky, perspire profusely, become confused, and suffer irritability, anxiety, restlessness, fatigue, sleep disturbances, nightmares, difficulty concentrating, moodiness, suspiciousness, depression, nausea, vomiting, and diarrhea. Survivors of a disaster often experience fear, anxiety, anger, guilt, shock, depression, denial, feelings of isolation, and vulnerability. All these reactions are normal. As soon as people begin working to remedy the disaster situation, their physical responses usually become less exaggerated, and they are able to work with less tension and fear.

Helping Disaster Patients

At high risk for severe emotional reactions are children, the elderly, those in poor physical or emotional health, individuals with disabilities, and those with a past loss or crisis.

The reactions of children depend on their age, individual disposition, family support, and community support:

- *Preschoolers* tend to cry, lose control of bowel and/or bladder, become confused, and suck their thumbs.
- *Elementary-age children* suffer extreme fears about their safety and show confusion, depression, headache, inability to concentrate, withdrawal, poor performance, and the tendency to fight with their peers.
- *Preadolescents and adolescents* may show the same reaction as elementary-age children, coupled with extreme aggression and stress that is severe enough to disrupt their lives.

While each disaster presents individual problems, the following general guidelines apply to any disaster:

- The families of patients need and deserve accurate information—something that is too often overlooked in the rush to begin emergency medical care. As soon as possible, assign several rescue workers to gather information and disseminate it to local radio and television stations so that psychological stress to other family members may be lessened.
- Reunite families as soon as possible. Emotional stress will be lessened once the patient is with family members, and family members may be able to provide you with critical medical history that may increase your ability to care for the patient.

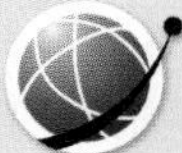

Media Resources

Go to www.bradybooks.com for mykit. Highlights:

- *Web Resource:* Resources for Emergency Workers
- *Video:* Responding to Children During Disasters

- If the disaster involved a large number of people, group the patients with their families and neighbors. This will help reduce feelings of fear and alienation.
- Encourage patients to do necessary chores. Work can be therapeutic and should be used to help the patients get over their own problems.
- Provide a structure for the emotionally injured, and let them know your expectations. Tell the patient exactly what is happening—that he is suffering a temporary setback and will probably recover rapidly, and that meanwhile, you expect certain minimal tasks to be performed. For instance, direct the emotionally traumatized with basic commands such as "Let's walk to the treatment unit."
- Help patients confront the reality of the disaster. Help them work through their feelings. Encourage them to talk about the disaster and its long-term effects. Arrange for a group discussion where patients can exchange ideas as soon as physical needs are taken care of. If you sense that any patients are not facing reality or that expectations are much worse than reality, help them adjust their views.
- Don't give false assurances. The patient needs help in facing problems and deciding how he will react to them, but he will need to face facts sooner or later. If the patient finds that you have lied, he may resist any further outside help, and the recovery period will probably be extensive.
- A patient may refuse offers of help because of cultural upbringing, threats to self-image, or an inaccurate concept of the seriousness of the situation. Explain that by accepting help no one is in any way admitting weakness. Make sure it is understood that the help (and, therefore, the patient's dependency) is only temporary and that as soon as things are under control the patient may be needed to help someone else.
- Identify high-risk patients: the elderly, children, the bereaved, those with prior psychiatric illness, those with multiple stresses, those with low or no support systems, those from low socioeconomic backgrounds, and those with severe injuries. Target these people for immediate crisis intervention care.
- Identify people who are in a unique position to help people in need, and recruit them for psychological emergency care.
- Arrange for all those involved in the disaster—including rescuers—to get good follow-up care and support.

CHAPTER REVIEW

SUMMARY

Response to a multiple-casualty incident (MCI) requires standardized preplanning and training in order for the incident to be managed effectively and efficiently. The National Incident Management System (NIMS) has been established to standardize many aspects of disaster and MCI response and activities. Part of the NIMS structure is an incident command system (ICS) that clearly identifies the authority and responsibilities for activities occurring at a disaster or MCI. There is only one designated incident commander at the scene. The incident commander may establish finance/administration, logistics, operations, and planning sections and chiefs as necessary. The section chiefs, in turn, can establish units and unit leaders. Most often in an MCI, EMS is part of the operations section and manages the triage, treatment, transport, and staging units. A morgue unit may be established if a large number of casualties have resulted in death.

Triage is a system of sorting patients based on the criticality of their injuries. The START triage system is commonly used to triage adults and young adults, while JumpSTART is used for children. Once triage has occurred, the patients are tagged according to their priority. Red identifies the highest-priority patients, yellow the next priority, and green the lowest priority. Patients tagged with a black tag are either already deceased or have mortal injuries with no chance of survival. Patients are moved into and out of the treatment unit based on their triage designation.

Multiple-casualty incidents and disasters could prove to be very stressful to emergency responders. Be sure to recognize signs of stress and seek assistance, if necessary.

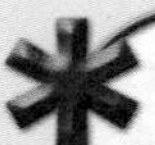

CASE STUDY FOLLOW-UP

SCENE SIZE-UP

You have been dispatched to the Firebird Raceway, where two race cars have crashed into a bleacher. As you arrive at the raceway, you perform a quick scene size-up. Raceway officials have extinguished the fires caused by the race cars. However, many people have been seriously burned. You decide the scene is safe to enter. You see bystanders are trying to give aid to the injured on the unstable bleachers. Using your vehicle's PA system, you direct the bystanders off the bleachers. You tell them rescue personnel will be here in moments.

Your local plan has predesignated you the incident commander during an MCI or disaster. You estimate at least 50 patients and begin to establish a mobile command center within a safe range of the crash. Next you and your partner, Judy Eibers, put on unit leader identification vests and set up the incident command center flag.

You confirm with dispatch the nature of the event, the precise location, and your best estimate of the total number of patients. You also request at least 20 ambulances. Because many of the patients appear entangled in the metal bleachers, you request at least 10 rescue units with medium to heavy extrication equipment. This may be more equipment and vehicles than you need, but you know it is better to have too many resources than not enough.

In preparation for arriving vehicles, equipment, and personnel, you establish an extrication unit, a treatment unit, a transport unit, a staging unit, a supply unit, and a triage unit.

Using your vehicle as the mobile command center, you contact incoming units and begin assigning a leader to each unit.

TRIAGE

While you are busy communicating with incoming emergency personnel, Judy has started initial triage, using the START system. Using a bullhorn, she directs those patients who are able to walk (green, or priority 3) to a safe area away from the bleachers. She counts at least 10 people who are able to walk away. She knows that, for now, these patients have adequate airways and circulation. Additional EMTs arrive and set up a treatment unit. You have the red, priority 1 patients, many of whom have severe burns and airway problems, moved to the triage/treatment unit first.

SUPPLY AND EXTRICATION UNITS

While the initial triage phase continues, you work closely with the supply and extrication leaders who have been assigned to determine the amount of medical materials and extrication equipment necessary to render care. The supply and extrication leaders then direct personnel and equipment to where the need is greatest during the initial triage phase.

TRIAGE AND TREATMENT UNITS

The initial triage is complete. You next work closely with Vinnie Lorenzo, the secondary triage leader, to further separate the triaged patients into treatment groups based on the priority tags attached to each patient. Unfortunately, there have been 10 deaths.

Vinnie has a total of 30 patients in the treatment unit. Harriet Lerner, the treatment leader, directs the EMTs to the red-tagged patients. In the red, priority 1 treatment unit, there are five patients with inadequate airways and severe burns. Harriet consults with the supply unit leader to request more blood pressure cuffs, bandages, and oxygen. The remaining 25 patients are classified as yellow, priority 2 patients and are moved to the priority 2 treatment unit. Some of these patients are suffering from burns without airway problems. Many have multiple bone and back injuries, with or without spinal cord damage.

STAGING AND TRANSPORT

The staging leader, Harold Walters, has been working closely with Harriet Lerner of the treatment unit to determine the number and priority of patients in need of transport. Harold has kept a record of the number of available ambulances and EMS personnel. Meanwhile, the transport leader, John Bukowski, has consulted with the receiving hospitals to determine the number of available beds and to make sure the hospitals have called in additional medical personnel.

John Bukowski contacts Harold Walters and requests three ambulances respond to the red, priority 1 treatment unit. All five patients with severe burns and inadequate breathing are then transported to the appropriate hospitals. Because of heavy radio communications, EMTs transporting priority 1 patients do not contact the hospital. John provides patient information and estimated times of arrival. Once the priority 1 patients are released to hospital personnel, the ambulances return with more medical supplies to the staging area.

John next requests 13 more ambulances from Harold Walters, the staging leader. Harold directs the ambulances to the yellow, priority 2 treatment units in a staggered sequence so as not to overload the treatment areas. Priority 2 patients are transported to the appropriate area hospitals.

Again, transporting EMTs do not contact the receiving hospitals. Maintaining only essential communications, John Bukowski has informed the receiving hospitals of only the number of patients and each patient's chief complaint.

Finally, John requests five ambulances from Harold Walters in staging to transport the remaining 10 green, priority 3 patients. Harold directs the ambulances to the priority 3 treatment unit. As incident manager, you keep a skeleton crew of EMTs to assist in cleanup and scene restoration. You direct remaining EMS personnel to the receiving hospitals to assist in further patient care.

Thoroughly exhausted from managing the MCI at Firebird, you take time to have something nourishing to eat and rest for a bit. An MCI is an incredibly stressful experience. Both you, as incident manager, and the EMTs providing direct patient care will inevitably be plagued by doubts and second-guessing in the time following the MCI: "Did I make the right triage decision?" "Should I have started CPR?" "How should I have dealt with the mother begging me to care for her dying child?" You know that the best way to minimize these doubts, and the stress they cause, is to routinely practice your MCI plan. Then, when the unexpected happens, as it did at Firebird Raceway, you know how to get the right patient to the right hospital in the right amount of time.

IN REVIEW

1. Name the criteria for determining that an emergency is a multiple-casualty incident.
2. List the responsibilities of an incident commander.
3. Define the role of the EMT in a multiple-casualty incident or a disaster operation.
4. Name the five basic units of an incident command system and describe their responsibilities.
5. Explain how to perform the primary assessment of a patient during initial triage.
6. Identify the appropriate triage level (in a system with three levels of triage) for each of the following: (a) a patient with inadequate breathing, (b) a patient who is in cardiac arrest with insufficient EMS personnel to provide care, (c) a patient found with a suspected fractured forearm, (d) a patient with a laceration to his back.
7. Explain the reasons for using a patient identification or tagging system and give the criteria for a successful patient identification system.
8. List guidelines for effective transport of patients in a multiple-casualty incident.
9. List at least five ways for reducing stress on EMTs during a multiple-casualty incident or disaster operation.

CRITICAL THINKING

You are responding to the scene of a natural gas explosion in a residential neighborhood. You are the first EMS unit to arrive on scene. You report to the incident commander and he indicates that so far approximately 30 patients have been identified. He designates you as the EMS branch director.

1. What responsibilities would you have as the EMS branch director?
2. What units would you establish?
3. How should triage be conducted?
4. What patients would be moved into the treatment unit first and moved out of the treatment unit first?
5. How would you manage all of the responding EMS units?

PEARSON

EXPLORE mybradykit™

Please go to **www.bradybooks.com** to access mykit for this text. You will find quizzes, critical thinking scenarios, weblinks, animations, and videos related to this chapter—and much more. Look for online information on resources for emergency workers and START as well as a video about responding to children during disasters.

Register your access code from the front of your book by going to **www.bradybooks.com** and selecting the mykit links.

CHAPTER 45

EMS Response to Terrorism Involving Weapons of Mass Destruction

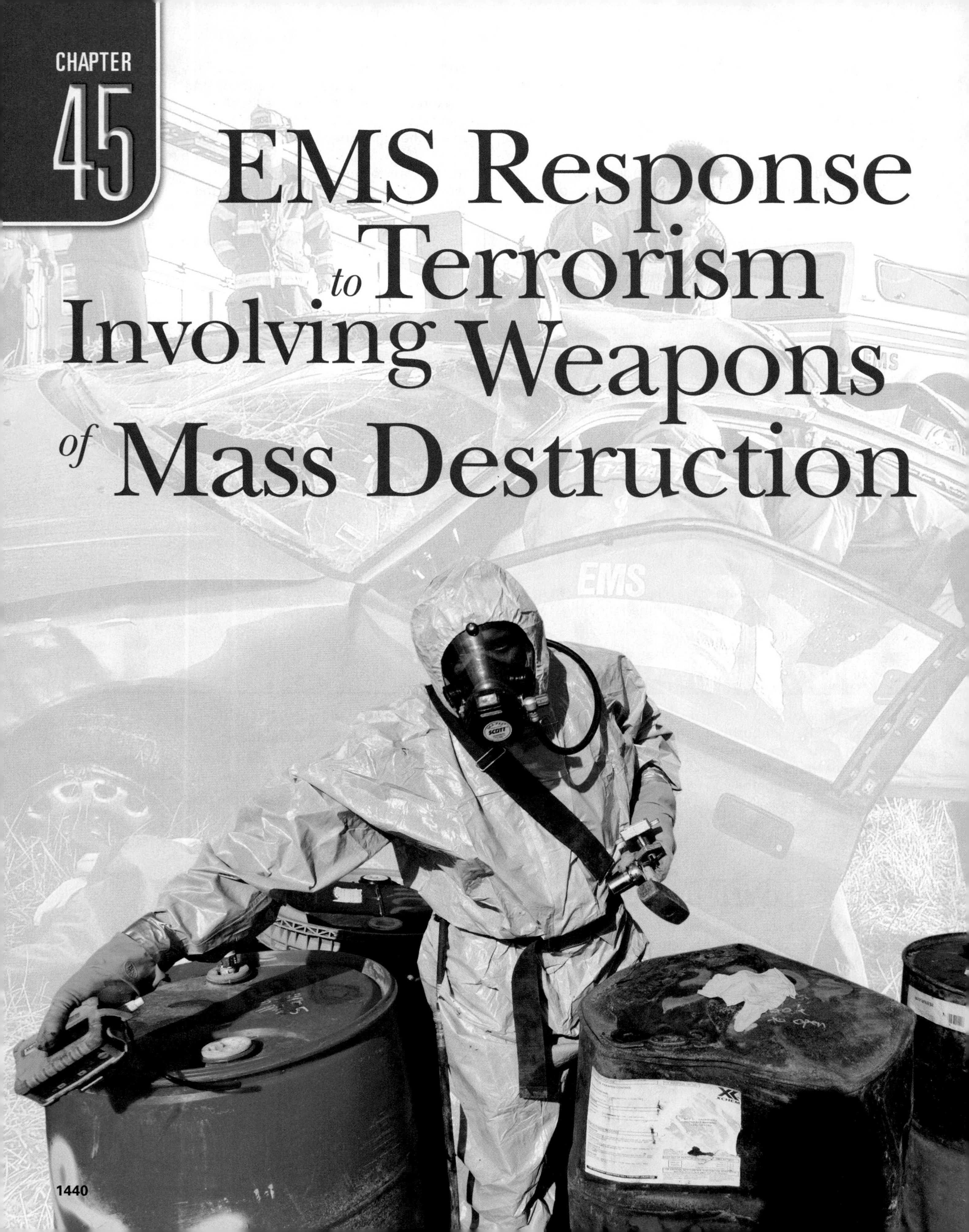

Navigation Guide

The following items provide an overview to the purpose and content of this chapter. The Standard and Competency are from the new National EMS Education Standards.

STANDARD **EMS Operations** (Content Area: Terrorism and Disaster)

COMPETENCY Applies knowledge of operational roles and responsibilities to ensure patient, public, and personnel safety.

OBJECTIVES: After reading this chapter, you should be able to:

45-1. Define key terms introduced in this chapter.

45-2. Explain the mnemonics CBRNE and B-NICE and describe the characteristics of the various types of weapons of mass destruction.

45-3. Explain the importance of preplanning a response to terrorism involving weapons of mass destruction.

45-4. Discuss the components that should be included in a plan for responding to terrorism involving weapons of mass destruction.

45-5. Recognize indications that a response may involve terrorism with weapons of mass destruction.

45-6. Describe the EMT's role when responding to terrorism involving weapons of mass destruction.

45-7. Describe types of injuries that may occur from conventional explosives and incendiary devices.

45-8. Discuss the effects of exposure to and explain the appropriate medical care for each of the following types of chemical agents:
- **a.** Nerve agents
- **b.** Vesicants
- **c.** Cyanide
- **d.** Pulmonary agents
- **e.** Riot-control agents
- **f.** Toxic industrial chemicals

45-9. Give examples of biological agents in each of the following categories and the appropriate medical care for exposure to biological agents:
- **a.** Pneumonia-like agents
- **b.** Encephalitis-like agents
- **c.** Biological toxins
- **d.** Other agents

45-10. Differentiate between the characteristics of the following types of radiation:
- **a.** X-ray and gamma radiation
- **b.** Neutron radiation
- **c.** Beta radiation
- **d.** Alpha radiation

45-11. Differentiate between primary exposure and fallout associated with a nuclear explosion.

45-12. Explain blast injuries and thermal burns as mechanisms of injury from nuclear explosions.

45-13. Differentiate between a nuclear weapon and a radiological dispersal device (RDD, or "dirty bomb").

45-14. Discuss assessment and care of patients affected by nuclear detonation and radiation injuries.

45-15. Explain issues of personal protection and patient decontamination in connection with chemical, biological, and radiological/nuclear weapons exposure.

KEY TERMS: Page references denote first major use in this chapter. For complete definitions, see the Glossary at the back of the book.

acetylcholine (ACh) p. 1449
acetylcholinesterase (AChE) p. 1449
biological agents p. 1452
cyanide p. 1451
fallout p. 1456
incendiary devices p. 1448
nerve agents p. 1449
nuclear radiation p. 1455
persistence p. 1448
primary effect p. 1447
primary exposure p. 1455
pulmonary agents p. 1451
secondary effects p. 1447
tertiary effects p. 1447
vesicants p. 1450
volatility p. 1448
weapons of mass destruction (WMD) p. 1442

MEDIA RESOURCES: Please go to www.bradybooks.com to access mykit for this text. You will find quizzes, critical thinking scenarios, weblinks, animations, and videos related to this chapter—and much more. Look for online information on terrorism and on the Department of Homeland Security.

continued

CASE STUDY

The Dispatch

EMS Unit 101—respond code 3 to the Stambaugh Stadium Complex for a possible explosion and multiple injuries. The fire department and law enforcement have been notified. Time out is 1504 hours.

En Route

You and your partner immediately get to the ambulance and respond. As you are en route, you remember that the local college football team is hosting a playoff game. You mention this to your partner. You put on gloves and eye protection. You also mentally review your triage protocols and the use of your additional personal protective equipment in case they are needed.

As you pull up to the stadium's north side, you notice that the fire department has one pumper on the scene. There are masses of people running from the stadium into the adjacent streets. You notice many appear to be injured and bleeding.

How Would You Proceed?

During this chapter, you will learn special considerations related to weapons of mass destruction. Later, we will return to the case and apply the procedures learned.

Introduction

Terrorism involving weapons of mass destruction (WMD) is a realistic threat that all EMS providers must be prepared to manage. Weapons of mass destruction—biological, nuclear/radiological, incendiary, chemical, and explosive, as well as unconventional weapons such as airplanes—can cause widespread, indiscriminate death and destruction. The best way to manage an attack is to be informed and prepared and to understand your limitations. The goal of emergency medical services is to successfully manage the patients affected by the attack.

The term *weapons of mass destruction* typically conjures thoughts of chemical, biological, and radiological/nuclear threats. However, conventional bombs, explosives, and incendiary devices are the most commonly used terror devices worldwide. An example is the Oklahoma City bombing in 1995. Unconventional weapons, such as the use of commercial airliners as in the attack on the World Trade Center and Pentagon on September 11, 2001, must also be considered. EMS providers must be prepared to deal with any type of WMD attack.

Weapons of Mass Destruction

Weapons of mass destruction (WMD) are intended to cause widespread and indiscriminate death and destruction. The mnemonic CBRNE is a useful way to remember the types of weapons of mass destruction: chemical, biological, radiological, nuclear, and explosive. Another useful mnemonic is B-NICE: biological, nuclear/radiological, incendiary, chemical, and explosive. These lists reflect the types of weapons or agents that might be employed in a terrorist attack. Because each of the agents has its own characteristics, this chapter introduces the EMT to these critical threats.

The destructive power of the weapon used to carry out the attack is dependent on the agent and the delivery method. A small amount of a chemical agent may kill hundreds or thousands of people if it is spread over a densely populated area, with minimal or no physical damage suffered to the structures in that area. On the other hand, a nuclear device that can fit inside a footlocker may have the power to obliterate ten city blocks and cause damage to many more. The subtle and gradual nature of biological weapons that can be spread by contact with a person or infected object leads to potentially huge numbers of possible deaths.

Nuclear and conventional bomb detonations last for only a brief moment and have immediate effects on the individuals involved in the attack. The fallout from a nuclear weapon may last for days to weeks, and it may have long-lasting effects. Chemical agents may take a few minutes to begin to show the effects, and those effects may last from minutes to hours. Biological weapons are the most insidious and may take hours to days for the onset of effects, and the duration may be days to weeks. The destructive power of conventional explosives is the lowest, yet they have the highest likelihood of being used as the primary weapon. Nuclear weapons carry the highest destructive capabilities, but because of the complexity of developing the devices and the special materials

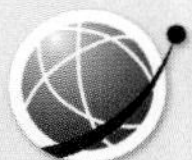

Media Resources

Go to www.bradybooks.com for mykit. Highlights:

- *Web Resource:* Department of Homeland Security
- *Web Resource:* Smallpox
- *Web Resource:* Anthrax

Objective 45-2
Explain the mnemonics CBRNE and B-NICE and describe the characteristics of the various types of weapons of mass destruction.

Objective 45-3
Explain the importance of preplanning a response to terrorism with weapons of mass destruction.

needed to build them, they have the lowest risk of use. Chemical and biological weapons have both a moderate likelihood of use and a moderate to high destructive power.

The greatest amount of structural damage is caused by nuclear weapons, which also carry a high risk of environmental contamination. Chemical and biological weapons cause minimal damage to structures; however, chemical weapons have a high impact on environmental contamination, whereas biological weapons have only a minimal effect on the environment. Do not underestimate the destructive power of weapons that do not produce massive structural damage. Conventional weapons, and unconventional ones such as jetliners, will cause a significant amount of damage. Response to such dramatic events may require such resources as heavy and confined-space rescue, whereas chemical and biological weapons may require more involvement from epidemiologists and other public health officials but less involvement of rescue personnel (Figure 45-1*).

Detection of weapons of mass destruction may also pose a problem. Biological agents, radiation, and even many chemical agents are typically colorless and odorless. They cannot be detected by human senses and are identified only after the clinical signs and symptoms become apparent. The subtle and silent nature of the agents leads to a delayed response. Until the deployment of such weapons is identified or their effects are recognized, response cannot begin. Combinations of weapons are also possible. Radiological dispersal devices (RDDs), also known as dirty bombs, are made by combining a conventional explosive with radioactive material. Detonation results not only in physical damage from the blast but also in a spread of the radioactive material, causing additional complications to the scene.

The general prehospital approach to an incident involving weapons of mass destruction is similar to that for any disaster involving mass casualties. The principles of the response are relatively the same with some additional considerations. All local, regional, and state disaster agencies should develop WMD disaster plans that are readily functional. This is important because prehospital providers often don't know the exact nature of a disaster when it first unfolds. A common approach to a disaster—whether it is caused by human accident, nature, or terrorist intent—serves to prepare the EMT for all of the possibilities. This general method of dealing with disasters and special situations is often termed the *all-hazards approach.*

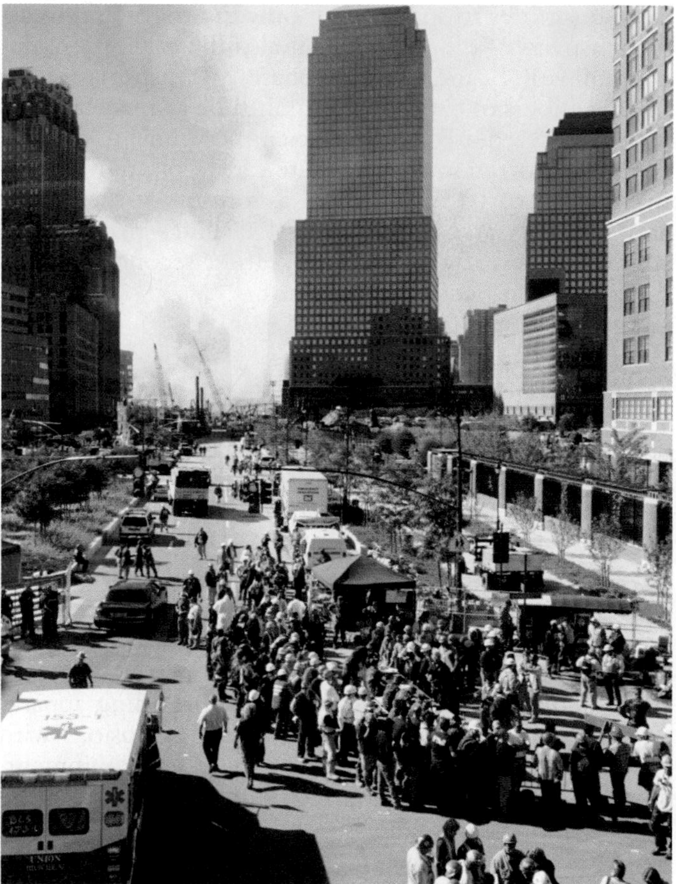

FIGURE 45-1 * The World Trade Center attack of September 11, 2001, required a massive coordinated effort for rescue and recovery operations. (© Stephanie Ruet/Corbis Sygma)

Prehospital Response to Terrorism Involving WMD

Terrorist attacks involving weapons of mass destruction can wrest you from your everyday, customary responsibilities to an incident that involves mass numbers of people over a prolonged period of time while working with limited resources. Response to a terrorist attack involving weapons of mass destruction requires specific planning and preparedness.

Planning for a WMD incident must encompass several aspects of preparation and response. Consider that incidents may require special protective equipment in

Key Terms

weapons of mass destruction (WMD) weapons intended to cause widespread and indiscriminate death and destruction.

Objective 45-4

Discuss components needed in a plan for responding to terrorism involving WMD.

Key Points

Be aware of the personal risks and dangers associated with responding to a WMD incident. Personal safety is the first priority for all EMS personnel.

large quantities to support not only the triage and treatment aspects of the incident but also the extrication, decontamination, and cleanup phases. Transportation of mass numbers of patients to a multitude of medical facilities may be required with sufficient personnel to provide both transportation and en-route care. Communications may be destroyed or disrupted as a result of the attack, and hospitals and other medical facilities may be destroyed or severely damaged, creating secondary treatment and transportation problems.

Supplies and Equipment

It is unrealistic to think that a single EMS agency will have the equipment necessary to manage a WMD incident. Rather, it is necessary to establish a community response to the disaster (Figure 45-2*).

Each type of WMD incident requires different types of specially trained personnel, equipment, and supplies. For example, nerve agents may require massive amounts of certain drugs along with a large number of ventilators. Chemical incidents may require special personal protective equipment such as self-contained breathing apparatus or hazardous materials suits. Large explosions with structural collapse may require heavy rescue equipment, specially trained search and rescue teams, electronic detection devices, and trained search dogs.

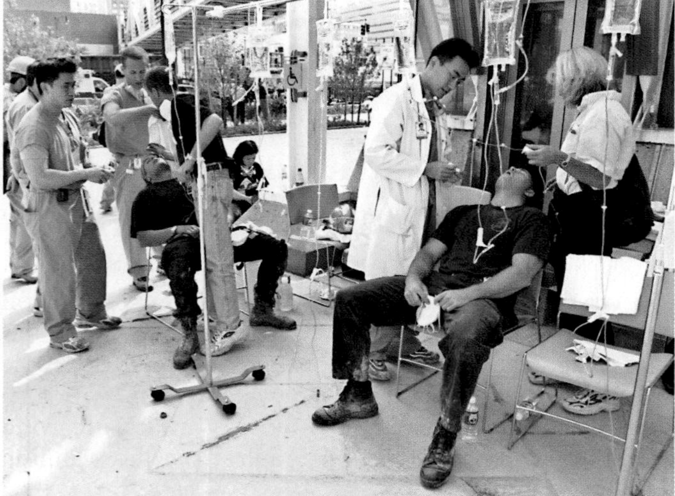

FIGURE 45-2 * Coordinated community medical response to the World Trade Center attack. Medical treatment is conducted on the sidewalk. (© Ellinguac Orjan/Corbis Sygma)

A plan must be in place that will allow the communications center immediate access to the individuals who are capable of deploying the equipment, supplies, and personnel. Mutual assistance agreements must also be in place to allow for neighboring departments to provide equipment, supplies, and personnel.

Medical Direction

There will be a multitude of EMS providers from a variety of systems responding to a multiple-casualty incident involving weapons of mass destruction. The response of providers from several areas may pose a problem with medical direction and the use of protocols from a different jurisdiction. A plan should address how medical direction will be provided to EMS personnel at the scene as well as how to confirm the credentials of EMS personnel from outside the area.

The communications system should not be relied on to provide on-line medical direction, since it will likely become overloaded. One possibility is to make all protocols standing orders in a case involving weapons of mass destruction. This would clear communications channels to allow for scene updates, incoming patient reports, and on-line orders for special medical treatment requests, such as medical personnel to perform a field amputation of an extremity of a trapped patient.

The protocol should address treatment for specific agents used in weapons of mass destruction. Triage protocols should ensure that minor injuries and walking wounded patients do not proceed to the nearest hospital. The closest hospitals should be reserved for the more seriously injured.

Provider Preparation

As an EMS provider, you must be aware of the personal risks and dangers associated with responding to a WMD incident. Personal safety is the first priority for all EMS personnel. As an example, coming into contact with sarin, a nerve agent, could result in immediate death or permanent disability. The presence of biological agents may not be immediately apparent, but in rare circumstances they may cause the slow, agonizing death of an EMS responder.

Understanding the threats and the potential consequences is vital. Rushing onto the scene of an explosion may cause the deaths of many rescuers, which may be the

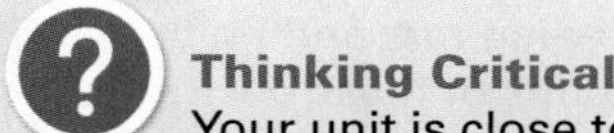

Thinking Critically
Your unit is close to the scene of an explosion and you respond immediately. Your first instinct is to rush in to save lives. What should you consider before proceeding into the scene?

Objective 45-5
Recognize indications that a response may involve terrorism with weapons of mass destruction.

secondary objective of the terrorist. This was seen in the World Trade Center attacks of September 11, 2001, where hundreds of firefighters, law enforcement officers, and EMS personnel were killed or injured as a result of the secondary effects of the attack. In some past incidents, secondary explosive devices were even planted and detonated with the specific purpose of injuring and killing rescue personnel and others who rushed to the scene.

In regard to patient care, you must be aware of the various agents that can be used as weapons of mass destruction and the signs and symptoms of the conditions that result from exposure. (See the discussion of specific agents and findings associated with these agents later in this chapter.) You should have specific guidelines on triage and management of these patients. As always, your personal safety is your first priority and requires that you be informed of the potential dangers to your health when you enter the scene, both during and after the incident.

Responding to the Scene

One of the most important aspects of a WMD incident is recognition. The earlier the incident and the weapon are recognized, the earlier you can protect yourself and contact the necessary resources to respond.

These incidents employ the same incident command system as does any multiple-casualty incident. If a chemical agent is involved, it is also similar to a hazardous materials incident. Thus, you may be required to establish an EMS command center if you are one of the first-arriving EMS crews on the scene, and you will be required to function within the incident command system throughout your time at the incident.

Be wary of the possibility of secondary explosions when conventional weapons are used. Booby traps may be used to injure and kill responders. Subsequent attacks may occur to inflict more damage, as in the 2001 World Trade Center attacks.

Issues of Scene Safety

There is a significant difference between the effects of conventional, chemical, and most biological weapons as compared to the death, injury, and mass destruction of nuclear weapons. Conventional, chemical, and most biological weapons cause a relatively small region of impact, yet place an extreme strain on the EMS system and medical care. On the other hand, the medical facilities and personnel are primarily intact after the attack.

By contrast, a large nuclear weapon will cause concentric rings of complete destruction, severe devastation, and areas of limited damage, with death and injury superimposed. Access to the scene is severely limited by the mass physical destruction. The nuclear weapon destroys emergency services, health care services, and facilities within the rings of the impact. Shelters, medical supplies, food, and clean water are also destroyed. Electrical equipment, including computers and radios, may be destroyed even when located relatively far from the center of the detonation, which may leave the entire response area without effective communication. About 1 hour after the detonation, radioactive fallout will begin to occur and will last for days to weeks. A sizable nuclear event will require extreme measures to evacuate, care for, and support the injured.

Chemical and biological weapons present a danger that is much more difficult to recognize and identify as compared to the nuclear or conventional blast. Chemical weapons may release gases or aerosols that are only recognized upon exposure or shortly thereafter. If numerous patients present with similar signs and symptoms with an unexplainable or unidentifiable cause, a chemical weapon should be suspected. Consider the environment to be toxic and unsafe. With chemical weapons, the patients will often complain of the following:

- Respiratory distress
- Dyspnea
- Cough
- Burning chest
- Burning eyes

If excessive salivation, loss of bowel and bladder control, and tearing are noted, suspect a serious chemical exposure. Inspect the scene for dead or incapacitated animals or insects. Odors of bitter almond, peaches, mustard, garlic, onions, or fresh-cut grass or hay may also be indications of deadly chemical weapons.

The exposure to a biological weapon will typically have occurred days before the first signs or symptoms appear. The contamination source may not be identified for days to weeks after the patients present with signs and symptoms. Biological weapons may also affect the EMS crews, hospital personnel, other rescue personnel, and their families. As an example, a patient exposed to and ill from smallpox who seeks medical treatment from EMS and is transported to a medical facility will contaminate the EMS crew and hospital personnel well before identification of the biological agent can be made. This may

Key Points
Enter the scene of a suspected chemical, biological, or nuclear incident only if you have the necessary specialized training and personal protective equipment, including self-contained breathing apparatus.

Objective 45-6
Describe the EMT's role when responding to terrorism involving weapons of mass destruction.

Objective 45-7
Describe types of injuries that may occur from conventional explosives and incendiary devices.

cripple the personnel in the systems that normally respond to these incidents. When presented with a patient with a suspected communicable disease, use a HEPA or N-95 mask, gloves, eye protection, and gown. Alert medical direction prior to transport to the medical facility so that the staff may prepare for immediate patient isolation.

When accessing the scene of a suspected chemical, biological, or nuclear weapon, approach from upwind. If the area is large or entry is limited, the best approach is from the side. Avoid confined spaces such as subways, basements, buildings, or low-lying areas. Chemical or biological agents may be harbored in these areas for longer periods of time because of poor ventilation. Entry must be made only by responders with specialized training and with the proper personal protection equipment, including self-contained breathing apparatus.

The target of terrorists is typically an area that is heavily populated or one that would have a great impact on the population. These areas might include airports, subways, schools, churches, government buildings, and large gatherings such as fairs, sporting events, and festivals.

If a WMD incident is suspected, stay away from the scene until the nature of the weapon is identified and you are able to take the necessary personal protection. Once the incident is recognized, employ the incident command structure to begin a careful and organized response to the scene. Similar to a hazardous materials incident, sectors of operations should be established. Coordinating efforts with law enforcement is necessary because of the increased security needs related to this type of incident. The individuals responsible for perpetrating the incident may be among the sick or injured; therefore, the EMT must be able to provide adequate care while maintaining a high index of suspicion. If a suspected perpetrator is located, law enforcement should be contacted immediately.

Whenever possible, all responders should enter the scene from a single staging or mobilization point in order to maintain security. An escape plan should be determined and communicated to all responders on the scene, with a predesignated responder collection point having been chosen so that all personnel can be accounted for if evacuation becomes necessary.

Role of the EMT at the Terrorist Incident Involving WMD

Upon arrival at the scene of a WMD incident, you may be required to fill one of three possible roles. If you are the first unit to arrive, you must establish incident command, quickly size up the scene, evaluate the need for additional resources, and begin to communicate the essential information to the communications center to organize an adequate response.

The scene size-up is of utmost importance, as it allows you to gather as much information as possible regarding the incident so that other incoming responders can be adequately warned of dangers. Perform a 360-degree assessment of the scene, keeping in mind all of the signs and characteristics of a terrorist-WMD incident. An estimate of the number of patients should be made, and multiple-casualty incident plans and protocols should be implemented as soon as possible.

If you are the second or third unit in, you may be asked to take on a sector-leader or officer role, such as triage, treatment, supply, or transportation officer. If you are in a unit that arrives after all sector officers have been assigned, you will likely be assigned to the triage or transportation sector to provide care and transportation of injured victims.

Regardless of your role, the overall goal is ensuring that the most good is done for the most people. Utilize triage principles when faced with challenging decisions. Patients must be protected from harm, informed of your actions, and cared for to the best of your ability despite the difficult situation.

Conventional Weapons and Incendiary Devices

Conventional explosives and incendiary devices remain the most widely used weapons of mass destruction by terrorists. EMS providers must be familiar with the effects of the various devices and the necessary treatments for their victims.

Explosives

Explosives work by igniting special fuels that burn extremely rapidly, causing hot gases to displace air in a violent fashion, creating a shock wave or a blast. The blast moves out in all directions at supersonic speed. This shock wave is what causes blast injury. As victims get farther from the explosion, the severity of blast injury will greatly diminish. Barriers may offer some protection from the

Key Terms

primary effect the blast of an explosion.

secondary effects effects from flying debris, shrapnel, and other projectiles in an explosion.

Key Terms

tertiary effects in an explosion, injuries produced by propulsion, for example when a person is propelled by a blast or shock wave and strikes the ground or other objects.

shock wave and lessen injuries. If a blast occurs in a closed room or space, the effects of the blast are amplified.

Primary, Secondary, and Tertiary Effects

The blast of an explosion is considered to be the **primary effect**. The **secondary effects** result from flying debris, shrapnel, and other projectiles. Flying debris can cause significant penetrating injury or blunt trauma. Flames and hot gases present in explosions also lead to secondary-effect injuries (Figure 45-3*).

The patient may be propelled by the blast or shock wave. As the body strikes the ground or other objects, blunt trauma may occur. The injuries produced by the propulsion are referred to as **tertiary effects**.

Body Position

Body position plays a role in determining the extent of the blast injury. Victims who are standing or lying perpendicular to the blast will suffer the greatest amount of injury, whereas victims lying directly toward or away from the blast will suffer the least amount of injury. If you know that a blast is imminent, drop to a prone position facing away from the detonation. This will reduce the shrapnel and blast injuries.

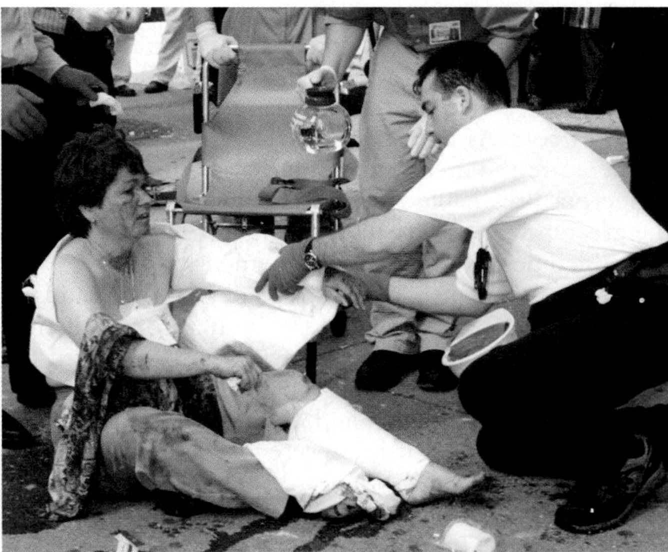

FIGURE 45-3 * Secondary-effect injuries at the World Trade Center attack occurred from flying and falling debris from both the initial impact and from the collapsing structures. (© Ciniglio Lorenzo/Corbis Sygma)

Types of Injuries

A wide variety of injuries may result from explosions and incendiary devices. The more common injuries are as follows:

Area/Type	Effects
Lungs	Lung injury may occur from primary blast effects, since the lung is an air-containing space. Look for evidence of lung injury such as altered mental status, dyspnea, blood-tinged sputum, respiratory distress, chest pain, and strokelike signs and symptoms. Be careful if positive pressure ventilation is needed, since it may convert a pneumothorax into a tension pneumothorax. Also, the blast may have caused injury to the alveolar-capillary wall, and positive pressure ventilation may force small air bubbles into the vessels, creating air emboli.
Abdomen	Blast injury may cause bleeding to the bowel or may allow a lacerated bowel to leak its contents into the abdominal cavity. If the victim is close to the detonation, he may suffer an evisceration. In this case, manage the evisceration (refer to Chapter 35, "Abdominal and Genitourinary Trauma") and transport rapidly.
Ears	The eardrum may rupture from the blast. The delicate bones inside the ear may fracture or dislocate. The patient may experience temporary or permanent hearing loss.
Crush injuries	Crush injuries may occur as a result of structural collapse. The weight of the debris on the patient may create excessive compression forces, causing a crush syndrome. In addition, the structural collapse may inflict direct blunt and penetrating injury, while dust and smoke can cause respiratory and eye injuries. Crush syndrome is associated with entrapment for 4 hours or more. The crushed tissue will produce harmful by-products. Once the pressure to the crushed area is relieved, the accumulated by-products are released into the systemic circulation, causing serious problems.

Objective 45-8

Discuss the effects of exposure to and explain the appropriate medical care for specific types of chemical agents.

Key Terms

incendiary devices devices using agents such as napalm, thermite, magnesium, and white phosphorus to cause injury by burning at high temperatures.

Key Terms

volatility the tendency of a chemical agent to evaporate and create a dangerous vapor.

Area/Type	Effects
Shrapnel injuries	Shrapnel may cause penetrating injury to the solid organs, hollow organs, connective tissue, and bone. Each may experience a different effect from the missile. Solid organ tissues are rapidly compressed and stretched. Contents of ruptured hollow organs will leak out into surrounding cavities. Connective tissue injuries are frequently limited to the shrapnel pathway because of their resiliency. Bones will fracture when struck by shrapnel.

Incendiary Devices

Incendiary devices create different injury patterns from conventional explosives. Incendiary devices include napalm, thermite, magnesium, and white phosphorus. Many are designed to be used against equipment, with the exception of napalm, which is used against personnel. The devices are designed to burn at extremely high temperatures. The primary injury is a burn.

A terrorist could possibly use any number of common flammable chemicals to make an improvised, yet devastating, incendiary device. Gasoline, propane, and natural gas are transported and stored around the United States in tremendous volumes. Virtually every community has tons of these chemicals within their boundaries at any given moment. The threat from a hijacked gasoline tanker or sabotaged natural gas pipeline should be considered when thinking of potential incendiary devices of mass destruction.

Incendiary-device burns are assessed in the same way as typical thermal burns. The same burn-depth classification system and rule of nines are used to determine extent of injury. The general management is the same as for a thermal burn (see Chapter 29, "Burns."). Be sure to pay particular attention to the airway and ventilation. Dress the burned areas.

Chemical Agents

Chemical weapons are among the most feared weapons of mass destruction. However, with proper training and equipment, it is possible to operate safely and effectively in a contaminated environment and perform basic emergency care. Terrorist groups can manufacture chemical agents with relative ease; therefore, it is imperative that EMS providers be familiar with the chemicals that are likely to be used and the necessary patient management.

Properties of Chemical Weapons

Most chemicals for military use are stored in munitions (shells, rockets, and bombs) as a liquid. When the munition explodes, the liquid is converted to an aerosol, or tiny droplets of liquid suspended in the air. Alternatively, a bomb may be attached to a liquid chemical agent canister that will break open and spread the chemical upon detonation of the bomb. Terrorists can acquire such munitions or design their own. They can also release the liquid chemical, perhaps enhanced with an aerosol device, into a closed building or simply into the air. Some riot-control agents are stored as solids, but become an aerosol once deployed.

Some chemical agents, such as hydrogen cyanide, chlorine, and phosgene, may be in the form of a gas in warm weather. Nerve and mustard agents typically remain a liquid at the same warm temperature but will evaporate similarly to a puddle of water. The tendency of the chemical agent to evaporate is called **volatility**. A volatile liquid evaporates easily and creates a dangerous breathable vapor. A characteristic of agents that do not evaporate quickly and tend to remain as a puddle for long periods of time is referred to as **persistence**. These chemicals remain concentrated and dangerous to touch for days to weeks. As a general rule, the warmer the ambient temperature the greater the evaporation and creation of dangerous breathable vapors; the colder the temperature the greater the persistence and danger from contact for a prolonged period following deployment.

Chemical agents in the form of aerosolized liquids or solids, vapor, or gas can enter the body through the respiratory tract (lungs), skin, and eyes. Entry through the lungs is by far the most critical, since a large quantity of chemical can be absorbed and dispersed throughout the body by this route, causing severe systemic effects.

Liquid agents are primarily absorbed through the skin and eyes. They may cause both severe local effects, such as chemical burns, and serious systemic effects. Accidental ingestion of chemical agents in contaminated food is possible, yet rare.

Key Terms

persistence a characteristic of agents that do not evaporate quickly and tend to remain as a puddle for long periods of time.

nerve agents agents that block the action of acetylcholinesterase (AChE) with severe effects to the nervous tissue.

Key Terms

acetylcholinesterase (AChE) an enzyme that stops the action of the neurotransmitter acetylcholine.

acetylcholine (ACh) a neurotransmitter necessary for normal function of the parasympathetic nervous system.

Types of Chemical Agents

There are six major types of chemical agents:

- Nerve agents
- Vesicants
- Cyanide
- Pulmonary agents
- Riot-control agents
- Toxic industrial chemicals (TICs)

Nerve Agents

Nerve agents are among the most deadly known chemicals (Table 45-1). These agents are extremely potent and are relatively easy to make; therefore, they are a significant threat and a deadly weapon in the hands of a terrorist. In most weather conditions, nerve agents are in liquid form. When released, the volatile agents become both a vapor and a liquid hazard.

Nerve agents block the action of an enzyme called **acetylcholinesterase (AChE)**. Acetylcholinesterase is found in the plasma of the blood, red blood cells, and nervous tissue. Its function is to stop the action of **acetylcholine (ACh)**, a neurotransmitter. When nerve agents block the action of acetylcholinesterase, acetylcholine is allowed to accumulate. The most severe effects will be to the nervous tissue. With the body's AChE being inactivated by the nerve agent, the skeletal muscles, smooth muscles, glands, and nerves remain in a steady "on" state, with uncontrolled and uncoordinated contraction of muscle fibers. This will be apparent in movements that are jerky. Seizures may also occur. The muscles eventually fatigue, stop working, and begin to die. Death usually results from inadequate breathing resulting from respiratory muscle failure.

TABLE 45-1 Nerve Agents

Nerve Agents
Tabun (GA)
Sarin (GB)
Soman (GD)
GF
Methylphosphonothioic acid (VX)

Signs and Symptoms The signs and symptoms depend on the amount of exposure, the dose, and the route. The larger the dose with direct respiratory inhalation of the nerve agent vapor, the quicker the onset and severity of the effects (Table 45-2). The most significant effects are on the nervous system, airway, and respiratory system. Large doses interfere with the brain's ability to function and will result in a rapid loss of consciousness, seizures, and apnea (lack of breathing). Lower doses may result in difficulty concentrating, inability to sleep, impaired judgment, and depression.

The pulmonary system is affected in two ways:

- Respiratory failure occurs as a result of the paralysis of respiratory muscles (diaphragm, intercostals, and abdominal).
- Copious (excessive) airway secretions lead to airway obstruction, while bronchoconstriction obstructs the lower airways.

The patient may be in respiratory distress or arrest. He may be drooling or may be found with a large amount of secretions in the oropharynx. You may also hear wheezing on auscultation of the lungs if he is moving air on respiration.

TABLE 45-2 Signs and Symptoms of Nerve Agent Exposure

	Small Exposure	Large Exposure
Vapor	Runny nose, mild dyspnea, pupillary constriction	Sudden onset of unresponsiveness, seizures, apnea, copious secretions, pupillary constriction
Liquid	Localized sweating, nausea, vomiting, fatigue	Sudden onset of unresponsiveness, seizures, apnea, paralysis, copious secretions

Key Points
Many EMS systems carry a nerve agent antidote in auto-injector form, as either a Mark I kit or a DuoDote.

Key Terms
vesicants chemical agents that damage exposed skin, lungs, and eyes, causing blistering, burning, and tissue damage as well as possible generalized illness.

Other signs and symptoms include miosis (pinpoint pupils), rhinorrhea (runny nose), excessive salivation, tearing in the eyes, blurry vision, nausea and vomiting, diarrhea, sweating, and loss of bladder control. The mnemonic SLUDGE (salivation, lacrimation, urination, defecation, gastric distress, emesis) is used to remember the signs and symptoms. Initially, the vital signs may show tachypnea (rapid breathing), tachycardia (rapid heart rate) or bradycardia (slow heart rate), and a normal blood pressure. As the patient's condition worsens, you may see apnea, tachycardia, and hypotension (low blood pressure).

Emergency Medical Care Initial care for nerve agent exposure should be directed at establishing an airway and, for inadequate breathing or apnea, providing positive pressure ventilation at 12 ventilations per minute in the adult. It may be necessary to suction the airway to clear the large amount of secretions. Position the patient in the lateral recumbent (coma or recovery) position. Monitor the airway and breathing status closely.

Administration of an antidote is the next step. Two drugs are used to counteract the effects of the nerve agent: atropine and pralidoxime (Protopam). Many EMS systems carry this nerve agent antidote in auto-injector form, either as a two-injector set known as the Mark I kit (Figure 45-4*), or as a single-injector containing both drugs known as the DuoDote (Figure 45-5*). EMS providers should administer these nerve agent antidotes, if available, to render care to themselves, their peers, or patients who have been affected by nerve agents. Standing orders for the approved use of these antidotes should be considered for addition to the disaster plan. These nerve agent auto-injectors function in exactly the same manner as epinephrine auto-injectors (see Chapter 21, "Anaphylactic Reactions"), and should be used and disposed of in the same way.

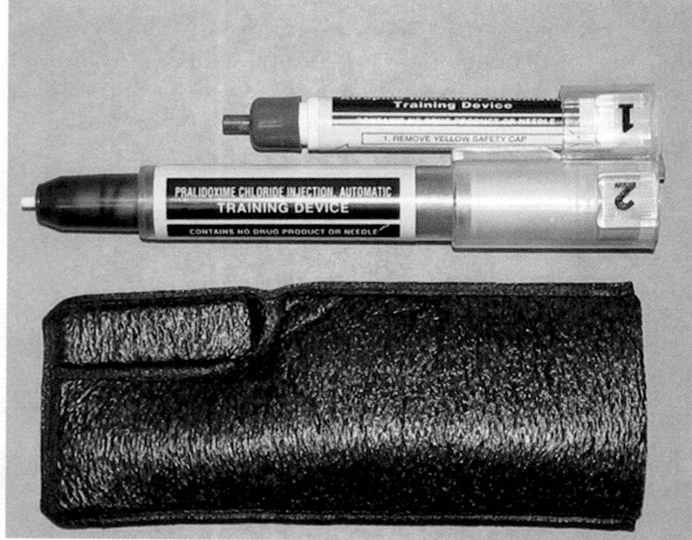

FIGURE 45-4 * The two-injector Mark I™ kit.

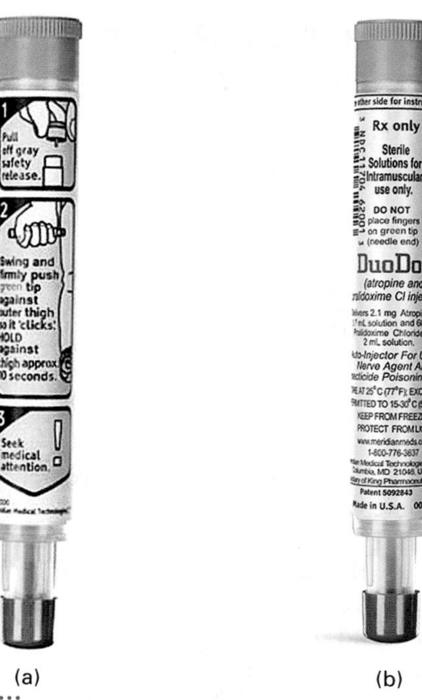

FIGURE 45-5 * The DuoDote™ auto-injector: **(a)** front view; **(b)** back view. (Both photos: DuoDote™ is a trademark of Meridian Medical Technologies™, Inc.)

To combat seizures, a third drug, diazepam (Valium), may also be used.

Wounds should be covered quickly to prevent further contamination and absorption of the nerve agent. Keep the patient warm and transport him as soon as possible.

Vesicants

Vesicants are another group of chemical agents that result in damage to exposed skin, lungs, and eyes. If a significant amount is absorbed, they may also produce systemic effects, including generalized illness. The currently known agents include sulfur and nitrogen mustards, lewisite, and phosgene oxime. These agents cause blistering, burning, and tissue damage on contact. The eyes, skin, and lungs are the organs most commonly affected. The onset of signs and symptoms may provide a

Key Terms
cyanide a rapid-acting agent that disrupts the ability of the cell to use oxygen, leading to severe cellular hypoxia and death.

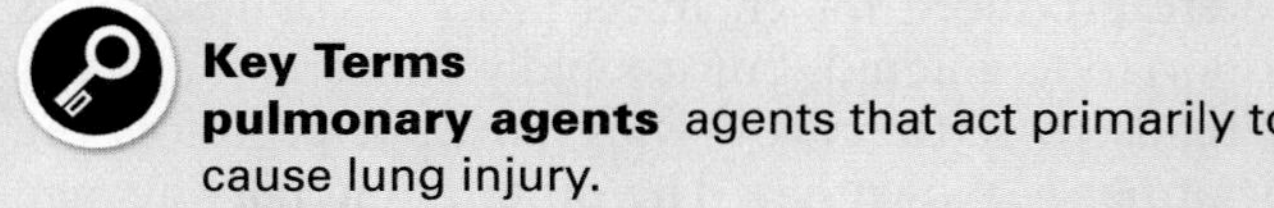

Key Terms
pulmonary agents agents that act primarily to cause lung injury.

clue to what agent was used. Mustard agents cause little initial discomfort but lead to severe damage in a matter of hours. Lewisite and phosgene oxime produce immediate discomfort and redness on contact.

Vesicant agents, with the exception of phosgene oxime, are thick, oily liquids. They have low volatility and tend to be persistent. In warm temperatures, vesicants pose a significant threat of vapor exposure. Mustard gas has a characteristic odor of onions, garlic, or mustard. Phosgene oxime smells like newly mown grass or hay.

Signs and Symptoms Vesicants were once referred to as "blister agents" because of their effects on the skin. These agents may have contact and systemic effects, depending on the exposure and the agent. Signs and symptoms of vesicant agents may include the following:

- Burning, redness, blistering, and necrosis of the skin (wheals or hives in the case of phosgene oxime)
- Stinging, tearing, and development of ulcers in the eyes
- Shortness of breath, coughing, wheezing, and pulmonary edema when inhaled
- Nausea and vomiting
- Fatigue

It may take 2–24 hours for mustard exposure to produce signs and symptoms. Eye damage may occur within 1–2 hours after exposure.

Emergency Medical Care The most important emergency care that can be provided for vesicant exposure is immediate irrigation. Treatment during the first few minutes after exposure is crucial to preventing damage. Irrigate with water or a chemical decontamination kit. Continue to irrigate the areas of exposure. Manage the blistering as chemical burns. Apply a dry, sterile dressing once the area has been adequately flushed. Patch eye injuries after adequate flushing has occurred.

Cyanide

Cyanide is a rapid acting agent that disrupts the ability of the cell to use oxygen, leading to severe cellular hypoxia and eventually death. It used to be referred to as a "blood agent," but its effects are on the cell and not the blood. Cyanide is relatively easy and inexpensive to produce.

Cyanide is absorbed by inhaling the vapor or by ingestion of contaminated food or water. Once in the body, the cyanide acts quickly. It targets the brain and heart. If a large concentration is inhaled, the patient may lose consciousness within 1 minute and die within 6–8 minutes. Even moderate exposure can lead to death. Low-dose exposures will lead to illness, but the patient would likely recover.

Signs and Symptoms Low concentrations of cyanide exposure cause milder signs and symptoms and a slower rate of onset. Signs and symptoms of cyanide exposure may include the following:

- Anxiety
- Weakness
- Dizziness
- Nausea
- Muscular trembling
- Tachycardia
- Tachypnea
- Pale, cyanotic, or normal color skin
- Seizures
- Apnea
- Unresponsiveness

Signs and symptoms that appear to be initially mild may progress and eventually lead to death. The classic cherry-red skin and lip color is an unreliable and very late sign. The pulse oximeter may provide a false sense of reassurance, since the blood is being oxygenated well, yet the cell cannot use the oxygen.

Emergency Medical Care Cyanide treatment must be initiated early to be effective. Manage the airway and provide positive pressure ventilation if the respiratory rate or tidal volume is inadequate. If an adequate respiratory rate and tidal volume are present, administer oxygen by a nonrebreather mask at 15 lpm. An antidote may be necessary to save the patient. It consists of a nitrite, such as amyl nitrite or sodium nitrite, and sodium thiosulfate. In 2006, the U.S. Food and Drug Administration (FDA) approved the injectable drug Cyanokit (hydroxocobalamin) for the treatment of cyanide poisoning, whether the cyanide has been inhaled or ingested. These agents work to remove the cyanide from the patient's system.

Pulmonary Agents

Pulmonary agents include phosgene (CG), other halogen compounds, and nitrogen-oxygen compounds. They act primarily to cause lung injury and are commonly referred to as "choking" agents. Large amounts of phosgene are produced for chemical processes. Phosgene is transported as a liquid, but it rapidly converts into a gas that tends to settle in low-lying areas. It produces the odor of newly mown hay. The other pulmonary agents, like chlorine, have similar characteristics and are treated the same as phosgene.

Phosgene directly attacks the airway and lung tissue. The smaller airways and alveoli are the most susceptible to injury. The damaged airways and alveoli will leak fluid, leading to pulmonary edema and inflammation. This leads to hypoxemia and, potentially, respiratory failure.

Signs and Symptoms Relatively small concentrations of phosgene irritate the mucous membranes of the mouth, eyes, nose, and throat. The initial signs and symptoms may reflect this irritation. Pulmonary edema may take several hours to develop after exposure. The mild symptoms may be a key indicator that the patient can progress to severe hypoxemia from pulmonary edema in a few hours. Exertion may worsen the condition. The typical signs and symptoms are as follows:

- Tearing
- Runny nose
- Throat irritation
- Dyspnea
- Wheezing
- Cough
- Crackles
- Stridor
- Secretions

Emergency Medical Care The priority in pulmonary agent exposure is to manage the airway and ensure the patient is breathing adequately. Tracheal intubation may be needed if airway obstruction is evident. Suction secretions, if necessary. If the respiratory rate or tidal volume is inadequate, begin positive pressure ventilation. Be sure to administer high concentrations of oxygen when ventilating. If the patient has adequate breathing, apply a nonrebreather mask at 15 lpm. Calm the patient and do not allow him to exert himself. If the patient is wheezing, a $beta_2$ agonist can be administered.

Riot-Control Agents

As noted earlier, some riot-control agents are solids that become an aerosol when deployed. Thus, "tear gas" is not a gas but an aerosolized solid. The most recent type of riot-control agent is derived from the capsicum family of peppers.

Signs and Symptoms Tear gas and capsicum-based "pepper spray" cause extreme irritation of the eyes, nose, mouth, skin, and respiratory tract. It may cause involuntary eye closing from the severe irritation or temporary blindness. The irritation usually lasts approximately 30 minutes after exposure.

Emergency Medical Care Emergency medical care is primarily supportive and should focus on removing the patient from the contaminated environment and irrigating the eyes with water or saline. If the patient is wearing contact lenses, remove them. If the patient presents with signs of respiratory distress, provide oxygen therapy via a nonrebreather mask at 15 lpm. If the patient is wheezing and has a metered-dose inhaler, administer the MDI according to your protocol. If the pain from skin exposure is prolonged, decontaminate with soap and water. Do not use bleach.

Toxic Industrial Chemicals

Any toxic chemical can potentially be exploited by a terrorist and used as a chemical weapon. Millions of tons of hazardous chemicals, such as chlorine and anhydrous ammonia, are transported by rail and truck across the United States every year, and tons more are stored at chemical and manufacturing facilities. The terrorist threat from hijacked or diverted industrial chemicals or the possibility of sabotage of a chemical plant or storage site must be considered when thinking about chemical agents of mass destruction.

Signs and Symptoms and Emergency Medical Care The effects of and emergency care for industrial chemicals are as diverse as the chemicals themselves. Many of the more potent chemicals behave like pulmonary agents; that is, they primarily attack the respiratory tract. Examples include chlorine, phosgene, and methyl isocyanate (the chemical that killed thousands in Bhopal, India). Others act like cyanide, including salts of cyanide and related compounds called cyanogens. Insecticides act similarly to nerve agents. It is important to utilize special resources to identify the exact chemicals involved, and this requires the expertise of a trained hazmat team. (Refer to Chapter 43, "Hazardous Materials.")

Biological Agents

Biological agents are made up of living organisms or the toxins produced by the living organisms and are used to cause disease in a target population. Diseases caused by these agents are no different from the naturally occurring diseases. The only difference is that, as weapons of mass destruction, the harm they cause is intentional. Biological agents lend themselves to use as weapons of mass destruction because small amounts can cause widespread disease and mass casualties. It may take several days to detect a biological assault. Viruses, bacteria, and fungi can be used to form the biological agents.

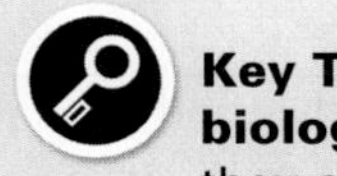

Key Terms

biological agents living organisms or toxins they produce used as weapons of mass destruction to cause disease in a target population.

Objective 45-9

Give examples of specific categories of biological agents and explain the appropriate medical care for exposure to biological agents.

To be effective as a WMD, the biological agent must reach the intended target. This is usually accomplished by spraying a liquid agent through a nozzle. Delivery can be accomplished by an airplane that can achieve widespread distribution of the agent. Wind speed and direction, rain, and sunlight can each have an effect on the delivery. High winds can disperse the agent and carry it over a long distance. Rain and sunshine will usually decrease the effectiveness of the agent. Ideal conditions for delivery are night and very early morning.

Far less effective but nearly as frightening is a simpler method of introducing a biological agent into the population by using one or more individuals infected with a highly contagious agent to come in close contact with members of the general public. This technique could take place in an airport or other transportation hub and result in widely dispersed emerging epidemics throughout the nation or the world. The anthrax attacks through the U.S. Postal Service demonstrate another uncomplicated method of dispersal that, while ineffective at producing massive casualties, resulted in widespread fear and disruption of people's lives in several locations.

The respiratory tract is the most common and efficient portal of entry for most biological agents. The size of the biological agent is also important. A particle that is between 1 and 5 microns in size can get lower in the respiratory tract and into the lungs. If it is too large, the particle will fall out of the air, or will stay in the upper respiratory tract and be less effective. If the particle is too small, it will be exhaled back out. The mucous membranes of the mouth, nose, and eye are also portals of entry. Biological agents can be ingested in contaminated food and water.

Most biological weapons are intended to kill the victims. They can be extremely potent weapons of mass destruction. Small amounts of these potent agents can lead to a horrible death. The biggest potential threat from biological agents comes from their ability to spread, much as natural infectious diseases do. Epidemics can race through unsuspecting and unprotected populations, infecting and killing thousands, if not millions. Fortunately, only a few agents possess this chilling capability to a strong degree: smallpox, ebola, and plague.

The key to recognition of a biological attack is to distinguish the number and timing of the cases from the isolated case of an expected illness. This may be difficult to do when other, naturally occurring incidents of mass food poisoning or epidemic meningitis occur. It is necessary to identify the commonality between those who are ill, such as a shared meal, living quarters, or water source. Because a biological incident may evolve slowly, initially occurring as individual cases throughout the community, the usual EMS notification and first response to the disaster may not occur. Instead, doctors' offices, emergency departments, and public health agencies may be the first to detect the outbreak. Traditional hazmat approaches of containment and isolation may be impractical when a single source cannot be located. Instead, a public health response may be more effective.

Specific Biological Agents

Several biological agents can be used as weapons of mass destruction and pose a serious threat. They are categorized into four groups:

- Pneumonia-like agents (presenting with fever and rapidly progressing dyspnea)
- Encephalitis-like agents (presenting with fever and altered mental status)
- Biological toxins
- Other agents

Pneumonia-Like Agents

Pneumonia-like agents include anthrax, plague, and tularemia. The common symptoms are cough, shortness of breath, fever, and malaise (a general feeling of illness). The specific findings for each are as follows:

Pneumonia-Like Agents

Agent	Specific Findings
Anthrax	Incubation period is 1–6 days. Fever, malaise, fatigue, nonproductive cough, mild chest discomfort with progressing dyspnea, diaphoresis, stridor, cyanosis, shock, and death can occur within 24–36 hours.
Plague	Incubation period is 2–3 days. Headache, hemoptysis (coughing up blood), severe dyspnea, high fever, stridor, cyanosis, and death from respiratory failure, circulatory collapse, and bleeding disorder.
Tularemia	Chest pain that worsens with breathing, headache, malaise, nonproductive cough, and weight loss.

Additional agents presenting with fever and pneumonia include *Q fever* and *glanders.*

Encephalitis-Like Agents

Encephalitis-like agents cause symptoms that resemble the flu, to include headache, fever, and malaise. These diseases are much more lethal than flu. They have a tendency to affect the brain and spinal cord; therefore, they are referred to as encephalitis-like agents.

The two most common encephalitis-like agents are smallpox and Venezuelan equine encephalitis. Common signs and symptoms are headache, fever, and malaise. The signs and symptoms are as follows:

Encephalitis-Like Agents

Agent	Specific Findings
Smallpox	Sudden onset of malaise, fever, headache, vomiting, and backache. Rash appears in 2–3 days.
Venezuelan equine encephalitis	Sudden onset with malaise, fever, severe headache, rigor, nausea, vomiting, cough, sore throat, and diarrhea, with recovery within 1–2 weeks.

Other agents with similar signs and symptoms include *brucellosis* and the *Eastern and Western equine encephalitis.*

Biological Toxins

Biological toxins are potentially the most significant threat of all the biological agents. Toxins are not living organisms but are products of living organisms. For this reason, toxins cannot be transmitted from one infected individual to another. This does not lessen the threat of these agents, however. Biological toxins are among the most dangerous compounds known to man.

The five most significant biological toxins are botulinum, ricin, staphylococcus enterotoxin 13 (SEB), epsilon toxin of clostridium perfringens, and trichothecene mycotoxins (T2). The signs or symptoms of the agents are as follows:

Biological Toxins

Agent	Specific Findings
Botulinum	Descending paralysis, which includes generalized weakness, ptosis (droopy eyelids), double vision, blurred vision, dry mouth and throat, dysphasia (difficulty speaking), dysphagia (difficulty swallowing), and dyspnea, leading to respiratory failure and death. Symptoms typically begin in 12–36 hours or may occur several days after inhalation or ingestion.
Ricin	Weakness, fever, cough, and hypothermia about 36 hours after inhalation, followed by death in the next 12 hours from hypotension and cardiovascular collapse.
Staphylococcus enterotoxin 13 (SEB)	Fever, chills, headache, body aches, and nonproductive cough will occur 3–12 hours after inhalation. Shock and death may occur at high doses.
Epsilon toxin	Cough, wheezing, and shortness of breath occur within 6 hours of exposure. Respiratory failure and death follow shortly from high exposure. Liver damage can also occur.
Trichothecene mycotoxins (T2)	Pain, itching, redness, and lesions on the exposed skin, nose, and throat; pain; runny nose and sneezing; skin may slough; nasal discharge; dyspnea; wheezing; chest pain; and hemoptysis (coughing up blood).

Other Agents

Other biological agents include cholera, brucellosis, and viral hemorrhagic fevers. Viral hemorrhagic fevers include the Ebola and Marburg viruses and the agents dengue and yellow fever. These agents are very lethal and result in a 5–50 percent death rate in infected individuals. Cholera is still seen in epidemic proportions in developing nations. The dehydration associated with cholera can easily lead to death. The signs and symptoms of these agents are as follows:

Other Biological Agents

Agents	Specific Findings
Cholera	Vomiting, abdominal distention, profuse watery diarrhea, severe dehydration, and little or no fever. Death results from severe dehydration and shock associated with hypovolemia.
Viral hemorrhagic fevers (VHFs)	Malaise, body aches, headache, vomiting, flushing of the face and chest, edema, petechiae (small pinpoint hemorrhages), easy bleeding (early), hypotension, and shock (late).
Brucellosis	Fever, malaise, body aches, joint pain, headache, and cough.

Emergency Medical Care for Biological Agents

The care for biological agents is primarily supportive. Recognition is extremely important to advanced management of the patient. In a WMD incident where biological weapons are used, a large number of patients can be expected. Contacting the necessary resources, including public health officials, early is crucial in providing the needed antibiotic and antitoxin treatments to reduce the number of deaths from exposure.

Objective 45-10
Differentiate between the characteristics of X-ray and gamma radiation, neutron radiation, beta radiation, and alpha radiation.

Objective 45-11
Differentiate between primary exposure and fallout associated with a nuclear explosion.

Key Terms
nuclear radiation energy released when an unstable atom breaks apart.

primary exposure radiation injury occurring during or shortly after a radioactive detonation.

Only a few of the biological agents are highly contagious and can be passed from an infected individual to another person. Smallpox, plague, and Ebola are all typically contagious. Isolate these patients, as best you can in the field, from those who are not affected. Response personnel should use personal protective equipment, including a HEPA respirator; head and face protection; and impervious boots, gloves, and body-splash protection.

The priorities in patient care include securing an adequate airway and ensuring that the patient is breathing adequately. If the breathing is adequate, administer oxygen by a nonrebreather mask at 15 lpm to any patient with mild to moderate respiratory distress. For patients who are breathing inadequately, provide positive pressure ventilation. Respiratory support is especially crucial in botulinum poisoning, since the cause of death is respiratory failure. If the respirations can be supported, the patient's chance of survival is good.

The use of antibiotics and antitoxins is imperative in the management of patients exposed to biological agents. It is important for the EMS provider to recognize a patient who may be in need of such treatment, summon the necessary medical personnel, and continue to assist with the treatment.

The best protection against biological weapons is prevention. A key to prevention is proper immunization and prophylaxis. Immunization involves taking substances related to the biological agent to develop a resistance or antibodies. Prophylaxis is taking antibiotics prior to exposure or during the incubation stage. Several effective immunizations and prophylaxis strategies are available and their use should be incorporated in the EMS response plan to a disaster.

Nuclear Weapons and Radiation

Nuclear weapons have been in existence since the United States developed the first atomic bomb in the 1940s. Nuclear weapons can cause extensive death by a variety of mechanisms and lead to severe destruction of buildings and other structures in the detonation area. There are three primary mechanisms of death or injury associated with nuclear detonation: radiation, blast, and thermal burns.

Radiation

When an unstable (radioactive) atom breaks apart, it releases energy in the form of rays and particles that travel at high speeds (**nuclear radiation**). It differs from other types of radiation (light, heat, sound) because it can change the structure of molecules it passes. These rays and particles damage the cells of the human body. The cells may die, repair themselves, or go on to produce damaged or mutated cells.

X-ray radiation and *gamma radiation* are the same type, although they are created by different processes. This is the most penetrating type of radiation and can travel long distances. This is the type of radiation that is generated in the reactor of a nuclear power plant, by a nuclear bomb, and through the decay of radioactive particles, as in fallout. Gamma radiation is the major external hazard and, to a lesser extent, internal hazard associated with a nuclear detonation or a reactor accident.

Neutron radiation is a powerful and very damaging particle that penetrates several hundred meters of air and easily passes through the body. Since it occurs infrequently outside of the nuclear chain reaction, its greatest threat to life occurs in close proximity to an active nuclear reactor or bomb explosion.

Beta radiation is a low-speed, low-energy particle that is easily stopped by 6–10 feet of air, clothing, or the first few millimeters of skin. It is a common product of fallout decay and is a serious threat from ingestion of contaminated foods and inhalation of airborne particles. Thus, it poses a great internal hazard.

Alpha radiation is a heavy and slow-moving particle that travels only inches in air and is stopped by clothing or the outer layer of the skin. It is a very serious internal contaminant because it causes a great amount of damage along its short course of travel. As in beta radiation, alpha radiation can be ingested or inhaled.

Radiation Exposure

There are two types of radiation exposure associated with a nuclear explosion: primary exposure and fallout.

Primary Exposure **Primary exposure** is the primary radiation injury occurs during or shortly after the detonation. The rising fireball draws the radioactive materials upward and away from the ground very quickly. The exposure only occurs for the first minute immediately after the detonation. Neutron and gamma radiation travel

Key Terms

fallout radioactive dust and particles that disperse far from the epicenter of a radioactive detonation.

Objective 45-12

Explain blast injuries and thermal burns as mechanisms of injury from nuclear explosions.

Objective 45-13

Differentiate between a nuclear weapon and a radiological dispersal device (RDD, or "dirty bomb").

1,000–2,000 meters through the air, so exposure is limited to the blast proximity. Thus, most injury and death in the nuclear blast is caused by the blast and burns and not from primary radiation. An exception is a small radiological dispersal device where the radiation doses are strong enough to cause illness or injury well beyond the blast radius.

In the case of a radioactive reactor accident involving radioactive materials where detonation does not occur, gamma radiation is the most serious hazard. This can result in severe and life-threatening injuries to persons near the radiation source. The radioactive source strength, duration of exposure, shielding, and distance from the source directly affect the potential for injury and death.

Fallout Fallout is the second form of radiation exposure. Fallout is radioactive dust and particles that may be life threatening to people far from the epicenter of the detonation. As the superheated products of nuclear detonation and surrounding debris are drawn up into the atmosphere, they are bombarded with nuclear reaction by-products, energized, and then distributed by wind. The closer the detonation occurs to the ground, the greater the updraft of particles, resulting in more fallout.

The radioactive material may be scattered anywhere from a few miles from the detonation site to around the world. The most immediate danger from fallout occurs within 48 hours and within close proximity to the blast. It contains intense ionizing radiation, since it has had very little time to decay, therefore making it the most hazardous.

Radiation injuries are different from burn injuries. The radiation travels through the body tissues and may alter some cell structures. The most common structure in the cell that is damaged is the DNA. The cells that are most sensitive to radiation injury are bone marrow, blood, bowel, skin, and nervous and cardiovascular tissue.

Blast Injuries

The nuclear detonation causes a rapid heating of air surrounding the nuclear ignition and an explosively expanding gas cloud. As the cloud movement reaches the speed of sound, it creates a shock wave, followed by a blast of wind. The shock wave and wind blast produce typical shock wave injuries as found in conventional weapons, although the intensity is much greater the closer the victims are to ground zero. The windblast may reach 160 miles per hour, displacing personnel and collapsing structures, leading to crush injuries and entrapment. The blast effects to the victims are reduced the farther they are from ground zero.

Thermal Burns

The mechanism that causes most deaths and injury associated with nuclear detonation is the thermal burn. A tremendous amount of thermal energy is released from the nuclear reaction and travels unimpeded through the air to its target. The heating is of very short duration, but it is extremely intense. Anything in close proximity to the detonation is incinerated. The heat energy is fairly easy to shield yourself against. Any opaque object captures the energy. White or light clothing will reflect a great deal of the energy. Flame burns may result from ignition of clothing and building materials. Often the burns of a patient far from the detonation seem very serious; however, they may be only superficial burns.

Eye injuries may be associated with the brilliant light flash. The patient may be blinded for a few seconds or minutes or longer. The retina can be permanently damaged if the person looks directly at the detonation and focuses on the intense light.

Radiological Dispersal Devices

A radiological dispersal device (RDD, also called a "dirty bomb") is a conventional explosive attached to radioactive materials. Such a device has none of the immense blast power of a nuclear weapon, since it cannot sustain a nuclear chain reaction. Instead, it gains its destructive power first by the blast of the conventional explosive, and second by the spread of radioactive material all around the blast site. Thus, the primary mass destruction threat of such a device is to contaminate a wide area with radioactive materials. Such a hazard could induce radiation illness in many persons while seriously contaminating the local environment.

Assessment and Care for Nuclear Detonation and Radiation Injuries

The closer the patient is to the detonation, the more severe the injuries expected.

Assessment

As the energy travels away from the blast center, it quickly dissipates. This is viewed as concentric circles of injury

Objective 45-15
Explain issues of personal protection and patient decontamination in connection with chemical, biological, and radiological/nuclear weapons exposure.

Objective 45-14
Discuss assessment and care of patients affected by nuclear detonation and radiation injuries.

and destruction. In the innermost circle of destruction, the buildings will be flattened and burned and no people will be found alive. The next circle will contain massive destruction to all structures. Most people will suffer lethal injuries from radiation, the blast wave, and burns. Some victims may survive if they are shielded from the heat and flying debris; however, they may die from a building collapse. The next circle has more survival with those patients exposed to the flash suffering from burns. The shock wave and radiation may cause serious injury, but thermal burns are the greatest cause of death. As the circles move farther from the site, the injuries and death from the radiation and blast wave are reduced, but burns remain the major cause of injury and death.

When assessing patients, it is important to realize that this is a multiple-casualty scene. The multiple-casualty incident management plan will be activated. Assessment and triage will be done quickly, using the same criteria as in other multiple-casualty incidents. Identify the time after exposure that the patient complains of any radiation-related signs and symptoms.

Radiation injury will cause the following signs and symptoms:

Bone marrow and blood cells	Nausea, fatigue, malaise, clotting disorders, and possible uncontrolled hemorrhage
Bowel	Nausea and vomiting, loss of appetite, diarrhea, fluid loss, malaise, and dehydration
Skin	Reddening (erythema)
Nervous and cardiovascular systems	Rapid onset of incapacitation, cardiovascular collapse, confusion, burning or "on fire" sensation with high doses

Emergency Medical Care

Victims of a nuclear incident will include patients suffering thermal burns, blunt trauma and pressure injuries from the explosive blast, and radiation exposure. Emergency medical care provided to these patients is primarily the same care provided to patients suffering such injuries from any cause.

Your primary concern is for your own and the patients' safety. Move the patients so that they are perpendicular to the wind direction. Be careful, since the wind direction shifts frequently. If transportation of the patients is not possible, shelter them from the radioactive contamination by putting as much distance and substance as possible between them and the radioactive material. If fallout is expected to be a hazard, a shelter should be constructed for protection. It takes 2 inches of steel, 6 inches of concrete, 8 inches of earth, or 22 inches of wood to serve as protection.

Manage the airway and ventilatory status of the patient. Be cognizant of upper airway burns. If necessary, perform tracheal intubation if you are permitted or summon ALS to provide intubation for patients with upper airway burns. If the patient is breathing adequately and shows evidence of trauma or respiratory distress, apply a nonrebreather mask at 15 lpm. If the patient is breathing inadequately, begin positive pressure ventilation. Pressure injuries to the lungs may have caused severe damage leading to swelling, fluid accumulation, and possible pulmonary emboli. Be aware of the potential for a pneumothorax to occur.

Manage burns as you would normally manage a thermal burn. Use sterile dressings and sterile burn sheets to cover the burned areas. Manage blunt trauma as you normally would in a trauma patient.

Radiation exposure injury will occur hours after the exposure. The damage is typically diffuse throughout the body. Keep all wounds clean to reduce the incidence of infection, since the radiation may alter the body's immune system and make the patient more susceptible to infection. Irrigate contaminated wounds and apply sterile dressings.

In an area of nuclear fallout or radioactive contamination, it is possible to prevent one of the long-term effects of the radiation by taking iodine tablets. If proper doses are taken before or immediately after the radiation exposure, future thyroid cancer risk can be reduced. This prophylactic measure should be considered in every EMS response plan to such a situation. It is important to remember that iodine only protects against one of the many harmful effects of radiation and its use does not reduce the need for proper shielding, personal protective equipment, decontamination, and long-term monitoring.

Personal Protection and Patient Decontamination

In chemical, biological, and radiological/nuclear weapons exposure, it is necessary for you to use personal protective equipment to reduce your risk of exposure and

Key Points
The same principles you use in dealing with hazardous materials can be applied to a chemical, biological, or nuclear incident.

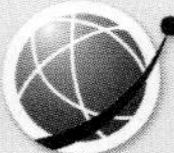

Media Resources
Go to www.bradybooks.com for mykit. Highlights:

- *Web Resource:* Terrorism
- *Web Resource:* Blast Injuries

subsequent illness or death. This may involve wearing specialized suits, gloves, boots, and breathing apparatus (Figure 45-6*). You must understand the agent you are dealing with in order to take the necessary precautions.

The same principles you use in dealing with hazardous materials can be applied to a chemical, biological, or nuclear incident. Zones should be established so that limited exposure occurs to rescuers. The principles of time, distance, and shielding should be used for personal protection. Patients may require decontamination. The same principles of decontamination used in a hazardous materials incident apply to patients exposed to chemical, biological, or radiological agents. (Refer to Chapter 43, "Hazardous Materials," for a detailed discussion of personal protective equipment and decontamination.) Typically, those specially trained in decontamination will perform this critical task. If you are not properly trained in specialized rescue when dealing with hazardous materials or the proper methods of decontamination, you should perform other tasks related to patient treatment or transportation.

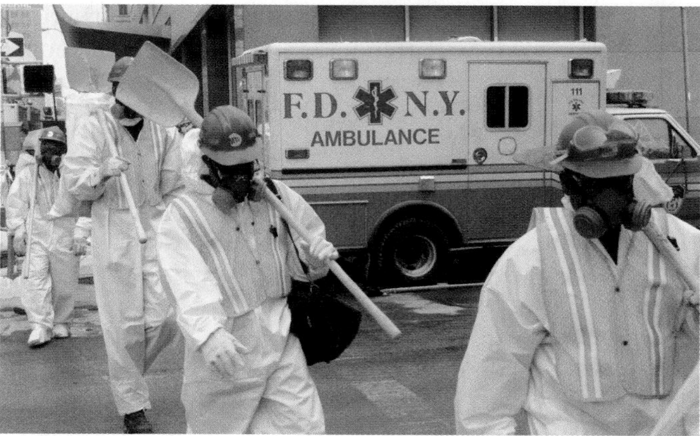

FIGURE 45-6 * Specialized personal protection equipment used at the World Trade Center attack. (© Szenes Jason/Corbis Sygma)

SUMMARY

Weapons of mass destruction (WMD) are intended to produce widespread death and destruction. The weapons may be chemical, biological, radiological, nuclear, or explosive agents. Conventional explosive agents have the greatest likelihood of being used in an attack.

Prehospital personnel must be prepared to respond to a WMD incident. Preplanning is crucial to effective management of the incident and the patients. In preplanning, consideration must be given to supplies and equipment, medical direction, provider education and preparation, response to the scene, and scene safety issues. Also, having a basic knowledge of the signs and symptoms and emergency care necessary for the various agents will better prepare the EMT to manage the patients who are victims of a WMD incident.

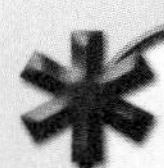

CASE STUDY FOLLOW-UP

SCENE SIZE-UP

You have been dispatched to the local college football stadium for an explosion with injuries. As you arrive on the scene, you note a large number of people running from the stadium. Some of the patients appear to have suffered some type of trauma.

Your partner finds an open parking lot next to the dormitories that is upwind and uphill from the stadium. He immediately contacts dispatch and indicates that there are a large number of possible patients and to implement the disaster plan with specification of an explosive agent. This triggers the response of the emergency management agency and local public health officials. He then sets up the EMS command center and erects the identification flag. Soon after, the assistant fire chief and police major converge on the parking lot and establish their respective command centers.

Meanwhile, you have immediately sought out the fire officer in charge at the stadium. He indicates the explosion appears to have been a conventional-type bomb that exploded under the east sector of the stands. He has fire personnel in the stadium and is beginning rescue operations. You put on your helmet, turnout coat and pants, leather gloves, and eye protection and proceed to the east side of the stadium. You see that the midsection of the stadium has collapsed. There are wounded people walking about and others trapped within the concrete rubble.

PRIMARY ASSESSMENT AND TRIAGE

Communicating with your partner, who is still the EMS incident commander, you approach the walking patients and instruct them all to move to the south side of the stadium. You instruct the next arriving EMT to go to the south side, gather all the walking injured patients, and take them to the practice field located just east of the stadium. You then pull out the colored ribbons from the multiple-casualty kit and begin to perform triage, using the START method.

As additional firefighters arrive, you instruct them to gather backboards and begin to move the red-tagged patients from the scene to the secondary triage and treatment area located on the soccer field west of the stadium.

As you continue to perform the primary triage, you note typical injuries to the patients from an explosive device. Many have penetrating injuries.

ESTABLISHING SECTORS

While you are conducting the initial triage, your partner, the EMS incident commander, establishes the secondary triage and treatment sector, supply sector, extrication sector, staging sector, and transportation sector. As the EMS units arrive, he appoints the EMTs as sector officers.

Before long, patients are moving quickly from the incident area to the secondary triage and treatment sectors. Arriving EMS units are now being directed toward the treatment sector for manpower or to the staging and transportation sectors. The red-tagged patients are being moved from the treatment sector to the local medical facilities. The operation appears to be going smoothly with an estimated 150 people injured.

ADDITIONAL THREATS

The specially trained experts in weapons of mass destruction are now on the scene, evaluating the situation for the possibility of chemical weapons used in conjunction with the explosive device, but there is no confirmation at this point. Also, there is concern that a secondary explosion may be set to go off.

You continue with initial triage of the patients as the fire department personnel continue with rescue. There are no further explosions, and the WMD experts indicate that this was only a conventional-type explosive device. No evidence of chemical, biological, or nuclear material is apparent. You continue to work until the scene is completely cleared of all patients.

IN REVIEW

1. Name the types of weapons of mass destruction.
2. Describe the safety issues to EMS providers when responding to a scene where weapons of mass destruction have been used.
3. Define a conventional weapon and incendiary device.
4. Describe the injuries expected from detonation of an explosive.
5. Explain the difference between a primary, secondary, and tertiary blast effect associated with an explosion.
6. List and describe the different types of chemical agents used as weapons of mass destruction.
7. Describe the emergency care for the different types of chemical agents.
8. List and describe the various biological agents that are used as weapons of mass destruction.
9. List the general principles of treatment of biological agent exposure.
10. List and describe the different types of radiation.
11. List the injuries that are most likely to occur with detonation of a nuclear device.
12. Describe the general emergency care of a radiation exposure patient.

CRITICAL THINKING

You are responding to the local mall for a large number of ill patients. You are the second EMS unit to arrive on the scene. You find a crowd of approximately 60 people huddled in the parking lot. They claim they heard a loud bang and then, within minutes, many of them started to cough and choke. Most of them are now complaining of shortness of breath and irritation of the throat. You note that most patients have a runny nose, tears, cough, and secretions. You also note wheezing and crackles on auscultation of the lungs of many of the patients.

1. What is the first action you would take?
2. How would you initially manage the patients?
3. What do you suspect they are suffering from?

PEARSON

EXPLORE mybradykit™

Please go to **www.bradybooks.com** to access mykit for this text. You will find quizzes, critical thinking scenarios, weblinks, animations, and videos related to this chapter—and much more. Look for online information on terrorism and on the Department of Homeland Security.

Register your access code from the front of your book by going to **www.bradybooks.com** and selecting the mykit links.

Appendix 1 ALS-Assist Skills

At times, Advanced EMTs or paramedics may ask that you assist in setting up equipment so that they can perform an advanced skill. Two of the most common advanced skills that EMTs assist with are intravenous (IV) therapy and ECG monitoring. Be sure to follow your local protocol when assisting with ALS skills.

Assisting in Intravenous Therapy

Intravenous therapy is a common advanced life support procedure that is initiated on many patients in the prehospital environment by Advanced EMTs and paramedics. An intravenous line is typically inserted to administer fluids or medication to the patient. A large number of the medications that the Advanced EMT and paramedic administer are given through an intravenous route.

In intravenous therapy, a catheter is inserted directly into a vein. The catheter is connected to intravenous tubing that allows the fluid to flow from the intravenous bag into the vein. The fluid in the bag is primarily composed of water and either electrolytes, such as sodium chloride or others (normal saline and lactated Ringer's), or sugar (5% dextrose in water, or D_5W). These solutions have specific purposes for different patient conditions. Pay close attention to the solution the Advanced EMT or paramedic is requesting when preparing to set up for intravenous therapy.

Intravenous Therapy Equipment Components

There are three major equipment components involved in intravenous therapy:

- Catheter
- Tubing
- Bag of fluid

Catheter

When assisting, you will typically be asked to set up or prepare the bag of fluid and the tubing. The Advanced EMT or paramedic may ask you to retrieve the catheter, or you may do nothing more than open the packaging. The catheters come in different sizes according to diameter and length. The diameter is identified by the gauge, and the length is in inches. A higher gauge number indicates a smaller diameter. Most often you will find 14-, 16-, 18-, 20-, and 22-gauge catheters. The catheters typically used in the prehospital setting are 2- to 1¼-inch in length.

Intravenous Tubing

The intravenous tubing is also called the administration set. It connects the fluid bag to the catheter. The tubing is typically identified by the number of drops per minute it takes to deliver 1 mL of fluid. For example, it may be a 10-, 15-, 20-, or 60-drop/mL administration set. The lower-drop tubings deliver fluid at a faster rate. The higher-drop tubings deliver fluid at a more controlled and slower rate. The drops/mL may also be referred to as gtt/mL. A mini-drip tubing is a 60 gtt/mL solution set, whereas the macro-drip tubing delivers more fluid through the 10-, 15-, and 20-gtt/mL sets.

The tubing has five major components:

- **Spike.** The spike is the pointed and angled hard plastic barrel at the top of the tubing. It is sterile and covered with a plastic cap or covering to protect it from being contaminated. The spike is used to puncture through the seal of the intravenous bag to allow fluid to flow into the tubing.
- **Drip chamber.** The drip chamber is near the top of the tubing. The size refers to the plastic or metal barrel contained in the chamber. The smaller the barrel, the higher the number of drops it will take to deliver 1 mL of fluid. Drip chambers deliver 10, 15, and 20 gtt/mL.
- **Flow control or regulator valve.** This device controls or regulates the rate at which the fluid is delivered through the tubing and into the vein. It can also completely stop the flow of fluid.
- **Drug or needle or needleless injection port.** The drug or needle or needleless injection port is located below the flow control valve. It is where the Advanced EMT or paramedic administers medication to the patient.
- **Hub connector.** The hub connector is where the tubing inserts into the hub of the catheter. This area of the tubing is protected by a plastic cover or cap to keep it sterile. This should only be removed immediately prior to insertion into the hub of the catheter to protect against the introduction of infection into the vein. The caps are perforated to allow fluid to escape when flushing the tubing.

Bag of Fluid

The bag of fluid comes in a protective outer package. On the front of the bag, the type of solution and the amount of solution in mL is clearly marked. An expiration date is also found on the bag. The bag has two pigtail devices. One has a pull-type cover and the other has an injection port. The pull-type-cover pigtail is where the spike will be inserted.

Preparing the Intravenous Setup ("Spiking the Bag")

Often the Advanced EMT or paramedic will ask you to "spike a bag" of an intravenous solution, typically normal saline, lactated Ringer's, or D_5W. He is referring to setting up the solution for use. To do so, perform the following steps (ALS-Assist Skills A1-1):

1. Remove the protective wrap (ALS-Assist Skills A1-1A).
2. Check the fluid for impurities, particulate matter, and discoloration. Check the expiration date (ALS-Assist Skills A1-1B).
3. Select the proper administration set based on the instructions from the Advanced EMT or paramedic. Tear open the packaging of the solution set and uncoil the tubing. Be careful not to let the ends of the tubing touch the ground. Close the flow regulator, if it is open, by rolling the stopcock valve away from the bag.
4. Remove the protective covering from the intravenous bag pigtail port. Be careful not to contaminate the inside of the port.
5. Remove the protective cap or covering from the spike (ALS-Assist Skills A1-1C). Be sure not to touch or drop the spike, since it is sterile. If you contaminate the spike, discard the tubing and use another administration set.
6. Insert the spike into the intravenous bag pigtail port (ALS-Assist Skills A1-1D).
7. Holding the bag higher than the drip chamber, squeeze the drip chamber once or twice to fill it to the marker line, which is about ⅓ full (ALS-Assist Skills A1-1E).
8. Open the flow regulator to "flush" the tubing of all of the air (ALS-Assist Skills A1-1F). Most devices will allow easy flushing without removing the hub connector cap; however, some tubing may require that you briefly remove the cap to allow the fluid to be released. Make sure the entire length of tubing has been flushed free of air. If the hub connector cap was removed, do not allow it to touch anything, since it is sterile. Be sure to replace it immediately without contaminating it. If it becomes contaminated by touching the ground, your gloves, or any other object, replace the tubing so that you don't introduce any bacteria or other microorganisms into the patient.

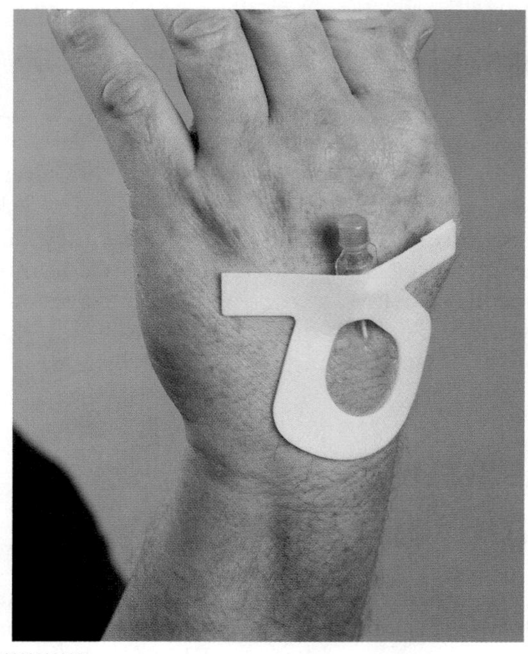

FIGURE A1-1 * Heparin lock. (© Scott Metcalfe)

At this point, the intravenous bag is "spiked" and prepared for insertion into the hub of the catheter.

Saline Lock or Heparin Lock

A saline lock or a heparin lock (Figure A1-1*) is used when a patient requires occasional IV medication but does not need continuous fluid. Each of these lock devices is a peripheral IV cannula with a distal medication port. In a saline lock, saline is injected into the device to maintain its patency. In a heparin lock, flushes of heparin solution, which inhibits coagulation, maintain patency.

ECG Lead Placement

An electrocardiogram (ECG) is a device that provides information about the electrical activity of the heart. This electrical activity may indicate to the Advanced EMT or paramedic that the patient is experiencing an abnormal rhythm (dysrhythmia) or, with more advanced monitoring techniques and equipment, that the patient is suffering a myocardial infarction.

You may be asked to place the electrodes and leads on the patient to assist the Advanced EMT or paramedic. To do so effectively, become familiar with the specific equipment used in your system. Some systems may use a form of combined monitoring electrodes and defibrillation pads, which are much larger than the standard ECG electrode. You may be asked to apply a "3-lead," "4-lead," or "12-lead" monitor. This will depend on local protocol and the scope of practice defined by your state.

3- or 4-Lead Electrode Placement

If asked to apply a 3- or 4-lead monitor, you will apply the three or four "limb leads" by performing the following steps (ALS-Assist Skills A1-2):

1. Cleanse the skin with alcohol or an abrasive pad to remove dirt, body oil, and other substances that may interfere with the conductivity between the electrode and the skin (ALS-Assist Skills A1-2A). If there is a significant amount of chest hair, shave it quickly. Dry the skin if there is a large amount of diaphoresis (sweat). Some systems use antiperspirant or tincture of Benzoin to keep the skin dry to allow for effective adhesion of the electrode.
2. Apply the electrodes to the skin. Some prefer to attach the lead or cable to the electrode prior to placing it on the skin. Others will apply the electrodes and then attach the leads. If three leads are used, apply the electrodes and leads as follows (ALS-Assist Skills A1-2B):
   a. Place one electrode to the right side of the anterior chest just under the clavicle at the midclavicular line. This is where the negative lead attaches. The lead is usually white and it has RA on the head of the lead—indicating "right arm" placement, even though the lead is being placed to the right chest.
   b. Apply the second electrode to the left anterior chest just under the clavicle at the midclavicular line. This is where the ground lead attaches. The lead is usually black, brown, or green and it has LA on the head of the lead—indicating "left arm" placement, even though the lead is being placed to the left chest. Since this is the ground electrode, it can be placed in other areas on the chest in the 3-lead configuration.
   c. Apply the third electrode to the left lower chest at about the seventh intercostal space on the anterior axillary line. This is where the positive lead attaches. The lead is usually red and it has RL on the head of the electrode—indicating "right leg" placement, even though the lead is placed on the lower left lateral chest.
   d. If a fourth lead is to be used, apply the electrode to the right lower lateral chest wall. This lead is often green in color and will have LL for "left leg" on the head of the electrode.

12-Lead Electrode Placement

A 12-lead ECG monitor will provide a much more detailed picture of the electrical activity of the heart than will a 3- or 4-lead application. The 12-lead arrangement requires placing 10 electrodes and leads on the patient (the four "limb leads" as just described plus six "precordial leads"). To apply the 12-lead ECG monitor, perform the following steps (ALS-Assist Skills A1-3):

1. Cleanse the skin with alcohol or an abrasive pad to remove dirt, body oil, and other substances that may interfere with the conductivity between the electrode and the skin. If there is a significant amount of chest hair, shave it quickly. Dry the skin if there is a large amount of diaphoresis (sweat). Some systems use antiperspirant or tincture of Benzoin to keep the skin dry to allow for effective adhesion of the electrode.
2. Place the four limb leads according to the manufacturer's recommendation. These are the right arm, right leg, left arm, and left leg electrodes and leads (ALS-Assist Skills A1-3A).
3. The precordial leads are V_1, V_2, V_3, V_4, V_5, and V_6. These are all placed on the anterior chest. The electrode heads are imprinted with the respective lead numbers.
4. Place lead V_1 to the immediate right of the sternum at the fourth intercostal space (ALS-Assist Skills A1-3B).
5. Place lead V_2 to the immediate left of the sternum at the fourth intercostal space (ALS-Assist Skills A1-3C).
6. Out of order, next place lead V_4 to the left midclavicular line at the fifth intercostal space (ALS-Assist Skills A1-3D).
7. Place lead V_3 midway between lead V_2 and V_4 on the left anterior chest (ALS-Assist Skills A1-3E).
8. Place lead V_5 to the left anterior axillary line at the same level as V_4 (ALS-Assist Skills A1-3F).

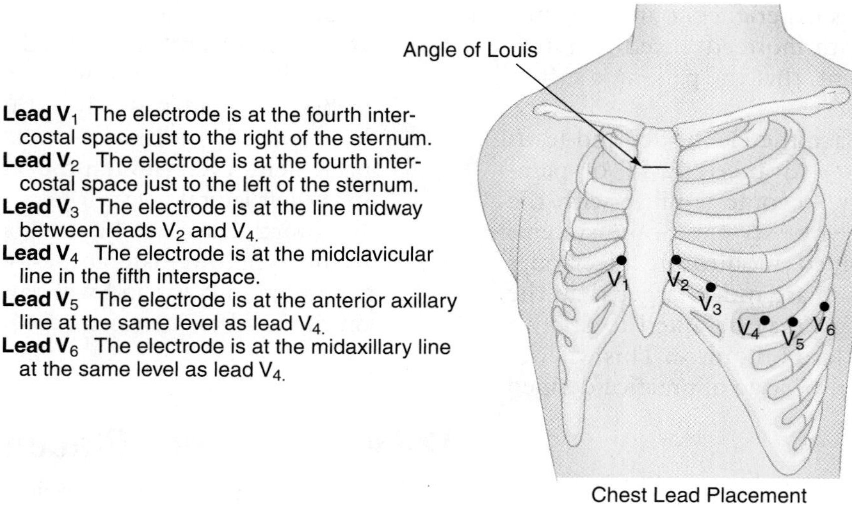

Angle of Louis

Lead V_1 The electrode is at the fourth intercostal space just to the right of the sternum.
Lead V_2 The electrode is at the fourth intercostal space just to the left of the sternum.
Lead V_3 The electrode is at the line midway between leads V_2 and V_4.
Lead V_4 The electrode is at the midclavicular line in the fifth interspace.
Lead V_5 The electrode is at the anterior axillary line at the same level as lead V_4.
Lead V_6 The electrode is at the midaxillary line at the same level as lead V_4.

V_1 V_2 V_3 V_4 V_5 V_6

Chest Lead Placement

FIGURE A1-2 * Proper placement of the precordial leads.

9. Place lead V_6 to the left midaxillary line at the same level as V_4 and V_5 (ALS-Assist Skills A1-3G).
10. Check to ensure that all leads are properly placed, especially the precordial leads (Figure A1-2*) and that all of the leads are properly adhering and are making good contact with the skin.

As an EMT, there may be other skills that you are asked to assist the Advanced EMT or paramedic with during the call. Be sure you are familiar with the equipment and that you have been properly trained in applying or setting up the equipment before doing so. The intent of your assistance is to save valuable time in providing an intervention, as with the intravenous line, or in gaining clinical information about the patient, as in the case of the ECG monitor. Follow your local protocols in determining what assistance you can provide.

ALS-Assist skills A1-1

Assisting with IV Administration

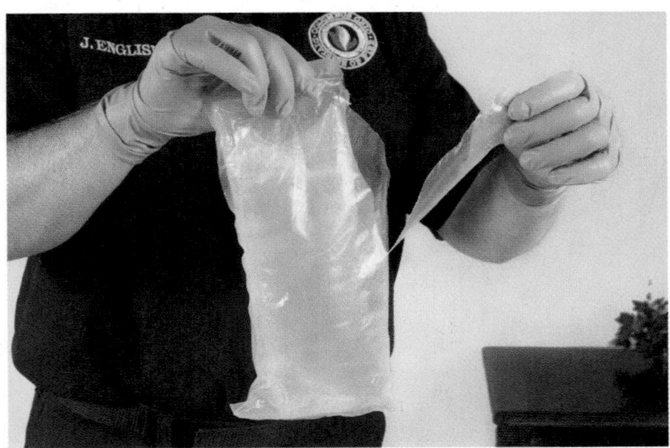

A1-1A ✱ Remove the protective covering from the IV bag.

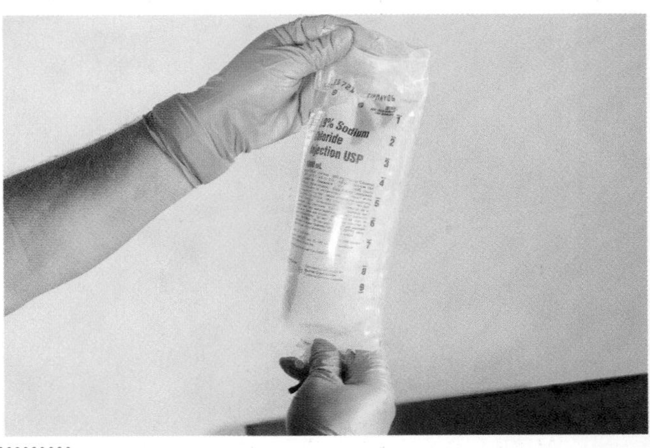

A1-1B ✱ Inspect the IV fluid for impurities, particulate matter, and discoloration and check the expiration date.

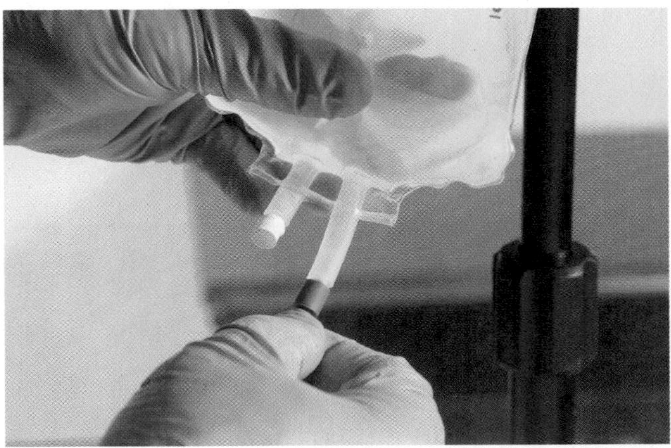

A1-1C ✱ Remove the protective covering from the spike.

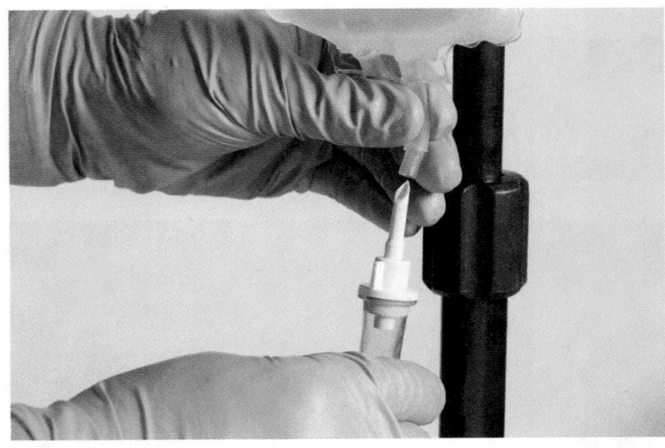

A1-1D ✱ Spike the IV bag.

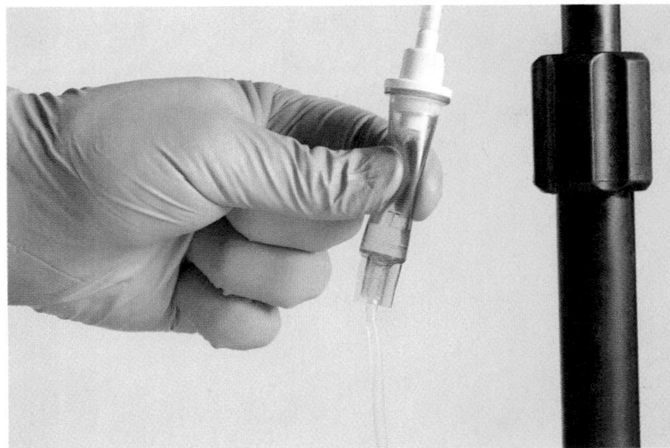

A1-1E ✱ Fill the drip chamber to the marker line.

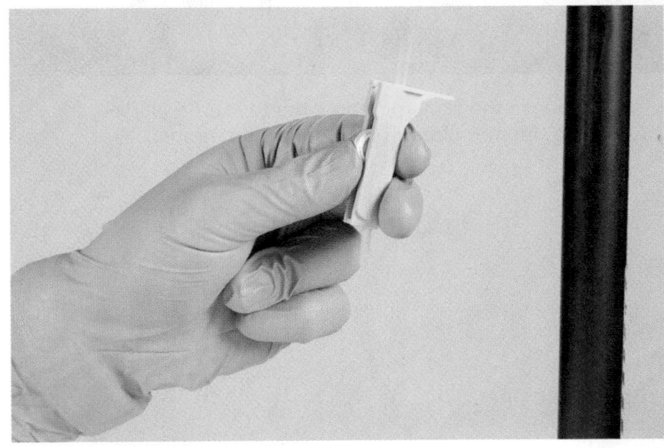

A1-1F ✱ Open the flow regulator to flush the IV tubing of all air.

ALS-Assist skills A1-2 ECG 3-Lead Placement

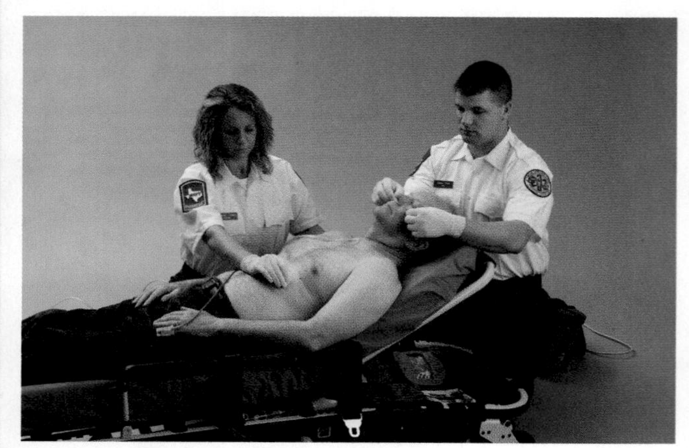

A1-2A ✻ Cleanse the skin.

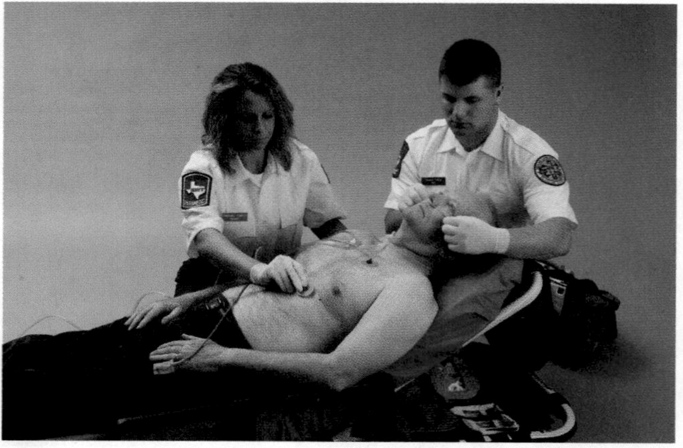

A1-2B ✻ Apply the limb-lead electrodes according to the manufacturer's recommendations.

ALS-Assist skills A1-3 ECG 12-Lead Placement

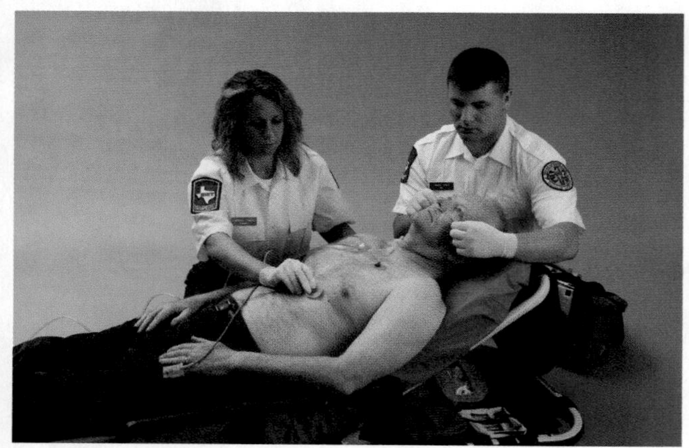

A1-3A ✻ Cleanse the skin and apply the four limb leads according to the manufacturer's recommendations.

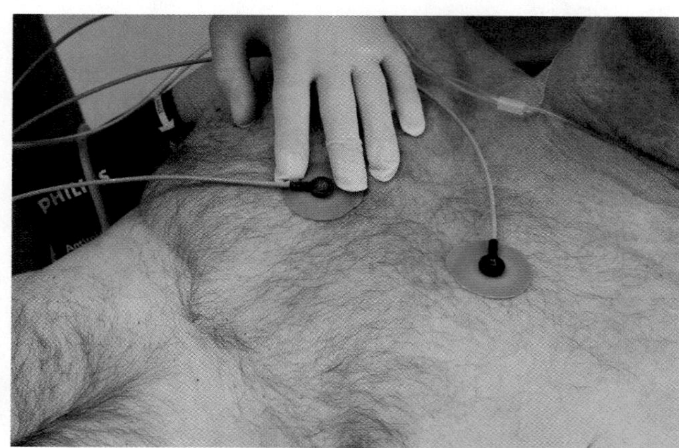

A1-3B ✻ Place lead V_1.

ECG 12-Lead Placement *continued*

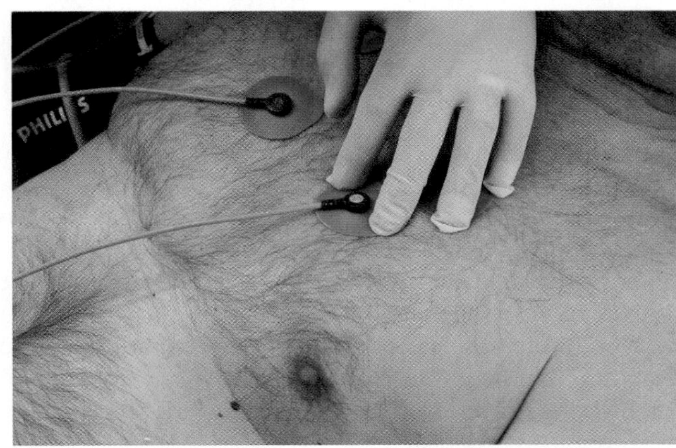

A1-3C * Place lead V_2.

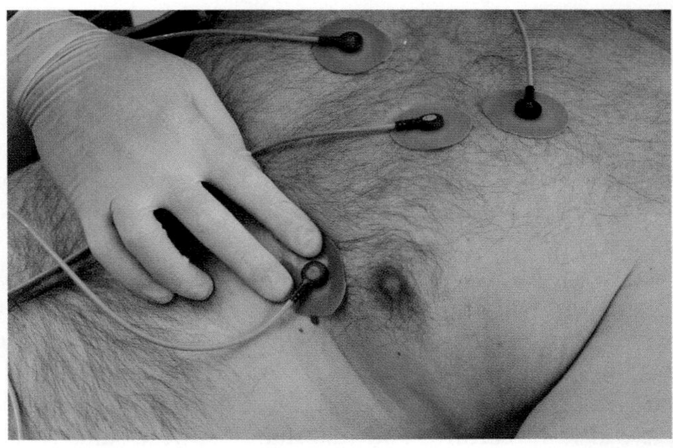

A1-3D * Place lead V_4.

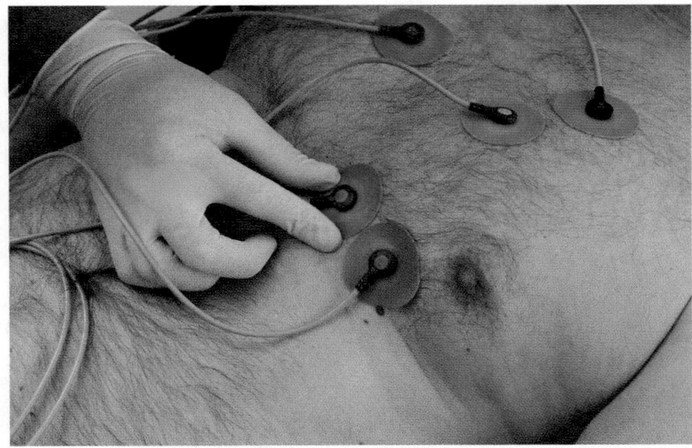

A1-3E * Place lead V_3.

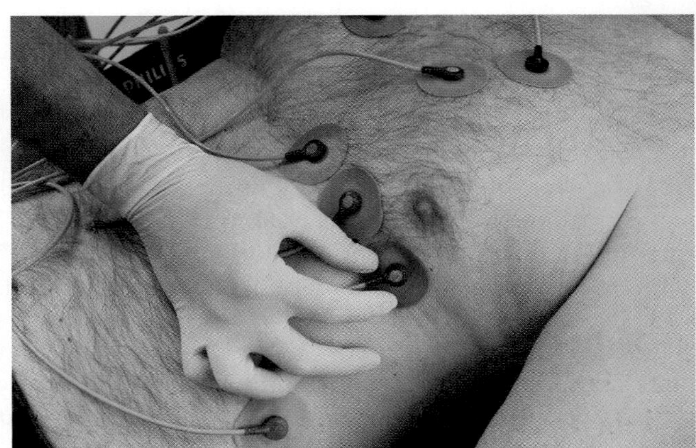

A1-3F * Place lead V_5.

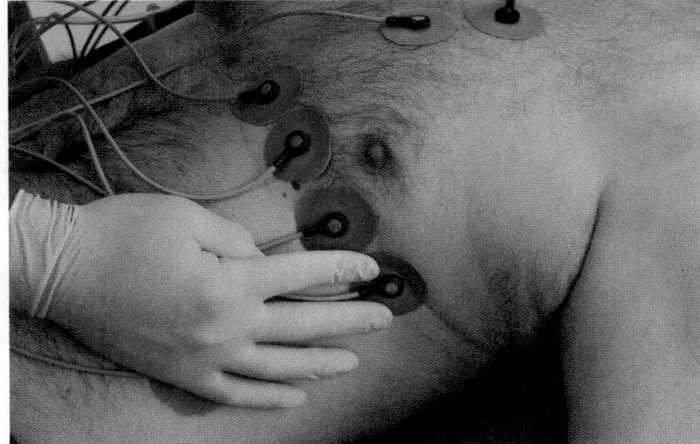

A1-3G * Place lead V_6.

Appendix 2 Advanced Airway Management

There are some situations in which manual maneuvers and basic airway adjuncts are not adequate to maintain or possibly even to establish an airway. In those situations, the use of advanced airway adjuncts is necessary.

Advanced airway skills are not included in the National EMS Scope of Practice for the EMT and can only be performed if the EMT is specifically trained and at the discretion of the medical director and local jurisdiction. If allowed by your medical director and local jurisdiction, you will find learning and maintaining these skills to be challenging.

Airway and Respiratory Anatomy and Physiology

The basic anatomy and physiology of the airway and respiratory system have already been discussed in Chapter 7, "Anatomy, Physiology, and Medical Terminology," Chapter 10, "Airway Management, Artificial Ventilation, and Oxygenation," and Chapter 16, "Respiratory Emergencies." However, advanced airway management requires a more detailed understanding of upper airway anatomy, because many anatomical landmarks there must be visualized and identified when performing certain maneuvers. Also, to use various pieces of equipment correctly, it is necessary to understand their relationship to the parts of the upper airway.

Airway Anatomy

The respiratory system is made up of the upper and lower airway. The upper airway extends from the opening of the nose and mouth down to the larynx. It includes the nasopharynx, oropharynx, and hypopharynx, which is also called the laryngopharynx. The lower airway continues from the inferior (lower) portion of the larynx and consists of the trachea and bronchi. The bronchi branch out, treelike, into the bronchioles and terminate at the alveoli of the lungs.

Nose, Mouth, and Pharynx

The nose is the superior (upper) part of the airway and has several functions: (1) it warms and humidifies the air, (2) it serves as a passageway for inhaled air, and (3) its nasal hairs serve as an initial filter of foreign bodies. The air entering the nose passes through the nasopharynx, the area of the throat just behind the nose.

The mouth also serves as a conduit for airflow. Air enters the mouth and passes into the oropharynx, the area of the throat just behind the mouth. The reflexes of the oropharynx protect the airway in the responsive patient; however, in the unresponsive patient, the mandibular and submandibular muscles relax and allow the tongue to drop into the posterior pharynx, causing a potentially life-threatening obstruction.

The openings of the esophagus and larynx begin at the level of the hypopharynx (or laryngopharynx). The esophagus is an oval, hollow, tubelike structure that lies posterior to (behind) the larynx and trachea. The openings to the esophagus (which leads to the stomach) and the larynx (which is part of the airway to the lungs) are very close together, and this—as you will learn during this chapter—is the reason for a number of the complications involved in establishing an airway and ventilating a patient.

Larynx

The larynx, which contains the vocal cords and is the major organ of speech, lies inferior to the pharynx and superior to the trachea. It connects and allows air to travel from the pharynx into the trachea. The larynx is composed of three cartilaginous structures: the thyroid cartilage, the cricoid cartilage, and the epiglottis.

The thyroid cartilage is the bulky, shieldlike structure—commonly known as the Adam's apple—that is found at the anterior (front) portion of the neck. The cricoid cartilage is a firm circle of cartilage that is located below the thyroid cartilage. The cricoid is attached by ligaments to the first ring of the trachea. Immediately posterior to the cricoid is the esophagus. When performing advanced airway techniques, it is sometimes useful to occlude, or close off, the esophagus. This can be accomplished by applying pressure directly to the cricoid ring to push it back against the esophagus.

The epiglottis is a leaf-shaped cartilaginous structure (consisting of cartilage, a gristlelike tissue) that covers the opening of the larynx during swallowing. When a person swallows, the muscles of the larynx contract and move the epiglottis downward and the larynx upward, closing the opening and preventing food and liquid from entering the trachea. A depression that is located between the base of the tongue and the epiglottis is known as the vallecula. The glossoepiglottic ligament, which helps support and suspend the epiglottis, is found in the center of the val-

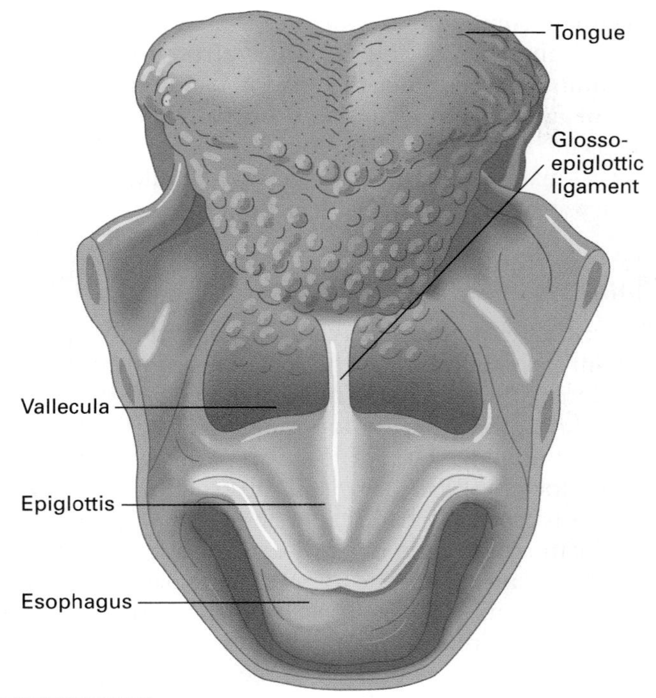

FIGURE A2-1 * The epiglottis.

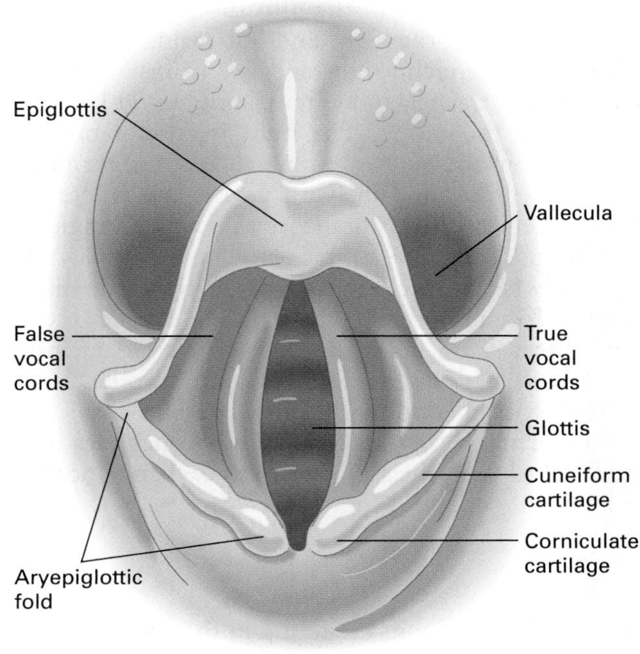

FIGURE A2-2 * The glottis.

lecula (Figure A2-1*). The vallecula and glossoepiglottic ligament are important anatomical structures that are sometimes manipulated to indirectly lift the epiglottis, making it possible to visualize the vocal cords and glottic opening during advanced airway management.

The vocal cords are located in the larynx. The true vocal cords, which are normally pale and pearly white, regulate the flow of air into the trachea and produce sounds by vibrating. The space between the true vocal cords is the glottis or glottic opening (Figure A2-2*). The glottic area is covered by the epiglottis during swallowing. The false vocal cords lie above the true vocal cords. The true and false vocal cords can close the glottic opening, preventing air or foreign bodies from entering the trachea. This serves a protective function but can also cause an obstruction by blocking airflow in some conditions.

The larynx also contains three sets of paired cartilages (Figure A2-2). The arytenoids are irregular, pyramid-shaped structures located on the superior aspect of the posterior cricoid ring. The corniculates are cone-shaped and are attached to the top of the arytenoids. The cuneiforms are more elongated and are attached to the posterior arytenoids. These structures are extremely important in advanced airway maneuvers where visualization of the glottic opening is required.

The pertinent glottic structures that the EMT should visualize and identify during intubation are (1) the epiglottis, which will comprise the anterior border of the glottic opening; (2) the true vocal cords, which form the lateral borders of the glottic opening; and (3) the arytenoid cartilages, which form the posterior border of the glottic opening. Additionally, the EMT should be able to see the cartilaginous rings, which comprise the trachea inferior to the glottic opening. Directly posterior to these structures, the EMT should also be able to visualize the esophagus.

As already noted, the openings of the larynx and of the esophagus are in close proximity, making incorrect placement of a tracheal tube a common error. It is also a *serious* error. Inadvertent placement of a tracheal tube in the esophagus instead of the trachea means that the stomach rather than the lungs will receive the air during ventilation.

Fortunately, the cartilaginous structures just described provide landmarks to differentiate the opening of the larynx from that of the esophagus. One key difference between the two openings is that the esophagus does not have cartilage surrounding its opening as does the larynx. Therefore, before inserting a tube into the larynx, it is imperative to identify the cartilaginous structures and vocal cords to ensure that you are directing the tube into the larynx and trachea, not the esophagus.

Trachea, Bronchi, and Bronchioles

The trachea extends from the lower portion of the larynx to the bronchi. The trachea has 16–20 incomplete C-shaped cartilage rings on its anterior surface that support the airway and prevent it from collapsing. The trachea is shaped like the letter D with the straight edge on the posterior side. The C-shaped cartilage rings are joined together by fibrous and elastic tissue. Posteriorly, the trachealis muscle, a muscular wall that closes the C-shaped rings, abuts the esophagus, which lies directly posterior.

At about the level of the fifth thoracic vertebra, the trachea splits into the right and left mainstem bronchi. This point, where the right and left mainstem bronchi split from the trachea and enter the right and left lungs, is known as the carina. The right mainstem bronchus branches from the trachea at a much lesser angle and appears to be almost in a line with the trachea, whereas the left mainstem bronchus branches at a greater angle. Because of this difference, aspiration of food, liquids, or foreign bodies is far more common on the right side than on the left. More important, the lesser angle makes it easier to misdirect a tracheal tube into the right mainstem bronchus than in the left if it is advanced too far.

The bronchi continue to subdivide into smaller passages known as the bronchioles. The bronchioles terminate at the alveoli, the sacs where gas exchange occurs in the lungs.

Lungs

The right and left lungs are found in the thoracic (chest) cavity. They are separated by the space called the mediastinum, which contains the heart and other structures and tissues. The right lung has three lobes and the left lung has two lobes. The lungs contain the alveoli and supporting tissue. Both lungs are covered by the pleura. The pleura consists of two layers, the inner visceral pleura and the outer parietal pleura. Between the layers of the pleura is a small amount of pleural fluid, which acts as a lubricant that reduces friction when the lungs move during respiration. There is also a negative (or subatmospheric) pressure between these layers, which causes the lungs to expand as the thoracic cavity expands from intercostal and diaphragmatic muscle contraction. The diaphragm is located at the base of the thoracic cavity and separates the chest from the abdominal cavity. The diaphragm is the major muscle of respiration, providing roughly 60 percent of the effort needed for normal breathing.

The mechanics and physiology of respiration were discussed in Chapter 7, "Anatomy, Physiology, and Medical Terminology," and Chapter 10, "Airway Management, Artificial Ventilation, and Oxygenation."

Airway Anatomy in Infants and Children

There are considerable differences between the airways of adults and those of infants and children. These differences are extremely important to remember when performing advanced airway maneuvers on patients in these age groups.

Head

The head of an infant is much larger in proportion to its body than that of an adult. Because the head is larger, especially the occiput (back of the head), when an infant is placed in a supine position its head tilts forward, flexing the neck and constricting the airway structures. Any type of padding placed under the head in children less than 9 years of age may cause an airflow obstruction. For infants and young children, in fact, it is commonly necessary to place a small, folded towel under the shoulders to keep the airway aligned and ensure airflow.

Mouth, Nose, and Pharynx

The structures in these areas are smaller and more pliable in infants and children and thus more easily obstructed by secretions, foreign objects, and swelling. The infant is basically a nose breather during much of his first year because of the more superior location of the epiglottis and anterior location of the larynx, so obstruction of the nasal passages is especially critical.

The most common cause of airway obstruction in the infant or young child is the tongue falling back and blocking the pharynx. This is an even greater problem in infants and children than in adults because the child's tongue is larger in proportion to the mouth and pharynx and the jaw is less prominent. When the muscles of the pharynx relax, the tongue is pulled back like a valve during inspiration, causing an obstruction. The larger tongue also interferes with visualization of anatomical structures during tracheal intubation.

Larynx

The airway of the infant and child is narrowest at the level of the cricoid cartilage. Also, that cartilage is less developed and less rigid than in adults. This is important to keep in mind during tracheal intubation. The tube may pass easily through the vocal cords but be too large to fit through the cricoid ring. Therefore, it is necessary to have tracheal tubes available that are at least one half-size larger and smaller than the one you estimate is correctly sized when performing this procedure. Pressure on the cricoid and overextension or overflexion of the neck can cause an obstruction.

Trachea and Bronchi

The major airways are narrower and shorter in infants and children. The trachea is also softer and more flexible. This means that the airway can be more easily occluded by swelling and other obstructions or kinked by flexion or extension of the neck. Small movements of the head or neck may also cause a tracheal tube to advance into the right mainstem bronchus or out of the glottis.

Chest Wall and Diaphragm

The chest wall in infants and children is softer and more flexible than in adults. Infants and children also have a tendency to rely more heavily on the diaphragm for breathing.

Summary of Pediatric Airway Considerations

As just discussed, there are important anatomical and physiological differences between the pediatric and adult airway that factor not only into how you assess the airway but also into how you manage the airway.

Remember that infants are obligate nose breathers, and therefore a nasal obstruction may be a critical airway occlusion. Recall also that the tongue is proportionally larger in the oral cavity, and the mandibular muscles that support it may not be fully developed. This combination allows the tongue to become a formidable obstruction in an unresponsive pediatric patient. These conditions, in conjunction with the larger occipital region of the head, easily allow the tongue to block the airway when the neck flexes in the supine, unresponsive pediatric patient. Additionally, the glottic opening is positioned more cephalad (toward the head) and more anterior than in the adult, which makes direct visualization of glottic structures more challenging during advanced airway procedures.

The ribs and intercostal muscles are usually more pliable and less developed than in the adult, so when there are increased demands on the pediatric pulmonary system, these muscles may fail to adequately support the lungs, which will allow a more rapid onset of respiratory distress and progression to respiratory failure. The pediatric patient consumes oxygen at a rate roughly double that of the adult patient, so hypoxemia occurs rapidly during periods of hypoventilation.

Recent studies have shown that pediatric patients under 14 years of age have better outcomes when managed with bag-valve-mask ventilation than with intubation. Therefore, pediatric patients should be intubated only when BVM is unsuccessful.

▶ Basic Airway Management

One of the situations in which advanced airway management techniques are of great use is when prolonged ventilation of a patient becomes necessary. Some advanced airways reduce problems of poor mask seal and of hand fatigue from holding a mask seal for a prolonged period or performing one- or two-handed bag-valve ventilation. Before using advanced airway management, however, you must first determine whether a patient is breathing adequately or inadequately.

Methods of assessing for adequate or inadequate breathing were discussed in Chapter 10, "Airway Management, Artificial Ventilation, and Oxygenation," and Chapter 16, "Respiratory Emergencies."

The first step in airway management is to establish a patent airway by using a manual maneuver. The head-tilt, chin-lift maneuver is used in the patient with no suspected spinal injury. The jaw-thrust maneuver is used in a trauma patient or any patient with suspected spinal injury. If any blood, secretions, vomitus, or other substances are in the airway, you must suction them immediately to prevent aspiration. Two basic mechanical airway adjuncts, the oropharyngeal and the nasopharyngeal airways, can be inserted to help maintain the airway. You can review these basic methods of establishing and maintaining an airway in Chapter 10.

Basic airway techniques must be employed prior to advanced airway management. There are some conditions where immediate use of an advanced airway technique is necessary, as in upper airway burns and in anaphylaxis, where swelling of the larynx requires immediate insertion of a tracheal tube through the larynx and into the trachea. In most situations, however, if the basic steps of airway management and ventilation are omitted and advanced procedures are performed instead, the patient can become dangerously hypoxic and suffer irreversible consequences. The patient can utilize the oxygen that was made available during basic airway management and ventilation during insertion of the advanced airway.

For the most part, advanced airway management techniques are used for the following reasons: when it is necessary to protect the patient from aspiration of secretions, blood, or vomitus; when prolonged ventilation by the EMT is necessary; or when basic airway management techniques are not adequate. Remember, though, that in these situations, the airway is initially controlled with basic techniques while the patient is being ventilated and oxygenated and the necessary equipment is being prepared.

Although advanced airway management is often performed under highly stressful circumstances when the patient's life is threatened by the compromised or potentially compromised airway, bear in mind that airway management procedures can be extremely frightening and uncomfortable to the patient (even if minimally responsive) or to the patient's family. These procedures are rarely performed in an awake patient without sedation.

Oropharyngeal Suctioning

Before you use any advanced airway techniques, remove any secretions, blood, vomitus, or other substances from the oropharynx with suction. If you hear a gurgling sound during ventilation, it is an indication that some liquid is in the airway and should be suctioned immediately. Some suction units cannot adequately remove heavy vomitus or solid objects, such as teeth, from the airway. You may have to sweep the mouth with your finger, a tongue blade, or the end of the rigid suction catheter to remove the vomitus or object.

A variety of suction units exist. It is vital that a portable suction unit, either electrical or hand operated, be available during airway management, especially when advanced airway procedures are to be performed. Hard, or rigid, suction catheters are used when suctioning the mouth and oropharynx. Soft, or French, suction catheters are useful for suctioning the nose and nasopharynx. Soft suction catheters are also used in clearing secretions from the trachea once a tracheal tube is in place (a technique that is discussed later in this appendix). Also note that as the lower structures are visualized, further suctioning may be required. Review oropharyngeal suctioning in Chapter 10.

Orotracheal Intubation

Orotracheal intubation (from *oro,* meaning "mouth," and *tracheal,* referring to the trachea) is the insertion of a tube through the mouth and along the oropharynx and larynx directly into the trachea. Because the distal end of the tube is designed to be placed in the trachea, it is referred to as a *tracheal tube* or *endotracheal tube* (from *endo,* meaning "into," and *tracheal,* referring to the trachea). The process of inserting the tube is known as intubation. The terms *orotracheal intubation, endotracheal intubation*, and *tracheal intubation* are often used almost interchangeably.

Orotracheal intubation requires the EMT to visualize anatomical landmarks with the use of a device called a *laryngoscope*. The laryngoscope, equipped with a light to aid in visualization, is inserted into the mouth and down into the pharynx. It is used to lift, either directly or indirectly, the epiglottis and to expose the vocal cords and glottic opening. The tracheal tube is then passed through the vocal cords and directly into the trachea.

Visualization of the tracheal tube as it enters and passes through the vocal cords is extremely important to reduce the risk of improper placement in the esophagus. The EMT must be completely familiar with techniques of properly placing the tracheal tube and must be able to differentiate immediately between a tracheal intubation and an esophageal intubation. If a tube is inadvertently placed in the esophagus, the patient's lungs will receive no ventilation or oxygen and the patient will die.

Advantages

Tracheal intubation is the most effective means of controlling the patient's airway. The following advantages make tracheal intubation the preferred method for controlling the airway in the apneic patient (patient who is not breathing):

- It provides complete control of the airway. The tracheal tube is placed into the trachea, establishing a direct route of ventilation and oxygenation. The tongue no longer threatens airway occlusion, so it is not necessary to maintain a head-tilt, chin-lift or jaw-thrust maneuver, allowing the EMT to focus on other critical tasks, such as ensuring that adequate tidal volumes are being delivered at an appropriate rate.
- The tracheal tube is designed to isolate the trachea, eliminating the risk of aspiration of material into the lower airways and lungs. Secretions, blood, vomitus, and other substances are blocked by the tracheal tube in the upper portion of the trachea and pharynx and kept from traveling farther down the airway. The substances can then be removed by suction.
- The tracheal tube permits better ventilation and oxygen delivery. The bag-valve device is connected directly to the tracheal tube, thus allowing more effective ventilation because air goes directly into the trachea and lungs. Because no mask seal is required, only one EMT is needed to perform two-handed bagging. Also, hazards associated with air entering the esophagus and subsequently the stomach are eliminated since the tube directs ventilation into the trachea and lungs.
- A suction catheter can be passed through the tracheal tube to allow for deeper suctioning of the trachea and bronchi. This removes secretions that the patient may not have been able to eliminate otherwise and effectively clears the airway.
- The tracheal tube with positive pressure ventilation can overcome both mechanical and physiological problems that compromise normal ventilation.

Indications

Not every patient requires tracheal intubation. It should be used only under certain conditions. Indications for its use include the following:

- *The EMT is unable to ventilate the apneic patient effectively with standard methods such as mouth-to-mask or bag-valve mask.* Establishing a good mask seal may be very difficult in some patients, especially those with trauma to the mouth or jaws. Sealing the mask may also be difficult in patients who have no teeth or dentures. A good seal is difficult to maintain during a long transport.
- *The patient cannot protect his own airway.* This includes patients who are unresponsive or in cardiac arrest. Whenever you determine that a patient is unable to protect his own airway, consider endotracheal intubation. Keep in mind that good basic airway maneuvers, basic airway devices, and suctioning are the preferred methods to manage the airway for the EMT. The patient who cannot protect his own airway is the patient who:
  - **Is unresponsive to any type of stimulus.** In a completely unresponsive patient, the muscles that control the tongue and epiglottis relax and easily occlude the airway. The patient cannot clear blood, vomitus, secretions, and other substances from his airway, and the risk of aspiration is high.
  - **Has no gag reflex or loses the cough reflex.** The gag and cough reflexes are very important in protecting the airway against foreign body occlusion and aspiration. The loss of these reflexes leaves the airway vulnerable to blockage or foreign body aspiration.

As a general rule, if you are able to insert an oropharyngeal airway in the patient without incident, you can assume that he has lost his gag reflex and cannot protect his airway; he is, therefore, a good candidate for tracheal intubation. Since the patient is unable to protect his own airway, have a suction device ready in case of vomiting. Provide adequate ventilation and oxygenation before any attempt at tracheal intubation.

Standard Precautions

When performing tracheal intubation, the EMT must get extremely close to the patient's open mouth and visualize deep into the airway. Contact with the patient's secretions, vomitus, and/or blood is likely during the intubation procedure. Put on gloves, eye protection, and a mask before attempting the procedure to avoid contact with body fluids.

Equipment

Several pieces of equipment are required for tracheal intubation. Check that the equipment is in proper working order before any attempt at intubation. The equipment needed for intubation includes the following:

- Laryngoscope (handle and blades)
- Tracheal tube
- Stylet
- Water-soluble lubricant
- 10 mL syringe
- Tracheal tube securing device
- Suction unit
- Towels or padding
- Stethoscope
- End-tidal CO_2 or esophageal detection device

Laryngoscope

The laryngoscope is inserted in the mouth and then into the hypopharynx where it is used to lift the epiglottis and provide visualization of the vocal cords and glottic opening. This procedure is known as laryngoscopy. Laryngoscopes may be reusable or disposable.

The laryngoscope has two components: the handle and the blade. The laryngoscope handle is a cylindrical device that contains batteries as a source of power. During intubation, the EMT holds the laryngoscope handle in his left hand and uses it to control the laryngoscope blade. The laryngoscope blade is the component that directly or indirectly lifts the epiglottis for visualization during intubation. A locking bar on the laryngoscope handle interfaces with a c-channel fitting at the base of the blade, which allows the two components to securely lock into each other, and which also enables the electrical circuit to the lighted end of the blade. A bulb is located in the distal third of the blade and serves as a light source to permit visualization of the glottic opening and the vocal cords. Fiber-optic laryngoscope handles have the light source in the handle and a fiber-optic strand in the blade to provide a bright light.

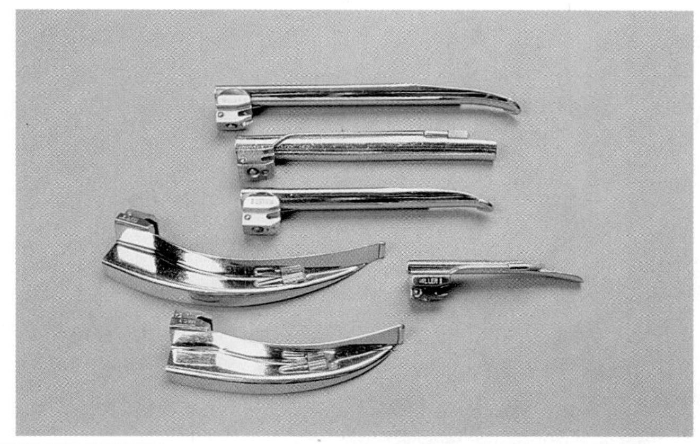

FIGURE A2-3 * Straight and curved laryngoscope blades.

Two types of laryngoscope blades are traditionally available: the straight blade (Miller, Wisconsin, or Flagg) or the curved blade (McIntosh) (Figure A2-3*). The name of the blade describes its shape. Both types of blades can lift the epiglottis, but each type does this differently. The choice of blade type is basically a matter of personal preference.

Straight Blade The straight blade is straight at the distal end and has a more rounded edge. The blade is narrower than the curved blade and has a hollow central channel. The straight blade comes in a variety of sizes ranging from 0, the smallest, to 4, the largest. A size 0 blade would be used on an infant, whereas a size 4 would be used to intubate a large adult.

The end (or distal edge) of the straight blade is fitted under (or posterior to) the epiglottis and directly lifts it to expose the vocal cords and glottic opening (Figure A2-4a*). During insertion, the rounded part of the blade is used to push the tongue over to the left side as the blade is brought into the midline of the mouth and oropharynx. The top of the straight blade is then used to gently lift the tip of the epiglottis. The hollow channel is used as a sight as the tracheal tube is advanced from the corner of the mouth and placed between the vocal cords and into the glottic opening. The channel is not used to advance the tube. Attempts to force the tracheal tube through the straight blade channel will likely result in damage to the tube and obstruct visualization of the vocal cords. If the tube is damaged, it is necessary to remove it and repeat the intubation process. During this time, the patient's airway is not protected.

The straight blade is preferred for performing intubation in infants and children. Because of the anatomical differences, the straight blade provides greater displacement of the tongue and better visualization of the vocal cords and glottic opening and causes less tissue damage in this age group. The straight blade is also preferred in larger patients with short, thick necks.

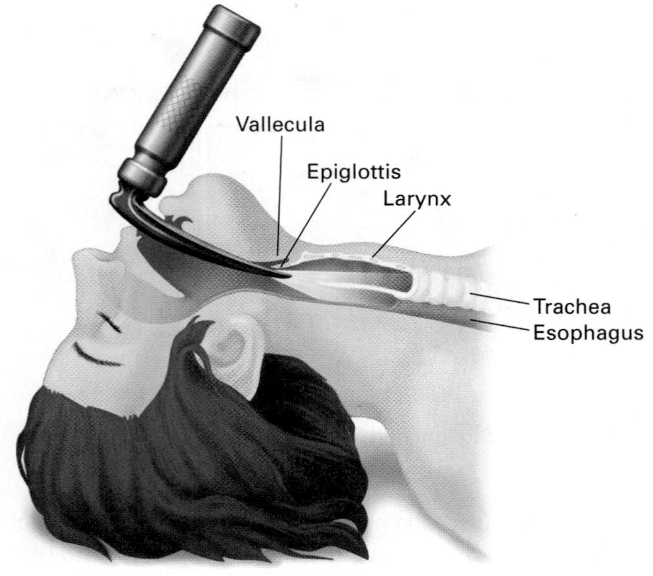

FIGURE A2-4a ✻ The straight blade is placed under the epiglottis. It directly lifts the epiglottis upward to expose the vocal cords and glottic opening.

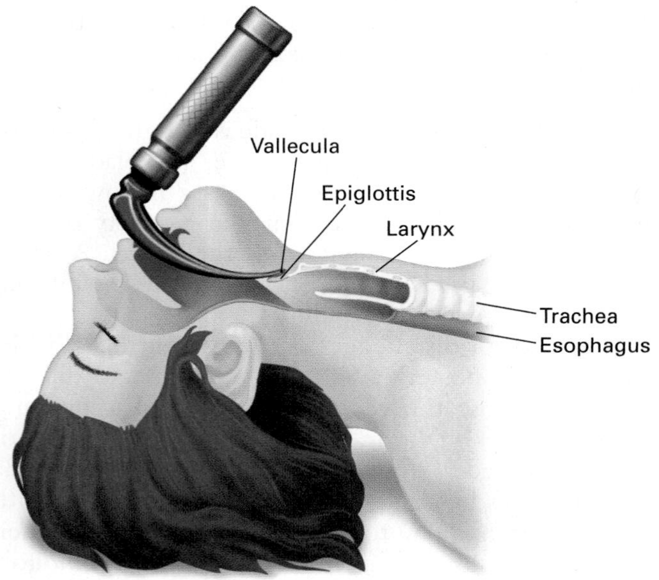

FIGURE A2-4b ✻ The curved blade is placed into the vallecula and indirectly lifts the epiglottis.

Curved Blade The curved blade is curved at the distal end and has a beaded or blunt edge. The blade has a broad surface and tall flange that is used to move and hold the tongue out of the way during intubation (Figure A2-4b✻). The curved blade also comes in a variety of sizes ranging from 0 for the infant to 4 for the large adult.

The beaded end of the curved blade is inserted into the vallecula, the space located between the epiglottis and base of the tongue. When the edge of the blade is placed in the vallecula it presses on the glossoepiglottic ligament, causing the epiglottis to be indirectly lifted upward and exposing the vocal cords and glottic opening.

Alternative Blades Newer, redesigned blades that share some of the features of the straight and curved blades have come to market in the past several years. These newer blades, as well as some adjunctive intubation equipment, are discussed later in this appendix.

Assembly The indentation on the laryngoscope blade is designed to lock onto the bar of the laryngoscope handle. The blade is lifted upward so it is at a right angle to the handle. The electrical connection is then made and the bulb at the end of the blade is lit. Check to be sure that it is on. The light should be tight, bright, and white. If it is not, check that the blade is securely locked. The bulb must be tightly screwed into the socket of the blade. If the bulb is loose, tighten it. If the light is not bright and white, it may also be necessary to change the batteries in the handle. It is best to check the equipment daily and always to have an extra bulb and batteries available in case of failure.

In fiber-optic laryngoscope handles and blades, the fiber-optic light source is located in the handle. The blade contains a fiber-optic strand, rather than a bulb, to provide illumination at the end of the blade. This provides a brighter light source for visualizing the glottic structures.

Tracheal Tubes

The tracheal tube is a flexible, translucent tube made of polyvinyl chloride that is open at both ends. Tracheal tubes come in a variety of sizes (Figure A2-5✻). The size noted on the outside of the tube is the tube's internal diameter (i.d.). The external diameter is estimated by adding 2–3 mm to the internal diameter size. In general, an adult male will require an 8.0–8.5 mm i.d. tube and the adult female will take a 7.0–8.0 mm i.d. tube. Tube sizes for infants and children range from 2.5–6.0 mm i.d.

If you are uncertain what size to use, it is prudent to select a smaller-sized tube. In an emergency, a 7.5 mm

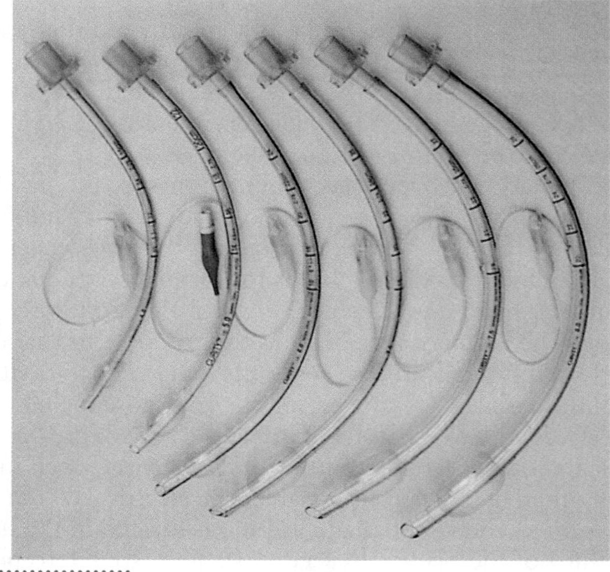

FIGURE A2-5 ✻ An assortment of tracheal tubes of different sizes.

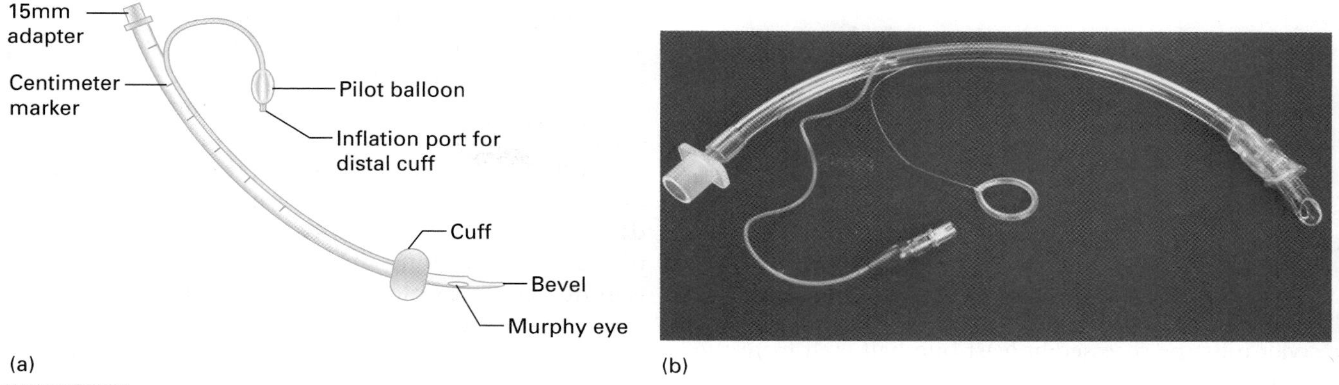

FIGURE A2-6 ✱ **(a)** Tracheal tube components. **(b)** An Endotrol tube has a trigger-type device that lifts the end of the tube upward to facilitate placement in the glottic opening.

i.d. tube will usually fit either an adult male or an adult female. When intubating, it is helpful to have available tubes one size smaller and one size larger than the estimated size.

The tracheal tube has several components (Figure A2-6✱). At the proximal end, a 15 mm connector allows attachment of a bag-valve and other ventilation devices. The distal end has a cuff that serves to seal off the trachea. An inflation line extends up the main tube to a pilot balloon that verifies that the cuff is inflated. A one-way inflation valve allows use of a syringe to inflate the cuff. The cuff will hold approximately 10 mL of air. The cuff should be inflated to prevent any leakage of air from around the cuff and the tracheal tube and between the tube and the tracheal wall. Typically, tubes for infants and children under 8 years of age have no cuff at the distal end and are referred to as uncuffed. The i.d. sizes for these uncuffed tracheal tubes are usually less than 6.0 mm. Uncuffed tubes are usually used in this age bracket because the narrowest portion of the airway is the cricoid ring and not the vocal cords as in an adult. In the hospital setting, it has been found that cuffed tracheal tubes can also be used safely for infants beyond the newborn age. In this environment, the use of a cuffed tracheal tube may be preferable in situations of poor lung compliance or high airway resistance. However, greater attention needs to be given to the selected tracheal tube size, the position of the cuff, and the pressure in the cuff once inflated. Because of these particularities, the use of a cuffed tracheal tube by the EMT in the prehospital environment may not be common practice.

At the distal end of the tracheal tube is a Murphy eye. This is a small hole on the side opposite the beveled side. The eye lessens the chance of complete tube obstruction. If the distal end of the tube becomes obstructed by the tracheal wall, blood clots, or secretions, the Murphy eye will still allow air to escape and ventilation to take place.

The length of the tube from the distal end is indicated in centimeter (cm) markings along the tube. The length of the tube for the adult is 33 cm. Following placement of the tube in the adult, the 22 cm marker is typically at the level of the teeth. The level should be documented on the prehospital report. This is only a general rule and does not apply to all patients because of variations in their sizes. Other standard measurements are: 15 cm from the teeth to the vocal cords; 20 cm from the teeth to the sternal notch; and 25 cm from the teeth to the carina.

The measurements are helpful, but you must rely on good clinical assessment skills to determine that the tube is properly placed. When properly placed, the distal tip of the tracheal tube is in the trachea and midway between the carina and the vocal cords and good equal breath sounds are heard over both lungs with rise of the chest observed. The tip of the tube must not extend past the carina. If the tube is inserted beyond the carina, it will most likely enter the right mainstem bronchus (because it is straighter and at a lesser angle from the trachea than the left mainstem bronchus) and only ventilate the right lung. This is referred to as a right mainstem intubation, a common complication of tracheal intubation.

Once you verify that the tube is correctly placed, it is extremely important to note the centimeter level marking on the tube at the teeth and record it on the prehospital report. This should be reverified any time the patient is moved or transferred. If at any time the level marking has changed, it is an indication that the tube has been inserted deeper or has been pulled back. *You must then immediately reassess tube placement.* The tube can become dislodged and end up either in the right mainstem bronchus if pushed farther down or, worse, in the esophagus if pulled upward and then pushed down again. Continuous reassessment of tube placement is necessary.

Stylet

The malleable stylet is a piece of pliable metal wire, typically coated with plastic, that is inserted into the tracheal tube to alter its shape and provide stiffness (Figure A2-7✱). The stylet should be lubricated with a water-soluble jelly prior to insertion in the tube to facilitate easy removal. The stylet should not be inserted beyond the Murphy eye and should never extend or project out of the distal end of the tracheal tube. This could lead to severe trauma to the

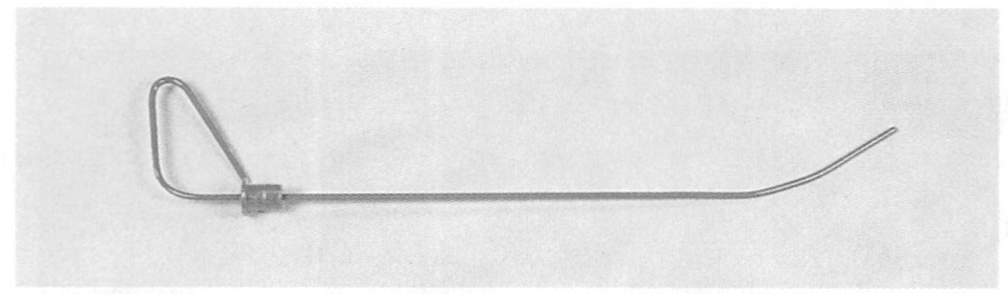

FIGURE A2-7 ✱ The stylet is inserted into the tube to provide stiffness and shape the tube. It should not extend past the end of the tube.

airway and trachea from accidental perforation. The end of the stylet must be recessed at least one-half inch from the distal end of the tube. To ensure proper stylet position, recess the stylet at least one-quarter inch from the cuff or proximal end of the Murphy eye. Once the stylet is in place, it can be used to form the tube into a "hockey stick" shape to aid in proper insertion. After the tube is passed through the vocal cords, carefully remove the stylet, holding the tube securely to avoid dislodging it.

Other Intubation Equipment

Water-soluble lubricant is applied to the end of the tracheal tube to facilitate insertion and to the stylet to allow for easy removal. Tube displacement may result from pulling out a stylet that is not lubricated. Do not use petroleum-based lubricants, because they may damage the tracheal tube and can irritate and inflame the tracheal lining.

A 10 mL syringe is used to inflate the cuff at the distal end of the tracheal tube. Prior to insertion, check the cuff to ensure it is working properly by injecting 10 mL of air into the inflation port. It is then necessary to deflate the cuff completely by pulling back on the plunger of the syringe while ensuring that the syringe is firmly engaged into the one-way inflation valve before inserting the tube. During intubation, leave the syringe attached to the inflation port. Once the tube is in place, use the syringe to inflate the cuff, and then immediately remove the syringe. The cuff can deflate if the syringe is left attached. Assess cuff inflation by checking the volume of air in the pilot balloon. Being able to seal the trachea through cuff inflation is a primary advantage of the tracheal tube. Monitor constantly to ensure that inflation is maintained. Keep the syringe near in case readjustment is needed.

Once the tracheal tube is properly positioned, you must secure it. Movement of the patient or attachment or removal of the ventilation device can cause the tube to become dislodged and end up in the esophagus or mainstem bronchus. The cuff on the tracheal tube seals the trachea; it does not secure the tube in place. There are, however, a variety of devices available to do this job. You can employ an elaborate commercial device or simply use tape. Follow your local protocol or medical direction's advice for securing the tube.

The tracheal tube is flexible enough so that if the patient should bite down or clench his teeth, the tube will be crimped and occluded. An oral airway or bite block should be inserted after the tracheal tube has been successfully placed to avoid this problem, especially if the patient begins breathing on his own or becomes more responsive after being intubated. Some commercially available securing devices contain a bite block.

A suction unit must be available during tracheal intubation to clear any fluid, vomitus, blood, secretions, or debris from the oral cavity. A large-bore catheter is needed for suctioning the oropharynx. Once the patient is intubated, a flexible French catheter is used for tracheal suction (as is described later).

Towels may be placed under the patient's shoulders or back of the head to help align the airway axis for easier visualization during intubation. In patients with suspected spinal injury, you must maintain stabilization of the head in a neutral, in-line position during intubation.

Ensuring proper tube placement is of utmost importance when performing this skill. The EMT should utilize both clinical assessment findings and confirmation devices to ensure that the tracheal tube is placed properly. Initially, tube placement should be confirmed during the intubation procedure. Since the EMT is only allowed to perform visual orotracheal intubation, the tip of the tracheal tube should have been seen passing between the vocal cords. Following placement, the tube is further assessed by auscultation of the epigastrium and the chest. An end-tidal CO_2 and esophageal detector device are additional tracheal tube confirmatory devices used after auscultation to ensure proper tube placement. Confirmation of tracheal tube placement occurs when the EMT *does not* hear sounds of air entering the stomach when listening over the epigastrium, and *does* hear sounds of air entering the lungs bilaterally. In addition, the end-tidal carbon dioxide detector should register the presence of exhaled carbon dioxide. If the esophageal detector is used, it should rapidly reinflate.

Cricoid Pressure

Cricoid pressure, also known as the Sellick maneuver (Figure A2-8✱), was once thought to effectively reduce complications associated with positive pressure ventilation with a pocket mask, bag-valve mask, or other device when the airway of an unresponsive patient is not protected by an advanced airway device. The technique was intended to reduce the incidence of gastric inflation, regurgitation, and aspiration of gastric contents.

According to the *2010 American Heart Association Guidelines for Cardiopulmonary Resuscitation and Emergency Cardiovascular Care*, cricoid pressure is not recommended for routine use, but it can be applied to facilitate insertion of an endotracheal tube in the adult patient. In the pediatric patient, cricoid pressure can be considered only if an extra EMT is available to apply the pressure without compromising the airway or effectiveness of ventilation and to guard against collapse of the trachea from excessive pressure.

Cricoid pressure may be applied to facilitate visualization of the glottic opening, the laryngeal opening that leads to the trachea, where an endotracheal tube is inserted during intubation (laryngoscopy). The backward pressure displaces the larynx posteriorly, allowing the intubator a better view of the opening. A paramedic or other advanced practitioner may ask you to apply cricoid pressure during laryngoscopy Once the endotracheal tube is in place, the cricoid pressure is released.

The technique to perform cricoid pressure is:

1. Locate the thyroid cartilage (Adam's apple) by starting at the chin and sliding your index and middle finger slowly toward the feet until you feel the obvious cartilage prominence.
2. Continue to slide your fingers downward until you feel the base of the thyroid cartilage and, below it, a small, soft midline indentation, the cricothyroid membrane. Immediately below the cricothyroid membrane is the bulky cricoid cartilage.
3. Place your index finger on one side of the cricoid cartilage, your thumb on the other side, and apply firm backward pressure.

The cricoid cartilage is the only complete cartilaginous ring (review Figure A2-8). When forced backward, it may collapse the esophagus behind it against the cervical vertebrae. A collapsed esophagus may prevent air from traveling down to inflate the stomach and may also prevent stomach contents from moving up. In this way, cricoid pressure protects the airway from regurgitation and consequent aspiration of stomach contents and also protects against gastric inflation. If the patient starts to regurgitate, release the cricoid pressure to prevent an esophageal tear. Immediately turn the patient onto his side, if possible, and suction the airway until clear.

Slow, sustained ventilation over a 1-second period with a controlled tidal volume is the best method to reduce the incidence of gastric inflation. Additionally, proper and adequate positioning of the airway with the head-tilt, chin-lift maneuver will reduce the amount of resistance in the airway and allow more of the ventilation to flow down the trachea and into the lungs instead of down the esophagus and into the stomach.

Tracheal Tube Insertion in an Adult

When properly placed, the tracheal tube is the only adjunct that will ensure an airway. However, if it is misplaced, the tube can contribute to rapid deterioration and death. You must become completely competent in orotracheal intubation during your education program. As a certified EMT, you must continuously review and practice the technique. This is one of the most critical and complicated skills that you will ever perform.

The steps for orotracheal intubation are as follows (Advanced Airway Management Skills A2-1A to A2-1H):

1. The person performing the intubation should take the necessary Standard Precautions, including wearing gloves, eye protection, and a mask.
2. Prior to any intubation attempt, the patient must be adequately ventilated with a bag-valve-mask device and a high concentration of supplemental oxygen to achieve hyperoxygenation of the patient.
3. Ventilate the patient for 2 minutes before the intubation attempt.
4. Gather the necessary equipment for inserting and securing the tube, assemble it, and test it.
   a. Test the cuff on the tracheal tube by injecting 10 mL of air into the inflation port with a syringe and feeling the cuff to ensure that it is inflated fully and does not automatically deflate. Then deflate the cuff by withdrawing all of the air with the syringe. Leave the syringe attached to the inflation port. The tracheal tube should be kept in its packaging, if possible, while checking the cuff to avoid any unnecessary contamination.

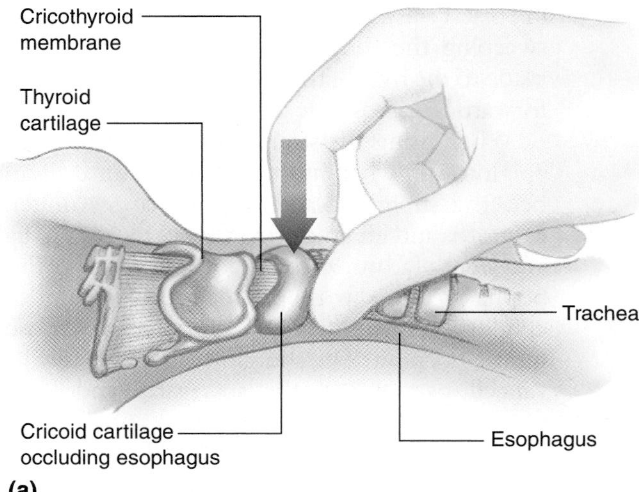

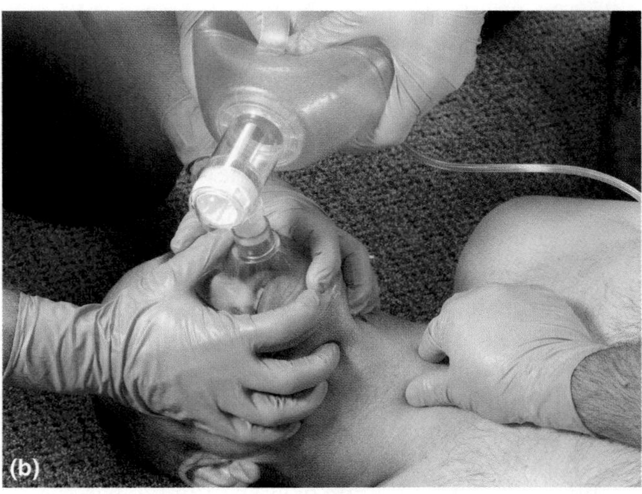

FIGURE A2-8 ✻ **(a)** To carry out cricoid pressure, locate the cricoid cartilage inferior to the thyroid cartilage (Adam's apple). **(b)** Apply firm posterior pressure with the thumb and index finger.

b. Assemble the laryngoscope blade and handle. Lift the blade to illuminate the bulb and check the brightness. Also check the bulb to ensure that it is tight and will not become dislodged during the intubation.
c. If a stylet is to be used, lubricate it with a water-soluble lubricant and insert it into the tube. Check the distal end of the stylet to ensure that it is not projecting out of the tracheal tube and is recessed adequately. Form the tube into a hockey-stick configuration.
d. Lubricate the distal end of the tracheal tube with a water-soluble lubricant.
e. Have a suction unit equipped with a large-bore catheter available. Check to make sure that the suction unit works adequately.
f. Prepare the device that will be used to secure the tube in place.

5. Position yourself at the patient's head. The tracheal tube and suction unit should be on your right and the laryngoscope on your left.
6. The patient's head must be positioned properly to permit maximum visualization of the vocal cords and glottic opening. The position of the head will depend on whether a spinal injury is suspected.
   - **No spinal injury suspected.** Tilt the head backward and lift the chin forward into a "sniffing position." The sniffing position is created by extension of the neck at cervical vertebrae 1 and 2 combined with flexion of cervical vertebrae 6 and 7. Do not hang the head over the end of a table or bed. If visualization is unsuccessful, it may be necessary to reposition the head. You can place folded towels of approximately 1-inch thickness under the shoulders or under the back of the head to adjust flexion or extension as necessary. The desired position aligns the mouth, pharynx, and trachea and permits better visualization during intubation.
   - **Suspected spinal injury.** If a spinal injury is suspected, maintain in-line spinal stabilization throughout the intubation procedure. One EMT should hold the head and neck stable from below while the EMT who is to intubate secures the head and neck with his thighs (Advanced Airway Management Skills A2-1D). The limited ability to align the head and neck will make visualization more difficult.
7. Stop ventilation and remove the oropharyngeal airway if one has been used. Ventilation must not be interrupted for more than 30 seconds while intubating. The 30-second period begins when positive pressure ventilation is stopped and ends when ventilation is resumed following placement of the tube. If you cannot intubate within 30 seconds, stop the procedure and immediately resume oxygenating the patient. After 2 minutes of ventilation and hyperoxygenation, try again to intubate. It is also desirable to monitor the pulse oximeter reading during the procedure for evidence of deoxygenation.
8. If enough personnel are available, one EMT should apply cricoid pressure to reduce the possibility of regurgitation during the intubation procedure. The intubator may use backward pressure on the thyroid cartilage to move the glottic opening slightly posterior and may make visualization of the vocal cords easier. The mnemonic BURP (backward, upward, rightward pressure) is often used to describe the thyroid pressure used to bring the glottic opening into the best position for visualization by the intubator. Cricoid pressure must be maintained until after the cuff of the tracheal tube is inflated. Cricoid pressure and BURP are two separate maneuvers.
9. Hold the laryngoscope in your left hand and insert the blade into the right corner of the mouth. You may need to use a crossed-finger (scissors-type) technique to separate the teeth, using the thumb and index finger of the right hand. Move the blade to the midline, gently sweeping the tongue to the left to allow for more room and better visualization. Advance the blade to the base of the tongue and place it in the proper position, depending on the type used:
   - **Curved blade.** The tip of the curved blade is inserted into the vallecula (the indentation between the base of the tongue and the epiglottis).
   - **Straight blade.** The tip of the straight blade is placed under the epiglottis.

   The handle and blade are lifted up and forward, away from the patient's teeth and gums and in the direction of the laryngoscope handle. Do not angle the handle backward in a prying motion or use the teeth as a fulcrum; such actions could cause trauma to the airway and teeth. Do not use a digging motion with the blade and handle in trying to expose the glottic opening. The movement should be smooth and controlled. Exposure should be achieved in three easy movements of the blade: (1) insert the blade in the right corner of the mouth, sweeping the tongue to the left; (2) advance the blade to the base of the tongue; (3) gently lift up and forward to expose the glottic opening.

   When using the straight blade, you may see the epiglottis tip when lifting up and forward. Remember, the straight blade is used to get under the epiglottis and lift it up. Drop the blade down slightly and gently advance the blade farther into the hypopharynx to slip the tip of the blade under the epiglottis. Again lift up and forward to expose the glottic opening. The straight blade can easily be advanced past the glottic structures and into the esophagus. This is why you should not just blindly insert the blade into the mouth and begin the lifting movement without properly identifying the structures. If, however, the blade is accidentally inserted too deep, pull back on the blade and again attempt to visualize the structures. This is the method preferred by some experienced intubators.

10. Identify the glottic opening by (1) cartilaginous structures surrounding it, (2) the fact that it is round—not oval like the esophageal opening, and (3) the fact that it contains the vocal cords. Once you identify the vocal cords and glottic opening, do not lose sight of them.
11. Insert the tracheal tube through the right side of the mouth. It may help to have an assistant lift upward and out on the patient's right cheek. Guide the tracheal tube through the vocal cords. *You must actually visualize the tube passing through the vocal cords.* Continue to insert the tube until the proximal end of the cuff is advanced about one-half to one inch beyond the vocal cords. This should place the tip of the tracheal tube about halfway between the carina and the vocal cords. This position will allow for some movement of the patient's head and neck without displacement of the tube out of the trachea or into a mainstem bronchus. Typically, the tube marker will be at about 19–23 cm at the level of the teeth.

    Do not attempt to advance the tube through the hollowed-out area of the blade. This space is for visualization only and will likely tear the cuff as well as obscure your view of the glottic opening.
12. Remove the laryngoscope blade and fold the blade down so that it is parallel with the handle. This will shut off the light. Hold the tube firmly at all times until it is properly secured in place.
13. If a stylet was used, remove it gently by pulling it out in the direction it was inserted. Hold the tube securely against the patient's cheek with one hand while removing the stylet with the other. Pulling the stylet out without holding the tube securely in place may cause accidental extubation, or removal of the tube. Reconfirm the marking at the corner of the mouth.
14. With the syringe attached to the inflation port, inflate the cuff by injecting 10 mL of air. Remove the syringe when you have completed inflation so that the cuff does not deflate.
15. Hold the tracheal tube in position at all times until it is properly secured. Once the tube is in place, do not let go until the securing device is applied.
16. Have your partner attach the bag-valve device to the tracheal tube and begin to deliver positive pressure ventilation.
17. Confirm correct tube placement. *This is one of the most important parts of the intubation process.* You must verify that the tube has been properly placed in the trachea. As the first ventilation is delivered, you must simultaneously confirm tube placement through these confirmatory techniques:
    - *Auscultate over the epigastrium.* Gurgling or rushing sounds heard while auscultating over the stomach during ventilation are an indication that the tube is improperly placed in the esophagus. Do not deliver any more ventilations. Deflate the cuff, and immediately remove the tube. Resume ventilating the patient with the bag-valve-mask device. It is common for the patient to vomit after esophageal placement of a tracheal tube, so have a suction unit ready. Ventilate for approximately 1–2 minutes and reattempt the intubation. If you are unsuccessful on the second attempt, resume ventilation and contact medical direction or follow your local protocol to determine if additional intubation attempts should be made.
    - *Watch for chest rise and fall* during ventilation.
    - *Auscultate breath sounds.* If there are no sounds over the epigastrium and the chest rises with ventilation, auscultate the breath sounds in both lungs. Listen to each apex (top) at about the second intercostal space, midclavicular. Compare the breath sounds heard over the left apex to the sounds over the right apex. Then auscultate at the fourth intercostal space midaxillary and over the bases at about the fourth intercostal space on the anterior side, again comparing the right and left sounds. Breath sounds should be equal on both sides. Patients with unilateral chest injury (e.g., pneumothorax) may have unequal breath sounds unrelated to tube placement.

      If breath sounds are heard on the right, but the breath sounds are diminished or absent on the left, the tube has likely been advanced into the right mainstem bronchus. The problem with a bronchial intubation is that only one lung is being ventilated, which could lead to hypoxia. If a right mainstem intubation is indicated, you should:

      a. Deflate the cuff and gently withdraw the tube slightly (1–2 cm) while continuing to ventilate the patient and to auscultate for breath sounds on the left side.
      b. Be careful not to pull the tube completely out of the trachea. Pull back on the tube only enough to restore breath sounds on the left.
      c. Once breath sounds become evident on the left, begin to compare the left and right breath sounds. When both sides are equal, reinflate the cuff, secure the tube, and resume positive pressure ventilation. If there is any doubt, use the laryngoscope to visualize whether the tube is passing through the vocal cords.

At least one other confirmatory method must be used to assess for proper tracheal tube placement. These are:

a. *Use of an end-tidal carbon dioxide detector* to measure the concentration of exhaled carbon dioxide. A lack of carbon dioxide indicates that the tube is improperly placed in the esophagus. There are several different types and models of detectors available, from simple colorimetric devices to more elaborate electronic devices with digital readout (Figure A2-9∗). The end-tidal carbon dioxide

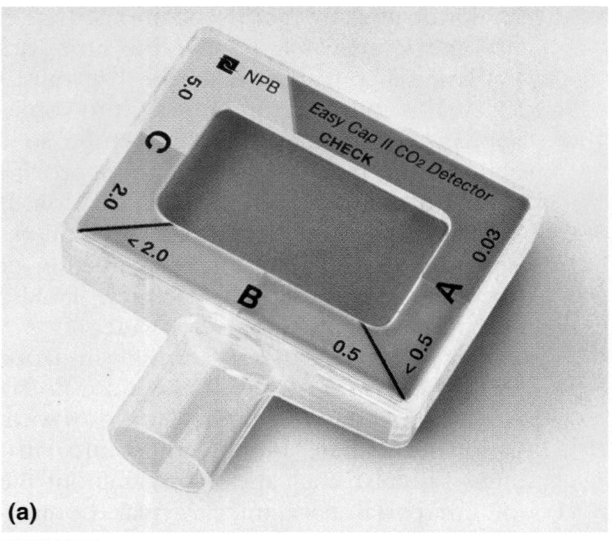

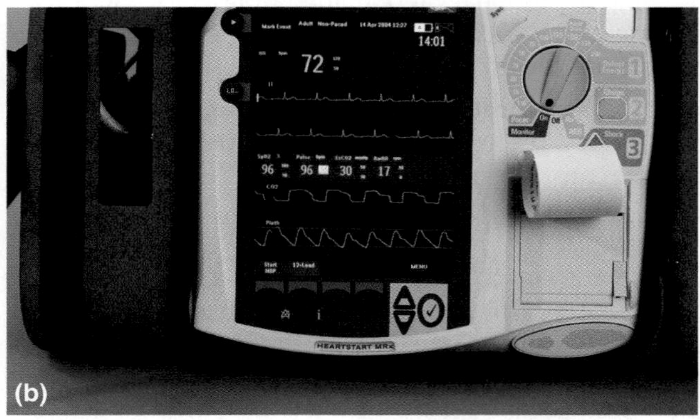

FIGURE A2-9 ✻ **(a)** Colorimetric end-tidal CO_2 detector. **(b)** Electronic end-tidal CO_2 detector. (Photo a: © Nellcor Puritan Bennett, Inc.; photo b: © Scott Metcalfe)

detector is used as an adjunct in assessment of tracheal tube placement, in addition to the methods that have been described. In some cardiac arrest patients, the extremely low blood flow to the lungs does not produce amounts of carbon dioxide adequate enough to be detected. An alternative device should be available to confirm tube placement when no CO_2 is found in the cardiac arrest patient. Capnometry will be discussed further later in this section.

b. *Use a bulb- or syringe-type esophageal intubation detection device* (Figure A2-10✻). The function of these devices depends on a key difference between the structure of the trachea and the structure of the esophagus. The trachea is surrounded by rigid cartilage and does not collapse when negative pressure is applied, whereas the esophagus is fibroelastic tissue and collapses easily when negative pressure is applied. The syringe and bulb devices connect to the end of the 15 mm adapter of the tracheal tube once the patient has been intubated and the cuff inflated. With the syringe device, the plunger is pulled back. If air enters the syringe, you can assume that the tracheal tube has been properly placed in the trachea. If resistance is met, you should suspect that the esophagus has been intubated and is collapsing as negative pressure is applied by the syringe. Remove the tube immediately. Similarly, with the bulb device, the bulb is squeezed, placed on the 15 mm adapter, and allowed to refill. If the refill is swift, you assume that the tube is properly placed in the trachea. If the bulb refills slowly or doesn't refill at all, you presume that the tube is in the esophagus. Immediately remove the tube and ventilate the patient with a bag-valve-mask device. Unlike the colorimetric device, the esophageal detector will generally provide reliable results in both the perfusing and the nonperfusing patient. The device may, however, provide inaccurate results in pa-

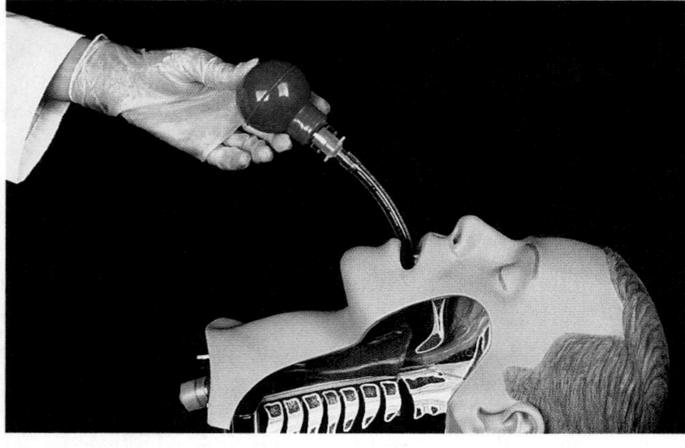

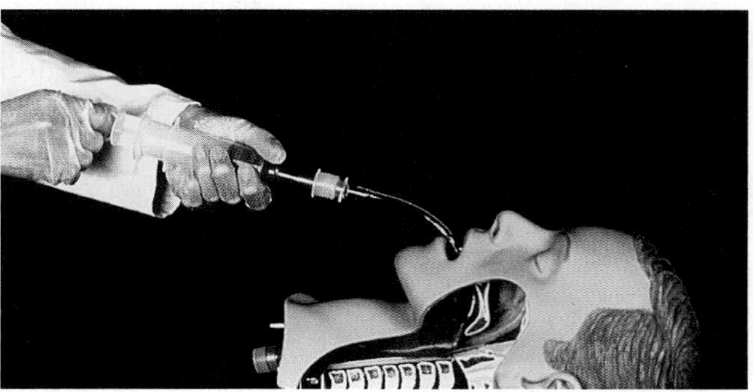

(a) (b)

FIGURE A2-10 ✻ **(a)** Bulb-type esophageal detection device. **(b)** Syringe-type esophageal detection device.

tients who are extremely obese, in late pregnancy, in status asthmaticus, or in patients with large amounts of secretions. In an obese patient or one in late pregnancy, the trachea will have a tendency to collapse when negative pressure is applied by the bulb syringe device. In the patient suffering from status asthmaticus or one who has copious amounts of secretions, the smaller airways may be blocked and prevent air from being aspirated from the lower airways, providing a false reading.

c. Exhaled condensation should be evident in the tracheal tube, although this is not completely reliable. Another clinical sign indicative of good placement is the presence of equal chest rise and fall and relative ease in ventilating the patient manually.

Indications that the tube is improperly placed are:

a. Inability to visualize the tracheal tube passing into the glottic opening.
b. Presence of air passing into the stomach with ventilation, as heard upon auscultation.
c. Lack of carbon dioxide when an end-tidal carbon dioxide detector is used.
d. Inability to rapidly aspirate air when using an esophageal detector device.
e. Absence of bilateral breath sounds upon auscultation, or unilateral breath sounds.

The following are indications that the tracheal tube may have become displaced:

a. *A sudden drop in pulse oximeter reading may indicate a misplaced tracheal tube.* (A pulse oximeter is a device attached to a patient's finger or earlobe that "reads" the oxygen saturation of the blood.) Immediately use conventional methods to assess for proper tube placement.
b. *A patient who begins to deteriorate rapidly, becomes combative, or begins to exhibit cyanosis or cardiac arrest could be suffering from tracheal tube misplacement.* Again, you should immediately use conventional methods including direct visualization to check tube placement.

18. If no sounds are heard over the epigastrium, the chest rises and falls with each ventilation, the breath sounds are equal bilaterally, and the tracheal confirmation device reads correctly, the tube should be secured in place with a tape or commercial securing device that has been approved by medical direction. Once the tube has been secured, you should do the following:
    a. Ventilate the patient at the appropriate rate based on his age.
    b. Note the centimeter marking on the tracheal tube at the level of the teeth. This should be included in your written documentation.
    c. Insert an oral airway or other appropriate device to serve as a bite block.
19. Reassess breath sounds as often as possible. It is necessary to reassess breath sounds following any movement of the patient, including movement onto a stretcher or out to the ambulance. If breath sounds are heard only on the right after a move, assume a right mainstem intubation and reposition the tube as described earlier to correct the placement. If no breath sounds are heard but sounds are heard over the epigastrium, suspect an esophageal intubation and immediately stop ventilation, remove the tube, and resume ventilation with the bag-valve-mask device. *If you are uncertain that the tube is properly placed after reassessment, remove it. Remember, an esophageal intubation is lethal. There is no room for error in judgment. Err to benefit the patient.*

Note: If you were the EMT who performed the intubation, it is necessary for you to confirm tube placement. Others, such as Emergency Medical Responders or other EMTs, can help you to check tube placement, but do not rely on them to confirm *your* placement; they may lack the necessary training. Likewise, if an inexperienced EMT has intubated the patient, you must confirm that the tracheal tube is properly placed. This is a critical skill that requires repetition and experience to produce true competence. Measuring and monitoring end-tidal carbon dioxide is recommended for ensuring correct placement.

Capnometry

Partial pressure of end-tidal carbon dioxide ($PETCO_2$) monitoring is a noninvasive method of measuring the levels of carbon dioxide (CO_2) in the exhaled breath, which is an excellent gauge of how well the lungs are being ventilated. Over time, numerous terms and labels have been associated with capnography, and a quick review of the following terms may help you understand the material in this section:

- *Partial pressure of end-tidal CO_2 ($PETCO_2$)* represents the measurement of the CO_2 concentration at the end of expiration, which correlates with the maximum CO_2 content in the exhaled gas.
- *$PaCO_2$* represents the partial pressure of CO_2 in the arterial blood, which is directly impacted by quality of alveolar ventilation.
- *Capnometry* is the measurement of expired CO_2. It typically provides a numeric display of the partial pressure of CO_2 in torr or mmHg.
- *Capnogram* refers to the visual representation of the expired CO_2 waveform throughout the phases of breathing.

CO_2, a normal by-product of cellular metabolism, is transported by the venous system to the right side of the heart. From there it is delivered to the capillary beds of the lungs so that the CO_2 can be off-loaded to the alveoli and exhaled. With normal cardiovascular and pulmonary function, there is a relatively reliable correlation between the $PETCO_2$ and the $PaCO_2$ (the concentration of CO_2 in the arterial blood). Capnometry is the process of monitoring the exhaled carbon dioxide in the body. This information is helpful in making clinical inferences as to the patient's status. Initially, a device that changed color according to the presence or absence of exhaled carbon dioxide (colorimetric) was used to help determine if the trachea was properly intubated by the EMS personnel. However, as the cost of electronic end-tidal CO_2 technology lowered and the use and familiarity of capnography expanded, so did the instances of clinical use.

In the prehospital setting, the use of continuous electronic capnometry (instead of single "snapshot" readings) has increased over the past several years. In fact, the EMT may be working in an ALS system that uses cardiac monitors or mechanical ventilators already equipped with this technology for both the breathing and nonbreathing patient. The advantage of monitoring the exhaled carbon dioxide levels is that it provides clinical information as to the degree of alveolar ventilation that is occurring. Since carbon dioxide is created by the peripheral tissues at a fairly constant rate and the venous blood is constantly being perfused to the lungs, elevations or depressions in the $ETCO_2$ levels will occur as changes in alveolar ventilation or tissue perfusion occur.

If perfusion to the lungs decreases, this may alter $PETCO_2$ as well, because venous blood rich in carbon dioxide is not being delivered to the lungs. Likewise, if for some reason the metabolic activity of the body increases, for example during a seizure or if the patient has a high temperature, the amount of carbon dioxide in the venous blood will increase or decrease in shock and will change the amount monitored by the electronic end-tidal CO_2 device. The normal physiological range for $PETCO_2$ is about 38–42 mmHg, although the acceptable range may be slightly wider.

Following are some possible reasons for changes in the $PETCO_2$ level:

- The $PETCO_2$ level may decrease if there is a rise in alveolar ventilation (increased ventilation lowers the $PETCO_2$), if there is diminished cardiac output, or if there is a decline in metabolic activity.
- The $PETCO_2$ level may increase if there is a drop in alveolar ventilation (because each exhaled breath will then contain more carbon dioxide) or if metabolic activity suddenly increases.

Capnometry provides a noninvasive measure of $PETCO_2$ levels, thus providing the EMT information not only about the degree of alveolar ventilation, but also about the status of systemic metabolism and the patient's circulatory status. The use of capnography is commonplace in the operating room, critical care departments, and emergency departments of the hospital and is increasingly common in the prehospital setting.

Complications of Orotracheal Intubation

Many complications, some severe, can occur from tracheal intubation. The complications are typically associated with either the laryngoscopy (the lifting of the epiglottis to expose the vocal cords and glottic opening with the laryngoscope) or actual tube placement. Some complications can be lethal if they are not recognized immediately and corrected; other complications are minor. Some of the more common complications of tracheal intubation include the following:

- *Hypertension (elevated blood pressure), tachycardia (increased heart rate), and dysrhythmias (irregular heart rhythms) may result from stimulation of the airway during intubation.* These conditions can occur during intubation of an adult patient who is not in cardiac arrest.
- *Bradycardia (decreased heart rate) and hypotension (decreased blood pressure) may be seen in infants and children and some adults,* particularly those who are hypoxic, because of stimulation of the airway during intubation, an opposite response from that in adults. Also, heart rates in infants and children may drop as they become hypoxic. Closely monitor the heart rate during intubation.
- Frequent complications include trauma to the lips, tongue, gums, teeth, and airway. The blade, the end of the tracheal tube, and an improperly positioned stylet projecting from the end of the tube can all perforate soft tissue.
- *Inadequate oxygenation and severe hypoxia can result from prolonged attempts at intubation, those lasting longer than 30 seconds.* The apneic patient has no other source of ventilation and oxygenation except what you are providing. Cessation of positive pressure ventilation during intubation can lead to hypoxia. Even 3 minutes without any ventilation may lead to irreversible brain damage in a patient. Therefore, it is important (a) to ventilate the patient before the intubation attempt, (b) not to exceed 30 seconds during an intubation attempt from the time you stop ventilating to the point when you resume ventilation, and (c) to oxygenate after either proper tube placement or a failed attempt. A properly oxygenated patient has a functional residual capacity in the lungs of 2,500 mL of oxygen, which can sustain the apneic patient for some time.
- *A right mainstem intubation may result in hypoxia, because only one lung is being ventilated.* Closely assess breath sounds and pull back on the tube until bilateral breath sounds are heard equally.
- *Absence of ventilation or oxygenation will result from misplacement of a tracheal tube in the esophagus.* ***This***

is a lethal complication if it is not immediately recognized and corrected. If you suspect an esophageal intubation, immediately deflate the tracheal tube cuff, remove the tube, and ventilate the patient with the bag-valve-mask device and high-concentration oxygen.

- *Vomiting may result from stimulation of the gag reflex during intubation.* Be sure to have a suction device readily available when intubating. If the patient begins to vomit and no spinal injury is suspected, turn him on his side to facilitate removal of the vomitus and suction to clear the airway. Prevention of aspiration should be a high priority.
- *The cuff may leak, requiring reinflation.* If the cuff does not stay inflated, extubation and insertion of a new tracheal tube will be required.
- *Stimulation of the epiglottis or vocal cords during intubation may cause laryngospasm.* The vocal cords will close completely and not allow air to pass through. The vocal cords will eventually relax and allow air to pass through again. Ventilation with a bag-valve-mask device may be necessary if the cords do not relax immediately.
- *The patient may be accidentally extubated during movement or ventilation.* To avoid accidental extubation, secure the tube adequately and limit any unnecessary pulling or pushing on it. If a bag-valve device is connected to the tube and is being used to ventilate the patient, do not drop it while it is still connected to the tube, as for example when clearing during defibrillation. Dropping the bag-valve device while it is connected to the tube puts the weight of the device directly on the tube, greatly increasing the risk of tube displacement. If you have to clear the patient or interrupt ventilations, remove the bag-valve device from the 15 mm adapter. Reconnect it when you are ready to resume ventilation. After every interruption, check tube placement by assessing chest rise, breath sounds, and gastric sounds during ventilation and the marking on the tube.
- *The patient may become responsive enough to extubate himself following resuscitation or intervention.* If the patient makes attempts to remove the tube, reassure the patient and restrain his hands.

Orotracheal Suctioning

Orotracheal suctioning is the process in which a long, soft suction catheter is inserted through the tracheal tube to clear secretions. The suction catheter is advanced down the tracheal tube and beyond its tip to the level of the carina. As the catheter is being withdrawn, suction is applied to remove any heavy secretions that could block the airway. In contrast to suctioning of the oropharynx or nasopharynx, where the catheter is never advanced beyond the posterior pharynx, this procedure allows for deep suctioning at the level of the trachea.

Indications

There are two major indications for performing orotracheal suctioning:

- **Obvious secretions in the tracheal tube.** While performing positive pressure ventilation, you may notice secretions in the tracheal tube. These secretions could reduce the effectiveness of ventilation or obstruct the tracheal tube.
- **Poor compliance or an increase in resistance when ventilating with the bag-valve device.** These may be signs of obstruction of the tracheal tube or trachea by heavy, thick secretions that should be cleared by orotracheal suctioning.

Many conditions or illnesses can produce secretions that require suctioning. Patients with respiratory conditions may have problems not only with bronchospasm or inflammation of the lower airways but also with overproduction of mucus. The secretions are usually very thick and heavy and can occlude the trachea and bronchi. The best method for removal, if the patient is unable to remove them himself by coughing, is through orotracheal suctioning. Also, trauma may cause bleeding in the trachea, bronchi, or lungs that may require suctioning.

Suctioning Technique

The procedure for performing orotracheal suctioning is as follows (Advanced Airway Management Skills A2-2A to A2-2F):

1. Take the necessary Standard Precautions, including gloves and eye protection.
2. Ventilate the patient using a high concentration of supplemental oxygen. The patient should be ventilated for 2 minutes before suctioning. This will build up his oxygen reserve and reduce the chances of severe hypoxia.
3. Assemble and check all equipment to be sure it is in working order. Orotracheal suctioning is a sterile procedure; do not contaminate the catheter while assembling or checking it. A sterile glove must be used to handle the catheter. The catheter should remain inside the sterile package until ready for use.
4. Measure the catheter length from the lips to the ear and down to the level of the nipple. This length of catheter should allow placement at about the level of the carina.

5. Set the suction between 80 and 120 mmHg (negative pressure).
6. Insert the catheter down the tracheal tube with no suction applied.
7. Advance the catheter to the carina or its approximate depth as previously measured.
8. Apply suction. While doing so, withdraw the catheter in a twisting motion. Do not apply suction for longer than 15 seconds in the adult patient.
9. Ventilate the patient for 2 minutes. The procedure can be repeated, if necessary, following the same steps.

Complications

As with any advanced invasive maneuver, complications can occur with orotracheal suctioning. Many of those complications result from the interruption of ventilation to perform the procedure. The following are common complications associated with orotracheal suctioning:

- Hypoxia can result from a decrease in lung volume during the application of suction, because you are removing residual air and also interrupting ventilation. (In other words, you are removing whatever air was left in the lungs, and you have stopped providing replacement air.) If hypoxia is severe, it could lead to cardiac arrest. Proper ventilation and the use of a high concentration of oxygen for 2 minutes before and after suctioning will reduce the possibility of severe hypoxia. Even more important, do not apply suction for a period greater than 15 seconds in the adult.
- Cardiac dysrhythmias can result from suctioning. Tachycardia may occur from stimulation of the airway (or bradycardia in infants and children). Other, more lethal cardiac dysrhythmias may result from a decrease in the supply of oxygen to the heart secondary to hypoxia. Or such dysrhythmias may result from an increase in the oxygen demand from hypertension and tachycardia. Stimulation of the vagus nerve during suctioning as a result of inserting the suction catheter too deeply into the trachea can cause bradycardia and hypotension.
- Coughing may be triggered by the catheter stimulating the mucosal lining. Coughing can increase pressure within the skull and decrease the blood flow to the brain. This is especially dangerous in a patient with a head injury, stroke, or other condition that had already caused an increase in pressure within the brain.
- The catheter may damage the mucosa, causing swelling, bleeding, and ulcerations that can lead to tracheal infections.
- Bronchospasm can occur if the catheter is inserted beyond the carina and into the bronchi.

Alternative Intubation Methods

Alternative Intubation Equipment

Grandview Intubation Blade

The *Grandview blade* (Figure A2-11*) is a redesigned blade that shares characteristics of both the curved and straight blades. It shows less curvature than a traditional curved blade and is designed with an 80 percent wider blade surface than standard blades. With the redesigned curve, which closely mirrors the normal human anatomy, and the wider width with a short flange, the blade is said to improve direct visualization. It also removes the need to choose between a straight or a curved blade, since the Grandview blade is designed with the best features of both. The adult blade is 165 mm in length to fit the majority of adult patients, creating a universal blade for most cases. A pediatric version is also available and measures 120 mm in length. The Grandview fits all standard laryngoscope handles with no special connections required.

Viewmax Intubation Blade

The *Viewmax blade* (Figure A2-12*) is shaped and used in a similar fashion to a traditional curved blade. The ad-

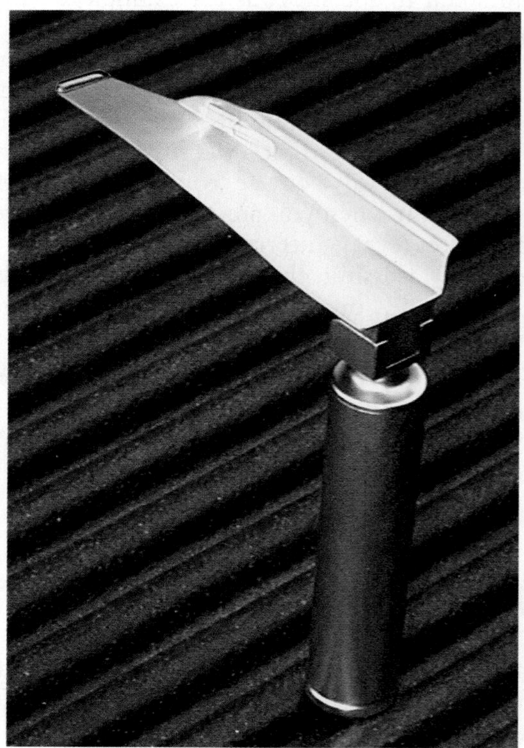

FIGURE A2-11 * Grandview laryngoscope blade. (© Hartwell Medical)

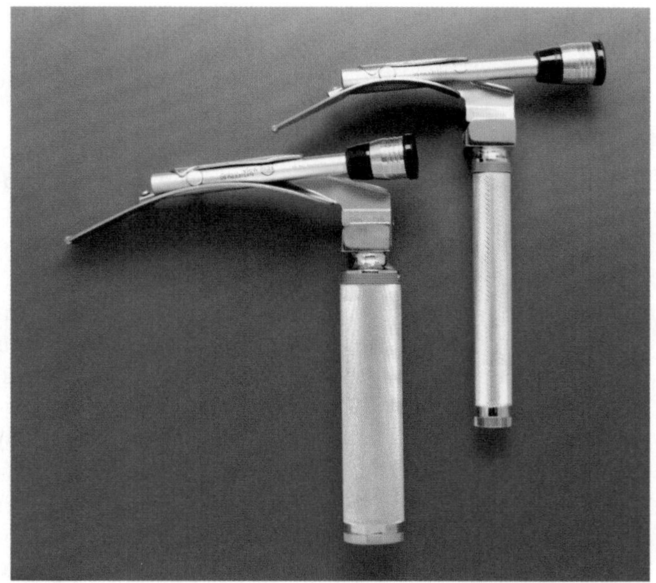

FIGURE A2-12 ✱ Viewmax laryngoscope blade. (Viewmax™, Rüsch Inc., a division of Teleflex Medical)

vantage to this blade is a patented viewing tube with a lens system that refracts the image approximately 20° from horizontal. This refraction allows better visualization of an anterior larynx through the eyepiece. This should improve intubation success rates in patients with an anterior larynx or otherwise difficult airway. The Viewmax blade is available in sizes for both adult and pediatric patients. Additionally, blades can be ordered to fit either a regular or a fiber-optic laryngoscope handle.

Gum Elastic Bougie

The *gum elastic bougie* (also referred to as an Eschmann tracheal tube introducer) (Figure A2-13✱) is used to facilitate tracheal intubations when intubation is (or is anticipated to be) difficult because of incomplete visualization of the glottic opening. It is a 60–70 cm long, semirigid, styletlike device with the tip bent at about a 35° angle, 2.5 cm from the distal end. The device is suitable for use with tracheal tubes that have an internal diameter of 6.0 mm or greater. The longer (70 cm) version is easier to thread the tracheal tube over.

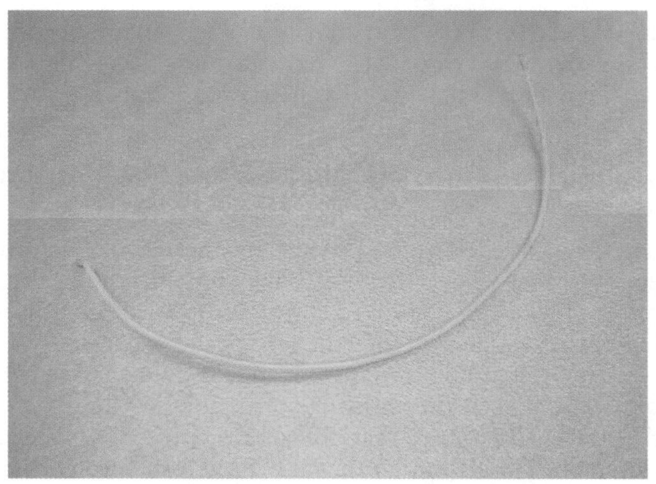

FIGURE A2-13 ✱ Gum elastic bougie. (© Roy Alson, MD)

During laryngoscopy, prior to tube insertion, the bougie is carefully advanced so that the bent tip is in contact with the posterior surface of the epiglottis. It is then advanced into the larynx and through the cords until the tip enters the trachea. When the bougie enters the trachea, the EMT should be able to feel "bumps" as the curved tip of the bougie slides over the tracheal rings bordering the anterior trachea. The bougie should be advanced to about the 25 cm mark at the corner of the mouth. When the tip arrives at the carina, usually at about 27 cm, the EMT will note that the bougie is "held up," and any further advancement will not be possible. By interpreting the combination of "bumps" and "hold-up," the EMT confirms that the bougie is in the trachea. If the EMT identifies that the bougie can be advanced farther than about 27 cm, or there is an absence of the "bumping" and "holding-up," the bougie is probably in the esophagus.

If the device is in its correct position, the first EMT will maintain the laryngoscope in position and hold the inserted bougie. A second EMT can then pass the tracheal tube over the end of the bougie and into the larynx. Once the tracheal tube is in place, the bougie is removed. Normal confirmation procedures for the tracheal tube should then proceed.

Alternative Intubation Techniques

You may encounter situations in which you are unable to intubate a patient using the standard techniques already described. There are, however, several ways of inserting a tracheal tube orally that employ different techniques and equipment. To use these techniques, some of which are described in the following sections, you must be completely familiar with them and the equipment they require. You must also have approval from medical direction before attempting any of the alternative intubation techniques. Remember that any method for inserting the tracheal tube into the trachea that does not employ direct visualization of the glottic opening is associated with a higher rate of tube misplacement and other complications. If the EMT does not utilize direct visual orotracheal intubation, it is a step backward in accuracy of placement. Remember that the laryngoscope can also be used after insertion of the endotracheal tube to confirm placement. Orotracheal intubation is still the preferred method for intubating adults or pediatrics.

Digital Intubation

In digital intubation, the EMT inserts his fingers into the patient's hypopharynx and uses them to lift the epiglottis.

The tracheal tube is then passed through the glottic opening with the help of the fingers. Digital intubation may be used in a patient who is in cardiac arrest or is unresponsive, has no gag reflex, and is in a position where direct visual orotracheal intubation is impossible. It may also be considered for patients with distortions to the necessary visual landmarks.

Digital intubation is referred to as a "blind" technique, because you do not actually visualize the tracheal tube passing through the vocal cords. As already stated, standard intubation using a laryngoscope is preferred because it permits such visualization. However, you may encounter situations where the patient's position or condition precludes tracheal intubation with a laryngoscope—for example, when you cannot manipulate the head and neck of an immobilized patient with suspected spinal injury. It is very difficult in such a case to achieve an axis that allows for proper visualization without moving the patient's head and neck. Because digital intubation can be performed without visualizing the vocal cords, it eliminates the need to manipulate the head or neck.

Another situation in which digital intubation might be used is with a patient trapped in a wrecked vehicle. The patient's immediate airway problem may be severe, but the time required for extricating him from the wreck may be long and the position in which he is trapped makes standard intubation with a laryngoscope virtually impossible. Digital intubation may be helpful in such a case.

Digital intubation would allow you to insert a tracheal tube even if the laryngoscope was not working properly or if its batteries or bulb failed and no spares were available. This should not be performed if the patient has an intact gag reflex or has the ability to bite.

Equipment The equipment needed to perform digital intubation includes the following:

- Appropriately sized tracheal tube
- Malleable stylet
- Water-soluble lubricant
- 10 mL syringe
- Bite block
- Device to secure the tracheal tube

Procedure Follow these steps to perform a digital intubation (Advanced Airway Management Skills A2-3A and A2-3B):

1. Take the necessary Standard Precautions. Gloves, eye protection, and a mask are recommended.
2. Ventilate the patient for approximately 2 minutes while delivering a high concentration of supplemental oxygen.
3. Check the tracheal tube as you normally would. Lubricate the tube with a water-soluble lubricant. Lubricate the stylet and insert it to form the tube into an open J shape.
4. If the patient is suspected of having a spinal injury, have an EMT or other properly trained rescuer manually stabilize the patient's head and neck. Face the patient and kneel at his left shoulder.
5. Instruct the person ventilating the patient to stop. Quickly place a bite block between the patient's molars to prevent him from biting down on your fingers during the procedure. Ideally, the technique should be reserved for the unresponsive patient only.
6. Insert the middle and index fingers of your nondominant hand into the patient's mouth. Advance your fingers down the midline while simultaneously lifting the tongue up and out of the way. Palpate the epiglottis with your middle finger (Advanced Airway Management Skills A2-3A).
7. Press upward and move the epiglottis forward. Insert the tracheal tube into the mouth with your dominant hand and advance the tube using your index finger to maintain the tip of the tube against the middle finger. The tip will be directed upward toward the epiglottis. Guide the tip of the tube into the glottic opening with the index finger by sliding it alongside your middle finger that is retracting the epiglottis (Advanced Airway Management Skills A2-3B).
8. Remove your fingers while holding the tube in place with your other hand. Inflate the cuff with 5–10 mL of air. Attach a bag-valve device to the tube. Artificial ventilation must not be interrupted for more than 30 seconds during the insertion.
9. As with any tracheal intubation, ensure that the tube is not misplaced in the esophagus or mainstem bronchus. Auscultate over the epigastrium (gurgling should not be heard) and at the apices laterally and at the bases of the lungs (breath sounds should be present and equal). Watch for equal rise and fall of both sides of the chest with each ventilation. Take the steps described earlier in this appendix to correct any misplacement of the tube. Ventilate the patient between attempts to intubate.
10. When correct placement is confirmed, secure the tube as described earlier. Reassess tube position whenever the patient or the ventilating device is moved.

Transillumination (Lighted Stylet) Intubation

Another method of inserting a tracheal tube is transillumination, or the "lighted stylet" technique. In this procedure, a special lighted stylet is inserted into the tracheal tube, which is then inserted through the mouth, into the hypopharynx, and on into the larynx and trachea.

The trachea is anterior to the esophagus, so the bright light seen through the soft tissues at the front of the neck will indicate that the tube is correctly placed in the trachea. This means that the EMT can pass the tracheal tube through the glottic opening without visualizing the structures directly to ensure correct placement.

There is no need to manipulate the head or neck during this procedure. Thus, the transillumination technique can be an effective means of intubating a trauma patient.

The stylet used in this technique is a special device with a high-intensity bulb at the distal end. A small battery housed at the proximal end supplies power for the light and is controlled by an on-off switch. Because tube placement with this method requires seeing the light through the tissues of the neck, the technique is best performed in a darkened room or, if in the sunlight, with the neck shielded or in a shadow. A major problem with this technique is the inability to see the stylet light well in bright ambient light.

Equipment The equipment needed to perform transillumination tracheal intubation includes the following:

- Appropriately sized tracheal tube
- Lighted stylet
- Water-soluble lubricant
- 10 mL syringe
- Scissors (to trim the tube if necessary)
- Securing device for the tracheal tube

Procedure To perform a transillumination intubation:

1. Take the necessary Standard Precautions including gloves, eye protection, and a mask.
2. Ventilate the patient for approximately 2 minutes while delivering a high concentration of supplemental oxygen.
3. Assemble and check the equipment. The tracheal tube should be between 7.5 and 8.5 mm i.d. Some older tubes will need to be cut to 25 to 27 cm to accommodate the stylet. (Some newer devices do not require cutting the tube.) Place the stylet into the tube and bend it just proximal to the cuff.
4. Kneel on one side of the patient, facing his head.
5. Turn on the stylet light.
6. With your index and middle fingers inserted deeply into the patient's mouth and your thumb on the chin, lift the patient's tongue and jaw forward. Insert the tube/stylet combination and advance it through the oropharynx and into the hypopharynx along the midline. Using a "hooking" motion, lift the epiglottis out of the way (Figure A2-14✱).
7. When you see a circle of light at the level of the larynx on the anterior neck, hold the stylet stationary (Figure A2-15✱). Advance the tube off the stylet into the larynx approximately 1/2 to 1 inch. Indications of misplacement of the stylet and tube are as follows:
   - *If the light at the front of the neck is diffuse, dim, or hard to see—or not visible at all—this indicates that the tube/stylet combination is incorrectly placed in the esophagus.* The tube should be withdrawn immediately and hyperventilation resumed.
   - *A bright light appearing lateral to the upper aspect of the thyroid cartilage (Adam's apple) indicates that the tube/stylet is placed in the right or left pyriform fossa (furrow).* Immediately withdraw the tube and resume hyperventilation. Make another attempt after a few minutes.
8. Hold the tube in place with one hand and remove the stylet.
9. Inflate the cuff with 5–10 mL of air and attach the bag-valve device to the end of the tube.

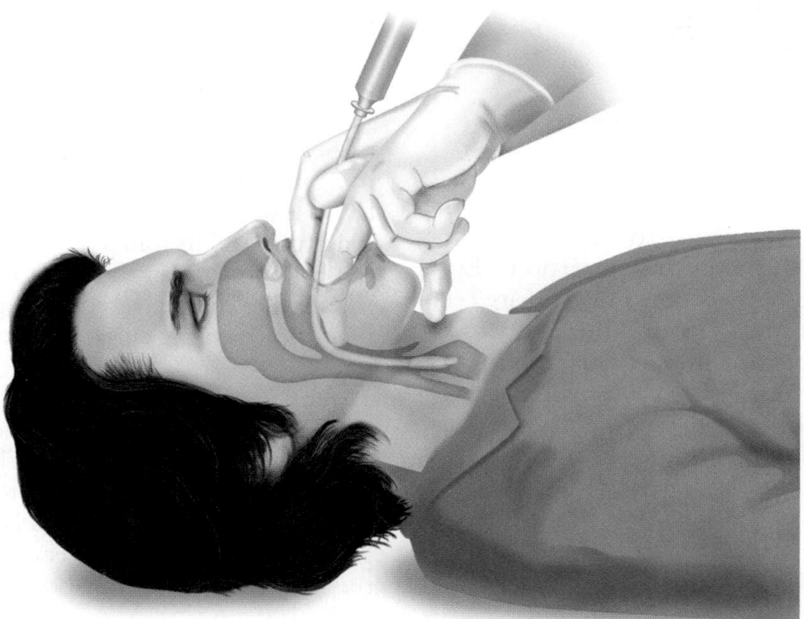

FIGURE A2-14 ✱ Lighted stylet (transillumination) tracheal tube in position.

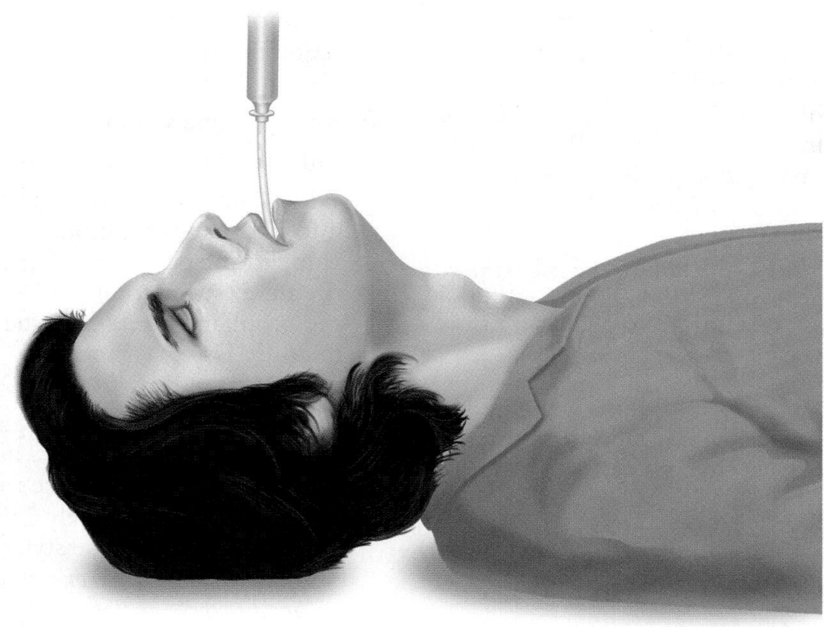

FIGURE A2-15 ✱ The properly positioned stylet should be visible at the front of the patient's neck.

10. As with any tracheal intubation, ensure that the tube is not misplaced in the esophagus or mainstem bronchus. Auscultate over the epigastrium and at the apices and bases of the lungs and watch for equal rise and fall of both sides of the chest with each ventilation. Take the steps described earlier in this appendix to correct any misplacement. Ventilate the patient between attempts to intubate. Do not interrupt ventilation for more than 30 seconds.
11. When correct placement is confirmed, secure the tube. Reassess tube position whenever the patient or the ventilating device is moved.

Alternative Advanced Airway Adjuncts

Several other devices are available to help control the airway. Some serve a similar purpose to the tracheal tube but require no visualization during insertion. Even though insertion techniques with these devices are relatively simple, just as with any intubation the ability to assess and differentiate tube placement is the key to using them effectively. Note that the tracheal tube is preferred over all of the devices described in the next sections. Medical direction is required prior to use of any of these devices.

Pharyngeo-Tracheal Lumen (PTL) Airway

The Pharyngeo-tracheal Lumen (PtL) airway is a dual-lumen, or two-tube, device designed to be inserted into the airway without direct visualization (Figure A2-16✱). Actually, the PtL is a tube within a tube. A long, clear tracheal-type tube with a cuff at the distal end is situated inside a shorter, wider tube that is designed to fit just proximal to the glottic opening. The shorter tube has a large balloon cuff on the distal third of the device. The balloon is inflated to seal the entire pharynx. The proximal end of the shorter tube is green in color. The longer tube has a cuff at the distal end that can be inserted into either the trachea or the esophagus. That distal cuff is then inflated to seal the trachea or the esophagus. The proximal end of this tube is longer, is clear in color, and contains a semi-rigid plastic stylet.

When the long, clear tube has been inserted into the trachea, the plastic stylet is removed and ventilation is performed through that tube with a bag-valve or other ventilation device attached to its proximal end. However, if the long tube is placed in the esophagus, as occurs in most instances, the plastic stylet is left in place and ventilation is delivered through the short green tube. Since the long tube and its inflated cuff seal off the esophagus, and the balloon cuff on the short tube seals off the pharynx, the ventilations delivered through the short tube into the space between the cuffs have nowhere to go but into the trachea.

Inflation lines are provided to inflate the two cuffs—the one on the long tube and the one on the short tube—simultaneously or separately. The oropharyngeal cuff on the short tube can be deflated to allow for orotracheal intubation if the long tube has been placed in the esophagus. The short tube also serves as a bite block that keeps the patient from biting down and occluding the tube with his teeth.

This device is only used in an adult patient. Only one size is available.

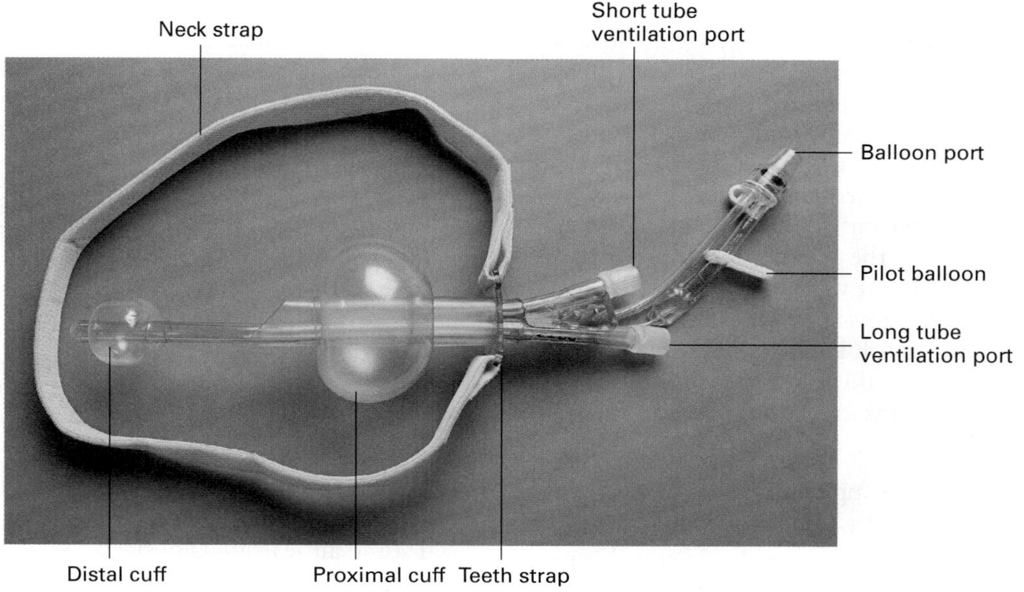

FIGURE A2-16 ✻ The Pharyngeo-tracheal Lumen (PtL) airway. (Photo: © Michal Heron)

Advantages Advantages of the PtL airway over standard tracheal intubation include the following:

- The PtL cannot be improperly placed. It can function when placed in either the trachea or esophagus.
- A mask seal is not required because the large pharyngeal cuff seals the upper airway and does not allow air to escape.
- Insertion is a blind technique that does not require visualization at the level of the glottic opening. Thus, less skill is required for the insertion technique.
- It can be used in a trauma patient with suspected spinal injury because the head or neck does not need to be moved during insertion.
- The pharyngeal cuff helps protect the lower airway from secretions and from blood coming from the nasopharynx or mouth.
- It can be inserted following failed attempts at tracheal intubation when visualization is hampered by difficult anatomy or position.

Disadvantages Disadvantages of the PtL airway include the following:

- The tube requires accurate assessment of tracheal versus esophageal placement for appropriate ventilation.
- The patient must be completely unresponsive and cannot have a gag reflex.
- It cannot be used in a patient younger than 16 years of age or less than 5 feet tall.
- It must be removed when the patient starts becoming responsive or regains a gag reflex.
- If the pharyngeal cuff deflates and the longer tube is in the esophagus, the tube loses its effectiveness.

Indications Standard tracheal intubation is the preferred method of airway control. However, you can consider using the PtL in the following circumstances:

- Tracheal intubation is not successful after two attempts.
- Tracheal intubation is indicated but is not allowed or cannot be performed immediately.
- Tracheal intubation cannot be performed or is unsuccessful because the patient's head is immobilized in a neutral position because of possible spinal injury.
- The patient's anatomy or profuse bleeding or vomiting are obstructing direct visualization.

Contraindications The PtL airway should not be inserted in any of the following situations:

- The patient is younger than 16 years of age.
- The patient is less than 5 feet tall.
- The patient is responsive or has a gag reflex.
- The patient has swallowed a caustic substance.
- Esophageal disease is present.

Equipment The following equipment is necessary for PtL insertion:

- Pharyngeal-tracheal lumen (PtL) airway
- Water-soluble lubricant
- Suction unit

Insertion Before inserting the PtL airway, you must ensure that the patient is being adequately ventilated with a bag-valve mask or other acceptable ventilation device.

Gather and prepare the equipment that will be used in insertion. Make sure that both the pharyngeal and distal tube cuffs are completely deflated. The tubes and inflation ports are marked as follows: The inflation port is designated as #1, the green shorter tube is #2, and the long clear tube is #3. Be sure that the white inflation port cap is closed. If the cuffs require further deflation, remove this white cap and compress the cuffs until they are completely flat. A clamp is located on the inflation port allowing deflation of the pharyngeal cuff while the cuff on the distal end of the longer tube remains inflated. Lubricate the long clear #3 tube with a water-soluble lubricant. An adjustable cloth strap is used to secure the PtL airway in place.

Follow these steps to insert the PtL airway:

1. Ventilate the patient for 2 minutes while delivering a high concentration of supplemental oxygen.
2. Place the patient's head into a hyperextended position if no spinal injury is suspected. If a spinal injury is suspected, maintain the head in a neutral, in-line position.
3. Insert your thumb deep into the mouth, grasping the tongue and lower jaw between the thumb and index finger, and lift the tongue and lower jaw forward.
4. Insert the PtL airway into the mouth with your free hand while maintaining the tongue-jaw lift with the other hand. Insert the airway so that it follows the natural curvature of the oropharynx. Insert the tip into the patient's mouth and advance it carefully beyond the tongue until the teeth strap touches the patient's teeth. You will feel modest resistance when passing the tube at the correct angle in the oropharynx. Do not use force during insertion. If the tube is not advancing, either redirect the tip or withdraw it and attempt insertion a second time, following 2 minutes of ventilation. Do not interrupt artificial ventilation for more than 30 seconds when inserting the device.
5. When the flange that holds the strap meets the teeth, the tube is in the proper position. Slide the neck strap over the patient's head and tighten it with the hook-and-tape closures on both sides.
6. Inflate both cuffs simultaneously by blowing into the main inflation valve #1 with a sustained breath. If the cuffs are not inflated properly, the pilot balloon will not be inflated or air will rush from the mouth during ventilation. These may be indications that one of the cuffs is defective and the device needs to be replaced. If the pilot balloon is inflated, puffs of air delivered through inflation port #1 can improve the seal if some air leakage is noticed.
7. Attach the bag-valve device to the shorter green #2 tube and deliver a ventilation. If the chest rises with the ventilation and breath sounds are heard over the chest in the apex and base of each lung, you know that the longer #3 tube has been placed in the esophagus and ventilations through the shorter tube are being directed into the trachea. Continue to ventilate through the shorter green #2 tube with a bag-valve or other ventilation device (Figure A2-17✱).
8. If the chest fails to rise or no breath sounds are heard upon ventilation through the short green #2 tube, you will assume that the longer #3 tube has been placed in the trachea and is blocking ventilations delivered through the short tube. Detach the bag-valve

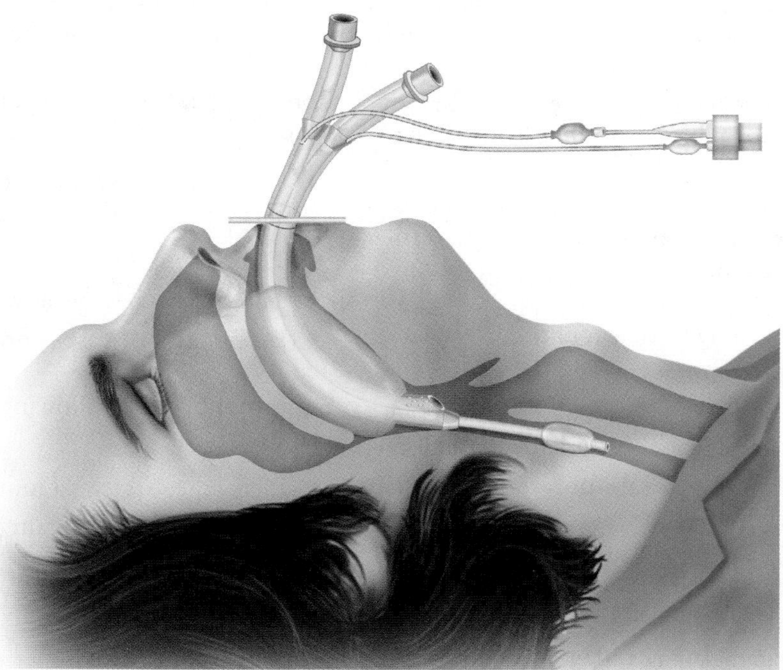

FIGURE A2-17 ✱ The PtL airway in place. The longer tube is shown placed in the esophagus while ventilations delivered through the shorter tube are directed into the trachea.

from the #2 tube, remove the plastic stylet from the #3 tube, attach the bag-valve device to the #3 tube, and deliver ventilations through the #3 tube.

Auscultate the chest for breath sounds, auscultate the epigastrium for gurgling sounds in the stomach, and watch the chest for rise and fall with each breath. Breath sounds should be equal bilaterally, no gurgling sounds should be heard over the stomach, and the chest should rise and fall with each ventilation. If these conditions apply, you have confirmed that the longer #3 tube has been placed in the trachea and is functioning much like a tracheal tube.

9. After insertion, resume ventilation. Continuously reassess the breath sounds and chest rise and fall to ensure correct tube placement. Check the pilot cuff periodically to ensure that the cuffs are adequately inflated.

Removal If either the patient regains responsiveness or his gag reflex returns, the PtL airway must be removed. Tracheal intubation is very difficult to perform around the PtL airway; therefore, in some cases it may be necessary to remove it to achieve proper visualization and oral placement of a tracheal tube. Follow these steps when removing the PtL airway:

1. Take the necessary Standard Precautions including gloves, eye protection, and a mask. Splatters of secretions and vomitus should be expected.
2. If the patient is not suspected of having any spinal injury, turn him on his side into the lateral recumbent position. If the patient has a suspected spinal injury and is properly secured to a long backboard, turn the entire board on its side.
3. A gastric tube can be inserted through the tube not being used for ventilation and passed on into the stomach. In this way, you can decompress and evacuate the stomach contents prior to PtL removal. This should only be done if you are properly trained in the procedure and have received approval from medical direction. You may be asked to remove the PtL airway in the medical facility, where you can suggest that personnel decompress the stomach by insertion of a Levine (gastric) tube down the nonventilation tube.
4. Remove the white cap from the inflation port #1 to simultaneously deflate both cuffs.
5. Have suction ready. Remove the PtL gently and discard it. Be alert for vomiting.
6. Reassess the patient's breathing status and resume positive pressure ventilation, if necessary.

Esophageal Tracheal Combitube (ETC) Airway

The esophageal tracheal Combitube airway, simply known as the Combitube or the ETC, is a double-lumen airway that is structurally and functionally similar to the PtL airway. Unlike the PtL lumens, however, the ETC lumens are not placed one inside the other. Instead, the lumens are side by side and separated by a partition wall within a single larger tube (Figure A2-18*).

The distal end of the ETC tube has a cuff that is used to seal either the trachea or the esophagus, depending on placement. A proximal pharyngeal cuff is used to seal the pharynx. The #1 tube is slightly longer and is used to deliver ventilations through holes located between the two cuffs. These holes are located just proximal to the glottic opening when the tube is placed in the esophagus. At the proximal end, the #2 tube is slightly shorter than the #1 tube and provides ventilation from the end of the tube below the distal cuff, similar to a tracheal tube. This tube is used when the device has been placed in the trachea. It is more likely that the device will be placed in the esophagus.

Advantages The advantages of the ETC airway over standard tracheal intubation are similar to those of the PtL airway. They include the following:

- No visualization is required during insertion, allowing for rapid insertion.
- The device is properly placed whether it is in the esophagus or trachea.
- The inflated pharyngeal cuff prevents ventilations delivered through the tube from escaping through the nose and mouth. This eliminates the need to maintain a mask seal.
- The pharyngeal balloon (cuff) is self-adjusting and self-positioning, an advantage over the PtL.
- There is no stylet in the distal lumen, allowing for immediate suctioning of the gastric contents. This is another advantage over the PtL airway.

Disadvantages The complication rate reported with use of the ETC in one limited study group was low. However, complications do exist. Disadvantages to ETC use include the following:

- The ETC requires accurate assessment of tracheal versus esophageal placement.
- Tracheal intubation is difficult to achieve when the ETC airway is in the esophagus.
- The ETC cannot be used in responsive patients or those with a gag reflex.
- Tracheal suctioning cannot be done with the device in the esophagus.
- The device cannot be used in patients younger than 16 years old or less than 5 feet tall.

Indications Standard tracheal intubation is the preferred method of controlling the airway. However, as with the PtL, you can consider using the ETC when tracheal intubation is not successful after two attempts,

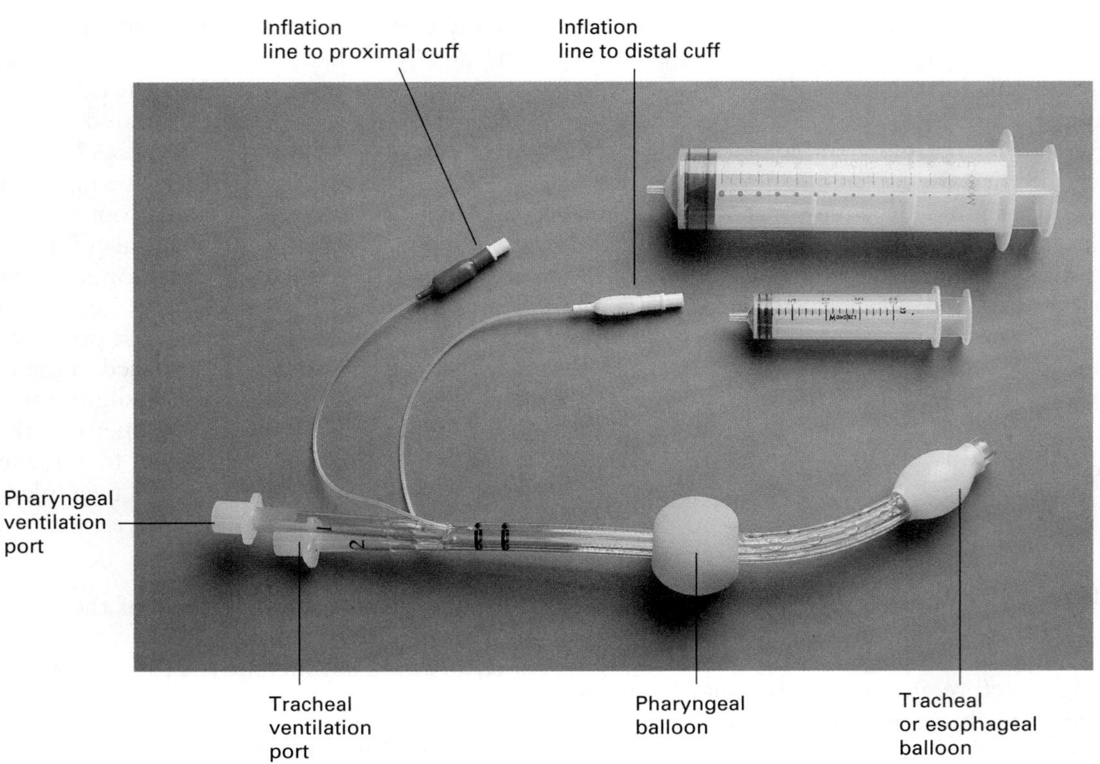

FIGURE A2-18 ✱ The Combitube airway.

when tracheal intubation is not allowed or cannot immediately be performed although indicated, when in-line immobilization of the patient with possible spine injury prevents successful tracheal intubation, or when the patient's anatomy, bleeding, or vomiting obstruct the direct visualization required for tracheal intubation.

Contraindications As with the other airway adjuncts, there are times when the ETC should not be used. Do not use an ETC if the patient is younger than age 16 or less than 5 feet tall, if the patient is responsive or has a gag reflex, if the patient has swallowed a caustic substance, or if esophageal disease is present.

Insertion ETC insertion should be attempted only after the patient has been well ventilated and hyperoxygenated with an appropriate device. Take Standard Precautions. Because this is an invasive procedure, you should use gloves, eye protection, and a mask. The procedure for insertion of the ETC is as follows:

1. Ventilate the patient for at least 2 minutes while delivering a high concentration of oxygen.
2. Assemble and check the equipment. Ensure that the cuffs on the ETC are not leaking. Lubricate the distal end of the tube with a water-soluble lubricant.
3. Place the patient's head and neck in a neutral position. If a spinal injury is suspected, maintain the head in a neutral, in-line position.
4. Perform a tongue-jaw-lift maneuver and insert the device to the level of the black rings. The teeth should be between the two black rings. If the patient has no teeth, use the gum line where the bony structure once held the teeth.
5. Use the large syringe to inflate the pharyngeal cuff with 100 mL of air. The pharyngeal balloon will self-position behind the hard palate in the posterior pharynx. The pharynx will be sealed once the cuff is inflated. For proper placement of the device, the pharyngeal cuff must be inflated prior to the distal cuff.
6. Inflate the distal cuff with 10–15 mL of air with the smaller syringe.
7. Attach the ventilation device to tube #1, the longer of the two tubes. This is the esophageal tube. It is ventilated first because the tube has most likely been placed in the esophagus (directing ventilations through the holes above the sealed-off esophagus and into the trachea—Figure A2-19✱). During the ventilation, auscultate over the epigastrium and listen for gurgling sounds. If no sounds are heard, watch for chest rise and auscultate for breath sounds. If equal chest rise and breath sounds are present bilaterally and no gastric sounds are heard over the stomach, continue to ventilate through tube #1.
8. If you hear gurgling sounds in the stomach over the epigastrium, assume that the device has been placed in the trachea and the ventilations exiting through the holes are going into the esophagus. Cease ventilation immediately and reposition the ventilation device on the shorter #2 tube, which will direct the

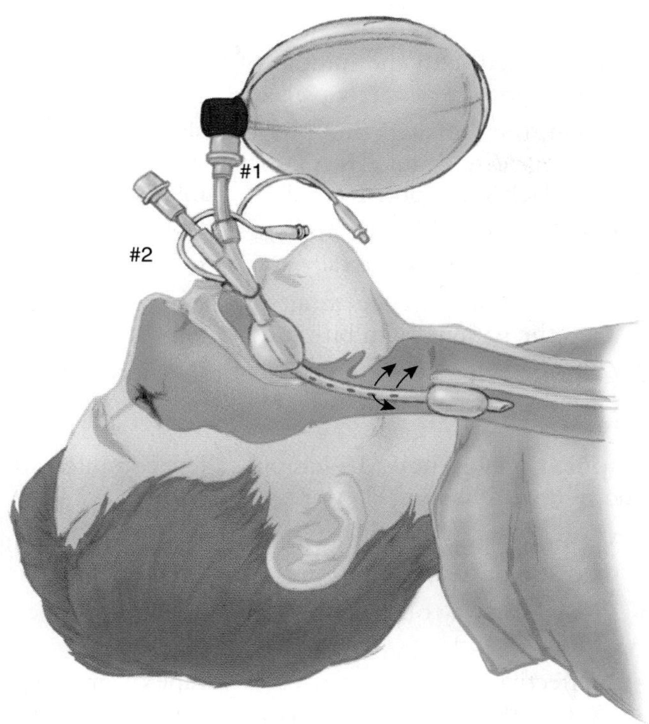

FIGURE A2-19 * Combitube airway. First ventilate through the longer, blue tube (#1). Ventilation will be successful if the tube has been placed (as is most common) in the esophagus.

ventilations into the trachea (Figure A2-20*). Auscultate over the epigastrium and listen for gurgling. If gurgling is present, remove the tube. If no gurgling is heard, assess the breath sounds. If the breath sounds are equal bilaterally, continue to ventilate through tube #2.

9. Resume ventilation. Reassess tube placement after each move involving the patient. Periodically check the pilot balloon located on each tube to ensure the cuffs are adequately inflated.

Removal If the patient regains responsiveness or his gag reflex returns, the ETC airway must be removed. As with the PtL, removal of the ETC is likely to be followed by vomiting. Remove the tube gently and discard it. Be alert for vomiting. If the patient is not suspected of having any spinal injury, place him in a lateral recumbent position. If the patient has a suspected spinal injury and is properly secured to a long backboard, turn the entire board on its side. Have suctioning equipment ready for use. Reassess the patient's breathing status and resume positive pressure ventilation, if necessary.

Laryngeal Mask Airway (LMA)

The laryngeal mask airway (LMA) (Figure A2-21*) was developed by a British anesthesiologist in 1981 and has been widely used by anesthesiologists and prehospital

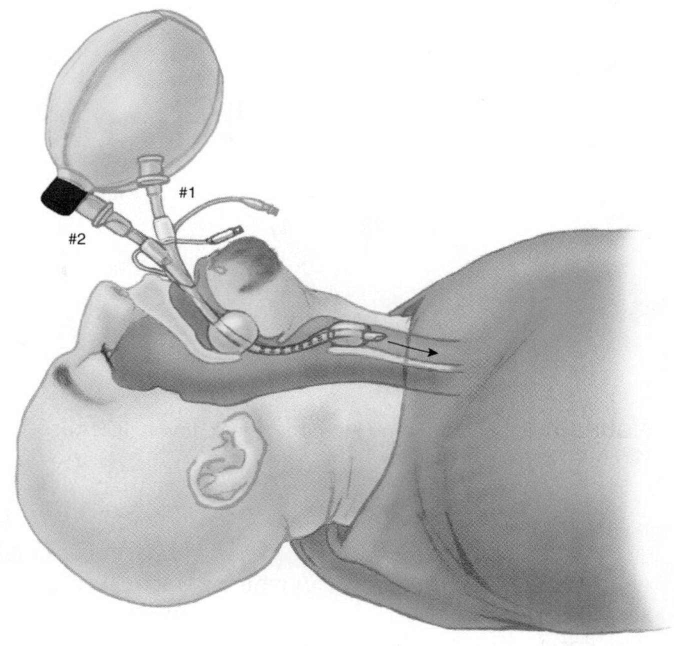

FIGURE A2-20 * Combitube airway. If ventilation through tube #1 is not successful, then ventilate through the shorter clear tube (#2). Ventilation will be successful if the tube has been placed in the trachea.

providers in the United Kingdom for several years. For the past few years, the LMA has been used more widely in the United States. The LMA is gaining popularity as an emergency adjunct airway device that may be considered for prehospital airway management when difficult tracheal intubation is encountered or as a primary adjunct to control the airway.

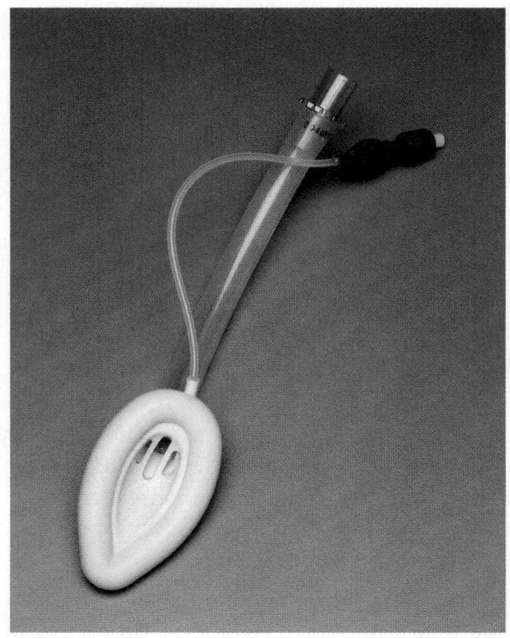

FIGURE A2-21 * The laryngeal mask airway (LMA). (© LMA North America, Inc.)

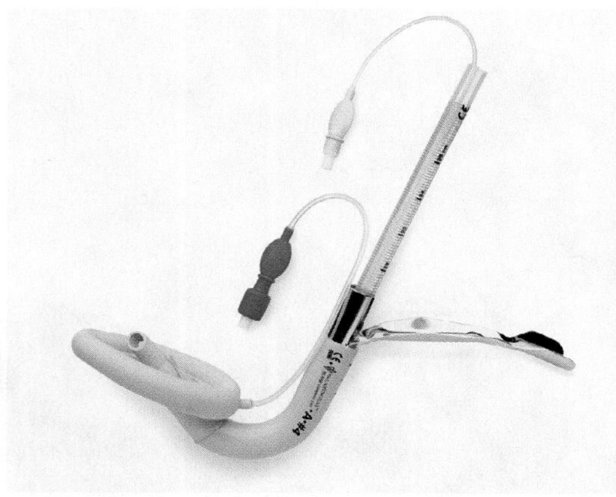

FIGURE A2-22 ∗ Intubating laryngeal mask airway (LMA). (© LMA North America, Inc.)

An intubating LMA (ILMA or LMA FasTrach) (Figure A2-22∗) is available in which a tracheal tube is inserted through the LMA once it is properly positioned. This intubating LMA device is also equipped with a handle, which allows one-handed insertion, removal, or manipulation to ensure proper alignment with the glottic opening. This does not require visualization of the vocal cords and is performed as a blind tracheal-tube insertion technique.

The LMA consists of a tube similar to a tracheal tube connected to a cufflike mask at the distal end of the tube. An inflation line is used to inflate the mask, and a pilot balloon monitors the mask inflation. The tube is connected to the mask at a 30° angle. Two vertical bars inside the inflatable mask support the epiglottis and prevent it from falling into the opening of the tube. The tube is inserted in the hypopharynx, and the cuff-like mask forms a seal around the laryngeal opening. The LMA comes in a variety of sizes from 1 for neonates to 5 for adults.

Insertion Insert the LMA, following these steps (Figure A2-23∗):

1. Ventilate the patient for 2 minutes while delivering a high concentration of oxygen.
2. Check the LMA mask for leaks. Be sure to completely deflate the mask prior to insertion.
3. Lubricate the posterior portion of the mask with a water-soluble lubricant.
4. If no cervical injury is suspected, place the patient's head in a sniffing position with the head hyperextended and the neck flexed. Hold the occiput of the head with your free hand to ensure the correct position. Another EMT may assist in opening the patient's mouth by lifting the chin forward.
5. Hold the LMA device like a dart as you insert it into the patient's mouth. Make sure the opening of the mask is anterior with the black line on the tube aligned with the middle of the patient's nose.
6. Advance the LMA into the hypopharynx until resistance is met. Do not rotate the tube. Keep the black line aligned with the middle of the nose. The tube should now be properly placed.
7. Inflate the cuff with the proper volume of air. The tube may rise about 1.5 cm once the mask is inflated. The black line should be midline against the upper lip.
8. Confirm tube placement by assessing for the presence of breath sounds bilaterally and no epigastric sounds.
9. Insert an oropharyngeal airway or a bite block to keep the patient from biting down on the tube.
10. Once you have confirmed proper tube placement, secure the device in place.

Complications The LMA has only a few complications associated with its use. They are:

- Vomiting during the insertion when used in a patient who still has a gag reflex
- Possible airway obstruction if the mask is improperly aligned in the hypopharynx
- Ineffective ventilation caused by escape of air around the mouth resulting from mask deflation or improper mask seal
- Aspiration (Remember that the LMA does not protect the patient from aspiration like an appropriately placed tracheal tube.)

Alternative Supraglottic Airway Devices

Cobra Perilaryngeal Airway (PLA)

The Cobra perilaryngeal airway (PLA) (Figure A2-24∗) is similar to the LMA in its basic design. It is inserted into a supraglottic location where the "cobra head" of the device holds the epiglottis and surrounding soft tissue out of the way to allow airway patency. Ventilations are then provided through the hollow tube of the airway from the proximal 15/22 mm adapter, and exit the airway through the fenestrated openings at the distal end. Like the LMA, it comes in a variety of sizes from pediatric to adult. After ensuring medical direction will allow use of the device, the EMT should be completely familiar with the indications, contraindications, insertion, and removal techniques prior to use.

King LT-D Airway

The King LT-D Airway (Figure A2-25∗) is another supraglottic airway that is gaining popularity in emergency prehospital care. It is a tubular device with a large pharyngeal cuff that disperses pressure over a large surface area at the pharyngeal level to stabilize the airway at the base of the tongue and minimize the risk to the vocal cords and trachea. The distal end of the tube is also equipped with a

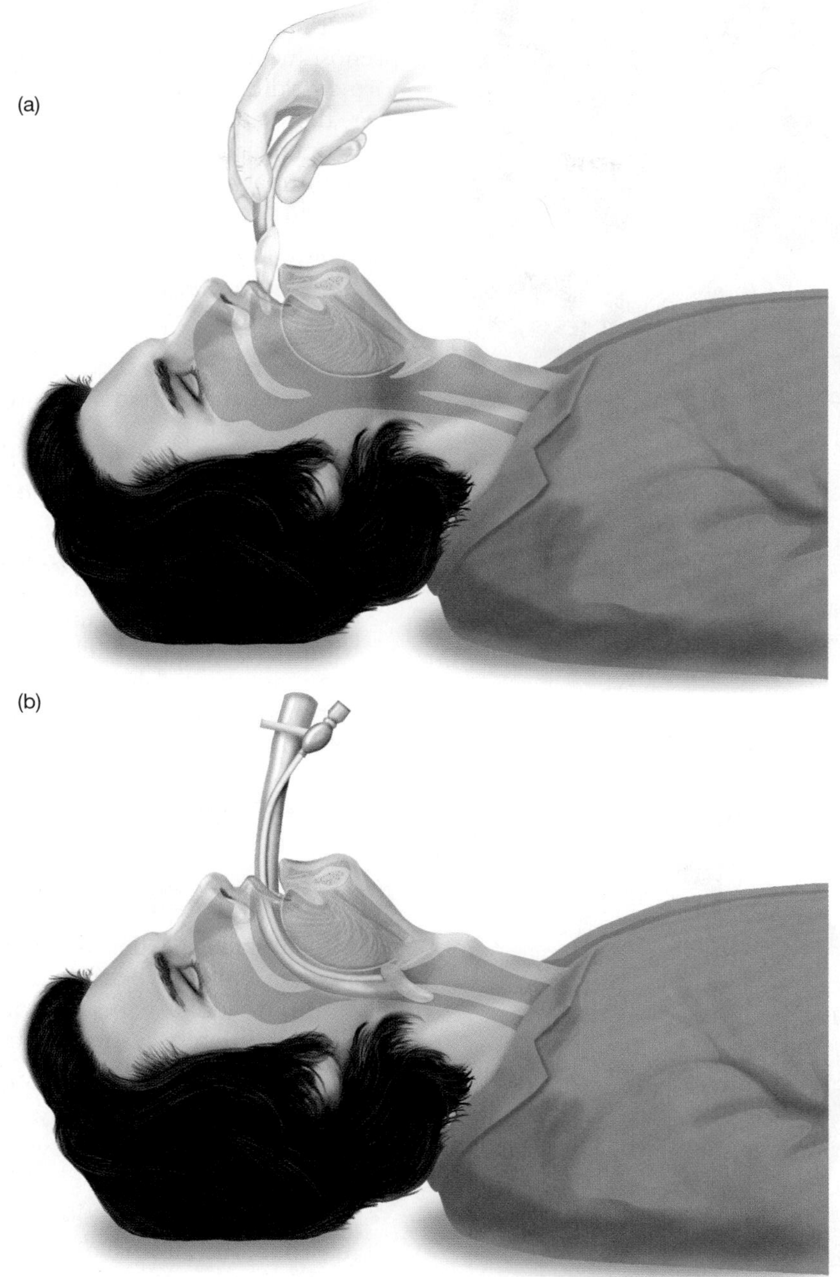

FIGURE A2-23 * (a) Inserting the laryngeal mask airway. (b) The laryngeal mask airway in place.

smaller cuff that provides occlusion to the esophagus. Between the cuffs is a large opening that is continuous with the lumen of the tube. Upon providing ventilations through the proximal end of the device, the ventilation exits through the port between the cuffs. Since the airway has been isolated between the cuffs, the ventilation is directed through the glottic opening and into the lungs. The King LT airway is supplied in three sizes, and both disposable (King LT-D) and reusable (King LT) models are available. After ensuring that medical direction will allow use of the device, the EMT should be completely familiar with the indications, contraindications, insertion, and removal techniques prior to use.

Orotracheal Intubation in Infants and Children

The procedure for pediatric intubation is much the same as in adults. However, there are special considerations with infants and children about when and how to intubate.

Indications in Infants and Children

The airway in an infant or child should be managed with the proper manual position and an airway adjunct. Most

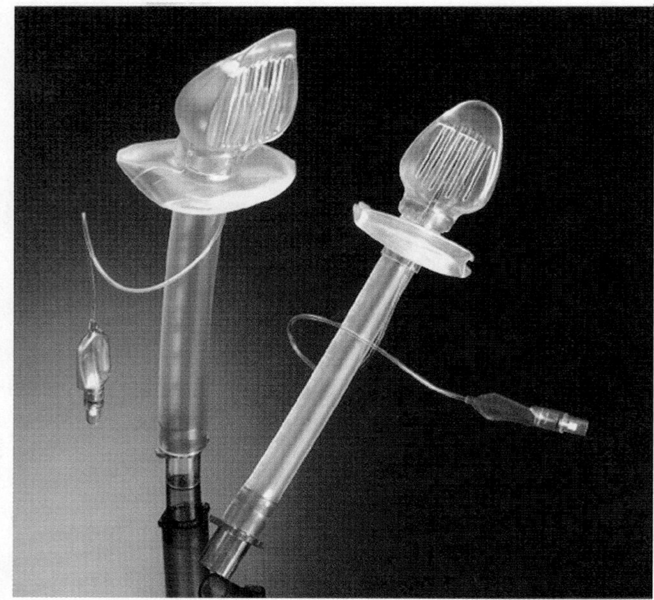

FIGURE A2-24 ✱ Cobra perilaryngeal airway (PLA).
(© Engineered Medical Systems, Inc., Indianapolis, IN)

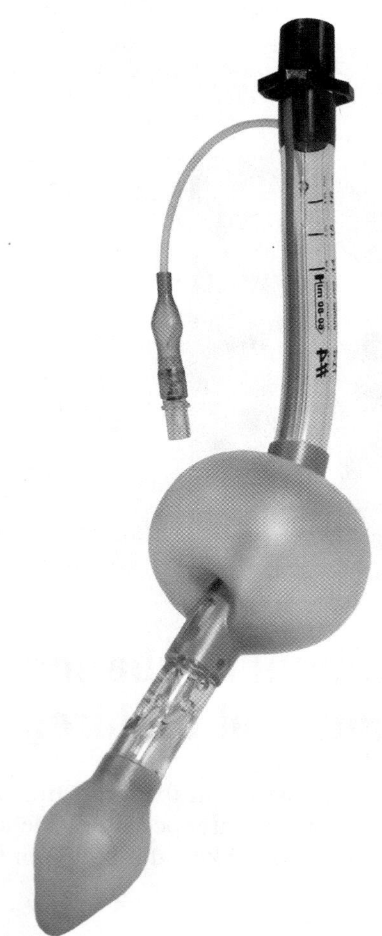

FIGURE A2-25 ✱ The King LT-D (disposable model) airway.
(© Tracey Lemons/King Systems Corporation)

often, a bag-valve-mask device is all that is needed to ventilate the patient adequately. Research has shown that prehospital pediatric intubation is an infrequently performed skill, which may lead to poor outcomes. However, there are some situations where ventilation cannot be properly achieved without tracheal intubation. Tracheal intubation for the infant and child should be considered in the following circumstance:

- *Artificial ventilation cannot be delivered adequately when using other airway maneuvers and adjuncts.*

Tracheal intubation may be considered in the following circumstances; however, a person with experience intubating pediatric patients should perform the intubation.

- *Prolonged positive pressure ventilation is required.*
- *The patient is completely apneic.* The patient in respiratory arrest or cardiac arrest should be intubated.
- *The patient is unresponsive, with no gag or cough reflex.* If the unresponsive patient accepts an oropharyngeal airway without gagging, consider tracheal intubation. The infant or child has the same risk of aspiration as the adult in this circumstance. Tracheal intubation minimizes the risk of aspiration by sealing off the trachea at the level of the cricoid cartilage. Cricoid pressure can be used to reduce the chances of aspiration during the intubation procedure.

Anatomical Considerations

Additional skill is needed when performing intubation in infants and children because of their anatomical differences from adults. Special considerations related to anatomical differences include the following:

- In general, infants' and children's noses, mouths, and jaws are smaller and their tongues are disproportionately larger. This makes visualization of the glottic opening and the vocal cords more difficult.
- Sizing of tracheal tubes for infants and children is based on the internal diameter of the cricoid cartilage and not the glottic opening. Most often, tracheal tubes used in infants and in children less than 8 years of age do not have cuffs; the tubes are sealed by the narrow cricoid cartilage. Therefore, ensuring a proper fit of a tracheal tube is vital.
- The vocal cords and glottic opening are typically more anterior and cephalad (toward the head), making visualization more difficult. It is difficult to create a single, clear visual plane from the mouth through the pharynx to the glottic opening during intubation.
- Bradycardia may result from stimulation of the airway during intubation. The onset of bradycardia may limit your intubation attempt to even less than 30 seconds. Infants and children are extremely sensitive to hypoxia, which normally results in bradycardia.

Equipment for Infants and Children

The same basic equipment is used for intubating adults, infants, and children. However, because of the anatomical differences, the equipment has some variations and must be carefully sized prior to the intubation procedure. One aid to determining the proper equipment necessary to perform tracheal intubation in the infant and child is a resuscitation tape. Refer to Figure A2-26* to see an example of a resuscitation tape (the Broselow tape), which is commercially available. The tape is stretched from the head to the feet of the patient and provides information regarding appropriate tube sizes and drug dosages as well as other information necessary in the emergency management of the pediatric patient.

Suction Devices

A suction device should be readily available during the pediatric intubation procedure. As in the adult, there may be fluid, blood, or heavy secretions obstructing your view of the landmarks and increasing the patient's risk of aspiration. Any substance must be removed immediately. A suction unit with an adjustable regulator that can tailor the negative pressure used to between 80 and 120 mmHg is warranted. Ensure that the appropriate suction catheter and noncollapsible suction tubing are available.

Laryngoscope Handles and Blades

The same laryngoscope handle used in adult intubation is also used interchangeably with the infant and child laryngoscope blades. A smaller-diameter laryngoscope handle is available, if necessary, for infant intubation. The locking mechanism and assembly are the same as in adult equipment.

A straight laryngoscope blade is preferred in infants because it provides greater displacement of the tongue and better visualization of the glottic opening, which is more anterior and cephalad. It also causes less damage to the soft tissues. The straight blade is fitted under the epiglottis and directly lifts it up and forward to expose the vocal cords and glottic opening. The straight blade comes in sizes from 0 to 4. A size 0 blade is usually used in premature infants, whereas a full-term infant would require a 0 or 1. A size 2 blade is usually used to intubate children from 2 to 8 years old. A size 3 straight blade is typically used in adolescent patients.

The curved blade is preferred in older children because its broader base and flange provide better displacement of the tongue in this age group. Curved blades also come in a size range of 0 to 4. A size 2 curved blade is typically used in 8- to 12-year-olds. A size 3 curved blade is used for 12-year-olds and adolescents. The curved blade is inserted into the vallecula and indirectly lifts the epiglottis with an upward and forward movement of the handle.

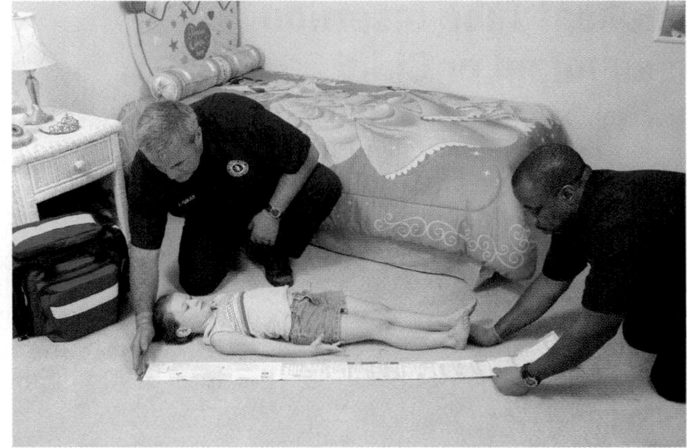

FIGURE A2-26 * A resuscitation tape (Broselow tape) can be used to estimate appropriate tube sizes, drug dosages, and other information based on the child's height.

Tracheal Tubes

When intubating an infant or child, tubes at least one-half size above and below the selected size must be immediately available. The tube should be of uniform diameter and not tapered. It should have centimeter distance markings along its length for use as reference points. Some tubes have a vocal cord marker at the distal end to ensure that the tip of the tube is midway between the carina and the level of the vocal cords.

Tracheal tubes used in infants and children under age 8 are typically uncuffed, with no inflation cuff at the distal end of the tube (Figure A2-27*). The cricoid ring is the narrowest portion of the upper airway in infants and children and serves as a functional cuff to seal off the trachea. Therefore, sizing the tube is extremely critical. Cuffed tubes should be used for children older than 8 years. When a cuffed tube is inserted into the trachea, the proximal end of the cuff is inserted approximately one-half inch beyond the level of the vocal cords, since no vocal cord marker may be available on the tube. The use of cuffed tracheal tubes in pediatrics, as discussed earlier, is becoming more common in the hospital. Your medical director may allow the use of cuffed tracheal tubes in this

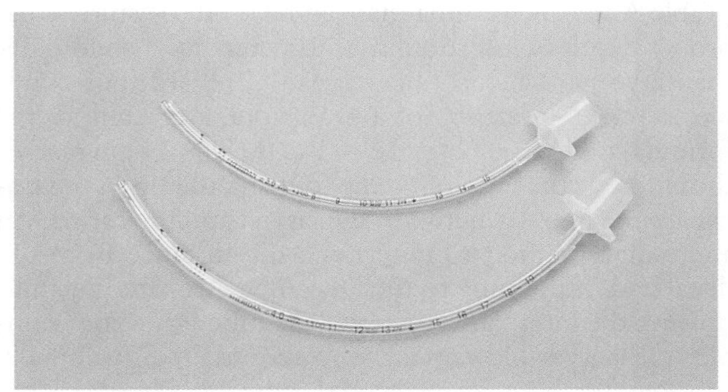

FIGURE A2-27 * Uncuffed tracheal tubes.

age range. Always use the equipment recommended by your medical director when you perform this skill.

The best, most accurate method of selecting the appropriate-sized tracheal tube for infants and children is to refer to a sizing chart. You should carry a copy of the chart or keep one in the airway kit containing the infant and child intubation equipment. A commercially available resuscitation tape can be used to determine the appropriate-sized tracheal tube. The tape, which is stretched out alongside the infant or child, has reference areas corresponding to the height of the infant or child.

Several formulas can be used to estimate the correct size of tracheal tube for children. For a child 1–10 years of age, the formula for an uncuffed tracheal tube is: tube size = 4 + (age in years/4). For example, the formula for a 4-year-old child would be: 4 + (4/4) = 5.0 mm i.d. tracheal tube. A half size above and below this range (4.5 and 5.5) should also be available. If the EMT is using a cuffed tracheal tube, per medical direction protocol, the formula becomes: tube size = 3 + (age in years/4). This formula will result in a tube size that is slightly smaller than the uncuffed version. This is to allow the cuff at the distal end adequate space to inflate to secure the airway. When inflating the cuff of a small tracheal tube such as this, you should inflate with no more air than is needed to make the inflation port mildly tense after inflation, yet enough to prevent air or fluid from passing by the inflated cuff.

Other methods for estimating the size of the uncuffed tracheal tube can be used. One method calls for choosing a tracheal tube with the same outside diameter as the child's little finger. Another method is to select a tube with an outside diameter that is the same as the internal diameter of the child's nares, or nostrils. These methods at best are estimations; therefore, it is vital to have tubes one-half size larger and one-half size smaller than the one you select available during intubation.

Newborn infants typically require a 3.0–3.5 mm tracheal tube. A 1-year-old usually requires a 4.0–4.5 mm tube size. An 8-year-old child usually requires a 6.0 mm cuffed or uncuffed tracheal tube. Refer to Table A2-1 for other tracheal tube sizes.

Both infant- and child-sized tracheal tubes have centimeter markers as reference points to monitor the depth of tube insertion. The depth also corresponds with age (Table A2-2). A formula that can be used to estimate the proper depth of insertion in centimeters for a child older than 2 years of age is: (age in years/2) + 12. For example, depth of insertion for a 4-year-old, according to the formula, is (4 years/2) + 12 = 14 cm. The 14 cm marker should be at the level of the lip, putting the tip of the tracheal tube midway between the larynx and the carina. An alternative method to determine the distance from the distal end of the tube to the lip can be estimated by multiplying the internal diameter of the tube by 3. For example, the 4-year-old patient who requires a 5.0 mm i.d. tube would have an estimated tube length of 15 cm (5.0 mm i.d. × 3 = 15 cm). Thus, the tube marking at the level of the lips should be approximately 15 cm.

TABLE A2-1 Tracheal Tube Sizes Based on Age

Age	Uncuffed Tracheal Tube Size in Millimeters (i.d.)
Premature	2.5–3.0 uncuffed
Newborn	3.0–3.5 uncuffed
6 months	3.5–4.0 uncuffed
1 year	4.0–4.5 uncuffed
2 years	4.5 uncuffed
4 years	5.0 uncuffed
6 years	5.5 uncuffed
8 years	6.0 cuffed
10 years	6.5 cuffed
12 years	7.0 cuffed
Adolescent	7.0–8.0 cuffed

TABLE A2-2 Measuring the Tracheal Tube

Distance from Tube Tip Placed Mid-Trachea to Level of the Teeth

Age	Centimeter Marking at the Level of the Teeth
Premature	8
Newborn	9–10
6 months	10.5–12
1 year	13.5
2 years	13.5
4 years	15
6 years	16.5
8 years	18
10 years	19.5
12 years	21
Adolescent	21

Tracheal Tube Insertion in an Infant or Child

Orotracheal intubation in infants and children is basically the same as in adults except for some variations caused by anatomical differences in the upper airway and by the size of the laryngoscope blades and tracheal tubes. Some research suggests that bag-valve-mask ventilation is as effective as ventilation with a tracheal tube in place in pediatric patients. Refer to the step-by-step procedure for orotracheal intubation in adults described earlier, plus the following special considerations for intubating infants and children:

- The patient must be ventilated and hyperoxygenated.
- The heart rate should be continuously monitored during the intubation attempt. Bradycardia is an early sign of hypoxia. (Interruption of ventilation to intu-

bate can drastically reduce the oxygen level and cause severe hypoxia, especially if the intubation attempt lasts longer than 30 seconds.) Stimulation of the airway in infants and young children can also cause bradycardia. If the heart rate drops below 80 beats per minute in an infant or below 60 beats per minute in a child, the intubation procedure should be stopped and the patient ventilated with a bag-valve-mask device with supplemental oxygen. Continuously monitor the pulse oximeter reading.

- Align the axes of the mouth, pharynx, and trachea to achieve better visualization of the glottic opening. This can be done by tilting the patient's head back, flexing the neck forward, and lifting the chin to place him in a "sniffing position." This should only be done if there is no suspicion of spinal injury. If spinal injury is suspected, the head and neck must be stabilized manually in an in-line position during the intubation attempt. If you are unable to visualize the cords, raise the patient's shoulders 1 inch by placing a folded towel or sheet under them. The height required will vary with the age of the patient and will need to be adjusted accordingly. (Remember that the larger occipital region of the pediatric head may result in flexion of the neck when the patient is supine, making the intubation procedure more difficult.)
- The laryngoscopy should be very gentle. Never use force. Do not use the handle in a prying or levering motion as if digging in the airway. Doing so could cause extensive damage to the upper airway. Do not use the teeth or upper gums as a fulcrum. Pull in the direction of the handle to get better visualization.
- The epiglottis is more flexible and less developed in infants and young children. As a result, it is more likely to cause obstruction of your view and may require extra effort to control when using the straight blade.
- Application of cricoid pressure during intubation will reduce the risk of vomiting and aspiration. Pressure on the cricoid and thyroid cartilage will move the glottic opening slightly posterior, making visualization easier.
- Insert the tube until the vocal cord or glottic marker on the uncuffed tube, if available, is at the level of the vocal cords. If a cuffed tube is being used, insert the tube until the proximal end of the cuff is approximately one-half inch beyond the vocal cords.
- The tracheal tube must be held in place until it is properly secured. Any movement could easily dislodge it.
- Confirm tracheal tube placement using the methods described earlier for adults, including use of end-tidal CO_2 detection devices. An esophageal detection device may be less reliable in infants and children. If corrective action is necessary, follow the procedures that were described. Be aware, however, that observing symmetrical rise and fall of the chest is the best indicator of proper placement in infants and children. Breath sounds could be misleading because sounds are easily referred and transmitted to the other side of the chest and epigastrium because of the small size of the chest cavity.
- Improvement in heart rate and skin color should occur after intubation. If the tube is not placed properly, the patient's heart rate may continue to deteriorate and the cyanosis may worsen.
- If the tube is properly placed, secure it with tape or a commercial device approved by medical direction. Insert an oropharyngeal airway as a bite block.
- Note the centimeter marker at the level of the patient's teeth or gums when the tube is properly positioned. If at any time you note a change in insertion depth, immediately reassess tube placement. Remember that small movements of the head or neck of the child can dislodge the tube.
- Once tube placement is confirmed and the tube secured, the patient's head should be immobilized to limit movement that might dislodge the tube. Remember that flexion or extension of the neck in an infant or child can displace the tube. Consider immobilizing the neck, even if no trauma is suspected.
- If the tube is properly placed but inadequate lung expansion or tidal volume is noted, assess for one of the following causes:
  - **The tube is too small and there is an air leak around the cricoid cartilage.** Such a leak can be heard when auscultating over the neck. If a leak is detected, the tube should be replaced with a larger one. If using a cuffed tube, inflate the cuff until the air leak is eliminated. Check the pilot balloon to determine if the cuff is still working properly. A defective cuff may leak and deflate.
  - **The pop-off valve on the bag-valve device is not deactivated (as it should be) and air is escaping with ventilation.** This is a problem particularly in children with poor lung compliance or high airway resistance.
  - **The bag-valve device has a leak or is not functioning properly.** Check all its parts, especially the valves, to be sure they are working properly. Remove the bag-valve device from the tube and occlude the tube connection while squeezing the bag to check for any leaks or malfunctions.
  - **The EMT performing ventilation is not delivering an adequate volume with each squeeze of the bag.** Have the ventilator increase the volume delivered by squeezing more air out of the bag. Be careful, however, because a pneumothorax can result from overly aggressive ventilation.
  - **The tube has become blocked with secretions or has kinked.** Perform tracheal suctioning to remove any secretions. Visualize the tube with the laryngoscope to detect any kinks. If the tube remains occluded, remove it and begin positive pressure ventilation by bag-valve mask. After ventilation for 2–5 minutes, attempt intubation again.

- Excessive force and/or volume in ventilating an infant or child can easily cause rupture of a lung (barotrauma) and a subsequent pneumothorax (leakage of air into the chest cavity—an extremely dangerous condition). Carefully inspect the chest with each ventilation and watch for rise. As soon as the chest rises adequately, cease your ventilation.

Once the patient is intubated, it is necessary to continuously monitor the patient for deterioration that may result from a problem associated with the tracheal tube or ventilation device. A common mnemonic that can be used to determine possible causes for deterioration in the patient's oxygenation or ventilation status is DOPE (displacement, obstruction, pneumothorax, and equipment failure).

The tube may be displaced from the trachea or may have been pushed farther into the trachea, creating a right or left mainstem bronchus intubation. Auscultate the lungs carefully to check for tube placement and, if necessary, perform a laryngoscopy to be sure the tube has not been displaced into the esophagus. A right or left mainstem bronchus intubation can be corrected by pulling back on the tube. If the tube is in the esophagus, it must be immediately removed and ventilation with a bag-valve-mask device or other ventilation device immediately initiated with a manual airway maneuver.

The tracheal tube may become obstructed with secretions, pus, blood, or a foreign body, or it may kink. Pass a suction catheter through the tube to ensure that it is free of any obstructions. If the tube is obstructed and cannot be unobstructed with suction applied via a catheter, remove the tube immediately and provide positive pressure ventilation with a bag-valve-mask device or other ventilation device with a manual airway maneuver.

The patient may have suffered a pneumothorax, which can lead to rapid deterioration of the patient. If you suspect a tension pneumothorax, expedite transport and contact an ALS unit for thoracic decompression.

Equipment failure must be considered in acute deterioration of the intubated patient. Check to be sure the oxygen has not become disconnected from the ventilation device, the oxygen source has not run out, and the ventilation device is still working properly.

Nasogastric Insertion in Infants and Children

Gastric distention (air in the stomach) tends to be a greater problem in infants and children than in adults. Because of their small airway structures, it is easy to ventilate them too quickly or too hard, causing air to enter the esophagus and be forced into the stomach. The child's less-developed diaphragm is easily pushed upward by the air in the stomach, compressing the small chest cavity to the point where effective ventilation is impossible, leading to hypoxia. The risk of regurgitation and aspiration of gastric contents is also increased.

In this instance, the gastric air pressure must be relieved by inserting a nasogastric (NG) tube, a specialized catheter that is inserted through the nose and down the esophagus into the stomach (Figure A2-28∗). The NG tube may also be used to dilute or lavage ingested poisons in the stomach, to remove blood associated with internal gastrointestinal bleeding, or to introduce medications. However, relief of gastric distention in an infant or child patient is the most common purpose for nasogastric intubation by the EMT.

Indications

The indications for insertion of an NG tube in infants and children include the following:

- You are unable to provide effective positive pressure ventilation because of gastric distention.
- The patient is unresponsive and at risk of vomiting gastric contents or developing gastric distention.

Contraindications

An NG tube should not be inserted in a patient who has suffered major facial, head, or spinal trauma. Consult medical direction about using oral insertion with such trauma patients. Do not insert the NG tube if you suspect an airway disease such as epiglottitis or croup unless the patient is intubated. This can cause spasms or exacerbate swelling to the point of occluding the airway. The NG tube is also contraindicated if the patient has ingested certain caustic substances (alkalis) and some hydrocarbons.

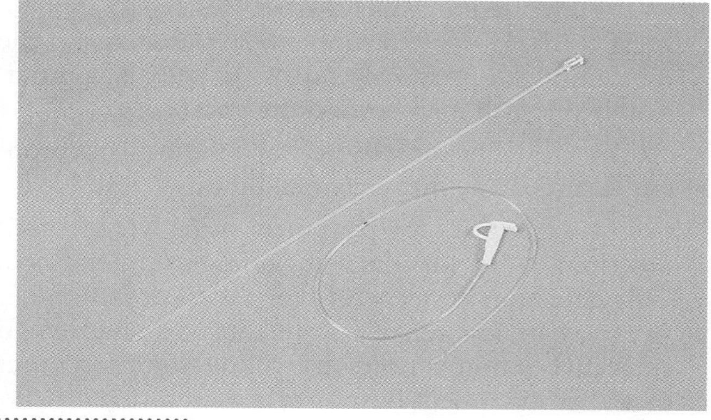

FIGURE A2-28a ∗ Nasogastric tubes.

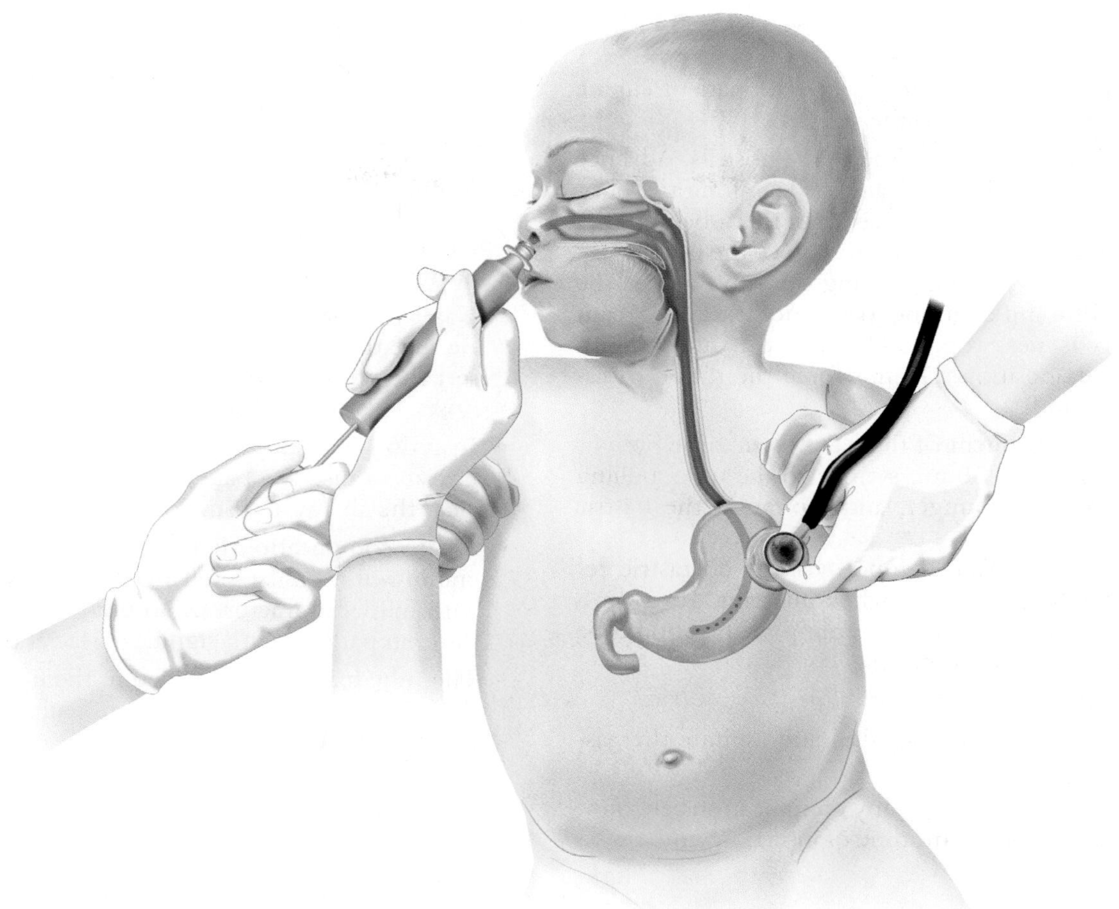

FIGURE A2-28b ✱ Nasogastric tube placed in an infant.

Equipment

The equipment for nasogastric intubation includes the following:

- A nasogastric tube (NG tubes come in a variety of sizes and are measured in units called French. Newborns and infants typically take an 8.0 French; toddlers or preschool children, a 10 French; school-age children, a 12 French; and adolescents, a 14–16 French.)
- 20 mL syringe to check tube placement
- Water-soluble lubricant to facilitate insertion of the tube
- An emesis basin, in case the patient vomits
- Tape to secure the tube
- Stethoscope to check for proper placement
- Suction unit and suction catheters in case of vomiting and to evacuate the stomach contents following tube placement

Insertion

Before beginning insertion, take Standard Precautions. Gloves, eye protection, and a mask should be worn because of the potential for splatters of secretions, blood, and vomitus. Then insert the NG tube using the following procedure (Advanced Airway Management Skills A2-4A to A2-4F):

1. Prepare and assemble the equipment.
2. Determine which nostril appears more patent. If obstruction or other deformity is present in one nostril, select the other.
3. Measure the tube by placing it at the tip of the nose, around the ear, and extending it until the most proximal of the holes at the distal end is just below the xiphoid process. Mark the tube with a piece of tape at the level of the tip of the nose; the tape will serve as a guide, indicating when an adequate length of tube has been inserted to enter the stomach.

4. Lubricate 6–8 inches of the distal end of the tube with water-soluble lubricant.
5. If trauma is not suspected, place the patient supine with the head turned to the side.
6. Insert the tube gently in one of the nostrils. Advance the tube straight back toward the ear along the floor of the nostril. Continue to advance the tube until the tape marker is at the level of the tip of the nose. If resistance is met when advancing the tube, rotate the tube slightly and continue to advance it. If significant resistance is met, stop, pull back on the tube, and reevaluate its position. Do not force the tube if resistance is found.
7. Check the placement of the nasogastric tube by:
   a. Attaching the 20 mL syringe to the tube, pulling back on the plunger, and aspirating the gastric contents.
   b. Placing your stethoscope over the epigastric region and auscultating while injecting 10–20 mL of air into the tube. A gurgling sound should be heard over the stomach.
8. Secure the tube in place with tape.
9. Attach the tube to low suction and aspirate the gastric contents.
10. Document the tube size, any complications encountered during placement, time of insertion, and assessment of placement.

Complications

There are several possible complications associated with placement of the nasogastric tube:

- Tracheal intubation is possible, with the NG tube entering the larynx and trachea instead of the esophagus. The patient will typically begin severe coughing and choking. Pull back on the tube until it is at the posterior pharynx and reattempt insertion.
- Nasal trauma can occur from insertion of the tube. Be sure the tube is adequately lubricated. Do not insert the tip of the tube in an upward direction in the nose. This commonly causes pain and bleeding.
- Insertion of the NG tube may stimulate the gag reflex and cause the patient to vomit. Be prepared to clear the airway and suction.
- A rare complication is passage of the tube into the cranium if a basilar skull fracture exists, particularly with midfacial fractures. Do not attempt this procedure on patients with significant facial trauma.
- The tube may become curled in the nose, mouth, or trachea. If insertion becomes difficult, inspect inside the mouth and withdraw the tube to determine its position.
- Perforation of the esophagus may occur with an overly aggressive insertion technique.

Medical direction or your local protocol may allow insertion of the NG tube only after tracheal intubation. Once the airway is secured with a tracheal tube, the risks of misplacing the NG tube in the trachea or of vomiting and aspiration are greatly reduced.

Orotracheal Intubation

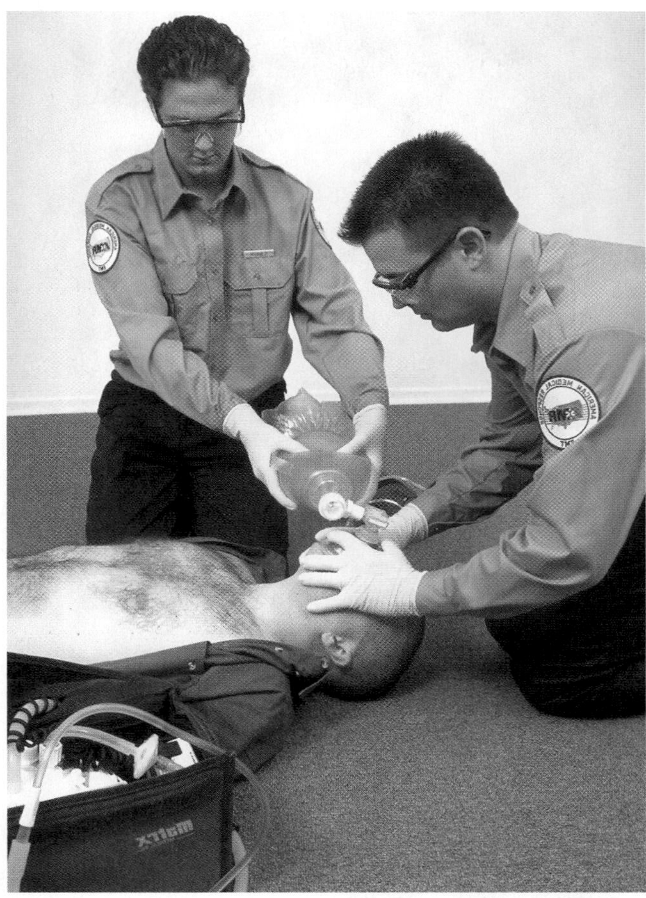

A2-1A ✻ Ensure adequate ventilation and oxygenation. Prior to any intubation attempt, ventilate and hyperoxygenate the patient.

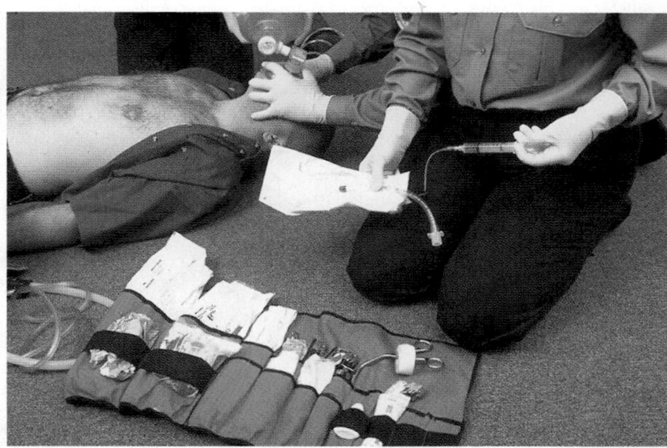

A2-1B ✻ Assemble and test the equipment.

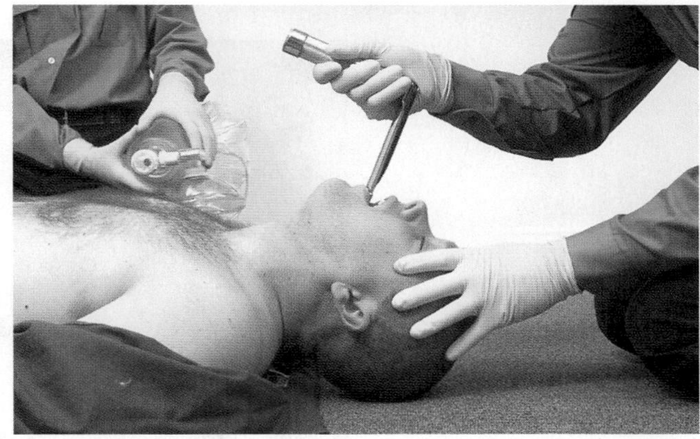

A2-1C ✻ In the nontrauma patient, tilt the head and lift the chin into a "sniffing position." Insert the blade on the right and sweep the tongue to the left until the blade is midline.

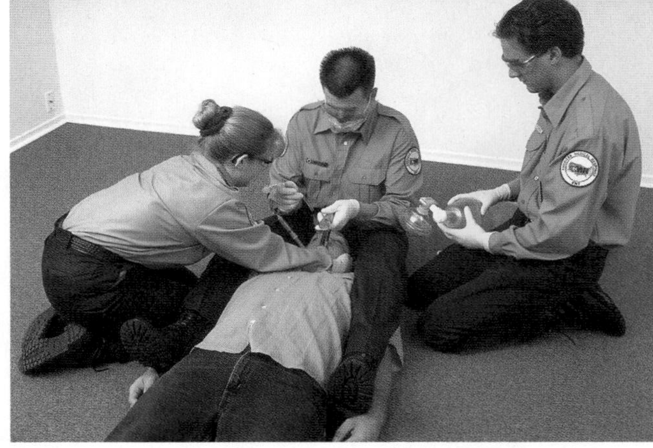

A2-1D ✻ The trauma patient with suspected spinal injury must be intubated with in-line spinal stabilization maintained. The EMT intubating secures the patient's head with his thighs while the second EMT holds the head from a position below the patient's neck.

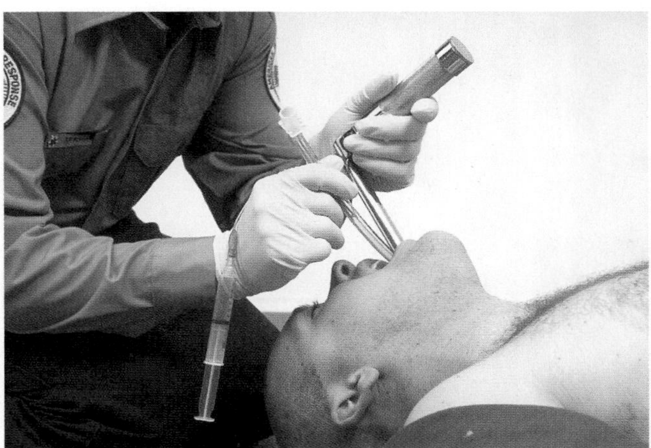

A2-1E ✻ Visualize the vocal cords and glottic opening and insert the tracheal tube through the vocal cords. Lift in the direction of the blade handle.

continued

Orotracheal Intubation *continued*

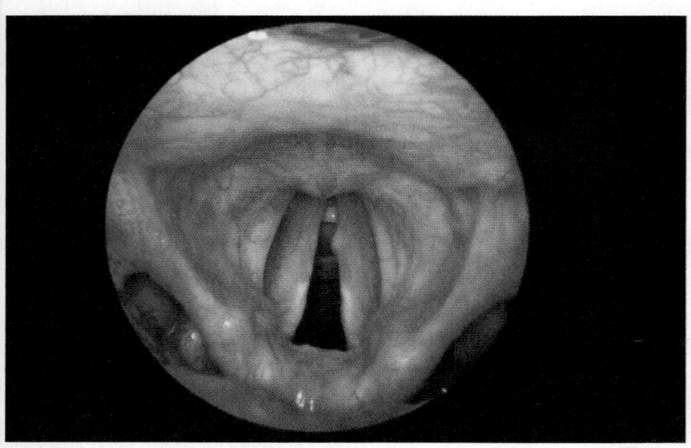

A2-1F ✱ To visualize the glottic opening (shown here), lift the laryngoscope in the direction of the handle.
(CNRI/Photo Researchers, Inc.)

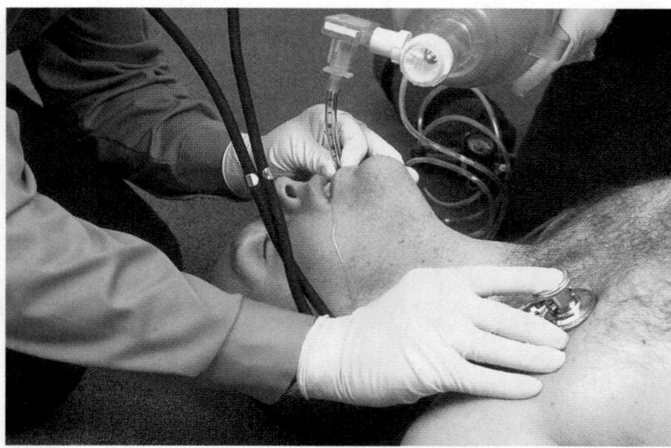

A2-1G ✱ Confirm tube placement.

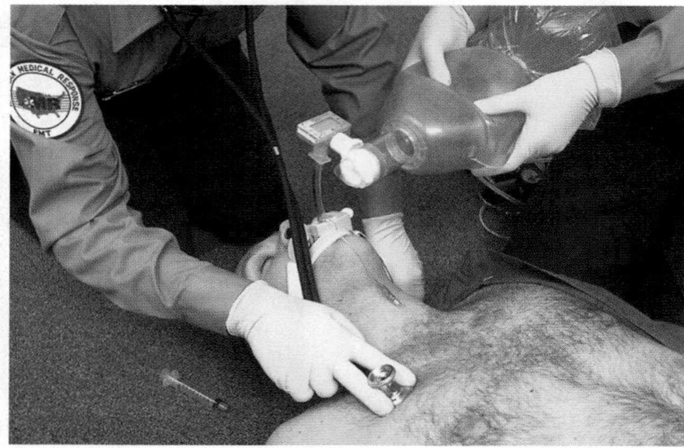

A2-1H ✱ Secure the tube and reassess for tube placement.

ADVANCED AIRWAY skills A2-2 Orotracheal Suctioning

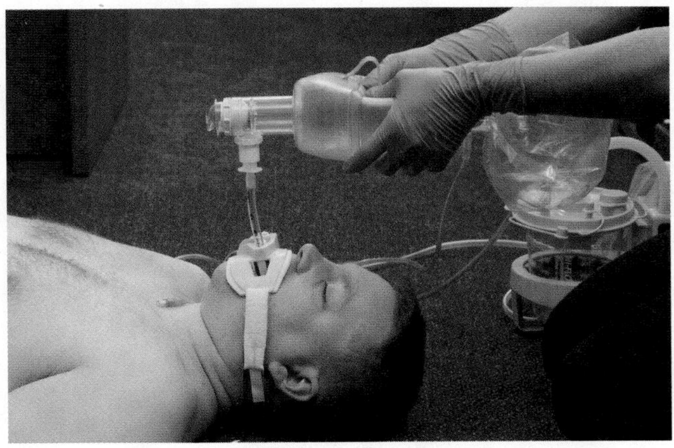

A2-2A ✻ Preoxygenate the patient for 2 minutes prior to orotracheal suctioning.

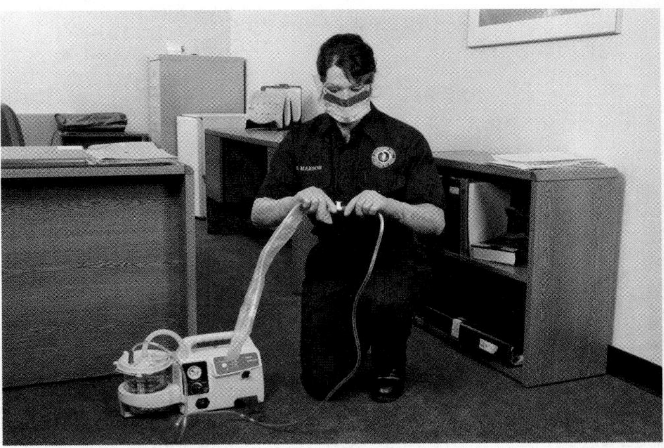

A2-2B ✻ Check the suction equipment. Orotracheal suctioning is a sterile procedure; therefore, do not contaminate the suction catheter.

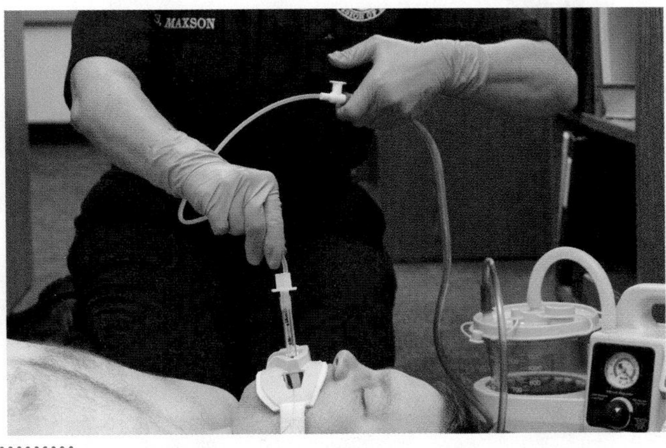

A2-2C ✻ Insert and advance the catheter without suction being applied.

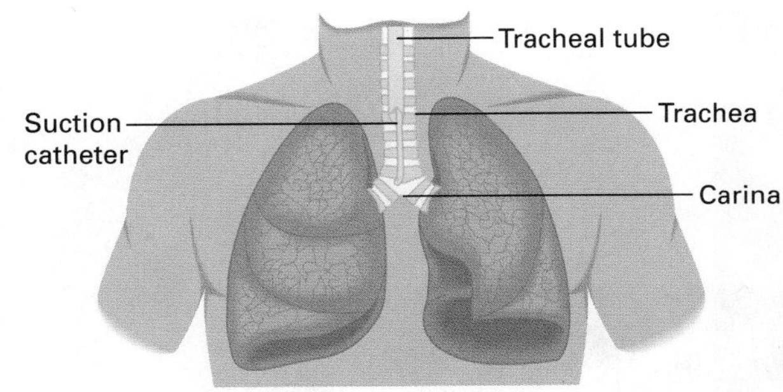

A2-2D ✻ Continue to advance the catheter to the level of the carina.

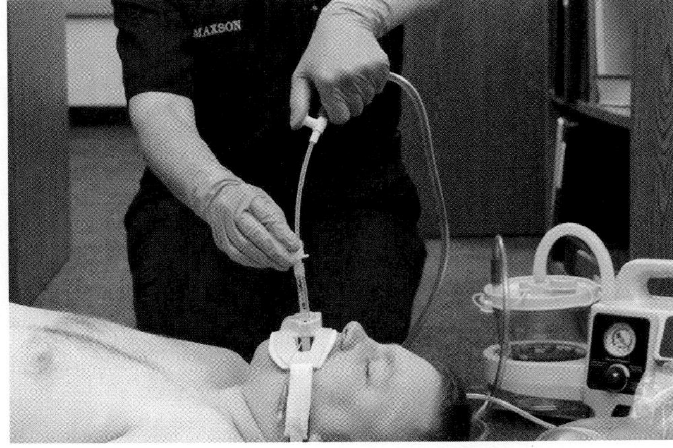

A2-2E ✻ Apply suction by covering the open part on the catheter. Using a twisting motion, withdraw the catheter with suction.

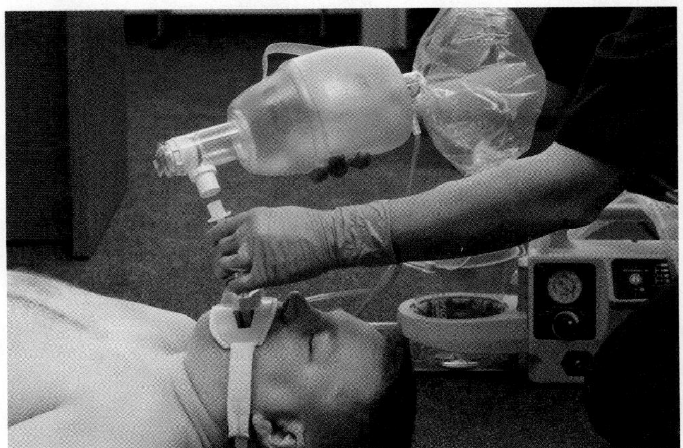

A2-2F ✻ Resume ventilation of the patient for 2 minutes following suctioning.

ADVANCED AIRWAY *skills* A2-3 Digital Intubation

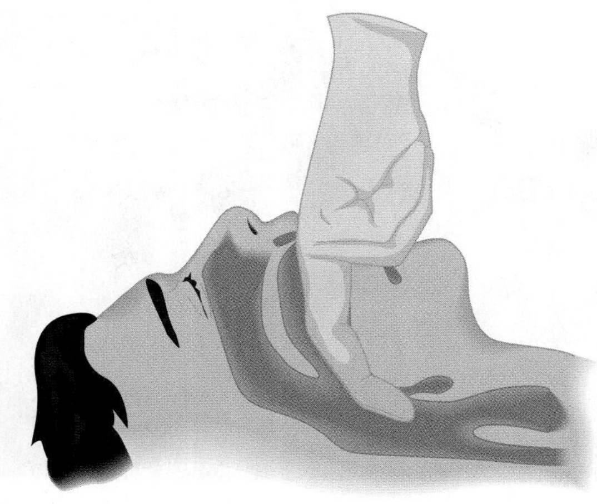

A2-3A * Insert your index and middle finger into the patient's mouth. Elevate the epiglottis with your middle finger.

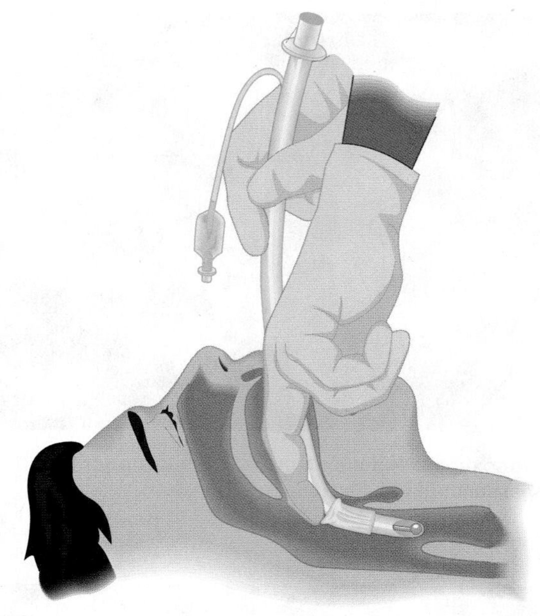

A2-3B * Guide the tube forward and into the glottic opening with your index and middle fingers.

ADVANCED AIRWAY *skills* A2-4 Nasogastric Intubation

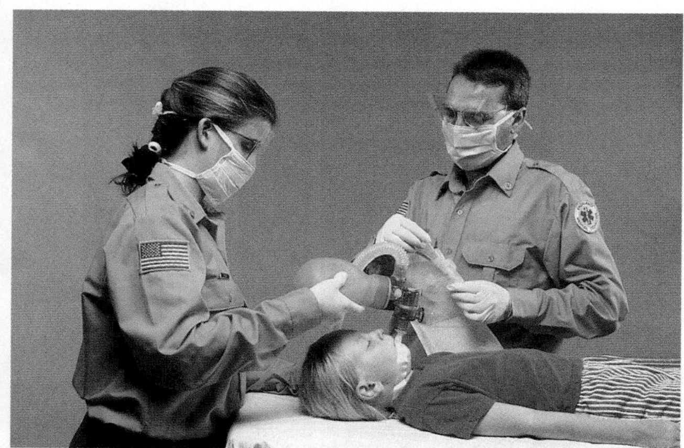

A2-4A * Oxygenate the patient.

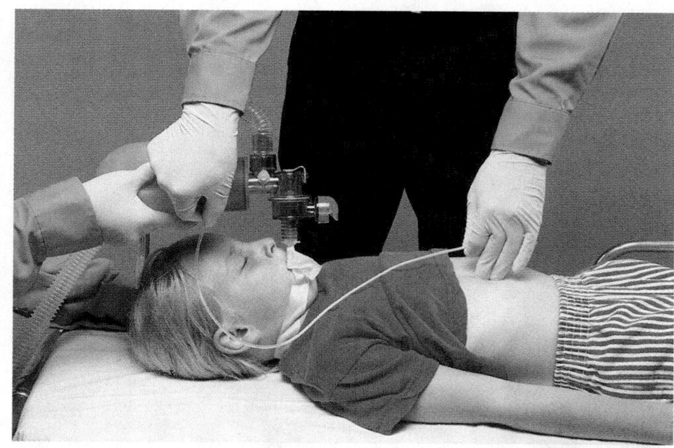

A2-4B * Determine the proper length by measuring from the tip of the nose, over the ear, to just below the xiphoid process.

Nasogastric Intubation *continued*

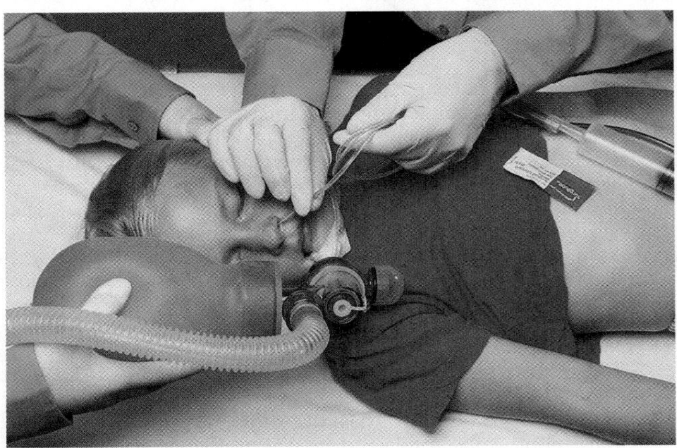

A2-4C ✱ Slightly flex the neck by supporting the head with your hand. Advance the tube straight back, not toward the head.

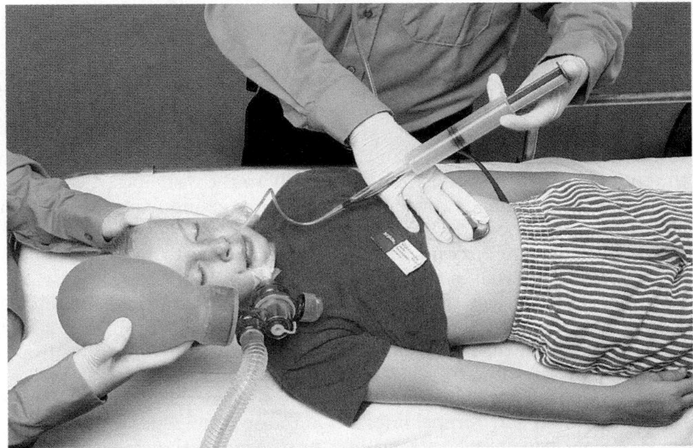

A2-4D ✱ Confirm placement by injecting 15–20 mL of air into the tube while auscultating over the stomach. If air is heard entering the stomach, proper placement is confirmed.

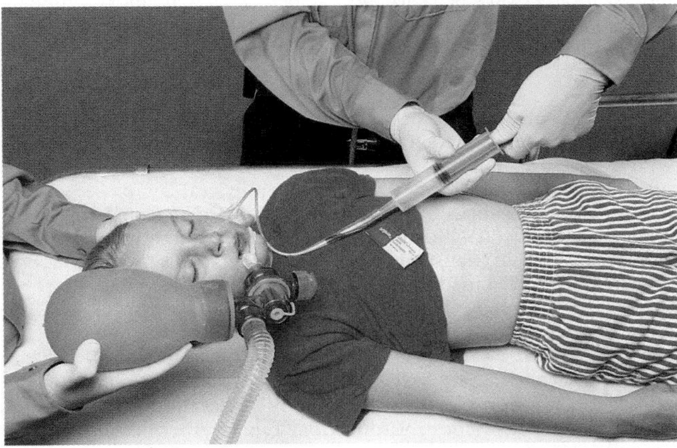

A2-4E ✱ Apply negative pressure to the syringe to aspirate gastric material and air.

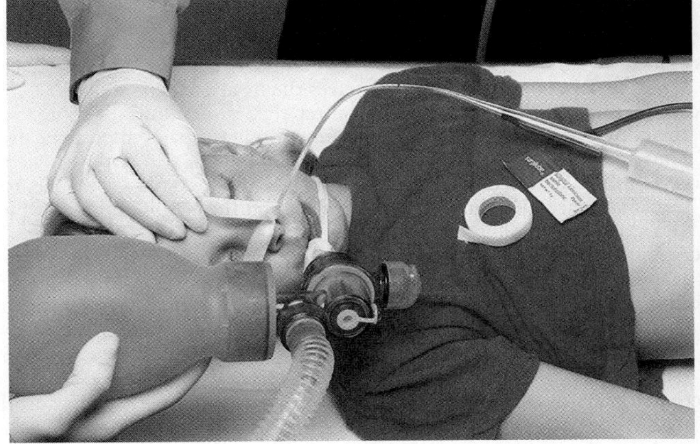

A2-4F ✱ Tape the NG tube in place.

Glossary

abandonment the act of discontinuing emergency care without ensuring that another health care professional with equivalent or better training will take over.
abdominal aorta the portion of the descending aorta that extends from the thoracic portion of the aorta proximally to the distal point where the aorta divides into the iliac arteries. Arteries branching from the abdominal aorta supply the abdominal organs.
abdominal aortic aneurysm (AAA) a weakened, ballooned, and enlarged area of the wall of the abdominal aorta.
abdominal cavity the space located below the diaphragm that extends to the pelvis.
abdominal evisceration abdominal organ protrusion through an open wound to the abdomen.
abdominal quadrants the four parts of the abdomen as divided by imaginary horizontal and vertical lines through the umbilicus.
abrasion an open injury to the outermost layer of the skin (epidermis) caused by a scraping away, rubbing, or shearing away of the tissue.
abruptio placentae the premature separation of the placenta from the uterine wall.
absorbed passed through skin or mucous membranes on contact.
absorption passage of a substance through skin or mucous membranes upon contact.
abuse *see* physical abuse.
acceleration/deceleration injury a head injury typical of a car crash in which the head comes to a sudden stop, but the brain continues to move back and forth inside the skull, resulting in bruising to the brain.
acetabulum (AS-i-TAB-u-lum) the rounded cavity or socket on the external surface of the pelvis that receives the head of the femur.
acetylcholine (ACh) a neurotransmitter that is distributed throughout the body and is necessary for normal function of the parasympathetic nervous system.
acetylcholinesterase (AChE) an enzyme that breaks down the neurotransmitter acetylcholine. Nerve agents inhibit the action of this enzyme, allowing acetylcholine to accumulate.
acromion (ah-KRO-me-on) the lateral triangular projection of the scapula that forms the point of the shoulder.
action the effect a drug has on the body. The *therapeutic effect* is the intended positive response by the body. The *mechanism of action* is how the drug works to create its effect on the body. For example, an action of nitroglycerin is dilation of the blood vessels.
activated charcoal a distilled charcoal in powder form that can adsorb many times its weight in contaminants to prevent their absorption by the body; no longer commonly administered in the emergency care of patients who have ingested a poison.
active rewarming technique of aggressively applying external sources of heat to a patient to rewarm his body.
acute with rapid onset.
acute abdomen a sharp, severe abdominal pain with rapid onset. Acute abdomen can have a number of causes. Also called *acute abdominal distress.*
acute coronary syndrome (ACS) a group of signs and symptoms resulting from any of a variety of conditions that can affect the heart in which the coronary arteries are narrowed or occluded by fat deposits, clots, or spasm.
acute renal failure (ARF) a rapid loss of renal function that results in poor urine production, electrolyte disturbance, and fluid balance disturbance.
Adam's apple *see* thyroid cartilage.
administration the route and form by which a drug is given.
adolescent a child 12 to 18 years of age.
advance directive instructions, written in advance, such as a do not resuscitate (DNR) order, a living will, or a durable power of attorney.
Advanced Emergency Medical Technician (AEMT) the level of EMS practitioner who performs the responsibilities of an EMT with the addition of the use of advanced airway devices, monitoring of blood glucose levels, initiation of intravenous and intraosseous infusions, and administration of a select number of medications.
aerobic (eh-ROB-ik) metabolism chemical and physical changes that take place within the cells in the presence of oxygen.
afterbirth the placenta and other tissues that are expelled after the delivery of the fetus.
afterload the force of contraction that the left ventricle has to generate to overcome the resistance in the aorta to eject the blood.
ageism stereotyping or discrimination against old people.
agitated delirium a mental and physiological state of arousal that is usually characterized by extreme strength and endurance, tolerance to pain, hostility, and hyperactive behavior; may result in sudden cardiac death; also called *excited delirium.*
agonal respirations gasping-type respirations that have no pattern and occur very infrequently; a sign of impending cardiac or respiratory arrest. Also called *agonal breathing.*
air embolism an air bubble that enters the bloodstream and obstructs a blood vessel.
airway resistance the restriction of airflow that is related to the diameter of the airways.
allergen a substance (antigen) that enters the body by ingestion, injection, inhalation, or absorption and triggers an allergic reaction. *See also* antigen.
allergic reaction a misdirected and excessive response by the immune system to a foreign substance or an allergen.
alpha radiation a very heavy and slow-moving particle that travels only inches in air and is stopped by clothing or the outer layer of the skin. It is a very serious internal contaminant and can be ingested or inhaled.
altered mental status a variation from normal function of the mind as judged by a person's behavior, appearance, speech, memory, judgment, or responsiveness to stimuli; altered mental status may range from disorientation to total unresponsiveness or unconsciousness.
alveolar ventilation the amount of inspired air that reaches the alveoli of the lungs.
alveoli (al-VE-oh-le) the air sacs of the lungs. *Pl.* of alveolus.
Alzheimer disease disease characterized by cerebral function loss as seen with diseases that affect the brain.
Americans with Disabilities Act (ADA) a federal law passed in 1990 that protects individuals with a documented disability from being denied initial or continued employment based on their disability.
amniotic sac a thin, transparent membrane that forms the sac that holds the fetus suspended in amniotic fluid. Also called *bag of waters.*
amputation an open injury caused by the ripping or tearing away of a limb, body part, or organ.
anaerobic (AN-eh-ROB-ik) metabolism chemical and physical changes that take place within the cells without the presence of oxygen.
anaphylactic reaction a reactive release of chemical mediators that produce bronchoconstriction, vasodilation, capillary permeability, and increased mucus production leading to airway and respiratory compromise and hypoperfusion. Also called *anaphylaxis.*
anaphylactic shock a shock (hypoperfusion) state that results from dilated and leaking blood vessels related to severe allergic reaction. Also called *anaphylaxis* or *anaphylactic reaction.*
anaphylactoid reaction a reaction to a foreign substance that resembles an anaphylactic reaction that may occur on first exposure to the substance, without immune system sensitization.
anaphylaxis another term for anaphylactic reaction. *See* anaphylactic reaction.
anatomical planes imaginary divisions of the body.
anatomical position a position in which the patient is standing erect, facing forward, with arms down at the sides and palms forward.
anatomy the study of the structure of the body and the relationship of its parts to each other.
antepartum the period of pregnancy prior to the onset of labor.
anterior toward the front. Opposite of *posterior.*
anterior chamber the front chamber of the eye containing the aqueous humor.
anterior cord syndrome loss of most function below the site of injury to the anterior portion of the spinal cord.
anterior plane the front, or abdominal side of the body.
anterograde amnesia inability to remember circumstances after an incident.
antibodies special proteins produced by the immune system that search out antigens and combine with and help to destroy them.
antidote a substance that neutralizes the effects of a poison or a toxic substance.

antigen a foreign substance that enters the body and triggers an immune response. *See also* allergen.
anxiety a state of painful uneasiness about impending problems characterized by agitation and restlessness.
aorta (ay-OR-tah) the major artery from the heart.
apnea absence of breathing; respiratory arrest.
apnea monitor device that monitors breathing and emits a warning signal if breathing stops.
apneustic center the respiratory center in the brainstem that intensifies and prolongs inhalation.
appendicitis inflammation of the appendix.
aqueous humor the watery fluid that fills the anterior chamber of the eye.
arachnoid middle layer of protective brain tissue (meninges).
arteriole (ar-TE-re-ol) the smallest branch of an artery, which at its distal end leads into a capillary.
arteriosclerosis disease process that causes the loss of elasticity in the vascular walls from thickening and hardening of the vessels.
artery blood vessel that carries blood away from the heart.
aspiration breathing a foreign substance into the lungs.
aspiration pneumonia inflammation of the lungs caused by the aspiration of vomitus or other foreign matter.
aspirin a common household medication that will keep platelets from clumping together to form clots; also used as a pain reliever, as an anti-inflammatory agent, and to reduce fever; often administered to the patient suspected of having a heart attack.
assault a willful threat to inflict harm on a person.
asystole a heart rhythm indicating absence of any electrical activity in the heart. Also known as *flatline*.
atria (AY-tre-uh) the two upper chambers of the heart. *Pl.* of atrium.
aura an unusual sensory sensation that may precede a seizure episode by hours or only a few seconds.
auscultation listening for sounds within the body with a stethoscope.
auto-injector a device with a concealed, spring-loaded needle, used for injecting a single dose of medication. An epinephrine auto-injector is often prescribed to patients with a history of anaphylactic reaction.
automated external defibrillator (AED) a device that can analyze the electrical activity or rhythm of a patient's heart and deliver an electrical shock (defibrillation) if appropriate.
automatic transport ventilator (ATV) a positive pressure ventilation device that delivers ventilations automatically.
automaticity the ability of cells within the cardiac conduction system to generate a cardiac impulse on their own.
autonomic nervous system part of the nervous system that influences involuntary muscles and glands.
AVPU a mnemonic for alert, responds to verbal stimulus, responds to painful stimulus, unresponsive, to characterize levels of responsiveness.
avulsion an open injury characterized by a loose flap of skin and soft tissue that has been torn loose or pulled completely off.
bag-valve-mask (BVM) device a positive pressure ventilation device that consists of a bag with a nonrebreather valve and a mask. The bag-valve device is connected to the mask or other airway. The bag is squeezed to deliver a ventilation to the patient.
bandage any material used to secure a dressing in place.
bariatrics medical management of obese patients.
baroreceptors stretch-sensitive receptors located in the aortic arch and carotid bodies that constantly measure the blood pressure.
base station the central dispatch and coordination area of an EMS communications system that ideally is in contact with all other elements of the system.
baseline vital signs the first set of vital sign measurements to which subsequent measurements can be compared.
basilar skull floor of the skull.
battery the act of touching a person unlawfully without his consent.
Battle sign discoloration of the mastoid suggesting basilar skull fracture.
behavior the way a person acts or performs.
behavioral emergency a situation in which a person exhibits abnormal behavior.
beta radiation a low-speed, low-energy particle that is easily stopped by 6–10 feet of air, clothing, or the first few millimeters of skin. It is a common product of fallout decay and is a serious threat from ingestion of contaminated foods and inhalation of airborne particles.
bilateral on both sides.
bilevel positive airway pressure (BiPAP) device that provides back pressure, higher during inhalation and lower during exhalation, to keep bronchioles open and improve ventilation and oxygenation.
biological agents agents that are made up of living organisms or the toxins produced by the living organisms that are used as weapons of mass destruction to cause disease in a target population.
bipolar disorder a psychiatric condition, also known as *manic-depressive disorder*, characterized by wide swings between periods of depression and periods of elation and manic behavior.
birth defect a variation from normal structure or function that is present at birth.
blood pressure the force exerted by the blood on the interior walls of the blood vessels.
bloody show the mucus and blood that are expelled from the vagina as labor begins.
blunt trauma a force that impacts or is applied to the body but is not sharp enough to penetrate it, such as a blow or a crushing injury.
body mechanics application of the study of muscles and body movement (kinesiology) to the use of the body and to the prevention and correction of problems related to posture and lifting.
Boyle law the concept that the volume of a gas is inversely proportionate to the pressure.
brachial (BRAY-ke-al) artery the major artery of the upper arm.
bradycardia a heart rate less than 60 beats per minute.
bradypnea a breathing rate that is slower than the normal rate.
brain herniation a protrusion, or pushing, of a portion of the brain through the cranial wall or tentorium.
brainstem the funnel-shaped inferior part of the brain that controls most automatic functions of the body. It is made up of the pons, the midbrain, and the medulla, which is the brain's connection to the spinal cord.
breech birth a common abnormality of delivery in which the fetal buttocks or both lower extremities are low in the uterus and are the first to be delivered.
bronchi (BRONG-ke) the two main branches leading from the trachea to the lungs, providing the passageway for air movement. *Pl.* of bronchus.
bronchioles (BRONG-ke-olz) small branches of the bronchi.
bronchoconstriction constriction of the smooth muscle of the bronchi and bronchioles causing a narrowing of the air passageway.
bronchodilator a drug that relaxes the smooth muscle of the bronchi and bronchioles and reverses bronchoconstriction.
bronchospasm spasm or constriction of the smooth muscle of the bronchi and bronchioles.
Brown-Séquard syndrome loss of different functions on opposite sides of the body from injury to one side of the spinal cord.
bundle of His a band of cardiac muscle fibers that originates in the atrioventricular node and passes through the atrioventricular junction and carries the electrical impulse from the atria and, by connecting to the Purkinje fibers, to the ventricles.
burn sheet commercially prepared sterile, particle-free, disposable sheet used to cover the entire body in severe burn injuries.
burn shock a form of nonhemorrhagic hypovolemic shock resulting from a burn injury.
burnout a condition resulting from chronic job stress, characterized by a state of irritability and fatigue that can markedly decrease effectiveness.
calcaneus (kal-KAY-ne-us) the heel bone.
capillary (KAP-i-lair-e) tiny blood vessel that connects an arteriole to a venule.
capillary refill the amount of time it takes for capillaries that have been compressed to refill with blood.
cardiac arrest the cessation of cardiac function with the patient displaying no pulse, no breathing, and unresponsiveness.
cardiac compromise reduced heart function caused by any of a variety of conditions, diseases, or injuries affecting the heart.
cardiac conduction system the specialized contractile and conductive tissue of the heart that generates electrical impulses and causes the heart to beat. Also called the *coronary conduction system*.
cardiac contusion a bruise to the heart wall caused by severe blunt trauma to the chest where the heart is violently compressed between the sternum and the spinal column.
cardiac hypertrophy an increase in the size of the heart from a thickening of the heart wall, without a parallel increase in the size of the cavity.
cardiac muscle a type of involuntary muscle found only in the walls of the heart. Cardiac muscle has the property of automaticity, the ability to generate an impulse on its own, separately from the central nervous system.
cardiac output the volume of blood ejected from the left ventricle in one minute.
cardiogenic shock poor perfusion resulting from an ineffective pump function of the heart, typically the left ventricle.
cardiovascular system *see* circulatory system.
carina the point at which the trachea splits into the right and left mainstem bronchi.
carotid (kah-ROT-id) artery one of two major arteries of the neck, which supply the brain and head with blood.

carpals (KAR-pulz) the eight bones that form the wrist.

cataract clouding of the lens of the eye from pathologic changes within the lens.

cavitation a cavity formed by a pressure wave resulting from the kinetic energy of a bullet traveling through body tissue; also called *pathway expansion*.

central chemoreceptors receptors located in the medulla that are most sensitive to changes in carbon dioxide and the pH. *See also* chemoreceptors.

central cord syndrome loss of function in upper extremities caused by injury to the middle portion of the spinal cord.

central intravenous catheter a catheter that is designed to deliver medication into the central circulation of the body.

central nervous system (CNS) the brain and the spinal cord.

cerebellum part of the brain controlling equilibrium and muscle coordination.

cerebrospinal fluid (CSF) a clear fluid that surrounds and cushions the brain and the spinal cord.

cerebrum largest part of the brain, responsible for most conscious and sensory functions, the emotions, and the personality.

cervical (SER-vi-kal) spine the first seven vertebrae, or the neck.

cervix the neck of the uterus.

Chain of Survival term used by the American Heart Association for the series of four interventions—early access, early CPR, early defibrillation, and early ACLS (advanced cardiac life support)—that provides the best chance for successful resuscitation of a cardiac arrest patient.

chemoreceptors receptors that constantly monitor the arterial content of oxygen, carbon dioxide, and the blood pH and stimulate a change in respiratory rate and depth. *See also* central chemoreceptors *and* peripheral chemoreceptors.

chief complaint the patient complaint that is the primary reason why the EMS crew was called to the scene.

child abuse physical, emotional, or sexual mistreatment or neglect of a child from newborn to 18 years of age.

cholecystitis inflammation of the gallbladder.

chronic long term, progressing gradually.

chronic kidney disease (CKD) a progressive loss of kidney function over a period of months to years.

chronic obstructive pulmonary disease (COPD) umbrella term used to describe pulmonary diseases such as emphysema or chronic bronchitis.

chronic renal failure (CRF) *see* chronic kidney disease.

circulatory system system composed of the heart and blood vessels that brings oxygen and nutrients to and takes wastes away from body cells. Also called the *cardiovascular system*.

circumferential burn burn that encircles a body area (e.g., arm, leg, or chest).

clammy a moist, or a cool and moist, condition; a skin condition often characteristic of shock.

clavicle (KLAV-i-kul) the collarbone, attached to the superior portion of the sternum.

cleaning the process of washing a soiled object with soap and water.

closed injury any injury in which there is no break in the continuity of the skin.

closed-ended question a question that requires only a "yes" or "no" answer.

CNS depressants substances that inhibit or decrease central nervous system functions.

CNS stimulants substances that excite or increase central nervous system functions.

coccyx (KOK-siks) the four fused vertebrae that form the most distal end of the spine; the tailbone.

cold zone the area adjacent to the warm zone in a hazardous materials emergency. Normal triage, treatment, and stabilization are performed here. Also called *support zone*.

colloid oncotic pressure *see* plasma oncotic pressure.

coma an unconscious state in which a person does not respond to any stimulus, including pain.

combining form word part that carries the word's essential meaning.

commotion cordis sudden cardiac arrest caused by a projectile, such as a baseball, striking the anterior chest.

communication a dynamic process that incorporates verbal and nonverbal expressions into meaningful messages that are received and interpreted by others.

compartment syndrome a condition in which increased tissue pressure in a confined space causes decreased blood flow, leading to hypoxia and possible muscle, nerve, and vessel impairment, which may be permanent if the cells die.

compensated respiratory distress *see* early respiratory distress.

compensatory shock the stage of shock in which a cascade of organ and gland stimulation and hormones occurs to increase the blood pressure, restore arterial wall tension, and maintain a near normal blood pressure and perfusion of the vital organs. Also called *compensated shock*.

complete spinal cord injury injury to the spinal cord that results in a complete loss of motor, sensory, and autonomic function below the level of injury.

complex access a way to gain access to a patient that requires the use of tools and specialized equipment.

compliance the measure of the ability of the chest wall and lungs to stretch, distend, and expand.

compression of morbidity the concept of maximizing the number of healthy years in one's life while simultaneously minimizing the number of years of disease/disability at the end of life.

concussion temporary loss of brain function.

conduction transfer of heat through direct physical touch with nearby objects.

congestive heart failure (CHF) a cardiac disease in which the heart cannot pump blood sufficiently to meet the needs of the body.

conjunctiva the thin covering of the inner eyelids and exposed portion of the sclera of the eye.

consensual reflex same or similar reaction of the unstimulated pupil when the other pupil is stimulated, as when a light is shined into one pupil and both pupils contract.

consent permission that must be obtained before care is rendered.

Consolidated Omnibus Budget Reconciliation Act (COBRA) a federal regulation that ensures the public's access to emergency health care regardless of ability to pay.

constricted narrowed, made small.

contamination reduction zone *see* warm zone.

continuous positive airway pressure (CPAP) device that provides a constant level of back pressure during inhalation and exhalation to keep bronchioles open and improve ventilation and oxygenation.

contraindications situations in which a medication should not be used; for example, because nitroglycerin lowers blood pressure, existing low blood pressure in a patient is a contraindication for nitroglycerin.

contusion a closed injury to the cells and blood vessels contained within the dermis that is characterized by discoloration, swelling, and pain; a bruise; bruising or swelling of the brain.

convection loss of body heat to the atmosphere when air passes over the body.

convulsion unresponsiveness accompanied by a generalized jerky muscle movement affecting the entire body.

cornea the clear front portion of the eye that covers the pupil and the iris.

coronal plane *see* frontal plane.

coronary (KOR-o-nair-e) arteries blood vessels that supply the heart with blood.

coup/contrecoup injury a brain injury in which there may be damage at the point of a blow to the head and/or damage on the side opposite the blow as the brain is propelled against the opposite side of the skull.

cranial skull bones fused together to form a helmet-like covering over the brain.

cranium (KRAY-ne-um) the bones that form the top, back, and sides of the skull plus the forehead.

crepitus the sound or feel of broken fragments of bone grinding against each other. Also called *crepitation*.

cricoid (KRIK-oyd) cartilage the most inferior portion of the larynx and only full cartilaginous ring of the upper airway. It is felt immediately below the thyroid cartilage.

cricoid pressure pressure applied to the cricoid cartilage to compress the esophagus. Also called *Sellick maneuver*.

critical incident any situation that causes unusually strong emotions that interfere with the ability to function.

critical incident stress debriefing (CISD) a session usually held within 24 to 72 hours of a critical incident, where a team of peer counselors and mental health professionals help emergency service personnel work through emotions that normally follow a critical incident.

crossed-finger technique a technique in which the thumb and index finger are crossed with the thumb on the lower incisors and the index finger on the upper incisors. The fingers are moved in a snapping or scissor motion to open the mouth.

crowing a sound similar to that of a cawing crow that indicates that the muscles around the larynx are in spasm and beginning to narrow the opening into the trachea.

crowning the stage in delivery when the fetal head presents at the vagina.

crush injury an injury in which tissues are compressed by high-pressure forces; the injury may be open or closed.

culture the thoughts, communications, actions, and values of a racial, ethnic, religious, or social group.

Cushing reflex a protective reflex by the body to maintain perfusion of the brain in a head-injured patient with increased intracranial pressure. The systolic blood pressure increases, heart rate decreases, and the respiratory pattern changes.
cyanide a rapid-acting agent that disrupts the ability of the cell to use oxygen, leading to severe cellular hypoxia and eventual death.
cyanosis a blue-gray color of the mucous membranes and/or skin, which indicates inadequate oxygenation or poor perfusion.
dead air space (V_D) anatomical areas in the respiratory tract where no gas exchange occurs but air collects during inhalation.
decerebrate posturing *see* extension posturing.
decoder device that recognizes and responds to only certain codes imposed on radio broadcasts.
decoding process by which a received message is translated and interpreted.
decompensated respiratory failure when the respiratory compensatory mechanisms have begun to fail and respiration becomes inadequate.
decompensatory shock an advanced stage of shock in which the body's compensatory mechanisms are no longer able to maintain a blood pressure and perfusion of the vital organs. Also called *decompensated shock* or *progressive shock.*
decorticate posturing *see* flexion posturing.
defamation an intentional false communication that injures another person's reputation or good name.
defense mechanisms psychological coping strategies individuals use to protect themselves from unwanted feelings or thoughts.
defibrillation electrical shock or current delivered to the heart through the patient's chest wall or internally from an implanted device to help the heart restore a normal rhythm.
defusing a session held prior to a critical incident stress debriefing (CISD) for emergency service personnel most directly involved to provide an opportunity to vent emotions and get information before the CISD.
delirium sudden-onset altered mental status that may involve illusions, disjointed thought processes, incoherent speech, and increased or decreased psychomotor activity.
dementia chronic condition resulting in the malfunctioning of normal cerebral processes.
deoxygenated containing low amounts of oxygen, as with venous blood.
deoxyhemoglobin hemoglobin that does not have any oxygen molecules attached to it.
depression one of the most common psychiatric conditions, one characterized by deep feelings of sadness, worthlessness, and discouragement, feelings that often do not seem connected to the actual circumstances of the patient's life.
dermis the second layer of the skin. *See also* epidermis, subcutaneous layer.
diabetes mellitus (DM) a disease in which the normal relationship between glucose and insulin is altered. *See also* type 1 diabetes *and* type 2 diabetes.
diabetic ketoacidosis (DKA) a condition typically found in type 1 diabetics where the blood glucose level is excessively elevated and insulin level is extremely-low-to-absent, which causes glucose to be excreted in the urine, dehydrating the patient, and causes the body to metabolize fat for energy, producing ketones and creating an acidic environment.
diabetic retinopathy damage to the small blood vessels of the eye from the long-term effects of diabetes mellitus.
dialysate a special fluid used for dialysis.
dialysis an artificial process used to remove water and waste substances from the blood when the kidneys fail to function properly.
dialysis shunt a joining of arterial and venous systems in such a way that the repeated needlesticks required for dialysis cause a minimal amount of damage to the patient's body.
diaphragm (DI-ah-fram) the major muscle of respiration that separates the chest cavity from the abdominal cavity.
diastolic (di-as-TOL-ik) blood pressure the pressure exerted against the walls of the arteries when the left ventricle is at rest. *See also* systolic blood pressure.
digestive (di-JES-tiv) system the structures and organs that ingest and carry food so that absorption and waste elimination can occur.
dilated expanded, made large.
diplopia double vision.
direct force direct blow. Injuries from direct force occur at the point of impact.
disaster a sudden catastrophic event that overwhelms natural order and causes great loss of property and/or life.
disk fluid-filled pad of cartilage between two vertebrae.
disinfecting in addition to cleaning, this process involves using a disinfectant such as alcohol or bleach to kill many of the microorganisms that may be present on the surface of an object.
dissipation of energy the way energy is transferred to the human body by the forces acting upon it
distal distant, or far from the point of reference. Opposite of *proximal.*
distributive shock shock associated with a decrease in intravascular volume caused by massive systemic vasodilation and an increase in the capillary permeability.
do not resuscitate (DNR) order a legal document, usually signed by the patient and his physician, that indicates to medical personnel which, if any, life-sustaining measures should be taken when the patient's heart and respiratory functions have ceased.
dorsal toward the back or spine. Opposite of *ventral.*
dorsal respiratory group (DRG) respiratory rhythm center located in the brainstem that controls the rate and depth of normal quiet respiration.
dorsalis pedis (dor-SAL-is PED-is) artery an artery of the foot, which can be felt on the top surface of the foot.
dose the amount of a medication that is given to a patient at one time; for example, a dose of nitroglycerin may be one tablet and a dose of epinephrine may be the contents of one auto-injector.
downtime the time from when the patient goes into cardiac arrest until CPR is effectively being performed.
drag the factors that slow a projectile.
dressing a sterile covering for an open wound that aids in the control of bleeding and prevention of further damage and contamination.
drowning an incident in which someone is submerged or immersed in a liquid that prevents the person from breathing air and that results in a primary respiratory impairment, whether the person lives or dies after this process.
drug a chemical substance that is used to treat or prevent a disease or condition.
drug abuse self-administration of drugs (or a single drug) in a manner that is not in accord with approved medical or social patterns.
drug toxicity an adverse or toxic reaction to a drug or drugs.
dura mater outer layer of protective brain tissue (meninges).
durable power of attorney a legal document that designates a person who is legally empowered to make health care decisions for the signer of the document if he is unable to do it himself. Also called a *health care proxy.*
duty to act the obligation to care for a patient who requires it.
dysarthria defective speech caused by impairment of the tongue or other muscles necessary for speech.
dysbarism a medical condition that results from pressure changes that occur when a person descends in water or ascends in altitude.
dysmenorrhea severe pain or cramps during menstruation.
dyspnea shortness of breath or perceived difficulty in breathing.
dysrhythmias irregular contractions of the myocardium secondary to electrical disturbances in the heart.
early respiratory distress increased respiratory effort caused by impaired respiratory function.
ecchymosis black and blue discoloration.
edema (uh-DEE-muh) swelling caused by fluid accumulating in the tissues.
elder abuse neglect or physical, sexual, financial, or emotional/mental mistreatment of an elderly person.
embolic stroke a type of ischemic stroke caused by plaque or other material that lodges in and blocks a cerebral artery.
Emergency Medical Responder (EMR) the level of EMS practitioner who is likely to be the first person on the scene with emergency care training.
Emergency Medical Technician (EMT) the level of EMS practitioner who provides basic emergency medical care and transportation to patients who access the EMS system including oxygen therapy and ventilation equipment, pulse oximetry, use of automatic blood pressure monitoring equipment, and limited medication administration.
Emergency Medical Treatment and Active Labor Act (EMTALA) a federal regulation that ensures the public's access to emergency health care regardless of ability to pay. Also known as the "anti-patient-dumping statute," forbidding turning a patient away at the door or sending him to a public hospital because of inability to pay.
emergency move a patient move that should be performed when there is immediate danger to the patient or to the rescuer.
EMS system Emergency Medical Services system.
encoder device that breaks down sound waves into unique digital codes for radio transmission.
encoding process of converting information into a message.
endocrine (EN-do-krin) system a system of ductless glands that produce hormones that regulate body functions.
endometriosis the condition in which endometrial tissue grows outside of the uterus.

endometritis inflammation of the endometrium.
endotracheal intubation placement of a tube down the trachea to facilitate airflow into the trachea and lungs.
enteral feeding provision of nutrition through a tube inserted through the nose, the mouth, or a surgical opening in the abdomen into the gastrointestinal system.
epidermis (EP-i-DER-mis) the outermost layer of the skin. *See also* dermis, subcutaneous layer.
epidural between the dura mater and the skull.
epidural hematoma bleeding between the dura mater and the skull.
epiglottis (EP-i-GLOT-is) a small, leaf-shaped flap of cartilaginous tissue, located immediately posterior to the root of the tongue, that covers the opening of the larynx to keep food and liquid from entering the trachea and lungs.
epilepsy a medical disorder characterized by recurrent seizures.
epinephrine a natural hormone that, when used as a medication, constricts blood vessels to improve blood pressure, reduces leakage from blood vessels, relaxes smooth muscle in the bronchioles (causes bronchodilation), and increases the heart rate and force of ventricular contractions.
epistaxis bleeding from the nose resulting from injury, disease, or environment; a nosebleed.
eschar the hard, tough, leathery dead soft tissue formed as a result of a full-thickness burn.
esophageal varices bulging, engorgement, or weakening of the blood vessels in the lining of the lower part of the esophagus.
esophagus (es-AH-fuh-gus) passageway at the lower end of the pharynx that leads to the stomach.
ethnocentrism the view that one culture's way of doing things is the right way and any other way is inferior.
evaporation conversion of a liquid or solid into a gas; evaporation of sweat is a means by which the body is cooled.
evidence-based medicine medical practice based on scientific evidence that certain procedures, medications, and equipment improve patient outcome.
evisceration a protrusion of organs from a wound.
excited delirium *see* agitated delirium.
exclusion zone *see* hot zone.
exhalation the passive process of breathing air out of the lungs. Also called *expiration.*
expiration *see* exhalation.
expressed consent permission that must be obtained from every conscious, mentally competent adult before emergency treatment may be provided.
extension posturing a posture in which the patient arches the back and extends the arms straight out parallel to the body. A sign of serious head injury. Also called *decerebrate posturing.*
external respiration gas exchange process that occurs between the alveoli and the pulmonary capillaries.
extremities the limbs of the body. The lower extremities include the hips, thighs, legs, ankles, and feet. The upper extremities include the shoulders, arms, forearms, wrists, and hands.
eyelids movable protective folds that can cover the eyes.
face the area of the skull between the brow and the chin.
fallopian tubes thin, flexible structures that extend from the uterus to the ovaries. Also called *uterine tubes.*
fallout radioactive dust and particles that may be life-threatening to people far from the epicenter of a radioactive detonation.
false imprisonment the intentional and unjustifiable detention of a person without his consent or other legal authority.
feedback any information that an individual receives about his behavior.
femoral (FEM-or-al) artery the major artery of the thigh that supplies the groin and leg with blood.
femur (FE-mer) the thighbone.
fetus the child in the uterus from the third month of pregnancy to birth; prior to that time it is called an embryo.
fibula (FIB-u-lah) the lateral, smaller long bone of the lower leg.
flail segment two or more adjacent ribs that are fractured in two or more places and thus move independently from the rest of the rib cage.
flexion posturing a posture in which the patient arches the back and flexes the arms inward toward the chest. A sign of serious head injury. Also called *decorticate posturing.*
flow-restricted, oxygen-powered ventilation device (FROPVD) a device that consists of a ventilation valve and trigger or button and is driven directly by oxygen. It is used to provide positive pressure ventilation.
flushing abnormally red skin color due to vasodilation.
fontanelle the "soft spot" on the top of an infant's head where the bony plates of the skull have not yet fused together.
form the size, shape, consistency, or appearance of a medication; for example, nitroglycerin may be in pill or spray form; oral glucose is in gel form.
Fowler position a position in which the patient is lying on the back with the upper body elevated at a 45° to 60° angle. *See also* semi-Fowler position.
fragmentation the breaking up of a bullet into small pieces on impact.
Frank-Starling law of the heart the concept that the stretch of the muscle fiber in the left ventricle at the end of diastole determines the force necessary to eject the blood contained within it.
French catheter *see* soft catheter.
frequency of ventilation (f) the number of ventilations in one minute.
frontal plane a plane that divides the body into anterior and posterior halves. Also called *coronal plane.*
full-thickness burn burn that involves all the layers of the skin and can extend beyond the subcutaneous layer into the muscle, bone, or organs below; also called a *third-degree burn.*
gamma radiation *see* X-ray radiation.
gastric distention inflation of the stomach.
gastroenteritis inflammation of the stomach and small intestines.
generalized cold emergency *see* generalized hypothermia.
generalized hypothermia an overall reduction in body temperature, affecting the entire body; also called *hypothermia* or *generalized cold emergency.*
generalized tonic-clonic seizure a common type of seizure that produces unresponsiveness and a convulsion that exhibits generalized jerky muscle activity. Also known as a *grand mal seizure.*
genitourinary system male organ system that includes both the reproductive and urinary structures.
gestures nonverbal body movements that convey meaning to others.
glaucoma an abnormal increase in intraocular pressure that damages the optic nerve, resulting in loss of peripheral vision and eventual blindness.
globe the eyeball.
glucagon a hormone secreted by the pancreas that raises the blood glucose level by stimulating the liver to convert stored glycogen and other substances into glucose.
glucose a form of sugar that is the body's basic source of energy.
glycolysis the breakdown of glucose into pyruvic acid in the cells.
Good Samaritan law a law that provides immunity from liability for acts performed in good faith to assist at the scene of a medical emergency unless those acts constitute gross negligence.
guarded position a position generally assumed by patients with acute abdominal pain with knees drawn up and hands clenched over the abdomen.
gurgling a gargling sound that indicates a fluid is in the mouth or pharynx.
gynecology branch of medicine that studies health of the female patient and her reproductive system.
hallucinogens substances that cause hallucinations, or false perceptions not based on reality. Also called *psychedelics.*
haptics the study of touching.
hard catheter *see* rigid catheter.
hazardous material material that in any quantity poses a threat or unreasonable risk to life, health, or property if not properly controlled during manufacture, processing, packaging, handling, storage, transportation, use, and disposal.
head-tilt, chin-lift maneuver a manual technique used to open the airway. The head is tilted back by one hand. The tips of the fingers of the other hand are placed under the chin and used to lift the mandible up and forward.
Health Insurance Portability and Accountability Act (HIPAA) a federal law enacted in 1996 that protects the privacy of patient health care information and gives the patient control over how the information is distributed and used.
heart the muscular organ that contracts to force blood into circulation through the body.
heel drop test *see* Markle test.
hematemesis vomiting of blood.
hematochezia bright red blood in the stool.
hematoma a closed injury to the soft tissues characterized by swelling and discoloration caused by a mass of blood beneath the epidermis.
hematuria blood in the urine.
hemoglobin a complex protein molecule found on the surface of the red blood cell that is responsible for carrying a majority of oxygen in the blood.
hemoptysis coughing up blood or blood-stained sputum.
hemorrhagic hypovolemic shock shock from the loss of whole blood from the intravascular space. Often called just *hemorrhagic shock.*
hemorrhagic stroke a stroke caused by rupture of a blood vessel in the brain that allows blood to leak and collect in or around the brain tissue.
hemothorax blood in the pleural space, causing collapse of the lung.
hernia protrusion or thrusting forward of a portion of the intestine through an opening or weakness in the abdominal wall.

high-pressure regulator a one-gauge regulator that is used to power the flow-restricted, oxygen-powered ventilation device. The flow rate cannot be adjusted.
histamine the primary chemical mediator released from the mast cells in an anaphylactic reaction.
hives raised, red blotches associated with allergic and anaphylactic reactions.
horizontal plane *see* transverse plane.
hospice a philosophy of care that is aimed at providing relief of symptoms for the patients and support for their families during the late stages of a terminal condition.
hot zone the area where contamination is actually present. It generally is the area that is immediately adjacent to the accident site and where contamination can still occur. Also called *exclusion zone.*
huffers people who inhale vapors in order to "get high."
humane restraints padded soft leather or cloth straps used to tie a patient down to keep him from hurting himself or others.
humerus (HU-mer-us) the largest bone in the upper extremity, located in the proximal portion of the upper arm.
hydrostatic (HY-dro-STAT-ik) pressure the blood pressure or force exerted against the inside of vessel walls; the "push" effect that forces fluid out of a capillary.
hypercarbia increased carbon dioxide levels in the blood. Also called *hypercapnia.*
hyperglycemia high blood sugar. A blood glucose level greater than 120 mg/dL.
hyperglycemic hyperosmolar nonketotic syndrome (HHNS) a condition typically found in type 2 diabetics where the blood glucose level rises excessively, causing loss of large amounts of fluid from glucose spilling into the urine, leading to severe dehydration.
hypersensitivity a state of altered reactivity to an antigen, or foreign substance, that causes allergic reactions to that substance. *See also* sensitization.
hyperthermia abnormally high core body temperature; core body temperature above the normal 37°C (98.6°F).
hypoglycemia low blood sugar. A blood glucose level of 60 mg/dL with signs or symptoms of hypoglycemia or a blood glucose level of less than 50 mg/dL with or without signs or symptoms of hypoglycemia.
hypoperfusion (HY-po-per-FU-zhun) *see* shock.
hypopnea inadequate tidal volume in a breathing patient.
hypothermia abnormally low core body temperature; core body temperature under 35°C (95°F). *See also* generalized hypothermia.
hypovolemic shock shock caused by the loss of blood or fluid from the intravascular space resulting in a low blood volume.
hypoxemia decreased oxygen levels in the blood.
hypoxia the absence of sufficient oxygen in the body cells.
iliac (IL-i-ak) crest the upper margin of the bones of the pelvis.
immune response production of antibodies by the immune system to fight off invasion by foreign substances.
immune system the body's defense mechanism against invasion by foreign substances.
impaled object an object embedded in an injury to the body.
implied consent the assumption that, in a true emergency where a patient who is unresponsive or unable to make a rational decision is at significant risk of death, disability, or deterioration of condition, that patient would agree to emergency treatment. Also called the *emergency doctrine.*
incendiary devices devices including napalm, thermite, magnesium, and white phosphorus that are designed to cause injury by burning at high temperatures.
incident command system (ICS) the standardized incident management concept that has become the standard for on-scene management of disasters and multiple-casualty incidents.
incident commander the person who is responsible for coordinating all aspects of a disaster or multiple-casualty incident.
incomplete spinal cord injury injury to the spinal cord that does not affect all spinal cord tracts: motor, light touch, and pain. May produce conflicting and confusing assessment findings as some motor and sensory functions remain intact while others do not.
index of suspicion an anticipation that certain types of accidents and mechanisms will produce specific types of injuries.
indications the common reasons for using a medication to treat a specific condition; for example, chest pain is an indication for nitroglycerin.
indirect force a force that causes injury some distance away from the point of impact.
infant a child from birth to 1 year old. The infant during the first month is often referred to as a neonate.
inferior beneath, lower, or toward the feet. Opposite to of *superior.*
inferior plane everything below the transverse line (below the waist). Opposite of *superior plane.*
informed consent consent for treatment that is given by a competent patient based on full disclosure of possible risks and consequences.
ingestion swallowing.
inhalation the active process of breathing air into the lungs. Also called *inspiration.*
injection forced introduction into the body through the skin, possibly into a muscle or blood vessel, usually via a syringe, a bite, or a sting.
in-line stabilization bringing the patient's head into a neutral position in which the nose is in line with the navel and the neck is not flexed or extended and holding it there manually.
inspiration *see* inhalation.
insulin a hormone secreted by the pancreas that lowers the blood glucose level by promoting the movement of glucose from the blood into the cells.
integumentary (in-teg-yu-MENT-uh-re) system the skin.
intentional tort a wrongful act, injury, or damage that is committed knowingly.
intercostal (in-ter-KOS-tal) muscles the muscles between the ribs.
internal respiration the gas exchange process that occurs between the cells and the capillaries.
intestinal obstruction blockage that interrupts the normal flow of intestinal contents.
intimate zone in American culture, the space within less than 1½ feet of an individual.
intracranial pressure (ICP) the amount of pressure within the skull.
intrapartum the period of time from the onset of labor to delivery of the infant.
intraventricular shunt a tube surgically placed in a ventricle of the brain that extends to a blood vessel in the neck, the heart, or the abdomen, or to an external collector to drain excess cerebrospinal fluid from the brain and keep intracranial pressure at an acceptable level.
involuntary consent consent that is assumed when the patient is either mentally incompetent or legally not permitted to make his own medical decisions.
involuntary guarding abdominal wall muscle contraction caused by inflammation of the peritoneum that the patient cannot control. Also called *rigidity.*
involuntary muscle *see* smooth muscle.
iris the colored portion of the eye that surrounds the pupil.
irreversible shock the stage of shock in which interventions are unable to prevent the advance of shock to death.
irritant receptors receptors that are found in the airways and are sensitive to irritating gases, aerosol, and particles and result in a cough, bronchoconstriction, and increased ventilatory rate when stimulated.
ischemic stroke a stroke caused by a clot obstructing a blood vessel in the brain, resulting in an inadequate amount of blood being delivered to a portion of the brain distal to the blocked vessel.
ischium (IS-ke-um) the posterior and inferior portion of the pelvis.
jaundice a condition characterized by yellowness of the skin, sclera of the eyes, mucous membranes, and body fluids. It typically indicates liver failure or disease.
jaw-thrust maneuver a manual technique used to open the airway in the patient with a suspected spinal injury. The fingers are placed at the angles of the jaw and used to lift the mandible up and forward.
joint a place where one bone meets another.
J-receptors receptors that are found in the capillaries surrounding the alveoli and are sensitive to increases in the pressure in the capillary and cause rapid, shallow ventilation when stimulated.
Kehr sign shoulder pain referred from the diaphragm when it is irritated by blood within the abdominal cavity.
kinetic energy the energy contained by an object in motion. Kinetic energy equals mass (weight in pounds), times the velocity (feet per second) squared, divided by two.
kinetics the branch of mechanics dealing with the motions of material bodies.
kinetics of trauma the science of analyzing mechanism of injury.
kyphosis abnormal curvature of the spine with convexity backward. Also called *slouch.*
labor the physiological process by which the fetus is expelled from the uterus into the vagina and then to the outside of the body. Also called *childbirth.*
laceration an open injury usually caused by forceful impact with a sharp object and characterized by a wound whose edges may be linear (smooth and regular) or stellate (jagged and irregular) in appearance; a wound that penetrates the brain.
laryngeal spasm a contraction of the vocal cords that causes them to close and prevents air from passing through into the trachea. Also called *laryngospasm.*
laryngectomy a surgical procedure in which a patient's larynx is partially or completely removed. A stoma is created for the patient to breathe through.

larynx (LAIR-inks) structure that houses the vocal cords and is located inferior to the pharynx and superior to the trachea.

lateral (LAT-er-al) refers to the left or right of the midline, or away from the midline, or to the side of the body. *See also* medial.

lateral recumbent a position in which the patient is lying on the left or right side. Also called *recovery position.*

leading questions questions that suggest an answer guided by the individual who is asking the question.

left refers to the patient's left.

left plane everything to the left of the midline.

lens the portion of the eye behind the pupil that focuses light on the retina.

libel the act of injuring a person's reputation or good name in writing or through the mass media with malicious intent or reckless disregard for the falsity of those statements.

life expectancy the average length of years of life remaining based on the individual's year of birth.

ligaments bands of fibrous tissue that connect bones about a joint and support organs.

limb presentation an abnormal obstetric presentation when an arm or single leg is the first fetal part to protrude from the vaginal opening.

living will a legal document that delineates the signer's wishes about general health care issues such as the use of long-term life support measures.

local cold injury damage to body tissues in a specific part of the body resulting from exposure to cold.

lordosis abnormal anterior convexity of the spine. Also called *swayback.*

lower airway the portion of the respiratory system that extends from the trachea to the alveoli of the lungs.

lumbar (LUM-bar) spine the five vertebrae located between the sacral and the thoracic spine that form the lower back.

lungs the principal organs of respiration.

malaise a general feeling of weakness or discomfort.

malleolus (mal-E-o-lus) the knobby surface landmark of the ankle. There is a medial malleolus and a lateral malleolus.

mammalian diving reflex the body's natural response to submersion in cold water in which breathing is inhibited, the heart rate decreases, and blood vessels constrict in order to maintain cerebral and cardiac blood flow.

mandible (MAN-di-bl) the lower movable portion of the jaw.

manubrium (ma-NU-bre-um) the superior portion of the sternum where the clavicle is attached.

Markle test a test for the presence of peritonitis in which the patient stands on his toes, then drops to his heels, or in which the heels are struck together or struck on the bottom. The jarring of the torso will elicit pain when the peritoneal linings are inflamed. Also called the *heel drop test.*

maxilla the fixed upper portion of the jaw.

maximum life span theoretically the longest period of time for an organism to live.

mechanism of injury (MOI) the factors and forces that cause traumatic injury.

meconium staining a greenish or brownish yellow staining of the amniotic fluid, caused by a fetal bowel movement resulting from distress.

medial toward the midline or center of the body. *See also* lateral.

median plane *see* sagittal plane.

medical concerning illness.

medical direction medical policies, procedures, and practices that are available to EMS providers either off-line or on-line.

medical director physician who is legally responsible for the clinical and patient care aspects of an EMS system.

medical oversight the medical director's broad responsibilities, including all clinical and administrative functions and activities necessary to exercise ultimate responsibility for the emergency care provided by individual personnel and the entire emergency medical services (EMS) system.

medical oxygen oxygen administered as a medication or to support or improve a patient's oxygenation.

medical patient a patient with a condition brought on by illness or by substances or by environmental factors that affect the function of the body.

medication a drug or other substance that is used as a remedy for illness.

melena dark tarry stools containing decomposing blood normally from the upper gastrointestinal system.

menarche onset of menses.

meninges layers of tissue protecting the brain. They include the dura mater, the arachnoid, and the pia mater.

menopause the permanent end of menstruation and fertility, which usually occurs in a woman's late 40s or 50s.

menses menstrual period in which the endometrium is sloughed off.

metacarpals (MET-uh-KAR-pulz) the bones of the hand.

metatarsals (MET-uh-TAR-sulz) the bones that form the arch of the foot.

metered-dose inhaler (MDI) device consisting of a plastic container and a canister of medication that is used to form an aerosolized medication that a patient can inhale.

microcirculation the flow of blood through the arterioles, capillaries, and venules that is the site of exchange of gases, nutrients, and waste products with the cells.

midaxillary (mid-AX-uh-lar-e) refers to the center of the armpit (axilla).

midaxillary line an imaginary line that divides the body into anterior and posterior planes; the imaginary line from the middle of the armpit to the ankle.

midclavicular (mid-klav-IK-u-ler) refers to the center of the collarbone (clavicle).

midclavicular line the imaginary line from the center of either clavicle down the anterior thorax.

midline an imaginary line drawn vertically through the middle of the patient's body, dividing it into right and left planes.

midsagittal (mid-SAJ-i-tul) plane a vertical plane that divides the body into equal right and left halves. *See also* sagittal plane.

minimum data set the minimum information the U.S. Department of Transportation has determined should be included on all prehospital care reports.

minor consent permission obtained from a parent or legal guardian for emergency treatment of a minor or a mentally incompetent adult.

minute ventilation the amount of air moved in and out of the lungs in one minute. Also called *minute volume.*

minute volume *see* minute ventilation.

miscarriage *see* spontaneous abortion.

mittelschmerz abdominopelvic pain during the middle of a menstrual cycle that is associated with ovulation.

mobile data terminal device that is mounted in the cab of an ambulance, receives a signal from a digital radio, and displays the information on the terminal screen. Some mobile data terminals will also print a hard copy of the information.

modified secondary assessment a physical exam that is focused on a specific injury site, performed on a responsive patient with no significant mechanism of injury or critical injuries; or on a medical patient who is alert, oriented, and stable.

mottling a skin discoloration similar to cyanosis but occurring in a blotchy pattern; a possible sign of shock.

mucous membrane a thin layer of tissue that lines various structures within the body.

multiple birth the delivery of more than one baby during a single birth, for example, twins or triplets.

multiple-casualty incident (MCI) an event that places excessive demands on EMS personnel and equipment.

multisystem trauma trauma in which more than one major body system is involved.

musculoskeletal (MUS-kyu-lo-SKEL-uh-tul) system the system of bones and muscle plus connective tissue that provides support and protection to the body and permits motion.

myxedema coma a life-threatening late complication of hypothyroidism that may be precipitated by exposure to cold temperatures as well as to illness, infection, trauma, or certain drugs.

narcotics central nervous system depressants that are derived from opium (opiates) or from synthetic opium (opioids).

nasal airway a nasopharyngeal airway.

nasal bones the bones that form the bed of the nose.

nasal cannula an oxygen delivery device that consists of two prongs that are inserted into the nose of the patient. The oxygen concentration delivered is from 24–44%.

nasopharyngeal airway a curved, hollow rubber tube with a flange or flare at the top end and a bevel at the distal end that is inserted into the nose. It fits in the nasopharynx and extends into the pharynx providing a passage for air.

nasopharynx (NA-zo-FAIR-inks) the portion of the pharynx that extends from the nostrils to the soft palate.

National Incident Management System (NIMS) a system administered by the U.S. Secretary of Homeland Security to provide a consistent approach to disaster management by all local, state, and federal employees who respond to such incidents.

nature of illness (NOI) the type of medical condition or complaint a patient is suffering from.

neglect the provision of insufficient attention or respect to someone who has a claim to that attention.

negligence the act of deviating from an accepted standard of care through carelessness, inattention, disregard, inadvertence, or oversight, which results in further injury to the patient.
neonate a child from birth to 1 month of age.
nerve agents agents that block the action of acetylcholinesterase (AChE) in the plasma of the blood, red blood cells, and nervous tissue. The most severe effects are those to the nervous tissue.
nervous system the body system including the brain, spinal cord, and nerves that controls the voluntary and involuntary activity of the human body.
neurogenic hypotension condition associated with injury to the spinal cord that results in vasodilation and relative hypovolemia. Also called *spinal-vascular shock* or *neurogenic shock*. *See also* spinal shock.
neurogenic shock a type of distributive shock that results from massive vasodilation. Also called *vasogenic shock*.
neurological deficit any deficiency in the nervous system's functioning, typically exhibited as a motor, sensory, or cognitive deficit.
neuropathy any disease of the nerves. *Peripheral neuropathy* is a syndrome in which weakness, numbness, tingling, or other neuropathic symptoms are experienced in the extremities, especially the hands and feet.
neutron radiation a powerful and very damaging particle that penetrates several hundred meters of air and easily passes through the body. Its greatest threat to life occurs in close proximity to an active nuclear reactor or nuclear bomb ignition.
nitroglycerin medication that dilates the blood vessels, increasing blood flow through the coronary arteries and decreasing the workload of the heart; often prescribed for patients with a history of chest pain.
nocturnal enuresis involuntary bed-wetting at night.
nonhemorrhagic hypovolemic shock shock caused by loss of fluid from the intravascular space with red blood cells and hemoglobin remaining within the vessels.
nonrebreather mask an oxygen delivery device that consists of a reservoir and one-way valve. It can deliver up to 95 to 98% oxygen to the patient.
nontraumatic brain injury a medical injury to the brain that is not caused by external trauma. Stroke is an example of a nontraumatic brain injury.
nonurgent move a patient move made when no immediate threat to life exists.
nuchal cord an umbilical cord that is wrapped around the infant's neck during the delivery.
nuclear radiation energy released when an unstable atom breaks apart.
obstetric having to do with pregnancy or childbirth.
obstructive shock a poor perfusion state resulting from a condition that obstructs forward blood flow.
occluded closed or blocked; not patent, as an occluded airway.
occlusive dressing a dressing that can form an airtight seal over a wound.
off-line medical direction medical policies, procedures, and practices that medical direction has established in written guidelines.
olecranon (o-LEK-ran-on) the part of the ulna that forms the bony prominence of the elbow.
oncotic pressure *see* plasma oncotic pressure.
on-line medical direction direct orders from a physician to a prehospital care provider given by radio or telephone.
open injury any injury in which the skin is broken as a result of trauma.
open pneumothorax an open wound to the chest that allows air to enter the pleural space and cause lung collapse.
open-ended questions questions that allow the patient to give a detailed response in his own words.
oral airway an oropharyngeal airway.
oral glucose a form of sugar often given as a gel, by mouth, to raise the blood glucose level.
orbits the bony structures that surround the eyes; the eye sockets.
oropharyngeal airway a semicircular hard plastic device that is inserted in the mouth and holds the tongue away from the back of the pharynx.
oropharynx (OR-o-FAIR-inks) the central portion of the pharynx lying between the soft palate and the epiglottis with the mouth as the opening.
orthopnea shortness of breath while lying flat.
orthostatic vital signs an increase in heart rate of 10–20 bpm and a decrease in systolic blood pressure of 10–20 mmHg when a patient moves from a supine to an upright or standing position; a positive finding for orthostatic hypotension. Also called a *tilt test*.
osteoporosis a degenerative bone disorder associated with an accelerated loss of minerals, primarily calcium, from the bone.
ostomy bag a pouch or bag that is attached outside the body to collect feces that are removed from the body through an opening in the abdominal wall.
ovaries the female gonads or sex glands.
overdose an emergency that involves poisoning by drugs or alcohol.
oxygen a gaseous element required by the body's tissues and cells to sustain life; often provided as a medication.
oxygen humidifier a container that is filled with sterile water and connected to the oxygen regulator to add moisture to the dry oxygen prior to being delivered to the patient.
oxygenated containing high amounts of oxygen, as with arterial blood.
oxygenation the form of respiration in which oxygen molecules move across a membrane from an area of high oxygen concentration to an area of low oxygen concentration, as when oxygen moves out of a blood vessel into a cell; the process by which the blood and the cells become saturated with oxygen.
oxyhemoglobin hemoglobin that has at least one oxygen molecule attached to it.
pallor pale or abnormally white skin color.
palmar relates to the palm of the hand.
palpation feeling, as for a pulse.
pancreatitis inflammation of the pancreas.
paradoxical movement a section of the chest that moves in the opposite direction to the rest of the chest during the phases of respiration. Typically seen with a flail segment.
Paramedic the level of EMS practitioner who provides the highest level of prehospital care, including advanced assessments and care, formation of a field impression, and invasive and drug interventions.
paranoia a highly exaggerated or unwarranted mistrust or suspiciousness.
paraplegic paralysis from the waist down.
paresthesia a prickling or tingling feeling that indicates some loss of sensation.
parietal pain localized, intense, sharp, constant pain associated with irritation of the peritoneum. Also called *somatic pain*.
parietal pleura the outermost pleural layer that adheres to the chest wall.
partial-thickness burn burn that involves the epidermis and portions of the dermis; also called a *second-degree burn*.
passive rewarming the use of the patient's own heat production and conservation mechanisms to rewarm him, for example, simply placing the patient in a warm environment and covering him with blankets.
patella the kneecap.
patent open; not blocked.
patent airway an airway that is open and clear of any obstructions.
pathogens microorganisms such as bacteria and viruses that cause disease.
pathologic fracture a broken bone resulting from a disease that causes degeneration and dramatic weakening of the bone, making it prone to fracture.
patient assessment procedures performed to determine immediate life threats and injuries sustained or the condition of the patient, on which decisions about emergency medical care and transport will be based.
pelvic inflammatory disease inflammation of the female reproductive tract.
pelvis the bones that form the floor of the abdominal cavity: the sacrum and coccyx of the spine, the iliac crests, the pubis, and the ischium.
penetrating trauma a force that pierces the skin and body tissues, for example, a knife or gunshot wound.
penetration/puncture an open injury caused by a sharp, pointed object being pushed into the soft tissues.
perfusion the delivery of oxygen and other nutrients to the cells of all organ systems, which results from the constant adequate circulation of blood through the capillaries.
pericardial tamponade blood or fluid filling the fibrous sac around the heart, causing compression of the heart and decreasing the ability of the ventricles to effectively fill and eject blood.
perineum the area of skin between a female's vagina and anus.
peripheral chemoreceptors receptors located in the aortic arch and the carotid bodies that are somewhat sensitive to CO_2 and pH but are most sensitive to the level of oxygen in the arterial blood. *See also* chemoreceptors.
peripheral nervous system that portion of the nervous system located outside the brain and spinal cord. *Abbr.* PNS.
peripheral neuropathy *see* neuropathy.
peritoneal space the anterior abdominal cavity that houses the majority of the abdominal organs and is lined by the peritoneum.
peritoneum the lining of the abdominal cavity.
peritonitis irritation and inflammation of the abdominal lining.
persistence a characteristic of agents that do not evaporate quickly and tend to remain as a puddle for long periods of time.
personal protective equipment (PPE) equipment worn to protect against injury and disease.
pertinent negatives signs or symptoms that might be expected in certain circumstances, based on the chief complaint or physical exam, but are denied by the patient or not found on examination.

phalanges (fa-LAN-jez) bones of the fingers, thumbs, and toes. *Pl.* of phalanx.

pharmacology the study of drugs.

pharming raiding others' home medicine supplies or using faked prescriptions to obtain drugs.

pharynx (FAIR-inks) the throat, or passageway for air from the nasal cavity to the larynx and passageway for food from the mouth to the esophagus; the common passageway for the respiratory and digestive tracts.

phobia an irrational fear of specific things, places, or situations.

physical abuse improper or excessive action taken so as to injure or cause harm.

physician orders for life-sustaining treatment (POLST) orders that identify the desired level of life-sustaining treatment in patients with a terminal or life-threatening illness who are not likely to survive.

physiology (FIZ-e-OL-o-je) the study of the function of the living body and its parts.

pia mater inner layer of protective brain tissue (meninges).

placenta the fetal organ through which the fetus exchanges nourishment and waste products during pregnancy.

plantar refers to the sole of the foot.

plasma the liquid part of the blood.

plasma oncotic pressure the force created by the presence of large molecules that tends to keep fluid inside a capillary by exerting a "pull" effect. Also called *colloid oncotic pressure* or *oncotic pressure*.

platelets (PLATE-lets) components of blood that are essential to the formation of blood clots.

pleura two layers of connective tissue that surround the lungs.

pleural space a small space between the visceral and parietal pleura that is at negative pressure and filled with serous fluid.

pneumonia infection of the lungs, usually from a bacterium or virus.

pneumotaxic center located in the brainstem, it sends inhibitory impulses to the apneustic center to turn off the inhalation before the lungs are too full.

pneumothorax air in the pleural space causing collapse of the lung.

pocket mask a plastic mask placed over the patient's nose and mouth through which ventilations can be delivered.

poison any substance—liquid, solid, or gas—that impairs health or causes death by its chemical action when it enters the body or comes into contact with the skin.

positive pressure ventilation (PPV) method of aiding a patient whose breathing is inadequate by forcing air into his lungs.

postterm pregnancy gestation of the fetus that extends beyond 42 weeks. *See also* postmaturity syndrome.

posterior (pos-TE-re-or) toward the back. Opposite of *anterior*.

posterior plane the back or dorsal side of the body.

posterior tibial artery a major artery that travels from the calf to the foot and that can be felt on the medial surface of the ankle bone.

postictal state the recovery period that follows the clonic phase of a generalized seizure. In a postictal state the patient commonly appears weak, exhausted, confused and disoriented and progressively improves.

postmaturity syndrome condition that occurs during pregnancy when gestation of the fetus extends beyond 42 weeks, leading to reduced oxygen and nutrient delivery to the fetus. *See also* postterm pregnancy.

postpartum the period following delivery of the infant.

postpartum hemorrhage the loss of greater than 500 mL of blood following delivery of the infant.

power grip recommended gripping technique. The palm and fingers come in complete contact with the object and all fingers are bent at the same angle.

power lift recommended technique for lifting. Feet are apart, knees bent, back and abdominal muscles tightened, back as straight as possible, lifting force driven through heels and arches, upper body rising before hips.

precipitous delivery birth of the fetus after less than 3 hours of labor.

prefix a word part added to the beginning of a word to modify its meaning or to give additional or specific meaning to the word.

pregnancy-induced hypertension (PIH) in a pregnant woman, a blood pressure greater than 140/90 mmHg on two or more occasions at least 6 hours apart, or an increase from prepregnancy of greater than 30 mmHg in systolic pressure and greater than 15 mmHg in diastolic pressure.

prehospital care emergency medical treatment given to patients before they are transported to a hospital or other facility. Also called *out-of-hospital care*.

prehospital care report (PCR) documentation of an EMT's contact with a patient.

preload the pressure generated in the left ventricle at the end of diastole (resting phase of the cardiac cycle).

premature infant an infant weighing less than 5 pounds, or an infant born before its 38th week of gestation.

premature rupture of membranes (PROM) spontaneous rupture of the amniotic sac prior to the onset of true labor and before the end of the 37th week of gestation.

preschooler a child 3 to 6 years of age.

preterm labor labor that occurs after the 20th but prior to the 37th week of gestation. Also called *premature labor*.

priapism a persistent erection of the penis resulting from injury to the spinal nerves to the genitals.

primary assessment patient assessment conducted immediately after scene size-up to discover and treat immediately life-threatening conditions, determine whether the patient is injured or ill, and establish priorities for further assessment, care, and transport.

primary effect the blast of an explosion.

primary exposure primary radiation injury that occurs during or shortly after a radioactive detonation.

primary triage evaluation of patients that occurs immediately upon arrival of the first EMS crew at the actual site of the incident to quickly categorize the severity of a patient's condition and priority for treatment and transport.

profile the size and shape of a bullet's point of impact; the greater the point of impact the greater the injury.

progressive shock *see* decompensatory shock.

prolapsed cord when the umbilical cord, rather than the head of the fetus, is the first part to protrude from the vagina.

prone lying face down.

protocols the policies and procedures for all components of an EMS system. Also called *orders* or *standing orders*.

proximal (PROK-sim-al) near the point of reference. Opposite of *distal*.

proximate cause the act of deviating from an accepted standard of care through carelessness, inattention, disregard, inadvertence, or oversight, which results in further injury to the patient.

psychosis state of delusion in which a person is out of touch with reality.

puberty the period in which the sexual organs mature during adolescence.

pubis (PYU-bis) bone of the groin.

pulmonary agents agents that act primarily to cause lung injury and are commonly referred to as choking agents, including phosgene (CG), other halogen compounds, and nitrogen-oxygen compounds.

pulmonary artery artery that carries deoxygenated blood from the right ventricle of the heart to the lungs.

pulmonary contusion bleeding within the lung tissue that causes a disturbance in gas exchange between the alveoli and capillaries.

pulmonary edema fluid in and around the alveoli in the lungs.

pulmonary embolism blockage in the pulmonary arteries of the lungs.

pulmonary vein vein that carries oxygenated blood from the lungs to the left atrium of the heart.

pulse the wave of blood propelled through the arteries as a result of the contraction of the left ventricle.

pulse oximeter electronic device used to determine the oxygen concentration in arterial blood.

pulse oximetry measurement of blood oxygen saturation.

pulse pressure the difference between the systolic blood pressure and the diastolic blood pressure.

pulseless electrical activity (PEA) a condition in which the heart generates relatively normal electrical rhythms but fails to perfuse the body adequately because of a decreased or absent cardiac output from cardiac muscle failure or blood loss.

pulsus paradoxus a decrease in pulse strength during inhalation; a drop in blood pressure of more than 10 mmHg during inhalation resulting from increased pressure within the chest that suppresses the filling of the ventricles of the heart with blood.

pupil the dark center of the eye; the opening that expands or contracts to allow more or less light into the eye.

purified protein derivative (PPD) tuberculin test a test to determine the presence of a tuberculosis infection based on a person's positive reaction to tuberculin, a substance prepared from the tubercle bacillus.

quadriplegic paralysis from the neck down.

quality improvement (QI) a system of internal and external reviews and audits of an EMS system to ensure a high quality of care. Also known as *continuous quality improvement (CQI)*.

raccoon sign discoloration of tissue around the eyes suggestive of basilar skull injury.

radial artery a major artery of the arm, distal to the elbow joint.

radiation transfer of heat from the surface of one object to the surface of another without physical contact between the objects.

radius the lateral bone of the forearm.

rapid extrication a technique using manual stabilization rather than application of an immobilization device for the purpose of speeding extrication when the time saved will make the difference between life and death.

rapid secondary assessment a head-to-toe physical exam that is swiftly conducted on a trauma patient who is unresponsive or who has a significant mechanism of injury, has altered mental status, responds to verbal or painful stimuli, or is unresponsive; or on a medical patient who is not alert, is disoriented, does not respond to verbal or painful stimuli, or is unresponsive.

reasonable force the minimum amount of force required to keep a patient from injuring himself or others.

reassessment the continuous assessment that is conducted following the secondary assessment to detect any changes in the patient's condition, to identify any missed injuries or conditions, and to adjust emergency care as needed.

red blood cells part of the blood that gives it its color, carries oxygen to body cells, and carries carbon dioxide away from body cells.

referred pain pain that is felt in a body part removed from the point of origin of the pain.

reflex an instantaneous and involuntary movement resulting from a stimulus.

renal (RE-nuhl) referring to the kidneys.

renal calculi kidney stones.

renal system *see* urinary system.

repeaters devices that receive transmissions from a relatively low-powered source such as a mobile or portable radio and rebroadcast them at another frequency and a higher power.

reproductive system the male or female organs that function to accomplish human reproduction, the creation of offspring.

residual volume the air remaining in the lungs after a maximal exhalation.

respiration the exchange of gases between an organism and its environment; the taking in of oxygen and giving off of carbon dioxide.

respiratory arrest complete stoppage of breathing. Also called *apnea*.

respiratory distress increased respiratory effort resulting from impaired respiratory function, while tidal volume and respiratory rate are still adequate.

respiratory failure insufficient respiratory rate and/or tidal volume.

respiratory rate the number of breaths taken in one minute. Also called *frequency*.

respiratory system the organs involved in the exchange of gases between an organism and the atmosphere.

resuscitation an attempt to restore normal or adequate physiologic function.

reticular activating system (RAS) a network of specialized nerve cells within the brainstem that controls states of arousal and consciousness including wakefulness, attentiveness, and sleep.

retina the structure at the back of the eye that is responsible for vision.

retractions depressions seen in the neck, above the clavicles, between the ribs, or below the rib cage from excessive muscle use during breathing. It is an indication of respiratory distress.

retrograde amnesia inability to remember circumstances prior to an incident.

retroperitoneal cavity the space located behind the peritoneal cavity.

return of spontaneous circulation (ROSC) return of a spontaneous pulse during the cardiac resuscitation.

right refers to the patient's right.

right plane everything to the right of the midline.

rigid catheter a rigid plastic tube that is part of a suctioning system, commonly referred to as a *tonsil tip* or *tonsil sucker*.

rigidity *see* involuntary guarding.

route the means by which a medication is given or taken; for example, sublingual (under the tongue), oral (by mouth), inhalation (breathed in), or injection (inserted by needle into a muscle or vein).

rule of nines standardized format to quickly identify the amount of skin or body surface area (BSA) that has been burned.

rule of ones the concept that the area of a patient's palm is equal to about 1% of his body surface area (BSA); a way to quickly identify the amount of skin or body surface area that has been burned. Also called the *rule of palms*.

rule of palms *see* rule of ones.

sacral (SAY-krul) spine five vertebrae that are fused together to form the rigid part of the posterior side of the pelvis. Also called the *sacrum*.

safety zones areas surrounding an accident involving hazardous materials, designated for specific rescue operations. *See also* hot zone, warm zone, and cold zone.

sagittal (SAJ-i-tul) plane a vertical plane that divides the body into right and left segments. Also called *median plane*. *See also* midsagittal plane.

SAMPLE history a format for taking a patient history. SAMPLE is an acronym used to remember categories of information necessary to the patient history: signs and symptoms, allergies, medications, pertinent past history, last oral intake, and events leading to the injury or illness.

SBAR acronym for *situation, background, assessment, and recommendation*; a method of organizing communications about a patient.

scapula (SKAP-u-la) the shoulder blade.

scene safety steps taken to ensure the safety and well-being of the EMT, his partners, patients, and bystanders.

scene size-up an assessment of the scene for safety hazards and to determine the nature of the patient's problem and the number of patients.

schizophrenia the name given to a group of mental disorders characterized by debilitating distortions of speech and thought, bizarre delusions, hallucinations, social withdrawal, and lack of emotional expressiveness.

school-age child a child 6 to 12 years of age.

sclera the outer coating of the eye; the exposed portion is "the white of the eye."

scope of practice the actions and care that an EMT is legally allowed to perform, as typically defined by state laws.

secondary assessment the portion of patient assessment conducted after the primary assessment, for the purpose of identifying additional serious or potentially life-threatening injuries or conditions and as a basis for further emergency care.

secondary effects effects from flying debris, shrapnel, and other projectiles. In an explosion, the flying debris can cause significant penetrating injury or blunt trauma. Flames and hot gases present in explosions also result in secondary effect injuries.

secondary triage re-evaluation that takes place in the triage unit of the severity of a patient's condition and priority for treatment and transport.

seizure a sudden and temporary alteration in the mental status caused by massive electrical discharge in a group of nerve cells in the brain.

Sellick maneuver *see* cricoid pressure.

semi-Fowler position a position in which the patient is lying on the back with upper body elevated at less than 45°. *See also* Fowler position.

sensitization exposure to an allergen that results in hypersensitivity to that allergen. *See also* hypersensitivity.

septic shock a type of distributive shock caused by an infection that releases bacteria or toxins into the blood.

serous fluid fluid that acts as a lubricant to reduce the friction between the parietal and visceral pleura.

shock the insufficient delivery of oxygen and other nutrients to some of the body's cells and inadequate elimination of carbon dioxide and other wastes that results from inadequate circulation of blood. Also called *hypoperfusion*.

shock position elevation of the legs of a supine patient approximately 12 inches; an alternative to the Trendelenburg position; sometimes useful for treating a simple faint but no longer recommended in the treatment of shock.

shoulder dystocia abnormal delivery when the fetal shoulders are larger than the fetal head and the head delivers but the shoulders are caught between the symphysis pubis and the sacrum.

side effects the undesired effects of a medication; for example, side effects of epinephrine are increased heart rate and anxiety.

signs any objective evidence of medical or trauma conditions that can be seen, heard, felt, or smelled in a patient.

silent heart attack a myocardial infarction (heart attack) that does not cause chest pain or discomfort.

simple access a way to gain access to a patient that does not require specialized tools.

skeletal muscle any muscle that can be consciously controlled by the individual. Also called *voluntary muscle*.

skeletal system the bony framework of the body.

skull the bony structure at the top of the spinal column that houses and protects the brain. The skull has two parts, the cranium and the face.

slander the act of injuring a person's reputation or good name through spoken statements with malicious intent or reckless disregard for the falsity of those statements.

small-volume nebulizer (SVN) a device that uses compressed air or oxygen to nebulize a liquid medication into a mist that a patient can inhale.

smooth muscle muscle that carries out the automatic muscular functions of the body. Also called *involuntary muscle*.

snoring a sound that is heard when the base of the tongue or relaxed tissues in the pharynx partially block the upper airway; also called a *sonorous sound*.

soft catheter flexible tubing that is part of a suctioning system, also called a *French catheter*.

somatic pain *see* parietal pain.

spacer a chamber that is connected to the metered-dose inhaler to collect the medication until it is inhaled.

sphygmomanometer instrument used to measure blood pressure. Also called a *blood pressure cuff.*

spinal column the column of 33 vertebrae that enclose and protect the spinal cord. Also called the *vertebral column.*

spinal cord a column of nervous tissue that exits from the brain and extends to the level of L2 within the spinal column. All nerves to the trunk and extremities originate from the spinal cord.

spinal shock shock caused by injury to the spinal cord, causing paralysis and loss of sensation below the level of the spinal cord injury. Signs include motor and sensory dysfunction. Normal to low heart rate and warm, dry, pink skin may occur if vasodilation and relative hypovolemia (neurogenic hypotension) are present.

splint any device used to immobilize a body part.

spontaneous abortion without apparent cause, the termination of a pregnancy before the fetus reaches the stage of viability, generally before the 20th week of pregnancy. Also called *miscarriage.*

staging unit in a multiple-casualty incident, the unit that monitors, inventories, and directs available ambulances to the treatment unit at the request of the transport officer.

standard of care emergency care that would be expected to be given to a patient by any trained EMT under similar circumstances.

Standard Precautions a method of preventing infection by disease organisms based on the premise that all blood and body fluids are infectious. Formerly called *body substance isolation.*

standing orders preauthorized treatment procedures; a type of treatment protocol. *See also* off-line medical direction, protocols.

status epilepticus a seizure lasting longer than 5 minutes or seizures that occur consecutively without a period of responsiveness between them. This is a serious medical emergency that may be life threatening.

stenosis constriction or narrowing of a passage or opening, for example of the valves of the heart.

sterile free from living microorganisms such as bacteria, viruses, or spores that may cause infection.

sterilization the process by which an object is subject to certain chemical or physical substances (typically, superheated steam in an autoclave) that kill all microorganisms on the surface of an object.

sternum the breastbone.

stoma a surgical opening into the neck and trachea. *See also* tracheostomy.

stretch receptors receptors found in the smooth muscle of the airways that monitor the size and volume of the lungs. These receptors stimulate a decrease in the rate and volume of ventilation when stretched by high tidal volumes to protect against lung overinflation.

stridor a harsh, high-pitched sound heard on inspiration that indicates swelling of the larynx or obstruction of the upper airway.

stroke a sudden disruption in blood flow to the brain that results in brain cell damage. Blood flow might be interrupted by a ruptured artery or blocked by a clot or other foreign matter in an artery that supplies the brain.

stroke volume the volume of blood ejected by the left ventricle with each contraction.

subarachnoid hemorrhage bleeding that occurs between the arachnoid membrane and the surface of the brain.

subarachnoid space a lattice of fibrous, spongy tissue filled with cerebrospinal fluid that separates the arachnoid membrane and the pia mater.

subcutaneous (SUB-kyu-TAY-ne-us) layer a layer of fatty tissue just below the dermis. *See also* dermis, epidermis.

subdural beneath the dura mater.

subdural hematoma bleeding between the brain and the dura mater.

sucking chest wound an open wound to the chest that permits air to enter into the thoracic cavity.

sudden death death of a patient within one hour of the onset of signs and symptoms.

sudden infant death syndrome (SIDS) the sudden and unexpected death of an infant or young child in which an autopsy fails to identify the cause of death. SIDS typically occurs while the infant is asleep.

suffix a word part added to the end of a word to modify its meaning or to give additional or specific meaning to the word.

suicide a willful act designed to end one's own life.

superficial burn burn that involves only the epidermis, also called a *first-degree burn.*

superior above; toward the head. Opposite to of *inferior.*

superior plane everything above the transverse line (above the waist). Opposite of *inferior plane.*

supine lying face up.

supine hypotensive syndrome inadequate return of venous blood to the heart, reduced cardiac output, and lowered blood pressure resulting from pressure on the inferior vena cava, caused by the weight of the uterus and fetus when the patient in late pregnancy is in a supine position.

support zone *see* cold zone.

surfactant a substance responsible for maintaining surface tension in the alveoli.

surgically implanted medication delivery devices medication administration devices that are surgically placed beneath the skin outside the rib cage.

survival term applied to a patient who survives cardiac arrest to be discharged from the hospital.

symptoms conditions that must be described by the patient because they cannot be observed by another person.

syncope brief period of unresponsiveness caused by a lack of blood flow to the brain; fainting.

systemic vascular resistance the resistance of blood flow through a vessel based on the diameter of the vessel.

systolic (sis-TOL-ik) blood pressure the pressure exerted against the walls of the arteries when the left ventricle contracts. *See also* diastolic blood pressure.

tachycardia a heart rate greater than 100 beats per minute.

tachypnea a breathing rate that is faster than the normal rate.

tarsals the bones of the ankle, hindfoot, and midfoot.

tenderness pain in response to palpation.

tension pneumothorax a condition in which the buildup of air and pressure in a hemothorax associated with an injured lung is so severe that it begins to shift to the uninjured side, resulting in compression of the heart, large vessels, and the uninjured lung.

terminally ill the condition of an individual who has a disease process that is realistically expected to result in the death of the patient, despite current medical treatment designed to halt or reverse the condition.

tertiary effects in an explosion, injuries produced by propulsion, for example when a person is propelled by a blast or shock wave and strikes the ground or other objects, resulting in blunt trauma.

therapy regulator a device that controls the flow and pressure of oxygen from the tank to allow for a consistent delivery of oxygen by liters per minute.

thermoreceptor a sensory receptor that is stimulated by temperature.

thoracic (tho-RAS-ik) spine the 12 vertebrae directly below the cervical vertebrae that comprise the upper back.

thorax (THO-raks) the chest, or that part of the body between the base of the neck and the diaphragm.

thrombotic stroke a type of ischemic stroke caused by a stationary clot that forms in and blocks a cerebral artery.

thyroid cartilage the bulky cartilage that forms the anterior portion of the larynx. Also called the *Adam's apple.*

tibia the medial, larger bone of the lower leg; the shinbone.

tidal volume the amount of air breathed in and out in one normal respiration.

tilt test *see* orthostatic vital signs.

toddler a child 1 to 3 years of age.

tonsil tip or tonsil sucker *see* rigid catheter.

tort a wrongful act, injury, or damage. *See also* intentional tort.

total downtime the total time from when a patient goes into cardiac arrest until he is delivered to the emergency department.

totally implantable venous access system (TIVAS) *see* surgically implanted medical delivery device.

toxicology the study of toxins, antidotes, and the effects of toxins on the body.

toxins drugs or substances that are poisonous to humans and will cause certain adverse effects that may ultimately lead to death. *Toxin* is sometimes considered a synonym to *poison,* sometimes defined more narrowly as a poisonous substance of plant or animal origin.

trachea (TRAY-ke-ah) the tubelike structure that leads from the larynx to the lungs.

tracheostomy a surgical opening in the trachea.

tracheostomy tube a hollow tube that is inserted into a tracheostomy to allow the patient to breathe.

trajectory the path of a projectile during its travel; a trajectory may be flat or curved.

transient ischemic attack (TIA) brief, intermittent episode with stroke-like symptoms that typically disappear within minutes, but usually last no longer than 1 hour. TIAs are caused by an oxygen deficit in the brain tissue (ischemia) and are often a precursor to a stroke.

transport unit in a multiple-casualty incident, the unit that coordinates patient transportation with the triage and staging units. Its officer communicates with the hospitals involved.

transverse line an imaginary line drawn horizontally through the waist.

transverse plane a plane that divides the body into superior and inferior segments. Also called *horizontal plane.*

trauma concerning injury.

trauma patient a patient who has a physical injury or wound caused by external force or violence.

traumatic asphyxia a severe and sudden compression of the thorax that causes a rapid increase in pressure within the chest that affects blood flow, ventilation, and oxygenation.

treatment unit in a multiple-casualty incident, the unit that is responsible for collecting and treating patients in a centralized treatment area.

Trendelenburg (tren-DEL-en-burg) position lying on the back with the lower part of the body elevated higher than the head on an inclined plane.

triage the process of sorting patients to determine the order in which they will receive care or transportation to definitive care.

triage tag a tag containing key information that is attached to a patient during a multiple-casualty incident.

triage unit in a multiple-casualty incident, the unit that is responsible for prioritizing patients for emergency medical care and transport.

tripod position a position in which the patient sits upright, leans slightly forward, and supports the body with the arms in front and elbows locked. This is a position commonly found in respiratory distress.

twisting force a force that twists a bone while one end is held stationary.

type 1 diabetes a form of diabetes in which the patient's pancreas typically does not produce or secrete any insulin. Also called *insulin-dependent diabetes mellitus (IDDM). See also* diabetes mellitus (DM).

type 2 diabetes a form of diabetes where the pancreas continues to produce and secrete insulin; however, the insulin is not completely effective in controlling the blood glucose level. Type 2 diabetes does not usually require the patient to take insulin and can, instead, be regulated by diet, exercise, and drugs other than insulin. Also called *non-insulin-dependent diabetes mellitus (NIDDM). See also* diabetes mellitus (DM).

ulcers open wounds or sores within the digestive tract.

ulna the medial bone of the forearm.

umbilical cord an extension of the placenta through which the fetus receives nourishment while in the uterus.

umbilicus the navel.

upper airway the portion of the respiratory system that extends from the nose and mouth to the larynx.

urban hypothermia hypothermia precipitated by cold environments such as with persons who live on the streets in cold weather or whose indoor environment is too cool.

urgent move a patient move made because there is an immediate threat to life because of the patient's condition and the patient must be moved quickly for transport.

urinary (YUR-in-air-e) system the organs and structures responsible for filtering and excreting wastes from the blood. Also called the *renal system.*

urinary catheter a device that is used to divert urine out of the bladder.

urology branch of medicine that studies the urinary system in females and the genitourinary system in males.

uterus an organ of the female reproductive system for containing and nourishing the embryo and fetus from the time the fertilized egg is implanted to the time of birth.

vagina the passageway through which the fetus is delivered. The lower part of the birth canal.

valves structures within the heart and circulatory system that keep blood flowing in one direction and prevent backflow.

vascular access device (VAD) a medical device that is used when a patient is in need of ongoing intravenous medications.

vein vessel that carries blood toward the heart.

venae cavae the principal veins that carry deoxygenated blood to the heart. *Pl.* of vena cava. The superior vena cava carries blood from the upper body; the inferior vena cava carries blood from the lower body.

ventilation the mechanical process by which air is moved in and out of the lungs, primarily caused by changes in pressure inside the chest.

ventilation/perfusion (V/Q) ratio the dynamic relationship between the amount of ventilation the alveoli receive and the amount of perfusion through the capillary surrounding the alveoli.

ventral toward the front, or toward the anterior portion of the body. Opposite of *dorsal.*

ventral respiratory group (VRG) respiratory rhythm center located in the brainstem that has both inspiratory and expiratory neurons. It becomes active and stimulates accessory muscles when an increase in ventilatory effort is necessary.

ventricles the two lower chambers of the heart.

ventricular fibrillation (VF or V-Fib) a continuous, uncoordinated, chaotic rhythm that does not produce pulses.

ventricular tachycardia (VT or V-Tach) a very rapid heart rhythm that may or may not produce a pulse and is generally too fast to adequately perfuse the body's organs.

venule the smallest branch of a vein.

vertebrae (VER-tuh-bray) the 33 bony segments of the spinal column. *Pl.* of vertebra.

vertebral (VER-tuh-bruhl) column *see* spinal column.

vesicants chemical agents that cause blistering, burning, and tissue damage on contact as well as causing generalized illness if a significant amount is absorbed. Vesicants include sulfur and nitrogen mustards, lewisite, and phosgene oxime.

visceral pain poorly localized, intermittent, crampy, dull, or aching pain associated with ischemia, tearing, or distention of an organ.

visceral pleura innermost layer of the pleura that covers the lung.

vital signs the traditional signs of life; assessments related to breathing, pulse, skin, pupils, and blood pressure.

vitreous body the large chamber of the eye, containing the vitreous humor.

vitreous humor the clear jelly that fills the large chamber of the eye.

volatile inhalants substances that are easily vaporized and inhalable.

volatility the tendency of a chemical agent to evaporate. A volatile liquid evaporates easily and creates a dangerous, breathable vapor.

voluntary guarding a deliberate abdominal wall muscle contraction.

voluntary muscle *see* skeletal muscle.

voluntary nervous system part of the nervous system that influences voluntary muscles and movements of the body.

warm zone the area that is established surrounding or immediately adjacent to the hot zone in a hazardous materials emergency, the purpose of which is to prevent the spread of contamination. Lifesaving emergency care is performed here. Also called *contamination reduction zone.*

water chill the increase in rate of cooling in the presence of water or wet clothing.

weapons of mass destruction weapons intended to cause widespread and indiscriminate death and destruction.

white blood cells the part of the blood that helps the body's immune system defend against infection.

wind chill the combined cooling effect of wind speed and environmental temperature.

withdrawal a syndrome that occurs after a period of abstinence from the alcohol or drugs to which a person's body has become accustomed.

xiphoid (ZI-foyd) process inferior portion of the sternum.

X-ray radiation X-ray radiation and *gamma radiation* are the same type of powerful and penetrating radiation that may be generated in the reactor of a nuclear bomb or through the decay of radioactive particles, as in fallout. Gamma radiation is both an external and an internal hazard associated with a nuclear detonation or reactor accident.

zygomatic (ZI-go-MAT-ik) bones the cheekbones.

Index

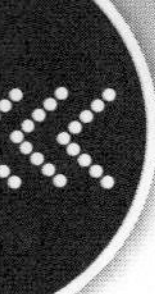